PSYCHIATRIC & MENTAL HEALTH NURSING
FOR CANADIAN PRACTICE

FIFTH EDITION

PSYCHIATRIC & MENTAL HEALTH NURSING FOR CANADIAN PRACTICE

FIFTH EDITION

DIANE KUNYK, PhD, MSc, BScN, RN

Professor
Faculty of Nursing and the Dossetor Health Ethics Centre
University of Alberta
Edmonton, Alberta, Canada

CINDY PETERNELJ-TAYLOR, MSc, BScN, RN, DF-IAFN

Professor
College of Nursing
University of Saskatchewan
Saskatoon, Saskatchewan, Canada

WENDY AUSTIN, PhD, MEd (Counselling), BScN

Professor Emeritus
Faculty of Nursing and the Dossetor Health Ethics Centre
University of Alberta
Edmonton, Alberta, Canada

MARY ANN BOYD, PhD, DNS, BC, APRN

Professor Emeritus
Southern Illinois University Edwardsville
Edwardsville, Illinois

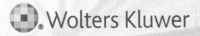

. Wolters Kluwer

Philadelphia • Baltimore • New York • London
Buenos Aires • Hong Kong • Sydney • Tokyo

Vice President and Publisher: Julie K. Stegman
Senior Acquisitions Editor: Jodi Rhomberg
Director of Product Development: Jennifer Forestieri
Director of Content Development: Jamie Blum
Development Editor: Beck Rist/Chelsea Neve
Editorial Coordinator: Remington Fernando
Senior Marketing Manager: Sarah Schuessler
Editorial Assistant: Phoebe Jordan-Reilly
Manager, Graphic Arts & Design: Stephen Druding
Art Director: Jennifer Clements
Production Project Manager: Kirstin Johnson
Manufacturing Coordinator: Margie Orzech-Zeranko
Prepress Vendor: Straive

Fifth Edition

Cataloging-in-Publication Data available on request from the Publisher

ISBN: 978-19751-7904-5

shop.lww.com

This book is dedicated to our nursing students and colleagues
who are so bravely serving to care for those with a deadly viral disease,
COVID-19. Knowingly, nurses are risking their lives—and mental wellbeing—
to uphold their commitment to patients and clients, families, and communities.

It is with gratitude that we acknowledge the loving support
(and patience) of our families across this project.

Diane, Cindy, and Wendy

Contributors

Simon Adam, PhD, MA, BScN, RN
Assistant Professor
Faculty of Health, School of Nursing
York University
Toronto, Ontario, Canada

Wendy Austin, PhD, MEd (Counselling), BScN
Professor Emeritus
Faculty of Nursing and the Dossetor Health Ethics
    Centre
University of Alberta
Edmonton, Alberta, Canada

Geertje Boschma, PhD, MSN, MA, BSN, RN
Professor
School of Nursing
University of British Columbia–Vancouver
Vancouver, British Columbia, Canada

Katherine S. Bright, PhD, MN, BN, BSc Kin, RN
Postdoctoral Fellow in Community Health Sciences
    (University of Calgary)
Triage Coordinator and Outpatient Psychiatric
    Consultation Liaison at the Women's Mental Health
    Clinic (Alberta Health Services)
Cumming School of Medicine (University of Calgary)
    and Psychiatry (Alberta Health Services)
University of Calgary and Alberta Health Services
Calgary, Alberta, Canada

Anne Marie Creamer, PhD, MSN, BN, RN
Nurse Practitioner
Addictions and Mental Health Program
Horizon Health Network
Saint John, New Brunswick, Canada

Cheryl Forchuk, PhD, MScN, RN, FCAHS,
    O Ont
Distinguished University Professor
Beryl and Richard Ivey Research Chair in Aging, Mental
    Health, Rehabilitation and Recovery
Parkwood Institute Research
Lawson Health Research Institute, Western University
London, Ontario, Canada

Holly Graham, PhD, MN, BScN, BA, RN, R. D.
    Psychologist
Associate Professor
College of Nursing
University of Saskatchewan
Saskatoon, Saskatchewan, Canada
Member, Thunderchild First Nation, Saskatchewan

Marlee Groening, MSN, BSN, RN
Regional Tertiary Clinical Nurse Specialist
Tertiary Mental Health and Substance Use
Vancouver Coastal Health
Vancouver, British Columbia, Canada

Catherine A. Hamilton, PhD, MSc, BScN, CNM
Assistant Professor
Nursing and Health Sciences
University of New Brunswick Saint John
Saint John, New Brunswick, Canada

Saima Hirani, PhD, MScN, BScN, RN
Assistant Professor
School of Nursing
University of British Columbia
Vancouver, British Columbia, Canada

Kathleen F. Hunter, PhD, MN, BSCN, RN, NP,
    GNC(C), NCA
Professor
Faculty of Nursing
University of Alberta
Edmonton, Alberta, Canada

Carmen Hust, PhD, MScN, BScN, RN CPMHN(C)
Professor
Nursing
Algonquin College
Ottawa, Ontario, Canada

Jean Daniel Jacob, PhD, MScN, BScN, RN
Director and Associate Dean, Full Professor
School of Nursing, Faculty of Health Sciences
University of Ottawa
Ottawa, Ontario, Canada

Emily Jenkins, PhD, MPH, BSN, RN
Associate Professor
School of Nursing
University of British Columbia
Vancouver, British Columbia, Canada

Cindy Jiang, MPH, PhD student
Research Assistant
Faculty of Health, Critical Disability Studies
York University
Toronto, Ontario, Canada

Kristen Jones-Bonofiglio, PhD, MPH, BScN, RN
Director & Associate Professor, School of Nursing
Director, Centre for Health Care Ethics
Faculty of Health & Behavioural Sciences
Lakehead University
Thunder Bay, Ontario, Canada

Arlene Kent-Wilkinson, PhD, MN, BSN, RN,
  CPMHN(C)
Associate Professor
College of Nursing
University of Saskatchewan
Saskatoon, Saskatchewan, Canada

Patricia M. King, MN, BN, RN
Instructor
College of Nursing
University of Saskatchewan
Saskatoon, Saskatchewan, Canada

Diane Kunyk, PhD, MSc, BScN, RN
Professor and Acting Dean
Faculty of Nursing and the Dossetor Health Ethics
  Centre
University of Alberta
Edmonton, Alberta, Canada

Gerri C. Lasiuk, PhD, MN, BA, RPN RN,
  CPMHN(C)
Assistant Dean & Associate Professor
College of Nursing
University of Saskatchewan
Regina, Saskatchewan, Canada

Hua Li, PhD, MPH, BSN, RN
Assistant Professor
College of Nursing
University of Saskatchewan
Saskatoon, Saskatchewan, Canada

Duncan Stewart MacLennan, MN, NP
Associate Teaching Professor
Faculty of Nursing
University of Alberta
Edmonton, Alberta, Canada

Shelley Marchinko, MN, BN, RN, CPMHN(C)
Instructor
College of Nursing
University of Manitoba
Winnipeg, Manitoba, Canada

Mary-Lou Martin, MScN, MEd, RN
Clinical Nurse Specialist/Associate Clinical Professor
St. Joseph's Healthcare Hamilton
Hamilton, Ontario, Canada

Lynn C. Musto, PhD, RPN, RN
Assistant Professor
School of Nursing
Trinity Western University
Langley, British Columbia, Canada

Tanya Park, PhD, MMid, GDMHN, BNSc, RN
Associate Professor
Faculty of Nursing
University of Alberta
Edmonton, Alberta, Canada

Cindy Peternelj-Taylor, MSc, BScN, RN, DF-IAFN
Professor
College of Nursing
University of Saskatchewan
Editor-in-Chief, *Journal of Forensic Nursing*
Saskatoon, Saskatchewan, Canada

Nicole Snow, PhD, MN, BN, RN, CPMHN(C)
Assistant Professor
Faculty of Nursing
Memorial University of Newfoundland
St. John's, Newfoundland and Labrador, Canada

Barbara Tallman, PhD, MN, BSc, RN
Instructor II
College of Nursing, Faculty of Rady Health Science
University of Manitoba
Winnipeg, Manitoba, Canada

Amanda Vandyk, PhD, MScN, BScN, RN
Associate Professor and Assistant Director for
  Undergraduate Programs
School of Nursing
University of Ottawa
Ottawa, Ontario, Canada

Colleen Varcoe, PhD, MSN, MEd, BSN, RN
Professor
School of Nursing
University of British Columbia
Vancouver, British Columbia, Canada

Kathryn Weaver, PhD, MN, BN, RN
Professor
Faculty of Nursing
University of New Brunswick
Fredericton, New Brunswick, Canada

Preface

In this, the fifth edition of *Psychiatric & Mental Health Nursing for Canadian Practice*, we are pleased to continue to present a Canadian approach to psychiatric and mental health (PMH) nursing practice. This edition was developed amidst the COVID-19 pandemic, which continues to plague the world as we write these words. We wish to acknowledge our nurse colleagues who contributed their expertise to the textbook during such challenging times. Along with them, we hope our efforts will support students of nursing, and those already practicing, to serve Canadians well in the area of mental health care. Although mental health nursing is a specialty area, eligible for certification by the Canadian Nurses Association, it remains a crucial aspect of all nursing. We hope this text will be a useful resource for nurses wherever they practice.

Across the world, the pandemic has strengthened the realization that we live together in a global community. Unfortunately, within this community, individuals and entire groups of people remain excluded from full participation in their society. Such exclusion negatively impacts mental health and wellbeing significantly. To increase nurses' awareness of and to inform their response to such impacts, this edition has a new chapter: *Identity, Inclusion, and Society*, contributed by Simon Adam and Cindy Jiang. As well as presenting the mental health sources and ramifications of social exclusion, the chapter will inform nurses of ways to address it.

This text continues to focus on contemporary mental health care and its foundations. Assessment and interventions (from psychopharmacology to psychological health and safety in the workplace) are presented, as are specific challenges to mental health: trauma, crisis, and disasters; anger, aggression, and violence; self-harm and suicide. The nursing care of and support for recovery of persons with a psychiatric disorder is comprehensively addressed. A lifespan perspective is offered with a focus on children and adolescents and on the older adult. The final unit provides key aspects of care for persons with additional vulnerabilities: those with experience of abuse, those with concurrent disorders, and those who are under forensic purview. Our focus across all the chapters has been to create a resource that truly enables excellence in psychiatric and mental health practice. A new feature is *Thinking Challenges*, which includes questions to assist you in reflecting upon what you have just learned. Answers are found on ThePoint, often with further questions to test your "know-how." All the pedagogical features that support us in doing so are listed below, as are further teaching and learning resources.

As in the previous editions, the terminology used to identify individual recipients of nursing care (e.g., individual, client, patient) has been left to the preference of the chapter contributors and the context in which this term is used.

Features

- Chapters open with **Learning Objectives**, **Key Terms**, and **Key Concepts** that cue students to the material they will encounter.
- **Research for Best Practice boxes** focus on specific studies, primarily Canadian, which contribute to improving nursing practice in PMH care. The selected studies reflect the broad range of research methods used to inform practice.
- The **In-a-Life feature** illustrates the way the topic of the chapter has shaped or been played out in a particular person's life.
- **Therapeutic Dialogue boxes** encourage the comparison of therapeutic and nontherapeutic communication by giving relevant examples of both.
- **Drug Profile boxes** present a profile of specific psychotropic medications, commonly prescribed in the treatment of mental disorders.
- **Psychoeducation Checklists** identify content areas for the education of persons with specific disorders and their families.
- **Summary of Key Points** encapsulates core chapter content to facilitate assimilation and review.
- **Thinking Challenges** include questions to reflect upon the material, with suggested answers found on ThePoint.
- **Web Links** connect to sites of relevance to the chapter content, including key documents, professional practice organizations, national and international institutions and groups, such as the Government of Canada,

the International Council of Nurses, and the World Health Organization.

Teaching and Learning Resources

To facilitate mastery of this text's content, a comprehensive teaching and learning package has been developed to assist faculty and students.

Resources for Instructors

Tools to assist you with teaching your course are available upon adoption of this text at http://thePoint.lww.com/Austin5e

- A **Test Generator** lets you put together exclusive new tests from a bank containing hundreds of questions to help you in assessing your students' understanding of the material. Test questions link to chapter learning objectives.
- **PowerPoint Presentations** provide an easy way for you to integrate the textbook with your students' classroom experience, either via slide shows or handouts. Multiple-choice and true/false questions are integrated

into the presentations to promote class participation and allow you to use i-clicker technology.
- An **Image Bank** lets you use the photographs and illustrations from this textbook in your PowerPoint slides or as you see fit in your course.
- **Case Studies** with related questions (and suggested answers) give students an opportunity to apply their knowledge to a client case similar to one they might encounter in practice.
- Answers to Thinking Challenges from the text are available for download

Resources for Students

Free resources are available to help students review material and become even more familiar with vital concepts. Students can access these resources at http://thePoint.lww.com/Austin5e using the codes printed in the front of their textbooks.

- **Journal Articles** provided for each chapter offer access to current research available in Wolters Kluwer journals.

Contents

Contributors vi
Preface viii

UNIT 1 Contemporary Canadian Mental Health Care 1

1   **Psychiatric and Mental Health Nursing: From Past to Present 2**
    Geertje Boschma and Marlee Groening

    Early Forms of Institutional Care 2
    A Revolutionary Idea: Humane Treatment 3
    Canadian Trends in the 19th and Early
       20th Centuries: An Era of Asylum
       Building 5
    Modern Thinking 8
    The Late 20th and Early 21st Century 12

2   **Mental Health, Mental Disorder, Recovery, and Wellbeing 20**
    Wendy Austin

    Mental Health 20
    Wellbeing 21
    Mental Disorders 23
    The Mental Health of Canadians 25
    Research-Based Care 25
    Global Mental Health 26

3   **Identity, Inclusion, and Society 29**
    Simon Adam and Cindy Jiang

    Identity and Social Exclusion 29
    Medicalization as a Form of Exclusion in
       Psychiatric Practice 36
    Global Responses to Social Exclusion 37
    Implications for Mental Health Nursing
       Practice 38
    Future Directions: Beyond Identity 39

4   **The Context of Mental Health Care: Cultural, Socioeconomic, and Geographic 42**
    Arlene Kent-Wilkinson and Wendy Austin

    Cultural Context of Mental Health Care 42
    Religion as a Cultural System 45
    Aboriginal or Indigenous Peoples in
       Canada 46
    Stereotyping, Prejudice, Discrimination, and
       Stigma 51
    Cultural Competence and Cultural Safety 53
    Socioeconomic Context of Mental Health
       Care 55
    Geographic Context of Mental Health Care 59

5   **The Continuum of Canadian Mental Health Care 66**
    Nicole Snow

    Primary Healthcare Approach 67
    Defining the Continuum of Care 68
    Comprehensive Mental Health System: Core
       Programs and Services 71

UNIT 2 Foundations of Psychiatric and Mental Health Nursing Practice 81

6   **Contemporary Psychiatric and Mental Health Nursing Practice 82**
    Carmen Hust and Cindy Peternelj-Taylor

    The Bio/Psycho/Social/Spiritual Model 82
    Entry-to-Practice Mental Health
       Competencies 84
    Standards of Professional Practice 95
    Key Components of PMH Nursing Practice 96
    Challenges of PMH Nursing 99
    PMH Nursing in a Global Community 101

7   **Communication and the Therapeutic Relationship 105**
    Cheryl Forchuk

    Self-Awareness 105
    The Bio/Psycho/Social/Spiritual Self 106
    Understanding Personal Feelings and Beliefs
       and Changing Behaviour 106
    Communication 106
    Using Verbal Communication 107
    Using Nonverbal Communication 108
    Recognizing Empathic Linkages 109
    Selecting Communication Techniques 111
    Applying Communication Concepts 111

Analyzing Interactions   114
The Nurse–Client Relationship   115
Nontherapeutic Relationships   118
Strategies Within the Therapeutic
    Relationship   119

**8   Legal and Ethical Aspects of
     Practice   125**
Wendy Austin and Arlene Kent-Wilkinson

Human Rights, the Law, and Psychiatric and
    Mental Health Care   126
Ethics and Psychiatric and Mental Health
    Nursing Care   133
Codes of Ethics for Nurses   135
Approaches to Ethics   136
Ethical Practice Environments   141
Moral Dilemmas and Moral Distress   141
Ethical Issues in Psychiatric and Mental
    Healthcare Settings   142

9   Theoretic Basis of Practice   153
Wendy Austin

Nursing Theories   153
Biologic Theories   159
Psychological Theories   160
Social Theories   167
Spiritual Theories   169
Recovery as a Framework for Mental Health
    Care   169

10   Biologic Basis of Practice   173
Catherine A. Hamilton

Foundational Concepts   173
Current Research Approaches and
    Advances   178
Neuroanatomy of the Central Nervous
    System   183
Neurophysiology of the Central Nervous
    System   190
Endocannabinoid System   200
Other   200
Related Fields of Study   200
Diagnostic Approaches   203
Integration of the Biologic, Psychologic, Social,
    and Spiritual Domains   204

UNIT
3
**Interventions in Psychiatric
and Mental Health Nursing
Practice   207**

11   The Assessment Process   208
Gerri C. Lasiuk

Assessment as a Process   208
Types of Assessment   209
Bio/Psycho/Social/Spiritual Psychiatric/Mental
    Health Nursing Assessment   216

**12   Care Planning and Implementation
     in Psychiatric and Mental Health
     Nursing   229**
Nicole Snow

Collaborative, Person-Centred Nursing
    Practice   229
Deriving a Nursing Focus of Care   232
Developing Individual Goals of Care   233
Nursing Interventions   234
Evaluation of Care Goals   246

**13   Psychopharmacology and Other
     Biologic Treatments   248**
Duncan Stewart MacLennan

Pharmacodynamics   249
Pharmacokinetics: How Drugs Move Through
    the Body   253
Phases of Drug Treatment   259
Antipsychotic Medications   261
Mood Stabilizers (Antimania Medications)   269
Antidepressant Medications   273
Phases of Mood Stabilizing and Antidepressant
    Therapy   278
Antianxiety and Sedative–Hypnotic
    Medications   278
Stimulants   281
New Medications and Emerging Therapies   283
Other Biologic Treatments   284
Psychosocial Issues in Biologic Treatments   285

**14   Cognitive–Behavioural
     Interventions   290**
Wendy Austin

The Cognitive Model   291
Levels of Cognition   293
Principles of Cognitive–Behavioural
    Therapy   294
Treatment Strategies   295
Mindfulness-Integrated CBT   299
Conclusion   299

15   Interventions With Groups   301
Shelley Marchinko

Group: Definitions and Concepts   301
Group Leadership   308
Types of Groups   311
Common Nursing Intervention Groups   313
Self-Care Groups   315

**16   Family Assessment and
     Interventions   319**
Cindy Peternelj-Taylor and Patricia M. King

Characteristics of Canadian Families   320
Family Caregivers   322
Contextual Issues to Consider When Working
    With Families   324

Family Assessment 325
Family Assessment in the Bio/Psycho/Social/
    Spiritual Domains 329
The Pyramid of Family Care Framework 335
Family Interventions 335

**17 Psychological Health and Safety
in the Workplace 341**
Diane Kunyk

Work 342
Healthy Workplaces 344
Threats to Workplace Psychological Health and
    Safety 347
Mental Health Problems and Disorders in the
    Workplace 349
Nurses and Workplace Psychological Health
    and Safety 350

UNIT

4 Challenges to Mental Health 357

18 Stress, Trauma, Crisis, and Disaster 358
Holly Graham and Wendy Austin

Stress 358
Crisis 375
Disaster 380

19 Anger, Aggression, and Violence 394
Mary-Lou Martin

Anger 395
Aggression and Violence 396
Models of Anger, Aggression, and Violence 397

20 Self-Harm and Suicidal Behaviours 420
Kristen Jones-Bonofiglio

Common Myths 420
Effects of Suicide 422
Epidemiology of Suicidal Behaviours 424
Holistic Risk Factors 429
Nursing Assessment and Interventions 434

UNIT

**5 Care and Recovery for Persons
With a Psychiatric Disorder 447**

**21 Schizophrenia Spectrum and Other
Psychotic Disorders 448**
Wendy Austin and Tanya Park

Schizophrenia 449
Epidemiology 455
Aetiology of the Schizophrenia Spectrum
    Disorders 457
Interdisciplinary Treatment 462
Priority Care Issues 462
Family Response to Disorder 462
Nursing Management: Human Response to
    Disorder 463

Schizoaffective Disorder 491
Delusional Disorder 494
Other Psychotic Disorders 494

**22 Depressive, Bipolar, and Related
Disorders 501**
Katherine S. Bright

Depressive Disorders 503
Bipolar Disorders 519

**23 Anxiety, Obsessive–Compulsive, and
Related Disorders 544**
Emily Jenkins and Lynn C. Musto

Normal Versus Abnormal Anxiety
    Response 545
Overview of Anxiety Disorders 545
Aetiologic Theories of Anxiety
    Disorders 552
Evaluation and Treatment Outcomes 563
Continuum of Care 563
Assessment and Treatment Issues Specific to
    Obsessive–Compulsive Disorder 566
Assessment and Treatment Issues Specific to
    Hoarding Disorder 568

**24 Somatic Symptom and Related
Disorders 573**
Duncan Stewart MacLennan

Somatization 574
Somatic Symptom Disorder 574
Other Somatic Symptom and Related
    Disorders 588
Psychological Factors Affecting Other Medical
    Conditions 589
Factitious Disorders 589

25 Eating Disorders 594
Kathryn Weaver

Anorexia Nervosa 596
Bulimia Nervosa 628
Binge-Eating Disorder 636
Prevention of Eating Disorders 643
Future Directions in Eating Disorder
    Knowledge 644

**26 Substance-Related and Addictive
Disorders 653**
Diane Kunyk

Definition 654
Neurobiology 654
Diagnostic Criteria 655
Epidemiology 656
Alcohol 656
Aetiologic Theories 658
Prevention 659
Interdisciplinary Treatment 660
Nursing Interventions for Specific Substance-
    Related Disorders 667

Special Populations and Situations   681
Nurses as Health Advocates   683

27 Personality Disorders and Disruptive, Impulse Control, and Conduct Disorders   687
Jean Daniel Jacob and Amanda Vandyk

Personality Disorders   688
Specific Personality Disorders   694
Cluster B Disorders   696
Cluster C Disorders   721
Other Personality Disorders   723
Disruptive, Impulse Control, and Conduct Disorders   723

28 Sleep–Wake Disorders   729
Anne Marie Creamer

Historical Perspectives on Sleep and Dreams   729
What Is Sleep?   730
Dreaming   731
Biologic Processes   732
Epidemiology: Canadian Sleep Habits   738
Overview of Sleep–Wake Disorders   738
Comorbid Mental Illnesses and Mental Health Problems   741
Insomnia   741
Obstructive Sleep Apnea   749
Common Circadian Rhythm Sleep–Wake Disorders   751

UNIT
6
Mental Health Across the Lifespan   755

29 Mental Health Promotion and Assessment: Children and Adolescents   756
Patricia M. King and Cindy Peternelj-Taylor

Childhood and Adolescent Mental Health   756
Common Childhood Stressors   757
Development of Child Psychopathology   765
Addressing Risks and Challenges to Children's and Adolescents' Mental Health   773
Mental Health Assessment of Children and Adolescents   776
Collection of Assessment Data   777
Bio/Psycho/Social/Spiritual Psychiatric Nursing Assessment of Children and Adolescents   785

30 Psychiatric Disorders in Children and Adolescents   803
Hua Li

Schizophrenia Spectrum and Other Psychotic Disorders   804
Bipolar and Related Disorders   805
Depressive Disorders   806

Anxiety Disorders   808
Obsessive–Compulsive Disorder   810
Trauma- and Stressor-Related Disorders   811
Neurodevelopmental Disorders of Childhood   814
Disruptive, Impulse Control, and Conduct Disorders   825
Motor Disorders: Tourette Disorder   827
Elimination Disorders   829
Spiritual Domain of Nursing Care   831

31 Mental Health of Older Adults: Promotion and Assessment   837
Barbara Tallman and Wendy Austin

Mental Health Promotion of the Older Adult   838
Bio/Psycho/Social/Spiritual Mental Health Nursing Assessment: The Older Adult   841
The Bio/Psycho/Social/Spiritual Domains and the Older Adult   844

32 Neurocognitive Disorders: Delirium and Dementia   861
Kathleen F. Hunter

Delirium   862
Mild Cognitive Impairment   872
Dementia   872
Dementia and Alzheimer Disease   872
Other Major NCDs (Dementias)   896

UNIT
7
Care of Persons With Additional Vulnerabilities   903

33 Care of Persons With Concurrent Substance-Related, Addictive, and Other Mental Disorders   904
Diane Kunyk

Epidemiology of Concurrent Disorders   905
Development of Concurrent Disorders   906
Assessment Approaches Specific to Concurrent Disorders   907
Care and Treatment Approaches Specific to Concurrent Disorders   907
Implementing Interventions for Specific Concurrent Disorders   909
Nursing Management: Summary   911
Where Do We Go From Here?   912

34 Care of Persons With Experiences of Abuse   915
Saima Hirani and Colleen Varcoe

The Social Context of Abuse   915
Forms of Abuse   918
The Health Impacts of Abuse   919
The Nursing Role: Recognizing and Responding to Abuse   921

35 **Care of Persons Under Forensic Purview** 933

Cindy Peternelj-Taylor

Criminalization of the Mentally Ill 933
The Paradox of Custody and Caring 934
Forensic Nursing: A Model for Care 935

Appendix A
Brief Psychiatric Rating Scale 953

Appendix B
Simpson-Angus Rating Scale 954

Appendix C
Abnormal Involuntary Movement Scale (AIMS) 956

Appendix D
Simplified Diagnoses for Tardive Dyskinesia (SD-TD) 958

Appendix E
Hamilton Rating Scale for Depression 960

Index 961

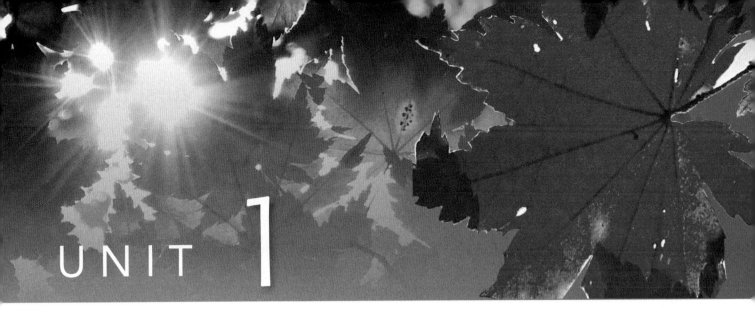

Contemporary
Canadian
Mental Health
Care

Psychiatric and Mental Health Nursing: From Past to Present

Geertje Boschma and Marlee Groening

Until the 19th century, people with mental disorders were mainly kept at home and cared for by their families. Sometimes, their legal guardians boarded them with other families for a fee as part of a broader poor relief system. Only the most seriously afflicted people, whose behaviour was severely disturbing or who were considered a danger to themselves, their families, or other citizens were often locked in prisons or poorhouses. Indigent people with mental disorders were grouped with old, sick, orphaned, or convicted people, and the circumstances in these scanty public facilities were most basic and often harsh. For those who could afford it, privately maintained institutions emerged as well (Boschma, 2003; Moran & Wright, 2006).

Early Forms of Institutional Care

Around the turn of the 15th century—the beginning of the European Renaissance—some towns in Europe established small-scale asylums as charitable enterprises, each one initially housing about 10 people. Most often, they were civilian, charitable initiatives in which neither the church nor doctors were involved. London's Bethlehem Hospital (famously known as Bedlam) (Fig. 1.1), founded in 1371, and the Reinier van Arkel asylum, founded in 1442 in the Dutch town of Den Bosch, are early examples of the insane asylums or "mad houses"

that would over the next centuries spread throughout Europe and, in the wake of colonialism, other parts of the world. These asylums were managed as large households, like other guesthouses or poorhouses, and administered by a board of noted citizens, with a steward and matron, often a married couple, taking charge of day-to-day management with the assistance of a few servants. With the social and economic changes of the 18th and 19th centuries, these homes grew into larger institutions (Boschma, 2003).

Religious orders, often under the protection or authority of the church, also involved themselves with charitable work and poor relief. Roman Catholic orders, for example, reemerged in 17th-century France during the Counter-Reformation, and many of them managed the care in small-scale premodern hospitals. The orders themselves sometimes owned the houses. Influential cases in point were the male order of the Congregation of Lazarists and the female congregation of the Sisters of Mercy (or Daughters of Charity), founded by Vincent de Paul in 1625 and 1633, respectively (Jones, 1989). These orders produced early models for nursing work as a socially respectable endeavour at a time when medical care had barely developed and was scarcely available (Nelson, 1999, 2001). In the Americas, one of the first institutions that took in people with mental disorders was San Hipólito in Mexico City, which opened

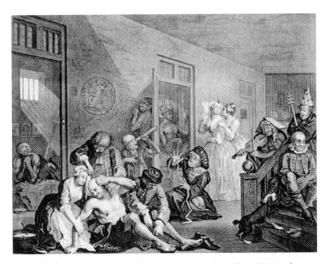

Figure 1.1 Interior of Bethlehem Asylum ("Bedlam"), London, as depicted by William Hogarth in his series *A Rake's Progress*. (From U.S. National Library of Medicine. Images from the history of medicine. National Institutes of Health, Department of Health and Human Services.)

in 1589 as a hospital for the insane, under the auspices of the Roman Catholic Church. It was run by the brothers of the order of La Caridad y San Hipólito, who, vowing poverty and charity, relied on alms to support themselves and worked as attendants in the institution (Leiby, 1992). The earliest forms of **institutional care** in Canada date back to the 19th century.

Diverse beliefs and approaches to deal with mental illness or attempts to treat it have been employed and must be understood in their historical context. Spiritual, biologic, and social explanations commonly were intertwined in popular perceptions of causes of mental illness. Evil spirits, sin, demonic possession, fears, contagious environments, or brain disturbances have figured in explanations of mental disorders and accordingly shaped people's responses, community resources, and medical treatment. History reflects that, generally, social fears and tolerance for what is deemed as "deviant behaviour" are related to social stability and availability of resources. In periods of relative social stability, individuals with mental disorders often have a better chance to live safely within their communities. During periods of rapid social change and instability, there are more general anxieties and fears, and subsequently, more intolerance and ill treatment of people with mental disorders.

As industrialization and urbanization increased during the 18th and 19th centuries, the rising middle class became concerned about a growing number of poor and deviant people who were not able to work and sustain themselves. At the same time, medical and social ideas about mental illness changed under the influence of ideas associated with the Enlightenment, and medical concerns with the treatment of mental illness increased. The insight gained ground that, rather than being

afflicted by loss of reason or evil spirits, people with mental disorders were rational beings with a human nature common to all human beings and should be treated humanely. As a result, the idea of a moral pedagogical treatment emerged that allegedly would help the suffering restore their innate capacity for self-control (Boschma, 2003; D'Antonio, 2006).

KEY CONCEPT

Social change, the structural and cultural evolution of society, is constant but often erratic. Psychiatric and mental health care has evolved within a historical context of social, economic, and political influences and cannot be separated from such realities.

A Revolutionary Idea: Humane Treatment

By the height of the French Revolution in 1792, **moral treatment** became an influential idea that altered the care of the mentally ill and gave rise to important initiatives in which reform-minded physicians had an influential role. During this time, Philippe Pinel (1745–1826) was appointed physician to Bicetre, a hospital for men, which had a very poor reputation. Pinel, influenced by Enlightenment ideals, believed that the insane were sick patients who needed humane treatment. He ordered the removal of the chains, stopped the abuses of drugging and bloodletting, and introduced exercises for patients and more appropriate medical care. Three years later, the same standards were extended to Salpetrière, the asylum for patients who were women. At about the same time in England, William Tuke (1732–1822), a Quaker tea merchant in York and a member of the Society of Friends, raised funds for a retreat for members of his Quaker community with mental disorders. The York Retreat, which opened in 1796, became another influential example for reform initiatives, introducing a regimen of humane, moral treatment, a pedagogical approach of kind supervision, proper medical treatment, and meaningful activities and distractions. Those reformers believed that a purposefully designed asylum that supported an environment that allowed for sympathetic care in quiet, pleasant surroundings with some form of useful occupation such as weaving or farming would cure people with mental disorders (D'Antonio, 2006). Based on these ideals, purposefully designed asylums were established throughout the Western world. In the United States, the Quaker Friends Asylum, which opened in 1817 in Frankford, Pennsylvania (now Philadelphia), was an example of this trend to humanize the care of people with mental disorders (D'Antonio, 2006). Despite these influential trends, however, public funds for state asylums were often insufficient to fully implement these ideals and

IN-A-LIFE

Boarding People With Mental Disorders With Families (12th to 19th Centuries)

THE GEEL LUNATIC COLONY, BELGIUM

The Legend of Saint Dymphna

According to legend, Dymphna, an Irish princess, came to Geel in the 6th century. Her father, the king of Ireland, disappointed that she was not a son and left her and her mother in the care of a priest who converted them to Christianity. After Dymphna's mother died, the king became filled with grief and wanted another woman just like his former wife. His advisors decided that only his own daughter could match the queen. However, when her pagan father wanted to marry Dymphna, she fled out of fear with the priest and came to Geel. When the Irish king eventually found Dymphna and the priest, he beheaded them. In some sources, the legend tells that several lunatics witnessing this frightful scene suddenly became cured. Dymphna became patron of lunatics due to her symbolic resistance to the spirit of evil and the site of her death a place of miraculous healing. Some sources tell how the Saint Dymphna Guesthouse and chapel were built at this place, becoming a place of pilgrimage.

A Powerful Example of Family Care in Geel, Belgium

Since the Middle Ages (1286), the Saint Dymphna Guesthouse and chapel have existed in Geel,

Belgium, eventually with a separate sick room for so-called lunatic pilgrims. Patients chronic with mental disorders who came to the Guesthouse as pilgrims seeking healing were often boarded out to families, and the Geel Lunatic Colony came into being. In the 19th century, the place became a formal institution with a strong emphasis on boarding outpatients with foster families, which became a model for many countries to follow and has lasted into the the 21st century. The legend of Saint Dymphna illustrates mythical and religious beliefs, explanations, and practices that have lost their meaning today; however, the cultural heritage of the Geel Colony demonstrates how powerful past ideas and beliefs can be in structuring creative and humane solutions to the care of people with mental disorders.

References
Compiled (with an update) from Parry-Jones, W. L. L. (1981). The model of the Geel Lunatic Colony and its influence on the nineteenth-century asylum system in Britain. In A. Scull (Ed.), *Madhouses, mad-doctors, and madmen. The social history of psychiatry in the Victorian Era* (pp. 201–217). The Athlone Press.
    Boschma, G. (2003). *The rise of mental health nursing: A history of psychiatric care in Dutch asylum, 1890–1920.* Amsterdam University Press.
    Goldstein, J. L., & Godemont, M. M. L. (2003). The legend and lessons of Geel: A 1500-year-old legend, a 21st-century model. *Community Mental Health Journal, 39*(5), 441–458.

living conditions in the emerging public state institutions remained constrained whereas the common practice to confine mentally afflicted people in poorhouses and jails also remained in place.

A Social Reformer: Dorothea Lynde Dix

An ardent advocate for reform of state-supported public care was Dorothea Lynde Dix (1802–1887). Her crusade for more humane treatment strongly influenced reform of public asylums in North America in the 19th century (Fig. 1.2). At age 40, Dix, a retired school teacher living in Massachusetts, was solicited by a young theology student to help with a Sunday school class for women inmates at the East Cambridge jail. Dix herself led the class and was shocked by living conditions in the jail. She was particularly struck by the treatment of inmates with mental disorders. It was the dead of winter, and the jail was providing no heat. When she questioned the jailer about this, he replied that "the insane need no heat." The prevailing myth was that the insane were insensible to extremes of temperature.

Dix's outrage initiated a long struggle in institutional reform (Lightner, 1999).

Dix followed patterns of new women's activism that emerged in the 19th century, similar to social reformers

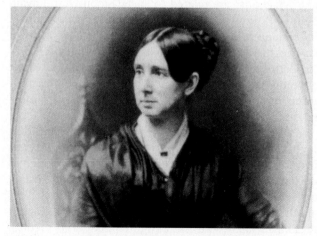

Figure 1.2 Dorothea Lynde Dix. (From U.S. National Library of Medicine Digital Collections. National Institutes of Health, Department of Health and Human Services.)

such as Elizabeth Fry in prison reform and Josephine Butler in protecting women against prostitution (Van Drenth & De Haan, 1999). Dix diligently investigated the conditions of jails and the plight of people who were mentally ill while promoting the building of mental hospitals. Her influence extended into Canada, where she was instrumental in advocating for mental institutions in Halifax and St. John's (Hurd, 1973/1916–17; Lightner, 1999).

Canadian Trends in the 19th and Early 20th Centuries: An Era of Asylum Building

In Canada, New Brunswick was the first of the former British North American province to open a mental institution. In 1835, a committee was appointed to prepare a petition to the provincial legislature proposing the establishment of a provincial asylum. Until then, counties had carried the responsibility under the Poor Laws system, typically confining indigent "insane" in local jails or in poorhouses. As the population increased in the early 1800s, so did the number of people with mental disorders who were in need of publicly provided care. In that same year, the provincial government approved the conversion of a building in Saint John, formerly a hospital for cholera patients, to a Provincial Lunatic Asylum until a new facility could be built. By 1848, this new facility was ready for use (Fig. 1.3) (Hurd, 1973/1916–17; Sussman, 1998).

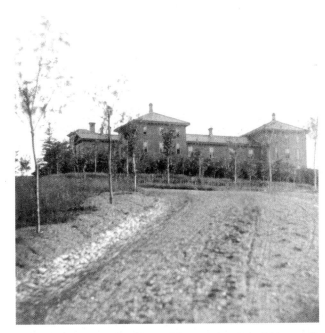

Figure 1.3 Canada's first hospital for people who were mentally ill, Saint John, New Brunswick, ca. 1885. (From Provincial Archives of New Brunswick, Saint John Stereographs—P86-67.)

During the latter half of the 19th century and beginning of the 20th century, each Canadian province established a publicly funded asylum (Table 1.1). Involuntary confinement and institutional care became the dominant treatment modality for people who were mentally ill, replacing older forms of familial care and Poor Law–based approaches (Moran, 2000; Moran & Wright, 2006). Some private institutions were also

Table 1.1	The First Asylums in British North America and Canada	
Province	**Date**	**Notes**
Quebec	1845	• Beauport, or the Quebec Lunatic Asylum, was opened. • A small dwelling for 12 mentally ill women was erected by Bishop St. Vallier.
	1714	• The Hotel Dieu cared for indigents, the crippled, and "idiots."
New Brunswick	1848	• The Provincial Lunatic Asylum was erected.
	1835	• Canada's first mental hospital opened in a small wooden building, a former cholera hospital, and was used as a temporary asylum.
Ontario	1850	• The Provincial Lunatic Asylum in Toronto admitted patients.
	1841	• People who were mentally ill were placed in county jails until 1841, after which the Old York Jail served as a temporary asylum.
Newfoundland	1854	• An asylum for patients with mental illness was erected and admitted its first patients.
Nova Scotia	1857	• The first patients were admitted to the Provincial Hospital for the Insane.
British Columbia	1872	• A remodelled provincial general hospital (the old Royal Hospital) was opened as the Asylum for the Insane in British Columbia.
Prince Edward Island	1877	• The Prince Edward Island Hospital for the Insane was built.
Manitoba	1886	• The Selkirk Lunatic Asylum was opened.
Saskatchewan	1914	• The Saskatchewan Provincial Hospital admitted the first patients.
Alberta	1911	• The Provincial Asylum for the Insane opened in Ponoka.
Yukon and Northwest Territories		• These districts had no asylums in the early 20th century. The Royal North West Mounted Police assisted in transporting mentally ill patients to asylums in neighbouring provinces.

Adapted from Sussman, S. (1998). The first asylums in Canada: A response to neglectful community care and current trends. *Canadian Journal of Psychiatry, 43*, 260–264; Hurd, H. M. (Ed.). (1973, originally printed 1916–1917). *The institutional care of the insane in the United States and Canada* (Vol. IV). Arno Press.

established, such as the Homewood Retreat in Ontario, although circumstances mirrored the conditions in public asylums (Warsh, 1989). An analysis of the British Columbia psychiatric system revealed that as of the late 19th century, patients who were Indigenous Peoples were also admitted to the provincial asylum (Menzies & Palys, 2006). The poorly resourced and physical conditions in these asylums were such that at the turn of the 20th century, many patients once admitted died from tuberculosis.

The Legal Basis for Mental Health Care

Following the terms established by the British North America Act of 1867, the organization of mental health care in Canada became provincially based, and each province developed its own legislation to deal with problems created by mental illness. In the late 19th century, all provinces passed legislation, most often called an Insanity Act, to provide a legal basis to publicly support hospitalization of mentally ill persons. In the course of the 20th century, legislation has been updated several times and eventually renamed a provincial Mental Health Act (MHA), reflecting changing views and a stronger medical influence on the care and treatment of people with mental illness. In the beginning of institutional psychiatric care in Canada, all patients admitted to public institutions were certified patients and no provisions existed for voluntary admission. In the course of the 20th century, voluntary admission became possible. Today, patients are being admitted to an institutional facility on either a voluntary or a certified basis. MHAs are purposefully designed legal procedures that provide authority and criteria that must be followed for patients admitted as certified patients, although criteria may differ between provinces. In several provinces, the use of community treatment or extended leave orders is a more recent development under the MHA (see Chapter 4 for the current legal context of mental health care).

Life Within Early Institutions

Despite the good intentions of early reformers, the approach inside the institution was one of custodial care and practical management, and treatment rarely occurred. The major concern was the management of a large number of people, many of whom exhibited disruptive or difficult to manage behaviours. Similar to trends in other countries, patient numbers in Canadian institutions grew rapidly, particularly after provinces became legally responsible for financing care of the people who were mentally ill, and more families opted to make use of them (Boschma, 2008). Institutions soon experienced severe overcrowding and had little more to offer than food, clothing, pleasant, but often remote, surroundings, and perhaps some means of employment

and exercise. Limited resources made life in these institutions difficult. Although they were typically under the direction of a medical superintendent, overcrowding and resource shortages created rowdy, dangerous, and often unbearable situations. Use of restraints or isolation continued to be common practices. Quiet, calm patients were involved in work as institutions grew into self-contained communities that produced their own food and made their own clothing. Day-to-day care was in the hands of lay personnel who shared with patients the routines of eating, sleeping, and working. Once admitted, many patients were cut off from society, in part due to remote settings. As part of the wider social reforms referred to above, reform-minded citizens and psychiatrists began to activate for change and better professional care, including the introduction of trained nurses.

Psychiatrist Charles K. Clarke (1857–1924) was an influential mental healthcare reformer in Ontario. As superintendent of various Ontario **psychiatric hospitals** (e.g., Rockwood Hospital, 1881–1905), he was well aware of the existing problems (Brown, 2000). He introduced nurse training for asylum personnel to improve matters. Supported by university-based scientific research, he also advocated for an urban centre for the treatment of acute mental illness, which was eventually established in 1925 as the Toronto Psychiatric Hospital.

The deplorable state of large mental institutions also gave rise to public attention and objection. In 1908, the American Clifford Beers (1876–1943) published an autobiography, *A Mind That Found Itself*, depicting his 3-year experience of admissions to both private hospitals and a state institution (Beers, 1908). He reported that in each facility, he had been beaten, choked, and imprisoned for long periods in dark, dank, padded cells and for many days had been confined in a straitjacket. He became an ardent advocate of the reform of psychiatric care. Beers' cause was supported by a prominent neuropathologist, Adolf Meyer (1866–1950), who suggested the term "mental hygiene" for bringing about improvement of people's mental health care in a manner similar to other public health initiatives. In 1909, they established a National Committee for Mental Hygiene in the United States, through whose efforts there developed child guidance clinics, prison clinics, and industrial mental health approaches. Beers and Meyer found a close Canadian ally in Clarence Hincks, a leading Toronto psychiatrist who was instrumental in founding the Canadian National Committee for Mental Hygiene (CNCMH) in 1918, together with his colleague Charles Clarke.

The appalling situation of Canadian provincial mental hospitals triggered particular political concern following World War I, when returning veterans suffering from shell shock had to rely on existing psychiatric facilities in their home provinces. A new belief gained ground in scientific approaches and reliance on expert knowledge in the prevention of mental illness. Compounding with ideas of prevention were class-based concerns about an alleged weak-mindedness among lower social classes and the need for betterment of the human race, influenced by eugenic ideas of the time (Dyck, 2013). This context of change provided a climate for expanding professionalism of many groups, including psychiatrists, psychologists, and nurses. The CNCMH keenly promoted improvement of mental hospitals. Introducing a trained nursing staff was part of this strategy. Voluntary admission controlled by physicians was supported, thus advancing the view that mental illness was similar to any physical illness.

Development of Psychiatric and Mental Health Nursing

Early Developments

As part of psychiatric reform, the CNCMH promoted the introduction of training schools for mental nurses similar to nurse training schools in general hospitals (Boschma et al., 2005; Tipliski, 2004). These nurses were later called psychiatric nurses. During his tenure as superintendent of Rockwood Mental Hospital (1881–1905), Charles Clarke was instrumental in establishing one of the first nurse training schools for female personnel

at this hospital and then at the Provincial Hospital in Toronto (Brown, 2000). Well-educated women with a sense of order and compassion had been essential in the introduction of training schools in general hospitals. In their efforts to model psychiatric hospitals after the general hospitals, psychiatrists took that ideal and geared the training of mental nurses toward women. The trained nurses provided them with the assistance they needed for new therapies and enhanced the hospital's reputation (Boschma, 2003; Brown, 2000). It was thought that women had the right moral and feminine characteristics for good patient care. The care of male patients was put in the hands of female nurses assisted by male orderlies in general hospitals; however, this shift was less common in psychiatry. While male attendants still retained a prominent place in the care of patients who were mentally ill, their training typically obtained a lower status, or they initially did not receive any training at all, as was the case in Ontario mental hospitals (Tipliski, 2002). See Box 1.1 for historical highlights.

Regional Influences

In western Canada, which had a stronger orientation to British traditions of institutional care, the introduction of mental nurse training schools did not occur until the

---

BOX 1.1 Highlights From Psychiatric Mental Health Nursing History

1888	The first mental nurse training school established at Kingston's Rockwood Asylum
1918	Foundation of the Canadian National Committee of Mental Hygiene
1920	First psychiatric nursing text published, *Nursing Mental Diseases*, by Harriet Bailey
1922	First Registration of Nurses Act passed in Ontario including nurse training schools at the mental hospitals
1930s	Mental hospitals in western Canada established schools for mental nurses and attendants
1950	Psychiatric Nurses Association of Canada (PNAC) founded
1952	Publication of Hildegard E. Peplau's *Interpersonal Relations in Nursing*
1963	*Perspectives in Psychiatric Care* and *Journal of Psychiatric Nursing* first issued
1979	PNAC working paper on Standards of Practice for Psychiatric Nurses published
1986	The Canadian Nurses Association establishes a national certification program for specialty nursing practice
1988	Canadian Federation of Mental Health Nurses (CFMHN) founded
1995	CFMHN *Standards of Psychiatric and Mental Health Nursing Practice* published
2006	CFMHN *Standards for Psychiatric-Mental Health Nursing*, 3rd edition published
2014	CFMHN *Standards for Psychiatric-Mental Health Nursing*, 4th edition, provides direction to all nurses and to the public on acceptable practices of psychiatric–mental health nurses (http://cfmhn.ca/professionalPractices)
2015	*Canadian Association for Schools of Nursing (CASN) and Canadian Federation of Mental Health Nurses (CFMHN)* jointly developed Entry-to-Practice Mental Health and Addiction Competencies for Undergraduate Nursing Education in Canada

1930s, by which time male attendants were also being trained. In Alberta, for example, the Department of Health hired psychiatrist Charles A. Barager in 1932, to implement reform. Barager came from Manitoba, where as superintendent at the Brandon Asylum, he introduced a nurse training school (Dooley, 2004). He had a strong belief in the ability of compassion in women: "The nursing of mental patients requires women of finer personality, of wider sympathies, greater self-control and higher intelligence than even the nursing of those who are physically ill" (Tipliski, 2002, p. 95).

Barager's term in Alberta was short lived (he died in 1936), but the training for nurses and attendants that he initiated in the Alberta Hospital at Ponoka had a lasting influence. Despite opposition to his ideas from the Registered Nurses Association in Alberta, which had controlled the registration of nurses since 1916, he was able to secure approval for a new diploma in mental nursing through the Alberta Department of Health. He also established arrangements with general hospitals so that, after 2 years of training in the mental hospital, female nurse students could undertake an additional 18 months of training at a general hospital and take licensing exams for registered nurses, after which they would return to the mental hospital. For male attendants, a 3-year certificate course was implemented, leading to a diploma in mental nursing. Graduates who were men did not obtain registered nursing status, reflective of the gendered context in which mental nurse training emerged. These trained and skilled nurses were essential for new therapies, such as electroshock and insulin coma therapy introduced in the 1940s requiring more skilled nursing. Medical care needs also shifted. Alberta Hospital at Ponoka also had a large infirmary with many frail and sick older adult patients (Boschma et al., 2005).

This climate of change created many new opportunities for working- and middle-class men and women to pursue careers as psychiatric nurses, and nurses began to articulate **psychiatric nursing** knowledge in nursing textbooks. The first psychiatric and mental health (PMH) nursing textbook that appeared in North America was *Nursing Mental Diseases*, written by Bailey (1920). The content of the book reflected an understanding of mental disorders of the times and set forth nursing care in terms of appropriate procedures.

Modern Thinking

As PMH nursing began to develop as a profession in the early 20th century, it incorporated new perspectives on mental illness that were emerging, particularly ideas on prevention as well as **biologic views** on mental illness. These new theories would profoundly shape the future of mental health care for all practitioners. Chapter 9 examines the underlying ideologies, but it is important to understand their development within the social and

historical context to appreciate fully their impact on treatment approaches.

Evolution of Scientific Thought

In the early 1900s, there were two opposing views of mental illness: the belief that mental disorders had biologic origins and the belief that the problems were attributed to environmental and social stresses. **Psychosocially oriented ideas** proposed that mental disorders resulted from environmental and social deprivation. Moral treatment grew out of this idea, and the notion of prevention advocated by the mental hygiene movement also reflected a psychosocial orientation. The biologic view held that mental illnesses had a biologic cause and could be treated with physical interventions. Biologic approaches and physical treatments such as bed rest; wet packs, which entailed wrapping patients in wet sheets; and prolonged baths became popular around 1900 as part of the rise of scientific psychiatry. They were grounded in the idea that overstrained nerves should obtain rest. Such treatments turned out to be largely ineffective.

Meyer and Psychiatric Pluralism

Adolf Meyer (1866–1950) bridged the ideological gap between the two approaches by introducing the concept of **psychiatric pluralism**, an integration of human biologic functions with the environment. He focused on investigating how organic functions related to the person and how the person, constituted of these organs, related to the environment (Neill, 1980). Unfortunately, this included the surgical treatment of psychosis by one of his disciples, Henry Cotton, who believed infection caused insanity and attempted to cure patients by removing sites of sepsis such as the teeth, tonsils, and colon (Scull, 2005). Meyer's ideas had little chance to evolve and flourish as the emerging psychoanalytic theories would soon dominate the psychiatric world in North America for a long time to come. It was not until after World War II, when a new emphasis on community-based care evolved, that environmental views and psychosocial approaches gained renewed prominence with the application of psychosocial rehabilitation models for people living with severe and persistent mental illness (Shepherd et al., 2008).

Freud and Psychoanalytic Theory

Sigmund Freud (1856–1939) and the **psychoanalytic movement** of the early 1900s promised a radically new approach to PMH care. Trained as a neuropathologist, Freud developed a personality theory based on unconscious motivations for behaviour, or drives. Using a new technique called psychoanalysis, he delved into the patient's feelings and emotions regarding past experiences, particularly early childhood and adolescent memories, to explain the basis of aberrant behaviour. He showed that symptoms of hysteria could be produced and made to disappear while patients were in a subconscious state of hypnosis.

According to the Freudian model, normal development occurred in stages, with the first three—oral, anal, and genital—being the most important. The infant progressed through the oral stage, experiencing the world through symbolic oral ingestion; into the anal stage, in which the toddler developed a sense of autonomy through withholding; and on to the genital stage, in which a beginning sense of sexuality emerged within the framework of the oedipal relationship. Freud posited that any interference in this normal development, such as psychological trauma, would give rise to neurosis or psychosis. Primary causes of mental illnesses were viewed as psychological, and any physical manifestations or social influences were considered secondary (Malamud, 1944). Psychoanalysts believed that mental illnesses originated from disturbed personality development and faulty parenting. They categorized mental illnesses either as a psychosis (severe) or as a neurosis (less severe). A psychosis impaired daily functioning because of breaks in contact with reality. A neurosis was less severe, but individuals were often distressed about their problems. The terms psychosis and neurosis entered common everyday language and added credibility to Freud's conceptualization of mental disorders. Freud's ideas would soon represent the forefront of psychiatric thought, and they shaped society's view of mental health care. Freudian ideology dominated psychiatry well into the 1970s. Intensive psychoanalysis, aimed at repairing the trauma of the original psychological injury, was the treatment of choice. Psychoanalysis was costly and time consuming and required lengthy training; few could perform it, and as a result, thousands of patients in state institutions with severe mental illnesses were essentially ignored.

Integration of Biologic Theories Into Psychosocial Treatment

Until the 1940s, the biologic understanding of mental illness did not result in effective treatment. Early somatic treatments based on these views often were unsuccessful because of the lack of understanding and knowledge of the biologic basis of mental disorders. As discussed, the use of hydrotherapy, or baths, was an established procedure in mental institutions. The use of warm baths and, in some instances, ice cold baths were thought to produce calming effects for patients with mental disorders. Still, baths often ended up as a form of restraint rather than as a therapeutic practice, and the physiologic responses were poorly understood. During the 1930s and 1940s, other biologic treatments

emerged, which sparked new hope that they would result in effective treatment, such as insulin coma therapy and electroconvulsive therapy (ECT) (Boschma, 2019a; Shorter & Healy, 2007). Yet, often, these biologic procedures were applied either indiscriminately or inappropriately with substantial side effects including psychosurgery and ECT (see Chapter 13). ECT, the application of a short (1 to 2 s) electrical current to the brain in order to generate a convulsion for an allegedly healing effect, was first used around 1940. Unlike the original procedure, contemporary ECT is modified by being applied under anaesthesia. Psychosurgical treatment, direct surgical intervention in lobes of the brain, also called lobotomy, began to be applied as of the late 1940s. Results from such brain therapies were mixed, and by the 1970s, the use of lobotomy became increasingly controversial; the use of ECT as treatment across a broad range of disorders was also questioned, but in its modified form, it is now widely used for the treatment of depression (Boschma, 2019b; Pressman, 2002). Recent insights resulting from brain research and new technologic advancements such as electromagnetic brain-stimulating techniques have generated a renewed interest in biologic treatments, offering new possibilities for treatment of depression and other neurophysiologic disorders (George, 2003). Thanks to modern technology and improved methods, neurosurgical techniques, such as deep brain stimulation, as well as ECT and transcranial magnetic stimulation can now be applied more humanely with positive therapeutic outcomes for some psychiatric disorders (George, 2003; Rai et al., 2010; Sadowsky, 2006).

Support for the biologic approaches received an important boost in the early 1950s with the introduction of psychotropic medications. Psychopharmacology revolutionized the treatment of mental illness and led to an increased number of patients discharged into the community as symptoms became more manageable. The eventual focus on brain research became a key to understanding psychiatric disorders. Chlorpromazine was an early neuroleptic drug that became widely used. Profound behavioural changes observed as a result of this medication in patients who experienced long-term mental illness created an enormous enthusiasm about the potential of new medications. Understanding of the working of these drugs was in infancy, however, and their side effects soon became serious drawbacks. As knowledge increased and the management of side effects improved, psychopharmacotherapeutics obtained a central place in the treatment of mental illness. The introduction of lithium in the early 1970s brought a lasting change in the treatment of bipolar disorder, as did antidepressants in the treatment of mood disorders (LaJeunesse, 2000). Nurses obtained an essential role in administering medications, monitoring their effects, and teaching patients about their effects.

New Trends in Post–World War II Mental Health Care

Following the experiences of World War II, insight grew among governments, as well as health professionals, that psychiatric services had to be placed on a new footing and new attention began to be paid to patient rights. By the end of the 1940s, patients in overcrowded and isolated psychiatric hospitals outnumbered the number of patients in other healthcare facilities, including general hospitals. Increased federal funding for health services and training of healthcare personnel created new opportunities. The implementation of universal health insurance for hospital care and medical services during the 1950s and 1960s, based on a 50/50 cost sharing between federal and provincial governments, generated funding for the establishment of psychiatric departments in general hospitals, shifting the focus of services away from large provincial institutions (Ostry, 2009). The downsizing of mental hospitals began.

The Canadian Mental Health Association (CMHA), renamed from the earlier CNCMH, had an instrumental role in policy development for new services in general hospitals and the community. In its influential 1963 report, *More for the Mind*, the CMHA argued that mental illness had to be dealt with similarly to physical illness, and it argued for the application of multiple perspectives—medical, social, and familial—in multidisciplinary services and community treatment. A critical social movement emerged, protesting the poor circumstances in large mental hospitals, the frequent use of seclusion, and the lack of patient rights. Psychiatry became the target of fierce debate and antipsychiatric critique in the 1970s (Crossley, 2006). Power relationships and the dominance of the medical model were questioned, and an emerging **patient movement** obtained a new voice and presence in mental health.

KEY CONCEPT

Deinstitutionalization involves the downsizing or elimination of psychiatric hospitals with a new orientation to community-based mental health services and general hospital departments of psychiatry.

The shift in 20th century mental health policy resulted in deinstitutionalization, the downsizing of the large provincial psychiatric hospitals, and a new orientation on community-based services to support people with mental illness within their own communities (Boschma, 2011; Dyck, 2011). Initially, no services in the community were available for the large number of people discharged from mental hospitals. They had to adjust to community living with little support. A new patient liberation movement emerged in response and was fueled by an antipsychiatric critique of the

mental health system. Canada saw its first patient-led community mental health initiative with the foundation of the Mental Patient Association (MPA) of Vancouver in 1971, a unique organization that transformed Canada's psychiatric landscape (MPA Founders Collective, 2013). The MPA formed as a patient driven, grassroots response to deinstitutionalization and to tragic gaps in community mental health, thereby inverting traditional mental health hierarchies (Boschma et al., 2014; Davies, 2014). The MPA members started to offer community living in several communal houses, offering housing, work, support, and community activities organized by and for mental patients (Fig. 1.4). Soon similar groups followed, such as Phoenix Rising in Toronto, established by former patients, purposefully calling themselves psychiatric survivors. Improving support and resources for people with mental illness within the community became a key mental health target (Fingard & Rutherford, 2011).

Mental hospitals began to reduce their size and, over the course of the next decades, many closed or changed their focus—a process that in Canada would last until the end of the 20th century. In British Columbia, for example, the provincial mental hospital, Riverview, closed its doors permanently in 2012 (Hall, 2012). During the second half of the 20th century, funding for mental health care became part of the larger healthcare system, with a stronger emphasis on general hospital–based psychiatry and community-based care. Nurses had an essential role in this transformation in the emerging field of **community mental health nursing** (Boschma, 2012).

In the late 1970s, the federal government modified the funding structure for health care, reducing its share in the cost. Services and treatments diversified. Provinces developed different models and strategies to fund specialized services such as alcohol and substance abuse treatment programs, which following World War II were pressing mental healthcare needs. Biologic approaches, such as use of psychopharmacology and, eventually, safer application of ECT, were complemented by new rehabilitative services, the use of group therapy and other psychotherapies, as well as the provision of day treatment. To address the needs of different population groups, subspecialties also emerged, such as child psychiatry, forensic, and geriatric services. The perception of health care as a human right enhanced consumer and volunteer involvement, as well as public education on mental illness, and it increased the demand for patient autonomy.

Continued Evolution of Psychiatric and Mental Health Nursing

The new multidisciplinary approaches and services emerging in the postwar era generated a pressing need for more and better trained mental healthcare

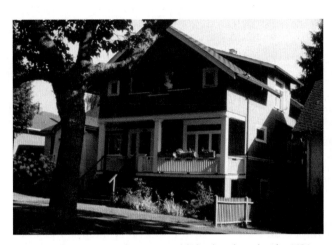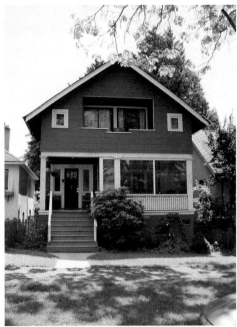

Figure 1.4 Original community homes established and run by the MPA members in Vancouver in the 1970s. (Courtesy of David MacIntyre.) For a full documentary of Vancouver's Mental Patient Association (MPA), see: *MPA Founders Collective (2013)*. Retrieved from https://oralhistorycentre.ca/2014/01/16/dr-megan-davies-the-inmates-are-running-the-asylum-stories-from-mpa

personnel, including nurses. The changes created a context for new developments in PMH nursing education. Organized responses of provincial professional nurses' organizations, and the initial efforts of hospital administrators and psychiatrists to continue staffing psychiatric hospitals through hospital-based nurse training programs, resulted in a diverse pattern of PMH nurse education. As of the 1950s, Canada entertained two models of education for PMH nursing, resulting in the preparation of two different professional nursing groups for nursing care in mental health services. Regional influences played a large role in the generation of the two models. On the one hand, general hospital–based schools of nursing, especially in eastern Canada, began to integrate psychiatric nursing into their curriculum. In Ontario, for example, under the influence of the mental hygiene movement, general hospital nurse training schools had included care of mentally ill patients into their training as early as the 1930s. Student nurses attended the provincial psychiatric hospitals for a brief period of training, called an affiliation program. Conversely, mental nurse trainees, mostly women, from the psychiatric hospital–based nurse training programs opted for an affiliation to the general hospital, resulting in both groups obtaining the title of registered nurse. After World War II, the provincial government and the provincial association of registered nurses in Ontario formalized this pattern into a permanent structure. Gradually, the psychiatric hospital–based programs decreased in number and size, and the registered nurse became the main nursing care provider in mental health services (Tipliski, 2004).

In the less densely populated western Canadian provinces, the pattern emerged of general hospital nurse trainees choosing affiliation experiences at the psychiatric hospitals, but the bulk of nursing care in the provincial hospitals continued to be provided by nurses and attendants graduated from psychiatric hospital–based nurse training programs (Hicks, 2011). As noted previously of Alberta Hospital in Ponoka, some western provinces established an affiliation program for mental nurse trainees who were women, and its graduates obtained the title of registered nurse. The program was limited in size, however, and psychiatric hospital–based training schools remained the norm, graduating large numbers of psychiatric nurses, whereas many women also worked in the institution as untrained attendants to meet demands for personnel. Trainees who were men received a diploma in mental nursing. In British Columbia, a training school for mental nurses (who were later called psychiatric nurses) was established in 1930 at Essondale, which eventually became Riverview Hospital (Fig. 1.5).

In the western provinces, the government had less control over nurse training than in the eastern province of Ontario. Provincial associations of registered nurses in western provinces also failed to support affiliation for psychiatric hospital–based nurse trainees, and medical superintendents of psychiatric hospitals continued to retain much of their influence over psychiatric nurse education (Boschma et al., 2005; Tipliski, 2004).

Around 1950, psychiatric attendants in the province of Saskatchewan took the lead in obtaining political support for a different pattern of nurse education that would lead to a separate Psychiatric Nurses Act and related training acts independent of provincial registered nurse practice acts. In Saskatchewan, registered

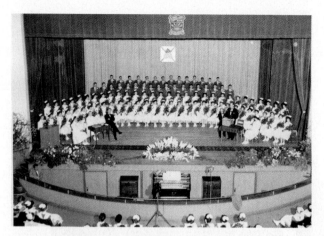

Figure 1.5 Graduation ceremony, School of Psychiatric Nursing, Essondale (Riverview Hospital), ca. 1950s. (From Historical collection, Riverview Hospital Historical Society, Coquitlam, BC.)

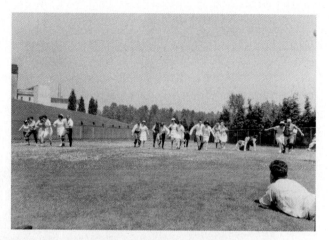

Figure 1.6 Sports Day on Riverview Hospital grounds, nurses and patients, 1966. (From Historical collection, Riverview Hospital Historical Society, Coquitlam, BC.)

nurses had never successfully integrated into the mental hospitals. Although a psychiatric nurse training program had existed for Saskatchewan for asylum attendants since the 1930s and was expanded after World War II to address the new need for psychiatric nursing expertise, it never resulted in registration as a nurse. Dissatisfied with their exclusion from any professionally recognized nursing title, provincial hospital attendants, who in Saskatchewan had obtained the right to unionize after the election of the new Co-operative Commonwealth Federation government in 1944, became instrumental in generating union support, as well as backing from the new government, for legislation of a separate psychiatric nurses act, which passed Parliament in 1948. In 1950, the Psychiatric Nurses Association of Canada was formed. Their action resulted in a distinct professional group of psychiatric nurses (Hicks, 2011; Tipliski, 2004). During the 1950s, all four western Canadian provinces passed acts that entitled graduates of western Canadian psychiatric hospital–based nurse training programs to receive the title of psychiatric nurse. Eventually, these programs moved into the college system. The two separate models of psychiatric nursing education still exist today and have been integrated into the regular education system over the past decades. This resulted in baccalaureate education programs in generic and psychiatric nursing education.

The Late 20th and Early 21st Century

In the post–World War II era, nurses facilitated the therapeutic climate within psychiatric hospitals (Fig. 1.6). The shift to community mental health and deinstitutionalization generated many new functions for PMH nurses (Boschma et al., 2005). Nurses obtained a central role in supporting large numbers of discharged patients in their transition to living in the community. In the psychiatric hospitals and general hospital units, nurses obtained new therapeutic roles in group therapies, and their work in community mental health services expanded (oschma, 2012). New theoretical models became available that emphasized building therapeutic nurse–patient relationships and holistic nursing approaches. Hildegard Peplau, who in recent scholarship was considered one of the most influential psychiatric nurses of the 20th century, proved to be a strong leader in the development of these new therapeutic frameworks for psychiatric nursing (Boschma et al., 2005; Calaway, 2002).

Expansion of Holistic Nursing Care

In 1952, Peplau published the landmark work *Interpersonal Relations in Nursing*. It introduced PMH nursing practice to the concepts of interpersonal relations and the importance of the therapeutic relationships. In fact, the nurse–patient relationship was defined as the very essence of PMH nursing and supported a holistic perspective on patient care (see Chapters 5, 6, and 7). These new frameworks underscored a new professional and disciplinary independence for nurses.

By 1963, two U.S.-based nursing journals, the *Journal of Psychiatric Nursing* (now the *Journal of Psychosocial Nursing and Mental Health Services*) and *Perspectives in Psychiatric Care*, as well as the *Canadian Journal of Psychiatric Nursing* (1975–1990), focused on psychiatric nursing. Also, the *Canadian Journal for Nursing Research* began to publish PMH nursing research. During the 1980s, the Canadian Federation of Mental Health Nurses (CFMHN) formed as an interest group of the Canadian Nurses Association with a view to promoting the interests of mental health nurses and bringing matters of mental health nursing interest and psychiatric patient care to the attention of the public at large. In 1995, this group published the Canadian Standards of Psychiatric and Mental Health Nursing Practice. Based on the influential work of Patricia Benner (1984), the standards were written within a framework of "domains of practice." This promoted a holistic perspective on nursing care, with PMH nurses practicing in a variety of settings with a variety of clientele. The emphasis was on activities ranging from health promotion to health restoration. The standards reflected the belief that PMH nursing should be research driven, continually incorporating new findings into nursing practice. Relying on these standards, the Canadian Nurses Association created the opportunity to become certified in mental health nursing as part of their larger certification program of specialty nursing areas established during the 1980s.

Wrinkles in the System—Rethinking Mental Health Care in the 1980s

During the 1980s, wrinkles in the emerging social fabric of downsizing mental hospitals, general hospital psychiatric departments, and community mental health care emerged. The mixed results of deinstitutionalization became apparent and generated a series of government-commissioned reports in all provinces to improve mental health services. Enormous variation existed among provinces in the extent and timing in which they implemented deinstitutionalization policies. People with mental disorders were discharged into communities that were often ill prepared to offer community support programs, housing, or vocational opportunities. Communities were sometimes hesitant in accepting people with persistent mental illness in their midst, and stigma remained attached to mental health services (Hector, 2001; Sealy & Whitehead, 2004). The 1981 Charter of Rights and Freedoms reflected a public statement intended to counter such responses (Greenland et al., 2001).

Self-help groups and family and consumer organizations, such as the Schizophrenia Society of Canada and the Mood Disorder Society of Canada, voiced critique and asserted themselves as active participants in improving mental healthcare services during the past decades. Moreover, the self-formed patient organizations generated new and participatory caring roles as peers using their lived experience with mental illness as a resource for others. **Peer support** work became a new and relied upon form of advocacy and peer help (See Box 1.2).

Outreach and mobile crisis response teams emerged to address problems people with severe mental illness experienced in the community. Multiple admissions of patients, sometimes referred to as "revolving door" patients, signified that long-term severe mental illness remained a persistent problem, with patients continuously moving in and out of the acute care system. More and better equipped community supports were needed. Also, the interconnected issues of severe mental illness, substance dependency, and inadequate community resources and housing have resulted in a growing number of people with mental illness who were experiencing homelessness, as well as a large population of people who were mentally ill winding up in the criminal justice systems. Within these groups, the specific mental health needs of women remain poorly addressed. While the threat of suicide is increasingly recognized as a severe mental health concern for women and men alike; men diagnosed with depression are found to have higher suicide rates than women (Gagnon & Oliffe, 2015).

The insight grew that mental health services were still fragmented and not sufficiently developed to meet the needs of diverse populations as the 20th century drew to a close. Disability resulting from mental illness affected millions of adults and children every year. When compared with all other diseases, at the turn of the

---

BOX 1.2 Changing Directions, Changing Lives: The Mental Health Strategy for Canada

Six key strategic directions to address the mental health needs for Canadians.

- *Promote* mental health across the lifespan in homes, schools, and workplaces, and *prevent* mental illness and suicide wherever possible.
- Foster *recovery* and wellbeing for people of all ages living with mental health problems and illnesses, and uphold their *rights*.
- Provide *access* to the appropriate combination of services, treatments, and supports, when and where people need them.

- Reduce *disparities* in risk factors and access to mental health services, and strengthen the response to the needs of *diverse* communities and Northerners.
- Work with *First Nations, Inuit, and Métis* to address their mental health needs, acknowledging their distinct circumstances, rights, and cultures.
- Mobilize *leadership*, improve knowledge, and foster *collaboration* at all levels.

From Mental Health Commission of Canada. (2012). *Changing directions, changing lives: The mental health strategy for Canada*. http://strategy.mentalhealthcommission.ca/pdf/strategy-text-en.pdf

21st century, mental illness ranked first in terms of causing disability in North America and Western Europe (Hart Wasekeesikaw, 2006; Morrow, 2002; World Health Organization, 2001).

A New Era of Healthcare Reform at the Turn of the 21st Century

Although public and private expenditures for health care services have increased in North America, still, financial and social barriers continued to affect the overall funding for mental health service and generated inequity. By the 1990s, new federal initiatives in mental health policy were urgently needed to address systemic issues of fragmentation. In 1998, the Canadian Alliance on Mental Illness and Mental Health (CAMIMH) was formed as a conjoint initiative of the Canadian Psychiatric Association, the CMHA, the Mood Disorder Association of Canada, the National Network for Mental Health, and the Schizophrenia Society of Canada. Consumers and service providers jointly began to lobby the federal government to develop an action plan and a new national agenda for mental health care (Beauséjour, 2001). Two years later, the CAMIMH joined the Canadian Collaborative Mental Health Initiative, which was formed to focus specifically on the improvement of mental health care in the primary healthcare setting. Collaboration of consumers and caregivers remains a vital and significant strategy in mental health care (see Chapters 7 and 11).

In 2002, the CAMIMH published its first report, a collation of the latest Canadian data on mental illness, with assistance from Health Canada (2002). Among other aspects of mental health care, the report revealed that 86% of hospitalizations for mental illness in Canada occurred in general hospitals. This profound change from traditional institutional care to general hospital care underscored the need for additional and improved acute and community-based mental health services. A senate-commissioned review of the Canadian health care system resulted in a call for better service: *Out of the Shadows at Last: Transforming Mental Health, Mental Illness and Addiction Services in Canada* (Kirby & Keon, 2006). The report highlighted the need to counter fragmentation and to address the disparate services provided across the provinces and between rural and urban regions, complicated by unique regional multicultural needs. Stories of Canadians suffering from mental illness illustrated the complex issues of stigmatization and discrimination. The report also drew attention to the determinants affecting health, such as health care, housing, employment, social welfare, as well as the justice system for Canadians with mental health concerns. The report also included stories of patients themselves (Kirby & Keon, 2006). The lack of a nationwide mental health strategy and the inconsistency between provincial jurisdictions that determine mental health policies

and service delivery were key findings that called for **mental healthcare reform**. Some critics of the report, however, noticed a lack of emphasis on "preventative determinants" and recognition of the depth of disability caused by mental illness (Arboleda-Flórez, 2005), and some women's advocate groups challenged the report's "silence" on the disparities between mental health and addiction services for men and women (Canadian Women's Health Network, 2006). In the end, the findings and recommendations from the CAMIMH and Kirby reports became the impetus for the establishment in 2007 of the Mental Health Commission of Canada mandated to develop a national mental health strategy.

Public awareness arose that continued impact of stigmatization and discrimination had to be countered by targeted prevention strategies to address historical injustice. There was recognition that diverse ethnic and cultural populations and different age groups had distinctive mental health needs and different social and mental pressures placed upon them. Also, continued consumer input from patients themselves as active participants in their care resulted in the recognition of the important role of peer support (Boschma & Devane, 2019; Murphy & Higgins, 2018). Peer support, typically defined "support provided by peers, for peers; or any organized support provided by and for people with mental health problems and illnesses," has become an integrated part of mental health services (Cyr et al., 2016, p. 45).

Various groups experience inequity in a mental healthcare system that is not adequately geared to meeting diverse needs or address historical injustice. Mental health of Indigenous Peoples is a critical issue in Canada because communities of Indigenous Peoples experience disproportionate rates of both physical and mental illness (Varcoe et al., 2015). Enhancing historical understanding of the health issues and inequities affecting Indigenous Peoples has been central to the work of the Truth and Reconciliation Commission (TRC), which was established in 2008 to address and acknowledge the detrimental impact and consequences of Canada's residential school system imposed upon families of Indigenous Peoples until 1984 (The Truth and Reconciliation Commission of Canada, 2015). Closely intertwined with the residential school system were Canada's Indian Hospitals, established for treatment of tuberculosis among Indigenous Peoples (Meijer Drees, 2013). The effects of these institutions and the very nature of the colonial structure of the Indian Health Services have been detrimental and a major source of mental health trauma. An unbalanced healthcare system that has not been adaptive to the specific health needs of Indigenous Peoples, therefore, is in need of urgent attention (see Chapters 3 and 4). Healing efforts to include voices and stories of Indigenous Peoples and to acknowledge historical injustice and trauma in ways that foster awareness and provide nurses with tools to strengthen their professional ability for health care of Indigenous Peoples are a key and much needed focus in current health research (MacNaughton, 2015).

To better meet needs of diverse populations and accommodate to new demands for care and treatment, the PMH nursing organizations regularly renew their professional standards. The CFMHN updated its standards in 2006 and again in 2014 to incorporate the most recent perspectives on PMH care. For the first time, the 2006 revisions sought input from former patients, who were typically identified as mental healthcare consumers (Beal et al., 2007). This trend reflected the new patient voice and consumer input in mental health care. In 2015, the CFMHN joined the Canadian Association for Schools of Nursing to jointly develop entry-to-practice mental health and addiction competencies for undergraduate nursing education in Canada for the first time. These provided much needed guidance for both practice and education (see Chapter 6).

New Demand for a National Mental Health Strategy

A national *health* strategy was first adopted in 1984 through the Canada Health Act, which set out the values, principles, and guidelines for health care. While mental healthcare principles were ensconced in the overall Act to some degree, there continued to be significant gaps and inconsistencies in *mental health* care across the country. Canada continued to be the only one of the eight wealthiest nations without a national mental health strategy (Kirby, 2009). System inadequacies, including stigmatization and questionable use of controversial interventions such as seclusion, continued to draw public attention and pressure the government to address injustices and outmoded forms of treatment (Dyck & Deighton, 2017).

To address service gaps, Health Canada funded the Mental Health Commission of Canada in 2007.

The commission was established outside the federal health mandate, but with a structure that mirrored inclusiveness with regard to membership and stakeholder participation (Goldbloom & Bradley, 2012). The MHCC was originally assigned three primary objectives: to develop a mental health strategy for Canada, begin an antistigma campaign, and create a knowledge exchange centre to promote research and build capacity and opportunities in evidence-based mental health strategies. In 2012, the Commission issued a comprehensive national mental health strategy with six strategic directions (Box 1.3). It further initiated several research projects to enhance evidence-based practice of which two are highlighted here: the *At Home/Chez Soi* initiative, a mental health research project examining housing for individuals who are mentally ill in five large urban settings and a Mental Health First Aid project, involving provision of training to the public on how to identify the early signs and symptoms of mental illness and suitable interventions for the unique needs of youth or adults (Hwang et al., 2012). An issue of concern of the *At Home/Chez Soi* project, ending in 2013, was that financial support to consolidate their novel approaches was not guaranteed (Goldbloom & Bradley, 2012). Affordable low-cost housing for people living with mental illness remains a key health issue and a persistent point of policy debate (Nelles & Spence, 2013).

Many insights have been gained through the MHCC initiatives, and its contributions are ongoing. In their strategic plan for 2017–2022, the MHCC identified key strategic priority areas to meet mental health needs of Canadians (Box 1.4).

A series of fundamental and persistent challenges stay on the policy agenda, however, forming key focus areas requiring attention of policy makers and health professionals, including needs of youth and seniors, housing, stigma, suicide prevention among all age groups, and workplace issues. Also, mental health of immigrants and refugees is on the mental health policy agenda (see Chapter 4) (Agic et al., 2016).

BOX 1.3 The MHCC's 2017–2022 Strategic Plan: Strategic Objectives and Priorities

Strategic Objective 1: **Leadership, Partnership, and Capacity Building**

Increasing the effectiveness of Canada's mental health system by convening stakeholders, developing and influencing sound public policy, and inspiring collective action.

Strategic Objective 2: **Promotion and Advancing of *The Mental Health Strategy for Canada***

Encouraging actions that advance *the Strategy*.

Strategic Objective 3: **Knowledge Mobilization**

Developing and sharing effective and innovative knowledge.

From Mental Health Commission of Canada. (2016). http://www.mentalhealthcommission.ca/English/mhcc-strategic-plan-2017-2022

BOX 1.4 Research for Best Practice

THE ART OF PEER SUPPORT

Boschma, G., & Devane, C. (2019). The art of peer support: Work, health, consumer participation and new forms of citizenship in late twentieth century mental health care in British Columbia. *BC Studies, 202*(Summer issue), 65–98. https://doi.org/10.14288/bcs.v0i202.190414

Background: Within a new discourse of self-help, patient rights, rehabilitation, and recovery peer support emerged as a new field of work and imagination in post-1970s Canadian mental health care.

Purpose: This historical research paper explores peer support as it originally evolved within the patient liberation movement and the way it became incorporated as an accepted form of work in British Columbia's (BC) evolving mental healthcare system as of the 1990s.

Methods: Historical research methods included analysis of relevant archival documents, published sources and reports, and oral history.

Findings: Patients had an essential role in imagining, creating, and enacting new forms of citizenship that critiqued and provided new alternatives for health and healing in the new context of community mental health. They engaged with policy development, advisory, and advocacy work and developed new forms of peer help. Their contributions not only shifted patient *and* professional identities but also raised new questions about the way peer help should be incorporated and acknowledged: contradictory visions of citizenship, of patients versus workers, of productive versus social citizenship, and of communal versus individualized forms of peer support had to be negotiated. As of the 1990s, peer support became an accepted form of mental health work and an integral part of mental health services.

Implications: The creative idea that patients can help each other has found a cultural niche and social acknowledgement as an enduring part of mental health service in BC. Peer support continues to be recognized as empowering and destigmatizing—peer support roles divert from a preoccupation with diagnosis and illness and construct experiential expertise as a resource and strength, albeit that careful negotiation of the (work) conditions of peer support remain vital.

While mental illness is no longer kept from sight, we still need to work on ways to provide permanent and persistent support for the most vulnerable populations. These challenges are not unique to Canada and have been recognized at a global level by the World Health Organization (WHO). This respected organization has focused its leadership on four key areas of mental health and substance use policies and services:

- Promotion of rights-based policy and law for mental health
- Coordination of effective mental health response in emergencies
- Prioritization of care for mental, neurological, and substance use disorders
- Improvement of mental and brain health of children and adolescents

Mental health and human right violations are known to have significant impacts on the overall health and economic wellbeing of people around the world. To address this need, the WHO (2019) is taking the lead to support access to quality and affordable health care for 12 priority countries (for 100 million more people) by aiming to raise 60 million dollars (U.S.) over 4 years (2019–2023) in their Special Initiative: Universal Health Coverage for Mental Health. This initiative has highlighted two strategic actions. The first is to advance mental health policies, advocacy, and human rights, and the second is to scale up services and interventions in the community, general health, and specialty settings.

The challenge before Canadian nurses at this time is to strive to support and address these national and global goals. We must work with a view to include mental health while working within existing constraints to provide cost-effective and equitable services. To address pressing mental healthcare needs, nurses must continue to participate in devising and implementing a continuum of mental health services that provides access for all and develop appropriate partnerships with other health professionals and diverse consumer groups.

Summary of Key Points

- Throughout history, attitudes and treatment toward those with mental disorders have drastically changed as a result of the changing socioeconomic backdrop of our society and the development of new theories and study by key individuals and groups.

- During the 1800s, as mental illness began to be viewed as an illness, more humane and moral treatments began to develop.
- Social reformers such as Dorothea Dix, Charles Clarke, Clifford Beers, and Clarence Hincks dedicated their efforts to raising society's awareness and advocating public responsibility for the proper treat-

ment of persons with mental illness. At the turn of the 19th century, mental hospitals started implementing Schools of Nursing to build psychiatric nursing capacity and quality within the hospitals.

- Theoretic arguments characterized the evolution of scientific thought and psychiatric practice. Gradually, the importance of the biologic aspect of mental disorders was recognized while psychosocial approaches were also developed. After the 1950s, the discipline of nursing began to add to the theoretical basis of mental health practice, adding holistic and interpersonal frameworks of psychiatric nursing.

- Although the need for PMH nursing was recognized near the end of the 19th century, initially, there was resistance to training attendants for the care of the insane. At the initiative of Charles Clarke, medical superintendent of Rockwood Hospital (1881–1905), the first Training School for Mental Nurses was established in 1888.

- All provinces gradually adapted to education for PMH nurses. By the 1930s, all provinces had established training schools for asylum attendants and nurses. In the era following World War II, provinces started to downsize mental hospitals in a process of deinstitutionalization and a shift to community-based care. Two models of education for psychiatric nurses emerged, leading to two distinct professional groups.

- Key federal and provincial reform initiatives generated political support and funding for mental health services, but many pressing issues and system inadequacies remain, requiring strategic action and policy initiative of professionals and consumers alike.

- The establishment of the Mental Health Commission of Canada in 2007 has generated a series of projects to fill the gaps in the system by initiating national mental health strategies and is moving beyond its original mandate to address ongoing mental health issues affecting Canadians.

 ## Thinking Challenges

1. Social change has been a driving force in adapting mental health services to adequately meet social demand for public mental health care. One of these historical changes was to move away from large mental institutions toward smaller scale community-based services.

   a. What were some of the key arguments (or theoretical insights) emerging in the 1970s that made the system of large mental institutions obsolete and fostered a policy of deinstitutionalization?

   b. What theoretical insights about patient participation and mental illness drove the shift to community mental health services?

   c. As a nurse, how are you able to contribute to the ongoing development of community mental health services?

Visit the Point to view suggested responses. Go to thePoint.lww.com/activate and use the activation code found in the front of this text to unlock answers to the "Thinking Challenges" and other online resources.

 ## Web Links

nfb.ca/interactive/here_at_home The National Film Board of Canada presents this clever interactive Web documentary on the radical research project that is revealing the true cost of homelessness in Canada.

cpa.ca/docs/File/Practice/strategy-text-en.pdf In 2012, the government of Canada presented "Changing directions, changing lives: The mental health strategy for Canada," a culmination of the policy work conducted by the Mental Health Commission of Canada established in 2007. It provides direction for mental health services at a national level.

cna-aiic.ca/en/on-the-issues/national-expert-commission The Canadian Nurses Association (CNA) published the 2012 CNA National Experts Commission report *A Nursing Call to Action: The Health of Our Nation, The Future of Our Health System* (with a discussion of mental health and disabilities on page 10) to inform health policy from a nursing point of view.

cna-aiic.ca/~/media/cna/page-content/pdf-en/ps85_mental_health_e.pdf?la=en CNA's statement on mental health can be found here. It is another policy tool.

cfmhn.ca/professional/practice This website of the Canadian Federation of Mental Health Nurses lists the Canadian standards of mental health nursing.

rpnc.ca/history This website gives background on the foundations of the Registered Psychiatric Nurses Associations existing in western Canadian provinces. It also lists national regulations for Registered Psychiatric Nurses.

cmha.ca/about-cmha/history-of-cmha The history of the Canadian Mental Health Association highlights this organization's long-standing role in mental health policy.

nctr.ca/map.php The Truth and Reconciliation Commission's reports have been transferred to the National Centre for Truth and Reconciliation at the University of Manitoba. This site provides important background information and historical context to the work of the TRC. Final Report, Volume 5, deals specifically with the legacy of Canada's residential schools and its impact on the health of Indigenous Peoples.

madnesscanada.com This public Canadian website offers digital archive and resources, educational tools, and historical research findings on the history of mental health care, created to enhance critical thinking, heritage preservation, and historical research in the fields of psychiatric medicine and mental health. The site has a special section "Caring Minds" on histories of mental health for the class room.

References

Agic, B., McKenzie, K., Tuck, A., & Antwi, M. (2016). *Supporting the mental health of refugees to Canada*. Report of the Mental Health Commission of Canada.

Arboleda-Flórez, J. (2005). The epidemiology of mental illness in Canada. *Canadian Public Policy: Analyse de Politique, 31*(s1), 13–16.

Bailey, H. (1920). *Nursing mental diseases*. Macmillan.

Beal, G., Chan, A., Chapman, S., Edgar, J., McInnis-Perry, G., Osborne, M., & Mina, E. S. (2007). Consumer input into standards revisions: Changing practice. *Journal of Psychiatric and Mental Health Nursing, 14*, 13–20.

Beauséjour, P. (2001). Advocacy and misadventures in Canadian Psychiatry. In Q. Rae-Grant (Ed.), *Psychiatry in Canada: 50 years, 1951–2000* (pp. 137–148). Canadian Psychiatric Association.

Beers, C. (1908). *A mind that found itself*. Longmans, Green, & Co.

Benner, P. (1984). *From novice to expert: Excellence and power in clinical nursing practice*. Addison-Wesley.

Boschma, G. (2003). *The rise of mental health nursing: A history of psychiatric care in Dutch asylum, 1890–1920*. Amsterdam University Press.

Boschma, G. (2008). A family point of view: Negotiating asylum care in Alberta, 1905–1930. *Canadian Bulletin of Medical History, 25*(2), 367–389.

Boschma, G. (2011). Deinstitutionalization reconsidered: Geographic and demographic changes in mental health care in British Columbia and Alberta, 1950–1980. *Histoire Sociale/Social History, 44*(88), 223–256.

Boschma, G. (2012). Community mental health nursing in Alberta, Canada: An oral history. *Nursing History Review, 20*, 103–135.

Boschma, G. (2019a). Electroconvulsive therapy (ECT) and nursing practice in the Netherlands, 1940–2010. *European Journal for Nursing History and Ethics, 1*, 17–39. https://doi.org/10.25974/enhe2019-7en

Boschma, G. (2019b). Negotiating Electroconvulsive Therapy (ECT) in Dutch psychiatry: Cultural and intra-professional tension over biological psychiatry, 1950–2010. In P. Pfütsch (Ed.), *Marketplace, power, prestige: The healthcare professions' struggle for recognition* (pp. 98–136). Franz Steiner Verlag.

Boschma, G., Davies, M., & Morrow, M. (2014). "Those people known as mental patients…": Professional and patient engagement in community mental health in Vancouver, BC in the 1970s. *Oral History Forum d'histoire orale, 34.* http://www.oralhistoryforum.ca/index.php/ohf/issue/current

Boschma, G., & Devane, C. (2019). The art of peer support: Work, health, consumer participation and new forms of citizenship in late twentieth century mental health care in British Columbia. *BC Studies, 202*(Summer issue), 65–98.

Boschma, G., Yonge, O., & Mychajlunow, L. (2005). Gender and professional identity in psychiatric nursing practice in Alberta, Canada, 1930–1975. *Nursing Inquiry, 12*(4), 243–255.

Brown, W. H. (2000). Dr. C. K. Clarke and the training school for nurses. In E. Hudson (Ed.), *The provincial asylum in Toronto: Reflections on social and architectural history* (pp. 167–180). Toronto Region Architectural Conservancy.

Calaway, B. J. (2002). *Hildegard Peplau: Psychiatric nurse of the century*. Springer.

Canadian Association for Schools of Nursing & Canadian Federation of Mental Health Nurses. (2015). *Entry-to-practice mental health and addiction competencies for undergraduate nursing education in Canada*. https://www.casn.ca/2015/11/entry-to-practice-mental-health-and-addiction-competencies-for-undergraduate-nursing-education-in-canada/

Canadian Women's Health Network. (2006). *Women, mental health, mental illness and addiction in Canada*. Response to out of the shadows at last. http://www.cwhn.ca/resources/cwhm/mentalHealth.html

Crossley, M. L. (2006). *Contesting psychiatry: Social movements in mental health*. Routledge.

Cyr, C., McKee, H., O'Hagan, M., & Priest, R. (2016). *Making the case for peer support: Report to the peer support project committee of the Mental Health Commission of Canada* (2nd ed., pp. 10, 45). http://www.mentalhealth-commission.ca

D'Antonio, P. (2006). *Founding friends: Families, staff, and patients at the Friends Asylum in early nineteenth century Philadelphia*. Lehigh University Press.

Davies, M. (2014). MPA lecture and documentary. *The Inmates are Running the Asylum: Stories from the MPA*. https://oralhistorycentre.ca/2014/01/16/dr-megan-davies-the-inmates-are-running-the-asylum-stories-from-mpa/

Dooley, C. (2004). "They gave their care, but we gave loving care": Defining and defending boundaries of skill and craft in the nursing service of a Manitoba Mental Hospital during the Great Depression. *Canadian Bulletin of Medical History, 21*(2), 229–251.

Dyck, E. (2011). Dismantling the asylum and charting new pathways into the community: Mental health care in twentieth-century Canada. *Histoire Sociale/Social History, 44*(88), 181–196.

Dyck, E. (2013). *Facing eugenics: Reproduction, sterilization, and the politics of choice*. University of Toronto Press.

Dyck, E., & Deighton, A. (2017). *Managing madness: Weyburn mental hospital and the transformation of psychiatric care in Canada*. University of Manitoba Press.

Fingard, J., & Rutherford, J. (2011). Deinstitutionalization and vocational rehabilitation for mental health consumers in Nova Scotia since the 1950s. *Histoire Sociale/Social History, 44*(88), 385–408.

Gagnon, M., & Oliffe, J. L. (2015). Male depression suicide: What NPs should know. *The Nurse Practitioner, 40*(11), 50–55.

George, M. S. (2003). Stimulating the brain: The emerging new science of electrical brain stimulation. *Scientific American, 289*(3), 66–73.

Goldbloom, D., & Bradley, L. (2012). The Mental Health Commission of Canada: The first five years. *Mental Health Review Journal, 17*(4), 221–228.

Goldstein, J. L., & Godemont, M. M. L. (2003). The legend and lessons of Geel: A 1500-year-old legend, a 21st-century model. *Community Mental Health Journal, 39*(5), 441–458.

Greenland, C., Griffin, J., & Hoffman, B. F. (2001). Psychiatry in Canada from 1951–2000. In Q. Rae-Grant (Ed.), *Psychiatry in Canada: 50 years, 1951–2001* (pp. 1–16). Canadian Psychiatric Association.

Hall, N. (2012). Closure of Riverview Hospital marks end of era in mental health treatment. Vancouver Sun. http://www.vancouversun.com/index.html

Hart Wasekeesikaw, F. (2006). Challenges for the new millennium: Nursing in First Nations. In M. McIntyre, E. Thomlinson, & C. McDonald (Eds.), *Realities of Canadian nursing: Professional, practice and power issues* (pp. 415–433). Lippincott Williams & Wilkins.

Health Canada. (2002). A report on mental illnesses in Canada. https://www.phac-aspc.gc.ca/publicat/miic-mmac/pdf/men_ill_e.pdf

Hector, I. (2001). Changing funding patterns and the effect on mental health care in Canada. In Q. Rae-Grant (Ed.), *Psychiatry in Canada: 50 years, 1951–2001* (pp. 59–76). Canadian Psychiatric Association.

Hicks, B. (2011). Gender, politics, and regionalism: Factors in the evolution of registered psychiatric nursing in Manitoba, 1920–1960. *Nursing History Review, 19*, 103–126.

Hurd, H. M. (Ed.). (1973, originally printed 1916–17). *The institutional care of the insane in the United States and Canada* (Vol. IV). Arno Press.

Hwang, S. W., Stergiopoulos, V., O'Campo, P., & Gozdzik, A. (2012). Ending homelessness among people with mental illness: The At Home/Chez Soi randomized trial of a Housing First intervention in Toronto. *BMC Public Health, 12*(1), 787–802.

Jones, C. (1989). *The charitable imperative: Hospitals and nursing in ancien régime and revolutionary France*. Routledge.

Kirby, M. (2009). *Key note address*. Mental Health Commission of Canada National Child and Youth Mental Health Day.

Kirby, M. J. L., & Keon, W. J. (2006). Out of the shadows at last: Transforming mental health, mental illness and addiction services in Canada. http://www.parl.gc.ca/39/1/parlbus/commbus/senate/com-e/soci-e/rep-e/rep02may06-e.htm

LaJeunesse, R. A. (2000). *Political asylums*. Muttart Foundation.

Leiby, J. S. (1992). San Hipólito's treatment of the mentally ill in Mexico City, 1589–1650. *The Historian, 54*(3), 491–498.

Lightner, D. L. (Ed.). (1999). *Asylum, prison, and poorhouse: The writings and reform work of Dorothea Dix in Illinois*. Southern Illinois University Press.

MacNaughton, A. (2015). *Tuberculosis (TB) storytelling: Improving community nursing TB program delivery [Master's Thesis, Nursing]*. University of British Columbia. https://open.library.ubc.ca/cIRcle/collections/ubctheses/24/items/1.0223067

Malamud, W. (1944). The history of psychiatric therapies. In J. K. Hall, G. Zilboorg, & H. Bunker (Eds.), *One hundred years of American psychiatry* (pp. 273–323). Columbia University Press.

Meijer Drees, L. (2013). *Healing histories: Stories from Canada's Indian Hospitals*. The University of Alberta Press.

Menzies, R., & Palys, T. (2006). Turbulent spirits: Aboriginal patients in the British Columbia psychiatric system, 1879–1950. In J. E. Moran & D. Wright (Eds.), *Mental health and Canadian society: Historical perspectives* (pp. 149–175). McGill-Queen's University Press.

Moran, J. E. (2000). *Committed to the state asylum: Insanity and society in nineteenth-century Quebec and Ontario*. McGill-Queen's University Press.

Moran, J. E., & Wright, D. (Eds.). (2006). *Mental health and Canadian society: Historical perspectives*. McGill-Queen's University Press.

MPA Founders Collective. (2013). "The inmates are running the asylum: Stories from the MPA [Mental Patient Association]": A documentary about the group that transformed Canada's psychiatric landscape. DVD, 36-minutes. Producer: Megan Davies, Co-Producer: Marina Morrow,

Associate Co-Producer: Geertje Boschma. © History of Madness Productions 2013. https://oralhistorycentre.ca/2014/01/16/dr-megan-davies-the-inmates-are-running-the-asylum-stories-from-mpa/

Morrow, M. (2002). *Violence and trauma in the lives of women with serious mental illness: Current practices in service provision in British Columbia.* Centre of Excellence for Women's Health.

Murphy, R. & Higgins, A. (2018). The complex terrain of peer support in mental health: What does it all mean? *Journal of Psychiatric Mental Health Nursing, 25*(7), 441–448. https://doi.org/10.1111/jpm.12474

Neill, J. (1980). Adolf Meyer and American psychiatry today. *American Journal of Psychiatry, 137*(4), 460–464.

Nelles, H., & Spence, A. (2013). *Blended financing for impact: The opportunities for social finance in supportive housing.* Report commissioned by the Mental Health Commission of Canada and stakeholders. http://www.marsdd.com/wp-content/uploads/2013/03/MaRS_BlendedFinancing-forImpact_2013.pdf

Nelson, S. (1999). Entering the professional domain: The making of the modern nurse in 17th century France. *Nursing History Review, 7,* 171–187.

Nelson, S. (2001). *Say little, do much: Nursing, nuns, and hospitals in the nineteenth century.* University of Pennsylvania Press.

Ostry, A. (2009). The foundations of national public hospital insurance. *Canadian Bulletin of Medical History, 26*(2), 261–282.

Parry-Jones, W. L. L. (1981). The model of the Geel Lunatic Colony and its influence on the nineteenth-century asylum system in Britain. In A. Scull (Ed.), *Madhouses, mad-doctors, and madmen. The social history of psychiatry in the Victorian Era* (pp. 201–217). The Athlone Press.

Peplau, H. (1952). *Interpersonal relations in nursing.* Putnam.

Pressman, J. D. (2002). *Psychosurgery and the limits of medicine.* Cambridge University Press.

Rai, S., Kivisalu, T., Rabheru, K., & Kang, N. (2010). Electroconvulsive therapy clinical database: A standardized approach in tertiary care psychiatry. *Journal of Electro-Convulsion-Therapy (ECT), 26*(4), 304–309.

Sadowsky, J. (2006). Beyond the metaphor of the pendulum: Electroconvulsive therapy, psychoanalysis, and the styles of American psychiatry. *Journal of the History of Medicine, 61,* 1–25.

Scull, A. (2005). *Madhouse: A tragic tale of megalomania and modern medicine.* Yale University Press.

Sealy, P., & Whitehead, P. C. (2004). Forty years of deinstitutionalization of psychiatric services in Canada: An empirical assessment. *Canadian Journal of Psychiatry, 49,* 249–257.

Shepherd, G., Boardman, J., & Slade, M. (2008). *Making recovery a reality.* http://www.centreformentalhealth.org.uk/publications/making_recovery_a_reality.aspx?ID=578

Shorter, E., & Healy, D. (Eds.). (2007). *Shock therapy: A history of electroconvulsive treatment in mental illness.* University of Toronto Press.

Sussman, S. (1998). The first asylums in Canada: A response to neglectful community care and current trends. *Canadian Journal of Psychiatry, 43,* 260–264.

The Truth and Reconciliation Committee of Canada. (2015). *Honoring the truth, reconciling for the future: Summary of the final report of the Truth and Reconciliation Commission of Canada.* www.trc.ca

Tipliski, V. M. (2002). *Parting at the crossroads: The development of education for psychiatric nursing in three Canadian provinces, 1909–1955.* Ph.D. thesis, University of Manitoba, Winnipeg, MB.

Tipliski, V. M. (2004). Parting at the crossroads: The emergence of education for psychiatric nursing in three Canadian provinces, 1909–1955. *Canadian Bulletin of Medical History, 21*(2), 253–279.

Van Drenth, A., & De Haan, F. (1999). *The rise of caring power: Elizabeth Fry and Josephine Butler in Britain and the Netherlands.* Amsterdam University Press.

Varcoe, C. M., Browne, A. J., & Einboden, R. (2015). *Prince George: Socio-historical, geographical, political and economic context profile.* EQUIP Healthcare: Research to equip primary healthcare for equity, in partnership with Central Interior Native Health Society, University of British Columbia. Posted on UBC Circle: https://circle.ubc.ca/bitstream/handle/2429/52327/EQUIP_Report_PrinceGeorge_Sociohistorical_Context_2015.pdf?sequence=1

Warsh, C. K. (1989). *Moments of unreason: The practice of Canadian psychiatry and the Homewood Retreat, 1883–1923.* McGill-Queen's University Press.

World Health Organization. (2001). The world health report: Mental health 2001. In Mental health: New understanding, new hope. https://www.who.int/whr/2001/en/

World Health Organization. (2019). The WHO Special Initiative for Mental Health (2019–2023): Universal Health Coverage for Mental Health. https://apps.who.int/iris/bitstream/handle/10665/310981/WHO-MSD-19.1-eng.pdf

2

Mental Health, Mental Disorder, Recovery, and Wellbeing

Wendy Austin

LEARNING OBJECTIVES

After studying this chapter, you will be able to:

- Recognize the integral relationship between mental and physical health.
- Define mental health and mental illness.
- Explain the concepts of recovery and wellbeing.
- Define mental health literacy and the role of mental health first aid.
- Describe the purpose of the *Diagnostic and Statistical Manual of Mental Disorders*, 5th edition (*DSM-5*).
- Identify the role of research in psychiatric and mental health nursing.
- Name four issues affecting mental health care at the global level.

KEY TERMS

- Canadian Index of Wellbeing (CIW) • gender differences • mental health literacy • social progress

KEY CONCEPTS

- mental disorder • mental health • recovery
- wellbeing

This chapter presents and explores concepts foundational to psychiatric and mental health (PMH) nursing practice. While these key concepts may appear to be straightforward and even obvious at first glance, their meaning continues to evolve. For instance, nurses, other healthcare professionals, and the public have for some time viewed "recovery" as the restoration of health. The concept, however, embraces more. Recovery related to mental health is envisioned as gaining hope and purpose; understanding one's abilities, disabilities, rights and resources; and living a meaningful, satisfying life even with mental health problems or illnesses (Mental Health Commission of Canada [MHCC], 2009, 2015; World Health Organization [WHO], 2013). It is important that nurses have a deep understanding of these basic terms, as such knowledge will explicitly and implicitly shape their practice.

Mental Health

Mental health, as defined by the Mental Health Commission of Canada (MHCC, 2013), is "a state of wellbeing in which the individual realizes his or her own potential, can cope with the normal stresses of life, can work productively and fruitfully, and is able to make a contribution to his or her own community" (p. 3). Mental health is not the polar opposite of

mental illness. In fact, one can experience mental health while one is living with a severe mental disorder. Envision mental health and mental illness as existing on two separate and simultaneously occurring continua (Epp, 1988). Optimal mental health and minimal mental health represent the extremes on one continuum, while maximal mental disorder and absence of mental disorder represent the extremes on the other continuum (Fig. 2.1). It is possible that a person with a mental disorder can experience optimal mental health (quadrant A), and a person without a mental disorder can experience minimal mental health (quadrant D). This situation is similar to that of a person with diabetes who, using diet, exercise, and medication, is healthy and symptom free, and a person without a diagnosable medical condition who, eating a diet of "fast food," avoiding exercise, and smoking cigarettes daily, can be unhealthy. Both the level of mental health and the severity of a mental disorder can vary over a person's lifetime.

Mental health and physical health are integrated, not distinct. The separation of the mental and physical aspects of health is highly problematic. Since the first Director-General of the World Health Organization (WHO), the Canadian psychiatrist Brock Chisholm, stipulated that there is no true physical health without mental health, this has been the WHO's position.

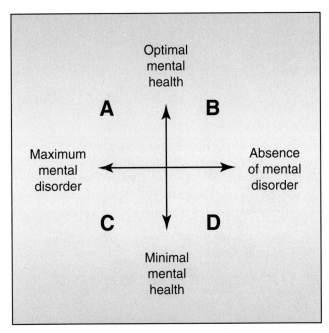

Figure 2.1 Diagram of mental health and mental disorder continua. (Adapted from Epp, J. (1988). *Mental health for Canadians: Striking a balance* (Cat. H39-128/1988E). Supply and Services Canada.)

 KEY CONCEPT

Mental health is a state of wellbeing in which individuals realize self-potential, cope with life stresses, and are able to work productively and contribute to their society. It is integral to general health and can be possessed and enhanced, including in the presence of mental illness.

Canadians' mental health and its determinants are appraised using the *Positive Mental Health Surveillance Framework*. This work was developed by The Public Health Agency of Canada using five indicators of positive mental health and 25 risk and protective factors across individual, family, community, and society domains (Orpana et al., 2016). See Figure 2.2.

The International Council of Nurses Policy Statement on Mental Health

The International Council of Nurses (ICN) (2020) "Policy Statement on Mental Health" makes it clear that nurses' roles in the promotion and maintenance of mental health and wellbeing are essential. As promoted in this text, ICN specifies that nursing practice must be grounded in the lived experience of individuals with mental disorders and their families, and shaped by the concept of recovery that places the person at the centre of care. It identifies a global emergency in mental health: one in ten persons has a mental disorder, which contributes to 10% of the global burden of disease. The number

of mental health professionals equates to one per every 10,000 people. ICN notes that such shortages are exacerbated when psychiatric and mental health nursing is undervalued, including in nursing education when there is insufficient attention to it in the curriculum. This situation must improve if the global emergency is to be successfully addressed.

ICN calls upon each nurse to address stigma and discrimination as it contributes to marginalization and poor quality of care for persons with mental disorders, to advocate for policies to reduce such stigma, to contribute to research in mental health, to recognize the nursing relationship as foundational to care, to educate others regarding person-centred services based on health literacy and informed decision-making, to support community actions that promote social connectedness and reduce loneliness and isolation, and to participate in climate change–related planning and interventions (ICN, 2020).

Wellbeing

Mental health is considered a state of wellbeing, but what does "wellbeing" mean? The Oxford English Dictionary (OED Online, 2014) defines wellbeing as: "the state of being healthy, happy, or prosperous; physical, psychological, or moral welfare." A Canadian phenomenological study suggests that wellbeing is not a purposeful quest but experienced as coming home to self with harmony and balance at its foundation (Healey-Ogden & Austin, 2011).

Canadian Index of Wellbeing

The Canadian Index of Wellbeing (CIW) is used as a measure of the quality of life in Canada. With data primarily from Statistics Canada, the CIW is calculated using 64 indicators across eight interconnected quality-of-life domains: community vitality, democratic engagement, education, environment, healthy populations, leisure and culture, living standards, and time use (CIW, 2016). Using measures of wellbeing to examine our national status is important. The Gross Domestic Product (GDP) is a measure of national income, but growth in the GDP is affected by all goods and service activities (including smoking, overharvesting our forests, increasing use of fossil fuels): it is like a giant calculator with an addition but no subtraction button. Measures of wellbeing allow a broader depth of understanding that, when used with GDP, will allow Canadians to move towards a society with a quality of life that all may enjoy.

Social Progress Index

"**Social progress** is the capacity of a society to meet the basic human needs of its citizens, establish the building blocks that allow citizens and communities to enhance

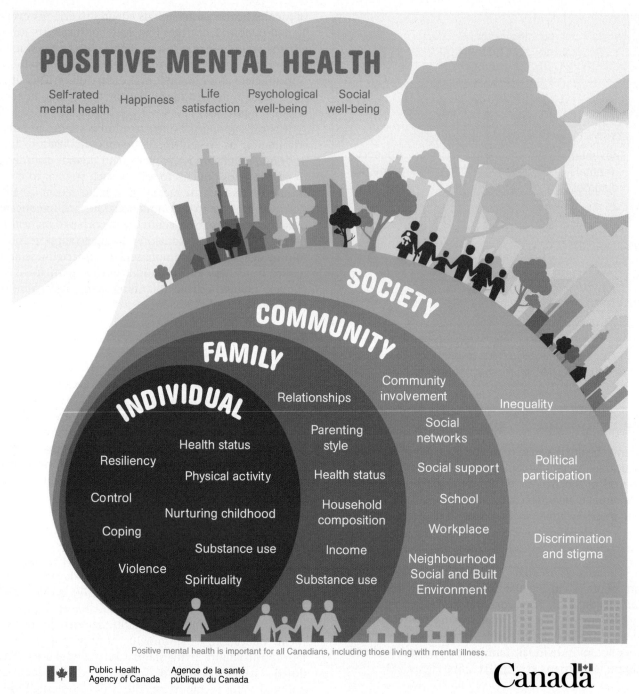

Positive mental health is important for all Canadians, including those living with mental illness.

Public Health Agency of Canada   Agence de la santé publique du Canada

Canada

Figure 2.2 Positive Mental Health Surveillance Framework. (©All Rights Reserved. *Monitoring positive mental health and its determinants in Canada: the development of the Positive Mental Health Surveillance Indicator Framework.* Public Health Agency of Canada, 2016. Reproduced with permission from the Minister of Health, 2021.)

and sustain the quality of their lives, and create the conditions for all individuals to reach their full potential" (Green et al., 2020, p. 3). The Social Progress Index (SPI) measures a nation's progress in delivering social and environmental value. It was created to complement the GDP index to give a more holistic picture of a country's overall performance. A country can be economically wealthy without its citizens being able to achieve a high quality of life.

The SPI represents components of *basic human needs* (i.e., nutrition and basic medical care, water and sanitation, shelter, personal safety), *foundations of wellbeing* (i.e., access to basic knowledge, access to information and communication, health and wellness, environmental quality), and *opportunity* (i.e., personal rights, personal freedom and choice, tolerance and inclusion, access to advance education). Canada's 2020 SPI rank is 7th of the 163 nations ranked, while our GDP per capita is 18/163. An area for improvement for Canada in the dimension of wellbeing is environmental quality related to greenhouse gas emissions and protection of our biome (forests, tundra, grasslands and desert). See https://www.socialprogress.org/?tab=2&code=CAN for Canada's complete rating.

KEY CONCEPT

Wellbeing is an individual's sense of being content and happy with life and life situation; a sense of flourishing.

Mental Disorders

Each year, one in five Canadians will be living with a mental health problem or illness; this translates to nearly 7.5 million people. The annual cost of mental health problems and disorders is estimated at $50 billion (MHCC, 2020). Mental disorder is the medical term for mental illness and refers to a diagnosable health condition based on an accepted classification system with criteria related to alterations in mood and affect, behaviour, and thinking and cognition. These alterations are beyond the parameters of psychological states such as sadness and grief that may be encountered in life. In deriving mental disorder diagnoses, cultural definitions of responses need to be considered. When a particular culture sees certain behaviours as normal, its members will not view the behaviour as a symptom of a mental disorder. For example, it is common in some religious groups to "speak in tongues." To an observer, it may appear that the individuals are experiencing hallucinations (see Chapter 11), a psychiatric symptom, but this behaviour is usual for this group within a particular setting.

KEY CONCEPT

Mental disorders are health conditions characterized by alteration in a variety of factors that include mood and affect, behaviour, and thinking and cognition. The disorders are associated with various degrees of distress and impaired functioning.

Diagnosing Mental Disorders

Classification systems for medical diagnoses are guidelines that identify the criteria required for a particular condition to be diagnosed and provide a common language for healthcare professionals to use. It is important to note that clinical judgment must inform the use of such criteria. The two most accepted psychiatric classifications are the Mental and Behavioural Disorders

Section of the WHO's *International Statistical Classification of Diseases and Related Health Problems (ICD)*, 11th edition (*ICD-11*) (WHO, 2018), and the American Psychiatric Association's (APA, 2013) *Diagnostic and Statistical Manual of Mental Disorders (DSM)*. In its fifth edition, the *DSM-5* includes the equivalent *ICD-11* Codes for reference. These two systems are compatible, but the DSM is commonly used in North America.

The *DSM-5*

The *DSM-5* has three sections: (I) an introduction and explanation of its use, including a caution regarding its forensic use; (II) the diagnostic criteria and codes; and (III) emerging measures (assessment) and models (e.g., cultural formulation), an alternative model for personality disorders, and conditions for further study (e.g., internet gaming disorder). For clinical utility, the *DSM-5* is organized along development and life span lines (e.g., diagnoses reflecting developmental processes appearing early in life are at the beginning). Mental disorders are delineated in a way such that cultural, social, and familial norms and values can be recognized as influencing the expression and experience of symptoms, signs, and behaviours addressed in the criteria (APA, 2013). See Box 2.1 for *DSM-5* diagnostic categories and Box 2.2 for other conditions that may be a focus of clinical attention or may affect diagnosis, course, prognosis, or treatment.

Concerns do exist that some aspects of everyday life may be transformed into illness by a *DSM-5* classification, for example, if grief is "medicalized," then the dignity of grief's pain may be diminished, interfering with processing the loss and reducing the use of rituals that can console the person experiencing it. Grieving persons could become at risk if prescribed unnecessary medication. Shyness, too readily, becomes "social phobia" and an ardent interest in something (e.g., chocolate, the internet) becomes considered an addiction (Frances, 2013).

Gender Differences and the DSM-5

The *DSM-5* notes the influence of **gender differences** (or the lack thereof) for several disorders. Gender differences are defined in the *DSM-5* as "variations that result from biological sex as well as an individual's self-representation that includes the psychological, behavioral, and social consequences of one's perceived gender" (APA, 2013, p. 15). The variations may result from only biologic sex differences, self-representation of gender, or both. Gender influences illnesses in several ways, including: risk for a disorder, symptom presentation, and willingness to endorse symptoms (which impacts willingness to seek help for them). Events related to reproductive life cycle (e.g., postpartum period) affect risk and symptom expression.

BOX 2.1 *DSM-5* Diagnostic Categories

Neurodevelopmental Disorders
Schizophrenia Spectrum and Other Psychotic Disorders
Bipolar and Related Disorders
Depressive Disorders
Anxiety Disorders
Obsessive–Compulsive and Related Disorders
Trauma- and Stressor-Related Disorders
Dissociative Disorders
Somatic Symptom and Related Disorders
Feeding and Eating Disorders
Sleep–Wake Disorders
Sexual Dysfunctions

Gender Dysphoria
Disruptive, Impulse Control, and Conduct Disorders
Substance-Related and Addictive Disorders
Neurocognitive Disorders
Personality Disorders
Paraphilic Disorders
Other Mental Disorders
Medication-Induced Movement Disorders
Other Adverse Effects of Medication

Source: American Psychiatric Association. (2013). *Diagnostic and statistical manual of mental disorders* (5th ed.). https://doi.org/10.1176/appi.books.9780890425596

BOX 2.2 *DSM-5* and Other Conditions That May Be a Focus of Clinical Attention or May Affect Diagnosis, Course, Prognosis, or Treatment

Relationship Problems
Abuse and Neglect
Educational and Occupational Problems
Housing and Economic Problems
Other Problems Related to Social Environment (e.g., phase of life problem, problems related to living alone)
Problems Related to Crime or Interaction With the Legal System

Other Health Service Encounters for Counselling and Medical Advice
Problems Related to Other Psychosocial, Personal, and Environmental Circumstances (e.g., unwanted pregnancy, experience with war, victim of torture)
Other Circumstances of Personal History (e.g., self-harm, nonadherence to medical treatment)

Source: American Psychiatric Association. (2013). *Diagnostic and statistical manual of mental disorders* (5th ed.). https://doi.org/10.1176/appi.books.9780890425596

Culture and the DSM-5

The *DSM-5* uses three concepts to point to ways culture influences the illness experience, including symptom presentation, help-seeking behaviours, expectations of and response to treatment, and adaptation to living with the illness (APA, 2013). These concepts are *cultural syndrome, cultural idiom of distress,* and *cultural explanation or perceived cause* (APA, 2013, p. 14). See Chapter 4 for a discussion of culture and mental illness.

Diagnosis as Labelling

Receiving a diagnosis can be a relief for an individual and their family if it allows for better understanding of symptoms, signs, and behaviour and means that treatment can begin. As a way of labelling a particular

person's illness, however, diagnosis can have negative consequences, such as the loss of personal identity if the labelled person becomes viewed as the disease and experiences stigma associated with mental illness. The fear of this can cause "label avoidance" in which a person does not accept their health issue as a mental health one or does not seek help in order to avoid stigmatization by others (Horsfield et al., 2020).

To avoid labelling a person, refer to individuals using person-first language. For example, refer to someone with diabetes mellitus as a "person with diabetes" rather than as a "diabetic." Likewise, someone with a mental disorder should be referred to as a "person with schizophrenia" or as a "person living with bipolar disorder" rather than as "schizophrenic" or as "bipolar." Understanding labelling processes can allow nurses and other healthcare professionals to help others and themselves avoid the pitfalls of negative labelling and stigmatization.

Mental Health Literacy

A strategic way to decrease stigma and discrimination related to mental illness is to increase **mental health literacy (MHL)**. MHL is being knowledgeable about mental health; being able to recognize mental health problems and symptoms; being comfortable speaking with others about mental health, and being willing and able to provide to someone experiencing a mental health issue initial support and guidance, such as ways to seek appropriate professional assistance. An initiative of the MHCC, MHL resources are available, such as *Mental Health First Aid Canada* which provides the awareness, knowledge, and skills to help people cope with potential or developing mental health problems in themselves or others. MHL actions need to be attentive to context and adapted to fit the needs and situation of the participants (Kutcher et al., 2016).

Research indicates that a focused approach to MHL with specific population groups works. For instance, a mental health literacy program for Ontario farmers taught by a mental health professional with farming experience, "In the Know," significantly improved and sustained all elements of participant mental health literacy (Hagen et al., 2020). This is a meaningful achievement as farmers in Canada (and other nations) are reported to experience mental illness more frequently than general populations and non-farming rural residents and are less likely to seek help for mental health concerns. MHL needs to evolve in conjunction with Canada's overall efforts in health literacy.

Recovery, viewed as an active process unique to each individual, is a cornerstone of Canada's approach to mental health care. Conceptually, this process is broader than clinical recovery (i.e., remission or cure) and, although persons with mental illness certainly can experience clinical recovery, recovery is viewed as learning how to live alongside of one's illness to have a satisfying and hopeful life. A recovery orientation for nurses and other healthcare professionals means that engagement with those in their care involves a focus on strengths, values, resources, and rights and is shaped by culturally safe and competent practices. This orientation requires a less medically centred approach and a wider perspective on what constitutes positive outcome measures (see Chapter 12).

A recovery approach is appropriate for all users of mental health services. Studies examining the use of this approach for individuals diagnosed with a severe mental health disorder (e.g., schizophrenia) show promising results (Bitter et al., 2020); useful strategies have been identified, such as care partner support when new behaviours/activities are tried (Holttum, 2020).

Recovery practices when working with youth are evolving. Considerations of developmental processes, of a youth's view of recovery (which may develop along with their self-understanding), and of goal differences that may exist between a teen and parents are integral to meaningful recovery approaches (Khoury, 2020).

The WHO (2019a) has an excellent training guide for healthcare practitioners: *Recovery practices for mental health and well-being.* For those using mental health services, *Short Guide to Personal Recovery in Mental Health* (2019) from Mental Health Europe is a good resource. (See "References" for the URLs to these guides.)

KEY CONCEPT

Recovery related to mental illness means "gaining and retaining hope, understanding of one's abilities and disabilities, engagement in an active life, personal autonomy, social identity, meaning and purpose in life and a positive sense of self." It is not synonymous with "cure" (WHO, 2013, p. 39).

The Mental Health of Canadians

Nurses need to be actively engaged in addressing the mental health of Canadians. The MHCC takes a strategic focus on promoting mental health across the life span, including in the workplace; fostering recovery and wellbeing for those living with mental health problems and illnesses and upholding their rights; providing appropriate services and reducing disparities in access to them; working with First Nations, Inuit, and Métis peoples to address their needs; and mobilizing collaboration and leadership at all levels (see Chapter 1, Box 1.3). The MHCC plays a catalytic role in promoting positive change through sharing knowledge.

Research-Based Care

In the continuing quest to improve the lives of Canadians living with a mental health problem or illness, research will be a major tool. Nurses are challenged to generate evidence for best care interventions; to use methods of inquiry that allow a better understanding of the experiences of mental health, mental illness, recovery, and wellbeing; and to translate new knowledge into better care. For instance, the science related to decreasing the use of seclusion and restraint or that which underscored the need to determine an individual's trauma-related experiences when diagnosing, as well as research showing the efficacy of new approaches to mental health community services, have transformed care in positive ways. In most chapters of this textbook,

BOX 2.3 Research for Best Practice

MENTAL DISORDER SYMPTOMS AMONG CANADIAN NURSES

Stelnicki, A. M., Carleton, R. N., & Reichert, C. (2020). *Mental disorder symptoms among nurses in Canada.* Canadian Federation of Nurses Union.

Question: What is the prevalence of mental disorder symptoms among nurses across Canada?

Method: A web-based, self-report survey was distributed in 2019 by the Canadian Federation of Nurses' Unions (CFNU) to member unions, nonmember unions in BC and Quebec, and unions whose members included nurses, as well as nurses' associations, and colleges. Sample = 7,358 nurses (RNs, RPNs, LPN, NPs) with 43.6% completing all survey questions. Survey questions queried nurses' trauma experiences, symptoms of PTSD, depression, anxiety, and potentially harmful alcohol use. Burnout and stressors measures were included.

Findings: The three most frequent trauma exposures (direct, witnessed, or learned about) were physical assault (92.7%); the death of an individual after extraordinary efforts were made to save their life (88.9%); and death of an individual who reminded the nurse of family or friends (86.0%).

The positive screens for disorders revealed PTSD at 23.0%; major depressive disorder, 36.4%; generalized anxiety disorder, 26.1%; panic disorder, 20.3%. Suicidal behaviour (over lifetime) involves suicidal ideation, 33.0; plans to commit suicide, 17.0; and suicide attempts, 8.0%. Burnout symptom severity was 29.3% at clinically significant level; at level of some symptoms only, 63.2%.

Implications: The work of nurses involves high-stress situations, some of which are traumatic. Such exposure to stress can have a cumulative effect and be linked to the development of mental disorder symptoms. CFNU developed recommendations for employers based on this study's findings that included increasing support to nurses after a critical incident and the creation of evidence-based return-to-work programs.

Note: To view the complete study, findings, and recommendations, please go to https://nursesunions.ca/research/mental-disorder-symptoms/

"Research for Best Practice" is featured. As well as noting the implications research findings have for practice, attention should be paid to the various research methods that are being utilized. In this chapter, web-based survey research of mental disorder symptoms among Canadian nurses is featured (see Box 2.3).

Global Mental Health

The need to improve mental health and the care and treatment of mental disorders is global in scope. Severe stigma, discrimination, and human rights violations are experienced by persons with mental health conditions around the world. The WHO reports that depression and anxiety disorders cost the global economy one trillion U.S. dollars per year and that deaths from suicide number 800,000 annually (WHO, 2019b). Mental health conditions, including substance use and neurological disorders, substantially increase in times of crises and disasters (e.g., the COVID-19 pandemic). Although evidence-based interventions and treatments are known, their availability is significantly lacking in many low- and middle-income countries (LMICs).

In a special initiative for mental health, the WHO is working to increase access to care for more than 100 million people by raising 60 million U.S. dollars for universal coverage of mental health care in 12 LMICs by 2023. Two strategic actions are being implemented. The first actions include advancing mental health policies, advocacy, and human rights. The second strategic actions include improving interventions and services in community-based, general health, and specialist settings. As nine out of ten of the world's children live in LMIC, evidence-based mental health services for children and youth will be particularly important. See Figure 2.3.

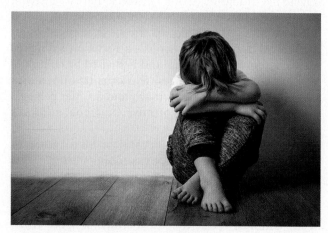

Figure 2.3 Distressed child. (Source: shutterstock.com/Sharomka.)

Summary of Key Points

- Four complex concepts are the cornerstone of Canada's mental health strategy and fundamental to psychiatric and mental health nursing practice: mental health, wellbeing, mental illness, and recovery.
- "There is no health without mental health." Mental health needs to be integrated into general health in all areas of practice and around the world.
- ICN takes the position that all registered nurses must have the knowledge and skills to respond to mental health needs, including their own. The ICN 2020 Policy Statement on Mental Health delineates expectations for individual nurses, ranging from working to address stigma and discrimination to promoting social connectedness.
- Measures used to explore wellbeing include the CIW and the SPI.

- The medical term for mental illness is mental disorder. In Canada, the *DSM-5* is the most commonly used classification of mental disorders. The Mental and Behavioural Disorders section of the ICD classification of the WHO is an alternative but compatible system.
- Diagnosis can be used in a way that increases negative labelling of persons living with mental health problems or illnesses. It is important not to use language such as, "they are a schizophrenic," but rather say, "they have schizophrenia."
- Nurses need to play a role in increasing the mental health literacy of Canadians.
- Affordable and accessible mental health care is lacking in many areas of the world. The WHO aims to change this reality through its special initiative to achieve universal coverage of mental health care for over 100 million people by 2023.

Thinking Challenges

Nick is finishing high school. He's a good student and a member of the school's football team. Around November, Nick's parents became worried about mood and behaviour changes they noticed in their child. Nick quit playing football, and he sleeps a lot but is low in energy. He used to have a hearty appetite but is now disinterested in food. Teachers have called Nick's parents because he is not doing assignments and missed several classes. Nicks parents noticed that his friends have stopped calling him. Nick is reluctantly taken to a family medical clinic, where he is diagnosed with a major depressive episode and placed on antidepressant medication.

a. Although he agrees to take the medication, Nick tells the clinic nurse he feels that going through this not only confirms he is a "loser," but now he'll

be labelled as a "psycho," too. If you were this nurse, how would you respond to Nick?

b. Although several students at Nick's school have mental health problems, a strong negative attitude prevails among the student body toward mental health issues. The principal wants this attitude to change. What intervention(s) might create a positive change among the student body?

c. Name indicators in a psychiatric setting that would provide clues to whether patient recovery is viewed as more than "being cured."

> Visit the Point to view suggested responses.
> Go to thePoint.lww.com/activate and use the activation code found in the front of this text to unlock answers to the "Thinking Challenges" and other online resources.

Web Links

https://www.camimh.ca This site of the Canadian Alliance on Mental Illness and Mental Health offers resources, such as its *Mental Health Now!* policy document that calls on governments in Canada to improve mental health care through such actions as increased funding, acceleration of mental health innovation, and investment in social infrastructure.

https://hc-sc.gc.ca Health Canada provides information on primary health care, healthcare systems, mental health and wellness, and the health of Indigenous Canadians.

https://www.mentalhealthcommission.ca/English The MHCC's website has information on its strategies and programs. For information about its Mental Health First Aid program, see: https://www.mentalhealthcommission.ca/English/resources/mental-health-first-aid

https://phac-aspc.gc.ca The Public Health Agency of Canada's website provides links to mental health reports and best practices. Statistics from the Positive Mental Health Surveillance Indicator Framework can be found here.

https://www.socialprogress.org The SPI data for 163 countries is available here.

uwaterloo.ca/canadian-index-wellbeing/resources Information and resources on the CIW can be found at this University of Waterloo site.

https://www.who.int/mental_health/mindbank/en/here Comprehensive information regarding national and international mental health resources can be found. This resource is one means of supporting the enactment of best practice standards and human rights.

References

American Psychological Association. (2013). *Diagnostic and statistical manual of mental disorders* (5th ed.).

Bitter, N., Roeg, D., van Hieuwenhuizen, C., & van Weeghel, J. (2020). Recovery in supported accommodations: A scoping review and synthesis of interventions for people with severe mental illness. *Community Mental Health Journal, 56*, 1053–1076. https://doi.org/10.1007/s10597-020-00561-3

Canadian Index of Wellbeing. (2016). *How are Canadians really doing? The 2016 Canadian Index of Wellbeing report.* Canadian Index of Wellbeing & University of Waterloo. https://uwaterloo.ca/canadian-index-wellbeing/resources

Epp, J. (1988). *Mental health for Canadians: Striking a balance* (Cat. H39-128/1988E). Supply and Services Canada.

Frances, A. (2013). *Saving normal: An insider's revolt against out-of-control psychiatric diagnosis, DSM-5, Big Pharma, and the medicalization of ordinary life.* Harper Collins.

Green, M., Harmacek, J., & Krylova, P. (2020). *2020 Social Progress Index Executive Summary.* Social Progress Imperative. https://www.social-progress.org/search/?q=2020-Social-Progress-Index-Executive-Summary

Hagen, B. N. M., Harper, S. L., O'Sullivan, T. L., & Jones-Bitton, A. (2020). Tailored mental health literacy training improves mental health knowledge and confidence among Canadian farmers. *International Journal of Environmental Research and Public Health, 17*(11), 3807. https://www.mdpi.com/1660-4601/17/11/3807

Healey-Ogden, M., & Austin, W. (2011). Uncovering the lived experience of well-being. *Qualitative Health Research, 21*, 85–98. https://doi/10.1177/1049732310379113

Holttum, S. (2020). Research Watch: What really helps recovery in relation to severe mental health difficulties. *Mental Health and Social Inclusion, 24*(6), 8–12. https://doi/10.1108/MHSI-11-2019-0037

Horsfield, P., Stolzenburg, S., Hahm, S., Tomczyk, S., Muehlan, H., Schmidt, S., & Schomerus, G. (2020). Self-labeling as having a mental or physical illness: The effects of stigma and implications for help-seeking. *Social Psychiatry and Psychiatric Epidemiology, 55*(7), 907–916. https://doi.org/10.1007/s00127-019-01787-7

International Council of Nurses. (2020). *Policy statement on mental health.* https://www.icn.ch/sites/default/files/inline-files/PS_A_Mental%20Health_1.pdf

Khoury, E. (2020). Narrative matters: Mental health recovery—Considerations when working with youth. *Child and Adolescent Mental Health, 25*(4), 473–276. https://doi.org/10.1111/camh.12419

Kutcher, S., Wei, Y., & Coniglio, C. (2016). Mental health literacy: Past, present, future. *Canadian Journal of Psychiatry, 61*(3), 154–158. https://doi.org/10.1177/0706743715616609

Mental Health Commission of Canada. (2009). *Toward recovery & well-being: A framework for a Mental Health Strategy for Canada.* http://www.mentalhealthcommission.ca/English/document/241/toward-recovery-and-well-being

Mental Health Commission of Canada. (2013). *Making the case for investing in mental health in Canada.* https://www.mentalhealthcommission.ca/sites/default/files/2016-06/Investing_in_Mental_Health_FINAL_Version_ENG.pdf

Mental Health Commission of Canada. (2015). *Guidelines for recovery-oriented practice. Hope. Dignity. Inclusion.*

Mental Health Commission of Canada. (2020). *Hidden Heroes: Annual report 2019–2020.* https://www.mentalhealthcommission.ca/sites/default/files/2020-08/annual_report_2019_2020_eng.pdf

Mental Health Europe. (2019). *Short guide to personal recovery in mental health.* https://www.mhe-sme.org/guide-to-personal-recovery

OED Online. (2014). "well-being." *Oxford University Press.* Retrieved August 11, 2021, from University of Alberta Libraries. https://www.oed.com/oed2/00282689;jsessionid=6C04BC77AD21CC7D7034E3096CDC0AD4

Orpana, H., Vachon, J., Dykxhoorn, J., McRae, L., & Jayaraman, G. (2016). Monitoring positive mental health and its determinants in Canada: The development of the Positive Mental Health Surveillance Indicator Framework. *Health Promotion and Chronic Disease Prevention in Canada: Research, Policy and Practice, 36*(1), 1–10. https://doi.org/10.24095/hpcdp.36.1.01

Stelnicki, A. M., Carleton, R. N., & Reichert, C. (2020). *Mental disorder symptoms among nurses in Canada.* Canadian Federation of Nurses Union. https://nursesunions.ca/research/mental-disorder-symptoms/

World Health Organization. (2013). *Mental health action plan 2013–2020.* https://www.who.int/publications/i/item/9789241506021

World Health Organization. (2018). *International Statistical Classification of Diseases and Related Health Problems* (11th rev.) (ICD-11).

World Health Organization. (2019a). *Recovery practices for mental health and well-being: WHO QualityRights Specialized training. Course guide.* https://apps.who.int/iris/handle/10665/329602

World Health Organization. (2019b). *The WHO Special Initiative for Mental Health (2019–2023): Universal Health Coverage for Mental Health.* https://apps.who.int/iris/handle/10665/310981

CHAPTER 3

Identity, Inclusion, and Society

Simon Adam and Cindy Jiang

Exclusion is a major health problem globally, and it impacts almost every population, community, and individual. It is a contemporary issue of concern for mental health nursing because it carries mental health consequences on a mass scale, ranging from mild depression to suicide. Exclusion stems from the creation of the category of "difference," where difference is seen as inferior and those assigned this category are seen as inadequate and labeled "the other." This is also known as **othering**. The process of othering has two steps. First, a group of people are identified by their perceived differences (e.g., race, sexual orientation, ethnicity, disability, illness, social class), and second, they are categorized as inferior (Montréal Holocaust Museum, 2019). A complex, multifaceted phenomenon, othering does not occur in a vacuum but rather evolves within relationships of power (Peternelj-Taylor, 2004). For instance, forensic psychiatric facilities are settings where the dual nursing responsibilities of caring and custody can amplify the dangers of othering (see Chapter 35). The consequences of othering can include "alienation, marginalization, stigmatization, oppression, internalized oppression, and decreased social and political opportunities" (Peternelj-Taylor, 2004, p. 133). The marginalized "other" can be so reduced in status as to be perceived as less than human and disposable (Braidotti, 2013). **Structural othering** has been introduced by Jacob and colleagues (2021) as a dimension of othering that focuses on the way structural processes can give rise to exclusionary practices (e.g., arising from past decisions, historical issues, economics) and limit opportunities for those

that foster inclusion. They point to the need to examine structural influences to determine whether they enable or limit nursing practice and the possibilities of practices of inclusion.

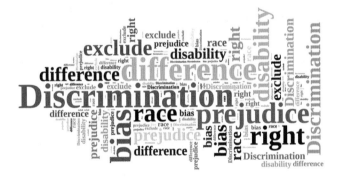

Identity and Social Exclusion

Identity is defined as the characteristics, attributes, beliefs, assumptions, and expressions that define an individual or group (Leary & Tangney, 2003). Ward (2009) further defines identity in two ways: self-identity and ascribed identity. **Self-identity** is understood as what the individual feels and believes about themselves. It includes the person's perceptions, emotions, thoughts, and behaviours as they become organized in a definable way of characterizing that part of themselves. **Ascribed identity** refers to the characteristics that others assign to the person, based on who the person is perceived to be. For example, a man who is identified as gay may be ascribed the characteristics of effeminate and flamboyant. Thus, identity ascription can be positive, negative, or neutral, depending on its context. People simultaneously embody multiple identities and often go about everyday life negotiating the multiplicity of their identities. This is because people often "exist within multiple, intersecting, and competing identity categories" (Roof, 2003, p. 2). For example, in answer to the question "Tell me a little bit about yourself," a person might respond that she is a 23-year-old Black lesbian woman. This short response incorporates four identities related to age, race, sexuality, and gender. Identity formation is largely unconscious and gradual. The more complex a society is, the more differentiation will exist among and between its various communities. The more differentiation that exists, the more socially stratified a society is said to be. Therefore, it is more likely that such a society will experience not only diversity in identities but also a wide range of degrees of inclusion and exclusion based on these very identities. This can be true of Canada, despite national efforts such as the affirmation of multiculturalism in 1982 (made into law by The Canadian Multicultural Act of 1988) and the Equality Rights stipulated in our Charter of Rights and Freedoms.

KEY CONCEPT

Identity, the characteristics, attributes, beliefs, assumptions, and expressions that define an individual or group, may be in the form of self-identity, a person's or group's view of themselves, or of ascribed identity, the characteristics that others, based on their perceptions, assign to a person or group (Leary & Tangney, 2003; Ward, 2009).

Social Exclusion

In the instances when the person's identity is a source of ongoing stress and hardship, that identity can take on a central role in the person's life and can become a basis for persistent marginalization and **social exclusion**. Such exclusion can deny or limit the individual's access to resources, rights, and goods and services, and negatively affect their ability to participate in their society as others do. Such exclusion impacts not only the individual's quality of life but also the cohesion of the society.

KEY CONCEPT

Social exclusion is the lack of or denial of resources, rights, and goods and services, and the inability to participate in the normal relationships and activities available to the majority of people in a society, whether in economic, social, cultural, or political arenas. It affects both the quality of life of individuals and the equity and cohesion of society as a whole (Levitas et al., 2007, p. 9).

Many communities and groups of people experience social exclusion based simply on how they identify. Those most negatively impacted are groups with historically marginalized identities, such as Black, Indigenous, people of colour (BIPoC), and lesbian, gay men, bisexual, transgender, queer (or questioning), intersex, two-spirit, and asexual (LGBTQI2SA+) people. Coined by Crenshaw (1991), **intersectionality** shows how people's lives are better understood by looking at the multiple social identities they inhabit. A person embodying a number of marginalized identities (e.g., a disabled Black lesbian woman) is likely to experience multiple, intersecting oppressions simultaneously. An intersectionality approach to mental health care reveals the complex interactions among social categories of difference and the systems and processes of domination and oppression (Crenshaw, 1991; Hankivsky, 2011; Hankivsky & Jordan-Zachery, 2019; Morrow & Malcoe, 2017) (Fig. 3.1).

KEY CONCEPT

Intersectionality is a framework that reveals the way in which social categories (e.g., race, gender) applied to an individual or group interconnect, creating systems of discrimination or privilege.

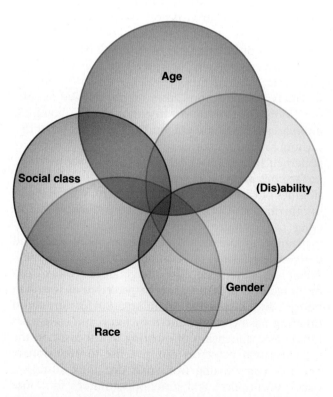

Figure 3.1 Intersectionality. Personal identities are not independent, but overlapping.

Identity-based Exclusion

Exclusion occurs for a variety of reasons and is motivated and maintained by various social, political, and historical events and structures. A great number of communities have been, and continue to be, marginalized and socially excluded, and it is beyond the scope of this chapter to discuss them all. Instead, we focus on several communities that have enduringly experienced exclusion both historically and currently within contemporary society. These are:

- people with a mental illness diagnosis,
- racialized communities,
- sexualized groups,
- people who identify as disabled,
- groups with a low socioeconomic status, and
- those excluded based on their age.

Mental Illness Diagnosis

A diagnosis of a mental illness, particularly one with a chronic trajectory, such as schizophrenia, may become incorporated within one's identity and substantially impact one's quality of life. The marginalization and exclusion of people based on their mental health status can be traced as far back as antiquity, although depending on how mental health is defined, this could be dated much earlier. In the 17th century, people who were identified as "insane," "morally inappropriate," or "mentally unhygienic" (e.g., prostitutes, vagrants, nonbelievers, as well as those ill with what we now recognize as neurobiological and other disorders) were framed as "mad" and were shunned from mainstream society and indefinitely confined to "madhouses" (Foucault, 1988). This exclusion was largely based on European Christian ideology that demanded, by way of reward and punishment, the reversal of such unwanted behaviour. Such shunning, however, occurred globally across many religious and cultural communities when an individual's behaviour seemed strange or was deemed "possessed."

Today, a substantial body of evidence points to a growing global problem of social exclusion related to mental health (Morgan et al., 2007), and Canada is no exception. Livingston (2013), in a report for the Mental Health Commission of Canada, observed that "insufficient funding of mental health services and research, the coercive philosophy of care that underpins the delivery of mental health services, and the unprofessional practices of mental health professionals" (p. 13) are manifestations of structural stigma in mental health. Stigma is the process of disapproving or rejecting a person or group of people by another person or group of people based on a perceived inferior characteristic or identity. Such disapproval or rejection does not need to be blatant to be powerful; it can be more subtly, but constantly and callously, conveyed. See Box 3.1, Research for Best Practice.

Structural stigma refers to the perpetuation of this disapproval or rejection by way of laws, policies, and practices, which create a systemic and enduring process of oppression and exclusion. When the individual internalizes and believes this disapproval or rejection, it is known as self-stigma. Much of the development of structural stigma owes its origin to historical practices of exclusion and oppression, which have impacted the development of contemporary law and policies and influenced professional practice (e.g., nursing, medicine, social work, etc.).

Although Canada uses the *National Standard for Psychological Health and Safety in the Workplace*—a voluntary set of guidelines, tools, and resources to guide organizations in promoting mental health and preventing psychological harm at work (see Chapter 17)—individuals with a mental illness diagnosis continue to report experiencing barriers to becoming employed and to obtaining employment commensurate with their education and experience. Although such stigma violates the values of equity, diversity, and inclusion in the Canadian workplace, it exists through "unspoken resistance, resentment, confusion, and prejudices" (Krupa et al., 2009, p. 418).

Racialized Communities

Race has been one of the most common indicators of identity-based exclusion, and BIPoC communities have a long history of exclusion based strictly on their racial identity. Owing its origin to the legacy of European colonization, assimilation, and ongoing oppression perpetuated by settler ideology, Indigenous Peoples continue to experience alarmingly high rates of exclusion with consequences to their physical and mental health. For example, resulting from feelings of depression, substance use, and a history of abuse, Canadian Inuit youth have one of the highest suicide rates globally (Karl, 2016). Indigenous people are 90 times more likely than the general Canadian population to lack safe piped water (Hanrahan, 2017). This troubling example is one of the many inadequacies in health services, social programming, and infrastructure experienced by Indigenous communities across Canada (Nesdole et al., 2014).

A study that examined Indigenous-specific racism in British Columbia's healthcare system found that Indigenous communities experienced ongoing widespread racism within the system, which limits access to medical care and treatment (Turpel-Lafond, 2020). A recent example of nursing's participation in anti-Indigenous racism was demonstrated in the actions of one Canadian nurse that led to the unfortunate iatrogenic death of an Indigenous woman (Hill Times, 2020; see Box 4.4 in Chapter 4). Exclusionary practices within healthcare systems in Canada are intolerable and must be identified and effectively addressed.

BOX 3.1 Research for Best Practice

UNDERSTANDING AND ADDRESSING STIGMA/DISCRIMINATION RELATED TO MENTAL HEALTH AND SUBSTANCE USE.

Murney, M. A., Sapag, J. C., Bobbili, S. J., & Khenti, A. (2020). Stigma and discrimination related to mental health and substance use issues in primary healthcare in Toronto, Canada: A qualitative study. *International Journal of Qualitative Studies on Health and Well-being, 15,* 1–13. https://doi.org/10.1080/17482631.2020.1744926

The Aim: To explore the experiences of healthcare practitioners in three Community Health Centres (CHCs) in Toronto, Ontario, regarding stigma and discrimination related to mental health and substance use issues, and to discover their perspectives re: interventions for addressing it.

Methods: The researchers identified their method as phenomenological in nature. Three focus groups with frontline providers and 23 senior staff members interviews were conducted. The primary research questions were "What are practitioners' understandings of the problem?" and "What are providers' ideas for an intervention?" Thematic analysis of data involved emergent and *a priori* coding.

Findings: Research participants described their clients, who included Indigenous Peoples, immigrants and refugees, street-involved youth, and transgender people, as facing multiple forms of stigma that created health service barriers, including accessibility to the neighbourhood surrounding the CHCs. For instance, immigrants faced language barriers and fears regarding their citizenship status; clients struggling with drug addiction faced being viewed as criminals, and sex workers were at risk for rape, assault, and robbery. Clients were dealing daily with personal, economic, and social adversities. The social norms and behavioural expectations of the CHCs (e.g., maintaining appointments; sitting quietly in the waiting room; being involved in care decisions) were alienating for some clients. Systematic efforts to mitigate stigma were negatively affected by related proximal factors. The stigma/discrimination related to mental health and substance use concerns intersected with that of gender, race, class, age, and other issues including the degree and visibility of distress. Participants looked to find practical solutions, including training to help tend to the distress and health conditions of their clients; development of more communicative and connected working environments; and creation of antistigma campaigns to address client–client stigma/discrimination in the CHCs, and to mitigate negative interactions with the neighbourhood.

Implications: Stigma/discrimination associated with mental health and substance use may be affected by contextual complexities, such as poverty, income insecurity, housing, food, racism, ethnocentrism, language barriers, and histories of trauma, abuse, and violence.

As an essential element of primary healthcare, CHCs can be a starting place for meaningful interventions.

Black communities and people of colour continue to endure exclusionary experiences, most often rooted in ongoing histories of racism, cultural imperialism, and migration policies that perpetuate racist practices, with some experiencing poor working and living conditions and high levels of stress and inadequate social support (Vahabi & Wong, 2017). Race has been specifically identified as a mechanism of exclusion among Canadian Black and Muslim communities (Reitz et al., 2017), African and Caribbean Black women (Logie et al., 2016), and immigrants from China, Hong Kong, and the Philippines (Oxman-Martinez et al., 2012). Racial and ethnic stereotypes (e.g., the "model minority" myth) also perpetuate racism (Chou, 2008). The effects of racial exclusion can also be seen in the areas of employment and income. A study conducted in Canada found that people with ethnic names, particularly South and East Asian names, received fewer interviews (Banerjee et al., 2018; Oreopoulos, 2011) and racialized women earn less and are less likely to be promoted (Beck et al., 2002; Yap & Konrad, 2009).

It has been well established that the social determinants of health (SDoH) are key to a thriving and inclusive society (Government of Canada, 2020; see Box 3.2 for the Canadian Government's list of the *Social Determinants of Health and Health Inequalities*). However, whereas some groups enjoy the privilege of accessing the SDoH, others, such as BIPoC communities, continue to be excluded and experience major and direct negative impacts on their mental health (McGibbon & Mbugua, 2020; Statistics Canada, 2016; Tisdale & Campbell McArthur, 2020). Although a substantial part of exclusionary practices can be identified, researched, and mitigated, also of major concern to BIPoC communities are the subtle and less noticeable forms of racism and exclusion, marked by daily verbal and behavioural discriminatory gestures known as **racial microaggressions**. For example, asking a person of colour "But where are you *really* from?" infers they are not from the country where they live and questions their belonging and social inclusion. Given its subtle nature, microaggression has been identified as one of the most dangerous forms of daily racism and racially based exclusion because it often goes unnoticed and unacknowledged by mainstream society.

Sexualized Groups: Gender and LGBTQI2SA+ Identity

The World Health Organization (WHO) (2021) defines **gender identity** as "a person's deeply felt, internal and

BOX 3.2 Social Determinants of Health

Determinants of health are the broad range of personal, social, economic, and environmental factors that determine individual and population health. The main determinants of health are:

1. Income and social status
2. Employment and working conditions
3. Education and literacy
4. Childhood experiences
5. Physical environments
6. Social supports and coping skills
7. Healthy behaviours
8. Access to health services
9. Biology and genetic endowment
10. Gender
11. Culture
12. Race and racism

individual experience of gender, which may or may not correspond to the person's physiology or designated sex at birth" (para. 3). Gender identity, much like race, has been a determining barrier to inclusion and the overall attainment of health. Gender as an influential factor for inclusion is rather complex. This is because gender itself is complex, as are theories about gender. For instance, some individuals may identify as being on a gender spectrum rather than possessing a specific gender identity. Therefore, efforts to understand gender identity and put forward gender-specific interventions may not prove helpful to those who do not conform to the category stratifications of gender, such as male, female, transgender, and so on. Moreover, identities continue to be redefined as they evolve and incorporate more complex notions of identity and human characteristics within them, as suggested by the acronym LGBTQI2SA+, where "+" implies that other identities may be subsumed under this growing category in the future.

Gender-based exclusion results in significant negative mental health consequences (van Daalen-Smith & Dosani, 2020). Some gender-specific communities may experience more pronounced barriers than others, but at some point, all genders face some form of exclusion. For example, it is a common understanding that men's perspectives and worldviews have dominated various facets of society, including the degree to which medical research disproportionately supports men's health relative to that of women. Notwithstanding this reality, men also experience unique male-based exclusion that centrally places them at risk for violence and criminal activity. Baker (2005) identified that young men engage in risky behaviour (e.g., driving a motorcycle too fast or participating in gang activity) to demonstrate to others such masculinist ideals as strength and fearlessness.

In Canadian nursing, males make up only 9% of regulated nurses (Canadian Institute for Health Information [CIHI], 2019 cited in Canadian Nurses Association, 2021); CIHI's data are by sex, so nurses' gender expressions have not been captured. Exclusionary elements affecting entry of nonfemale individuals into nursing do not appear to be situated in the profession nor in healthcare services: active recruitment of males for entry into nursing, although unsuccessful,[1] does occur. The exclusion of nonfemales appears to reside in societal attitudes: the caring work of nurses is a "transgression of heteronormativity" when carried out by males (Jamieson et al., 2019, p. 25). Societal change, so that gender is not considered binary and gender, ethnicity, and sexuality are not viewed as inclusion/exclusion factors for professions, needs to occur (Trueland, 2020).

Gender- and sexual-based phobias, such as homophobia, transphobia, and so on, occurring within healthcare services create barriers and cause negative experiences for LGBTQI2SA+ communities (Colpitts & Gahagan, 2016; Scheim et al., 2017). This harm is perpetuated by the social stigma that is ascribed to these groups and the assumption that all nonmale genders and nonheterosexual identities are inferior (Ward, 2009). The mental health consequences of exclusion to LGBTQI2SA+ communities are not only troubling but also have been linked to an increased rate of suicide among transgender people (Bauer et al., 2015). If such exclusion occurs in Canadian healthcare systems, despite expectations that dignity, equity, and justice be upheld, sensitivity education for healthcare staff regarding gender and sexual identity is required. Members of LGBTQI2SA+ communities are entitled to be safe and respected in healthcare services (Webster, 2021).

---

[1]Lack of success may lie in approaches taken. A video clip ad of England's National Health Services (with 9% male regulated nurses in 2020) shows a young man as he works out, plays soccer, and cares for patients, as a voiceover states: "We are not who you think we are. We're not embarrassed by what we do. We're proud of our work." (Trueland, 2020, p. 27). Not embarrassed?

Disability

Disability can be visible (e.g., mobility) or invisible (e.g., mental health, learning, memory) and can impact a significant portion of Canadians, where one in five self-report as having a disability (Morris et al., 2018). Disability has historically been framed as a problem located within the body (e.g., missing limb, blindness) and understood as a problem of the body that must be corrected (Titchkosky, 2011). This is known as the medical model of disability. The social model of disability, however, suggests that disability is the result of social, political, and structural forces that impose restrictions on people with disabilities, and these restrictions disable such people and prevent their full participation in society (Oliver, 1996). For example, if all buildings were accessible, then buildings would not be disabling for someone with mobility issues, or if all web pages were coded so they can be used by screen readers, then reading web pages would not be disabling for someone with visual impairments. Khanlou and colleagues (2021) completed a study grounded in the social model of disability to look at technology access for young people with developmental disabilities. Their scoping review of the literature found that multiple factors create barriers to technology access related to education (e.g., training), to daily living and integration (e.g., inadequate support for parents, low levels of literacy, lack of fit with the young adults' unique needs, and social exclusion), and to employment (e.g., a lack of availability of the technology, poor design, and inadequate accommodation). Barriers to equitable use of technology negatively impact the inclusion and social integration of this group of young adults.

Ableism is a term used to identify discrimination in favour of able-bodied people. An example of ableism occurs when people with disabilities experience exclusion in schools (e.g., segregation in the classroom), workplaces (e.g., stigma in finding employment; higher unemployment rates), and in social settings (e.g., inaccessible places) (Oliver, 1996; Prince, 2009). Income, education, and employment are key SDoH, and people with disabilities often have limited access to them.

Disability-based exclusion has been associated with psychological distress with an overall negative impact on mental health and wellbeing (Temple & Kelaher, 2018). The problem grows in magnitude relative to the intersections of oppressed identities the person possesses. For example, when a mental health disability intersects with criminalization, the exclusion is compounded. This complication can lead to the individual being caught in a cycle of incarceration and re-incarceration (Dowse et al., 2009) and never able to break free from the "criminal justice" system. When disability intersects with ethnicity and sexual orientation, for example, it can result in a person experiencing triple or quadruple oppressions simultaneously.

Socioeconomic Status

Social class as an identity is a powerful—and consequential—predisposition to exclusion. Of people with an ascribed low socioeconomic status and at high risk for exclusion are those living in poverty. Poverty is a determinant of social class and is highly contingent on the SDoH, such as income, education, and social supports. Stewart and colleagues (2009) noted that those with lower income experienced greater isolation and a lesser sense of belonging. Much like people with disabilities, those experiencing poverty are at high risk for intersectional oppression, social exclusion, and mental health challenges. For example, people most likely to experience poverty tend also to be those with disabilities, people who are homeless or lack adequate housing, single mothers, and those with an Indigenous identity (Canada Without Poverty/Canada Sans Pauverté, 2020). This serves as an example that not one specific identity predisposes people to a negative life trajectory or poor mental health; rather, it is the interaction of multiple identities that can lead to marginalization and exclusion.

Communities identified as having a low socioeconomic status become marginalized on two levels. First, because they lack the instrumental resources (e.g., income), they are predisposed to barriers that those with a stable income do not necessarily experience. Second, by way of stigma and structural exclusion, such as in policy and poor funding to social supports and programming, these communities experience ongoing systemic oppression and exclusion from full participation in society. Box 3.3 outlines a number of salient facts about poverty in Canada that directly impact social exclusion and mental health.

Chronological Age

Much like gender, one's age is also an identity that has been used to exclude people from social life, with negative consequences on their mental health. Although any age group can experience unique challenges leading to their exclusion from society, children and older adults are at a particularly high risk (see Chapter 29 for children's mental health; Chapter 31 for that of older adults).

Children and Youth

"There is a huge gap between what should happen to children and the real-life situation of children" (Emilia, 2010, p. 1781). Recognition of this moved the world in 1989 to create the United Nations (UN) Convention on the Rights of the Child, a treaty which, by 2021, had been signed by all UN members (except the United States). Rights range from the right to life and protection to the right to leisure and play, with emphasis

BOX 3.3 Poverty and Demographics: Marginalized Communities

Some members of society are particularly susceptible to the effects of poverty. The following statistics suggest groups who are particularly likely to experience poverty.

- People living with disabilities (both mental and physical) are *twice* as likely to live below the poverty line.
- Nearly *15%* of people with disabilities live in poverty; *59%* of these are women.
- Estimates place the number of people who are homeless and living with a disability or mental illness as high as *45%* of the overall homeless population.
- Children with disabilities are *twice* as likely to live in households relying on social assistance.
- Regarding single parents in Canada, *21%* of single mothers raise their children while living in poverty; *7%* of single fathers raise their children in poverty.
- Women parenting on their own enter shelters at *twice* the rate of two-parent families.
- Indigenous Peoples (including First Nations, Métis, and Inuit Peoples) are *overrepresented*

among the homeless population in virtually all urban centres in Canada.
- *28% to 34%* of people who use housing shelters are Indigenous.
- *1 in 5 racialized* families lives in poverty in Canada, as opposed to *1 in 20* nonracialized families.
- Racialized women living in poverty were almost *twice* as likely to work in manufacturing jobs as other women living in poverty.
- Overall, racialized women earn *32%* less at work.
- Nearly *15%* of older single individuals live in poverty.
- Nearly 2 million older adults receive the Guaranteed Income Supplement and live on about *$17,000* per year. However, the most basic standard of living in Canada is calculated at $18,000 per year for a single person.

Adapted from Canada Without Poverty/Canada Sans Pauverté. (2020). *Just the facts.* https://cwp-csp.ca/poverty/just-the-facts/

on a child's right to health, to good education, and to safety from abuse and exploitation in all forms. Further, a child's right to information, to express their opinion on matters that affect them, and to be heard and taken seriously—in other words, to participate, shaped by their age and maturity—is recognized. In places of great poverty and in times of war, famine, and disaster, upholding children's rights can be incredibly challenging for parents and other adults; however, it is the right to participate that has not been achieved for most children (Lansdowne, 2011). In many nations, upholding such rights involves significant cultural change, as well as new services, policies, and laws. Given, however, that children's participation protects them, facilitates their personal development (including that of tolerance and respect for others), strengthens a sense of accountability, and prepares them for societal roles, it is a worthy global goal (Emilia, 2010).

The "imagination, ideals and energies of young people are vital for the continuing development of the societies in which they live" (UN, 2010, p. i). Youth aspire to meaningful participation in their societies, including to transform what they regard as negative aspects of social life. The United Nations is working to support such aspirations, developing a UN Youth Strategy "Youth 2030." In many respects, however, youths' authentic participation in their societies remains aspirational. Strategies for engaging youth include The World Youth Report (WYR), a UN publication facilitating dialogue with youth to

promote their social participation (e.g., role of inclusive social policies in youth mental health), and The World Future Council led project to identify laws/policies that foster environments where youths' contributions to Youth 2030 goals can be realized. (See Web Links for Youth Strategy 2030 and resources on youth participation.)

Nurses have a role in implementing children's and youths' participation in healthcare settings (see Web Links to access a child-friendly version of the Convention). Upholding their rights encompasses inclusion in decisions and discussions about their care, time for information and questions about treatments, freedom to voice fears, and explanations when their choices cannot be realized (Lansdowne, 2011).

Older Adults

Older adults can experience marginalization and exclusion based on their age. Given that aging has been accelerated by a decline in the birth rate and by the fact that the majority of people now live to be "old" (UN, 2015), this is a significant global concern. Canada in mid-2020 had nearly 7 million people who were 65 years of age or older (Statistics Canada, 2020). In a literature review examining the state of determining the prevalence of ageism, Wilson and colleagues (2019) found that ageism prevalence studies involved few subjects and often convenience sampling. Two distinct types of prevalence were considered: ageism as reported by older persons and ageist attitudes and/or behaviours self-reported by younger people. Because both approaches require self-awareness as well as self-disclosure, the validity of the results are questionable. These researchers concluded that further development of ageism measurement tools is required and that ageism needs to be studied in developing and developed populations and in such subpopulations as healthcare professionals.

Social isolation may occur for older adults, caused or exacerbated by the death of friends and partners and the loss of the individual's sensorium (e.g., hearing loss, vision loss, etc.) (Nicolson, 2012). **Social isolation** is defined as the loss or breakdown of relationships deemed important to the individual, leading to an absence or near-absence of contact with people. One of the consequences of social isolation is depression, which is a common mental health challenge for the older adult population (Canadian Coalition for Seniors' Mental Health [CCSMH], 2021). Depression may be triggered not only by social isolation but also by various forms of social exclusion, such as loss of independence and confinement to long-term care institutions (e.g., nursing homes). Negative stereotypes perpetuate the idea that older individuals are excessive users of the healthcare system and thus economically and socially burdensome to society (McPherson & Curry, 2020).

The WHO (2002) has advanced the idea of **active aging**, defined as "the process of optimizing opportunities for health, participation and security in order to enhance quality of life as people age" (p. 12). The WHO suggests that, to help achieve active aging, older adults should be supported to engage in civic and social participation and that strategies and resources for social inclusion also be implemented. See Box 3.4 for an example of healthcare organizational outreach enabling participation in health services by marginalized communities in its region.

Medicalization as a Form of Exclusion in Psychiatric Practice

Psychiatric diagnosis has been critiqued as problematic on the grounds that it can create labeling and stigma out of otherwise normal human behaviour (Burstow, 2005, 2015; Hagen, 2007; Hagen & Nixon, 2011). The process by which human issues are "described using medical language, understood through the adoption of a medical framework, or 'treated' with a medical intervention" (Conrad 2007, p. 5) is known as **medicalization**. When such issues happen to be behavioural or emotional in nature, resulting in a mental illness diagnosis, the process is known as **psychiatrization**. For example, an individual is considered to be psychiatrized when their suffering from prolonged grief and sadness related to the loss of their partner is subsequently misdiagnosed as major depression and treated with antidepressants. (See Chapter 2 for concerns about aspects of everyday life being transformed into illness and about labeling by diagnostic classification.)

The history of psychiatry includes the designation of human behaviours as mental illnesses, which were later discredited as unscientific and removed from psychiatric practice. Psychiatric diagnoses based on other than medical science, but rather on racial, sexual, and gender biases, are harmful. Some examples follow.

Diagnosis Impacted by Racial Identity

A review of empirical literature spanning a 24-year period demonstrated that members of a Black community were three to four times more likely to be diagnosed with a

---

BOX 3.4 Addressing Exclusion of Marginalized Communities from Healthcare Services

Montesanti, S. R., Abelson, J., Lavis, J. N., & Dunn, J. R. (2017). Enabling the participation of marginalized populations: Case studies from a health service organization in Ontario, Canada. *Health Promotion International, 32,* 636–664. https://doi.org/10.1093/heapro/dav118

Healthcare organizations need to ensure members of marginalized communities can participate in healthcare services. In an Ontario health service organization, strategies were enacted for engaging marginalized populations (including Low-German–speaking Mennonites in a rural town, newly arrived immigrants and refugees in an urban downtown area, immigrant and French-speaking older adults in an inner city, and women who were refugees in an inner city). Based in a community development approach, these strategies involved time spent in building trust with the communities and achieving incremental success around small issues, while identifying the barriers that constrained participation (e.g., language barriers for newly arrived and established immigrants and refugees, French-speaking older adults, and Low-German–speaking Mennonites). Addressing barriers occurred through such strategies as training peer leaders and community stakeholder partnerships, as the capacity building of community members' skills and abilities evolved.

psychotic disorder than Euro-Americans (Schwartz & Blankenship, 2014). Moreover, among individuals diagnosed with schizophrenia, Black people were more likely than non-Black people to be diagnosed with major depression as well (Gara et al., 2018). Racial bias, thus, can influence diagnostic decisions and, even when unconsciously acted upon, can cause medical harm and social suffering to an individual, their family, and their community. An early example is that of *drapetomania*, an 1851 diagnosis given to enslaved Africans who attempted to flee their captivity. Even some contemporary primary providers saw this "diagnosis" as more political than medical (Bynum, 2000). While Black communities are used here as an example of identity-based exclusion in psychiatric practice, it is important to note that other racialized groups have experienced similar problems—for example, Indigenous populations (Turpel-Lafond, 2020) and Chinese immigrant communities (Cheng et al., 2013).

Exclusion Based on Sexual Identity

Exclusion based on sexual identity is another example of psychiatric diagnosis being used to further societal biases. This use contributed to the stigmatization, marginalization, and the exclusion of gay men and lesbian women from mainstream society by way of medicalizing their experiences. In 1968, with the publication of the second edition of the *Diagnostic and Statistical Manual of Mental Disorders*, homosexuality was classified as a mental illness, although it was later dropped from the third edition, in 1973. During this development, the gay liberation movement was gaining momentum, and riots, demonstrations, and calls to action for gay men, lesbian, and transgender people's rights took hold. This marked an important moment in North American history for LGBTQI2SA+ people and serves as a good example of community-based resistance and activism that led to the demedicalization of sexual identity.

Exclusion Based on Gender Identity

Experience of and access to healthcare is influenced by one's gender (WHO, 2020;2021). Gender inequality, revealed in mobility restrictions, lack of decision-making power, and lower literacy, creates healthcare barriers for women, who face greater risk of malnutrition, poor vision, respiratory infections, and elder abuse than men, as well as risk of harmful practices such as female genital mutilation and early (childhood) forced marriage. Gender norms related to notions of masculinity (e.g., smoking, risk-taking, misuse of alcohol, and avoidance of help and healthcare) have serious consequences on men's health, including mental health. Those with

gender identities other than "male" or "female" too often face stigma and discrimination, including in healthcare, placing them at significant risk for mental health issues, such as suicide.

Gender identity has been addressed in contemporary psychiatric discourse and practice. "Gender identity disorder" was included in the revised fourth edition of the *DSM* (APA, 2000, 2020) and replaced by "gender dysphoria" in the 5th edition of the manual (APA, 2013). These concepts medicalize gender and label nonconforming gender-identified groups (e.g., transgender) as in need of treatment and other medical intervention. Gender-identified underrepresented groups and sexualized minorities find that they must lobby for gender equity and inclusion into mainstream society.

▌ Global Responses to Social Exclusion

Given the longstanding critical movements and calls to action for equity, diversity, and inclusion, a global response has been established in an effort to close social gaps impacting various marginalized groups and populations. To that effect, the UN has been a forceful global advocate for the rights of people with disabilities (UN, 2007a), Indigenous people (UN, 2007b), and children (UN, 1990). For example, in an effort to support equity for persons with disabilities, in 2007, the UN launched a global symposium known as The UN *Convention on the Rights of Persons with Disabilities* (2007a), which has as its purpose to "promote, protect and ensure the full and equal enjoyment of all human rights and fundamental freedoms by all persons with disabilities, and to promote respect for their inherent dignity" (UN, 2007a, art. 1). This event and the subsequent documents that emerged from it mark a historic moment in the global advocacy for social inclusion of persons with disabilities.

During the same year, recognizing the widespread racism that Indigenous communities face globally, the UN published its *United Nations Declaration on the Rights of Indigenous Peoples* (UNDRIP), outlining steps towards the recognition, promotion, and protection of the rights and freedoms of Indigenous communities (2007b). The UNDRIP has been adopted by 148 countries, including Canada, as a guide to help ensure that the rights of Indigenous people are protected in accordance with international human rights legislation. A third example of the UN's global advocacy efforts for social inclusion is the *Convention on the Rights of the Child*, noted previously (UN, 1990). Nations possess varying levels of resources to implement human rights legislation and inclusion strategies, revealing the need for equity within and among countries. The UN's global response to social exclusion and human rights is one of the largest equity-seeking global projects.

Implications for Mental Health Nursing Practice

Allman (2013) states:

> Exclusion societies are identifiable at different places in time, space, and geography. Such societies tend to be associated with differential access to social and economic wellbeing, and differential proximity to illness and disease. Inclusion societies, however, evolve from within such contexts. They are characterized by movements towards greater social justice, equality, and collectivism in response to the kinds of global oppressions exclusion societies embody and perpetuate. (p. 2)

To contribute to the creation of sustainable and inclusive societies, nurses must uphold their ethical codes that repudiate discrimination based on identity in the provision of care. They need to go further and recognize and expose identity-based marginalization. Developing their understanding of the larger social structures and power relations that create oppression, marginalization, and exclusion located in "the political, economic, and social structure of society and of the culture that informs them" (Navarro, 2007, p. 2) will facilitate an effective response. While some of these structures may be more easily identified, such as sexist policies, biased laws, or inaccessible healthcare services, others, such as microaggressions, will be less obvious and can continue undetected and unremedied. Engaging in "big-picture" (or macro) critical thinking (Adam & Juergensen, 2019), such as asking the "yes-but-why?" question, will be important. Informed, just practice requires nurses to recognize that one's society and its institutions, such as healthcare, are shaped by social, political, and economic factors that can be oppressive if individuals or communities are marginalized by them.

When caring for individuals diagnosed with mental illness, as when caring for those with any illness, it is crucial to truly "see" the person beyond the diagnosis. Nurses require in their practice an understanding of the complexity of identity and an awareness that each individual embodies multiple identities that take on various degrees of importance at various times. Box 3.5 lists strategies to consider in identifying structural exclusionary factors, which can inform inclusive, antioppressive nursing care. Healthcare environments are to be inclusive communities where it is actively recognized that all people are joined by the common experience of the human condition, where differences are not highlighted and constructed as binary opposition to one another, such as disabled/able-bodied, gay/straight, Black/White, and so on.

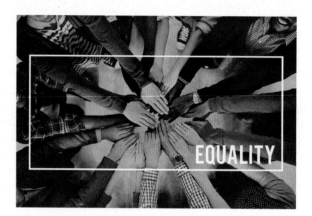

BOX 3.5 Antioppressive and Structural Analysis Strategies for Nursing Practice

1. Partner with individuals and communities in providing relational antioppressive care.
2. Provide a safe space for the individual, including those in extreme states of distress, to contribute to their own care.
3. Acknowledge that the nurse cannot know all identities and all experiences, and thus, is not an expert in that regard.
4. Make careful use of language that does not psychiatrize or medicalize human behaviour.
5. Ask questions that direct attention to the structural causes of mental illness diagnoses, such as:
   - What historical events led to the individual experiencing mental distress?
   - What issues of access to health and social services require attention at this time?
   - How have health and social policies contributed to the mental distress of this individual?
   - What other societal exclusionary practices have contributed to this individual's mental distress?
   - How can the nurse intervene to disrupt the social, political, and economic events that have contributed to this individual's mental health issues?
6. Engage in political and activist efforts to achieve social justice and health equity. Some specific strategies may involve:
   - Lobbying local politicians;
   - Writing to the media on issues related to equity in mental health, including the critical use of sensitive and inclusive language;
   - Generating position statements directed at nursing and other health professional organizations; and
   - Working with individuals and mental health communities for health equity and social justice.

Future Directions: Beyond Identity

Theories about identity and identity politics are extensive and have been developing for many decades now. It remains challenging to understand any one identity, much less all the complex identities embodied within one person. The effort to do so, however, is vital, especially for caring professions such as nursing, given that safe, competent, compassionate, and ethical care is contingent on understanding the individual and their community. Identities "have a real, material role in subject formation, the production of community, and the assignment of rights and access to privilege," but they are also "constructions" (Roof, 2003, p. 2). A shift to a postidentity practice may be a promising direction for contemporary nursing. That is, while acknowledging that individuals possess important experiences that culminate in identity formation (e.g., excellent care in a first episode of psychosis that shapes one's identity as a healthy individual with a controlled health issue [see Fig. 2.1 in Chapter 2] or poor mental healthcare, resulting in the formation of a psychiatric survivor identity), nursing can move beyond the fragmenting of the human experience towards a holistic and unstratified approach to healthcare.

Summary of Key Points

- Identity is a complex concept. Individuals often embody a number of identities simultaneously, gradually incorporating and relinquishing various identities as they gain or lose relevance to their lives. Identity can be self-created (by the individual) or ascribed (by others towards the individual) and can be negative, positive, or neutral.
- Identity can be made a source of oppression and social exclusion. This is especially evident in individuals or groups who possess marginalized identities, such as BIPoC communities or sexualized communities, who in turn become othered, stigmatized, and socially excluded. This has substantial negative impacts on their mental health, ranging from depression to suicide. The combination of multiple marginalized identities within one individual or community often results in compounding oppressions, known as intersectionality.
- The process of medicalization contributes to stigma and a marginalized identity, as demonstrated by historical and contemporary examples of psychiatric diagnoses that medicalize race, gender, sexuality, and the overall human condition. The classification of human traits and behaviours as mental illnesses is termed psychiatrization.
- Nurses need to be vigilant regarding the effect of exclusionary attitudes and discriminatory practices and be strategically informed and responsive to the individuals and communities affected by them. In mental healthcare, such vigilance involves respecting the viewpoint and concerns of those who identify as survivors not of an illness, but of the system itself.

Thinking Challenges

1. How can you as a nurse incorporate an intersectional perspective within a mental health assessment?
2. What other structural barriers to inclusion can you identify for the communities discussed in this chapter?
3. Provide three examples of how a nurse can advocate for the promotion of the SDoH in marginalized communities.

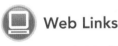

Web Links

Persons With Disabilities
https://www.un.org/development/desa/disabilities/convention-on-the-rights-of-persons-with-disabilities/convention-on-the-rights-of-persons-with-disabilities-2.html *The UN Convention on the Rights of Persons with Disabilities.*

Children, Youth, and Older Adults
https://www.ohchr.org/EN/ProfessionalInterest/Pages/CRC.aspx *The UN Convention on the Rights of the Child*

https://www.unicef.org/sop/convention-rights-child-child-friendly-version *A child-friendly version of the Convention on the Rights of the Child.*

https://www.un.org/youthenvoy/wp-content/uploads/2018/09/18-00080_UN-Youth-Strategy_Web.pdf United Nations' *Youth Strategy 2030: Working with and for Youth.*

http://www.youthpolicypress.com/ The site of the Publishing House on Youth, Research & Policy, which features news, magazines, research books, podcasts, and documentaries.

https://www.google.com/search?q=Lisbon+Declaration+on+Youth+Policies+and+Programmes+2019&rlz=1C1SQJL_enCA877CA877&oq=lis&aqs=chrome.0.69i59j69i57j46i433j46i131i433j46i433j46i131i433j46i433l3j0i271.7377j0j15&sourceid=chrome&ie=UTF-8 At this site is the *Lisboa+21 Declaration on Youth Policies and Programmes 2019* from the World Conference of Ministers Responsible for Youth, 2019, in Portugal.

https://www.who.int/ageing/features/attitudes-quiz/en/ The World Health Organization's *Ageing Attitudes Quiz* is available at this site.

Gender
https://www.who.int/health-topics/gender#tab=tab_1 WHO: "Gender and Health"

Indigenous Peoples

https://www.un.org/development/desa/indigenouspeoples/
wp-content/uploads/sites/19/2018/11/UNDRIP_E_web.pdf
The UN Declaration on the Rights of Indigenous Peoples.

Healthcare Inclusion Issues

https://engage.gov.bc.ca/app/uploads/sites/613/2020/11/In-Plain-Sight-Full-Report.pdf A report commissioned by the BC Ministry of Health that outlines systemic healthcare racism against Indigenous communities and recommendations to redress it.

https://madnesscanada.com A teaching/learning resource in mad studies. This website is a rich source of materials ranging from visual arts to poetry created by people who self-identify as mad people and psychiatric survivors.

https://www.mentalhealthcommission.ca/sites/default/files/MHCC_OpeningMinds_MentalIllness-RelatedSructuralStigmaReport_ENG_0_0.pdf A report by the Mental Health Commission of Canada that examines structural stigma in mental health.

References

Adam, S., & Juergensen, L. (2019). Toward critical thinking as a virtue: The case of mental health nursing education. *Nurse Education in Practice, 38*, 138–144. https://doi.org/10.1016/j.nepr.2019.06.006

Allman, D. (2013). The sociology of social inclusion. *Sage Open*, 1–16. https://doi.org/10.1177/2158244012471957

APA. (2000). *Diagnostic and statistical manual of mental disorders: DSM-IV-TR.*

APA. (2013). *Diagnostic and statistical manual of mental disorders* (5th ed.).

APA. (2020). *DSM history.* https://www.psychiatry.org/psychiatrists/practice/dsm/history-of-the-dsm

Baker, G. (2005). *Youth, masculinity and social exclusion.* Routledge.

Banerjee, R., Reitz, J. G., & Oreopoulos, P. (2018). Do large employers treat racial minorities more fairly? An analysis of Canadian field experiment data. *Canadian Public Policy, 44*(1), 1–12. https://doi.org/10.3138/cpp.2017-033

Bauer, G. R., Scheim, A. I., Pyne, J., Travers, R., & Hammond, R. (2015). Intervenable factors associated with suicide risk in transgender persons: A respondent driven sampling study in Ontario, Canada. *BMC Public Health 15*, 525. https://doi.org/10.1186/s12889-015-1867-2

Beck, J., Reitz, J., & Weiner, N. (2002). Addressing systemic racial discrimination in employment: The Health Canada case and implications of legislative change. *Canadian Public Policy/Analyse De Politiques, 28*(3), 373–394. https://doi.org/10.2307/3552228

Braidotti, R. (2013). *The posthuman.* Polity.

Burstow, B. (2005). A critique of posttraumatic stress disorder and the DSM. *Journal of Humanistic Psychology, 45*(4), 429–445. https://doi.org/10.1177/0022167805280265

Burstow, B. (2015). *Psychiatry and the business of madness: An ethical and epistemological accounting.* Palgrave.

Bynum, B. (2000). Discarded diagnoses: Drapetomania. *The Lancet, 356*, 1615.

Canada Without Poverty/Canada Sans Pauverté. (2020). *Just the facts.* https://cwp-csp.ca/poverty/just-the-facts/

Canadian Nurses Association. (2021, June 1). *Nursing statistics.* https://www.cna-aiic.ca/en/nursing-practice/the-practice-of-nursing/health-human-resources/nursing-statistics

Canadian Coalition for Seniors' Mental Health. (2021). *Canadian guidelines on prevention, assessment, and treatment of depression among older adults.* https://ccsmh.ca/wp-content/uploads/2021/06/CCSMH_Depression_Guidelines_FINAL_EN.pdf

Cheng, F-P., Lai, G. Y-C., & Yang, L. (2013). Mental illness disclosure in Chinese immigrant communities. *Journal of Counseling Psychology, 60*(3), 379–391. https://doi.org/10.1037/a0032620

Chou, C. C. (2008). Critique on the notion of model minority: An alternative racism to Asian American? *Asian Ethnicity, 9*(3), 219–229. https://doi.org/10.1080/14631360802349239

Conrad, P. (2007). *The medicalization of society.* Johns Hopkins University Press.

Crenshaw, K. (1991). Mapping the margins: Intersectionality, identity politics, and violence against women of colour. *Stanford Law Review, 43*(6), 1241–1299. https://doi.org/10.2307/1229039

Colpitts, E., & Gahagan, J. (2016). "I feel like I am surviving the health care system": Understanding LGBTQ health in Nova Scotia, Canada. *BMC Public Health, 16*, 1005. https://doi.org/10.1186/s12889-016-3675-8

Dowse, L., Baldry, E., & Snoyman, P. (2009). Disabling criminology: Conceptualising the intersections of critical disability studies and critical criminology for people with mental health and cognitive disabilities in the criminal justice system. *Australian Journal of Human Rights, 15*(1), 29–46. https://doi.org/10.1080/1323238X.2009.11910860

Emilia, C. (2010). Promotion and protection of the rights of the child. *Procedia Social and Behavioral Sciences, 2*, 1781–1785. https://doi.org/10.1016/j.sbspro.2010.03.984

Foucault, M. (1988). *Madness and civilization: A history of insanity in the age of reason.* Vintage.

Gara, M. A., Minsky, S., Silverstein, S. M., Miskimen, T., & Strakowski, S. M. (2018). A naturalistic study of racial disparities in diagnoses at an outpatient behavioral health clinic. *Psychiatric Services, 70*(2), 130–134. https://doi.org/10.1176/appi.ps.201800223

Government of Canada. (2020). *Social determinants of health and health inequalities.* https://www.canada.ca/en/public-health/services/health-promotion/population-health/what-determines-health.html

Hagen, B. (2007). Measuring melancholy: A critique of the Beck Depression Inventory and its use in mental health nursing. *International Journal of Mental Health Nursing, 16*, 108–115. https://doi.org/10.1111/j.1447-0349.2007.00453.x

Hagen, B., & Nixon, G. (2011). Spider in a jar: Women who have recovered from psychosis and their experience of the mental health care system. *Ethical Human Psychology and Psychiatry, 13*(1), 47–63. https://doi.org/10.1891/1559-4343.13.1.47

Hankivsky, O. (Ed.). (2011). *Health inequities in Canada: Intersectional frameworks and practices.* UBC Press.

Hankivsky, O., & Jordan-Zachery, J. S. (Eds.). (2019). *The Palgrave handbook of intersectionality in public policy.* Springer.

Hanrahan, M. (2017). Water (in)security in Canada: National identity and the exclusion of Indigenous peoples. *British Journal of Canadian Studies, 30*(1), 69–89. https://doi.org/10.3828/bjcs.2017.4

Hill Times. (2020, October 5). *Joyce Echaquan's degrading treatment a national disgrace* [Editorial]. https://www.hilltimes.com/2020/10/05/echaquans-death-a-national-disgrace/266290

Jacob, J. D., Gagnon, M., Perron, A., & Canales, M. K. (2021, June). Revisiting the concept of othering: A structural analysis. *Advances in Nursing Science, 44*, 280–290. https://doi.org/10.1097/ANS.0000000000000353

Jamieson, I., Harding, T., Withington, J., & Hudson, D. (2019). Men entering nursing: Has anything changed? *Nursing Praxis in New Zealand, 35*, 18–29.

Karl, M. (2016). Suicide and suicide prevention among Inuit in Canada. *Canadian Journal of Psychiatry, 6*(11), 688–695. https://doi.org/10.1177/0706743716661329

Khanlou, N., Khan, A., Vasquez, L. M., & Zangeneh, M. (2021). Digital literacy, access to technology and inclusion for young adults with developmental disabilities. *Journal of Developmental and Physical Disabilities, 33*, 1–25. https://doi.org/10.1007/s10882-020-09738-w

Krupa, T., Kirsh, B., Cockburn, L., & Gewurtz, B. (2009). Understanding the stigma of mental illness in employment. *Work, 33*, 413–425. https://doi.org/10.3233/WOR-2009-0890 IOS

Lansdowne, G. (2011). Every child's right to be heard: A resource guide on the UN Committee on the Rights of the Child general comment no.12. Save the Children UK.

Leary, M. R., & Tangney, J. P. (2003). *Handbook of self and identity.* Guilford Press.

Levitas, R., Pantazis, C., Fahmy, E., Gordon, D., Lloyd, E., & Patsios, D. (2007). *The multi-dimensional analysis of social exclusion.* Department of Sociology and School for Social Policy Townsend Centre for the International Study of Poverty and Bristol Institute for Public Affairs, University of Bristol.

Livingston, J. D. (2013). Mental illness-related structural stigma: The downward spiral of systemic exclusion. *Mental Health Commission of Canada.* https://www.mentalhealthcommission.ca/sites/default/files/MHCC_OpeningMinds_MentalIllness-RelatedStructuralStigmaReport_ENG_0_0.pdf

Logie, C. H., Jenkinson, J. I. R., Earnshaw, V., Tharao, W., & Loutfy, M. R. (2016). A structural equation model of HIV-related stigma, racial discrimination, housing insecurity and wellbeing among African and Caribbean Black women living with HIV in Ontario, Canada. *PLoS One, 11*(9), e0162826. https://doi.org/10.1371/journal.pone.0162826

McGibbon, E., & Mbugua, J. (2020). Race, culture, and health. In L. Leeseberg Stamler, L. Liu, A. Dosani, J. Etowa, & C. van Daalen-Smith (Eds.), *Community health nursing: A Canadian perspective* (pp. 168–182). Pearson Canada.

McPherson, G., & Curry, K. (2020). Older adult health. In L. Leeseberg Stamler, L. Liu, A. Dosani, J. Etowa, & C. van Daalen-Smith (Eds.), *Community health nursing: A Canadian perspective* (pp. 391–405). Pearson Canada.

Montesanti, S. R., Abelson, J., Lavis, J. N. & Dunn, J. R. (2017). Enabling the participation of marginalized populations: case studies from a health service organization in Ontario, Canada. *Health Promotion International, 32*, 636–664. https://doi.org/10.1093/heapro/dav118

Montréal Holocaust Museum. (2019). *Us vs. Them: Creating the other.* Government of Canada.

Morgan, C., Burns, T., Fitzpatrick, R., Pinfold, V., & Priebe, S. (2007). Social exclusion and mental health: Conceptual and methodological review. *British Journal of Psychiatry, 191*(6), 477–483. https://doi.org/10.1192/bjp.bp.106.034942

Morris, S., Fawcett, G., Brisebois, L., & Hughes, J. (2018). *A demographic, employment and income profile of Canadians with disabilities aged 15 years and over, 2017.* Canadian Survey on Disability. Statistics Canada. https://www150.statcan.gc.ca/n1/en/pub/89-654-x/89-654-x2018002-eng.pdf?st=4voFwbam

Morrow, M., & Halinka Malcoe, L. (Eds.). (2017). *Critical inquiries for social justice in mental health.* University of Toronto Press.

Murney, M. A., Sapag, J. C., Bobbili, S. J., & Khenti, A. (2020). Stigma and discrimination related to mental health and substance use issues in primary health care in Toronto, Canada: A qualitative study. *International Journal of Qualitative Studies on Health and Well-Being, 15*, 1–13. https://doi.org/10.1080/17482631.2020.1744926

Navarro, V. (2007). What is national health policy? *International Journal of Health Services, 37*(1), 1–14. https://doi.org/10.2190/H454-7326-6034-1T25

Nesdole, R., Voigts, D., Lepnurm, R., & Roberts, R. (2014). Reconceptualizing determinants of health: Barriers to improving the health status of First Nations peoples. *Canadian Journal of Public Health, 105*(3), 209–213. https://doi.org/10.17269/cjph.105.4308

Nicolson, N. (2012). A review of social isolation: An important but unaddressed condition in older adults. *Journal of Primary Prevention, 33*, 137–152. http://dx.doi.org/10.1007/s10935-012-0271-2

Oliver, M. (1996). *Understanding disability.* Macmillan.

Oreopoulos, P. (2011). Why do skilled immigrants struggle in the labor market? A field experiment with thirteen thousand resumes. *American Economic Journal: Economic Policy, 3*(4), 148–171. https://doi.org/10.1257/pol.3.4.148

Oxman-Martinez, J., Rummens, A. J., Moreau, J., Choi, Y. R., Beiser, M., Ogilvie, L., & Armstrong, P. (2012). Perceived ethnic discrimination and social exclusion: Newcomer immigrant children in Canada. *American Journal of Orthopsychiatry, 3*, 376–388. https://doi.org/10.1111/j.1939-0025.2012.01161.x

Peternelj-Taylor, C. (2004). An exploration of othering in forensic psychiatric and correctional nursing. *Canadian Journal of Nursing Research, 36*, 130–146.

Prince, M. J. (2009). *Pride and prejudice: The ambivalence of Canadian attitudes toward disability and inclusion.* Institute for Research and Development on Inclusion and Society. https://irisinstitute.ca/wp-content/uploads/sites/2/2016/07/Pride-and-prejudice_prince_iris_cr2.pdf

Reitz, J. G., Simon, P., & Laxer, E. (2017). Muslims' social inclusion and exclusion in France, Québec, and Canada: Does national context matter? *Journal of Ethnic and Migration Studies, 43*(15), 2473–2498. https://doi.org/10.1080/1369183X.2017.1313105

Roof, J. (2003). Thinking post-identity. *The Journal of the Midwest Modern Language Association, 36*(1), 1–5. http://www.jstor.org/stable/1315394

Scheim, A. I., Bauer, G. R., & Shokoohi, M. (2017). Drug use among transgender people in Ontario, Canada: Disparities and associations with social exclusion. *Addictive Behaviors, 72*, 151–158. https://doi.org/10.1016/j.addbeh.2017.03.022

Schwartz, R., & Blankenship, D. M. (2014). Racial disparities in psychotic disorder diagnosis: review of empirical literature. *World Journal of Psychiatry, 4*(4), 133–140.

Statistics Canada. (2016). *Aboriginal peoples survey, 2012. Social determinants of health for the off-reserve First Nations population, 15 years of age and older, 2012.* https://www150.statcan.gc.ca/n1/en/pub/89-653-x/89-653-x2016010-eng.pdf?st=lgVdi8DX

Statistics Canada. (2020). Population estimates on July 1st, by age and sex [Table: 17-10-0005-01]. https://www150.statcan.gc.ca/t1/tbl1/en/tv.action?pid=1710000501

Stewart, M. J., Makwarimba, E., Reutter, L. I., Veenstra, G., Raphael, D., & Love, R. (2009). Poverty, sense of belonging and experiences of social isolation. *Journal of Poverty, 13*(2), 173–195. https://doi.org/10.1080/10875540902841762

Temple, J. B., & Kelaher, M. (2018). Is disability exclusion associated with psychological distress? Australian evidence from a national cross-sectional survey. *BMJ Open, 8*, e020829. http://dx.doi.org/10.1136/bmjopen-2017-020829

Tisdale, D., & Campbell McArthur, G. (2020). Indigenous health. In L. Leeseberg Stamler, L. Liu, A. Dosani, J. Etowa, & C. van Daalen-Smith (Eds.), *Community health nursing: A Canadian perspective* (pp. 406–425). Pearson Canada.

Titchkosky, T. (2011). *The question of access: Disability, space, meaning.* University of Toronto Press.

Trueland, J. (2020, December). Odd man out: Weighing up the profession's gender. *Nursing Standard, 35*, 26–29. http://dx.doi.org/10.7748/ns.35.12.26.s14

Turpel-Lafond, M. E. (2020). *In plain sight: Addressing Indigenous-specific racism and discrimination in BC health care.* https://engage.gov.bc.ca/app/uploads/sites/613/2020/11/In-Plain-Sight-Full-Report.pdf

United Nations. (1990). *Convention on the Rights of the Child.* https://www.ohchr.org/EN/ProfessionalInterest/Pages/CRC.aspx

United Nations. (2007a). *Convention on the rights of persons with disabilities.* https://www.un.org/development/desa/disabilities/convention-on-the-rights-of-persons-with-disabilities.html

United Nations. (2007b). *United Nations Declaration on the Rights of Indigenous Peoples.* https://www.un.org/development/desa/indigenouspeoples/declaration-on-the-rights-of-indigenous-peoples.html

United Nations, Economic and Social Affairs. (2010). *The World Programme of Action for Youth.* https://www.un.org/esa/socdev/unyin/documents/wpay2010.pdf

United Nations, Economic and Social Affairs, Population Division. (2015). *World Population Ageing 2015 (ST/ESA/SER.A/390).* https://www-un-org.login.ezproxy.library.ualberta.ca/en/development/desa/population/publications/pdf/ageing/WPA2015_Report.pdf

Vahabi, M., & Wong, J. (2017). Caught between a rock and a hard place: Mental health of migrant live-in caregivers in Canada. *BMC Public Health, 17*, 498–512. http://dx.doi.org/10.1186/s12889-017-4431-4

van Daalen-Smith, C., & Dosani, A. (2020). Gender and community health. In L. Leeseberg Stamler, L. Liu, A. Dosani, J. Etowa, & C. van Daalen-Smith (Eds.), *Community health nursing: A Canadian perspective* (pp. 365–379). Pearson Canada.

Ward, N. (2009). Social exclusion, social identity, and social work: Analysing social exclusion from a material discursive perspective. *Social Work Education, 28*(3), 237–252. https://doi.org/10.1080/02615470802659332

Webster, A. (2021). The concept of vulnerability among black and latina transgender women in the United States. *Advances in Nursing Science, 44*, 136–147. http://dx.doi.org/10.1097/ANS.0000000000000354

World Health Organization. (2002). *Active ageing: A policy framework.*

World Health Organization. (2020). *Gender and women's mental health.* https://www.who.int/mental_health/prevention/genderwomen/en/

World Health Organization. (2021). *Gender and health.* https://www.who.int/health-topics/gender#tab=tab_1

Wilson, D., & Errasti-Ibarrondo, B., & Low, G. (2019). Where are we now in relation to determining the prevalence of ageism in this era of escalating population ageing? *Ageing Research Reviews, 51*, 78–84. https://doi.org/10.1016/j.arr.2019.03.001

Yap, M., & Konrad, A. M. (2009). Gender and racial differentials in promotions: Is there a sticky floor, a mid-level bottleneck, or a glass ceiling? *Relations Industrielles/Industrial Relations, 64*(4), 593–619. https://doi.org/10.7202/038875

CHAPTER 4

The Context of Mental Health Care: Cultural, Socioeconomic, and Geographic

Arlene Kent-Wilkinson and Wendy Austin

LEARNING OBJECTIVES

After studying this chapter, you will be able to:

- Identify cultural, socioeconomic, and geographical challenges to the provision of mental health care across Canada.
- Explore the cultural roots of mental illness and its relationship to beliefs of religion and spirituality.
- Relate the concepts of cultural identity, cultural competence, and cultural safety to the role of the nurse in mental health care.
- Consider the unique culture of Aboriginal people or Indigenous Peoples in Canada and their health beliefs.
- Describe factors related to the pre- and postmigration mental health of immigrants and refugees to Canada.
- Identify the influence of socioeconomic factors on the mental health of Canadians.
- Describe the mental healthcare delivery issues related to providing services in Canada's many geographic areas.

KEY TERMS

- Aboriginal or Indigenous • assimilation • colonialism • cultural diversity • cultural identity • ethnocentrism • health disparity • historical trauma • prejudice • racism • religion • residential school syndrome • spirituality • stereotyping • telehealth

KEY CONCEPTS

- cultural competence • cultural humility • cultural safety • culture • discrimination • diversity • poverty • stigma

Health, including the mental health, of any human population is the product of a complex web of cultural, environmental, historical, physiologic, psychological, spiritual, and socioeconomic factors. Cultural, socioeconomic, and geographical contexts of mental health in Canada are the focus of this chapter. Culture with regard to cultural identity and diversity as well as the cultural roots of spirituality and religion is examined. The unique culture of Indigenous Peoples in Canada will be a focus, as will be the factors that influence the mental wellness of immigrants and refugees to Canada. Socioeconomic factors that influence mental health and the geographic context of mental health care will be explored. The role and the responsibility of the nurse is emphasized in meaningfully addressing the contexts shaping Canadian mental health care.

Cultural Context of Mental Health Care

Culture is the "learned values, beliefs, norms and way of life that influences an individual's thinking, decisions and actions in certain ways" (Canadian Nurses Association [CNA], 2017, p. 21). Culture reflects the basic values and biases through which we interpret the world around us and make decisions about our own behaviour and our relationships with others. Our culture shapes our perceptions and attitudes—from our personal space comfort zones to our attitudes toward mental health and mental disorders. Culture is reflected in an individual's symptom expression, the meaning ascribed to disorder and treatment choices (National Collaborating Centre for Aboriginal Health [NCCAH], 2016). A challenge to all individuals is to gain insight into their own culturally learned ideas and values and to guard against an assumption that these are the correct and proper ones for everyone. This assumption is termed **ethnocentrism**.

KEY CONCEPT

Culture is the "learned values, beliefs, norms and way of life that influence an individual's thinking, decisions and actions in certain ways" (CNA, 2017, p. 21).

Cultural Diversity in Canada

Canada is a culturally diverse nation. If a Canadian is not an Indigenous person, then they are descendants of immigrants or are immigrants themselves. According to the 2016 Census in Canada, more than one-fifth of Canadians are born in foreign countries, which is the highest rate of all the G8 countries (Statistics Canada, 2016a; 2016b). Many of Canada's largest cities are among the most diverse in the world.

Diversity is "the variation between people in terms of a range of factors such as ethnicity, national origin, race, gender, gender identity, gender expression, ability, age, physical characteristics, religion, values and beliefs, sexual orientation, socio-economic class or life experiences" (CNA, 2017, p. 21). Overall, Canadians have a positive view of immigration and **cultural diversity** and consider both as assets to Canada. The 2016 Social Progress Index placed Canada second among 133 nations, citing among other aspects tolerance for minority communities (Social Progress Imperative, 2020).

KEY CONCEPT

Diversity is "the variation between people in terms of a range of factors such as ethnicity, national origin, race, gender, gender identity, gender expression, ability, age, physical characteristics, religion, values and beliefs, sexual orientation, socio-economic class or life experiences" (CNA, 2017, p. 21). It is both a source of richness and a distinct challenge to civil society (Kirmayer, 2019; Kirmayer & Jarvis, 2019).

Canadian Multiculturalism Policy

In 1971, Canada became the first country to adopt a policy of multiculturalism as an official government policy (Canadian Museum of Immigration at Pier 21, 2017). *The Canadian Multiculturalism Policy, 1971*, advocated support for the maintenance and development of heritage cultures and the reduction of barriers to full and equitable participation of all Canadians in the life of the larger society (Government of Canada, 2020a). The *Multiculturalism Policy of Canada, 1971*, affirmed the rights, dignity, and value of all Canadians regardless of ethnic, linguistic, or religious background. The policy confirmed the rights of Indigenous peoples in Canada and recognized Canada's two official languages as well as the need to preserve and enhance the use of other languages. Canada's multicultural policy has encouraged broad immigration (Government of Canada, 2020b).

Cultural Roots of Mental Health and Illness

The experience of mental disorders is influenced by culture. Symptoms of a disorder that are prominent in one culture may be insignificant or absent in another and may be interpreted as normal in a third. Some mental disorders may be a recent development in response to cultural change. For example, posttraumatic stress disorder (PTSD) can be manifested in the plight of refugees coming to a new country and to the effects of government policies of colonization (i.e., residential school syndrome) resulting in intergenerational trauma, as will be discussed later in the chapter.

Cultural Identity

Culture is strongly linked to identity; the suppression or marginalization of one's **cultural identity** has a negative impact on self-worth. However, when a culture is valued and supported, individuals and communities self-identifying with that culture will experience a sense of belonging and value. Shared cultural beliefs, practices, and language create social cohesion in communities, which can positively influence the health of individuals. Culture is the foundation of both individual and collective identity, and its erosion can adversely affect mental health and wellbeing, leading to depression, anxiety, substance abuse, and even suicide (Kirmayer et al., 2000a, 2000b; NCCAH, 2016). When cultural practices and language are denied to communities, as historically occurred with many communities of Indigenous Peoples in Canada, social cohesion and health are negatively affected (Brascoupé & Waters, 2009).

Cultural Beliefs About Health

Every culture has a conception of what constitutes health and disorders and how disorders should be treated. It is crucial to understand how the relationship between culture and health influences health behaviours in individuals. The "healthy immigrant effect" identifies that the health of new immigrants is generally better than that of the Canadian born but tends to decline as years lived in Canada increase (Statistics Canada, 2015). There are many factors contributing to this, one being the loss of social connections in one's home country. Transnational ties occur when immigrants can maintain a connection with their country of origin (Statistics Canada, 2015). This bond helps to maintain social connections and cultural identity. In the context of populations of Indigenous Peoples, moving off reserve and into urban areas can make the maintaining of traditional cultural ties difficult, thereby affecting cultural identity and social connections.

Cultural beliefs influence the ways both health professionals and patients view health, disorders, diseases and their causes, treatment options, how and where they seek help, and their views about dying and death (Mayhew, 2018). It influences beliefs about the choice to engage in health-promoting behaviours, whether to seek advice about concerns from a traditional healer or a medical doctor as well as whether to follow treatment options.

Beliefs about mental disorders are intimately linked with concepts of religion, social values, norms, and ideals of human relationships. These shared beliefs determine the nature of traditional medicine and provide the framework for interpreting symptoms and guiding action in response to them. Western medicine and psychiatry are premised on the belief that mental disorder is caused by biologic and experiential events; many other cultures ascribe a metaphysical or spiritual cause as well.

Traditional medical practices of Indigenous Peoples are closely related to other aspects of the culture, especially their **spirituality**. Getting in touch with one's own spirituality is identified as a key to recovery or healing. There is a holistic approach taken and, although spiritual rites have been modified throughout the years, they continue to be practiced. Spirituality is linked to a sense of life purpose and personal identity and is seen as a key element for finding one's place in the world. To most Indigenous Peoples, the concept of spirituality refers to a sense of direction: it is not a religion but a way of life. The Royal Commission of Aboriginal Peoples (1996) noted spirituality as a critical component of health for Indigenous Peoples because it permeates every aspect of life. Health to Indigenous Peoples is ultimately the achievement of equilibrium, whereby a state of harmony connects to health and disharmony to disorders.

Cultural Beliefs and the Mental Health of Immigrants and Refugees to Canada

Perceptions of health and wellbeing and of mental health differs across and within societies. For example, some immigrants may not be familiar with Western ideas about mental health and mental disorders nor with Western-style health services. They may use informal support systems, such as family and friends, rather than formal services to deal with mental health problems (Chaze et al., 2015). Mental disorders may be conceptualized differently by immigrant groups. Depression may not be a term familiar to some groups as it was not used in their prior communities, nor did people there seek out medical help for symptoms we identify here as "depression" (Chaze et al., 2015).

Thus, cultural beliefs and practices can be barriers to identifying symptoms of mental illness and to mental health service utilization (Chaze et al., 2015). It can affect the adoption of preventive and health promotion measures such as vaccination, birth control, and pre-natal care and influence health-related choices (Mayhew, 2018). Just as linguistic accommodation through interpreters is important to safe care, cultural brokers may assist in the provision of services to diverse ethnoracial clients (Kirmayer et al., 2011). Assessment of each patient's cultural beliefs related to health can be essential. Ensuring cultural safety for patients is critical to overall safe nursing care and necessary to improving patient outcomes.

Immigrants and refugees have different migrant trajectories. Immigrants usually made a choice to move to another country, even if economic, family, and other factors played a role in that decision. Refugees fled their country of origin due to a natural disaster, war, or persecution. As well as the trauma that forced their migration, refugees may have lived for months or years in crowded refugee camps, uncertain of any future home. Research with refugees, in recipient countries, reveals that prolonged detention, insecure residency status, restricted access to services, and inability to access work or education exacerbate the effects of depression and PTSD related to past trauma (Silove et al., 2017). For PTSD among refugees, the strongest predictor is exposure to torture; for depression, it is a number of different traumas (Silove et al., 2017).

While premigration factors influencing mental health may differ for immigrants and refugees, postmigration determinants of mental health are similar. A scoping review of Canadian studies (all situated in Ontario and Quebec) was conducted from 1990 to 2013 regarding the mental health of immigrant and refugee youth. Guruge and Butt (2015) found that determinants of mental health among immigrants and refugees have been identified as "individual (e.g., age, gender, language fluency, ethnicity, knowledge of the healthcare system); familial (e.g., family [in]stability, socio-economic status, intergenerational conflict); institutional (e.g., availability or lack of access to appropriate care and services, [non] acceptance of foreign credentials); and societal (e.g., discrimination, **racism**, poverty)" (pp. e72–e73). The authors of this review note that for the mental health of youth, family involvement was important; the first year in Canada was a critical period; and schools are a strategic point for services. The Mental Health Commission of Canada (MHCC, 2016) is working to support the mental health of immigrants and refugees who have come to Canada. (See Box 4.1 for Research for Best Practice—Women Who Are Immigrants and Mental Health.)

Diagnostic Cultural Formulations

In 2013, the American Psychiatric Association (APA) published the *Diagnostic and Statistical Manual of Mental Disorders*, 5th edition, or *DSM-5* (APA, 2013a). The fifth edition explicitly seeks to provide culturally appropriate diagnosis by incorporating cultural sensitivity throughout the manual (APA, 2013a). In the introduction of the *DSM-5*, mental disorders are defined "in relation to cultural, social, and familial norms and values. Culture provides interpretive frameworks that shape the experience and expression of the symptoms, signs, and behaviors that are criteria for diagnosis" (APA, 2013b, p. 13). The *DSM-5* provides criteria reflecting cross-cultural variation, outlines cultural concepts of distress, and offers an

BOX 4.1 Research for Best Practice

WOMEN WHO ARE IMMIGRANTS AND MENTAL HEALTH CARE: FINDINGS FROM AN ENVIRONMENTAL SCAN IN INTERIOR BC CANADA

O'Mahony, J., & Clark, N. (2018). Immigrant women and mental health care: Findings from an environmental scan. *Issues in Mental Health Nursing, 39*(11), 924–934. https://doi.org/10.1080/01612840.2018.1479903

Research Questions: (a) What are the reproductive and mental healthcare services within the Interior Health Region? (b) How are women who are immigrants screened for and referred to follow-up care and treatment of postpartum depression? and (c) What policies influence the reproductive mental health care of women who are immigrants in rural settings? These questions arise as new mothers who are immigrants may be vulnerable to mental health issues after childbirth due to such factors as cultural and geographic isolation, socioeconomic status, gender roles, and language difficulties that may shape and influence their postpartum experiences.

Method: Grounded in a critical social theoretical perspective which aims toward positive social change, data were collected within the Interior Health Authority of British Columbia from July 2016 to June 2017. Three

types of data were collected: (a) hospital and community profiles, regional health policies, and literature regarding reproductive mental health of immigrants (e.g., culturally tailored approaches); (b) open-ended interviews with 10 key informants regarding research questions 1 and 2; (c) an opinion survey (*n* = 100) of public health nurses and mental health professionals regarding the Edinburgh Postnatal Depression Scale (EPDS) and referral practices. Thematic analyses were completed across the data sets.

Findings: Four interrelated themes that impact the maternal mental health of women who are immigrants were identified: (a) community capacity building, (b) facilitators of mental health support and care, (c) barriers of mental health promotion and support, and (d) public policy and postpartum depression. There is a need for culture- and gender-sensitive training and support of healthcare staff to promote the maternal mental health of women who are immigrants and for the development of accessible pathways for their maternal health care. Further evaluation of the EPPD scale as a tool for universal screening is required.

---

interview tool. The criteria are designed to be as universally valid across different cultures as possible. For example, "offending others" has been added to the criteria for social anxiety disorder to better reflect the appearance of social anxiety disorder in Japan, where avoiding harm to others is of greater concern than avoiding harm to oneself (APA, 2013b).

Because symptoms manifest and are understood differently across cultures, clinicians must attend to relevant aspects of a patient's context when making a diagnosis. For instance, depending on the patient's culture, panic attacks may manifest as uncontrollable crying and headaches or as difficulty breathing. Clinician awareness of cultural, ethnic, and linguistic differences allows for more accurate diagnoses and more effective treatment.

Religion as a Cultural System

Culture, spirituality, and religion are central and interconnecting components of human societies (Chaze et al., 2015). **Religion** (from the Latin *religare*, to bind) can be defined as an organized set of beliefs providing answers to questions about life through sacred texts, rituals, and practices usually experienced within a community (Chaze et al., 2015). Spirituality when considered "meaning making" helps individuals to achieve personal understanding of life and their circumstances (Ameling & Povilonis, 2001, p. 16). Prior to the advent of modern medicine, when praying and offerings to the divine were often all

that could be done, illness and recovery were inescapably linked with spirituality or faith (Skip Knox, 1999).

Religions in Canada

Canada aims to be a nation of tolerance, respect, and religious harmony with support for religious pluralism important to our political culture. The majority of Canadians are people who identify as Christian, although this number has been decreasing since 2001. Those with no religious affiliation formed the second largest and youngest group (Statistics Canada, 2018). Similar to trends in the United States and Western Europe, the Pew Research Center's most recent survey in Canada conducted in 2018 found that a slim majority of Canadian adults (55%) say they identify as Christian, including 29% who are Catholic and 18% who are Protestant. About a third (29%) of Canadians say they identify as either atheist (8%), agnostic (5%), or "nothing in particular" (16%) (Lipka, 2019). People who identify as Muslim came third with the greatest increase in numbers. The numbers of persons identifying as Hindu, Sikh, and Buddhist religions are increasing as well, with the number of Jewish people slightly decreasing (Statistics Canada, 2018). The religious, as well as the racial, ethnic, and linguistic, diversity of the Canadian population continues to grow, presenting unique challenges to social institutions and governments as well as opportunity to embrace tolerance.

Religious Beliefs and Approaches to Mental Disorder

The Canadian Mental Health Strategy (MHCC, 2012) recognizes the vulnerability of immigrants, refugees, and racialized groups in relation to mental health and mental health service utilization; improving services to them is a priority. A challenge is to understand the role of religion, culture, and spirituality in a person's life without stereotyping them. Religious and spiritual beliefs can play a role in coping with illness, improving quality of life, and sustaining recovery. Activities and worshipping practices such as praying, spiritual reading, meditation, and repeating God names are described by some immigrants as spiritual resources for mental health care (Chiu et al., 2005). If one believes, however, that mental health symptoms are wholly spiritual in nature, help will not be sought in health services. For instance, a study by Okpalauwaekwe et al. (2017) found that some people from Nigeria attribute mental disorder to supernatural causes or believe that the person is being punished for bad deeds. Such beliefs have them seeking help from traditional healers or religious groups rather than physicians. If depression is understood from within a religious context, individuals may seek solace in prayer; fortunately, they may also take strength from their faith to seek other forms of help, including health care (Chaze et al., 2015). It is important that information regarding mental health and mental health services are available to new immigrants in an accessible form so that lack of knowledge about them is not a factor.

Although religion and spirituality may be important components of health and healing for immigrants, they may encounter in Canada a healthcare system that is science-based and not sufficiently acknowledging the spiritual aspects of care. A review of evidence-based literature concluded that many health practitioners are reluctant to incorporate spirituality into their practice because of the historical belief that it is antithetical to science. Other reasons include the ambiguity of their understandings of spirituality and lack of training in implementing spirituality in patient care. As well, health practitioners can allow their own religious beliefs to impact their provision of care (Chaze et al., 2015). (See Chapter 12 for interventions in the spiritual domain.)

Religious Freedoms and Practices

Canada has low levels of government restrictions on religion, according to a Pew Research Center study using data from 2016. The country's constitution protects the freedom of religion (Lipka, 2019). This is evident in basic ways. For example, men who identify as Sikh in the Royal Canadian Mounted Police are exempt from wearing hats as part of the uniform and wear turbans, which are required by their faith. Further, in 2018, a Quebec court ruled that a woman who identified as Muslim was wrongly told to remove her hijab in a courtroom and that head scarves should be allowed in court if they do not harm the public interest (Lipka, 2019).

Most Canadians say religion's influence in public life is waning in their country. The 2018 Pew survey found that roughly two thirds of Canadian adults (64%) say religion has a less important role in their country than it did 20 years ago (Lipka, 2019). Relatively, few Canadians engage frequently in traditional religious practices, such as daily prayer or weekly worship. While two thirds of Canadians (67%) say it is *not* necessary to believe in a higher power in order to be moral and have good values, about 3 in 10 Canadians take the opposite view, saying that in order to have good values, belief in a higher power is essential (Lipka, 2019).

Aboriginal or Indigenous Peoples in Canada

The term "Aboriginal" or "Indigenous" refers to individuals identifying themselves as First Nations, Métis, or Inuit peoples in Canada (Statistics Canada, 2020b). According to the 2016 Canadian census, 1,673,785 people in Canada (4.9% of the total population) self-identify as First Nation, Métis, or Inuit peoples (Statistics Canada, 2020b). There are more than 600 communities of First Nations Peoples in Canada, which represent more than 50 Nations and 50 Indigenous Peoples' languages (Government of Canada, 2018). Although often treated as a single group, there are many Indigenous cultures in Canada, each having a unique heritage, language, set of cultural practices, and spiritual beliefs that are woven into the fabric of Canada. (See Box 4.2 for Definitions of the three groups of Indigenous Peoples in Canada: First Nations, Inuit, and Métis peoples.)

Cultural Diversity Among Indigenous Peoples of Canada

The cultural and linguistic differences among Indigenous groups in Canada are greater than the differences that divide European nations. In addition to intergroup social, cultural, and environmental differences, there is an enormous diversity of values, lifestyles, and perspectives within any community or urban populations of Indigenous Peoples. Issues of cultural identity and community are especially salient for Indigenous Peoples who have sustained deliberate efforts by the state to suppress their cultures. Although they recognize themselves as having distinctive cultures, they also internalize the status of nations (Kirmayer, 2019).

Colonialism, Assimilation, and Historical (Intergenerational) Trauma

Colonialism is the institutionalized, political domination of one nation over another, including when one

BOX 4.2 Definitions: Aboriginal or Indigenous Peoples of Canada

Indigenous Peoples is a collective name for the original peoples of North America and their descendants. The term "Indigenous" is increasingly replacing the term "Aboriginal" as the former is recognized internationally; for instance, it is used with the United Nations' Declaration on the Rights of Indigenous Peoples (Charron, 2019). *Aboriginal peoples* is a collective name for all the original peoples of Canada and their descendants. Section 35 of the Constitution Act of 1982 specifies that Aboriginal peoples in Canada consist of three groups: First Nations, Inuit, and Métis.

First Nation(s). In Canada, the accepted term for people who are Indigenous and who do not identify as Inuit or Métis is *First Nations*. In the past, these people were referred to as "Indians." Today, *Indian* is considered an offensive colonial term and should not be used under any circumstances (Caldwell, 2019). First Nations Peoples have lived and thrived for hundreds of years on this land now called Canada. They have many different languages, cultures, traditions, and spiritual beliefs. Historically, First Nations managed their lands and resources with their own governments, laws, policies, and practices. Their societies were very complex and included systems for trade and commerce, building relationships, managing resources, and spirituality (Caldwell, 2019). Today, there are around 630 different First Nation communities across Canada—about half of which are in British Columbia and Ontario (Caldwell, 2019). According to the 2016 Census (Statistics Canada, 2017c), there

are over 70 distinct Indigenous languages recognized across the country.

Inuit. The Inuit people are Indigenous Peoples in Northern Canada who live above the tree line in Nunavut, the Northwest Territories, Northern Quebec, and Labrador. The word Inuit means *people* in the Inuit language—*Inuktitut*. The singular of Inuit is Inuk. The Inuit people are a circumpolar group, inhabiting regions in Russia, Alaska, Canada, and Greenland, united by a common culture and language. There are approximately 65,000 Inuit living in Canada (Statistics Canada, 2017b).

Métis. People of mixed European and Indigenous ancestry are Métis; they are one of the three recognized Aboriginal peoples in Canada (The Canadian Encyclopedia, 2019). The use of the term Métis is complex, contentious, and has different historical and contemporary meanings. The term is used to describe communities of mixed European and Indigenous descent across Canada, and a specific community of people, defined as the Métis Nation, which originated largely in Western Canada and emerged as a political force in the 19th century, radiating outwards from the Red River Settlement. While the Canadian government politically marginalized the Métis after 1885, they have since been recognized as an Aboriginal people with rights enshrined in the Constitution of Canada and more clearly defined in a series of Supreme Court of Canada decisions (The Canadian Encyclopedia, 2019).

---

nation overthrows another for the purpose of domination (Paquette et al., 2017). Colonialism involves direct political administration by the colonial power, control of all economic relationships, and a systematic attempt to transform the culture. Colonialism involves the exploitation or subjugation of people by a larger or wealthier power (Peters, 2017).

Before confederation and up through the first half of the 20th century, the strategy of the government of Canada toward the First Nations was a colonial one. **Assimilation** was the government policy to "Canadianize" Indigenous Peoples to the extent that they would abandon their own culture and adopt the dominant culture (i.e., French or British Canadian) and religion (i.e., Catholic or Protestant) (Thira, 2005). Populations of Indigenous Peoples in Canada have been subjected to **historical trauma**, which is the cumulative effect of maltreatment across generations and which results in the reproduction of maladaptive social and cultural patterns with each generation (see Chapter 18).

Effects of Colonialism

Colonialism in Canada had significant negative mental health effects for Indigenous Peoples, as well as causing intergenerational trauma (Roy, 2014). These mental health issues include "depression, alcoholism, suicide, and violence" (Kirmayer et al., 2000a, 2000b). Fetal alcohol spectrum disorder and **residential school syndrome**, a form of PTSD with a significant cultural component and impacting children (Douglas, 2020), affect Communities of Indigenous Peoples.

A case study of 95 Indigenous Peoples survivors of residential schools who had undergone a clinical assessment and possessed existing mental health profiles revealed that all but two people had a mental disorder. The most common being PTSD, substance abuse disorder, and major depression. All had experienced sexual abuse (Corrado & Cohen, 2010). Further, trauma is perpetuated today in the form of suicide and family violence, which then significantly contribute to substance abuse and major depression. Substance abuse is a major health issue. Alcohol-related deaths of Indigenous Peoples are almost double that of the Canadian population who are not Indigenous Peoples; drug-related overdose rates are two to five times higher (Russell et al., 2016). Further, perceptions of negative media coverage of events related to substance abuse have reinforced racism and negative stereotypes (Richmond & Cook, 2016). Perpetual trauma has left many communities in social and mental distress, where anger, hopelessness, lack of purpose, and pessimism have become the norm. Suicides have become the way to "communicate distress and escape when these seem to be few other options" (Government of Canada, 2020e, p. 8). These detrimental effects of colonialism on Populations of Indigenous Peoples are not unique to Canada but are experienced by many Indigenous Peoples around the globe.

Residential Schools

From first contact, the European missionaries sought to convert local Indigenous Peoples and save their souls. The Indian Residential School (IRS) system arose out of this history. In 1874, the federal government began to develop and administer the IRS (Government of Canada, 2020e). The schools were located in every province and territory except Newfoundland (where the entire population of Indigenous Peoples had been decimated), New Brunswick, and Prince Edward Island. Approximately 150,000 children, some as young as 4, were taken to these schools between 1896 and 1996, when the last one (on the Gordon Reserve in Saskatchewan) was closed (Joseph, 2014). Most of the federally run residential schools were closed by the mid-1970s. An estimated 80,000 people alive today attended an IRS in Canada (Government of Canada, 2020e).

The loss of their cultural identity, including seasonal ceremonies, storytelling, rituals, and health beliefs, and of knowledge of their languages affected the children's relationships with their own families and communities. They were to assimilate into the mainstream culture and its dominant religions and ways of life (Kuhl, 2017). The effects of this racist-based forced assimilation have had lasting and profound effects on Indigenous Peoples that persist to present day (McNally & Martin, 2017; Truth and Reconciliation Commission of Canada [TRCC], 2015a). That many of the children experienced physical, psychological, and/or sexual abuse greatly deepened this traumatic legacy (Government of Canada, 2020e). It can be linked to the high suicide rates, mental disorders, inadequate parenting skills, and sexual/physical violence to be found in some communities (Kumar & Nahwegahbow, 2016). Beyond the importance of culture for health and wellbeing, the ability to participate in one's own culture and transmit it to future generations is a basic human right (Kirmayer & Jarvis, 2019).

Effects on Mental Health and Addiction

The IRS is recognized as a contributing factor to the poorer health status seen in many populations of Indigenous Peoples today. Survivors face various health problems such as poorer general and self-rated health, increased rates of chronic and infectious diseases, and mental and emotional wellbeing including mental distress, depression, addictive behaviours and substance misuse, stress, and suicidal behaviours (Wilk et al., 2017). Research indicates that exposure to the IRS system along with a history of abuse is associated with suicidal thoughts and behaviours (Elias et al., 2012). In fact, researchers using data from the *2012 Aboriginal Peoples Survey (APS)* examined the relationship of IRS attendance of a previous generation family member and the current health of off-reserve First Nations, Métis, and Inuit Canadians in terms of five outcomes: self-perceived health, mental health, distress, suicidal ideation, and suicide attempt. All outcomes were directly affected: lower self-perceived physical and mental health and higher risk for distress and suicidal thoughts and behaviours, with the odds of a suicide attempt within the past 12 months twice as high for those with familial attendance in the IRS (Hackett et al., 2016). Suicide has been, at times, an emergency-level public health issue for a community (Rutherford, 2016). Suicide rates are twice as high in populations of Indigenous Peoples than in populations of non-Indigenous Peoples (McQuaid et al., 2017).

A growing concern is gang activity among the youth of Indigenous Peoples (Preston et al., 2012). Group membership can bring young people a sense of belongingness and purpose. Although gangs can promote such feelings, their members are more susceptible to making poor life decisions (Kyoung et al., 2015). Research suggests such gang formation, too, has its roots in the legacy of aggressive assimilation and colonization, as well as the challenges of adapting to contemporary society, and a lack of positive coping mechanisms (Mercredi, 2015).

National Efforts to Make Amends and Support Recovery From the IRS System

In 1996, the Canadian government published the report of the *Royal Commission on Aboriginal Peoples (RCAP): People to People, Nation to Nation* (Government of Canada, 2010) with recommendations about a wide range of social and economic issues. Less than 1% of health care workers in Canada are of Indigenous Peoples ancestry, which affects the provision of health services to this population, so it was recommended this number be increased. Federal and provincial initiatives were implemented.

In 1998, the Indian Affairs Minister, Jane Stewart, apologized to the Indigenous Peoples in Canada for the IRS system, announcing a $350-million healing fund

(O'Hara & Treble, 2000). The fund's mandate was to "encourage and support Indigenous Peoples in building and supporting sustainable healing processes that address the legacy of physical and sexual abuse in the residential school system, including intergenerational impacts" (Waldram et al., 2006, p. 19). The 2002 report of the *Commission on the Future of Health Care in Canada, the Romanow Report,* addressed the necessity for health care and policy improvements for populations of Indigenous Peoples, including importance of transferring responsibilities to Indigenous Peoples for the management and delivery of their health care.

Then, in September 2007, the largest class action settlement in Canadian history, the IRSs Settlement Agreement, came into effect, recognizing the damage inflicted by the IRS system and establishing a multibillion-dollar fund to help former students in their recovery (Government of Canada, 2016a). The IRS Settlement Agreement has five main components: Common Experience Payment, Independent Assessment Process, Truth and Reconciliation Commission (TRC), Commemoration, and Health and Healing Services (Government of Canada, 2016a). The Government of Canada (2020d) and Indian and Northern Affairs Canada (INAC, 2020) have developed a series of services to support IRS survivors and their families.

In 2008, the government of Canada apologized to Indigenous Peoples for the harmful effects of assimilation policies that resulted in the IRS system (King et al., 2009). In 2009, the TRCC (2015a, 2015b) began a 5-year process of gathering and preserving information from former students and their families about the effects of IRS system to ensure Canadian society recognized what happened and its long-term impact and to support reconciliation with Indigenous Peoples. The TRCC records are housed at the University of Manitoba. (See Box 4.3 for results of a *Confederation of Tomorrow Survey* that reports the opinions of a representative sample of Indigenous and non-Indigenous Canadians on issues such as reconciliation.)

Health Care of Indigenous Peoples in Canada

Diversity of social, economic, and political circumstances among communities of Indigenous Peoples in Canada means that there are many different approaches to health and healing. Many people are raised to believe that the body is governed by four elements comprising the spiritual, emotional, mental, and physical. Traditionally, Indigenous Peoples have a holistic view of health that is based on ways of knowing and being, wherein mental health is considered a part.

BOX 4.3 The Confederation of Tomorrow Survey: Relations With Indigenous and Non-Indigenous Peoples

A national survey of public opinion of a representative sample of Canadians, aged 18 and over (*n* = 5,152; 603 identified as Indigenous Peoples), from every province/territory was conducted from January 13, 2020 to February 20, 2020, just prior to the COVID-19 pandemic reaching Canada. In the previous survey (December 2018 to February 2019), upon which this survey builds, the majority surveyed believed that they had a role to play in the reconciliation (i.e., the establishment of mutual, respectful relationships) of the Indigenous and non-Indigenous Peoples of Canada. In this 2020 survey, there was less public consensus, with views ranging from a pro-Indigenous Peoples perspective to those taking the opposite view to those with no opinion. Overall, however, it was found that Canadians were dissatisfied with the status quo, that they supported increased action to address the issues facing Indigenous Peoples, and that they believed that not enough has been done to advance and strengthen reconciliation. At a ratio of three to one, respondents believed that people like themselves had a role to play

in reconciliation with most, especially respondents who are Indigenous Peoples, being more optimistic than pessimistic about progress in their lifetimes. Two of one Canadians preferred measures to increase representation of Indigenous Peoples in federal government (e.g., a seat in the federal cabinet) with most Canadians agreeing that Indigenous Peoples should have the final say over resource development on traditional lands.

References
The survey was conducted (online and by telephone) by the *Environics Institute for Survey Research,* in partnership with these public policy organizations: the *Canada West Foundation,* the *Centre D'Analyse Politique—Constitution et Fédéralisme,* the *Institute for Research on Public Policy,* and the *Brian Mulroney Institute of Government* at Saint Francis Xavier University.

Environs Institute for Survey Research. (2020, December). *Survey of Canadians: Indigenous-Non-Indigenous Relations (Report 4).* https://www.environicsinstitute.org/docs/default-source/project-documents/cot-2020---indigenous-non-indigenous-relations/confederation-of-tomorrow-2020---indigenous-non-indigenous-relations---final-report.pdf?sfvrsn=ac064ead_2

Mental Health Views of Indigenous Peoples

To be ill, including mental disorders, is to be out of balance in one of these elements (Douglas, 2020). The holistic view of health goes beyond the four identified elements to include the value of the collective group over the individual, an approach contrary to individualistic Western thinking (Little Bear, 2012). Notions of sanity and insanity and of personality disorders are not defined. These differences in views may present challenges to Indigenous Peoples accessing care and in caregiver's delivery of care, including system barriers such as institutional policy.

A literature review of the knowledge of Indigenous Peoples (Marsh et al., 2015) reveals that most Indigenous scholars propose that the wellness of a community of Indigenous Peoples can only be adequately measured from within a framework of Indigenous People's knowledge that is holistic, inclusive, and respectful of the balance between the spiritual, emotional, physical, and social realms of life. Treatment interventions need to honour the historical context and history of Indigenous Peoples. Cultural identity, community involvement, and empowerment are seen as important to health outcomes (see Fig. 4.1).

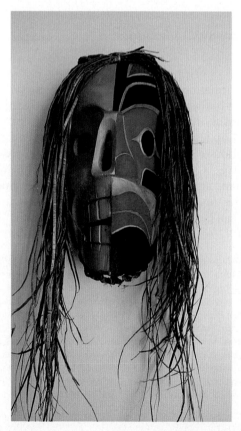

Figure 4.1 Life and Death transformation mask, by Kurtis Anton of the Squamish Tribe of the Coast Salish Nation. (Courtesy of Wendy Austin.)

The Indian Act, 1876

The Indian Act of 1876 is the only national-level legislative act for the First Nations still in effect. It ascribes health and health care of Indigenous Peoples to the federal government, while health care for non-Indigenous Peoples is under provincial purview (Richmond & Cook, 2016). (It also established the IRS system.) It formalized the reserve system, assigning financial responsibility and power over band administration, education, and health care to the federal government (Boksa et al., 2015). As these historical documents and organizations are discussed in the text, their original names will be preserved. It is important to recognize that this language is no longer acceptable in addressing the Indigenous Peoples of Canada and is under no circumstances condoned.

Health Services to Populations of Indigenous Peoples

During the time of early settlement and once the Indian Act of 1876 was signed, the Canadian government felt a moral and obligatory responsibility to the health of those considered Status Indian (Reading, 2018a, 2018b). Assimilation was reinforced with an increase in diseases and a belief that assimilation (from the Latin *assimilationem*, "similarity"; taking into the community) was the only way to guarantee good health (Reading, 2015), along with the signing of Treaty 6 in which the government guaranteed to provide medicine (Douglas, 2020). The responsibility of health services for Indigenous Peoples has been shuffled through different departments since 1904: from the "Department of Indian Affairs" to the "Medical Services Branch," which changed names in 2000 to the "First Nations and Inuit Health Branch" (Government of Canada, 2020c). The NCCAH (2011c) suggested that due to the lack of clarity within the Indian Act, in combination with the British North America Act, which assigned health to provincial control and Indian Affairs to federal control, the health of Indigenous Peoples at times falls between cracks in health services.

Indigenization of Curricula

Curriculum changes in schools to teach younger generations about the IRS system have been introduced using resource guides prepared by educators to the First Nations to ensure that all generations understand the historical context of residential schools and to develop student awareness about the reconciliation process (First Nations Education Steering Committee, 2017). This is a response, in part, to a call from the TRC, which also called upon Canadian medical and nursing schools to have a required course on health issues for Indigenous Peoples. Such a course should include the history and legacy of residential schools and indigenous teachings and practices. The *United Nations Declaration on the Rights of Indigenous Peoples*, as well as other treaties and documents pertaining to rights of Indigenous Peoples, need to be in the curriculum, as do skills in intercultural competency, conflict resolution, human rights, and anti-racism. Nursing curricula have had some content related to Indigenous cultures, including elective courses on health of Indigenous Peoples (Kent-Wilkinson, 2009), but more must be achieved to answer the call of the TRC.

Trauma-Informed Care in Services

Trauma-informed care (TIC) has evolved in Canadian health services as a means of establishing a safe environment for all patients, impacted by historical violence such as residential schooling (Browne & Baker, 2016; see Chapter 18).

Mental Health Strategy for Canada

Canada's first national mental health strategy, *Changing Directions, Changing Lives: Mental Health Strategy for Canada, 2012* (MHCC, 2012), identifies six strategic directions, including one focused on mental health of Indigenous Peoples, with First Nations, Métis, and Inuit peoples each identified as separate priorities. Rural, urban, and remote challenges of populations of Indigenous Peoples and social determinants of health issues are prioritized.

Strength-Based Approach

Government policies related to populations of Indigenous Peoples have too often used a deficit- or problem-focused approach (Paraschak & Thompson, 2013). Such an approach identifies barriers to good health without identifying strengths. Indigenous Peoples, however, focus on cultural strengths and bring resilience to the forefront (Graham & Martin, 2016). Ensuring a strength-based focus is taken with individuals who are an Indigenous person is important to the provision of culturally safe care (Douglas, 2020).

Stereotyping, Prejudice, Discrimination, and Stigma

For one cultural group to understand the values, beliefs, and patterns of accepted behaviour of a different cultural group is challenging. This can be especially true regarding mental disorders. Some cultures view mental health disorders as a condition for which the person with the disorder must be punished or ostracized from society; other cultures believe that family and community members are key to the care and treatment of persons with mental disorders.

The effects of mental disorders reach beyond the individual with the disorder; mental health conditions, including addictions, also impact families, communities, and healthcare systems. Mental disorders indirectly affect all Canadians through family members, friends, and colleagues. Families may become casualties under the stress of caring for relatives with acute mental disorders, especially within a rejecting community. Thus, the concepts of stereotyping, prejudice, discrimination, and stigma are important in understanding the lives of people with mental disorders, their families, and cultural groups. They are important to this "global, multifaceted problem" (Gronholm et al., 2017, p. 1341).

Stereotyping

Stereotyping occurs when individuals are expected to act in a characteristic manner that conforms, most often, to a negative perception of their cultural group. Stereotyping occurs because of lack of exposure to sufficient members of the group in question. Media representations of people with mental disorders (e.g., movies, television, magazines, and newspapers) help perpetuate negative stereotypes of those with this type of medical disorder. When stereotyping occurs by healthcare practitioners, patients and families are put at risk. Not only will they not be culturally safe but their care will be put in jeopardy. Stereotyping associated with Indigenous cultures can create barriers to access, resulting in poor health outcomes. For example, in 2008 in Winnipeg, an Indigenous man, Brian Sinclair, died of sepsis while sitting in his wheelchair for 34 hours in an emergency room as the hospital failed to provide him with medical care. The staff assumed that he was intoxicated or homeless rather than in need of medical care. When he was found, his body was entering the stage of rigor mortis (National Post, 2014; Sinclair Working Group, 2017, September 15).

Prejudice

Prejudice is a hostile attitude toward others simply because they belong to a group that is considered to have objectionable characteristics. Everyone has some biases and prejudices, but healthcare personnel need to acknowledge and examine their biases in preparation for safe, competent, compassionate, and ethical care for all patients and families. If they do not address their biases in a meaningful way, their ability to form trusting, healing relationships will be affected, and patients and families will be put at risk for receiving substandard care. Racism is a too common basis for prejudice (see Chapter 3 where racism is defined, described, and discussed). There is evidence that racism occurs in Canadian healthcare systems (see Box 4.4 for the 2020 Joyce Echaquan Case).

Discrimination

Discrimination is the negative differential treatment of others because they are members of a certain group or identified as being negatively different. Discrimination can include ignoring, derogatory name-calling, denying services, and threatening. Discrimination arises from a

---

BOX 4.4 **The Joyce Echaquan Case: Racism in Health Care (2020)**

Joyce Echaquan, a 37-year-old Atikamekw woman, mother of seven, from the Manawan reserve in Quebec was admitted to the Centre hospitalier de Lanaudière in Joliette, Quebec, on Saturday, September 26, 2020, due to stomach pains that may have been related to an existing heart condition. Her family believes that she may have reacted to the morphine she received once in the hospital as well. Joyce Echaquan died on Monday, September 28. Her final moments were captured in a video she took on her phone that revealed her to be in great distress, crying out, and asking for help as hospital staff insulted and sweared at her. This shocking revelation led to a Quebec coroner investigation and an administrative inquiry of her death and care. A nurse and orderly were fired. It sparked national protests and a call for addressing racism in our country.

For nurses, this is a highly disturbing incident, given that the Canadian Nurses Association's (CNA)

Code of Ethics stipulates that nurses are to uphold the dignity of all persons in their care and, in upholding justice, "do not discriminate on the basis of a person's race, ethnicity, culture, political and spiritual beliefs, social or marital status, gender, gender identity, gender expression, sexual orientation, age, health status, place of origin, lifestyle, mental or physical ability, socio-economic status, or any other attribute" (CNA, 2017, p. 15). A further responsibility is to promote healthcare environments as moral communities.

Sources: Canadian Broadcasting Corporation. (2020, September 29). Investigations launched after Atikamekw woman records Quebec hospital staff uttering slurs before her death (By B. Shingler). *CBC News.* https://www.cbc.ca/news/canada/montreal/quebec-atikamekw-joliette-1.5743449

Lowrie, M., & Malone, K. (2020, October 4). Joyce Echaquan's death highlights systemic racism in health care, experts say. *CTV News.* https://www._ctvnews.ca/health/joyce-echaquan-s-death-highlights-systemic-racism-in-health-care-experts-say-1.5132146

---

lack of understanding and appreciation of differences among people, but it can be overcome.

Nurses, too, can experience subtle discrimination from patients and families. Patients may express a desire to have a nurse "more like them" assigned to their care. Alberta Pasco's (2004) study of the experience of Canadians who are Filipino in hospital care found that her participants initially desired nurses who were "one of us" (*hindi ibang tao*). However, nurses who were not of Filipino descent became "one of us" as the patient came to know the nurse as a caring person who was kind, respectful, and trustworthy.

KEY CONCEPT

Discrimination is negative differential treatment of others because they are members of a certain group or identified as being negatively different.

Stigma

Stigma is negative, discriminatory, and rejecting attitudes and behaviour toward a characteristic or element exhibited by an individual or group. It can occur at three levels: self, public, and structural (MHCC, 2013a). The stigma of mental disorders is evident across history (see Chapter 1) and still exists as a significant and problematic issue. Self-stigma occurs when a person with a mental health disorder internalizes the negative views of others and feels ashamed about his condition.

This not only seriously diminishes their sense of self-worth but can prevent them from seeking help. Public stigma is influenced by cultural misbeliefs about those with a mental disorder: they will never recover; they are dangerous, unpredictable, and violent; they should not be around other people; they are flawed as human beings. Such stigma is oppressive and alienating. Stigma can act as a barrier in all aspects of life: housing, education, employment, and health care. The stigma of mental disorders can affect families of persons with mental disorders, as well. Their status in their community can be affected; they may be assigned blame for the presence of the disorder in a family member. Stigma can affect health professionals who choose to practice in psychiatric and mental health settings (Harrison & Hauck, 2017). Such a career choice can be silently queried: Lack of "real" skills? Personal psychological problems? It is evident in its effects upon recruitment and retention to this clinical area. Stigma occurring at the institutional level is evident when persons with a mental disorder are denied their basic rights. Bias against mental disorders can also affect funding for health services and research.

KEY CONCEPT

Stigma is negative, discriminatory, and rejecting attitudes and behaviour toward a characteristic or element exhibited by an individual or group. It can occur at three levels: self, public, and structural.

Reducing Stigma and Discrimination

The Senate Canada's (2006) report, *Out of the Shadows at Last, 2006*, indicated that the stigma of mental disorders pervades all levels of Canadian society. In response, the *Opening Minds* program was initiated by the MHCC in 2009 with the goal of changing Canadian behaviour and attitude toward mental disorders and making the acknowledgment of having a mental health disorder and the seeking mental health care more socially acceptable (MHCC, 2009; 2013a). *Opening Minds* promotes contact-based education that involves individuals with a lived experience of a mental disorder sharing their experiences of the disorder and recovery. When possible, it builds on existing programs, sharing resources such as toolkits, and aims to replicate successful programs and best practices (MHCC, 2013a). Interventions to reduce the discrimination and stigma of mental disorders are being conducted within many countries and globally (Gronholm et al., 2017).

Triple Stigma in Corrections in Canada

In 2012, the *Mental Health Strategy for Corrections in Canada* pointed out the double stigmatization of having a mental disorder and being an offender (Correctional Services Canada, 2012). A triple stigmatization has been since identified in a Saskatchewan needs assessment of mental health services in corrections: having a mental disorder, being an offender, and being an Indigenous person by racial descent (Kent-Wilkinson et al., 2012a; 2012b).

Role of Nursing and Nursing Education

Every nursing student brings with them to their new profession the attitudes and beliefs of their family and culture. It can initially be a challenge to live fully up to the demand that "Nurses do not discriminate on the basis of a person's race, ethnicity, culture, political and spiritual beliefs, social or marital status, gender, gender identity, gender expression, sexual orientation, age, health status, place of origin, lifestyle, mental or physical ability, socio-economic status, or any other attribute" (CNA, 2017, p. 15). As a student gains clinical practice and experience in the role of a nurse, this challenge becomes more easily met.

This approach is advocated by the Canadian Association of Schools of Nursing (CASN) and the Canadian Federation of Mental Health Nurses (CFMHN) in their joint publication, *Entry-to-Practice Mental Health and Addiction Competencies for Undergraduate Nursing Education* (CASN & CFMHN, 2015) (see Chapter 6). As well, the CFMHN's 2016 position paper on *Mental Health and Addiction Curriculum in Undergraduate Nursing Education in Canada* (Kent-Wilkinson et al., 2016) advocates that the most effective response to increasing knowledge of mental health and disorder and decreasing the stigma of mental disorders is to ensure evidence-informed nursing education through a significant increase of psychiatric mental health theory and practice in undergraduate nursing curricula.

Although Canada has maintained a benign self-image as an inclusive society, racism and discrimination play an important role as causes of disorder and as barriers to seeking help and appropriate care (Kirmayer & Jarvis, 2019), "Lack of familiarity with the experiences of discrimination by minority groups limits clinicians' ability to understand patients' predicaments and deliver culturally responsive care pointing to the need for specific training in anti-racist approaches to care" (Kirmayer & Jarvis, 2019, p. 17).

Antiracism education involves integrating an analysis of history and systemic/institutional processes with personal and particular (often emotional) experiences. An effective, brief definition of racism that works very well as a visual aid and focal point for discussion is *Racism = Racial Prejudice + Power* (ACLRC, 2021). The head of the Canadian Association of Schools of Nursing (CASN) notes that "Tackling racism isn't a 'flash-in-the-pan kind of thing'" (Beaulne-Stuebing, 2021), which means that it takes a sustained effort with collaboration on every front. Important initiatives and research have taken place in some provinces. (See Box 4.5, Research for Best Practice—In Plain Sight: Addressing Racism and Discrimination Specific to Indigenous Peoples In Health Care.)

Cultural Competence and Cultural Safety

Cultural competency and cultural safety are critical components of undergraduate and postgraduate education of healthcare practitioners and provide a foundation for what will be a continuous learning process. Opportunities for students to share their own cultural backgrounds with each other and to interact with various cultural groups are strategies that support the development of competence (Repo et al., 2017).

Cultural Competence

Cultural competence is considered an entry-to-practice competence (CNA, 2018) that is evident in quality practice environments and improves health outcomes. For nurses, it is the application of respect, equity, and cultural sensitivity and the valuing of diversity to the knowledge, skills, and attitudes required to provide appropriate care in relation to cultural characteristics of their clients. It is both process and outcome oriented (Alexander, 2008). Obtaining cultural competence is an ongoing, lifelong process, not an end. Cultural competence has been the dominant approach to address

BOX 4.5 Research for Best Practice

IN PLAIN SIGHT: ADDRESSING RACISM AND DISCRIMINATION SPECIFIC TO INDIGENOUS PEOPLES IN HEALTH CARE

In Plain Sight: Addressing Indigenous-Specific Racism and Discrimination in B.C. Health Care. (November 2020). https://engage.gov.bc.ca/app/uploads/sites/613/2020/11/In-Plain-Sight-Full-Report.pdf

A summary of the report is at: https://engage.gov.bc.ca/app/uploads/sites/613/2020/11/In-Plain-Sight-Summary-Report.pdf

Question: Are Indigenous Peoples experiencing racism and discrimination in British Columbia's healthcare system?

Method: Launched in June 2020, an independent review into discrimination specific to Indigenous Peoples in British Columbia's healthcare system analyzed health data (e.g., utilization of services and outcomes of approximately 185,000 patients who are First Nations and Métis) and heard from (e.g., through surveys) patients who are Indigenous Peoples, their families, healthcare workers, and third-party witnesses (numbering nearly 9,000 individuals).

Findings: Evidence of pervasive interpersonal and systemic racism, adversely affecting patient and family experiences, as well as long-term health outcomes for Indigenous Peoples, were found. Over two thirds of respondents to the Indigenous Peoples Survey noted that they had experienced discrimination based on their ancestry, with only 16% reporting "never" experiencing it. More than one third of healthcare workers who are non-Indigenous Peoples reported witnessing interpersonal racism or discrimination against Indigenous patients or their visitors. Healthcare data analysis revealed that racism limited access to medical treatment and negatively affected the health and wellness of Indigenous Peoples who experienced it. Women who are Indigenous Peoples were disproportionately impacted.

Implications: There is a serious systemic problem in BC health services that requires remedy. The 24 recommendations based on the review include that the BC government lead/co-ordinate apologies for racism specific to Indigenous Peoples in its healthcare system; develop cultural safety and humility training for health care workers, and implement a comprehensive system-wide approach (policies and practices) to address the issues that aligns with the *UN Declaration on the Rights of Indigenous Peoples* and the *Declaration on the Rights of Indigenous Peoples Act* of BC.

Source: Government of British Columbia. (2020, November 30). *Review recommends steps to solve widespread racism in B.C. health care.* https://engage.gov.bc.ca/addressingracism/review-recommends-steps-to-solve-widespread-racism-in-b-c-health-care/

Note: The *In Plain Sight* report can be found at: https://engage.gov.bc.ca/app/uploads/sites/613/2020/11/In-Plain-Sight-Full-Report.pdf

A summary of the report is at: https://engage.gov.bc.ca/app/uploads/sites/613/2020/11/In-Plain-Sight-Summary-Report.pdf

diversity in Canada, the United States, and other countries. This approach focuses on healthcare professionals understanding the cultural background of their clients and, ideally, begins with a process of self-reflection (Kirmayer & Jarvis, 2019). Cultural competence involves an appreciation of diversity and its influence on relationships and situations (CNA, 2018). Practitioners need to recognize the attributes of their own culture and the way in which it shapes their own beliefs and behaviours. Then, there is need to acknowledge their knowledge deficits regarding the cultures of others. The CNA (2018) suggests that this part of cultural competence involves understanding cultural diversity through an "atmosphere of respect" (p. 1). As awareness, knowledge, and skill evolve, cultural competence develops (Purnell, 2016).

Exposure and face-to-face encounters, along with keeping an open mind to the individuals' experiences, can contribute to this development. For instance, nurses can become culturally competent when working in communities of Indigenous Peoples by being open to learning about their culture, beliefs, and practices. They may participate in cultural ceremonies when invited, learn a few words of the language, gain knowledge of traditional events, and attend conferences or classes that focus on Indigenous culture.

Cultural competence is particularly important to understanding the way in which culture is influencing perceptions of health needs and ensuring this understanding influences nursing practice. Cultural competence also involves collaborative approach with other specialists (CNA, 2014). Nurses not only act as advocates but also strive to promote accessible and culturally friendly services in the areas of health promotion and education (MHCC, 2016). Being culturally competent is a strategy in addressing racial and ethnic health disparities in health care by ensuring services are culturally safe and meeting patient needs (McCalman et al., 2017).

KEY CONCEPT

Cultural competence is "a set of consistent behaviors, attitudes, and policies that enable a system, agency, or individual to work within a cross-cultural context or situation" (Watt et al., 2016).

Cultural Humility

"Cultural humility," first outlined in 1998, incorporates:

- Lifelong commitment to critical self-reflection
- Redressing power imbalances
- Institutional accountability (Tervalon & Murray-Garcia, 1998)

Rather than a focus on increasing "competence" and expert knowledge of the cultural "other," MacKenzie and Hatala (2019) note that cultural humility focuses the attention toward healthcare providers in clinical settings and critical self-reflection by "stepping back to understand one's own systematic biases, values, and cultural assumptions, and the politics and institutionalized power dynamics latent within biomedical context" (pp. e126–e127).

KEY CONCEPT

Cultural humility is a lifelong commitment to self-evaluation and self-critique to redress power imbalances and to develop and maintain mutually respectful dynamic partnerships based on mutual trust (CNA, 2018).

Cultural Safety

Cultural safety, a concept developed originally by Maori nurses in New Zealand (Papps & Ramsden, 1996), "focuses on ways in which lack of knowledge of history and social context, along with power disparities, racism and discrimination, makes mainstream institutions unsafe for minorities" (Kirmayer & Jarvis, 2019, p. 15). It is both a process and an outcome with the goal of greater equity and the promotion of integrity, social justice, and respect (McGough et al., 2018).

KEY CONCEPT

Cultural safety comes from recognizing colonial histories and systems of racialized identity and discrimination, domination, marginalization, and exclusion. Cultural safety works to redistribute power to achieve equity (Kirmayer, 2019; Kirmayer & Jarvis, 2019).

Role of Nursing, Healthcare Professionals, and Education

Healthcare practitioners, the institution, and the patient are all key players in the creation and maintenance of cultural safety as a reciprocal process. Each accommodates the other's values and culture within the clinical setting (Douglas, 2020). Many healthcare organizations are insufficiently equipped to provide cultural safety, given that it requires engagement with communities, including Indigenous Peoples, immigrants, and refugees. Such engagement allows a space to be created in which patients and families feel safe to be open and express their concerns.

Strategies a healthcare organization can implement include the provision of information and training sessions on cultural safety, individual practitioners (or a team) choosing to learn more about a specific cultural group, and the use of cultural brokers, persons knowledgeable about a culture, its language, and the healthcare organization, who offer guidance and assistance in patient care situations. Cultural safety, competence, and antiracism training needs to be systematically incorporated into professional education and corresponding accreditation standards developed and applied to the governance of healthcare institutions and delivery of services (Kirmayer & Jarvis, 2019).

The CASN (2020) *Framework of Strategies for Nursing Education to Respond to the Calls to Action of Canada's Truth and Reconciliation Commission* paper was created in partnership with the Canadian Indigenous Nurses Association and with cross-country input. It identifies two calls to action that schools of nursing can make a reality: increasing the number of professionals who are Indigenous Peoples working in health care and creating a requirement for nursing and medical students to take a course on health issues of Indigenous Peoples, including the legacy of residential schools, treaties, rights and teachings and practices of Indigenous Peoples. The CASN 2020 document states that many universities and colleges in Canada have already begun to respond to the TRC's calls to action and that nursing schools are "well-positioned" to address and accomplish these goals (Beaulne-Stuebing, 2021). (See Box 4.6, TRCC 2015 Calls to Action.)

Strengthening diversity and inclusion is fundamental to building a consciously more inclusive society where everyone is able to participate fully. Racism and all forms of discrimination are some of the main causes of social and economic barriers for many Canadians. While progress has been made, much more remains to be done (Government of Canada, 2020a).

Socioeconomic Context of Mental Health Care

Socioeconomic circumstances influence our health status. Factors such as income and social status, social support networks, education, employment and working

BOX 4.6 Truth and Reconciliation Commission of Canada (2015b) TRCC: Calls to Action

23. We call upon all levels of government to:
    i. Increase the number of Aboriginal professionals working in the healthcare field.
    ii. Ensure the retention of Aboriginal healthcare providers in Aboriginal communities.
    iii. Provide cultural competency training for all healthcare professionals.
24. We call upon medical and nursing schools in Canada to require all students to take a course dealing with Aboriginal health issues, including the history and legacy of residential schools, the United Nations Declaration on the Rights of Indigenous Peoples, Treaties and Aboriginal rights, and Indigenous teachings and practices.
    i. This will require skills-based training in intercultural competency, conflict resolution, human rights, and antiracism (TRCC, 2015a).

Source: Truth and Reconciliation Commission of Canada. (2015b). *Truth and Reconciliation Commission of Canada: Calls to action.* http://trc.ca/assets/pdf/Calls_to_Action_English2.pdf

conditions, physical environment, and available health services affect one's wellbeing. People living in poverty are no longer a problem of developing regions only; it is on the rise in developed countries (UN Development Programme [UNDP], 2020). Although Canada has consistently ranked in the top five on the UN Human Development Index, it has slipped down in recent years (UNDP, 2020). The wellbeing of Indigenous Peoples in Canada plays a role in this. In 2014, the report of the UN Special Rapporteur on the rights of Indigenous Peoples regarding Canada noted that Canada has yet to close the wellbeing gap between Indigenous Peoples and other Canadians. Urgent action, he stated, was needed to address a housing crisis and to provide sufficient funding for education, health care, and child welfare; better coordination in the delivery of services was required (Anaya, 2014).

Disadvantageous socioeconomic circumstances and social exclusion can increase the likelihood of adopting unhealthy or risky behaviours and create feelings of hopelessness and helplessness among those affected and vulnerable (Statistics Canada, 2013, para 12). Vulnerable groups are groups in society who are "systematically disadvantaged in a way that leads to a risk of emotional or physical harm; in health care, harms are related to diminished health and wellbeing" (CNA, 2017, p. 27).

Social Determinants of Health

Social determinants of health are defined as "the conditions in which peoples are born, grow, live, work, and age, including the health system. These circumstances are shaped by the distribution of money, power and resources at global, national or local levels, which are themselves influenced by policy choices" (World Health Organization [WHO], 2017, para 1). Healthy child development is among the most important determinants of health. Preconception to the age of 6 is a critical time for a child's brain development, as positive stimulation during these years influences learning, behaviour, and health into adulthood, as well as a child's sense of identity (Douglas, 2020).

COVID-19 Pandemic

The social determinants of health are front and center as the public health community works to address the coronavirus, COVID-19. The COVID-19 pandemic has exposed some of the gaps in the social safety net, exacerbating key social determinants of health that make it hard for people to be healthy. There are clear delineations between different social groups and how they are faring in the new normal that the coronavirus has dawned. The issue of social distancing, coupled with questions about access to care and other health resources, has specifically highlighted disparities for individuals who are experiencing homeless or housing insecurities, who experience limited food security, and who live in rural regions.

Poverty

Poverty is associated with the undermining of a range of key human attributes, including health. People experiencing poverty are exposed to greater personal and environmental health risks, are less well-nourished, have less information, and are less able to access health care; thusly, they experience a higher risk of illness and disability. Conversely, illness can reduce household savings, lower learning ability, reduce productivity, and lead to a diminished quality of life, thereby perpetuating or even increasing poverty (WHO, 2017). Those living with the experience of extreme poverty around the world have the worst health. The evidence shows that within countries in general, the lower an individual's socioeconomic position, the worse their health (WHO, 2017

Poverty creates hopelessness (endPoverty.org, 2020). In the day-to-day lives of people experiencing extreme poverty, it becomes a network of disadvantages. The result is generation after generation of people who lack access to education, health care, adequate housing, proper sanitation, and good nutrition. They are the most vulnerable to disasters, armed conflict, and systems of political and economic oppression, and they lack basic resources and control to improve their circumstances. These conditions often carry with them dysfunctional family and societal relationships, paralyzingly low self-esteem, mental health disorders, and spiritual darkness.

KEY CONCEPT

Poverty is the lack of income and access to essential goods and services, housing, and employment required to meet the necessities of life relative to one's society.

Poverty and Mental Health

Poverty and mental health (as well as overall health) are linked such that "the lower an individual's socio-economic status, the worse their health" and *vice versa* (WHO, 2017). Understanding this relationship is key to addressing poverty, promoting mental health, and supporting the recovery of persons with mental disorders. For persons who are experiencing poverty and predisposed to developing a mental disorder, a loss of income, employment, and housing can increase the chance of developing a mental disorder or, if recovered, of relapsing. Further, developing mental disorders can seriously interrupt a person's education or career path, leading to fewer and less secure employment opportunities and, correspondingly, a lower income. As a result, a drift into poverty can occur, particularly for those with recurrent mental disorders.

Investment in Mental Health

The economic burden of mental health and addiction in Canada is estimated at $51 billion per year. This cost to the Canadian economy includes healthcare dollars spent, lost productivity, and reductions in health-related quality of life (MHCC, 2013b; Mood Disorders Society of Canada [MDSC], 2014). If one in five Canadians lives with a mental health or an addiction problem, then 20% of the healthcare budget is needed to address this reality. Nurses must be prepared to provide preventative mental health education to reduce the increasing costs associated with mental health

conditions as well as to promote quality of life (Kent-Wilkinson et al., 2016).

Strong evidence for the value of mental health interventions comes from work with children and youth in such areas as conduct disorders, depression, parenting, and suicide awareness and prevention (Roberts & Grimes, 2011). Nurses prepared in mental health assessment and care of children and youth can thus serve as an investment in the mental health (Kent-Wilkinson et al., 2016; see Chapters 29 and 30). Work is being done to examine what is needed for the future. *Life and Economic Impact of Major Mental Illnesses in Canada* is an examination of the economic impact of major mental disorders in Canada, beginning in 2011 and annually over the next three decades (Smetanin et al., 2011). In 2011, the direct cost of mental disorders was $42.3 billion and, indirectly, $6.3 billion. By 2041, it is predicted that costs will be magnified due to an increase in the number of those with mental disorders (due to population growth and aging). In 2016, *Mental Health Now! Advancing the Mental Health of Canadians: The Federal Role*, prepared by the Canadian Alliance on Mental Illness and Mental Health (CAMIMH, 2016), identified five recommendations to improve access to mental health care for Canadians: increase federal funding for access to mental health services to 25% of the total cost; create a Mental Health Innovation Fund to support mental healthcare innovation; measure and monitor mental health by creating pan-Canadian indicators; establish an expert advisory panel; and invest in social infrastructure. Such work, along with Canada's mental health strategy, is contributing to the improvement of mental health care.

Socioeconomic Influences on the Mental Health of Indigenous Peoples

Health of Indigenous Peoples in Canada is impacted by 13 determinants of health, but the social support determinant is one that affects both the individual and the community. The wellbeing of individuals can be shaped by relationships, and the caring and respect involved (Douglas, 2020). Relationships assist in safeguarding against both physical and mental disorders, by providing "feelings of belonging and being cared for, loved, respected and valued" (NCCAH, 2012, p. 38). Many traditional Indigenous societies have strong family and community supports, which can offer a sense of social inclusion and, therefore, improve recovery rates when illness does occur (Douglas, 2020). Indigenous heritage and geographic location are also factors affecting this social support determinant, as there are many access inequities within this population that influence individual and community health. (See Box 4.7, Determinants of Health in Analyzing Indigenous Health in Canada.)

> **BOX** 4.7 **Determinants of Health in Analyzing Indigenous Health in Canada**
>
> 1. Income and Social Status
> 2. Social Support Systems
> 3. Education and Literacy
> 4. Employment and Working Conditions
> 5. Social Environment
> 6. Personal Health Practices
> 7. Healthy Child Development
> 8. Biology and Genetic Endowment
> 9. Health Services
> 10. Gender
> 11. Culture
> 12. Physical Environment
> 13. Ecosystem Health
>
> Douglas, V. (2020). *Introduction to Indigenous health and health care in Canada: Bridging health and healing* (2nd ed.). Springer Publishing Company.

Poverty and Mental Health of Indigenous Peoples

As poverty rates are high among populations of Indigenous Peoples, poor mental health is also common. Approximately "60% of First Nation children on reserves live in poverty" (Kirkup, 2016), while 40% of Indigenous children living off reserves do so (NCCAH, 2010). Children who are born into poverty are at higher risk for negative outcomes of low birth weight, learning disabilities, mental health problems, burns and injuries, and other health conditions such as asthma, obesity, and iron deficiency anemia (Conroy et al., 2010). Poverty is linked, as well, to violence (Douglas, 2020). Children who are exposed to violence, especially from loved ones, and experience attachment issues are more likely to participate in acts of violence as adults, creating a cycle of violence (Macinnes et al., 2016). Children learn to internalize their environments, assume them as normal, and pass such experiences along to their own children (Douglas, 2020).

Disparities in Mental Health Outcomes

There are substantial differences among communities of Indigenous peoples, including in relation to mental health issues. Suicide rates reported within populations of Indigenous peoples, however, are in general double that of the rest of the Canadian population (Crawford, 2016). Suicide rates are five to seven times higher for First Nations youth as for non-Indigenous youth; Inuit youth have rates among the highest in the world, at 11 times the national average (Government of Canada, 2020c). Alcohol-related deaths of Indigenous peoples are nearly twice that of non-Indigenous Canadians (43.7 vs. 23.6 per 100,000), with Indigenous youth at two to six times at greater risk for alcohol-related problems than their non-Indigenous counterparts (Russell et al., 2016). Fetal alcohol spectrum disorders (FASD) in Indigenous women is found to be about 16 times higher than in the general public (Popova et al., 2017).

Factors that create **health disparity** between populations of Indigenous Peoples and the general population of non-Indigenous Canadians include reduced and impeded access to health services. The lack of clarity on whom delivers health services and who is responsible financially can be a barrier to accessing treatment (NCCAH, 2011a, 2011b, 2011c; Richmond & Cook, 2016). This barrier has led to limited health services, resulting for some in death (Douglas, 2020). Significant gaps still exist in primary care on reserves, despite significant financial investment in millions of dollars. Such gaps were made highly visible in the case of a boy who is an Indigenous person that resulted in *Jordan's Principle*. Jordan River Anderson was a child with complex medical needs, who was hospitalized and unable to access home care due to a dispute between the federal and Manitoba governments over allocation of home care costs. Jordan died at age 5, in hospital. Jordan's principle, passed in December 2007, calls on the government of first contact to pay for services and seek reimbursement later so no child's health and wellbeing is tangled in red tape (Blackstock, 2012). The Canadian Human Rights Tribunal in 2016 ordered the federal government to implement the full scope of Jordan's Principle (Galloway, 2017).

Other factors of health disparity include the negative impacts on healthy child development due to intergenerational trauma and the negative impacts of colonization on Indigenous cultural identity (Aguiar & Halseth, 2015; Douglas, 2020). The diverse nature of factors that create health disparities indicates that addressing health inequities cannot be achieved by the health sector alone but needs a collaborative, multisectoral approach (Reading & Halseth, 2013).

Role of Nursing and Healthcare Professionals

Nurses are responsible to maintain "an awareness of major health concerns, such as *poverty*, inadequate shelters, food insecurity and violence, while working for *social justice* (individually and with others) and advocating for laws, policies and procedures that bring about equity" (CNA, 2017, p. 19). Social justice is defined as "the fair distribution of society's benefits and responsibilities and their consequences. Social justice focuses on the relative position of one social group in relations to others in society as well as on the root causes of disparities and what can be done to eliminate them" (CNA, 2017, p. 26).

Mental disorders put a person at greater risk to experience poverty and homelessness, which, in turn, places serious constraints on regaining and maintaining health. While addressing poverty and homelessness is outside the realm of healthcare systems, nurses should be aware of their impact on mental health and be able to identify relevant policy changes that could be enacted in both public and private spheres (MHCC, 2012).

Geographic Context of Mental Health Care

Although comprehensiveness, universality, portability, and accessibility are key components of the *Canada Health Act* getting mental health services to rural and remote communities continues to be a challenge. Most mental health services are in urban areas, with access for people in the far North being very different from that of people living in the more highly populated areas of Canada. All age groups in rural and remote areas have limited access to health care, but the lack of resources is particularly problematic for children and older adults, who have specialized needs.

"Rural" is defined by Statistics Canada (2017b) as an area with a population of under 1,000 people and a population density of less than 400 inhabitants per square kilometre. The rural population of Canada has been declining since 1851, when 9 in 10 Canadians lived in rural areas (Statistics Canada, 2017a). Today, more than

80% of Canadians live in metropolitan areas, with over one in three Canadians living in Toronto, Montréal, or Vancouver (Statistics Canada, 2020a).

"Remoteness" involves a community's proximity to other places and services, such as health services, with proximity being measured by such metrics as travel time and travel cost (Alasia et al., 2017). Figure 4.2 is a map of the geographic distribution of accessibility to health services in Canada. Many remote communities are home to Indigenous Peoples. Healthcare services in remote communities have a strong focus on prevention; utilize smaller, integrated teams with a broad scope of practice; and look to visiting services for specialized treatment (Wakerman et al., 2017). Being the second largest country in the world with a diverse population of over 37 million requires ongoing dedication and innovation in the provision of health care.

Availability, accessibility, acceptability, and quality of health services are key elements of the right to health (United Nations Development Programme, 2020) (see Fig. 4.3). These elements are useful in considering health services in rural and remote communities in Canada.

Availability

Nurses and nurse practitioners (NPs) play key roles in making health care available in rural and remote areas or in Canada's north, where the nursing station is often the first point of contact and nurses may be the only

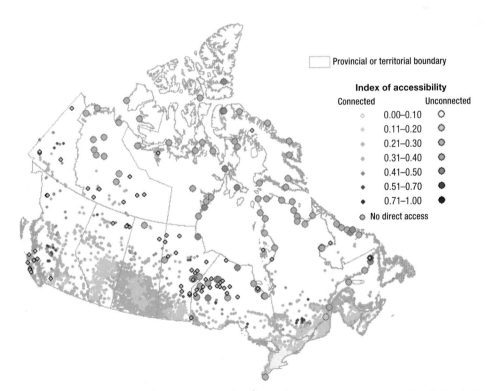

Figure 4.2 Geographic distribution of accessibility measures to health services. (Reprinted from Statistics Canada. (2017). *Measuring remoteness and accessibility: A set of indices for Canadian communities* (p. 31). Statistics Canada Catalogue no. 18-001-x. Statistics Canada. Accessed September 25, 2017.)

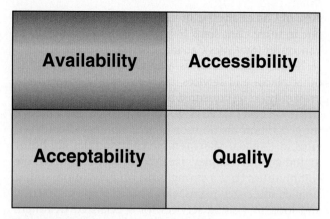

Availability	Accessibility
Acceptability	Quality

Figure 4.3 Elements of the right to health.

healthcare professionals and thus the primary health care providers. Nurses may be required to work outside their scope of practice in certain circumstances in order to provide essential services and need to have supportive mechanisms in place to authorize them to do so (Auditor General of Canada, 2015). They may act as advocates, collaborators, or mediators in encouraging the development of public policies and resources for their region.

For persons with mental health problems or mental disorders, including addiction, a shared care approach to services may be used in which specialists support the integration of mental health services in primary care (Kates et al., 2011). The Canadian Collaborative Mental Health Initiative provides a "Rural and Isolated Toolkit" to support such collaboration (Haggarty et al., 2010).

Accessibility

"Despite universal healthcare coverage and community-based clinics in many regions of Canada, significant structural barriers exist in access to healthcare" (Kirmayer & Jarvis, 2019, p. 13). Transportation is a major barrier to the receipt of health services in rural areas. Costs of travel and accommodation for patients and families can be high, in dollars and energy. Services should be delivered in communities where possible, but the small population of some rural communities can be a deterrent. As well, specialized services are in large urban centres. Mobile service delivery and specialist circuits are options used to address this issue.

Persons with severe and persistent mental disorders may be able to remain within their community if such approach is used, providing they have sufficient social support and continuing access to services. Local health care situations are shaped by their own unique social and structural factors, which need to be addressed if availability is to be optimized (Fitzpatrick et al., 2017). Despite shared care approaches, access to care can be a serious problem. A Canadian needs assessment survey of rural/remote physicians regarding access to child and adolescent mental health services revealed that there are issues with long waiting lists, a lack of child/adolescent psychiatrists,

and the need of other disciplinary services (e.g., paediatricians, psychologists, and social workers). System issues, such as a need for a more systematized, transparent referral process, were also noted (Zayed et al., 2016).

Telehealth (e.g., telepsychiatry) is an effective tool that can reduce wait times and travel time and costs. Telehealth is the use of electronic information and communication technologies to support healthcare services over distance. It ranges from the retrieval of laboratory results or other health records posted on a network to the direct assessment and treatment of an individual by primary care providers to consultation with specialists through videoconferencing. In fact, in specialized care through telehealth, mental health is a top area of consultation (Caxaj, 2016).

Telehealth emerged as an essential tool in combating the coronavirus outbreak regardless of rurality. Telehealth can help connect people to a qualified provider; however, the internet is necessary to connect to telehealth. When the COVID-19 pandemic took hold in early 2020, connecting virtually became a necessity in all aspects of life including health care. This change appears likely to be sustained with benefits in the promotion and development of better virtual resources that will help overcome the geographic challenges.

Acceptability

In rural and remote areas, there may be a lack of information regarding mental health and psychiatric care. Help-seeking behaviours may be affected by an expectation that one should be self-reliant and independent. As well, social and cultural aspects of a community can increase risk for mental health stigma and diminish anonymity. First Nations Peoples may be unable to find health services that they find culturally appropriate (Caxaj, 2016). The high staff turnover that tends to exist in health services in remote communities can impede the ability of practitioners to engage in the community and establish trusting relationships, essential to working within rural and remote communities (Davy et al., 2016).

While preparation for nursing in remote areas usually involves mandatory advanced life support training, adequate preparation for mental health care seems essential, as well. NPs, for instance, should be skilled in this area (Creamer & Austin, 2017). A survey study of NPs across Canada revealed that the majority of NPs would like more theoretical and/or clinical preparation in mental health. They rated their existing mental health educational preparation at a mean of 2.6 on a scale of 1 to 5, with "5" equaling "very well prepared" (Creamer et al., 2014).

Quality

Quality health care involves effectiveness, efficiency, equity, safety, timeliness, and patient-centredness (Institute of Medicine, 2001). From a clinical care perspective, quality means the treatment and care provided will be evidence-based and shaped by best practices. While individuals and their families may not be able to critically evaluate clinical care, they will have their own perceptions of the quality of care based on their subjective experiences (Hanefeld et al., 2017). Responsiveness (i.e., access to treatment, confidentiality, privacy, being treated with respect and cultural appropriateness) is a significant component of perceptions of quality care, as is the assurance that one's care will be culturally responsive (Hanefeld). In rural and remote communities, there can be high annual turnover of healthcare practitioners (Wakeman et al., 2019) that may, at times, create continuity of care issues, particularly challenging when ongoing mental health care is required.

Geographic location remains a significant factor in the challenge to provide mental health services to all Canadians who require them. Technologic innovations can make a positive difference, but attention must continue to be paid to the social and cultural aspects of mental health care and to the sufficient preparation of health professionals in mental health care.

Summary of Key Points

- *Culture* is defined as a way of life that manifests the learned beliefs, values, and accepted behaviours that are transmitted socially within a specific group.
- Diversity is both a source of richness and a distinct challenge to civil society.
- Religious beliefs are closely intertwined with beliefs about health and mental disorder.
- There are many cultures of the Indigenous Peoples in Canada, with unique heritages, languages, cultural practices, and spiritual beliefs. Treatment interventions need to honour the historical context and history of Aboriginal or Indigenous Peoples. Cultural identity, community involvement, and empowerment can be important to health outcomes. Stigmatization occurs as a result of prejudice, discrimination, and stereotyping. Cultural groups and people with mental illness are often stigmatized.

- Cultural competence is an entry-to-practice nursing competence.
- Cultural competence is a dominant approach to address diversity in many countries.
- Mental health services should be integrated as completely as possible into the helping systems currently accepted by the culture.
- All of the common social determinants of health are related to cultural issues. Culture may also be a determinant of mental health in its own right.
- Racism and discrimination play an important role as causes of disorders and as barriers to access health care services.
- Access to mental health treatment is particularly limited for those living in rural, remote, and northern areas or for those living in poverty.

Thinking Challenge

A nurse is caring for a client who is a person of Indigenous origin. Cultural roots of all populations should be respected.

a. What are some cultural influences of Indigenous Peoples that affect mental health care?

b. How does the nurse demonstrate cultural competence, cultural safety, and cultural humility with this client's population?

Visit the**Point** to view suggested responses.
Go to **thePoint.lww.com/activate** and use the activation code found in the front of this text to unlock answers to the "Thinking Challenges" and other online resources.

Web Links

https://www.camimh.ca *The Canadian Alliance on Mental Illness and Mental Health (CAMIMH)* is Canada's largest mental health advocacy group. It is an alliance of mental health organizations composed of healthcare providers as well as people with mental disorders and their families.

http://cmha.ca *The Canadian Mental Health Association (CMHA)* is a national voluntary organization that promotes mental health and serves consumers and others through education, public awareness, research, advocacy, and direct services.

disabilityrightsintl.org / *Disability Rights International (DRI)* is an advocacy organization dedicated to the recognition and enforcement of rights of people with mental disabilities.

https://www.mentalhealthcommission.ca/English *The Mental Health Commission of Canada (MHCC)* is a nonprofit organization created to focus national attention on mental health issues, to work to improve the mental health of Canadians, and to reduce the stigma associated with these disorders.

www.shared-care.ca This website of the Canadian Collaborative Mental Health Initiative has toolkits that are useful to healthcare professionals.

https://www150.statcan.gc.ca/n1/daily-quotidien/130508/dq130508b-eng.htm?HPA The 2011 National Household Survey: Immigration, place of birth, citizenship, ethnic origin, visible minorities, language, and religion in Canada can be found at this site.

https://wfmh.global *The World Federation for Mental Health (WFMH) is the only international, multidisciplinary, grassroots advocacy and education mental health organization.*

https://www.who.int/about The World Health Organization (WHO) is the United Nations agency for health. The objective set out in its constitution is the attainment, by all peoples, of the highest possible level of health.

References

Aguiar, W., & Halseth, R. (2015, April 29). *Aboriginal peoples and historic trauma: The processes of intergenerational transmission.* National Collaborating Centre for Aboriginal Health. http://www.nccah-ccnsa.ca/Publications/Lists/Publications/Attachments/142/2015-04-28-Aguiar-Halseth-RPT-IntergenTraumaHistory-EN-Web.pdf

Alasia, A., Bédard, F., Bélanger, J., Guimond, G., & Penney, C. (2017). *Measuring remoteness and accessibility: A set of indices for Canadian communities.* Statistics Canada Catalogue no. 18-001-x. https://www150.statcan.gc.ca/n1/pub/18-001-x/18-001-x2017002-eng.pdf

Alberta Civil Liberties Research Centre. (2021). *Racism.* http://www.aclrc.com/racism

Alexander, G. R. (2008). Cultural competence models in nursing. *Critical Care Nursing Clinics of North America, 20*(4), 415–421. https://doi.org/10.1016/j.ccell.2008.08.012

Ameling, A., & Povilonis, M. (2001). Spirituality, meaning, mental health and nursing. *Journal of Psychosocial Nursing and Mental Health Services, 39*(4), 14–20. https://pubmed.ncbi.nlm.nih.gov/11324173/

American Psychiatric Association. (2013a). *Cultural concepts in DSM-5.* file:///C:/Users/aek587/Downloads/APA_DSM_Cultural-Concepts-in-DSM-5%20(7).pdf

American Psychiatric Association. (2013b). *Diagnostic and statistical manual of mental disorders* (DSM-5, 5th ed.). https://www.psychiatry.org/psychiatrists/practice/dsm

Anaya, J. (2014, July 4). *Report of the special rapporteur on the rights of Indigenous peoples.* Human Rights Council, United Nations, General Assembly. http://unsr.jamesanaya.org/docs/countries/2014-report-canada-a-hrc-27-52-add-2-en.pdf

Auditor General of Canada. (2015, Spring). *Report 4: Access to health services for remote First Nations communities.* http://www.oag-bvg.gc.ca/internet/English/parl_oag_201504_04_e_40350.html#hd3a

Beaulne-Stuebing, L. (2021, January 15). *Canada's nursing programs address racial prejudice in the profession.* University Affairs. https://www.universityaffairs.ca/news/news-article/canadas-nursing-programs-address-racial-prejudice-in-the-profession/

Blackstock, C. (2012, August). Jordan's Principle: Canada's broken promise to First Nations children? *Paediatrics Child Health, 17*(7), 368–370. https://www.ncbi.nlm.nih.gov/pmc/articles/PMC3448536/

Boksa, P., Jooper, R., & Kirmayer, L. J. (2015). Mental wellness in Canada's Aboriginal communities: Striving toward reconciliation. *Journal of Psychiatry and Neuroscience, 40*(6), 363–365. https://doi.org/10.1503/jpn.150309

Brascoupé, S., & Waters, C. (2009). Cultural safety: Exploring the applicability of the concept of cultural safety to Aboriginal health and community wellness. *Journal of Aboriginal Health, 5*(2), 6–41. https://journals.uvic.ca/index.php/ijih/article/view/12332

Browne, S. M., & Baker, C. N. (2016). Measuring trauma-informed care: The attitudes related to trauma-informed care (ARTIC) Scale. *Trauma Psychology News, 12*(1). http://traumapsychnews.com/2016/03/measuring-trauma-informed-care-the-attitudes-related-to-trauma-informed-care-artic-scale/

Caldwell, A. (2019). Two spirt Indigenous offenders in the Correctional Service of Canada: Cultural reclamation and need for a healing approach to policies and programs. Major paper submitted in partial fulfillment of the requirement for the Masters of Arts (Criminal Justice) in the School of Criminology and Criminal Justice, University of the Fraser Valley. https://themicahmission.org/wp-content/uploads/2020/08/Caldwell_Andrew-2019-TwoSpiritIndigenousOffendersCanada.pdf

Canada Association of Schools of Nursing. (2020). *CASN framework of strategies for nursing education to respond to the calls to action of Canada's Truth and Reconciliation Commission.* https://www.casn.ca/wp-content/uploads/2020/11/EN-TRC-RESPONSE-STRATEGIES-FOR-NURSING-EDUCATIONTRC-Discussion-Paper-Revised-Final.pdf

Canadian Alliance on Mental Illness and Mental Health. (2016, September 6). *Mental health now! Advancing the mental health of Canadians: The federal role.* http://www.camimh.ca/wp-content/uploads/2016/09/CAMIMH_MHN_EN_Final_small.pdf

Canadian Association of Schools of Nursing & Canadian Federation of Mental Health Nurses. (2015). *Entry-to-practice mental health and addiction competencies for undergraduate nursing education.* https://www.casn.ca/2015/11/entry-to-practice-mental-health-and-addiction-competencies-for-undergraduate-nursing-education-in-canada/

Canadian Broadcasting Corporation. (2020, September 29). Investigations launched after Atikamekw woman records Quebec hospital staff uttering slurs before her death (By B. Shingler). *CBC News.* https://www.cbc.ca/news/canada/montreal/quebec-atikamekw-joliette-1.5743449

Canadian Museum of Immigration at Pier 21. (2017). *Canadian multiculturalism policy, 1971.* http://www.pier21.ca/research/immigration-history/canadian-multiculturalism-policy-1971

Canadian Nurses Association. (2014). *Aboriginal health nursing and Aboriginal health: Charting policy direction for nursing in Canada.* https://www.cna-aiic.ca/~/media/cna/page-content/pdf-en/aboriginal-health-nursing-and-aboriginal-health_charting-policy-direction-for-nursing-in-canada.pdf?la=en

Canadian Nurses Association. (2017). *Code of ethics for registered nurses.* https://www.cna-aiic.ca/~/media/cna/page-content/pdf-en/code-of-ethics-2017-edition-secure-interactive

Canadian Nurses Association. (2018). *Promoting cultural competence in nursing* [Position statement]. https://www.cna-aiic.ca/-/media/cna/page-content/pdf-en/position_statement_promoting_cultural_competence_in_nursing.pdf?la=en&hash=4B394DAE5C2138E7F6134D59E505DCB059754BA9

Caxaj, C. S. (2016). A review of mental health approaches for rural communities: Complexities and opportunities in the Canadian context. *Canadian Journal of Community Mental Health, 35*(1), 29–45. https://doi.org/10.7870/cjcmh-2015-023

Charron, M. C. (2019, March 6). *No perfect answer: Is it First Nations, Aboriginal or Indigenous?* National Public Relations, Indigenous Affairs. https://www.national.ca/en/perspectives/detail/no-perfect-answer-first-nations-aboriginal-indigenous/

Chaze, F., Thomson, M. S., George, U., & Guruge, S. (2015). Role of cultural beliefs, religion, and spirituality in mental health and/or service utilization among immigrants in Canada: A scoping review. *Canadian Journal of Community Mental Health, 34*(3), 87–101. https://doi.org/10.7870/cjcmh-2015-015

Chui, L., Ganesan, S., Clark, N., & Morrow, M. (2005). Spirituality and treatment choices by South and East Asian women with serious mental illness. *Transcultural Psychiatry, 42*(4), 630–656.

Conroy, K., Sandel, M., & Zuckerman, B. (2010). Poverty grown up: How childhood socioeconomic status impacts adult health. *Journal of Developmental and Behavioural Pediatrics: JDBP, 31*(2), 154–160. https://doi.org/10.1097/DBP.0b013e3181c21a1b

Corrado, R. R., & Cohen, I. M. (2010). Mental health profiles for a sample of British Columbia's Aboriginal survivors of the Canadian residential school system. In *Aboriginal Health Foundation's a compendium of Aboriginal healing foundation research* (pp. 5–6). Aboriginal Health Foundation. http://www.ahf.ca/downloads/research-compendium.pdf

Correctional Service Canada. (2012). *Mental health strategy for corrections in Canada: A Federal-Provincial-Territorial Partnership.* Correctional Service Canada, Government of Canada. http://www.csc-scc.gc.ca/health/092/MH-strategy-eng.pdf

Crawford, A. (2016). Suicide among Indigenous Peoples in Canada. *The Canadian Encyclopedia.* http://www.thecanadianencyclopedia.ca/en/article/suicide-among-indigenous-peoples-in-canada/

Creamer, A. M., & Austin, W. (2017). Canadian nurse practitioner core competencies identified: An opportunity to build mental health and illness skills and knowledge. *The Journal for Nurse Practitioners, 13*(5), e231–e236. https://doi.org/10.1016/j.nurpra.2016.12.017

Creamer, A. M., Mill, J., Austin, W., & O'Brien, B. (2014). Canadian nurse practitioners' therapeutic commitment to persons with mental illness. *Canadian Journal of Nursing Research, 46*(4), 13–32. http://cjnr.archive.mcgill.ca/article/viewFile/2464/2458

Davy, C., Hartfield, S., McArthur, A., Munn, Z., & Brown, A. (2016). Access to primary health care services for Indigenous peoples: A framework synthesis. *International Journal for Equity in Health, 15*, 163. https://doi.org/10.1186/s12939-016-0450-5

Douglas, V. (2020). *Introduction to Indigenous health and health care in Canada: Bridging health and healing* (2nd ed.). Springer Publishing Company.

Elias, B., Mignone, J., Hall, M., Hong, S. P., Hart, L., & Sareen, J. (2012). Trauma and suicide behaviour histories among a Canadian Indigenous population: An empirical exploration of the potential role of Canada's residential school system. *Social Science and Medicine, 74*(10), 1560–1569. http://doi.org/10.1016/j.socscimed.2012.01.026

endPoverty.org. (2020). *endPoverty is committed to help the most vulnerable in these unprecedented.* https://www.endpoverty.org/

Environs Institute for Survey Research (2020, December). *Survey of Canadians: Indigenous-Non-Indigenous Relations (Report 4).* https://www.environicsinstitute.org/docs/default-source/project-documents/cot-2020---indigenous-non-indigenous-relations/confederation-of-tomorrow-2020---indigenous-non-indigenous-relations---final-report.pdf?sfvrsn=ac064ead_2

First Nations Education Steering Committee. (2017). *Indian residential schools and reconciliation resources.* http://www.fnesc.ca/irsr/

Fitzpatrick, S. J., Perkins, D., Luland, T., Brown, D., & Corvan, E. (2017). The effect of context in rural mental health care: Understanding integrated services in a small town. *Health and Place, 45*, 70–76. https://doi.org/10.1016/j.healthplace.2017.03.004

Galloway, G. (2017). Ottawa still failing to provide adequate health care on reserves: Report. *The Globe and Mail.* https://www.theglobeandmail.com/news/politics/ottawa-still-failing-to-provide-adequate-health-care-on-reserves-report/article33746065/

Government of British Columbia. (2020, November 30). *Review recommends steps to solve widespread racism in B.C. health care.* https://engage.gov.bc.ca/addressingracism/review-recommends-steps-to-solve-widespread-racism-in-b-c-health-care/

Government of Canada. (2010). *Highlights from the Report of the Royal Commission of Indigenous Peoples RCAP 1996: People to people, nation to nation.* Indigenous and Northern Affairs Canada. https://static1.squarespace.com/static/562e7f2ae4b018ac41a6e050/t/59d0024a9f74567b7ee58b43/1506804313123/RCAP_reading.pdf

Government of Canada. (2016a). *Archived-Indian residential schools settlement agreement-Health support component.* Indigenous and Northern Affairs Canada. https://www.aadnc-aandc.gc.ca/eng/1466537513207/1466537533821

Government of Canada. (2018, October 15). *About Indigenous peoples and culture.* https://www.canada.ca/en/services/culture/canadian-identity-society/indigenous-peoples-cultures.html

Government of Canada. (2020a, November 9). *Building a more inclusive Canada: The Government of Canada supports anti-racism projects in Manitoba, Saskatchewan, and Alberta.* Canadian Heritage. https://www.canada.ca/en/canadian-heritage/news/2020/11/building-a-more-inclusive-canada-the-government-of-canada-supports-anti-racism-projects-in-manitoba-saskatchewan-and-alberta.html

Government of Canada. (2020b). *Canadian Multiculturalism Act* (R.S.C., 1985, c. 24, 4th Supp.). Justice Laws Website. http://laws-lois.justice.gc.ca/eng/acts/C-18.7/

Government of Canada. (2020c). *First Nations and Inuit health: Suicide prevention.* Indigenous Services Canada. https://www.sac-isc.gc.ca/eng/1576089685593/1576089741803

Government of Canada. (2020d). *Health care services for First Nations people and Inuit.* https://www.sac-isc.gc.ca/eng/1581895601263/1581895825373

Government of Canada. (2020e). *Indian residential schools resolution support program.* Indigenous Services Canada. https://www.sac-isc.gc.ca/eng/1581971225188/1581971250953

Graham, H., & Martin, S. (2016). Narrative descriptions of miyo-mahcihoyān (physical, emotional, mental, and spiritual well-being) from a contemporary Néhiyawak (Plains Cree) perspective. *International Journal of Mental Health Systems, 10*, 58. https://doi.org/10.1186/s13033-016-0086-2

Gronholm, P. C., Henderson, C., Deb, T., & Thornicroft, G. (2017). Interventions to reduce discrimination and stigma: The state of the art. *Social Psychiatry and Psychiatric Epidemiology, 52*(3), 249–258. http://doi.org/10.1007/s00127-017-1341-9

Guruge, S., & Butt, H. (2015). A scoping review of mental health issues and concerns among immigrant and refugee youth in Canada: Looking back, moving forward. *Canadian Journal of Public Health, 106*(2), e72–e78. https://doi.org/10.17269/CJPH.106.4588

Hackett, C., Feeny, D., & Tompa, E. (2016). Canada's residential school system: Measuring the intergenerational impact of familial attendance on health and mental health outcomes. *Journal of Epidemiology and Community Health, 70*(11), 1096–1105. https://doi.org/10.1136/jech-2016-207380

Haggarty, J. M., Ryan-Nicholls, K. D., & Jarva, J. A. (2010). Mental health collaborative care: A synopsis of the Rural and Isolated Toolkit. *Rural and Remote Health, 10*(1314), 1–10. https://www.researchgate.net/publication/45437770_Mental_health_collaborative_care_A_synopsis_of_the_Rural_and_Isolated_Toolkit

Hanefeld, J., Powell-Jackson, T., & Balabanova, D. (2017). Understanding and measuring quality of care: Dealing with complexity. *Bulletin of the World Health Organization, 98*, 368–374. http://dx.doi.org/10.2471/BLT.16.179309

Harrison, C. A., & Hauck, Y. H. (2017). Breaking down the stigma of mental health nursing: A qualitative study reflecting opinions from western Australian nurses. *Journal of Psychiatric and Mental Health Nursing, 24*(7), 513–522. https://doi.org/10.1111/jpm.12392

Indian and Northern Affairs Canada. (2020). *A history of Indian and Northern Affairs Canada.* https://www.aadnc-aandc.gc.ca/DAM/DAM-INTER-HQ/STAGING/texte-text/ap_htmc_inaclivr_1314920729809_eng.pdf

Institute of Medicine. (2001). *Crossing the quality chasm: a new health system for the 21st century.* National Academy Press.

Joseph, B. (2014). *What is residential school syndrome?* https://www.ictinc.ca/blog/what-is-residential-school-syndrome

Kates, N., Mazowita, G., Lemire, F., Jayabaratham, A., Bland, R., Selby, P., Isomura, T., Craven, M., Gervais, M., & Audet, D. (2011). The evolution of collaborative mental health care in Canada: A shared vision for the future. Position paper of the Canadian Psychiatric Association, The College of Family Physicians of Canada. *Canadian Journal of Psychiatry, 56*(5), 1–10. http://www.shared-care.ca/files/2011_Position_Paper.pdf

Kent-Wilkinson, A. (2009). *Aboriginal health issues* (online elective, 2009-current). College of Nursing, University of Saskatchewan.

Kent-Wilkinson, A., Blaney, L., Groening, M., Santa Mina, E., Rodrigue, C., & Hust, C. (2016). *CFMHN's 3rd Position paper 2015: Mental health and addiction curriculum in undergraduate nursing education in Canada.* Prepared by members of the Canadian Federation of Mental Health Nurses' Education Committee. https://www.cfmhn.ca/2019/05/14/cfmhn-2016-position-paper/

Kent-Wilkinson, A., Sanders, S. L., Mela, M., Peternelj-Taylor, C., Adelugba, O., Luther, G., & Wormith, J. S. (2012a). *Needs assessment of forensic mental health services and programs for offenders in Saskatchewan: Executive summary.* Study conducted by Forensic Interdisciplinary Research: Saskatchewan Team (FIRST) Centre for Forensic Behavioural Sciences and Justice Studies. University of Saskatchewan. https://cfbsjs.usask.ca/documents/2.%20EXECUTIVE%20SUMMARY_Nov%2029,%202012.pdf

Kent-Wilkinson, A., Sanders, S. L., Mela, M., Peternelj-Taylor, C., Adelugba, O., Luther, G., & Wormith, J. S. (2012b). *Needs assessment of forensic mental health services and programs for offenders in Saskatchewan: Condensed Report.* Conducted by Forensic Interdisciplinary Research: Saskatchewan Team (FIRST). Centre for Forensic Behavioural Sciences and Justice Studies. University of Saskatchewan. https://cfbsjs.usask.ca/documents/research/research_papers/3_Condensed_FINAL_REPORT_Dec_3_2012.pdf

King, M., Smith, A., & Gracey, M. (2009). Indigenous health part 2: The underlying causes of the health gap. *The Lancet, 374*(9683), 76–85. https://doi.org/10.1016/S0140-6736(09)60827-8

Kirkup, K. (2016, May 17). *60% of First Nation children on reserve live in poverty, institute says.* The Canadian Press. http://www.cbc.ca/news/indigenous/institute-says-60-percent-fn-children-on-reserve-live-in-poverty-1.3585105

Kirmayer, L. J. (2019). The politics of diversity: Pluralism, multiculturalism and mental health. *Transcultural Psychiatry, 56*(6). https://doi.org/10.1177/1363461519888608https://doi.org/10.1177/1363461519888608

Kirmayer, L. J., & Jarvis, G. E. (2019). Culturally responsive services as a path to equity in mental healthcare. *HealthcarePapers, 18*(2), 11–23. https://www.academia.edu/40493134/Culturally_Responsive_Services_as_a_Path_to_Equity_in_Mental_Healthcare?email_work_card=reading-history

Kirmayer, L. J., Brass, G. M., & Tait, C. L. (2000a). The mental health of Aboriginal peoples: Transformations of identity and community. *Canadian Journal of Psychiatry, 45*(7), 607–616. https://doi.org/10.1177/070674370004500702

Kirmayer, L. J., Dandeneau, S., Marshall, E., Phillips, M., & Williamson, K. (2011). Rethinking resilience from Indigenous perspectives. *Canadian Journal of Psychiatry, 56*(2), 84–91. http://indigenouspsych.org/Interest%20Group/Kirmayer/2011_CJP_Resilience.pdf

Kirmayer, L. J., Macdonald, M. E., & Brass, G. M. (2000b, May 29). The mental health of Indigenous peoples. *Culture & Mental Health Research Unit, Report No. 10.* Proceedings of the Advanced Study Institute The Mental Health of Indigenous Peoples. McGill Summer Program in Social & Cultural Psychiatry and the Aboriginal Mental Health Research Team (May 29–May 31, 2000). Montréal, Québec https://www.mcgill.ca/tcpsych/files/tcpsych/Report10.pdf

Kuhl, J. L. (2017). Putting an end to the silence: Educating society about the Canadian residential school system. *Bridges: An Undergraduate Journal of Contemporary Connections, 2*(1). http://scholars.wlu.ca/cgi/viewcontent.cgi?article=1013&context=bridges_contemporary_connections

Kumar, M. B., & Nahwegahbow, A. (2016). Aboriginal peoples survey, 2012 past-year suicidal thoughts among off-reserve First Nations, Metis and Inuit adults aged 18 to 25: Prevalence and associated characteristics.

Statistics Canada. http://www.statcan.gc.ca/pub/89-653-x/89-653-x2016011-eng.htm

Kyoung, J. Y., Landais, E., Kolahdooz, F., & Sharma, S. (2015). Framing health matters. Factors influencing the health and wellness of urban Aboriginal youths in Canada: Insights of in-service professionals, care providers, and stakeholders. *American Journal of Public Health, 105*(5), 881–890. https://https://doi.org/10.2105/AJPH.2014.302481

Lipka, M. (2019, July 1). *5 facts about religion in Canada. FactTank: News in numbers.* Pew Research Center. https://www.pewresearch.org/fact-tank/2019/07/01/5-facts-about-religion-in-canada/

Little Bear, L. (2012). Traditional knowledge and humanities: A perspective by a Blackfoot. *Journal of Chinese Philosophy, 39*(4), 518–527. https://https://doi.org/10.1111/j.1540-6253.2012.01742.x

Lowrie, M., & Malone, K. (2020, October 4). Joyce Echaquan's death highlights systemic racism in health care, experts say. *CTV News.* https://www._ctvnews.ca/health/joyce-echaquan-s-death-highlights-systemic-racism-in-health-care-experts-say-1.5132146

Macinnes, M., Macpherson, G., Austin, J., & Schwannauer, M. (2016). Examining the effect of childhood trauma on psychological distress, risk of violence and engagement, in forensic mental health. *Psychiatry Research, 246,* 314–320. https://https://doi.org/10.1016/j.psychres.2016.09.054

MacKenzie, L., & Hatala, A. (2019). Addressing culture within healthcare settings: The limits of cultural competence and the power of humility. *Canadian Medical Education Journal, 10*(1), e124–e127. https://doi.org/10.36834/cmej.52966

Marsh, T. N., Coholic, D., Cote-Meek, S., & Najavits, L. M. (2015). Blending Aboriginal and Western healing methods to treat intergenerational trauma with substance use disorder in Aboriginal peoples who live in Northeastern Ontario, Canada. *Harm Reduction Journal, 12,* 14. https://http://doi.org/10.1186/s12954-015-0046-1

Mayhew, M. (2018). *How culture influences health.* Canadian Paediatric Society. http://www.kidsnewtocanada.ca/culture/influence

McCalman, J., Jongen, C., & Bainbridge, R. (2017). Organizational systems' approaches to improving cultural competence in healthcare: A systematic scoping review of the literature. *International Journal for Equity in Health, 16,* 78. https://equityhealthj.biomedcentral.com/articles/10.1186/s12939-017-0571-5

McGough, S., Wynaden, D., & Wright, M. (2018). Experience of providing cultural safety in mental health to Aboriginal patients: A grounded theory study. *International Journal of Mental Health Nursing, 27*(1), 204–213. http://onlinelibrary.wiley.com/doi/10.1111/inm.12310/ful

McNally, M., & Martin, D. (2017). First Nations, Inuit and Métis health: Considerations for Canadian health leaders in the wake of the Truth and Reconciliation Commission of Canada report. *Healthcare Management Forums, 3*(2), 117–122. http://journals.sagepub.com/doi/abs/10.1177/0840470416680445

McQuaid, R. J., Bombay, A., McInnis, O. P., Humeny, C., Matheson, K., & Anisman, H. (2017). Suicide ideation and attempts among First Nations peoples living on reserve in Canada: The intergenerational and cumulative effects of Indian residential schools. *The Canadian Journal of Psychiatry, 62*(6), 422–430. https://https://doi.org/10.1177/0706743717702075

Mental Health Commission of Canada. (2009, November). *Toward recovery and wellbeing.* https://www.mentalhealthcommission.ca/sites/default/files/FNIM_Toward_Recovery_and_Well_Being_ENG_0_1.pdf

Mental Health Commission of Canada. (2012). *Changing directions, changing lives: The mental health strategy for Canada.* https://www.mentalhealthcommission.ca/sites/default/files/MHStrategy_Strategy_ENG.pdf

Mental Health Commission of Canada. (2013a). *Opening minds: Interim report.* https://www.mentalhealthcommission.ca/sites/default/files/opening_minds_interim_report_0.pdf

Mental Health Commission of Canada. (2013b). *Why investing in mental health will contribute to Canada's economic prosperity and to the sustainability of our health care system.* https://www.mentalhealthcommission.ca/sites/default/files/MHStrategy_CaseForInvestment_ENG_0_1.pdf

Mental Health Commission of Canada. (2016, January). *Supporting the mental health of refugees to Canada.* https://ontario.cmha.ca/wp-content/files/2016/02/Refugee-Mental-Health-backgrounder.pdf

Mercredi, O. W. (2015). *Aboriginal initiatives: Aboriginal gangs a report to the Correctional Service of Canada on Aboriginal youth gang members in the federal corrections system.* http://www.csc-scc.gc.ca/aboriginal/5-eng.shtml

Mood Disorders Society of Canada. (2014). *Workplace mental health.* http://www.mooddisorderscanada.ca/documents/WorkplaceHealth_En.pdf

National Collaborating Centre for Aboriginal Health. (2010). *Poverty as a social determinant of First Nations, Inuit, and Métis health.* http://www.nccah-ccnsa.ca/docs/fact%20sheets/social%20determinates/NCCAH_fs_poverty_EN.pdf

National Collaborating Centre for Aboriginal Health. (2011a). *Access to health services as a social determinant of First Nations, Inuit and Métis health.* Social determinants of health. http://www.nccah-ccnsa.ca/docs/fact%20sheets/social%20determinates/Access%20to%20Health%20Services_Eng%202010.pdf

National Collaborating Centre for Aboriginal Health. (2011b). *Looking for Aboriginal health in legislation and policies, 1970 to 2008: The policy synthesis project.* Prepared by J. Lavoie, L. Gervais, J. Toner, O. Bergeron, & G. Thomas for the NCCAH. http://www.nccah-ccnsa.ca/Publications/Lists/Publications/Attachments/28/Looking%20for%20Aboriginal%20Health%20in%20Legislation%20and%20Polcies%20(English%20-%20Web).pdf

National Collaborating Centre for Aboriginal Health. (2011c). *The Aboriginal health legislation and policy framework in Canada.* Setting the context. http://www.nccah-ccnsa.ca/docs/Health%20Legislation%20and%20Policy_English.pdf

National Collaborating Centre for Aboriginal Health. (2012). *The state of knowledge of Aboriginal health: A review of Aboriginal public health in Canada.* https://www.ccnsa-nccah.ca/docs/context/RPT-StateKnowledgeReview-EN.pdf

National Collaborating Centre for Aboriginal Health. (2016). *Culture and language as social determinants of First Nations, Inuit, and Metis health.* Social Determinants of Health. http://www.nccah-ccnsa.ca/Publications/Lists/Publications/Attachments/15/NCCAH-FS-CultureLanguage-SDOH-FNMI-EN.pdf

National Post. (2014, June 14). *Man's death after 34-hour ER wait must be ruled homicide, family's lawyers tell inquest.* The Canadian Press. https://nationalpost.com/news/canada/mans-death-after-34-hour-er-wait-must-be-ruled-homicide-familys-lawyers-tell-inquest

O'Hara, J., & Treble, P. (2000, June 26). Abuse of trust: What happened behind the walls of residential church schools is a tragedy that has left native victims traumatized. *Maclean's, 6,* 16. https://www.proquest.com/docview/218482842/fulltext/761876F25D644CE6PQ/1?accountid=14739

O'Mahony, J., & Clark, N. (2018). Immigrant women and mental health care: Findings from an environmental scan. *Issues in Mental Health Nursing, 39*(11), 924–934. https://doi.org/10.1080/01612840.2018.1479903

Okpalauwaekwe, U., Mela, M., & Oji, C. (2017). Knowledge of and attitude to mental illness in Nigeria: A scoping review. *Integrative Journal of Global Health, 1*(1). http://www.imedpub.com/articles/knowledge-of-and-attitude-to-mental-illnesses-in-nigeria-a-scoping-review.php?aid=18642

Papps, E., & Ramsden, I. (1996). Cultural safety in nursing: The New Zealand experience. *International Journal for Quality in Health Care, 8*(5), 491–497. http://doi:10.1093/intqhc/8.5.491

Paquette, J., Beauregard, D., & Gunter, C. (2017). Settlers colonialism and cultural policy: The colonial foundation and refoundation of Canadian cultural policy. *International Journal of Cultural Policy, 23*(3), 269–284. https://doi.org/10.1080/10286632.2015.1043294

Paraschak, V., & Thomson, K. (2013, October 18). Finding strength(s): Insights on Aboriginal physical cultural practices in Canada. *Sport in Society, 17*(8). https://doi.org/10.1080/17430437.2013.838353

Pasco, A. (2004). Cross-cultural relationships between nurses and Filipino Canadian patients. *Journal of Nursing Scholarship, 36*(3), 239–246. https://doi.org/10.1111/j.1547-5069.2004.04044.x

Peters, J. (2017). Impact: Colonialism in Canada. *CM: Canadian Review of Materials, 23*(30), 231.

Popova, S., Lange, S., Probst, C., Parunashvili, N., & Rehm, J. (2017). Prevalence of alcohol consumption during pregnancy and fetal alcohol spectrum disorders among the general and Aboriginal populations in Canada and the United States. *European Journal of Medical Genetics, 60*(1), 32–48. http://doi.org/10.1016/j.ejmg.2016.09.010

Preston, J. P., Carr-Stewart, S., & Bruno, C. (2012). The growth of Aboriginal youth gangs in Canada. *Canadian Journal of Native Studies, 32*(2), 193–207. file:///C:/Users/aek587/Downloads/169-Article%20Text-253-1-10-20140105%20(1).pdf

Purnell, L. (2016). Are we really measuring cultural competence? *Nursing Science Quarterly, 29*(2), 124–127. http://doi.org/10.1177/0894318416630100

Reading, C. (2015). Structural determinants of Aboriginal peoples' health. In M. Greenword, S. de Leeuw, N. M. Lindsay, & C. Reading (Eds.), *Determinants of Indigenous peoples' health in Canada* (pp. 3–15). Canadian Scholars Press Inc.

Reading, C. (2018). Structural determinants of Aboriginal peoples' health. In M. Greenwood, S. de Leeuw, N. M. Lindsay, & C. Reading (Eds.), *Determinants of Indigenous peoples' health in Canada* (2nd ed., pp. 3–15). Canadian Scholars' Press Inc. https://www.canadianscholars.ca/books/determinants-of-indigenous-peoples-health

Reading, J., & Halseth, R. (2013). *Pathways to improving wellbeing for Indigenous peoples: How living conditions decide health.* National Collaborating Centre for Aboriginal Health. http://www.nccah-ccnsa.ca/en/publications.aspx?sortcode=2.8.10&publication=102

Repo, H., Vahlberg, T., Salminen, L., Papadopoulos, I., & Leino-Kilpi, H. (2017). The cultural competence of graduating nursing students. *Journal of Transcultural Nursing, 28*(1), 98–107. https://doi.org/10.1177/1043659616632046

Richmond, C. A. M., & Cook, C. (2016). Creating conditions for Canadian Aboriginal health equity: The promise of healthy public policy. *Public Health Reviews, 37*(2). http://doi.org.cyber.usask.ca/10.1186/s40985-016-0016-5

Roberts, G., & Grimes, K. (2011). Return on investment: Mental health promotion and mental illness prevention. *Canadian Institute for Health Information.* http://tools.hhr-rhs.ca/index.php?option=com_mtree&task=viewlink&link_id=6080&lang=en

Roy, A. (2014). Intergenerational trauma and Aboriginal women: Implications for mental health during pregnancy. *First Peoples Child and Family Review, 9*(1). http://journals.sfu.ca/fpcfr/index.php/FPCFR/article/view/189

Russell, C., Firestone, M., Kelly, L., Mushquash, B., & Fischer, C. (2016). Prescription opioid prescribing, use/misuse, harms and treatment among Aboriginal people in Canada: A narrative review of available data and indicators. *Rural and Remote Health, 16*(4), 3974. http://www.rrh.org.au/articles/subviewnew.asp?ArticleID=3974

Rutherford, K. (2016, April 9). Attawapiskat declares state of emergency over spate of suicide attempts. *CBC News.* https://www.cbc.ca/news/canada/sudbury/attawapiskat-suicide-first-nations-emergency-1.3528747

Silove, D., Ventevogel, P., & Rees, S. (2017). The contemporary refugee crisis: An overview of mental health challenges. *World Psychiatry, 16*(2), 130–139. http://doi.org/10.1002/wps.20438

Sinclair Working Group. (2017, September 15). *Systemic racism: Interim report of the Sinclair Working Group.* http://ignoredtodeathmanitoba.ca/index.php/2017/09/15/out-of-sight-interim-report-of-the-sinclair-working-group/

Skip Knox, E. L. (1999). *Western civilization.* https://www.arlima.net/the-orb/textbooks/westciv/civindex.html

Smetanin, P., Stiff, D., Briante, C., Adair, C. E., Ahmad, S., & Khan, M. (2011). *The life and economic impact of major mental illnesses in Canada: 2011 to 2041.* RiskAnalytica, on behalf of the Mental Health Commission of Canada. https://www.mentalhealthcommission.ca/sites/default/files/MHCC_Report_Base_Case_FINAL_ENG_0_0.pdf

Social Progress Imperative. (2020). *Social progress index: Canada.* https://www.socialprogress.org/?tab=3

Statistics Canada. (2013). *Canadian community health survey: Mental health, 2012.* Government of Canada. http://www.statcan.gc.ca/daily-quotidien/130918/dq130918a-eng.htm

Statistics Canada. (2015). *2011 National Household Survey (NHS).* Survey guide. http://www12.statcan.gc.ca/nhs-enm/2011/ref/nhs-enm_guide/index-eng.cfm

Statistics Canada. (2016a). *2011 National Household Survey.* Data tables. Immigration and ethno-cultural diversity. http://www12.statcan.gc.ca/nhs-enm/2011/dp-pd/dt-td/index-eng.cfm

Statistics Canada. (2016b). *Immigration and ethnocultural diversity in Canada. 2011 National Household Survey.* Archived content. http://www12.statcan.gc.ca/nhs-enm/2011/as-sa/99-010-x/99-010-x2011001-eng.cfm

Statistics Canada. (2017a). *Canadian demographics at a glance* (2nd ed., Cat. No. 91-003-X). www.statcan.gc.ca/pub/91-003-x/91-003-x2014001-eng.pdf

Statistics Canada. (2017b). *Population centre and rural area classification 2016.* http://www23.statcan.gc.ca/imdb/p3VD.pl?Function=getVD&TVD=339235

Statistics Canada. (2017c, October 25). *The Aboriginal languages of First Nations people, Métis and Inuit.* Census in Brief. https://www12.statcan.gc.ca/census-recensement/2016/as-sa/98-200-x/2016022/98-200-x2016022-eng.cfm

Statistics Canada. (2018, July 25). *Religions in Canada. 2011 National Household Survey.* http://www12.statcan.gc.ca/nhs-enm/2011/as-sa/99-010-x/99-010-x2011001-eng.cfm#a6

Statistics Canada. (2020a). *Census Profile, 2016 Census.* http://www12.statcan.gc.ca/census-recensement/2016/dp-pd/prof/index.cfm?Lang=E

Statistics Canada. (2020b, November 2). *Statistics on Indigenous people.* https://www.statcan.gc.ca/eng/subjects-start/indigenous_peoples

Tervalon, M., & Murray-Garcia, J. (1998). Cultural humility versus cultural competence: A critical distinction in defining physician training outcomes in multicultural education. *Journal of Health Care for the Poor and Underserved, 9*(2), 117–125. http://doi.org/10.1353/hpu.2010.0233

The Canadian Encyclopedia. (2019). *Métis.* https://www.thecanadianencyclopedia.ca/en/article/metis

The Senate Canada. (2006). *Out of the shadows at last: Transforming mental health, mental illness and addiction services in Canada.* Final Report of the Standing Senate Committee on Social Affairs, Science and Technology. http://www.parl.gc.ca/Content/SEN/Committee/391/soci/rep/pdf/rep-02may06part1-e.pdf

Thira, D. (2005). *Beyond the four waves of colonization.* https://thira.ca/files/2014/08/Colonization-Article-CNPR-Revised1.pdf

Truth and Reconciliation Commission of Canada. (2015a). *Honoring the truth, reconciling for the future: Summary of the final report of the Truth and Reconciliation Commission.* McGill-Queen's University Press. https://www.queensu.ca/provost/sites/webpublish.queensu.ca.provwww/files/files/Comittees/TRC%20Reports/Summary%20of%20TRC%20Final%20Report.pdf

Truth and Reconciliation Commission of Canada. (2015b). *Truth and Reconciliation Commission of Canada: Calls to action.* http://trc.ca/assets/pdf/Calls_to_Action_English2.pdf

United Nations Development Programme. (2020). *Planning for an uncertain future. UNDP annual report 2020.* https://www.undp.org/

Wakeman, J., Humphreys, J., Russell, D., Guthridge, S., Bourke, L., Dunbars, T., Zhao, Y., Ramjan, M., Murakami-Gold, L., & Jones, M.P. (2019). Remote health workforce turnover and retention: what are the policy and practice priorities? *Human Resources for Health, 17*(99), 1–8. https://doi.org/10.1186/s12960-019-0432-y

Wakerman, J., Bourke, L., Humphreys, J. S., & Taylor, J. (2017). Is remote health different to rural health? *Rural and Remote Health, 17*(3832), 1–8. https://doi.org/10.22605/RRH3832

Waldram, J. B., Herring, D. A., & Young, T. K. (2006). *Aboriginal health in Canada: Historical, cultural and epidemiological perspectives* (2nd ed.). University of Toronto Press. https://www.ncbi.nlm.nih.gov/pmc/articles/PMC1949183/

Watt, K., Abbott, P., & Reath, J. (2016). Developing cultural competence in general practitioners: An integrative review of the literature. *BMC Family Practice, 17*(158). https://bmcfampract.biomedcentral.com/articles/10.1186/s12875-016-0560-6

Wilk, P., Maltby, A., & Cooke, M. (2017). Residential schools and the effects on Indigenous health and wellbeing in Canada-a scoping review. *Public Health Reviews, 38*, 8. https://doi.org/10.1186/s40985-017-0055-6

World Health Organization. (2017). *Social determinants of health.* http://www.who.int/social_determinants/en/

Zayed, R., Davidson, B., Nadeau, L., Callanan, T. S., Fleisher, W., Hope-Ross, L., Espinet, S., Spenser, H. R., Lipton, H., Srivastava, A., Lazier, L., Doey, T., Khalid-Khan, S., McKerlie, A., Stretch, N., Flynn, R., Abidi, S., St. John, K., Auclair, G., Liashko, V., … Steele, M. (2016). Canadian rural/remote primary care physicians' perspectives on child/adolescent mental health care service delivery. *Journal of the Canadian Academy of Child and Adolescent Psychiatry, 25*(1), 24–34. https://www.ncbi.nlm.nih.gov/pmc/articles/PMC4791103/

CHAPTER 5

The Continuum of Canadian Mental Health Care

Nicole Snow*

*Adapted from the chapter "The Continuum of Psychiatric and Mental Health Care" by Diane Kunyk

LEARNING OBJECTIVES

After studying this chapter, you will be able to:

- Identify the different treatment settings and associated programs along the continuum of care.
- Discuss the role of the nurse along the continuum of care.
- Describe current healthcare trends in psychiatric and mental health services.
- Describe the importance of integrated services for people with mental illness or mental health concerns.

KEY TERMS

- assertive community treatment • case management • community-based residential services • community treatment orders • e-mental health • empowerment • illness prevention • integrated approach • intensive outpatient program • intensive residential services • mental health promotion • mobile crisis response • partnership • primary care • primary health care • referral • reintegration • relapse • stabilization • supportive employment

KEY CONCEPTS

- collaborative practice • continuum of care

Healthcare systems need to have well-integrated psychiatric and mental health (PMH) care across the continuum, from health promotion to recovery and rehabilitation. It is well recognized that most mental illnesses are not caused by a single factor but are a result of a combination of factors. These causative factors relate to the complex interactions between biologic, social, psychological, and spiritual aspects of people's lives. Effective PMH care must be able to people's needs across these areas. However, it must also move upstream to develop and implement mental health wellness policies and programs. In its fullest conceptual understanding, the scope of care ought to be similar to those incorporated for physical health and include support for health promotion, disease prevention, early intervention, disease treatment, and recovery management. In their position statement, the Canadian Public Health Association (2021) has called upon governments to develop a national strategy for population mental wellness that incorporates personal, social, and ecological determinants of health and that addresses the effects of racism, colonialism, and social exclusion on mental health and wellness, using a life-course approach (Box 5.1). Here is a call for the continuum of PMH care to include not only a range of services but the inclusion of mental wellness strategies.

Health professionals across all aspects of the Canadian healthcare system, oftentimes nurses, are expected to provide health promotion interventions through to appropriate care for individuals with mental health concerns and/or mental disorders. PMH services offer more specialized expertise in meeting their individualized needs. Resources that foster people's sense of self, social inclusion and belonging, meaning, and purpose, and that empower individuals to develop their capacity for wellbeing are important components of the PMH care continuum. Many of these resources are "outside" the formal healthcare system and are provided in the community by educational institutions, employers, nonprofit organizations, religious or other groups, as well as family and peers.

A comprehensive approach to mental health requires the provision of quality care that not only meets the needs of communities but continuously improves the care provided in all healthcare settings. HealthCare*CAN* and the

---

BOX 5.1 Public Health Approach to Population Mental Wellness

In 2021, the Canadian Public Health Association called upon the federal government to take action on developing a national strategy for population mental wellness. More specifically, this document drew attention to the following actions:

- develop and implement a health/mental-health-in-all-policies approach to policy and program development;
- establish a life-course, culturally sensitive approach when developing mental wellness programs, with special emphasis on:
  - perinatal, postpartum, infant, child and youth programming;
  - senior adults;
  - gender;
  - LGBTQ2S+ communities;
  - Black and racialized communities;
  - refugees;
  - people experiencing homelessness;
  - Indigenous Peoples; and
  - peoples with disabilities, including those with chronic health conditions;
- develop adaptable approaches for addressing mental health that are appropriate to diverse situations;

- make programs universal in nature but proportionate to meet the requirements of those who have the greatest need;
- provide universally available, affordable, high-quality, developmentally appropriate early childhood education and care [that is culturally sensitive];
- develop poverty reduction programs that meet the needs of those who need them most;
- continue efforts to address the needs of Indigenous Peoples by acting on the Calls to Action of the Truth and Reconciliation Commission and supporting strength-based approaches to mental wellness that include Indigenous mental wellness models;
- support the development of provincial, territorial, and regional/community PMW planning and performance measurement activities;
- recognize and develop approaches to address anxiety and grief resulting from climate change, COVID-19, and the opioid poisonings crisis; and
- continue efforts to support and enhance workplace mental health programs.

Source: Canadian Public Health Association. (2021). *A Public Health Approach to Population Mental Wellness*. https://www.cpha.ca/public-health-approach-population-mental-wellness

---

Mental Health Commission of Canada have collaborated to develop the Quality Mental Health Framework. It describes ten key elements to address quality mental health care for patients and providers (see Fig. 5.1).

Primary Healthcare Approach

Primary health care (not to be confused with "primary care") was adopted by the World Health Organization (WHO) in 1978 as the basis for the delivery of health services (WHO, 2008b). It is an approach that encompasses five types of health care: promotive, preventive, curative, rehabilitative, and supportive/palliative. It is based on the principles of accessibility, public participation, health promotion, appropriate technology (i.e., adapted to the community's social, economic, and cultural developments), and intersectoral cooperation (necessary as health and wellbeing are linked to social and economic policies).

Since the release of this document, the WHO has begun further strategizing how to provide these services to ensure that all people have access to universal health coverage. In doing so, health must also be considered in light of the socioeconomic, environmental, and climate factors that influence it (WHO, 2013). There are numerous exemplars of individuals, families,

and populations who have inequitable access to mental health services. Services must be available in numbers to address this need and to be of a high-quality standard to achieve universal health coverage (WHO, 2013).

Canadian nurses are expected to apply primary healthcare principles in their practice across the continuum of mental health care (Canadian Nurses Association [CNA], 2012). The Mental Health Commission of Canada (MHCC, 2012) has put forward recommendations for action that closely align with the principles of primary health care and have incorporated them into their *Framework for Action* (2016).

Defining the Continuum of Care

The continuum of care represents the complex, integrated system of services provided by health professionals in general and by those with specialized psychiatric and mental expertise, as well as the supports provided by informal providers and organizations within the community that help people to maintain and to restore their mental health and wellbeing.

The continuum of care begins with health promotion strategies for preventing people from experiencing mental health problems or becoming mentally ill, as well as improving the mental health status of the whole population. When people do experience a mental health problem or a mental illness, most of the services in Canada are situated in community settings. Inpatient care (hos-pitalization) may be periodically necessary, but it is typically of very short duration. There are also components of the continuum that are focused on the PMH care needs of specific patient populations, such as children

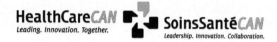

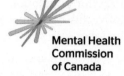

The Quality Mental Health Care Framework

The Quality Mental Health Care Framework builds on the Health Standards Organization/Canadian Patient Safety Institute Canadian Quality and Patient Safety Framework for Health and Social Services and includes the Institute for Healthcare Improvement's Framework for Safe, Reliable, and Effective Care and Quadruple Aim approaches to the inclusion of providers in quality care.

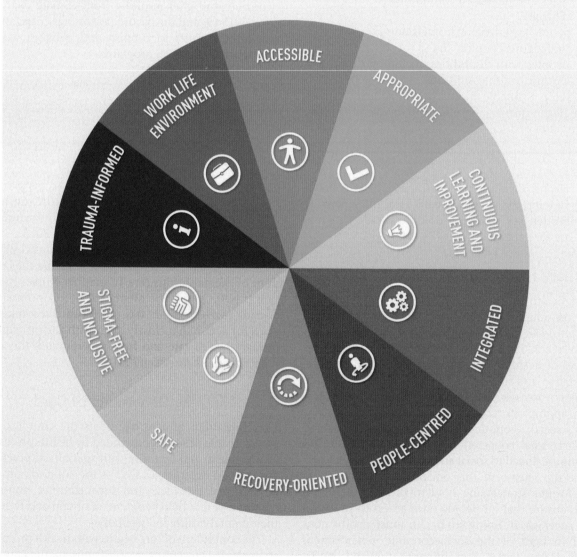

Figure 5.1 The Quality Mental Healthcare Framework. (Source: Mental Health Commission of Canada. (2021). Quality Mental Health Care Network: Infographic. https://www.mentalhealthcommission.ca/English/media/4475)

	DIMENSION	DESCRIPTION
	ACCESSIBLE	Having timely and equitable care across the continuum. Promotes prevention and early intervention. Community-based interventions are available.
	APPROPRIATE	Care is evidence-informed and culturally competent.
	CONTINUOUS LEARNING AND IMPROVEMENT	Knowledge sharing and capacity building among members of the healthcare workforce. Innovative care is encouraged and supported.
	INTEGRATED	Care is continuous across the continuum. Transition into community settings is smooth. Family and/or patient's support system is involved. Integration with services that address social determinants of health.
	PEOPLE-CENTRED	Care that is focused and organized around the health needs and expectations of people and communities rather than on disease.
	RECOVERY-ORIENTED	Living a satisfying, hopeful, and meaningful life, even when there may be ongoing limitations related to mental health problems and illnesses.
	SAFE	Keeping people and providers safe from preventable harm. Care is culturally safe across the continuum for individuals and community.
	STIGMA-FREE AND INCLUSIVE	Care addresses drivers of mental health stigma and prevents stigma practices in mental health care. Health providers are comfortable in coming forward with their mental health problems and illnesses at work. Addresses multiple layers of stigma (individual, interpersonal, intersectoral, and structural). A need to better support individuals who have experienced stigma and discrimination. Individuals feel respected and valued.
	TRAUMA-INFORMED	Recognizes the impacts of trauma and violence on individuals receiving mental health care services.
	WORK LIFE ENVIRONMENT	A healthy workplace environment supports provider wellness and promotes psychological safety.

Financial contribution from

 Health   Santé
Canada   Canada

Figure 5.1 *(Continued)*

and families, seniors, military personnel, people with brain injuries, people who are involved with the legal system, people with addictions, and people with developmental challenges. Such services are often provided by specially trained mental health professionals.

The continuum of care extends beyond the services for acute events to support recovery. The MHCC (2021)

defines the concept of recovery as "living a satisfying, hopeful, and contributing life, even when a person may be experiencing a mental health problem or illness" (p. 1). Recovery also includes the concept of wellbeing—individuals realizing their potential. In order to facilitate recovery and wellbeing for individuals, family, groups, or communities, the MHCC has concluded that care provision must be founded on core principles. These include hope and optimism, focused on the individual, occurring in the context of the individual's life, and responsive to diversity among individuals. Working with people who are First Nations, Inuit, and Métis, and transforming existing services and systems are also considered fundamental (MHCC, 2015).

The goal of PMH care is to deliver the right care (appropriate medical, nursing, psychological, social, and spiritual services), by the right person, to the right person and/or family members, at the right time and in the right place. By doing so, this continuum facilitates the stability, continuity, and comprehensiveness of service provision to individuals over their lifetime. Further components of the continuum of care range from supportive interventions by informal community support providers to professional service providers delivering clinical treatment in the community to professional services being provided in a hospital setting. Due to the complexity of the continuum of care, individuals and families may require assistance with the coordination of their care, services, and supports. The preconditions to continuity of care include such elements as ease of access to, adequate information about, and availability of services.

KEY CONCEPT

A continuum of care consists of an integrated health system of supports and services designed to maximize people's health and wellbeing across the life span that is provided by health professionals (some who offer specialized services, such as psychiatric mental health services), as well as by nonprofessional caregivers.

Coordination of Care

Coordination of care is the integration of appropriate services so that individualized person-centred care and treatment is provided. Appropriate services are those that are tailored to promote recovery and wellbeing of the individual and family (when appropriate) through holistic care that supports and develops an individual's strengths, addresses vulnerabilities, promotes cultural competency and safety, inspires hope, facilitates empowerment, and offers choice and responsibility. People's input and opinions need to be solicited, including what they require in terms of knowledge, skills, and support to make decisions as well as their ability to participate in their own care. Person-centered care promotes the needs of people and does not hold disease as the focus of healthcare services and supports. As such, individuals, families, and communities are encouraged to participate in the decisions surrounding their care. In taking this approach, an integrated health system is needed to ensure that people receive needed services and that the collaboration and coordination of these services can be enhanced (WHO,

2021). Improved coordinated care is hinged on effective collaboration amongst everyone involved and is particularly important for those who have complex mental and physical healthcare needs (Evidence Exchange Network for Mental Health and Addictions, 2017).

There are many terms that are used to describe the types of coordinating services. They include the following: **case management**, service coordination, care management, care coordination, service navigation, and transition care services. Although the terms may be different, the services provided can be described as a collaborative, patient-driven process designed to support the patient's achievement of goals within a complex health, social, and fiscal environment. To meet patient goals, the coordinator of services for patients and families may need to liaise and develop collaborative and cooperative relationships among many different service partners, such as primary care services, public health, mental health, social services, housing, education, the workplace, and the criminal justice system, to name but a few. See Box 5.2 for principle functions of case management and Box 5.3 for dimensions of recovery-oriented practice.

The Nurse as Manager of Patient Services

Nurses serve in various pivotal functions across the continuum of care due to the oftentimes cyclical nature of serious mental illness. These functions can involve both direct care and coordination of the care delivered by others. The role of manager of patient services (also referred to as case manager or care coordinator) does not refer to the client or patient but to service provision. When functioning in this position, the nurse must have commanding knowledge of the patient's and family's needs, areas of strengths, and the available community resources. In order for nurses to be successful, they must practice with the philosophy that recovery is defined by the patient, not the service provider, and a belief that wellbeing is possible for all people living with a mental illness. The nurse must also have expertise in working with the family as a unit. The repertoire of required skills includes collaboration, teaching, management, leadership, followership, as well as group, critical thinking, and research skills. A nurse working as a case manager arguably has one of the most diverse roles within the psychiatric services continuum.

What is becoming increasingly apparent is the critical and important role that the nurse has in developing therapeutic relationships with patients. While contemporary models of mental health care strive to promote inclusion and **empowerment** and to recognize the preferences of individuals, there are challenges to accomplish this within the constraints of current mental health system structures (Kingston & Greenwood, 2020). This requires that relationships must be built with patients and their families to meet their needs and expectations. The nurse–patient relationship is not only foundational for including patients in their care planning but also

BOX 5.2 Principle Functions of Case Management

- **Assessment**
  Case management includes conducting a comprehensive assessment of the patient's mental and physical health needs.
- **Patient-centred**
  Case management is patient/caregiver centred, involves the patient in the decision-making process, and is sometimes driven or provided by the patient.
- **Navigation**
  Case management provides navigation through the wide spectrum of services to meet patient needs. It moves beyond the boundaries of programs and service sectors, and includes assisting patients with transitioning their care.
- **Collaboration/coordination**
  Case management strategies include developing and carrying out a care plan collaboratively with patients, their families, primary healthcare providers, and others. It builds upon clinical expertise and the collaborative relationships/formalized partnerships among healthcare professionals, patients, and their caregivers.
- **Health promotion/illness prevention**
  Case management strategies enhance health promotion, illness prevention, and risk mitigation through patient education and emphasis on enhancing patient self-care capacity. Case management incorporates the principles of population health and the broad determinants of health.
- **Quality of care**

Case management incorporates evidence-based practice to promote quality of care, problem solving, and exploring options for planning and improving care.
- **Communication**
  Case management requires facilitating effective communication and coordination between the patient, the patient's family, primary healthcare providers, and others to minimize fragmentation and maximize evidence-based care delivery.
- **Advocating**
  Case management advocates on behalf of patients to receive quality care, the healthcare team to be supported in providing quality services, and effective use of health resources. The case manager also promotes the patient to similarly self-advocate and to achieve independence.
- **Flexibility**
  Case management considers alternative plans, when necessary, to achieve desired outcomes.
- **Education**
  Case management provides patients and their families with the education and support that enables patients to understand their care needs, to make informed decisions, and to be confident in providing self-care.

Adapted from: System case management for continuing care clients: Prepared for Continuing Care Leaders Council. Edmonton, AB; Kathol, R., Perez, R., & Cohen, J. (2010). *The integrated case management manual* (p. 4). Springer Publishing Company

Victoria Government Australia. (2021). *Mental health services- case managers.* https://www.betterhealth.vic.gov.au/health/ConditionsAndTreatments/mental-health-services-case-managers

influences patient engagement in ongoing mental health care (Newman et al., 2015).

Comprehensive Mental Health System: Core Programs and Services

Each Canadian province has slightly different services to promote mental health, prevent mental illness, and provide treatment services and/or community supports to people with a mental health problem or mental illness. All, however, should be based on a commitment to patient-centred care (CNA, 2012; MHCC, 2012).

Mental Health Promotion and Illness Prevention

Effective and efficient mental health service delivery systems have integrated **mental health promotion** and **illness prevention** into all aspects of the system. Mental

health promotion strategies are directed toward addressing the determinants of health that can impact the population's mental health. These strategies recognize and address the broader issues, which include the promotion of mental health, but which are largely dependent on intersectoral approaches. Several mental health promotion policies and programs have been mainstreamed into Canada's government and business sectors. A few examples of these include early childhood intervention programs, nutritional and psychosocial interventions for vulnerable populations, and community-based violence prevention that involves community policing initiatives. See Box 5.4 for a summary of best practices related to mental health promotion.

Mental illness prevention strategies are designed to keep something from happening. This something may be the development of a disorder itself, the severity or duration of the disorder, or a disability associated with the disorder. The WHO has identified three categories of prevention strategies that will reduce the risk of experiencing

BOX 5.3 Six Dimensions of Recovery-Oriented Practice

1 **Creating a Culture and Language of Hope.** Recovery is possible and is essentially about hope. Hope stimulates recovery and acquiring the capabilities to nurture hope is the starting point for building a mental health system geared to fostering recovery.

2 **Recovery Is Personal.** Each person is unique and has a right to determine, to the greatest extent possible, their own path to mental health and wellbeing. Recovery acknowledges the individual nature of each person's journey of wellness and their right to find their own way to living a life of value and purpose.

3 **Recovery Occurs in the Context of One's Life.** Most of a person's recovery journey occurs outside the mental health system. Therefore, fostering recovery necessitates understanding people within the context of their lives. Family, friends, neighbours, local community, schools, workplaces, and spiritual and cultural communities all influence mental health and wellbeing and have an important role in recovery.

4 **Responding to the Diverse Needs of Everyone Living in Canada.** Recovery-oriented practice is grounded in principles that encourage and enable respect for diversity and that are consistent with culturally safe, responsive, competent practice.

5 **Working with First Nations, Inuit and Métis.** There is common ground between recovery principles and shared Indigenous understandings of wellness that provides a rich opportunity for learning and strengthening mental health policy and practice.

6 **Recovery Is About Transforming Services and Systems.** Achieving a fully integrated recovery-oriented mental health system is an ongoing process. The commitment to recovery needs to find expression in everything a health organization does including ensuring support for a workforce that has the skills and resources required to deliver recovery-oriented practice.

From Mental Health Commission of Canada. (2015). *Guidelines for recovery-oriented practice: Hope, dignity, inclusion* (pp. 15–17).

BOX 5.4
BEST PRACTICES

MENTAL HEALTH PROMOTION

- early childhood interventions
- support to children
- socioeconomic empowerment of women
- social support for older adult populations
- programs targeted at vulnerable groups, including minorities, Indigenous peoples, migrants, and people affected by conflicts and disasters
- mental health promotional activities in schools
- mental health interventions at work
- housing policies
- violence prevention programs
- community development programs
- poverty reduction and social protection for the poor
- antidiscrimination laws and campaigns
- promotion of the rights, opportunities, and care of individuals with mental disorders

Adapted from World Health Organization. (2018, March 30). *Mental health: Strengthening our response.* https://www.who.int/news-room/fact-sheets/detail/mental-health-strengthening-our-response

an illness: (a) universal prevention, targets the general population; (b) selective prevention, targets groups or individuals at higher risk for a specific illness than the general population; and (c) indicated prevention, targets people at high risk for mental illness (WHO, 2002). An important example of illness prevention services is respite services for family caregivers of persons with a mental illness. The goals of respite programs are typically threefold:

- to validate and reinforce the necessity and value of informal caregiving within the continuum of care;
- to provide support and advocacy to informal caregivers; and
- to prevent unnecessary long-term care placements and hospitalizations due to informal caregiver burnout. Respite services can be provided within the home or within a community living option (group home or supportive living setting) or may be provided within an inpatient setting.

Another example of a mental illness prevention strategy is the practice of providing critical incident stress debriefings. For example, if a volunteer fire crew responded to the scene of a very gruesome accident, then the community mental health services may offer a critical incident stress debriefing. This intervention strategy is provided as a means to help the fire crew members avoid the potential onset of posttraumatic stress disorder.

Consumer Self-Help and Consumer/ Survivor Initiatives

The knowledge and experiences of people living with mental illness are recognized and supported as part of a comprehensive mental healthcare system. In 2012, the MHCC identified six strategic directions to achieve its vision that "All people living in Canada have the opportunity to achieve the best possible mental health and wellbeing" (MHCC, 2012, p. 10). Half of these strategic directions require the direct involvement of people with or who have experienced a mental illness. For example, patients and their families need to be actively involved in decisions about services which uphold patient rights and foster recovery and wellbeing (MHCC, 2012). The importance of input from patients goes beyond decisions about their own care; it extends to the broader healthcare system. Expanding the "leadership role of people living with mental health problems and illnesses, and their families, in setting mental health related policy" (MHCC, 2012, p. 19) will improve knowledge and foster collaboration, which will ultimately have significant positive effects on decision making within the mental healthcare system. Research supports that individuals with mental health concerns, along with their families, need to be encouraged to become active decision makers in their recovery. Concerns with engaging in this process often revolve around the amount of time involved in collaborative efforts with the individual and other healthcare professionals, as well as determining the individual's competency (Huang et al., 2020).

Almost half of Canadians report having their mental health needs partially met with some help or fully unmet (Statistics Canada, 2019a). Canadians who needed help for their mental health but were without a regular healthcare provider were more likely to report unmet or partially met needs (60.3%) compared to those who did have a regular healthcare provider (41.2%). The most frequently reported reasons for having unmet or partially met needs were related to not knowing where to go, being too busy, or not being able to afford to pay.

One strategy that is used to extend assistance to people with mental health concerns or disorders is through peer support organizations. These initiatives are operated exclusively by and for people with serious mental illness. Rather than focusing on treatment, they offer various services such as education and peer support that are delivered through clients engaging with individuals who have also experienced mental illness. The overall goal of these initiatives is to promote recovery. This can be measured through reductions in the need for hospitalization, improved quality of life.

Crisis Response Systems and Psychiatric Emergency Services

Crisis intervention measures are needed to reduce the likelihood of a person developing mental health vconcerns in response to frightening, stressful, or potentially life-threatening events. Crisis intervention services are an important part of a comprehensive mental health system and can be found from a variety of sources. These include telephone crisis services, **mobile crisis response**, access to crisis emergency residential services, or psychiatric emergency services in hospitals (National Alliance on Mental Health, 2018). This type of short-term intervention care focuses on de-escalation, **stabilization**, symptom reduction, and prevention of **relapse** requiring inpatient services.

Crisis intervention units can be found in the emergency department of a general or psychiatric hospital or in crisis centres within a community mental health centre. Patients in crisis demonstrate severe symptoms of acute mental illness, including labile mood swings, suicidal ideation, or self-injurious behaviours. This treatment option therefore demands a high degree of nursing expertise. Patients in crisis usually require medications such as anxiolytics or benzodiazepines for symptom management. Key nursing roles include making an accurate assessment, delivering short-term therapeutic interventions, and administering medication. For example, there are opportunities for nurses to be members of mobile crisis response units. Such services include the collaboration of various health professionals who have experience in crisis intervention including nurses, social workers, and police who can respond to individuals who are experiencing crisis. Once there, the clinician, such as the nurse, will assess the person and make a clinical judgment regarding the need for further intervention. In Canada, under provincial mental health acts, peace officers, including police, can detain individuals who are experiencing a mental health crisis and who are at risk to harm self or others. The officer in this case can aid in ensuring that the individual is safely transported to a mental health facility or other service for further assessment if needed. Nurses will also facilitate **referrals** for increased community services or support, for admission to the hospital, or for outpatient services. See Box 5.5 for a systematic review of research that explored how housing, mental health, substance use, and family cohesion are affected by homelessness.

Crisis Stabilization

When the immediate crisis does not resolve quickly, the next step is crisis stabilization. The primary purpose of stabilization is to control precipitating symptoms through medications, behavioural interventions, and coordination with other agencies for appropriate aftercare. The major focus of nursing care in a short-term inpatient setting is symptom management and linkage to community resources. During stabilization, the major components of nursing care are ongoing assessment; short-term, focused interventions; and medication administration while monitoring efficacy and side effects. Nurses may also provide focused group psy-

BOX 5.5 **Research for Best Practices**

RELATIONSHIP BETWEEN HOUSING, MENTAL HEALTH, SUBSTANCE ABUSE, AND FAMILY COHESION ON THE MENTAL HEALTH OF HOMELESS YOUTH

Wang, J. Z., Mott, S., Magwood, O., Matthew, C., Mclellan, A., Kpade, V., Gaba, P., Kozloff, N., Pottie, K., & Andermann, A. (2019). The impact of interventions for youth experiencing homelessness on housing mental health, substance abuse, and family cohesion: A systematic review. *BMC Public Health, 19*, 1528–1550.

Background: There is a need for a greater understanding of youth experiencing homelessness. These individuals are vulnerable to becoming homeless as a result of family issues, abuse, and neglect, which involves different pathways than adults.

Method: Databases (including Medline, Embase, PsycINFO, and others) were searched for randomized controlled trials (RCTs) and systematic reviews regarding youth interventions. The PRISMA-E approach was used to review the articles obtained.

Findings: The systematic review yielded 11,936 results. Four systematic reviews and 18 articles on RCTs met the criteria after screening. Major categories explored include individual and family therapy, cognitive behavioural therapy, motivational interviewing, skill building, case management, structural support (housing programs, drop-in and shelter services), and gender and equity analysis.

Implications: Cognitive behavioural interventions and family therapy have promise with addressing depression and substance use, respectively. Housing initiative models, such as Housing First, have been helpful in providing reliable shelter. Some of the interventions explored yielded inconsistent results and more study is needed in gender and ethnicity considerations. A more holistic, flexible approach is needed to explore and understand the processes by which youth find themselves homeless and survive.

chotherapy designed to develop and strengthen patients' personal management strategies.

Psychosocial Emergency Preparedness and Response

A national priority is to be prepared for emergencies (e.g., transportation accidents, power outages, terrorist threats) and disasters (e.g., floods, fires, tornadoes, outbreaks of disease). Most local emergencies are handled at that level; however, **partnership** is a key principle of Canada's emergency management directorate (Emergency Management Policy and Outreach Directorate, 2017). When assistance is requested or when an emergency involves more than one province or territory, the federal government mobilizes resources and coordinates federal response in the health sector through Public Safety Canada. Health Canada and the Public Health Agency of Canada play critical roles in emergency response to risks to public health. The psychosocial aspect of preparedness and response is recognized as an essential component (Health Canada, 2021).

In times of major emergencies and disasters, individuals, families, and entire communities face severe risks to psychosocial (as well as physical) wellbeing, and the mental health system can be overwhelmed. Some individuals are resilient and can adapt to find ways of coping after emergencies and disasters; however, the longer that significant sequelae impact individual, family, and community personal and socioeconomic wellbeing, the greater the risk for distress to occur (see Chapter 18). This is particularly evident in the COVID-19 pandemic. There have been increasing concerns in mental health and wellness due to extended restrictions on personal freedoms, regulations on social interactions, worry regarding contracting the illness, and other deleterious socioeconomic outcomes permeating the population's consciousness (Pan et al., 2020; Pfefferbaum & North, 2020). Canada's psychosocial preparedness and response initiative offers services to help Canadians better prepare for disasters and emergencies (e.g., resiliency building) as well as consultation during disaster response.

Primary Care

Primary care refers to the first point of access to the healthcare system. Provincial healthcare planning has typically divided the delivery of the services for physical illness and mental illness. This has resulted in a system that fragments people's needs, which is both counterproductive and harmful. An **integrated approach** is required that assists people in managing illness, regardless of its origin. The integrated approach begins with ensuring that the services and supports that are delivered are done so in a patient-centred manner. This means that people are empowered: choice is promoted, they remain in control, and they remain in their community when possible. A patient-centred approach emphasizes the partnership that the person with mental illness has with the service providers. This model does not place blame on the affected individual; rather, people with mental illness are true partners in their recovery. Although the extent of a person's involvement will depend on their particular circumstances, it is only through involvement in their own recovery that people who experience a mental illness can expect the best possible health and wellbeing.

Collaborative mental healthcare models have been established in response to specialist mental health service provider shortages, access issues, and the recognition that family primary providers are the first point of contact. These models have been described using a variety of terms: integrated care, shared care, collaborative care, and managed care, among others. In essence, collaborative care recognizes that primary care for mental health is essential, but to be fully effective, it must be supported by additional levels of care as no single service setting, or provider, can meet everyone's mental health needs (WHO, 2008b). See Box 5.6 for best practices related to the goals and potential activities of collaborative mental healthcare services. See Box 5.7 related to the benefits of integrating mental health into primary care.

KEY CONCEPT

The World Health Organization defines collaborative practice as health care that occurs when "multiple health workers from different professional backgrounds provide comprehensive services by working with patients, their families, carers and communities to deliver the highest quality of care across settings" (2010, p. 13).

The other levels of care required to support primary care providers include secondary service components.

These components include opportunities for consultation and support through referrals regarding patient care needs outside the primary care provider's current competency level, as well as supervision and support to facilitate further skill development and education of the primary care provider. Collaborative mental health care also extends to include formal and informal community supports for people with mental illness, such as housing, education, and recreational organizations. It has been demonstrated that people with mental illness who receive good community care services and support have better health and mental health outcomes, and better quality of life, than do those people who were treated in psychiatric hospitals (WHO, 2008b). However, there is a small proportion of the population that requires very specialized services. These are people who have treatment-resistant or very complex presentations of illness, those who lack community support, and/or those requiring forensic services.

Outpatient Care

Outpatient care is a level of care that occurs outside of a hospital or institution. Outpatient services usually are less intensive and are provided to patients who do not require inpatient services. Many patients enroll in outpatient services immediately upon discharge from an inpatient setting. Others are enrolled as a means of providing treatment services when hospitalization is not required. This promotes a continued connection with

BOX 5.6 BEST PRACTICES

GOALS AND POTENTIAL ACTIVITIES OF COLLABORATIVE MENTAL HEALTHCARE SERVICES

Goals

- Improve access to a comprehensive range of high-quality and effective healthcare services.
- Improve outcomes for people who use the mental health system.
- Integrate community services across sectors.

Potential Activities

- Regular visits by a mental healthcare worker to a primary care setting
- Unified programs that offer mental health and physical health care through one administration and financial entity
- Regular telephone consultation between primary care and mental health providers
- Integration of specialized care providers such as psychiatrists, psychologists, nurses, social workers,

pharmacists, occupational therapists, and dietitians within primary care settings
- Joint development of treatment plans by consumers and providers
- Incorporation of mental health interventions into the management of general medical conditions (e.g., diabetes)
- Meeting the primary healthcare needs of individuals with severe and persistent mental illness
- Strategies to improve access to community mental health services
- Development of more formal partnerships with specialized service providers

Reference: Kates, N., Mazowita, G., Lemire, F., Jayabarathan, A., Bland, R., Selby, P., & Audet, D. (2011). The evolution of collaborative mental health care in Canada: A shared vision for the future. *The Canadian Journal of Psychiatry, 56*(5), 1–10.

BOX 5.7 Benefits of Integrating Mental Health Into Primary Care

1 **The burden of mental disorders is great.** Mental disorders are prevalent in all societies. They create a substantial personal burden for affected individuals and their families, and they produce significant economic and social hardships that affect society as a whole.

2 **Mental and physical health problems are interwoven.** Many people suffer from both physical and mental health problems. Integrated primary care services help ensure that people are treated in a holistic manner, meeting the mental health needs of people with physical disorders, as well as the physical health needs of people with mental disorders.

3 **The treatment gap for mental disorders is enormous.** In all countries, there is a significant gap between the prevalence of mental disorders and the number of people receiving treatment and care. Primary care for mental health helps close this gap.

4 **Primary care for mental health enhances access.** Integrating mental health into primary care is the best way of ensuring that people get the mental health care they need. When mental health is integrated into primary care, people can access mental health services closer to their homes, thus keeping their families together and maintaining their daily activities. Primary care services also facilitate community outreach and mental health promotion, as well as long-term monitoring and management of affected individuals.

5 **Primary care for mental health promotes respect of human rights.** Mental health services delivered in primary care minimize stigma and discrimination. This also removes the risk of human rights violations that occur in psychiatric hospitals.

6 **Primary care for mental health is affordable and cost-effective.** Primary mental healthcare services are less expensive than are psychiatric hospitals, for patients, communities, and governments alike. In addition, patients and families avoid indirect costs associated with seeking specialist care in distant locations. The treatment of common mental disorders is very cost-effective, and even small investments by governments can bring important benefits.

7 **Primary care for mental health generates good health outcomes.** The majority of people with mental health disorders treated in primary care have good outcomes, particularly when linked to a network of services at secondary level and in the community.

From World Health Organization and World Organization of Family Doctors. (2008). *Integrating mental health into primary care: A global perspective.*

their community and community **reintegration**, medication management and monitoring, and symptom management. Patients and their families have the right to choose their home or community as the site for service provision. When remaining at home with their families and other supports, individuals with mental health concerns or mental illnesses are more socially integrated into society (Hair et al., 2013). Outpatient services are provided by private practices, clinics, and community mental health centres.

Intensive Outpatient Programs and Approaches

The primary focus of **intensive outpatient programs** is on stabilization and relapse prevention for highly vulnerable individuals who can function autonomously on a daily basis. People who meet these criteria have returned to their previous lifestyle although their quality of life is still impacted by their mental illness (e.g., interacting with family, resuming work, or returning to school). Participation in outpatient programs is a benefit to individuals who still require frequent monitoring and support within a therapeutic milieu that enables them to remain connected to the community. The duration of treatment and level of services rendered are based on the patient's immediate needs. Treatment duration usually is time limited, with sessions offered 3 to 4 hours per day and 2 to 3 days per week for 6 to 12 weeks. See Box 5.8 for best practices related to bridging the gaps in inpatient care and outpatient care.

Housing and Community Support

With the focus on community-based care, there has also been increasing attention to housing and community support. As people have transitioned from primarily receiving services as an inpatient for serious mental illness to receiving those services within their community, there have been increased demands on families, communities, local mental health workers, and other community agencies (Sealy, 2012). Consequently, as symptoms wax and wane over the course of a chronic mental illness, families, caregivers, and workers in non–health community agencies often experience caregiving fatigue. Despite

---

BOX 5.8 Bridging the Gaps in Inpatient and Outpatient Care

Research Evidence

Well-designed follow-up studies show the following:

- Barriers to mental health services impede access to care.
- Psychological barriers include fear of public rejection (stigmatization) and participant's judgments of the therapist.
- Physical barriers include travel barriers that are caused by restricted finances, physical abilities, geographical location, or personal responsibilities (work, school, childcare).

Preliminary study results suggest that Web- and telephone-based interventions can address a number of barriers to mental health services that are traditionally delivered.

Key Elements of Best Practice

- Distance mental health delivery systems (web- and telephone-based) can be used to overcome physical and psychological access barriers.
- Regardless of service delivery system, establishing an effective therapeutic relationship is critical to the success of therapy.
- People with mental health problems or illness continue to experience social alienation and stigma. Care providers, whether they are providing care in person or in another manner, must be aware of the potential fear of public rejection.
- The ability of the care provider to create an environment with a sense of social presence and belonging is critical to potential success of the interventions.

Reference: Lingley-Pottie, P., McGrath, P., & Andreou, P. (2013). Barriers to mental health care: Perceived delivery system differences. *Advances in Nursing Science, 36*(1), 51–61. doi: 10.1097/ ANS.0b013e31828077eb

---

the challenges for the caregivers, one of the largest hurdles to overcome for people living with a serious and chronic mental illness is finding appropriate housing to meet their immediate social, financial, and safety needs. Compounding this situation is the positive correlation between individuals with severe mental illness, the presence of stigma, and housing instability (Mejia-Lancheros et al., 2021). Most individuals with severe forms of mental illness live in some form of supervised or supported community living situation, which ranges from highly supervised congregate settings to independent apartments. Without the presence of safe, affordable housing, the ability to recover from mental illness is impaired (Centre for Addiction and Mental Health, 2014).

Supported Housing

There has been a paradigm shift from the earlier reliance on the residential continuum to what is now known as supported housing. The focus of supportive housing is on rehabilitation and community integration (Canadian Mental Health Association-Ontario, 2021). **Community-based residential services** provide a place for people to reside during a 24-hour period or any portion of the day on an ongoing basis. A residential facility can be publicly or privately owned. **Intensive residential services** are staffed for patient treatment. These services may include medical, nursing, psychosocial, vocational, recreational, or other support services. Combining residential care and mental health services, this treatment

form offers rehabilitation and therapy to people with serious and persistent mental illnesses, including chronic schizophrenia, bipolar disorder, and unrelenting depression. These services may provide short-term treatment for stays from 24 hours to 3 or 6 months or long-term treatment for several months to years.

Nursing has an important role in the care of people who have severe and persistent mental illnesses and who require long-term stays at residential treatment facilities. Nurses provide PMH nursing care with a focus on psychoeducation, basic social skills training, aggression management, activities of daily living training, and group living. Education on symptom management, understanding mental illnesses, and medication management is essential to recovery. *The Canadian Standards for Psychiatric-Mental Health Nursing* guides the nurse in delivering patient care (Canadian Federation of Mental Health Nurses, 2014) (see Chapter 5).

Supportive Employment

A key component in a comprehensive mental health system is also the provision of supports for employment. Employment is strongly linked to a person's sense of self-worth and personal environment. Having a mental illness increases the risk for reduced employment, sick leave, and reliance on disability benefits (Jarl et al., 2020). **Supportive employment** services assist individuals to find work; assess individuals' skills, attitudes, behaviours, and interest relevant to work; offer vocational rehabilitation or other training; and provide work opportunities. Supportive employment programs—individual placement and support services—are highly individualized and competitive. Service providers deliver on-site support and job-coaching services on a one-to-one basis. They occur in real work settings and are used for patients with severe mental illnesses. The primary focus is to maintain attachment between the person who is mentally ill and the workforce (see Chapter 17).

Acute Inpatient Care

Acute inpatient hospitalization involves the most intensive treatment and is considered the most restrictive setting in the continuum. Inpatient treatment is reserved for patients who are acutely ill who, because of a mental illness, meet one or more of three criteria: high risk for harming oneself, high risk for harming others, or inability to care for one's basic needs. The delivery of inpatient care can occur in a psychiatric hospital or psychiatric unit within a general hospital. Admission to inpatient environments can be voluntary or involuntary (see Chapter 4). Provincial legislation (mental health acts) describes conditions that warrant hospitalization. Length of inpatient stay is kept as short as possible without harmful effects on patient outcomes.

Assertive Community Treatment and Community Treatment Orders

The goal of **assertive community treatment** (ACT) is to "provide intensive treatment, rehabilitation and support services for individuals with serious mental illness and complex needs who find it difficult to engage in other mental health services. The goal is to support these individuals in their recovery and their desire to live in the community" (Canadian Mental Health Association-Toronto, 2012). This treatment approach is used to aid individuals to recover from mental use disorders, including substance use disorders (Penzenstadler et al., 2019). This treatment is provided by multidisciplinary teams who work to support clients in a variety of wellness enhancing activities, such as monitoring medication administration, accompanying individuals to appointments, acting as client advocates, and aiding the individual to develop skills related to activities of daily living. The benefits of ACT approaches are well documented and are identified in the list of recommendations for Canadian practice guidelines for severe and persistent mental illnesses (Addington et al., 2017).

Community treatment orders (CTOs) are included under the ACT umbrella. CTOs are not forms of treatment, *per se*, but are legislative means of ensuring that an individual continues to receive treatment in the community as much as possible. Many Canadian jurisdictions have CTOs included in their mental health legislation.

The criteria for enacting a CTO vary but usually involve an individual who, for whatever reason, has a repeated history of involuntary admissions to hospital under mental health legislation, recovery that allows for hospital discharge, and subsequent treatment nonadherence and mental deterioration while at home, thus necessitating repeated admissions. The individual is considered an involuntary client while under the CTO and certain stipulations are put in place as consequences of nonadherence to treatment (such as readmission to hospital if the person refuses to take prescribed medication). In Canada, CTOs are initiated by clinicians, often psychiatrists, as opposed to the United States where they are ordered by judges. Other countries, such as Britain and Australia, have CTO legislation in place (Canadian Mental Health Association [CMHA], 2012; Jobling, 2014; O'Reilly et al., 2009).

The use of CTOs is well disputed in literature. There is conflicting evidence of their effectiveness in reducing hospital readmission rates (Kallapiran et al., 2010). One recent study found that individuals on CTOs were readmitted more quickly than those who were not on CTOs (Barkhuizen et al., 2020). This could be attributable to the fact that individuals who receive more intensive monitoring have the potential to be identified at an earlier point in a relapse than others. Lengths of stay in hospital have also been studied with variances noted (Awar et al., 2013; Hunt et al., 2007). In terms of treatment, medication adherence appears to be positively correlated with the amount of time one is on a CTO (Maughan et al., 2014). Families tend to be more approving of the use of CTOs versus affected clients, speaking to the challenges that families face in supporting loved ones with severe mental illness. However, the success of CTO use must be considered in terms of its ethics, again with arguments made for and against.

e-Mental Health

The offering of mental health services via electronic means is not entirely new. Christensen et al. (2002, p. 3) defined **e-mental health** as "…mental health services and information delivered or enhanced through the Internet and related technologies." In Canada, the Mental Health Commission of Canada developed a briefing document to guide the incorporation of technology into mental health service delivery (MHCC, 2014). A key component of this transformation was client empowerment as individuals may have greater access to information and peer support through online connections. Mental health interventions are being adapted for online access in, for example, the forms of mobile and smart watch apps, telehealth, games that promote health and wellbeing, learning modules, and virtual reality for role playing scenarios.

While very promising, the use of internet technologies has a number of pragmatic considerations. People need access to computers and internet. According to the *Canadian Internet Use Survey* by Statistics Canada (2019a, 2019b), 94% of Canadian households have internet access. Reasons for not having internet access at home included the cost of internet service and equipment and a lack of internet services in their home community. Healthcare providers require the necessary infrastructure and expertise to operate the technology and their appropriate involvement will need to be considered from a professional regulatory perspective. Certain populations are at greater risk for lacking access. Individuals in rural and remote locations, including communities of Ingenious Peoples, often lack the needed internet bandwidth. Any online supports will also need to take culture into consideration and represent the diversity of the population. The incorporation of these services into the existing mental healthcare delivery structure might meet resistance, particularly from the associated costs. More research is needed into the effectiveness of these approaches as they are integrated into the system. Finally, internet security is a significant concern. Data breaches are ongoing threats to confidentiality and online monitoring of service use could have ethical and legal implications for individuals seeing insurance reimbursement (MHCC, 2014).

An example of an initiative that incorporates e-mental health is the Newfoundland and Labrador Stepped Care 2.0 demonstration project. The goal of this approach is to identify the most appropriate service (and its intensity level) the client needs at a given time and help the individual access these services quickly. After connecting with a healthcare provider, the two collaboratively work on an individualized plan of care that can include brief, (sometimes single session) counseling sessions, peer support, specialist care, and acute care. Some of these interventions can be provided via distance using devices that can utilize the technology. Stepped Care 2.0 aims to distribute care "more impartially and systematically across the whole population to help reach the right balance on wellness promotion, illness prevention, low-intensity supports, recovery-oriented care, intensive treatment, and risk management" (Mental Health Commission of Canada, 2019, p. 9). After evaluating the implementation of the program, the preliminary results were promising. Healthcare providers generally reported positive experiences with e-mental health services, wait times were reduced considerably, and more individuals gained faster access to services.

Summary of Key Points

- The continuum of PMH care must be well integrated within the overall healthcare system and shaped by the principles of primary health care: accessibility, public participation, health promotion, appropriate technology, and intersectoral cooperation.
- The continuum of care is a comprehensive system of services and programs spanning the range from mental health promotion and illness prevention to very specialized services designed to match the needs of the individuals and populations with the appropriate care and treatment, which vary according to levels of service, structure, and intensity of care.
- The nurse's specific responsibilities vary according to the setting. In most settings, nurses function as members of an interprofessional team. Consumers of mental health services and their families should be considered as core members of that team.
- An integrated approach to delivering a patient-centred mental health care is required to ensure effective and efficient services.

Thinking Challenge

Most of the mental health services available are in the community setting. The continuum of care is provided by both professional and nonprofessional healthcare clinicians.

a. What are some of the various nursing roles involved in the continuum of care?
b. How are current trends in psychiatric–mental health care evolving?

Visit thePoint to view suggested responses. Go to **thePoint.lww.com/activate** and use the activation code found in the front of this text to unlock answers to the "Thinking Challenges" and other online resources.

Web Links

https://cmha.ca The Canadian Mental Health Association advocates leadership by the federal and provincial governments to ensure equitable access to services and treatment across Canada.

https://hc-sc.gc.ca The Health Canada website provides current information about federal initiatives in mental health policy and practice.

https://mindyourmind.ca This is a website for youth, young adults, and the professionals who work with them to access information about resources and tools related to mental health and mental illness. These resources are designed to reduce the stigma associated with mental illness and increase access and use of community support, both professional and peer-based.

References

Addington, D., Anderson, E., Kelly, M., Lesage, A., & Summerville, C. (2017). Canadian practice guidelines for comprehensive community treatment for schizophrenia and schizophrenia spectrum disorders. *The Canadian Journal of Psychiatry, 62*(9), 662–672.

Awar, M. A., Jaffar, K., & Roberts, P. (2013). Effectiveness of the community treatment order in streamlining psychiatric services. *Journal of Mental Health, 22*(2), 191–197.

Barkhuizen, W., Cullen, A. E., Shetty, H., Pritchard, M., Stewart, R., McGuire, P., & Patel, R. (2020). Community treatment orders and associations with readmission rates and duration of psychiatric hospital admission: A controlled electronic case register study. *BMJ Open, 10*, e035121.

Canadian Federation of Mental Health Nurses. (2014). *Canadian standards of psychiatric and mental health nursing: Standards of practice* (4th ed.). http://cfmhn.ca/professionalPractices?f=7458545122100118.pdf&n=212922-CFMHN-standards-rv-3a.pdf&inline=yes

Canadian Mental Health Association. (2012). *Community committal.* https://www.cmha.ca/public_policy/community-committal/#.VXncFGDDlGg

Canadian Mental Health Association-Ontario. (2021). *Types of housing.* https://ontario.cmha.ca/documents/types-of-housing/

Canadian Mental Health Association-Toronto. (2012). *Assertive community treatment (ACT) teams.* https://toronto.cmha.ca/programs-services/assertive-community-treatment-act-teams/

Canadian Nurses Association. (2012). *Position statement on mental health services.*

Canadian Public Health Association. (2021). *A Public Health Approach to Population Mental Wellness.* https://www.cpha.ca/public-health-approach-population-mental-wellness

Centre for Addictions and Mental Health. (2014). *Housing policy framework.*

Christensen, H., Griffiths, K., & Evans, K. (2002). *E-mental health in Australia: Implications of the internet and related technologies for policy.* Commonwealth Department of Health and Ageing.

Emergency Management Policy and Outreach Directorate. (2017). *An emergency management framework for Canada* (3rd ed.). https://www.publicsafety.gc.ca/cnt/rsrcs/pblctns/2017-mrgnc-mngmnt-frmwrk/2017-mrgnc-mngmnt-frmwrk-en.pdf

Evidence Exchange Network for Mental Health and Addictions. (2017). *Effective care coordination approaches for individuals with mental health and substance use concerns.* Provincial System Support Program & Centre for Addictions and Mental Health. https://www.eenet.ca/resource/effective-care-coordination-approaches-individuals-mental-health-and-substance-use-concerns

Hair, H., Shortall, R., & Oldford, J. (2013). Where's help when we need it? Developing responsive and effective brief counseling services for children, adolescents, and their families. *Social Work in Mental Health, 11*(1), 16–33. https://doi.org/10.1080/15332985.2012.716389

Health Canada. (2021). *Emergency preparedness.* https://www.canada.ca/en/health-canada/services/health-concerns/emergencies-disasters/emergency-preparedness.html

Huang, C., Plummer, V., Lam, L., & Cross, W. (2020). Perceptions of shared decision-making in severe mental illness: An integrative review. *Journal of Psychiatric and Mental Health Nursing, 27*, 103–127.

Hunt, A. M., daSilva, A., Lurie, S., & Goldbloom, D. S. (2007). Community treatment orders in Toronto: The emerging data. *The Canadian Journal of Psychiatry, 52*(10), 647–656.

Jarl, J., Linder, A., Busch, H., Nyberg, A., & Gerdtham, U. (2020). Heterogeneity in the associations between common mental disorders and labour outcomes—A population study from southern Sweden. *BMC Public Health, 20*, 1285–1297

Jobling, H. (2014). Using ethnography to explore causality in mental health policy and practice. *Qualitative Social Work, 13*(1), 49–68.

Kallapiran, K., Sankaranarayanan, A., & Lewin, T. (2010). A pilot investigation of the relationship between community treatment orders and hospital utilization rates. *Australasian Psychiatry, 18*(6), 503–505.

Kates, N., Mazowita, G., Lemire, F., Jayabarathan, A., Bland, R., Selby, P., & Audet, D. (2011). The evolution of collaborative mental health care in Canada: A shared vision for the future. *The Canadian Journal of Psychiatry, 56*(5), 1–10.

Kathol, R., Perez, R., & Cohen, J. (2010). *The integrated case management manual.* Springer Publishing Company.

Kingston, M. A., & Greenwood, S. (2020). Therapeutic relationships: Making space to practice in chaotic institutional environments. *Journal of Psychiatric and Mental Health Nursing, 27*, 689–698.

Lingley-Pottie, P., McGrath, P., & Andreou, P. (2013). Barriers to mental health care: Perceived delivery system differences. *Advances in Nursing Science, 36*(1), 51–61. https://doi.org/10.1097/ANS0b013e31828077eb

Maughan, D., Molodynski, A., Rugkåsa, J., & Burns, T. (2014). A systematic review of the effect of community treatment orders on service use. *Social Psychiatry and Psychiatric Epidemiology, 49*, 651–663.

Mejia-Lancheros, C., Lachaud, J., Woodhall-Melnik, J., O'Campoa, P., Hwang, S. W., & Stergiopoulos, V. (2021). Longitudinal interrelationships of mental health discrimination and stigma with housing and well-being outcomes in adults with mental illness and recent experience of homelessness. *Social Science and Medicine, 268*, 113463. https://doi.org/10.1016/j.socscimed.2020.113463

Mental Health Commission of Canada. (2012). *Changing directions, changing lives: The mental health strategy for Canada.*

Mental Health Commission of Canada. (2014). *E-mental health in Canada: Transforming the mental health system using technology.* https://www.mentalhealthcommission.ca/sites/default/files/MHCC_E-Mental_Health-Briefing_Document_ENG_0.pdf

Mental Health Commission of Canada. (2015). *Guidelines for recovery-oriented practice, Hope, Dignity, Inclusion.*

Mental Health Commission of Canada. (2016). *Advancing the mental health strategy for Canada: A framework for action (2017–2022).*

Mental Health Commission of Canada. (2019). *Newfoundland and Labrador Stepped Care 2.0 e-mental health demonstration project.*

Mental Health Commission of Canada. (2021). *What is recovery?*

National Alliance on Mental Health. (2018). *Navigating mental health crisis: A NAMI resource guide for those experiencing a mental health emergency.*

Newman, D., O'Reilly, P. L., Lee, S. H., & Kennedy, D. (2015). Mental health service users' experiences of mental health care: An integrative literature review. *Journal of Psychiatric and Mental Health Nursing, 22*, 171–182. https://doi.org/10.1111/jpm.12202View

O'Reilly, R. L., Brooks, S. A., Chaimowitz, G. A., Neilson, G. E., Carr, P. E., Zikos, E., Leichner, P. P., & Beck, P. R. (2009). *CPA position paper: Mandatory outpatient treatment.* http://publications.cpa-apc.org/media.php?mid=912

Pan, K. Y., Kok, A. A. L., Eikelenboom, M., Horsfall, M., Jorg, F., Luteijn, R. A., et al. (2020). The mental health impact of the COVID-19 pandemic on people with and without depressive, anxiety, or obsessive-compulsive disorders: A longitudinal study of three Dutch case-control cohorts. *The Lancet Psychiatry, 8*(2), P121–P129.

Penzenstadler, L., Soares, C., Anci, E., Molodynski, A., & Khazaal, Y. (2019). Effect of assertive community treatment for patients with substance use disorder: A systematic review, *European Addiction Research, 25*, 56–67.

Pfefferbaum, B., & North, C. S. (2020). Mental health and the COVID-19 pandemic. *The New England Journal of Medicine, 383*, 510–512.

Sealy, P. (2012). The impact of the process of deinstitutionalization of mental health services in Canada: An increase in accessing of health professionals for mental health concerns. *Social Work in Public Health, 27*(3), 229–237. https://doi.org/10.1080/19371911003748786

Statistics Canada. (2019a). *Mental health care needs, 2018.* https://www150.statcan.gc.ca/n1/pub/82-625-x/2019001/article/00011-eng.htm

Statistics Canada. (2019b). *The Canadian internet use survey.* https://www150.statcan.gc.ca/n1/daily-quotidien/191029/dq191029a-eng.htm

Victoria Government. (2021). *Mental health services-case managers.* https://www.betterhealth.vic.gov.au/health/ConditionsAndTreatments/mental-health-services-case-managers

Wang, J. Z., Mott, S., Magwood, O., Matthew, C., Mclellan, A., Kpade, V., Gaba, P., Kozloff, N., Pottie, K., & Andermann, A. (2019). The impact of interventions for youth experiencing homelessness on housing mental health, substance abuse, and family cohesion: A systematic review. *BMC Public Health, 19*, 1528–1550.

World Health Organization. (2002). *Prevention and promotion in mental health.*

World Health Organization. (2008b). *The world health report 2008: Primary health care—Now more than ever.*

World Health Organization. (2010). *Framework for action on interprofessional education and collaborative practice.*

World Health Organization. (2013). *The world health report 2013: Research for universal health coverage.*

World Health Organization. (2021). *What are integrated people-centered health services?* https://www.who.int/servicedeliverysafety/areas/people-centred-care/ipchs-what/en/

https://www.mind.org.uk This is the website of Mind, the leading mental health charity in England and Wales. Inspiring the development of quality services that reflect expressed need and diversity is among its objectives.

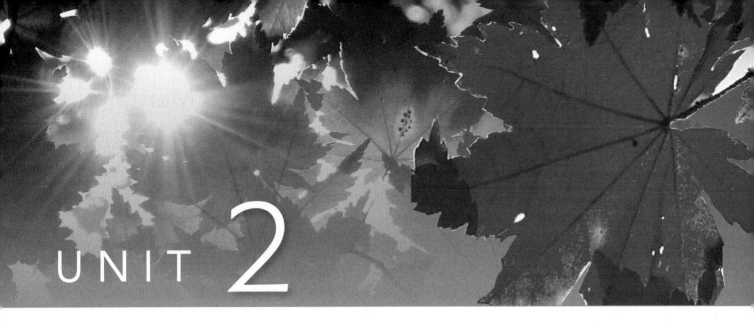

UNIT 2

Foundations
of Psychiatric and Mental Health Nursing Practice

Contemporary Psychiatric and Mental Health Nursing Practice

Carmen Hust and Cindy Peternelj-Taylor*

After studying this chapter, you will be able to:

- Explain the bio/psycho/social/spiritual model as a conceptual framework for understanding and responding to mental health problems and disorders.
- Explain the scope of psychiatric and mental health nursing practice.
- Classify current and emerging roles and responsibilities of psychiatric and mental health nurses across Canada.
- Describe entry-to-practice mental health nursing competencies.
- Discuss the role of standards of practice for Canadian nurses.
- Specify six key components of psychiatric and mental health nursing.
- Discuss current challenges of psychiatric and mental health nursing.
- Identify national and international organizations with relevance to psychiatric and mental health nursing practice.

- clinical decision-making • collaborative care • critical pathways • domains of practice • e-Mental health • harm reduction • recovery model • trauma-informed care

- bio/psycho/social/spiritual model • competency • standards of practice

This chapter introduces the bio/psycho/social/spiritual model as an approach to understanding human health that informs psychiatric and mental health (PMH) nursing practice. The scope of PMH nursing is explained, entry-to-practice competencies for mental health nursing outlined, and standards of practice explicitly describing the obligations of nurses in Canadian PMH care settings presented. The discussion of the challenges of PMH nursing sets the stage for the rest of the textbook through an overview of the dynamic nature of this aspect of nursing.

The Bio/Psycho/Social/Spiritual Model

Contemporary PMH nursing uses theories from the biologic, psychological, and social sciences as a basis of practice, as well as knowledge of the spiritual aspects of human life. This holistic approach, referred to as the bio/psycho/social/spiritual model, is necessary to guide understanding of the individual who is experiencing mental health problems or a mental disorder. Holism joins the biologic, psychological, social, and spiritual domains in an integrated, dynamic conceptualization of human health. The model provides a basis for the organization of nursing care and is used throughout this text for integrating theoretic knowledge and the nursing process (Fig. 6.1).

KEY CONCEPT

The bio/psycho/social/spiritual model consists of separate but interacting domains that can be understood independently but that are interdependent with the other domains.

Biologic Domain

The *biologic* domain consists of the biologic theories related to mental disorders and problems as well as all of the biologic processes related to other health problems.

---

*Adapted from the chapter "Contemporary Psychiatric and Mental Health Nursing Practice" by Wendy Austin.

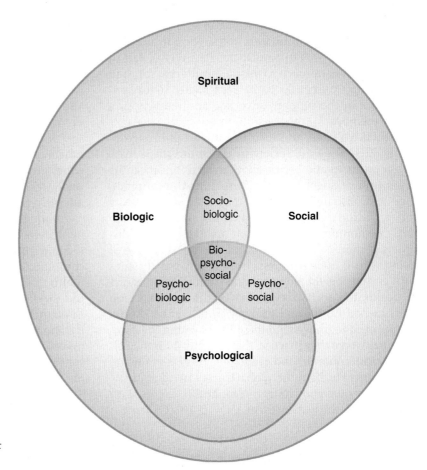

Figure 6.1 Bio/psycho/social/spiritual model of psychiatric and mental health nursing. (Adapted from Abraham, I., Fox, J., & Cohen, B. (1992). Integrating the bio into the biopsychosocial: Understanding and treating biological phenomena in psychiatric–mental health nursing. *Archives of Psychiatric Nursing, 6*(5), 296–305.)

For instance, there is evidence of neurobiologic changes in some mental disorders that informs our understanding of possible causes and/or presentation of those disorders. Within this domain, theories and concepts shape interventions that focus on an individual's physical functioning, such as exercise, relaxation, sleep, and nutrition. Neurobiologic theories inform understanding of such biologic treatments as pharmacologic agents and electroconvulsive therapy (ECT) (see Chapter 13).

Psychological Domain

The *psychological* domain contains the theoretical basis of the psychological processes: thoughts, feelings, and behaviours (intrapersonal dynamics) that influence one's emotions, cognitions, and actions. The psychological and nursing sciences generate theories and research that are critical to understanding an individual's symptoms and responses to mental disorders. Although some mental disorders have been found to have a biologic component, symptoms manifest in the psychological domain. The person with a thought disorder may express atypical behaviour that can be interpreted within the context of the neurobiologic dysfunction of the mental disorder.

Many PMH nursing interventions are based on knowledge generated within this domain, such as cognitive approaches, behavioural therapies, and client education. These interventions are explained in Unit 3 of this textbook. PMH interventions are also based on the use of interpersonal communication techniques, which require nurses to develop awareness of their own, as well as their client's, internal thoughts, feelings, and behaviours. Such understanding is necessary for the development of therapeutic relationships and for helping clients learn about their lived experience and to participate in their treatment and its management. Motivating clients to engage in learning activities occurs within the context of a therapeutic relationship (see Chapter 7).

Social Domain

The *social* domain includes theories that account for the influence of social forces (including economic, political, and cultural forces) encompassing the client, family, and community. This knowledge base is generated from social and nursing sciences and delineates the connections within families and communities that affect the health and treatment of people with mental disorders. Understanding family factors, including origin, extended family, and other significant relationships, contributes to the total understanding and treatment of individual clients. Family-based interventions can reduce rates of relapse, improve client recovery, and improve the wellbeing of their family (MacCourt et al., 2013). Families need to receive information and support in addition to services if they are to participate effectively as part of a collaborative approach to mental health care for their relative (MacCourt et al., 2013). See Chapter 16 for families' roles in the support, advocacy, and recovery of a family member.

Mental disorders and their treatment can be significantly affected by the society in which the client lives. Public attitudes and beliefs about mental illness can be supportive or stigmatizing and isolating due to prejudice and discrimination (see Fig. 6.2). Community forces, including cultural and ethnic groups within larger communities, shape clients' manifestation of disorders, response to treatment, and overall experience of living with a mental illness. Community-based issues such as housing, employment opportunities, and access to health and social services have a broad impact on both mental health and recovery from mental illness. Nurses need to understand these forces within the communities where they practice. (See Chapter 4 for the cultural, socioeconomic, and geographic context of mental health care.) Furthermore, global forces can significantly affect individual and family mental health, as seen with the negative consequences of COVID-19 (Gaderman et al., 2021).

Spiritual Domain

The spiritual domain encompasses the bio/psycho/social domains. Spirituality relates to the core of whom we are; one definition of spirituality is "the essence of our being, which permeates our living and infuses our unfolding awareness of who and what we are, our purpose in being, and our inner resources; and shapes our life journey" (Dossey et al., 2004, p. 91). Spirituality

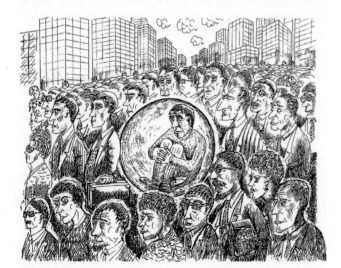

Figure 6.2 Negative public attitudes and beliefs about mental illness can stigmatize and isolate people with mental health problems. (Drawing by Al Mier. Used with permission.)

comprises the connections within and among self, others, and the universe over time and space. Spirituality is a complex, even mysterious, concept: it may be regarded as the driving force that pervades all aspects of and gives meaning to an individual's life. Hope, trust, reconciliation, and inspiration are associated with the spiritual domain (Barss, 2012). Spiritual activity involves introspection, reflection, and a sense of connectedness to others or to the universe. For many people, this connectedness focuses ultimately on a Supreme Being. God, Allah, Jehovah, and Creator are among the names that refer to a worshipped Supreme Being.

Although there remains a lack of agreement concerning the way spirituality should be defined, a review of the interprofessional literature on spirituality reveals common themes: everyone has the potential for spirituality and spiritual growth; the way one lives one's life is reflective of spirituality; spirituality is relational in nature; and there is a link among religion, spirituality, and moral norms (Catalano, 2015). Religion differs, however, from spirituality. Religion involves organized systems of rituals, patterns of beliefs, and groups of people usually congregating around the worship of a deity. A religious person may or may not be spiritual; a person's spirituality may or may not involve religion.

Spiritual growth may be stimulated by pivotal life events, including distressing ones like being diagnosed with a mental disorder. It can be difficult, however, to transcend one's current reality and the suffering it may entail. Individuals living with a mental illness often struggle with loss of meaning and purpose and wonder, "Why has this happened to me?" They may be affected by religious or cultural beliefs that view mental illness as a form of punishment. The nurse can help those who are experiencing spiritual distress by supporting their efforts to find meaning in their circumstances, which may include meditation, contemplation, prayer, and other spiritual practices that may give comfort. The relationship of the body, mind, and spirit in the context of human health is holistic, synergistic, and unifying. It is central to the process of recovery and wellbeing. Including the spiritual domain in care planning is the responsibility of the healthcare team (Michael, 2019; Saiz et al., 2021).

Entry-to-Practice Mental Health Competencies

Nursing education is guided in part by the practice competencies expected of a credentialed nurse upon entry to practice. The competencies are identifiable, measurable descriptions of the knowledge, skills, and attitudes deemed essential to the particular nursing role (e.g., registered nurse, registered psychiatric nurse, licensed/registered practical nurse [LPNs/RPNs], nurse practitioner [RN-NP], and more recently nurse authorized prescriber [RN-AP]). These regulated designations delineate roles and mandates in each province where the regulated mental health professional is practicing. Almost (2021) notes the importance of recognizing nursing as a nonhomogeneous group and the centrality of intraprofessional education for collaboration and practice. As students study and gain practice experiences, the entry-to-practice competencies of their future occupation are helpful guides. Those of Canadian registered nurses (RNs) and RPNs follow. The competency profiles for LPNs/RPNs are delineated by provincial and territorial jurisdictions. These can be located through the Canadian Council for Practical Nurse Regulators (CCPNR) (see Web Links). The scope of practice for nurse practitioners is also outlined by provincial and territorial jurisdictions. Typically, the role of the RN (NP) has a broader scope of practice, in which the nurse can independently prescribe medication and order and manage the results of screening and diagnostic tests. An emerging role for RNs in Canada is that of the RN-AP in which the RN with a specific scope of practice can prescribe certain medications or order and receive diagnostic tests in the specific area of practice (College of Registered Nurses of Manitoba, 2021). This evolving nursing role in response to increased healthcare needs across Canada stirred the Canadian Nurses Association (CNA) to develop the RN Prescribing Framework to guide the implementation of Authorized Prescribing regulation (CNA, 2015).

KEY CONCEPT

Competencies are a set of specific areas of competence that accord a person the capability to act appropriately and effectively in a role. Competencies involve the effective use of internal resources (e.g., knowledge, skills, attitudes) and external resources (e.g., policies, interprofessional and intraprofessional teams, research).

CASN/CFMHN Entry-to-Practice Mental Health and Addiction Competencies

The competencies expected of all Canadian RNs upon entry to practice have been delineated by the Canadian Association of Schools of Nursing (CASN) in partnership with the Canadian Federation of Mental Health Nurses (CFMHN). *Entry-to-Practice Mental Health and Addiction Competencies for Undergraduate Nursing Education in Canada* (CASN with CFMHN, 2015) is a national framework that outlines essential knowledge, attitudes, and skills all RNs should possess as they begin to practice. The competencies are organized within domains (identified by provincial/territorial nursing regulatory bodies) along with achievement indicators. See Boxes 6.1 to 6.5.

BOX 6.1 **CASN and CFMHN Entry-to-Practice Mental Health and Addiction Competencies for Undergraduate Nursing Education in Canada**

DOMAIN 1 PROFESSIONAL RESPONSIBILITY AND ACCOUNTABILITY

Competency 1

The nurse provides care in accordance with professional and regulatory standards when promoting mental health and preventing or managing mental health conditions and/or addiction.

Indicators

1.1 Understands and applies mental health–related legislation, and upholds the rights and autonomy of persons with a mental health condition and/or addiction.

1.2 Therapeutically engages with persons experiencing a mental health condition and/or addiction, with dignity and respect.

1.3 Recognizes stigmatizing and discriminating attitudes regarding mental health conditions and addiction in healthcare professionals and/or

self, as well as the detrimental impact of such attitudes on healthcare outcomes and responds therapeutically.

1.4 Applies policies related to principles of health promotion and prevention of injury (i.e., least restraint) in caring for persons with a mental health condition and/or addiction.

1.5 Demonstrates knowledge related to the process of voluntary and involuntary care.

1.6 Protects clients, self, and others from harm in situations where a person with a mental health condition and/or addiction poses a safety risk while maintaining the client's dignity and human rights.

Canadian Association of Schools of Nursing with the Canadian Federation of Mental Health Nurses. (2015). *Entry to practice mental health and addiction competencies for undergraduate education in Canada.* Canadian Association of Schools of Nursing. Used with permission.

BOX 6.2 CASN and CFMHN Entry-to-Practice Mental Health and Addiction Competencies for Undergraduate Nursing Education in Canada

DOMAIN 2 KNOWLEDGE-BASED PRACTICE

Competency 2

The nurse uses relational practice to conduct a person-focused mental health assessment and develops a plan of care in collaboration with the person, family, and health team to promote recovery.

Indicators

Knowledge

2.1 Demonstrates an understanding of the concepts of mental health, developmental, and situational transitions and the spectrum of mental health conditions and addictions as they are manifested in individuals across the life span.

2.2 Demonstrates an understanding of how mental health comorbidities increase severity, levels of disability, and use of mental health services.

2.3 Describes key elements of relevant theories, including but not limited to stress, coping, adaptation, development, harm reduction, crisis intervention, recovery, loss, and grief, and articulates their implications for clinical practice.

2.4 Demonstrates knowledge of the possible effects of complementary therapies on mental health conditions and addiction.

2.5 Understands the complex interrelationship of physiology, pathophysiology, and mental health (e.g., neuroleptic malignant syndrome, delirium, hypertension, etc.).

2.6 Demonstrates knowledge of medications used to treat addiction and withdrawal, including opiate replacement medications.

Assessment

2.7 Conducts a mental status examination.

2.8 Uses a range of relational and therapeutic skills including listening, respect, empathy, reaffirmation, mutuality, and sensitivity in assessments and care planning for persons experiencing a mental health condition and/or addiction.

2.9 Demonstrates the ability to identify clients' emotional, cognitive, and behavioural states, as well as level of anxiety, crisis states, indices of aggression, self-harm, suicide, risk to others, competency to care for self, and signs of substance abuse, addiction, and withdrawal.

Planning Care

2.10 Plans care in partnership with clients to promote mental health, prevent a mental health condition and addiction, minimize negative effects on physical health, manage or reduce symptoms of mental health conditions, and foster recovery and resilience.

2.11 Recognizes the role of social determinants of health on mental health outcomes and incorporates this when planning care of persons experiencing a mental health condition and/or addiction.

2.12 Uses a trauma-informed approach to plan care and recognizes the negative effects of violence, abuse, racism, discrimination, colonization, poverty, homelessness, and early childhood maltreatment (such as neglect) on mental health.

Competency 3

Provides and evaluates person-centred nursing care in partnership with persons experiencing a mental health condition and/or addiction, along the continuum of care and across the life span.

Indicators

3.1 Communicates therapeutically with persons and families who are experiencing a range of mental health conditions and/or addiction, abuse, bereavement, or crisis.

3.2 Uses self therapeutically in providing health-promoting, preventive, and supportive care for persons experiencing a mental health condition and/or addiction.

3.3 Engages clients in strengths-based care that promotes resilience.

3.4 Advocates for persons experiencing a mental health condition and/or addiction.

3.5 Demonstrates basic knowledge of psychobiology in relation to psychopharmacology and the therapeutic dose range, side effects, interactions, and adverse effects of psychotropic medications across the life span.

3.6 Engages individuals and families in learning about a mental health condition and/or addiction and its management.

3.7 Provides care to persons experiencing a mental health condition and/or addiction that is recovery oriented and trauma-informed and uses principles of harm reduction and addresses social determinants of health.

3.8 Administers medication used to treat a mental health condition and/or addiction safely; monitors clients for therapeutic effects, side effects, and adverse reactions to medications; and intervenes effectively when side effects and adverse effects of medications occur.

Canadian Association of Schools of Nursing with the Canadian Federation of Mental Health Nurses. (2015). *Entry to practice mental health and addiction competencies for undergraduate education in Canada.* Canadian Association of Schools of Nursing. Used with permission.

BOX 6.3 CASN and CFMHN Entry-to-Practice Mental Health and Addiction Competencies for Undergraduate Nursing Education in Canada

DOMAIN 3 ETHICAL PRACTICE

Competency 4
Acts in accordance with the CNA Code of Ethics when working with persons experiencing a mental health condition and/or addiction

Indicators
4.1 Provides a safe and respectful environment to voluntary and involuntary clients seeking or receiving treatment for a mental health condition and/or addiction.

4.2 Assists persons with a mental health condition and/or addiction in making informed decisions about their health care and symptom management.

4.3 Demonstrates cultural competency and cultural safety when caring for diverse persons with a mental health condition and/or addiction.

Canadian Association of Schools of Nursing with the Canadian Federation of Mental Health Nurses. (2015). *Entry to practice mental health and addiction competencies for undergraduate education in Canada.* Canadian Association of Schools of Nursing. Used with permission.

BOX 6.4 CASN and CFMHN Entry-to-Practice Mental Health and Addiction Competencies for Undergraduate Nursing Education in Canada

DOMAIN 4 SERVICE TO THE PUBLIC

Competency 5
The nurse works collaboratively with partners to promote mental health and advocate for improvements in health services for persons experiencing a mental health condition and/or addiction.

Indicators
5.1 Demonstrates knowledge of the healthcare system in order to contribute to the improvement of mental health and addiction services.

5.2 Recognizes the impact of the organizational culture on the provision of mental health care to persons experiencing mental health conditions and addiction, and acts to ensure appropriate services are delivered safely.

5.3 Facilitates and engages in collaborative, inter- and intraprofessional, and intersectoral practice when providing care for persons with a mental health condition and/or addiction.

Canadian Association of Schools of Nursing (CASN) with the Canadian Federation of Mental Health Nurses (CFMHN). (2015). *Entry to practice mental health and addiction competencies for undergraduate education in Canada.* Canadian Association of Schools of Nursing. Used with permission.

BOX 6.5 CASN and CFMHN Entry-to-Practice Mental Health and Addiction Competencies for Undergraduate Nursing Education in Canada

DOMAIN 5 SELF-REGULATION

Competency 6
Develops and maintains competencies through self-reflection and new opportunities working with persons experiencing a mental health condition and/or addiction

Indicators
6.1 Evaluates one's individual practice and knowledge when providing care to persons with a mental health condition and/or addiction, and seeks help as required.

6.2 Identifies one's own morals, values, attitudes, beliefs, and experiences related to mental health conditions and/or addiction and the effect these may have on care.

6.3 Identifies learning needs related to mental health conditions and addiction.

6.4 Seeks new knowledge, skills, and supports related to mental health conditions and addiction.

6.5 Evaluates self-learning related to mental health conditions and addiction.

Canadian Association of Schools of Nursing (CASN) with the Canadian Federation of Mental Health Nurses (CFMHN). (2015). *Entry to practice mental health and addiction competencies for undergraduate education in Canada.* Canadian Association of Schools of Nursing. Used with permission.

Registered Psychiatric Nursing Entry-to-Practice Competencies

The client-centred competency framework for RPNs was approved by the Registered Psychiatric Nurse Regulators of Canada (RPNRC) in 2014. There are seven categories with key and enabling competencies. The competencies are considered equal in importance and are to be viewed as an integrated whole. Evolving these competencies and acquiring further ones occur in practice and through orientation, continuing education, and professional development (RPNRC, 2014). Along with the approved standards of practice and code of ethics, the competencies delineate the safe, competent, and ethical practice expected of RPNs in Canada. See Boxes 6.6 to 6.12.

BOX 6.6 **Registered Psychiatric Nurses Entry-to-Practice Competencies**

Competency 1

Therapeutic Relationships and Therapeutic Use of Self

Therapeutic use of self is the foundational instrument that registered psychiatric nurses use to establish therapeutic relationships with clients to deliver care and psychosocial interventions.

1.1 Apply therapeutic use of self to inform all areas of psychiatric nursing practice.

1.1.1 Utilize one's personality consciously and with full awareness in an attempt to establish relationships.

1.1.2 Assess and clarify the influences of one's personal beliefs, values, and life experiences on interactions.

1.1.3 Differentiate between a therapeutic relationship and a social, romantic, sexual relationship.

1.1.4 Recognize, identify, and validate the feelings of others.

1.1.5 Recognize and address the impact of transference and countertransference in the therapeutic relationship.

1.1.6 Demonstrate unconditional positive regard, empathy, and congruence in relationships.

1.1.7 Monitor the communication process and adapt communication strategies accordingly by using a variety of verbal and nonverbal communication skills.

1.1.8 Critique the effectiveness of therapeutic use of self on others.

1.1.9 Engage in personal and professional development activities to enhance the therapeutic use of self.

1.1.10 Engage in self-care activities to decrease the risk of secondary trauma and burnout.

1.2 Establish a therapeutic relationship with the client.

1.2.1 Develop a rapport and promote trust through mutual respect, genuineness, empathy, acceptance, and collaboration.

1.2.2 Establish and negotiate boundaries (e.g., role and service offered, length and frequency of meetings, responsibilities) to clarify the nature, content, and limits of the therapeutic relationship.

1.2.3 Engage with the client to explore goals, learning, and growth needs (e.g., problem identification, thought exploration, feelings, and behaviours).

1.2.4 Differentiate between therapeutic and nontherapeutic communication techniques.

1.2.5 Apply therapeutic communication strategies and techniques to reduce emotional distress, facilitate cognitive and behavioural change, and foster personal growth (e.g., active listening, clarifying, restating, reflecting, focusing, exploring, therapeutic use of silence).

1.3 Maintain the therapeutic relationship.

1.3.1 Engage in ongoing assessment, planning, implementation, and evaluation over the course of the psychiatric nurse–client relationship.

1.3.2 Apply strategies, techniques, and resources to meet client goals (e.g., conflict resolution, crisis intervention, counseling, clinically appropriate use of self-disclosure).

1.3.3 Collaborate with the client to help achieve client-identified goals.

1.3.4 Adapt therapeutic strategies when encountering resistance and ambivalence.

1.3.5 Provide teaching and coaching around client goals and evaluate learning.

1.3.6 Dedicate time to maintain the relationship with the client.

1.3.7 Engage in systematic review of progress with the client.

1.3.8 Address the impact of transference and countertransference in the therapeutic relationship.

1.3.9 Engage in consultation to facilitate, support, and enhance the therapeutic use of self.

BOX 6.6 Registered Psychiatric Nurses Entry-to-Practice Competencies (*Continued*)

1.4 Terminate the therapeutic relationship.

1.4.1 Identify the end point of the therapeutic relationship.

1.4.2 Summarize the outcomes of the therapeutic relationship with the client.

1.4.3 Evaluate the therapeutic process and outcomes of the interventions.

1.4.4 Establish the boundaries of the posttherapeutic relationship.

1.4.5 Determine the need for follow-up and establish referral(s) accordingly.

Registered Psychiatric Nurse Regulators of Canada. (2014). *Registered psychiatric nurse-entry level competencies.* Used with permission.

BOX 6.7 Registered Psychiatric Nurses Entry-to-Practice Competencies

Competency 2

Body of Knowledge and Application

Registered psychiatric nurses' practice is composed of foundational nursing knowledge and specialized psychiatric nursing knowledge. RPNs integrate general nursing knowledge and knowledge from the sciences, humanities, research, ethics, spirituality, and relational practice with specialized knowledge drawn from the fields of psychiatry and mental health. RPNs use critical inquiry and apply a decision-making process in providing psychiatric nursing care for clients. There are two categories under this competency: evidence-informed knowledge and application of body of knowledge.

Evidence: Informed Knowledge

2.1 Demonstrate knowledge of the health sciences, including anatomy, physiology, microbiology, nutrition, pathophysiology, psychopharmacology, pharmacology, epidemiology, genetics, and prenatal and genetic influences on development.

2.2 Demonstrate knowledge of social sciences and humanities, including psychology, sociology, human growth and development, communication, statistics, research methodology, philosophy, ethics, spiritual care, determinants of health, and primary health care.

2.3 Demonstrate knowledge of nursing science: conceptual nursing models, nursing skills, procedures, and interventions.

2.4 Demonstrate knowledge of current and emerging health issues (e.g., end-of-life care, substance use, vulnerable or marginalized populations).

2.5 Demonstrate knowledge of community, global, and population health issues (e.g., immunization, disaster planning, pandemics).

2.6 Demonstrate knowledge of applicable informatics and emerging technologies.

2.7 **Demonstrate evidence-informed knowledge of psychopathology across the life span.**

2.7.1 Demonstrate knowledge of disorders of developmental health and mental health.

2.7.2 Demonstrate knowledge of resources and diagnostic tools (e.g., standardized assessment scales, the *Diagnostic and Statistical Manual of Mental Disorders*).

2.8 **Demonstrate knowledge of the disorders of addiction, as well as relevant resources and diagnostic tools (e.g., standardized screening tools, detoxification, and withdrawal guidelines).**

2.9 **Demonstrate knowledge of therapeutic modalities (e.g., individual, family, and group therapy and counseling, psychopharmacology, visualization, consumer-led initiatives).**

2.10 **Demonstrate knowledge of how complementary therapies can impact treatment (e.g., naturopathy, acupuncture).**

2.11 **Demonstrate knowledge of conceptual models of psychiatric care (e.g., trauma-informed care, recovery model, psychosocial rehabilitation).**

2.12 **Demonstrate evidence-informed knowledge of the impact of social, cultural, and family systems on health outcomes.**

2.13 **Demonstrate knowledge of interpersonal communication, therapeutic use of self, and therapeutic relationships.**

2.14 **Demonstrate knowledge of the dynamic of interpersonal abuse (e.g., child, spousal, or elder abuse).**

(Continued)

2.15 Demonstrate knowledge of mental health legislation and other relevant legislation (e.g., privacy laws).

Application of Body of Knowledge

2.16 Conduct a comprehensive client assessment.

2.16.1 Select an evidence-informed framework applicable to the type of assessments required (e.g., biopsychosocial, cultural model, community assessment model, multigenerational family assessment).

2.16.2 Perform holistic assessment (e.g., physical, mental, social, spiritual, developmental, and cultural).

2.16.3 Perform an in-depth psychiatric evaluation (e.g., suicide, history of violence, trauma, stress, mental status, self-perception, adaptation and coping, substance use and abuse).

2.16.4 Collaborate with the client to identify health strengths and goals.

2.17 Formulate a clinical judgment based on the assessment data (e.g., nursing care focus, psychiatric nursing diagnosis).

2.17.1 Identify psychiatric signs and symptoms that are commonly associated with psychiatric disorders, using current nomenclature (e.g., the *Diagnostic and Statistical Manual of Mental Disorders*).

2.17.2 Identify clinical indicators that may negatively impact the client's wellbeing (e.g., pain, hyperglycemia, hypertension).

2.17.3 Incorporate data from other sources (e.g., laboratory tests, collateral information).

2.17.4 Use critical thinking to analyze and synthesize data collected to arrive at a clinical judgment.

2.18 Collaborate with the client to develop a treatment plan to address identified problems, minimize the development of complications, and promote functions and quality of life.

2.18.1 Discuss interventions with the client to achieve client-directed goals and outcomes (e.g., promote health, prevent disorder and injury, foster rehabilitation, and provide palliation).

2.18.2 Plan care using treatment modalities such as psychotherapy and psychopharmacology.

2.18.3 Propose a plan for self-care that promotes client responsibility and independence to the maximum degree possible (e.g., relaxation techniques, stress management, coping skills, community resources, complementary and alternative therapies).

2.19 Implement a variety of psychiatric nursing interventions with the client, according to the plan of care.

2.19.1 Assess the ethical and legal implications of the interventions before providing care.

2.19.2 Perform required nursing interventions to address physical conditions, including, but not limited to, intravenous therapy and drainage tubes, skin and wound care, metabolic screening, and management of withdrawal symptoms.

2.19.3 Perform safe medication administration by a variety of methods (e.g., oral, parenteral).

2.19.4 Provide complex psychiatric nursing interventions (e.g., facilitating group process, conflict resolution, crisis interventions, individual, group and family counseling, assertiveness training, somatic therapies, pre- and post-ECT [electroconvulsive therapy] care, milieu therapy, and relaxation).

2.19.5 Provide ongoing health education and teaching to promote health and quality of life, minimize the development of complications, and maintain and restore health (e.g., social skills training, anger management, relapse prevention, assertiveness training, and communication techniques).

2.19.6 Coordinate appropriate referrals and liaise to promote access to resources that can optimize health outcomes.

2.20 Use critical thinking and clinical judgment to determine the level of risk and coordinate effective interventions for psychiatric and nonpsychiatric emergencies.

2.20.1 Intervene to minimize agitation, de-escalate agitated behaviour, and manage aggressive behaviour in the least restrictive manner.

2.20.2 Intervene to prevent self-harm or minimize injury related to self-harm.

2.20.3 Conduct an ongoing suicide risk assessment and select an intervention from a range of evidence-informed suicide prevention strategies (e.g., safety planning, crisis intervention, referral to alternative level of care).

BOX 6.7 Registered Psychiatric Nurses Entry-to-Practice Competencies (*Continued*)

2.20.4 Apply crisis intervention skills with clients experiencing acute emotional, physical, behavioural, and mental distress (e.g., loss, grief, victimization, trauma).

2.20.5 Recognize and intervene to stabilize clients experiencing medical emergencies (e.g., shock, hypoglycemia, management of neuroleptic malignant syndrome, cardiac events).

2.21 Collaborate with the client to evaluate the effectiveness and appropriateness of the plan of care.

2.21.1 Collect, analyze, and synthesize data to evaluate the outcomes from the plan of care.

2.21.2 Use a critical inquiry process to continuously monitor the effectiveness of client care in relation to anticipated outcomes.

2.21.3 Solicit the client's perception of the nursing care and other therapeutic interventions that were provided.

2.21.4 Modify and individualize the plan of care in collaboration with the client and according to evaluation findings.

Registered Psychiatric Nurse Regulators of Canada. (2014). *Registered psychiatric nurse entry-level competencies.* . Used with permission.

BOX 6.8 Registered Psychiatric Nurses Entry-to-Practice Competencies

Competency 3

Collaborative Practice

RPNs work in collaboration with team members, families, and other stakeholders to deliver comprehensive psychiatric nursing care in order to achieve the client's health goals.

3.1 Establish and maintain professional relationships that foster continuity and client-centred care.

3.1.1 Use interpersonal communication skills to establish and maintain a rapport among team members.

3.1.2 Share relevant information with team members, clients, and stakeholders in a timely manner.

3.1.3 Promote collaborative and informed shared decision-making.

3.2 Partner effectively with team members in the delivery of client-centred care.

3.2.1 Demonstrate knowledge of the roles, responsibilities, and perspectives of team members and stakeholders.

3.2.2 Inform stakeholders of the roles and responsibilities of psychiatric nursing and the perspectives of the RPN when required.

3.2.3 Engage participation of additional team members as required.

3.2.4 Accept leadership responsibility for coordinating care identified by the team.

3.3 Share responsibility for resolving conflict with team members.

3.3.1 Identify the issues that may contribute to the development of conflict.

3.3.2 Recognize actual or potential conflict situations.

3.3.3 Employ effective conflict resolution and reconciliation approaches and techniques.

3.3.4 Negotiate to mitigate barriers in order to optimize healthcare outcomes.

Registered Psychiatric Nurse Regulators of Canada. (2014). *Registered psychiatric nurse entry-level competencies.* Used with permission.

BOX 6.9 Registered Psychiatric Nurses Entry-to-Practice Competencies

Competency 4

Advocacy

Registered psychiatric nurses use their expertise and influence to support their clients to advance their health and wellbeing on an individual and community level.

4.1 Collaborate with clients to take action on issues that may impact their health and wellbeing.

    4.1.1 Advocate for needed resources that enhance the client's quality-of-life services and social inclusion (e.g., housing, accessibility, treatment options, basic needs).

    4.1.2 Inform clients of their rights and options (e.g., appeals, complaints).

    4.1.3 Support the client's right to informed decision-making (e.g., treatment plan, treatment orders).

    4.1.4 Support client autonomy and right to choice (e.g., right to live at risk).

    4.1.5 Promote the least restrictive treatment and environment.

4.2 Promote awareness of mental health and addictions issues by providing accurate information and challenging negative attitudes and behaviour that contribute to stigma and discrimination.

4.3 Collaborate with others to take action on issues influencing mental health and addictions.

    4.3.1 Demonstrate knowledge and understanding of demographic and sociopolitical environments.

    4.3.2 Recognize the impact of mental illness and stigma on society and the individual.

    4.3.3 Recognize attitudes and behaviours that contribute to stigma.

    4.3.4 Provide education to the community about mental health and addictions.

    4.3.5 Engage with stakeholders and the community to promote mental health and wellness.

    4.3.6 Engage in addressing social justice issues at an individual or community level (e.g., poverty, marginalization).

Registered Psychiatric Nurse Regulators of Canada. (2014). *Registered psychiatric nurse entry-level competencies.* Used with permission.

BOX 6.10 Registered Psychiatric Nurses Entry-to-Practice Competencies

Competency 5

Quality Care and Client Safety

Registered psychiatric nurses collaborate in developing, implementing, and evaluating policies, procedures, and activities that promote quality care and client safety.

5.1 Use reflective practice and evidence to guide psychiatric nursing practice.

    5.1.1 Reflect on and critically analyze practice (e.g., journaling, supervision, peer review) to inform and change future practice.

    5.1.2 Reflect on current evidence from various sources and determine relevance to client need and practice setting (e.g., published research, clinical practice guidelines, policies, decision-making tools).

    5.1.3 Integrate evidence into practice decisions to maximize health outcomes.

    5.1.4 Evaluate the effectiveness of the evidence in practice.

5.2 Engage in practices to promote physical, environmental, and psychological safety.

    5.2.1 Recognize potential risks and hazards, including risk for suicide and violence.

    5.2.2 Use recognized assessment tools to address potential risks and hazards (e.g., medication reconciliation, client falls assessment tool).

    5.2.3 Implement interventions to address potential risks and hazards (e.g., protocols, clinical practice guidelines, decision-making tools).

    5.2.4 Evaluate the effectiveness of the interventions in practice.

    5.2.5 Report and document safety risks and hazards.

    5.2.6 Identify and address occupational hazards related to working with unpredictable behaviours, such as violence and suicide (e.g., burnout, secondary traumatization).

BOX 6.10 **Registered Psychiatric Nurses Entry-to-Practice Competencies** (*Continued*)

5.3 Integrate cultural awareness, safety, and sensitivity into practice.

  5.3.1 Evaluate personal beliefs, values, and attitudes related to own culture and others' culture.

  5.3.2 Explore the client's cultural needs, beliefs, practices, and preferences.

  5.3.3 Incorporate the client's cultural preferences and personal perspectives into the plan of care when applicable.

  5.3.4 Adapt communication to the audience while considering social and cultural diversity based on the client's needs.

  5.3.5 Engage in opportunities to learn about various cultures (e.g., talking to client, attending cultural events, and courses).

  5.3.6 Incorporate knowledge of culture and how multiple identities (e.g., race, gender, ethnicity, sexual orientation, disability) shape one's life experience and contribute to health outcomes.

Registered Psychiatric Nurse Regulators of Canada. (2014). *Registered psychiatric nurse entry-level competencies.* Used with permission.

BOX 6.11 **Registered Psychiatric Nurses Entry-to-Practice Competencies**

Competency 6

Health Promotion

Registered psychiatric nurses use their expertise to promote the physical and mental health of clients to prevent disease, illness, and injury.

6.1 Engage in health promotion and the prevention of disease, illness, and injury.

  6.1.1 Integrate knowledge of the determinants of health, health disparities, and health inequities when assessing health promotion needs.

  6.1.2 Develop and implement evidence-informed health promotion strategies and programs based on a range of theories and models (e.g., Stages of Change, Health Belief Model, Social Learning Theory).

  6.1.3 Select and implement evidence-informed interventions to promote health and prevent disease, illness, and injury (e.g., health communication, health education, community action, immunization, harm reduction).

  6.1.4 Engage clients to seek out or develop resources that promote health (e.g., support groups, exercise programs, spiritual organizations).

  6.1.5 Contribute to the development of policies and standards that support health promotion, and prevent disease, illness, and injury (e.g., falls prevention, medication reconciliation, prevention and management of aggressive behaviour, cultural sensitivity).

  6.1.6 Advocate for health-promoting healthcare systems and environments.

6.2 Engage in mental health promotion when collaborating with clients.

  6.2.1 Integrate knowledge of determinants of health in the assessment process (e.g., social inclusion, discrimination, economic resources, violence).

  6.2.2 Recognize the impact that the interrelationship of comorbid physical and mental health issues have on overall health (e.g., diabetes, cardiovascular disease, cancer, obesity).

  6.2.3 Gather information about biologic, psychological, spiritual, social, and environmental risk and protective factors specific to mental health during the assessment process (e.g., metabolic status, exposure to violence, support systems).

  6.2.4 Incorporate strategies into healthcare planning that strengthen protective factors and enhance resilience (e.g., principles of recovery, psychosocial rehabilitation, holistic care, cultural continuity).

  6.2.5 Contribute to the development of policies and standards that support mental health promotion (e.g., preventing and minimizing restraint and seclusion, promoting client autonomy).

6.3 Engage in the prevention of mental illness, and substance-related and behavioural addictions, when collaborating with clients.

  6.3.1 Use a variety of strategies to address stigma and discrimination around mental health and addictions issues (e.g., acting as a positive role

(Continued)

BOX 6.11 Registered Psychiatric Nurses Entry-to-Practice Competencies (*Continued*)

model, reflective practice, engaging communities in dialogue, responding to media portrayal of mental illness, addressing stigmatizing and discriminatory language, promoting social change, participation, and inclusion).

6.3.2 Recognize and address the impact of societal factors that contribute to mental health and addictions issues (e.g., abuse, poverty, trauma).

6.3.3 Incorporate strategies into healthcare planning that reduce risk (e.g., smoking cessation, responsible substance use, strengthening community networks, violence prevention, healthy childhood development, stress management, increasing social capital, responsible gambling).

6.3.4 Incorporate trauma-informed philosophies and best practices into healthcare planning.

6.3.5 Assist clients to gain insight into the relationship between mental illness and addictions.

6.3.6 Integrate harm reduction philosophies and best practices into healthcare planning (e.g.,

methadone maintenance, needle exchange, safe sex, nicotine replacement therapy).

6.3.7 Engage and empower clients to seek out and/or develop resources that support relapse prevention (e.g., self-help groups, Alcoholics Anonymous, Narcotics Anonymous, Gamblers Anonymous).

6.3.8 Contribute to the development of policies and standards that support the prevention of mental illness and addictions (e.g., alcohol use during life stages, smoke-free environment, workplace health, suicide awareness).

6.4 **Engage in suicide prevention when collaborating with clients.**

6.4.1 Identify individuals, groups, communities, and special populations that are at risk for suicide.

6.4.2 Collaborate with communities in suicide prevention and postvention activities (e.g., skill building, antibullying programs, school-based education).

Registered Psychiatric Nurse Regulators of Canada. (2014). *Registered psychiatric nurse entry-level competencies.* Used with permission.

BOX 6.12 Registered Psychiatric Nurses Entry-to-Practice Competencies

Competency 7

Ethical, Professional, and Legal Responsibilities
Registered psychiatric nurses (RPNs) practice within legal requirements, demonstrate professionalism, and uphold professional codes of ethics, standards of practice, bylaws, and policies.

7.1 **Practice in compliance with federal and provincial/territorial legislation and other legal requirements.**

7.1.1 Demonstrate knowledge of the legislation governing psychiatric nursing practice.

7.1.2 Adhere to the psychiatric nursing code of ethics, standards of practice, and bylaws of the regulatory authority.

7.1.3 Practice within the jurisdiction's legislated scope of practice for psychiatric nurses and understand that the scope of practice may be influenced by limits and conditions imposed by the regulatory authority, employer policies, and the limits of individual competence.

7.1.4 Adhere to and apply the jurisdiction's mental health legislation.

7.1.5 Adhere to and apply other relevant legislation that has an impact on practice.

7.1.6 Protect client confidentiality and adhere to relevant legislation that governs the privacy, access, use, retention, and disclosure of personal information.

7.1.7 Adhere to legal requirements regarding client consent.

7.1.8 Adhere to any legislated duty to report, including the duty to report abuse or to report unprofessional or unsafe practice, or the risk of such.

7.1.9 Adhere to standards and policies regarding proper documentation, including being timely, accurate, clear, concise, and legible.

7.2 **Assume responsibility for upholding the requirements of self-regulation in the interest of public protection.**

BOX 6.12 Registered Psychiatric Nurses Entry-to-Practice Competencies (*Continued*)

7.2.1 Accept responsibility for own actions, decisions, and professional conduct.

7.2.2 Practice within own level of competence and use professional judgment when accepting responsibilities, including seeking out additional information or guidance when required.

7.2.3 Demonstrate an understanding of the regulatory purpose of own governing body and the significance of participating in professional activities of a regulatory nature.

7.2.4 Demonstrate an understanding of the significance of fitness to practice in the context of public protection, and strive to maintain a level of personal health, mental health, and wellbeing in order to provide safe, competent, and ethical care.

7.2.5 Question orders, decisions, or actions that are unclear or inconsistent with positive client outcomes, best practices, health and safety standards, or client wishes.

7.2.6 Protect clients and take steps to prevent or minimize harm from unsafe practices.

7.2.7 Engage in a process of continuous learning and self-evaluation, including following the requirements of the regulatory authority's continuing competence program.

7.3 **Demonstrate a professional presence and model professional behaviour.**

7.3.1 Conduct oneself in a manner that promotes a positive image of the profession.

7.3.2 Respond professionally, regardless of the behaviour of others.

7.3.3 Articulate the role and responsibilities of an RPN.

7.3.4 Practice within agency policies and procedures, and exercise professional judgment when using these, or in the absence of agency policies and procedures.

7.3.5 Organize and prioritize own work and develop time management skills for meeting responsibilities.

7.3.6 Demonstrate initiative, curiosity, flexibility, creativity, and beginning self-confidence.

7.3.7 Demonstrate professional leadership (e.g., act as a role model, coach, and mentor to others; support knowledge transfer; engage in professional activities).

7.4 **Uphold and promote the ethical values of the profession.**

7.4.1 Conduct oneself in a manner that reflects honesty, integrity, reliability, and impartiality.

7.4.2 Avoid situations that could give rise to a conflict of interest and ensure that the vulnerabilities of others are not exploited for one's own interest.

7.4.3 Identify the effects of one's own values, biases, and assumptions on interactions with clients and other members of the healthcare team.

7.4.4 Recognize ethical dilemmas and implement steps toward a resolution.

7.4.5 Differentiate between personal and professional relationships and maintain the boundaries of the psychiatric nurse–client relationship (e.g., addressing power differentials, use of personal disclosure).

Registered Psychiatric Nurse Regulators of Canada. (2014). *Registered psychiatric nurse entry-level competencies.* Used with permission.

Standards of Professional Practice

As regulated health professions, nurses are given the authority to practice under provincial or territorial laws that set out governance, registration, and discipline requirements as a means of protecting the public. These laws require provincial or territorial nursing regulatory bodies to set, monitor, and enforce standards of practice that, along with a code of ethics (see Chapter 8), articulate a profession's values, knowledge, and skills. Such standards facilitate a profession's self-governance because they make explicit the profession's expectations of its members' competency and performance.

KEY CONCEPT

Standards of practice are used by self-regulating professional groups to identify their expected and achievable competencies and to make explicit their obligations to the public.

CFMHN Standards of Practice

PMH nursing has been a designated CNA specialty since 1995. The Canadian Federation of Mental Health Nurses (CFMHN) is the national association for the specialty and sets PMH nursing standards for RNs. The *Canadian Standards of Psychiatric–Mental Health Nursing* was developed by expert PMH nurses in 1996 (Austin et al., 1996), revised in 1998, 2006, and 2014 (CFMHN, 2014) and is under revision and expected to be published in early 2022. The Standards of Practice document is freely available at the CFMHN Web site (see Web Links). The standards are organized by a **domains of practice** framework, as identified by Patricia Benner (1984) through research determining the way in which nurses describe their clinical practice, with competencies classified within the seven domains (see Web Links).

It is acknowledged that nurses' achievement of competent practice is shaped by the nursing model they practice as well as by the social, cultural, economic, and political factors impacting healthcare provision in their jurisdiction. Values underlying the CFMHN standards include the belief that the therapeutic nurse–client relationship, based on trust and mutual respect, is at the core of PMH nursing practice and holistic, ethical, and culturally competent care. Collaborative relationships with individuals, families, communities, and different populations, as well as with interprofessional and intraprofessional colleagues, are highly valued. Key practice foci are the alleviation of stigma and discrimination, the protection of human rights, and the promotion of recovery and wellbeing for those living with mental illness. Advocacy for equitable access to healthcare resources, for practice environments that promote safe and positive work environments and relationships, for research and its application to improve care, treatment, and sustained recovery, and for nursing action to promote political and social awareness that impacts healthcare policy, is considered part of the nursing role.

National certification in this specialty from the CNA can be achieved by nurses who have either a minimum of 1,950 h of experience within PMH nursing within the last 5 years or 1,000 h of experience in PMH nursing within the last 5 years plus 300 h of formal education, which can be specialty postbasic course or program at a college/university. As well, verification by a supervisor/consultant that the practice experience was acquired and successful completion of the CNA's PMH nursing certification examination is required. Recertification is necessary every 5 years, either by submitting a list of continuous learning experiences or by rewriting the certification examination. Registered nurses, registered psychiatric nurses, and nurse practitioners with certification in PMH nursing include "CPMHN(C)," [Certified in Psychiatric and Mental Health Nursing Canada] with their signature.

Registered Psychiatric Nurses Standards of Practice

In Western Canada (Manitoba, Saskatchewan, Alberta, and British Columbia) and the Yukon, the distinct profession of Registered Psychiatric Nursing is regulated by separate provincial/territorial associations and regulatory bodies. In 2019, the Standards of Psychiatric Nursing Practice were published collaboratively by the College of Registered Psychiatric Nurses of Alberta (CRPNA); British Columbia College of Nursing Professionals (BCCNP); The College of Registered Psychiatric Nurses of Manitoba (CRPNM); and the Registered Psychiatric Nurse Association of Saskatchewan (RPNAS). Refer further to Web Links.

The Canadian Council for Practical Nurse Regulators (CCPNR) Standards of Practice

The CCPNR (2021), a federation of provincial and territorial members who are legislated as responsible to the public for safe practice of licensed practical nurses and registered practical nurses, oversees and approves the standards of LPN/RPN practice in Canada (see Web Links).

Key Components of PMH Nursing Practice

Clinical Decision-Making

Decision-making involves critical thinking and is at the core of clinical practice. **Clinical decision-making** focuses on choices made in clinical settings. In addition to complex decisions, such as collecting, processing, and organizing information and formulating nursing approaches, many moment-to-moment decisions are made, such as deciding whether a client should receive a PRN medication. The development and implementation of efficacious interventions involves critical analysis of client, family, and community data. Such decision-making should involve the client, family, and other significant stakeholders as much as ethically, legally, and logistically possible. Reflective thinking about the client's illness experience and personal response to the treatment and care situation is an important aspect of choosing interventions. The nurse needs to have a thorough understanding of the rationale and the theoretical underpinnings of the client's care plan.

Critical Pathways in Care Planning

Many healthcare facilities use **critical pathways** (CPW), also known as clinical pathways, multidiscipline pathways, or care maps, to ensure a quality level of care in a cost-effective way. These pathways are similar to individual treatment plans in that all the disciplines' interventions are included on one plan. Critical pathways, however, are designed for a hypothetical client who has typical symptoms and who follows an expected course of treatment. Such pathways are not developed for each individual client nor tailored for specific settings and thus can be difficult to implement and evaluate (McCabe et al., 2019). This unification of care can be helpful if it means that best practices shape the care received by all clients and if it facilitates the use of expert knowledge by all those providing care. The implementation of CPWs has shown the potential to reduce inconsistencies between client care and to improve client outcomes (Nielsen & Nielsen, 2015). However, CPWs are not helpful if the unique needs and situation of each client and family are overlooked, or if nurses are restrained in their provision of thoughtful, sensitive, and personal care at the expense of following the standardized CPW. Pathways which identify key interventions and related best practices for a typical client with a specific mental disorder can, however, be helpful study tools for students.

Recovery as the Framework for Mental Health Care

Recovery, defined as "a process in which people with mental health problems and illnesses are empowered and supported to engage actively in their own journey of wellbeing," has been placed at the centre of Canada's national mental health strategy (Mental Health Commission of Canada [MHCC], 2009, p. 122). In *Changing Directions, Changing Lives* (2012, p. 15), The Mental Health Commission of Canada further clarifies that "recovery refers to living a satisfying, hopeful and contributing life, even when there are on-going limitations caused by mental health problems and illness." Key components of recovery are individualized/person-centred care, person empowerment, and finding purpose and hope (Ellison et al., 2018). The recovery process is envisioned as enabling individuals to have a meaningful, fulfilling life and is supported by the strengths of the individual, family, and community (see Chapter 9). It requires an interdisciplinary approach, valuing the lived experience of persons with mental health concerns, and advocating for the rights of people with mental health concerns. "Cure" is not implied, but full remission is held as likely for some people living with mental health concerns (MHCC, 2012). In 2015, the MHCC released guidelines for recovery-oriented practice as a way to promote and advance the consistent application of recovery principles across clinical settings in Canada (MHCC, 2015).

This vision of "recovery" that focuses on quality of life, rather than the narrower notion of clinical recovery, challenges nurses and other health professionals to reassess their practice. Nursing associations (e.g., CFMHN, RPNC) are ensuring that a **recovery model** of practice informs practice standards. Standards are therefore excellent resources for identifying ways to enact a recovery framework in mental health care.

The World Health Organization (WHO) (2019), in a specialized training guide entitled *Recovery Practices for Mental Health and Well Being*, acknowledges the importance of promoting and enhancing recovery and identifying the need for community-based mental health services. In this important document is included the role of practitioners and support systems in promoting recovery, inclusive recovery communication skills, explanation of the way recovery approaches differ from clinical approaches, and the CHIME framework (Connectedness, Hope, Identity, Meaning and Empowerment) as a means of providing healthcare practitioners worldwide with the tools to incorporate recovery into mental health care. See also Chapter 5.

Trauma-Informed Care

Traumatic events experienced across the life span can have lasting adverse effects on a person's bio/psycho/social/spiritual functioning. It is important that treatment and care of any individual be carried out with awareness that the person may have a trauma history (see Chapter 18), in what is known as **trauma-informed care**. Extreme behaviours and distress could be misinterpreted as symptoms of mental illness rather than a coping response to past or current trauma (Sweeney et al., 2018). Events that can be traumatic include abuse (physical, psychological, or sexual), assault, community violence, combat, torture, suicide of a significant other, neglect, natural or human-caused disasters, forced displacement, witnessing death, destruction, or suffering, and other similar occurrences. Persons with such experiences can become distressed or retraumatized. Re-traumatization "occurs when something in the present experience is redolent of past trauma, such as the inability to stop or escape a perceived or actual personal threat" (Sweeney et al., 2018, p. 322). In healthcare settings, re-traumatization may be sparked by certain procedures, such as the application of restraints (Reeves, 2015), seclusion, forced medication, and round-the-clock observation (Sweeney et al., 2018). Controlling practices may also traumatize staff, thus the need for adapting alternative and less traumatizing care approaches in healthcare settings cannot be underestimated. Nurses must understand that re-traumatization can relate to a person's experience of historic or cultural trauma, substantiating the need for nurses to diligently practice cultural humility and cultural safety at all times.

Protecting clients and staff from trauma, re-traumatization, and vicarious trauma is paramount in today's health care. The Substance Abuse and Mental Health Services Administration purports that a trauma-informed organizational approach to care is grounded in four assumptions, often referred to as the four Rs (SAMHSA, 2014, pp. 9–10):

- Realization—of the widespread impact of trauma on individuals, families, groups, and communities
- Recognize—the signs of trauma
- Respond—by integrating knowledge about trauma all areas of functioning (e.g., policies, procedures, and practices)
- Resist Re-traumatization—of clients and of staff, and prevent triggering painful memories.

A healthcare setting that uses universal trauma precautions with all clients can mitigate the consequences of trauma (Raja et al., 2015). Precautions are based on the knowledge that in healthcare settings, trauma survivors need to have a sense of control, to utilize personal coping mechanisms (e.g., holding onto a particular object, such as a purse), and may have a fear of being physically exposed or touched. These precautions involve simple actions. Staff should wear clearly visible identification that specifies their names and roles, and they should introduce themselves to their clients and family members. When carrying out procedures, clients should be informed of the time and steps involved and asked if they have any questions, worries, or preferences regarding the process. It is important to determine if there is something that would make them more comfortable (Raja et al., 2015).

As well as understanding the potential impact of traumatic events and the ways in which traumatic memories may be triggered in healthcare settings, nurses need to recognize their own trauma histories (Reeves, 2015). This history may include personal adverse experiences, those gained in their nursing role, vicarious knowledge of horrors revealed in clients' trauma disclosures, and their own experiencing or witnessing of tragic incidents. Self-understanding and attention to one's own wellbeing are important to sustaining one's capacity for competent and compassionate care.

Compassion fatigue, secondary traumatic stress, and vicarious trauma can be experienced by nurses and refers to the effect that working with traumatized persons can have on the practitioner (Walsh et al., 2017). Refer to Chapter 18 for further discussion of these and related concepts.

Harm Reduction

Contemporary nursing practice includes an understanding of **harm reduction** no matter the healthcare setting. In regard to substance use, the Canadian Nurses Association (2018) asserts that harm reduction is an evidence-based approach for mitigating the adverse biologic, psychologic, social, and economic effects of substance use (legal or illicit) without requiring abstinence. A harm reduction approach is nonjudgmental, human rights–affirming, and consistent with the values in the CNA Code of Ethics for Registered Nurses. Harm reduction practice is value-neutral with respect to substance use and focuses on the importance of treating all people with respect, dignity, and compassion. The key principles of a harm reduction approach are pragmatism, humanistic values, reducing harm and risk, using cost-effective, evidence-based science, empowering human rights, focusing on immediate goals, acknowledging incremental change, challenging policies and practices that maximize harm, assuring transparency, and meaningful participation of those with lived experience with substance use in policy making and program development (CNA, 2018, p. 17; Thomas, 2005). Nurses play an important role in lessening the health-related harm associated with substance use. Adopting a harm-reduction framework of practice, advocating for the urgent need for health and social services that are culture and gender sensitive, and providing trauma-informed care are all essential actions in contemporary nursing practice.

Collaborative Care

PMH care has a long tradition of using a dynamic interprofessional and interdisciplinary approach, with several disciplines working together in the provision of quality client care. In practice, **collaborative care** varies among healthcare settings depending on models of practice in use. While collaborative care is fundamental to continuity of care (diagnosis to discharge), especially for clients with chronic, severe mental illness, it has been cited as one of the major issues in mental healthcare delivery (Nicaise et al., 2021). Nurses play an important role in improving collaborative practice. For instance, a nurse and a psychologist, simultaneously working with a client on changing a behaviour related to medication adherence, need to take a congruent, integrated approach and to share information regarding client needs and progress. A coordinator, "case manager," or "patient/client navigator" may be effective in supporting collaborative care (Kates et al., 2011)—a role often held by a nurse (see Chapter 5).

Collaborative care extends beyond healthcare professionals. According to the WHO (2010), collaborative care is defined as diverse disciplines working together with clients, families, care providers, and communities to deliver quality care. Researchers have shown that effective collaboration benefits the health outcomes of people living with mental health concerns, particularly when clients are involved in the collaboration because this decreases feelings of stigmatization and powerlessness (Hackmann et al., 2019; Nicaise et al., 2021; Tippin et al., 2017). In a study by Barr and colleagues (2020), clients expressed the need for improved communication between mental health professionals and described feeling disappointed with the care they received when professionals did not act on the recommendation of other team members, especially when the person was experiencing a crisis. Clients want better communication among professionals and the sharing of resources between professionals and themselves so that they can be empowered and their recovery fostered.

A Canadian study that explored new graduates' experiences of interprofessional collaboration found that organizational environments where the nurses found relationships to be respectful and supportive and where they had opportunities for collaborative experiences and knowledge of others' roles, and of how and when to collaborate, fostered confidence in interprofessional work; a challenge was to balance self and others' expectations (Pfaff et al., 2014).

Challenges of PMH Nursing

The challenges of PMH nursing are shaped by new knowledge arising from research, new dimensions of health care generated by biotechnologic advances, the reality that nursing practice is becoming more specialized and autonomous and is situated within a global context. This section discusses a few of the challenges.

Knowledge Development, Dissemination, and Application

Results of new research efforts continually redefine our knowledge base relative to mental disorders and their treatment. Consider the significant advances in neurobiologic knowledge. In the 1970s, the cause of schizophrenia was hypothesized to be overactivity of dopamine. Later, it was discovered that other neurotransmitters seemed to play a role as well. Such knowledge resulted in new medications becoming available with various side effect profiles, requiring nurses to redefine their monitoring and interventions related to medication administration. Advances over the last decade in our understanding of genetics and epigenetics are, bringing new knowledge, controversy and new ethical issues. A literature review of publications between 2008 and 2018 showed that maternal prenatal stress could affect fetal brain development and program risk for emotional dysregulation over a lifetime and across generations (DeSocio, 2019). On the other hand, Cromby and colleagues (2019) undertook a systematic review of schizophrenia and epigenetics and found their results to be inconclusive because of the complexity of the disorder in relation to environmental influences. Developments in genetic and epigenetic data protection are of particular ethical concern, along with confidentiality, because these findings may have implications on "deep seated distinction between natural and social deprivations and inequalities that have structured much political science as well as policy work" (Melonia & Testac, 2014, p. 447).

Comorbid medical disorders are significant to the treatment of mental disorders. For example, hypertension, hypothyroidism, hyperthyroidism, and diabetes mellitus can each affect the disease trajectory of mental disorders. In some settings, the nurse may be the only healthcare provider on the collaborative team who has a background in such medical disorders, such as metabolic syndrome, human immunodeficiency viral illness, acquired immunodeficiency syndrome, and other somatic health problems. Thus, the nurse's contribution to the care of the individual is invaluable.

The challenge for nurses today is to stay abreast of the advances in holistic health care in order to provide safe, competent, evidence-based care. This requires ongoing knowledge development across one's career. Accessing up-to-date information and research through journals, electronic databases, and continuing education programs is a recognized responsibility. Evaluating the usefulness of research studies is required. For instance, one research project supporting a particular treatment approach may not be as meaningful as several statistically significant studies, assessed in systematic reviews. The results of qualitative research studies, although not generalizable, can have important implications for practice, such as insights that can deepen understanding of client experiences. Resources such as the International Knowledge Exchange Network for Mental Health (IKEN-MH), evolving through the Mental Health Commission of Canada (MHCC), with a current focus on innovative practices and systematic evidence for the design and management of mental health services and the WHO's MiNDbank are important to the improvement of care (see Web Links).

Healthcare Delivery System Challenges

Continuing challenges for Canadian nurses include supporting the integration of mental health care within primary health care, articulating the influence of the determinants of health on mental health and advocating to municipal, provincial, and federal authorities to address inequities, as well as playing a strong, effective role in the enactment of Canada's national strategy for mental health.

Consumers of mental health services and their families are gaining voice and calling for meaningful changes in the delivery of services. Inequities in health care for marginalized populations, such as those living with a chronic mental illness, are being challenged, as are paternalistic approaches to the delivery of care. One source of this challenge is the Canadian Alliance on Mental Illness and Mental Health (CAMIMH). The CAMIMH, created in 1998, consists of consumers, their families, researchers, and care providers from numerous professions. Their mission is to influence national policy, to speak in a unified voice, and to focus strategically on mental health and mental illness. Active partnership among users of services, nurses and other health providers, and the community at large is necessary to effect the positive changes initiated by our national strategy in mental health.

Recently research has turned its gaze from the consumer mental health experience to the mental health and wellbeing of providers of healthcare services, and to the consequences of workplace environment and policies impacting the mental health of frontline staff. For example, the Federation of Canadian Nurses Unions (Stelnicki et al., 2020a) has used research to substantiate recommendations for healthcare employers, provincial governments, and the federal government. Their recommendations highlight the need for funding for evidence-based training, resources, and supports for nurses, and federal funding for Canadian Institutes of Health Research (CIHR) to build national research capacity to mitigate occupational stress injury for nurses.

Overcoming Stigma, Discrimination, and Racism

Overcoming the stigma, discrimination related to mental illness, and racism in Black, Indigenous, and racialized communities is a priority of the MHCC and must occur within healthcare systems. Not only do persons with mental health disorders and their families experience stigmatization due to some healthcare professionals' avoidance, discomfort, or even disdain, but professionals who practice in PMH settings may also experience stigma by association. Psychiatry has a dark history reflected in images of asylums with chained inmates (e.g., Bedlam), negative media portrayals (e.g., "One Flew Over the Cuckoo's Nest"), and lack of recognition of the scientific basis of contemporary psychiatric care. Mental health professionals may be seen as less skilled than their colleagues in other areas and be less respected (Bhugra et al., 2015). This can result in health science students, including those in nursing, not considering mental health care as a career choice.

Cénat (2020) explains that racial discrimination, racial profiling, racism, and microaggressions exist in health care. Nurses must make racial issues a priority and be vigilant regarding its potential impact on care and treatment (e.g., racial and ethnic disparities in pharmacologic treatment), as well as being culturally competent. Nurses need to practice from a place of recognizing uniqueness and diversity. Addressing racism in PMH nursing begins with an authentic exploration of each nurse's personal ideas, beliefs, privileges, and attitudes as the foundation to providing meaningful mental health care. See Chapters 3 and 4.

e-Mental Health

e-Mental health is the name given to mental health services and education delivered across distances using communication and information technologies. The MHCC's (2014) briefing paper, *E-Mental Health in Canada: Transforming the Mental Health System Using Technology*, notes that such services (which can be self-guided or partly self-guided) can be as effective as those provided face-to-face. As cost-effective alternatives to traditional mental health care, e-Mental health approaches are particularly useful across Canada's vast geography. Services range from information and advocacy to assessment, intervention, monitoring, and evaluation. The technologies involved include telephones, mobile devices, emailing, videoconferencing, social media, as well as Web-based software programs (see Fig. 6.3).

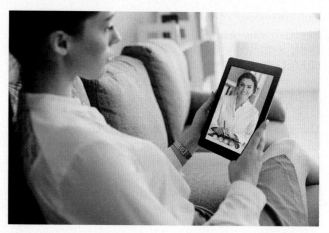

Figure 6.3 An example of e-Mental health. A client has a consult with a PMH nurse at a remote location via a personal digital device.

Increasingly human–computer interactions, such as online digital interventions and mobile applications for support, are being used to promote mental health (Schueller et al., 2017). Neilson and Wilson (2019) found that human–computer interaction can be helpful for individuals to engage in treatment on their own, in the form of self-help or as guided treatment to strengthen mental and emotional resilience and health promotion and prevention strategies. However, the authors warn that nurses must carefully assess the therapeutic purposes to assure quality and safety of e-mental health interventions. And although there is great variety in e-mental health products, not all are well suited for persons with mental health concerns.

An evolving, related area is that of gamification, which involves interactive (including online) computer games as an engaging means of offering education and training (Ricciardi & De Paolis, 2014). Simulation platforms are increasingly being developed for education in nursing and other healthcare professions and for mental health promotion (Hopia & Raitio, 2016). The College and Association of Registered Nurses of Alberta, for example, explored the use of gamification as a way to teach RNs about jurisprudence and to confirm their competence in this registration requirement. Evaluation of the project revealed that nurses did learn about jurisprudence, felt engaged, and appreciated the ease of participation; 97% believed what they learned would influence their practice (Lemermeyer & Sadesky, 2016).

COVID-19 and Beyond

Healthcare providers across the globe were significantly impacted by the COVID-19 pandemic, and the lingering impact on the mental health of individuals, families, and healthcare providers (Foye et al., 2021; Havaei et al., 2021) quickly emerged. Increased workload, lack of access to usual supports due to isolation requirements, risk of infection, and lack of personal protective equipment (PPE) all had a significant negative impact on the mental wellbeing of nurses across Canada. In a study of workplace conditions impacting nurses' mental health during the COVID-19 pandemic (*n* = 3,676), Havaei and colleagues (2021) found prevalence rates for posttraumatic stress disorder were 47%, anxiety 38%, depression 41%, and emotional exhaustion 60%. Frequent changes in COVID policies and procedures were related to high scores on posttraumatic stress disorder, anxiety, and depression. However, in the face of COVID-19, nurses also demonstrated resilience: Ward–Miller and colleagues (2021) observed that nurses worked to their full scope of practice and adapted to their new reality in innovative ways. Nurses' responses to the pandemic will create research opportunities aimed at improving both client and workforce outcomes. Learning from the resourcefulness and resiliency of nurses will help prepare for future crises.

Maintaining Nurses' Mental Health and Wellbeing

Nurses are "witnesses of human tragedy and stewards for the healing of deep suffering" (Lauerer, 2020, p. 339), and this affects them at the core of what it is to be human, their bio/psycho/social/spiritual selves. A pan-Canadian Survey of more than 7,000 nurses (Stelnicki et al., 2020b) demonstrated that there is a significant need to pay attention to the mental health needs of nurses across Canada. The researchers found that nearly half of the nurses surveyed screened positive for a mental disorder; that 63.2% experienced some signs of burnout, and the rates of suicidal behaviours were much higher than in the general Canadian population. Protecting the mental wellbeing of nurses involves the adoption of evidence-based and workplace-specific psychological health and safety policies and interventions (see Chapter 17).

Nurse Stress and Substance Use

If care is not taken to manage work-related stresses, nurses are vulnerable to problematic substance use (Foli et al., 2020), leading to potential negative impacts on client care, public trust, and the nursing profession (CNA, 2009). Grissinger (2018) reported that rates of substance misuse, abuse, and addiction in nurses could be as high as 20%, a fact that further emphasizes the importance of

healthy workplaces that support psychological wellbeing and provide resources to respond to substance misuse, as well as training and recovery. Nurse managers have a role to play in supporting the recovery of nurses should substance use develop (Foli et al., 2020). Those who have engaged in substance misuse often experience stigma from their peers, underscoring the importance of changing the conversation from shame and blame to trauma- and substance use-informed models of care (Carter et al., 2019; Grissinger, 2018). All too often, biases manifest in a lack of support, coupled with practice and professional barriers, which include actual or potential disciplinary actions from licensing boards and impair the implementation of recovery-oriented models of care for nurses (Carter et al., 2019; Ross et al., 2018) (see Chapter 26).

PMH Nursing in a Global Community

As members of a global community, Canadian nurses recognize their role in achieving "health for all." Mental health is a particularly disadvantaged aspect of health care around the world, so capacity building for mental health care is a pressing priority (Kakuma et al., 2011). Mental health care can be effectively delivered in primary care settings through collaboration among skilled, nonspecialist professionals, trained lay workers, consumer representatives, and caregivers when supported by mental health specialists in consultative roles for services and training (Kakuma et al., 2011). There is a great need, as well, to ensure that all delivery of mental health care upholds the dignity and human rights of those receiving it (Austin, 2017).

The International Society of Psychiatric–Mental Health Nurses (ISPN), an organization with student members, works to unite and strengthen the presence and voice of PMH nurses and to promote quality care for individuals and families with mental health problems. The World Federation for Mental Health (WFMH), an organization to which nurses belong, has as its mission, since its founding in 1948, the advancement of mental health promotion, prevention, and care among all people. It works with governments from more than 100 countries and nongovernment groups. WFMH sponsors World Mental Health Day, which occurs annually on October 10. Organizations are an important pathway for nurses' contribution to the improvement of mental health and mental health care across the globe.

Summary of Key Points

- The bio/psycho/social/spiritual model focuses on separate but interdependent dimensions of biologic, psychological, social, and spiritual factors in the assessment and treatment of mental disorders. This comprehensive and holistic approach to mental disorders is the foundation for effective PMH nursing practice and is used as the basic organizational framework for this text.
- Entry-to-practice competencies outline the essential knowledge, skills, and attitudes required at the onset of a credentialed nursing role.

- Standards of practice set out the explicit responsibilities and competencies of a profession.
- Nurses practicing in psychiatric and mental health settings collaborate interprofessionally and intraprofessionally and many times act as coordinators in the delivery of care.
- PMH nurses need to be aware of team dynamics and their impact on care. When nurses practice in interprofessional and intraprofessional settings, there may be an overlapping of professional roles. Nurses are accountable for both discrete and shared functions that they perform in their practice.

- Challenges facing nurses practicing in PMH settings include knowledge development dissemination, and application; e-Mental Health; addressing stigma and discrimination within healthcare systems; and working to make the healthcare system more collaborative and responsive to the mental health needs of Canadians.
- Provincial, national, and global organizations are important pathways for nurses' contributions to improving mental health and mental health care worldwide.

 Thinking Challenges

John is a new nursing graduate who has secured a position on an inpatient acute mental health unit in his hometown. Although he completed a 3-credit theory course in psychiatric and mental health nursing in his baccalaureate program and completed two clinical rotations in mental health nursing, he wants to learn more about being a professional in his new role and provide safe, competent, ethical care. He notices that some nurses sign their name BSN, RN, CPMHN(C), and has talked to staff about joining the Canadian Federation of Mental Health Nurses, and work toward certification.

a. What are some reasons to join a professional nursing association or organization?

b. What benefits would John gain from joining a professional organization such as the Canadian Federation of Mental Health Nurses?
c. What are the advantages of becoming certified as a PMH nurse with the Canadian Nurses Association?

> Visit thePoint to view suggested responses. Go to thePoint.lww.com/activate and use the activation code found in the front of this text to unlock answers to the "Thinking Challenges" and other online resources.

 Web Links

camimh.ca   The Canadian Alliance on Mental Illness and Mental Health provides key reports, news, and information regarding mental illness and its treatment on its website.

ccmhi.ca   Canadian Collaborative Mental Health Initiative, a consortium of 12 national organizations, including CNA, CFMHN, and RPNC, seeks to improve the delivery of mental health services within primary care through interdisciplinary collaboration. A series of papers and toolkits related to collaborative care can be found here.

ccpnr.ca   This site of the Canadian Council for Practical Nurse Regulators offers links to the provincial and territorial regulators that have information on the competency profiles for LPNs/RPNs.

cfmhn.ca   The Canadian Federation of Mental Health Nurses website has the complete standards of practice document, hosts a biennial national conference, and is a source of national psychiatric and mental health nursing initiatives.

cna-aiic.ca/   The Canadian Nurses Association website has information regarding certification as a PMH nurse in Canada.

cpa-apc.org   The Canadian Psychiatric Association, a voluntary organization of psychiatrists, publishes the *Canadian Journal of Psychiatry* among other periodicals and information. Clinical practice guidelines and position and discussion papers are available here.

ispn-psych.org   The International Society of Psychiatric–Mental Health Nurses website has links to their publications, including position statements and psychiatric nursing journals.

mentalhealthcommission.ca/English/initiatives/11859/iken-mh   The MHCC's International Knowledge Exchange Network for Mental Health facilitates searching of focus areas, such as mental health and the law, First Nations, Inuit, and Métis, peer support.

porticonetwork.ca   An e-Mental health resource, the *Portico Network*, is a trustworthy website created by the Centre for Addiction and Mental Health in Toronto. It is an excellent resource, offering information re: disorders, treatment options, and primary care toolkits; opportunities for training or consultation; and links to partner sites. It is open to the public.

rpnrc.ca   The Registered Psychiatric Nurse Regulators of Canada. Here you will find the registered psychiatric nurse entry-level competencies, position statements, RPN organizations and publications, and links to other provincial associations. The 2019 Registered Psychiatric Nurses Standards of Practice can be found athttps://crpnm.mb.ca/wp-content/uploads/2019/10/Standards-of-Psychiatric-Nursing-Practice-FINAL-October-2019.pdf

https://www.mindbank.info/   This WHO online platform provides access to international resources related to mental health, disability, and general health, including policies and law and service standards. Browsing by country and region is possible.

wfmh.com   This World Federation for Mental Health site gives information about World Mental Health Day (October 10) and free access to the WFMH Bulletin.

References

Abraham, I., Fox, J., & Cohen, B. (1992). Integrating the bio into the bio-psychosocial: Understanding and treating biological phenomena in psychiatric–mental health nursing. *Archives of Psychiatric Nursing, 6*(5), 296–305. https://doi.org/10.1016/0883-9471(92)90041-G

Almost, J. (2021). *Regulated nursing in Canada: The landscape in 2021.* Canadian Nurse Association.

Austin, W. (2017). Global health ethics and mental health. In E. L. Yearwood & V. P. Hines-Martin (Eds.), *Routledge handbook of global mental health nursing* (pp. 71–90). Routledge.

Austin, W., Gallop, R., Harris, D., & Spencer, E. (1996). A domains of practice approach to the standards of psychiatric and mental health nursing. *Journal of Psychiatric and Mental Health Nursing, 3,* 111–115.

Barr, K. R., Jewell, M., Townsend, M. L., & Grenyer, B. F. (2020). Living with personality disorder and seeking mental health treatment: patients and family members reflect on their experiences. *Borderline Personality Disorder and Emotion Dysregulation, 7*(1), 1–11. https://doi.org/10.1186/s40479-020-00136-4

Barss, K. S. (2012). T.R.U.S.T.: An affirming model for inclusive spiritual care. *Journal of Holistic Nursing, 30*(1), 24–34. https://doi.org/10.1177/0898010111418118

Benner, P. (1984). *From novice to expert: Excellence and power in clinical nursing practice.* Addison-Wesley.

Bhugra, D., Sartorius, N., Fiorillo, A., Evans-Lacko, S., Ventriglio, A., Hermans, M. H. M., Vallon, P., Dales, J., Racetovic, G., Samochowiec, J., Bennemar, M. R., Becker, T., Kuimay, T., & Gaebel, W. (2015). EPA guidance on how to improve the image of psychiatry and of the psychiatrist. *European Psychiatry, 30*(3), 423–430. https://doi: 10.1016/j.eurpsy.2015.02.003

Canadian Association of Schools of Nursing with Canadian Federation of Mental Health Nursing. (2015). *Entry to practice mental health and addiction competencies for undergraduate nursing education in Canada.* http://www.casn.ca/wp-content/uploads/2015/11/Mental-health-Competencies_EN_FINAL-3-Oct-26-2015.pdf

Canadian Council Practical Nurse Regulators. (2021). *2020 standards of practice for licensed practical nurses in Canada.* https://www.anblpn.ca/wp-content/uploads/2021/04/CCPNR-2020-Standard_ENG.pdf

Canadian Federation of Mental Health Nurses. (2014). *The Canadian standards of psychiatric-mental health nursing* (4th ed.). http://cfmhn.ca/

Canadian Nurse Association. (2009). *Fact sheet: Problematic substance use by nurses.* https://www.cna-aiic.ca/~/media/cna/page-content/pdf-fr/problem_substance_abuse_fs_e.pdf?la=en

Canadian Nurses Association. (2015). *Framework for registered Nurse Prescribing in Canada.* ISBN 978-1-55119-427-1. https://www.cna-aiic.ca/~/media/cna/page-content/pdf-en/cna-rn-prescribing-framework_e.pdf?la=en

Canadian Nurses Association. (2018). *Joint position statement: Harm reduction and substance use.* https://www.cna-aiic.ca/-/media/cna/page-content/pdf-en/joint_position_statement_harm_reduction_and_substance_use.pdfCanadian

Carter, T. A., McMullan, S. P., & Patrician, P. A. (2019). Barriers to reentry into nurse anesthesia practice following substance use disorder treatment: A concept analysis. *Workplace Health & Safety, 67*(4), 189–199. https://doi: 10.1177/2165079918813378

Catalano, J. T. (2015). *Nursing now: Today's issues, tomorrow's trends* (7th ed.). F. A. Davis Company.

Cénat, J. M. (2020). How to provide anti-racist mental health care. *The Lancet Psychiatry, 7*(11), 929–931. https://doi.org/10.1016/S2215-0366(20)30309-6

College of Registered Nurses of Manitoba. (2021). https://www.crnm.mb.ca/about/registered-nursing/registered-nurse-authorized-prescriber

Cromby, J., Chung, E., Papadopoulos, D., & Talbot, C., (2019). Reviewing the epigenetics of Schizophrenia. *Journal of Mental Health, 28*(1), 71–79. https://doi.org/10.1080/09638237.2016.1207229

DeSocio, J. E. (2019). Epigenetics, maternal prenatal psychosocial stress, and infant mental health. *Archives of Psychiatric Nursing, 33,* 232–237. https://doi.org/10.1016/j.apnu.2019.05.001

Dossey, B. M., Keegan, L., & Guzzetta, C. E. (2004). *Holistic nursing: A handbook for practice* (4th ed.). Aspen.

Ellison, M. L., Belanger, L. K., Niles, B. L., Evans, L. C., & Bauer, M. S. (2018). Explication and definition of mental health recovery: A systematic review. *Administration and Policy in Mental Health and Mental Health Services Research, 45*(1), 91–102. https://doi.org/10.1007/s10488-016-0767-9

Foli, K. J., Reddick, B., Zhang, L., & Krcelich, K. (2020). Substance use in registered nurses: "I Heard About a Nurse Who…". *Journal of the American Psychiatric Nurses Association, 26*(1), 65–76. https://doi.org/10.1177/1078390319886369

Foye, U., Dalton-Locke, C., Harju-Seppänen, J., Lane, R., Beames, L., Vera San Juan, N., Johnson, S., & Simpson, A. (2021). How has COVID-19 affected mental health nurses and the delivery of mental health nursing care in the UK? Results of a mixed-methods study. *Journal of Psychiatric and Mental Health Nursing, 28*(2), 126–137. https://doi.org/10.1111/jpm.12745

Gaderman, A. C., Thomson, K. C., Richardson, C. G., Gagné, M., McAuliffe, C., Hirani, S., & Jenkins, E. (2021). Examining the impacts of the COVID-19 pandemic on family mental health in Canada: Findings from a national cross-sectional study. *BMJ Open, 11*(1), e04287. https://doi.org/10.1136/bmjopen-2020-042871

Grissinger M. (2018). Partially filled vials and syringes in sharps containers are a key source of drug diversion. *Pharmacy and Therapeutics: A Peer-Reviewed Journal for Formulary Management, 43*(12), 714–717.

Hackmann, C., Wilson, J., Perkins, A., & Zeilig, H. (2019). Collaborative diagnosis between clinician and patient: Why to do it and what to consider. *BJPsych Advances, 25*(4), 214–222.

Havaei, F., Ma, A., Staempfli, S., & MacPhee, M. (2021, January). Nurses' workplace conditions impacting their mental health during COVID-19: A cross-sectional survey study. *Healthcare, 9*(1), 84. https://doi.org/10.3390/healthcare9010084

Hopia, H., & Raitio, K. (2016). Gamification in healthcare: Perspectives of mental health services users and health professionals. *Issues in Mental Health Nursing, 37*(12), 894–902. https://doi.org/10.1080/01612840.2016.1233595

Kakuma, R., Minas, H., van Ginneken, N., Dal Paz, M. R., Desiraju, K., Morris, J. E., Saxena, S., & Scheffler, R. M. (2011). Human resources of mental health care: Current situation and strategies for action. *The Lancet, 378,* 1654–1663. https://doi.org/10.1016/S0140-6736(11)61093-3

Kates, N., Mazowita, G., Lemire, F., Jayabarathan, A., Bland, R., Selby, P., Isomura, T., Craven, M., Gervais, M., & Audet, D. (2011). The evolution of collaborative mental health care in Canada: A shared vision for the future: Position paper of the Canadian Psychiatric Association & the College of Family Physicians of Canada. *The Canadian Journal of Psychiatry, 56*(5), 1–10.

Lauerer, J. A. (2020). Caring for Nursing. *Journal of American Psychiatric Nurses Association, 26*(4), 339. https://doi.org/10.1177/1078390320917750

Lemermeyer, G., & Sadesky, G. (2016). The gamification of jurisprudence: Innovation in registered nurse regulation. *Journal of Nursing Regulation, 7*(3), 4–10. https://doi.org/10.1016/S2155-8256(16)32314-6

MacCourt, P.; Family Caregivers Advisory Committee & Mental Health Commission of Canada. (2013). *National guidelines for a comprehensive service system to support family caregivers of adults with mental health problems and illnesses.* https://www.mentalhealthcommission.ca/sites/default/files/Caregiving_MHCC_Family_Caregivers_Guidelines_ENG_0.pdf

McCabe, E. M., Lightbody, T. K., Mummery, C., Coloumbe, A., GermAnn, K., Lent, B., Black, L., Graham, K. E. R., Gross, D. P., & Miciak, M. (2019). Implementing a clinical pathway for paediatric mental health care in the emergency department. *Canadian Journal of Community Mental Health, 38*(4), 1–18. https://doi.org/10.7870/cjcmh-2019-015

Melonia, M., & Testac, G. (2014). Scrutinizing the epigenetics revolution. *BioSocieties, 9,* 431–456. https://doi.org/10.1057/biosoc.2014.22

Mental Health Commission of Canada. (2009). *Toward recovery and well-being: A framework for a mental health strategy for Canada.* https://www.mentalhealthcommission.ca/sites/default/files/FNIM_Toward_Recovery_and_Well_Being_ENG_0_1.pdf

Mental Health Commission of Canada. (2012). *Changing directions, changing lives: The mental health strategy for Canada.* https://www.mentalhealthcommission.ca/sites/default/files/MHStrategy_Strategy_ENG.pdf

Mental Health Commission of Canada. (2014). *E-Mental health in Canada: Transforming the mental health system using technology.* http://www.mentalhealthcommission.ca/English/document/27081/e-mental-health-canada-transforming-mental-health-system-using-technology

Mental Health Commission of Canada. (2015). Guidelines for recovery-oriented practice. Hope. Dignity. Inclusion. https://www.mentalhealthcommission.ca/sites/default/files/MHCC_Recovery-Guidelines_ENG_0.pdf

Michael, L. (2019). Spirituality as agency and restoration in existential recovery. *Journal of Spirituality in Mental Health, 21*(3), 206–214. https://doi.org/10.1080/19349637.2018.1458690

Nicaise, P., Grard, A., Leys, M., Van Audenhove, C., & Lorant, V. (2021). Key dimensions of collaboration quality in mental health care service networks. *Journal of Interprofessional Care, 35*(1), 28–36. https://doi.org/10.1080/13561820.2019.1709425

Nielsen, A. S., & Nielsen, B. (2015). Implementation of a clinical pathway may improve alcohol treatment outcome. *Addiction Science & Clinical Practice, 10*(1), 1–7. https://doi.org/10.1186/s13722-015-0031-8

Neilson, A. S., & Wilson, R. (2019). Combining e-mental health intervention developed with human computer interaction (HCI) design to enhance technology-facilitated recovery for people with depression and/or anxiety conditions: An integrative literature review. *International Journal of Mental Health Nursing, 28*(1), 22–39. https://doi.org/10.1111/inm.12527

Pfaff, K. A., Baxter, P. E., Jack, S. M. & Ploeg, J. (2014). Exploring new graduate nurse confidence in interprofessional collaboration: A mixed methods study. *International Journal of Nursing Studies, 51*(8), 1142–1152. https://doi.org/10.1016/j.ijnurstu.2014.01.001

Raja, S., Hasnain, M., Hoersch, M., Gove-Yin, S., & Rajagopalan, C. (2015). Trauma-informed care in medicine: Current knowledge and future research directions. *Family Community Health, 38*(3), 216–226. https://doi.org/10.1097/FCH.0000000000000071

Reeves, E. (2015). A synthesis of the literature in trauma-informed care. *Issues in Mental Health Nursing, 36*(9), 698–709. https://doi.org/10.3109/01612840.2015.1025319

Registered Psychiatric Nurse Regulators of Canada. (2014). *Registered psychiatric nurse entry-level competencies.* http://www.rpnc.ca/sites/default/files/resources/pdfs/RPNRC-ENGLISH%20Compdoc%20%28Nov6-14%29.pdf

Ricciardi, F., & De Paolis, L. T. (2014). A comprehensive review of serious games in health professions. *International Journal of Computer Games Technology, 14*, 11. https://doi.org/10.1155/2014/787968

Ross, C., Berry, N. S., Smye, V., Goldner, E. M. (2018). A critical review of knowledge on nurses with problematic substance use: The need to move from individual blame to awareness of structural factors. *Nursing Inquiry, 25*(2), e12215. https://doi.org/10.1111/nin.12215

Saiz, J., Chen-Chen, X., Mills, P. J. (2021). Religiosity and spirituality in the stages of recovery from persistent mental disorders. *Journal of Nervous & Mental Disease, 209*(2), 106–113. https://doi.org/10.1097/NMD.0000000000001271

Schueller, S. M., Stiles-Shields, C., & Yarosh, L. (2017). Online treatment and virtual therapists in child and adolescent psychiatry. *Child and Adolescent Psychiatric Clinics of North America, 26*(1), 1–12. https://doi.org/10.1016/j.chc.2016.07.011

Stelnicki, A. M., Carleton, N., & Reichert, C. (2020a). *Mental disorder symptoms among nurses in Canada.* Canadian Federation of Nurses Unions. https://www.nsnu.ca/sites/default/files/OSI_report_final.pdf

Stelnicki, A. M., Jamshidi, L., Ricciardelli, R., & Carleton, N. (2020b). Exposures to potentially psychologically traumatic events among nurses in Canada. *Canadian Journal of Nursing Research, 53*, 277–291. https://doi.org/10.1177/0844562120961988

Substance Abuse and Mental Health Services Administration. (2014). SAMHSA's Concept of Trauma and Guidance for a Trauma-Informed Approach (HHS Publication No. (SMA) 14-4884). https://ncsacw.samhsa.gov/userfiles/files/SAMHSA_Trauma.pdf

Sweeney, A., Filson, B., Kennedy, A., Collinson, L., & Gillard, S. (2018). A paradigm shift: relationships in trauma-informed mental health services. *BJPsych Advances, 24*(5), 319–333. https://doi.org/10.1192/bja.2018.29

Thomas, G. (2005). *Harm reduction policies and programs for persons involved in the criminal justice system.* https://www.academia.edu/5670450/Harm_reduction_policies_and_programs_for_persons_involved_in_the_criminal_justice_system

Tippin, G. K., Maranzan, K. A., & Mountain, M. A. (2017). Client outcomes associated with interprofessional care in a community mental health outpatient program. *Canadian Journal of Community Mental Health, 35*(3), 83–96. https://doi.org/10.7870/cjcmh-2016-042

Walsh, C. R., Mathieu, F., Hendricks, A. (2017). Report from the secondary traumatic stress San Diego think tank. *Traumatology, 23*(2), 124–128. http://dx.doi.org/10.1037/trm0000124

Ward-Miller, S., Farley, E. M., Espinosa, L., Brous, M. E., Giorgi-Cipriano, J., & Ferguson, J. (2021). Psychiatric mental health nursing in the international year of the nurse and COVID-19: One hospital's perspective on resilience and innovation-Past, present and future. *Archives of Psychiatric Nursing, 35*(3), 303–310. https://doi.org/10.1016/j.apnu.2020.11.002

World Health Organization. (2010). *Framework for action on interprofessional education and collaborative practice.* http://apps.who.int/iris/bitstream/handle/10665/70185/WHO_HRH_HPN_10.3_eng.pdf;jsessionid=5D60291A224267D5C521733DE52FE343?sequence=1

World Health Organization. (2019). *Recovery practices for mental health and well-being.* WHO QualityRights specialized training. https://apps.who.int/iris/bitstream/handle/10665/329602/9789241516747-eng.pdf

Communication and the Therapeutic Relationship

Cheryl Forchuk

LEARNING OBJECTIVES

After studying this chapter, you will be able to:

- Identify the importance of self-awareness in nursing practice.
- Develop a repertoire of verbal and nonverbal communication skills.
- Develop a process for selecting effective communication techniques.
- Explain how nurses can establish therapeutic relationships with clients by using rapport and empathy.
- Examine the physical, emotional, social, and spiritual boundaries of the nurse–client relationship.
- Discuss the significance of defence mechanisms.
- Explore each of the three phases of the nurse–client relationship: orientation, working, and resolution.
- Describe motivational interviewing (MI), including assumptions and techniques.
- Describe the transitional relationship model (TRM), including assumptions and components.

KEY TERMS

- active listening • boundaries • communication blocks
- content themes • countertransference • defence mechanisms • empathic linkages • empathy
- motivational interviewing • nontherapeutic relationships • nonverbal communication • orientation phase • passive listening • process recording • rapport
- resolution phase • self-disclosure • symbolism
- telehealth • therapeutic relationships • transference
- validation • verbal communication • working phase

KEY CONCEPTS

- nurse–client relationship • self-awareness
- therapeutic communication

Clients with mental health concerns may have special communication and relationship needs that require advanced therapeutic communication skills. In psychiatric and mental health (PMH) nursing, the nurse–client relationship is an important tool used to reach treatment goals. The purposes of this chapter are to (a) help nurses develop self-awareness and communication techniques needed for therapeutic nurse–client relationships, (b) examine the specific stages or steps involved in establishing the relationship, (c) explore the specific factors that make a nurse–client relationship successful and therapeutic, and (d) differentiate therapeutic from nontherapeutic relationships.

Self-Awareness

Self-awareness is the process of understanding one's own beliefs, thoughts, motivations, biases, and limitations and recognizing how they affect others. Without self-awareness, nurses will find it impossible to establish and maintain therapeutic relationships with clients. "Know thyself" is a basic tenet of PMH nursing (see Box 7.1).

To come to self-awareness, nurses can carry out self-examination. Self-examination involves reflecting on the personal meaning of the current nursing situation. This reflection can relate to similar past situations and issues related to personal values and beliefs. Self-examination can provoke anxiety and is rarely comfortable; it can occur alone or with help from others. Self-examination without the benefit of another's perspective can lead to a biased view of self. Conducting self-examination is best with a trusted individual who can give objective but realistic feedback. The development of self-awareness requires a willingness to be introspective and to examine personal beliefs, attitudes, and motivations.

KEY CONCEPT

Self-awareness is the process of understanding one's own beliefs, thoughts, motivations, biases, and limitations and recognizing how they affect self and others.

BOX 7.1 "Know Thyself"

- Do you have any physical problems or illnesses?
- Have you had significant traumatic life events (e.g., divorce, death of a significant person, abuse, disaster)?
- Do your family or significant others have prejudiced or embarrassing beliefs and attitudes about groups different than yours?
- Would sociocultural factors in your background contribute to being rejected by members of other cultures?
- Do you have strong religious beliefs that shape your daily life?

If your answer to any of these questions is yes, then how would these experiences and beliefs affect your ability to care for clients with these characteristics?

The Bio/Psycho/Social/Spiritual Self

Each nurse brings a bio/psycho/social/spiritual self to nursing practice. The client perceives the biologic dimension of the nurse in terms of physical characteristics: age, gender, body weight, height, ethnic or racial background, and any other observed physical characteristics. The nurse can have a certain genetic composition, illness, or unobservable physical disability that may influence the quality or delivery of nursing care. The nurse's psychological state also influences how they analyze client information and select treatment interventions. An emotional state or behaviour can inadvertently influence the therapeutic relationship. For example, a nurse who has just learned that their child is misusing drugs and who has a client with a history of drug use may inadvertently project a judgmental attitude toward the client, which would interfere with the formation of a therapeutic relationship. Nurses need to examine underlying emotions, motivations, and beliefs and determine how these factors shape behaviour.

The nurse's social biases can be particularly problematic for the nurse–client relationship. Although the nurse may not verbalize these values to clients, some are readily evident in the nurse's behaviour and appearance, such as how the nurse acts or appears at work. The nurse's religious beliefs or feelings can also affect interactions. For instance, beliefs about divorce, abortion, or same-sex relationships can affect how the nurse interacts with a client who is undergoing such experiences.

Understanding Personal Feelings and Beliefs and Changing Behaviour

Nurses must understand their own personal feelings and beliefs and try to avoid projecting them onto clients. This is not an easy task. For instance, due to ethnocentrism, our own sociocultural values may not be readily apparent. It takes effort to develop self-awareness, but it will enhance the nurse's objectivity and foster a nonjudgmental attitude, which is so important in building and maintaining trust throughout the nurse–client relationship. Soliciting feedback from colleagues and supervisors about how personal beliefs or thoughts are being projected onto others is a useful self-assessment technique. One of the reasons that ongoing clinical supervision is so important is that the supervisor often knows the nurse well and is able to continually observe for inappropriate communication and question assumptions that the nurse may hold, as well as reinforce helpful behaviour.

Once a nurse has identified and analyzed personal beliefs and attitudes, prejudicial behaviours may change. The change process requires introspective analysis that may result in viewing the world differently. Through self-awareness and conscious effort, the nurse can change learned behaviours to engage effectively in therapeutic relationships with clients. Nevertheless, a nurse may realize that some attitudes are too ingrained to support a therapeutic relationship with a client with different beliefs. In such cases, the nurse should refer the client to someone who may be better able to be therapeutically helpful.

Communication

Effective communication skills, including verbal and nonverbal techniques, are the building blocks for all successful relationships. The nurse–client relationship is built on therapeutic communication, the ongoing process of interaction through which meaning emerges (see Box 7.2). **Verbal communication**, which is principally achieved by spoken words, includes the underlying emotion, context, and connotation of what is actually said. **Nonverbal communication** includes gestures, expressions, and body language. Both the client and the nurse use verbal and nonverbal communication. **Empathic linkages** are the direct communication of feelings. To respond therapeutically in a nurse–client relationship, the nurse is responsible for assessing and interpreting all forms of client communication.

Therapeutic and social relationships are very different. In a **therapeutic relationship**, the nurse focuses on the client and client-related issues, even when engaging in social activities with that client. For example, a nurse may take a client shopping and out for lunch. Even though the nurse is engaged in a social activity,

BOX 7.2 Principles of Therapeutic Communication

1. The client should be the primary focus of the interaction.
2. A professional attitude sets the tone of the therapeutic relationship.
3. Use self-disclosure cautiously and only when the disclosure has a therapeutic purpose.
4. Avoid social relationships with clients.
5. Maintain client confidentiality.
6. Assess the client's intellectual competence to determine the level of understanding.
7. Implement interventions from a theoretic base.
8. Maintain a nonjudgmental attitude. Avoid making judgments about the client's behaviour and giving advice. By the time the client sees the nurse, they have had plenty of advice.
9. Guide the client to reinterpret their experiences rationally.
10. Track the client's verbal interaction through the use of clarifying statements. Avoid changing the subject unless the content change is in the client's best interest.

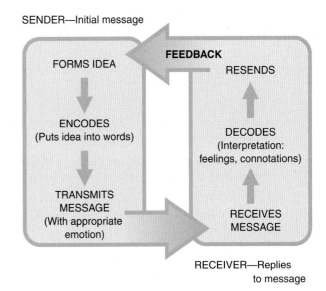

Figure 7.1 The communication process. (Adapted from Boyd, M. (1995). Communication with clients, families, health care providers, and diverse cultures. In M. Strader & P. Decker (Eds.), Role transition to patient care management (p. 431). Appleton & Lange.)

ent. On the surface, this interaction is deceptively simple, but unseen complexities lie beneath. Is the message that the nurse receives consistent with the client's original idea? Did the nurse interpret the message as the client intended? Is the verbal message consistent with the nonverbal flourishes that accompany it? Validation is essential to ensure that the nurse has received the information accurately. (See section "Validation" later in this chapter for further discussion.)

Self-Disclosure

One of the most important principles of therapeutic communication for the nurse to follow is to focus the interaction on the client's concerns. **Self-disclosure**, or telling the client personal information, is generally not a good idea since the conversation should focus on the client, not the nurse. If a client asks the nurse personal questions, the nurse should elicit the underlying reason for the request. The nurse can then determine how much, if any, personal information to disclose. In revealing personal information, the nurse should be purposeful and have identified therapeutic outcomes. For example, a client struggling with the implications of marriage and fidelity asks a nurse if they have had an extramarital affair. The nurse interprets the client's statement as seeking role-modeling behaviour for an adult and judges self-disclosure in this instance to be therapeutic. The nurses respond honestly that they do not engage in affairs and redirect the discussion back to the client's concerns.

Nurses may feel uncomfortable avoiding client questions for fear of seeming rude. Sometimes they disclose too much personal information because they are trying

that trip should have a definite purpose, and conversation should focus only on the client. The nurse must not attempt to meet their own social or other needs during the activity.

KEY CONCEPT

Therapeutic communication is the ongoing process of interaction through which meaning emerges.

Using Verbal Communication

The process of verbal communication involves a sender, a message, and a receiver. The client is often the sender, and the nurse is often the receiver (Fig. 7.1), but communication always works two ways. The client formulates an idea, encodes a message (puts ideas into words), and then transmits the message with emotion. The client's words and their underlying emotional tone and connotation communicate their needs and emotional problems or issues. The nurse receives the message, decodes it (interprets the message, including its feelings, connotation, and context), and then responds to the cli-

Table 7.1 Self-Disclosure in Therapeutic Versus Social Relationships		
Situation	Appropriate Therapeutic Response	Inappropriate Social Response With Rationale
A client asks the nurse if they had fun over the weekend.	"The weekend was fine. How did you spend your weekend?"	"It was great. My boyfriend and I went to dinner and a movie." (This self-disclosure has no therapeutic purpose. The response focuses the conversation on the nurse, not the client.)
A client asks a student nurse if they have ever been to a particular bar.	"Many people go there. I'm wondering if you have ever been there."	"Oh yes—all the time. It's a lot of fun." (Sharing information about outside activities is inappropriate.)
A client asks a nurse if mental illness is in his family.	"Mental illnesses do run in families. I've had a lot of experience caring for people with mental illnesses."	"My sister is being treated for depression." (This self-disclosure has no purpose, and the nurse is missing the meaning of the question.)
While shopping with a client, the nurse sees a friend who approaches them.	To their friend: "I know it looks like I'm not working, but I really am. I'll see you later."	"Hi, Bob. This is Jane Doe, a client." (Introducing the client to the friend is very inappropriate and violates client confidentiality.)

to be nice; however, being nice is not necessarily therapeutic. As appropriate, redirecting the client, giving a neutral or vague answer, or saying, "Let's talk about you" may be all that is necessary to limit self-disclosure. In some instances, nurses may need to tell the client directly that they will not share personal information (Table 7.1).

Verbal Communication Techniques

Nurses use many verbal techniques in establishing relationships and helping clients focus on their problems and goals. Asking a question, restating, and reflecting are examples of such techniques. These techniques may seem artificial at first, but with practice, they can be useful.

One of the most difficult, but often most effective, techniques is the use of silence during verbal interactions. By maintaining an open silence, the nurse allows the client to gather thoughts and to proceed at their own pace.

Listening is another valuable tool. Silence and listening differ in that silence consists of deliberate pauses to encourage the client to reflect and eventually respond. Listening is an ongoing activity by which the nurse attends to the client's verbal and nonverbal communication. The art of listening is developed through careful attention to the content and meaning of the client's speech. There are two types of listening: passive and active. **Passive listening** involves sitting quietly and letting the client talk. A passive listener allows the client to ramble and does not focus or guide the thought process. Passive listening does not foster a therapeutic relationship. Through **active listening**, the nurse focuses on what the client is saying to interpret and respond to the message objectively. While listening, the nurse concentrates on the underlying meaning of what the client says. The nurse's verbal and nonverbal behaviours indicate active listening. The nurse usually responds indirectly, using techniques such as open-ended statements, reflection (Table 7.2), and questions that elicit additional responses from the client. In active listening, the

nurse should avoid changing the subject and instead follow the client's lead, although at times, it is necessary to respond directly to help a client focus on a specific topic or to clarify content, thoughts, or beliefs.

Some verbal techniques, however, block interactions and inhibit therapeutic communication (Table 7.3). One of the biggest blocks to communication is giving advice, particularly that which others likely have already given. Giving advice is different from supporting clients through decision-making. The therapeutic dialogue presented in Box 7.3 differentiates between advice (telling clients what to do or how to act) and therapeutic communication, by which the nurse and client explore alternative ways of viewing the client's world. The client then can reach their own conclusions about the best approaches to use.

Using Nonverbal Communication

Gestures, facial expressions, and body language actually communicate more than do verbal messages. Under the best circumstances, body language mirrors or enhances verbal communication; however, if verbal and nonverbal messages are conflicting, the listener likely will believe the nonverbal message since it functions on a more basic level. For example, if a client says they feel fine but has a sad facial expression and is slumped in a chair away from others, a message of sadness will more likely be received than the client's words. The same is true of a nurse's behaviour. If a nurse tells a client they are happy to see them, but their facial expression communicates indifference, the client will receive the message that the nurse is indifferent. At times, people with mental health concerns have difficulty verbally expressing themselves and interpreting the emotions of others. Nurses therefore need to continually assess the nonverbal communication needs of clients. Eye contact (or lack thereof), posture, movement (e.g., shifting in chair, pacing), facial expressions, and gestures are nonverbal behaviours that communicate thoughts and feelings. A client with low self-esteem may be unable to maintain eye contact and

Table 7.2 Verbal Communication Techniques

Technique	Definition	Example	Use
Acceptance	Encouraging and receiving information in a nonjudgmental and interested manner	*Client*: I have done something terrible. *Nurse*: I would like to hear about it. It's OK to discuss it with me.	Used in establishing trust and developing empathy
Confrontation	Presenting the client with a different reality of the situation	*Client*: My best friend never calls me. They hate me. *Nurse*: I was in the room yesterday when they called.	Used cautiously to immediately redefine the client's reality However, it can alienate the client if used inappropriately. A nonjudgmental attitude is critical for confrontation to be effective
Doubt	Expressing or voicing doubt when a client relates a situation	*Client*: My best friend hates me. They never call me. *Nurse*: From what you have told me, that does not sound like them. When did they call you last?	Used carefully and only when the nurse feels confident about the details It is used when the nurse wants to guide the client toward other explanations
Interpretation	Putting into words what the client is implying or feeling	*Client*: I could not sleep because someone would come in my room and rape me. *Nurse*: It sounds like you were scared last night.	Used in helping the clients identify underlying thoughts or feelings
Observation	Stating to the client what the nurse is observing	*Nurse*: You are trembling and perspiring. When did this start?	Used when a client's behaviours (verbal or nonverbal) are obvious and unusual for that client
Open-ended statements	Introducing an idea and letting the client respond	*Nurse*: Trust means…. *Client*: That someone will keep you safe.	Used when helping the client explore feelings or gain insight
Reflection	Redirecting the idea back to the client	*Client*: Should I go home for the weekend? *Nurse*: Should you go home for the weekend?	Used when the client is asking for the nurse's approval or judgment. Use of reflection helps the nurse maintain a nonjudgmental approach
Restatement	Repeating the main idea expressed; lets the client know what was heard	*Client*: I hate this place. I don't belong here. *Nurse*: You don't want to be here.	Used when trying to clarify what the client has said
Silence	Remaining quiet but nonverbally expressing interest during an interaction	*Client*: I am angry!! *Nurse*: (Silence) *Client*: My partner had an affair.	Used when the client needs to express ideas but may not know quite how to do it. With silence, the client can focus on putting thoughts together
Validation	Clarifying the nurse's understanding of the situation	*Nurse*: Let me see if I understand.	Used when the nurse is trying to understand a situation the client is trying to describe

thus may spend a great deal of time looking toward the floor. A client who is pacing and restless may be agitated or having a reaction to medication. A clenched fist may indicate that a person feels angry or hostile.

Nonverbal behaviour is culturally specific. The nurse must therefore be careful to understand their own cultural context as well as that of the client. For example, in some cultures (e.g., First Nations, Métis, and Inuit Peoples of Canada), it is considered disrespectful to look directly into another person's eyes. Other cultures may see a person who makes little eye contact as "hiding something" or having low self-esteem. Other examples of nonverbal communication that may vary considerably among cultures are whether one points with the finger, nose, or eyes and how much hand gesturing one uses.

Nurses should use positive body language, such as sitting at the same eye level as the client with a relaxed posture that projects interest and attention. Leaning slightly forward helps engage the client. Generally, nurses should not cross their arms or legs during therapeutic communication because such postures erect barriers to interaction. Uncrossed arms and legs project openness and a willingness to engage in conversation (Fig. 7.2). Verbal responses should be consistent with nonverbal messages.

Recognizing Empathic Linkages

Empathic linkages are the communication of feelings (Peplau, 1952/1988). This form of communication commonly occurs with anxiety. Nurses may become aware of subjective feelings of anxiety. It may be difficult for nurses to determine whether the anxiety is communicated interpersonally or whether they are personally reacting to some of the content of what the client is

Table 7.3   Techniques That Inhibit Communication

Technique	Definition	Example	Problem
Advice	Telling a client what to do	*Client*: I can't sleep. It is too noisy. *Nurse*: Turn off the light and shut your door.	The nurse solves the client's problem, which may not be the appropriate solution and encourages dependency on the nurse.
Agreement	Agreeing with a particular viewpoint of a client	*Client*: Abortions are sinful. *Nurse*: I agree.	The client is denied an opportunity to change their view now that the nurse agrees.
Challenges	Disputing a client's beliefs with arguments, logical thinking, or direct order	*Client*: I'm a cowboy. *Nurse*: If you are a cowboy, then what are you doing in the hospital?	The nurse belittles the client and decreases self-esteem. The client will avoid relating to the nurse who challenges.
Disapproval	Judging a client's situation and behaviour	*Client*: I'm so sorry. I did not mean to kill my mother. *Nurse*: You should be. How could anyone kill their mother?	The nurse belittles the client. The client will avoid the nurse.
Reassurance	Telling a client that everything will be OK	*Client*: Everyone thinks I'm bad. *Nurse*: You are a good person.	The nurse makes a statement that may not be true. The client is blocked from exploring feelings.

BOX 7.3 THERAPEUTIC DIALOGUE

Giving Advice Versus Recommendations

Salma has just received a diagnosis of phobic disorder and been given a prescription for fluoxetine. Salma was referred to the primary care unit because of reluctance to take this medication due to a fear of becoming suicidal.

Two approaches are given below.

Ineffective Communication (Advice)

Nurse: Salma, the doctor has ordered the medication because it will help you.

Salma: I don't want to take the medication because I am afraid of becoming suicidal. I heard that some of this psychiatric medication does that. I haven't had any attacks for 2 weeks.

Nurse: This medication has rarely had that side effect. You should try it and see if you have any suicidal thoughts.

Salma: OK. (The nurse leaves and Salma does not take the medication. Within a week, Salma is taken to the emergency room with a panic attack.)

Effective Communication (Recommendations)

Nurse: Salma, how have you been doing?

Salma: So far, so good. I haven't had any attacks for 2 weeks.

Nurse: I understand that the doctor gave you a prescription for medication that may help with the panic attacks.

Salma: Yes, but I don't want to take it because I am afraid of becoming suicidal. I heard that some of this psychiatric medication does that.

Nurse: Have you ever had feelings of hurting yourself?

Salma: Not really.

Nurse: If you took the medication and had thoughts like that, what would you do?

Salma: I don't know.

Nurse: I think I see your dilemma. This medication may help your panic attacks, but the suicidal thoughts are a real fear. Is that it?

Salma: Yeah, that's it.

Nurse: Are there any circumstances under which you would be able to try the medication?

Salma: If I knew that I would not have suicidal thoughts.

Nurse: I can't guarantee that but I could call you every few days to see if you are having any of these thoughts and help you deal with them.

Salma: Oh, that will be OK.

(Salma continued with taking the medication.)

CRITICAL THINKING CHALLENGE

- Contrast the communication in the first scenario with that in the second.
- What therapeutic communication techniques did the second nurse employ that may have contributed to a better outcome?
- Are there any cues in the first scenario that indicate that the client will not follow the nurse's advice? Explain.

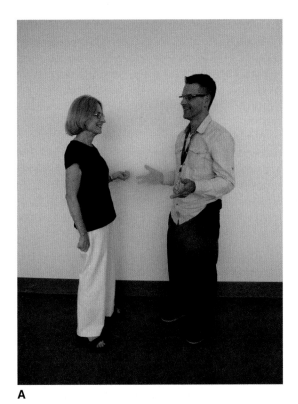
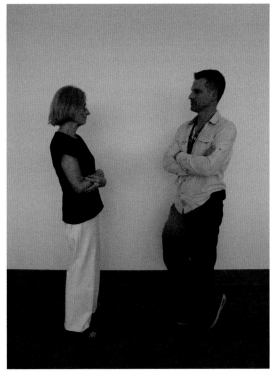

A   B

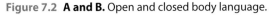

Figure 7.2 A and B. Open and closed body language.

communicating. Being aware of one's own feelings and analyzing them is crucial to determining the source of the feelings.

Selecting Communication Techniques

In therapeutic communication, nurses choose the best words to say and use nonverbal behaviours that are consistent with these words. If a client is angry and upset, should the nurse invite the client to sit down and discuss the problem, walk quietly with the client, or simply observe the client from a distance and not initiate conversation? Choosing the best response begins with assessing and interpreting the meaning of the client's communication—both verbal and nonverbal.

Nurses should not necessarily take verbal messages literally, especially when clients are upset or angry. For example, a nurse enters the room of a newly admitted client who accusingly says, "You locked me up and threw away the key." The nurse could respond defensively that they had nothing to do with the client being admitted; however, that response would end in an argument and communication would be blocked. It would be more appropriate for the nurse to recognize that the client is communicating frustration at being in a locked psychiatric unit and not take the accusation personally.

Nurses also need to identify desired client outcomes. To do so, nurses should engage clients with eye contact (if culturally appropriate) and quietly try to interpret clients' feelings. In the example just discussed, the desired

outcome is for the client to clarify the hospitalization experience. The nurse responds by saying, "It must be frustrating to feel locked up." The nurse focuses on the client's feelings rather than the accusations, which reflects an understanding of the client's feelings. The client knows that the nurse accepts these feelings, which leads to further discussion. It may seem impossible to plan reactions for each situation, but with practice, the nurse will begin to respond consistently in a therapeutic way.

Applying Communication Concepts

When nurses are interacting with clients, additional considerations can enhance the quality of communication. This section describes the importance of rapport, validation, empathy, and the role of boundaries and body space in nurse–client interactions.

Rapport

Rapport, interpersonal harmony characterized by understanding and respect, is important in developing a trusting, therapeutic relationship. Nurses establish rapport through interpersonal warmth, a nonjudgmental attitude, and a demonstration of understanding. A skilled nurse will establish a rapport that alleviates the client's anxiety in discussing personal problems.

People with mental health problems often feel alone and isolated. Establishing a rapport helps lessen those feelings. When a rapport develops, a client feels comfortable with the nurse and finds self-disclosure easier. The nurse also feels comfortable and recognizes that an interpersonal bond or alliance is developing. All these factors—comfort, sense of sharing, and decreased anxiety—are important in establishing and building the nurse–client relationship.

Validation

Validation is explicitly confirming with another person one's own thoughts or feelings with respect to a specific event or behaviour. To do so, the nurse must own their own thoughts or feelings by using "I" statements. Validating communication generally refers to observations, thoughts, or feelings and seeking explicit feedback. For example, a nurse who sees a client pacing the hallway before a planned family visit may question whether the client is anxious. Validation may occur with a statement such as, "I noticed you pacing the hallway. I wonder if you are feeling anxious about the family visit?" The client may agree, "Yes. I keep worrying about what is going to happen!" or disagree, "No. I have been trying to get into the bathroom for the last 30 minutes, but my roommate is still in there!"

Empathy

The use of empathy in a therapeutic relationship is central to PMH nursing. **Empathy** is the ability to experience, in the present, a situation as another did at some time in the past. It is the ability to put oneself in another person's circumstances and feelings. The nurse does not need to have actually had the experience but has to be able to imagine the feelings associated with it. Empathic communication involves the nurse receiving information from the client with open, nonjudgmental acceptance and communicating this understanding of the experience and feelings so that the client feels understood.

Bio/Psycho/Social/Spiritual Boundaries and Body Space Zones

Boundaries are the defining limits of individuals, objects, or relationships. Boundaries mark territory, identifying what is "mine" from what is "not mine." Human beings have many different types of boundaries. Material boundaries, such as fences around property, artificially imposed territorial lines, and bodies of water, can define territory as well as provide security and order. Within the bio/psycho/social/spiritual model, personal boundaries have physical, psychological, social, and spiritual dimensions. Physical boundaries are those established in terms of physical closeness to others—whom we allow to touch us or how close we want others to stand near us. Psychological boundar-

ies are established in terms of emotional distance from others—how much of our innermost feelings and thoughts we want to share. Social boundaries, such as norms, customs, and roles, help us establish our closeness and place within the family, culture, and community. Spiritual boundaries, related to such things as our understanding of the meaning of life, our religious values, and/or our sense of relationship with a greater power, shape our way of being in the world. Boundaries are not fixed but dynamic. When boundaries are involuntarily transgressed, the individual can feel threatened and may respond to the perceived threat. Nurses must elicit permission before implementing interventions that invade personal boundaries.

Personal Boundaries

Every individual is surrounded by four different body zones. These were identified by Hall (1990) as the intimate zone (e.g., whispering and embracing), the personal zone (e.g., for close friends), the social zone (e.g., for acquaintances), and the public zone (e.g., usually for interacting with strangers). These zones provide varying degrees of protection against unwanted physical closeness during interactions. The breadth of each zone varies according to culture. Some cultures define the intimate zone narrowly and the personal zones widely. Friends in these cultures stand and sit close while interacting. While other cultures may define the intimate zone widely and are uncomfortable when others stand close to them, the variability of intimate and personal zones has implications for nursing. For a client to be comfortable with a nurse, the nurse needs to protect the intimate zone of that individual. The client usually will allow the nurse to enter the personal zone but will express discomfort if the nurse breaches the intimate zone. For the nurse, the difficulty lies in differentiating personal and intimate zones for each client.

The nurse's awareness of their own need for intimate and personal space is another prerequisite for therapeutic interactions with the client. It is important that nurses feel comfortable when interacting with clients. Establishing a comfort zone may entail fine-tuning the size of body zones. Recognizing this will help nurses understand occasional inexplicable reactions to the proximity of clients.

Professional Boundaries

For nurses, professional boundaries are essential to consider in the context of the nurse–client relationship. Clients often enter such relationships at a very vulnerable point, and nurses need to be aware of professional boundaries to avoid exploitation of clients. For example, in a friendship, there is a two-way sharing of personal information and feelings, but as mentioned previously, the focus is on the client's needs, and the nurse generally does not share personal information or attempt to meet their own needs through the relationship. The client may seek a friendship or sexual relationship with the nurse (or vice versa), which would be a violation of the professional role. Although professional boundaries are about power, influence, and control, they are not clear and precise. Professional boundaries can become blurred and ambiguous, given the familiarity, trust, and emotional intensity often involved in therapeutic relationships. Nurses can address boundary concerns by examining risk factors for boundary crossings and boundary violations, identifying how to appropriately respond when encountering these situations, and discussing any perceived challenges with a supervisor or senior colleague (Valente, 2017).

There are several indicators that a nurse–client relationship may be crossing professional boundaries. These include gift-giving by either party, a nurse spending inordinate time with a particular client, a nurse strenuously defending or explaining a client's behaviour in team meetings, a nurse feeling that they are the only one who truly understands the client, a nurse and client keeping secrets, and a nurse thinking frequently about a client outside of work (College of Nurses of Ontario [CNO], 2019; Forchuk et al., 2006; Gallop et al., 2002). Provincial regulatory bodies may have guidelines or firm rules, such as stipulating how long following the termination of a therapeutic relationship before one may engage in a romantic or sexual relationship. Within psychiatric disciplines, a romantic or sexual relationship with a former client is considered inappropriate, regardless of the length of time since the professional relationship was terminated. In nursing, the guidelines are generic and do not identify differences between specialties. Nevertheless, the professional implications of a personal relationship following a nursing relationship that involved

psychotherapy are serious and must be carefully considered. Guidelines are generally quite vague regarding when friendships would be appropriate, but such relationships are not appropriate when nurses are actively providing care to clients. An exceptional case could be a relationship that preexisted that of a nurse with a client, for which another nurse is unavailable, such as in a nursing outpost (CNO, 2019). Similarly, relationships to meet the nurse's needs that are acquired through the nursing context, such as a relationship with a client's family member, also breach professional boundaries. It is important that nurses be familiar with the standards of practice related to boundaries and therapeutic relationships of their provincial regulatory and professional associations. When concerns arise related to therapeutic boundaries, nurses must seek clinical supervision or transfer care of the client immediately. The therapeutic dialogue presented in Box 7.4 illustrates how to respond to a client's request for the nurse's personal contact information.

Defence Mechanisms

Defence mechanisms (or coping mechanisms) are defined in the fifth edition of the *Diagnostic and Statistical Manual of Mental Disorders* (DSM-5) as "mechanisms that mediate the [client's] reaction to emotional conflicts and to external stressors. Some defense mechanisms (e.g., projection, splitting, acting out) are almost invariably maladaptive. Others (e.g., suppression, denial) may be either maladaptive or adaptive, depending on their severity, their inflexibility, and the context in which they occur" (American Psychiatric Association, 2013, p. 819). The concept of defence mechanisms originated with Freud's psychoanalytic theory and was conceived as the way the ego protected the individual from

BOX 7.4 THERAPEUTIC DIALOGUE

Client Request for a Nurse's Contact Information
How should a nurse respond when a client asks for their phone number or Facebook contact? Politely clarify that the relationship is professional and that the nurse will not share this information.

Context: The client located the nurse on Facebook and submitted a friend request. The nurse did not accept the friend request and did not message the client online to explain why.

At the next meeting with the client, the nurse brought up the Facebook request.

Nurse: "I noticed that you sent a friend request to me over Facebook."
Client: "Yes, I did. I was wondering why you didn't accept my friend request."

Nurse: "I did not accept it because what we have is a professional relationship, and it would not be appropriate for me to have social contact with clients outside of the therapeutic setting."
Client: "Oh. I was hoping to contact you if I had some questions after discharge."
Nurse: "Your discharge date is approaching. We have discussed community resources that are available, and follow-up appointments will continue with your physician. How are you feeling about discharge?"

overwhelming anxiety (see Chapter 9). Healthy individuals use various defence mechanisms throughout their lives. A defence mechanism becomes pathologic when it is used so persistently that it becomes maladaptive. Suppression or denial, for instance, involves a process where anxiety-provoking information is not accepted (for suppression, this is conscious, and for denial, this is unconscious). These two defence mechanisms may be either maladaptive or adaptive depending on their severity and the context in which they occur. Other defence mechanisms such as projection (attributing one's own feelings onto another), splitting (self or others viewed as all bad or all good), and acting out (expressing unconscious feelings in actions rather than words), however, are almost invariably maladaptive.

As nurses develop therapeutic relationships, they will recognize their clients, and perhaps themselves, using defence mechanisms. As defence mechanisms are almost always used unconsciously, it will be difficult for nurses to readily identify their own without reviewing the relationship with someone else. With experience, nurses will evaluate the purpose of a defence mechanism and then determine whether it should be discussed with the client. For example, if a client is using humour to alleviate an emotionally intense situation, it may be very appropriate. On the other hand, if someone continually rationalizes antisocial behaviour, the use of the defence mechanism should be discussed.

Analyzing Interactions

It is not unusual for people with mental health concerns to have difficulty communicating. For example, perceptual, cognitive, and information-processing deficits, typical of people with schizophrenia, can interfere with the person's ability to express ideas, understand concepts, and accurately perceive the environment. Because of the complexity of communication, mental health professionals monitor their interactions with clients using various methods, including audio recording, video recording, and process recording (writing a verbatim transcript of the interaction). A video or audio recording of an interaction provides the most accurate monitoring but is cumbersome to use. Process recording, one of the easiest methods to use, is adequate in most situations. Nurses should use it when first learning therapeutic communication and during times when communication becomes problematic. In a **process recording**, the nurse records, from memory, the verbatim interaction immediately after the communication (Box 7.5). The nurse then analyzes the content of the interaction in terms of the words and their meaning for both the client and the nurse. The analysis is especially important because the ability to communicate verbally is often compromised in people with mental health disorders.

Words may not have the same meaning for the client as they do for the nurse. Clarification of meaning becomes especially important. The analysis can identify symbolic meanings, themes, and blocks in communication. **Symbolism**, the use of a word or phrase to represent an object, event, or feeling, is used universally. For example, automobiles are named for wild animals that represent speed, prowess, and beauty. In people with mental health disorders, the use of words to symbolize events, objects, or feelings is often idiosyncratic, and they cannot explain their choices. For example, a person who is feeling scared and anxious may tell the nurse that bombs and guns are exploding. It is up to the

---

BOX 7.5 Process Recording

Setting: The living room of a teenage client's home. Their parents are in the room but cannot hear the conversation. The client is sitting on the couch and the nurse is sitting on a chair. This is the nurse's first visit after the client's discharge from the hospital.

Client	Nurse	Comments/Interpretation
	How are you doing, Alex?	*Plan*: Initially develop a sense of trust and initiate a therapeutic relationship.
I'm fine. It's good to be home. I really don't like the hospital.	You didn't like the hospital?	*Interpretation*: Alex does not want to return to the hospital. Use reflection to begin to understand his experience.
NO. The nurses lock you up. Are you a nurse?	Yes. I'm a nurse. I'm wondering if you think that I will lock you up.	*Interpretation*: Alex is wondering what my role is and whether I will put him back in the hospital.
You could tell my mom to put me back in the hospital.	Any treatment I recommend I will thoroughly discuss with you first. I am here to help you stay out of the hospital. I will not discuss anything with your mother unless you give me the permission to do so.	Use interpretation to clarify Alex's thinking. Alex is wondering about my relationship with his mother. Explain my role.

nurse to make the connection between the bombs and guns and the client's feelings and then validate this with the client. Because of the client's cognitive limitations, the individual may express feelings only symbolically.

Some clients, for example, who have developmental disabilities or neurocognitive challenges, may experience difficulties with abstract thinking and symbolism. Conversations may be interpreted literally. For example, in response to the question, "What brings you to the hospital?," a client might reply, "The ambulance." In these situations, the nurse must be cautious to avoid using symbols or metaphors. Concrete language—that is, language reflecting what can be observed through the senses—will be more easily understood.

Verbal behaviour is also interpreted by analyzing **content themes**. Clients often express concerns or feelings repeatedly in several different ways. After a few sessions, a common theme emerges. Themes may emerge symbolically, as in the case with the client who constantly talks about the "guns and bombs." Alternatively, a theme may simply be identified as a recurrent thread of a story that a client retells at each session. For example, a client who always explained their early abandonment by their family led the nurse to hypothesize that this client had an underlying fear of rejection. The nurse was then able to test whether there was an underlying fear and to develop strategies to help the client explore the fear (Box 7.6). It is important to involve clients in analyzing themes so that they may learn this skill. Within the therapeutic relationship, the person who does the work is the one who develops the competencies, so the nurse must be careful to share this opportunity with the client (Peplau, 1952/1988).

Communication blocks are identified by topic changes that either the nurse or the client makes. Topics are changed for various reasons. A client may change the topic from one that does not interest them to one that they find more meaningful. However, an individual often changes the topic because they are uncomfortable with a particular subject. Once a topic change is identified, the nurse or client hypothesizes the reason for it. If the nurse changes the topic, they need to determine why. The nurse may find that they are uncomfortable with the topic or may not be listening to the client. Beginning mental health nurses who are uncomfortable with silences or trying to elicit specific information from the client often change topics.

The nurse must also record and interpret the client's nonverbal behaviour in light of the verbal behaviour. Is the client saying one thing verbally and another nonverbally? The nurse must consider the client's cultural background. Is the behaviour consistent with cultural norms? The nurse must also record and interpret the client's nonverbal behaviour in light of the verbal behaviour. Is the client saying one thing verbally and another nonverbally? Is the person's nonverbal behaviour inconsistent with what is normal behaviour for that person? Is it inconsistent with the person's cultural norms as previously expressed in their everyday life?

The Nurse–Client Relationship

The nurse–client relationship is a dynamic process that changes with time. It can be viewed in steps or phases with characteristic behaviours for both the client and the nurse. Chapter 9 provides a description of Hildegard Peplau's (1952/1988) model that was introduced in the seminal work, *Interpersonal Relations in Nursing*. The nurse–client relationship is conceptualized in three overlapping phases that evolve with time: orientation phase, working phase, and resolution phase. Research for Best Practice Box 7.7 describes factors that facilitate and interfere with the development of the nurse–client relationship from the client perspective.

The **orientation phase** is the phase during which the nurse and client get to know each other. During this phase, which can last from a few minutes to several months, the client develops a sense of trust in the nurse. The second phase is the **working phase**, in which the client uses the relationship to examine specific problems and learn new ways of approaching them. The final stage, the **resolution phase**, is the termination stage of the relationship and lasts from the time the problems are actually resolved to the close of the relationship. The relationship does not develop in a linear manner; rather, the relationship may be predominantly in one phase, but reflections of all phases can be seen in most nurse–client relationships.

BOX 7.6 Themes and Interactions

Session 1	Client discusses the death of their mother at a young age.
Session 2	Client explains that their sister is now married and never visits them.
Session 3	Client says that their best friend in the hospital was discharged and is someone they really miss.
Session 4	Client cries about a lost kitten.

Interpretation: Theme of loss is pervasive in several sessions.

KEY CONCEPT

The nurse–client relationship is a dynamic process that changes with time. It can be viewed in steps or phases with characteristic behaviours for both the client and the nurse.

BOX 7.7 Research for Best Practice

CLIENT PERSPECTIVE OF FACTORS THAT FACILITATE AND INTERFERE WITH INTERPERSONAL RELATIONSHIPS WITH CARE PROVIDERS

Bacha, K., Hanley, T., & Winter, L. A. (2020). 'Like a human being, I was an equal, I wasn't just a patient': Service users' perspectives on their experiences of relationships with the staff in mental health services. *Psychology and Psychotherapy: Theory, Research and Practice, 93*(2), 367–386. https://doi. org/10.1111/papt.12218

Purpose: This article positions the therapeutic relationship as being "at the heart of psychological change." It reports on experiences of mental health service users who are in therapeutic relationships with mental health practitioners and the impact of these relationships on the view of self and treatment outcomes.

Methods: The authors used an interpretive phenomenological analysis to explain how people make sense of their experiences. Data were collected in the United Kingdom through in-depth interviews with eight service user participants who experienced severe psychological distress and had been in a therapeutic relationship with a mental health practitioner.

Findings: Participants described factors that made service providers effective and helpful. These factors include being treated as a human being, feeling safe within the relationship, the attuned practitioner, and receiving effective treatments. In transformative relationships, practitioners provided a secure and consistent relationship that reinforced a positive sense of self and included a "protective power and empowerment" element, which supported movement toward recovery. Traumatic relationships involved service users being treated as an illness and not as a person, having feelings of disempowerment, and receiving threatening and oppressive treatment.

Implications for Practice: Interactions between service users and mental health practitioners can either be effective and helpful or harmful and traumatizing for clients. Practitioners can enhance the therapeutic relationship by treating clients with dignity, creating a safe and trusting space, and listening to clients describe personal needs in care for effective interventions.

Orientation Phase

The orientation phase begins when the nurse and client meet and ends when the client begins to identify problems to be examined within the relationship. During the orientation phase, the nurse discusses the client's expectations, explains the purpose of the relationship and its boundaries, and facilitates the development of the relationship. It is natural for the nurse and client to be more nervous during the first few sessions. The goal of the orientation phase is to develop trust and security within the nurse–client relationship. During this initial phase, the nurse listens intently to the client's history and perception of problems and begins to understand the client and identify themes. The use of empathy facilitates the development of a positive therapeutic relationship.

First Meeting

During the first meeting, it is important to outline both nursing and client responsibilities. The nurse is responsible for providing guidance throughout the therapeutic relationship, protecting confidential information, and maintaining professional boundaries. The client is responsible for attending agreed-upon sessions, interacting during the sessions, and participating in the nurse–client relationship. The nurse should also explain

clearly to the client the role of the nurse as well as pragmatic issues, such as meeting times, handling of missed sessions, and the estimated length of the relationship. Issues related to recording information and how the nurse will work within the interprofessional team should also be made explicit.

It is not unusual for both the nurse and the client to feel anxious at the first meeting. The nurse should recognize the anxieties and attempt to alleviate them before the meeting. The client's behaviour during this first meeting may indicate to the nurse some of the client's problems in interpersonal relationships. For example, a client may talk nonstop for 15 minutes or may boast of sexual conquests. What the client chooses to tell or not to tell is significant. What a client first does or says may not accurately indicate their true feelings or the situation. In the beginning, clients may deny problems or choose not to discuss them as defence mechanisms or to prevent the nurse from getting to know them. The client is usually nervous and insecure during the first few sessions and may exhibit behaviour reflective of these emotions, such as rambling. Often by the third session, the client can better focus on a topic.

Confidentiality in Treatment

Ideally, nurses include people who are important to the client in planning and implementing care. The nurse and client should discuss the issue of confidentiality in the first session. The nurse should be clear about any information that is to be shared with anyone else. Usually, the nurse shares significant assessment data and client progress with supervisors and interprofessional team members, including physicians. Most clients expect the nurse to communicate with other mental health professionals and are comfortable with this arrangement. Boundaries around what information can be shared with whom, and under what circumstances, are covered under provincial/territorial legislation, such as mental health acts and health information acts. Appropriate behaviour regarding confidentiality and social media is important to address. Nurses, including nursing students, are prohibited from discussing client information through any form of social media (e.g., personal blogs, Facebook, Instagram, TikTok, Tumblr, etc.). It is therefore important that each nurse be aware of the legislation in the province or territory in which they are practicing.

Testing the Relationship

This first part of the orientation phase, called the "honeymoon phase," is usually pleasant. However, the therapeutic team typically hits rough spots before completing this phase. The client begins to test the relationship to become convinced that the nurse will really accept them. Typical testing behaviours include forgetting a scheduled session or being late. Clients may also express anger at something a nurse says or accuse the nurse of breaking confidentiality. Another common pattern is for the client to introduce a relatively superficial issue first as if it is the major problem. Nurses must recognize that these behaviours are designed to test the relationship and establish its parameters, not to express rejection or dissatisfaction with the nurse. Nursing students often feel personally rejected when clients engage in testing and may even become angry with the client. It is important

for nurses and nursing students alike to understand the behaviour as testing and continue to be available to the client. With the adoption of consistent responses, these behaviours usually subside. Testing needs to be understood as a normal way that human beings develop trust.

Some issues specific to mental health clients can occur. For example, a client experiencing paranoia, by definition, is going to have difficulty establishing trust and may require a longer orientation phase. A client who is depressed may have difficulty expressing needs and may require periods of silence to feel comfortable in moving forward in the relationship.

Working Phase

When the client begins identifying problems to work on, the working phase of the relationship has started. Problem identification can yield a wide range of issues, such as managing symptoms of a mental health issue, coping with chronic pain, examining issues related to sexual abuse, and dealing with problematic interpersonal relationships. Through the relationship, the client begins to explore the identified problems and develop strategies to resolve them. By the time the working phase is reached, the client has developed enough trust that they can examine the identified problems within the security of the therapeutic relationship. In the working phase, the nurse can use various verbal and nonverbal techniques to help the client examine problems and support the client to plan strategies to address concerns.

Transference (unconscious assignment to others of the feelings and attitudes that the client originally associated with important figures) and **countertransference** (the provider's emotional reaction to the client based on personal unconscious needs and conflicts) become important issues in the working phase (refer to Box 7.8). For example, a client could be hostile to a nurse because of the underlying resentment of authority figures; the nurse, in turn, could respond defensively because of earlier experiences of

---

BOX 7.8 THERAPEUTIC DIALOGUE

Countertransference in the Nurse–Client Relationship

A client and nurse are having a formal talk therapy session. The nurse is grieving the recent loss of their father after a prolonged illness. The client is an adolescent who lives at home with their parents and is having challenges in the area of family relationships.

Client: "I am having problems with my dad again."
Nurse: "What sort of problems?"
Client: "He just won't leave me alone. When I'm in my room, he walks in whenever he wants and doesn't give me privacy."
Nurse: "That sounds like it is frustrating for you."

Client: "It is. I get so mad! I even threw a book at him once so he would get out."
Nurse: "Was he hurt?"
Client: "I didn't care."
Nurse: "Well, your dad will not be around forever. It is important to have a good relationship with your parents."

anger. The client uses transference to examine problems. During this phase, the client is psychologically vulnerable and emotionally dependent on the nurse. The nurse needs to recognize countertransference and prevent it from eroding professional boundaries.

Many times, nurses are eager to implement rehabilitation plans. However, implementation of such plans requires the clients' trust and an ability to identify what issues they wish to work on within the context of the relationship. Nurses can facilitate the development of trust by displaying positive qualities that many clients value in the therapeutic relationship, such as respect, empathy, honesty, companionship, and friendliness (Moreno-Poyato et al., 2016).

Resolution Phase

The final stage of the nurse–client relationship is the resolution phase, which begins when the actual problems are resolved and ends with the termination of the relationship. During this phase, the client is redirected toward a life without this specific therapeutic relationship. The client connects with community resources, solidifies a newly found understanding, and practices new behaviours. The client takes responsibility for follow-up appointments and interacts with significant others in new ways. New problems are not addressed during this phase, except in terms of what was learned during the working stage. The nurse assists the client in strengthening relationships, making referrals, and recognizing and understanding signs of future relapse.

Termination begins on the first day of the relationship when the nurse explains that this relationship is time limited and is established to help manage and resolve the client's problems. Because a therapeutic relationship is dependent, the nurse must constantly evaluate the client's level of dependence and continually support the client's move toward independence. Termination is usually stressful for the client who must sever ties with the nurse and who has shared thoughts and feelings and given guidance and support over many sessions. Depending on previous experiences with terminating relationships, some clients may not handle their emotions well during termination. Some may not show up for the last session to avoid their feelings of sadness and separation. Many clients will also display anger about the relationship ending. Clients may express anger toward the nurse or displace it onto others. One of the best ways to handle the anger is to help the client acknowledge it, to explain that anger is a normal emotion when a relationship is ending, and to reassure the client that it is acceptable to feel angry. The nurse should also reassure the client that anger subsides once the relationship is over.

Another typical termination behaviour is raising old problems that have already been resolved. The nurse may feel frustrated if clients in the termination phase present resolved problems as if they were new. The nurse may feel

that the sessions were unsuccessful. In reality, clients are unconsciously attempting to prolong the relationship and avoid its ending. Nurses should avoid addressing these problems. Instead, they should reassure clients of having already covered those issues and learned methods to control them. They should explain that the client may be feeling anxious about the relationship ending and redirect the client to newly acquired skills and abilities in forming new relationships, including support groups and social groups. The final meeting should focus on the future (see Box 7.9). The nurse can reassure the client that the nurse will remember them, but the nurse should not agree to see the client outside the relationship. Many clients who have difficulty establishing relationships may similarly have difficulty letting go of supportive relationships. The ending of the therapeutic relationship is a significant opportunity for client learning, including the opportunity for healthy closure to relationships. The nurse needs to plan for and to support this learning.

Nontherapeutic Relationships

Although it is hoped that all nurse–client relationships will go through the phases as described in the previous section, this is not always the case. **Nontherapeutic relationships** also go through predictable phases (Forchuk et al., 2000). These relationships also start in the orientation phase. However, trust is not established, and the relationship moves to a *phase of grappling and struggling*. The nurse and client both feel very frustrated and keep varying their approach with each other in an attempt to establish a meaningful relationship. This is different from a prolonged orientation phase in that the efforts are not sustained; they vary constantly. The nurse may try having longer or shorter meetings, being more or less directive, and varying the therapeutic stance from warm and friendly to aloof. Clients in this phase may try to talk about the past but then change to discussions of the here and now. They may try talking about their family and in the next meeting talk about their work goals. Both the client and the nurse grapple and struggle to come to a common ground, and both become increasingly frustrated with each other. Eventually, the frustration becomes so great that the pair gives up on each other and moves to a *phase of mutual withdrawal*. The nurse may schedule seeing this client at the end of the shift and "run out of time" so that the meeting never happens. The client will leave the unit or otherwise be unavailable during scheduled meeting times. If a meeting does occur, the nurse will try to keep it short, rationalizing, "What's the point— we just cover the same old ground anyway." The client will attempt to keep it superficial and stay on safe topics, "You can always ask about your medications—nurses love to teach health, you know." Obviously, no therapeutic progress can be made in such a relationship. The nurse may be hesitant to ask for a therapeutic transfer, assuming that a relationship would similarly fail with

BOX 7.9 THERAPEUTIC DIALOGUE

The Last Meeting

Ineffective Approach

Nurse: "Today is my last day."

Client: "I need to talk to you about something important."

Nurse: "What is it?"

Client: "I have been hearing voices again."

Nurse: "Oh, how often?"

Client: "Every night. You are the only one I'm going to tell."

Nurse: "I think you should tell the new nurse."

Client: "That nurse is too new and won't understand. I feel so bad about your leaving. Is there any way you can stay?"

Nurse: "Well, I could check on you tomorrow."

Client: "Oh, would you? I would really appreciate it if you would give me your new telephone number."

Nurse: "I don't know what the number will be, but it will be listed in the telephone book."

Effective Approach

Nurse: "Today is my last day."

Client: "I need to talk to you about something important."

Nurse: "We talked about that. Anything 'important' needs to be shared with the new nurse."

Client: "But, I want to tell you."

Nurse: "Saying good-bye can be very hard."

Client: "I will miss you."

Nurse: "Your feelings are very normal when relationships are ending. I will remember you in a very special way."

Client: "Can I please have your telephone number?"

Nurse: "No, I can't give that to you. It is important that we say good-bye today."

Client: "OK. Good-bye. Good luck."

Nurse: "Good-bye."

CRITICAL THINKING CHALLENGE

- What were some of the mistakes the nurse in the first scenario made?
- In the second scenario, how does therapeutic communication in the termination phase differ from effective communication in the working phase?

---

another nurse. However, each relationship is unique, and difficulties in one relationship do not predict difficulties in the next. Clinical supervision early on may assist the development of the relationship, but often, a therapeutic transfer to another nurse is required.

A narrative review by Moreno-Poyato and colleagues (2016) identified several factors that may interfere with the establishment of the therapeutic relationship from the perspectives of nurses and clients. For instance, nurses may face multiple barriers, including increasing administrative responsibilities, shortened length of inpatient stay, fear of causing harm, lack of experience individualizing client care, organizational structure and policy, and negative perceptions of the workplace environment. Clients, on the other hand, found that the amount of time allotted to interactions was the most prominent factor impeding the relationship. Other limitations perceived by clients include inaccessible nursing staff, insufficient involvement in care, being treated as an object or a problem to solve, authoritarian or paternalistic staff, and a tense or unsafe atmosphere.

Strategies Within the Therapeutic Relationship

Motivational Interviewing

One evidence-based strategy is motivational interviewing. **Motivational interviewing** (MI) is a clinical method designed to facilitate change in client behaviour by engaging a client's own autonomous decision-making ability. Practitioners of MI seek to selectively elicit and reinforce the client's own arguments for change. Carried out in a collaborative manner, MI encourages the client to make their own decisions through directed counseling that addresses increasing preferred behaviours and decreasing nonpreferred behaviours. MI is inherently exploratory and adaptive.

MI involves at least two processes: increasing preferred behaviours and decreasing nonpreferred behaviours. Ambivalence is an expected part of the process of change, and resistance to change is to be expected. In the efforts to help clients, two critical components emerge that are iteratively assessed for their influence. These are *conviction* (importance) and *confidence*. Strategies for increasing the client's conviction include asking questions regarding the relative importance of changing behaviour, examining the risks and benefits of the particular behaviour and of changing, exploring concerns about behaviour, having the "hypothetical look over the fence," and exploring possible next steps. Enhancing confidence also includes brainstorming solutions, focusing on successful past efforts, and serial reassessment and repetition of the process. Asking the client open-ended questions, listening reflectively, issuing affirming and summarizing statements, and eliciting self-motivational statements from the client are conducive strategies to building motivation for change. These include problem recognition, expression of concern, the

BOX 7.10 The Principles of Motivational Enhancement

1. **Avoid Arguing:** Generally, the more the therapist tells a client, "You can't do this," the more likely they will respond, if unconsciously, with, "I will." Resistance to change is influenced by how the therapist responds to the client's ambivalence.

2. **Express Empathy:** The attitude underlying empathy might also be called acceptance, and it is not the same as approval of harmful behaviour, but rather an unconditional acceptance of where the client is in terms of the behaviour. Through skillful reflective listening, the therapist can seek to understand the client's feelings and perspectives without judging, criticizing, or blaming. Paradoxically, this kind of acceptance of people appears to free them to change, whereas insistence on change and non-acceptance of "where they are at" in the process of change can have the effect of keeping people as they are. It is not helpful to view the client as "problematic," "pathologic," "unwilling to change," or "incapable of change"; rather, the client's situation is understood as one of being "stuck."

3. **Develop Discrepancy:** Motivation for change is created when people perceive a discrepancy between their present behaviour and important personal goals. Thus, MI aims at developing discrepancy until it overrides attachment to the present behaviour. This is accomplished without coercion. It is the client who gives voice to concerns and intentions to change.

4. **Roll With Resistance:** When encountering resistance, the therapist acknowledges ambivalence as natural. The client is invited to consider new information and perspectives. The responsibility for change is repeatedly handed back to the client, but with the offer of help and support. It is not the therapist's role to generate all solutions or to tell the client what to do. Directive approaches may elicit, "Yes, but…" responses from the client, with little or no change following and often a disengagement and dropping out of treatment.

5. **Support Self-efficacy:** This refers to the reinforcement of the client's belief in their ability to carry out and succeed. Change is a stepwise approach, and each small step along the journey should be reinforced and supported. The therapist's expectations about a client's chances for recovery can have a powerful impact on outcome.

Source: Miller, W. R., & Rollnick, S. (2002). *Motivational interviewing: Preparing people for change.* Guilford Press.

---

intention to change, and a sense of optimism. Refer to Box 7.10 for the principles of MI.

Some of the signals of successful MI are the following: the nurse is speaking slowly, the client is doing much more of the talking than the nurse, the client is actively talking about behaviour change, and finally, the nurse is listening very carefully and gently directing the interview at appropriate moments. The acronym FRAMES (*feedback, responsibility, advice, menu, empathy, self-efficacy*) was coined by Miller and Sanchez (1994) to summarize elements of brief interventions with clients using MI (refer to Box 7.11).

Effective practice of MI requires ongoing instruction and feedback. Topics discussed in this chapter, such as self-awareness, empathic linkages, active listening, and avoidance of defence mechanisms, will all have to be effectively employed to achieve MI's desired results. Techniques of MI may be combined with other interventions, such as mindfulness and self-regulation, to achieve optimal client outcomes (Sohl et al., 2016). According to Miller and Moyers (2006, p. 3), these techniques are as follows:

- Openness to collaboration with clients' own expertise
- Proficiency in client-centred counseling, including accurate empathy

- Recognition of key aspects of client speech that guide the practice of MI
- Eliciting and strengthening client change talk
- Rolling with resistance
- Negotiating change plans
- Consolidating client commitment
- Switching flexibly between MI and other intervention styles

Transitional Relationship Model

The transitional relationship model (TRM) evolved from the transitional discharge model, originally developed to help people through the discharge process. An extension of Peplau's theory, TRM is based on the assumption that people heal in relationships and require both professional and therapeutic peer relationships. The TRM was developed to sustain therapeutic relationships throughout the client's transition from hospital to the community. There are two essential components to this model: professional support and peer support. The professional's role is to bridge the therapeutic relationship over the discharge (or other transition) process so that the therapeutic relationship with the client is not terminated until the client enters another professional

---

BOX 7.11 FRAMES: Effective Elements of Brief Intervention

Feedback

Provide clients with personal feedback regarding their individual status, such as personal alcohol and other substance consumption relative to norms, information about elevated liver enzyme values, and so forth.

Responsibility

Emphasize the individual's freedom of choice and personal responsibility for change. General themes are as follows:

1. It's up to you; you're free to decide to change or not.
2. No one else can decide for you or force you to change.
3. You're the one who has to do it if it's going to happen.

Advice

Include a clear recommendation or advice on the need for change, typically in a supportive and concerned, rather than in a judgmental, manner.

Menu

Provide a menu of treatment options, from which clients may pick those that seem more suitable or appealing.

Empathic Counseling

Show warmth, support, respect, and understanding in communication with clients.

Self-Efficacy

Reinforce self-efficacy or an optimistic feeling that they can change.

---

relationship with a care provider (e.g., a nurse staying involved after discharge until a community relationship is established). The peer support component is essential during the transition from hospital to community. Peer supporters are generally trained and supported through a consumer–survivor group. In other words, people need both professionals and an experienced friend. Studies have found that this approach reduces the time in hospital (Forchuk, 2015; Forchuk et al., 2005) and reduces readmissions (Forchuk, 2015; Reynolds et al., 2004).

While TRM had previously been shown to be an effective model of discharge (Forchuk et al., 1998), the most recent evaluation in 36 tertiary care psychiatric wards examined the facilitators and barriers to successful implementation (Forchuk et al., 2013). The results of the study demonstrated that a complex relationship existed between a variety of factors necessary for successful implementation. Of the implementation strategies offered to wards, which included educational modules, on-ward champions, and documentation systems, the effectiveness of implementation varied as a result of the staff feeling overwhelmed, poor group dynamics, and unforeseen losses of on-ward champions. This suggests the need for careful introduction of TRM in order to continually foster ongoing support, education, and communication.

Technology and the Therapeutic Relationship

Traditionally, the nurse–client relationship has been face-to-face. However, changes to information and

communication technologies, particularly in the past decade, have significantly changed how health professionals and their clients interact. **Telehealth** is the extension of healthcare service delivery across distance by use of information and communication technologies such as telephone, video, and the internet. Telehealth in Canada has been particularly effective in improving access to health professionals by clients in rural locales (Jong et al., 2019). In the instance of *telenursing*, telehealth can involve something as basic as a phone call between a nurse and client or something as complex as assisting with a remote surgical procedure. For the purposes of PMH nursing in particular, there are important things to consider about the communicative aspect of the therapeutic relationship in situations mediated by communication technology. Nonverbal communication, which makes up so much of an interaction between nurse and client, is lessened or largely absent; access to necessary technology may also be difficult for some clients; it can be difficult to ensure that health providers do not step outside the scope of their practice; and issues of privacy, security, and consent can be more complicated in these situations. In order to address the latter issues, many agencies presently do not allow e-mail communication. A system can be set up behind a secure hospital firewall (Forchuk et al., 2013), but access control is always a concern with sensitive information. It is important to be aware of agency policy and security before using any Web-based communication. Public platforms, such as Facebook, do not allow privacy, sufficient security, or confidentiality for use in healthcare communication.

BOX 7.12 **Research for Best Practice**

FACILITATORS AND BARRIERS TO TELEHEALTH APPLICATIONS

Koivunen, M., & Saranto, K. (2018). Nursing professionals' experiences of the facilitators and barriers to the use of telehealth applications: A systematic review of qualitative studies. *Scandinavian Journal of Caring Sciences, 32*(1), 24–44. https://doi.org/10.1111/scs.12445

Study Aim: To synthesize evidence on nurses' experiences of facilitators and barriers to using telehealth services in practice.

Methods: The authors completed a thematic synthesis following the Johanna Briggs' Institute protocol for systematic reviews of qualitative studies. Articles were reviewed against inclusion and exclusion criteria and appraised using the Critical Appraisal Skills Program for Qualitative Studies. A total of 25 papers were included in the review.

Findings: Facilitators and barriers were grouped into five main categories: (a) nurses' skills and attitudes, (b) nurses' work and operations, (c) organizational factors, (d) patients, and (e) technology. Nurses perceived that telehealth increased job satisfaction, decreased workload, and reduced stress; however, negative attitudes of nurses toward telehealth created barriers to implementation. Inadequate support and training, lack of coordination of services, and lack of resources (e.g., budget, time, technical support) were also barriers for nurses.

Implications for Practice: Nurses need to be trained and supported to use telehealth applications, with organizations having a role in providing such support. To facilitate online communication between clients and nurses, it is important that nurses also attend to client knowledge, skills, and attitudes toward telehealth applications.

The internet can be a useful tool for health teaching or for finding resources, but its increasing use in mediating relationships, including those between healthcare providers and clients, raises issues of personal autonomy and consent (e.g., how clients' data are stored, exchanged, and used), persistent threats to privacy and confidentiality, and other issues of risk management. Refer to the Box 7.12, Research for Best Practice for a summary of a systematic review on the facilitators and barriers to nurses using telehealth applications.

Remote Delivery of Therapeutic Communication

In the advent of the COVID-19 pandemic, more providers are integrating synchronous and asynchronous technologies to deliver mental health care. Synchronous technologies involve communication that occurs in real time (e.g.,

video conferencing). Asynchronous technologies allow communication to happen between visits (e.g., e-mail). In addition to applying the communication techniques outlined in this chapter, considerations for communicating virtually have been published by the College of Nurses of Ontario (2020) and Harvard Medical School (James, 2020). Common strategies include asking open-ended questions, avoiding premature conclusions, attending to verbal and nonverbal cues, using active listening techniques, asking clients if they have anything to add, and providing clients with a telephone or e-mail contact. It may be helpful to set up virtual meetings in a room where the nurse can remove their face mask to facilitate communication. In virtual health care, empathy must be conveyed verbally and visually, so using empathetic statements that address the client's feelings and expressing empathy by touching one's own hand to the heart are strategies to employ (Cleveland Clinic, 2020).

Summary of Key Points

- To deal therapeutically with the emotions, feelings, and problems of clients, nurses must understand their own cultural values and beliefs and interpersonal strengths and limitations.
- The nurse–client relationship is built on therapeutic communication, including verbal and nonverbal interactions between the nurse and client. Some communication skills include active listening, positive body language, appropriate verbal responses, and the ability of the nurse to interpret appropriately and analyze the client's verbal and nonverbal behaviours.
- Two of the most important communication concepts are empathy and rapport.
- Defence mechanisms, used by all individuals, can be adaptive or maladaptive depending on factors like context, inflexibility, and severity.
- In the nurse–client relationship, as in all types of relationships, certain physical, psychological, social, and spiritual boundaries and limitations need to be observed.

- The therapeutic nurse–client relationship consists of three major and overlapping stages or phases: the orientation phase, in which the client and nurse meet and establish the parameters of the relationship; the working phase, in which the client identifies and explores problems; and the resolution phase, in which the client learns to manage the problems and the relationship is terminated.
- The nontherapeutic relationship also consists of three major and overlapping phases: the orientation phase,

the grappling and struggling phase, and the phase of mutual withdrawal.
- Strategies that can be used within therapeutic relationships include MI and TRM.
- Synchronous and asynchronous remote delivery of mental health care is evolving due to constraints revealed through the COVID-19 pandemic and brings new challenges to therapeutic communication.

Thinking Challenges

a. Nurses are in the unique role of establishing a strong relationship with their clients. In psychiatric–mental health nursing, this relationship is used to meet and evaluate treatment goals.

b. How does self-awareness influence the therapeutic relationship and its associated outcome?

c. What is the nurse's role in the therapeutic relationship?

> Visit thePoint to view suggested responses. Go to **thePoint.lww.com/activate** and use the activation code found in the front of this text to unlock answers to the "Thinking Challenges" and other online resources.

Web Links

https://www.cna-aiic.ca/-/media/cna/page-content/pdf-en/telehealth-fact-sheet.pdf This link takes you to the 2017 Canadian Nurses Association *Fact Sheet: Telehealth*, which provides a definition of telehealth; outlines its facilitators, barriers, and benefits; and discusses registration and insurance protection for nurses.

https://www.bccnp.ca/Standards/RN_NP/PracticeStandards/Lists/GeneralResources/RN_NP_PS_Boundaries.pdf At this site is the practice standard (2020) of the British Columbia College of Nursing Professionals for *Boundaries in the Nurse-Client Relationship*.

www.cno.org/globalassets/4-learnaboutstandardsandguidelines/prac/learn/modules/tncr/pdf/tncr-chapter3.pdf

The College of Nurses of Ontario's (2006) *Therapeutic Nurse-Client Relationship Practice Standard: Therapeutic Communication and Client-Centred Care*, can be found here.

http://publish.uwo.ca/~cforchuk/peplau/discusses nurse theorist, *Hildegard Peplau.*

www.youtube.com/watch?v=J_EJQgKihvk&feature=youtu.be Video by L. Killam re: *Therapeutic Relationships in Nursing: The Profession's Perspective Part 1 of 2*. www.youtube.com/watch?v=wN9bf7L_9oY *Part 2 of 2* is here.

https://rnao.ca/bpg/guidelines/establishing-therapeutic-relationships The Registered Nurses Association of Ontarios guideline, *Establishing Therapeutic Relationships*, is here.

References

American Psychiatric Association. (2013). *Diagnostic and statistical manual of mental disorders* (5th ed.).

Bacha, K., Hanley, T., & Winter, L. A. (2020). 'Like a human being, I was an equal, I wasn't just a patient': Service users' perspectives on their experiences of relationships with staff in mental health services. *Psychology and Psychotherapy: Theory, Research and Practice, 93*(2), 367–386. https://doi.org/10.1111/papt.12218

Boyd, M. (1995). Communication with clients, families, healthcare providers, and diverse cultures. In M. Strader & P. Decker (Eds.), *Role transition to patient care management* (p. 431). Appleton & Lange.

Cleveland Clinic. (2020). *Communicating with patients in a new world of virtual visits.* https://consultqd.clevelandclinic.org/communicating-with-patients-in-a-new-world-of-virtual-visits/

College of Nurses of Ontario. (2019). *Practice standard: Therapeutic nurse-client relationship* (rev. ed.). https://www.cno.org/globalassets/docs/prac/41033_therapeutic.pdf

College of Nurses of Ontario. (2020). *Practice guideline: Telepractice.* https://www.cno.org/globalassets/docs/prac/41041_telephone.pdf

Forchuk, C. (2015). Implementing the transitional discharge model: Final report—Prepared for the Council of Academic Hospitals of Ontario (CAHO) adopting research to improve care (ARTIC). https://www.opdi.org/de/cache/resources/1/rs_CAHO-TDM-FINAL%20REPORT-February132015.pdf

Forchuk, C., Carmichael, C., Golea, G., Johnston, N., Martin, M.-L., Patterson, P., Ray, K., Robinson, T., Sogbein, S. A., Srivastava, R., & Skov,

T. (2006). *Nursing best practice guideline: Establishing therapeutic relationships* (rev. suppl.). Registered Nurses Association of Ontario. https://rnao.ca/bpg/guidelines/establishing-therapeutic-relationships

Forchuk, C., Jewell, J., Schofield, R., Sircelj, M., & Valledor, T. (1998). From hospital to community: Bridging therapeutic relationships. *Journal of Psychiatric and Mental Health Nursing, 5*(3), 197–202. https://doi.org/10.1046/j.1365-2850.1998.00125.x

Forchuk, C., Martin, M.-L., Chan, Y. C., & Jensen, E. (2005). Therapeutic relationships: From psychiatric hospital to community. *Journal of Psychiatric and Mental Health Nursing, 12*(5), 556–564. https://doi.org/10.1111/j.1365-2850.2005.00873.x

Forchuk, C., Martin, M.-L., Jensen, E., Ouseley, S., Sealy, P., Beal, G., Reynolds, W., & Sharkey, S. (2013). Integrating an evidence-based intervention into clinical practice: 'transitional relationship model'. *Journal of Psychiatric and Mental Health Nursing, 20*(7), 584–594. https://doi.org/10.1111/j.1365-2850.2012.01956.x

Forchuk, C., Westwell, J., Martin, M.-L., Bamber-Azzapardi, W., Kosterewa-Tolman, D., & Hux, M. (2000). The developing nurse–client relationship: Nurses perspectives. *Journal of the American Psychiatric Nurses Association, 6*(1), 3–10. https://doi.org/10.1177%2F107839030000600102

Gallop, R., Choiniere, J., Forchuk, C., Golea, G., Johnston, N., Levac, A. M., Martin, M.-L., Robinson, T., Sogbein, S., Sutcliffe, H., & Wynn, F. (2002). *Nursing best practice guideline: Establishing therapeutic relationships.* Registered Nurses Association of Ontario. https://rnao.ca/sites/rnao-ca/files/Establishing_Therapeutic_Relationships.pdf

Hall, E. T. (1990). *The hidden dimension.* Anchor Books.

James, T. (2020). *Best practices for patient engagement with telehealth.* Harvard Medical School. https://leanforward.hms.harvard.edu/2020/06/04/best-practices-for-patient-engagement-with-telehealth/

Jong, M., Mendez, I., & Jong, R. (2019). Enhancing access to care in northern rural communities via telehealth. *International Journal of Circumpolar Health, 78*(2). https://doi.org/10.1080/22423982.2018.1554174

Koivunen, M., & Saranto, K. (2018). Nursing professionals' experiences of the facilitators and barriers to the use of telehealth applications: A systematic review of qualitative studies. *Scandinavian Journal of Caring Sciences, 32*(1), 24–44. https://doi.org/10.1111/scs.12445

Miller, W. R., & Moyers, T. B. (2006). Eight stages in learning motivational interviewing. *Journal of Teaching in the Addictions, 5*(1), 3–17. https://doi.org/10.1300/J188v05n01_02

Miller, W. R., & Rollnick, S. (2002). *Motivational interviewing: Preparing people for change.* Guilford Press.

Miller, W. R., & Sanchez, V. C. (1994). Motivating young adults for treatment and lifestyle change. In G. S. Howard & P. E. Nathan (Eds.), *Alcohol use and misuse by young adults* (pp. 55–81). University of Notre Dame Press.

Moreno-Poyato, A. R., Monteso-Curto, P., Delgado-Hito, P., Suarez-Perez, R., Acena-Dominguez, R., Carreras-Salvador, R., Leyva-Moral, J., Lluch-Canut, T., & Roldan-Merino, J. F. (2016). The therapeutic relationship in inpatient psychiatric care: A narrative review of the perspective of nurses and patients. *Archives of Psychiatric Nursing, 30*(6), 782–787. https://doi.org/10.1016/j.apnu.2016.03.001

Peplau, H. E. (1952/1988). *Interpersonal relations in nursing.* MacMillan.

Reynolds W., Lauder W., Sharkey, S., Maciver S., Veitch T., & Cameron, D. (2004). The effect of a transitional discharge model for psychiatric patients. *Journal of Psychiatric and Mental Health Nursing, 11*(1), 82–88. https://doi.org/10.1111/j.1365-2850.2004.00692.x

Sohl, S. J., Birdee, G., & Elam, R. (2016). Complementary tools to empower and sustain behavior change: Motivational interviewing and mindfulness. *American Journal of Lifestyle Medicine, 10*(6), 429–436. https://doi.org/10.1177/1559827615571524

Valente, S. M. (2017). Managing professional and nurse-patient relationship boundaries in mental health. *Journal of Psychosocial Nursing and Mental Health Services, 55*(1), 45–51. https://doi.org/10.3928/02793695-20170119-09

Legal and Ethical Aspects of Practice

Wendy Austin and Arlene Kent-Wilkinson

LEARNING OBJECTIVES

After studying this chapter, you will be able to:

- Identify the ways in which mental health legislation protects and promotes the wellbeing of Canadians.
- Discuss the way that the *UN Charter* and international agreements provide a foundation for mental health legislation.
- Explain the key components of your provincial/ territorial Mental Health Act, including the criteria and processes for voluntary and involuntary admission and for mandatory outpatient treatment.
- Discuss the determination of "competency."
- Identify the ways a substitute decision-maker can be chosen.
- Describe the role of the nurse in upholding the rights of persons whose care and treatment is regulated by mental health legislation.
- Explain the phrase, "not criminally responsible due to a mental disorder."
- Define ethics.
- Distinguish between the domains of ethics and law.
- Describe the nurse as a moral agent and the resources available to support this role.
- Identify the most common approaches to ethics that inform health ethics.
- Describe the components of an ethical practice environment.
- Distinguish between a moral dilemma and moral distress.
- Consider the components of an ethical decision-making framework.
- Identify and discuss key ethical issues in psychiatric and mental health nursing.

KEY TERMS

- admission certificate • beneficence • best interests • capable wishes • casuistry • community treatment order • competence • conditional leave • conscientious objection • deontology • ethics of care • feminist ethics • formal patient • human rights • involuntary admission • justice • mandatory outpatient treatment • modified best interests • nonmaleficence • practical wisdom • principlism • relational ethics • renewal certificate • respect for autonomy • review panel • substitute decision-maker • utilitarianism • virtue

KEY CONCEPTS

- ethics • mental health act • moral agent • moral dilemma • moral distress

This chapter presents the legal and ethical aspects of mental healthcare practice. Although both are essential to the creation and maintenance of a just society, the law and ethics are separate domains. In a perfect world, societal laws would be totally compatible with ethical behaviours in every situation. In the real world, however, this is not always the case. Citizens may need to work to change laws that they believe do not support ethical action. In serving and protecting the public, it is crucial that nurses know and understand the laws relevant to nursing and can enact their code of ethics in daily practice. Codes are aspirational in nature but also have a regulatory purpose and a role in ensuring that the Canadian public receives quality nursing care.

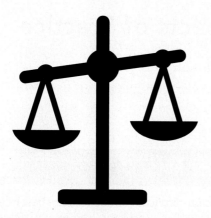

Human Rights, the Law, and Psychiatric and Mental Health Care

Every society needs laws to protect the security and well-being of its citizens and to achieve its collective objectives. Human rights law allows for international scrutiny of a nation's health policies and practices (Gostin, 2001). Mental health legislation is a means to protect and promote the mental wellbeing of citizens, codifying the fundamental protection of the rights of persons with psychiatric illnesses while providing a mechanism for the care and treatment of those whose illness significantly interferes with their ability to recognize their need for medical assistance and/or their ability to seek it. The absence of such protection would put them and others at risk and limit their right to the best available health care.

Recognition of Mental Health as a Human Right

Set out in prescriptive documents, **human rights** are recognition of the dignity and worth of every human being. Rights are delineated in such documents as the *Canadian Charter of Rights and Freedoms, 1982,* and the United Nations *Universal Declaration of Human Rights, 1948.* Key rights and principles include equality and nondiscrimination, the right to privacy and individual autonomy, freedom from inhuman and degrading treatment, the principle of the least restrictive environment, and the rights to information and participation. The Canadian Nurses Association (CNA) has a position statement, *Registered Nurses, Health and Human Rights, 2018,* that is a helpful reference for nurses. (See Web Links.)

"Health" as a human right means that every person has a right to the highest attainable level of health (including a standard of living that is adequate for health) and access to health care and social services as needed. There are tangible connections between health and human rights (Mann et al., 1999).

First, *health policies and practices have an impact on human rights.* For instance, mandatory outpatient treatment (MOT) for persons with a mental illness is an infringement on individual rights. This infringement can only be justified if it is in the person's best interests or for the necessary protection of the public.

Second, *human rights violations impact health.* The International Council of Nurses (ICN) in its 2020 position statement, *Mental Health,* "endorses human rights as foundational to freedom from discrimination for those with mental and/or substance use disorders, a prerequisite to access high-quality, evidence-based treatment and linked to social services and basic survival resources to support recovery" (p. 2; see Web Links).

Third, *health professionals have a responsibility to protect human rights by helping the public identify rights violations.* The World Health Organization (WHO) has noted that some of the most serious human rights violations against persons with mental illness and substance abuse problems occur in healthcare settings. In 2021, WHO guidance on community mental health services and the promotion of person-centred and rights-based approaches was released. It complements WHO's global QualityRights initiative that aims to transform health services across the world so all are in line with the United Nations' *Convention on the Rights of Persons with Disabilities (CRPD), 2006.* (See Web Links for access to WHO resources on these initiatives.)

In 2010, Canada ratified the CRPD. As a signatory of the Convention, Canadians are committed to ensuring the promotion and protection of the human rights of all persons with disabilities. Disability in the CRPD is understood from a social perspective as arising from the way in which the environment interacts with a person's condition rather than the condition itself. It provides a basis for legislation, policies, and regulations for eliminating barriers to the societal participation of those with a mental illness. A resource provided by the WHO is MiNDbank, an online platform that brings together international and national policies, strategies, laws, and standards for mental health and disability and promotes dialogue, debate, and research for the purposes of achieving national reforms that conform to international human rights and best practice standards. (See Web Links.)

Significant Canadian and international rights documents are listed in Table 8.1. The rights of people who have mental illness, as put forth in the *Principles for the Protection of Persons with Mental Illness and the Improvement of Mental Health Services,* adopted in 1991 by the United Nations, are outlined in Box 8.1. Information regarding national and international advocacy organizations is to be found in the Web Links section at the end of this chapter.

A rights approach is not without its critics. Some find that such an approach is too legalistic and the law too slow and ineffective in addressing rights violations and that this approach is too individualistic, placing the individual in an antagonistic position against the community (Austin, 2001). In 2005, bioethics and human

Table 8.1 Canadian and International Rights Agreements Relevant to Mental Health

Year	Agreement
1948	Universal Declaration of Human Rights
1966	The International Covenant on Economic, Social, and Cultural Rights
1966	The International Covenant on Civil and Political Rights
1982	Canadian Charter of Rights and Freedoms
1984	Canada Health Act
1986	Canada Employment Equity Act
1990	Declaration of Caracas
1991	Principles of Protection of Persons With Mental Illness
2007	United Nations Declaration on the Rights of Indigenous Peoples
2016	MAID Medical Assistance in Dying
2017	MAID Medical Assistance in Dying Revised

rights were brought together in the *Universal Declaration on Bioethics and Human Rights*, adopted by United Nations Educational, Scientific and Cultural Organization (UNESCO, 2019). Among other things, its principles uphold respect for autonomy, solidarity among human beings, and the need for sharing the benefits of scientific research and for protecting future generations and the planet itself. Across its history, the profession of nursing has held human rights to be central to

BOX 8.1 Rights of Persons with Mental Illness

- Right to medical care (Principle 1.1)
- Right to be treated with humanity and respect (Principle 1.2)
- Equal protection right (Principle 1.4)
- Right to be cared for in the community (Principle 7)
- Right to provide informed consent before receiving any treatment (Principle 11)
- Right to privacy (Principle 13)
- Freedom of communication (Principle 13)
- Freedom of religion (Principle 13)
- Right to voluntary admission (Principles 15 and 16)
- Right to judicial guarantees (Principle 17)

From United Nations. (1991). *Principles for the protection of persons with mental illness and the improvement of mental health care, 1991.* Adopted by General Assembly resolution 46/119 of 17 December 1991, Office of the United Nations High Commissioner for Human Rights. http://www.unhchr.ch/html/menu3/b/68.htm

its practices, as evident in its scholarship and codes of ethics (Tisdale & Symenuk, 2020). This remains true of the Canadian Nurses Association Code of Ethics (2017).

Human Rights and Mental Health Legislation

ICN recognizes the call from the United Nations Human Rights Council (2017), which states that mental health is a priority and needs to be integrated with physical health, "professionally, politically and geographically" (p. 18). The report of the Special Rapporteur to the Council noted that power imbalances are a greater problem in mental health care than chemical imbalances and recommends that care be recovery- and community-based, promoting social inclusion, and that promotion and prevention be a focus. Further, the need for rights-based treatments and psychosocial support is emphasized.

Mental Health Legislation in Canada

Legislation in Canada strongly influences the context of our mental health care. Each province and territory is guided by its own Mental Health Act, which provides a framework for the delivery of mental health services and establishes rules and procedures governing the commitment of persons suffering from mental disorders. Each Act permits certain infringements upon a person's rights and freedoms only to the extent necessary to ensure that the person receives required care and treatment. Procedural safeguards are outlined, which must be followed when such curtailment of a person's rights becomes temporarily necessary. Each Act must be congruent with the rights stipulated under the *1982 Charter of Rights and Freedoms* (Butler & Phillips, 2013), and the resources to enforce the Act must be in place. Internet access information for the various *Mental Health Acts* can be found in Table 8.2. A nonlegal element of the protection for persons whose rights are temporarily curtailed due to a mental disorder is the recovery-oriented approach to care expected of Canadian mental health services (Mental Health Commission of Canada [MHCC], 2009; see Chapter 2).

Mental Health Acts within Canada can allow **involuntary admission** of a person to a designated facility. Although the language varies by province and territory, the conditions that must be met are usually that an examination by a physician (note: the Nunavut Mental Health Act uses the term "mental health practitioner" rather than "physician"; psychologists can play a role in the involuntary process in Nunavut) indicates that the person has a mental disorder, is likely to cause harm to self or others or to suffer substantial mental or physical deterioration or serious physical impairment, and is unsuitable for admission to a facility other than as a **formal patient**. An **admission certificate** allows the person to be conveyed to a mental health facility and to

Table 8.2	Mental Health Acts
Province/Territory	**Website Addresses of Mental Health Acts in Canada**
Alberta	Mental Health Act www.albertahealthservices.ca/info/mha.aspx
British Columbia	Mental Health Act www2.gov.bc.ca/gov/content/health/managing-your-health/mental-health-substance-use/ mental-health-act
Manitoba	Mental Health Act web2.gov.mb.ca/laws/statutes/ccsm/m110e.php
New Brunswick	Mental Health Act www.canlii.org/en/nb/laws/stat/rsnb-1973-c-m-10/latest/rsnb-1973-c-m-10.html
Newfoundland and Labrador	Mental Health Care and Treatment Act www.gov.nl.ca/hcs/mentalhealth-committee/mentalhealth/mental-health-care-and-treatment-act/
Northwest Territories	Mental Health Act www.canlii.org/en/nu/laws/stat/rsnwt-nu-1988-c-m-10/latest/rsnwt-nu-1988-c-m-10.html
Nova Scotia	Mental Health Act nslegislature.ca/legc/bills/59th_1st/1st_read/b109.htm
Nunavut	Mental Health Act www.canlii.org/en/nu/laws/stat/rsnwt-nu-1988-c-m-10/latest/rsnwt-nu-1988-c-m-10.html
Ontario	Mental Health Act www.ontario.ca/laws/statute/90m07
Prince Edward Island	Mental Health Act www.princeedwardisland.ca/sites/default/files/legislation/M-06-1-Mental%20Health%20Act.pdf
Quebec	Act Respecting the Protection of Persons Whose Mental State Presents a Danger to Themselves or to Others www.canlii.org/en/qc/laws/stat/cqlr-c-p-38.001/latest/cqlr-c-p-38.001.html
Saskatchewan	Mental Health Services Act www.publications.gov.sk.ca/details.cfm?p=626
Yukon	Mental Health Act www.gov.yk.ca/legislation/acts/mehe.pdf

be detained and cared for during a 24-h period. Within that time, the person must be assessed by a physician (usually staff of that facility).

Two admission certificates are required for the person to remain a formal patient; otherwise, they must be released at the end of the 24-h period. These two admission certificates are sufficient to detain the person as a formal patient for a period of 1 month. **Renewal certificates** can extend the formal patient designation for another month. There must be two renewal certificates completed, each by a physician (usually, one of the physicians must be a psychiatrist) after an independent examination of the person. See Figure 8.1 for an example of the process of formal patient certification, that of Alberta.

The **competence** of the person to make decisions regarding treatment, and thus to give consent, must be assessed. Competence in this respect means being able to be informed and to understand (at a basic level) matters relevant to the decision and to understand the consequences of the decision. Competence is not a fixed capacity; it changes over time. There are specific provisions within mental health acts regarding the evaluation of competency and what action may be taken if a person is deemed not competent.

When a person is unable to consent to treatment, consent from a **substitute decision-maker** may be

sought. Depending on the jurisdiction, these substitute decision-makers can be state appointed, appointed by the person when competent, or be a guardian or relative. There are different criteria to guide substitute decision-making: **best interests** (e.g., treatment will make the person less ill, the person will get more ill without treatment, the benefits outweigh any risks), **capable wishes** (what the person expressed while capable, even if not in current best interests), and **modified best interests** (follow expressed wishes except if they would endanger the person or others) (Gray et al., 2016). Figure 8.2 shows a flowchart of competency and consent for treatment in the province of Alberta.

KEY CONCEPT

A *Mental Health Act* is a law that gives certain powers and sets the conditions (including time limits) for those powers to stipulated healthcare professionals and designated institutions regarding the admission and treatment of individuals with a mental disorder. The Act also provides a framework for mental health delivery of services and establishes rules and procedures that govern the commitment of persons suffering from mental disorders (Government of Saskatchewan, 2018).

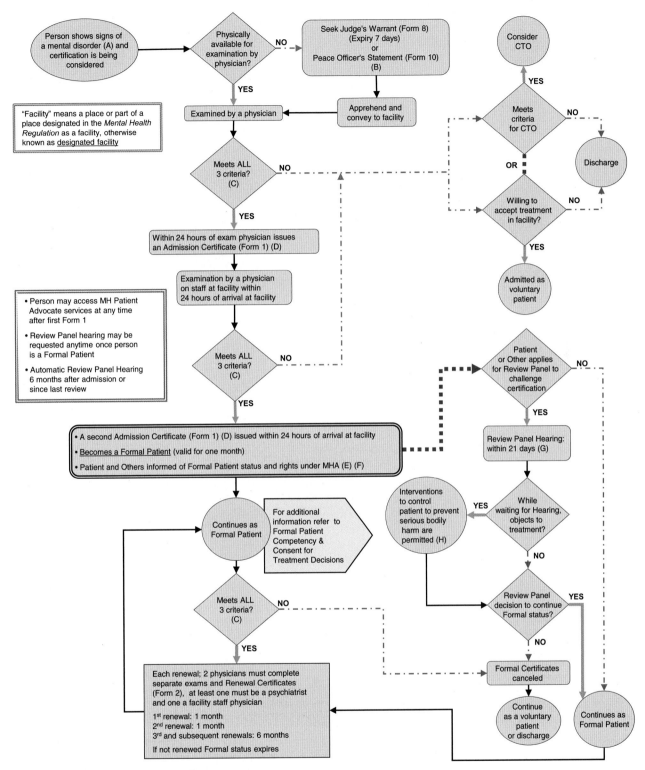

Figure 8.1 Process of Formal Patient Certification, Mental Health Act of Alberta. (Source: Alberta Health Services. (2021, February). *Guide to the mental health act and community treatment order legislation* (p. 41). https://www.albertahealthservices.ca/ MHA.asp.)

In a review of the Mental Health Act provisions in all Canadian jurisdictions, significant differences were found among the provinces and territories (Gray et al., 2016). See Box 8.2 for an overview of basic criteria for involuntary admission in the various jurisdictions, based on this review.

Mandatory Outpatient Treatment

In some jurisdictions, an involuntary patient may return to the community on a **conditional leave** if the admission criteria are still met and if stipulations for treatment are followed. If the stipulations (e.g., taking medication

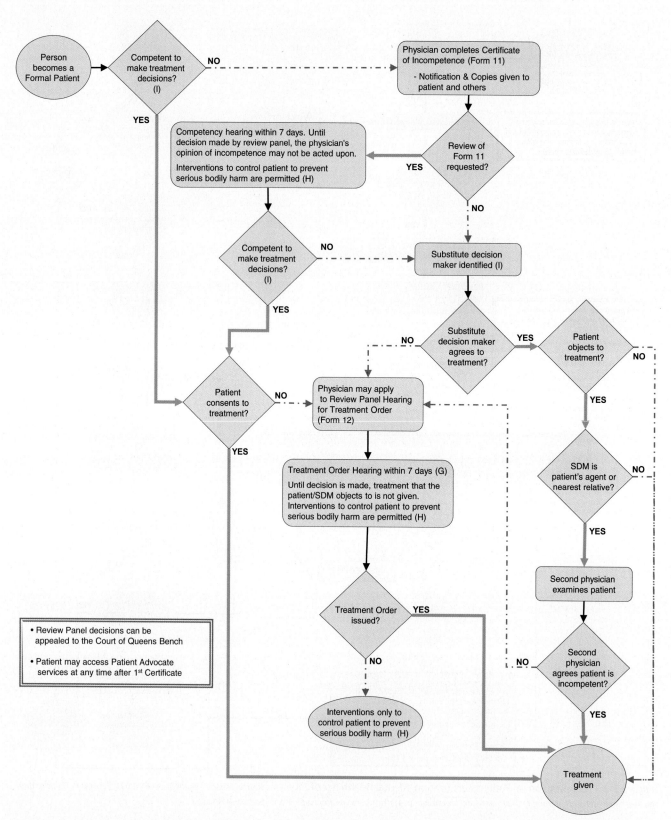

Figure 8.2 Process of Formal Patient Competency & Consent for Treatment Decisions, Mental Health Act of Alberta. (Source: Alberta Health Services. (2021, February). *Guide to the mental health act and community treatment order legislation* (p. 41). http://www.albertahealthservices.ca/MHA.asp.)

BOX 8.2 Involuntary Admission Criteria in Provincial and Territorial Mental Health Acts

Is not suitable as a voluntary inpatient: A person who is willing and capable of consenting to a voluntary admission cannot be admitted with an involuntary status anywhere in Canada.

Meets the definition of mental disorder: The person must have a mental disorder. In many, but not all of the jurisdictions, it is specified that the disorder must seriously impair the person's functioning.

Meets the criteria for harm: In most jurisdictions, this is not limited to serious bodily harm; non-bodily harms are acceptable. The criterion of "danger" stipulated in some acts has been interpreted by the courts to mean bodily harm.

Likely to suffer substantial mental or physical deterioration: This is included in some provinces (British Columbia, Saskatchewan, Manitoba, and Ontario) as an alternative to the harm criterion.

In need of psychiatric treatment: This is a criterion in British Columbia, Saskatchewan, and Ontario. It is possible in other jurisdictions to commit a person with a mental disorder who is dangerous, but for whom there is no treatment (e.g., antisocial personality disorder) for the purpose of preventive detention.

Refusal of treatment: By the person after admission: This is allowed in some jurisdictions but not others. In some jurisdictions, a refusal can be overruled in the person's best interests.

Review and appeal procedures regarding the validity of involuntary hospitalization: These are found in all jurisdictions.

Source: Adapted from Gray, J. E., Hastings, T. J., Love, S., & O'Reilly, R. L. (2016). Clinically significant differences among Canadian Mental Health Acts: 2016. *Canadian Journal of Psychiatry, 61*(4), 222–226. https://doi.org/10.1177/0706743716632524

---

and meeting with a physician) are not followed, the person can be returned to the hospital. **Mandatory outpatient treatment** (MOT) involves legal provisions requiring people with a mental illness to comply with a treatment plan while living in the community. A **community treatment order** (CTO), a form of MOT, is an order to provide a comprehensive plan of community-based treatment to someone with a serious mental disorder. They are only issued for persons with severe mental illness and, in most provinces, with a history of hospitalization who have been examined by a physician and been deemed in need of continuing treatment and care while residing in the community. Generally, CTOs are less restrictive than being detained in a psychiatric facility and serve as an alternative to hospitalization. The CTO plan identifies the conditions that must be met by the individual and support system (e.g., family, friends, and healthcare professionals) for the individual to stay out of the hospital. The CTOs often involve intense case management support provided by nurse managers. Research by Snow (2015) regarding CTO use in one Canadian province concluded that too often the care of persons with severe mental illness is socially organized to fall upon family members; this occurs with CTOs at times.

Physicians and psychiatrists in most provinces and territories in Canada are able to issue CTOs requiring mentally ill patients to accept treatment, medication, and supervision as a condition of living in the community (Rynor, 2010). All Canadian jurisdictions, with the exception of the three territories, authorize the use of CTOs or variations, such as extended leave provisions (Rynor). For instance, in 2017, New Brunswick introduced Community Support Orders (CSOs), a form of supervised community care ordered by a physician and agreed to by the patient (Government of New Brunswick, 2017). See Figure 8.3 for a flowchart of the CTO process in the province of Alberta.

Review Panels

All jurisdictions have a check on the involuntary aspects of mental health legislation. Usually, a **review panel** (court or tribunal), chaired by a lawyer and composed of four or five persons with representative expertise (e.g., a lawyer, a psychiatrist, a physician, and a member of the public), accepts applications for review by formal patients in designated facilities, persons subject to a CTO, and physicians of a formal patient. The panel will review whether formal patients are competent or should continue to be detained in the facility or have treatment decisions made for them. Usually, for formal patients who have been detained for 6 months through renewal certificates, some form of review is conducted by the panel without an application from the patient. Decisions of review panels may be appealed at the highest level of provincial court (Court of Queen's Bench).

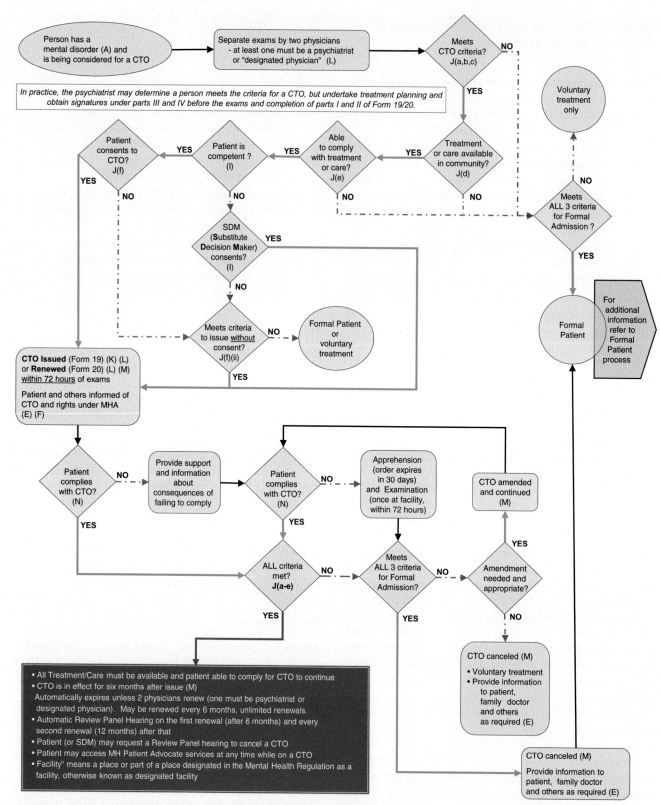

Figure 8.3 Community Treatment Orders (CTO). (Community Source: Alberta Health Services. (2021, February). *Guide to the mental health act and community treatment order legislation* (p. 41). https://www.albertahealthservices.ca/MHA.asp.)

Canadian Nurses' Responsibility Regarding Mental Health Legislation

It is the responsibility of nurses to understand the *Mental Health Act* of their province/territory. Nurses need to be able to explain the Act's basic provisions to people with mental illness and their families. In the province of Saskatchewan, for instance, their *Guide to Mental Health Service Act* outlines other functions of nurses, such as explaining patient and family rights, keeping track of certificate expiry dates, reporting to review panels, supervising CTOs and providing information to other clinicians and family members (Government of Saskatchewan, 2015, p. 125). These functions are similar to those expected of nurses in other provinces and territories.

In some jurisdictions, amendments to their Mental Health Acts have expanded the role of nurses when particular criteria are met. For example, in Saskatchewan, a nurse in a mental health centre may detain a voluntary patient requesting discharge if the nurse has reasonable grounds to believe that the patient now meets the criteria for involuntary status and needs to be examined by a physician. If this detention occurs, the medical examination must happen within 3 h. As well, in this province, a nurse may be deemed a "prescribed health professional" in some circumstances and permitted to complete and issue a certificate that enables a person to be taken for examination by a physician with admitting privileges to a mental health centre. In every jurisdiction, nurses have an important advocacy role ensuring that the rights of persons coming under a mental health act are protected.

The Criminal Code and Mental Disorders

Separate from mental health legislation are the legal provisions that can require people to follow treatment as a condition of probation. The Criminal Code of Canada allows for persons to be found *Not Criminally Responsible due to a Mental Disorder* for an offence if they are suffering from a mental disorder that makes them incapable of appreciating the nature of the act or knowing that what they did was wrong. In these cases, the offender with mental illness needs to comply with treatment monitored by the Criminal Code Review Boards (see Chapter 35).

Mental Illness and Medical Assistance in Dying

In June 2016, an amendment to the Criminal Code made medical assistance in dying (MAID) legal in Canada, provided all required conditions are met (Government of Canada, 2016). According to an Act to amend the Criminal Code, Section 241.1, MAID is defined as "(a) the administering by a medical practitioner or nurse practitioner of a substance to a person, at their request, that causes their death or (b) the prescribing or providing by a medical practitioner or nurse practitioner of a substance to a person, at their request, so that they may self-administer the substance and in doing so cause their own death" (Government of Canada, 2016). At that time, criteria included that the person was in an irreversible decline in capability and their natural death was reasonably foreseeable. This criterion was removed when the Act was amended as of March 17, 2021, and eligibility requirements for MAID changed, such that persons who wish to receive MAID must:

a. have a serious and incurable illness, disease, or disability (*excluding a mental illness until March 17, 2023*),
b. be in an advanced state of irreversible decline in capability,
c. have enduring and intolerable physical or psychological suffering that cannot be alleviated under conditions the person considers acceptable.

The temporary (2-year) exclusion for persons with a mental illness as the sole serious and incurable disease underlying their request for MAID was to allow the Canadian government time to address how MAID can be provided safely to these individuals.

Those who argued for the amendment to include mental illness as a sole and incurable disease point to the Charter rights of persons with mental illness. They contended, rightfully so, that mental illness can cause terrible suffering to the extent that life can seem not worth living. Those who disagree with the amendment are concerned that the decline and suffering may be related more to lack of access to effective treatment and social support, and to the stigma associated with mental illness that still pervades society, than to the state of the disease. Mental health care is significantly underfunded: countries on the average spend only 2% of their healthcare budget on mental health. (See Web Links.) Just as access to good pain control and palliative care should occur before a request for MAID due to severe pain is acted upon, access to holistic treatment and quality of life measures needs to occur for persons with mental illness.

Ethics and Psychiatric and Mental Health Nursing Care

Ethics is about how we should live; it is *"aiming at the 'good' with and for others in just institutions"* (Ricouer, 1992, p. 172). Ethics is about learning how to reach our potential as human beings, and so it is about values, relationships, principles, duties, rights, and responsibilities. In writing about ethics in *On Equilibrium*, Saul (2001) noted that, although we may think about ethics as something exotic or romantic, for heroes or saints, ethics is actually down to earth and practical: it needs to be an everyday part of our lives and built into our society.

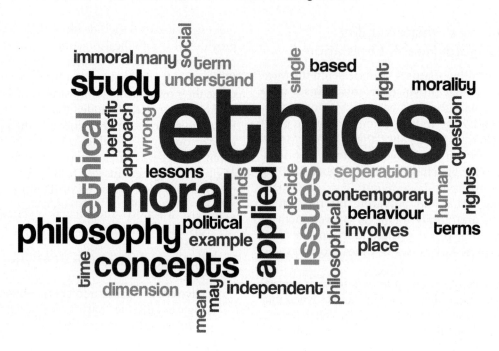

Moral philosophy considers ways that individuals may approach decisions about how to act and how to be. The work of moral philosophers offers guidance in ethical actions. Although some philosophers differentiate ethics from morality, ethics and morals can be used as interchangeable terms (ethics comes from *ethos*, Greek for *custom*; *morals* comes from *mores*, Latin for *custom*) and are so used here.

KEY CONCEPT

Ethics is consideration of the way a person should act to live a good life with and for others. Moral philosophy offers ideas about how to decide this. Just institutions enable and support ethical actions.

Health Ethics

Somerville (2000) describes Canada as a secular society, with diverse religious groups: we have no common, external, absolute moral authority. She asks, how can we know, as a society, how to respond to new approaches to science, technology, and health care? Contemporary ethics is shaped by factors such as intense individualism (the individual coming before the common good), corporatism (dominance of business interests), unprecedented advances in science and technology, the power of the media, the increased use of law as a means to resolve disputes that are inherently about values, and a loss of a sense of the sacred. She proposes that two absolute values, *profound respect for life* and *commitment to the human spirit*, will allow us to make ethical societal choices.

Somerville (2000, p. xii) uses the metaphor of a canary to signify key issues that "test the ethical air in our societal mineshaft." As canaries once served to detect toxic gas in underground mines (i.e., sick or dead canaries warned miners that the air was unsafe), these issues warn us that the ethical tone of our society is putting us at risk. The way in which Canadians address the wellbeing of those living with mental illness is recognizable to those practicing in mental health care as an ethical canary in the coal mine.

It is an ethical responsibility for nurses to keep abreast of societal issues, at a local, national, or global level, and to respond to those that may be informed by nursing expertise. The Canadian Nurses Association's (CNA) *Code of Ethics for Registered Nurses* identifies ethical actions that nurses can do to address social issues that affect health and wellbeing (CNA, 2017).

The Ethical Nurse

Stating "I am a nurse" is a form of moral claim. Nurses have a fiduciary relationship with the public (*fiducial* comes from the Latin, *fidere*, to trust). Nurses, as professionals, profess or claim that they will use their specialized knowledge and skills for the benefit of the public in a trustworthy way. Nurses are trusted to be ethical (Austin, 2006). In polls, nurses are consistently rated the most trusted and ethical professionals (Gallup, 2021, January). Whenever nurses enact their professional responsibilities, they are active as moral agents. As a recent example, nurses were a critical group in call for and recommendation of vaccines for COVID-19 and critical to the vaccines' implementation. They had, too, a responsibility to advocate for the necessary, proven, scientific restrictions to prevent the spread of the novel coronavirus in the global pandemic. Being ethical as a nurse requires more than having moral courage in times of crises (although it may require this): it requires the everyday expression of a commitment to the wellbeing of those in their care (Levine, 1977).

BOX 8.3 Research for Best Practice

CANADIAN NURSING STUDENTS' PERSPECTIVES: PROFESSIONAL VALUES AND ETHICAL IDEOLOGY

Arries, E. J. (2020). Professional values and ethical ideology: Perceptions of nursing students. *Nursing Ethics, 27,* 726–740. https://doi.org/10.1177/0969733019889396

Question: How do Canadian undergraduate nursing students perceive professional values and ethical ideology?

Method: In this descriptive, questionnaire survey study, participants were a convenient sample of nursing baccalaureate students at a Canadian university who had completed at least one clinical rotation in any practice area. (Note: Use of convenient samples can negatively affect generalizability of results.) The questionnaires measured ethical ideology using Forsyth's Ethics Position Questionnaire (two domains: idealism and relativism) and the Ethics Position Questionnaire (5-point Likert-type scale: strongly agree to strongly disagree). Values were assessed using the Nurses Professional Values Scale (NPVS-R) (5 domains: caring, activism, trust, professionalism, and justice corresponding to the CNA's Code of Ethics for Registered Nurses' values). Responses were anonymous and entered through a secure inhouse portal.

Findings: Idealism scored stronger than relativism as an ethics position (4.02 to 3.18). Third year students scored highest in idealism (mean: 4.10) and 4th year, the lowest (mean: 3.90). The professionalism scores were high: mean of 4.55; trust (highest), justice, and caring dimensions were higher than professionalism and activism (lowest).

Implications: The positive association between idealism and professional values of the nursing student participants in this study is a promising outcome given that it is known that idealism significantly impacts care outcomes in practice.

 KEY CONCEPT

A moral agent is a person engaged in determining or expressing a moral (ethical) choice.

Codes of Ethics for Nurses

To guide nurses in enacting their moral agency, codes of ethics have been developed by nursing associations. These are statements of the shared values and recognized duties and commitments of the profession. They set the ethical standards for practice and inform other disciplines and the public about the ethical commitments of nurses. (See Box "IN-A-LIFE".)

Although codes of ethics in nursing are for registered or licensed professionals, students are expected to be in compliance with their relevant code. Persons cared for by students should know the student status of the caregiver; students' caregiving should be congruent with their level of learning.

In 2018, CNA, with overwhelming support from its registered nurse members, opened CNA membership to all regulated nursing professionals in Canada (Almost, 2021). CNA is the global professional voice of Canadian nurses: registered nurses (RNs), registered psychiatric nurses (RPNs) (regulated to practice in British Columbia, Alberta, Saskatchewan, Manitoba, and the Yukon Territory), registered practical nurses (RPNs) (in Ontario only), and licensed practical nurses (LPNs). It may be that one code of ethics will evolve for Canadian nursing professionals. For now, the separate codes of ethics for Canadian registered nurses and RPNs are discussed below.

The Canadian Nurses Association's (CNA's) *Code of Ethics for Registered Nurses*

The CNA (2017) *Code of Ethics for Registered Nurses* is framed by seven values with related ethical responsibilities: providing safe, compassionate, competent, and ethical care; promoting health and wellbeing; promoting and respecting informed decision-making; honouring dignity; maintaining privacy and confidentiality; promoting justice; and being accountable. The code document includes "ethical endeavours related to broad societal issues," ways that RNs may strive, on their own and collectively, to change systems and social structures to promote greater equity for all. There is a glossary of pertinent terms and an example of an ethical model to help with reflection and decision-making (the Oberle and Raffin model), as well as reference to other models. Delineated, too, are ways to apply the code in certain circumstances, for example, responding to incompetent, noncompassionate, unsafe, or unethical care and ethical consideration in relationships with nursing students.

Nurses' right to follow their conscience is identified in the code, with steps in declaring a conflict with conscience outlined. **Conscientious objection** is defined as "a situation in which a nurse informs their employer about a conflict of conscience and the need to refrain from providing care because a practice or pro-

Patricia (Paddy) Anne Rodney

CANADIAN NURSE ETHICIST

A nurse with a strong clinical background in critical care, Paddy Rodney, BSN, MSN, PhD, RN, has contributed to Canadian health ethics as an educator, researcher, mentor, and leader. Her career reveals her deep commitment to the promotion of ethical nursing practice and to ensuring social justice within our healthcare system.

As an associate professor of nursing, first at the University of Victoria (UV) (1997–2005) and then at the University of British Columbia (UBC) (2005–2020), she has guided and supervised/co-supervised over 70 graduate students, many of whom continue to make their own contributions to nursing ethics. A selected sample of Paddy's research includes such issues as "Towards professional accountability: An observational study of nurses' experiences dealing with ethical problems" (NHRDP-funded); "Leadership for policy and practice" (CHSRF-funded); "Ethics in action: Strengthening nurses' enactment of their moral agency within the cultural context of health care delivery" (SSHRC-funded), and Constructing bioethics policy through consensus building and community participation (AMS).

Paddy has held several key leadership roles in health ethics, including as Chair, Canadian Nurses' Association Ethics Committee; as President, Canadian Nurses Interested in Ethics (a Canadian Nurses Association interest group); and as President of the Canadian Bioethics Society, a national interdisciplinary body of healthcare professionals, academics, researchers, practicing ethicists, public policy experts, and students interested in ethical issues in health, biology, and the environment. Her published works include several books used in ethics education: *Toward a Moral Horizon: Nursing Ethics for Leadership and Practice* (with Janet Storch and Rosalie Starzomski; 3rd edition in 2022) and *Concepts and Cases in Nursing Ethics* (with Michael Yeo, Anne Moorhouse, and Pamela Khan; 4th edition in 2020), as well as articles with colleagues in such journals as *Advances in Nursing Science, Journal of Nursing Philosophy, Nurse Education Today, American Journal of Nursing*, and the *Canadian Journal of Nursing Research* to name only a few.

Paddy retired from UBC in 2020, becoming an Associate Professor Emerita, but she continues to enrich and enhance health ethics through her work and example but has more time to enjoy life and travels with her husband, John Thomasson.

cedure conflicts with the nurse's moral beliefs" (British Columbia College of Nurses and Midwives [BCCNM], 2017; CNA, 2017, p. 21). It is important to recognize that the objection to a procedure or an aspect of care must be a moral concern and not due to fear, convenience, or prejudice and that the nurse must maintain the safety of the person receiving care until other nursing is available.

Ethics Guidelines for Registered Psychiatric Nurses

RPNs in Canada are guided by codes of ethics designated by their provincial colleges or association. RPNs in Alberta, for instance, follow a provincial code of ethics (congruent with Alberta's Health Professions Act) with the principles of beneficence, nonmaleficence, integrity, fidelity, respect for autonomy, and justice (College of RPNs of Alberta, 2013). For RPNs in Manitoba and the Yukon (and congruent with their applicable health professions legislation), the values framing their code of ethics are "safe, competent, and ethical practice to ensure the protection of the public"; "respect for the

inherent worth, right of choice, and dignity of persons"; "health, mental health, and wellbeing"; and "quality practice" (College of RPNs of Manitoba, 2017). In September 2020, the RPNs in British Columbia became part of the British Columbia Colleges of Nurses and Midwives. As this text goes to press, the ethical guidelines for RPNs in British Columbia remain those previously established (RPNC, 2010) based on four core values: "safe, competent, and ethical practice"; "respect for the inherent worth, right of choice, and dignity of persons"; "health, mental health, and wellbeing"; and "quality practice" (p. 3). The values of the code of the RPN Association of Saskatchewan (2020) are "professional accountability, unconditional respect, wholistic health, and quality practice milieu." See Web Links for access to the various RPN codes of ethics.

Approaches to Ethics

Nurse philosopher Sally Gadow describes the way societies have evolved their approach to ethics. She notes that communities in *premodern times* were immersed in the tradition and religion of their family and community. There was "ethical immediacy," a *subjective certainty* about what was moral and what was not, no shades of grey about right and wrong. In *modern times*—the era encompassing the 1800s to the 1990s—there was a search for *objective certainty*, for reason-based universal principles and a generally applicable ethical theory (e.g., utilitarianism; deontology). In our postmodern times, Gadow finds a *relational narrative* exists in which contingency is embraced, certainties refused, and the modern drive for unity, order, and foundations resisted. Intersubjectivity predominates and an individual's existential self is situated not only in rationality but also in emotion, imagination, memory, language, and the body, with the uniqueness of an individual and their essential feature. She envisions these not as stages but as elements that coexist within our clinical practice (Gadow, 1999).

An argument made from a cognitive science perspective by Rosenberg (2021) notes that the way an ethical dilemma is framed has incredible influence on the judgment made. For instance, an example of research revealing this *framing effect* was a simple one in which physicians were randomly assigned to two different groups and directed to decide if they would recommend a surgical procedure. One group was told the 1-month survival rate of the surgery was 90%; the other told the 1-month mortality rate was 10%: equal statements. When framed in terms of survival for a group, 86% of the members recommended the surgery; when framed in terms of mortality, only 50% would. Much of the time our brains operate without our conscious attention (i.e., we make fast, efficient judgments using affective associations) and need to do so to get us through the day. Our brains, however, also operate with our conscious attention (i.e., logical, requiring effort). Understanding these two approaches may help us make better ethical decisions, suggests Rosenberg, and to consciously consider a diversity of frames and be aware of our affective response.

Thus, there are several theoretical approaches (frames) to ethical knowledge that inform ethical action in health care, grounded in moral philosophy. Human rights may be used, as well, to guide ethical decisions. A brief outline of the most common approaches follows. See Table 8.3 for a summary.

Virtue Ethics

Virtue ethics, emphasizing the character of the moral agent, was the earliest approach to ethics used in nursing (Fowler, 1997). A virtuous person is one who, without

Table 8.3	Approaches to Ethics		
Approach	Core Elements	Proponents	Critiques
Virtue ethics	Character of the moral agent Some virtues: honesty, courage, compassion, practical wisdom	Aristotle Alasdair MacIntyre	Exclusive focus on the agent
Deontology	Duty based Some acts are wrong in themselves Universality Do not treat others as a means to an end (respect)	Immanuel Kant	Disregard of consequences Impartiality over relationship Emotion = irrationality
Utilitarianism	Consequence based Actions are right if they promote the best outcome (e.g., happiness, pleasure, satisfaction) for most people	Jeremy Bentham John Stuart Mill	Utility as the only principle Majority rules
Principlism	Based on a set of principles compatible with most moral theories Nonmaleficence, beneficence, respect for autonomy, justice	Tom Beauchamp James Childress	Too abstract Which has priority when principles compete?
Casuistry	Case based Use of paradigm cases to identify issues and courses of action for a new case	Albert Jonsen Stephen Toulmin	Keeps the status quo Can miss the broad issues
Ethics of care	Care based Connection/responsibility for others Emotional responsiveness	Carol Gilligan Nel Noddings	Creates a dichotomy between "care" (feminine) and "justice" (masculine) approaches to ethics Valorizes women as caregivers
Feminist ethics	Addresses power inequities, dominance, and oppression	Annette Baier Susan Sherwin	Lacks impartiality Lacks universal norms
Relational	Ethical action involves relationships Context matters; emotion accepted Dialogue is supported Aims for the "fitting" response	Vangie Bergum John Dossetor	Too relativistic Lacks impartiality Lacks universality
Human rights	Rights based (negative and positive) Every person is entitled to certain basic rights	John Locke Thomas Paine United Nations	As a concept, it is "nonsense" Too legalistic Too individualistic

strict reliance on rules, is wise enough to perceive how to act well in a particular situation. Lists of the virtues vary, but they include compassion, courage, tolerance, prudence, honesty, humility, justice, temperance, and trustworthiness. Aristotle (1996), the Greek philosopher whose works most inform virtue theory, believed that acquiring the virtues would assist a person to flourish as a human being. He found our moral upbringing to be important: we learn the virtues through our relationships. Observing compassion in others, for instance, can help us to develop a compassionate disposition. Although we need to comprehend key concepts to enact the virtues (e.g., justice and the notion of fairness), the ability to describe and discuss these abstractly is insufficient. One only masters the virtues through practice over one's lifetime (Darr, 2020). To acquire a virtue, it must become habitual; it is not enough, for instance, to be occasionally honest.

Aristotle's concept of the virtue of *phronesis* or **practical wisdom** seems particularly relevant to nurses. It means having the sensitivity, imagination, and experience to do what is ethically fitting in difficult situations (Austin, 2007a). In a profession with role-specific duties and responsibilities (evidenced by such things as a code of ethics), a trait that supports the good of that practice acquires the status of a moral virtue. A professional's virtues, in that sense, are necessary to their role (Radden & Sadler, 2008). In *After Virtue*, MacIntyre (1984) raises a question worthy of reflection: What would a person (nurse) lack, who lacked the virtues?

Deontology

Deontology (from the Greek *deon* or *duty*) postulates duty or obligation as the basis of doing right. This is duty not as in following external orders but as self-imposed obligation. This approach is also termed *Kantian ethics* because the work of Kant (1996), an 18th-century philosopher, laid its foundation. Kant believed that we should use reason alone to determine how to act. Reason unhampered by emotions or desires allows us to determine the types of acts that are wrong in themselves, no matter how good their consequences might be. Kant stipulated that a criterion (a *categorical imperative*) for judging the reason (or "maxim") for one's actions is universality: one should act only on a choice that one can conceive of as a universal law. Is a lie acceptable if it saves someone from danger? No, because lying cannot be willed as a universal principle. If we lie to help a person in trouble, truth will be subverted and society corrupted. In Kantian ethics, the moral worth of a person's action is determined by the intent of the person, not the effects of the action. If you act rightly, you are not responsible for bad effects.

Kant (1996) stipulated a second imperative: act so that you treat others always as an end and never as a means. Kant argued that we must treat one another with

dignity and respect; it is wrong to use other people for our own purposes. Informed consent is grounded on this belief. For instance, individuals should not be used as research subjects unless they understand what will happen and agree to it. Nor should we, according to Kantian ethics, place individuals at risk in research by depriving them of the best-known treatment in order to carry out a placebo-controlled study, even though this would provide the most valid evidence.

Kant's emphasis on rationality is such that he viewed it as necessary for personhood. This is sometimes known as "the Kantian line." It excludes those who are considered nonrational—children, those with dementia, and those experiencing psychosis—from being "persons." However, it has been argued that Kant's moral demand that all be treated with dignity and respect means that the rational and nonrational must be regarded as alike (Kahn, 2019). Kant's (1996) emphasis on the individual's rational capacity can be seen as highly relevant to psychiatric ethics, because it is the impairment of rational capacity alone that justifies coercive or involuntary psychiatric treatment (Robertson et al., 2007). It necessitates, as well, the moral responsibility of respect for persons if such action occurs. Kantian ethics supports the quest for universal ethical principles, such as the efforts of the United Nations Educational, Scientific, and Cultural Organization (UNESCO). A major problem with deontology is its disregard for the role of consequences in ethical action. Consequences, however, are the sole focus of the next approach.

Utilitarianism

The principle of utility is the foundation of **utilitarianism**: actions are right in proportion to their tendency to promote happiness or, as usually termed today, wellbeing. What is right to do is what gives the best consequences (e.g., happiness, wellbeing, pleasure, preference, satisfaction) for the greater number of people. Bentham (1983) and Mill (2002), philosophers of the 18th and 19th centuries, originated this theory that uses a type of cost/benefit analysis to determine the moral worth of an action. In their time, a theory where everyone's wellbeing counted equally was highly progressive and radical. This was an era where many citizens were disenfranchised and the upper classes' privilege institutionalized. This utilitarian approach to ethics has contributed to antislavery, women's liberation, and the animal rights movements. Most recently, it was a meaningful approach to the difficult decision-making related to resource allocation in the COVID-19 pandemic (Savulescu et al., 2020).

The principle of utility can also be applied to determining which moral rules to follow. This is termed rule utilitarianism and holds that once we decide on the best rules, we should follow them, even if in some situations, happiness is not maximized. A rule utilitarian might determine that a good rule for a nurse is not to go against hospital policies except if it is necessary for the best interests of a patient. Covertly putting an anti-psychotic medication in an acutely ill person's food, for instance, might be regarded as ethically acceptable in a special circumstance when such an action causes the least suffering to the ill person (Ipperciel, 2003). A Kantian would never approve of this, and despite ethical justification from a utilitarian perspective, such an act can result in a disciplinary or legal action.

Principlism

In the **principlism**, it is believed that a few moral principles (ethical norms) can provide a basis for moral reasoning in health ethics (Beauchamp, 1994). Four *prima facie* (at first sight) principles are widely accepted: non-maleficence, beneficence, respect for autonomy, and justice (Beauchamp & Childress, 2019). **Nonmaleficence** as a principle means that one should do no harm. **Beneficence** means that one should do, or attempt to do, good and make things better (promote benefit) for others when one can. **Respect for autonomy** (also considered as respect for persons) means an obligation to respect a person's right to be self-governing and their ability to make decisions. **Justice** is conceived as obligations of fairness in the distribution of benefits and risks. Criticisms of principlism include that the claim the four principles are grounded in the common morality does not hold up (Trotter, 2020). Critics have also noted that the principle of autonomy is too individualistic and better conceived as "relational autonomy," given the interdependence of human beings and the sociocultural nature of their choices (Walker, 2020). Another common criticism is that when principles compete, as they will in complex situations, there is no framework for settling the conflict.

The nature of mental illness creates situations in which respect for autonomy and beneficence conflict. How should one act when persons with a mental illness choose to act in ways that bring them harm? For instance, what if a person with schizophrenia is living homeless on the streets? Should respect for autonomy be upheld or should there be a beneficent intervention to bring the person to shelter? Respect for autonomy depends on a person's competence to make their own informed decisions, and evaluating such competence can be difficult.

Casuistry or Case-Based Ethics

Casuistry (pronounced kăzh' ū-ĭ;-strē), from the Latin *casus* for *case*, is the use of case comparisons to facilitate moral reasoning and decision-making. It is a bottom-up approach in which one starts with the details of the present case and locates that case in a taxonomy of cases as a way to identify the pertinent ethical concerns and responses (Jonsen, 1991; Jonsen & Toulmin, 1988). The focus in casuistry is on agreement about cases, not nec-

essarily principles or theories, and precedents are central to this approach. Past decisions about what was right or wrong in significant cases serve to inform decisions about the new case. (This is similar to what happens in legal judgments.) It supports learning how to analyze a situation into its key components, in a step-by-step way, and then to compare and evaluate it in relation to other relevant situations (Bleyer, 2020). The nurse using this approach will need to decide how the "case" does and does not fit paradigmatic cases. Suggested steps to use in doing this follow (Strong, 2000):

1. Identify the main ethical values and concerns relevant to the case.
2. Identify the main alternative courses of action that can be taken.
3. Identify the casuistic factors (i.e., the morally relevant ways the cases of this type differ).
4. Compare the case with relevant paradigm cases that have been identified.

Casuistry seems congruent with the way nurses think in practice. When a clinical situation confronts us, we often think of similar situations that we have experienced, or we turn to paradigm cases to guide us. This can become problematic, however, if we do not question prevalent beliefs and practices, preventing our thinking from evolving beyond past ethical deliberations and decisions. Other criticisms of casuistry are that it is not grounded in an understanding of "the good" (Robertson et al., 2007) and that there is a risk that one will miss the broader issues.

The Ethics of Care and Feminist Ethics

The **ethics of care** can be viewed as a feminine approach to ethics (Sherwin, 1992). Gilligan (1982), in researching moral development, found that females seemed to differ from males in their approach to ethical decision-making. Females focused on caring, connectedness, and responsibility rather than the deductive reasoning and abstract principles preferred by males. She argued that women are different from men in their approach to moral decisions, not inferior to them. (Aristotle and Kant both assumed that the moral agent was male.) The perspective of the world as a web of interdependent relationships in which our responsibility to one another is implicit is increasingly predominant in health ethics, as is the recognition that receptivity, relatedness, and responsiveness, as well as emotions, like compassion, are important components of ethical responses (Noddings, 1984; Sherwin, 1992). Branicki (2020), for instance, offers an ethics of care and feminist crisis management approach to addressing the COVID-19 pandemic, comparing it to a rationalist approach, typified by utilitarian logic.

Feminist ethics differs from the ethics of care in that it comes from a political perspective, offering insight into oppression (unjust, unwarranted use of power) and dominance in individual and societal-level relationships.

Using understandings gained from the analysis of women's oppression, feminist ethicists illuminate negative power differentials that may be so inherent as to be invisible and remain unquestioned. Because feminist ethics combines political dimensions with the core values of care and commitment, it offers a constructive framework for challenging the oppression of people with mental illness.

Relational Ethics

Relational ethics is based on the assumption that all ethical actions are situated in relationship. Ideas of duty and utility, principles, and the character of the moral agent are accepted as important in informing action, but relationship is taken as foundational. Ethics is about how we treat one another, individually and within society, as well as how we resolve moral problems. Ethical situations are encompassed by complexity, vulnerability, and uncertainty, and understanding this reality is necessary to ethical action.

Within this perspective, one strives to be responsive to the situation at hand in such a way that genuine dialogue is opened and mutual respect fostered among those involved. Feelings and emotions are viewed as a component of rational thinking and are explored, not ruled out as too subjective or confusing. Context matters. Not anything goes, but one's actions need not only to be shaped by ethical knowledge but also to be adapted to the specific circumstances of the situation. In relational ethics, one aims for the fitting response (Niebuhr, 1963/1999). Questions can be raised within this approach (e.g., issues of power and control) that may not be raised in approaches that focus primarily on moral reasoning (Bergum & Dossetor, 2020). Refer, for example, to relational ethics perspectives on responses to nurses who have an addiction (Kunyk & Austin, 2012), on nurses' responsibilities during an epidemic (Austin, 2008), and on hope in palliative care (Olsman et al., 2016). Core elements of relational ethics are mutual respect, engagement, embodied knowledge, attention to the interdependent environment, and uncertainty/vulnerability (Austin et al., 2003a; Bergum & Dossetor, 2020). Relational ethics provides a framework for a communities-of-practice approach for healthcare professionals as they address their own vulnerability arising from witnessing and engaging with fragility, suffering, pain, and dying in their practice (Delgado et al., 2021). A relational ethics decision-making framework is outlined in Box 8.4.

BOX 8.4 **A Relational Ethics Decision-Making Framework**

KEY QUESTIONS

1. What is happening here?
2. What are the alternatives for ethical action?
3. What is the most fitting thing to do?
4. What happened as the result of our action?

Question 1: What Is Happening Here?

- What are the ethical questions? Their context?
- Who is involved? (Who are the moral agents?) What are their commitments to one another?
- What further information do we need?
- Are there legal, organizational, professional, cultural, religious, or any other aspects to consider? Are values in conflict?
- What resources do we have? Need?
- Patient and family resources (e.g., personal directive)?
- Healthcare resources (e.g., access to home care)?
- Ethics resources: principles, precedents, codes, policies, guidelines, ethicists/ethics committees, etc.?
- To what, in particular, do we need to attend?

Question 2: What Are the Alternatives for Ethical Action?

- What are the consequences for each alternative?
- What might constrain ethical action?

- What, if anything, makes me or others uncomfortable in regard to a potential action?
- Remember: refraining from making a decision is still a decision.

Question 3: What Is the Most Fitting Thing to Do?

- What is the best way to carry out the decision (or plan)?
- Who is affected? Who needs to be involved?
- How may disparate views be bridged?

TAKE ACTION

Question 4: What Happened as the Result of Our Action?

- What concerns remain?
- Is anyone distressed about the result?
- Is further action desirable?
- Do we need to address systemic factors that gave rise to the situation?
- Would we act in the same way again?
- What did we learn?

©: Wendy Austin, University of Alberta, Canada.

Ethical Practice Environments

Healthcare environments need to be understood as moral communities where practice is grounded in compassion, empathy, and professionalism (Austin, 2012). For psychiatric and mental health (PMH) settings to be morally habitable, a "culture of questioning" must be actively nurtured (Austin et al., 2004). This means that ethical questions are to be expected as an everyday aspect of practice, not perceived as challenging or troublesome. Consultation with a clinical ethicist or ethics committee should be viewed as an acceptable option, a common use of an ethics resource.

Interprofessional communication, collaboration, and conflicts are critical factors in the ethical climate of healthcare areas (Austin, 2007b). Research in PMH settings has revealed for some time that the desire to get along with colleagues can trump "doing the right thing" (Carpenter, 1991; Fisher, 1995) and that staff conflict influences the way an ethical situation is resolved (Forchuk, 1991). Institutional policies, demands, and supports also play a role. Institutional constraints on a nurse's ability to advocate for patients have been identified as a common contributor to nurses' moral distress (Rittenmeyer & Huffman, 2009). A Canadian study of practitioners enacting their moral agency in acute mental healthcare settings described the process as "risking vulnerability" within a context of "systemic inhumanity" in which the healthcare system was unable to consistently respond to those requiring care with respect, dignity, and compassion (Musto et al., 2021, p. 2464). How can this be? The researchers concluded that policies and practices shaped by discourses of scarcity and efficiency undermined ethical practice (Musto et al., 2021).

Moral Dilemmas and Moral Distress

A moral dilemma is a morally relevant conflict (Audi, 1995). It may be defined more narrowly as a situation in which one has an obligation to act but must choose between two incompatible alternatives. In health ethics, frameworks have been developed to facilitate the decision-making process. Decision-making frameworks are tools to guide ethical deliberation, based on particular or composite approaches (see Box 8.4).

A definition of moral distress, composed by incorporating elements from the work of experts (Austin, 2016), is:

the *embodied response* (e.g., frustration, anger, sleeplessness, headache, nausea, anxiety, anguish, etc.) of an individual to a moral problem for which the individual assumes some *moral responsibility* makes *a moral judgment* about the appropriate ethical action to be taken but, due to real or perceived constraints, participates by act or omission in what they regard as *moral wrongdoing* (Jameton, 1984, 2013; Nathaniel, 2006; Wilkinson, 1987–1988).

Moral distress is a risk component of healthcare provision and its associated responsibility. It is not a sign of weakness, but rather an indication of one's sensitivity to the ethics of practice and a commitment to public trust (Austin, 2016). An example of the moral distress of nurses in an acute care psychiatric setting is shared in a study situated in a setting where patients' dignity and participation, as well as minimal use of coercion, were stated values. Determined sources of moral distress were identified as inadequate time, resources, and competency (use of untrained staff) that led to less than quality care. Researchers concluded that the act of voicing moral concerns may have been affected by nurses' moral doubt, loyalty, and lack of courage and energy (Jansen et al., 2020). Other earlier studies of the moral distress of nurses and other healthcare professionals in PMH settings showed that lack of resources, institutional demands, and unrealistic demands on the part of society that deviant behaviour be controlled are contributing factors (Austin et al., 2003b, 2005, 2008).

Research indicates that when nurses experience moral distress, they either choose to continue giving voice to their ethical concerns or they withdraw—from ethically challenging situations, from their position, or entirely from the discipline of nursing (Pauly et al., 2012). Opportunities for discussing and processing care situations that are ethically challenging (e.g., informal or formal debriefings, ethics consultation, ethics rounds, ethics committees) are important to the prevention and resolution of moral distress (Austin, 2017). Nursing leaders play a key role in supporting such opportunities, as well as in creating positive ethical climates where voicing ethical concerns is an expectation of members of interprofessional teams rather than viewed as problematic (Schick Makaroff et al., 2014).

Nursing's approach to moral distress has evolved since it was first described in the 1980s: moral distress has become a common term with healthcare team members using it to name their experience. The need for speaking up, dialogue, cooperation, and moral resilience is recognized (Jameton, 2017), although not without familiar barriers. Research examining the relationship between resilience factors and moral distress among nursing students indicates that higher social support and sense of efficacy correlate with lower levels of moral distress. This suggests that an emphasis in nursing education on developing teamwork capacities, collegial communications, and ways of addressing interdisciplinary conflict, along with ethics education that involves rehearsal of ethical situations to nurture moral sensitivity and understanding of ethical action, may better prepare nurses for moral distressing situations in practice (Krautscheid et al., 2020). Ethics education should be core to nursing curricula, not "threaded" across a program (Jones-Bonofiglio, 2020) nor offered only as an elective.

KEY CONCEPT

A moral dilemma is a conflict in which one feels a moral obligation to act but must choose between incompatible alternatives.

KEY CONCEPT

Moral distress is an embodied response that occurs when one acknowledges an ethical obligation, makes a moral choice regarding fitting ethical action, but is then unable to act on this moral choice because of internal or external constraints.

Ethical Issues in Psychiatric and Mental Healthcare Settings

It is not possible in this chapter to identify all the complex ethical issues of PMH settings; rather, selected significant ones are discussed. Although some issues may not be unique to this specialty area (e.g., confidentiality), all are shaped by the PMH context and by the potential vulnerability of individuals living with a stigmatized illness. Such vulnerability is increased for those who have a mental disorder that can sometimes affect their competency to give informed consent to treatment and who may thus receive treatment involuntarily.

Threats to Dignity

An important aspect of ethical nursing care involves safeguarding the dignity of patients, as violated dignity can lead to suffering and a loss of self-worth. Nurses in PMH settings, when asked about experiences that involved preserving patient dignity, described being genuinely "present" with patients (e.g., supporting the individual through emotions like anger) and being their advocate. Issues of dignity arising for those who have been a patient in PMH settings have been identified through study of their experiences. For instance, persons with experience of a coercive intervention (e.g., seclusion, restraints, or rapid tranquillization) describe feeling powerless and/or hopeless as they felt neither sufficiently informed about, nor involved in, their treatment plan, including medications and being held within a hospital environment, which seemed prison-like (Chambers et al., 2014).

It can be in the "small things" where dignity resides: awareness of individuals as more than their illness, in

choice and tone of language, and in gestures and courtesies associated with acts of daily living (Skorpen et al., 2015). When nurses described their experiences of violations to the dignity of those who had an involuntary PMH treatment status, they noted these individuals being ignored or not taken seriously, being physically "violated" through restraints, being betrayed by broken promises, and being exposed (e.g., medication given in front of others; personal history shared with the entire team). They identified the power differential between staff and patients as a potential source of loss of dignity, as was predefining individuals by their diagnosis (Gustafsson et al., 2014).

Maureen Foy (2007), mother of a young woman with a severe and persistent mental illness, described her experience as a family member. One example she offered occurred when her daughter was admitted to a crisis unit in a Canadian general hospital:

> Over a period of two to three hours of waiting, the staff did not speak to us or look at us once. It was as though we were not there, we were invisible. There were no words of comfort or care. There was no information given and we were left to wonder on our own what or whom we were waiting for…. Staff looked through us, around us, above us, below us, but they did not look at us. At a time of crisis and in a place where you go for help and maybe even care, this is hard to bear. This behaviour silences you. (p. 1).

She notes that advancements in brain imaging, psychotropic drugs, and models of therapy are nothing if comfort and compassion are not shown to the persons needing care. Nurses and other healthcare professionals must consistently ask: What is it like to use our mental health services? What is it like to be in our care or to be a patient's family member? The value of respect, integral to the support of dignity, is very evident in policy documents and the literature of PMH nursing, but too frequently, there is a disconnect between what is espoused and what occurs in practice; ongoing attentiveness to nursing actions that may convey disrespect is crucial to ethical practice (Cutcliffe & Travale, 2013).

Behaviour Control, Seclusion, and Restraint

Recovery-oriented, trauma-informed mental health care demands that the least intrusive and restrictive interventions are used in protecting and reducing risk to patients. This means that individual rights, dignity, and autonomy are respected and that there is "the least possible recourse" to measures (mechanical, chemical, environmental, or physical) to limit a person's activity or to control behaviour (MHCC, 2009, p. 121). Restrictive measures are to be used only when absolutely necessary and then with sensitivity and great caution. They can have serious relational consequences (see Chapter 12).

Coercion and control in PMH care are abiding ethical and clinical issues. The healthcare team must continually evaluate whether these measures equate with best practice when being considered as an intervention. Expressing moral doubt about such clinical interventions, however, can be difficult. It can delay rapid response to a crisis situation, can be viewed as professional inexperience or weakness, or can be taken as criticism of one's colleagues or leaders (Molewijk et al., 2017). Nevertheless, as coercion involves limiting the autonomy of an individual through institutional power, it seems important that the query, "Is this the right action?" gets raised (Molewijk et al., 2017). Ethical reflexivity and dialogue can help nurses and other team members to ensure that whatever form such measures take that they are clinically and morally justified. Institutional support for staff's ethical questioning, ongoing evaluation of its policies and practices, and training to increase of staff's competence in dealing with aggression, distress, and psychoses can lead to greater use of alternatives to coercion and control (Norvoll et al., 2017). Ethical consultation, for instance, with a clinical ethicist, can help healthcare teams to engage in meaningful dialogue regarding the use of coercive measures and increase their capacity for dealing with such ethical issues (Austin, 2017). PMH settings should be well-designed healing places with sufficient numbers of competent, compassionate staff. When this is not so, it is an ethical issue.

Psychiatric Advance Directives

Psychiatric advance directives (PADs) are a legal resource for people to use for times when their decision-making ability is compromised by a mental illness (MHCC, 2009). An advance directive (also known as a personal directive) allows for designation of a surrogate decision-maker who can act on one's behalf when one is not competent to do so. It can delineate one's preferred choices to guide the surrogate and the healthcare team. Provincial governments have a personal directive registry where one indicates that they have a personal directive and the name of the surrogate decision-maker.

As an individual with a bipolar disorder noted, "It will give me peace of mind to know that if I get to the point where I can't say anything, there is something in place that will represent myself" (Ambrosini et al., 2012, p. 4). PADs are a useful tool in communicating with physicians, avoiding side effects by identifying specific medications that an individual wishes to avoid, and preventing involuntary treatment. Research indicates that PADs not only give patients a sense of control and increase the use of treatments congruent with patient preferences but also lower the need for coercive interventions

(Olsen, 2017). Nurses can support patients in their preparation of PADs and can actively and consistently foster autonomy through learning patient preferences and helping reduce constraints to independence. (See Web Links to connect to a provincial Advance Health Care Directive Act, that of Newfoundland and Labrador.)

Relational Engagement: Boundaries

Engagement in therapeutic relationships is an important aspect of most, if not all, PMH care, and complex ethical issues are situated in the boundaries of these relationships (see Chapter 7). Although "boundary," the term commonly used to describe the limits of therapeutic relationships, implies clear, firm borders that should not be crossed, actual practice can be more complicated. Gift giving is an example. Although accepting a gift from a patient can be seen as an initial step down the "slippery slope" toward a boundary violation and something to be always avoided, a particular situation may be more complex (Austin et al., 2006). Refusing a small, homemade gift from a grateful patient may be a hurtful act. Accepting a significant gift from a vulnerable patient, on the other hand, may be viewed as theft (Griffith, 2016). Nurses need to be thoughtful about the meaning of a gift and seek out knowledgeable advice from members of the team and clinical supervisors.

Not unlike refusal of a gift, declining a "friend invitation" on a social networking site such as Facebook can be a complex ethical issue and requires similar thoughtful deliberation (Ginory et al., 2012). In fact, "breaching patient confidentiality and privacy has become increasingly common for nurses and students since the advent of social media" (Smith & Knudson, 2016, p. 911). In a study of student nurses' unethical behaviour, use of social media was found to positively correlate with students' unethical behaviour (as did year of birth, with younger students having a greater degree of unethical behaviour) (Smith & Knudson, 2016).

The use of e-mail for therapeutic communication and patient-centred care raises similar issues, as does other uses of health information technology, which soon may be commonplace, such as virtual home visits to patients (a form of telehealth) and patients' submission of health data (e.g., stress measures) through their smartphones. Internet security will be a dominant concern. Interacting online with patients is challenging and requires that professional boundaries be maintained, including the avoidance of dual relationships; nurses and health care staff need to monitor their online presence (Ginory et al., 2012).

One of the most serious types of boundary violation is the sexual harassment and abuse of patients. Despite policies of zero tolerance, abuse occurs and is known to be significantly underreported. Professionals who commit serious boundary violations at times argue that it was a mutual decision made with the patient.

This "defence" does not hold up because "consent" is not applicable, given the significant disparities in status, power, and vulnerability that exist between patient and healthcare professional (DuBois et al., 2019).

Transgressions of boundaries are most often discussed as *overinvolvement. Under involvement* can also be an ethical issue. Lack of time to engage with patients has been found to contribute to nurses' moral distress (Austin et al., 2003a). Countertransference experienced by the nurse may affect therapeutic availability if the nurse fails to address it appropriately (see Chapter 7). A negative response may be evoked as well, when a patient rejects care, is abusive, or is guilty of a morally reprehensible act, such as child abuse (Liaschenko, 1994). Liaschenko found that when nurses had difficulty connecting with a patient, they chose among three options: to emotionally distance themselves from the patient, to transfer the patient to another nurse, or to make a conscious effort to be respectful and provide good care. The nurses in this study recognized difficulties in "bridging the gap" to a patient as an ethical issue.

To engage ethically with patients, nurses must attend to their own personal and professional boundaries and must respect those of others. Education about boundaries is helpful, as are strategies such as clinical supervision and resources such as *Professional Boundaries: Guidelines for the Nurse–Client Relationship* (College and Association of Registered Nurses of Alberta, 2020) and the practice standard, *Boundaries in the Nurse Client Relationship* of the Colleges of Registered Licensed Practical Nurses, Registered Nurses, and Registered Psychiatric Nurses of British Columbia (BCCNM, 2017, 2020).

Confidentiality and Privacy

Maintaining privacy and confidentiality is an ethical responsibility of nurses. See the ethical responsibilities related to upholding this value in the CNA (2017, p. 14) *Code of Ethics for Registered Nurses*. Privacy is a basic human right, and individuals may not wish their personal information disclosed to others or for others to intrude upon their personal space. Legislation at the federal and provincial/territorial levels protects personal health information, and there are regulations that allow individuals to access and request correction of their personal information. Privacy laws in Canada include the *Privacy Act* (Government of Canada, 2020d), which limits the collection, use, and disclosure of personal information in federal government agencies, and the *Personal Information Protection and Electronic Documents Act* (PIPEDA) (Government of Canada, 2020c) with which all provinces and territories must comply. The PIPEDA regulates personal information collection, use, and disclosure that occur in commercial activities (including personal health information), requiring that organizations obtain informed consent to use individuals' personal information, secure it, and provide them with

access to their own information, which they may request to have corrected. CNA has a *Privacy of Personal Health Information* fact sheet for nurses. (See Web Links.)

Canada has a Privacy Commissioner who advocates for privacy rights and is able to publicly report on the handling of personal information from public and private organizations, to investigate complaints, and to promote public awareness of privacy issues (Office of the Privacy Commissioner of Canada [OPCC], 2015). A priority concern of the OPCC is that information about our bodies is merging with information technology. Digital measurement of vital signs; collection of biometric data for recreational, forensic, and commercial purposes; implantable sensors that communicate internal status (e.g., blood pressure; glucose levels); biomedical electronics (e.g., implants that read brain activity; genetic testing); and automated medical records have brought us to a place where we have an incredible level of intimate information about our bodies and our health status. The risk to the privacy of our health information is similarly amplified (OPCC). Nurses will need to keep informed on the risks and ways to counter them as this most personal of private information increasingly exists in digital form.

Privacy can be particularly important in PMH settings, given the stigma and discrimination attached to mental disorders and to psychiatric care. Consent is a central factor in decisions related to privacy and confidentiality, and this factor becomes more complicated when the person involved has an illness that affects their ability to give consent. Overall, nurses safeguard the information learned in the context of their professional relationships, sharing it outside the healthcare team only with the patients' permission or as legally required.

Disclosure of information within the healthcare team occurs as necessary for treatment and care, but when patients confide information that is not relevant to the patient's health and wellbeing, this type of information is not shared. Patients and families need to be made aware that health information and care decisions are shared among the team. This is particularly important as there can be misconception that anything communicated to a health professional is protected as confidential, even within legal testimony. Such communication, however, cannot be presumed privileged in the way that attorney–client communication is held to be. As well, there are situations that legally require the reporting of information received in a patient care situation. Mandatory reporting of child abuse and abuse of adults in care are examples (refer to provincial and territorial legislation for reporting requirements). Nurses are expected to intervene if others within the healthcare system fail to meet obligations regarding confidentiality and privacy (CNA, 2017).

Too strict observation of privacy and confidentiality rules can create problems if it means that families and other caregivers are excluded from knowledge that can help them protect and support persons with a mental disorder when they are at risk. A balance needs to be found between respecting the person's privacy and facilitating family assistance (MHCC, 2009). The PADs are a way to address this potential problem.

Spiritual Care

Spirituality can be a source of comfort and hope, and most individuals want a spiritual component included in their care (Sager, 2020). Nevertheless, spiritual care is neglected in psychiatric treatment settings (Neathery et al., 2020). Avoidance of spiritual care may be due to uncertainty regarding how to ethically engage with diverse spiritual practices while maintaining professional boundaries (Sager, 2020). In an American survey study, psychiatric mental health nurses ($n = 159$) identified barriers to spiritual care as apprehension regarding triggering negative religious thoughts and their own lack of educational preparation in spiritual care. A small number of nurses ($n = 7$) indicated internal barriers (e.g., "personal trigger for me"; "how can I support something I do not believe in?") or an external one ($n = 2$; e.g., "not important in my institution") (Neathery et al., 2020). In other nations, such as Ghana, nurses report that many patients identify mental illness as having a spiritual cause (e.g., spiritual punishment), not a biomedical one. Some Ghanaian nurses may share this belief and view spiritual care as a genuine approach to healing an individual's experience of mental illness (Koduah et al., 2019).

Nurses need to reflect on their own spiritual beliefs and consider what may inhibit their ability to understand or support patients in their beliefs. Consider that, in addressing the clients' spiritual needs, it is unnecessary to use terms like "spiritual" or "religious." Instead, the nurse can express the concepts of hope, values, comfort, and strength (Ramluggun et al., 2021). In these situations, nursing care can involve exploring an individual's fears and concerns and ways of coping with distress. Asking clients open questions such as "What gives you strength in difficult times?" or "What gives you hope?" or "Are there beliefs or ideas that bring you comfort?" may be a means for nurses to more comfortably engage with the spiritual aspect of those in their care.

Advances in Neurotechnology

Advances in neurotechnology reveal new insights into human brain functioning and are creating ways of altering it. Not only does this bring new threats to privacy (e.g., uses being explored include detection of lying and prediction of violent or criminal behaviour), but it brings possible threats to autonomy through invasive and noninvasive ways of influencing the brain (Beauvais et al., 2021; Ryberg, 2017). Will the use of such technologies be a threat to personhood (Racine & Affleck, 2016)?

Neuroethics is the area of health ethics exploring such ethical issues.

The uses of neurotechnology have clinical implications for the mental health field. There are implications, for instance, in memory manipulation, made possible through such procedures as transcranial magnetic stimulation, transcranial direct current stimulation, deep brain stimulation, and the use of pharmacologic agents (e.g., donepezil and propranolol). While this manipulation may have treatment benefits for such disorders as posttraumatic stress, anxiety dementia, and drug abuse (Agren, 2014; Cestari et al., 2014), there are fundamental ethical implications to be considered. Will using neurotechnology in such ways alter an individual's perception of "true self"? Will only pleasant memories be deemed acceptable? Will those unable to afford enhancements be at a great disadvantage in education and the workplace? In other words, what will such technology do to us? To date, there is limited evidence that treatments using such neurotechnology have caused loss of personal identity. But there remains a need for continued evaluation of neurotechnology and oversight to ensure that research and clinical guidelines are followed (Racine & Affleck, 2016) and that social dialogue and adequate policies are developed as the science evolves (Robillard & Illes, 2016).

Further, global cooperation and Open Science, a movement that aspires to make scientific research data accessible to all, are creating extraordinary possibilities for scientific advancement, along with complex ethical risks. Canada's scientific initiatives, such as the Canadian Brain Research Strategy and the Canadian Open Neuroscience Platform, will benefit from open collaboration and data sharing with other nations, but inherent risks will be shared as well. Sharing neurological data, for instance that of schizophrenia research, has implications for participants' anonymity (individuals and identifiable groups) and, given the stigma associated with this disease, potential social risk. Beauvais and colleagues (2021) advance the need for a principle such as solidarity that can encompass both the right to benefit from scientific progress and the right to be protected from unjustified harms, involving legal prohibitions on re-identification, disallowing the use of datasets for nonscientific purposes, and a harm mitigation fund.

Advances in Genetics

Advances in genetics raise other concerns, given events in history. Eugenics (Greek for "wellborn") was once a worldwide movement, beginning at the onset of the 20th century aimed at improving the human race. In 1939, in Nazi Germany, a program was initiated that lead to the killing of thousands of "incurable" psychiatric patients deemed to have a life "not worth living" that weakened their society. Nurses actively participated in this program (Aly & Roth, 1984; Benedict & Kuhla,

1999; McFarland-Icke, 1999). For the most part, however, eugenics involved preventing the physically and mentally disabled from reproducing; sterilization was a favoured strategy.

With contemporary advances in genetic engineering, a new eugenics is evolving. Genetic testing may make possible prenatal selection and termination of a pregnancy when the fetus is at risk for a mental disorder. (Many of the common mental health disorders have a known genetic component. It is doubtful, however, that direct linkages between a given gene and a psychiatric disorder exist; see Chapter 10.) Genetic profiles of individuals may lead to discrimination and to "genetic essentialism" (i.e., a person is defined by their genes). In considering the ethical acceptability of clinical genetic testing, questions should be asked, such as: What is the purpose of the test? How stigmatized is the condition being tested for? Do effective interventions exist for it? Will the testing affect third parties, such as family members? Increasingly, others' access to one's genetic information is a realistic concern. Private companies and researchers, hoping to develop new treatments, are seeking legal access to medical records from governments. Although data are anonymized in such cases, confidentiality remains at issue.

These concerns have increased with the current development of "personalized medicine." Described often as adapting treatment to the individual patient's needs and preferences, personalized medicine is, at its basics, medicine adapted to a person's genomic makeup. Its success is evident in oncology, most dramatically in the treatment of lung cancer. It has the potential to predict, for instance, a person's response to a specific treatment and vulnerability to adverse events (Perna & Nemcroff, 2017). This individualizing of treatment fits well with psychiatry's original approach (Perna & Nemcroff, 2017). A journal, *Personalized Medicine in Psychiatry*, was created in 2017 and continues to support dialogue and communication of research with this approach. To evolve the genetic evidence that is the basis of personalized medicine, significant genetic research needs to occur. Its risks and benefits will need to be continually assessed and monitored, but there is much promise for better care.

Social Justice

Nursing has a long history of promoting health equity and social justice (Rudner, 2021). Optimal mental health requires conditions of fundamental equality and justice. Justice, a principle of fair treatment of individuals and groups and of promotion of the common good within society, is a core value underpinning the CNA (2017) *Code of Ethics for Registered Nurses*. It is acknowledged that broad societal issues affect health and wellbeing, and thus, nurses need to be cognizant of these issues, including at the global level, and to safeguard human

rights, equity, and fairness in their practice, acting as advocates for positive change. Part II of the CNA Code describes examples of what nurses can do to address social inequities, using the principles of primary health care for the benefit of patients and the public, as well as working for social justice, advocating for policies and laws that support equity, and promoting environmental preservation and restoration (CNA, 2017).

Although nursing codes of ethics indicate that nurses have a role in social justice, nursing education programs do not necessarily address this role significantly. The International Society of Psychiatric-Mental Health Nurses (Raphel et al., 2021), in its commitment to global social justice, identifies among its strategies advocating for culturally competent nursing educators who are literate in social justice and health equity. Other strategies are advocating for human rights, reducing barriers to health service utilization, and engaging in consumer-driven and community-generated research. The social injustices related to mental illness due to stigma and discrimination are global. The Global Burden of Diseases, Injuries, and Risk Factors Study (GBD), a systematic scientific assessment of public data on incidence, prevalence, and mortality, indicates that depressive disorders are in the top 10 of global burdens of disease from teenage years into old age and that mental disorders are a major contributor to disability globally (GBD 2019 Diseases and Injuries Collaborators, 2020). Nevertheless, mental health care remains a poorly resourced area of health care worldwide.

Research Ethics

Research is vitally important to improving the lives of persons with mental illness and their families, and determining ways to prevent mental illness and foster mental health and wellbeing. However, it is vital that risks and benefits be identified, ensuring individuals are never exploited. Canada has delineated ethics policies for federal research funding agencies in the *Tri-Council Policy Statement: Ethical Conduct of Research Involving Humans* guided by the core principles of respect for persons and concern for welfare and justice (Government of Canada, 2018).

Informed consent is key to the protection of research subjects. The Tri-Council policy requires that consent to participate in research must be voluntary, ongoing, and informed. A person who lacks capacity to make an informed decision is not necessarily deprived of the right to participate in research. Participation may occur if the person is involved in the decision-making process as much as possible, with consent given by an authorized third party that is based on the best interests of the person. In the area of psychiatry, however, there is some debate over whether the research participation of hospitalized persons who are currently deemed not competent to make decisions due to a mental disorder is ethical. The high level of vulnerability of such persons and their dependence on the healthcare system and its personnel calls their involvement in research into question (Elliott & Lankin, 2016).

Informed consent in addiction research has also been queried. Research on cravings (intense desires for a drug) for the purpose of understanding their neuro-biologic and cognitive bases may allow development of better treatment for addiction. However, the ability of substance-dependent research participants to give genuinely informed consent, based on understanding the risks, may be diminished by potential access to their drug of addiction.

Clinical trials research can raise significant research ethics issues. Such research is needed, however, if effective treatments are to evolve. A review of the evidence regarding risks suggests that it is possible to conduct research in this area safely, even with drug withdrawals

and placebo controls (Nugent et al., 2017). Ongoing attention to the balance of risks and benefits, however, remains essential.

In the history of psychiatric research in Canada, there is a strong reminder that vigilance in terms of ethics is necessary. In the 1950s and early 1960s, the "depatterning" experiments of Dr. Ewen Cameron at the Allen Memorial Institute, McGill University (partially funded by the U.S. Central Intelligence Agency), attempted to erase the memories of patients and insert new "positive" ideas. Without their consent, patients were "brainwashed," with many permanently losing their memories. Although Dr. Cameron was an international leader in psychiatric medicine with the reputation of being a humanitarian, his research caused great harm (Collins, 1988). Remembering that such serious violations of research ethics have occurred can act as a safeguard against future contraventions.

🍁 Summary of Key Points

- Ethics and law are separate domains. Nurses must understand and be vigilant about the laws that affect their practice.
- Human rights are prescriptive and delineated in such documents as the *Canadian Charter of Rights and Freedoms, 1982* and the United Nations *Universal Declaration of Human Rights, 1948*.
- Each province and territory has its own Mental Health Act, congruent with the Canadian *Charter of Rights and Freedoms,* that includes the rules and procedures governing the commitment of persons suffering from mental disorders. Nurses need to be knowledgeable regarding the Mental Health Act in the province where they practice. The Criminal Code of Canada has a provision in which an individual may be deemed not criminally responsible for an act due to a mental disorder.
- Canadians may be eligible for medical assistance in dying (MAID) if they meet the criteria. In 2023, this eligibility will be extended to persons on the basis of a mental disorder.
- Key issues can warn us about the ethical tone of our society; many of these issues are situated in health care. The way in which Canadians address the wellbeing of persons living with mental illness is one of these issues.
- Whenever nurses enact their professional responsibilities, they are active as moral agents. Nursing practice

involves an attentiveness and responsiveness to duties and commitments.
- Nurses' regulatory bodies support ethical practice through codes of ethics, position statements, and resources.
- There are theoretical approaches to ethical knowledge (based on moral philosophy and concepts such as human rights) that inform health ethics. These include virtue ethics, deontology, utilitarianism, principlism, casuistry, ethics of care, feminist ethics, relational ethics, and human rights.
- Practice environments need to be morally habitable and support ethical questioning and dialogue.
- Frameworks for ethical decision-making are available to assist in resolving moral dilemmas.
- Moral distress occurs when one is unable to act on an ethical judgment and/or fulfill one's ethical obligations as one believes one should.
- There are many complex ethical issues in PMH settings. These include issues related to threats to dignity, including behaviour control and restraint, relational engagement ("boundaries"), aspects of spiritual care, confidentiality and privacy, genetics, research ethics, and social justice.
- PADs are a tool intended to support the autonomy of patients. They have been found to facilitate therapeutic alliance and promote treatment integration.

🧠 Thinking Challenges

1. Facebook Posting by a Registered Nurse: Professional Misconduct or Freedom of Expression?
   In 2015, a registered nurse (RN) in Prince Albert, Saskatchewan, posted comments on Facebook regarding the concern over the poor quality of palliative care

that their grandfather was receiving in an unidentified long-term care home. The Saskatchewan Registered Nurses Association (SRNA) evaluated this posting as a violation of confidentiality and found the guilty of professional misconduct. In 2016, the RN was fined

$26,000, a decision that was upheld by a Queen's Bench Justice. In 2019, the decision was appealed by the nurse and overturned by the Saskatchewan Court of Appeal in 2020 on the basis of freedom of expression. It was found that the SRNA erred in their decision: a Facebook post by an RN about the need to improve quality of care (that did not identify the institution) did not justify a ruling of misconduct. In the Justice's ruling, it was noted that the right to criticize public services is essential to freedom of expression in a democracy (Hicks, 2020).

a. Identify possible rationales for
  i. the nurse's action to post the concerns on social media.
  ii. the SRNA's judgment of such behaviour as professional misconduct.
b. Describe your own response to the nurse's decision to post the criticism of care on Facebook: was it ethical or unethical in your opinion?

c. What are some alternative actions that the nurse might have taken to address the concerns regarding the poor quality of care?
d. Are there resources that could be put in place to allow healthcare practitioners to report their concerns regarding quality of care without fear of formal (or informal) repercussions?
2. What would your answer be to MacIntyre's (1984) question in *After Virtue,* when phrased in terms of a nurse: What would a nurse lack who lacked the virtues?
3. Outline three qualities necessary to a morally habitable healthcare environment.

Visit thePoint to view suggested responses. Go to **thePoint.lww.com/activate** and use the activation code found in the front of this text to unlock answers to the "Thinking Challenges" and other online resources.

 ## Web Links

Advocacy Organizations for Persons With Mental Illness and Their Families

camimh.ca Canadian Alliance on Mental Illness and Mental Health (CAMIMH)
cmha.ca Canadian Mental Health Association (CMHA)
driadvocacy.org/ Disability Rights International (DRI)
icn.ch/sites/default/files/inline-files/PS_A_Mental%20Health_1.pdf International Council of Nurses' Position Statement: Mental Health
mdsc.ca Mood Disorders Society of Canada (MDSC)
mentalhealthcommission.ca Mental Health Commission of Canada (MHCC)
schizophrenia.ca Schizophrenia Society of Canada
wfmh.org World Federation for Mental Health (WFMH)
who.int/en World Health Organization (WHO)

Codes of Ethics for Nurses in Canada

cna-aiic.ca/on-the-issues/best-nursing/nursing-ethics The Canadian Nurses Association *Code of Ethics for Registered Nurses.*
bccnm.ca/RPN/Pages/Code_of_Ethics.aspx British Columbia College of Nurses and Midwives' Code of Ethics for Registered Psychiatric Nurses.
crpnm.mb.ca/wp-content/uploads/2019/03/CRPNM-Code-of-Ethics-Adopted-May-2017.pdf College of Registered Psychiatric Nurses of Manitoba. (2017). *Code of ethics.*
https://www.rpnas.com/members/code-of-ethics/ Registered Psychiatric Nurses of Saskatchewan. (2020). *Code of ethics.*

Resources Related to Mental Health Acts

albertahealthservices.ca/MHA.asp An excellent resource for understanding a provincial mental health act (Alberta's) and such processes as community treatment orders and formal certification of patients. Educational resources include videos, flowcharts, and links to related sites.
psychdb.com/teaching/on-mha/home Created and maintained by Canadian resident physicians in psychiatry, this site introduces Ontario's mental health laws and provides information about substitute decision-makers, etc.
parl.ca/LegisInfo/BillDetails.aspx?Language=E&billId=10875380 The amended Medical Assistance in Dying law (2021-03-17) is available here.
canada.ca/en/health-canada/services/medical-assistance-dying.html Information on MAID can be found at this government website.

Health Ethics Centres and Related Resources

bioethics.ca Canadian Bioethics Society
bioethics.georgetown.edu The Bioethics Research Library at Georgetown University
bioethics.medicine.dal.ca Dalhousie University, Department of Bioethics
ethics.ubc.ca The W. Maurice Young Centre for Applied Ethics, University of British Columbia
fabnet.org International Network of Feminist Approaches to Bioethics
mcgill.ca/biomedicalethicsunit McGill University Biomedical Ethics Unit
ualberta.ca/john-dossetor-health-ethics-centre/index.html Dossetor Health Ethics Centre, University of Alberta
jcb.utoronto.ca University of Toronto Joint Centre for Bioethics

National Resources for Relevant to Legal and Ethical Aspects of Practice

<u>assembly.nl.ca/legislation/sr/statutes/a04-1.htm</u> Advance Health Care Directive Act of Newfoundland and Labrador.

<u>cna-aiic.ca/~/media/cna/page-content/pdf-en/ps85_mental_health_e.pdf?la=en</u> CNA position paper on *Mental Health Services.*

<u>cna-aiic.ca/-/media/cna/page-content/pdf-en/nurses-health-and-human-rights-position-statement_dec-2018.pdf</u> CNA position paper on *Registered Nurses, Health and Human Rights.*

<u>cna-aiic.ca/~/media/cna/page-content/pdf-fr/fs28_privacy_personal_health_info_2011_e.pdf</u> CNA's Fact Sheet on *Privacy of Personal Health Information.*

<u>mindbank.info/collection/country/canada</u> Access links to Canadian resources related to human rights, mental health strategies and polices, disability legislation, and much more. A valuable resource.

<u>pre.ethics.gc.ca</u> The Interagency Panel on Research Ethics website provides access to the *Tri-Council Policy Statement on Ethical Conduct for Research Involving Humans* and links to other research ethics websites.

<u>priv.gc.ca</u> Office of the Privacy Commissioner of Canada.

<u>elearning.rcpsych.ac.uk/learningmodules/exploringspiritualitywithpe.aspx</u> A free e-learning module on spiritual care for those using mental health services by the Royal College of Psychiatrists in Britain. Other e-learning modules related to psychiatric services are also available at this site.

United Nations

<u>equalrightstrust.org/sites/default/files/ertdocs//UN_Resolution_on_protection_of_persons_with_mental_illness.pdf</u> United Nations' *Principles for the Protection of Persons with Mental Illness and for the Improvement of Mental Health Care* 1991 can be found here.

<u>unesco.org/new/en/social-and-human-sciences/themes/bioethics</u> UNESCO's bioethics site, where the UNESCO Declaration of Bioethics and Human Rights can be found, also provides access to the Global Ethics Observatory (GEObs) with worldwide databases in ethics (e.g., environmental ethics).

<u>unesco.org/new/en/communication-and-information/portals-and-platforms/goap/open-science-movement/</u> The Global Open Access Portal for the Open Science Movement aimed at making scientific research and data accessible to all.

<u>who.int/mental_health/mindbank/en</u> The World Health Organization's MiNDbank is a repository of national and international resources related to mental health, addiction, disability, and human rights.

<u>who.int/activities/transforming-services-and-promoting-human-rights-in-mental-health-and-related-areas</u> WHO's QualityRights initiative aims to ensure that mental health care is rights-based and recovery-oriented, such that coercive interventions are not tolerated, autonomy and choice are supported, and the right to informed consent respected.

References

Agren, T. (2014). Human reconsolidation: A reactivation and update. *Brain Research Bulletin, 105,* 70–82. https://doi.org/10.1016/j.brainresbull.2013.12.010

Aly, G., & Roth, K. H. (1984). The legalization of mercy killings in medical and nursing institutions in Nazi Germany from 1938 to 1941. *International Journal of Law and Psychiatry, 7,* 145–163. https://doi.org/10.1016/0160-2527(84)90029-3

Almost, J. (2021). Regulated nursing in Canada: The landscape in 2021. *Canadian Nurses Association.* cna-aiic.ca/-/media/cna/page-content/pdf-en/regulated-nursing-in-canada_e.pdf

Ambrosini, D., Bemme, D., Crocker, A., & Latimer, E. (2012). Narratives of individuals concerning psychiatric advanced directives: Qualitative study. *Journal of Ethics in Mental Health, 6,* 1–9. https://jemh.ca/issues/v6/documents/JEMH_Vol6_SupplementArticle-Narrativesofindividualsconcerningpsychiatricadvancedirectives.pdf

Aristotle. (1996). *Nicomachean ethics.* H. Rackham (Trans.). Wordsworth Classics.

Audi, R. (Ed.). (1995). *The Cambridge dictionary of philosophy.* Cambridge University Press. https://doi.org/10.1017/CBO9781139057509

Austin, W. (2001). Using the human rights paradigm in health ethics: The problems and the possibilities. *Nursing Ethics, 8*(13), 183–195. https://doi.org/10.1177/096973300100800304

Austin, W. (2006). Toward an understanding of trust. In J. Cutcliff & H. McKenna (Eds.), *The essential concepts of nursing* (pp. 317–330). Churchill Livingstone.

Austin, W. (2007a). The terminal: A tale of virtue. *Nursing Ethics, 14*(1), 54–61. https://doi.org/10.1177/0969733007071358

Austin, W. (2007b). The ethics of everyday practice: Healthcare environments as moral communities. *Advances in Nursing Science, 30*(1), 81–88. https://journals.lww.com/advancesinnursingscience/Fulltext/2007/01000/The_Ethics_of_Everyday_Practice__Healthcare.9.aspx

Austin, W. (2008). Ethics in a time of contagion: A relational perspective. *Canadian Journal of Nursing Research, 40*(4), 10–24. https://europepmc.org/article/MED/19186783

Austin, W. (2012). Moral distress and the contemporary plight of health professionals. *HEC Forum, 24*(1), 27–38. https://link.springer.com/article/10.1007/s10730-012-9179-8

Austin, W. (2016). Contemporary healthcare practice and the risk of moral distress. *Healthcare Management Forum, 29*(3), 131–133. https://doi.org/10.1177/0840470416637835

Austin, W. (2017). What is the role of ethics consultation in the moral habitability of health care environments? *AMA Journal of Ethics, 19*(6), 595–600. https://doi.org/10.1001/journalofethics.2017.19.6.pfor1-1706

Austin, W., Bergum, V., & Dossetor, J. (2003a). Relational ethics: An action ethic as foundation for health care. In V. Tschudin (Ed.), *Approaches to ethics: Nursing beyond boundaries* (pp. 45–52). Butterworth-Heinemann.

Austin, W., Bergum, V., & Goldberg, L. (2003b). Unable to answer the call of our patients: Mental health nurses' experiences of moral distress. *Nursing Inquiry, 10*(3), 177–183.

Austin, W., Bergum, V., & Nuttgens, S. (2004). Addressing oppression in psychiatric care: A relational ethics perspective. *Ethical Human Psychology and Psychiatry, 6*(1), 69–78. researchgate.net/publication/8025780_Addressing_oppression_in_psychiatric_care_A_relational_ethics_perspective

Austin, W., Bergum, V., Nuttgens, S., & Peternelj-Taylor, C. (2006). A re-visioning of boundaries in professional helping relationships: Exploring other metaphors. *Ethics & Behaviour, 16*(2), 77–94. https://doi.org/10.1207/s15327019eb1602_1

Austin, W., Kagan, L., Rankel, M., & Bergum, V. (2008). The balancing act: Psychiatrists' experience of moral distress. *Medicine Health Care and Philosophy, 11,* 89–97. https://doi.org/10.1007/s11019-007-9083-1

Austin, W., Rankel, M., Kagan, L., Bergum, V., & Lemermeyer, G. (2005). To stay or to go, to speak or stay silent, to act or not to act: Moral distress as experienced by psychologists. *Ethics & Behavior, 15*(3), 197–212. https://doi.org/10.1207/s15327019eb1503_1

Beauchamp, T. (1994). The "four principles" approach. In R. Gillon (Ed.), *Principles of health care ethics* (pp. 3–12). John Wiley & Sons. https://doi.org/10.1002/9780470510544

Beauchamp, T., & Childress, J. (2019). *Principles of biomedical ethics* (8th ed.). Oxford University Press.

Beauvais, M. J. S., Knoppers, B. M., & Illes, J. (2021). A marathon, not a sprint—neuroimaging, Open Science and ethics. *NeuroImage, 236*, 1–7. https://doi.org/10.1016/j.neuroimage.2021.118041

Benedict, S., & Kuhla, J. (1999). Nurses' participation in the euthanasia programs of Nazi Germany. *Western Journal of Nursing Research, 21*(2), 246–263. https://doi.org/10.1177/01939459922043749\

Bentham, J. (1983). *Deontology together with a table on the springs of action and the article on utilitarianism.* Oxford University Press. https://www.ucl.ac.uk/bentham-project/publications/collected-works-jeremy-bentham/deontology-together-table-springs-action-and-article

Bergum, V., & Dossetor, J. (2020). *Relational ethics: The full meaning of respect* (2nd ed.). https://www.amazon.com/Relational-Ethics-Full-Meaning-Respect/dp/1555720609

Bleyer, B. (2020). Casuistry: On a method of ethical judgement in patient care. *HEC Forum, 32*, 211–226. https://doi.org/10.1007/s10730-020-09396-7

Branicki, L. J. (2020). COVID-19, ethics of care and feminist crisis management. *Gender, Work, & Organization, 27*, 872–883. https://doi.org/10.1111/gwao.12491

British Columbia College of Nurses and Midwives. (2017). *Practice standard: Boundaries in the nurse client relationship.* https://www.bccnm.ca/NP/PracticeStandards/Pages/boundaries.aspx

British Columbia College of Nurses and Midwives. (2020). *Registered Nurses: Practice standards.* https://www.bccnm.ca/RN/PracticeStandards/Pages/Default.aspx

Butler, M., & Phillips, K. (2013, August 15). *In brief: Current issues in mental health in Canada: The federal role in legal and social affairs in mental health.* Publication No, 2013-75-e. Library of the Parliament of Canada. https://lop.parl.ca/staticfiles/PublicWebsite/Home/ResearchPublications/InBriefs/PDF/2013-76-e.pdf

Canadian Nurses Association. (2017). *Code of ethics for registered nurses.* https://cna-aiic.ca/-/media/cna/page-content/pdf-en/code-of-ethics-2017-edition-secure-interactive.pdf?la=en&hash=09C348308C44912AF216656BFA31E33519756387

Carpenter, M. (1991). The process of ethical decision making in psychiatric nursing practice. *Issues in Mental Health Nursing, 12*(2), 179–191. https://doi.org/10.3109/01612849109040513

Cestari, V., Rossi-Arnaud, C., Saraulli, D., & Constanzi, M. (2014). The MAP(K) of fear: From memory consolidation to memory extinction. *Brain Research Bulletin, 105*, 8–16. https://doi.org/10.1016/j.brainresbull.2013.09.007

Chambers, M., Gallagher, A., Borschmann, R., Gillard, S., Turner, K., & Kantaris, X. (2014). The experience of detained mental health service users: Issues of dignity in care. *BMC Medical Ethics, 15*(50), 1–8. https://doi.org/10.1186/1472-6939-15-50

College and Association of Registered Nurses of Alberta. (2020). *Professional boundaries: Guidelines for the nurse–client relationship.* https://www.nurses.ab.ca/docs/default-source/document-library/guidelines/rn_professional-boundaries.pdf?sfvrsn=cc43bb24_2

College of Registered Psychiatric Nurses of Alberta. (2013, September). *Code of ethics and standards of psychiatric nursing practice.* https://www.crpna.ab.ca/CRPNAMember/CRPNA_Member/CRPNA_Code_of_Ethics_and_Standards_of_Practice.aspx

College of Registered Psychiatric Nurses of Manitoba. (2017). *Code of ethics.* https://crpnm.mb.ca/wp-content/uploads/2019/03/CRPNM-Code-of-Ethics-Adopted-May-2017-1.pdf

Collins, A. (1988). *In the sleep room: The story of the CIA brainwashing experiments in Canada.* Lester & Orpen Dennys. https://digitalcommons.osgoode.yorku.ca/cgi/viewcontent.cgi?referer=https://www.google.com/&httpsredir=1&article=1157&context=jlsp

Cutcliffe, J. R., & Travale, R. (2013). Respect in mental health: Reconciling the rhetorical hyperbole with the practical reality. *Nursing Ethics, 20*(3), 273–284. https://doi.org/10.1177/0969733012462055

Darr, R. (2020). Virtues as qualities of character: Alasdair MacIntyre and the situationist critique of virtue ethics. *Journal of Religious Ethics, 48*, 7–25.

Delgado, J., de Groot, J., McCaffrey, G., Dimitropoulos, G., Sitter, K. C., & Austin, W. (2021). Communities of practice: acknowledging vulnerability to improve resilience in healthcare teams. *Journal of Medical Ethics, 47*, 488–493. https://doi.org/10.1136/medethics-2019-10586

DuBois, J. M., Walsh, H. A., Chibnall, J. T., Anderson, E. E., Eggers, M. R., Fowose, M., & Ziobrowski, H. (2019). Sexual violation of patients by physicians: A mixed-methods, exploratory analysis of 101 cases. *Sexual Abuse, 31*, 503–523. https://doi.org/10.1177/1079063217712217

Elliott, C., & Lankin, M. (2016). Restrict the recruitment of involuntarily committed patients for psychiatric research. *JAMA Psychiatry, 73*(4), 317–318. https://doi.org/10.1001/jamapsychiatry.2015.3117

Fisher, A. (1995). The ethical problems encountered in psychiatric nursing practice with dangerous mentally ill persons. *Scholarly Inquiry for Nursing Practice: An International Journal, 9*(2), 193–208. https://pubmed.ncbi.nlm.nih.gov/7667570/

Forchuk, C. (1991). *Ethical problems encountered by mental health nurses. Issues in Mental Health Nursing, 12*, 375–383. https://doi.org/10.3109/01612849109010018

Fowler, M. (1997). Nursing's ethics. In A. Davis, J. Liaschenko, M. Aroskar, & T. Drought (Eds.), *Ethical dilemmas and nursing practice* (pp. 17–34). Appleton & Lange. https://www.pearson.com/us/higher-education/product/Davis-Ethical-Dilemmas-and-Nursing-Practice-4th-Edition/9780838522837.html

Foy, M. (2007). Thoughts on the ethics of compassion. *Journal of Ethics in Mental Health, 2*(1), 1–2. https://jemh.ca/issues/v2n1/documents/JEMH_V2N1_InMyLife_Thoughts_on_Ethics_of_Compassion.pdf

Gadow, S. (1999). Relational narrative: The postmodern turn in nursing ethics. *Scholarly Inquiry for Nursing Practice: An International Journal, 13*, 59–67.

Gallup Poll. (2021, January). *Honesty/ethics in professions.* Accessed July 25, 2021. https://news.gallup.com/poll/1654/honesty-ethics-professions.aspx

GBD 2019 Diseases and Injuries Collaborators. (2020, October 17). Global burden of 369 diseases and injuries in 204 countries and territories, 1990–2019: A systematic analysis for the Global Burden of Disease Study 2019. *The Lancet, 396*, 1204–1222.

Gilligan, C. (1982). *In a different voice: Psychological theory and women's development.* Harvard University Press. researchgate.net/publication/275714106_In_A_Different_Voice_Psychological_Theory_and_Women's_Development

Ginory, A., Sabatier, L. M., & Eth, S. (2012). Addressing therapeutic boundaries in social networking. *Psychiatry, 75*(1), 40–48. https://doi.org/10.1521/psyc.2012.75.1.40

Gostin, L. (2001). Beyond moral claims: A human rights approach in mental health. *Cambridge Quarterly of Healthcare Ethics, 10*, 264–274. https://doi.org/10.1017/S0963180101003061

Government of Canada. (2016). *Chapter 3, An Act to amend the criminal code and to make related amendments to other Acts (medical assistance in dying),* S. C. 2016, c. 3. Statutes of Canada, Parliament of Canada. http://laws-lois.justice.gc.ca/PDF/2016_3.pdf

Government of Canada. (2018). *Tri-council policy statement: Ethical conduct for research involving humans, TCPS 2 (2018).* Research Panel. https://ethics.gc.ca/eng/policy-politique_tcps2-eptc2_2018.html

Government of Canada. (2020c). *Personal Information Protection and Electronic Documents Act.* [S.C. 2000, c. 5; Act current to 2020-12-02, last amended 2019-06-21]. Justice Laws website. http://laws-lois.justice.gc.ca/eng/acts/p-8.6/

Government of Canada. (2020d). *Privacy Act,* R.S.C. 1985, c. P-21. https://laws-lois.justice.gc.ca/PDF/P-21.pdf

Government of New Brunswick. (2017, February 14). *News release: Revised. Community support orders introduced to help those suffering from mental illness.* https://www2.gnb.ca/content/gnb/en/news/news_release.2017.02.0203.html

Government of Saskatchewan. (2015). *Guide to the Mental Health Services Act of Saskatchewan.* https://www.ehealthsask.ca/services/resources/Resources/GuidetoTheMentalHealthServicesAct-Nov-2015.pdf

Government of Saskatchewan. (2018). *Mental Health Services Act of Saskatchewan.* M-13.1. Publications Centre. http://www.publications.gov.sk.ca/details.cfm?p=626

Gray, J. E., Hastings, T. J., Love, S., & O'Reilly, R. L. (2016). Clinically significant differences among Canadian Mental Health Acts: 2016. *Canadian Journal of Psychiatry, 61*(4), 222–226. https://doi.org/10.1177/0706743716632524

Griffith, R. (2016). When accepting a gift can be professional misconduct and theft. *British Journal of Community Nursing, 21*(7), 365–367. https://doi.org/10.12968/bjcn.2016.21.7.365

Gustafsson, L-K., Wigerblad, Å., & Lindwall, L. (2014). Undignified care: Violation of patient dignity in involuntary psychiatric hospital care from a nurse's perspective. *Nursing Ethics, 21*(2), 176–186. https://doi.org/10.1177/0969733013490592

Hicks, G. (2020, October 6). *P. A. nurse wins appeal regarding health care social media.* SaskNOW. [Freedom of Speech]. https://sasknow.com/2020/10/06/p-a-nurse-wins-appeal-regarding-health-care-social-media-comments/

Ipperciel, D. (2003). Dialogue and discussion in a moral context. *Nursing Philosophy, 4*, 211–224. https://doi.org/10.1046/j.1466-769X.2003.00141.x

Jameton, A. (1984). *Nursing practice: The ethical issues.* Prentice Hall. https://www.jstor.org/stable/27799853?seq=1#metadata_info_tab_contents

Jameton, A. (2013). A reflection on moral distress in nursing together with a current application of the concept. *Bioethical Inquiry, 10*, 297–308. https://link.springer.com/article/10.1007/s11673-013-9466-3

Jameton, A. (2017). What moral distress in nursing history could suggest about the future of health care. *AMA Journal of Ethics, 19*(6), 617–628. https://journalofethics.ama-assn.org/article/what-moral-distress-nursing-history-could-suggest-about-future-health-care/2017-06

Jansen, T-L., Hem, M. H., Dambolt, L. J., & Hanssen, I. (2020). Moral distress in acute psychiatric nursing: Multifaceted dilemmas and demands. *Nursing Ethics, 27,* 1315–1326. https://doi.org/10.1177/0969733019877526

Jones-Bonofiglio, K. (2020). *Health care ethics through the lens of moral distress.* Springer.

Jonsen, A. (1991). Casuistry as methodology in clinical ethics. *Theoretical Medicine, 12,* 295–307. https//doi.org/10.1007/BF00489890

Jonsen, A., & Toulmin, S. (1988). *The abuse of casuistry: A history of moral reasoning.* University of California Press. www.thefreelibrary.com/The+Abuse+of+Casuistry%3A+a+History+of+Moral+Reasoning.-a09331013

Kahn, S. (2019). The problem of the Kantian line. *International Philosophical Quarterly, 59,* 193–217. https://doi.org/10.5840/ipq2019311128

Kant, I. (1996). *Practical philosophy.* M. Gregor (Trans.). Cambridge University Press. https://b-ok.global/book/1104106/dd1366

Koduah, A. O., Leung, A. M., Leung, D. Y. L., & Liu, J. Y. W. (2019). "I sometimes ask patients to consider spiritual care": Health literacy and culture in mental health nursing practice. *International Journal of Environmental Research and Public Health, 16,* 1–13. https://doi.org/10.3390/ijerph16193589

Krautscheid, L., Mood, L., McLennon, S. M., Mossman, T. C., Wagner, M., & Wode, J. (2020). Examining relationships between resilience protective factors and moral distress among nursing students. *Nursing Education Perspectives, 41,* 43–45. digitalcommons.georgefox.edu/cgi/viewcontent.cgi?article=1026&context=sn_fac

Kunyk, D., & Austin, W. (2012). Nursing under the influence: A relational ethics perspective. *Nursing Ethics, 19*(3), 380–389. https://doi.org/10.1177/0969733011406767

Levine, M. (1977). Nursing ethics and the ethical nurse. *American Journal of Nursing, 77*(5), 845–849. https://doi.org/10.2307/3461709

Liaschenko, J. (1994). Making a bridge: The moral work with patients we do not like. *Journal of Palliative Care, 10*(3), 83–89. https://doi.org/10.1177/082585979401000318

MacIntyre, A. (1984). *After virtue* (2nd ed.). University of Notre Dame. https://www3.nd.edu/~undpress/excerpts/P01162-ex.pdf

Mann, J., Gostin, L., Gruskin, S., Brennan, T., Lazzarini, Z., & Fineberg, H. (1999). Health and human rights. In J. Mann, S. Gruskin, M. Grodin, & G. Annas (Eds.), *Health and human rights: A reader* (pp. 7–20). Routledge. https://www.routledge.com/Health-and-Human-Rights-in-a-Changing-World/Grodin-Tarantola-Annas-Gruskin/p/book/9780415503990

McFarland-Icke, B. R. (1999). *Nurses in Nazi Germany: Moral choice in history.* Princeton University Press. https://www.thelancet.com/pdfs/journals/lancet/PIIS0140-6736(05)73327-4.pdf

Mental Health Commission of Canada. (2009). *Toward recovery & well-being: A framework of a mental health strategy for Canada.* https://www.mentalhealthcommission.ca/sites/default/files/FNIM_Toward_Recovery_and_Well_Being_ENG_0_1.pdf

Mill, J. S. (2002). *The basic writings of John Stuart Mill: On liberty, the subjection of women and utilitarianism.* Modern Library. https://read.amazon.com/kp/embed?asin=B004A8ZWIS&tag=bing08-20&linkCode=kpp&resharelId=0CHKGPK33QVY7B9RJGEX&reshareChannel=system

Molewijk, B., Kok, A., Husum, T., Pedersen, R., & Aasland, O. (2017). Staff's normative attitudes towards coercion: The role of moral doubt and professional context—A cross-sectional survey study. *BMC Medical Ethics, 18*(37), 1–14. https://doi.org/10.1186/s12910-017-0190-0-0

Musto, L., Schreiber, R., & Rodney, P. (2021). Risking vulnerability: Enacting moral agency in the is/ought gap in mental health care. *Journal of Advanced Nursing, 77,* 2458–2471. https://doi.org/10.1111/jan.14776

Nathaniel, A. (2006). Moral reckoning in nursing. *Western Journal of Nursing Research, 28*(4), 419–438. https://doi.org/10.1177/0193945905284727

Neathery, M., Taylor, E. J., & He, Z. (2020). Perceived barriers to providing spiritual care among psychiatric mental health nurses. *Archives of Psychiatric Nursing, 34,* 572–579. https://doi.org/10.1016/j.apnu.2020.10.004

Niebuhr, H. R. (1963/1999). *The responsible self: An essay in Christian moral philosophy.* Harper & Row. https://coorleeufourgetan.files.wordpress.com/2016/11/mew.pdf

Noddings, N. (1984). *Caring: A feminine approach to ethics and moral education.* University of California Press. file:///C:/Users/aek587/Downloads/Noddings%20Caring%20(1).pdf

Norvoll, R., Hem, M. H., & Pedersen, R. (2017). The role of ethics in reducing and improving the quality of coercion in mental health care. *HEC Forum, 29*(1), 59–74. https://doi.org/10.1007/s10730-016-9312-1

Nugent, A. C., Miller, F. G., Henter, I. D., & Zarate, C. A. Jr. (2017). The ethics of clinical trials research in severe mood disorders. *Bioethics, 31*(6), 443–453. https://doi.org/10.1111/bioe.12349

Office of the Privacy Commissioner of Canada. (2015). *Setting the priorities for the Office of the Privacy Commissioner: A conversation with stakeholders/ summaries of privacy issues for discussion/the body as information.* https://priv.gc.ca/en/about-the-opc/opc-strategic-privacy-priorities/pp_bg/

Olsen, D. (2017). Increasing the use of psychiatric advance directives. *Nursing Ethics, 24*(3), 265–267. https://doi.org/10.1177/0969733017708881

Olsman, E., Willems, D., & Leget, C. (2016). Solicitude: Balancing compassion and empowerment in a relational ethics of hope—An empirical-ethical study in palliative care. *Medicine Health Care and Philosophy, 19*(1), 11–20. https://doi.org/10.1007/s11019-015-9642-9

Pauly, B. M., Varcoe, C., & Storch, J. (2012). Framing the issues: Moral distress in health care. *HEC Forum, 24*(1), 1–11. https://doi.org/10.1007/s10730-012-9176-y

Perna, G., & Nemcroff, C. B. (2017). Personalized medicine in psychiatry: Back to the future. *Personalized Medicine in Psychiatry, 1–2,* 1. https://doi.:org/10.1016/j.pmip.2017.01.001

Racine, E., & Affleck, W. (2016). Changing memories: Between ethics and speculation. *AMA Journal of Ethics, 18*(12), 1241–1248. https://journalofethics.ama-assn.org/article/changing-memories-between-ethics-and-speculation/2016-12

Radden, J., & Sadler, J. (2008). Character virtues in psychiatric practice. *Harvard Review of Psychiatry, 16*(6), 373–380. https://doi.org/10.1080/10673220802564194

Ramluggun, P., Idowu, C., Sandy, P., & Wright, S. (2021, May). Supporting mental health nurses to meet patients' spiritual needs. *Mental Health Practice.* https://doi.org/10.7748/mhp.2021.e1549

Raphel, S., Black, K., Peterson, B., Galehouse, P., Handrup, C. & Yearwood, E. L. (2021). Social justice & social responsibility an official statement from The International Society of Psychiatric-Mental Health Nurses. *Archives of Psychiatric Nursing, 35,* 111–112. https://doi.org/10.1016/j.apnu.2020.10.015

Registered Psychiatric Nurses Association of Saskatchewan. (2020). *Code of ethics.* https://www.rpnas.com/members/code-of-ethics/

Registered Psychiatric Nurses of Canada (RPNC). (2010). *Code of ethics & standards of psychiatric nursing practice.* https://unalocal183.com/wp-content/uploads/2018/06/CRPNA.pdf

Ricouer, P. (1992). *Oneself as another.* K. Blamey (Trans.). University of Chicago Press. (Original work published 1990). https://www.goodreads.com/book/show/125875.Oneself_as_Another

Rittenmeyer, L., & Huffman, D. (2009). How professional nurses working in hospital environments experience moral distress: A systematic review. *JBI Library of Systematic Reviews, 7*(28), 1233–1290. https://doi.org/10.11124/jbisrir-2009-209

Robertson, M., Morris, K., & Walter, G. (2007). Overview of psychiatric ethics V: Utilitarianism and the ethics of duty. *Australasian Psychiatry, 15*(5), 402–410. https://doi.org/10.1080/10398560701439640

Robillard, J. M., & Illes, J. (2016). Manipulating memories: The ethics of yesterday's science fiction and today's reality. *AMA Journal of Ethics, 18*(12), 1225–1231. https://doi.org/10.1001/journalofethics.2016.18.12.msoc1-1612

Rosenberg, N. (2021). A cognitive science approach to bioethics [Perspective]. *European Journal of Emergency Medicine, 28,* 90–91. https://doi.org/10.1097/MEJ.0000000000000797

Rudner, N. (2021). Nursing is a health equity and social justice movement. *Public Health Nursing, 38,* 87–691. https://doi.org/10.1111/phn.12905

Ryberg, J. (2017). Neuroethics and brain privacy: Setting the stage. *Res Publica, 23,* 153–158. https://doi.org/10.1007/s11158-016-9340-3

Rynor, B. (2010). Value of community treatment orders remains at issue. *Canadian Medical Association Journal, 182*(8), E337–E338. https://doi.org/10.1503/cmaj.109-3237

Sager, G. (2020). Components of successful spiritual care. *Journal of Religion and Health.* https://doi.org/10.1007/s10943-020-01089-2

Saul, J. R. (2001). *On equilibrium.* Penguin/Viking. https://www.penguinrandomhouse.ca/books/375931/on-equilibrium-by-john-ralston-saul/9780140288032

Savulescu, J., Wilkinson, I., & Perrson, D. (2020). Utilitarianism and the pandemic. *Bioethics, 34,* 620–632. https://doi.org/10.1111/bioe.12771

Schick Makaroff, K., Storch, J., Pauly, B., & Newton, L. (2014). Searching for ethical leadership in nursing. *Nursing Ethics, 21*(6), 642–658. https://doi.org10.1177/0969733013513213

Sherwin, S. (1992). *No longer patient: Feminist ethics and health care.* Temple University Press. https://www.researchgate.net/publication/235800732_No_Longer_Patient_-_Feminist_Ethics_and_Health_Care_Book_Review

Skorpen, F., Rehnsfeldt, A., & Thorsen, A. A. (2015). The significance of small things for dignity in psychiatric care. *Nursing Ethics, 22*(7), 754–764. https://doi.org/10.1177/0969733014551376

Smith, G. C., & Knudson, T. K. (2016). Student nurses' unethical behavior, social media, and year of birth. *Nursing Ethics, 23*(8), 910–918. https://doi.org/10.1177/0969733015590009

Snow, N. (2015). *Exploring community treatment orders: An institutional ethnographic study.* Unpublished doctoral dissertation, University of Alberta, Edmonton, AB. https://era.library.ualberta.ca/items/471b5287-2dcf-45db-8e64-b36ccd11f584/view/4f41e3d3-17af-43c9-8c3b-38546b58900d/Snow_Nicole_201509_PhD.pdf

Somerville, M. (2000). *The ethical canary: Science, society and the human spirit.* Penguin Books. https://bookreviews.bbcf.ca/2012/10/somerville-margaret-the-ethical-canary-science-society-and-the-human-spirit-penguin-books-toronto-on/

Strong, C. (2000). Specified principlism: What is it, and does it really resolve cases better than casuistry? *Journal of Medicine and Philosophy, 25*(3), 323–341. https://doi.org/10.1076/0360-5310(200006)25:3;1-H;FT323

Tisdale, D., & Symenuk, P. M. (2020). Human rights and nursing codes of ethics in Canada 1953–2017. *Nursing Ethics, 27*(4), 1077–1088. https://doi.org/10.1177/0969733020906606

Trotter, G. (2020). The authority of the common morality. *Journal of Medicine and Philosophy, 45*, 427–440. https://doi.org/10.1093/jmp/jhaa015

United Nations. (1991). *Principles for the protection of persons with mental illness and the improvement of mental health care.* Adopted by General Assembly resolution 46/119 of 17 December 1991, Office of the United Nations High Commissioner for Human Rights. https://www.who.int/mental_health/policy/en/UN_Resolution_on_protection_of_persons_with_mental_illness.pdf

United Nations Educational, Scientific and Cultural Organization. (2019). *Universal declaration on bioethics and human rights, 2005.* Adopted by UNESCO. https://en.unesco.org/themes/ethics-science-and-technology/bioethics-and-human-rights#:~:text=UNESCO%20has%20contributed%20to%20the,in%201998%2C%20and%20the%20International

United Nations Human Rights Council. (2017, June 6–23). *Thirty-fifth session, Agenda item 3: Report of the Special Rapporteur on the right of everyone to the enjoyment of the highest attainable standard of physical and mental health.* https://www.ohchr.org/en/issues/health/pages/srrighthealthindex.aspx

Walker, R. (2020). The unfinished business of respect for autonomy: Persons, relationships, and nonhuman animals. *Journal of Medicine and Philosophy, 45*, 521–539. https://doi.org/10.1093/jmp/jhaa016

Wilkinson, J. M. (1987–1988). Moral distress in nursing practice: Experience and effect. *Nursing Forum, 23*(1), 16–29. https://doi.org/10.1111/j.1744-6198.1987.tb00794.x

Theoretic Basis of Practice

Wendy Austin

LEARNING OBJECTIVES

After studying this chapter, you will be able to:

- Explain the need for theory-based psychiatric and mental health (PMH) nursing practice.
- Compare the key elements of theories that provide a basis for such practice.
- Describe the common nursing theories used in PMH nursing.
- Identify theories that contribute to understanding human beings and their mental health.

KEY TERMS

- anima • animus • archetype • behaviourism
- change • classical conditioning • cognition • collective unconscious • conscious • countertransference
- disinhibition • ego • elicitation • empathy • extrovert
- id • interpersonal relations • introvert • modeling
- need • object relations • operant behaviour
- preconscious • persona • reclamation • role • self-actualization • self-efficacy • self-system • shadow
- superego • transaction • transference • unconditional positive regard • unconscious

KEY CONCEPTS

- recovery • theory

This chapter presents an overview of some of the nursing and other theories that serve as the knowledge base for psychiatric and mental health (PMH) nursing practice. Many of the theories underlying this practice are evolving, and only some have research support to date. As acknowledged in the *Canadian Standards of Psychiatric-Mental Health Nursing* (2014), PMH nurses use knowledge from nursing, the health sciences, and related mental health disciplines in their practice. The chapter begins, then, with selected nursing theories and moves to some of the many theories that underlie our understanding of the biologic, psychological, social, and spiritual aspects of human knowledge and experience.

Nursing Theories

Nursing theories are essential in conceptualizing nursing practice. Some theories described here are commonly referred to as models, not as theories, and we have followed common practice. We are not, however, differentiating between a model and a theory, as this remains an area of some debate within nursing.

A nurse may choose to base their practice consistently on one nursing theory or may choose to use a specific theory depending on the care situation. For example, in nursing a person with schizophrenia who has problems related to maintaining self-care, Dorothea Orem's deficit theory (1991) may be particularly useful. Peplau's model (1952) may be more helpful in addressing relationship issues. The theory or theories used by a nurse reveal the way that this nurse conceives their practice.

KEY CONCEPT

A theory "is an imaginative grouping of knowledge, ideas, and experience that are represented symbolically and seek to illuminate a given phenomenon" (Watson, 1988, p. 1).

Theories as Maps

The study of theories in the health sciences can be experienced as an oppressive task by students unless the meaningful link between theory and practice is made evident (Georges, 2005). If it is recognized that theories are maps that orientate us to our care environments and guide our practice, then their relevance becomes apparent. Like a map, a theory is an attempt to represent the real world and is only as useful as its correspondence to the terrain to be travelled. Just as maps need to be redrawn when the landscape changes, theories need to change with our knowledge of the human condition and the world.

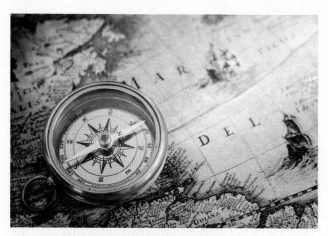

Figure 9.1 Theories help nurses navigate the unique province of each patient's needs. (Shutterstock.com/Triff.)

The Visionary: Nightingale

Florence Nightingale, the founder of modern nursing, is recognized as the first nurse researcher and the pioneer of theory development in nursing. The patterns of knowing of contemporary nursing are to be found in her work begun in the 1800s (Clements & Averill, 2006). The respect for her legacy is apparent: International Nurses Day is celebrated on her birthday, May 12, and Canada's National Nursing Week occurs that same week. Nightingale's model emerged from her clinical work in hospitals and in the Crimean War, where unhealthy physical environments for the sick prevailed (Nightingale, 1859). This is the reason that the primary focus of her model, although not neglecting psychosocial and spiritual needs, is on improving environmental conditions. Nightingale's intent was to create healthy surroundings that help alleviate suffering and promote wellbeing. Health, for her, included the ability to use "every power we have." For example, she considered that giving false reassurance to sick people was an unacceptable behaviour. For Nightingale, the curative process was accomplished by nature alone: medicine and nursing do not cure. Nursing activities, therefore, were to put patients in the best state for nature to act upon them.

Interpersonal Relations Models

Interpersonal Relations: Hildegard Peplau

Hildegard Peplau introduced the first systematic framework for PMH nursing in her book *Interpersonal Relations in Nursing* (1952). A major contribution was her conceptualization of the nurse–patient relationship and its phases (see Chapter 7). Although her work continues to stimulate debate, she led PMH nursing out of the confinement of custodial care into a unique model for practice.

Peplau (1992) believed in the importance of **interpersonal relations**, which included interactions between person and family, parent and child, or patient and nurse. She emphasized empathic linkage, the ability to feel in oneself the feelings experienced by another person or people. The interpersonal transmission of anxiety or panic is the most common empathic linkage, but other feelings, such as anger, disgust, and envy, can also be communicated nonverbally to others. Peplau believed that if nurses pay attention to what they feel during a relationship with a patient, then they can gain invaluable observations of feelings a patient is experiencing, even those the patient has not yet recognized. Peplau's theory has been identified as a useful framework for educating nursing students on communicating holistically with older adults (Deane, 2015).

The **self-system** is an important concept in Peplau's model. Peplau defined the self as an "antianxiety system" and a product of socialization. The self proceeds through personal development that is always open to revision but tends toward stability. For example, in parent–child relationships, patterns of approval, disapproval, and indifference are used by children to define themselves. If the verbal and nonverbal messages have been derogatory, then children incorporate these messages and also view themselves negatively. The concept of **need** is also important to Peplau's model. Needs are primarily of biologic origin but are met within a sociocultural environment. When a biologic need is present, it gives rise to tension that is reduced and relieved by behaviours meeting that need. According to Peplau, nurses should strive to recognize patients' patterns and style of meeting their needs in relation to their health status and help them to identify available resources, such as food and interpersonal support.

Anxiety is an important concept for Peplau, who contended that unless anxiety is understood, professional practice is unsafe. There are various levels of anxiety (mild, moderate, severe, and panic levels), each having observable behavioural cues. These cues Peplau considered "relief behaviours." For example, some people may relieve their anxiety by yelling and swearing, whereas others seek relief by withdrawing. In both instances, anxiety, according to Peplau, is generated by an unmet self-system security need.

The Dynamic Nurse–Patient Relationship: Ida Jean Orlando

In 1954, Ida Jean Orlando studied the factors that enhanced or impeded the integration of mental health principles in the basic nursing curriculum. From this study, she published *The Dynamic Nurse–Patient Relationship* (1961). A nursing situation for Orlando (1961, 1972) involves the patient's behaviour, the nurse's reaction, and anything that does not relieve the distress of the patient, which Orlando understands as related to the individual's inability to meet or communicate their own needs. She focuses on the whole patient, rather than on disease or institutional demands. Her ideas continue

Hildegard Peplau (1909–1999)

PSYCHIATRIC NURSE OF THE CENTURY

Peplau became a nurse in 1931 in Pennsylvania. During World War II, she joined the Army Nurse Corps and worked in a neuropsychiatric clinic in London. She obtained a Master's Degree (1947) and a PhD (1953) from Columbia University. Peplau took the lead in the development of psychiatric nursing as a specialty at the Master's level and developed the Theory of Psychodynamic Nursing. Peplau has numerous publications, with her most influential works being *Interpersonal Relations in Nursing* (1952), *Aspects of Psychiatric Nursing* (1957), and *Principles of Patient Counselling* (1964).

Peplau's ideas regarding the centrality of relationship to nursing practice and the efficacy of the use of self as a nursing tool have had far-reaching effects. She envisioned nursing as a discipline independent from medicine and worked to ensure that this was so. She deeply influenced nursing's professional and scientific development by drawing on interdisciplinary knowledge from psychology, education, and pragmatic educational philosophy. Her achievements occurred during a time when strong leadership from women was frowned upon, and she faced many conflicts and controversies throughout a 50-year career that included being President of the American Nurses Association and consultant to the World Health Organization in psychiatric nursing. She was named one of 50 Great Americans by Marquis' *Who's Who*. Hildegard Peplau was an honorary member of the Canadian Federation of Mental Health Nurses.

Reference: Calaway, B. J. (2002). *Hildegard Peplau: Psychiatric nurse of the century*. Springer.

to be useful today with research supporting her model (Olson & Hanchett, 1997). Orlando's model has been used, for example, as a framework for guiding nurses in addressing patient risk for falls, which can be higher on psychiatric units than on acute medical care areas due to patient experiences with cognitive disturbances and the side effects of some psychotropic medication (Abraham, 2011).

Existential and Humanistic Theoretic Perspectives

Seeking Life Meaning: Joyce Travelbee

Influenced by Peplau and Orlando, Joyce Travelbee provided an existential perspective on nursing based on the works of Viktor Frankl, an existential philosopher (see Spiritual Theories section in this chapter). Existentialists believe that humans seek meaning in their life and experiences. Travelbee believed that the nurse's spiritual values and philosophical beliefs about suffering would determine the extent to which the nurse could help ill people find meaning in their situation. She understood "suffering" as a feeling of displeasure ranging from simple and transitory mental, physical, or spiritual discomfort to extreme anguish and beyond to the malignant phase of despair (Travelbee, 1971). Travelbee expanded the area of concern of mental illness to include long-term physical illnesses. Overall, her use of the interpersonal process as a nursing intervention (Travelbee, 1969) and her focus on suffering and illness helped to define areas of concern for nursing.

Humanbecoming: Rosemarie Rizzo Parse

Quality of life as perceived by a person and their family is the focus of the nurse within the humanbecoming model. When Parse (2007) was asked what the practice of nurses using this model would be like in 2050, she imagined that their repertoire would remain focused on enhancing quality of life and attending to human freedom and dignity. While the quality of life will be different in 2050, it will still be unique to the individual. The individual (not to be understood as reducible to qualities or traits) is perceived as open and free to ascribe meaning to life (through values and beliefs developed) and to bear responsibility for choices (Parse, 1987). Reality for an individual is cocreated with the environment. It is in the rhythm of moving closer and away from others where creativity and change (becoming different) occur (Leddy & Pepper, 1998). Three principles structure Parse's model:

- meaning: "Structuring meaning is the imaging and valuing of language";
- rhythmicity: "Configuring rhythmical patterns of relation is the revealing–concealing and enabling–limiting of connecting–separating"; and
- transcendence: "Cotranscending with possible is the powering and originating of transforming" (Parse, 2007, p. 309).

Permeating these three principles are the postulates of *illimitability* (indivisible, unbounded knowing extending to infinity), *paradox* (rhythm expressed as pattern preference), *freedom* (contextually construed liberation), and *mystery* (the unexplainable). The language of humanbecoming can be challenging, but the vision of personhood that it offers can richly inform nursing practice. For instance, it can be applied when caring for a family experiencing a stillbirth or loss of a newborn. It helps guide the nurse to support the family's understanding of paradoxical feelings (such as simultaneous guilt and powerlessness) rather than attempting to make them "feel better" (Wilson, 2016) or to an exploration of the human experience of hope (Doe, 2021).

Primacy of Caring: Patricia Benner

Patricia Benner has developed a particular notion of nursing as a caring relationship. As a caring profession, nursing "is guided by the moral art and ethics of care and responsibility" (Benner & Wrubel, 1989, p. xi), and nursing practice is based upon "the lived experience of health and illness" (p. 8). Based upon Heidegger's phenomenologic philosophy, Benner describes the person as "a self-interpreting being ... (who) gets defined in the course of a life ... (and) has an effortless and nonreflective understanding of the self in the world" (p. 41). Wellbeing (the human experience of health or wholeness) is, as is being ill, a distinct way of being in the world. With a phenomenologic view, Benner believes the environment situates meaning. People enter situations with their own sets of meanings, habits, and perspectives, and their personal interpretations affect the way they respond in those situations. Benner and Wrubel's identification of the domains of nursing practice, as described in *The Primacy of Caring*, was used to frame the original Canadian standards of PMH nursing practice (Austin et al., 1996).

Benner's model, with its vision of the evolution of a nurse's practice as knowledge and experience is gained and integrated, has proven effective in increasing the retention of nurses (Davis & Maisano, 2016) and as a framework for leadership development and mentoring programs (Titzer et al., 2014).

Caring: Jean Watson

The science of caring was initiated by Jean Watson (1979) based on the belief that caring is the foundation of nursing. Watson (2005) recommends that specific theories of caring be developed in relation to specific human conditions and health and illness experiences. The science of caring is based on 7 assumptions and 10 "carative" factors (Barnhart et al., 1994). One of the assumptions is that "effective caring promotes health and individual or family growth" (p. 153); another of the carative factors is that "a trusting relationship ... involves congruence, empathy, nonpossessive warmth, and effective communication" (p. 152). The model has evolved to address more specifically the spiritual dimension of the nurse's role, including helping the patient to grow spiritually (Watson, 1988). For Watson, spiritual wellbeing is the foundation of human health, and she suggests that a troubled soul can lead to illness and disease.

Watson's view is applicable to the care of those who seek help for mental illness. This model emphasizes the importance of sensitivity to self and others; the development of helping and trusting relations; the promotion of interpersonal teaching and learning; and provision for a supportive, protective, and corrective mental, physical, sociocultural, and spiritual environment. The application of Watson's caring model to the environmental transformation of a unit with a history of disengaged, dissatisfied nurses and poor clinical practice indicators was significantly successful in measurable ways, such as health system employee engagement scores (from 35th to 85th percentile) and specialty certification (from 6% to 64% of staff) (Summerell, 2015).

The Tidal Model of Mental Health Recovery and Reclamation: Philip Barker

Philip Barker's Tidal Model (Barker & Buchanan-Barker, 2005) incorporates Barker and colleagues' Model for Empowering Interactions. It emphasizes the centrality of the lived experience of the person in care and is based on the assumption that people are their life stories and that they generate meaning through such stories (Barker, 2001a). It is focused on helping people to recover their lives after an arrest in development, a breakdown, or a disruption in the flow of life. This **reclamation** of one's own life story is necessary to recovery. The nurse's role is envisioned as helping the persons seeking care to discover, identify, and address the problems or challenges affecting them at this point in life. Nurses are to foster the creation of a safe haven in which the persons can recuperate and recover. Recovery is clarified by each person in a particular way but is defined in this model generally as "getting going again" (Barker & Buchanan-Barker, 2010, p. 171).

Change (i.e., becoming different) is a core element in this model (hence the metaphor of the tide), and the nurse's role will be shaped by the changing needs of patients across the continuum of care (e.g., critical, transitional, or developmental care) and the provision of interdependent services (Barker, 2001b). Box 9.1 outlines the Tidal Model's "10 commitments" of care.

The Tidal Model considers the domains of self, world, and others. They are metaphorical settings for the unfolding of the person's story. The process of exploring the person's experience may begin within any of the domains (Barker & Buchanan-Barker, 2010). Tidal processes, used with much flexibility, assist in exploring the person's experience within each domain. A personal security plan is considered in the self-domain to help the person to feel as safe as possible. A holistic assessment is an aspect of the world domain as a means of more deeply exploring the person's lifework and

---

BOX 9.1 **Ten Commitments of the Tidal Model**

1. *Value the voice*: The person's own account of their story is the beginning and end point of the helping encounter. Records of care should represent the patient's own voice.
2. *Respect the language*: People develop their own unique way of telling their story. It is not necessary to "rewrite" the story in the language of psychiatry and psychiatric nursing.
3. *Develop genuine curiosity*: Those who seek to be of assistance to the person need to develop ways of expressing genuine interest in the story so that they might better understand the storyteller.
4. *Become the apprentice*: One is the authority on one's own life story. Professionals learn from the person what needs to be done, rather than leading.
5. *Use the available toolkit*: The person's story contains examples of "what has worked" or "what might work" for this person. These are the main tools to use in helping the person's recovery.
6. *Craft the step beyond*: The professional helper and the person work together to construct an appreciation of what needs to be done *now*.

The first step is the crucial step, revealing the power of change and pointing toward the ultimate goal of recovery.

7. *Give the gift of time*: There is no value in asking "How much time do we have?" The question is "How do we use this time?"
8. *Reveal personal wisdom*: One of the key tasks for the helper is to assist in revealing the person's life wisdom that will sustain and guide their recovery.
9. *Know that change is constant*: The professional helper needs to become aware of how change is happening and discover the way that knowledge may steer the person out of danger and distress and help remain on the journey to recovery.
10. *Be transparent*: Both the person and the professional embody the opportunity to become a team. The professional can support this by being transparent at all times, helping the person understand *what* is being done and *why*.

Source: Buchanan-Barker, P., & Barker, P. (2008). The Tidal Commitments: Extending the value base of mental health recovery. *Journal of Psychiatric and Mental Health Nursing, 15*, 93–100.

---

problems in living. Group work in various forms is part of the process in the others domain in order to encourage individuals to share aspects of themselves as persons rather than patients (Barker & Buchanan-Barker, 2010). Box 9.2, Research for Best Practice presents an analysis of the Tidal Model.

The first Canadian application of this model was at the Royal Ottawa Mental Health Centre. In their evaluation of its implementation, they found that stories were captured in the holistic assessments of patients and that risk incidents (e.g., restraint use) decreased (Brookes et al., 2008).

Systems Models

Health Promotion: The McGill Model of Nursing

This model was developed under the guidance of Dr. Moyra Allen by the students and faculty of McGill University School of Nursing. It distinguishes nursing from other health disciplines but also identifies their complementary relationships (Allen, 1977). The model's four major concepts are health, family (person), collaboration, and learning (Gottlieb & Rowat, 1987). Health is considered the focus of the practice of nursing and is seen as coexisting with illness. Coping and development are health processes that facilitate functioning and

satisfaction with life; family (person) is viewed as the unit of concern. The person is perceived through their web of significant relationships. Family and person are considered open systems in constant interaction with their environment. The environment is viewed "as the context within which health and healthy ways of living are learned" (p. 56). Collaboration and learning are essentials for the nurse to structure a learning environment to meet "the needs, goals, and problem-solving styles of the family (person) … based upon the family (person's) strengths and resources" (p. 51). This strength-based component (rather than a deficit focus) of the McGill model makes it particularly useful in assessment, planning, and intervention with families (Feeley & Gottlieb, 2000).

Goal Attainment: Imogene M. King

The theory of goal attainment developed by Imogene M. King is based on a model that includes three interacting systems: personal, interpersonal, and social (King, 1971). King believed that human beings interact with the environment and that the individual's perceptions influence reactions and interactions. For King, nursing involves caring for the human being, with the goal of health defined as adjusting to the stressors in both internal and external environments. She defines nursing as a "process of human interactions between nurse

BOX 9.2 Research for Best Practice

ANALYZING THE TIDAL MODEL AND APPLYING IT TO CARE OF THE OLDER ADULT AT RISK FOR SUICIDE

Sagna, A. O., & Walker, L. O. (2020). Analysis of the tidal model and its implications in late-life suicidality. *Nursing Science Quarterly, 33,* 315–321. https://doi.org/10.1177/0894318420943139/10

Research Question: What is the scope, context, and content of the Tidal Model theory, as well as itsapplication in the care of older adults at risk for suicide?

Method: The Fawcett and DeSanto-Madeya framework for theory analysis was used to objectively examine and describe this middle-range theoretical model. Three categories are examined: theory scope (unique focus), theory context (its evolution); motivation of author(s), and theory content (concepts, metaparadigm, propositions, and competencies.)

Findings: *Theory scope:* A model for psychiatric nursing practice created by nursing professor and psychotherapist, Phillip Barker, and social worker and therapist, Poppy Buchanan-Barker. Now used across other disciplines. Interventions and tools are adapted to the person's life situation.

Theory context: Perspective shaped by chaos theory: small change in initial conditions can produce unpredictable changes in later conditions.

Theory content:
- **Concepts:** *person* with domains of need; *world* (for validation and understanding); *self* (for physical and emotional safety); *other* (supports and services for everyday life); *life* as a journey on an ocean of experience; *recovery* as returning to the course of life; the *practitioner* as lifeguard who, with understanding of person's stories, helps build a safety plan
- **Metaparadigm:** caring with not caring for; understanding the person in the "now" and their interpretation of experience
- **Propositions and competencies:** focused on the person, recovery (redesign of one's life), environment (context of lived experience and space for growth)

The Tidal Model grounds care on attention to emotional and physical safety with a focus on the person's story. This enables understanding of aspects of their distress and move toward suicide not readily known from the checklist inventories commonly used. The Model outlines potential reasons for an older adult's decision to end life: escape from despair (e.g., depression), escape from pain or bodily deterioration (e.g., physical pain), to transcend life (e.g., to be with a loved one), to "follow orders" (delusional ideas), and to save others. This model promotes the creation of an open dialogue to help the person explore how they might overcome their distress and problems in living and whether they want support for this effort from others. As the person overcomes or faces their current life problems, it is movement to recovery.

As presented in Fawcett, J., & DeSanto-Madeya, S. (2013). *Contemporary nursing knowledge: Analysis and evaluation of nursing models and theories* (3rd ed.). F.A. Davis Company.

---

and patient whereby each perceives the other and the situation; and through communication, they set goals, explore means, and agree on means to achieve goals" (King, 1981, p. 144). The process is initiated to help the patient cope with a health problem that compromises the ability to maintain social roles, functions, and activities of daily living (King, 1992). In this theory, the person is goal oriented and purposeful, is reacting to stressors, and is viewed as an open system interacting with the environment. It is within an interpersonal system of nurse and client that the healing process is performed. Interaction is depicted in which the outcome is a **transaction**, which is defined as the transfer of value between two or more people. The transaction process is what occurs in nursing situations. In the past, King's theory has been applied to group therapy for inpatient juvenile offenders, maximum security state offenders, and community parolees (Laben et al., 1991) and as a nursing framework for individual psychotherapy (DeHowitt,

1992). It continues to be used to investigate the effectiveness of clinical pathways for a surgical procedure in terms of clinical quality, cost, and patient and staff satisfaction (Knowaja, 2006).

Systems and Stress: Betty Neuman

The purpose of Neuman's (1989) systems model is to guide the actions of the professional caregiver through the assessment and intervention processes by focusing on two major components: the nature of the relationship between the nurse and patient and the patient's response to stressors. The patient may be an individual, group (e.g., a family), or community. The nurse is an "intervener" who attempts to reduce an individual's encounter with stress and to strengthen the person's ability to deal with stressors. The patient is viewed as a collaborator in setting healthcare goals and determining interventions. Neuman was one of the first PMH nurses to include the concept of stressors in understanding nursing care.

The Neuman systems model has been applied in diverse settings, including community health, family therapy, renal nursing, perinatal nursing, and mental health nursing of older adults (DeWan & Ume-Nwagbo, 2006; Neuman et al., 2000; Olowokere & Okanlawon, 2015; Partlak Günüşen et al., 2009). More recently, in a randomized control study (*n* = 72) to determine the effect of a Neuman systems model-based "coping with depression" program (that utilized individual psycho education and cognitive–behavioural techniques), it was found that the level of depression and use of avoidance strategies for intervention group participants decreased, while self-esteem and problem-solving skills increased. The results were sustained when measured 2 months later (Başoğul & Buldukoğlu, 2020).

Self-Care: Dorothea Orem

Self-care is the focus of the general theory of nursing initiated by Dorothea Orem in the early 1960s. The theory has three main focuses: self-care, self-care deficit, and a theory of nursing systems (Orem, 1991). Self-care is defined as those activities performed independently by an individual to promote and maintain personal wellbeing throughout life. Self-care deficits occur when an individual has a deficit in attitude (motivation), knowledge, or skill that impedes the meeting of self-care needs. Nurses can help individuals meet self-care requisites through five approaches: acting or doing for, guiding, teaching, supporting, and providing an environment to promote the patient's ability to meet current or future demands. The nursing systems theory refers to a series of actions a nurse takes to meet patient self-care requirements, which vary from patients totally dependent on the nurse for care to those who need only some education and support. For example, Orem's model has been viewed as a means of empowering individuals with chronic illness. In an experimental study in which participants with multiple sclerosis (*n* = 63) were randomly assigned to treatment and control groups, eight sessions of nursing interventions that were tailored to each participant's self-care requisites were carried out with the treatment group. Significant improvement in balance and motor function measures were observed for treatment participants. Enabling self-care in this way can prevent early disabilities and impact quality of life (Afrasiabifar et al., 2020).

Orem's emphasis on promoting independence of the individual and on self-care activities is of particular importance to PMH nursing (Biggs, 2008). This emphasis fits well with recovery principles, and it has potential use in moving inpatient psychiatric cultures toward a recovery focus and in guiding research that explores patient self-care agency to recovery outcomes (Seed & Torkelson, 2012). See, for instance, Pickens' (2012) exploration of nursing strategies to enhance motivation of persons with schizophrenia to engage in self-care activities.

Adaptation: Callista Roy

Callista Roy's nursing model is often selected by nurses working in inpatient psychiatric units because they find its concepts particularly relevant to their practice. Roy's adaptation model (1974), originating in 1964, describes humans as living adaptive systems with two coping mechanisms: the regulator and the cognator. The regulator copes with physiologic stimuli and the cognator with psychosociocultural stimuli. Manifestations of the coping mechanisms can be assessed by four adaptive modes: physiologic needs, self-concept, role function, and interdependence. In this model, the nursing process has six steps: "assessment of behaviour, assessment of stimuli (focal, contextual, and residual), nursing diagnosis, goal setting, intervention, and evaluation" (Lutjens, 1991a, p. 10). Research informed by this model includes a study of the sharing of the experience of a traumatic event from both the storyteller's and the listener's perspectives (Cummins, 2011).

Unitary Human Beings: Martha Rogers

The central concept of nursing for Martha Rogers is energy fields, which are open systems (Rogers, 1970). Her abstract system offers a perspective of change as continuous and evolutionary with its principles of homeodynamics—integrality, resonancy, and helicy (Rogers, 1994). Health and nonhealth are considered value laden, with the purpose of nursing being the promotion of human betterment. Important concepts are accelerating change, paranormal phenomena, and rhythmic manifestation of change. Rogers' science enables us to see human phenomena differently (Lutjens, 1991b), including a psychiatric disorder (Thompson, 1990). Her influence on other nursing perspectives, such as Rosemarie Parse's health as human-becoming, is evident. According to Lego (1973), the holistic, unitary human beings approach differentiates a nurse psychotherapist from other psychotherapists. An example of research based on Roger's theory is Coakley and colleagues (2016) study of the experience and impact of therapeutic touch (TT) treatments for nurse colleagues. TT, based on Roger's understanding of energy fields as interactive, involves the transfer of energy through the hands of one person to another for the purpose of healing. It was found that changes in heart rate, blood pressure, cortisol levels, and perceived levels of comfort of nurse participants, whom provided and received TT, indicated that a sense of wellbeing was promoted.

Biologic Theories

Biologic theories are clearly important in understanding the manifestations of mental disorders and caring for people with these illnesses. This importance is growing as we gain further knowledge of the brain, and Chapter 10 is decidedly dedicated to the biologic foundations of PMH nursing. This chapter addresses many of the important neurobiologic theories and introduces other new fields of study. Further knowledge about the biologic domain can be found in Chapter 13, which focuses on psychopharmacology and other biologic treatments. Many of the biologically focused nursing interventions can be found in Chapter 12.

Psychological Theories

Psychodynamic Theories

Psychodynamic theories explain human development processes, especially in early childhood, and their effects on thought and behaviour. The study of the unconscious

is a key aspect of psychodynamic theory (Ellenberger, 1970). Many important concepts in PMH nursing began with the Austrian physician, Sigmund Freud (1856–1939). Psychodynamic theories initially attempted to explain the cause of mental disorders, but etiologic explanations have not been consistently supported by empiric research. These theories, however, proved to be especially important in the development of therapeutic relationships, techniques, and interventions (Table 9.1).

Psychoanalytic Theory

Study of the Unconscious

In Sigmund Freud's psychoanalytic model, the human mind was conceptualized in terms of **conscious** mental

Table 9.1 Psychological Theories: Psychodynamic and Humanistic

Theorist	Overview	Major Concepts	Applicability
Psychoanalytic			
Sigmund Freud (1856–1939)	Founder of psychoanalysis. Believed that the unconscious could be accessed through dreams and free association. Developed a personality theory and theory of infantile sexuality.	Id, ego, superego Consciousness Unconscious mental processes Libido Object relations Anxiety and defence mechanisms Free associations, transference, and countertransference	Individual therapy approach used for enhancement of personal maturity and personal growth
Anna Freud (1895–1982)	Application of ego psychology to psychoanalytic treatment and child analysis with emphasis on the adaptive function of defence mechanisms	Refinement of concepts of anxiety, defence mechanisms	Individual therapy, childhood psychoanalysis
Neo-Freudian			
Alfred Adler (1870–1937)	First defected from Freud Founded the school of individual psychology.	Inferiority	Added to the understanding of human motivation
Carl Gustav Jung (1875–1961)	After separating from Freud, founded the school of psychoanalytic psychology. Developed new therapeutic approaches.	Redefined libido Introversion Extroversion Persona	Personalities are often assessed on the introversion and extroversion dimensions.
Karen Horney (1885–1952)	Opposed Freud's theory of castration complex in women and his emphasis on the Oedipus complex. Argued that neurosis was influenced by the society in which one lived.	Situational neurosis Character	Beginning of feminist analysis of psychoanalytic thought
Humanistic			
Abraham Maslow (1921–1970)	Concerned himself with healthy rather than sick people. Approached individuals from a holistic–dynamic viewpoint.	Needs Motivation	Used as a model to understand how people are motivated and needs that should be met
Frederick S. Perls (1893–1970)	Awareness of emotion, physical state, and repressed needs would enhance the ability to deal with emotional problems.	Reality Here and now	Used as a therapeutic approach to resolve current life problems that are influenced by old, unresolved emotional problems
Carl Rogers (1902–1987)	Based theory on the view of human potential for goodness. Used the term *client* rather than *patient*. Stressed the relationship between the therapist and the client.	Empathy Positive regard	Individual therapy approach that involves never giving advice and always clarifying client's feelings

processes (an awareness of events, thoughts, and feelings with the ability to recall them) and **unconscious** mental processes (thoughts and feelings that are outside awareness and are not remembered). Freud believed that the unconscious part of the human mind is only rarely recognized by the conscious part, which is remembered dreams. The term **preconscious** was used to describe unconscious material that is capable of entering consciousness. Uncovering unconscious material to help patients gain insight into unresolved issues was basic to the psychotherapy Freud developed.

Personality and Its Development

Freud's personality structure consists of three parts: the id, ego, and superego (Freud, 1927). According to Freud, the **id** is formed by unconscious desires, primitive instincts, and unstructured drives, including sexual and aggressive tendencies that arise from the body. The **ego** consists of the sum of certain mental mechanisms, such as perception, memory, and motor control, as well as specific defence mechanisms. The ego controls movement, perception, and contact with reality. The capacity to form mutually satisfying relationships is a fundamental function of the ego, which is not present at birth but is formed throughout a child's development. The **superego** is that part of the personality structure associated with ethics, standards, and self-criticism. A child's identification with important and esteemed people in early life, particularly parents, helps form the superego.

Object Relations and Identification

Freud introduced the concept of **object relations**, the psychological attachment to another person or object. He believed that the choice of a love object in adulthood and the nature of the relationship depend on the nature and quality of the child's object relationships during the early formative years. A child's first love object is the mother, who is the source of nourishment and the provider of pleasure. Gradually, as the child separates from the mother, the nature of this initial attachment influences any future relationships. The development of the child's capacity for relationships with others progresses from a state of narcissism to social relationships, first within the family and then within the larger community. Although the concept of object relations is fairly abstract, it can be understood in terms of a child who imitates their mother and then becomes like their mother in adulthood. This child has incorporated their mother as a love object, identifies with her, and becomes like her as an adult. This process becomes especially important in understanding an abused child who, under certain circumstances, becomes the adult abuser.

Anxiety and Defence Mechanisms

For Freud, anxiety was a specific state of unpleasantness accompanied by motor discharge along definite pathways, the reaction to danger of object loss. Defence mechanisms protected a person from unwanted anxiety. Although they are defined differently than in Freud's day, defence mechanisms still play an explanatory role in contemporary PMH practice. Defence mechanisms are discussed in Chapter 7.

Sexuality

According to Freud, the energy or psychic drive associated with the sexual instinct, called the *libido*, translated from Latin as "pleasure" or "lust," resides in the id. Tension results and is transformed into anxiety when sexual desire is controlled and not expressed (Freud, 1905). Freud believed that adult sexuality is an end product of a complex process of development that begins in early childhood and involves a variety of body functions or areas (oral, anal, and genital zones) that correspond to stages of relationships, especially with parents.

Psychoanalysis

Freud (1949) developed *psychoanalysis*, a therapeutic process of accessing the unconscious and with the mature adult mind resolving the conflicts that originated in childhood. As a system of psychotherapy, psychoanalysis attempted to reconstruct the personality by examining free associations (spontaneous, uncensored verbalizations of whatever comes to mind) and the interpretation of dreams (Freud, 1955). Freud believed that therapeutic relationships had their beginnings within the psychoanalytic framework.

Transference and Countertransference

Transference is the displacement of thoughts, feelings, and behaviours originally associated with significant others from childhood onto a person in a current therapeutic relationship (Moore & Fine, 1990). For example, a woman's feelings toward her parents as a child may be transferred to the therapist. If she were unconsciously angry with her parents, then she may feel inexplicable anger and hostility toward her therapist. In psychoanalysis, the therapist uses transference as a therapeutic tool to help the patient understand emotional problems and their origin. It is considered an essential aspect of therapy. **Countertransference,** on the other hand, is defined as the direction of all the therapist's feelings and attitudes toward the patient. Feelings and perceptions caused by countertransference may interfere with the therapist's ability to understand the patient.

Neo-Freudian Models

Many of Freud's followers ultimately established their own forms of psychoanalysis. The various psychoanalytic schools have adopted other names because their doctrines deviated from Freudian theory.

Adler's Foundation for Individual Psychology

Alfred Adler was a Viennese psychiatrist, founder of the school of individual psychology, and an early colleague of Freud who disagreed with Freud's focus on instinctual determination. He focused instead on the social aspects of human existence. Adler believed mental health involves love, work, and community. For Adler (1963), the motivating force in human life is a striving for superiority. Seeking perfection and security while trying to avoid feelings of inferiority can lead the individual to adopt a life goal that is unrealistic and frequently expressed as an unreasoning desire for power and dominance (i.e., *inferiority complex*). Inferiority is intolerable, so the compensatory mechanisms set up by the mind may result in self-centred attitudes, overcompensation, and a retreat from life's problems.

Adler focused on growth, lifestyle, and becoming: humans are looking to realize their potential and flourish within their community. Adlerian theory is based on principles of mutual respect, choice, responsibility, consequences, and belonging. It informs both psychotherapy (e.g., family therapy and Ellis' (1973) Rational Emotive Therapy) and education.

Jung's Analytical Psychology

One of Freud's earliest colleagues, Carl Gustav Jung, a Swiss psychoanalyst, created a model called *analytical psychology*. For Jung, humans were influenced not only by their past but also by their hopes for the future. He not only supported the idea of a personal unconscious but also proposed a second psychic system, inherited and universal to all humans, the **collective unconscious**. Within the collective unconscious are **archetypes**, symbols common to all cultures. Images such as "mother" or "hero" or "trickster," for instance, have forms common to every society (Jung, 1959). Jung described humans as having both feminine and masculine characteristics. Therapy may help an individual develop more fully as a person by embracing both aspects of themselves. The feminine side of men is the **anima**; the masculine side of women is the **animus**. The concept of **persona** (the mask one wears in society or one's public self) is similar to Freud's superego (Jung, 1966). The **shadow** is Jung's image for the dark side of every person. It is the side we do not like to recognize or show to others. One needs to become aware of and integrate the shadow into one's personality to evolve as an individual.

Jung believed in the existence of two psychological types: the **extrovert** (who finds meaning in the world) and the **introvert** (who finds meaning within). He also described four primary modes of orientation to the world: *thinking, feeling, intuition,* and *sensation.* Although he argued that each of these functions exists in an individual, certain preferences will dominate. Our unconscious is revealed often through our least developed mode. The Myers-Briggs Type Indicator test is based on Jung's personality theory.

Horney's Feminine Psychology

Karen Horney, a German American psychiatrist, challenged many of Freud's basic concepts and introduced principles of feminine psychology. Recognizing a male bias in psychoanalysis, Horney questioned the psychoanalytic belief that women felt disadvantaged because of their genital organs, and she rejected Freud's concept of "penis envy." She argued that there are significant cultural reasons for women to strive to obtain qualities or privileges that are defined by a society as masculine and that women truly were at a disadvantage in a paternalistic culture (Horney, 1939). She observed that men have a deep-seated dread of women that is revealed in analysis (Horney, 1932). Her primary concept was that of basic anxiety: early (childhood) feelings of helplessness and isolation which one strives to cope with and resolve. According to Horney, this anxiety underlies all of an individual's relationships and can help explain behaviour. Horney (1950) named the unrealistic expectations that one puts on oneself "tyranny of the should." With other Neo-Freudians, such as Eric Fromm, she introduced sociocultural dimensions of human behaviour into the psychoanalytical model.

Humanistic Theories

Humanistic theories were generated as a reaction against psychoanalytic premises of instinctual drives and are based on the views of human potential for goodness. Humanist therapists focus on one's ability to learn about oneself, acceptance of self, and exploration of personal capabilities. Within the therapeutic relationship, the patient begins to develop positive attitudes and views them as a person of worth. The focus is not on investigation of repressed memories but on learning to experience the world in a different way.

Rogers' Client-Centred Therapy

Carl Rogers, an American psychologist, developed new methods of client-centred therapy. Rogers (1980) defined **empathy** as the capacity to assume the internal reference of the individual in order to perceive the world in the same way as the individual does. The counsellor must be nondirective but not passive to use empathy in the therapeutic process. Thus, the counsellor's attitude and nonverbal communication are crucial. He advocated that the therapist develops **unconditional positive regard**, a nonjudgmental caring, for the client (Rogers, 1980) and believed that the therapist's emotional investment (i.e., true caring) in the client is essential to the therapeutic process. Genuineness on the part of the therapist, in contrast with the passivity of the psychoanalyst, is seen as key.

Gestalt Therapy

Another humanistic response to the psychoanalytic model was Gestalt therapy, developed by Frederick S. (Fritz) Perls. Perls believed that modern civilization inevitably produces neurotic anxiety because it forces people to repress natural desires and frustrates an inherent human tendency to adjust biologically and psychologically to the environment. For a person to be cured, unmet needs must be brought back to awareness. Perls rejected the notion that intellectual insight enabled people to change. His individual and group exercises aimed to enhance a person's awareness of emotions, physical state, and repressed needs as well as physical and psychological stimuli in the here-and-now environment (Perls, 1969).

Maslow's Hierarchy of Needs

Abraham Maslow developed a humanistic model that is used in PMH nursing today (Maslow, 1998). His major contributions were to the understanding of human needs and motivation (Maslow, 1970). He studied exemplary healthy individuals (e.g., Albert Einstein) whom he saw as self-actualizing and described their characteristics. For instance, he noted that they were creative, had a deep sense of kinship with others, and had a strong sense of ethics. People are self-actualized when they are making the most of their unique human potential. Maslow's view of human motivation was based on a hierarchy of needs, ranging from lower-level survival needs, such as air, water, basic food, and shelter; to higher-level needs, such as those for belonging and esteem; and to achieve **self-actualization**. One must meet lower-level needs before moving to the higher-level ones (see Fig. 9.2). According to Maslow's model, values such as truth, beauty, and justice are aspects of our metaneeds, and their persistent deprivation can lead to spiritual–existential ailments often expressed as apathy, boredom, hopelessness, and powerlessness (Hoffman, 1996). Maslow's model offers a framework for assessment.

Applicability of Psychodynamic Theories to PMH Nursing

Several concepts in psychodynamic models are core elements in PMH nursing practice, such as interpersonal

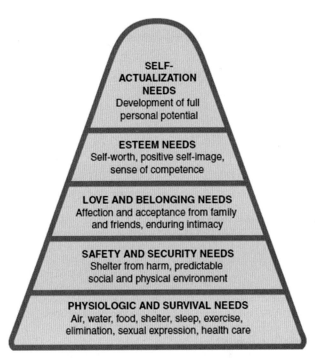

Figure 9.2 Maslow's hierarchy of needs.

relationships, needs, anxiety, defence mechanisms, transference, and countertransference. Many of these concepts are further developed within nursing theories. A key psychodynamic concept, the therapeutic relationship, is recognized as a core of PMH nursing intervention.

Behavioural Theories

Behavioural theories, with roots in the discipline of psychology, offer important explanatory models for PMH nursing in terms of the way in which people act and learn (Table 9.2).

Early Stimulus–Response Theories

Pavlovian Theory

One of the earliest behavioural theorists was Ivan P. Pavlov, who was studying the gastric functioning of dogs when he noticed that stomach secretions of dogs were stimulated by triggers other than food, such as the sight and smell of food. He became interested in this anticipatory secretion. Through his experiments, he was able to stimulate secretions with a variety of other laboratory nonphysiologic stimuli. Thus, a clear connection was made between thought processes and physiologic responses.

In Pavlov's model, there is an unconditioned stimulus (not dependent on previous training) that elicits an unconditioned (i.e., specific) response. Meat was the unconditioned stimulus in his experiments, and salivation was the unconditioned response. Pavlov would then select other stimuli, such as a bell, a ticking metronome,

Table 9.2 Psychological Theories: Behavioural, Cognitive, and Developmental

Theorist	Overview	Major Concepts	Applicability
Stimulus–Response Theories			
Ivan P. Pavlov (1849–1936)	Classical conditioning	Unconditioned stimuli Unconditioned response Conditioned stimuli	Important in understanding learning of automatic responses such as habitual behaviours
John B. Watson (1878–1958)	Introduced behaviourism, believed that learning was classical conditioning called *reflexes*; rejected distinction between the mind and the body	Principle of frequency Principle of recency	Focuses on the relationship between the mind and the body
Reinforcement Theories			
B. F. Skinner (1904–1990)	Developed an understanding of the importance of reinforcement and differentiated types and schedules	Operant behaviour Respondent behaviour Continuous reinforcement Intermittent reinforcement	Important in behaviour modification
Edward L. Thorndike (1874–1949)	Believed in the importance of effects that followed behaviour	Reinforcement	Important in behaviour modification programs
Cognitive Theories			
Albert Bandura (b. 1925)	Developed social cognitive theory, a model for understanding how behaviour is learned from others	Modeling Disinhibition Elicitation Self-efficacy	Important in helping individuals learn appropriate behaviours
Aaron Beck (b. 1921)	Conceptualized distorted cognitions as a basis for depression	Cognitions Beliefs	Important in cognitive therapy
Kurt Lewin (1890–1947)	Developed field theory, a system for understanding learning, motivation, personality, and social behaviour	Life space Positive valences Negative valences	Important in understanding motivation for changing behaviour
Edward Chace Tolman (1886–1959)	Introduced the concept of cognitions; believed that human beings act on beliefs and attitudes and strive toward goals	Cognition	Important in identifying the person's beliefs
Developmental Theories			
Erik Erikson (1902–1994)	Viewed psychosocial development as influenced by environment and occurring in stages, each one having a task to resolve	Eight stages Trust vs. mistrust Autonomy vs. shame/doubt Initiative vs. guilt Industry vs. inferiority Identity vs. role diffusion Intimacy vs. isolation Generativity vs. stagnation Ego integrity vs. despair	Allows unresolved developmental tasks to be identified
Jean Piaget (1896–1980)	Viewed intelligence as adaptation to the environment. Understood cognitive development in children to be like embryonic development: increasing differentiation in structure	Children learn particular concepts only when they have reached the appropriate stage of development	Important in assessment of children Useful in age-appropriate health education for children
Carol Gilligan (1936–)	Gender differences in moral development	Found a tendency for women to be more focused in relationships and issues of care in resolving moral problems, while men tend to apply abstract principles such as justice	Important in the evolution of gender studies

and a triangle drawn on a large cue card, and present this conditioned stimulus just before the meat (the unconditioned stimulus). If the conditioned stimulus was repeatedly presented before the meat, then eventually salivation was elicited by the conditioned stimulus. This phenomenon was called **classical** (Pavlovian) **conditioning** (Pavlov, 1927/1960).

John B. Watson and the Behaviourist Revolution

At about the same time Pavlov was working in Russia, John B. Watson initiated the psychological revolution known as **behaviourism** in the United States. He developed two principles: frequency and recency. The principle of frequency states that the more often a given response is made to a given stimulus, the more likely the response to that stimulus will be repeated. The principle of recency states that the more recently a given response to a particular stimulus is made, the more likely it will be repeated. Watson's major contribution was the rejection of the distinction between body and mind and his emphasis on the study of objective behaviour (Watson & Rayner, 1917).

Reinforcement Theories

Edward L. Thorndike

A pioneer in experimental animal psychology, Edwin L. Thorndike, studied the problem-solving behaviour of cats to determine whether animals solved problems by reasoning or instinct. He found that neither choice was completely correct; animals gradually learn the correct response by "stamping in" the stimulus–response connection. The major difference between Thorndike and behaviourists such as Watson was that Thorndike believed in the importance of the effects that followed the response or the reinforcement of the behaviour. He was the first reinforcement theorist, and his view of learning became the dominant view in learning theory (Thorndike, 1916, c.1906).

B. F. Skinner

One of the most influential behaviourists, B. F. Skinner, recognized two different kinds of learning that each involved a separate kind of behaviour. *Respondent behaviour*, or the end result of **classical conditioning,** is elicited by specific stimuli. The response occurs automatically given the stimulus. The other kind of learning is referred to as **operant behaviour**. In this type of learning, the distinctive characteristic is the consequence of a particular behavioural response not a specific stimulus. The learning of operant behaviour is also known as *conditioning*, but it is different from the conditioning of reflexes. If a behaviour occurs and is followed by reinforcement, then it is probable that the behaviour will

recur. For example, if a child climbs on a chair, reaches the faucet and is able to get a drink of water successfully, then it is more likely that the child will repeat the behaviour (Skinner, 1935). Skinner wrote a book about a utopian community based on the principles of behaviourism that he titled *Walden II* (Skinner, 1976).

Cognitive Theories

The initial behavioural studies focused attention on human actions without attention to the internal thinking process. As complex behaviour was examined and could not be accounted for by strictly behavioural explanations, thought processes became new subjects for study. Cognitive theories, an outgrowth of different theoretic perspectives including the behavioural and the psychodynamic, attempted to link internal thought processes with human behaviour.

Albert Bandura's Social Cognitive Theory

Acquiring behaviours by learning from other people is the basis of social cognitive theory developed by the psychologist Albert Bandura, born in Mundare, Alberta. Bandura developed his ideas after being concerned about violence on television contributing to aggression in children. He believes that important behaviours are learned by internalizing behaviours of others. His initial contribution was identifying the process of **modeling**: pervasive imitation or one person trying to be like another. According to Bandura, the model may not need to be a real person but could be a character in history or generalized to an ideal person (Bandura, 1977).

The concept of **disinhibition** is important to Bandura's model and refers to the situation in which someone has learned not to make a response; then, in a given situation, when another is making the inhibited response, the individual becomes disinhibited and also makes the response. Thus, the response that was "inhibited" now becomes disinhibited through a process of imitation. For example, during severe dieting, an individual may have learned to resist eating large amounts of food. However, when at a party with a friend who eagerly fills a plate at a buffet, the person also eats large amounts of food.

In the instance of disinhibition, the desire to eat is already there, and the individual indulges that desire. However, in another instance called **elicitation**, there is no desire present, but when one person starts an activity, others want to do the same. An example of this occurs when a child is playing with a toy and the other children now want to play with the same toy even though they showed no interest in it before that time.

An important concept of Bandura's model is **self-efficacy**, a person's sense of their ability to deal effectively with the environment, which he develops in his work, *Self-Efficacy: The Exercise of Control* (1997). Efficacy beliefs influence how people feel, think, motivate themselves, and behave. The stronger the self-efficacy, the higher the goals people set for themselves and the firmer their commitment to them. Social cognitive theory extends to understanding collective efficacy and the way in which people strive to shape and control their lives.

Aaron T. Beck: Thinking and Feeling

American psychiatrist, Aaron T. Beck of the University of Pennsylvania, devoted his career to understanding the relationship between **cognition** and mental health. For Beck, cognitions are verbal or pictorial events in the stream of consciousness. He realized the importance of cognitions when treating people with depression, finding that the depression improved when patients began thinking differently. He believed that people with depression had faulty information-processing systems that led to biased cognitions. These faulty beliefs cause errors in judgment that become habitual errors in thinking. When individuals incorrectly interpret life situations, they judge themselves too harshly and jump to inaccurate conclusions. Individuals may, for example, truly believe that they have no friends and therefore no one cares. On examination, the evidence for the beliefs is faulty. For instance, it may be that there has been no contact with anyone because of moving from one city to another or because calls are not returned nor invitations accepted. Thus, distorted beliefs are the basis of the cognitions. Beck et al. (2003) developed cognitive therapy, a successful approach for the treatment of depressive disorders (Chapter 22). Beck (2011) continues to develop cognitive–behavioural therapy at *The Beck Institute of Cognitive Behavior Therapy*, which he established in collaboration with his daughter, Judith Beck. See Chapter 14 for an overview of cognitive–behavioural interventions.

Applicability of Cognitive and Behavioural Theories to PMH Nursing

Interventions based on cognitive and behavioural theories are important in nursing. For example, patient education interventions are usually based on learning principles derived from these theories, and the teaching of new coping skills for patients in their recovery is usually based on them. Changing an entrenched habit involves helping people to identify what motivates them, recognize cues that precede the behaviour they desire to change, and create new lifestyle habits. Examples of cognitive and behavioural interventions used on inpatient hospital units include privilege systems and token economies and the application of cognitive–behavioural interventions (see Chapter 14).

Developmental Theories

Developmental theories explain normal human growth and development and focus on change over time. Many are presented in terms of stages based on the assumption that normal development proceeds stage-by-stage longitudinally. Human development, however, does not necessarily unfold sequentially and in the same way for each person.

Erik Erikson: Psychosocial Development

Erik Erikson's psychosocial developmental model, an expansion of Freud's psychosexual development theory, is commonly used in nursing. Each of Erikson's eight stages is associated with a specific task that can be successfully or unsuccessfully resolved. The model is organized according to developmental conflicts by age: basic trust versus mistrust, autonomy versus shame and doubt, initiative versus guilt, industry versus inferiority, identity versus role diffusion, intimacy versus isolation, generativity versus stagnation, and ego integrity versus despair. Erikson's wife, Joan Serson Erickson, extended his theory to include old age as a ninth stage, gerotranscendence (Erikson & Erikson, 1997). Gerotranscendence theory focused on the continued growth in dimensions such as spirituality and inner strength (see Chapter 31).

Successful resolution of a crisis leads to essential strength and virtues within Erickson's theory. For example, a positive outcome of the trust versus mistrust crisis is the development of a basic sense of trust. If the crisis is unsuccessfully resolved, then the infant moves into the next stage without a sense of trust. According to this model, a child who is mistrustful will have difficulty completing the next crisis successfully and, instead of developing a sense of autonomy, will more likely be full of shame and doubt (Erikson, 1963). One of Erikson's major contributions was the recognition of the turbulence of adolescent development. Erikson wrote extensively about adolescence, youth, and identity formation. Childhood ways must be given up when adolescence begins, and body changes must be reconciled with the individual's social position, previous history, and identifications. An identity is formed. This task of reconciling how young people see themselves and how society perceives them can become overwhelming and lead to role confusion and alienation (Erikson, 1968).

Research has explored developmental stages of this model with mixed results. For instance, in an early study, male college students who measured low on identity also scored low on intimacy ratings (Orlofsky et al., 1973), lending support to the idea that identity precedes intimacy. Yet in another study, intimacy was found to begin developing early in adolescence, prior to the development of identity (Ochse & Plug, 1986). Studying fathers with young children, Christiansen and Palkovitz (1998) found that *generativity* (defined as the need or drive to produce, create, or effect a change) was associated with a paternal identity, psychosocial identity, and psychosocial intimacy. In a longitudinal study testing Erikson's model, 86 men were assessed at

21 years of age and then at 52 years. Fifty-six percent of the men achieved generativity, which was associated with work achievement, close friendships, successful marriage, altruistic behaviours, and mental health.

Favourable predictors in young adulthood included a warm family environment and good peer relationships (Westermeyer, 2004). Research also suggests that gender influences development. One study found generativity to be associated with wellbeing; however, in men, generativity seems related to the urge for self-protection, self-assertion, self-expansion, and mastery, while in women, the antecedents may be the desire for contact, connection, and union (Ackerman et al., 2000). A Canadian study that investigated grandparents' role in the socialization of children within the family queried whether midlife generativity would predict parents' descriptions of grandparenting problems. It did: generative fathers were more optimistic that problems with grandparents would be solved. Both generative mothers and fathers showed higher levels of forgiveness of grandparents (Pratt et al., 2008).

Jean Piaget: Learning in Children

One of the most influential people in child psychology was Jean Piaget, who was the first to make a systematic study of cognitive development (Piaget, 1936). Piaget viewed intelligence as an adaptation to the environment. He proposed that cognitive growth is like embryologic growth: an organized structure increasingly differentiates over time. He determined that readiness is an important consideration in children's learning. According to Piaget, a particular concept should be taught to children only when they have reached an appropriate stage of development. Piaget developed a system that explains how knowledge develops and changes. Each stage of cognitive development represents a particular structure with major characteristics (Piaget, 1957). Piaget tested his theory through observation of his own children; the theory was never subjected to formal testing.

The major strength of his model was its recognition of the central role of cognition in development and the discovery of surprising features of young children's thinking. Piaget's model provides a framework in nursing to define different levels of thinking and use the data in the assessment and intervention processes.

Carol Gilligan: Gender Differentiation

Psychologist Carol Gilligan studied the ways men and women approached moral problems and identified differences (Gilligan, 1982). She wrote about these differences in moral development in her 1982 landmark work, *In a Different Voice: Psychological Theory and Women's Development*. Men tended to approach moral problems by applying abstract rules such as those related

to justice. Women in her study were more likely to be concerned with preserving the relationships of those involved and with responsibilities related to care. For Gilligan, attachment within relationships is the important factor for successful development in women. Thus, women were set at a disadvantage in traditional models of development that advocate separation as a primary goal of human development, such as Erikson's. They can be viewed as impaired by the importance placed on attachments. According to Gilligan, development in women does not follow a progression of stages but is based on experiences within relationships. This may be the case for men, as well, in their development of a strong sense of self (Nelson, 1996).

The scientific merit of Gilligan's work has been challenged by many critics, but it has had a significant impact on the development of gender studies (Graham, 2012).

Applicability of Developmental Theories to PMH Nursing

Developmental theories are used in understanding childhood and adolescent experiences and their manifestations as adult problems. When working with children, nurses can use developmental models to help gauge development and mood. However, because most of the models are based on the assumptions of the linear progression of stages and have not been adequately tested, applicability has limitations. In addition, these models were based on a relatively small number of children who typically were raised in a Western middle-class environment. Most do not account for gender differences and diversity in lifestyles and cultures.

Social Theories

Numerous social theories underlie PMH nursing practice, and the nursing profession itself serves a specific societal function. This section represents a sampling of important social theories that nurses may use. This discussion is not exhaustive and should be viewed by the student as including only some of the theoretic perspectives that may be applicable.

Family Dynamics

Family dynamics are the patterned interpersonal and social interactions that occur within the family structure over the life of a family. Family dynamics models are based on systems theory describing a phenomenon in terms of a set of interrelated parts, in which the change of one part affects the total functioning of the system. A system can be "open" and interacting in the environment or "closed," completely self-contained, and not influenced by the environment. The family is viewed organizationally as an open system in which one member's actions influence the functioning of the total system. Most of the theoretic explanations have emerged from treatment case studies, rather than from systematic development of theory based on generalizable research. Consequently, the limitation of available research should be considered when these models are used to understand family interactions and plan patient care (see Chapter 16).

Applicability of Family Theories to PMH Nursing

Family theories are especially useful to nurses who are assessing family dynamics and planning interventions (Wright & Leahey, 2013). Family systems models are used to help nurses form collaborative relationships with individuals and families dealing with health problems. While only nurses with specialized training in family therapy will be engaged in it, understanding family dynamics is important in every nurse's practice, and family theories must inform a nurse's family interventions (see Chapter 16). The mental health problems or mental illness of a family member will have important implications for the entire family system.

Role Theories

A **role** describes an individual's social position and function within an environment. Anthropologic theories explain members' roles that relate to a specific society. For example, the universal role of healer may be assumed by a nurse in one culture and a spiritual leader in another. Societal expectations, social status, and rights are attached to these roles. Psychological theories, which are concerned about roles from a different perspective, focus on the individual and the self. The responsibilities of a parent are often in conflict with the personal needs for time alone. All of the Neo-Freudian and humanist models that have been discussed focus on reciprocal social relationships or interactions that determine how the mind develops.

Applicability of Role Theories to PMH Nursing

Role theories emphasize the importance of social interaction in either the individual's choice of a particular role or society's recognition of it. Several nursing models have role as a major concept, including King (1971), Roy (1974), and Peplau (1952). PMH nursing uses role concepts in understanding group interaction and the role of the individual in the family and community (see Chapters 15 and 16). In addition, milieu therapy approaches discussed in later chapters are based on the individual's assumption of a role within the psychiatric care environment.

Sociocultural Perspectives

Gender and culture are now recognized as significant in determining human behaviour, including the

manifestation of mental health problems and illness, as well as in shaping our understanding of health and disease. Critical and emancipatory scholarship is furthering our understanding of the way power differences can stigmatize and marginalize underrepresented groups and can take institutionalized form. Canadian society is addressing these issues in our national mental health strategy that stresses the importance of healthcare services that are gender and culturally sensitive.

Gender

There is no foundational figure in the application of feminist approaches to psychotherapy, but rather many scholars who used feminist theory to inform and advance practice (Truscott, 2010).

From Horney's (1932) *Feminine Psychology* to Chesler's (1972) *Women and Madness* to Brown's (2010) *Feminist Therapy*, feminist therapists have been challenging societal, political, and medical conventions that frame gender in oppressive and discriminatory ways. They have reintroduced validity to concepts such as emotions and embodied knowledge that were previously deemed irrational and thus dysfunctional. Throughout the development of feminist approaches to therapy, a constant has been that the constructs of gender, power, and powerlessness inform the therapy process; feminist therapy is not just for women (Brown, 2010).

Since the 1970s, gender identity and sexual orientation studies have been bringing together scholarship from areas such as biology, psychology, sociology, science, philosophy, political science, and ethics to further understanding and knowledge of lesbian, gay, bisexual, transgender, intersex, two spirit, ally (and/or asexual), etc. (LGBTQI2SA+) identities. Such knowledge is important to the competent and ethical practice of nurses and other health professionals, but significant gaps remain. Research indicates, for instance, that nurses lack knowledge regarding the nursing needs of transgendered persons and experience uncertainty regarding how to interact with them and their families (Carabez et al., 2016). Further, nursing curricula needs to better address LGBTQI2SA+health (Carabez et al., 2015). There is a pressing need for nursing research, scholarship, and education to advance our understanding in this area.

Culture

Likewise, postcolonial theories and Marxist approaches have been introduced and call on nurses to attend to the ways that the various notions of race and class function in our understanding of psychiatric illness and mental health, respectively. "The social and moral mandate of nursing is now seen to include illumination of the experiences of those marginalized within society and within health care" (Kirkham & Anderson, 2002, p. 2).

Madeleine Leininger: Transcultural Health Care

Concern about the impact of culture on the treatment of children with psychiatric and emotional problems led Madeleine Leininger, a nurse anthropologist, to develop a new field called transcultural nursing, which is directed toward holistic, congruent, and beneficent care. She used concepts from anthropology and nursing (from such theorists as [Henderson, 1966; Rogers, 1970; Watson, 1979]) to depict universal and diverse dimensions of human caring. Caring is culturally based because caring is an integral part of being human, as well as a learned behaviour (Leininger, 1991, 1999). Care is considered the essence of nursing, and caring manifestations include compassion, presence, and enabling (Leininger, 1993). Leininger developed a model to depict her theory symbolically. The model depicts the "world view, religion, kinship, cultural values, economics, technology, language, ethnohistory, and environmental factors that are predicted to explain and influence culture care" (p. 27).

Applicability of Sociocultural Theories to PMH Nursing

Sociocultural theories are important to PMH nursing practice as the sociocultural aspect is integral to mental health. Adequate nursing assessments and interventions are not possible without consideration of the role of the individual within the family and within society and the significance of familial and cultural norms. Understanding cultural values is crucial to meaningful interactions with persons, families, and communities (see Chapter 4). Healthcare systems have their own cultures, as well, and it is necessary for nurses to ensure that the care environment is safe and conducive to healing and recovery (see Chapter 12). Sociocultural theories inform many group interventions (see Chapter 15).

Spiritual Theories

Frankl's Logotherapy

Viktor Frankl was an Austrian psychiatrist who survived being a prisoner in Nazi concentration camps during World War II. In his book, *Man's Search for Meaning*, he describes the way he discovered the importance of meaning to human existence (Frankl, 1992). Frankl wrote that each of us needs to find a reason to live. Otherwise, life can seem empty. Logotherapy is an existentialist theory and is focused on helping a person find meaning in life. Based on his experience, Frankl concluded that love was the greatest salvation. Even when one's only option is to endure suffering, contemplation of a beloved enables suffering to be endured in an honourable way (Frankl, 1992).

Yalom's Existential Psychotherapy

Influenced by Frankl's work, Irving Yalom grounds his existential psychotherapy upon what he considers central or ultimate life concerns: death, freedom, isolation, and meaninglessness. Conflicts may arise as each person attempts to confront these concerns. In his theory, Yalom (1980) describes how life concerns play a role in psychopathology and psychotherapy. For instance, "fear of death plays a major role in our internal experience; it haunts as does nothing else" (p. 27). A childhood developmental task is to deal with this fear. Often, however, we use denial to keep awareness of death at bay. Ineffective modes of facing our mortality can result in psychopathology; psychotherapy, therefore, may need to be aimed at death awareness. Yalom (a talented novelist as well as therapist) addresses this topic in *The Schopenhauer Cure* (2005). His central character, group psychotherapist Julius Hertzfeld, is diagnosed with a terminal illness and must confront his own mortality. Fact, fiction, and philosophy (that of Arthur Schopenhauer) are woven into this tale.

Yalom does not claim the existential orientation is *the* paradigm from which to understand all behaviour: the human being is too complex for this to be possible. However, existential psychotherapy is a useful, systematic approach for addressing many people's clinical situation or symptoms (Box 9.2).

Applicability of Spiritual Theories to PMH Nursing

These theoretic perspectives allow nurses to explore the way that the search for meaning in life and death shapes human development, experience, and understanding, as well as directly influence nurse theorists such as Travelbee. The existential suffering of individuals with serious and persistent mental illness (SPMI) can go unacknowledged in mental health care. Directly related to their illness, symptoms and treatment, and/or indirectly to the stigma, loneliness, and loss of autonomy and self-esteem associated with SPMI, it may fully encompass their illness experience. Nurses can support such individuals through the development of a caring, trust-based relationship and by being aware of the universal need of all humans to find purpose and meaning in their lives (Moonen et al., 2016).

Recovery as a Framework for Mental Health Care

In the Canadian Senate report *Out of the Shadows at Last: Transforming Mental Health, Mental Illness and Addiction Services in Canada*, recovery is placed at the centre of mental health reform. It is acknowledged that recovery is an active process rather than an end point and that each individual's path to recovery is unique (Kirby & Keon, 2006, p. 5). When the framework for such a transformation of the healthcare system was presented (Mental Health Commission of Canada [MHCC], 2009), recovery was conceived of as broader than *clinical* recovery (remission or cure). While persons with mental illness do experience clinical recovery, recovery is better understood as living a satisfying and hopeful life, even with mental health problems or illness. The MHCC created tools to facilitate recovery-oriented practice: The Recovery Declaration, which organizations and individuals may sign online (see Web Links); an online inventory of recovery resources (see www.mentalhealthcommission.ca/inventory); and Guidelines for Recovery-Oriented Practice: Hope, Dignity, Inclusion (MHCC, 2015).

Recovery

A recovery orientation is a significant shift from the medically centred approach to mental health care. Persons with mental illness and their families are to be engaged in such a way that strengths, resources, and rights are acknowledged. Health professionals are to practice in culturally safe ways that respond meaningfully to diversity, address complex mental health needs in the least restrictive ways possible, and broaden the types of evidence they use to evaluate individual improvements in health and wellbeing. Like other health professionals, nurses will need to assess, and perhaps adapt, their current theoretical perspectives in regard to the centrality of recovery.

KEY CONCEPT

Recovery is "a process in which people living with mental health problems and illnesses are empowered and supported to be actively engaged in their own journey of wellbeing. The recovery process builds on individual, family, cultural, and community strengths and enables people to enjoy a meaningful life in their community while striving to achieve their full potential" (Mental Health Commission of Canada, 2009, p. 122).

Summary of Key Points

- Nursing theories form the conceptual basis for nursing practice and are useful in a variety of PMH settings.
- The Tidal Model and its focus on the person's experience and on recovery are increasingly used as an approach to care in PMH settings.
- The traditional psychodynamic framework helped form the basis of early nursing interpersonal interventions, including the development of therapeutic relationships and the use of such concepts as transference, countertransference, empathy, and object relations.

- The cognitive and behavioural theories are often used in strategies that help individuals change behaviour and thinking.
- Sociocultural theories remain important in understanding and interacting with individuals as members of families, cultures, and society.
- Spiritual theories offer a way to consider the human search for meaning in life and how an individual's view of life can affect their health and wellbeing.
- The recovery orientation approach of Canada's mental health strategy is key to effective and ethical mental health care.

Thinking Challenges

1. Emma, an RN, practices on an acute care psychiatric unit that uses an interdisciplinary, patient-centred approach to care. This works well in the planning and implementation of treatment and care, but Emma wants to use a nursing theory to guide her thinking re: nursing care. It will enable her to better contribute to the overall plan of care of a patient. *What are the factors Emma should consider in choosing a theory?*
2. The Alcott family has brought their 18-year-old son, Ethan, to the emergency room. He has been increasingly agitated over the past month, quietly talking to himself, and has become worried that others are thinking bad thoughts about him. Yesterday, he accused his sister of causing his favourite hockey team to lose when she changed the TV channel away from the game. Today he spread flour around the edge of their property to keep others' mean thoughts about him away. *At what level of need would you place Ethan in Maslow's hierarchy? Ensure that you can explain your rationale.*
3. Describe a recovery orientation to care as envisioned by the MHCC.

Visit the**Point** to view suggested responses.
  Go to **thePoint.lww.com/activate** and use the activation code found in the front of this text to unlock suggested answers to the "Thinking Challenges," as well as find recommendations for "Movies and Other Things."

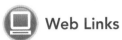 **Web Links**

ww w.florence-nightingale.co.uk This is the site of the Florence Nightingale Museum.

feministvoices.com/profiles/carol-gilligan This site, Psychology's Feminist Voices, provides a brief overview of Carol Gilligan, a video-taped interview with her, and links to other media. www.fre ud.o rg.uk This is the website of the Freud Museum in London. It has pictures, publications, and links to other relevant sites.

www.humanbecoming.org The International Consortium of Parse Scholars' website has an overview of the humanbecoming theory and related research.

www.jungianstudies.org This is the site of the International Association of Jungian Studies, which will be of interest to those wanting to learn more about his work.

www.mcgill.ca/nursing/about/model This site offers information about the McGill model and its origins and examples of its application in nursing practice.

www.mentalhealthcommission.ca/English/recovery-signatories#anchor-indv-A The Recovery Declaration is here and may be signed at this site.

www.tidal-model.com The evolution of the Tidal Model and its core concepts are presented.

References

Abraham, S. (2011). Fall prevention conceptual framework. *The Health Care Manager, 30*(2), 179–184.

Ackerman, S., Zuroff, D. C., & Moskowitz, D. S. (2000). Generativity in midlife and young adults: Links to agency, communion, and subjective well-being. *International Journal of Aging and Human Development, 5*(1), 17–41.

Adler, A. (1963). *The practice and theory of individual psychotherapy.* Littlefield, Adams.

Afrasiabifar, A., Mehri, Z., & Shirazi, H. R. G. (2020). Orem's self-care model with multiple sclerosis patients' balance and motor function. *Nursing Science Quarterly, 33*, 46–54. https://doi.org10.1177/0894318419881792

Allen, M. (1977). Comparative theories of the expanded role in nursing and its implications for nursing practice: A working paper. *Nursing Papers/Perspectives in Nursing, 9*, 38–45.

Austin, W., Gallop, R., Harris, D., & Spencer, E. (1996). A domains of practice approach to the standards of psychiatric and mental health nursing practice. *Journal of Psychiatric and Mental Health Nursing, 3*, 111–115.

Başoğul, C., & Buldukoğlu, K. (2020). Neuman systems model with depressed patients: a randomized controlled trial. *Nursing Science Quarterly, 33*, 148–158. https://doi.org/10.1177/0894318419898172

Bandura, A. (1977). *Social learning theory.* Prentice-Hall.

Bandura, A. (1997). *Self-efficacy: The exercise of control.* W. H. Freeman and Company.

Barker, P. (2001a). The Tidal Model: The lived-experience in person-centred mental health nursing care. *Nursing Philosophy, 2*, 213–223.

Barker, P. (2001b). The Tidal Model: Developing a person-centred approach to psychiatric and mental health nursing. *Perspectives in Psychiatric Care, 37*, 79–87.

Barker, P., & Buchanan-Barker, P. (2005). *The Tidal Model: A guide for mental health professionals.* Brunner-Routledge.

Barker, P., & Buchanan-Barker, P. (2010). The Tidal Model of mental health recovery and reclamation: Application in acute care settings. *Issues in Mental Health Nursing, 31*, 171–180.

Barnhart, D. A., Bennett, P. M., Porter, B. D., & Sloan, R. S. (1994). Jean Watson: Philosophy and science of caring. In A. Marriner-Tomey (Ed.), *Nursing theorists and their work* (3rd ed., pp. 148–162). Mosby.

Beck, J. (2011). *Cognitive behavior therapy: Basics and beyond.* Guilford Press.

Beck, A. T., Thase, M. D., & Wright, J. H. (2003). Cognitive therapy. In R. E. Hales & S. C. Ydofsky (Eds.), *Textbook of clinical psychiatry* (4th ed., pp. 1245–1283). American Psychiatric Publishers, Inc.

Benner, P., & Wrubel, J. (1989). *The primacy of caring: Stress and coping in health and illness.* Addison-Wesley.

Biggs, A. (2008). Orem's self-care deficit nursing theory: Update on the state of the art and science. *Nursing Science Quarterly, 21*(3), 200–206.

Brookes, N., Murata, L., & Tansey, M. (2008). Tidal waves: Implementing a new model of mental health recovery and reclamation. *Canadian Nurse, 104*(8), 23–27.

Brown, L. (2010). *Feminist therapy.* American Psychiatric Association.

Buchanan-Barker, P., & Barker, P. (2008). The Tidal commitments: Extending the value base of mental health recovery. *Journal of Psychiatric and Mental Health Nursing, 15*, 93–100.

Calaway, B. J. (2002). *Hildegard Peplau: Psychiatric nurse of the century.* Springer.

Canadian Federation of Mental Health Nurses (CFMHN). (2014). *The Canadian standards of psychiatric and mental health nursing* (4th ed.).

Carabez, R., Eliason, M. J., & Martinson, M. (2016). Nurses' knowledge about transgender patient care: A qualitative study. *Advances in Nursing Science, 39*(3), 257–271.

Carabez, R., Pelligrini, M., Mankovitz, A., Eliason, M., Ciano, M., & Scott, M. (2015). "Never in all my years…": Nurses' education about LGBT Health. *Journal of Professional Nursing, 31*(4), 323–329.

Chesler, P. (1972). *Women and madness.* Doubleday.

Christiansen, S. L., & Palkovitz, R. (1998). Exploring Erikson's psychosocial theory and development: Generativity and its relationship to paternal identity, intimacy, and involvement in childcare. *Journal of Men's Studies, 7*(1), 133–156.

Clements, P., & Averill, J. (2006). Finding patterns of knowing in the work of Florence Nightingale. *Nursing Outlook, 54*, 268–274.

Coakley, A. B., Barron, A. M., & Annese, C. D. (2016). Exploring the experience and impact of therapeutic touch treatments for nurse colleagues. *Visions: The Journal of Rogerian Nursing Science, 22*(1), 13.

Cummins, J. (2011). Sharing a traumatic event. The experience of the listener and the storyteller within the dyad. *Nursing Research, 60*(6), 386–392.

Davis, A., & Maisano, P. (2016, November). Patricia Benner: Novice to expert—A concept whose time has come (Again). *The Oklahoma Nurse, 61*, 13–14.

Deane, W. H. (2015). Incorporating Peplau's theory of interpersonal relations to promote holistic communication between older adults and nursing students. *Journal of Holistic Nursing, 34*(1), 35–41.

DeHowitt, M. (1992). King's conceptual model and individual psychotherapy. *Perspectives in Psychiatric Care, 28*(4), 11–14.

DeWan, S. A., & Ume-Nwagbo, P. N. (2006). Using the Neuman systems model for best practices. *Nursing Science Quarterly, 19*(1), 31–35.

Doe, M. J. (2021). A Parsesciencing inquiry on hope. *Nursing Science Quarterly, 34*, 139–148. https://doi.org/10.1177/0894318420987187

Ellenberger, H. (1970). *The discovery of the unconscious: The history and evolution of dynamic psychiatry.* Penguin Press.

Ellis, A. (1973). *Humanistic psychotherapy: The rational-emotive approach.* McGraw-Hill.

Erikson, E. (1963). *Childhood and society* (2nd ed.). Norton.

Erikson, E. (1968). *Identity: Youth and crisis.* Norton.

Erikson, E., & Erikson, J. (1997). *The lifecycle completed, extended version.* Norton.

Feeley, N., & Gottlieb, L. (2000). Nursing approaches for working with family strengths and resources. *Journal of Family Nursing, 6*(1), 9–24.

Frankl, V. (1992). *Man's search for meaning: An introduction to logotherapy* (4th ed.). Beacon Press.

Freud, S. (1905). Three essays on the theory of sexuality (1953). In J. Strachey, A. Freud, A. Strachey, & A. Tyson (Eds.), *The standard edition of the complete psychological works of Sigmund Freud* (pp. 135–248). Hogarth Press.

Freud, S. (1927). The ego and the id (1957). In E. Jones (Ed.), *The international psycho-analytical library* (No. 12). Hogarth Press.

Freud, S. (1949). *An outline of psychoanalysis.* Norton.

Freud, S. (1955). *The interpretation of dreams.* Hogarth Press.

Georges, J. (2005). Linking nursing theory and practice: A critical-feminist approach. *Advances in Nursing Science, 28*(1), 30–57.

Gilligan, C. (1982). *In a different voice: Psychological theory and women's development.* Harvard University Press.

Gottlieb, L., & Rowat, K. (1987). The McGill model of nursing: A practice-derived model. *Advances in Nursing Science, 9*(4), 51–61.

Graham, R. (2012). Carol Gilligan's persistent "voice": Thirty years after the feminist classic "In a Different Voice" shook up psychology, do its claims hold up at all? *In the Boston Globe.* http://www.bostonglobe.com/

Henderson, V. (1966). *The nature of nursing: A definition and its implications for practice, research, and education.* Macmillan.

Hoffman, E. (Ed.). (1996). *Future visions: The unpublished papers of Abraham Maslow.* Sage Publications, Inc.

Horney, K. (1932). *Feminine psychology.* Norton.

Horney, K. (1939). *New ways in psychoanalysis.* Norton.

Horney, K. (1950). *Neurosis and human growth*. Norton.

Jung, C. G. (1959). *The basic writings of C. G. Jung*. Modern Library.

Jung, C. G. (1966). On the psychology of the unconscious: The personal and the collective unconscious. In C. Jung (Ed.), *Collected works of C. G. Jung* (2nd ed., Vol. 7, pp. 64–79). Princeton University Press.

King, I. M. (1971). *Toward a theory for nursing: General concepts of human behavior*. John Wiley and Sons.

King, I. M. (1981). *A theory for nursing: Systems, concepts, process*. John Wiley and Sons.

King, I. M. (1992). King's theory of goal attainment. *Nursing Science Quarterly, 5*(1), 19–26.

Kirby, M. J. L., & Keon, W. J. (2006). *Out of the shadows at last: Transforming mental health, mental illness and addiction services in Canada*. http://www.parl.gc.ca/39/1/parlbus/commbus/senate/com-e/soci-e/rep-e/rep02may06-e.htm

Kirkham, S. R., & Anderson, J. M. (2002). Postcolonial nursing scholarship: From epistemology to method. *Advances in Nursing Science, 25*(1), 1–17.

Knowaja, K. (2006). Utilization of King's interacting systems framework and theory of goal attainment with new multidisciplinary model: Clinical pathway. *Australian Journal of Advanced Nursing, 24*(2), 44–49.

Laben, J., Dodd, D., & Snead, L. (1991). King's theory of goal attainment applied in group therapy for inpatient juvenile sexual offenders, maximum security state offenders, and community parolees, using visual aids. *Issues in Mental Health Nursing, 12*(1), 51–64.

Leddy, S., & Pepper, J. M. (1998). *Conceptual basis of professional nursing* (4th ed.). Lippincott Williams & Wilkins.

Lego, S. (1973). Nurse psychotherapists: How are we different? *Perspectives in Psychiatric Care, 11*, 144–147.

Leininger, M. (1991). *Culture care diversity and universality: A theory of nursing*. National League for Nursing.

Leininger, M. (1993). Assumptive premises of the theory. In C. Reynolds & M. Leininger (Eds.), *Madeleine Leininger: Cultural care diversity and universality theory. Notes on nursing theories* (Vol. 8, pp. 15–30). Sage Publications, Inc.

Leininger, M. (1999). What is transcultural nursing and culturally competent care? *Journal of Transcultural Nursing, 10*(1), 9.

Lutjens, L. R. (1991a). *Callista Roy: An adaptation model*. Sage Publications, Inc.

Lutjens, L. R. (1991b). *Martha Rogers: The science of unitary human beings*. Sage Publications, Inc.

Maslow, A. (1970). *Motivation and personality* (rev. ed.). Harper & Brothers.

Maslow, A. (1998). *Toward a psychology of being* (3rd ed.). John Wiley & Sons.

Mental Health Commission of Canada. (2009). *Toward recovery and well-being: A framework for a mental health strategy for Canada*.

Mental Health Commission of Canada. (2015). *Guidelines for recovery-oriented practice: Hope. Dignity, Inclusion*. https://www.mentalhealthcommission.ca/sites/default/files/MHCC_RecoveryGuidelines_ ENG_0.pdf

Moonen, C., Lemiengre, J., & Gastmans, C. (2016). Dealing with existential suffering of patients with severe, persistent mental illness: Experiences of psychiatric nurses in Flanders (Belgium). *Archives of Psychiatric Nursing, 30*(2), 219–225.

Moore, B., & Fine, B. (Eds.). (1990). *Psychoanalytic terms and concepts*. American Psychoanalytic Association and Yale University Press.

Nelson, M. (1996). Separation versus connection, the gender controversy: Implications for counseling women. *Journal of Counseling and Development, 74*(4), 339–344.

Neuman, B. (1989). *The Neuman systems model* (2nd ed.). Appleton & Lange.

Neuman, B., Newman, D. M. L., & Holder, P. (2000). Leadership and scholarship integration: Using the Neuman system model for 21st-century professional nursing practice. *Nursing Science Quarterly, 13*(1), 60–63.

Nightingale, F. (1859). *Notes on nursing: What it is and what it is not*. Harrison, Bookseller to the Queen.

Ochse, R., & Plug, C. (1986). Cross-cultural investigation of the validity of Erikson's theory of personality development. *Journal of Personality and Social Psychology, 50*(6), 1240–1252.

Olowokere, A. E., & Okanlawon, F. A. (2015). Application of Neuman system model to psychosocial support of vulnerable school children. *West African Journal of Nursing, 26*(1), 14–25.

Olson, J., & Hanchett, E. (1997). Nurse-expressed empathy, patient outcomes, and the development of a middle-range theory. *Image: The Journal of Nursing Scholarship, 29*(1), 71–76.

Orem, D. (1991). *Nursing concepts of practice* (4th ed.). Mosby–Year Book.

Orlando, I. J. (1961). *The dynamic nurse–patient relationship*. G. P. Putnam's Sons.

Orlando, I. J. (1972). *The discipline and teaching of nursing process*. G. P. Putnam's Sons.

Orlofsky, J., Marcia, J., & Lesser, I. (1973). Ego identity status and the intimacy versus isolation crisis of young adulthood. *Journal of Personality and Social Psychology, 27*(2), 211–219.

Parse, R. R. (1987). *Nursing science: Major paradigms, theories, and critiques*. Saunders.

Parse, R. R. (2007). The humanbecoming school of thought in 2050. *Nursing Science Quarterly, 20*, 308–311.

Partlak Günüşen, N., Üstün, B., & Gigliotti, E. (2009). Conceptualization of burnout from the perspective of the Neuman systems model. *Nursing Science Quarterly, 22*(3), 200–204.

Pavlov, I. P. (1927/1960). *Conditioned reflexes*. Dover Publications.

Peplau, H. (1952). *Interpersonal relations in nursing*. G. P. Putnam & Sons.

Peplau, H. (1992). Interpersonal relations: A theoretical framework for application in nursing practice. *Nursing Science Quarterly, 5*(1), 13–18.

Perls, F. (1969). *In and out of the garbage pail*. Real People Press.

Piaget, J. (1936). *Origins of intelligence in the child*. Routledge & Kegan Paul.

Piaget, J. (1957). *Construction of reality in the child*. Kegan Paul.

Pickens, J. (2012). Development of self-care agency through enhancement of motivation in people with schizophrenia. *Self-Care, Dependent-Care & Nursing, 19*(1), 47–52.

Pratt, M., Norris, J., Cressman, K., Lawford, H., & Hebblethwaite, S. (2008). Parents' stories of grandparenting concerns in the three-generational family: Generativity, optimism, and forgiveness. *Journal of Personality, 76*(3), 581–604.

Rogers, M. E. (1970). *An introduction to the theoretical basis of nursing*. F.A. Davis.

Rogers, C. (1980). *A way of being*. Houghton Mifflin.

Rogers, M. E. (1994). The science of unitary human beings: Current perspectives. *Nursing Science Quarterly, 7*(1), 33–35.

Roy, C. (1974). The Roy adaptation model. In J. P. Riehl & C. Roy (Eds.), *Conceptual models for nursing practice* (pp. 135–144). Appleton-Century-Crofts.

Sagna, A. O., & Walker, L. O. (2020). Analysis of the Tidal Model and its implications in late-life suicidality. *Nursing Science Quarterly, 33*, 315–321. https://doi.org/10.1177/0894318420943139/10

Seed, M., & Torkelson, D. (2012). Beginning the recovery journey in acute psychiatric care: Using concepts from Orem's self-care deficit nursing theory. *Issues in Mental Health Nursing, 33*, 394–398.

Skinner, B. F. (1935). The generic nature of the concepts of stimulus and response. *Journal of General Psychology, 12*, 40–65.

Skinner, B. F. (1976). *Walden II*. Macmillan.

Summerell, P. (2015). P. Jean Watson's caritas processes: A model for transforming the nursing practice environment. *Critical Care Nurse, 35*(2), e66–e67.

Thompson, J. E. (1990). Finding the borderline's border: Can Martha Rogers help? *Perspectives in Psychiatric Care, 26*(4), 7–10.

Thorndike, E. L. (1916, c.1906). *The principles of teaching, based on psychology*. A. G. Seiler.

Titzer, J. L., Shirey, M. R., & Hauck, S. (2014). A nurse manager succession planning model with associated empirical outcomes. *Journal of Nursing Administration, 44*, 37–46. http://dx.doi.org/10.1097/NNA.0000000000000019

Travelbee, J. (1969). *Intervention in psychiatric nursing: Process in the one-to-one relationship*. F.A. Davis.

Travelbee, J. (1971). *Interpersonal aspects of nursing* (2nd ed.). F.A. Davis.

Truscott, D. (2010). *Becoming an effective psychotherapist: Adopting a theory of psychotherapy that is right for you and your client*. American Psychological Association.

Watson, J. (1979). *Nursing: The philosophy and science of caring* (2nd ed.). Little, Brown.

Watson, J. (1988). *Nursing: Human science and human care: A theory of nursing*. National League for Nursing.

Watson, J. (2005). *Caring science as sacred science*. F.A. Davis.

Watson, J. B., & Rayner, R. (1917). Emotional reactions and psychological experimentation. *American Journal of Psychology, 28*, 163–174.

Westermeyer, J. (2004). Predictors and characteristics of Erikson's Life Cycle Model among men: A 32-year longitudinal study. *International Journal of Aging and Human Development, 58*(1), 29–48.

Wilson, D. R. (2016). Parse's nursing theory and its application to families experiencing empty arms. *International Journal of Childbirth Education, 31*(2), 29–33.

Wright, L., & Leahey, M. (2013). *Nurses and families: A guide to family assessment and intervention* (6th ed.). F.A. Davis.

Yalom, I. D. (1980). *Existential psychotherapy*. Basic Books.

Yalom, I. D. (2005). *The Schopenhauer Cure*. Harper Collins.

10

Biologic Basis of Practice

Catherine A. Hamilton*

LEARNING OBJECTIVES

After studying this chapter, you will be able to:

- Identify ways in which the brain changes across the life span and affects behaviour.
- Describe the association between biologic functioning and symptoms of psychiatric disorders.
- Describe the approaches researchers have used to study the central nervous system and the significance of each approach.
- Locate the brain structures primarily involved in psychiatric disorders and describe the primary functions of these structures.
- Assess symptoms of common psychiatric disorders in terms of central nervous system functioning.
- Describe the mechanisms of neuronal transmission.
- Identify the location and function of neurotransmitters significant to hypotheses regarding major mental disorders.
- Discuss the basic utilization of new knowledge gained from fields of study, including psychoendocrinology, psychoimmunology, and chronobiology.
- Discuss the role of genetics in the development of psychiatric disorders.
- Describe the role of early adverse childhood experiences on brain development.

KEY TERMS

- adverse childhood experiences (ACES) • autonomic nervous system • basal ganglia • biogenic amines • biologic markers • chronobiology • cortex • epigenetics • frontal, parietal, temporal, and occipital lobes • genome • hippocampus • limbic system • neurohormones • neuroimaging • neuroplasticity • neuropeptides • polymorphism • psychoendocrinology • psychoneuroimmunology • receptors • symptom expression • synapse • zeitgebers

KEY CONCEPTS

- neurotransmitters • plasticity

All behaviours recognized as human result from actions that originate in the brain and its dense interconnection of neural networks. Modern research has increased understanding of how the complex circuitry of the brain interacts with the external environment, memories, and experiences. Through the spinal column and peripheral nerves, along with other systems, such as the endocrine and immune systems, the brain constantly receives and processes information. As the brain shifts and sorts through the profound amount of information it processes every hour, it decides on actions and initiates behaviours that allow each person to act in entirely unique and very human ways. As we age, our brain changes and, in turn, impacts our behaviour. See Table 10.1 for examples.

Foundational Concepts

This chapter is a review of the basic information necessary for understanding neuroscience as it relates to the role of the psychiatric and mental health (PMH) nurse. The review includes basic central nervous system (CNS) structures and functions, basic mechanisms of neurotransmission, general functions of the major neurotransmitters, basic structure and function of the endocrine system, genetic research, circadian rhythms, neuroimaging techniques, biologic tests, and how the environment influences brain development. This chapter was written with the assumption that the reader has a basic knowledge of human biology, anatomy, and pathophysiology.

*Adapted from the chapter "The Biologic Basis of Practice" by Anne Marie Creamer

Table 10.1	Brain Changes Across the Life Span	
Developmental Period	Some Brain Changes	Some Behavioural Changes
Gestational	By 3rd week gestation: formation of liquid-filled neural tube. First month: neuron production occurring at a maximum of 250,000 per minute. Around 14 weeks, neurons begin to migrate to form different brain areas, yet around 20 weeks, half of the cells are pruned. By birth, 100 billion neurons developed. Neural connections are immature but developing.	At birth, babies can hear, smell, see, and respond to touch. Prenatal stress, drugs, alcohol, and smoking impact brain development.
Early childhood to preschool	Rapid increase in synapses with strengthening in connections of those frequently used. Elimination of unused connections. Number of white matter neurons in the motor nervous system increases.	There is increasing range of more complex actions (e.g., lifting head to crawling to running).
School age	Growth to peak volume in some parts of the temporal lobes. Between 5 and 11 years, neural connections increase, especially in frontal, parietal, and temporal lobes associated with language and cognition.	The capacity to manage social situations increases. Many language and cognition milestones are reached between 5 and 11 years of age.
Adolescence	Continuing frontal lobe development. Areas involved in reward, motivation, and emotion developing. Unused connections are pruned.	Abstract reasoning develops. Intensity and urgency of emotions are heightened.
Young adulthood	Frontal lobe development involved in goal-directed behaviour matures. White matter connections increasing.	Mastery of impulse control and planning abilities occurs, and the ability to integrate information improves.
Pregnancy	Grey matter reductions in areas of social cognition lasting at least 2 years after birth. Hippocampus loses volume.	Promotes maternal attachment
Middle age	White matter connections strengthen. Temporal lobe white matter increases.	Abstract reasoning, math and special reasoning, and verbal abilities increase. Optimism and social appropriateness increase.
Menopause	Estrogen impacts neuron and synapse development; prefrontal cortex and hippocampus especially impacted.	Variable, but modest verbal memory loss. If ovaries removed surgically, more severe consequences
Old age	Some structures and areas shrink and less white matter.	Complex mental processes may be negatively affected. Speed of processing decreases. Vocabulary and experience-based knowledge remain strong.

Adapted from Rojahn, S. (2013). *Tracking brain connections in utero.* https://www.technologyreview.com/s/511551/tracking-brain-connections-in-utero/; Northeastern University. (2010). *Traumatic brain injury resource for survivors and caregivers.* http://www.northeastern.edu/nutraumaticbraininjury/braintbi-anatomy/brain-changes-over-the-lifespan/; Hara, Y., Waters, E., McEwen, B., & Morrison, J. (2015). Estrogen effects on cognitive and synaptic health over the lifecourse. *Physiological Reviews, 95,* 785–807. https://doi.org/10:1152/physrev.00036.2014; Sanders, L. (2016). Pregnancy linked to long-term changes in mom's brain: Loss of gray matter may aid in caring for baby. *Science News.* https://www.sciencenews.org/article/pregnancy-linked-long-term-changes-moms-brain

It is not intended as a full presentation of neuroanatomy and physiology but rather as an overview of the structures and functions most critical to the role of the PMH nurse.

The Biologic Basis of Behaviour, Emotions, and Cognition

As our understanding of the brain grows, evidence accumulates that most human behaviours, thoughts, and emotions have a biologic basis. Whether it is responding angrily to someone, impulsively making a purchase, or struggling to make a decision, behaviours are in large part rooted in the neurocircuitry of the brain. So, when maladaptive psychiatric symptoms manifest, for example, hallucinations, self-harm, talking in odd or unusual ways, we look to the brain. **Symptom expression** is a term referring to the behavioural symptoms seen in mental health disorders and the link to the neurobiologic basis of those symptoms. Because symptoms of

mental health disorders are expressed mainly through maladaptive behavioural symptoms and these symptoms are often linked to anomalies in brain functioning, nurses need to understand disease symptoms in relation to brain function.

Just as a breathing problem is often a symptom of a respiratory disorder, symptoms of mental health disorders often indicate CNS problems. Understanding this fundamental concept makes it much easier to understand the scientific rationale for many of the nursing care and treatment decisions presented in this book.

As you read this chapter, think about what you know about the symptoms of mental health disorders. Nurses must be able to make the connection between (a) a person's psychiatric symptoms, (b) the possible alteration in brain functioning linked to those symptoms, and (c) the rationale for treatment and care practices. Knowledge of the CNS is an essential aspect of modern PMH nursing.

IN-A-LIFE

Sidney Crosby and a Life-Changing Concussion

PUBLIC PERSONA

Called "the best player in the world," Sidney Crosby has played in the National Hockey League since he was 18 years old. In January 2011, attention was drawn to the risk of contact sports when, while playing for the Pittsburgh Penguins, he was struck on the head during a game. Later he described feeling "off, headaches, a little sick." Shortly after this, he was sidelined for the rest of the season because of a concussion, a form of traumatic brain injury (TBI). At the time of the injury, he was leading the NHL in scoring.

REALITIES

Concussions are a common sports injury, but they are not detectable by x-rays, magnetic resonance imagings (MRIs), or computed tomography (CT) scans. They occur when the person is hit on the head or face or through a whiplash injury. When this happens, the brain strikes the inside of the skull and is bruised by hitting the inside of the skull on one side and then again on the opposite side when the brain bounces back from the initial jostle. As a result, the

person may suffer physical, cognitive, or emotional symptoms after the injury. In some cases, the symptoms can last for years. In 2010–2011, there were 2,766 hospitalizations in Canada for concussion-related injuries (Morrish & Carey, 2013). During 2016–2017, approximately 46,000 children and youth were diagnosed with concussion in Canadian hospital ERs (Government of Canada, 2018). June is declared Brain Injury Awareness Month in Canada because of the high rate of incidence. Sidney Crosby, after missing 2 years of play, is back in the game.

Sources: Government of Canada. (2018). *Concussion in sport: Sport and recreation-related traumatic brain injuries among Canadian children and youth.* For excellent information on "Concussion in Sport" see: https://www.canada.ca/en/public-health/services/diseases/concussion-sign-symptoms/concussion-sport-infographic. Retrieved February 6, 2021.

Graves, W. (2013, January 15). *Sidney Crosby says he's free of concussion symptoms.* Associated Press. http://www.cbc.ca/sports/hockey/nhl/sidney-crosby-says-he-s-free-of-concussion-symptoms-1.1400543

Morrish, J., & Carey, S. (2013). *Concussions in Canada. Canada injury compass.* Parachute.

Wyshynski, G. (2011). *Sidney Crosby talks concussion, "irresponsible" blind side hits and when Penguins knew about injury.* http://ca.sports.yahoo.com/nhl/blog/puck_daddy/post/Sidney-Crosby-talks-concussion-irresponsible-?urn=nhl-305051

The Role of Genetics in Mental Health Disorders

It has long been observed that family members of persons with a major mental health disorder, such as schizophrenia, bipolar disorder, and panic disorder, have an increased risk for the same disorder. As early as 1823, the archives of London's Bethlehem Royal Hospital (Bedlam) note physicians needed to identify whether there was a hereditary component to the person's illness (McGuffin & Southwick, 2003). Animal models have greatly increased the ability of researchers to understand the influence of genetics on symptom expression in mental health disorders, and many of the common mental health disorders that nurses encounter have a known genetic component. As knowledge of the **genome** increases, treatments that work at the genetic level are being developed (Oedegaard et al., 2016).

Genetic *processes* control how humans develop from a single-cell egg into an adult human. Genes control the regrowth of hair and skin cells, the growth and connection of nervous system cells, and our biologic reaction to stress, among other processes. Genes make humans dynamic organisms, capable of growth, change, and development. The Human Genome Project, completed in 2003, mapped the complete set of human genes, or **H**,

carried by all of us and transmitted to our offspring. There are approximately 30,000 genes in the human genome, with the brain accounting for only about 1% of the body's DNA. The completed human genome provides researchers with a map of the exact sequence of the 3 billion nucleotide bases that make up human organisms. If printed out, the entire human genome sequence would fill approximately a million pages. The genome map is used to study the function of specific genes and their disease-inducing capacity when they malfunction. Also to come from the Human Genome Project is a catalogue of common human genetic variations, called the HapMap (short for "haplotype map") that will help researchers understand the common genetic patterns related to human health and disease.

A single gene is made of short segments of DNA packed with the "instructions" for making proteins that have a specific function. Genes do not directly control nerve function on a cellular level. Rather the genes control the proteins that regulate neural functioning. This allows nerve function to change as individual nerve cells respond to neurochemical changes outside the cell and produce different proteins in adaptation to the new environment. This dynamic nature of gene function highlights the way in which the body and the environment interact and how environmental factors influence gene expression. The diathesis–stress model holds that the diathesis (derived from a Greek word for "disposition" or "vulnerability") or biologic risk(s) interacts with environmental stressors and, depending on how successful the compensatory mechanisms work, a mental health disorder may or may not develop.

When genes are absent or malfunction, protein production is altered, and bodily functions are disrupted. A gene or part of a gene can be altered and, when this change occurs commonly and affects human behaviour, it is called a **polymorphism** (Quigley, 2015). For example, recent research demonstrates persons with schizophrenia are at risk for a genetic subtype of schizophrenia called 22q11.2 deletion syndrome, in which there is a deletion on part of chromosome 22 (Merico et al., 2015). This deletion has been linked to other abnormalities, including craniofacial and cardiovascular alterations and behavioural and learning disorders.

Population Genetics

Much of what we know about the genetics of mental health disorders is from studies that trace given disorders within groups of people. This technique, called population genetics, involves the analysis of genetic transmission of a trait within families and populations to determine risks and patterns of transmission. This is achieved by comparing the occurrence of a given disorder in the general population to the occurrence of that disorder within families and between groups of relatives. These studies rely on the initial identification of an individual who has the disorder and include the following principal methods:

- **Family studies** analyze the occurrence of a disorder in first-degree relatives (biologic parents, siblings, and children), second-degree relatives (grandparents, uncles, aunts, nieces, nephews, and grandchildren), and so on.
- **Twin studies** analyze the presence or absence of the disorder in pairs of twins. The *concordance rate* is the measure of similarity of occurrence in individuals with similar genetic makeup.
- **Adoption studies** compare the occurrence of a disorder in separated siblings raised in different environments. The strongest inferences may be drawn from studies that involve children separated from their parents at birth.

Some traits are completely inheritable. For example, monozygotic (identical) twins have identical genetic contributions, and therefore, both would have the same blood type, if they expressed that gene. This is 100% concordance. If a disorder is unrelated to genetics, then monozygotic twins would have the same concordance rates as dizygotic (fraternal) twins, who share roughly 50% of genes, as do ordinary siblings. If the environment influences the genetic contribution, the concordance rates would be less than 100% for monozygotic twins but significantly greater than for dizygotic twins.

Although no conclusive evidence exists for a complete genetic cause of most mental health disorders, significant evidence suggests that strong genetic contributions exist for most (Pirooznia et al., 2012). It is likely that mental health disorders are *polygenic*. This means that more than one gene is involved in producing the disorder and the disorder develops from genes interacting with each other, which produces a risk factor, and from environmental influences that lead to the expression of the illness. The environmental factors include conditions such as stress, infections, poor nutrition, catastrophic loss, complications during pregnancy, and exposure to toxins. Thus, in the at-risk individual, genetic composition creates vulnerability, or a risk for the disorder, and the environmental factors are present for the disease to develop. Additionally, specific genes may convey risk for more than one disorder (Agius & Aquilina, 2014).

Using the human genome map and databases containing human samples of DNA sequences, markers for genetic variations associated with particular disorders can be identified. Research studies using these tools are called genome-wide association studies. For example, APOE 4, a genetic polymorphism, is found in approximately 15% of the population and is linked to increased risk for atherosclerosis and Alzheimer disease. The next step in making this research applicable is to find out whether one treatment works better in those with different genetic profiles. However, these studies remain controversial, and it is important to keep in mind that mental health disorders are not determined by one polymorphism but rather by a complex interaction between the multiple genes and the environment.

When considering information regarding risks for genetic transmission of mental health disorders, it is important to remember several key points:

- Mental health disorders have been described and labeled differently across generations, and errors in diagnosis may occur.
- Similar psychiatric symptoms may arise from different causes, just as chest pain may originate in cardiac or gastrointestinal conditions.
- Even though a gene may be present, the expression of that trait may not occur.
- A gene alteration may express as different symptoms in different people.
- Several genes work together in an individual to produce a given trait or disorder.
- A mental health disorder is not always only genetic in origin. Environmental influences alter the body's function and often mediate or worsen genetic risk factors.

As public awareness of genetic evidence grows, it is likely that nurses will be faced with persons and/or family members requesting genetic testing or needing information regarding their risk for a mental health disorder. As a result, nurses increasingly require a greater understanding of the role genetics play in mental health disorders.

Epigenetics

Epigenetics (*epi* meaning "above") is the study of the mechanisms by which gene expression is modified without changes in an organism's genetic (DNA) sequence. The term was first coined in 1942 by Conrad Waddington (1957), with 21st-century science making significant advances in this area. The long-held nature versus nurture debate is now known to be not about "either/or," but rather about the interaction between the two. Stem cell and other research reveals cell development is highly flexible and plastic (Shah & Allegrucci, 2013).

It has been known for some time that all cells in an individual organism have the identical genetic makeup (genotype) but can function in radically different ways (e.g., as a heart cell, a skin cell, a brain cell, etc.). As influences (environmental, lifestyle) on the genotype occur prenatally and across the life span, cell genes are distinctively expressed (phenotype) (Marques & Fleming Outeiro, 2013). An individual's *epigenome* is a set of chemicals that may dynamically alter the person's genome (complete set of DNA) in a way that determines genetic expression (how gene information is used) (National Human Genome Research Institute, 2013). Epigenetic phenomena are related to chromatin structure and organization, chromatin being the protein–DNA complex that makes up the nucleus of a cell. The epigenome "marks" (meaning turns on or off) the genome through a variety of processes such as DNA methylation and histone acetylation, which may down-regulate or up-regulate gene expression, respectively, or histone methylation and phosphorylation, which may activate or repress protein transcription; gene expression can also be silenced by RNA, a nucleic acid (Tafet & Nemeroff, 2016). Additionally, it is now understood these epigenetic alterations to the genome do not only affect the person in whom the changes originally occur but also may affect their offspring through transgenerational inheritance (Legoff et al., 2019).

Epigenetic changes are necessary to development and health, but some may trigger disease. It was in 1983 that evidence of a link between epigenetic changes and disease was first noted when persons with colorectal cancer were found to have less DNA methylation in their diseased tissue than in their normal tissue (Simmons, 2008).

Epigenetics is a key research area in the quest to understand health, aging, and disease (Kundu, 2013), as these mechanisms are now recognized as affecting individuals across the life span. The Genome Canada and Canadian Epigenetics, Environment and Health Research Consortium, as an initiative of Canadian Institutes of Health Research (CIHR), supports research on the role of DNA

and environment interactions in human health and disease (Canadian Institutes of Health Research, 2020; Genome Canada, 2017). The growing understanding of these interactions has sparked an expansion of studies that link epigenetic changes to areas of health care as diverse as cancer, dementia, human reproduction, neurodegenerative disease, and aging (Fenoglio et al., 2018; Franzago et al., 2019; Gangisetty et al., 2018; Joosten et al., 2018). Also emerging as an area of debate is Social Epigenetics, which evaluates the effect of social inequality, including poverty, food insecurity and inadequate housing, on the epigenome of the individual (Loi et al., 2013).

Epigenetic research in the field of psychiatry and mental health is abundant. Early on, Labonté et al. (2013) identified that there were DNA methylation changes in the hippocampal DNA of individuals who had completed suicide. Emerging science indicates that relationships between epigenetic marks and mental health may occur over the life course; however, the sensitive developmental stages, such as the prenatal, early life, and adolescence periods, are most vulnerable (Szyf, 2019). The impact of adverse early life epigenetic marks, which when later in life are triggered by stress, may increase the risk of psychopathic behavioral phenotypes, such as schizophrenia, bipolar disorder, and PTSD (DeSocio, 2018; Kim et al., 2018). More positively, evidence that damage of early adversity may be mediated has sparked research aimed at early epigenetic detection, prevention, and intervention to more effectively address mental health disorders (Kumsta, 2019; Rodriguez-Paredes & Esteller, 2011). See Box 10.1 for information on the effects of adverse childhood experiences.

Risk Factors

The concept of genetic susceptibility suggests that an individual may be at increased risk for a mental health disorder. Research into risk factors is an important avenue of study. Just as knowledge of risk factors for diabetes and heart disease led to the development of preventive interventions, learning more about risk factors for mental health disorders will lead to prevention, detection, and interventional care practices. Specific risk factors for mental health disorders are becoming more understood, and some of the environmental influences listed previously may be examples of risk factors. These events, circumstances, or demographic features are more likely to occur in individuals who experience a particular mental health disorder. In the absence of one specific gene for major mental health disorders, risk factor assessment may be a logical alternative for predicting who is more likely to experience psychiatric disorders or certain conditions such as aggression or suicidality. This is a growing area of PMH nursing; nurses serve an important role in mental health promotion, illness prevention, care delivery, and research.

BOX 10.1 Adverse Childhood Experiences (ACEs)

Don't ask "What's wrong with you?," ask "What has happened to you?"

The Brain

The phenomenon of **adverse childhood experiences** (ACEs) was described by Drs. Felitti and Anda and their team in 1998 and is based on research into how the brain changes due to early life adversity and the resultant health and behavioral effects of this adversity. At birth, neuronal networks in the infant brain are sparse. As children grow and develop in the world around them, these networks become more complex and specialized in response to what they most experience. Over time, the most stimulated networks become more robust, and those that are least used withdraw around the time of puberty.

The Adversity

In this model, adversity is defined by types of neglect, abuse, and household dysfunction. If children have experienced adversity in their early environment, then pathways of fear and trauma are reinforced, and their developing brain cells and connections are damaged. Additionally, the brain is bathed in stress hormones, such as cortisol, which can cause the brain cells to die. When impaired, neuronal pathways and development of the limbic system, which includes the amygdala and **hippocampus**, may result in heightened fight-or-flight response, difficulties learning, poor executive function, and difficulties forming relationships. These maladaptive behaviours, among others that may also result, can last a lifetime.

The Consequences

Types of ACEs most often occur together. Research has found resounding positive associations between the number of ACEs experienced by the individuals in a population and many varied chronic physical and mental health disorders in children and adults, such as depression, anxiety, obesity, heart disease, diabetes, and suicide. Social challenges such as homelessness and poverty are also significant. These findings have led some experts to view ACEs as the root cause of many of the health and social conditions faced in society today. In response, three mediating factors are identified: individual capabilities, attachment and belonging, and community, faith and cultural processes. In our nursing practice, we must be diligent in our understanding of the profound, and sometimes unrelenting, effects of a person's early childhood experiences on their mental health and behaviour.

References

Anda, R. F., Felitti, V. I., Brenner, J. D., Walker, J. D., Whitfield, C., Perry, B. D., Dube, S. R., & Giles, W. H. (2006). The enduring effects of abuse and related adverse experiences in childhood: A convergence of evidence from neurobiology and epidemiology. *European Archives of Psychiatry and Clinical Neuroscience, 256*(3), 174–186.

Felitti, V. I., Anda, R. F., Nordenburg, D., Williamson, D. F., Spitz, A. M., Edwards, V., Koss, M. P., & Marks, J. S. (1998). Relationship of childhood abuse and household dysfunction to many of the leading causes of death in adults: The adverse childhood experiences (ACE) study. *American Journal of Preventative Medicine, 14*(4), 245–258.

Current Research Approaches and Advances

Neuroscience researchers have applied several approaches to the study of the CNS structure and function. These approaches occur with both human research and animal models. The approaches, highlighted in Table 10.2, include the following:

- Comparative
- Developmental
- Chemoarchitectural
- Cytoarchitectural
- Functional

These different approaches to studying the CNS have significantly increased our understanding of its normal functioning and how a disease affects behaviour and contributes to the development of psychiatric disorders.

Research shows that areas of the brain, and the groups of nerve cells that constitute that area, often work together as functional units. A hierarchy of function exists in which primary sensory input is used in an increasingly more complex and integrated manner across areas of the brain. In addition, some areas of the brain, such as those that control basic levels of alertness and attention, must work correctly for information to be received, understood, and used by higher levels of the brain to organize a response. The brain's functional units work together to control or contribute to specific behaviours or emotions.

The *integrated approach* to brain development is the term used to describe the interactive working of brain areas and function. Understanding the work as an integration of parts allows us to understand that specific areas of the brain control specific functions. For example, there is a speech area in the brain, a mood area, an

Table 10.2   Approaches to the Study of Neuroanatomy

Approach	Purpose	Potential Limitations
Comparative	Explores and compares behaviour across animal nervous systems, from a simple primitive cordlike structure in some species to the large complex structure of the human brain	Difficult to correlate animal behaviour to human, especially emotional New brain structures do not necessarily correlate to new behaviour.
Developmental	Studies nervous system structure within an individual or species of animal across different stages of development	Impossible to follow one human being's neuronal development Individual variation in development complicates comparisons of individuals across a specific point of time in development.
Chemoarchitectural	Identifies differences in location of neurochemicals such as neurotransmitters throughout the brain	Boundaries between regional changes are subtle and may vary across individuals.
Cytoarchitectural	Identifies differences or variations in cell type, structure, and density throughout the brain, mapping these variations by location	Boundaries between regional changes are subtle and may vary across individuals.
Functional	Identifies location of predominant control over various behavioural functions within the brain Studies often conducted based on dysfunction from a localized injury to the brain	Several regions or structures within the brain may contribute to one behaviour, making predominant control difficult to assign. Controversy exists in correlating normal brain function to damaged brain tissue.

appetite area, and so on. Understanding the functions of areas of the brain allows nurses to assess a person's symptoms largely as the expression of a problem in a specific brain area. Just as a person with an irregular heartbeat is experiencing disruption in normal cardiac function, a person who fails to eat because of depression is experiencing a disruption in the brain's normal appetite and mood function.

Neuroplasticity is an important concept when describing brain function. The changes in neural environment can come from internal sources such as a change in electrolytes or from external sources such as exercise, toxins, and viruses. With neuroplasticity, nerve signals may be rerouted, cells may learn new functions and gain sensitivity, the number of cells may increase or decrease, and some nerve tissue may, to some extent, be regenerated. Neuroplasticity contributes to understanding how

function may be restored over time after brain damage occurs or how an individual may react over time to psychotherapy or a continuous pharmacotherapy regimen.

There are several behavioural principles that may impact brain plasticity (see Table 10.3). For example, brains are most plastic during infancy and early childhood, when large adaptive learning tasks should normally occur. With age, brains become less plastic, which explains why it is easier to learn a second language at the age of 5 years than at 55 years. Brains are still capable of change, though; when nurses teach mindful attention to breathing, they are promoting positive brain change, likely in the amygdala–dorsal prefrontal cortex pathways (Doll et al., 2016). Understanding these principles provides a framework for nurses coaching new emotional, cognitive, and behavioural skills.

Table 10.3   Principles of Experience-Derived Brain Plasticity

Principle	Example
1. Use it or lose it	Brain circuits not used in task performance over time can decay.
2. Use it and improve it	Through extended training, brain plasticity can be induced.
3. Learning something new	Repeating something already learned does not induce plasticity but learning something new will.
4. Repeat, repeat, repeat	Repeating a new or relearned skill may be needed to induce long-term changes.
5. Be intense but not too intense	Training too intensely can worsen things; balance is needed.
6. Brain age matters	Plasticity occurs more easily in a younger brain.
7. Timing matters	Certain types of plasticity change follow a pattern.
8. A little can go a long way	Plasticity in one set of neurons can promote ongoing development in the same or other areas of the brain.
9. Make it important	Motivation and attention are important mediators.
10. Plasticity in one form can block a different plasticity within the same circuit	Developing brain circuits to do one skill may block learning another.

Adapted from Kleim, J., & Jones, T. (2008). Principles of experience-dependent neural plasticity: Implications for rehabilitation after brain damage. *Journal of Speech, Language, and Hearing Research, 51*, S225–S239.

KEY CONCEPT

Plasticity is the ability of the brain to change its structure and function in response to internal and external pressures.

Neuroimaging

Since the 1980s, technologic advances in **neuroimaging** techniques have been a major aid to the current understanding of how the human brain functions. As knowledge grows, neuroimaging techniques are moving from research to routine clinical use, requiring nurses to understand this technology. Two basic neuroimaging methods are structural and functional neuroimaging. See Table 10.4 for methods of neuroimaging.

Structural Neuroimaging

Structural neuroimaging techniques were the first form of neuroimaging that allowed visualization of brain structures. Structural images show what normal structures of the brain look like and allow clinicians to identify tissue abnormalities, changes, or damages. Commonly used structural neuroimaging techniques include computed

Table 10.4	Methods of Neuroimaging		
Method	**Description**	**Considerations**	
Structural Imaging			
Computed tomography (CT), also called computed axial tomography (CAT)	Uses x-ray technology to measure tissue density; is readily available; can be completed quickly, and less costly; may be used for screening, but many disease states are not clearly seen; use of contrast medium improves resolution	Contrast medium may produce allergic reactions; individuals with increased risk for contrast media complications include those with: History of previous reactions Cardiac disease Hypertension Diabetes Sickle cell disease Contraindications for use of contrast: Iodine/shellfish allergies Renal disease Pregnancy	
Magnetic resonance imaging (MRI)	Uses a magnetic field to magnetize hydrogen atoms in soft tissue, changing their alignment—this creates a tiny electric signal, which can be received to produce an image; produces greater resolution than a CT, diagnosing more subtle pathologic changes	Individuals may experience headaches, dizziness, and nausea; symptoms of anxiety, claustrophobia, or psychosis can increase; contraindicated when the person has aneurysm clips, internal electrical, magnetic, or mechanical devices such as pacemakers, metallic surgical clips, sutures, or dental work, which distort the image; claustrophobia.	
Functional Neuroimaging			
Positron emission tomography (PET)	Uses positron emitting isotopes (very short-lived radioactive entities such as oxygen-15) to image brain functioning; isotopes are incorporated into specific molecules to study cerebral metabolism, cerebral blood flow, and specific neurochemicals	Images appear blurry, lacking anatomic detail, but have been extremely useful in research to study distribution of neuroreceptors and the action of pharmacologic agents; invasive procedure, use of radioactivity limits the number of scans done with a single individual	
Single-photon emission computed tomography (SPECT)	Like PET, SPECT uses radioisotopes that produce only one photon; data are collected as a three-dimensional volume, and two-dimensional images can be constructed on any plane; less expensive than PET technology	Less resolution and sensitivity than the PET, but inhalation methods may be used, allowing for some repeated studies; useful in drug dependency research	
Functional magnetic resonance imaging (fMRI)	Combines spatial resolution of MRI with the ability to image neural activity; can show sequential, movie-type images of blood flow in the brain as it is happening; shows whether brain activity occurs simultaneously or sequentially in different areas of the brain while engaged in selected activities	Requires no radiation and can be completely noninvasive; individual can be imaged many times, in different clinical states, before or after treatments; removes many of the ethical constraints when studying children and adolescents with psychiatric disorders	
Magnetic resonance spectroscopy (MRS)	Uses the same imaging equipment as the fMRI; by altering scanning parameters, signals represent specific chemicals in the brain	Noninvasive, repeatable, may be ideal for longitudinal studies, but has limited spatial resolution, especially with molecules that occur in low concentrations	

tomography (CT) scanning and magnetic resonance imaging (MRI). Although these techniques are useful in identifying what the brain looks like, they do not reveal anything about how the brain works.

Computed Tomography

CT (also referred to as computed axial tomography or CAT) scanning first allowed scientists and clinicians to see structures inside the brain without more invasive and potentially dangerous methods. CT scans still use an x-ray beam passed through the head in serial slices. High-speed computers measure the decreased strength in the x-ray beam that results from absorption, and the computer assigns a shade of grey that reflects that change. The degree of energy absorbed by a tissue is proportionally related to its density. For example, cerebrospinal fluid (CSF) absorbs the least, so it appears the darkest, whereas bone absorbs the most and appears light. The computer then develops a 3D x-ray image. This technique is good at detecting skull fractures and injuries or abnormalities such as a subdermal hematoma requiring surgery. White matter and grey matter are more difficult to discriminate with CT technology.

CT scans can be done with or without contrast material. Contrast materials are used to increase the visibility of certain tissues or blood vessels. If a contrast agent is used, an iodinated or other material is intravenously administered to enhance the CT image. Although CT scanning is a relatively safe, noninvasive procedure, the contrast material may have some adverse side effects in some individuals. Some receiving contrast materials report a metallic taste in the mouth, mild nausea, rashes, or joint pain. In rare instances, severe allergic responses, including anaphylaxis, may develop, so nurses must closely monitor individuals who have received contrast materials. Radiation exposure by a CT scan is approximately 400 times that of a standard chest x-ray (Miglioretti & Simth-Bindman, 2011). In addition, because the CT equipment itself may be frightening, prior to the scan, the nurse should educate the person about what to expect. Some may need to be accompanied by a nurse during the procedure for ongoing reassurance.

Magnetic Resonance Imaging

MRI is performed by placing the individual into a long tube that contains powerful magnets. The magnetic field causes hydrogen-containing molecules (primarily water) to line up and move in symmetric ways around their axes. The magnetic field is then interrupted in pulses, causing the molecules to turn 90 or 180 degrees. Electromagnetic energy is released when the molecules return to their original position. The energy released is related to the density of the tissue and is detected by the MRI device, resulting in a scan measurement of the density of the examined tissue. The MRI can produce

three-dimensional images extremely clearly, allowing for gross discrimination of white and grey matters, detection of subacute hemorrhages, and rough areas of white matter damage. Sometimes, contrast material is used.

MRI scans produce more information than CT images, but MRI scans are more complicated and costly. In addition, MRI scans cannot be used for all people. Because MRI uses magnet energy, individuals with pacemakers, aneurysm clips, or other metal in their body may not be able to undergo the procedure; pregnant women also cannot have MRI scans. The loud noise of the equipment and the very narrow tube in which the person must lie still can trigger claustrophobic responses in some people. Adequate preparation of the person by the nurse should eliminate any surprises. Assistance with shallow breathing techniques, mental distractions, or other anxiety-reducing strategies may help. Many MRI facilities are equipped with music to mask the whirring of the equipment and provide a distraction through the lengthy testing period. Some tubes are now being made of clear plastic to decrease the claustrophobic sensation.

Diffusion Tensor Magnetic Resonance Imaging

This special type of MRI produces information on white matter not presently available through any other techniques (Fig. 10.1). It cannot show what is happening to individual neurons, but it can identify what is happening at the fibre bundle level. The images are based on microscopic movement of water protons in tissues (Shenton et al., 2012). Water moves freely in CSF but is more restricted by other structures such as axons and myelin sheaths. Water can move more freely in a direction parallel to the axon but less freely perpendicular to the axon. Therefore, the directions of the axons will determine the direction of the water diffusion. If, for

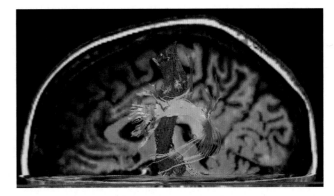

Figure 10.1 Diffusion tensor imaging (DTI). DTI is specifically useful in evaluating white matter tracts because of the highly directional diffusion in normal white matter bundles. Diffusion tractography can be used to visualize specific white matter tracts. Here, a sagittal 3D view shows corticospinal tracts (*blue*) and superior longitudinal fasciculus (*green*) tracts in a normal subject.

example, diffusion in the white matter is found to be less restricted than expected, it can mean that the myelin sheaths or axons are damaged or less dense. Diffusion tensor imaging cannot identify the cause of the diffusion changes. This technology is being used to investigate white matter changes in schizophrenia, dementia, and other mental health disorders. Ongoing developments in this technique will allow scientists to visualize and measure damage in fibre tracts connecting different brain regions.

Functional Neuroimaging

Although structural imaging identifies what the brain looks like, the scans do not show how the brain is working. Functional neuroimaging techniques measure physiologic activities, providing insight into how the brain works. These methods let researchers study such activities as cerebral blood flow, neuroreceptor location and function, and distribution patterns of specific chemicals within the brain. Single-photon emission computed tomography (SPECT) and positron emission tomography (PET) are the primary methods used to observe metabolic functioning.

Both procedures require administering radioactive substances that emit charged particles, which are then measured by scanning equipment. SPECT and PET differ in the type of isotopes used, the method of measuring isotope uptake, and therefore the equipment used. Because these procedures measure function, the person is usually asked to perform specific tasks during the test. The commonly used Wisconsin Card Sorting Test requires the individual to sort cards with different numbers, colours, and shapes into piles based on specified rules. This task requires the use of the brain's frontal lobe, an important area for concept formation and decision making and an area that often is disrupted in many psychiatric disorders.

CAUTION: Pregnant healthcare workers should avoid caring for individuals who have had a nuclear scan for 24 hr after the scan. Caregivers need to check their institution's guide for other safety precautions when caring for individuals who have been exposed to nuclear material.

Single-Photon Emission Computed Tomography

SPECT is a nuclear imaging scan that integrates CT and a radioactive tracer that may be applied to measure regional cerebral blood flow. SPECT scans have been shown to be effective in evaluating blood flow in the brains of individuals with Parkinson disease (PD) and depression. Researchers have been able to identify brain areas that were perfused differently in individuals with depression when compared to the brains of those who had PD but were not depressed (Kim et al., 2016). SPECT scans are also used to confirm changes in cerebral blood

flow caused by certain drugs. For example, caffeine and nicotine cause a generalized decrease in cerebral blood flow. Additionally, compounds have been developed to visualize the numbers or density of receptors in various areas of the brain, which may assist in understanding the effects of psychopharmacologic medications and neuroplastic changes in brain tissue over time.

Positron Emission Tomography

PET uses a radioactively charged particle (most commonly glucose) to measure that particle's activity in various brain regions. Because cells use glucose as fuel for cellular action, the higher the rate of glucose use detected by the PET scan, the higher the rate of metabolic activity in different areas of the brain. Abnormalities in glucose consumption, indicating more or less cellular activity, are found in Alzheimer disease, seizures, strokes, malignancies, and a number of mental health disorders. Scanning may be performed while the individual is at rest or performing a cognitive task. PET scans are often used to measure regional cerebral blood flow and neurotransmitter system functions.

Bridging the Structure–Function Gap

As structural and functional neuroimaging techniques advance, attempts are being made to develop imaging procedures that detail structure and function at the same time. Magnetic resonance spectroscopy (MRS) and functional magnetic resonance imaging (fMRI) are examples. The fMRI is useful for showing structure while localizing function and providing high-resolution images. Similar to other forms of neuroimaging, the fMRI is noninvasive, but it requires no radioactive agent, making it economical and safer than PET and SPECT.

MRS uses the same machinery as fMRI and provides precise and clear images of neuronal membranes as well as measures of metabolic cellular function (Currie et al., 2013). In addition to these procedures, magnetoencephalography (MEG) is being used. MEG testing records magnetic fields generated by neuronal activity. These results are paired with a technique that images anatomical information such as MRI, to provide both the structural and functional information. Table 10.4 summarizes these neuroimaging methods. These neuroimaging procedures are becoming useful in clinical practice.

Transcranial magnetic stimulation (TMS) is a treatment tool that painlessly delivers an alternating current through a metal coil placed around the scalp. The current causes a magnetic field to be generated, and this induces an electrical current that changes firing along neurons. Depending on where and at what frequency the treatment is applied, areas of the brain may be inhibited or excited. TMS is approved in Canada for treatment-resistant depression and in the United States for depression, obsessive–compulsive disorder, migraine, and smoking cessation. It is found to be well tolerated; however, adverse effects can include skin burns and lesions and, in some, depression may switch to mania (Holtzheimer, 2013). TMS has been used to investigate plasticity, medication effects, and nervous propagation along nerves. Additionally, it has been used in rehabilitation and operative settings.

Neuroanatomy of the Central Nervous System

With advances in brain science comes greater understanding of the biologic basis of mental illnesses. Therefore, nurses must increasingly be aware of the anatomic intricacy of the CNS as a foundation for modern psychiatric nursing assessments and interventions.

Although this section discusses each functioning area of the brain separately, each area is intricately connected and functions interactively with the others. The CNS contains the brain, brainstem, and spinal cord, whereas the total human nervous system includes the peripheral nervous system (PNS) as well. The PNS consists of the neurons that connect the CNS to the muscles, organs, and other systems in the periphery of the body. Whatever affects the CNS may also affect the PNS, and vice versa.

Cerebrum

The largest part of the human brain, the cerebrum, fills the entire upper portion of the cranium. The **cortex,** or outermost surface of the cerebrum, makes up about 80% of the human brain. The cortex is several millimetres thick and is composed of cell bodies mixed with capillary blood vessels. This mixture makes the cortex grey-brown, hence the term *grey matter*. The cortex contains bumps and grooves in a fully developed adult brain, as shown in Figure 10.2. This "wrinkling" allows for a large amount of surface area to be confined in the limited space of the skull. The increased surface area allows for more potential connections between cells within the cortex. The grooves are called *fissures* if they extend deep into the brain and *sulci* if they are shallower. The bumps or convolutions are called *gyri*. Together, they provide many of the landmarks for the subdivisions of the cortex. The longest and deepest groove, the longitudinal fissure, separates the cerebrum into left and right hemispheres. Although these two divisions are nearly symmetric, there is some variation in the location and size of the sulci and gyri in each hemisphere. Substantial variation in these convolutions is found in the cortex of different individuals.

Left and Right Hemispheres

The cerebrum can be roughly divided into two halves, or hemispheres. Each hemisphere controls functioning mainly on the opposite side of the body. For about 95% of people, the left hemisphere is dominant, whereas about 5% of individuals have mixed dominance. The right hemisphere provides input into receptive nonverbal communication, spatial orientation, and recognition;

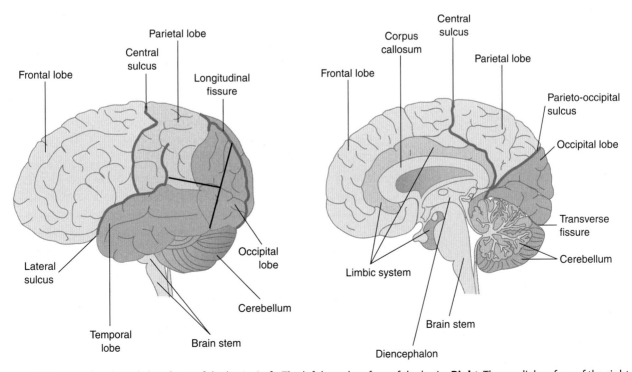

Figure 10.2 Lateral and medial surfaces of the brain. **Left.** The left lateral surface of the brain. **Right.** The medial surface of the right half of a sagittally hemisected brain.

intonation of speech and aspects of music; facial recognition and facial expression of emotion; and nonverbal learning and memory. In general, the left hemisphere is more involved with verbal language function, including areas for both receptive and expressive speech control. In addition, the left hemisphere provides strong contributions to temporal order and sequencing, numeric symbols, and verbal learning and memory. However, the intact brain may not be neatly organized with one side being the dominant because the degree of lateralization differs across individuals. The two hemispheres are connected by the corpus callosum, a bundle of neuronal tissue that allows information to be exchanged quickly between the right and left hemispheres. An intact corpus callosum is required for the hemispheres to function in a smooth and coordinated manner.

Lobes of the Brain

The lateral surface of each hemisphere is further divided into four lobes: the **frontal, parietal, temporal, and occipital lobes** (Fig. 10.3). The lobes work in coordinated ways, but each is responsible for specific functions. Knowledge of these unique functions is helpful for understanding how damage to these areas produces the symptoms of mental illness and how medications that affect the functioning of these lobes can produce certain effects.

Frontal Lobes

The right and left frontal lobes make up about one fourth of the entire cerebral cortex and are proportionally larger in humans than in any other mammal. The precentral gyrus, the gyrus immediately anterior to the central sulcus, contains the primary motor area. Damage to this gyrus, or to the anterior neighbouring gyri, causes

spastic paralysis in the opposite side of the body. The frontal lobe also contains Broca area, which controls the motor function of speech. Damage to Broca area produces expressive aphasia or difficulty with the motor movements of speech. The frontal lobes are also thought to contain the highest or most complex aspects of cortical functioning: personality, working memory, executive function, intellect, and speech. Working memory is an important aspect of frontal lobe function, including the ability to plan and initiate activity with future goals in mind. Insight, judgement, reasoning, concept formation, problem-solving skills, abstraction, and self-evaluation are all abilities that are modulated and affected by the action of the frontal lobes. These skills are often referred to as *executive functions* because they modulate more primitive impulses through numerous connections to other areas of the cerebrum.

When normal frontal lobe functioning is altered, executive functioning is decreased, and modulation of impulses can be lost, leading to changes in mood and personality. The importance of the frontal lobe and its role in the development of symptoms common to psychiatric disorders are emphasized in later chapters that discuss disorders such as schizophrenia, attention deficit hyperactivity disorder, and dementia. Box 10.2 describes how altered frontal lobe function can affect mood and personality.

Parietal Lobes

The postcentral gyrus, immediately behind the central sulcus, contains the primary somatosensory area (Fig. 10.2). The posterior areas of the parietal lobe appear to coordinate visual and somatosensory information. Damage to this area produces complex sensory deficits, including neglect of contralateral sensory stimuli and spatial relationships. The parietal lobes contribute to the ability to recognize objects by touch, calculate, write, recognize fingers of the opposite hands, draw, and organize spatial directions, such as how to travel to familiar places. They are important for speech and maintaining focused attention.

Temporal Lobes

The temporal lobes contain the primary auditory and olfactory areas. Wernicke area, located at the posterior aspect of the superior temporal gyrus, is primarily responsible for receptive speech. The temporal lobes also integrate sensory and visual information involved in the control of written and verbal language skills, as well as visual recognition. The hippocampus, an important structure discussed in its own section later in this chapter, lies in the internal aspects of each temporal lobe and contributes to memory. Other internal structures of this lobe are involved in the modulation of mood and emotion.

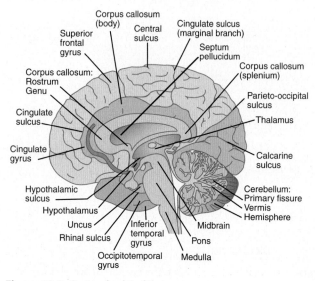

Figure 10.3 Gyri and sulci of the cortex.

BOX 10.2 Frontal Lobe Syndrome

In the 1860s, Phineas Gage became a famous example of frontal lobe dysfunction. Mr. Gage was a New England railroad worker who had a thick iron-tamping rod propelled through his frontal lobes by an explosion. He survived but suffered significant changes in his personality. Mr. Gage, who had previously been a capable and calm supervisor, began to show impatience, labile mood, disrespect for others, and frequent use of profanity after his injury (Harlow, 1868). Similar conditions are often called *frontal lobe syndrome*. Symptoms vary widely among individuals. In general, after damage to the dorsolateral (upper and outer) areas of the frontal lobes, the symptoms include a lack of drive and spontaneity. With damage to the most anterior aspects of the frontal lobes, the symptoms tend to involve more changes in mood and affect, such as impulsive and inappropriate behaviour.

The rendering shows the route the tamping rod took through Gage's skull. The angle of the rod's entry shot it behind the left eye and through the front part of the brain, sparing regions that are directly concerned with vital functions like breathing and heartbeat.

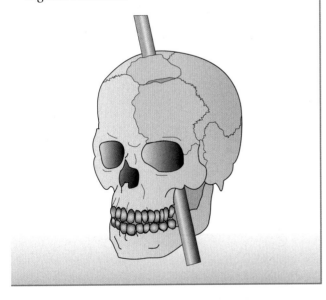

Occipital Lobes

The primary visual area is in the most posterior aspect of the occipital lobes. Damage to this area results in a condition called *cortical blindness*. In other words, the retina and optic nerve remain intact, but the individual cannot see. The occipital lobes are involved in many aspects of visual integration of information, including colour vision, object and facial recognition, and the ability to perceive objects in motion and judge distance.

Association Cortex

Although not a lobe, the association cortex is an important area that allows the lobes to work in an integrated manner. Areas of one lobe of the cortex often share functions with an area of the adjacent lobe. When these neighbouring nerve fibres are related to the same sensory modality, they are often referred to as *association* areas. For example, an area in the inferior parietal, posterior temporal, and anterior occipital lobes integrates visual, somatosensory, and auditory information to provide the abilities required for basic academic skills. These areas, along with numerous connections beneath the cortex, are part of the mechanisms that allow the human brain to work as an integrated whole.

Subcortical Structures

Beneath the cortex are layers of tissue composed of the axons of cell bodies. The axonal tissue forms pathways that are surrounded by glia, a fatty or lipid substance, which has a white appearance and gives these layers of neuron axons their name—*white matter*. Structures inside the hemispheres, beneath the cortex, are considered subcortical. Many of these structures, essential in the regulation of emotions and behaviours, play important roles in our understanding of mental disorders. Figure 10.4 provides a coronal section view of the grey matter, white matter, and important subcortical structures.

Basal Ganglia

The **basal ganglia** are subcortical grey matter areas in both the right and left hemispheres that contain interconnected cell bodies or nuclei. These nuclei include the caudate nucleus, putamen, globus pallidus, claustrum, subthalamus, and substantia nigra. The basal ganglia are involved with motor functions and in association with both the learning and programming of behaviours or activities that are repetitive and that over time become automatic. The basal ganglia have many connections with the cerebral cortex, thalamus, midbrain structures, and spinal cord. Damage to portions of these nuclei may produce changes in posture or muscle tone. In addition, damage may produce abnormal movements, such as twitches or tremors. Parkinson disease is the most common disorder of the basal ganglia. They can be adversely affected by some of the medications used to treat psychiatric disorders, leading to side effects and other motor-related problems.

Pituitary

The pituitary gland, often called the *master gland*, has two distinct parts, the anterior pituitary and the posterior pituitary. Located just below the hypothalamus, the anterior

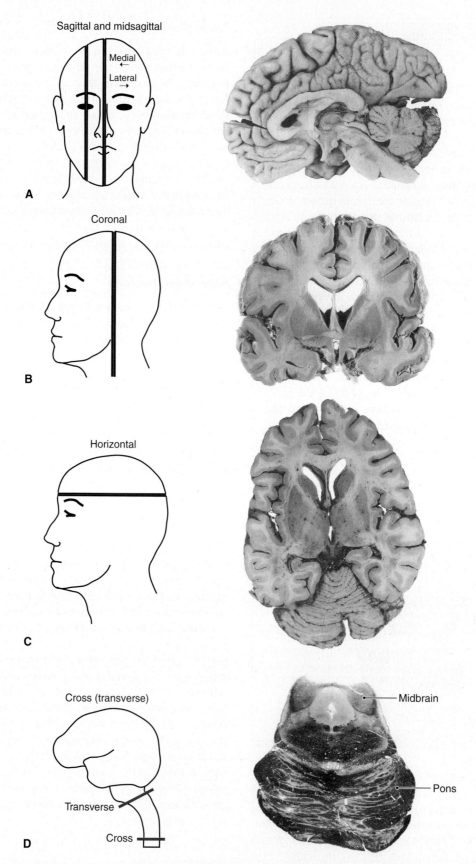

Figure 10.4 Three standard planes for visualizing brain structure: **(A)** sagittal, **(B)** coronal, and **(C)** horizontal cuts are made by physically slicing or rendered using imaging techniques. The transverse or crosscut **(D)** gives a view of subcortical structures. (Reprinted with permission from Bhatnagar, S. (2013). *Neuroscience for the study of communicative disorders.* Lippincott Williams & Wilkins.)

pituitary consists of glandular epithelial tissue and is connected to the hypothalamus by a vascular link. In contrast, the posterior pituitary is composed of neural tissue and is connected to the hypothalamus by a neural pathway. When stimulated, the posterior pituitary releases oxytocin or vasopressin (also known as antidiuretic hormone), two small peptide hormones that are produced in the hypothalamus. The anterior pituitary produces and releases seven different hormones—growth hormone (GH), thyroid-stimulating hormone (TSH), adrenocorticotropin hormone (ACTH), follicle-stimulating hormone (FSH), luteinizing hormone (LH), melatonin-stimulating hormone, and prolactin—when stimulated by a corresponding hormone from the hypothalamus (e.g., corticotrophin-releasing hormone stimulates secretion of ACTH). Together with the pituitary gland, the hypothalamus functions as one of the primary regulators of many aspects of the endocrine system. Its functions are involved in the control of visceral activities, such as body temperature, arterial blood pressure, hunger, thirst, fluid balance, gastric motility, and gastric secretions.

Of note, increased release of prolactin can result from blockade of naturally occurring dopamine by various medications, including antipsychotics, antidepressants, opiates, and cocaine. This can result in galactorrhea, menstrual irregularities in women, erectile dysfunction in men, and loss of libido and infertility in both men and women.

Limbic System

The **limbic system** is essential to understanding the many hypotheses related to psychiatric disorders and emotional behaviour in general. Basic emotions, needs, drives, and instinct begin and are modulated in the limbic system. Hate, love, anger, aggression, and caring are basic emotions that originate within the limbic system. Not only does the limbic system function as the seat of emotions but also, because emotions are often generated based on our personal experiences, the limbic system is involved with aspects of memory. Hypothesized changes in the limbic system play a significant role in many theories of major mental disorders, including schizophrenia, depression, and anxiety disorders (see Chapters 21, 22, 23). The limbic system is called a "system" because it comprises several small structures that work in a highly organized way. These structures include the hippocampus, thalamus, hypothalamus, amygdala, and limbic midbrain nuclei. See Figure 10.5 for identification and location of the structures within the limbic system and their relationship to other common CNS structures.

Hippocampus

The hippocampus is involved in forming and storing memories, especially the emotions attached to a memory. Our emotional response to memories and our

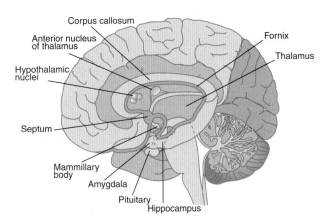

Figure 10.5 The structures of the limbic system are integrally involved in memory and emotional behaviour. Theories link changes in the limbic system to many major mental disorders, including schizophrenia, depression, and anxiety disorders.

association with other related memories are functions of how information is stored within the hippocampus. While most neurons are formed from before birth, the neurons in the hippocampus continue to form throughout life. Although memory storage is not limited to one area of the brain, destruction of the left hippocampus impairs verbal memory, and damage to the right hippocampus results in difficulty with recognition and recall of complex visual and auditory patterns. The main body of the hippocampus extends into the temporal lobe. Deterioration of the nerves of the hippocampus and other related temporal lobe structures found in Alzheimer disease produces the disorder's hallmark symptoms of memory dysfunction.

Thalamus

The thalamus is composed of several distinct subnuclei, each with its own specialized connections to many regions in the cerebral cortex. Sometimes called the "relay-switching centre of the brain," the thalamus functions as a regulatory structure to relay all sensory information, except smell, sent to the CNS from the PNS. The thalamus also relays memory, emotions, cognitions, behaviours, and motor functions. It regulates by filtering incoming information and determining what to pass on or what not to pass on to the cortex. In this fashion, the thalamus prevents the cortex from becoming overloaded with sensory stimulus. The thalamus is thought to play a part in controlling electrical activity in the cortex. Parts of the thalamus are involved in alertness, awareness, and memory. Injury to the anterior medial thalamus can cause alterations in autonomic functions, mood, and the sleep–wake cycle.

Hypothalamus

Basic human activities, such as sleep–rest patterns, body temperature, and physical drives (e.g., hunger and sex), are regulated by the hypothalamus, which rests deep within the brain. In emotional situations, the hypothalamus perceives changes and stimulates a visceral response through the **autonomic nervous system**, such as an increase in heart rate when we feel angry. Dysfunction of this structure, whether from disorders or because of the adverse effects of drugs used to treat mental illness, produces common psychiatric symptoms, such as appetite and sleep problems.

Nerve cells within the hypothalamus secrete hormones such as antidiuretic hormone, which when sent to the kidneys accelerates the reabsorption of water, and oxytocin, which acts on smooth muscles to promote contractions, particularly within the walls of the uterus. Because cells within the nervous system produce these hormones, they are often referred to as **neurohormones** and form a communication mechanism through the bloodstream to control organs that are not directly connected to nervous system structures.

Deregulation of the hypothalamus can be manifested in symptoms of certain psychiatric disorders.

Amygdala

The amygdala has numerous connections to the hypothalamus and lies adjacent to the hippocampus. It provides an emotional component to memory and is involved in modulating aggression, fear, anxiety, and sexuality. It is directly connected to more primitive centres of the brain involving the sense of smell, which serves to trigger these emotions. Impulsive acts of aggression and violence have been linked to dysregulation of the amygdala, and erratic firing of the nerve cells in the amygdala is a focus of investigation in bipolar mood disorders (see Chapter 22). The amygdala is also the part of the brain most affected by psychoactive drugs.

Limbic Midbrain Nuclei

The limbic midbrain nuclei are a collection of neurons (including the ventral tegmental area and the locus coeruleus) that appear to play a role in the biologic basis of addiction. Sometimes referred to as the pleasure centre or reward centre of the brain, the limbic midbrain nuclei function to chemically reinforce certain behaviours, ensuring their repetition. Emotions such as feeling satisfied with good food, the pleasure of nurturing, and the enjoyment of sexual activity originate in the limbic midbrain nuclei. The reinforcement of activities such as nutrition, procreation, and nurturing young are all primitive aspects of ensuring the survival of a species. When functioning in abnormal ways, the limbic midbrain nuclei can begin to reinforce unhealthy or risky behaviours, such as substance use and gambling. Exploration of this area of the brain is in its infancy but offers potential insight into addictions and their treatment.

Glymphatic System

The glymphatic system is a perivascular network distributed throughout the brain. This system, first described in 2012, travels through the parivascular space surrounding the blood vessels of the brain where it collects and then clears metabolic waste products and solutes. Almost all the clearance occurs during sleep; therefore, sleep disorders, such as insomnia and sleep apnea, may lead to an accumulation of toxic materials in the brain. Most notably this material may include the proteins involved in the pathogenesis of neurodegenerative diseases, such as amyloid-beta plaques and neurofibrillary tangles of Alzheimer disease (Reddy & van der Werf, 2020).

Other Central Nervous System Structures

Extrapyramidal tracts are part of the neuronal pathways through which motor signals are sent from the brain to lower motor neurones. Muscle tone, common reflexes, and automatic voluntary motor functioning, such as walking, are controlled by this nerve tract that is regulated through processing centres located in multiple brain regions such as parts of the cerebral cortex, the cerebellum, thalamus, reticular substance, and several basal ganglia. Dysfunction of this tract can produce hypertonicity in muscle groups. In Parkinson disease, the cells that compose the extrapyramidal motor system are severely affected, producing many involuntary motor movements. Various pharmacotherapies, which are discussed in Chapter 13, also affect this system.

The *pineal body* is a pinecone-shaped organ, measuring just 5 to 8 mm in length and 3 to 5 mm in width. It is located above and medial to the thalamus. Because the pineal gland easily calcifies, it can be visualized by neuroimaging and often is a medial landmark. Its functions remain somewhat of a mystery, despite long knowledge of its existence. It contains secretory cells that release the neurohormone melatonin and other substances. These hormones are thought to have various regulatory functions within the endocrine system. Darkness and hypoglycemia increase the release of melatonin. Melatonin has been associated with sleep and emotional disorders. In addition, it has been postulated that melatonin has a role in modulating immune function.

The *locus coeruleus* is a tiny cluster of norepinephrine-containing neurons that fan out and innervate almost every part of the brain, including most of the cortex, the thalamus and hypothalamus, the cerebellum, and the spinal cord. Just one neuron from the coeruleus can connect to more than 250,000 other neurons. Although it is very small, because of its wide-ranging neuronal connections, this tiny structure has influence in the regulation of attention, time perception, sleep–rest cycles, arousal, learning, pain, and mood, and it seems most involved with information processing of new, unexpected, and novel experiences. Some think its function/dysfunction may explain why individuals become addicted to substances and seek risky behaviours, despite awareness of negative consequences.

The *brainstem*, located beneath the thalamus, is composed of the midbrain, pons, and medulla and has important life-sustaining functions. Nuclei of numerous neural pathways to the cerebrum are in the brainstem. They are significantly involved in mediating symptoms of emotional dysfunction. These nuclei are also the primary source of several neurochemicals, such as serotonin, that are commonly associated with psychiatric disorders. Table 10.5 summarizes some of the key related nuclei.

Table 10.5 Classic and Putative Neurotransmitters, Their Distribution and Proposed Functions

Neurotransmitter	Cell Bodies	Projections	Proposed Function
Acetylcholine			
Dietary precursor: choline	Basal forebrain Pons Other areas	Diffuse throughout the cortex, hippocampus Peripheral nervous system	Important role in learning and memory Some role in wakefulness and basic attention Peripherally activates muscles and is the major neurochemical in the autonomic system
Monoamines			
Dopamine Dietary precursor: tyrosine	Substantia nigra Ventral tegmental area Arcuate nucleus Retina olfactory bulb	Striatum (basal ganglia) Limbic system and cerebral cortex Pituitary	Involved in involuntary motor movements Some role in mood states, pleasure components in reward systems, and complex behaviour such as judgement, reasoning, and insight
Norepinephrine Dietary precursor: tyrosine	Locus coeruleus Lateral tegmental area and others throughout the pons and medulla	Very widespread throughout the cortex, thalamus, cerebellum, brainstem, and spinal cord Basal forebrain, thalamus, hypothalamus	Proposed role in learning and memory, attributing value in reward systems; fluctuates in sleep and wakefulness Major component of the sympathetic nervous system responses, including "fight or flight"
Serotonin Dietary precursor: tryptophan	Raphe nuclei Others in the pons and medulla	Widespread throughout the cortex, thalamus, cerebellum, brainstem, and spinal cord	Proposed role in the control of appetite, sleep, mood states, hallucinations, pain perception, and vomiting
Histamine Dietary precursor: histidine	Hypothalamus	Cerebral cortex Limbic system Hypothalamus Found in all mast cells	Control of gastric secretions, smooth muscle control, cardiac stimulation, stimulation of sensory nerve endings, and alertness
Amino Acids			
GABA	Derived from glutamate without localized cell bodies	Found in cells and projections throughout the CNS, especially in intrinsic feedback loops and interneurons of the cerebrum Also in the extrapyramidal motor system and cerebellum	Fast inhibitory response postsynaptically, inhibits the excitability of the neurons and therefore contributes to seizure, agitation, and anxiety control
Glycine	Primarily the spinal cord and brainstem	Limited projection, but especially in the auditory system and olfactory bulb Also found in the spinal cord, medulla, midbrain, cerebellum, and cortex	Inhibitory Decreases the excitability of spinal motor neurons but not cortical
Glutamate	Diffuse	Diffuse, but especially in the sensory organs	Excitatory Responsible for the bulk of information flow
Neuropeptides			
Endogenous opioids, (e.g., endorphins, enkephalins)	A large family of neuropeptides, which has three distinct subgroups, all of which are manufactured widely throughout the CNS	Widely distributed within and outside the CNS	Suppresses pain, modulates mood and stress Likely involvement in reward systems and addiction Also may regulate pituitary hormone release Implicated in the pathophysiology of diseases of the basal ganglia
Melatonin One of its precursors: serotonin	Pineal body	Widely distributed within and outside the CNS	Secreted in dark and suppressed light, helps regulate the sleep–wake cycle as well as other biologic rhythms
Substance P	Widespread, significant in the raphe system and spinal cord	Spinal cord, cortex, brainstem, and especially sensory neurons associated with pain perception	Involved in pain transmission, movement, and mood regulation
Cholecystokinin	Predominates in the ventral tegmental area of the midbrain	Frontal cortex where it is often colocalized with dopamine Widely distributed within and outside the CNS	Primary intestinal hormone involved in satiety, also has some involvement in the control of anxiety and panic

The *cerebellum* is in the posterior aspect of the skull, beneath the cerebral hemispheres. This large structure controls movements and postural adjustments. To regulate postural balance and positioning, the cerebellum receives information from all parts of the body, including muscles, joints, skin, and visceral organs, as well as from many parts of the CNS.

Closely associated with the spinal cord, but not lying entirely within its column, is the autonomic nervous system, a subdivision of the PNS. It was originally given this name for being independent of conscious thought, that is, automatic. However, it does not necessarily function as autonomously as the name indicates. This system contains efferent (nerves moving away from the CNS) or motor system neurons, which affect target tissues such as cardiac muscle, smooth muscle, and the glands. It also contains afferent nerves, which are sensory and conduct information from these organs back to the CNS. The two main neurotransmitters of the ANS are acetylcholine (ACh) and norepinephrine. It is important for nurses to recognize that any medication that impacts these neurotransmitters can have far-reaching effects on the body.

The autonomic nervous system is further divided into the sympathetic and parasympathetic nervous systems. These systems, although peripheral, are included here because they are involved in the emergency, or "fight-or-flight," response as well as the peripheral actions of many medications (see Chapter 12). Figure 10.6 illustrates the innervations of various target organs by the autonomic nervous system. Table 10.6 identifies the actions of the sympathetic and parasympathetic nervous systems on various target organs.

Neurophysiology of the Central Nervous System

At their most basic level, the human brain and connecting nervous system are composed of billions of cells (Fig. 10.7). There are two main types of brain cells: glia and neurons.

Glial Cells

There are three types of glial cells: astrocytes, oligodendrocytes, and microglial cells. There are five times the number of astrocytes in the brain as neurons. Astrocytes are involved in regulating blood flow in the brain and forming the blood–brain barrier and "scaffolding" of the CNS (Sofroniew & Vinters, 2010). Controlled intracellular calcium concentrations are involved in astrocyte-to-astrocyte communication and astrocyte-to-neuron communication. Astrocytes do not initiate or pass electrical potentials along their processes. Astrocyte dysfunction may be related to anxiety, addiction behaviours, depression, and schizophrenia, and future

treatments may target these cells. Other studies are looking at the link between astrocyte dysfunction and other CNS conditions, including Alzheimer disease, Parkinson syndrome, neuropathic pain, and migraine.

Oligodendrites produce the myelin sheath, which speeds electrical conduction over the axons. In multiple sclerosis, the myelin sheath is thought to be damaged by an immune system attack and conduction of the action potential fails. Microglia are the immune cells of the brain, constantly scanning for threats like damaged cells and infection.

Neurons and Nerve Impulses

About 100 billion cells are nerve cells, or neurons, responsible for receiving, organizing, and transmitting information. Neurons come in many sizes, shapes, and lengths. These factors and their location in the brain determine how they function (Fig. 10.8). Each neuron has a cell body, or soma, which holds the nucleus containing most of the cell's genetic information. The soma also includes other organelles, such as ribosomes and endoplasmic reticulum, both of which carry out protein synthesis; the Golgi apparatus, which contains enzymes to modify the proteins for specific functions; vesicles, which transport and store proteins; and lysosomes, responsible for degradation of these proteins. Located throughout the neuron, mitochondria, containing enzymes and often called the "cell's engine," are the site of many energy-producing chemical reactions. These cell structures provide the basis for secreting numerous chemicals by which neurons communicate.

It is not just the vast number of neurons that accounts for the complexities of the brain but also the enormous number of neurochemical interconnections and interactions between neurons. A single motor neuron in the spinal cord may receive signals from more than 10,000 sources of interconnection with other nerves. Although most neurons have only one axon, which varies in length and conducts impulses away from the soma, each has numerous dendrites, receiving signals from other neurons. Because axons may branch as they terminate, they also have multiple contacts with other neurons.

Nerve signals are prompted to fire by a variety of chemical or physical stimuli. This firing produces an electrical impulse. The cell's membrane is a double layer of phospholipid molecules with embedded proteins. Some of these proteins provide water-filled channels through which inorganic ions may pass. Each of the common ions—sodium, potassium, calcium, and chloride—has its own specific molecular channel. These channels are voltage gated and thus open or close in response to changes in the electrical potential across the membrane. At rest, the cell membrane is polarized with a positive charge on the outside and about a 270-mV charge on the inside, owing to the

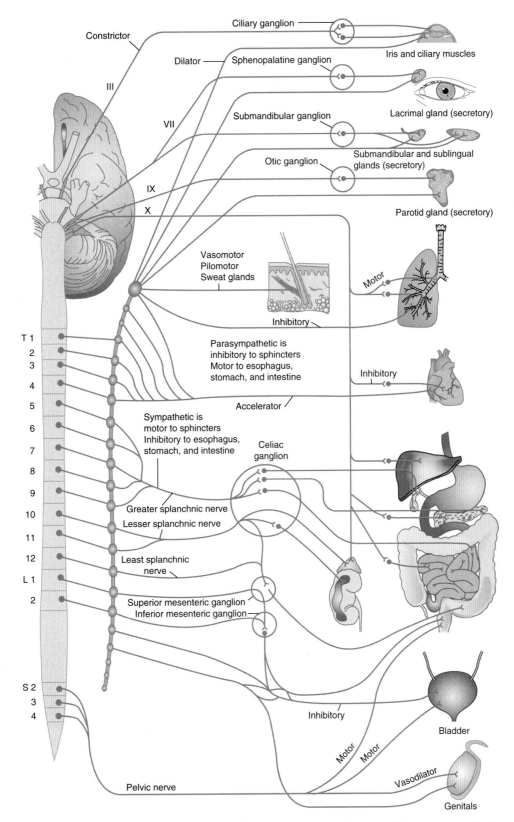

Figure 10.6 Diagram of the autonomic nervous system. Note that many organs are innervated by both sympathetic and parasympathetic nerves. (Adapted from Schaffe, E. E., & Lytle, I. M. (1980). *Basic physiology and anatomy.* J.B. Lippincott.)

Table 10.6   Peripheral Organ Response in the Autonomic Nervous System

Effector Organ	Sympathetic Response	Parasympathetic Response (Acetylcholine)
Eye		
• Iris sphincter muscle	Preganglionic neurons—acetylcholine	Constriction to normal
• Ciliary muscle	Postganglionic neurons—mostly norepinephrine Dilation Relaxation	Accommodation for near vision
Heart		
• Sinoatrial node	Increased rate	Decrease rate to normal
• Atria	Increased contractility	Decrease in contractility
• Atrioventricular node	Increased contractility Decrease in conduction velocity	
Blood vessels	Depending on type of sympathetic receptor, stimulation can cause constriction or dilation.	Dilation of vessels supplying penis and clitoris only
Lungs		
• Bronchial muscles	Relaxation	Constriction to normal
• Bronchial glands		Secretion
Gastrointestinal Tract		
• Motility and tone	Relaxation (decreased peristalsis)	Increased (for normal peristalsis)
• Sphincters	Contraction	Relaxation
• Secretion glands	Decrease secretion	Stimulation
Urinary Bladder		
• Detrusor muscle	Relaxation	Contraction
• Trigone and sphincter	Contraction	Relaxation
Uterus	Contraction (pregnant) Relaxation (nonpregnant)	Variable
Skin		
• Pilomotor muscles	Contraction	No effect
• Sweat glands	Increased secretion	No effect
Glands		
• Salivary	Stimulation of small volume of thick saliva	Stimulation of large volume of watery saliva
• Sweat	Increased secretion	None
• Adrenal medulla	Stimulation of epinephrine and norepinephrine secretion	None
• Endocrine pancreas	Inhibition of insulin secretion; stimulation of glucagon secretion	Stimulation of insulin and glucagon secretion

resting distribution of sodium and potassium ions. As potassium passively diffuses across the membrane, the sodium pump uses energy to move sodium from the inside of the cell against a concentration gradient to maintain this distribution. An action potential, or nerve impulse, is generated as the membrane is depolarized and a threshold value is reached, which triggers the opening of the voltage-gated sodium channels, allowing sodium to surge into the cell. The inside of the cell briefly becomes positively charged and the outside negatively charged. Once initiated, the action potential becomes self-propagating, opening nearby sodium channels. This electrical communication moves into the soma from the dendrites or down the axon by this mechanism.

Synaptic Transmission

For one neuron to communicate with another, the electrical process must change to a chemical communication. The synaptic cleft, a junction between one nerve and another, is the space where the electrical intracellular signal becomes a chemical extracellular signal.

Various substances are recognized as the chemical messengers between neurons.

Neurotransmitters are small molecules that directly and indirectly control the opening or closing of ion channels. Neuromodulators are chemical messengers that make the target cell membrane or postsynaptic membrane susceptible to the effects of the primary neurotransmitter. Some of these neurochemicals are synthesized quickly from dietary precursors, such as tyrosine or tryptophan, or enzymes inside the cytoplasm of the neuron, but most synthesis occurs in the ends of the axons, called *terminals*, or the neuron itself. Some neurochemicals can reduce the membrane potential and enhance the transmission of the signal between neurons. These chemicals are called *excitatory neurotransmitters*. Other neurochemicals have the opposite effect, slowing down nerve impulses, and these substances are called *inhibitory neurotransmitters*.

As the electrical action potential reaches the terminals, calcium ion channels are opened, causing an influx of Ca^{++} ions into the neuron. This increase in calcium stimulates the release of neurotransmitters into the **synapse**. Rapid signaling between neurons requires a ready supply

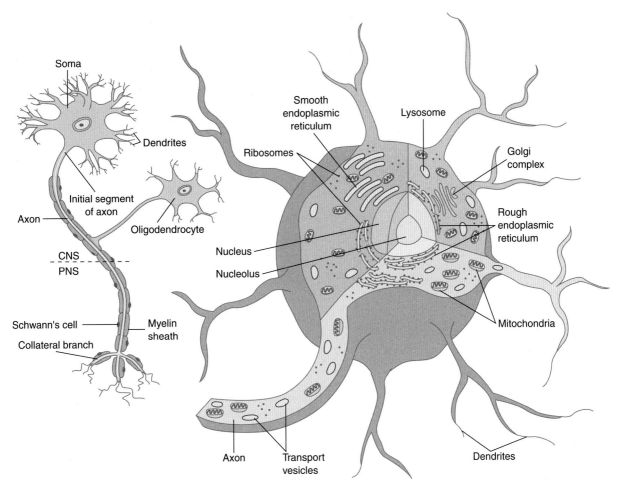

Figure 10.7 Cell body and organelles of an axon.

of neurotransmitters. These neurotransmitters are stored in small vesicles grouped near the cell membrane at the terminals. Because nerve terminals do not have the ability to manufacture proteins, the transmitters that fill these vesicles are small molecules, such as the bioamines (dopamine and norepinephrine) or the amino acids (glutamate or γ-aminobutyric acid [GABA]). Actions of these small molecules are discussed in the neurotransmitters section later in this chapter. When stimulated, the vesicles containing the neurotransmitter fuse with the cell membrane, and the neurotransmitter is released into the synapse (Fig. 10.9). The neurotransmitter then crosses the synaptic cleft to a **receptor** site on the postsynaptic neuron and stimulates adjacent neurons. This is the process of neuronal communication.

Embedded in the postsynaptic membrane are several proteins that act as receptors for the released neurotransmitters. The "lock-and-key" analogy has often been used to describe the fit of a given neurotransmitter to its receptor site. Each neurotransmitter has a specific receptor, or protein, for which it and only it will fit. The target cell, when stimulated by the neurotransmitter, will respond by evoking its own action potential and either producing some action common to that cell or acting as a relay

to keep the messages moving throughout the CNS. This pattern of the electrical signal from one neuron, converted to chemical signal at the synaptic cleft, picked up by an adjacent neuron, and again converted to an electrical action potential and then to a chemical signal, occurs billions of times a day in billions of different brain cells. It is this electrical–chemical communication process that allows the structures of the brain to function together in a coordinated and organized manner.

When the neurotransmitter has completed its interaction with the postsynaptic receptor and stimulated that cell, its work is done, and it needs to be removed. It can be removed by natural diffusion away from the area of high neurotransmitter concentration at the receptors by being broken down by enzymes in the synaptic cleft or through reuptake through highly specific mechanisms into the presynaptic terminal.

Many psychopharmacologic agents, particularly antidepressants, act by blocking the reuptake of the neurotransmitters, thereby increasing the available amount of chemical messenger. Presynaptic binding sites for neurotransmitters may serve not only as reuptake mechanisms but also as autoreceptors to perform various regulatory functions on the flow of neurotransmitters into

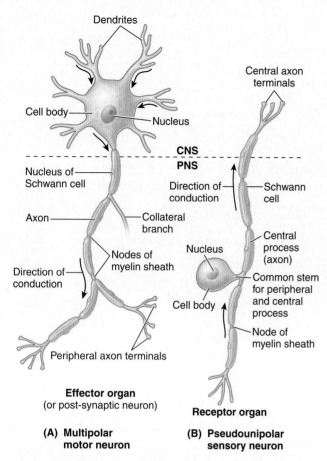

Figure 10.8 The two most common neurons are the **(A)** motor and **(B)** sensory neuron. (Reprinted with permission from Moore, K. L., Agur, A. M. R., & Dalley, A. F. (2014). *Clinically oriented anatomy.* Lippincott Williams & Wilkins.)

the synapse. When these presynaptic autoreceptors are saturated, the neuron slows down or stops releasing neurotransmitters. The neurotransmitters taken back into the presynaptic neuron may be stored in vesicles for rerelease, or they may be broken down by enzymes, such as monoamine oxidase, and removed entirely.

The primary steps in synaptic transmission are summarized in Figure 10.9. The preceding discussion contains only the basic mechanisms of neuronal communication. Many other factors that modulate or contribute to the communication between neurons are only beginning to be discovered. Examples include peptides that are released into the synapse and thought to behave like neurotransmitters or that also can appear in combination with another neurotransmitter. These peptides, known as *cotransmitters*, are believed to have a modulatory effect on the primary neurotransmitter.

KEY CONCEPT

Neurotransmitters are small molecules that directly and indirectly control the opening or closing of ion channels.

Receptor Activity

Both presynaptic and postsynaptic receptors have the capacity to change, developing either a greater than usual response to the neurotransmitter, known as *supersensitivity*, or a less than usual response, called *subsensitivity*. These changes represent the concept of neuroplasticity of brain tissue, which was discussed earlier in the chapter. The change in sensitivity of the receptor is most caused by the effect of a substance, such as a drug, on a receptor site or by disease that affects the normal functioning of a receptor site. Drugs can affect the sensitivity of the receptor by altering the strength of attraction or affinity of a receptor for the neurotransmitter, by changing the efficiency with which the receptor activity translates the message inside the receiving cell, or by decreasing over time the number of receptors.

These mechanisms may account for the long-term, sometimes severely adverse, effects of psychopharmacologic drugs, the loss of effectiveness of a given medication, or the loss of effectiveness of a medication after repeated use in treating recurring episodes of a psychiatric disorder. A disease may cause a change in the normal number or function of receptors, thereby altering their sensitivity. It has been hypothesized that depression is caused by a reduction in the normal number of certain receptors, leading to an abnormality in their sensitivity to neurotransmitters such as serotonin and norepinephrine. A decreased response to continued stimulation of these receptors is usually referred to as desensitization or *refractoriness*. This suspected subsensitivity is referred to as *down-regulation* of the receptors.

Receptor Subtypes

The nervous system uses many different neurochemicals for communication, and each specific chemical messenger requires a specific receptor on which the chemical can act. More than 100 different chemical messengers have been identified, with new ones being uncovered frequently as research on the functioning of the brain becomes more and more precise. In addition to the sheer number of receptors needed to accommodate these chemicals, the neurotransmitters may produce different effects at different synaptic sites. The ability of a neurotransmitter to produce different actions is, in part, because of the specialization of its receptors. The different receptors for each neurochemical messenger are referred to as *receptor subtypes* for the chemical. Each major neurotransmitter has several different subtypes of receptors, allowing the neurotransmitter to have different effects in different areas of the brain. For example, dopamine, a common neurotransmitter discussed in the next section, has five different subtypes of receptors that have been identified. Numbers usually name the receptor subtypes. In the example of dopamine, the various subtypes of receptors are called D_1, D_2, D_3, and so on.

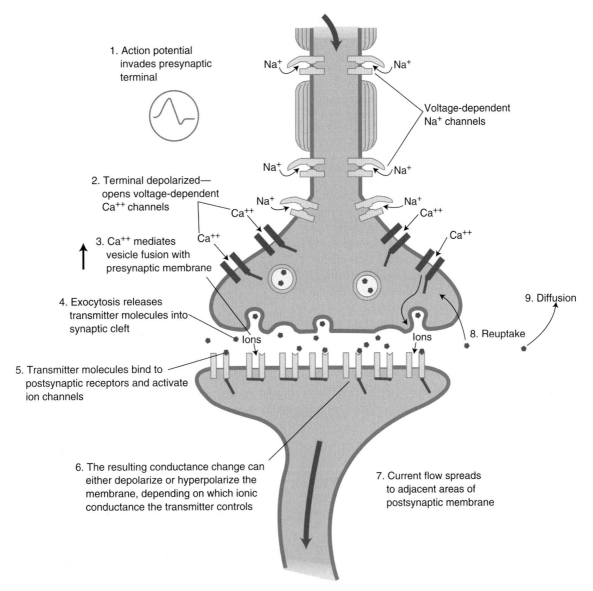

1. Action potential invades presynaptic terminal

Na⁺   Na⁺

Voltage-dependent
Na⁺ channels

Na⁺   Na⁺

2. Terminal depolarized—opens voltage-dependent Ca⁺⁺ channels

Na⁺   Na⁺
Ca⁺⁺   Ca⁺⁺
Ca⁺⁺   Ca⁺⁺

3. Ca⁺⁺ mediates vesicle fusion with presynaptic membrane

9. Diffusion

4. Exocytosis releases transmitter molecules into synaptic cleft

Ions   Ions

8. Reuptake

5. Transmitter molecules bind to postsynaptic receptors and activate ion channels

6. The resulting conductance change can either depolarize or hyperpolarize the membrane, depending on which ionic conductance the transmitter controls

7. Current flow spreads to adjacent areas of postsynaptic membrane

Figure 10.9 Synaptic transmission. The most significant events that occur during synaptic transmission: (*1*) the action potential reaches the presynaptic terminal; (*2*) membrane depolarization causes Ca⁺⁺ terminals to open; (*3*) Ca⁺⁺ mediates fusion of the vesicles with the presynaptic membrane; (*4*) transmitter molecules are released into the synaptic cleft, by exocytosis; (*5*) transmitter molecules bind to postsynaptic receptors and activate ion channels; (*6*) conductance changes cause an excitatory or inhibitory postsynaptic potential (excitatory and inhibitory processes are alternately referred to as depolarization and hyperpolarization), depending on the specific transmitter; (*7*) current flow spreads along the postsynaptic membrane; and (*8*) transmitter remaining in the synaptic cleft returns to the presynaptic terminal by reuptake or (*9*) diffuses into the extracellular fluid. (Adapted and reproduced from Schauf, C., Moffett, D., & Moffett, S. (1990). *Human physiology.* Times Mirror/Mosby, with permission.)

Knowledge of the different subtypes helps in understanding both the effects and side effects of medications used to treat mental health disorders.

Neurotransmitters

Many substances have been identified as possible chemical messengers, but not all chemical messengers are neurotransmitters. Classic neurotransmitters are those that meet certain criteria agreed on by neuroscientists. The traditional criteria include the following:

- The chemical is synthesized inside the neuron.
- The chemical is present in the presynaptic terminals.
- The chemical is released into the synaptic cleft and causes a particular effect on the postsynaptic receptors.
- An exogenous form of the chemical administered as a drug causes identical action.
- The chemical is removed from the synaptic cleft by a specific mechanism.

Neurotransmitters can be grouped into categories that reflect chemical similarities of the neurotransmitter.

Common practice classifies certain chemicals as neurotransmitters even though their ability to meet the strict traditional definition may be incomplete. For the purposes of this section, the classification of neurotransmitters will use this common system of classifying neurotransmitters. Common categories of neurotransmitters include the following:

- Cholinergic neurotransmitters
- Biogenic amine neurotransmitters (sometimes called *monoamines* or *bioamines*)
- Amino acid neurotransmitters
- Neuropeptide neurotransmitters

Neurotransmitters are also classified by whether their action causes physiologic activity to occur or to stop occurring. All the neurotransmitters commonly involved in the development of mental health disorders or affected by the drugs used to treat these disorders are excitatory except one, GABA, which is inhibitory. The significance of this concept is discussed in the section on amino acids below. Neurotransmitters are found wherever there are neurons, and neurons are contained in both the CNS and PNS. Because mental health disorders occur in the CNS, the following sections discuss neurotransmitters from the perspective of the CNS.

Cholinergic

Acetylcholine (ACh) is a primary cholinergic neurotransmitter. Found in the greatest concentration in the PNS, ACh provides the basic synaptic communication for the parasympathetic neurons and part of the sympathetic neurons, which send information to the CNS. Understanding both the action of ACh and the receptor subtypes for this neurotransmitter assists nurses in understanding the complex side effects of common medications used to treat mental disorders.

Cholinergic neurons, so named because they contain ACh, follow diffuse projections throughout the cerebral cortex and limbic system, arising primarily from cell bodies in the base of the frontal lobes. Pathways from this region also project throughout the hippocampus (Fig. 10.10). These connections suggest that ACh is involved in higher intellectual functioning and memory. Individuals who have Alzheimer disease or Down syndrome often exhibit patterns of cholinergic neuron loss in regions innervated by these pathways (such as the hippocampus), which may contribute to their memory difficulties and other cognitive deficits. Some cholinergic neurons are afferent to these areas bringing information from the limbic system, highlighting the role that ACh plays in communicating emotional state to the cerebral cortex. ACh is an excitatory neurotransmitter, meaning that when released into a synapse, it causes the postsynaptic neuron to initiate some action.

The subtypes of ACh receptors are divided into two groups: the muscarinic receptors and the nicotinic

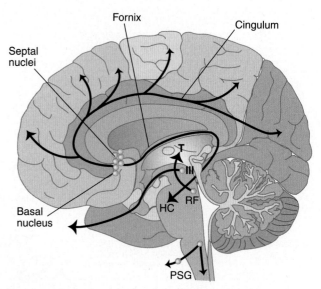

Figure 10.10 Cholinergic pathways. HC, hippocampal formation; PSG, parasympathetic ganglion cell; RF, reticular formation; T, thalamus. (Adapted from Nolte, J., & Angevine, J. (1995). *The human brain: In photographs and diagrams.* Mosby.)

receptors. Many psychiatric medications are anticholinergic agents, which block the effects of the muscarinic ACh receptors. This blocking effect of ACh causes common side effects, such as dry mouth, blurred vision, constipation, urinary retention, and tachycardia, which are seen in many psychotropic medications. Excessive blockade of ACh can cause confusion and delirium, especially in older individuals, as discussed in Chapter 32. Table 10.5 lists the effects of ACh on various organs in the parasympathetic system. Awareness of what organs are impacted by different medications that impact ACh and other neurotransmitters will help nurses link medications with their effects.

Biogenic Amines

The **biogenic amines** (bioamines) consist of small molecules manufactured in the neuron that contain an amine group. These include dopamine, norepinephrine, and epinephrine, which are all synthesized from the amino acid tyrosine; serotonin, which is synthesized from tryptophan; and histamine, manufactured from histidine. Of all the neurotransmitters, the biogenic amines are most central to current hypotheses of psychiatric disorders and hence are described individually in more detail.

Dopamine

Dopamine is an excitatory neurotransmitter found in distinct regions of the CNS, and it is involved in cognitive, motor, and neuroendocrine functions. Dopamine levels are decreased in Parkinson disease, and abnormal dopaminergic activity has been associated with schizophrenia (see Chapter 20). Dopamine is also the neurotransmitter that stimulates the body's natural "feel good" reward pathways, producing pleasant euphoric sensation under certain conditions. Abnormalities of dopamine use within the reward system pathways are suspected to be a critical aspect of the development of substance-related and addictive disorders. The dopamine pathways are distinct neuronal areas within the CNS in which the neurotransmitter dopamine predominates. Three major dopaminergic pathways have been identified.

The mesocortical and mesolimbic pathways originate in the ventral tegmental area and project into the medial aspects of the cortex (mesocortical) and the medial aspects of the limbic system inside the temporal lobes, including the hippocampus and amygdala (mesolimbic). Sometimes, they are considered to be one pathway and at other times two separate pathways. The mesocortical pathway has major effects on cognition, including such functions as judgement, reasoning, insight, social conscience, motivation, the ability to generalize learning, and reward systems in the human brain. It contributes to some of the highest seats of cortical functioning. The mesocortical system may be linked to the negative symptoms of schizophrenia. The mesocortical pathway also strongly influences emotions and has projections that affect memory and auditory reception. Abnormalities in the mesolimbic system may be linked with symptoms of schizophrenia.

Another major dopaminergic pathway begins in the substantia nigra and projects into the basal ganglia, parts of which are known as the *striatum*. This pathway, called the *nigrostriatal pathway*, influences the extrapyramidal motor system, which serves the voluntary motor system and allows involuntary motor movements. Destruction of dopaminergic neurons in this pathway has been associated with Parkinson disease.

The last dopamine pathway originates from projections of the mesolimbic pathway and continues into the hypothalamus, which then projects into the pituitary gland. Therefore, this pathway, called the *tuberoinfundibular pathway*, has an impact on endocrine function and other functions, such as metabolism, hunger, thirst, sexual function, circadian rhythms, digestion, and temperature control. Figure 10.11 illustrates the dopaminergic pathways.

As noted previously, researchers have identified at least five subtypes of dopamine receptors in the CNS. These subtypes are distributed differently throughout the brain. For example, the D_1 subtype receptor and its related receptor subtype, D_5, predominate in areas that affect memory and emotions, such as the cortex, hippocampus, and amygdala. They have not been detected in the substantia nigra. D_2 receptors are richly distributed throughout the neurons in the extrapyramidal motor system, whereas D_4 receptors are richly distributed in the frontal cortex, with few in the nigrostriatal system. Antipsychotic medications, discussed in Chapter 13, act by blocking the effects of dopamine at the receptor sites.

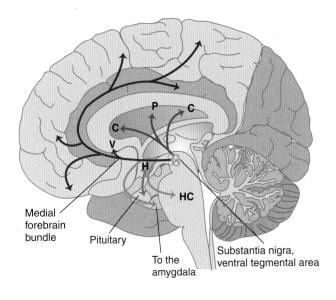

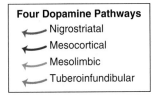

Figure 10.11 Dopaminergic pathways. C, caudate nucleus; H, hypothalamus; HC, hippocampal formation; P, putamen; V, ventral striatum. (Adapted from Nolte, J., & Angevine, J. (1995). *The human brain: In photographs and diagrams.* Mosby.)

Many of the medications that are most effective on the acute symptoms of psychosis have a strong attraction or affinity for D_2 receptors and a weaker but modest correlation with D_1 receptors. Because D_2 receptors predominate in the nigrostriatal pathway, medications that have a weaker blockade of D_2 will have fewer extrapyramidal motor system effects. Side effects and adverse effects from the involuntary motor system are at times extremely debilitating to individuals. Based on the assumption that these dopamine receptor subtypes have different functions in the CNS, medications have been designed to affect more predominantly one subtype than another, presumably avoiding effects on systems containing other subtypes and thus avoiding potential side effects of the medication. Researchers have reduced the occurrence of extrapyramidal effects through the development of so-called second generation antipsychotics; however, they continue to work to develop newer formularies that will avoid or minimize the effects on D_2 to further diminish the occurrence of these effects.

Norepinephrine

Norepinephrine was first demonstrated to be the primary neurotransmitter of the PNS in 1946. Although commonly found in the PNS, norepinephrine is also critical to CNS functioning. Norepinephrine is an excitatory neurochemical that plays a major role in generating and maintaining mood states. Decreased norepinephrine has been associated with depression, and excessive norepinephrine has been associated with manic symptoms. Because norepinephrine is so heavily concentrated in the terminal sites of sympathetic nerves, it can be released quickly to ready the individual for a fight-or-flight response to threats in the environment. For this reason, norepinephrine is thought to play a role in the physical symptoms of anxiety.

Nerve tracts and pathways containing predominantly norepinephrine are called *noradrenergic* and are less clearly delineated than the dopamine pathways. In the CNS, noradrenergic neurons originate in the locus coeruleus, where more than half of the noradrenergic cell bodies are located. Because the locus coeruleus is one of the major timekeepers of the human body, norepinephrine is involved in sleep and wakefulness. From the locus coeruleus, noradrenergic pathways ascend into the neocortex, spread diffusely (Fig. 10.12), and enhance the ability of neurons to respond to whatever input they may be receiving. In addition, norepinephrine appears to be involved in the process of reinforcement, which facilitates learning. Noradrenergic pathways innervate the hypothalamus and thus are involved to some degree in endocrine function. Anxiety disorders and depressive disorders are examples of mental health disorders in which dysfunction of the noradrenergic neurons may be involved.

Epinephrine

Epinephrine is very similar to norepinephrine chemically; however, in contrast to norepinephrine, only very small amounts of epinephrine are produced and released in the brain. Relatively few neurons, located in the caudal pons and the medulla in the brain, use epinephrine as a neurotransmitter. Epinephrine is found in much higher concentrations in the rest of the body, where it is secreted directly from the adrenal gland into the blood circulation.

Serotonin

Serotonin (also called 5-hydroxytryptamine or 5-HT) is primarily an excitatory neurotransmitter that is diffusely distributed within the cerebral cortex, limbic system, and basal ganglia of the CNS. Serotonergic neurons also project into the hypothalamus and cerebellum. Figure 10.13 illustrates serotonergic pathways. Serotonin plays a role in emotions, cognition, sensory perceptions, and essential biologic functions, such as sleep and appetite. During the rapid eye movement (REM) phase of sleep, or the dream state, serotonin concentrations decrease, and muscles subsequently relax. Serotonin is also involved in the control of food intake, hormone secretion, sexual behaviour, thermoregulation, and cardiovascular regulation. Some serotonergic fibres reach the cranial blood vessels within the brain and the pia mater, where they have a vasoconstrictive effect. The potency of some new medications for migraine headaches is related to their ability to block serotonin transmission in the cranial

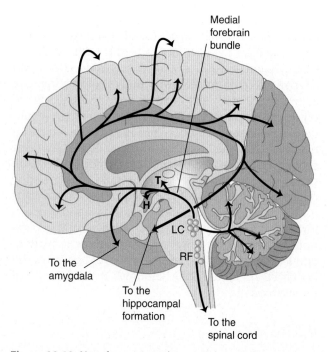

Figure 10.12 Noradrenergic pathways. H, hypothalamus; LC, locus coeruleus; RF, reticular formation; T, thalamus. (Adapted from Nolte, J., & Angevine, J. (1995). *The human brain: In photographs and diagrams.* Mosby.)

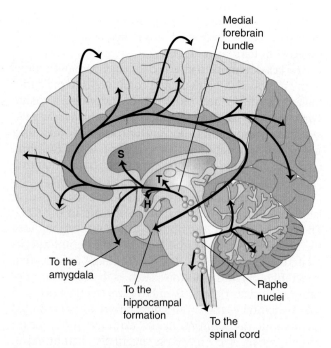

Figure 10.13 Serotonergic pathways. H, hypothalamus; S, septal nuclei; T, thalamus. (Adapted from Nolte, J., & Angevine, J. (1995). *The human brain: In photographs and diagrams.* Mosby.)

blood vessels. Descending serotonergic pathways are important in central pain control. Depression and insomnia have been associated with decreased levels of serotonin, whereas mania has been associated with increased serotonin. Some of the most well-known antidepressant medications, such as fluoxetine (Prozac) and sertraline (Zoloft), which are discussed in more depth in Chapter 13, function by raising serotonin levels within certain areas of the CNS. Obsessive–compulsive disorder, panic disorder, and other anxiety disorders are believed to be associated with dysfunction of the serotonin pathways, explaining why antidepressant medications have several uses in treating mental disorders.

Numerous subtypes of serotonin receptors also exist, and each of these appears to have a distinct function. 5-HT_{1a} is involved in the control of anxiety, aggression, and depression. Drugs such as lysergic acid diethylamide affect 5-HT_2 and produce hallucinatory effects.

Histamine

Histamine neurons originate predominantly in the hypothalamus and project to all major structures in the cerebrum, brainstem, and spinal cord. Exerting an influence in autonomic and neuroendocrine function, it is associated with many activities, including arousal, cognition, learning and memory, sleep, appetite, and seizures. Many psychiatric medications can block the effects of histamine postsynaptically and produce side effects such as sedation, weight gain, and hypotension.

Amino Acids

Amino acids are the building blocks of proteins and have many roles in intraneuronal metabolism. In addition, amino acids can function as neurotransmitters in up to 70% of the synaptic sites in the brain. Amino acids are the most prevalent neurotransmitters. Virtually, all neurons in the CNS are activated by excitatory amino acids, such as glutamate, and inhibited by inhibitory amino acids, such as GABA and glycine. Many of these amino acids coexist with other neurotransmitters.

γ-Aminobutyric Acid

GABA is the primary inhibitory neurotransmitter for the CNS. The pathways of GABA exist almost exclusively in the CNS, with the largest GABA concentrations in the hypothalamus, hippocampus, basal ganglia, spinal cord, and cerebellum. GABA functions in an inhibitory role in control of spinal reflexes and cerebellar reflexes. It has a major role in the control of neuronal excitability through the brain. In addition, GABA has an inhibitory influence on the activity of the dopaminergic nigrostriatal projections. GABA also has interconnections with other neurotransmitters. For example, dopamine inhibits cholinergic neurons, and GABA provides feedback and balance.

Decreased GABA activity is involved in the development of seizure disorders. Three specific subtype receptors have been identified for GABA: A, B, and C. Alcohol, certain anaesthetics, benzodiazepine antianxiety drugs, and sedative–hypnotic barbiturate drugs work because of their affinity for $GABA_A$ receptor sites. Interest in the beneficial effects of these drugs has led to increased interest in GABA receptor sites. Healthcare professionals frequently see alcohol used to self-treat anxiety; understanding how alcohol impacts the GABA receptors helps to explain this behaviour. Military combat experience increases the risk for posttraumatic stress disorder with and without depressive and substance use disorders among veterans. One recent American study found polymorphisms in a GABA transporter mechanism place veterans at risk for these disorders (Bountress et al., 2017).

Glutamate

Glutamate, the most widely distributed excitatory neurotransmitter, is the main transmitter in the associational areas of the cortex. Glutamate can be found in several pathways from the cortex to the thalamus, pons, striatum, and spinal cord. In addition, glutamate pathways have connections with the hippocampus. Some glutamate receptors may play a role in the long-lasting enhancement of synaptic activity. In the hippocampus, this enhancement may have a role in learning and memory.

An imbalance in glutamate is harmful to neurons. Considerable interest has emerged regarding its neurotoxic effects. Conditions that produce an excess of endogenous glutamate can cause neurotoxicity by overexcitation of the neuronal tissue. This process, called excitotoxicity, increases the sensitivity of glutamate receptors, produces overactivation of the receptors, and is increasingly being understood as a critical piece of the cascade of events involved in physical symptoms of alcohol withdrawal in dependent individuals. Excitotoxicity is also believed to be part of the pathology of conditions such as ischemia, hypoxia, hypoglycemia, and hepatic failure. Dysfunction of the glutamate system may be involved in depression, drug addiction, psychosis, fragile X syndrome, and Parkinson disease (Ouellet-Plamondon & George, 2012). A reduction in glutamate is seen in individuals with chronic pain and is significantly associated with emotional dysregulation, such as depression, anxiety, and high levels of harm avoidance characteristics (excessive worry, pessimism, fear, doubt, and fatigue) (Naylor et al., 2019).

Neuropeptides

Peptides are short chains of amino acids. **Neuropeptides** exist in the CNS and have several important roles as neurotransmitters, neuromodulators, or neurohormones. Neuropeptides were first thought to be pituitary hormones, such as adrenocorticotropin, oxytocin, and vasopressin, or hypothalamic-releasing hormones, such as corticotropin-releasing hormone and thyrotropin-releasing hormone (TRH). However, when an endogenous morphine-like substance was discovered in the 1970s, the term endorphin, or endogenous morphine, was introduced. Although amino acids and monoamine neurotransmitters can be produced directly from dietary precursors in any part of the neuron, almost without exception, neuropeptides are synthesized from messenger RNA in the cell body. To date, two types of neuropeptides have been identified: opioid and nonopioid. Opioid neuropeptides, such as endorphins, enkephalins, and dynorphins, act in endocrine functioning and pain suppression. Nonopioid neuropeptides, such as substance P and somatostatin, play roles in pain transmission and endocrine functioning.

There are considerable variations in the distribution of individual neuropeptides, but some areas are especially rich in cell bodies containing neuropeptides. These areas include the amygdala, striatum, hypothalamus, raphe nuclei, brainstem, and spinal cord. Many of the interneurons of the cerebral cortex contain neuropeptides, but there are considerably fewer in the thalamus and almost none in the cerebellum.

Endocannabinoid System

The endocannabinoid system (ECS) regulates diverse types of neurons throughout the body and plays important roles in CNS development, synaptic plasticity, and the response to insults originating inside (endogenous) and outside (exogenous) the body. The ECS comprises cannabinoid receptors, naturally occurring endogenous cannabinoids (endocannabinoids), and the enzymes responsible for the synthesis and degradation of the endocannabinoids. The most abundant cannabinoid receptor is the CB1 cannabinoid receptors. Exogenous cannabinoids, such as tetrahydrocannabinol, derived from marijuana, produce their biological effects through their interactions with cannabinoid receptors within this system. These compounds are degraded by distinct enzymatic processes, which determines the different physiological and pathophysiological effects they have on the body (Griffing & Thai, 2018).

It is suspected that cannabis use increases the risk for schizophrenia and may elicit psychotic symptoms in susceptible individuals (Lu & Mackie, 2016). With the legalization of cannabis in Canada and its purported therapeutic and deleterious effects, there is increased research in this area intended to provide a greater understanding of the ECS system.

Other

The complexities of neuronal transmission are enormous. Nurses have a significant role in assessing symptoms and administering and monitoring medications

for individuals with mental health disorders. Knowledge of neurotransmitters is essential because even a single dose of a drug affecting this system may cause relief of symptoms or have adverse effects. The actions of psychopharmacologic agents and related nursing responsibilities are discussed more fully in Chapter 13. In addition, many nursing interventions designed to effect changes in such functions as sleep, diet, stress management, exercise, and mood modulation affect these neurotransmitters and neuropeptides, directly or indirectly. More research is needed to understand the bio/psycho/social/spiritual aspects of nursing care.

Related Fields of Study

Fields of study related to neuroscience have emerged as the complexity of the nervous system and its interrelationship with other body systems and the environment have become more fully understood. From the discussion of neuroanatomy and neurotransmitters, it is logical to deduce that understanding the endocrine system and its interrelationship with the nervous system is essential. Although it has long been observed that individuals under stress have compromised immune systems and are more likely to acquire common diseases, only recently have changes in the immune system been linked to some mental health disorders (Capuron & Miller, 2011; Tafet & Nemeroff, 2016). In addition, as biologic rhythms have become more fully understood and defined, new information suggests that dysfunction of these rhythms may not only result from a mental health disorder but also contribute to its development. The following sections provide a brief overview of psychoendocrinology, psychoneuroimmunology, and chronobiology.

Psychoendocrinology

Psychoendocrinology examines the relationships among the nervous system, endocrine system, and mental health disorders. Messages are conveyed within the endocrine system mainly by hormones, and neurohormones are those substances excreted by special neurons within the nervous system. Neurohormones are cellular substances and are secreted into the bloodstream and transported to a site where they exert their effect. Of the several types of hormones, peptides are the most common hormones in the CNS.

The hypothalamus sends and receives information through the pituitary, which then communicates with structures in the peripheral aspects of the body. Figure 10.14 presents an example of the communication of the anterior pituitary with many organs and structures. Axes, the structures within which the neurohormones are providing messages, are the most often studied aspect of the neuroendocrine system. These axes always involve a feedback mechanism. For example,

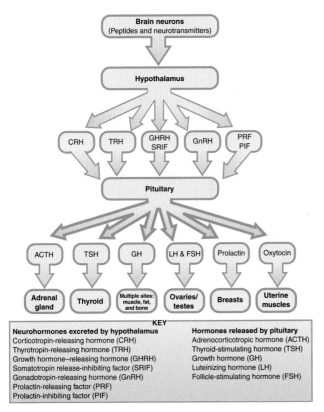

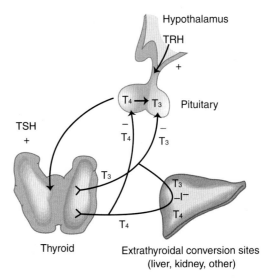

Figure 10.15 Hypothalamic–pituitary–thyroid axis. The regulation of thyroid-stimulating hormone (TSH or thyrotropin) secretion by the anterior pituitary. Positive effects of thyrotropin-releasing hormone (TRH) from the hypothalamus and negative effects of circulating triiodothyronine (T_3) and T_3 from intrapituitary conversion of thyroxine (T_4).

Figure 10.14 Hypothalamic and pituitary communication system. The neurohormonal communication system between the hypothalamus and the pituitary exerts effects on many organs and systems.

the hypothalamic–pituitary–thyroid axis regulates the release of thyroid hormone by the thyroid gland using TRH hormone from the hypothalamus to the pituitary and TSH from the pituitary to the thyroid. Figure 10.15 illustrates the hypothalamic–pituitary–thyroid axis. The hypothalamic–pituitary–gonadal axis regulates estrogen and testosterone secretion through LH and FSH.

Interest in psychoendocrinology is heightened by various endocrine disorders that produce psychiatric symptoms. Addison disease (hypoadrenalism) produces depression, apathy, fatigue, and occasionally psychosis. Hypothyroidism produces depression and some anxiety. Administration of steroids can cause depression, hypomania, irritability, and, in some cases, psychosis. Some psychiatric disorders have been associated with endocrine system dysfunction. For example, some individuals with mood disorders show evidence of dysregulation in the adrenal, thyroid, and GH axes.

Psychoneuroimmunology

Psychoneuroimmunology is the study of the interaction between the nervous system and the immune system. The immune system protects the body from foreign pathogens. Overactivity of the immune system can occur in autoimmune diseases such as systemic lupus erythematosus, allergies, or anaphylaxis. Too little activity may

result from cancer and its treatment and serious infections, such as AIDS. Evidence suggests that communication between the nervous system and the immune system is bidirectional. Specific immune system dysfunctions may result from damage to the hypothalamus, hippocampus, or pituitary and may produce symptoms of psychiatric disorders. Negative events and emotions influence catecholamines (norepinephrine and epinephrine), ACTH, cortisol, GH, and prolactin. Each of these hormones can affect the immune function. Figure 10.16 illustrates the interaction between stress and the immune system. This figure also demonstrates the true bio/psycho/social/spiritual nature of the complex interrelationship of the nervous system, the endocrine system, the immune system, and environmental or emotional stress.

Immune dysregulation may also be involved in the development of mental health disorders. This can occur by allowing neurotoxins to affect the brain, damaging the neuroendocrine tissue or damaging tissues in the brain at locations such as the receptor sites. Some antidepressants have been thought to have antiviral effects. Symptoms of diseases such as depression may follow an occurrence of serious infection, and prenatal exposure to infectious organisms may be associated with the development of schizophrenia. Stress and conditioning have specific effects on the suppression of immune function.

Cytokines are hormone-like proteins that control the intensity and duration of the body's immune response. An example of a cytokine is interferon alpha, a medication used in the treatment of cancer and hepatitis. Unfortunately, up to 45% of people treated with interferon develop major depression (Capuron & Miller, 2011). Depression and anxiety are linked to cytokines that

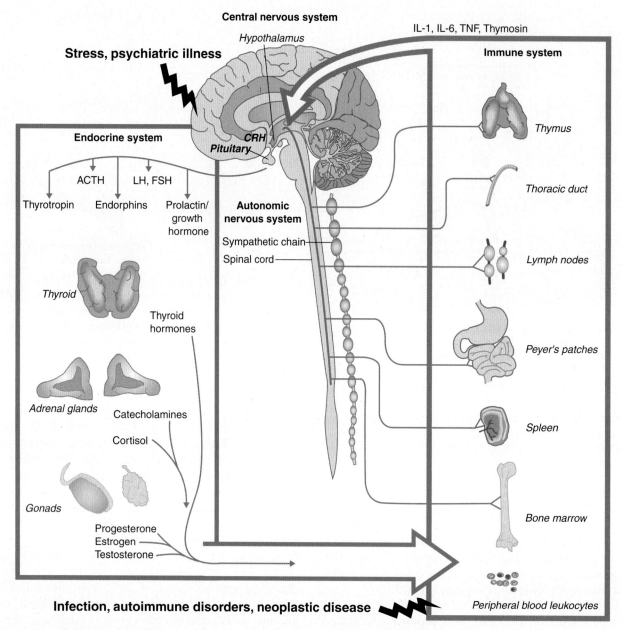

Figure 10.16 Examples of the interaction between stress or psychiatric illness and the immune system through the endocrine system. ACTH, adrenocorticotropic hormone; CRH, corticotropin-releasing hormone; FSH, follicle-stimulating hormone; IL, interleukin; LH, luteinizing hormone; TNF, tumour necrosis factor.

promote inflammation (Tafet & Nemeroff, 2016). The understanding of the relationship between the immune system and mental health disorders improves as our knowledge of the immune system continues to advance.

Chronobiology

Chronobiology involves the study and measure of time structures, or biologic rhythms that occur in living organisms. Examples of these include the circadian cycle, which is typically 24 hr, and the menstrual cycle, typically 28 days. Rhythms exist throughout the human body to control endocrine secretions, sleep–wake cycles, body temperature, neurotransmitter synthesis, and more. These cycles may become dysregulated and may

begin earlier than usual, known as a phase advance, or later than usual, known as a phase delay.

Zeitgebers are specific events that function as time givers or synchronizers and that set biologic rhythms. Light is the most common example of an external zeitgeber. The suprachiasmatic nucleus of the hypothalamus is an example of an internal zeitgeber. Some theorists think that psychiatric disorders may result from one or more biologic rhythm dysfunctions. For example, depression, in part, may be a phase advance disorder, including early-morning awakening and decreased time of onset of REM sleep. Seasonal affective disorder may be the result of shortened exposure to light during the winter months. Exposure to specific artificial light often relieves symptoms of fatigue, overeating, hypersomnia, and depression.

Diagnostic Approaches

Previously, mental health disorders were thought to have only a psychological component. With increasing knowledge of neural transmission, brain functioning, and psychopharmacology, however, research focus is shifting to the identification of **biologic markers** for mental health disorders. Biologic markers are diagnostic test findings that occur only in the presence of the mental health disorders and include findings of laboratory and other diagnostic tests and neuropathologic changes noticeable on assessment. Reliable markers increase diagnostic certainty, which allows for accurate and earlier treatment, increases the possibility of preventive interventions to forestall or avoid the onset of illness, and determines the expected prognosis for given conditions. Nurses should be aware of the most current information on biologic markers so that information, limitations, and results can be discussed knowledgeably with the individual.

Laboratory Tests and Neurophysiologic Procedures

For many years, laboratory tests have been used in the attempt to measure levels of neurotransmitters and other CNS substances in the bloodstream. Many of the metabolites of neurotransmitters can be found in the urine and CSF as well. However, these measures have had only limited utility in elucidating what is happening in the brain. Levels of neurotransmitters and metabolites in the bloodstream or urine do not necessarily equate with levels in the CNS. In addition, availability of the neurotransmitter or metabolite does not predict the availability of the neurotransmitter in the synapse, where it must act or directly relate to the receptor sensitivity. Studies of fresh brain tissue removed in neurosurgery and postmortem studies have helped localize neurotransmitters, their function, and pharmacologic properties. However, although these studies have provided diagnostic clues, they are not conclusive and therefore are not routinely used.

Although no commonly used laboratory tests exist that directly confirm a mental disorder, laboratory tests are still an active part of care and assessment of people with mental health disorders. Many physical conditions mimic the symptoms of mental health disorders, and many of the medications used to treat these disorders can produce health problems as adverse side effects. For these reasons, the routine care of individuals with mental health disorders includes laboratory tests such as complete blood counts, thyroid studies, electrolytes, hepatic enzymes, and other evaluative tests. Nurses must be familiar with these procedures and assist individuals in understanding the use and implications of such tests.

Electroencephalography

Developed in the 1920s by Hans Berger, an electroencephalograph (EEG) measures electrical activity in the uppermost layers of the cortex. Electrodes are placed on 8 to 20 sites on the person's scalp. The EEG machine is equipped with graph paper and recording pens that trace the electrical impulses generated over each electrode. Until the use of CT scanning in the 1970s, the EEG was the only method for identifying brain abnormalities. It remains the simplest and least invasive method for identifying some disorders.

An EEG may be used in psychiatry to differentiate possible causes of a person's symptoms. For example, some types of seizure disorders, such as temporal lobe epilepsy, head injuries, or tumours, may present with predominantly psychiatric symptoms. In addition, metabolic dysfunction, delirium, dementia, altered levels of consciousness, hallucinations, and dissociative states may require EEG evaluation.

Normal patterns seen on EEGs are called alpha, beta, theta, and delta waves; the rhythms may vary depending on the age of the person. Factors that interfere with obtaining accurate results include inability to remain still or cooperate during the test, being hypoglycemic or hypothermic, and hair that is dirty, oily, or treated with hair products. Spikes and wave pattern changes on the tracing may be indications of brain abnormalities, such as seizure activity. Because abnormal activity often is not discovered on a routine EEG while the individual is awake, additional methods are sometimes used to provoke a response. Nasopharyngeal leads allow the electrodes to be closer to the limbic regions of the brain; flashing strobe light may stimulate activity that is not in phase with the flashing light; and hyperventilation for 3 min may induce abnormal activity, if it exists.

Abnormalities are more likely to occur when an individual is asleep. Sleep deprivation may be induced by keeping the individual awake throughout the night before the EEG evaluation. This way, the person may then be drowsy and fall asleep during the procedure. Sleep may also be induced using medication; however, EEG wave patterns can be affected by medications, such as anticonvulsants, anxiolytics, and other substances that act as sedatives or stimulants. For example, the benzodiazepine class of drugs increases the rapid and fast beta activity and lithium increases theta activity. In addition to reassuring, preparing, and educating the person for the examination, the nurse should carefully assess the history of substance use and report this information to the examiner. If a sleep deprivation EEG is to be done, caffeine or other stimulants that might help the person stay awake should be withheld as they may change the EEG patterns.

Polysomnography

Polysomnography is a special procedure that involves recording the EEG throughout a night of sleep. See Chapter 28 for a discussion of sleep studies.

Other Neurophysiologic Methods

Evoked potentials (EPs), also called event-related potentials, use the same basic principles as an EEG. They measure changes in electrical activity in the visual, somatosensory, and auditory pathways in response to a given stimulus. Electrodes placed on the scalp measure a large waveform that stands out after the administration of repetitive stimuli, such as a click or flash of light. There are several different types of EPs to be measured, depending on the sensory area affected by the stimulus, the cognitive task required, or the region monitored, any of which can change the length of time until the wave occurrence. EPs are used extensively in psychiatric research. In clinical practice, EPs are used primarily in the assessment of demyelinating disorders, such as multiple sclerosis.

Integration of the Biologic, Psychologic, Social, and Spiritual Domains

Basic knowledge in the neurosciences has become essential content for the practising nurse. In a truly holistic bio/psycho/social/spiritual model, all psychological and social influences interact with the complex human biologic system. For example, treatment of generalized anxiety disorder would involve addressing etiologies in each of these areas (see Fig. 10.17).

As research continues to increase our understanding of the biologic dimension of psychiatric disorders and mental health, nursing care will focus on human biology in increasingly sophisticated ways. Nurses must integrate this information into all aspects of nursing management, including:

- Assessment—genetic, physical, and environmental factors that contribute to the symptoms of psychiatric disorders; biologic rhythm changes; cognitive abilities that may affect or complicate interventions; and risk factors that may predict development of psychiatric symptoms or disorders
- Diagnosis—difficulties related to diet, exercise, or sleep that may change the individual's biology; quality of life difficulties based on biologic changes; and knowledge deficits concerning the biologic basis of psychiatric disorders or treatment
- Interventions—designed to modify biologic changes and physical functioning, designed to enhance biologic treatments, or modified to consider cognitive dysfunction related to psychiatric disorders

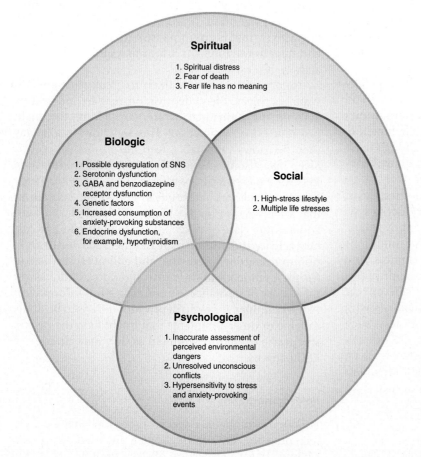

Figure 10.17 Bio/psycho/social/spiritual etiologies for patients with generalized anxiety disorders. GABA, γ-aminobutyric acid; SNS, sympathetic nervous system.

Summary of Key Points

- Neuroscientists now view behaviour and cognitive function as results of complex interactions within the CNS and its plasticity, or its ability to adapt and change, in both structure and function.
- Each hemisphere of the brain is divided into four lobes. The frontal lobe controls motor speech function, personality, and working memory—often called the executive functions that govern one's ability to plan and initiate action. The parietal lobe controls sensory functions. The temporal lobe contains the primary auditory and olfactory areas. The occipital lobe controls visual integration of information.
- The structures of the limbic system are integrally involved in memory and emotional behaviour. Dysfunction of the limbic system has been linked with major mental health disorders, including schizophrenia, depressive, and anxiety disorders.
- Neurons communicate with each other through synaptic transmission. Neurotransmitters excite or inhibit a response at the receptor sites and have been linked to certain mental health disorders. These neurotransmitters include ACh, dopamine, norepinephrine, serotonin, GABA, and glutamate.
- Psychoendocrinology examines the relationship between the nervous system and endocrine system and the effects of neurohormones excreted by special neurons to communicate with the endocrine system in effecting behaviour. Psychoneuroimmunology focuses on the nervous system as regulating immune function, which may play a significant role in effecting psychological states and psychiatric disorders. Chronobiology focuses on the study and measure of time structures or biologic rhythms occurring in the body and attributes dysregulation of these cycles to the development of mental health disorders.
- Biologic markers are physical indicators of disturbances within the CNS that differentiate one disease process from another, such as biochemical changes or neuropathologic changes. These biologic markers can be measured by several methods of testing, including electroencephalography, polysomnography, EPs, CT scanning, MRI, PET, and SPECT.

Thinking Challenge

1. The psychiatric–mental health nurse is caring for a client diagnosed with a depressive disorder. They lost their significant other 3 months ago and have not been able to leave their house because of their deep sadness. They are now receiving group counseling and have been placed on an antidepressant.

   a. What brain structures are involved in the development of depression?

   b. How are neurotransmitters implicated in this disease process?

   c. What genetic factors are associated with this mental health disorder?

   d. What biologic changes occur due to stressors and early life adversity that are associated with this mental health disorder?

> Visit the Point to view suggested responses.
> Go to **thePoint.lww.com/activate** and use the activation code found in the front of this text to unlock answers to the "Thinking Challenges" and other online resources.

Web Links

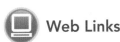

http://www.albertafamilywellness.org/brain-story-tookit Alberta Family wellness offers the Brain Story Toolkit. A library of brain-related resources addressing how early life experiences influences brain development, resilience, and later life behaviours. Also includes access to the free Brain Story certification course.

https://thebrain.mcgill.ca McGill University hosts this excellent presentation of "the brain from top to bottom," with the latest research informing explanations of the brain's anatomy and physiology, its relationship with mind and behaviour, and brain disorders from biologic, psychological, and social perspectives.

http://loni.usc.edu This is the site of the Laboratory of Neuro Imaging (LONI) at the University of Southern California. LONI is dedicated to the development of comprehensive brain mapping to improve understanding of the brain.

http://braintour.harvard.edu/click-watch-learn Several fascinating video talks about the brain are available at this site.

https://www.ted.com At this site, you can access many educational, entertaining talks on the brain, such as "Jocelyne Bloch: The brain may be able to repair itself—with help" and "Rebecca Brachman: Could a drug prevent depression and PTSD?"

https://alleninstitute.org/what-we-do/brain-science The Allen Institute for Brain Science has a site that posts many interesting interactive tools describing current areas of brain research.

References

Agius, M., & Aquilina, F. F. (2014). Comorbidities and psychotic illness. Part 1: Philosophy and clinical consequences. *Psychiatria Danubina, 26*(Suppl 1), 246–249.

Bhatnagar, S. (2013). *Neuroscience for the study of communicative disorders.* Lippincott Williams & Wilkins.

Bountress, K. E., Wei, W., Sheerin, C., Chung, D., Amstadter, A. B., Mandel, H., & Wang, Z. (2017). Relationships between GAT1 and PTSD, depression, and substance use disorder. *Brain Sciences, 7*(1), 6. http://dx.doi.org/10.3390/brainsci7010006

Canadian Institutes of Health Research. (2020). *Canadian epigenetics, environment and health research consortium.* https://cihr-irsc.gc.ca/e/43602.html

Capuron, L., & Miller, A. (2011). Immune system to brain signaling: Neuropsychopharmacological implications. *Pharmacology and Therapeutics, 130*, 226–238.

Currie, S., Hadjivassiliou, M., Crave, I., Wilkinson, I., Griffiths, P., & Hoggard, N. (2013). Magnetic resonance spectroscopy of the brain. *Postgraduate Medical Journal, 89*, 94–106.

DeSocio, J. E. (2018). Epigenetics, maternal prenatal psychosocial stress, and infant mental health. *Archives of Psychiatric Nursing, 32*, 901–906.

Doll, A., Hölzel, B. K., Mulej Bratec, S., Boucard, C. C., Xie, X., Wohlschläger, A. M., & Sorg, C. (2016). Mindful attention to breath regulates emotions via increased amygdala-prefrontal cortex connectivity. *NeuroImage, 134*, 305–313. https://doi.org/10.1016/j.neuroimage.2016.03.041

Fenoglio, C., Scarpini, E., Serpente, M., & Galimberti, D. (2018). Role of genetics and epigenetics in the pathogenesis of Alzheimer's disease and frontotemporal dementia. *Journal of Alzheimers Disorders, 62*(3), 913–932. https://doi.org/10.3233/JAD-170702

Franzago, M., La Rovere, M., Guanciali Franchi, P., Vitacolonna, E., & Stuppia, L. (2019). Epigenetics and human reproduction: The primary prevention of the noncommunicable diseases. *Epigenomics, 11*(12), 1441–1460. https://doi.org/10.2217/epi-2019-0163

Gangisetty, O., Cabrera, M. A., & Murugan, S. (2018). Impact of epigenetics in aging and age- related neurodegenerative diseases. *Frontiers in Bioscience, 23*, 1445–1464. https://doi.org/10.2741/4654

Genome Canada. (2017). *New funding opportunity—2017 Large-scale applied research project competition: Genomics and precision health.* https://www.genomecanada.ca/en/news-and-events/news-releases/new-funding-opportunity-2017-large-scale-applied-research-project

Government of Canada. (2018). *Concussion in sport: Sport and recreation-related traumatic brain injuries among Canadian children and youth.* https://www.canada.ca/en/public-health/services/diseases/concussion-sign-symptoms/concussion-sport-infographic

Griffing, G., & Thai, A. (2018). *Endocannabinoids.* Medscape. https://emedicine.medscape.com/article/1361971-overview#a2

Harlow, J. M. (1868). Recovery after severe injury to the head. *Publication of the Massachusetts Medical Society, 2*, 327.

Holtzheimer, P. E. (2013). Unipolar depression in adults: Treatment with transcranial magnetic stimulation (TMS). *UpToDate.* Retrieved from http://www.uptodate.com/index

Joosten, S. C., Smits, K. M., Aarts, M. J., Melotte, V., Koch, A., Tjan-Heijnen, V. C., & van Engeland, M. (2018). Epigenetics in renal cell cancer: Mechanisms and clinical applications. *Nature Reviews Urology, 15*(7), 430–451. https://doi.org/10.1038/s41585-018-0023-z

Kim, Y., Jeong, H. S., Song, I., Chung, Y., Namgung, E., & Kim, Y. (2016). Brain perfusion alterations in depressed patients with Parkinson's disease. *Annals of Nuclear Medicine, 30*(10), 731–737.

Kim, G. S., Smith, A. K., Nievergelt, C. M., & Uddin, M. (2018). Neuroepigenetics of post traumatic stress disorders. In B. P. F. Rutten (Ed.), *Progress in molecular biology and translational science* (Vol. 158, pp. 227–253). Academic Press. https://doi.org/10.1016/bs.pmbts.2018.04.001

Kumsta, R. (2019). The role of epigenetics for understanding mental health difficulties and its implications for psychotherapy research. *Psychology and Psychotherapy, 92*(2), 190–207. https://doi.org/10.1111/papt.12227

Kundu, T. K. (Ed.). (2013). *Epigenetics: Development and disease.* Springer.

Labonté, B., Suderman, M., Maussion, G., Lopex, J. P., Navarro-Sánchex, L., Yerko, V. G., Mechawar, N., Szyf, M., Meaney, M. J., & Turecki, G. (2013). Genome-wide methylation changes in the brains of suicide completers. *American Journal of Psychiatry, 170*(5), 511–520.

Legoff, L., D'Cruz, S. C., Tevosian, S., Primig, M., & Smagulova, F. (2019). Transgenerational inheritance of environmentally induced epigenetic alterations during mammalian development. *Cells, 8*(12), 1559. https://doi.org/10.3390/cells8121559

Loi, M., Del Savio, L., & Stupka, E. (2013). Social epigenetics and equality of opportunity. *Public Health Ethics, 6*(2), 142–153. https://doi.org/10.1093/phe/pht019

Lu, H. C., & Mackie, K. (2016). An introduction to the endogenous cannabinoid system. *Biological Psychiatry, 79*(7), 516–525. https://doi.org/10.1016/j.biopsych.2015.07.028

Marques, S., & Fleming Outeiro, T. (2013). Epigenetics in Parkinson's and Alzheimer's diseases. In T. K. Kundu (Ed.), *Epigenetics: Development and disease* (pp. 507–525). Springer.

McGuffin, P., & Southwick, L. (2003). Fifty years of the double helix and its impact on psychiatry. *Australian and New Zealand Journal of Psychiatry, 37*, 657–661.

Merico, D., Zarrei, M., Costain, G., Ogura, L., Alipanahi, B., Gazzellone, M. J., Butcher, N. J., Thiruvahindrapuram, B., Nalpathamkalam, T., Chow, E. W. C., Andrade, D. M., Frey, B. J., Marshall, C. R., Scherer, S. W., & Bassett, A. S. (2015). Whole-genome sequencing suggests schizophrenia risk mechanisms in humans with 22q11.2 deletion syndrome. *G3 (Bethesda, Md.), 5*(11), 2453–2461. https://doi.org/10.1534/g3.115.021345

Miglioretti, D., & Simth-Bindman, R. (2011). Overuse of computed tomography and associated risks. *American Family Physician, 83*, 1252–1254.

Moore, K. L., Agur, A. M. R., & Dalley, A. F. (2014). *Clinically oriented anatomy.* Lippincott Williams & Wilkins.

Morrish, J., & Carey, S. (2013). Concussions in Canada. *Canada injury compass.* Parachute.

National Human Genome Research Institute. (2013). *Fact sheets: Epigenomics.* National Institutes of Health. http://www.genome.gov/27532724

Naylor, B., Hesam-Shariati, N., McAuley, J. H., Boag, S., Newton-John, T., Rae, C. D., & Gustin, S. M. (2019). Reduced glutamate in the medial prefrontal cortex is associated with emotional and cognitive dysregulation in people with chronic pain. *Frontiers in Neurology, 3*(10), 1110. https://doi.org/10.3389/fneur.2019.01110.

Nolte, J., & Angevine, J. (1995). *The human brain: In photographs and diagrams.* Mosby.

Oedegaard, K. J., Alda, M., Anand, A., Andreassen, O. A., Balaraman, Y., Berrettini, W. H., Bhattacharjee, A., Bernnand, K. J., Burdick, K. E., Calabrese, J. R., Calkin, C. V., Claasen, A., Coryell, W. H., Craing, D., DeModena, A., Frye, M., Gage, F. H., Gao, K., Garnham, J., ... Kelsoe, J. R. (2016). The pharmacogenomics of bipolar disorder study (PGBD): Identification of genes for lithium response in a prospective sample. *BMC Psychiatry, 16*, 129. https://doi.org/10.1186/s12888-016-0732-x

Ouellet-Plamondon, C., & George, T. (2012). *Glutamate and psychiatry in 2012: Up, up and away!* Psychiatric times. http://www.psychiatrictimes.com/bipolar-disorder/glutamate-and-psychiatry-2012%E2%80%94-and-away

Pirooznia, M., Seifuddin, F., Judy, J., Mahon, P. B., Potash, J. B., & Zandi, P. P. (2012). Data mining approaches for genome-wide association of mood disorders. *Psychiatric Genetics, 22*(2), 55–61. https://doi.org/10.1097/YPG.0b013e32834dc40d

Quigley, P. (2015). Mapping the human genome: Implications for practice. *Nursing, 45*(9), 26–34. https://doi.org/10.1097/01.NURSE.0000470413.71567.fd

Reddy, O. C., & van der Werf, Y. D. (2020). The sleeping brain: Harnessing the power of the glymphatic system through lifestyle choices. *Brain Sciences, 10*(11), 868–883. https://doi.org/10.3390/brainsci10110868

Rodriguez-Paredes, M., & Esteller, M. (2011). Cancer epigenetics reaches mainstream oncology. *Nature Medicine, 17*, 330–339.

Schaffe, E. E., & Lytle, I. M. (1980). *Basic physiology and anatomy.* J.B. Lippincott.

Schauf, C., Moffett, D., & Moffett, S. (1990). *Human physiology.* Times Mirror/Mosby.

Shah, M., & Allegrucci, C. (2013). Stem cell plasticity in development and cancer: Epigenetic origin of cancer stem cells. In T. K. Kandu (Ed.). *Epigenetics: Development and disease* (pp. 545–565). Springer.

Shenton, M., Hamoda, H., Schneiderman, J., Bouiz, S., Pasternak, O., Rathi, Y., Vu, M. A., Purohit, M. P., Helmer, K., Koerte, I., Lin, A. P., Westing, C. F., Kikinis, R., Kubicki, M., Stern, R. A., & Zafonte, R. (2012). A review of magnetic resonance imaging and diffusion tensor imaging findings in mild traumatic brain injury. *Brain Imaging and Behavior, 6*, 137–192.

Simmons, D. (2008). *Epigenetic influence and disease.* Scitable by nature education. http://www.nature.com/scitable/topicpage/epigenetic-influences-and-disease-895

Sofroniew, M., & Vinters, H. (2010). Astrocytes: Biology and pathology. *Acta Neuropathologica, 119*, 7–35.

Szyf, M. (2019). The epigenetics of perinatal stress. *Dialogues in Clinical Neuroscience, 21*(4), 369–378. https://doi.org/10.31887/DCNS.2019.21.4/mszyf

Tafet, G. E., & Nemeroff, C. B. (2016). The links between stress and depression: Psychoneuroendocrinological, genetic, and environmental interactions. *The Journal of Neuropsychiatry and Clinical Neurosciences, 28*(2), 77–88. https://doi.org/10.1176/appi.neuropsych.15030053. http://www.nature.com/scitable/topicpage/epigenetic-influences-and-disease-895

Waddington, C. (1957). *The strategy of the genes: A discussion of some aspects of theoretical biology.* Allen & Unwin.

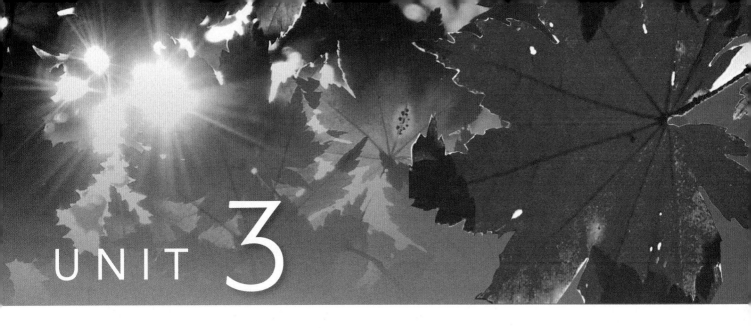

UNIT 3

Interventions in Psychiatric and Mental Health Nursing Practice

The Assessment Process

Gerri C. Lasiuk

The **nursing process** is a systematic and dynamic approach to collecting and analyzing client information and is the first step in providing nursing care. The four components of the nursing process are assessment, planning, implementation, and evaluation. This chapter deals with assessment—activities involved with the collection, validation, analysis, synthesis, and documentation of information concerning clients' responses to health and illness.

Assessment as a Process

Standard II of the *Canadian Standards of Psychiatric and Mental Health Nursing* states:

Effective assessment, diagnosis, and monitoring are central to the nurse's role and are informed by critical analyses and synthesis of evidence from multiple sources, including the client's lived experience. Working together, the client, family, nurse, and other members of the care team develop a client-centred plan of care.

The *Canadian Standards of Psychiatric and Mental Health Nursing Practice* (Canadian Federation of Mental Health Nurses [CFMHN], 2014) asserts that *assessment* is not a one-time activity; it is an ongoing, purposeful, systematic, and dynamic process in the nurse–client relationship. According to Standard II, effective assessment requires that the nurse:

1. Collaborates with clients and with other members of the healthcare team to gather holistic, client-centred assessments through observation, engagement, examination, interview (using respectful, recovery focussed language), and consultation while attending to confidentiality and pertinent legal statutes

2. Assesses, documents, and analyzes data to identify health status, potential for wellness, healthcare deficits, potential for risk to self and others; alterations in thought content and/or process, affect behaviour, communication and decision-making abilities; substance use and dependency; and history of trauma and/or abuse (emotional, physical, neglect, sexual, or verbal)

3. Formulates and documents a plan of care in collaboration with the client, family, and mental health team that supports recovery and reintegration/social inclusion in the community through discharge planning and provision for ongoing support, all while recognizing variability in the client's ability to participate in the process

4. Refines and expands client assessment information by assessing and documenting significant change(s) in the client's status and by comparing new data with the baseline assessment and client goals

5. Assesses and anticipates potential needs and risks continuously, collaborating with the client to

examine his/her environment for risk factors such as self-care, housing, nutrition, economic support, psychological state, and social interactions

6. Determines the most appropriate and available therapeutic modality that meets the client's needs, and assists the client to access necessary resources (p. 8)

KEY CONCEPT

Assessment is a purposeful, systematic, and dynamic process in nurses' relationships with clients. It involves the collection, validation, analysis, synthesis, organization, and documentation of client health–illness information.

Types of Assessment

Depending on the client's needs and the context of care, an assessment may be comprehensive or focused. A comprehensive assessment includes a complete health history (Table 11.1) and physical examination; considers the psychological, emotional, social, spiritual, and ethnocultural dimensions of health; attends to the client's lived experience; and is respectful of individuals who identify as LGBTQI2SA+ (Box 11.1). The purpose of a comprehensive assessment is to develop a holistic understanding of the individual's problems and needs as well as their strengths and resources. It is performed in collaboration with the client and other members of the care team and is the basis for establishing baseline information necessary to establish a diagnosis, identify treatment goals, and establish a plan of care.

Table 11.1 Health History and Significance to Psychiatric and Mental Health Problems	
Data	Considerations/Significance
Source of Information	Ideally, the client is the primary source of information; consultation with secondary sources is necessary with minors or when the client is unable to provide information.
	Note the apparent reliability and consistency of the information provided.
Identification/Biographic Information	Ask the clients how they wish to be addressed. This conveys respect and may elicit some information about their gender identity
	Legal name/nicknames/aliases, date and place of birth, address, telephone numbers, relationship status, next of kin, ethnicity, religious/spiritual affiliation, employer, education, and provincial/territorial health insurance number
	Once some rapport has been established, ask the persons about their gender identity and what pronouns they prefer. Inquiring in a matter-of-fact manner conveys acceptance and awareness of the importance of gender and gender identity to health
	Because this information is relatively nonthreatening, it is a safe place to begin an assessment. It also provides important clues about an individual's current living situation.
Primary Reason for Seeking Care	Record this verbatim because it speaks to the client and family perceptions of and insight into potential problems, judgement, and goals for treatment.
Past Health	
Past illness, injury, and/or hospitalization	Note positive history of childhood diseases, especially viral infection, which have been linked to some psychiatric disorders (e.g., schizophrenia).
	Inquire about surgeries and trauma, particularly those resulting in concussion or loss of consciousness.
	Ask about parental alcohol and drug use (especially during pregnancy), birth trauma, lengthy/repeated separation from parents/caregivers because of hospitalization, a pattern of injury suggestive of childhood abuse/neglect, and surgeries.
Chronic illnesses	Chronic illnesses (e.g., diabetes and thyroid dysfunction), even when well controlled, may affect mental status.
	Highlight known allergies, type of reaction, usual treatment, and effectiveness of treatment.
Family Health History	Record the name, age, and current health status of close relatives (spouse/partner, children, parents, siblings, grandparents, and aunts/uncles). If a family member is deceased, note the date and cause of death and indications of unresolved grief/loss.
	Inquire specifically about diseases/disorders that "run in the family," particularly mental disorders including substance-related and addictive disorders. A genogram is a useful tool for recording this information.
	Many mental disorders are influenced by genetics, so a family health history provides information about the client's risk factors. It also provides clues about social roles, the availability of social support, and family resources/stressors.
	Coping strategies, both effective and ineffective, are learned early in life from our family of origin. A family health history can help to identify these.
Developmental Considerations	Note achievement of important developmental milestones as well as social and educational difficulties. This information may be indicative of attentional or interpersonal deficits, behavioural problems, the nature and quality of the family environment, acquired brain injury, or childhood mental disorders.
	Ask about early parental death or separation because these may be associated with alterations in attachment and later relationship difficulties.
	The Canadian government's practice of removing Indigenous children to residential schools traumatized children, fragmented families, decimated cultures/languages, and contributed to serious social and psychological problems that still reverberate among First Nations people.

Table 11.1	Health History and Significance to Psychiatric and Mental Health Problems (*Continued*)
Data	Considerations/Significance
Immunization/HIV/Hepatitis Status	Individuals with severe and persistent mental disorders often live in severe poverty and lack resources for health promotion. In addition, many have lifestyles that put them at risk for a range of illnesses and communicable diseases.
Psychological Trauma	Ask: "Have you ever experienced or witnessed anything that threatened your life or safety or the life or safety of a loved one?" If yes, probe for details.
	Psychological trauma associated with natural disasters, motor vehicle crashes, combat, abuse/assault (physical or sexual), and childhood neglect is associated with a number of PMH problems (e.g., particularly posttraumatic stress disorder, other anxiety disorders, and depression).
Current Health Status	Provides information about medical conditions that affect mental status, global functioning, and quality of life.
	A systematic approach to performing a health history ensures thoroughness, helps the clinician to organize/cluster the data, and cues the informant's memory.
	Analyze significant symptoms (see Box 11.5).
Integument	Ask about problems/changes in the skin, hair, and nails. Note the presence of scars, piercings/body art, lesions/sores, rashes, discolouration, itching, or unusual sensations.
	Piercings and body art are expressions of one's personal aesthetic, which is part of self-concept. They may also indicate identification with particular social groups.
Sensory systems	Note sensory deficits and the presence of prescription lenses, contact lenses, hearing aids, and dentures.
	Uncorrected sensory deficits can affect an individual's day-to-day function and ability to communicate.
	Record the report of unusual perceptions or sensations because these may be related to perceptual or thought disturbances.
Respiratory	Note problems/disease, recurrent infections, cough, sputum, shortness of breath, noisy respirations, and smoking history.
Cardiovascular/haematologic	Inquire about history of cardiac disease/problems, palpitations, arrhythmias, murmurs, dizzy spells, coldness/blueness/swelling of extremities, and leg pain while walking.
	Individuals who experience panic episodes often present at emergency departments because their signs and symptoms mimic heart attack.
	Inquire about anemia, bleeding disorders, fatigue, blood transfusions, bruising, and cancers.
	Monitoring of some long-term neuroleptic medication use (e.g., lithium and clozapine) requires regular blood tests.
Gastrointestinal	Ask about changes in appetite, weight, and bowel patterns; nausea, vomiting, indigestion, and gastroesophageal reflux disease; antacid and laxative use; history of disease (e.g., ulcers, irritable bowel syndrome, and cancer); and rectal discharge/bleeding.
	Alterations in gastrointestinal function are implicated in some mental disorders and as a side effect of many psychotropic medications. For example, a person who is depressed may not have an appetite or the energy to prepare food. Others may respond to distressing emotions by eating more than usual. As well, the anticholinergic effects of antipsychotic medication can cause constipation, whereas lithium carbonate can cause diarrhea.
Genitourinary	Note pain/burning on urination, frequency, urgency, dribbling/incontinence, hesitancy, colour of urine, history of urinary tract infection/kidney disease, and frequent nighttime urination.
	Anticholinergic effects of antipsychotic medication can cause urinary hesitancy and/or retention.
Reproductive/breasts	Ask females about menarche; usual pattern of menses (frequency, duration, colour/amount of bleeding, and recent changes), obstetrical history (pregnancies, live births, miscarriages, abortions), infertility, dysmenorrhoea (pain, excessive bleeding), past or current infection/disease (e.g., sexually transmitted infections, sores/lesions, and unusual discharge or odour), date of last Pap smear, sexual orientation, sexual activity (including level of sexual desire, change in frequency of sexual activity, satisfaction with sexual relationships, painful intercourse), and contraceptive use.
	Ask males about number of children, infertility, past or current infection/disease (e.g., sexually transmitted infections, sores/lesions, and penile/rectal discharge), date of last testicular and prostate examinations, sexual orientation; sexual activity (including level of sexual desire, change in frequency of sexual activity, satisfaction with sexual relationships, painful intercourse, erectile/ejaculatory problems), and contraceptive use.
	Ask both men and women about past disease, changes in breasts or nipples (e.g., masses/lumps, pain, and discharge), and breast self-examination. Note the date of female clients' last mammogram.
	Attitudes, beliefs, and expressions of sexuality provide important information about an individual's self-concept, gender identity, sexual orientation, quality of relationships, overall satisfaction with life, and potential risk behaviours.
	Changes in level of desire and frequency of sexual activity are common in many psychiatric disorders, including depression, anxiety, and mania.
	Side effects of selective serotonin reuptake inhibitors are decreased sexual desire and erectile/ejaculatory dysfunction.
	Suicide rates among LGBTQ2S youth are higher than the national average.
Musculoskeletal	Note problems with mobility, limited range of motion, pain or weakness, joint problems, disease/injury (e.g., osteoporosis), use of prosthetics, and impairments to activities of daily living.

(Continued)

Table 11.1 Health History and Significance to Psychiatric and Mental Health Problems (*Continued*)	
Data	Considerations/Significance
Endocrine	Ask about disease/illness (e.g., diabetes, hypothyroidism/hyperthyroidism, and goiter); changes in height, weight, hair and skin, appetite, and energy level; excessive thirst; frequent urination; weakness; heat/cold intolerance; and current hormone therapy.
	Diseases of the endocrine system can imitate symptoms associated with psychiatric disorders (e.g., depression, anxiety, mania, eating disorders, and dementia).
Neurologic	Ask about head trauma, alterations in consciousness, seizures, headaches, changes in cognition and memory, and sensory and motor disturbances (numbness, tingling, loss of sensation, tremors, incoordination, balance problems, and pain). As well, inquire about alterations in personality, speech, or ability to manage activities of daily living.
	Neurologic signs and symptoms are associated with many psychiatric disorders as well as with side effects/toxicity of some neuroleptic medications (e.g., neuroleptic malignant syndrome [NMS], serotonin syndrome, and lithium toxicity).
Current Medications (including over-the-counter preparations and herbal remedies)	Specify the name of the medication, purpose, usual dose, frequency, effectiveness, side effects, prescriber, and the length of time the client has been taking it.
	This information helps to assess the client's health-promoting behaviours and potential knowledge deficits.
	Individuals with serious and persistent mental disorders often take several different medications, which puts them at risk for drug–drug and drug–food interactions.
Health/Lifestyle	
Health promotion/ maintenance	Ask individuals to evaluate their overall health and to describe what they do on a daily, weekly, and yearly basis to promote and maintain their health. Note the dates of their last physical examination, dental check-up, eye examination, and care from other providers.
Nutritional patterns	Ask about usual eating patterns and whether there have been any recent changes. Changes in eating patterns are associated with many affective states and psychiatric disorders.
	Particularly note dissatisfaction with weight and shape as well as activities aimed at weight loss. Body dissatisfaction is a factor in eating disorders and contributes to self-concept. It is particularly common among girls/women, elite athletes, and those with occupations that emphasize physical appearance (e.g., modeling and dancing).
	Psychiatric symptoms, neuroleptic medication, and poverty can all affect nutritional status.
	The weight gain associated with many neuroleptic medications increases individuals' risk for type II diabetes.
Sleep/rest patterns	Changes in sleep patterns can be a response to stress or symptoms of a psychiatric disorder.
	Probe a positive response about alterations in usual sleep patterns. Ask about *sleep onset* (latency between going to bed and falling asleep), *sleep maintenance* (frequency of wakening during the night and ease of falling back to sleep), and *early morning wakening* (consistently waking up before one needs to be up). Also, ask about whether the individual generally feels rested/refreshed.
	Alterations in sleep patterns are common in many psychiatric disorders (e.g., depression, mania, and schizophrenia). For many individuals with serious and persistent mental disorders, sleep disturbances are early signs of relapse.
Activity/exercise	Ask about usual activity level and type and amount of exercise.
	Involvement in social activities and hobbies enhances health and reduces stress. Withdrawal from these things may be early signs of illness.
	Two of the negative symptoms of schizophrenia are anhedonia (decreased ability to experience pleasure) and avolition (lack of motivational drive and energy). These explain why many individuals with schizophrenia sleep excessively.
	Alterations in usual activities are associated with many mental disorders including depression, mania, schizophrenia, and some eating disorders.
Tobacco, alcohol, cannabis and other nonprescription drug use, and problem gambling	*Tobacco.* Ask about tobacco use, including smoking, smokeless tobacco and other nicotine products (including vaping), from age of first use, frequency of use, and any recent changes to that pattern. If yes, probe for desire for change.
	Alcohol. Ask about age at first use, usual number of drinks per week, frequency of use, and any recent changes to that pattern. Probe for information about the effects of use (physical, psychological, emotional, social, legal, and economic). It is important to explore whether the individual or those close to them believe that alcohol is a problem in their lives. If yes, probe for details, desire for change, and any treatment received.
	Cannabis and nonprescription drugs. Similar to alcohol, ask about the age of first use, drug(s) of choice, dose, route, and frequency of nonprescription drug use, and changes to the pattern of use. Probe for information about the effects of drug use (physical, psychological, emotional, social, legal, and economic). It is important to explore whether the individual or those close to them believe that their drug use is a problem in their lives. If yes, probe for details, desire for change, and any treatment received.
	Problem gambling. Ask at what age it began, game(s) of choice, frequency, and average amount of money lost per month. Probe for information about the consequences (physical, psychological, emotional, social, legal, and economic). It is important to explore whether the individual or those close to them believe that their gambling is a problem in their lives. If yes, probe for details, desire for change, and any treatment received
	The co-occurrence of mental and substance-related/addictive disorders is well documented through research studies. Concurrent disorders are associated with more severe adverse outcomes than either condition alone, so their identification is of high priority.

BOX 11.1 Affirmative Care for Persons who identify as LGBTQI2SA+

Canadians who identify as lesbian, gay, bisexual, trans, queer, intersex, asexual, and two-spirit (LGBTQI2SA+) experience a number of health inequities (Government of Canada, 2019). From their literature review, Zeeman and her colleagues (2019) attribute these inequities to: (a) cultural and social norms that privilege heterosexual, cis-gender, and nonintersex individuals and ways of being; (b) minority stress associated with sexual orientation, gender identity, and sex characteristics; (c) victimization; (d) individual and institutional discrimination; and (e) stigma. Despite recent efforts to include sex and gender in research on health and disease, these phenomena have historically been underestimated, understudied, and underutilised (Mauvais-Jarvis et al., 2020). The consequence of these deeply entrenched hetero- and gender normative beliefs and practices is to render LGBTQI2SA+ individuals "invisible" in all facets of society, including health care (McCabe & Kinney, 2019). The default has been to assume that the lived experience, health and healthcare needs, and health outcomes of LGBTQI2SA+ individuals are the same as those of their heterosexual, cisgender counterparts (Colpitts & Gahagan, 2016). An additional problem is the assumption that LGBTQI2SA+ individuals belong to a single homogenous group when, in reality, they represent several unique and distinct communities composed of several sexual orientation and underrepresented gender identities (Government of Canada, 2019; McCabe & Kinney, 2019). It is only very recently that governments, healthcare systems, and researchers have begun to focus on understanding and responding to the needs of LGBTQI2SA+ individuals.

In Canada, the House of Commons Standing Committee on Health conducted a national study of LGBTQI2SA+ health. The Committee traveled across the country between February 2018 and May 2019 to collect information from 33 LGBTQI2SA+ serving organizations, academic researchers, provincial agencies, groups that offer peer support, and persons with lived experience. The Committee's findings were published in the *Health of LGBTQIA2 Communities in Canada Report* (Government of Canada, 2019).

The Report is an important first step to improving the health of Canadians who identify as LGBTQI2SA+ in that it: (a) establishes definitions related to LGBTQI2SA+ persons; (b) describes the mental, physical, and sexual health of LGBTQI2SA+ persons in Canada based on available evidence; (c) reveals ways that gender identity interacts with determinants of health to create health inequities among gender and sexual minorities; and (d) makes recommendations

about how the federal government can improve the health of LGBTQI2SA+ persons in Canada. Among its recommendations, the Committee calls on the Federal Government to "… work with the provinces, territories, and provincial health professional and regulatory bodies to establish a working group to identify ways to promote training and education of healthcare professionals about the health needs of sexual and gender minorities" (Government of Canada, 2019, p. 4).

It is critical for nurses and other healthcare providers to understand how sex, gender constructs, norms, policies, and practices influence LGBTQI2SA+ health, access to health care, help-seeking behaviours, health care service use, and adherence to treatment (Mauvais-Jarvis et al., 2020). As Zeeman et al. (2018) explain, the pervasive discrimination, prejudice, and social exclusion experienced by individuals who identify as LGBTQI2SA+ contributes to minority stress. **Minority stress** theory posits that marginalized individuals experience disproportionate levels of acute and chronic stress that can lead to increased incidence of physical and mental health problems (Meyer, 2003). This is borne out in recent research, which finds that, relative to their heterosexual and cisgender peers, individuals who identify as LGBTQI2SA+ have poorer physical and mental health including higher rates of anxiety, depression, substance misuse, self-harm, and suicide (Government of Canada, 2019; Mauvais-Jarvis et al., 2020).

Although nurses across all healthcare settings encounter persons who identify as LGBTQI2SA+, many of these individuals report feeling invisible in healthcare systems (Knox, 2019). In large part, this is because the health and health care of LGBTQI2SA+ persons is virtually absent in undergraduate nursing curricula (Greene et al., 2018). The little research that does exist on nurses' attitudes towards persons who identify as LGBTQI2SA+ demonstrates little overt bias (Greene et al., 2018). In one Canadian study, most participants argued "that differences such as sexual orientation and gender identity do not matter: Everyone should be treated as a unique individual" (Beagan et al., 2012, p. 44). As Knox (2019) explained in her presentation to the House of Commons Standing Committee on Health:

> "…while this attitude seems positive, it is ultimately not productive—since healthcare environments are overwhelmingly heteronormative, when queer patients are treated 'the same' as heterosexual patients, important parts of their lives, identities, and communities are denied. Structural inequalities LGBQ people experience and health disparities they are vulnerable to go unacknowledged." (p. 4)

(Continued)

This recognition has motivated LGBTQI2SA+-serving organizations and some healthcare systems to develop best practices for the affirmative care of LGBTQI2SA+ individuals that are informed, knowledgeable, respectful, and responsive (APA, 2015). Among other things, these affirmative practices begin with the recognition that sexual, gender diversity exists on a continuum, and that gender identity may not align with sex assigned at birth. They also require a commitment to recognizing and eliminating systemic barriers to equitable services by:

- Educating nurses and other healthcare providers about the unique lived experience and health and healthcare needs of LGBTQI2SA+ individuals

- Offering mandatory sensitivity training for all healthcare personnel
- Creating and enforcing policies and practices that safeguard LGBTQI2SA+ rights and advance their full participation in health care
- Learning and using appropriate and inclusive terminology and language
- Creating a welcoming environment for LGBTQI2SA+ patients
- Revising intake and assessment forms that include questions about sexual and gender diversity, use LGBTQI2SA+-sensitive language, and address relevant health issues
- Providing LGBTQI2SA+-specific education materials and resources

Because of its broad scope, and the time it takes to develop rapport, a comprehensive assessment may take days or even weeks to complete. Members of the care team collect information from multiple sources, including clients and their families, other healthcare providers, social service and justice personnel, educators, employers, and existing client records while attending to issues of confidentiality and legal requirements.

A **focused assessment** is the collection of specific information about a need, problem, or situation and may involve evaluation of such things as medication effects, risk for self-harm/suicide, knowledge deficits, or the adequacy of supports and resources. Focused assessments are briefer, narrower in scope, and more present oriented than are comprehensive assessments. They may be performed to screen individuals for particular problems or disorders and often employ standardized assessment tools (e.g., Glasgow Coma Scale [GCS], Mini-Mental Status Examination [MMSE], or Hamilton Rating Scale for Depression [HAM-D]).

The nurse determines the type of assessment required in light of two key factors: the immediate needs of the client and the practice setting. Efforts to perform a comprehensive assessment during a psychiatric emergency (e.g., when an individual is floridly psychotic or actively suicidal) can be both unsafe and futile. The quality and trustworthiness of the information collected in these circumstances are biased by the client's symptoms and the high emotionality of the situation. The priority in emergency situations is to perform a focused assessment to provide the treatment team with sufficient information to address the client's symptoms and to ensure the safety of all involved.

The type of assessment nurses perform is also largely determined by the setting in which they practice. The mandate of a psychiatric and mental health (PMH) facility or program determines the type of service it offers and the nature of the assessment required. During an initial admission to a psychiatric unit, for example, an individual is likely to undergo a comprehensive assessment. In contrast, nurses working with a telehealth line or with a mobile mental health crisis team will collect only the information required to address the immediate problem or crisis.

Assessment Techniques

PMH assessments involve observation of the individual at different times and in different circumstances, interviews with the individual and family members, consultation with other healthcare providers, and synthesis of findings from physical and mental status examinations.

Observation

Although verbal communication is vital to the assessment process, nonverbal cues also communicate important information about the client's health–illness experience (see Chapter 7). Nurses use their five senses to note and integrate mental health assessment during every encounter with clients. Attention to nuances of dress, behaviour, facial expression, gestures, and interactions with others (particularly when the client is not aware of being observed) provide important information about the client's mental status that may not be revealed through conversation. For example, as well as observing hygiene and personal grooming, the nurse considers whether the client's dress is appropriate to the season and situation. Other important observations include behavioural evidence of perceptual disturbances or disordered thoughts (e.g., listening or talking to unseen others) and apparent inconsistencies between what an individual reports and what the nurse observes.

Examination

A comprehensive health assessment includes a health history, a physical examination, and diagnostic testing. This is particularly important in the provision of holistic PMH care because, compared with the general population, individuals who live with serious mental disorders are at greater risk for developing a range of chronic physical conditions and have a shorter life expectancy (Byrne, 2018). Conversely, people who live with chronic physical illness often experience co-occurring mental health problems. For example, a recent systematic review and meta-analysis found that clients with irritable bowel syndrome (IBS) are three times more likely to have anxiety or depression compared with healthy individuals.

Persons living with a mental disorder can develop physical health problems related to the disorder itself and/or as a consequence of treatment. Mental disorders may disrupt hormone systems and sleep–wake cycles, while psychotropic medications (e.g., antipsychotics, mood stabilizers, and some antidepressants) are associated with insulin resistance, obesity, and dyslipidemia (Abosi et al., 2018), all of which can contribute to increased vulnerability to a range of physical conditions. Other risk factors that contribute to risk for physical illnesses include smoking, alcohol and drug use, obesity, poverty, and self-care deficits. It is also important to note that medical conditions can mask, imitate, or worsen psychiatric symptoms. The situation is further complicated because some mental disorders cause an individual to misattribute physical sensations, making it difficult to recognize and describe one's symptoms. For example, individuals who experience panic attacks often attribute their symptoms to a myocardial infarction or heart attack.

The mental status examination (MSE) is one type of focused assessment used to systematically assess an individual's psychological, emotional, social, and neurologic functioning. Although the components of the MSE are standard across clinical settings, the findings are highly subjective and rely heavily on the clinician's knowledge, communication skills, interpretation, and judgement. For this reason, it is important for clinicians to be reflective and to collaborate with colleagues to develop an unbiased understanding of the client's experience.

Interview

An assessment interview is a semi-structured conversation aimed at building rapport, obtaining information, clarifying perceptions and meanings, validating observations, and comparing understandings. Skillful interviewing is much more than asking a series of questions about signs and symptoms; it is both an art and a science and takes practice to develop (Box 11.2). Effective interviewers train themselves to be fully present in the

---

BOX 11.2 Factors That Facilitate Effective Interviewing

- As much as possible, **negotiate the terms of the interview with all participants** (e.g., choose a mutually agreeable time and place; clearly state your purpose; and continually invite the clients to express their thoughts, feelings, wants, and needs). This conveys respect, invites a collaborative alliance, and fosters rapport.
- **The environment.** Choose a private and comfortable setting that is free from interruption.
- **Realistic time management.** Be clear at the outset how much time you have available for an interview and make a realistic plan about what you can achieve.
- **Be attentive to your nonverbal communication.** Sit at the same level as the client and maintain an open body posture. If you make notes, inform the client at the beginning of the interview; keep your notes brief so you can attend to the conversation.
- **Avoid jargon** and choose language that is clear, simple, and developmentally and culturally appropriate. Repeatedly check with the clients to ensure that they understand what you are saying.
- **Begin with a less sensitive topic and move toward sensitive issues as rapport develops.**
- Leave some time at the end of the encounter for **closure and future planning**. This involves monitoring the available time and notifying the client when the interview is coming to an end.

---

situation and are genuinely warm and respectful and approach clients as collaborators working toward the same ends. Above all, competent interviewers engage in what Rogers (1975) referred to as empathic listening, which he describes as:

…being sensitive, moment by moment, to the changing felt meanings which flow in the other person and to the fear or rage or tenderness or confusion or whatever they are experiencing. It means temporarily living in the other's life, moving about in it delicately without making judgments (p. 4).

Because many psychiatric symptoms are outside of an individual's awareness, nurses may also interview family and friends to obtain relevant information. That being said, Canadian privacy legislation imposes obligations on government departments and public agencies, including health-serving facilities, to respect privacy rights and to limit the collection, use, and disclosure of

---

BOX 11.3 Barriers to Effective Interviewing

- **Lack of clarity about the purpose and parameters of the interview** is like embarking on a journey without a clear destination. A statement such as "Mrs. Woods, my name is Kate Donovan. I am a nurse on this unit and I would like to spend the next hour or so getting to know more about you and completing your admission assessment. Is that okay with you?" conveys respect, informs the client of your intent, and begins the process of negotiating a contract for the encounter.

- **Asking too many closed-ended questions.** Closed-ended questions invite brief responses and are most useful for eliciting specific facts, like those needed in a focused assessment. Heavy reliance on them tends to orient the interview around the interviewer's desire for information and prevents clients from introducing or expanding on topics of importance to them.

- **Avoiding silence.** Often in response to their own discomfort or anxiety, interviewers rush to fill all silences with words. Pauses in the conversation allow both the client and the interviewer time to reflect on their experience in the moment, to formulate or elaborate on their responses, to switch speakers, or to turn the conversation to a new topic.

- **Asking complex questions.** A complex question is really several questions presented as one, as in "Why did you come to the hospital today, who brought you, and how did you get here?" These types of questions are confusing to the respondent, who often does not know which to answer first. Successful interviewers ask one question at a time, listen carefully to the answer, and probe for more detail if it is not clear.

- **Making assumptions.** Effective interviewers are those who understand that all individuals experience and understand the world in their own unique ways. The failure to clarify and validate what the client means results in misunderstanding and inaccuracies.

- **Avoiding or ignoring expressions of emotion.** Emotions are rich communications. They provide insight into the meaning an individual assigns to an experience or event. Minimizing or ignoring an expression of emotion sends a powerful message. For example, "There are parts of you that I do not acknowledge" or "Your emotions are frightening or unimportant." Competent practitioners need to maintain a high level of self-awareness in order to remain grounded in their own experience so that they can bear witness to others.

---

personal information. In Canada, every province and territory has a commissioner or ombudsperson responsible for overseeing provincial and territorial privacy legislation. It is the responsibility of every nurse to know the limits of information sharing under that legislation (Office of the Privacy Commission of Canada, 2020).

It is often the case that novice interviewers are so overwhelmed by their own anxieties that they focus on their own experience and on asking questions to elicit needed information. When this happens, the client's needs and the relational nature of the interaction are forgotten. Box 11.3 identifies some interviewer behaviours that can impede effective interviewing.

Collaboration

A growing body of evidence stresses the importance of interprofessional collaboration in all healthcare settings. In their critical review of the literature, Pomare and colleagues (2020) found that interprofessional collaboration is associated with "improved clinical outcomes, patient satisfaction, staff satisfaction, post-discharge performance, quality of care, safety and efficiency, work engagement, and reduced staff burnout and stress, error rates, turnover, readmission rates, length of stay, morbidity or mortality rates, and review time" (p. 514). The impetus for interprofessional collaboration is further motivated by a shift toward primary health care and its emphasis on teams of health professionals who are accountable for providing comprehensive client care. Coordination of care among nurses, primary providers, and other practitioners and across care settings (e.g., in- and outpatient primary, secondary, and tertiary care), is particularly important for persons living with severe and persistent mental disorders and results in better health, improved access to services, more efficient use of resources, and higher levels of satisfaction for both consumers and health professionals (Nicaise et al., 2021).

PMH teams typically include clients and their families, nurses, primary providers, psychologists, social workers, pharmacists, occupational therapists, and recreational therapists. Depending on the treatment setting and the client's needs, other professionals (e.g., teachers, clergy or spiritual leaders, other medical specialists) may be regular contributors to the team or may participate on an *ad hoc* basis. In some settings, one member of the team may be assigned to be the client's primary therapist or case manager and takes on the role of coordinating team activities. Teams meet together frequently to share information, to develop and evaluate treatment goals, and to provide ongoing support.

In most North American PMH treatment facilities, the interdisciplinary team works to develop a psychiatric diagnosis based on the *Diagnostic and Statistical Manual of Mental Health Disorders*, 5th edition (*DSM-5*) (American Psychiatric Association, 2013). The *DSM-5* provides a common language and standard criteria for the classification of mental disorders.

Bio/Psycho/Social/Spiritual Psychiatric/Mental Health Nursing Assessment

A bio/psycho/social/spiritual PMH nursing assessment begins with the assumption that humans are whole, integrated beings who live in constant and reciprocal relationship with their physical and social environments (Fig. 11.1). The bio/psycho/social/spiritual model provides a framework for assessing the physical, psychological, emotional, social, and spiritual dimensions of health. Whereas the goal of medical assessment is the diagnosis and treatment of disease and illness, nursing assessment aims to develop a holistic understanding of the person's lived experience. In addition to identifying health problems and deficits, it attends to strengths and resources and evaluates how these affect the individual's quality of life and activities of daily living.

Types and Sources of Information

Client information (data) fall into two broad categories: objective and subjective. **Objective data** (signs) are directly observable and measurable. The physical examination, vital signs, and diagnostic tests all yield objective data. In contrast, subjective data (symptoms) are neither directly observable nor measurable. **Subjective data** are what the client and others report about their experiences, beliefs, emotions, perceptions, experiences, motivations, and observations. A health history provides this type of data. Subjective information provides a window into an individual's lifetime experiences and the meanings attached to those experiences. These are influenced by personal history and developmental stage, past learning, ethnicity and culture, and spirituality and offer insight into the sense an individual makes of the world. It is critical for nurses to remember that individuals act and react to the *meanings they assign* to events and experiences, rather than to the events or experiences themselves.

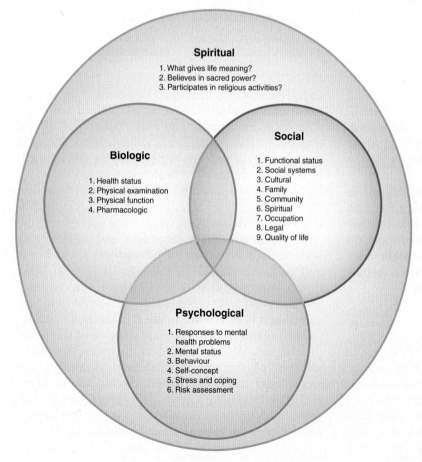

Figure 11.1 Bio/psycho/social/spiritual nursing assessment.

Both objective and subjective data are generated from *primary* or *secondary* sources. Clients are the primary sources of information about themselves. Secondary data, on the other hand, come from all other sources, including family, other healthcare providers, written reports, and client records.

Documentation

Healthcare records are important vehicles for communication as well as being legal documents. The type of information collected and how it is documented are regulated by the program or facility in which the nurse practices. In turn, programs and facilities develop documentation policies and procedures to comply with provincial and territorial legislation.

Generally speaking, there are two common approaches to documentation: *source-oriented* and *problem-oriented* documentations. In source-oriented documentation, each discipline is assigned a section of the client record (e.g., nurses' notes or primary providers' notes). Although this approach identifies the discipline of the person making the entry, it tends to fragment information and is antithetical to holistic care. In problem-oriented documentation, all team members make entries in the same section of the record. This not only facilitates interprofessional collaboration but also keeps team members oriented toward the client's identified goals, needs, and problems.

Information may be entered in the client record in several ways, including fillable forms, flow sheets, checklists, and narrative notes. Electronic health records are widely used because they are more efficient, save time, and facilitate sharing of client information. In many settings, practitioners use the SOAP (subjective data, objective data, assessment, and plan implementation/evaluation), DAR (data, action, and plan), or PIE (problem, implementation, and evaluation) methods to organize their notes. Another approach to documentation is *charting by exception*, which involves documenting only those client health–illness responses that deviate from well-articulated standards.

Biologic Domain

Health History

The health history establishes a subjective database about the client's current and past health–illness experience, identifies strengths and resources, suggests actual and potential health problems and deficits, and is an opportunity to build rapport. Depending on the practice setting, different members of the healthcare team may take responsibility for sections of the health history. For example, the social worker may perform the family and social assessments, the occupational therapist undertakes the occupational assessment, and the recreational therapist often assesses the individual's exercise and leisure activities. Table 11.1 outlines the components of a health history and relates the significance of important findings to mental health and illness.

Physical Examination

Physical examination is a process by which a clinician collects objective information about the client's health. Components include anthropomorphic measurements (e.g., height and weight), vital signs, an examination of all body systems, and diagnostic testing appropriate to the individual's age, level of risk, and sex. The physical examination aids in diagnosing disease or illness, establishes a baseline for evaluating change, and provides an opportunity to validate information provided in the health history. With respect to laboratory studies, particular attention is paid to any abnormalities of hepatic, renal, or urinary function because these systems metabolize or excrete many psychiatric medications. In addition, abnormal white blood cell (WBC) and electrolyte levels are noted. See Table 11.2 for selected haematologic measures and their relevance to psychiatric disorders.

Psychological Domain

The psychological domain includes manifestations of PMH problems/disorders; mental status; stress and coping; and risk assessment.

Responses to Mental Health Problems

The *DSM-5* (APA, 2013) describes mental disorders as patterns of thinking, feeling, and/or behaviour associated with significant distress, suffering, or impairment in one or more areas such (e.g., school, work, social and family interactions, or the ability to function independently). The identification and understanding of PMH conditions have varied throughout history and across cultures. Current thinking is that mental health–illness exists on a continuum such that mental health and mental disorder can coexist simultaneously within the same person. Like other illnesses, PMH disorders affect individuals and their families in many different ways. An important part of assessing the psychological domain is to explore the individual's experience of illness. Many fear being negatively stereotyped, discrimination in the workplace, or about their personal safety. It is important to identify the person's understanding of their disorder, their strategies for managing symptoms, and the effectiveness of those strategies. A simple question, such as "How do you deal with your voices when you are with other people?," may initiate a discussion about an experience or symptom.

Table 11.2   Selected Haematologic Measures and Their Relevance to Psychiatric Disorders

Test	Result	Implications
Complete Blood Count (CBC)		
Leucocyte count (WBC)	Leucopenia (↓ WBC)	May be a side effect of phenothiazines, clozapine, or carbamazepine
	Agranulocytosis (↓ granulocytic WBC)	Risk is 10–20 times greater with clozapine than with other antipsychotics. Lithium causes a benign mild to moderate increase (11,000–17,000/μL).
	Leucocytosis (↑ WBC)	NMS can be associated with increases of 15,000–30,000/mm^3 in about 40% of cases.
WBC differential	"Shift to the left"— from segmented neutrophils to band forms	This shift suggests a bacterial infection but has been reported in about 40% of cases of NMS.
Red blood cell (RBC) count	Polycythaemia (↑ RBC)	Primary form (true polycythaemia) is associated with several disease states; requires further evaluation.
		Secondary form is compensation for decreased oxygenation (e.g., chronic obstructive pulmonary disease).
		Blood is more viscous, which is exacerbated by being dehydrated.
	↓ RBCs	Associated with some types of anemia; requires further evaluation
Haematocrit (Hct)	↑ Hct	Associated with dehydration
	↓ Hct	Associated with anemia; may be related to alterations in mental status, including asthenia, depression, and psychosis
		20% of women of childbearing age in North America have iron deficiency anemia.
Haemoglobin (Hgb)	↓ Hgb	Indicative of anemia; evaluation of cause requires review of erythrocyte indices.
Erythrocyte indices, such as red cell distribution width (RDW)	↑ RDW	Finding suggests a combined anemia resulting from both vitamin B$_{12}$ and folic acid deficiencies and iron deficiency, as found in chronic alcoholism.
		Oral contraceptives also decrease vitamin B$_{12}$.
Other Haematologic Measures		
Vitamin B$_{12}$	Deficiency	May be associated with neuropsychiatric symptoms such as psychosis, paranoia, fatigue, agitation, marked personality change, dementia, and delirium
Folate	Deficiency	Associated with alcohol use and with medications such as phenytoin, oral contraceptives, and estrogens
Platelet count	Thrombocytopenia (↓ platelets)	Associated with use of some psychiatric medications, such as carbamazepine, phenothiazines, or clozapine and with other nonpsychiatric medications; may also cause thrombocytopenia
		Also, associated with some disease states; requires further evaluation
Serum Electrolytes		
Sodium	Hyponatraemia (serum sodium)	Associated with significant alterations in mental status. May be related to Addison disease, the syndrome of inappropriate secretion of antidiuretic hormone, polydipsia, and carbamazepine use
Potassium	Hypokalaemia (↓ serum potassium)	Associated with weakness, fatigue, electrocardiogram changes, paralytic ileus, and muscle paresis
		Common in individuals exhibiting bulimic behaviour, psychogenic vomiting, misuse of diuretics, and/or excessive laxative use. Hypokalaemia may be life threatening.
Chloride	Elevation	Chloride tends to increase to compensate for lower bicarbonate.
	Decrease	Associated with binging and purging behaviour
Bicarbonate	Elevation	Associated with binging and purging, disordered eating, excessive laxative use, and/or psychogenic vomiting
	Decrease	May develop in individuals who hyperventilate (e.g., panic disorder)
Renal Function Tests		
Blood urea nitrogen	Elevation	Associated with alterations in mental status (e.g., lethargy and delirium), dehydration, and medications excreted by the kidney, such as lithium and amantadine
Serum creatinine	Elevation	Indicative of decreased renal function; typically does elevate until 50% of nephrons in the kidney are damaged
Serum Enzymes		
Amylase	Elevation	Associated with the binging and purging behaviour in eating disorders; tends to decline when these behaviours stop
	Alanine aminotransferase (ALT) > aspartate aminotransferase (AST)	This disparity is common in acute forms of viral and drug-induced hepatic dysfunction.

(Continued)

Table 11.2 Selected Haematologic Measures and Their Relevance to Psychiatric Disorders (*Continued*)		
Test	Result	Implications
ALT (formerly serum glutamic pyruvic transaminase)	Elevation	Mild elevations are common with use of sodium valproate.
AST (formerly serum glutamic oxaloacetic transaminase)	AST > ALT	Severe elevations are associated with chronic hepatic disease and myocardial infarction.
Creatinine phosphokinase	Elevations of the isoenzyme related to muscle tissue	Associated with muscle tissue injury Level is elevated in NMS and by repeated intramuscular injections (e.g., depot antipsychotics).
Thyroid Function		
Serum triiodothyronine (T_3)	Decrease	Associated with hypothyroidism and other non–thyroid-related diseases Individuals with depression may convert less T_4 to T_3 peripherally, but not out of the normal range. Medications such as lithium and sodium valproate may suppress thyroid function, but clinical significance is unknown.
	Elevation	Indicative of hyperthyroidism; T_3 toxicosis is associated with alterations in mood, anxiety, and symptoms of mania.
Serum thyroxine (T_4)	Elevation	Indicative of hyperthyroidism
Thyroid-stimulating hormone	Elevation	Associated with hypothyroidism, which shares features of depression with the additional physical signs of cold intolerance, dry skin, hair loss, bradycardia, and so forth Lithium may also cause elevations.
	Decrease	Considered nondiagnostic; may be associated with hyperthyroidism, pituitary hypothyroidism, or even euthyroid status

Mental Status Examination

The mental status examination (MSE) (Box 11.4) is a systematic assessment of an individual's appearance, affect, behaviour, and cognitive function. It provides "a snapshot" of the client's experience and the examiner's observations and impressions at the time of the interview. The MSE is an approach used by practitioners across several disciplines and in many clinical settings to evaluate developmental, neurologic, and psychiatric disorders.

The MSE should not to be confused with the *Mini-Mental State Examination* (MMSE; Folstein et al., 1975), which is a screening tool used to evaluate cognitive impairment.

KEY CONCEPT

The mental status examination is a systematic assessment of an individual's appearance, affect, behaviour, and cognitive processes. It provides "a snapshot" of the client's subjective report and experiences and the examiner's observations and impressions at the time of the interview. The MSE is an approach used by health practitioners across several disciplines and in many clinical settings to evaluate developmental, neurologic, and psychiatric disorders.

General Observations

This section of the MSE provides a brief narrative summary of the examiner's observations and impressions of the individual during the interview. Although an individual's health history remains relatively stable, their mental status is variable over time.

Appearance

Describe the person's general appearance and presentation. Note the manner and appropriateness of dress, personal hygiene, odours, pupil size, and obvious identifying characteristics, such as tattoos and piercings. Physical signs such as skin tone (e.g., duskiness, pallor, or flushing), nutritional status, and energy level (e.g., catatonia, lethargy, or restlessness) provide clues to the person's general level of health–illness.

Psychomotor behaviour/activity

Observe and note the individual's behaviour during the interview, including posture, gait, motor coordination, facial expression, mannerisms, gestures, and activity. Pay particular attention and document cues to the person's emotional state (e.g., muscle tension, purposeless repetitive movements, and restlessness).

Attitude toward interviewer

The individual's attitude toward the interviewer and the interview process may be described as accommodating, cooperative, open, friendly, apathetic, bored, guarded, suspicious, hostile, or evasive. The following is an example of how the nurse may document general observations:

Mr. D. is a tall, thin, White Canadian man, who looks older than his stated age of 47 years. He is unshaven, his hair is uncombed, and he has a strong body odour. His clothing (jeans, plaid shirt, and a black nylon jacket) are appropriate for his age, the situation, and season but seem too large, are stained, and are dishevelled. He

---

BOX 11.4 Components of the Mental Status Examination

1. General observations
   a. Appearance
   b. Psychomotor behaviour
   c. Attitude toward interviewer
2. Mood
3. Affect
4. Speech
5. Perception
6. Thought
   a. Content

   b. Process/form
7. Sensorium
   a. Level of consciousness
   b. Orientation (person, place, time)
   c. Memory (immediate retention and recall; recent, short term, and long term)
   d. Attention and concentration
   e. Comprehension and abstract reasoning
8. Insight
9. Judgement

---

reports feeling "jumpy," and he declined to sit during the interview, opting instead to pace around the interview room. His posture is erect and his movements are quick, purposeful, and well-coordinated; he displays no unusual mannerisms. Mr. D. was cooperative with the interview process, although his verbal responses were brief and he did not maintain eye contact.

Mood and Affect

In everyday usage, the terms mood and affect are used interchangeably. In the context of an MSE, however, these words refer to specific phenomena. **Mood** refers to a pervasive and sustained emotion and is what the persons report about their prevailing emotional state. Although mood does vary with internal and external changes, it tends to be stable over time and reflects the person's general disposition or worldview. Mood can be assessed by asking an open-ended question like "How have you been feeling over the past while?" The nurse should document the client's response verbatim and probe to find whether this is typical or is a response to some recent life event. A person who is generally positive and content will remain so even when bad things happen. They will tend to view adversity as a temporary period of unpleasantness in an otherwise happy life. In contrast, an individual whose mood tends to be negative or depressed views life through dark-coloured glasses. They experience life as difficult and see happiness as fleeting.

Mood may be sustained for days or weeks, or it may fluctuate during the course of a day. For example, some individuals who are depressed have a diurnal variation in their mood; they experience their lowest mood in the morning, but as the day progresses, their mood lifts, and they feel somewhat better in the evening. Terms used to describe mood include **euthymic** (calm, cheerful),

euphoric (elated), and **dysphoric** (depressed, distressed, disturbed).

Affect refers to the client's expressed or observed emotion and is inferred by the examiner from facial expressions, vocalizations, and behaviour. During the MSE, individuals' affect may change as they talk about a difficult experience or recent life events. Affect is described in terms of its range, intensity, appropriateness, and stability. Affective range can be full or constricted. Individuals who express several emotions that are consistent with their stated feelings and the content of their speech are described as having a full range of affect that is congruent with the situation. On the other hand, a person who speaks of the recent, tragic death of a loved one with little outward expression of their internal feeling state may be described as having constricted affect. In evaluating the appropriateness of a particular response, the nurse must consider both the meaning of the event to the individual and cultural norms. Descriptions of intensity attempt to quantify an affective response. Intensity may be characterized as heightened, blunted, or flat. The phrase blunted affect describes limited emotional expression, whereas flat affect is its near absence. The person whose affect is flat speaks in a monotone voice and has little or no facial expression. Stability of affect can be described as mobile (normal) or labile. If a person displays a wide range of strong emotions in a relatively short period of time, the affect is described as being labile.

Speech

Patterns and characteristics of speech provide clues about the client's thoughts, emotions, and cognitive processes. Speech also conveys information about the person's understanding of the situation and ability to read and respond to social cues. Speech is described in terms of its quantity, rate and fluency of production, and quality. In assessing speech quantity, the individual may be described as talkative, verbose, or expansive or as having paucity or poverty of speech. Rate of speech may be slow, hesitant, fast, or pressured, whereas fluency refers to the apparent ease with which speech is produced. Pressured speech is speech that is rapid, increased in amount, and difficult to understand; it is often associated with mania. Aphasic disturbances are problems of speech output and may be neurologic, cognitive, or emotional in origin. Speech quality refers to its characteristics, such as monotone, whispered, slurred, mumbled, staccato, or loud. During conversation, the interviewer also notes speech impediments (e.g., stuttering), response latency (the length of time it takes for the individual to respond to a question or comment), and repetition, rhyming, or unusual use of words.

Perception

Perception is the complex series of mental events involved with taking in of sensory information from the environment and the processing of that information into mental representations. Two perceptual disturbances commonly associated with mental disorders are hallucinations and illusions. **Hallucinations** are false sensory perceptions not associated with external stimuli and are not shared by others. Although auditory hallucinations are the most common, hallucinations may be experienced in any of the five major sensory modalities: auditory, visual, tactile, olfactory, or gustatory. Most people are familiar with hypnagogic hallucinations—false sensory perceptions that occur while falling asleep; these are not associated with mental disorder. Of particular concern are command hallucinations, the false perception of commands or orders that an individual feels obligated to obey. For example, a person may hear voices telling them to harm or kill oneself or someone else. **Illusions** are the misperception or misrepresentation of real sensory stimuli (e.g., misidentifying the wind as a voice calling one's name or thinking that a label on a piece of clothing is an insect).

Thought

Because thought is not directly observable, it is indirectly assessed through language with respect to its content and process (form). **Thought content** refers to the subject matter occupying a person's thoughts; **thought process** is the manner in which thoughts are formed and expressed. Some individuals are very forthcoming about the content of their thoughts, whereas others are more reticent to talk about them. Assessing thought requires the clinician to carefully attend to and explore unusual or recurring themes in the individual's conversation. Box 11.5 lists some common disturbances of thought

content, and Box 11.6 lists some common disturbances of thought process.

Sensorium

This portion of the MSE assesses brain function and cognitive abilities.

Level of consciousness

Evaluating **level of consciousness** (LOC) assesses arousal or wakefulness. If the client is nonresponsive, the nurse applies increasing levels of stimulation (e.g., verbal, tactile, and painful) to elicit a response. The GCS (Teasdale & Jennett, 1974) is often used to assess LOC. Terms commonly used to describe LOC include alert, awake, lethargic, somnolent, stuporous, or comatose.

Orientation

Orientation is a cognitive function involving awareness of time, person, and place. Alterations in orientation can be caused by a number of factors including injury, drugs, brain lesions, and dementia. The examiner determines orientation by asking questions about time, place, and person because impairments tend to exist in this order (i.e., a sense of time is impaired before a sense of place). Begin with specific questions about the date, time of day, location of the interview, and name of the interviewer and move to more general questions if necessary. For example, if the client knows the year, but not the exact date, the nurse can ask the season.

Memory

Memory function is traditionally divided into four spheres: immediate retention and recall; recent memory; short-term memory; and remote or long-term memory. To assess immediate retention and recall, the nurse gives the persons three unrelated words to remember and asks them to recite these words immediately and at 5- and 15-minute intervals during the interview. To test recent memory, the nurse asks questions about events of the past few hours or days. Short-term memory involves things that occurred within the past few weeks or months. The nurse assesses remote or long-term memory by asking about events of years ago. If these are personal experiences or events, the nurse may need to verify the client's responses with others to assess their accuracy.

Attention and concentration

To test attention and concentration, the nurse asks the client to count backward, aloud, from 100 by increments of 7 (e.g., 93, 86, 79, and so on) or to start with 20 and subtract 3. The nurse must decide which is most

BOX 11.5 Alterations in Thought Content

Delusion—a false, fixed belief, based on an incorrect inference about reality. It is not shared by others and is inconsistent with the individual's intelligence or cultural background and cannot be corrected by reasoning.

Delusions of control—the belief that one's thoughts, feelings, or will are being controlled by outside forces. The following are some specific examples of delusions of control:

- **Thought insertion**—the belief that thoughts or ideas are being inserted into one's mind by someone or something external to one's self.
- **Thought broadcasting**—the belief that one's thoughts are obvious to others or are being broadcast to the world.
- **Ideas of reference**—the belief that other people, objects, and events are related to or have a special significance for one's self (e.g., a person on television is talking to or about them).

Paranoid delusions—an irrational distrust of others and/or the belief that others are harassing, cheating, threatening, or intending one harm.

Bizarre delusion—an absurd or totally implausible belief (e.g., light waves from space communicate special messages to an individual).

Somatic delusion—a false belief involving the body or bodily functions.

Delusion of grandeur—an exaggerated belief of one's importance or power.

Religious delusion—the belief that one is an agent of or specially favoured by a greater being.

Depersonalization—the belief that one's self or one's body is strange or unreal.

Magical thinking—the belief that one's thoughts, words, or actions have the power to cause or prevent things to happen; similar to Jean Piaget's notion of preoperational thinking in young children.

Erotomania—the belief that someone (often a public figure) unknown to the individual is in love with them or involved in a relationship with them.

Nihilism—the belief that one is dead or nonexistent.

Obsession—a repetitive thought, emotion, or impulse.

Phobia—a persistent, exaggerated, and irrational fear.

BOX 11.6 Alterations in Thought Process

Loosening of association—the lack of a logical relationship between thoughts and ideas; conversation shifts from one topic to another in a completely unrelated manner, making it confusing and difficult to follow.

Circumstantiality—the individuals take a long time to make a point because their conversation is indirect and contains excessive and unnecessary detail.

Tangentiality—similar to circumstantiality, except that the speaker does not return to a central point or answer the question posed.

Thought blocking—an abrupt pause or interruption in one's train of thoughts, after which the individuals cannot recall what they were saying.

Neologisms—the creation of new words.

Flight of ideas—rapid, continuous verbalization, with frequent shifting from one topic to another.

Word salad—an incoherent mixture of words and phrases.

Perseveration—a persisting response to a stimulus even after a new stimulus has been presented.

Clang association—the use of words or phrases that have similar sounds but are not associated in meaning; may include rhyming or puns.

Echolalia—the persistent echoing or repetition of words or phrases said by others.

Verbigeration—the meaningless repetition of incoherent words or sentences; typically associated with psychotic states and cognitive impairment.

Pressured speech—speech that is increased in rate and volume and is often emphatic and difficult to interrupt; typically associated with mania or hypomania.

appropriate for the patient/client considering education and understanding; subtracting 3s from 20 is the easier of the two tasks. Another way to test these areas is to ask the client to spell a simple word, such as house, backward.

Insight and Judgement

Insight and judgement are related concepts that involve the ability to examine ideas, conceptualize facts, solve problems, and think abstractly. **Insight** refers to the client's awareness and understanding of their circumstances. It reflects awareness of their own thoughts and feelings and an ability to compare them with the thoughts and feelings of others. For example, persons with impaired insight may not recognize their experiences as a symptom of a mental disorder. They may have delusions and hallucinations or be hospitalized for bizarre and sometimes dangerous behaviour but do not grasp that this is unusual or abnormal.

Judgement is the ability to consider a situation and to determine a reasonable course of action after examining and analyzing various possibilities. Throughout the interview, the nurse evaluates the person's problem-solving abilities and capacity to learn from past experience. For example, a nurse might conclude that an individual who repeatedly chooses partners who are abusive demonstrates poor judgement in selecting partners. Another way to assess judgement is to give a simple scenario and ask the person to identify the best response. An example of such a scenario is "What would you do if you found a bag of money outside a bank on a busy street?" If the client responds, "spend it," their judgement is questionable.

Stress and Coping Patterns

Everyone lives with some degree of stress in their life (see Chapter 18 for a full discussion). For vulnerable individuals, however, stress may contribute to the development or worsening of PMH disorders. Identification of major stressors in an individual's life helps the nurse to develop and support the use of successful coping behaviours in the future. The nurse should identify the individual's current stressors, coping strategies, and evaluate the effectiveness of the latter. This information is vital to the overall plan of care because it highlights both problem areas and resources.

Assessing Risk and Protective Factors

An individual's mental health–illness is influenced by the complex interaction of characteristics, socioeconomic circumstances, and environmental factors that vary across the lifespan (National Research Council and Institute of Medicine, 2009) (Fig. 11.2). Assessment takes into account the presence and balance of risk factors, protective factors, and promotive factors. **Risk factors**

are characteristics, conditions, situations, and events that increase the individual's vulnerability. Throughout this text, assessment of risk factors focuses on risks to safety, risks for developing PMH disorders, and risks for increasing, or exacerbating, symptoms and impairment in individuals with an existing psychiatric disorder. **Protective factors** are attributes or conditions of an individual, family, and/or community that, when present, reduces, mitigates, or eliminates risk for an adverse outcome. **Promotive factors** are conditions or attributes of individuals, families, and/or communities that actively enhance wellbeing. Taken together, protective and promotive factors increase the probability of positive, adaptive, and healthy outcomes, even in the face of risk and adversity.

Assessing safety is a priority and a part of every encounter with clients. Examples include the risk for deliberate self-harm or suicide; risk for violence toward others; and risk for adverse events, such as falls, seizures, allergic reactions, or elopement. Nurses must assess these risk factors on a priority basis. For example, they must assess the risk for violence or suicide and take measures to prevent injury, such as implementing environmental constraints, before addressing other areas of assessment.

Suicide/Self-Harm

Suicide is "an intentional, self-inflicted act that results in death" (Emanuel et al., 2017, p. 2). In contrast, "self-harm," while purposeful, is often repetitive behaviour that involves the infliction of harm to one's body without suicidal intent" (Emanuel et al., 2017, p. 2) and is often used as a method to relieve psychological distress. A suicide risk assessment involving gathering specific details regarding:

Suicidal ideation—thoughts about deliberate self-harm or of self-inflicted death
Threats of suicide—a verbal or behavioural indication (direct or indirect) that an individual is planning to end their life
Suicide attempt—action taken with the intent of ending one's life
Self-harm—Thoughts of or deliberate self-injurious behaviours not intended to end one's life (e.g., carving, cutting, scratching, or burning one's skin; pulling one's hair; ingestion of toxic substances; or hitting oneself)

To ascertain this information, the nurse asks specific questions such as the following (see Chapter 20 for a full discussion):

• Have you ever tried to harm or kill yourself? If the answer is "yes," probe for details about precipitating circumstances, means, and outcome. If the individual has thought about suicide but not acted on these thoughts, determine why not.

INFANCY & EARLY CHILDHOOD

- Difficult temperament
- Insecure attachment
- Hostile to peers, socially inhibited
- Irritability
- Fearfulness
- Difficult temperament
- Head injury
- Motor, language, and cognitive impairments
- Early aggressive behavior
- Sexual abuse

- Parental drug/alcohol use
- Cold and unresponsive mother behavior
- Marital conflict
- Negative events
- Cold and unresponsive mother behavior
- Parental drug/alcohol use
- Family dysfunction
- Disturbed family environment
- Parental loss

- Poor academic performance in early grades
- Specific traumatic experiences
- Negative events
- Lack of control or mastery experiences
- Urban setting
- Poverty

- Self-regulation
- Secure attachment
- Mastery of communication and language skills
- Ability to make friends and get along with others

- Reliable support and discipline from caregivers
- Responsiveness
- Protection from harm and fear
- Opportunities to resolve conflict
- Adequate socioeconomic resources for the family

- Support for early learning
- Access to supplemental services such as feeding, and screening for vision and hearing
- Stable, secure attachment to childcare provider
- Low ratio of caregivers to children
- Regulatory systems that support high quality of care

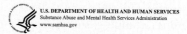
U.S. DEPARTMENT OF HEALTH AND HUMAN SERVICES
Substance Abuse and Mental Health Services Administration
www.samhsa.gov

Risk *and* Protective Factors *for* Mental, Emotional, *and* Behavioral Disorders Across *the* Life Cycle

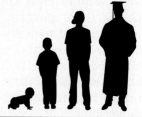

Disorders
- depression
- anxiety
- substance abuse
- schizophrenia
- conduct disorders

Type of Factor
- risk factor
- protective factor

Sources of Risk/Protective Factors
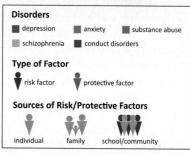
individual   family   school/community

MIDDLE CHILDHOOD

- Negative self-image
- Apathy
- Anxiety
- Dysthymia
- Insecure attachment
- Poor social skills: impulsive, aggressive, passive, and withdrawn
- Poor social problem-solving skills
- Shyness
- Poor impulse control
- Sensation-seeking
- Lack of behavioral self-control
- Impulsivity
- Early persistent behavior problems
- Attention deficit/hyperactivity disorder
- Anxiety
- Depression
- Antisocial behavior
- Head injury
- Self-reported psychotic symptoms

- Parental depression
- Poor parenting, rejection, lack of parental warmth
- Child abuse/maltreatment
- Loss
- Marital conflict or divorce
- Family dysfunction
- Parents with anxiety disorder or anxious childrearing practices
- Parental overcontrol and intrusiveness

(family risk factors continued)
- Parents model, prompt, and reinforce threat appraisals and avoidant behaviors
- Marital conflict; poor marital adjustments
- Negative life events
- Permissive parenting
- Parent-child conflict
- Low parental warmth
- Parental hostility
- Harsh discipline
- Child abuse/maltreatment
- Substance use among parents or siblings
- Parental favorable attitudes toward alcohol and/or drug use
- Inadequate supervision and monitoring
- Low parental aspirations for child
- Lack of or inconsistent discipline
- Family dysfunction

- Peer rejection
- Stressful life events
- Poor grades/achievements
- Poverty
- Stressful community events such as violence
- Witnessing community violence
- Social trauma
- Negative events
- Lack of control or mastery experiences

(school/community risk factors continued)
- School failure
- Low commitment to school
- Peer rejection
- Deviant peer group
- Peer attitudes toward drugs
- Alienation from peers
- Law and norms favorable toward alcohol and drug use
- Availability and access to alcohol
- Urban setting
- Poverty

- Mastery of academic skills (math, reading, writing)
- Following rules for behavior at home, school, and public places
- Ability to make friends
- Good peer relationships

- Consistent discipline
- Language-based rather than physically-based discipline
- Extended family support

- Healthy peer groups
- School engagement
- Positive teacher expectations
- Effective classroom management
- Positive partnering between school and family
- School policies and practices to reduce bullying
- High academic standards

Figure 11.2 Risk and protective factors for mental, emotional, and behavioral disorders across the life cycle. (Source: U.S. Department of Health and Human Services. (n.d.). Risk and protective factors for mental, emotional, and behavioral disorders across the life cycle. Substance Abuse and Mental Health Services Administration. https://iod.unh.edu/sites/default/files/media/Project_Page_Resources/PBIS/c3_handout_hhs-risk-and-proetctive-factors.pdf with data from National Research Council and Institute of Medicine. (2009). Preventing mental, emotional, and behavioral disorders among young people: Progress and possibilities. Washington, DC: The National Academies Press.)

Risk and Protective Factors for Mental, Emotional, and Behavioral Disorders Across the Life Cycle *(continued)*

ADOLESCENCE

- Female gender
- Early puberty
- Difficult temperament: inflexibility, low positive mood, withdrawal, poor concentration
- Low self-esteem, perceived incompetence, negative explanatory and inferential style
- Anxiety
- Low-level depressive symptoms and dysthymia
- Insecure attachment
- Poor social skills: communication and problem-solving skills
- Extreme need for approval and social support
- Low self-esteem
- Shyness
- Emotional problems in childhood
- Conduct disorder
- Favorable attitudes toward drugs
- Rebelliousness
- Early substance use
- Antisocial behavior
- Head injury
- Marijuana use
- Childhood exposure to lead or mercury (neurotoxins)

- Parental depression
- Parent-child conflict
- Poor parenting
- Negative family environment (may include substance abuse in parents)
- Child abuse/maltreatment
- Single-parent family (for girls only)
- Divorce

(family risk factors continued)

- Marital conflict
- Family conflict
- Parent with anxiety
- Parental/marital conflict
- Family conflict (interactions between parents and children and among children)
- Parental drug/alcohol use
- Parental unemployment
- Substance use among parents
- Lack of adult supervision
- Poor attachment with parents
- Family dysfunction
- Family member with schizophrenia
- Poor parental supervision
- Parental depression
- Sexual abuse

- Peer rejection
- Stressful events
- Poor academic achievement
- Poverty
- Community-level stressful or traumatic events
- School-level stressful or traumatic events
- Community violence
- School violence
- Poverty
- Traumatic event
- School failure
- Low commitment to school
- Not college bound
- Aggression toward peers
- Associating with drug-using peers
- Societal/community norms about alcohol and drug use

(school/community risk factors continued)

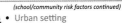
- Urban setting
- Poverty
- Associating with deviant peers
- Loss of close relationship or friends

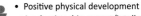
- Positive physical development
- Academic achievement/intellectual development
- High self-esteem
- Emotional self-regulation
- Good coping skills and problem-solving skills
- Engagement and connections in two or more of the following contexts: school, with peers, in athletics, employment, religion, culture

- Family provides structure, limits, rules, monitoring, and predictability
- Supportive relationships with family members
- Clear expectations for behavior and values

- Presence of mentors and support for development of skills and interests
- Opportunities for engagement within school and community
- Positive norms
- Clear expectations for behavior
- Physical and psychological safety

EARLY ADULTHOOD

- Early-onset depression and anxiety
- Need for extensive social support
- Childhood history of untreated anxiety disorders
- Childhood history of poor physical health
- Childhood history of sleep and eating problems
- Poor physical health
- Lack of commitment to conventional adult roles
- Antisocial behavior
- Head Injury

- Parental depression
- Spousal conflict
- Single parenthood
- Leaving home
- Family dysfunction

- Decrease in social support accompanying entry into a new social context
- Negative life events
- Attending college
- Substance-using peers
- Social adversity

- Identity exploration in love, work, and world view
- Subjective sense of adult status
- Subjective sense of self-sufficiency, making independent decisions, becoming financially independent
- Future orientation
- Achievement motivation

- Balance of autonomy and relatedness to family
- Behavioral and emotional autonomy

- Opportunities for exploration in work and school
- Connectedness to adults outside of family

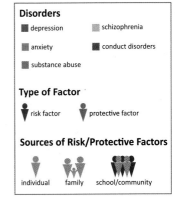

Disorders

- depression
- anxiety
- substance abuse
- schizophrenia
- conduct disorders

Type of Factor

- risk factor
- protective factor

Sources of Risk/Protective Factors

- individual
- family
- school/community

Figure 11.2 *(Continued)*

- Do you have a plan for how you might kill yourself? If the answer is "yes," ask for details (e.g., when and by what means).
- Do you have the things you need to carry out this plan?
- Have you made preparations for your death (e.g., writing a good-bye note, putting finances in order, and/or giving away possessions)?
- What does the future hold for you? Probe for indications of hopelessness, a sense of helplessness, a loss of enjoyment in life, guilt or shame, anger, or impaired judgement.

From this assessment, the nurse and other members of the team determine the individual's level of risk for self-harm and intervene as necessary. Most PMH programs and facilities use rating scales to quantify an individual's risk for self-harm.

It is important to note that nurses and other health care providers are often not very accurate at predicting suicide risk. Evidence for this comes from the work of Large and colleagues (2016) in Australia who conducted a systematic review of prospective studies of risk factors and risk assessment tools to predict suicide following an incident of self-harm. The researchers found that 95% of clients assessed as being high-risk for suicide did not die by suicide and that 50% of completed suicides involved clients assessed as being at lower risk. Large's group also concluded that the accuracy of predicting suicide has not improved over the past 40 years no matter what assessment tool is used. These findings are sobering and should remind us to listen carefully to clients and to remain cognizant that safety is always a concern.

Assaultive or Homicidal Ideation

A safety assessment also includes an evaluation of the level of threat an individual poses to others. Of particular importance are delusions or hallucinations that involve harming or killing others. Questions to ask to ascertain assaultive or homicidal ideation are as follows:

- Do you intend to harm someone? If yes, whom?
- Do you have a plan for how you might do this? If yes, what are the details of the plan?
- Do you have the things that you need to carry out your plan? (If the plan requires a weapon, is it readily available?)

Social Domain

A **comprehensive assessment** also attends to social dimensions of an individual's life. Much of this information is elicited during the health history and the MSE, and it includes information about the individual's current living situation, the family of origin, and the existence and quality of significant relationships (see Chapter 16). The treatment team also assesses work, education, and social and leisure activities. As well, the team observes the individual's interactions with others. This component of the assessment helps to identify important strengths and resources as well as problems and deficits.

Functional Status

Understanding how an individual functions in day-to-day life is a vital part of assessment. The *DSM-5* recommends clinicians use the *Cross-Cutting Symptom Measure* at the initial interview and over time to follow changes in status and treatment response (APA, 2013). Level 1 of the adult version of this tool is a self-rated survey of 13 symptom domains for adults. For children and adolescents, level 1 has 12 domains to be rated by a parent/guardian. Level 2 of the tool allows for more in-depth assessment of some domains.

The *DSM-5* also provides a *Clinician-Rated Dimension of Psychosis Symptom Severity* scale in which clinicians rate the severity (0 to 4) of eight symptom domains (e.g., hallucinations, delusions, negative symptoms, etc.) experienced by the client over the past 7 days. The *World Health Organization Disability Assessment Schedule 2.0* (WHODAS 2.0; Üstün et al., 2010), a self-administered tool, is recommended for assessing the difficulties experienced over the past 30 days due to health (including mental health) conditions. It explores six domains: understanding and communicating (cognition); moving and getting around (mobility); hygiene, dressing, eating, and staying alone (self-care); interacting with other people (getting along); domestic responsibilities, leisure, work, and school (life activities); and joining in community activities (participation). If the individual is unable to complete the questionnaire, a knowledgeable informant is asked to complete it. (See Web Links for the site where the WHODAS 2.0 can be found.)

Ethnic and Cultural Assessment

Ethnicity and culture profoundly affect an individual's worldview and frame their beliefs about life, death, health and illness, and roles and relationships. As part of a comprehensive assessment, the nurse must consider ethnic and cultural factors that influence health and illness (see Chapter 4). To understand these, the nurse might ask the following questions:

- Do you identify as belonging to a particular ethnic or cultural group? If yes, which one(s)?
- What parts of your culture are most important to you? (Probe for details about values, beliefs, personal practices, social customs, behaviours, etc.)
- What does health mean to you?
- What does illness mean to you?
- What things do you do to make yourself physically and mentally healthy?
- To whom do you turn when you feel physically or mentally ill?

The *DSM-5* offers a *Cultural Formulation Interview* schedule for clinicians' use in obtaining information about the way culture may be influencing important aspects of an individual's clinical presentation (American Psychiatric Association, 2013).

Spiritual Assessment

Nurses must be aware of their own spirituality and religious beliefs to ensure that these do not interfere with assessment of the client's spirituality. See Chapter 4 for a definition and discussion of spirituality. Examples of questions that may foster an understanding of an individual's spirituality include the following:

- What gives your life meaning?
- What brings joy to your life?
- Do you believe in God or a higher power?
- Do you participate in any religious activities? If yes, which ones?
- Do you feel connected with the world?

🍁 Summary of Key Points

- Assessment is a purposeful, systematic, and dynamic process that is ongoing throughout the nurse–client relationship. It involves the collection, validation, analysis, synthesis, organization, and documentation of the client's health–illness information.
- A comprehensive assessment includes a health history and physical examination; considers the psychological, emotional, social, spiritual, ethnic, and cultural dimensions of health; attends to the meaning of the client's health–illness experience; and evaluates how all this affects the individual's daily living.
- A focused assessment is the collection of specific information about a particular need, problem, or situation. It is briefer, narrower in scope, and more present oriented than is a comprehensive assessment.
- Techniques of data collection include observation, interview, physical and mental examinations, and collaboration.
- Biologic assessment includes health history, physical examination, and diagnostic testing.
- Assessment of the psychological domain includes understanding the individual's response to mental health problems, MSE, evaluation of stress and coping, and risk/protective factor assessment.
- The MSE is a systematic assessment of an individual's appearance, affect, behaviour, and cognitive function. It provides "a snapshot" of the person's experiences and the examiner's observations and impressions at the time of the interview. It is performed by health practitioners across several disciplines and clinical settings to evaluate developmental, neurologic, and psychiatric disorders.
- Risk factors are those characteristics, conditions, situations, or events that increase the individual's vulnerability to threats to safety or wellbeing. Examples include the risk for self-harm or suicide, violence toward others, and the risk for adverse events, such as falls, seizures, allergic reactions, or elopement.
- Protective factors are attributes or conditions of an individual, family, and/or community that reduce, mitigate, or eliminate risk.
- Promotive factors are conditions or attributes of individuals, families, and/or communities that actively enhance wellbeing.
- The social assessment involves a family and relationship assessment, evaluation of functional status, and information about the individual's ethnicity and culture.
- Nurses must be aware of their own spiritual beliefs and ensure that those beliefs do not affect their spiritual assessment of their clients.

🧠 Thinking Challenges

A nurse is completing a comprehensive assessment on a client newly diagnosed with bipolar disorder. The client is being seen in the local clinic and is quite anxious about the outcome of the treatment.

a. How does a comprehensive assessment differ from a focused assessment?
b. What would be important components of data collection specific to this client?
c. How is observation an important assessment technique in the treatment of mental health disorders?

Visit thePoint to view suggested responses.
Go to thePoint.lww.com/activate and use the activation code found in the front of this text to unlock answers to the "Thinking Challenges" and other online resources.

💻 Web Links

http://www.glma.org/index.cfm?fuseaction=Page.viewPage&pageId=1025&grandparentID=534&parentID=940&nodeID=1 The Gay & Lesbian Medical Association (GLMA) is committed to ensuring health equity for lesbian, gay, bisexual, transgender, queer (LGBTQ) and all sexual and gender minority (SGM) individuals, and equality for LGBTQ/SGM health professionals in their work and learning environments. They have created a four-part video series titled Quality *Healthcare for Lesbian, Gay, Bisexual & Transgender People* https://live-cfmhn.pantheonsite.io/wp-content/uploads/2019/05/2014-Standards-of-Practice-Final-1.pdf The Canadian Federation of Mental Health Nurses is the national voice for PMH nursing in Canada. The Standards of Practice are available on their website.

https://www.patientsafetyinstitute.ca/en/toolsResources/SuicideRisk/Documents/MHCC-CPSI- Suicide Risk Assessment Toolkit EN.pdf The World Health Organization website where the WHODAS2.0, its manual, and the user agreement can be found.

References

Abosi, O., Lopes, S., Schmitz, S., & Fiedorowicz, J. G. (2018). Cardiometabolic effects of psychotropic medications. *Hormone Molecular Biology and Clinical Investigation, 36*(1). https://doi.org/10.1515/hmbci-2017-0065

American Psychiatric Association. (2013). *Diagnostic and statistical manual of mental disorders* (5th ed.). Washington, DC.

American Psychological Association (APA). (2015). Guidelines for psychological practice with transgender and gender nonconforming people. *American Psychologist, 70*(9), 832–864. http://dx.doi.org/10.1037/a0039906

Beagan, B. L., Fredericks, E., & Goldberg, L. (2012). Nurses' work with LGBTQ patients: "They're just like everybody else, so what's the difference?" *Canadian Journal of Nursing Research, 44*(3), 44–63.

Byrne, P. (2018). Physical health in psychiatric patients. *Medicine, 46*(12), 725–730. https://doi.org/10.1016/j.mpmed.2018.09.002

Canadian Federation of Mental Health Nurses. (2014). *Canadian standards of psychiatric and mental health nursing* (4th ed.). https://live-cfmhn.pantheonsite.io/wp-content/uploads/2019/05/2014-Standards-of-Practice-Final-1.pdf

Colpitts, E., & Gahagan, J. (2016). "I feel like I am surviving the health care system": Understanding LGBTQ health in Nova Scotia, Canada. *BMC Public Health, 16*, 10005. https://doi.org/10.1186/s12889-016-3675-8

Emanuel, L. L., Taylor, L., Hain, A., Combes, J. R., Hatlie, M. J., Karsh, B., Lau, D. T., Shalowitz, J., & Shaw, T. (Eds.). (2017). *The patient safety education program—Canada (PSEP—Canada) curriculum.* http://www.patientsafetyinstitute.ca/en/education/PatientSafetyEducationProgram/PatientSafetyEducationCurriculum/Documents/Module%2013a%20Preventing%20Suicide%20and%20Self-Harm.pdf

Folstein, M. F., Folstein, S. E., & McHugh, P. R. (1975). Mini-mental state. A practical method for grading the cognitive state of patients for the clinician. *Journal of Psychiatric Research, 12*(3), 189–198.

Government of Canada. (2019). *The health of LGBTQIA2 communities in Canada: Report of the Standing Committee on Health* (42nd Parliament, 1st Session). https://www.ourcommons.ca/Content/Committee/421/HESA/Reports/RP10574595/hesarp28/hesarp28-e.pdf

Greene, M. Z., France, K., Kreider, E. F., Wolfe-Roubatis, E., Chen, K. D., Wu, A., & Yehia, B. R. (2018). Comparing medical, dental, and nursing students' preparedness to address lesbian, gay, bisexual, transgender, and queer health. *PLoS One, 13*(9), e0204104. https://doi.org/10.1371/journal

Knox, A. M. (2019). *LGBTQ2 Health in Hospital: A brief directed to the House of Commons Standing Committee on Health, study on LGBTQ2 Health in Canada.* https://www.ourcommons.ca/Content/Committee/421/HESA/Brief/BR10445091/br-external/KnoxAlyssa-e.pdf

Large, M., Kaneson, M., Myles, N., Myles, H., Gunaratne, P., & Ryan, C. (2016). Meta-analysis of longitudinal cohort studies of suicide risk assessment among psychiatric patients: Heterogeneity in results and lack of improvement over time. *PLoS One, 11*(6), e0156322. https://doi.org/10.1371/journal.pone.0156322

Mauvais-Jarvis, F., Bairey Merz, N., Barnes, P. J., Brinton, R. D., Carrero, J. -J., DeMeo, D. L., De Vries, G. J., Epperson, C. N., Govindan, R., Klein, S. L., Lonardo, A., Maki, P. M., McCullough, L. D., Regitz-Zagrosek, V., Regensteiner, J. G., Rubin, J. B., Sandberg, K., & Suzuki, A. (2020). Sex and gender: Modifiers of health, disease, and medicine. *Lancet, 396*(10250), 565–582. https://doi.org/10.1016/S0140-6736(20)31561-0

McCabe, H. A., & Kinney, M. K. (2019). LGBTQ+ individuals, health inequities, and policy implications. *Creighton Law Review, 52*(4), 427–450. http://hdl.handle.net/1805/23253

Meyer, I. H. (2003). Prejudice, social stress, and mental health in lesbian, gay, and bisexual populations: Conceptual issues and research evidence. *Psychological Bulletin, 129*(5), 674–697. https://doi.org/10.1037/0033-2909.129.5.674

National Research Council and Institute of Medicine. (2009). *Preventing mental, emotional, and behavioral disorders among young people: Progress and possibilities.* Washington, DC: The National Academies Press. https://iod.unh.edu/sites/default/files/media/Project_Page_Resources/PBIS/c3_handout_hhs-risk-and-proetctive-factors.pdf

Nicaise, P., Grard, A., Leys, M., Van Audenhove, C., & Lorant, V. (2021). Key dimensions of collaboration quality in mental health care service networks. *Journal of Interprofessional Care, 35*(1), 28–36. https://doi.org/10.1080/13561820.2019.1709425

Office of the Privacy Commission of Canada. (2020). *Provincial and territorial privacy laws and oversight.* https://www.priv.gc.ca/en/about-the-opc/what-we-do/provincial-and-territorial-collaboration/provincial-and-territorial-privacy-laws-and-oversight/

Pomare, C., Long, J. C., Churruca, K., Ellis, L. A., & Braithwaite, J. (2020). Interprofessional collaboration in hospitals: A critical, broad-based review of the literature. *Journal of Interprofessional Care, 34*(4), 509–519. https://doi.org/10.1080/13561820.2019.1702515

Rogers, C. R. (1975). Empathic: An unappreciated way of being. *The Counseling Psychologist, 5*(2), 2–10. http://tcp.sagepub.com/cgi/reprint/5/2/2-a

Teasdale, G., & Jennett B. (1974). Assessment of coma and impaired consciousness. A practical scale. *Lancet, 304*(7872), 81–84.

Üstün, T. B., Kostanjsek, N., Chatterji, S., & Rehm, J. (Eds.). (2010). *Measuring health and disability: Manual for WHO Disability Assessment Schedule* (WHODAS 2.0). Geneva, IL: World Health Organization.

Zeeman, L., Sherriff, N., Browne, K., McGlynn, N., Mirandola, M., Gios, L., Davis, R., Sanchez-Lambert, J., Aujean, S., Pinto, N., Farinella, F., Donisi, V., Niedźwiedzka-Stadnik, M., Rosińska, M., Pierson, A., Amaddeo, F., & the Health4LGBTI Network. (2018). A review of lesbian, gay, bisexual, trans and intersex (LGBTI) health and healthcare inequalities. *European Journal of Public Health, 29*(5), 974–980. https://doi.org/10.1093/eurpub/cky226

Care Planning and Implementation in Psychiatric and Mental Health Nursing*

Nicole Snow

After studying this chapter, you will be able to:

- Discuss the use of foci of nursing and goals related to psychiatric and mental health care.
- Discuss the way clinical knowledge and judgment and collaboration with individuals and families determine the selection of nursing interventions.
- Explain the use of best practice guidelines for psychiatric and mental health nursing care.
- Describe the application of nursing interventions for the biologic, psychological, social, and spiritual domains.
- Discuss the relationship between client-centred care, client goals of care, and quality care.
- Describe the process of developing and revising individualized outcomes of care.

- Automatic thinking • behaviour modification
- behaviour therapy • chemical restraint • cognitive interventions • conflict resolution • counselling • cultural brokering • de-escalation • discharge goals • distraction • guided imagery • home visits • indicators • initial goals • milieu therapy • observation • physical restraint • psychoeducation • recovery orientation • reminiscence • revised goals • seclusion • simple relaxation techniques • spiritual care • structured interaction

- best practice guidelines • collaboration • goals of nursing care • person- and family-centred care • nursing focus of care • nursing interventions

---

Care planning and its implementation in psychiatric and mental health nursing is client centred, collaborative, and evidence based. Given the complexity of mental health care, it can be challenging for the nurse to ensure that planning is grounded in the values of the client, their family, and all other stakeholders involved, including nurses (Beyene et al., 2019). The assessment process of the client who is to receive care was presented in the previous chapter. In this chapter, the next steps of the care planning process and its implementation are discussed. Nurses apply assessment data to determine the foci and goals of nursing care and its appropriate interventions. Evaluation of the outcomes of care determines whether revision of these goals and interventions are required (see Box 12.1). The nurse works in partnership with the client and/or their family throughout this process, making collaborative decisions that are shaped by the respect for and rights of the person receiving care.

Collaborative, Person-Centred Nursing Practice

Canadian nursing practice is grounded by an understanding of a person- and family-centred approach, recognizing that individuals are unique, make meaning of their own lived experiences, and should participate as they can in all aspects of their care. Thus, plans of care are created and provided with the preferences and particular needs of the person, the risks and benefits of proposed interventions discussed and considered, and then implemented as much as possible in partnership with the person and their family (Butcher et al., 2018).

This approach was fostered through the work of the Canadian Collaborative Mental Health Initiative [CCMHI], formed in 2004, with the goal of enhancing mental health services in primary care. As a consortium of 12 national organizations representing community

---

*Adapted from the chapter "Diagnosis, Interventions, and Outcomes in Psychiatric and Mental Health Nursing" by Nicole Snow, Christine Davis, and Wendy Austin

---

BOX 12.1 Nursing Care Planning
and Implementation

GOALS OF CARE

May include initial, revised, and long-term goals

Are person and family centred

NURSING FOCUS OF CARE

Interventions focus on the biological, psychological, social, and spiritual domains.

The client's needs, values, and preferred care goals and the *Canadian Standards of Psychiatric-Mental Health Nursing* guide the selection of interventions.

OUTCOME EVALUATION

Revised goals of care; revised intervention; re-evaluation, as necessary

Specific examples of Nursing Care Plans are provided within Unit 5 Care and Recovery for Persons with a Psychiatric Disorder.

---

services, consumer, family and self-help groups, dieticians, family physicians, nurses, occupational therapists, pharmacists, psychologists, psychiatrists, and social workers, the CCMHI's work centres on the needs of individual users of services (CCMHI, 2006a). The *Canadian Collaborative Mental Health Care Charter* (CCMHI, 2006b) was developed by national organizations of consumers and providers of mental health services (including the Canadian Nurses Association, the Registered Psychiatric Nurses of Canada, and the Canadian Federation of Mental Health Nurses). This chapter identifies seven principles of collaborative clinical decisions and interventions: health promotion and prevention of mental health problems, holistic promotion, collaboration, partnership, respect for diversity, information exchange, and resources.

KEY CONCEPT

A **person-** and **family-centred approach** to care places the person and their family members at the centre of health care, its practices, and services, to ensure that individuals are genuine partners with healthcare providers for their health.

KEY CONCEPT

Collaboration is the process of working together towards common goals. Sharing knowledge and information can be an important aspect of the process.

Culturally Safe and Trauma-Informed Care

Knowledge and competency related to the influence of culture and of trauma experience(s) on a client's health and wellbeing are required in care planning and its implementation. Culturally safe (see Chapter 4) and trauma-informed care (see Chapter 18) contribute to the trustworthiness of nursing services and client recovery. Clinical acumen in the provision of such care evolves with ongoing education and experience.

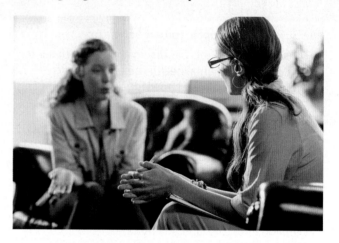

Canadian Federation of Mental Health Nursing's Scope of Practice

The *Canadian Standards of Psychiatric-Mental Health Nursing* (Canadian Federation of Mental Health Nurses [CFMHN], 2014), which have been recently under review, describe the scope of psychiatric and mental health (PMH) nursing practice, delineate nursing competencies, and guide the selection of interventions for implementation in the plan of care (see Web Links). PMH nursing interventions are actions that promote mental health, prevent mental illness, assess dysfunction, assist clients to regain or improve their coping abilities, and/or prevent further disabilities. (See Box 12.2 for *Standard III Administers and Monitors Therapeutic Interventions* of the CFMHN Standards document.) Based on clinical knowledge, judgment, and a commitment to collaboration and partnership with clients and their families, nursing interventions include any treatment that a nurse performs to enhance client goals of care. These interventions are direct (performed through interaction with the client) or indirect (performed away from but on behalf of the client) (Butcher et al., 2018). Interventions can be either nurse-initiated treatment, which is an autonomous action in response to a nursing focus of care, or treatment can be initiated by a nurse practitioner or physician. Physician-initiated treatment often requires an order.

After many factors are considered, including a client's self-care activities, the selection of nursing approaches involves integrating biologic, psychological, social, and spiritual interventions into a comprehensive plan of care with and for the client (Fig. 12.1). Nurses provide care in

---

BOX 12.2 CFMHN Standard III: Administers and Monitors Therapeutic Interventions

The nature of mental health problems and mental disorders raises specific practice issues for the psychiatric–mental health nurse in the assessment and the administration of therapeutic interventions. Many clients are at risk for harm to self or others, either directly or through neglect (including self-neglect). Every effort will be made to include the client in all aspects of decision-making. The PMH nurse will be alert and respond to adverse reactions. The nurse

1. Utilizes and evaluates evidence-based interventions to provide ethical, culturally competent, safe, effective, and efficient nursing care consistent with the mental, physical, spiritual, emotional, social, and cultural needs of the individual

2. Provides information to clients and families/significant others in accordance with relevant legislation

3. Assists, educates, and empowers clients to select choices which support informed decision-making and provides information about the possible consequence(s) of the choice

4. Supports clients to draw on their own assets and resources for self-care, daily living activities, resource mobilization, and mental health promotion

5. Determines clinical intervention, using knowledge of client's responses

6. Uses technology appropriately to perform safe, effective, and efficient nursing intervention

7. Uses knowledge of age-specific implications of psychotropic medications and administers medications accurately and safely, monitoring therapeutic responses, reactions, untoward effects, toxicity, and potential incompatibilities with other medications or substances and provides medication education with appropriate content

8. Utilizes therapeutic elements of group process

9. Incorporates knowledge of family dynamics, cultural values, and beliefs in the provision of care

10. Collaborates with the client, healthcare providers, and community members to access and coordinate resources such as employment, education, and volunteering, and seeks feedback from the client and others regarding interventions

11. Encourages and assists clients to seek out mutual support groups and to strengthen social support networks as needed

12. Seeks out the client's response to, and perception of, nursing and other therapeutic interventions and incorporates it into practice

13. Ensures care for individuals of different populations (e.g., incarcerated individuals, individuals with intellectual disabilities) from therapeutic and rehabilitative perspectives

---

various roles. In some settings, such as an acute care hospital or the home, the nurse provides direct nursing care. In other settings, such as the community, the nurse may assume the role of case manager, who primarily coordinates care for all disciplines, including nursing. In this instance, the nurse may be responsible for all or part of direct nursing care as well as for ensuring that agreed-on care is appropriate for the client, even if other providers deliver it. The nurse may also be the leader or manager of a nursing unit and thus responsible for delegating the care to paraprofessional and nonprofessional providers; however, the nurse remains accountable for the client's care.

Best Practices

Starting in 1999 in Canada, the Registered Nurses Association of Ontario (RNAO) was funded by the Ontario government to develop, implement, evaluate, and revise best practice guidelines (BPGs) that would inform nursing practice in a variety of settings. Successful integration of these best practice guidelines requires a concerted interprofessional approach and supportive work environments.

Box 12.3 provides examples of available RNAO guidelines. The purpose of BPGs is multifaceted: to deliver care that is effective and based on current evidence, to aid in seeking resolutions to clinical problems, to meet or exceed current quality standards in providing excellent care, to initiate use of innovations, to eliminate interventions that are not meeting best practice standards, and to foster clinical excellence through supportive work environments (RNAO, 2021a, 2021b).

KEY CONCEPT

Best practice guidelines (BPGs), also termed clinical practice guidelines, are broad or specific recommendations for health care based on the best current evidence.

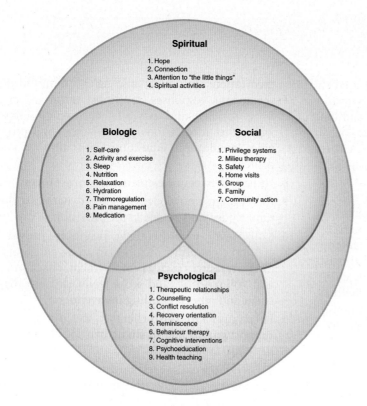

Figure 12.1 PMH nursing interventions.

Deriving a Nursing Focus of Care

Clusters of data lead the nurse to identify the focus on issues concerning the client, family, or group and form the basis for planning nursing interventions. For example, during assessment, the nurse observes that the client's responses are often self-negating (e.g., "I always mess things up," "I never get it right"). The nurse also observes that the client seems indecisive and lacking in problem-solving abilities (e.g., "I can never decide what

the right thing to do is, and when I do finally choose, it is always wrong"). Nonverbal and verbal information are used to identify defining characteristics. Observations of an individual sitting with their head down, making no eye contact, and appearing disheveled are important data points. Such observations raise nursing questions regarding the client's self-esteem. Further assessment will help the nurse determine whether there is a self-esteem concern and if so, whether it is chronic or situational.

BOX **12.3** BEST PRACTICES

EXAMPLES OF RNAO PRACTICE GUIDELINES

- Adopting eHealth solutions: Implementation strategies
- Assessment and care of adults at risk for suicidal ideation and behaviour
- Crisis intervention for adults using a trauma-informed approach: initial 4 weeks of management (3rd ed.)
- Delirium, dementia, and depression in older adults: assessment and care (2nd ed.)
- Engaging clients who use substances
- Enhancing healthy adolescent development
- Establishing therapeutic relationships
- Facilitating client-centred learning

- Implementing supervised injection services
- Integrating tobacco interventions into daily nursing practice
- Person- and family-centred care
- Preventing and addressing abuse and neglect of older adults: person-centred, collaborative, and system-wide approaches
- Promoting safety: alternative approaches to the use of restraints
- Women abuse: screening, identification, and initial response

BOX **12.4** Research for Best Practice

STAFF DEBRIEFING FOLLOWING SECLUSION OR RESTRAINT USE IN INPATIENT MENTAL HEALTH SETTINGS

Mangaoil, R. A., Cleverley, K., & Peter, E. (2020). Immediate staff debriefing following seclusion or restraint use in inpatient mental health settings: A scoping review. *Clinical Nursing Research, 29*(7), 479–495.

Purpose: To "synthesize the academic and gray literature on the use of immediate staff debriefing following seclusion or restraint events in inpatient mental health settings" (p. 479).

Method: The process of conducting the scoping review was guided by a framework initially developed by Arksey and O'Malley (2005) and further revised by Levac, Colquhoun, and O'Brien (2010) and the Joanna Briggs Institute (Pater et al., 2015). Multiple databases were searched, and all research, academic, and gray literature published from 1980 onward were considered. Articles were screened at various levels using two reviewers. The articles had to include definitions of restraint, identify the types used, and provide explanation as to how they are used within acute mental healthcare settings. Data were extracted from the sources using a tool developed by members of the research team and analyzed using content analysis. A total of 150 articles and 55 pieces of gray literature were initially screened. Subsequent re-screening according to inclusion and exclusion criteria yielded 31 academic journal articles and 11 gray literature sources.

Findings: Various definitions of debriefing were noted, with a common focus being on the importance of preventing further traumatization of staff and patients involved in restraint. Some sources considered debriefing as an opportunity to learn how to prevent or lessen the frequency of restraint use and to support staff in processing what happened. In addition, there was evidence of an interest to explore the importance of educating staff on how to conduct debriefing, what that process would involve, and how it can be documented.

Implications for Nursing: The authors conclude that a greater emphasis on debriefing is needed in organizational policy for staff at all levels of care, in conjunction with taking a proactive stance in working to reduce the actual use of restraint. To do this, more research in the area is needed. Multidisciplinary debriefing approaches, including considering the need for patient debriefing, can be explored. There are opportunities to consider researching organizational, and, in particular, unit dynamics and power differentials between staff and patients. The use of restraints invokes many emotions, and the ethical and professional considerations of its use need to be explored in more detail as well.

Related factors are those that influence or change the client's health status. To continue with the assessment example, the nurse learns that the client has lost three jobs within the past year, resulting in financial problems. These situation-related factors further support nursing care to place a focus on self-esteem.

KEY CONCEPT

A **nursing focus of care** is the identified issue concerning the client, family, or group and forms the basis for planning nursing interventions.

KEY CONCEPT

Goals of nursing care are the desired responses of an individual, family, or community in response to nursing care at a given point in time. They are to be written in a concise and neutral manner. Goals of care describe an individual's state, behaviour, or perception that is variable and can be measured.

Developing Individual Goals of Care

Goals of care should be individualized and linked to nursing care foci through the nursing process. By linking the goal to the nursing focus of care, it is possible to monitor nursing practice and facilitate clinical decision-making and knowledge development. Goals can be defined as an individual's response to care that is the end result of a process, a treatment, or a nursing intervention and should be monitored and documented over time and across clinical settings. Nursing focus-specific goals of care show that the intervention resolved the problem. At other times, the goal is nonspecific (i.e., not focus specific, meaning it does not show resolution of the focus). In that case, the outcome is abstract or general. Goals of care may be used to evaluate interventions by other healthcare disciplines as well as nursing. For example, occupational therapy may contribute significantly to an individual's psychosocial adaptation.

The process of working toward goals of care can be outlined in a systematic manner that identifies the required healthcare professionals and other supports and their actions. The Centre for Addictions and Mental Health (CAMH) is a Canadian leader in mental health treatment and research. It has identified a number of approaches (integrated pathways) to aid individuals in receiving treatment and support for their mental health concerns (CAMH, 2016). Integrated care pathways tend to have these characteristics:

* The focus is on the client's overall journey.
* Ensure clients receive the right care and treatment at the right time.
* Involve care decisions based on evidence.
* Effective teamwork among care providers (e.g., nurse, physician, psychologist, pharmacist, social worker).
* Empower and inform clients and their caregivers (CAMH, 2016, p. 3).

This process is mapped as *Admission > Assessment > Treatment (Medication and Nonmedication Treatment) > Planning for Discharge > Discharge* (CAMH, 2016, p. 6). Once this process is under way, there is a need to identify what indicators will indicate outcome attainment. **Indicators** answer the question "How close is the individual moving towards the outcome?" The indicator represents the dimensions of the outcome. Outcome indicators represent or describe individual status, behaviours, or perceptions evaluated during an individual's assessment. Indicators are a measurement of individual progress in relation to the individual's goals and can serve as intermediate goals in a clinical pathway or standardized care plan. In nursing care planning, these can be **initial goals** (written after the initial individual interview and assessment), **revised goals** (written after each evaluation), or **discharge goals** (goals to be met before discharge). Because of the decreased length of stay or days of service, discharge goals often are not met but are passed along to the community nurse. If these discharge goals continue to be relevant, then they become initial goals in community or home care.

Documentation of Goal Achievement

Nurses are accountable for documentation of individual goals of care, nursing interventions, and any changes in focus, care plan, or both. Individual responses to care are documented as changes in behaviour or knowledge and can include the degree of satisfaction with the health care provided. Care goals can be expressed in terms of the individual's actual responses (e.g., no longer reports hearing voices) or the status of a nursing focus at a point in time after implementation of nursing interventions, such as "caregiver role strain relieved." This documentation is important for understanding the client's current status.

Purposes of Individual Care Goals

The primary purposes of developing individual care goals are to ensure quality care is being provided and that the needs of the individual are being met. They provide consistent measures for what is happening with the individual and direction for the continuity of care that reflects the most current knowledge in the field of nursing. The measurement of individual care goals also helps meet the goal of continuous quality improvement.

Accountability is an important concept in health care. Nursing and other disciplines are being pressured within health service systems to justify their practice, to demonstrate to users of services that they deliver quality care, and to control healthcare costs. Measurement of care goals can be used to determine quality of care during a single episode of illness and across the continuum of care and can assist in discharge planning. Care goals can also be used to determine quality of care in different systems and between systems. Evaluation of individual care goals can help validate nursing interventions by identifying which interventions are effective. Goals can be an effective communication tool between nurses, and with case managers, caregivers, and policy makers. They can be used to conduct program evaluations and to develop research databases.

▌ Nursing Interventions

In Canada, the *Canadian Standards of Psychiatric-Mental Health Nursing* (CFMHN, 2014) provide a guide to the administration and monitoring of therapeutic interventions (see Web Links to connect to a free download of the standards). As stated in *The Standards*: "The nurse utilizes and evaluates evidence-based interventions to provide ethical, culturally competent, safe, effective, and efficient nursing care consistent with the mental, physical, spiritual, emotional, social, and cultural needs of the individual" (p. 9).

Another guide is the *Nursing Interventions Classification* (NIC) (Butcher et al., 2018), a system of specific interventions with discrete activities for each. The NIC system is based on data collected from surveys of nurses, who identified the interventions that were ultimately classified. The NIC taxonomy includes classes or groups of interventions categorized according to seven domains: physiologic basic, physiologic complex, behavioural, safety, family, health system, and community. The NIC taxonomy represents both basic and specialty advanced nursing practices. For example, both basic and specialist nurses use interventions such as reinforcing positive behaviour; however, the advanced practice psychiatric nurse may be the developer of the plan and use it as part of psychotherapy with the client.

KEY CONCEPT

Nursing interventions are treatments or activities, based upon clinical judgment and knowledge, that are used by nurses to enhance an individual's achievement of care goals (Butcher et al., 2018).

Interventions for the Biologic Domain

Biologic interventions focus on physical functioning and are directed towards the client's self-care, activities and exercise, sleep, nutrition, relaxation, hydration, and thermoregulation as well as pain management and medication management. In the NIC taxonomy, these interventions are found within the physiologic basic and physiologic complex domains.

Promotion of Self-Care Activities

Self-care is the ability to perform activities of daily living (ADLs) successfully. Many clients with PMH nursing focus or medical diagnoses can manage self-care activities such as bathing, dressing appropriately, selecting adequate nutrition, and sleeping regularly. (Although maintaining adequate nutrition and promoting normal sleep hygiene are considered self-care activities, they are discussed in separate sections because of their significance in mental health care.) Others, however, cannot manage such self-care activities either because of their symptoms, as a result of the side effects of medications, or due to a broad range of factors outside of their control (e.g., experiencing homelessness). Because nursing is concerned with maintaining the client's health and wellbeing, a focus on ADLs can become a nursing priority.

Orem's (1991) nursing model (see Chapter 9) identifies five nursing approaches to deficits in a client's self-care: acting or doing for, guiding, teaching, supporting, and providing an environment to promote the client's ability to meet current or future demands. The emphasis is on helping the individual develop independence. In the inpatient setting, the nurse works with the client so that basic self-care activities are completed. During acute phases of psychiatric disorders, the inability to attend to basic self-care tasks (e.g., getting dressed) is very common. Therefore, the ability to complete personal hygiene activities (e.g., dental care, grooming) is monitored, and clients are assisted in completing such activities. In a psychiatric facility, clients are encouraged and expected to develop independence in completing these basic self-care activities to the best of their ability. In the community, monitoring these basic self-care activities is a part of the nursing visit or clinic appointment but particularly one where socio–economic–political factors (e.g., housing, transportation, access to health care) becomes increasingly relevant for self-care and nursing advocacy.

Activity and Exercise Interventions

The nurse must attend to the client's level of activity. This is an area particularly impacted by global pandemic public health restrictions. Encouraging regular activity and exercise can improve general wellbeing and physical health. A healthy lifestyle that includes daily exercise can help clients deal with the weight gain and type II diabetes associated with many psychotropic medications. In some psychiatric disorders (e.g., schizophrenia and depression), people become sedentary and appear to lack the motivation to complete ADLs. This lack of motivation is part of the disorder and requires nursing intervention. In addition, side effects from the medication, sedation and lethargy, can compound the problem (Toups et al., 2017). It is possible for exercise behaviour to become an abnormal focus of attention, such as for some individuals with anorexia nervosa.

When assuming the responsibility of a direct care provider, the nurse can help clients identify realistic activities and exercise goals. Some institutions have other professionals (e.g., recreational therapists) available for the implementation of exercise programs. As a case manager, the nurse should consider the activity needs of individuals when jointly setting goals. As a leader or manager of a psychiatric unit, the nurse can influence ward routines that promote activity and exercise.

Sleep Interventions

Many psychiatric disorders and medications are associated with sleep disturbances. Sleep is also disrupted in clients with dementia. These clients may have difficulty falling asleep or may frequently awaken during the night. In dementia of the Alzheimer type, individuals may reverse their sleeping patterns by napping during the day and staying awake at night. In addition, there is increasing concern regarding the use of electronic devices such as computers and smartphones or playing video games prior to bedtime. There is evidence of a positive association between increased screen time and difficulty falling asleep (Jniene et al., 2019; Vallance et al., 2015).

Nonpharmacologic interventions are always used first for sleep disturbances (See Chapter 28) because of the side effect risks associated with the use of sedatives and hypnotics (see Chapter 13). Sleep interventions to communicate to clients include the following:

- Go to bed only when tired or sleepy.
- Establish a consistent bedtime routine.
- Avoid stimulating foods, beverages, or medications.
- Avoid naps in the late afternoon or evening.
- Eat lightly before retiring and limit fluid intake.
- Use the bed only for sleep or intimacy.
- Avoid emotional stimulation before bedtime.
- Use behavioural and relaxation techniques.
- Limit distractions.
- Reduce exposure to electronic devices prior to bedtime.

For some clients, disrupted sleep can become chronic and problematic. Obtaining adequate sleep is vital for optimal daily functioning, and it is imperative that nurses assess for sleep disturbances and possible disorders and intervene appropriately. More information about sleep disorders and the nursing process involved in caring for an individual with sleep disturbances is provided in Chapter 28.

Nutrition Interventions

Psychiatric disorders and medication side effects can affect eating behaviours. For varying reasons, some individuals eat too little, whereas others eat too much. For instance, individuals with mental illness who are experiencing homelessness have difficulty maintaining adequate nutrition because of their deprived circumstances. Substance abuse also interferes with maintaining adequate nutrition, through either stimulation or suppression of appetite or through neglecting nutrition because of drug-seeking behaviour. Nutrition interventions should, therefore, be specific and relevant to the individual's circumstances and mental health. In addition, recommended daily allowances are important in the promotion of physical and mental health, and nurses should consider them when planning care. Resources for planning include *Canada's Food Guide* and/or *Canada's Food Guide for First Nations, Inuit, and Métis* (Health Canada, 2019a, 2019b) (see Web Links).

Some psychiatric symptoms involve changes in perceptions of food, appetite, and eating habits. If a client believes that food is poisonous, then they may eat sparingly or not at all. Interventions are then necessary to address the suspiciousness as well as to encourage adequate intake of recommended daily allowances. It may be necessary for clients to examine foods, participate in preparation, and test the meal's safety by eating slowly or after everyone else.

A BMI of over 30, or obesity, can be a problem for individuals being treated for a mental disorder. Antipsychotics, antidepressants, and mood stabilizers are associated with weight gain, which is thought to be related to changes in metabolism and appetite caused by some of these medications. Many clients stop taking medications because of associated weight gain. Excessive weight gain can be especially stressful to the individual's emotional wellbeing, as well as detrimental to physical health. However, nurses should encourage clients to avoid quick weight loss programs because they are not effective. Furthermore, hypoglycaemia can exacerbate a depressed mood and lead to suicidal thoughts. If weight gain is a problem, then the best approach is to assist the client to monitor current intake and develop realistic strategies for changing eating patterns combined with a healthy lifestyle.

Relaxation Interventions

Relaxation promotes comfort, reduces anxiety, alleviates stress, eases pain, and prevents aggression. It can diminish the effects of hallucinations and delusions.

The many different relaxation techniques used as mental health interventions range from simple deep breathing to biofeedback to hypnosis. Although some techniques such as biofeedback require additional training, in some instances certification, nurses can easily apply simple relaxation, distraction, and imagery techniques.

Simple relaxation techniques encourage and elicit relaxation to decrease undesirable signs and symptoms. **Distraction** is the purposeful focusing of attention away from undesirable sensations. Distraction techniques include counting, exercising, reading, listening to music, watching television, or playing (e.g., video games). The important factor is that the particular distraction works for the person. Other factors in choice of technique involve its appropriateness based on energy level, age, developmental level, and literacy. Individuals should try out and practice the distraction technique of their choice before they need to use it (Butcher et al., 2018). **Guided imagery** is the purposeful use of imagination to achieve relaxation or to direct attention away from undesirable sensations. It is especially useful in stress management. With this technique, clients imagine themselves doing something pleasurable and relaxing, such as lying on the beach or watching snow fall. They are encouraged (with permissive directions from the nurse, such as "If you wish...") to slowly experience the scene and to express how they feel and think about it. Slow, deep breathing is also encouraged (Butcher et al., 2018). Guided imagery is an independent nursing intervention that can be used for such clients as those experiencing anxiety (Álvarez-García & Yaban, 2020). However, as clients may experience unexpected, albeit therapeutic, reactions (e.g., crying) during guided imagery, students should not attempt this technique with clients unless supervised.

As a direct care provider, the nurse may teach the client relaxation exercises. As a case manager, nurses can include relaxation exercises in the plan of care. The unit leader can be responsible for ensuring that appropriately prepared staff members implement relaxation exercises. Relaxation techniques that involve physical touch (e.g., back rubs) must be used particularly carefully, if at all, for people with mental disorders. Touching and massaging are often not appropriate for clients who have a history of physical or sexual abuse. Such clients may find touch too stimulating or misinterpret it as being sexual or aggressive. It is important for the nurse to maintain open communication with and elicit feedback from the client when providing physical interventions.

Hydration Interventions

Assessing fluid status and monitoring fluid intake and output are often important interventions. Overhydration or underhydration can be a symptom of a psychiatric disorder. For example, some clients with psychotic disorders experience chronic fluid imbalance. For these individuals, a treatment protocol that includes a target weight procedure can help prevent both overhydration and water intoxication and promote self-control. The nurse functions as the direct care provider (e.g., teaching the client), unit leader (e.g., delegating weighing of the client to staff), or coordinator of the protocol.

Many psychiatric medications affect fluid and electrolyte balance (see Chapter 13). For example, when taking lithium carbonate, clients must have adequate fluid intake, with special attention paid to serum sodium levels. When sodium levels drop through perspiration, lithium is used in place of sodium, which in turn leads to lithium toxicity. Many psychiatric medications cause dry mouth, which in turn causes individuals to drink fluids excessively. Interventions that help clients understand the relationship of medications to fluid and electrolyte balance are important in their overall care.

Thermoregulation Interventions

Many psychiatric disorders can disturb the body's normal temperature regulation. Thus, clients cannot sense temperature increases or decreases and consequently cannot protect themselves from extremes of hot or cold. This problem is especially problematic for people who are experiencing homeless or who live in substandard housing given the associated risk for flourishing and even survival. In addition, many psychiatric medications can also affect the ability to regulate body temperature. Interventions include educating clients about the problem of thermoregulation, identifying potential extremes in temperatures, and developing strategies to protect the client from the adverse effects of temperature changes. For example, community nurses often engage in active outreach to at-risk clients during extreme weather alerts and advocacy for adequate shelter/housing for vulnerable populations.

Pain Management

Emotional reactions are often manifested as pain. For instance, unexplained chronic pain can be a somatoform symptom (see Chapter 24). Chronic pain is particularly problematic when no cause for it is identified. Nurses in PMH settings are more likely to provide care to clients experiencing chronic pain than acute pain. A single intervention is seldom successful for relieving chronic pain. In some instances, pain is managed by medication; in other instances, nonpharmacologic techniques are used, such as relaxation techniques, distraction, or imagery. Indeed, relaxation is one of the most widely used cognitive and behavioural approaches to pain. Psychoeducation, stress management techniques, and biofeedback are also used in pain management.

The key to managing pain is engaging the client in identifying how it is disrupting their personal, social, professional, and family life. Education focusing on the pain, the use of medications for treatment, and the development of cognitive skills are important pain management components. In some cases, redefining treatment success as improvement in functioning, rather than alleviation of pain, may be necessary. The interaction between stress and pain is important; that is, increased stress leads to increased pain (Brataas & Evensen, 2016). Individuals can better manage their pain when stress is reduced.

Medication Management

Nurses use many medication management interventions to help clients maintain therapeutic regimens. Medication management involves more than the actual administration of medications. Nurses assess medication effectiveness and side effects and consider interactions with other drugs (including substances such as alcohol and cannabis), herbal remedies, or homeopathic preparations. In addition, nurses assess any factors that may affect the client's adherence to a medication regimen, such as concerns regarding weight gain or reproductive ability, attitude towards taking medication, or financial issues. Education regarding medication must be made available to the client in appropriate ways, including information regarding the importance of the recognition and reporting of side effects (Morrison et al., 2015). Guidance in ways to organize medication can be helpful to clients such as keeping medications in one safe place, out of the reach of children, and the use inexpensive pill organizers. When travelling out of the country, it is important to take prescription information (provided by the pharmacy with the medication) as this may be required by custom authorities. Suggesting strategies to assist the client in taking medication on time can be helpful, such as setting an alarm.

Treatment with psychopharmacologic agents can be lengthy because of the chronic nature of many disorders. Medication management occurs in both acute and community care settings, and medication follow-up may include home visits as well as telephone calls. Many clients remain on medication regimens for years and may never become medication free. Clients may require considerable support from nurses and other healthcare professionals that is focused on their individual needs and their context (Kauppi et al., 2015). Medication education is thus an ongoing intervention that requires careful documentation, monitoring, and engagement with the client.

Interventions for the Psychological Domain

Emphasis in the psychological domain is on emotion, behaviour, and cognition. The nurse–client relationship serves as the basis for interventions directed towards the psychological domain. Because the therapeutic relationship is discussed extensively in Chapter 7, it is not covered in this chapter. This section covers counselling, conflict resolution, recovery orientation, reminiscence, behaviour therapy, cognitive interventions, psychoeducation, health teaching, and spiritual interventions. Chapter 9 presents the theoretic basis for many of these interventions.

Nurses in the direct care role will use all of the psychological interventions to respond to the healthcare problems of their clients. Nurses in case manager roles will also frequently use interventions from the psychological domain in order to promote recovery and empower the client to make changes. The nurse manager oversees the use of the psychological interventions and evaluates the staff's ability to use the interventions and assess care goals.

Counselling Interventions

Counselling interventions are specific, time-limited interactions between a nurse and a client, family, or group experiencing immediate or ongoing difficulties related to their health or wellbeing. Counselling is usually short term and focuses on improving coping abilities, reinforcing healthy behaviours, fostering positive interactions, or preventing illnesses and disabilities. Counselling strategies are discussed throughout this text. Psychotherapy is generally a long-term approach aimed at improving or helping clients regain previous health status and functional abilities. Mental health specialists, such as advanced practice nurses, use psychotherapy.

An emerging intervention is the use of games to enhance the application of concepts learned in counselling sessions and for developing skills in managing mental health concerns. The use of video games is of particular note. For example, Pater et al. (2015) conducted an integrative literature review to identify whether gaming has potential as a therapeutic intervention. They found evidence of the use of video games to promote health and healthcare interventions since the 1970s. With gaming consoles becoming increasingly prevalent in private homes and healthcare facilities, there has been an increased awareness in their therapeutic use. These uses include cognitive–behavioural therapy for depression, anxiety, and anger management and interventions with veterans. Effective video games have the potential to "educate, empower, and encourage" (p. 159). Limitations and concerns include a dearth of information regarding nurses' attitudes towards the use of video games for therapeutic purposes, their affordability (e.g., program, equipment, and training costs), and a lack of nursing knowledge regarding how to therapeutically implement the games. The authors emphasized that nurses need to be aware of the availability of such

resources, their therapeutic usefulness, and to increase their skill in identifying patients for which gaming may be a particularly effective intervention.

Conflict Resolution

A conflict involves an individual's perceptions, emotions, and behaviours. In a conflict, a person believes that their own needs, interests, wants, or values are incompatible with someone else's (Boggs, 2020). The individual experiences fear, sadness, bitterness, anger, hopelessness, or some combination of these emotions in response to the perceived threat. Misunderstandings, poor communication, value or goal differences, personality issues, and stress can interplay to contribute to this conflict and impact its resolution (Boggs, 2020).

Conflict resolution is a specific type of intervention through which the nurse helps clients resolve disagreements or disputes with family, friends, or other individuals. Conflicts can be positive if individuals see the problem as solvable and providing an opportunity for growth and interpersonal understanding. The nurse may be in the position of resolving a family conflict or teaching family members how to resolve their own conflicts positively. In addition, because nurses are frequently in positions of leadership, they often need conflict resolution skills to settle employee conflicts.

Conflict Resolution Process

Calmness and objectivity are important in resolving any client or family conflict. The desired outcome of conflict resolution is a "win–win" situation in which each party feels positive about the outcome. The nurse will take the following steps in conflict resolution:

1. Identify conflict issues.
2. Know the nurse's own response to the conflict.
3. Separate the problem from the people involved.
4. Stay focused on the issue and the underlying motivations behind the position the other person took.
5. Identify available options.
6. Try to identify established standards to guide the decision-making process (Boggs, 2020).

It is important to be aware of what is causing the conflict. This can be difficult to discern at times, and open, honest, and respectful communication is necessary to facilitate this awareness. It is helpful when all parties involved reflect on their reactions to the conflict and what triggers their emotional responses. It is best and most constructive when all involved focus on the issue at hand and not be critical of the people involved. The focus needs to be on the here and now of the problem, without dwelling on issues that have occurred in the past. Once all parties understand the underlying reasons for the dispute, attention can be given to developing options on how to appropriately address it. As much as possible, this development should be a collaborative process with all parties contributing fairly to the outcome (Boggs, 2020).

Cultural Brokering in Client–System Conflicts

Clients may be marginalized within the healthcare system due to potentially stigmatizing factors, such as, amongst others, experiencing poverty, sexual orientation, lack of formal education, race, or ethnicity. Differences in cultural values and languages between clients and healthcare organizations can contribute to clients' feelings of powerlessness. For example, people who have recently immigrated, who are experiencing homelessness, or who need to make informed decisions under stressful conditions may be unable to navigate the healthcare system. The nurse can help through **cultural brokering** or the use of culturally appropriate strategies that aid in bridging or mediating between the client's culture and the healthcare system (Butcher et al., 2018). The healthcare system can be understood as a new and separate culture with culture shock being a potential experience for clients and families new to it.

For the "nurse as broker" to be effective, the nurse establishes and maintains a sense of connectedness or relationship with the client. In turn, the nurse also establishes and cultivates networks with other healthcare facilities and resources. Cultural sensitivity enables the nurse to be aware of and sensitive to the needs of clients from a variety of cultures. Cultural competence is necessary for the brokering process to be effective (see Chapter 4).

Recovery Orientation

Recovery-focused interventions are becoming more prevalent in PMH care. The Recovery Model comes out of the mental health consumer movement and the work of Dr. William Anthony (1993). Nurses apply this orientation to their everyday interactions with their clients. For example, in care of individuals with severe persistent mental illnesses such as schizophrenia, substance use disorder, or bipolar disorder, a **recovery orientation** means helping the person regain functioning or "get on with life," despite having ongoing symptoms of the psychiatric illness. Recovery may refer to what the client does, how the nurse functions, or how the mental health system is organized. There is recognition in this approach that a cure is not necessary for a sense of recovery for the individual with mental illness. At present, cure may not be possible for some mental disorders (Mental Health Commission of Canada, 2015). The Mental Health Commission of Canada (MHCC) has created guidelines for utilizing a recovery-oriented approach to mental health and illness in the Canadian context. These guidelines flow from six integral

dimensions of practicing with a recovery focus. These dimensions are as follows:

- Creating a culture and language of hope.
- Recovery is personal.
- Recovery occurs in the context of one's life.
- Responding to the diverse needs of everyone living in Canada.
- Working with People who are First Nations, Inuit, and Métis in origin.
- Recovery is about transforming services and systems (Mental Health Commission of Canada, 2015, pp. 15–17).

One approach to recovery, the Tidal Model, was created by nurses for use in mental health practice settings (Barker & Buchanan-Barker, 2010). The Tidal Model emphasizes the importance of a collaborative relationship between the nurse and the client. The client's perspectives and individual experiences are accepted and valued. Recovery is contingent on the health professional having a genuine interest in the client and their experiences. The process is open, transparent, and based on the mutual establishment of goals that both parties work together to achieve. It is recognized that recovery requires time and commitment from both the nurse and the client and that the process of change is enhanced through a genuine, nurturing therapeutic relationship. This approach has been used with success in a variety of contexts. For example, there is evidence of success in using the Tidal Model to aid women survivors of violence (Turgut & Çam, 2020). In addition, a recent critical analysis of the theory by Sagna and Walker (2020), exploring its applicability to guide care provision for older individuals experiencing suicidality, concluded that the Tidal Model takes a "pragmatic approach" (p. 319) to guiding recovery in mental health. Its patient-centred core concepts are relevant to mental health practice and facilitate clients to develop problem-solving and coping skills (see Chapter 9 for more information on this model).

Reminiscence

Reminiscence, the thinking about or relating of past experiences, is used as a nursing intervention to enhance life review particularly for older adults. Reminiscence encourages clients, either in individual or in group settings, to discuss their past and review their lives. Through reminiscence, individuals can identify past coping strategies that can support them in current stressful situations. Clients can also use reminiscence to maintain self-esteem, stimulate thinking, and support the natural healing process of life review (Djukanovic et al., 2016). Activities that facilitate reminiscence include writing an account of past events, making a tape recording and playing it back, explaining pictures in family albums, drawing a family tree, and writing to old friends (see Chapter 31 for health promotion with the older person).

Behaviour Therapy

Behaviour therapy interventions focus on reinforcing or promoting desirable behaviours or altering undesirable ones. The basic premise is that because most behaviours are learned, new functional behaviours can also be learned. Behaviours—not internal psychic processes—are the targets of the interventions. The models of behavioural theorists serve as a basis for these interventions (see Chapter 9).

Behaviour Modification

Behaviour modification is a specific, systematized behaviour therapy technique that can be applied to individuals, groups, or systems. The aim of behaviour modification is to reinforce desired behaviours and extinguish undesired ones. Desired behaviour is rewarded to increase the likelihood that clients will repeat it and, over time, replace the problematic behaviour with it. Behaviour modification is used for various problematic behaviours, such as dysfunctional eating and substance use, and often is used in the care of children and adolescents.

Cognitive Interventions

Cognitive interventions are verbally structured interventions that reinforce and promote desirable or alter undesirable, cognitive functioning. The belief underlying this approach is that thoughts guide emotional reactions, motivations, and behaviours. Cognitive interventions do not solve problems for clients but rather help clients develop new ways of viewing situations so that they can solve problems themselves (Beck, 2021). Nurses may use several models as the basis for cognitive interventions, but all models assume that by changing the cognitive appraisal of a situation (view of the world) and by examining the meaning of events, clients can reinterpret situations. In turn, emotional changes will follow the cognitive changes, and, ultimately, behaviours will change.

Because people develop their thinking patterns throughout their lifetime, many thoughts become so automatic that they are outside individuals' awareness. Thus, a person may be unaware of the automatic thoughts that influence their actions or other thoughts. **Automatic thinking** is often subject to errors or tangible distortions of reality that contradict objective appraisals. For example, a client with depression may be convinced that no one cares about them when, in fact, their family and friends are deeply concerned. Illogical thinking, another thinking error, occurs when a person draws a faulty conclusion. For example, a college student is so

devastated by failing an examination that it is perceived as catastrophic and that their college career is over.

To engage in cognitive treatment, the client must be capable of introspection and reflection about thoughts and fantasies. Cognitive interventions are used in a wide range of clinical situations, from short-term crises to persistent mental disorders. Cognitive interventions also include thought stopping, contracting, and cognitive restructuring. These specific interventions are discussed in Chapter 14.

Psychoeducation

Psychoeducation uses educational strategies to teach clients the skills they lack because of a psychiatric disorder. The goal of psychoeducation is a change in knowledge and behaviour. Nurses use psychoeducation to meet the educational needs of clients by adapting teaching strategies to their disorder-related issues. As clients gain skills, functioning improves. For example, some clients may need to learn how to maintain their morning hygiene. Others may need to understand their illness and cope with hearing voices that others do not hear.

Specific psychoeducation techniques are based on adult learning principles, such as beginning at the point the learner is currently at and building on their current experiences. Thus, the nurse assesses the client's current skills and readiness to learn. From there, the nurse individualizes a teaching plan for each client. The nurse can conduct such teaching in a one-to-one situation or in a group format.

Psychoeducation is a continuous process of assessing, setting goals, developing learning activities, and evaluating for changes in knowledge and behaviour. Nurses use it with individuals, groups, families, and communities. Psychoeducation serves as a basis for psychosocial rehabilitation, a service-delivery approach for those with severe and persistent mental illness (see Chapter 21).

Health Teaching

With health teaching–coaching, the nurse "attempts to understand the life experience of the client and uses this understanding to support and promote learning related to health and personal development" (CFMHN, 2014, p. 19). Based on the principles of teaching, health teaching involves collaborating with the client to determine learning needs and transmitting new information, "while considering the context of the client's life experiences. [The nurse] considers readiness, culture, literacy, language, preferred learning style, and resources available" (CFMHN, 2014, p. 9). According to the *Canadian Standards of Psychiatric-Mental Health Nursing*, "all interactions between the nurse and patient are potentially teaching/learning situations" (CFMHN, 2014, p. 9). Thus, in health teaching, the nurse attends holistically to potential healthcare problems. For example, if a person has diabetes mellitus and is taking insulin, the nurse provides healthcare teaching related to diabetes and the interaction of this problem with the mental disorder. Clients may need or want a family member or friend to be taught ways to assist and/or support them, as well. For instance, in the preceding example, teaching a family member or a friend of the client about diabetes and its treatment, including the administration of insulin, might be an important component of the health education.

There are many learning aids and tools that can assist individuals to increase their health literacy and understanding of their personal health situation. These range from pamphlets, diagrams, and books to websites, apps, and video gaming. Nurses have a role in helping clients identify appropriate resources and need to be aware that credibility (e.g., Is the source of a website reliable?), cost (e.g., Does the client have a mobile phone and is this app affordable?), accessibility (e.g., Does the client have internet access?), and ease of use (Is the client comfortable with video games?) will be factors in the effectiveness of a learning aid or tool.

Evaluation is a necessary aspect of teaching: has the client learned the knowledge and skills required to maintain their health? Evaluation is an ongoing process. While some information may be readily acquired, other knowledge and skills may need more time or teaching. Review of the material throughout the teaching–learning process is a good strategy, as is having the client "teach-back" what has been learned. Aids to retaining important information, such as written or audio materials that can be reviewed at home, are helpful (RNAO, 2021a).

Nurses need to be vigilant in the teaching–coaching role that they do not conflate the client's learning style with their own preferred way to learn. The nurse must also be aware of their own feelings when providing client education about what might be considered sensitive or culturally taboo topics. For example, some psychiatric medications have sexual side effects that significantly contribute to medication noncompliance. Nurses need to develop skills and confidence to educate clients about this important concern. Many clients are embarrassed to do so and are expecting the health professional to take the lead to initiate the discussion (Zhang et al., 2020) (see Fig. 12.2 for "EASE," a brief guide to health education with clients).

Interventions for the Social Domain

The social domain includes the individual's environment and its effect on their response to mental disorders and distress. Interventions within the social domain are geared towards couples, families, friends, and large and small social groups, with special attention given to ethnicity and community interactions. In some instances,

Health Education with Clients: EASE

ENGAGE
Collaborative approach
Learn about client's life situation
Learn client priorities and preferences

ASSESS
Health literacy needs
Client's learning style
Availability of learning resources

STRATEGIZE & START
Create learning goals and plan with client
Select or develop learning tools
Enact plan
Encourage

EVALUATE
Ongoing
Review
Client "teaches-back"

Figure 12.2 Health education with clients: EASE.

nurses design interventions that affect a client's environment, such as helping a family member decide to place a loved one in long-term care. In other instances, the nurse modifies the environment to promote positive behaviours through providing opportunities for clients to interact with others. For example, this can be accomplished through group or recreational activities for holidays or other special events, which clients can attend. Group and family interventions are discussed in Chapters 15 and 16.

Milieu Therapy

Milieu therapy provides a stable and coherent social organization to facilitate an individual's treatment. (The terms milieu therapy and *therapeutic environment* are often used interchangeably.) In milieu therapy, the design of the physical surroundings, structure of client activities, and promotion of a stable social structure and cultural setting enhance the setting's therapeutic potential. A therapeutic milieu facilitates client interactions and promotes personal growth. Although inpatient psychiatric units are increasingly used for intensive, short-term care of acutely and severely ill clients who are discharged as soon as possible to community care, milieu therapy remains important to these environments.

Milieu therapy is the responsibility of the nurse in collaboration with the client and other healthcare providers. The basic concepts of milieu therapy include safety and security, validation, open communication, and structured interaction.

Safety and Security

The milieu should be a healing place in which clients feel safe, secure, and cared for while dealing with their illness. The physical surroundings are important in this process and should be clean and comfortable, with special attention paid to promoting a noninstitutionalized environment. For in-patient and clinic settings, pictures on walls, comfortable furniture, and soothing colours help clients relax. Most facilities encourage clients and nursing staff to wear street clothes, which helps decrease the formalized nature of hospital settings and promotes nurse–client relationships. Clients need to feel that it is safe for them to be in hospital when they are most vulnerable. However, the stigma of mental illness can all too often exist within institutional walls. Clients have reported feeling stigma from health professionals, other clients, and themselves. The structure provided on units, while well intended, can leave some feeling dehumanized, shamed, and controlled (Eldal et al., 2019). On most inpatient psychiatric units, clients participate in maintaining the quality of the physical surroundings, such as assuming responsibility for making their own beds, attending to their own belongings, and keeping an acceptable living area. Families are viewed as a part of the client's life; family involvement is encouraged. Thus, family members should feel welcomed and safe in the milieu, as well.

Validation

In a therapeutic environment, validation is another process that affirms a client's individuality. Clients should feel validated as persons of worth and deserving of respect. Staff–client interactions should constantly reaffirm the client's humanity and their human rights. The importance of the client's personal story, history, experience, and understanding of their illness must be recognized in all aspects of care.

Open Communication

In open communication, health and treatment information is shared with clients and families. Client self-disclosure is invited within the support of a nurse–client relationship, with attention paid to the parameters of confidentiality that exist within that therapeutic relationship. These parameters may change with the care situation. For instance, if the client is undergoing a forensic assessment, information disclosed may be shared with the justice system (e.g., law courts). The client needs to understand this (see Chapter 35). Further, the environment is shaped to facilitate optimal interaction and resocialization. Support, attention, praise, and reassurance given to clients improve self-esteem and increase confidence. Client education is also a part of this support, including guidance regarding effective coping skills. Nurses and other team members should strive to role model effective communication when interacting with one another as well as with clients and families. The dynamics of team interactions can affect the milieu in both positive and negative ways.

Structured Interaction

Structured interaction is a purposeful interaction that is intended to help clients cope with particular behaviours or to learn better ways of interaction. For instance, the treatment team may assign structured interactions to specific clients as part of their treatment. Specific attitudes or approaches are assumed with individual clients or in response to particular client behaviour if beneficial to the client. These approaches include indulgence, flexibility, passive or active friendliness, matter-of-fact attitude, casualness, watchfulness, or kind firmness. For example, if and when a client becomes overexcited by daily events, the team may provide a matter-of-fact attitude when responding or if a client's illness includes delusions that lead them to engage in risky behaviour, the team may intervene with an attitude of kind firmness.

Milieu treatments are based on the individual needs of the clients and include relaxation groups, discussion groups, and medication groups. Spontaneous and planned activities are possible on a short-term unit as well as in a long-term setting. In the community, it is possible to apply milieu therapy approaches in day treatment centres, group homes, and single dwellings.

Promotion of Client Safety on Psychiatric Units

A critical aspect of nursing in PMH settings is the promotion of client safety, especially in inpatient units. It is critical because clients may be so severely ill that they engage in behaviours harmful to themselves or others. Clients experiencing delusions and hallucinations, for instance, can be responding to perceptions not based in reality. They can react with fear or in self-defence to dangers only they perceive. Sensitivity to the client's world as they are living it underlies nursing interventions used to keep the client safe. Interventions begin with observation and de-escalation and may evolve to the use of containment strategies, such as seclusion or physical or chemical (medication) restraints for clients with an involuntary status. See Chapter 8 for a discussion of ethical issues related to the use of behaviour control and restraint.

Psychiatric units vary in their rate of incidences of client behaviours such as aggression, self-harm, medication refusal, and suicide attempts that put both clients and care team at risk and frequently result in application of containment measures with the client. Key influences on these incidences have been identified as "the patient community, patient characteristics, the regulatory framework, the staff team, the physical environment, and outside hospital" (Bowers, 2014, p. 501). Examples in these domains include the following:

- Patient community: discord among patients, as when property is damaged; the contagion of emotions such as anxiety and noise levels within the community
- Patient characteristics: symptoms and their severity (e.g., hallucinations, delusions); staffing levels for care and support
- Outside hospital: tension in family, loss of accommodation or relationship, or bad news
- Physical environment: clean, tidy, respectful atmosphere and opportunities for client choice
- Staff team: levels of staff anxiety and frustration, ideology of care, rules, consistency
- Regulatory framework: legal status (e.g., involuntary admission); denial of an appeal

Recognition of these influences allows them to be addressed in ways that better promote client and staff safety.

Observation

Like all hospitalized clients, individuals hospitalized on a psychiatric unit are observed by the nurses caring for them. **Observation** is the ongoing assessment of the client's status to identify and subvert any potential problem. The nature of mental disorders shapes the focus of the nurses' observations. In psychiatric settings, for instance, clients are ambulatory and thus more susceptible to environmental hazards. In addition, judgment and cognition impairment are symptoms of many psychiatric disorders. The reason for the client's admission may be, in fact, that they pose a danger to themselves or others. When nursing in PMH settings, observation involves thoughtful, knowledgeable regard of the persons and consistent, responsible monitoring for any potential harm to themselves or others.

The intensity of the observation of the client depends on the assessed level of risk. Clients may be simply asked to "check in" at different times of the day, whereas other clients may be observed every 15 min by an assigned staff member. Some clients, such as those seen at a high risk for suicide, may be constantly observed by a staff member assigned to only them. Mental health facilities have policies that specify levels of observation for clients at varying degrees of risk.

De-escalation

De-escalation is an interactive process of calming and redirecting a client who has an immediate potential for violence directed towards self or others. This intervention involves assessing the situation and preventing it from escalating to one in which injury occurs to the client or others. Having assessed the situation, the nurse responds matter-of-factly to it, using various interventions that can include a request for the client and/or others to leave the situation, distraction, and conflict resolution. Psychiatric staff members are usually trained in responding to situations of aggression as a team and, thus, are often able to de-escalate such situations effectively (see Chapter 19 for information on the management of aggression and violence). Nurses can use various interventions in this situation, including distraction, conflict resolution, and cognitive interventions.

Seclusion

Seclusion is the process of removing a patient away from others and placing them into a locked room. The purpose of doing so is generally due to aggressive behaviour (Askew et al., 2019). A client is placed in seclusion for purposes of safety or behavioural management. The nature and physical content of the seclusion room can vary. It generally has no furniture except a mattress and a blanket. The walls may be padded. The room must be environmentally safe, with no hanging devices, electrical outlets, or windows from which the client could jump. Once placed in seclusion, the client is observed at all times (i.e., continuous or constant observation).

Research regarding the experiences of using seclusion rooms has yielded conflicting data. Seclusion can be an extremely negative client experience. Individuals who have been secluded have described feeling vulnerable, neglected, and shamed (Askew et al., 2019). Consequently, its use is seriously questioned, and many facilities have completely abandoned its practice. However, clients have also reported the use of seclusion rooms in aiding them feel safe and protected (Larue et al., 2013). Mental health staff appear to identify the potential for negative client perceptions and experiences regarding seclusion rooms and also experience the stress of facing the ethical challenges in using this approach. However, they also tend to feel that it can be beneficial for clients who demonstrate violent behaviour and need that high level of restriction (Haugom et al., 2019). If units are adequately staffed and personnel are trained in dealing with assaultive clients, then seclusion is rarely needed. If seclusion is used, then it must follow the same guidelines as the use of restraints.

Restraint

Restraint is the most restrictive safety intervention and is only used in the most extreme circumstances as a measure of last resort. Alternative approaches to the use of restraint include adjusting the environment in ways such as reducing stimulation, increasing or decreasing social interaction, providing access for the client to their preferred coping strategy, review of prescribed medication for potential change, use of appropriate distraction or relaxation techniques, and access to comfort zones or rooms (RNAO, 2021a). The Registered Nurses Association of Ontario's best practice guideline, "Promoting Safety: Alternative Approaches to the Use of Restraints," is an excellent resource (see Web Links). In Canada, the laws for restricting the freedom of clients against their will are specific to each province. Provincial mental health acts govern the situations under which restraint may be used in their jurisdiction.

Chemical restraint is the use of medication to manage or control client's behaviour. This is distinct from medication used to treat their psychiatric illness. A **physical restraint** is any human or mechanical method that restricts the freedom of movement or normal access to one's body, material, or equipment and cannot be easily removed. Different types of physical restraints are available. Wrist restraints restrict arm movement. Four-point restraints are applied to the wrists and ankles in bed. When five-point restraints are used, all extremities are secured, and another restraint is placed across the chest.

In addition to following provincial laws, the nurse must also adhere to hospital policies regarding restraint. A physician's order is necessary for restraint, and nurses should document all of the previously tried de-escalation interventions before the restraint was applied. Nurses should limit the use of restraints to times when an individual is judged to be a danger to self or others. As well, they should apply restraints only until the client has gained control over their behaviour. When a client is in physical restraints, the nurse should closely observe the client and protect them from self-injury. It is the nurse's responsibility to be aware of the institutional policies that govern this.

Research examining the experiences of nurses who have forcibly touched patients while physically restraining them sheds light into the "inconsistent thoughts, feelings, and perceptions of forcible touch" (Bailey et al., 2020, p. 405). Nurses have reported needing to justify why the forcible touch was needed. The lack of knowledge as to what it is like for the individual who is being touched, balanced with the assessments and mitigation of force, based on the information they receive via touching the patient, and the disconnect with having caring feelings towards the patient, shape the experience for nurses. They describe wanting to be compassionate. An issue, too, was the lack of time to care for oneself after an episode of using restraint (Bailey et al., 2020). Cusack and colleagues (2018) conducted an integrated literature review of physical and psychological harm in the use of physical restraint and a number of themes emerged: trauma/re-traumatization, distress, fear, feeling ignored, control, power, calm, and dehumanizing conditions. Given the negative consequences to the client and the impact on the nurse–client relationship, it is essential that nurses treat the client with respect and dignity at all times during a psychiatric emergency that necessitates seclusion or restraint.

Canadian nursing research (Larue et al., 2013) identified factors influencing client perspectives regarding seclusion: behaviour of the health professional upon entering the seclusion room, such as demonstrating understanding, listening, and reassurance; the offer of help in regaining control; and explanation of the situation to the client, such as seclusion as a means of addressing the need for calm, sleep, and safety. Some client participants voiced concerns regarding lack of alternatives to seclusion being offered and recommended changes to the physical environment.

Every incident of seclusion or restraint should be followed up by a thorough debriefing. In a systematic review of research in the area, debriefings were found to be reflective processes that were, in part, aimed in rebuilding trust with clients and staff, to reduce the traumatic effects of the events on staff and clients, and as a way to increase understanding of behaviours that could lead to restrained use. Some studies explored the learning potential that was possible with debriefing sessions. Individuals needed to feel open and supported in discussing the events and in identifying what lead to restraint use. Discussions of how to prevent restraint and seclusion from an organizational perspective were regarded as needed. Although less of a focus in the research reviewed, the need to ensure proper documentation of the events that occurred was noted; sources such as RNAO guidelines in the area were identified as possible resources to aid in this process (Mangaoil et al., 2020). In addition, education on the ethical, clinical, and legal issues related to restraint practices is essential (Hughes & Lane, 2016).

Home Visits

Clients usually have been hospitalized or have received treatment for acute psychiatric symptoms before being referred to a home care service. The goal of **home visits**, the delivery of nursing care in the client's living environment, is to maximize the client's functional ability within the nurse–client relationship and with the family or partner, as appropriate. The nurse who makes home visits needs to be able to work independently, is skilled in teaching clients and families, can administer and monitor medications, and uses community resources for the client's needs. Traditional home visits are regaining popularity, particularly when the client has concomitant psychiatric and physical illnesses.

Home visits can be especially useful when helping reluctant clients to enter therapy, conducting a comprehensive assessment, strengthening a support network, and maintaining clients in the community when their condition deteriorates. Home visits are also useful in helping individuals adhere to their medication regimen. The nurse, for instance, can gain a better understanding of the barriers to taking medication as prescribed and assist the client and family to address these. One major advantage of home visits is the opportunity to provide family members with information and education and to engage them in planning and interventions.

Home visits also offer the nurse an opportunity to develop cultural sensitivity to families from a variety of backgrounds. Home-based interventions require the nurse to gain an understanding, as much as possible, of the family structure and interactions, including the roles of various members, how the family functions in terms of responsibilities, and the family life cycle (see Chapter 16). A family's cultural background influences all of these factors and is important to consider when planning interventions. The home visit also allows the nurse to identify clients who lack support from others in their daily lives.

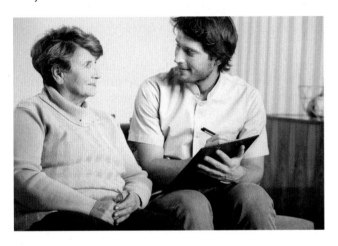

The home visit process consists of three steps: the previsit phase, the home visit, and the postvisit phase. During previsit planning, the nurse sets goals for the home visit based on data received from other healthcare providers or the client. Any safety precautions that should be taken for the visit should be identified and acted upon. For instance, winter road conditions for a rural home visit or crime levels in an urban district to be visited may need to be considered. The nurse and the client agree on the time of the visit. While the nurse travels to the home, a general assessment can be made of the neighbourhood for access to services, socioeconomic factors, safety, and other factors relevant to the client's wellbeing within the community.

The actual visit can be divided into four parts. The first is the greeting phase, usually brief, in which the nurse begins to connect with the client and family members in their home setting. Greetings are important as they set the atmosphere for the visit and, on the part of the nurse, should be friendly but professional. In some cultures, the greeting phase may involve more formal interactions, such as taking food or tea with family members. The second phase establishes the focus of the visit. Sometimes, the purpose of the visit is medication administration, health teaching, or counselling. The client and family must be clear regarding the purpose.

The implementation of the service is the next phase and should use most of the visit time. If the purpose of the visit is problem solving or decision-making, then the family's cultural values may determine the types of interaction and decision-making approaches. Closure is the last phase, the end of the home visit. It is a time to summarize and clarify important points. The nurse should also schedule any additional visits and reiterate client expectations between visits. Usually, the nurse is the only provider to see the client regularly. The nurse should acknowledge family members when leaving if they were not a part of the visit.

The postvisit phase includes documentation, reporting, and follow-up planning. This time is also when the nurse may meet with supervisors or colleagues and presents data from the home visit at the team meeting.

Community Action

Nurses have a unique opportunity to promote mental health awareness and support humane treatment for people with mental disorders including addiction. Activities range from being an advisor to support groups to participating in the political process through lobbying efforts and serving on community mental health boards. These unpaid activities are usually outside the realm of a particular job. However, an important role of professionals is to provide community service in addition to services through income-generating positions.

Interventions for the Spiritual Domain

Spiritual care cannot be readily separated from the bio/psycho/social components of care. It involves, rather, giving attention to all aspects of the individual's life and life circumstances and takes direction from their reality (Sawatzky & Pesut, 2005). In doing so, the nurse works with the client to identify their spiritual needs and facilitate a process by which the client can meet them. It is also important for the nurse to examine their own spirituality and how their beliefs influence the way that they help clients in this process (Rudolfsson et al., 2014). The integrative nature of spirituality, and therefore of spiritual care, can make it difficult to isolate and identify spiritual needs, document spiritual interventions, and stipulate care goals.

Times of illness and crisis can be opportunities for personal or spiritual growth for a person. The person may seek to connect or reconnect with others, with nature, with a power greater than themselves (that may be named in various ways, such as God, the Creator, or Allah, or not named out of respect), or with some aspect of the sacred. Nurses can support clients in their spiritual growth by listening to them as they describe their seeking; by responding to any requests for meeting with a religious leader/guide such as a minister, priest, rabbi, imam, lama, or elder; or by facilitating the use of religious ritual, such as a smudging ceremony for a client of Indigenous Peoples origin who requests it. Aspects of care for the spiritual domain relevant to particular disorders or age of human development may be found in this text in units *Care and Recovery for Persons With a Psychiatric Disorder* and *Mental Health Across the Lifespan*.

Evaluation of Care Goals

Evaluation of individual care goals involves answering the following questions:

• What were the benefits for the individual?
• What was the individual's level of satisfaction?
• Was the focus of care specific or nonspecific?
• What was the cost-effectiveness of the intervention?

Summary of Key Points

• Nurses should work collaboratively with clients and families in determining interventions.
• Nurses develop interventions from assessment data and may organize them around nursing care foci. The client's needs, values, and preferred care goals and the *Canadian Standards of Psychiatric-Mental Health Nursing* guide the selection of interventions.
• A client's ability to manage self-care activities can fluctuate with symptom severity. The Orem (1991) self-care model can be used to conceptualize client needs (related to attitude, knowledge, and skill) and choose appropriate interventions.
• The *Canadian Standards of Psychiatric-Mental Health Nursing* supports the importance of outcome identification.
• Care goals must be measurable and indicative of the individual's progress.
• More research is needed to identify individual care goals as they relate to nursing care foci and interventions.
• Nursing focus of care, nursing interventions, and individual care goals are initially derived from the assessment data.
• Initial, revised, and discharge care goals can be included in a nursing care plan.
• Care goal statements can cover the bio/psycho/social/spiritual domains.

When measuring care goals, nurses must consider the time frame. Identifying the intermediate goal indicators that may be achieved in one setting versus the indicators that can be achieved in a second setting provides for a measurement of progression and enhances continuity of care. Nevertheless, not until the individual is discharged or moved to a community setting can it be known if indicators (for instance, "demonstration of confidence when alone at home," "demonstration of confidence in role skills [worker/mother]," "demonstration of self-advocacy behaviour") are achieved. Care goals can be measured immediately after the nursing intervention or after time passes. However, care goals based on health prevention and health promotion care foci can be challenging to measure and may need to occur after considerable time has passed.

• Nursing care, from assessment to goal measurement, needs to be person and family centred. This means more than a recognition of the person's right to participate in healthcare decisions. It means genuine respect for the person's life experience and hopes for recovery.
• Interventions focusing on the biologic domain include activity and exercise; sleep, nutrition, relaxation, hydration, and thermoregulation interventions; pain management; and medication management. Nutritional interventions are used with most clients with psychiatric disorders. Medication management is a priority because of the long-term nature of the disorders and the importance of medication compliance.
• Interventions focusing on the psychological domain include counselling, behaviour therapy, cognitive interventions, psychoeducation, health teaching, and others. Implementation of these interventions requires a broad theoretic knowledge base.
• Interventions focusing on the social domain include group and family approaches, milieu therapy, safety interventions, home visits, and community action. On an inpatient psychiatric unit, the nurse uses milieu therapy to maximize the treatment effects of the client's environment.
• Interventions focusing on the spiritual domain involve a relationship and connection with the client that encompass the qualities of receptivity, humanity, competency, and positivity.

Thinking Challenges

A nurse is developing a plan of care for a client diagnosed with obsessive–compulsive disorder. The client washes their hands 34 times a day, reads 34 pages of their book, and brushes their hair 34 times. The client feels that everything has to be done 34 times, or something bad will happen to them.

a. What nursing interventions would be important from each of the interventional domains?

b. How are best practice guidelines used in mental health nursing?
c. How are interventions from the psychological domain important to this client?

Visit thePoint to view suggested responses.
Go to thePoint.lww.com/activate and use the activation code found in the front of this text to unlock answers to the "Thinking Challenges" and other online resources.

Web Links

beckinstitute.org/get-informed/what-is-cognitive-therapy
This site briefly describes the cognitive model and key terms
of CBT.

canada.ca/en/health-canada/services/canada-food-guides.
html Canada's food guides are available for download, free of
charge, at this Health Canada site.

www.canada.ca/content/dam/hc-sc/migration/hc-sc/fn-an/
alt_formats/pdf/food-guide-aliment/educ-comm/toolkit-
trousse/images-text-eng.pdf The *Eat well and Be Active Educational Toolkit* can be found at this Health Canada website,
a resource you can use to help educate adults and children
about eating healthy and being active.

www.cfmhn.ca/professional-practice The Canadian Federation of Mental Health Nurses' practice standards are freely
available at this link.

www.nursingcenter.com The Lippincott Nursing Center at
this site has student resources, including articles and information about nursing topics, such as patient education. Membership is free.

rnao.ca/bpg/guidelines The best practice guidelines of the
Registered Nurses Association of Ontario (RNAO) are found
here and may be downloaded free of charge.

rnao.ca/bpg/initiatives/mhaia The RNAO has a *Mental
Health & Addictions Initiative* aimed at enhancing evidence-
based care and services across all settings. This site includes
e-learning modules and other resources.

References

Anthony, W. A. (1993). Recovery from mental illness: The guiding vision of the mental health service system in the 1990's. *Psychosocial Rehabilitation Journal, 16*, 11–23.

Álvarez-García, C., & Yaban, Z. Ş. (2020). The effects of preoperative guided imagery interventions on preoperative anxiety and postoperative pain: A meta-analysis. *Complementary Therapies in Clinical Practice, 38*, 101077. https://doi.org/10.1016/j.ctcp.2019.101077

Arksey, H., & O'Malley, L. (2005). Scoping studies: Towards a methodological framework. *International Journal of Social Research Methodology, 8*, 19–32. doi:10.1080/1364557032000119616

Askew, L., Fisher, P., & Beazley, P. (2019). What are adult psychiatric inpatients' experience of seclusion: A systematic review of qualitative studies. *Journal of Psychiatric and Mental Health Nursing, 26*, 274–285.

Bailey, J., Nawaz, R. F., & Jackson, D. (2020). Acute mental health nurses' experience of forcibly touching service users during physical restraint. *International Journal of Mental Health Nursing, 30*(2), 401–412.

Barker, P. J., & Buchanan-Barker, P. (2010). The Tidal Model of mental health recovery and reclamation: Application in acute care settings. *Issues in Mental Health Nursing, 31*, 171–180.

Beck, J. S. (2021). *Cognitive therapy: Basics and beyond* (3rd ed.). Guilford Press. https://www.beckinstitute.org/get-informed/what-is-cognitive-therapy/

Beyene, L. S., Severinsson, E., Hansen, B. S., & Rørtveit, K. (2019). Being in a space of shared decision-making for dignified mental care. *Journal of Psychiatric and Mental Health Nursing, 26*, 368–376.

Boggs, K. U. (2020). Resolving conflicts between nurse and patient. In E. C. Arnold, & K. U. Boggs (Eds.), *Interpersonal relationships: Professional communication skills for nurses* (8th ed.). Elsevier.

Bowers, L. (2014). Safewards: A new model of conflict and containment on psychiatric wards. *Journal of Psychiatric and Mental Health Nursing, 21*, 499–508.

Brataas, H. V., & Evensen, A. E. (2016). Life stories of people on sick leave from work because of mild mental illness, pain, and fatigue. *Work, 53*(2), 285–291.

Butcher, H., Bulechek, G., Dochterman, J. M., & Wagner, C. M. (Eds.). (2018). *Nursing interventions classification (NIC)* (7th ed.). Elsevier.

Canadian Collaborative Mental Health Initiative (CCMHI). (2006a). *Canadian Collaborative Mental Health Charter.* http://www.shared-care.ca/files/EN_CharterDocument.pdf

Canadian Collaborative Mental Health Initiative (CCMHI). (2006b). *Principles and commitments.* http://www.shared-care.ca/files/Principles_and_Commitments.pdf

Canadian Federation of Mental Health Nurses (CFMHN). (2014). *Canadian standards of psychiatric-mental health nursing* (4th ed.).

Centre for Addiction and Mental Health. (2016). *Integrated care pathways.* http://www.camh.ca/en/hospital/care_program_and_services/ICPs/Pages/default.aspx

Cusack, P., Cusack, F. P., McAndrew, S., McKeown, M., & Duxbury, J. (2018). An integrative review exploring the physical and psychological harm inherent in using restraint in mental health inpatient settings. *International Journal of Mental Health Nursing, 27*(3), 1162–1176.

Djukanovic, I., Carlsson, J., & Peterson, U. (2016). Group discussions with structured reminiscence and a problem-based method as an intervention to prevent depressive symptoms in older people. *Journal of Clinical Nursing, 25*(7/8), 992–1000.

Eldal, K., Veseth, M., Natvik, E., Davidson, L., Skjølberg, A., Gytri, D., & Moltu, C. (2019). Contradictory experiences of safety and shame in inpatient mental health practice: A qualitative study. *Scandinavian Journal of Caring Sciences, 33*, 791–800.

Haugom, E. W., Ruud, T., & Hynnekliev, T. (2019). Ethical challenges of seclusion in psychiatric inpatient wards: A qualitative study of the experiences of Norwegian mental health professionals. *BMC Health Services Research, 19*, 879. https://doi.org/10.1186/s12913-019-4727-4

Health Canada. (2019a). *Eating well with Canada's Food Guide.* https://food-guide.canada.ca/en/

Health Canada. (2019b). *Eating well with Canada's Food Guide for First Nations, Inuit, and Métis.* https://www.canada.ca/en/health-canada/services/food-nutrition/reports-publications/eating-well-canada-food-guide-first-nations-inuit-metis.html

Hughes, L., & Lane, P. (2016). Use of physical restraint: Ethical, legal, and political issues. *Learning Disability Practice, 19*(4), 23–27.

Jniene, A., Errguig, L., El Hangouche, A. J., Rkain, H., Aboudrar, S., El Ftouh, M., & Dakka, T. (2019). Perception of sleep disturbances due to bedtime use of blue light-emitting devices and its impact on habits and sleep quality among young medical students. *BioMed Research International, 2019*, 7012350. https://doi.org/10.1155/2019/7012350

Kauppi, K., Hätönen, H., Adams, C. E., & Välimäki, M. (2015). Perceptions of treatment adherence among people with mental health problem and healthcare professionals. *Journal of Advanced Nursing, 71*(4), 777–788.

Larue, C., Dumais, A., Boyer, R., Goulet, M. H., Bonin, J. P., & Baba, N. (2013). The experience of seclusion and restraint in psychiatric settings: Perspectives of patients. *Issues in Mental Health Nursing, 34*, 317–324.

Levac, D., Colquhoun, H., & O'Brien, K. K. (2010). Scoping studies: Advancing the methodology. *Implementation Science, 5*(69), 1–9.

Mangaoil, R. A., Cleverley, K., & Peter, E. (2020). Immediate staff debriefing following seclusion or restraint use in inpatient mental health settings: A scoping review. *Clinical Nursing Research, 29*(7), 479–495.

Mental Health Commission of Canada. (2015). *Guidelines for recovery-oriented practice, hope, dignity, inclusion.*

Morrison, P., Meehan, T., & Stomski, N. J. (2015). Australian case managers' perception of mental health consumers use of anti-psychotic medications and associated side-effects. *International Journal of Mental Health Nursing, 24*, 104–111.

Orem, D. (1991). *Nursing concepts of practice* (4th ed.). Year Book.

Pater, P., Shattell, M. M., & Clary, M. (2015). Video games as nursing interventions. *Issues in Mental Health Nursing, 36*, 156–160.

Registered Nurses Association of Ontario. (2021a). *Clinical guidelines.* https://rnao.ca/bpg/guidelines/clinical-guidelines?items=75

Registered Nurses Association of Ontario. (2021b). *Clinical practice guidelines program.* https://rnao.ca/bpg/guidelines/clinical

Rudolfsson, G., Berggren, I., & da Silva, A. B. (2014). Experiences of spirituality and spiritual values in the context of nursing – An integrative review. *The Open Nursing Journal, 8*, 64–70.

Sagna, A. O., & Walker, L. O. (2020). Analysis of the Tidal Model and its implications in late-life suicidality. *Nursing Science Quarterly, 33*(4), 315–321.

Sawatzky, R., & Pesut, B. (2005). Attributes of spiritual care in nursing practice. *Journal of Holistic Nursing, 23*(1), 19–33.

Toups, M., Carmody, T., Greer, T., Rethorst, C., Grannemann, B., & Trivedi, M. H. (2017). Exercise as an effective treatment for positive valence symptoms in major depression. *Journal of Affective Disorders, 209*, 188–194.

Turgut, E. O., & Çam, M. O. (2020). The effect of Tidal Model-based psychiatric nursing approach on the resilience of women survivors of violence. *Issues in Mental Health Nursing, 41*(5), 429–437.

Vallance, J. K., Buman, M. P., Stevinson, C., & Lynch, B. M. (2015). Associations of overall sedentary time and screen time with sleep disorders. *American Journal of Health Behavior, 39*(1), 62–67.

Zhang, X., Sherman, L., & Foster, M. (2020). Patients' and providers' perspectives on sexual health discussion in the United States: A scoping review. *Patient Education and Counseling, 103*(11), 2205–2213.

Psychopharmacology and Other Biologic Treatments

Duncan Stewart MacLennan

LEARNING OBJECTIVES

After studying this chapter, you will be able to:

- Explain basic principles of pharmacokinetics and pharmacodynamics.
- Explain psychotropic drug actions by describing the role of neurotransmitter chemicals and their receptor sites.
- Explain the three major mechanisms of action of psychotropic medications in the central nervous system.
- Define the three properties that determine the strength and effectiveness of a medication.
- Describe more specific mechanisms of action for each of the major classes of psychopharmacologic medication.
- Describe the major therapeutic effects as well as prevalent side effects of various classes of psychotropic medications.
- Suggest appropriate nursing methods to administer medications.
- Implement interventions to minimize side effects of psychopharmacologic medications.
- Differentiate acute and chronic medication-induced movement disorders.
- Identify aspects of patient teaching that nurses must implement for successful maintenance of patients using psychotropic medications.
- Analyze the potential benefits and risks associated with other forms of somatic treatments, including electroconvulsive therapy, light therapy, and transcranial magnetic stimulation.
- Evaluate potential causes of nonadherence and implement interventions to improve adherence with treatment regimens.

KEY TERMS

- absorption • adherence • affinity • agonists • akathisia • antagonist • bioavailability • dystonia • efficacy • excretion • first-pass metabolism • half-life • intrinsic activity • kindling • metabolism • pharmacokenetics • phototherapy • potency • pseudoparkinsonism • selectivity • side effects • solubility • specificity • tardive dyskinesia • target symptoms • therapeutic index • tolerance • toxicity

KEY CONCEPTS

- psychopharmacology • receptors

In the early 1900s, Emil Kraeplin classified mental disorders based on clusters of observed symptoms, which provided the basic tenets of the contemporary biologic approach to understanding and treating psychiatric disorders. However, this approach fell out of favour as psychoanalytic, psychodynamic, interpersonal, and other therapies flourished, and mental disorders were increasingly assumed to have primarily a psychological aetiology.

In the 1950s, when it was discovered that the phenothiazine medications, such as chlorpromazine (Thorazine), relieved many of the symptoms of psychosis and that iproniazid, a medication for treating tuberculosis, elevated mood, there was renewed interest in neurophysiology and biologic treatments for treating mental disorders.

This chapter reviews the major classes of psychopharmacologic drugs used to treat psychiatric and mental health disorders, including antipsychotics, mood stabilizers, antidepressants, antianxiety medications, and stimulants. The biological basis for understanding the specific biologic treatments of psychiatric disorders are described more fully in later chapters. This chapter focuses on understanding the impact of psychotropic medications on the basic unit of central nervous system (CNS) functioning, the synapse, and on receptors embedded in neuronal cell membranes. This basic understanding allows the nurse to accept the roles and responsibilities of administering medications, proactively monitoring and treating side effects, and educating the patient and family, which are all crucial to successful psychopharmacologic therapy. As well as psychopharmacologic therapy, other biologic treatments—electroconvulsive therapy (ECT), light therapy, and nutritional therapy—are discussed in this chapter.

KEY CONCEPT

Psychopharmacology is a subspecialty of pharmacology that studies medications that affect behaviour through their actions in the CNS and that are used to treat psychiatric and neurodegenerative disorders. It is important to remember that many drugs used to treat other conditions, such as pain syndromes, heart disease, and autoimmune disease, may also have powerful effects in the brain.

Pharmacodynamics

A small amount of medication can have a significant and large effect on cellular function. When tiny molecules of medication are compared with the vast number of cells in the human body, the fraction seems disproportionate. Yet the drugs used to treat mental disorders often have profound effects on behaviour. To understand how this occurs, one needs to understand both *where* and *how* drugs work.

Targets of Drug Action: Where Drugs Act

Most drug molecules do not act on the entire cell surface, but rather at receptor sites, binding sites on enzymes, or transporters that remove neurotransmitter molecules from the synapse. Many psychopharmacologic drugs, especially older classes, act at multiple receptors. Newer agents are more specific to one type of receptor, but none act exclusively on one type of receptor. Understanding where receptors (and their subtypes), enzymes, and transporters are located within the body can be useful to explain the effects (including side effects) of specific drugs.

Consider diphenhydramine (Benadryl), a drug often used to treat allergic reactions, which works by interfering with histamine receptors (inverse agonist, discussed

below). As it turns out, the histamine 1 (H1) receptor is located in smooth muscles, in endothelial cells, and *in the brain*. When a person takes this drug to counter the effects of an allergic reaction (in the body tissues outside of the brain), the drug also has an effect on H1 receptors in the brain and causes sedation. Newer generation antihistamine drugs, such as loratadine (Claritin), will still have an effect on H1 receptors, but the drug molecules do not readily cross the blood–brain barrier. Little to no drug effect will occur at histamine receptors within the brain; thus, sedation is less likely to occur. The distribution of receptors in specific brain regions also plays a role in the side effect profile. For example, dopamine antagonists can produce dystonic movements because high concentrations of dopamine receptors are found in the region of the brain that controls fine motor movement.

Receptors are proteins that are embedded within the cell membrane and have binding sites for both naturally occurring chemicals (called *endogenous substances*) and drugs. Endogenous brain chemicals involved in neurotransmission, such as dopamine and serotonin, bind to specific groups of receptors. Administered drugs may compete with neurotransmitters for these receptors by mimicking or blocking the action of the neurotransmitter.

KEY CONCEPT

Receptors are associated with the work of German chemist Paul Erhlich, who in 1900 suggested that a receptive substance exists within the cell membrane. The biologic action of a drug depends on how its structure interacts with a specific receptor. Thus, a basic understanding of how receptors work is key to understanding how many drugs work in the body.

Receptors

Many drugs have been developed to act specifically at the receptor sites. When bound to the receptor, these drugs act as **agonists**—chemicals producing the same biologic action as the neurotransmitter itself—or as **antagonists**—chemicals blocking the biologic action of an agonist at a given receptor. Drugs that only produce a partial response are known as *partial agonists*. Figure 13.1 illustrates the action of an agonist, antagonist, and partial agonist drug at a receptor site. Not shown in Figure 13.1, an *inverse agonist* is a drug that produces an opposite response than what an endogenous neurotransmitter produces. As an example, all known H1-antihistamines are not receptor antagonists but inverse agonists. A drug's ability to interact with a given receptor type may be judged by three properties: selectivity, affinity, and intrinsic activity.

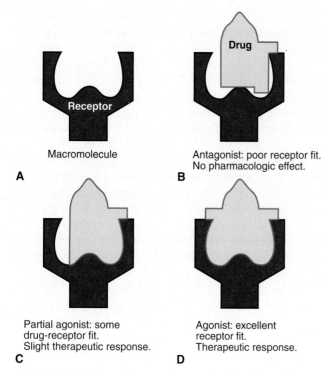

A Macromolecule

B Antagonist: poor receptor fit. No pharmacologic effect.

C Partial agonist: some drug-receptor fit. Slight therapeutic response.

D Agonist: excellent receptor fit. Therapeutic response.

Figure 13.1 A–D. Agonist and antagonist drug–receptor interactions at receptor sites.

Selectivity and Specificity

The first property, called **selectivity**, is the drug's ability to affect one receptor type over others. The more selective a drug is, the more likely it will affect only the specific receptors for which it is meant. A less selective drug will more likely bind to receptors intended for other neurochemicals and cause more unintended effects, or side effects. As an example, dopamine 2 (D2) receptors are the location of interest in treating the positive symptoms of schizophrenia. While haloperidol, an antipsychotic medication, does target these D2 receptors and reduces symptoms of schizophrenia, the drug will also interact (to varying degrees) with other receptors including H1 receptors, alpha 1 and 2 receptors, serotonin receptors, and other dopamine receptors. This lack of selectivity accounts for many side effects associated with this drug.

Specificity is the drug's ability to affect one receptor subtype over another. For example, a drug may be selective to adrenergic receptors but more specifically affect the beta-adrenergic receptor type 1 over other receptor subtypes (i.e., beta 2, beta 3). Drug specificity can further reduce drug side effects.

Affinity

The second property is that of **affinity**, which is the degree of attraction or strength of the bond between the drug and its receptor. Normally, these bonds are produced by relatively weak electrochemical attractions. Basic to the action of almost all CNS drugs within the body is their ability to bind to a receptor, produce a response, move off the receptor, and continue to repeat this binding/unbinding process until the drug is cleared from the body. There are some exceptions to this transient bond formation, such as is seen in a class of drugs that binds to an enzyme and is discussed in that section.

Intrinsic Activity

The final property of a drug's ability to interact with a given receptor is that of **intrinsic activity**, or the ability of the drug to produce a biologic response once it binds to a receptor. This is a measure of "how much response" a drug produces and ranges from maximal response (full agonist) to partial response (partial agonist) to no response (antagonist) to an inverse response (inverse agonist). Full agonists provide a maximal response, meaning that the biologic response from the receptor produced by the drug is the same as if it were stimulated by naturally occurring endogenous molecules. Partial agonists, while only capable of producing a partial response, may also be used to "block" the complete response produced by endogenous molecules (or other drugs). Buprenorphine, an opioid agent, is a partial agonist and can be used to decrease symptoms (or prevent) of an opioid overdose. Drugs that act as agonists have all three properties: selectivity, affinity, and intrinsic activity. However, antagonists have only selectivity and affinity because they produce no biologic response by attaching to that receptor. In complex biologic systems, such as the brain, preventing an agonist from binding can yield behavioural responses.

Ion Channels

Some drugs act directly on ion channels embedded in the nerve cell membrane. Examples include local anaesthetics that block the entry of sodium into the cell, preventing an action potential. The benzodiazepine drugs, frequently used in psychiatry for anticonvulsant, antianxiety and hypnotic properties, are an example of drugs that affect a specific ion channel of the nerve cell membrane. Benzodiazepine drug molecules, such as diazepam (Valium), work by binding to a region of the gamma-aminobutyric acid (GABAA) receptor–chloride channel complex. The binding site for these drugs is different from where GABA itself binds. When bound, these drugs increase the frequency and duration of chloride ion movement through GABA into the cell. This causes a decrease in the ability of that cell to conduct a nerve impulse. Thus, they are referred to as being indirect agonists or positive modulators of the GABA$_A$ channel.

Enzymes

Enzymes are complex proteins that catalyze specific biochemical reactions within cells and are the targets for some drugs used to treat mental disorders. For example, monoamine oxidase (MAO) is the enzyme required to break down most monoamine neurotransmitters, such as norepinephrine, serotonin, and dopamine, and can be inhibited by medications from a group of antidepressants called monoamine oxidase inhibitors (MAOIs). There are two types of MAO. MAO-A is more specific to norepinephrine, serotonin, and dopamine. MAO-A inhibition increases available monoamine neurotransmitter and is thought to initiate the cascade of cellular changes that ultimately relieve the symptoms of depression. MAO-B is more specific to dopamine metabolism, and MAO-B inhibition is used to treat Parkinson disorder, a neurodegenerative disorder where dopamine neurons die off.

Instead of the on–off property in relation to drugs that bind to receptors, the older MAOIs form a strong covalent bond with the enzyme. This causes irreversible changes to the enzyme, and more enzymes will need to be produced in order for further breakdown of neurotransmitters to occur. This irreversibility may contribute to serious side effects and is a major reason these drugs are seldom used in contemporary practice. Although they have similar effects, some MAOIs (e.g., moclobemide) do not form covalent bonds and so are called reversible. In this case, the enzymes are not reversibly changed and are thus available to be used to break down neurotransmitters (such as serotonin and norepinephrine) and other substrates such as tyramine during their unbound state. This flexibility significantly improves the drug safety profile for these novel MAOIs.

Carrier Proteins: Uptake Receptors

Neurotransmitters are small organic molecules that are released in response to a change in the polarity of the cell membrane (called an action potential), interact with receptors, and then are transported back into the neuronal cell by carrier proteins. These transporters have binding sites specific for the type of molecule to be transported. After a neurotransmitter, such as serotonin, has activated receptors in the synapse, its actions are terminated by these transporters that take serotonin back up into the presynaptic cell. Medications specific for this site may block or inhibit this transport and, therefore, increase the amount of the neurotransmitter in the synaptic space available for action on the receptors.

A primary action of most of the antidepressants is to increase the amount of neurotransmitters in the synapse

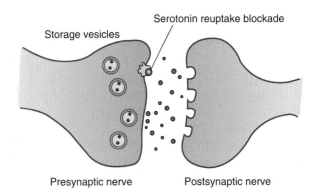

Figure 13.2 Reuptake blockade of a transporter for serotonin by an SSRI.

by blocking their reuptake. Older antidepressants, like the tricyclic antidepressants (TCAs), block the reuptake of more than one neurotransmitter and have affinity for other receptors, which produces increased side effects. Some antidepressants, such as fluoxetine (Prozac) and sertraline (Zoloft), are more selective for serotonin, whereas reboxetine (Endronax) is more selective for norepinephrine. These medications are called selective serotonin reuptake inhibitors (SSRIs) and norepinephrine reuptake inhibitors (NRIs), respectively. Newer antidepressants that are selective to both serotonin and norepinephrine are called SNRIs (e.g., venlafaxine [Effexor] and duloxetine [Cymbalta]). These more selective medications have reduced the number of side effects experienced by the patients. Figure 13.2 illustrates the reuptake blockade of serotonin by an SSRI.

Efficacy and Potency: How Drugs Act

Efficacy is the ability of a drug to produce a desired response. It is important to remember that the degree of receptor occupancy contributes to efficacy, yet it is not the only variable. A drug may occupy a large number of receptors but not produce a response. In contrast, **potency** considers the amount of drug required to produce the desired biologic response. One drug may be able to achieve the same clinical effect as another drug but at a lower dose, making it more potent. Although the drug given at the lower dose is more potent, they may be considered to have equal efficacy because both drugs achieve similar effects. The current opioid crisis in Canada is, in part, due to increasingly potent opioids (i.e., fentanyl, carfentanil) in the illicit drug supply.

Loss of Effect: Biologic Adaptation

In some instances, the effects of medications diminish with time, especially when they are given continuously,

BOX 13.1 Mechanisms Causing Decrease in Medication Effects

- Change in receptor density or affinity
- Depletion of neurotransmitter stores
- Increased metabolism of the drug
- Physiologic adaptation
- Interaction with female hormones

as in the treatment of chronic psychiatric disorders. This loss of effect can be a form of physiologic adaptation that may develop as the cell attempts to regain homeostatic control to counteract the effects of the drug. In responding to a prolonged drug exposure, an individual's body may increase (or decrease) the rate of receptor firing, the number of receptors on a cell's surface, or the quality of enzymes used to metabolize the drug. Cycling female hormones can also affect response to drugs. Progesterone and its metabolites bind to the same GABAA receptor as do the benzodiazepines and can affect the efficacy of benzodiazepines at certain stages of the menstrual cycle. In this instance, drug effect may be dependent on menstrual phase. These are only a few reasons for decreased drug effectiveness (Box 13.1). **Tolerance** is a gradual decrease in the action of a drug at a given dose or concentration in the blood. This decrease may take days or weeks to develop and results in the loss of therapeutic effect of a drug.

Other forms of physiologic adaptation result in a gradual tolerance that may be helpful in the case of unpleasant side effects, such as drowsiness or nausea. For example, the SSRIs can cause nausea and gastrointestinal upset when first started, but these side effects are short-lived. With forewarning about these temporary side effects, patients are more likely to stay on the medication and not discontinue the drug regime on their own. This information is important for the nurse to communicate to patients experiencing such side effects so that they can be reassured that the effects will subside.

Target Symptoms and Side Effects

Psychiatric medications are indicated for specific symptoms, referred to as target symptoms. **Target symptoms** are those measurable specific symptoms expected to improve with medication use. The target symptoms for each class of medication are discussed more fully in later sections of this chapter. Serotonin-related drugs produce widespread effects in many body systems because receptors for neurotransmitters (such as serotonin) are

found in all regions of the brain and in the periphery. For example, these drugs interact with receptors in the gastrointestinal tract and in facial motor nerves, causing gastrointestinal upset and bruxism (clenching and grinding of teeth). These unwanted effects of medications are called **side effects**.

Knowledge of a medication's affinity for receptors and subtypes of receptors may give some indication of the likelihood that specific target symptoms might improve and what side effects might be expected. Table 13.1 provides a brief summary of possible physiologic effects from drug actions on specific neurotransmitters. For example, antagonists with high affinity for acetylcholine receptors of the muscarinic subtype will be more likely to cause such side effects as dry mouth, blurred vision, constipation, urinary hesitancy or retention, and nasal congestion.

This information should serve only as a guide in predicting side effects because of considerable interindividual variability in drug responses, and not all underlying mechanisms have been elucidated. The nurse should use this information to focus assessment on these areas. If the symptoms are mild, then simple nursing interventions suggested in Table 13.2 should be implemented. If symptoms persist or are severe, then the prescriber should be notified immediately. Patients need to be encouraged to report side effects and to be aware that suggestions and solutions may be available to address the side effects. For example, changing from one drug to another within the same class of psychotropics can often decrease unwanted side effects.

Drug Toxicity

All drugs have the capacity to be harmful as well as helpful. Toxicity generally refers to the point at which concentrations of the drug in the body have gone beyond the safe range and may become harmful or poisonous to the body. However, what is considered harmful? Side effects can be harmful but not toxic, and individuals vary widely in their responses to medications. **Therapeutic index**, a concept often used to discuss the toxicity of a drug, is a ratio between median toxic dose and median effective dose (the dose at which 50% of the population will experience drug toxicity and drug effectiveness, respectively).

A high therapeutic index means that there is a large range between the dose at which the drug begins to take effect and a dose that would be toxic to the body. Drugs with a low therapeutic index have a narrow range and are often carefully monitored through blood levels. This concept has some limitations. The therapeutic index of a medication also may be greatly changed by the coadministration of other medications or drugs. For example, alcohol consumed with most CNS depressant

Table 13.1	Pharmacodynamic Properties of Antidepressants	
Neurotransmitter/ Receptor Action	Physiologic Effects	Examples of Drugs That Exhibit High Affinity
Reuptake inhibition blockade		
Norepinephrine reuptake inhibition	Antidepressant action Potentiation of pressor effects of norepinephrine Side effects: tachycardia, tremors, insomnia, erectile and ejaculation dysfunction, increased risk for suicidal ideation.	desipramine reboxetine
Serotonin reuptake inhibition	Antidepressant action Antiobsessional effect Antianxiety effect Side effects: gastrointestinal distress, nausea, headache, nervousness, motor restlessness, increased risk for suicidal ideation and sexual side effects, including anorgasmia	fluoxetine paroxetine escitalopram sertraline duloxetine
Receptor mediated		
Histamine (H_1) receptor antagonism	Side effects: sedation, drowsiness, hypotension	quetiapine amitriptyline imipramine olanzapine
Muscarinic Acetylcholine receptor antagonism	Side effects: anticholinergic (dry mouth, blurred vision, constipation, urinary hesitancy and retention, memory dysfunction) and sinus tachycardia	benztropine amitriptyline doxepin olanzapine chlorpromazine
Norepinephrine receptor (α_1 receptor) antagonism	Potentiation of antihypertensive effect of prazosin and terazosin Side effects: postural hypotension, dizziness, reflex tachycardia, sedation	amitriptyline clomipramine clozapine
Norepinephrine receptor (α_2 receptor) antagonism	Interactions with antihypertensive medications, blockade of the antihypertensive effects of clonidine Side effect: priapism	clomipramine clozapine trazodone
Norepinephrine receptor (β_1 receptor) antagonism	Antihypertensive action Side effects: orthostatic hypotension, sedation, depression, sexual dysfunction (including impotence and decreased ejaculation)	propranolol
Serotonin receptor ($5\text{-}HT_{1a}$) agonist	Antidepressant action Antianxiety effect Possible control of aggression	trazodone risperidone aripiprazole (partial agonist at 5-HT1a)
Serotonin receptor ($5\text{-}HT_2$) antagonism	Antipsychotic action Some antimigraine effect Decreased rhinitis Side effects: hypotension, ejaculatory problems, weight gain, metabolic disorders	aripiprazole risperidone clozapine olanzapine haloperidol ziprasidone
Dopamine receptor (D_2) antagonism	Antipsychotic action Side effects: extrapyramidal symptoms, such as tremor, rigidity (especially acute dystonia and parkinsonism); endocrine changes, including elevated prolactin levels, weight gain	aripiprazole (partial agonist at D2)

drugs will have added depressant effects, which greatly increases the likelihood of toxicity or death.

Despite the limitations of the therapeutic index, it is a helpful guide for nurses, particularly when working with potentially suicidal individuals. Nurses must be aware of the potential for overdose and closely monitor the availability of drugs for these patients. In some cases, prescriptions may have to be dispensed daily or weekly until a suicidal crisis has passed to ensure that patients do not have access to lethal doses of drugs. The choice of drug can also help address toxicity. For example, the TCAs can be lethal in overdose, whereas SSRIs are not; SSRIs are thus the safer choice for higher-risk patients and adolescents.

Pharmacokinetics: How Drugs Move Through the Body

The field of **pharmacokinetics** (PK) describes how a drug moves throughout the body to get to its target receptors and then is eliminated. The four processes of PK are Absorption, Distribution, Metabolism, and Excretion (ADME). Overall, the goal in PK is to describe and predict the time course of drug concentrations throughout the body and factors that may interfere with these processes. Together with the principles of pharmacodynamics, this information can be helpful to the nurse in ways such as facilitating or inhibiting drug effects and predicting behavioural response.

Table 13.2	Managing Common Side Effects of Psychiatric Medications
Side Effect or Discomfort	**Intervention**
Blurred vision	Reassurance (generally subsides in 2–6 weeks)
Dry eyes	Warn ophthalmologist; no eye examination for new glasses for at least 3 weeks after a stable dose
	Artificial tears may be required; an increased use of wetting solutions for those wearing contact lenses
Dry mouth and lips	Frequent rinsing of the mouth, good oral hygiene, sucking sugarless candies, lozenges, lip balm, lemon juice, and glycerin mouth swabs
Constipation	High-fibre diet; encourage bran, fresh fruits, and vegetables
	Metamucil (must consume at least 16 oz of fluid with dose)
	Exercise, increase fluids
	Mild laxative
Urinary hesitancy or retention	Monitor frequently for difficulty with urination, changes in starting or stopping stream
	Notify prescriber if difficulty develops
	A cholinergic agonist, such as bethanechol, may be required
Nasal congestion	Moisturizer, nasal rinse
Sinus tachycardia	Assess for infection
	Monitor pulse for rate and irregularities
	Withhold medication and notify prescriber if resting rate exceeds 100 bpm
Decreased libido and ejaculatory inhibition	Consider change to another drug in same class or change class of drug
Postural hypotension	Frequent monitoring of lying-to-standing blood pressure during dosage adjustment period, immediate changes and accommodation, measure pulse in both positions
	Advise the patient to get up slowly, sit for at least 1 min before standing (dangling legs over side of bed), and stand for 1 min before walking or until light-headedness subsides
	Increase hydration and avoid caffeine
	Notify prescriber if symptoms persist or significant blood pressure changes are present
Photosensitivity	Protective clothing
	Sunglasses
Dermatitis	Use of sun block; remember to cover *all* exposed areas
	Stop medication usage
	Consider medication change, may require a systemic antihistamine
	Initiate comfort measures to decrease itching
Impaired psychomotor functions	Advise the patient to avoid dangerous tasks, such as driving
	Avoid alcohol, which increases this impairment
Drowsiness or sedation	Encourage activity during the day to increase accommodation
	Avoid tasks that require mental alertness, such as driving
	May need to adjust dosing schedule or, if possible, give single daily dose at bedtime
	May need a cholinergic medication if sedation is the problem
	Avoid driving or operating potentially dangerous equipment
	May need change to less-sedating medication
	Provide quiet and decreased stimulation when sedation is the desired effect
Weight gain	Exercise and diet teaching; regular weighing
	Caloric control and regular monitoring of blood glucose levels
Edema	Check fluid retention
	Reassurance
	May need a diuretic
Irregular menstruation	Reassurance (reversible)
Amenorrhea	May need to change class of drug
	Reassurance and counselling (does not indicate lack of ovulation)
	Instruct the patient to continue birth control measures
Vaginal dryness	Instruct in use of lubricants

Absorption and Routes of Administration

Absorption

The first phase of PK is **absorption**, defined as the movement of the drug from the site of administration into the plasma. It is important to consider the impact of routes by which a drug is administered on the process of absorption. The primary routes available include oral (both tablet and liquid), sublingual, intramuscular (IM) (short- and long-acting agents), and intravenous (used

for rapid treatment of adverse reactions and rarely for the treatment of the primary psychiatric disorder). The nurse needs to know about the advantages and disadvantages of each route and the subsequent effects on absorption (Table 13.3).

Drugs taken orally are usually the most convenient for the patient; however, this route is also the most variable because absorption can be slowed or enhanced by a number of factors. Taking certain drugs orally with food or antacids may slow the rate of absorption or

Preparation and Route	Examples	Advantages	Disadvantages
Oral tablet	Basic preparation for most psychopharmacologic agents, including antidepressants, antipsychotics, mood stabilizers, anxiolytics, etc.	Convenience	Variable rate and extent of absorption, depending on the drug May be affected by the contents of the intestines May show first-pass metabolism effects May not be easily swallowed by some individuals
Oral liquid	Also known as concentrates Many antipsychotics, such as haloperidol, chlorpromazine, thioridazine, risperidone The antidepressant fluoxetine Antihistamines, such as diphenhydramine Mood stabilizers, such as lithium citrate	Ease of incremental dosing Easily swallowed In some cases, more quickly absorbed	More difficult to measure accurately Depending on drug: • Possible interactions with other liquids, such as juice, forming precipitants • Possible irritation to mucosal lining of the mouth if not properly diluted
Rapid-dissolving tablet	Atypical antipsychotics, such as olanzapine and risperidone Handy for people who have trouble swallowing or for patients who let medication linger in the cheek for later expectoration Can be taken when water or other liquid is unavailable	Dissolves almost instantaneously in the mouth	The patient needs to remember to have completely dry hands and to place tablet in the mouth immediately Tablet should not linger in the hand
Sublingual	Lorazepam	Rapid action, no first-pass metabolism	Increased risk for tolerance and psychological dependence
Intramuscular	Some antipsychotics, such as haloperidol, chlorpromazine, and risperidone Anxiolytics, such as lorazepam Anticholinergics, such as diphenhydramine and benztropine mesylate No antidepressants No mood stabilizers	More rapid acting than oral preparations No first-pass metabolism	Injection site pain and irritation Some medications may have erratic absorption if heavy muscle tissue at the site of injection is not in use High-potency antipsychotics in this form may be more prone to adverse reactions, such as NMS
IM depot	Haloperidol decanoate, fluphenazine decanoate, paliperidone palmitate	May be more convenient for some individuals who have difficulty following medication regimens	Significant pain at injection site
Intravenous	Anticholinergics, such as diphenhydramine, benztropine mesylate Diazepam used as an anticonvulsant	Rapid and complete availability to systemic circulation	Inflammation of tissue surrounding site Often inconvenient for the patient and uncomfortable Continuous dosage requires use of a constant-rate iv infusion

change the amount of the drug absorbed. For example, the β-receptor antagonist propranolol exhibits increased blood levels when taken with food. Antacids containing aluminum salts decrease the absorption of some antipsychotic drugs; thus, antacids must be given at least 2 h before administration or 1 h after.

Oral preparations absorbed from the gastrointestinal tract into the bloodstream first go to the liver through the portal vein. There, they may be metabolized in such a way that most of the drug is inactivated before it reaches the rest of the body—this is called **first-pass metabolism**. The consequence of first-pass metabolism is that the fraction of the drug reaching systemic circulation is reduced, sometimes substantially. First-pass metabolism explains why the dose of propranolol given intravenously is so much less than the oral dose. **Bioavailability** describes the amount of the drug that

actually reaches systemic circulation. With some oral drugs, the amount of drug entering the bloodstream is decreased by first-pass metabolism and bioavailability is lower.

Other factors affecting absorption should also be considered when administering drugs. Liver disease can decrease first-pass metabolism and result in increased drug levels and thus an increased risk for side effects. Gastric motility also affects how the drug is absorbed. Increasing age, many disease states, and concurrent medications can reduce gastrointestinal (GI) motility and slow absorption. Other factors, such as blood flow in the GI system, drug formulation, and chemical factors, may also interfere with absorption. Nurses must be aware of a patient's physical condition and use of medications or other substances that can interfere with drug absorption.

In full strength, many liquid preparations, especially antipsychotics, irritate the mucosal lining of the mouth, oesophagus, and stomach and must be adequately diluted. Nurses must be careful when diluting liquid medications because some liquid concentrate preparations are incompatible with certain juices or other liquids. If a drug is mixed with an incompatible liquid, then a white or grainy precipitant usually forms, indicating that some of the drug has bound to the liquid and inactivated. Thus, the patient actually receives a lower dose of the medication than intended. Therefore, some medications should be given at least an hour apart.

Novel administration routes and drug form arrive with the advent of new technologies. This includes rapidly dissolving tablets or wafers (i.e., Zyprexa Zydis, Risperdal M-tab), extended or slow-release oral tablets (paliperidone ER tablet—Invega), or the even slower release depot injection (Invega Sustenna, Abilify Maintena). Each of these dosage forms require special attention—for instance, the nurse must avoid touching rapidly dissolving tablets with moist hands and extended-release oral drugs generally should not be crushed, chewed, or divided. Similarly, depot injections should be administered in a single dose intramuscularly.

Distribution

Once a drug enters the bloodstream, several factors affect how it is distributed in the body. Distribution of a drug reflects how easy it is for a drug to pass out of the systemic circulation and move into other types of tissues, such as brain, abdominal organs, skin, or bone, where target receptors are found. Factors that affect medication distribution to specific tissues in the body include the amount of blood flow or perfusion within the tissue; how lipophilic ("fat-loving") the drug is; plasma protein binding; and anatomic barriers, such as the blood–brain barrier, that the drug must cross. Highly perfused organs like the heart, liver, kidney, and brain are quickly and extensively exposed to any drug. Almost all psychotropic drugs are lipophilic, making it easier for the drug to passively cross epithelial cell membranes that line blood vessels and to cross the blood–brain barrier. Table 13.4 provides a summary of how some significant factors affect distribution. Two of these factors, ionic characteristics and protein binding, warrant additional discussion with regard to how they relate to psychiatric medications.

Ionic Characteristics of Drugs

Drugs in the bloodstream can be charged or uncharged molecules in the form of positive or negative ions. There are many charged components within cell membranes. Thus, drugs that have an electrical charge cannot passively cross through a cell membrane; instead, they

Table 13.4	Factors Affecting Distribution of a Drug
Factor	Effect on Drug Distribution
Size of the organ	Larger organs require more drug to reach a concentration level equivalent to other organs and tissues.
Blood flow to the organ	The most important contributor to distribution, the major organs have the highest blood flow (heart, lung, liver, brain, kidney) and thus have the greatest drug exposure.
Ionic characteristics	Small drugs with no molecular charge move easily across cell membranes by passive transfer rather than needing active transport and thus will be widely distributed.
Plasma protein binding	If a drug binds well to plasma proteins, particularly to albumin, then it will stay in the body longer.
Anatomic barriers	Both the gastrointestinal tract and the brain are surrounded by layers of cells that control the passage or uptake of substances. Lipid-soluble substances are usually readily absorbed and pass the blood–brain barrier.

must be transported by carrier proteins. Uncharged drugs (also called lipophilic or "fat-loving" drugs) can move easily across cell membranes. Most psychiatric drugs are very lipophilic and can move into major organ systems, as well as cross the blood–brain barrier. However, this characteristic means that psychopharmacologic agents can also cross the placenta. It also means that these agents can be taken into fat stores. Drugs stored in fatty tissue are only slowly released back into the systemic circulation for eventual elimination. This is why a lipophilic drug can be detected long after discontinuation in older adults and overweight individuals. This effect may also account for unexpected drug–drug interactions when substitute drug regimens are initiated quickly.

Protein Binding

Many drugs bind to large carrier proteins, such as albumin, in the bloodstream, referred to as plasma protein binding. The degree to which a drug is bound to these plasma proteins affects the drug's ability to interact with receptors. Only unbound or "free" drugs can move across membranes to their target receptors or be excreted from the body. High protein binding prolongs the drug's duration of action, allowing for less frequent dosing. Many of the psychotropic drugs are more than 90% protein bound. Chronic disease and normal aging can decrease the amounts of plasma proteins, shifting the ratio of bound drug to free drug. For highly bound drugs like the classic antipsychotics, a decrease of only 10% of bound drug (e.g., from 90% to 80%) would translate into a doubling of free drug and significantly increase the risk for side effects and drug toxicity.

Metabolism

The duration of drug action also depends on the body's ability to change or alter a drug chemically. **Metabolism**, also called biotransformation, is the process by which the drug is altered, usually by adding to the drug molecule or breaking the drug molecule into smaller pieces, both processes make the molecule or the pieces more polar. Lipid-soluble drugs become more polar or hydrophilic so that they may be excreted more readily.

There are two types of metabolic transformation that occur in drug metabolism: phase 1 reactions (mostly using CYP enzymes) produce metabolites, and phase 2 reactions (mostly through the addition of chemical side chains) produce conjugates. In phase 1 metabolism, active, inactive, or toxic metabolites are produced. The PK and pharmacodynamics of each metabolite may either be similar or very different from their parent compound. For instance, the antidepressant imipramine (Tofranil) is metabolized to a pharmacologically active substance, desipramine, which also has antidepressant effects (desipramine is also available on its own as an antidepressant). Prozac (fluoxetine), an SSRI antidepressant, is metabolized in the liver and forms an active metabolite, norfluoxetine, which has a very long half-life. This is important when changing from fluoxetine to another antidepressant to avoid potential side effects from having two antidepressants still acting in the body.

Metabolism may also change an inactive drug (called a prodrug) to an active one, or it may an active drug to a toxic metabolite. Codeine is the classic example of a prodrug that must be metabolized before having analgesic properties. Lisdexamfetamine (Vyvanse) is also a prodrug requiring transformation using hydrolytic activity of the blood cells (not CYP enzymes) to slowly produce the active compound dextroamphetamine for the treatment of ADHD.

The cytochrome P-450 superfamily of metabolic enzymes (or CYP450s) is responsible for most drug metabolism. The classification of the CYP450 superfamily uses a combination of numbers and letters to denote families, subfamilies, and individual enzymes. Most psychiatric drugs are metabolized by members of the 1A, 2D, and 3A subfamilies of CYP450 enzymes. The 3A family is the most abundant, constituting more than 60% of the liver enzyme weight. The metabolizing activity of some of the CYP450 enzymes can be altered by drugs and environmental chemicals.

Some drugs, like phenobarbital, induce CYP450 activity. Drugs that induce enzyme activity are known as *CYP enzyme inducers*. This effect increases drug metabolism and thus decreases drug levels of any drug taken with phenobarbital. If the drug level fall below a therapeutic concentration, then the drug may be less effective. Other common substances, such as tobacco smoke, alcohol, and coal tar in charcoal-broiled foods, can induce specific CYP450 enzymes. Alternately, drugs can inhibit CYP450 activity (these are *CYP enzyme inhibitors*) and thus increase drug levels, potentially pushing drug concentrations into toxic ranges.

Antidepressants drug, such as fluoxetine (1A2, 2C19), nefazodone (3A3/4), and paroxetine (2D6), have substantial effects on CYP enzymes. Other drugs such as sertraline and citalopram have little to no inhibitory or inducer effect on CYP enzymes (Preskorn, 2020). Many anticonvulsant, benzodiazepine, antipsychotic, and antidepressant drugs are most frequently substrate of CYP enzymes 3A4, 1A2, and 2D6. CYP P-450 enzyme inhibition and induction is potentially the source for significant drug–drug and food–drug interactions.

The widespread use of herbal products has introduced another potential source of drug–drug interaction. A good example of this is St. John's wort, a botanical product used extensively in Europe for mild depression that is emerging as a potential therapy for depression (Galeotti, 2017). There are also drug–endogenous product interactions. The most notable examples are estrogens and progesterone. Through a pharmacodynamic mechanism, progesterone can decrease the effectiveness of the benzodiazepines, but it can also affect drug concentrations as it is an inhibitor of CYP3A enzymes. Estrogens inhibit CYP1A2. During periods of high hormone levels (ovulation, luteal phase of the menstrual cycle, and pregnancy), these interactions may become clinically significant for women.

There have been calls for increased genetic testing of CYP enzymes to identify genetic variants to individualize drug prescribing to improve therapeutic outcomes (Zanardi et al., 2020). This field is called precision medicine. For instance, people with a genetic variant producing higher than typical CYP1A2 enzyme activity were found to have fewer psychic side effects when treated for schizophrenia with antipsychotic drugs (Cendrós et al., 2020). Similarly, several practice guidelines now include drug dosing alterations based on patient-specific CYP genotype (Kam & Jeong, 2020). However, the science of precision medicine in psychiatry is in its infancy and further research, potentially using artificial intelligence, must be completed to further improve its clinical application (Fabbri & Serretti, 2020; Kam & Jeong, 2020).

Nurses should remain alert to the possibilities of drug–drug interactions when patients are receiving more than one medication, especially in older adults. Drug reference books and clinical practice guidelines are helpful sources. In addition, if an individual receiving a medication experiences an unusual reaction or suddenly loses effect from a medication that had previously been working, the nurse should carefully assess other substances that the person has recently consumed, including prescription medications, nonprescription remedies, dietary supplements or changes, and substances of abuse (including alcohol and tobacco).

Excretion

Excretion refers to the elimination of drugs from the body either unchanged or as metabolites. Clearance refers to the total volume of blood, serum, or plasma from which a drug is completely removed from the bloodstream per unit of time. The driving force that determines the time required to eliminate a drug is usually the concentration of drug and the clearance rate. The elimination **half-life ($t_{1/2}$)** refers to the time required for plasma concentrations of the drug to be reduced by 50%. For example, 50% of a drug is cleared in one $t_{1/2}$. In the next $t_{1/2}$, 50% of the remaining concentration would be eliminated (leaving 25% of the original concentration), then after the third $t_{1/2}$, there would be 12.5% of the initial concentration remaining. Thus, it usually takes five to seven half-lives for a drug to be completely eliminated from the body.

As indicated previously, the goal of most metabolic processes is to decrease the lipophilic nature of drugs by increasing their ionic characteristics. Drugs that are small or ionized in the bloodstream can be easily removed by the kidney and excreted through urine. Some drugs, like lithium, a mood stabilizer, is eliminated exclusively through the kidney. Any impairment in renal function or renal disease, or even temporary dehydration (e.g., from flu symptoms or even strenuous exercise), may lead to severe toxic symptoms (Ott et al., 2016). However, many psychiatric medications are large molecules and removed through bile and eliminated in feces. Biliary elimination can lead to enterohepatic recirculation, a process by which active drug or metabolites that were excreted in bile into the small intestine are reabsorbed into the portal circulation, go through the liver again, and end up back into the systemic circulation. Enterohepatic recirculation is important to maintain an effective serum concentration. A well-known example of this is oral contraceptives. Oral antibiotics change the intestinal environment, can decrease enterohepatic recirculation, and thus affect the contraceptive efficacy.

Dosing refers to the administration of medication over time so that a consistent drug concentration may be achieved or maintained without reaching toxic levels. With repeated dosing, a certain amount of the drug is accumulated in the body. This accumulation will reach a point where the quantity of drug entering the body is equal to that which is leaving the body. This is called *steady-state plasma concentration* or simply *steady state*. The rate of accumulation is determined by the half-life of the drug. Drugs generally reach steady state in five to seven times the elimination half-life. However, because elimination or excretion rates may vary significantly, fluctuations may still occur, and dose schedules may need to be individualized.

The nurse should remember that these principles can support best practice; however, they are not substitutes for ongoing individual assessment of indicators of treatment response or unwanted effects.

Individual Variations in Drug Effects

Many factors affect drug absorption, distribution, metabolism, and excretion. These factors may vary among individuals, depending on their age, genetics, and ethnicity. Nurses must be aware of and consider these individual variations in the effects of medications.

Age

PK is influenced by life cycle stages. For example, gastric absorption changes with age. Gastric pH in a newborn is 6 to 8 and decreases to 1 to 3 over the first 24 h (the pH remains elevated in a premature infant) (Nicolas et al., 2017). This significantly affects drug absorption. Changes in drug absorption are also seen in older adults because of increased gastric pH, decreased gastric emptying, slowed gastric motility, and reduced splanchnic circulation. Normally, these changes do not significantly impair the oral absorption of a medication, but addition of common conditions, such as diarrhoea, may significantly alter and reduce absorption.

Renal function is also altered in both very young and older adult patients. Infants who are exposed in utero to medications that are excreted through the kidneys may experience toxic reactions to these medications because renal function in the newborn is only about 20% of that of an adult. In less than a week, renal function develops to adult levels, but in premature infants, the process may take longer. Renal function also declines with age. Creatinine clearance in a young adult is normally 100 to 120 mL per minute, but after the age of 40, this rate declines by about 10% per decade. Medical illnesses, such as diabetes and hypertension, may further the loss of renal function. When creatinine clearance falls below 30 to 60 mL per minute, the excretion of drugs by the kidneys is significantly impaired, and potentially toxic levels may accumulate.

Metabolism changes across the life span, especially in infancy and childhood. At birth, many of the liver enzymes are not fully functional, whereas in early childhood, there is evidence of increased activity compared with adulthood. For example, CYP1A2 activity is reduced in the first 4 months but increased between ages 1 and 2 years; CYP2D6 activity is reduced until ages 3 to 5 years, and CYP3A4 is reduced in the first month of life but increased between ages 1 and 4 (Mahmood, 2016). Thus, pediatric pharmacotherapeutics cannot simply be based on relative dosing by weight. Blood flow to the liver and the mass of liver tissue both decrease with age. The activities of hepatic enzymes also slow with age. As a result, the ability of the liver to metabolize medications may show as much as a fourfold decrease between the ages of 20 and 70. Again, the use of multiple drugs in older adults adds to metabolic burden, potentially increasing drug levels of each individual drug.

Most psychiatric medications are bound to proteins. Albumin is one of the primary circulating proteins to which drugs bind. The production of albumin by the liver is lower in neonates, peaks in early childhood, and generally declines with age. In addition, a number of medical conditions change the ability of medications to bind to albumin. Malnutrition, cancer, and liver disease decrease the production of albumin, which translates to more unbound drug available to interact with target receptors and an increased risk for adverse or toxic effects.

Phases of Drug Treatment

The nurse is involved in all the phases of medication treatment. Considerations in terms of assessment, treatment issues such as **adherence** (keeping with the therapeutic regimen), prevalence and severity of side effects, and expected timelines for symptom relief vary across the phases of treatment, but all involve potential nursing actions. These phases include initiation, stabilization, maintenance, and discontinuation of the medication. Nurses must be concerned with treatment phases as a guide for what may be expected as they administer medications and monitor individuals receiving medications across each of these phases. The following subsections discuss some of the knowledge required and the assessments and interventions to be performed by the nurse within each phase.

Initiation Phase

Before beginning to take medications, patients must undergo several assessments.

- A psychiatric evaluation, including past health history and previous medication treatment response, will clarify diagnosis and determine target symptoms for medication use.
- An open discussion regarding adherence issues, such as attitudes toward drug treatments, patient-specific goals for the drug therapy, any lifestyle issues that affect the structuring of a drug regimen (e.g., shift work, type of occupation and current job responsibilities, reproductive issues), and any health insurance issues related to prescription benefits (ability to afford the drug), will help to identify barriers to the patient's willingness and ability to manage the medication regimen.
- Physical examination and laboratory tests, often including baseline tests such as complete blood count (CBC), liver and kidney function tests, electrolyte levels, urinalysis, and possibly thyroid function tests and electrocardiogram (ECG). This may be done to exclude other health issues presenting as psychiatric concerns or to detect any potential concerns with drug clearance or to evaluate for QT-prolongation. These tests and other assessments (such as tools to measure

depression) may be used to track progress of treatment and evaluate for potential drug complications.
- Any other current medications, including over-the-counter medications; herbal remedies and mixtures from health food stores; naturopathic or homoeopathic visitations; and alcohol, tobacco, marijuana, and illicit drug use should be identified to prevent harmful drug interactions.

Nurses should perform their own premedication evaluations, including baseline physical assessments that focus on preexisting symptoms, such as gastrointestinal distress, sexual function/libido, or restrictions in range of motion that may later be confused with side effects. Comparing future symptoms to a patient's baseline status may be useful in detecting if symptoms are improving or worsening and potentially detect drug side effects (e.g., extrapyramidal symptoms). An assessment of cognitive functioning will assist the nurse in assessing whether memory aids or other supports are necessary to assist the individual in safely taking medications. Information from the psychosocial and lifestyle assessment should be reviewed in consultation with the prescriber and other members of the interprofessional team to develop a plan that is acceptable to the patient and will improve functioning, minimize side effects, and improve quality of life.

Recommendations and treatment alternatives should be developed and reviewed with input from the individual seeking treatment in all situations. Doing so will allow the patient to ask questions and receive complete information about drug effects and the most common side effects. This allows for informed consent, strengthens the therapeutic relationships, and possibly improve therapeutic outcomes. Patients are often overwhelmed during the initial phases of treatment and may have symptoms that make it difficult for them to participate fully in treatment planning. Information is often forgotten or may need to be repeated and provided in written form for ongoing reference. Nurses must keep their detailed drug knowledge current to be able to answer questions and provide ongoing education.

When use of the medication is initiated, nurses should treat the first dose as if it were a "test" dose. They should observe the patient closely for sensitivity to the medication, such as changes in blood pressure, pulse, or temperature; changes in mental status; allergic reactions; dizziness; ataxia; or gastric distress. Other common side effects that may occur with even one dose of medication should also be closely monitored. A protocol for reporting side effects and determining which ones should trigger immediate urgent follow-up should be in place. In Canada, health professionals may report adverse drug reactions to Health Canada's MedEffect program online at www.canada.ca/en/health-canada/services/drugs-health-products/medeffect-canada.html

Stabilization Phase

During stabilization, the medication dosage is often adjusted to achieve the maximum amount of improvement with a minimum number of side effects. This process is sometimes referred to as *titration*. Nurses must continue to assess target symptoms by looking for change or improvement and side effects. If medications are being increased rapidly, such as in a hospital setting, then nurses must closely monitor temperature, blood pressure, pulse, mental status, common side effects, and unusual adverse reactions.

On an outpatient basis, nurses must provide both verbal and written materials to individuals who are receiving the medication as to the expected outcome and potential side effects. This educational support should include factors that may influence the effectiveness of the medication, such as whether to take the medication with food, common interventions that may minimize side effects if they develop, and what side effects require immediate attention. Again, a plan is needed to clearly identify what to do if adverse reactions develop and what adverse reactions should prompt immediate attention. The plan should include emergency contact information or available emergency treatment and should be reviewed frequently.

Therapeutic drug monitoring is important in this phase of treatment for drugs with a narrow therapeutic index, such as lithium, valproate, and carbamazepine. Nurses must be aware of when and how these levels are to be determined and assist patients in learning these procedures. Plasma levels of other psychiatric medications can be evaluated, for example, to rule them out as a potential source of treatment nonresponse related to increased metabolism.

Unfortunately, the first medication chosen may not adequately improve the patient's target symptoms. This can be very discouraging, particularly in a population where powerlessness and hopelessness are inherent in the disorder. This possibility must be discussed before initiating drug therapy. Most of the time, another drug from the same class or a drug from a new class will be prescribed. Medications may also be changed when adverse reactions or serious uncomfortable side effects occur, or if these effects substantially interfere with the individual's quality of life. Nurses should be familiar with the PK of both drugs to be able to monitor side effects and possible drug–drug interactions during this transition period.

At times, an individual may show only partial improvement from a medication, and the prescriber may try an augmentation strategy. *Augmentation* refers to the addition of another medication to enhance the effects of the first medication. For example, a prescriber may add a mood stabilizer, such as lithium, or antipsychotic agent, such as aripiprazole, to an antidepressant to improve treatment outcomes for unipolar depression

(Taylor et al., 2020). These strategies are often used in so-called treatment-resistant situations. *Treatment resistance* has various definitions, but it means most often that after several medication trials, the individual has gained only partial improvement at best. Treatment-resistant symptoms often require multiple medications. Multiple medications may affect different physiologic processes and, in combination, provide overall synergistic or additive pharmacologic effects. Nurses must be familiar with the potential effects, side effects, drug interactions, and rationale for this type of complex treatment regimen.

Maintenance Phase

Medications may be continued to prevent relapse or reoccurrence once the individual's target symptoms have improved. *Relapse* usually refers to reemerging symptoms in response to premature discontinuation of treatment, whereas *reoccurrence* refers to an entirely new episode that occurs over time after full remission was achieved. Other reasons for reemerging symptoms, despite continued use of medication, include the loss of drug efficacy, comorbid medical illness, psychosocial stressors, and concurrent use of prescription or nonprescription medications.

Whatever the reason, patients must be educated about their target symptoms and have a plan of action if the symptoms return. The nurse has a central role in assisting individuals to monitor their own symptoms, manage psychosocial stressors, and avoid other factors that may cause the exacerbation of symptoms that were previously under control. Some side effects or adverse reactions emerge only after the individual has been receiving the medication for an extended period. Specific examples are discussed in later sections of this chapter.

Discontinuation Phase

Many psychotropic drugs require a tapered discontinuation. Tapering involves slowly reducing dosage while monitoring closely for withdrawal symptoms and for the reemergence of key symptoms, such as a drop in mood, increased anxiety, sleep disturbance, thought disorder, or decreased level of self-care. Some mental illnesses, such as mild depression or adjustment disorder, may respond to several months of treatment and not reoccur. Other disorders, such as bipolar disorder, chronic major depressive disorder, and schizophrenia, usually require continued medication treatment for extended periods of time and in fact may never be discontinued.

A withdrawal syndrome, affecting up to 56% of individuals after abrupt cessation of the antidepressants (Davies & Read, 2019), has been described and includes such symptoms as influenza-like symptoms, headache, irritability, dizziness, low mood, GI disturbance, and electric shock sensations (Rizkalla et al., 2020).

The restoration of the drug therapy relieves the symptoms within 24 h. If the withdraw is untreated, then the symptoms can last 1 to 2 weeks or longer for some specific drugs such as paroxetine (Fava & Cosci, 2019). The abrupt discontinuation of benzodiazepine and barbiturate drugs can result in anxiety, elevated heart rate and blood pressure, and seizure.

Nurses must be aware of the potential for these symptoms, monitor them closely, and implement measures to minimize their effects. They should support individuals throughout this process, whether they can successfully stop taking the medication or must continue the treatment. Even if patients can successfully discontinue use of the medication without a return of symptoms, nurses may help implement preventive measures to avoid the reoccurrence of the psychiatric disorder. In the roles of advocate, patient educator, and provider of interpersonal support, nurses often have a central role in helping patients incorporate preventive mental health strategies into their daily routine.

Antipsychotic Medications

It is hard to imagine how psychiatric illnesses were treated before the development of psychopharmacologic medications. Antipsychotic medications were among the very first drugs ever used to treat psychiatric disorders. First synthesized by Paul Charpentier in 1950, chlorpromazine became the interest of Henri Lorit, a surgeon from France, who was attempting to develop medications that controlled preoperative anxiety. Administered in intravenous doses of 50 to 100 mg,

chlorpromazine produced drowsiness and indifference to surgical procedures. At Lorit's suggestion, a number of psychiatrists began to administer chlorpromazine to agitated psychotic patients. In 1952, Jean Delay and Pierre Deniker, two psychiatrists from France, published the first report of chlorpromazine's calming effects with psychiatric patients (Granger, 1999). They soon discovered it was especially effective in relieving hallucinations and delusions associated with schizophrenia. As more psychiatrists began to prescribe the medication, the use of restraints and seclusion in psychiatric hospitals dropped sharply, ushering in a revolution in psychiatric treatment.

Since that time, numerous antipsychotic medications have been developed. Older, typical antipsychotic medications that have been available since 1954 are equally effective and inexpensive drugs that vary in the degree to which they cause certain groups of side effects. Table 13.5 provides a list of selected antipsychotics grouped by the nature of their chemical structure and indicating the likelihood of certain side effects. These medications treat the symptoms of psychosis, such as hallucinations, delusions, bizarre behaviour, disorganized thinking, and agitation.

First- and Second-Generation Antipsychotics

Initially, the term *major tranquilizer* was applied to this group of medications. Later, major tranquilizers were known as *neuroleptics*, which more accurately describes the action of drugs such as chlorpromazine and haloperidol.

Table 13.5 Side Effect Comparison of Selected Antipsychotic Medications

Drug Category Drug Name	Sedation	Extrapyramidal	Anticholinergic	Orthostatic Hypotension	Metabolic Syndrome
First-Generation Antipsychotics					
Phenothiazines					
chlorpromazine (Thorazine)	+4	+2	+3	+4	+3
thioridazine (Mellaril)	+3	+1	+4	+4	+1
fluphenazine (Prolixin)	+1	+4	+1	+1	+1
perphenazine (Trilafon)	+2	+3	+2	+2	+1
trifluoperazine (Stelazine)	+1	+3	+1	+1	+1
Thioxanthenes					
thiothixene (Navane)	+1	+4	+1	+1	+1
Dibenzoxazepines					
loxapine (Loxitane)	+2	+3	+2	+3	+1
Butyrophenones					
haloperidol (Haldol)	+1	+4	+1	+1	0/+1
Second-Generation Antipsychotics					
clozapine (Clozaril)	+4	+/0	+4	+4	+3
risperidone (Risperdal)	+1	+/0	+/0	+2	+3
olanzapine (Zyprexa)	+4	+/0	+2	+1	+3
quetiapine fumarate (Seroquel)	+4	+/0	+/0	+3	+2
ziprasidone HCl (Geodon)	+1	+/0	+1	+2	0/+1
aripiprazole (Abilify)	+1	+/0	+/0	+1	0/+1
paliperidone (Invega)	0/+1	+2	+1	0/+1	+1

Neuroleptic means "to clasp the neuron." The term reflects the common and often significant neurologic side effects produced by these types of drugs. The development of newer antipsychotic drugs that have less significant neurologic side effects has led to these older agents being used as secondary, not first-line, drugs. The term *first-generation or typical antipsychotic* now identifies the older antipsychotic drugs with greater risk for neurologic side effects, and *second-generation or atypical antipsychotic* identifies the newer generation of antipsychotic drugs.

Indications and Mechanisms of Action

Antipsychotic medications are typically indicated for treating acute psychosis or severe agitation. In general, the older, first-generation antipsychotics such as haloperidol (Haldol), chlorpromazine, and thioridazine (Mellaril), are equally effective in relieving positive symptoms of psychosis including hallucinations, delusions, and bizarre ideation. The negative symptoms including blunted affect, social withdrawal, lack of interest in usual activities, lack of motivation, poverty of speech, thought blocking, and inattention do not respond as well to the first-generation antipsychotics and in some cases may even be worsened by such agents. Second-generation antipsychotics, such as clozapine (Clozaril), risperidone (Risperdal), olanzapine (Zyprexa), quetiapine (Seroquel), aripiprazole (Abilify), lurasidone (Latuda), and paliperidone (Invega), are more effective at improving negative symptoms and less likely to cause tardive dyskinesia and extrapyramidal side effect.

Although antipsychotic medications are the primary treatment for schizophrenia and related illnesses, they are increasingly being used to treat other psychiatric and medical illnesses. For example, antipsychotics have been found to be efficacious in the treatment of both positive and negative symptoms of amphetamine-induced psychosis (Fluyau et al., 2019). In contrast, despite the common use of antipsychotics for the treatment of delirium in the ICU, little evidence exists to support this practice (Pluta et al., 2020). Similarly, a recent study demonstrated that the use of antipsychotics among older people who are diagnosed with delirium is associated with poor clinical outcomes, such as long-term institutionalization (Egberts et al., 2020). In a systematic review, Rieck et al. (2020) recommend that low-dose antipsychotic drugs only be used as a secondary line of treatment for delirium and only in rare circumstances where agitated behaviours and distressing symptoms of psychosis cannot be managed using nonpharmacological approaches.

As discussed in Chapter 21, the D2 receptor (dopamine receptor subtype) and 5HT2A (serotonin receptor subtype) are the primary drug targets for the management of psychosis. With the exception of pimavanserin (Nuplazid), all antipsychotic agents decrease the positive symptoms of psychosis because they are potent postsynaptic D2-receptor antagonists (i.e., haloperidol, quetiapine) or partial agonists (i.e., aripiprazole). Most second-generation antipsychotic drugs have inverse agonist and/or antagonist pharmacological activity at 5HT2A receptors. In general, second-generation antipsychotic agents have stronger affinity for 5HT2a receptors than D2 receptors and preferentially bind to D2 receptors in the cortical region of the brain versus the striatal areas. These characteristics of second-generation antipsychotics contribute to increased control of negative symptoms of psychosis and a decreased risk of tardive dyskinesia and extrapyramidal side effects.

Pharmacokinetics

Most antipsychotic medications can be administered without regard to meals; however, there are exceptions. Lurasidone (Latuda) is best absorbed when taken with at least 350 calories of food. Serum quetiapine concentrations are increased, and aripiprazole absorption is delayed with high-fat meals. These drugs should be taken without food or a light snack. Risperidone is not compatible with tannin or pectinate, so tea and cola beverages should be avoided at the time of oral administration. In general, smoking cigarettes can increase drug metabolism and decrease antipsychotic serum concentrations, rendering the therapy less effective. Nurses need to review a reliable drug information database to verify the specific administration requirements, if any, prior to drug administration.

There are two forms of injectable antipsychotic drugs: long acting and immediate release preparations. The long-acting injectable antipsychotics are typically thick and oily substances intended to provide a slow release of the active drug in order to lengthen frequency of dosing to 2 to 12 weeks. Long-acting injectable antipsychotics are often provided in prefilled syringes and should be administered using a Z-track method in either the deltoid or gluteal sites. The nurse must ensure a proper length needle is used to deposit the injectable content into muscle versus subcutaneous tissue. Immediate release antipsychotic drugs are also injected intramuscularly and used for acute psychosis.

The metabolism of these drugs occurs almost entirely in the liver, where hepatic microsomal enzymes convert these highly lipid-soluble substances into water-soluble metabolites that can be excreted through the kidneys. Therefore, these medications are subjected to the effects of other drugs that induce or inhibit the cytochrome P-450 system described earlier. Genetic variances causing poor CYP 2D6 metabolism will increase serum concentrations of aripiprazole and clozapine at standard doses. A dose reduction of up to 50% has been recommended for these in people who have this genetic polymorphism. Table 13.6 summarizes many of the possible medication interactions with antipsychotics, including

Table 13.6 Chemical Interactions With Antipsychotic Medications

Agent	Effect
Alcohol	Phenothiazines potentiate CNS depressant effects
	Extrapyramidal reactions may occur
Barbiturates	Speed action of CYP enzymes so that antipsychotic is metabolized more quickly, reducing phenothiazine and haloperidol plasma levels; barbiturate levels may also be reduced by phenothiazines; potentiate CNS depressant effect
Tricyclic antidepressants	Can lead to severe anticholinergic side effects; some antipsychotics (especially phenothiazines or haloperidol) can raise the plasma level of the antidepressant, probably by inhibiting metabolism of the antidepressant
Hydrochlorothiazide and hydralazine	Can produce severe hypotension
Aluminum salts (antacids)	Impair gastrointestinal absorption of the phenothiazines, possibly reducing therapeutic effect
	Administer antacid at least 1 h before or 2 h after the phenothiazine
Tobacco	Heavy consumption requires larger doses of antipsychotic because of CYP enzyme induction. Similarly, when patients are restricting from smoking or quit, smaller doses may be required.
Charcoal (and charbroiled food)	Decreases absorption of phenothiazines
Anticholinergics	May reduce the therapeutic actions of the phenothiazines, increase anticholinergic side effects, lower serum haloperidol levels, worsen symptoms of schizophrenia, increase symptoms of tardive dyskinesia
Meperidine	May result in excessive sedation and hypotension when coadministered with phenothiazines
Fluoxetine	Case report of serious extrapyramidal symptoms when used in combination with haloperidol
Lithium	May induce disorientation, unconsciousness, extrapyramidal symptoms, or possibly the risk for NMS when combined with phenothiazines or haloperidol
Carbamazepine	Decreases haloperidol serum levels, decreasing its therapeutic effects
Phenytoin	Increase or decrease in phenytoin serum levels; thioridazine and haloperidol serum levels may be decreased
Methyldopa	May potentiate the antipsychotic effects of haloperidol or may produce psychosis
	Serious elevations in blood pressure may occur with methyldopa and trifluoperazine
General anaesthesia (barbiturates)	Antipsychotic may potentiate effect of anaesthetic; may increase the neuromuscular excitation or hypotension

those resulting from changes in hepatic enzymes. Careful observance of concurrent medication use, including prescribed, over the counter, and substances of abuse, is required to avoid drug–drug interactions.

Excretion of these substances tends to be slow because the drugs can easily accumulate in fat stores. Most antipsychotics have a half-life of 24 h or longer, but many also have active metabolites with longer half-lives. These two effects make it difficult to predict elimination time, and metabolites of some of these agents may be found in the urine months later. After discontinuation, drug accumulated in body fat will diffuse back into plasma. Over the course of several days, the drug concentration in the plasma will move below the minimum concentration required to produce a drug effect. At this point, the drug benefit or adverse drug event will typically disappear. In combination with a longer drug half-life, the long elimination time does allow the medication to be given in once-daily dosing. This schedule increases adherence and reduces the impact of the peak occurrence of some side effects, such as sedation during the day.

High lipid **solubility**, accumulation of the drug in the body, and other factors have also made it difficult to correlate blood levels with therapeutic effects. Although these can be measured for a number of antipsychotics, their correlation with therapeutic response has been inconsistent. Haloperidol and clozapine correlate well and may be helpful in determining whether an adequate blood level has been reached and maintained during a

trial of medication. Table 13.7 shows the therapeutic ranges available for some of the antipsychotic medications. Plasma levels may also be helpful in identifying absorption problems or metabolic differences (high or low metabolizer), determining adherence, and identifying adverse reactions from drug–drug interactions.

The potency of the antipsychotics also varies widely and is of specific concern when considering typical antipsychotic drugs. As Table 13.7 indicates, 100 mg chlorpromazine is roughly equivalent to 2 mg haloperidol and 5 mg trifluoperazine. Although drugs that are more potent are not inherently better than less potent drugs, differentiating low-potency versus high-potency antipsychotics may be helpful to estimate drug dosing if one antipsychotic drug is switched to another. Given that each antipsychotic agent has differing side effect profiles, a change in antipsychotic may be needed if patients are experiencing adverse drug effects.

Ultimately, selection of medication from the group of typical antipsychotics depends predominately on predicted side effects, prior history of treatment response, whether or not a depot preparation will be needed during maintenance, concurrent medications, and other medical conditions.

Drug Formulations: Long-Acting Preparations

In Canada, there are several different types of long-acting injectable antipsychotic agents, typically referred

Table 13.7 Antipsychotic Medications

Generic (Trade) Drug Name	Usual Dosage Range (mg/day)	Half-Life (hours)	Therapeutic Blood Level	Approximate Equivalent Dosage (mg)
First-Generation Antipsychotics				
Phenothiazines				
chlorpromazine (Thorazine)	50–1,200	2–30	30–100 mg/mL	100
thioridazine (Mellaril)	50–600	10–20	1–1.5 ng/mL	100
mesoridazine (Serentil)	50–400	24–48	Not available	50
fluphenazine (Prolixin)	2–20	4.5–15.3	0.2–0.3 ng/mL	2
perphenazine (Trilafon)	12–64	Unknown	0.8–12.0 ng/mL	10
trifluoperazine (Stelazine)	5–40	47–100	1–2.3 ng/mL	5
Thioxanthenes				
thiothixene (Navane)	5–60	34	2–20 ng/mL	4
Dibenzoxazepines				
loxapine (Loxitane)	20–250	19	Not available	15
Butyrophenones				
haloperidol (Haldol)	2–60	21–24	5–15 ng/mL	2
Dihydroindolones				
molindone (Moban)	50–400	1.5	Not available	10
Second-Generation Antipsychotics				
clozapine (Clozaril)	300–900	4–12	141–204 ng/mL	50
risperidone (Risperdal)	2–8	20	Not available	1
olanzapine (Zyprexa)	5–10	21–54	Not available	Not available
quetiapine fumarate (Seroquel)	150–750	7	Not available	Not available
ziprasidone HCl (Geodon)	40–160	7	Not available	Not available
aripiprazole (Abilify)	10–30	75–94	Not available	Not available

to as *depot preparations*. First-generation agents include haloperidol decanoate, flupenthixol decanoate (Fluanxol Depot), and zuclopenthixol decanoate (Clopixol Depot). Second-generation agents include aripiprazole monohydrate (Abilify Maintena), aripiprazole lauroxil (Abilify Aristada), olanzapine pamoate (Zyprexa Relprevv), paliperidone palmitate (Invega Sustenna, monthly; and Invega Trinza, 3 months), and risperidone microspheres (Risperdal Consta). Note that two different formulations of aripiprazole and paliperidone exist, and the dosing of each formulation differs. These antipsychotics may be administered by injection once every 2 to 12 weeks, depending on the formulation.

Because they bypass problems with gastrointestinal absorption and first-pass metabolism, use of long-acting drugs may enhance therapeutic outcomes for the patient by decreasing individual drug concentration variability due to kinetic differences. Long-acting injectable medications maintain a fairly constant blood level between injections, improve drug adherence, and reduce relapse risk and mortality in schizophrenia (Correll & Lauriello, 2020). Initiation of long-acting injectable antipsychotics, particularly in people with substance use disorder, decreases risk for relapse, increases relapse-free survival time, and decreases hospitalization (Abdel-Baki et al., 2020). Long-acting injectable antipsychotics as first-line therapy have demonstrated improved cognitive remediation, improved medication adherence (up to 78%), and improved quality of life and social functioning compared to daily oral therapy (Giordano et al., 2020;

Nuechterlein et al., 2020). Box 13.2 describes research exploring mode of delivery and drug adherence.

Nurses should be aware that the injection site may become sore and inflamed but should resolve within a few days. Do not massage the site of administration. The site of administration should be documented and injection sites rotated for subsequent doses. Administration of the injection is done with the supplies provided by the drug manufacturer. To avoid accidental injection of the drug into the systemic circulation, the nurse should aspirate the syringe to assess blood return.

Side Effects, Adverse Reactions, and Toxicity

Various side effects and interactions can occur with antipsychotics (see Tables 13.6 and 13.7), with the first-generation antipsychotics producing more significant side effects than the second-generation antipsychotics. The side effects vary largely based on their degree of affinity to different neurotransmitter receptors and their subtypes.

Cardiovascular Side Effects

Cardiovascular side effects, such as orthostatic hypotension, depend on the degree of blockade of α-adrenergic receptors. Low-potency, first-generation antipsychotics, such as chlorpromazine and thioridazine, and the second-generation antipsychotic clozapine have a high degree of affinity for α-adrenergic receptors and,

BOX **13.2** Research for Best Practice

SUBSTANCE USE, PSYCHOSIS, AND MORTALITY AMONG PEOPLE WITH UNSTABLE HOUSING IN VANCOUVER

Jones, A. A., Gicas, K. M., Seyedin, S., Willi, T. S., Leonova, O., Vila-Rodriguez, F., Procyshyn, R. M., Smith, G. N., Schmitt, T. A., Vertinsky, A. T., Buchanan, T., Rauscher, A., Lang, D. J., MacEwan, G. W., Lima, V. D., Montaner, J. S. G., Panenka, W. J., Barr, A. M., Thornton, A. E., & Honer, W. G. (2020). Associations of substance use, psychosis, and mortality among people living in precarious housing or homelessness: A longitudinal, community-based study in Vancouver, Canada. *PLOS Medicine*, 17(7), e1003172. https://doi.org/10.1371/journal.pmed.1003172

Question: What are the associations between substance use, psychosis, and mortality among people living in precarious housing or experiencing homelessness?

Method: This is a 17-year longitudinal study in Vancouver, Canada. Monthly follow-up occurred in a sample of 437 people with a median study retention of 6.3 years. Substance use was assessed by interview and urine drug screening. Psychosis severity was clinically assessed at each encounter.

Findings: The study found that 79 participants (18.1) died during the 2,481 total person-years of observation. The causes of death were physical illness (40.5%), accidental overdose (35.4%), trauma (5.1%), suicide (1.3%), and unknown (17.7%). Methamphetamine, alcohol, and cannabis use were associated with higher risk for psychosis. A history of psychosis was associated with greater mortality.

Implications for Practice: People with unstable housing and health challenges likely required integrated care across physical health, mental health, and substance use disorder care domains. Effective treatment of psychosis and reduction of risk factors may decrease high mortality rates in this group. Reducing substance use, particularly methamphetamine, cannabis, and alcohol, may decrease risk of psychosis.

---

therefore, produce considerable orthostatic hypotension. Most antipsychotic drugs cause QT prolongation, which may cause sudden cardiac death. An ECG may be used to determine the patient's QT interval, which may direct the nurse practitioner or primary provider to prescribe one type of antipsychotic over another. Nurses must be aware that other drugs may also lengthen the QT interval. The possibility of QT prolongation effects, particularly when new drugs are prescribed, needs to be examined and will involve collaboration with the pharmacist to determine overall risk profile.

Anticholinergic Side Effects

Anticholinergic side effects resulting from the blockade of muscarinic acetylcholine receptors are another common concern with the first-generation and some of the second-generation antipsychotic drugs. Dry mouth, slowed gastric motility, constipation, urinary hesitancy or retention, vaginal dryness, blurred vision, dry eyes, nasal congestion, and confusion or decreased memory are examples of these side effects. Interventions for decreasing the impact of these side effects are outlined in Table 13.2. This group of side effects occurs with many of the medications used for psychiatric treatment. Sometimes a cholinergic medication, such as bethanechol, may reduce the peripheral effects but not the CNS effects. Using more than one medication with anticholinergic effects often increases the symptoms. Older adult patients are often more susceptible to a potential toxicity that results from high blockade of acetylcholine. This toxicity is called an *anticholinergic*

crisis and is described, along with its treatment, in Chapter 21. The likelihood of anticholinergic side effects, along with sedation and extrapyramidal side effects, from antipsychotics is explored in Table 13.5.

Endocrine Side Effects

Metabolic syndrome is defined as a set of corelated conditions including weight gain, type 2 diabetes, and hyperlipidemia leading to cardiovascular complications. All antipsychotic drugs are associated with metabolic syndrome; however, some specific drugs, such as chlorpromazine, clozapine, olanzapine, and quetiapine, carry greater risk. Table 13.5 highlights the likelihood of selected antipsychotic agents to cause metabolic syndrome. Though metabolic syndrome is not well understood, it is believed that antipsychotic agents interfere with fat and cholesterol metabolism and produce central nervous system effects contributing to insulin resistance and obesity (Kornetova et al., 2019). The nurse should encourage diet and exercise interventions to manage weight gain. The patient may require a change in antipsychotic; aripiprazole is often used and may be associated with a subsequent loss of weight. The nurse must also encourage proper primary care follow-up with a physician or nurse practitioner for monitoring and pharmacological treatment of dyslipidemia, diabetes, and heart disease.

Prolactin elevations can occur with all antipsychotic drugs but are most notable in first-generation antipsychotics and specific second-generation drugs including risperidone and paliperidone. Elevated prolactin levels can cause menstrual irregularities, nipple discharge, and sexual dysfunction in women. Sexual dysfunction and breast development can occur in men. Changing antipsychotics will usually resolve the prolactin elevation and symptoms with resolve over several months.

Blood Disorders

Blood dyscrasias are rare but have received renewed attention since the introduction of clozapine. Agranulocytosis is an acute reaction that causes the individual's white blood cell count to drop to very low levels, and concurrent neutropenia, a drop in neutrophils in the blood, develops. Untreated agranulocytosis can be life threatening. Although agranulocytosis can occur with any of the antipsychotics, the risk with clozapine is far greater than with any other antipsychotics (Mijovic & MacCabe, 2020). For this reason, countries, including Canada, have introduced compulsory laboratory monitoring requirements for clozapine. Typically, weekly blood samples evaluating the absolute neutrophil count (ANC) are required for the first 6 months, every 2 weeks for the following 6 months, and then each 4 weeks thereafter if no agranulocytosis occurs. If sore throat or fever develops, then medications should be withheld until a leukocyte count can be obtained. Hospitalization, including reverse isolation to prevent infections, is usually required. Agranulocytosis is more likely to develop during the first 18 weeks of treatment.

Miscellaneous

Photosensitivity reactions to antipsychotics, including severe sunburns or rash, most commonly develop with the use of low-potency, first-generation antipsychotics. Sunblock must be worn on all areas of exposed skin when taking these drugs. In addition, sun exposure may cause pigmentary deposits to develop, resulting in the discoloration of exposed areas, especially the neck and face. This discoloration may progress from a deep orange colour to a blue grey. Skin exposure should be limited and skin tone changes reported to the prescriber. Pigmentary deposits may also develop on the retina of the eye, especially with high doses of thioridazine, even for a few days. This condition is called *retinitis pigmentosa* and can lead to significant visual impairment. Therefore, thioridazine should never be administered in doses greater than 800 mg per day.

Antipsychotics may also lower a patient's seizure threshold. Patients with an undetected seizure disorder may experience seizures early in treatment. Those who have a preexisting condition should be monitored closely.

Neuroleptic malignant syndrome (NMS) and water intoxication are two serious complications that may result from antipsychotic medications. Characterized by rigidity and high fever, NMS is a rare condition but a medical emergency that may occur abruptly with even one dose of medication. Temperature must always be monitored when administering antipsychotics, especially high-potency medications. Water intoxication may develop gradually with long-term use. This condition is characterized by the patient's consumption of large quantities of fluid (polydipsia) and the resulting effects of sodium depletion (hyponatremia).

Medication-Related Movement Disorders

Medication-related movement disorders are a group of side effects or adverse reactions that are commonly caused by first-generation antipsychotic medications but less commonly with second-generation antipsychotic drugs. These disorders of abnormal motor movements can be divided into two groups: acute extrapyramidal syndromes (EPSs), which are acute abnormal movements developing early in the course of treatment (sometimes after just one dose), and chronic syndromes, which develop from longer exposure to antipsychotic drugs.

Acute Extrapyramidal Syndromes

EPSs occurs in as many as 51.5% of all patients receiving first-generation antipsychotic medications and 24.4% taking second-generation drugs (Monteleone et al., 2021) and includes **dystonia**, pseudoparkinsonism, dyskinesia, and **akathisia** (an involuntary movement disorder). Despite an overall decrease in EPSs with second-generation antipsychotics, akathisia remains a concern and occurs at a rate of 2.9% to 13.0%. Higher doses of second-generation antipsychotics are more likely to cause akathisia. Quetiapine and clozapine are considered low risk, and only produce akathisia at a rate of 0% to 10% compared with placebo (Chow et al., 2020).

EPSs develop early in treatment, sometimes from as little as one dose. Although the abnormal movements are treatable, they are at times dramatic and frightening, causing physical and emotional impairments that often prompt patients to stop taking their medication. Some milder forms of EPS may occur with classes of medication other than antipsychotics, including the SSRIs. The acute EPS often are mistaken for aspects of anxiety, rather than medication side effects. Nurses play a vital role in the early recognition and treatment of these syndromes. Early recognition can save the patient considerable discomfort, fear, and impairment. All nurses must be aware of these symptoms, notifying the prescriber as soon as possible and implementing selected medication changes and other interventions. See Table 13.8 for several medications that can control acute EPS.

Dystonia, sometimes referred to as an *acute dystonic reaction*, is impaired muscle tone that generally is the first extrapyramidal symptom to occur, usually within a few days of initiating use of an antipsychotic. Dystonia is characterized by involuntary muscle spasms,

Table 13.8 Drug Therapies for Acute Medication-Related Movement Disorders

Agents	Typical Dosage Ranges	Routes Available	Common Side Effects
Anticholinergics			
benztropine (Cogentin)	2–6 mg/d	po, im, iv	Dry mouth, blurred vision, slowed gastric motility causing constipation, urinary retention, increased intraocular pressure; overdose produces toxic psychosis
trihexyphenidyl (Artane)	4–15 mg/d	po	Same as benztropine, plus gastrointestinal distress Older adults are most prone to mental confusion and delirium
biperiden (Akineton)	2–8 mg/d	po	Fewer peripheral anticholinergic effects Euphoria and increased tremor may occur
Antihistamines			
diphenhydramine (Benadryl)	25–50 mg q.i.d. to 400 mg daily	po, im, iv	Sedation and confusion, especially in older adults
Dopamine Agonists			
amantadine (Symmetrel)	100–400 mg daily	po	Indigestion, decreased concentration, dizziness, anxiety, ataxia, insomnia, lethargy, tremors, and slurred speech may occur on higher doses Tolerance may develop on fixed dose
β-Antagonist (Blockers)			
propranolol (Inderal)	10 mg t.i.d. to 120 mg daily	po	Hypotension and bradycardia Must monitor pulse and blood pressure Do not stop abruptly as this may cause rebound tachycardia
Benzodiazepines			
lorazepam (Ativan)	1–2 mg im 0.5–2 mg po	po, im	All may cause drowsiness, lethargy, and general sedation or paradoxical agitation Confusion and disorientation in older adults
diazepam (Valium)	2–5 mg t.i.d.	po, iv	Most side effects are rare and will disappear if dose is decreased
clonazepam (Rivotril)	1–4 mg/d	po	Tolerance and withdrawal are potential problems

especially of the head and neck muscles. Patients usually first complain of a thick tongue, tight jaw, or stiff neck. The syndrome can progress to a protruding tongue, oculogyric crisis (eyes rolled up in the head), torticollis (muscle stiffness in the neck, which draws the head to one side with chin pointing to the other), and laryngopharyngeal constriction. In severe cases, the spasms may progress to the intercostal muscles, producing more significant breathing difficulty for patients who already have respiratory impairment from asthma or emphysema.

Drug-induced parkinsonism is sometimes referred to as **pseudoparkinsonism** because its presentation is identical to Parkinson disease without the same destruction of dopaminergic cells. These symptoms include the classic triad of rigidity, slowed movements (bradykinesia), and tremor. The rigid muscle stiffness is usually seen in the arms. Bradykinesia can be observed by the loss of spontaneous movements, such as the absence of the usual relaxed swing of the arms while walking. In addition, masklike faces or loss of facial expression and a decrease in the ability to initiate movements also are present. Usually, tremor is more pronounced at rest, but it can also be observed with intentional movements, such as eating. If the tremor becomes severe, then it may interfere with the patient's ability to eat or maintain adequate fluid intake. Hypersalivation is possible as well. Pseudoparkinsonism symptoms may occur on one or both sides of the body and develop abruptly or subtly, but usually within the first 30 days of treatment.

Akathisia is characterized by the inability to sit still; there is profound restlessness. The person will pace, rock while sitting or standing, march in place, or cross and uncross the legs. All these repetitive motions have an intensity that is frequently beyond the explanation of the individual. In addition, akathisia may be present as a primarily subjective experience without obvious motor behaviour. This subjective experience includes feelings of anxiety, jitteriness, or the inability to relax, which the individual may or may not be able to communicate. It is extremely uncomfortable for a person experiencing akathisia to be forced to sit still or be confined. These symptoms are sometimes misdiagnosed as agitation or an increase in psychotic symptoms, but if the nurse administers an antipsychotic medication PRN (from the Latin, *pro re nata*, which roughly translated means "as needed"), the symptoms will not abate and will often worsen. Differentiating akathisia from agitation may be aided by knowing the person's symptoms before the introduction of medication. Psychotic agitation does not usually begin abruptly after antipsychotic medication use has been started, whereas akathisia may occur after administration. In addition, the nurse may ask the patient if the experience is felt primarily in the muscles (akathisia) or in the mind or emotions (agitation).

Akathisia is the most difficult acute medication-related movement disorder to relieve. It does not usually respond well to anticholinergic medications and is more common with second-generation antipsychotics than initially thought. It is thought that the pathology of akathisia may involve more than just the extrapyramidal motor system. It may include serotonin changes that also affect the dopamine system (Poyurovsky & Weizman, 2020). Switching to another antipsychotic agent is recommended. A number of medications have been used to reduce symptoms, including β-adrenergic antagonist (propranolol), anticholinergics (biperiden, benztropine), 5HT2A antagonist (mianserin, trazodone, mirtazapine), benzodiazepines (clonazepam), and vitamin B6 (Pringsheim et al., 2018).

Nurses must monitor for resolution of EPS symptoms and potential adverse effects from drugs used to manage EPS symptoms. For instance, nurses must monitor the patient's pulse and blood pressure because propranolol can cause hypotension and bradycardia. If the patient's pulse falls below 60 bpm, then propranolol should not be given and the prescriber should be notified. Normal signs of hypoglycaemia may be blocked by propranolol; therefore, patients with diabetes must monitor their blood or urine glucose levels carefully, especially because they are under physical stress from the disorder.

A number of nursing interventions may reduce the impact of these syndromes. Individuals with acute EPS need frequent reassurance that this is not a worsening of their psychiatric condition but instead is a treatable side effect of the medication. They also need validation that what they are experiencing is real and that the nurse is concerned and will be responsive to changes in these symptoms. Physical and psychological stress appears to increase the symptoms and further frighten the patient; therefore, decreasing stressful situations becomes important. These symptoms are often physically exhausting for the patient, and nurses should ensure that the patient receives adequate rest and hydration.

Risk factors for acute EPS include previous episodes of EPS and use of high-dose injected antipsychotics for acute psychotic symptoms or agitation. Listen closely when patients say they are "allergic" or have had "bad reactions" to antipsychotic medications. They are often describing one of the medication-related movement disorders, particularly dystonia or akathisia, rather than a rash or other allergic symptoms. About 90% of the individuals who have experienced EPS in the past will again have these symptoms if the use of an antipsychotic medication is restarted (Meyer, 2007). Age and gender appear to be risk factors for specific syndromes. Acute dystonia occurs most often in young men, adolescents, and children; akathisia is more common in middle-aged women. Older adult patients are at the greatest risk for experiencing pseudoparkinsonism.

Chronic Syndromes

First identified in 1957, **tardive dyskinesia** is the most well-known of the chronic syndromes. It involves irregular, repetitive involuntary movements of the mouth, face, and tongue, including chewing, tongue protrusion, lip smacking, puckering of the lips, and rapid eye blinking. Abnormal finger movements are common as well. In some individuals, the trunk and extremities are also involved, and in rare cases, irregular breathing and swallowing lead to belching and grunting noises. These symptoms usually begin no earlier than after 6 months of treatment or when the medication is reduced or withdrawn. Once thought to be irreversible, considerable controversy now exists as to whether or not this is true. Nurses in contact with individuals who are taking antipsychotic medications for months or years must be vigilant in monitoring for symptoms of these typical chronic conditions.

Part of the difficulty in determining the irreversibility of tardive dyskinesia is that any movement disorder that persists after the discontinuation of antipsychotic medication has been described as tardive dyskinesia. Atypical forms are now receiving more attention because some researchers believe that they may have different underlying mechanisms of causation. Some of these forms of the disorder appear to remit spontaneously. Symptoms of what is now called *withdrawal tardive dyskinesia* appear when use of an antipsychotic medication is reduced or discontinued abruptly. *Tardive dystonia* and *tardive akathisia* have also been described. Both appear in a manner similar to the acute syndromes but continue after the antipsychotic medication has been withdrawn. Collectively, these form potential unique chronic syndromes associated with antipsychotic use. Further research is needed to determine whether these syndromes are distinctly different in origin and outcome (Goff et al., 2017).

The risk for experiencing tardive dyskinesia increases with age and with higher rates during first-generation (30.0%) versus second-generation antipsychotic (20.7%) therapy. Despite a relatively lower overall prevalence rate of tardive dyskinesia in recent years, associated with increased use of second-generation antipsychotics, the global mean prevalence is 25.3% (Carbon et al., 2017). History of acute EPS, advancing age, smoking, diabetes, and history of organic brain injuries increased the risk of tardive dyskinesia. Women are at greater risk than men (Stegmayer et al., 2018). Individuals with affective disorders, particularly depression, are at higher risk than are those who have schizophrenia. Risk factors are summarized in Box 13.3.

BOX 13.3 Risk Factors for Tardive Dyskinesia

- Age older than 50 years
- Women
- Affective disorders, particularly depression
- Brain damage or dysfunction
- Increased duration of treatment
- Standard antipsychotic medication
- Use of acute higher doses of antipsychotic medication

Any individual receiving antipsychotic medication may experience tardive dyskinesia; therefore, nurses must be particularly alert and detect symptoms early. The causes of tardive dyskinesia remain unclear. Lack of a consistent theory of aetiology for the chronic medication-related movement disorder syndromes has led to inconsistent and disappointing treatment approaches. No one medication relieves the symptoms. Dopamine agonists, such as bromocriptine, and many other drugs have been tried. Clozapine slightly reduces symptoms in moderate to severe tardive dyskinesia (Mentzel et al., 2018). Even dietary precursors of acetylcholine, such as lecithin, and nutritional therapies, such as vitamin E supplements, may prove to be beneficial.

The best approach to treatment remains avoiding the development of the chronic syndromes. Preventive measures include use of second-generation antipsychotics, using the lowest possible dose of typical medication, minimizing use of PRN medication, and closely monitoring individuals in high-risk groups for development of the symptoms of tardive dyskinesia. All members of the mental health treatment team who have contact with individuals taking antipsychotics for longer than 3 months must be alert to the risk factors and earliest possible signs of chronic medication-related movement disorders. Abrupt discontinuation of an antipsychotic may worsen tardive dyskinesia and therefore should be avoided.

Monitoring tools, such as the Simpson-Angus Rating Scale (Simpson & Angus, 1970) and the Abnormal Involuntary Movement Scale (Guy, 1976), should be used routinely to standardize assessment and provide the earliest possible recognition of the symptoms. Standardized assessments should be performed at a minimum of 3- to 6-month intervals. The earlier the symptoms are recognized, the more likely they will resolve if the medication can be changed or its use discontinued. Second-generation antipsychotic medications have a lower risk for causing tardive dyskinesia and are increasingly being considered first-line medications for treating schizophrenia.

Mood Stabilizers (Antimania Medications)

Mood stabilizers, or antimania medications, are psychopharmacologic agents used primarily for stabilizing mood, particularly those of mania in bipolar disorders. For a number of years, lithium was the only drug known to stabilize the symptoms of mania. Although it remains the gold standard of treatment for acute mania and maintenance of bipolar disorders, not all individuals experience a positive response to lithium and other drugs are increasingly being used. Valproic acid, lamotrigine, and second-generation antipsychotic agents such as olanzapine and quetiapine are increasing being used either alone or in combination with lithium for improved efficacy in treatment-resistant cases. The combination of lithium and lamotrigine has demonstrated the highest efficacy in reducing suicidal symptoms and depressive relapse (Takeshima, 2017). Many other drugs, including other anticonvulsants, second-generation antipsychotics, and adrenergic blocking agents in conjunction with antidepressants, are used frequently to prevent episodes of hypomania or depression (Brunoni et al., 2017; Yatham & Kesavan, 2017). The first-line use of antidepressant agents to augment a drug response in bipolar depression is replaced with second-generation antipsychotic agents (Post, 2016).

Lithium

Lithium is a naturally occurring element and was first discovered in the early 1800s. In 1949, John Cade from Australia found that lithium reduced agitation in some patients experiencing psychosis, and in the 1950s, Schou (1978) published reports that lithium controlled and prevented the symptoms of mania. Since then, it has become a mainstay in psychopharmacology. Lithium is effective in only about 40% of patients with bipolar disorder; other agents may be coadministered to increase treatment efficacy among those with incomplete response to lithium alone (Bauer & Gitlin, 2016). Although lithium is not a perfect drug, a great deal is known regarding its use: it is inexpensive, it has restored stability to the lives of thousands of people, and it remains the gold standard of bipolar pharmacologic treatment.

Indications and Mechanisms of Action

The target symptoms for lithium are the symptoms of mania, such as rapid speech, jumping from topic to topic (flight of ideas), irritability, grandiose thinking, impulsiveness, and agitation. While lithium does seem to be effective in treating depressive disorders, caution is needed in interpreting these results. Specifically, depressive symptoms seen in hypomania may be mistakenly diagnosed as a depressive disorder—thus, lithium's efficacy in treating "depression" may actually point to a misdiagnosis (Takeshima, 2017). It has also been shown to be helpful in reducing impulsivity and aggression in certain psychiatric patients.

Lithium has been effective in treating several nonpsychiatric disorders, such as cluster headaches. Because lithium stimulates leukocytosis, it often improves the neutrophil counts of patients who are undergoing chemotherapy or who have other conditions that cause neutropenia. In addition, lithium has been investigated as an antiviral agent because it appears to inhibit the replication of several DNA viruses, including herpes virus. This research stalled due to the development of other effective antiviral medications. The antiviral properties of lithium have been reignited with the emergence of COVID-19 (Nowak & Walkowiak, 2020; Spuch et al., 2020).

Lithium is actively transported across cell membranes, altering sodium transport in both nerve and muscle cells. It replaces sodium in the sodium–potassium pump and is retained more readily than sodium inside the cell. Conditions that alter sodium content in the body, such as vomiting, diuresis, and diaphoresis, alter lithium retention. The results of lithium influx into the nerve cell lead to increased storage of catecholamines within the cell, reduced dopamine neurotransmission, increased norepinephrine reuptake, increased GABA activity, and increased serotonin receptor sensitivity. The specific mechanisms by which lithium improves the symptoms of mania are complex, most likely involving the sum of all or part of these actions and more.

Pharmacokinetics

Lithium carbonate is available orally in capsule, tablet, and liquid forms. Slow-release preparations are also available. Lithium is readily absorbed in the gastric system and may be taken with food, which does not impair absorption. Peak blood levels are reached in 1 to 4 h, and the medication is usually completely absorbed in 8 h. Slow-release preparations are absorbed at a slower, more variable rate.

Lithium is not protein bound, and its distribution into the CNS across the blood–brain barrier is slow. The onset of action is usually 5 to 7 days and may take as long as 2 weeks. The elimination half-life is 8 to 12 h, and 18 to 36 h in individuals whose blood levels have reached steady state. Lithium is almost entirely excreted by the kidneys. Conditions of renal impairment or decreased renal function in older adults decrease lithium clearance and may lead to toxicity. Several medications affect renal function and therefore change lithium clearance. See Chapter 22 for a list of these and other medication interactions with lithium. About 80% of lithium is reabsorbed in the proximal tubule of the kidney along with water and sodium. In conditions that cause sodium depletion, such as dehydration caused by fever, strenuous exercise, hot weather, increased perspiration, and vomiting, the kidney attempts to conserve sodium. Lithium is a salt, so the kidney retains lithium as well and can lead to increased blood levels and potential toxicity. Significantly increasing sodium intake causes lithium levels to fall.

Lithium is usually administered in doses of 300 mg two to three times daily. During the acute phases of mania, blood levels of 0.8 to 1.2 mEq/L are usually attained and maintained until symptoms are under control. During maintenance, the dosage is reduced, and dosages are adjusted to maintain blood levels of 0.8 to 1 mEq/L. Lithium toxicity can occur with serum concentrations of greater than 1.2 to 1.5 mEq/L. This is a drug with a narrow therapeutic index; blood levels are monitored frequently, usually every 3 to 5 days until stable.

These increases may be slower in older adults or patients who experience uncomfortable side effects. Blood levels should be monitored 8 to 12 h after the last dose of medication and around 5 days after any dose adjustment. In the hospital setting, nurses should withhold the morning dose of lithium until the serum sample is drawn to avoid falsely elevated levels. Individuals who are at home should be instructed to have their blood drawn in the morning about 8 to 12 h after their last dose and before they take their first dose of medication.

Lithium clears the body relatively quickly after the discontinuation of its use. It is important to remember that almost half of the individuals who discontinue lithium treatment abruptly experience a relapse of symptoms within a few weeks. A major recurrence after discontinuing lithium may cause a discontinuation-induced refractoriness leading to a nonresponse to lithium at previously effective doses. Lithium is also subject to nonresponse due to tolerance, where over time, symptoms of bipolar disorder reappear (Won & Kim, 2017). Patients should be warned of the risks in abruptly discontinuing their medication and should be advised to consider the options carefully, in consultation with their prescriber, if early symptoms of the illness occur.

Side Effects, Adverse Reactions, and Toxicity

At lower therapeutic blood levels, side effects from lithium are relatively mild. These reactions correspond with peaks in plasma concentrations of the medication after administration and most subside during the first few weeks of therapy. Frequently, individuals taking lithium complain of excessive thirst and an unpleasant metallic-like taste. Sugarless throat lozenges may be useful in minimizing this side effect. Other common side effects include an increased frequency of urination, fine head tremor, drowsiness, and mild diarrhoea. Weight gain occurs in about 20% of the individuals taking lithium. Nausea may be minimized by taking the medication with food or by use of a slow-release preparation. See Chapter 22 for a summary of selected nursing interventions to minimize the impact of common side effects associated with lithium treatment. Patients most frequently discontinued their own medication use because of concerns with mental slowness, poor concentration, and memory problems.

As blood levels of lithium increase, the side effects of lithium become more numerous and severe. Early signs of lithium toxicity include severe diarrhoea, vomiting, drowsiness, muscular weakness, and lack of coordination. Lithium should be withheld and the prescriber consulted if these symptoms develop. Lithium toxicity can easily be resolved in 24 to 48 h by discontinuing the medication, but haemodialysis may be required in severe situations. See Chapter 22 for a summary of the side effects and symptoms of toxicity associated with various blood levels of lithium.

Monitoring of serum creatinine concentration, thyroid-stimulating hormones, serum calcium, BMI, and waist circumference at a baseline of 6 months and then annually during maintenance therapy helps to assess the occurrence of other potential adverse reactions. An ECG is recommended to assess risk for QT prolongation at baseline. Kidney damage is considered an uncommon but potentially serious risk for long-term lithium treatment. This damage is usually reversible after discontinuation of the lithium use. A gradual rise in serum creatinine and decline in creatinine clearance indicate the development of renal dysfunction. Individuals with kidney dysfunction are susceptible to lithium toxicity.

Lithium may alter thyroid function, usually after 6 to 18 months of treatment. About 30% of the individuals taking lithium exhibit alterations in thyroid function, but most do not show the suppression of circulating thyroid hormone. Thyroid dysfunction from lithium treatment is more common in women and some individuals require the addition of thyroxine to their care. During maintenance, thyroid-stimulating hormone levels may be monitored. Nurses should observe for dry skin, constipation, bradycardia, hair loss, cold intolerance, and other symptoms of hypothyroidism. Other endocrine system effects result from hyperparathyroidism, which increases parathyroid hormone levels and calcium. Clinically, this change is not significant, but elevated calcium levels may cause mood changes, anxiety, lethargy, and sleep disturbances. These symptoms may erroneously be attributed to depression if hypocalcaemia is not investigated.

Lithium use must be avoided during pregnancy because it has been associated with birth defects, especially when administered during the first trimester. If lithium is given during the third trimester, then toxicity may develop in a newborn, producing signs of hypotonia, cyanosis, bradykinesia, cardiac changes, gastrointestinal bleeding, and shock. Diabetes insipidus may persist for months. Lithium is also present in breast milk; patients should not breastfeed while taking lithium. People expecting to become pregnant should be advised to consult with their healthcare provider before discontinuing the use of birth control methods.

Anticonvulsants

With the broader use of second-generation antipsychotics, anticonvulsants (with the exception of divalproex) are used as first-line monotherapy for acute mania. Carbamazepine is downgraded to a second-line therapy treatment option in acute mania due to safety concerns. Lamotrigine, despite risk for serious adverse reactions, is generally well tolerated and effective for the treatment of bipolar depression. Gabapentin has no role in the management of bipolar mania or depression (Yatham et al.,

2018). A group of researchers have found an increased risk of suicide among individuals taking anticonvulsant drugs for bipolar I disorders (Bellivier et al., 2017). However, the risk for suicide, particularly by self-poisoning, is significantly elevated during bipolar depression, thus clinical application of this finding is uncertain.

Indications and Mechanisms of Action

Anticonvulsant medications in general are primarily indicated for treating seizure disorders. Target symptoms for the use of anticonvulsants with bipolar disorder include all the symptoms of mania discussed earlier. However, anticonvulsants are often used for individuals who have not experienced response to lithium or who are identified as having rapid cycling. Studies have shown some common traits in these individuals. Those who do not experience response to lithium most often are those who have a dysphoric or mixed mania. These individuals experience an increase in physical activity during manic episodes without any elevation in mood. They often are referred to as *mixed states* because they have elements of both depression and mania. These individuals exhibit symptoms of high anxiety, agitation, and irritability, which are then target symptoms for the use of anticonvulsants. Empirical data show carbamazepine, lamotrigine, and valproic acid to be effective in mood stabilization.

The term *rapid cycling* is applied when individuals experience four or more episodes of either depression or mania during a 12-month period. This occurs more often in women than in men. These patients make up a group of individuals who experience poor response to lithium treatment. Mood instability is also a target symptom of anticonvulsant medications. The theory of the mechanism of action of the anticonvulsants involves the concept of kindling as it applies to mood disorders. **Kindling** refers to the emergence of spontaneous firing of nerve cells in response to repeated subthreshold electrical stimulation. Once brain regions, such as the amygdala, have been "kindled," it takes considerably less stimulation to initiate a seizure. In the case of mood disorders, it is hypothesized that "kindled" brain regions include the areas associated with emotional regulation. The stimulation of these regions by increasingly minor stressors or other environmental factors produces mood swings instead of a seizure.

Anticonvulsants have "antikindling" properties and decrease the sensitization of affected cells, making them less easy to stimulate. In general, the anticonvulsant mood stabilizers have many actions, but it is their effects on ion channels, reducing repetitive firing of action potentials in the nerves, that most directly decreases manic symptoms. In addition, drugs such as carbamazepine affect the release and reuptake of several neurotransmitters, including norepinephrine, GABA, dopamine, and glutamate. They also change several second messenger systems. No single mechanism has yet accounted for the anticonvulsant's ability to stabilize mood. Divalproex sodium also has been shown to have numerous neurotransmission effects. The most widely held theory of how it stabilizes mood swings relates to its effects on GABA. As the major inhibitory neurotransmitter in the CNS, increased levels of GABA and improved responsiveness of the neurons to GABA lead to the control of epileptic activity. Divalproex sodium increases levels of GABA in the CNS by activating its synthesis, inhibiting the catabolism (destructive metabolism) of GABA, increasing its release, and increasing receptor density (Solomon et al., 1998). However, it should be noted that suicide in bipolar depression occurs frequently by toxic ingestion of opioid and/or benzodiazepine agents. Thus, these drugs are typically avoided in this patient population (Yatham et al., 2018).

Pharmacokinetics

Carbamazepine is an unusual drug and is absorbed in a somewhat variable manner. The liquid suspension is absorbed more quickly than the tablet form, but food does not appear to interfere with absorption. Peak plasma levels occur in 2 to 6 h. Because high doses influence peak plasma levels and increase the risk for side effects, carbamazepine should be given in divided doses two or three times a day. The suspension, which has higher peak plasma levels and lower trough levels, must be given more frequently than the tablet form.

Valproic acid is more rapidly absorbed, but the enteric coating of divalproex sodium adds a delay of as long as 1 h. Peak serum levels occur in about 1 to 4 h. The liquid form (sodium valproate) is absorbed more rapidly and peaks in 15 minutes to 2 h. Food appears to slow absorption but does not lower bioavailability of the drug. Valproate is a good example of the importance of considering *bioequivalence*, a term referring to the abilities of two formulations of the same drug to induce a therapeutic response of similar magnitude and duration (Zintzaras, 2005). For example, divalproex, an enteric-coated formulation, has a half-life of 12 to 16 h. It is not affected by food intake and achieves more consistent plasma levels than valproic acid, which has a shorter half-life (8 h). Valproic acid should not be taken with food and produces gastrointestinal irritation in about 40% of patients.

Carbamazepine and valproic acid are highly protein bound; therefore, patients who are older, medically ill, or malnourished may experience the effects of increased unbound levels of both drugs. When given with other drugs that are competing for the same protein-binding sites, higher levels of unbound drug may occur. In both cases, these individuals risk more side effects and fluctuations in medication plasma levels. Carbamazepine and valproic acid also cross easily into the CNS and move

into the placenta as well. Both are associated with an increased risk for birth defects, including spina bifida, and carbamazepine accumulates in foetal tissue. Carbamazepine and valproic acid are metabolized by the cytochrome P-450 system of microsomal hepatic enzymes.

Carbamazepine activates its own metabolism through induction of the P-450 microsomal hepatic enzymes (CYP 3A4). Patients receiving carbamazepine may experience a precipitant drop in therapeutic blood levels and a relapse in symptoms, requiring a dosage increase for as long as 2 to 3 months after steady state has been achieved. Valproic acid is only minimally affected by other medications that stimulate the P-450 system; it does not enhance its own metabolism. Both carbamazepine and valproic acid are available in slow-release, extended-action forms, allowing for decreased daily dosing and improved adherence.

Nurses need to educate patients about potential drug interactions, especially with nonprescription medications. Nurses can also inform other healthcare practitioners who may be prescribing medication that these patients are taking carbamazepine. It is important to note that oral contraceptives may become ineffective, so patients taking oral contraceptives should be advised to use other methods of birth control. Valproic acid and carbamazepine can cause foetal malformation and should not be used in pregnancy.

Side Effects, Adverse Reactions, and Toxicity

The most common side effects of carbamazepine are dizziness, drowsiness, tremor, visual disturbance, nausea, and vomiting. These side effects may be minimized by initiating treatment in low doses. Patients should be advised that these symptoms will diminish, but care should be taken when changing positions or performing tasks that require visual alertness. Giving the drug with food may diminish nausea. Valproic acid also causes gastrointestinal disturbances, tremor, and lethargy. In addition, it can produce weight gain and alopecia (hair loss). These symptoms are transient and should diminish with the course of treatment. Dietary supplements of zinc and selenium may be helpful to patients experiencing hair loss. Constipation and urinary retention occur in some individuals. Nurses should monitor urinary output and assist patients to increase fluid consumption to decrease constipation.

Transient elevations in liver enzymes occur with both carbamazepine and valproic acid, but rarely do symptoms of hepatic injury occur. If the patient reports abnormal pain or shows signs of jaundice, then the prescriber should be notified immediately. Several blood dyscrasias are associated with carbamazepine, including aplastic anaemia, agranulocytosis, and leucopenia. Patients should be advised to report fever, sore throat, rash, petechiae, or bruising immediately. In addition, advise patients of the importance of completing routine blood tests throughout treatment (including complete blood cell count and liver function tests).

Both valproic acid and carbamazepine may be lethal if high doses are ingested. Toxic symptoms appear in 1 to 3 h and include neuromuscular disturbances, dizziness, stupor, agitation, disorientation, nystagmus, urinary retention, nausea and vomiting, tachycardia, hypotension or hypertension, cardiovascular shock, coma, and respiratory depression. Carbamazepine appears to be more lethal at lower doses, but valproic acid is absorbed rapidly, and gastric lavage may be ineffective, depending on time from ingestion.

Lamotrigine (Lamictal) in rare cases produces severe, life-threatening rashes that usually occur within 2 to 8 weeks of treatment. This risk is highest in children. The use of lamotrigine should be immediately discontinued if a rash is noted. Individuals of Asian origin should be tested by HLA-B*1502 allele prior to starting carbamazepine as this genetic variation significantly increases the risk of Stevens-Johnson syndrome, a rare but serious disorder of the skin and mucous membranes (Shnayder et al., 2020).

Topamax (topiramate) carries an increased risk for kidney stone formation. It can also cause a decrease in serum digoxin levels and may decrease effectiveness of oral birth control agents. In addition, ongoing ophthalmologic monitoring is required because of reports of acute myopia with secondary glaucoma. In some patients, these anticonvulsants may decrease the effectiveness of oral birth control agents. Careful patient teaching and monitoring are required because of the potentially significant adverse reactions that the anticonvulsants can produce.

Antidepressant Medications

Researchers in the 1950s who were investigating other drugs related to the phenothiazines for the treatment of psychosis discovered that imipramine, a related compound, relieved the symptoms of depression. Imipramine was the first of a number of medications that contained a three-ring structure in their chemical makeup and produced improvement in depression. These medications became known as TCAs. Table 13.9 lists other related TCAs still in use today.

Table 13.9 Antidepressant Medications

Generic (Trade) Drug Name	Usual Dosage Range (mg/day)	Half-Life (hours)	Therapeutic Blood Level (ng/mL)
Tricyclic			
amitriptyline (Elavil)	50–300	31–46	110–250
clomipramine (Anafranil)	25–250	19–37	80–100
doxepin (Sinequan)	25–300	8–24	100–200
imipramine (Tofranil)	30–300	11–25	200–350
amoxapine (Asendin)	50–600	8	200–500
desipramine (Norpramin)	25–300	12–24	125–300
nortriptyline (Aventyl)	30–100	18–44	50–150
protriptyline (Vivactil)	15–60	67–89	100–200
Selective Serotonin Reuptake Inhibitors			
fluoxetine (Prozac)	20–80	2–9 d	72–300
sertraline (Zoloft)	50–200	24	Not available
paroxetine (Paxil)	10–50	10–24	Not available
fluvoxamine (Luvox)	50–300	17–22	Not available
citalopram (Celexa)	20–50	35	Not available
escitalopram (Lexapro)	10–20	27–32	Not available
Norepinephrine Selective Reuptake Inhibitors			
reboxetine	12	12	Not available
Norepinephrine and Serotonin Selective Reuptake Inhibitors			
Venlafaxine (Effexor)	75–375	5–11	100–500
Desvenlafaxine (Pristiq)	50–100	10–11	Not available
Duloxetine (Cymbalta)	60–80	9–19	Not available
Other Antidepressant Medications			
trazodone (Desyrel)	150–600	4–9	650–1,600
nefazodone (Serzone)	100–600	2–4	Not available
bupropion (Wellbutrin)	200–450	8–24	10–29
mirtazapine (Remeron)	15–45	20–40	Not available
Monoamine Oxidase Inhibitors			
moclobemide (Manerix)	300–600	6–10	Not available
phenelzine (Nardil)	15–90	24 (effect lasts 3–10 d)	Not available
tranylcypromine (Parnate)	10–60	24 (effect lasts 3–10 d)	Not available

Concurrent with the discovery of TCAs, an antibiotic, iproniazid, used in treating tuberculosis, was found to alleviate the symptoms of depression. Iproniazid increased the monoamine neurotransmitters by inhibiting MAO, the enzyme that breaks down these neurotransmitters inside the nerve cell. Iproniazid is no longer used, but related, more effective drugs, phenelzine and tranylcypromine, make up a subgroup of antidepressants called the MAOIs. The Canadian clinical guidelines for the treatment of depressive disorders developed by the CANMAT Depression Working Group (Kennedy et al., 2016) as first-line treatment recommendations for a major depressive episode (based on level I evidence and little evidence of differences in efficacy or tolerability) include SSRIs, SNRIs, agomelatine, mirtazapine, vortioxetine, and bupropion. Box 13.4 describes factors influencing choice of antidepressants. These classes and specific drugs are described below.

TCAs, MAOIs, and More

Throughout the 1960s and 1970s, the TCAs and MAOIs were the primary medications for treating depression. Research continued to develop new agents with increased effectiveness, while decreasing the side effects and potential lethal effects. In the 1980s, several medications that were significantly different in chemical structure were introduced. Bupropion (Wellbutrin) was introduced in 1987 and had actions that were significantly different from those of previous antidepressants. Concern about the risk for seizures and other side effects limited initial excitement about its use. In 1988, the release of fluoxetine (Prozac) received much public attention and resulted in an increased awareness of depression and its treatment. Fluoxetine was the first of a class of drugs that acted "selectively" on one neurotransmitter, in this case serotonin. Other similarly selective medications, sertraline (Zoloft), paroxetine (Paxil), and fluvoxamine (Luvox), soon followed and together make up the SSRIs. The newest SSRIs include citalopram (Celexa) and escitalopram oxalate (Cipralex). Reboxetine and atomoxetine are examples of norepinephrine

selective reuptake inhibitors. Atomoxetine is commonly used in the treatment of attention deficit/hyperactivity disorder. Reboxetine is only available in Canada through special access programs. Two available drugs, venlafaxine (Effexor) and duloxetine (Cymbalta), are selective to both serotonin and norepinephrine. Agomelatine is a newer drug with targets at the melatonin and serotonin receptors. Vortioxetine is also a new SSRI-type drug with additional agonist at 5HT1A serotonin receptor subtypes and antagonist to 5-HT3. The TCAs are now considered as second-line treatments and the MAOIs as third-line treatments. Second-generation antipsychotics, such as aripiprazole, may be used to augment an antidepressant therapeutic response or as an adjunct when nonresponses occur (Kennedy et al., 2016).

Indications and Mechanisms of Action

The TCAs have multiple effects on a variety of receptors in the CNS, including reuptake inhibition at serotonin and norepinephrine transporters; down-regulation of specific serotonin and noradrenergic receptors; and blockade of cholinergic, adrenergic, and histamine receptors. On the other hand, the MAOIs are more specific in their actions. They inhibit MAO, an enzyme that breaks down monoamines, such as serotonin, thereby increasing synaptic neurotransmission, resulting in clinical improvement. SSRIs selectively inhibit the reuptake of serotonin, while NSRI inhibit the reuptake of norepinephrine and serotonin.

The primary indication for antidepressant medications is depression, thus the name "antidepressant." Antidepressants target symptoms such as loss of interest in the person's usual activities (anhedonia), depressed mood, lethargy or decreased energy, insomnia, decreased concentration, loss of appetite, and suicidal ideation (see Chapter 22 for a more complete discussion of the symptoms of depression). Antidepressants are also used to treat other symptoms and disorders, and increasingly the name antidepressant is somewhat misleading.

Antidepressants are prescribed to treat the whole range of anxiety disorders (see Chapter 23). Antidepressants are also used to treat eating disorders (see Chapter 25), depression in bipolar disorders, dysthymia, chronic pain disorders, premenstrual syndrome, and premenstrual dysphoric disorder. More sedating antidepressants are sometimes used in small doses to address sleep disturbances. Trazodone, amitriptyline, mirtazapine, and other agents have been used alone or as adjunctive interventions for sleep disturbance. Symptoms of some psychiatric disorders of childhood (see Chapter 30), such as attention deficit hyperactivity disorder (ADHD), enuresis (bed-wetting), and school phobia, often respond to antidepressant medication.

At times, the symptoms of depression present in an "atypical" manner, which is called *atypical depression*. There has been much debate concerning this form of depression over the past 60 years and controversy exists as to whether it is a bipolar or unipolar depression. Nonetheless, individuals with atypical depression have high levels of anxiety, increased appetite and sleep rather than the typical insomnia and loss of appetite, mood reactivity rather than consistent low mood, and oversensitivity to such interpersonal feelings of rejection (Brailean et al., 2019). Atypical depression remains an intriguing illness and is nonresponsive to most contemporary antidepressant drugs. The MAOIs, such as phenelzine (Nardil), have been effective (Łojko & Rybakowski, 2017). There is some evidence that electroconvulsive therapy and, more recently, ketamine infusions may be effective in treating atypical depression (Park et al., 2020).

Pharmacokinetics

All of the antidepressant medications are well absorbed from the gastrointestinal system; however, some individual variations exist. For example, food slightly increases the amount of trazodone absorbed but decreases its maximum blood concentrations and lengthens the time to peak effects from 1 h on an empty stomach to 2 h with food. Food also increases the maximum concentrations of sertraline in the bloodstream and decreases the time to peak plasma levels, whereas fluoxetine and fluvoxamine are unaffected, although food may delay the absorption of fluoxetine. Food has little effect on the TCAs.

Nurses should review pharmacokinetic information as it applies to each individual medication. They must consider how this information will affect the patient's use of the medication given the target symptoms for which the drug is intended. For example, if trazodone is being used on a continuous dose schedule for its antidepressant effect, the effects of food probably matter very little. However, if trazodone is being used in a small dose at bedtime to assist a patient to sleep, an empty stomach becomes important because food would lengthen the time of onset of clinical effects, in this case, sleep.

The TCAs undergo considerable first-pass metabolism but reach peak plasma concentrations in 2 to 4 h. The TCAs are highly bound to plasma proteins, which make the association between blood levels and therapeutic clinical effects difficult. However, some plasma ranges have been established. Table 13.9 includes the available ranges for therapeutic blood levels of the TCAs. In addition, times to steady-state plasma levels have wide variations, and the effective dose of medication must be individualized. Other antidepressants are also highly protein bound, which means that drugs that compete for these binding sites may cause fluctuations in blood levels of the antidepressants. Venlafaxine has the lowest protein binding; therefore, drug interactions of this type are not expected with this medication. Blood level changes caused by the presence of other drugs competing with binding sites are not expected.

The onset of action also varies considerably, depending on specific symptoms. For example, an improvement in sleep often occurs earlier than effects on overall mood or anhedonia. Complete relief of symptoms may take several weeks. Full enzyme inhibition with the MAOIs may take as long as 2 weeks, but the energizing effects may be seen within a few days. The variable onset of action may add to their sense of discouragement and powerlessness.

Although antidepressants are primarily excreted by the kidneys, their routes of metabolism vary. Most of the TCAs have active metabolites that act in much the same manner as the parent drug. Therefore, in determining the rate of elimination, one must consider the half-lives of these metabolites. Most of these antidepressants may be given in a once-daily single dose. If the medication causes sedation, then this dose should be given at bedtime. Fluoxetine causes more activation of energy and must be given in the morning. Venlafaxine, nefazodone, and bupropion are examples of antidepressants whose shorter half-life periods and other factors require administration two or three times per day. Extended-release venlafaxine formulation has allowed daily dosing with this drug. Fluoxetine and its active metabolite have particularly long half-lives, remaining present for as long as 5 to 6 weeks. This may affect a number of decisions. For example, people who wish to have children and are taking fluoxetine ideally should discontinue use of the agent at least 6 weeks before attempting to conceive. They should be advised to consult their prescriber before making this decision. Due to this long half-life, fluoxetine would also not be a good choice for intermittent use for premenstrual dysphoric disorder. Table 13.9 provides information about the average elimination half-lives of most of the antidepressants.

Most of the antidepressants are metabolized by the P-450 enzyme system so that drugs that induce this system tend to decrease blood levels of the antidepressants, and inhibitors of this system increase antidepressant blood levels. This effect varies according to the subfamily that is induced. For example, fluvoxamine (Luvox) substantially inhibits CYP1A2. Thus, other drugs that are metabolized by the system experience slower metabolism. These include such medications as agomelatine, clozapine, melotonin, olanzapine, theophylline, tobacco, and caffeine. Paroxetine, fluoxetine, and duloxetine are very potent inhibitors of CYP2D6, as well as being substrates for this CYP enzyme.

Side Effects, Adverse Reactions, and Toxicity

Side effects of the antidepressant medications vary considerably. Because the TCAs act at several types of receptors, in addition to serotonin and norepinephrine receptors, these drugs have many unwanted effects. Conversely, the SSRIs are more selective for serotonin and have comparatively fewer and better tolerated side effects. Attention to a patient's ability to tolerate side effects is critical because uncomfortable side effects are the primary reason patients discontinue medication treatment. With the TCAs, sedation, orthostatic hypotension, and anticholinergic side effects are the most common sources of discomfort for patients receiving these medications. See Chapter 22 for a comparison of side effects of antidepressant medications.

Receptor affinities may be helpful in predicting which side effects are most likely to occur with a given medication. Table 13.1 provides a summary of major receptor targets for common antidepressants. Using this table in conjunction with Chapter 22, nurses may be able to predict which side effects will be most common with each medication. Interventions to assist in minimizing these side effects are listed in Table 13.2.

Sexual dysfunction is a relatively common side effect, especially with the SSRIs. Erectile and ejaculation disturbances occur in men and anorgasmia in women. This side effect is often difficult to assess if the nurse has not obtained a sexual history before the initiation of use of the medication. Anorgasmia is particularly common with the SSRIs and often goes unreported, frequently because nurses and other healthcare providers do not ask. Bupropion and nefazodone (Serzone) appear to be least likely to cause sexual disturbance. In addition, when sexual dysfunction is related to the medication, several treatment options are available. These include a change in dose or type of antidepressant or, less frequently, using other medications to treat this side effect. Nurses must take responsibility for discussing the potential for sexual side effects before initiation of drug treatment and for continuing to reassess during follow-up visits.

The TCAs have the potential for cardiotoxicity, which limits their use in older adults. Symptoms include QT prolongation that may worsen preexisting cardiac conduction problems (such as second-degree heart block). The newer antidepressants, such as the SSRIs and bupropion, are less cardiotoxic, and nefazodone exhibits no evidence of cardiotoxicity at this time of writing this text. Antidepressants that block the dopamine receptor, such as amoxapine, have the potential to produce symptoms of NMS. Mild forms of extrapyramidal symptoms and endocrine changes, including galactorrhea and amenorrhea, may develop. Amoxapine should be avoided in older adult patients because it may be associated with the development of tardive dyskinesia with this age group. Antidepressant-associated bruxism is an underrecognized but significant complication of many antidepressants. This can affect dental health and contribute to temporomandibular disorders. A dose decrease may provide relief; however, buspirone may also be added to treat this condition (Singh et al., 2019).

The most common side effects of the SSRIs include headache, anxiety, insomnia, transient nausea, vomiting, and diarrhoea. Sedation may also occur, especially with fluvoxamine. Most often, these medications are given in the morning, but if daytime sedation occurs, they may be given in the evening. Venlafaxine (Effexor) has little effect on acetylcholine and histamine; thus, the risks for sedation and anticholinergic symptoms are low. However, higher doses are associated with sexual dysfunction, sedation, diastolic hypertension, increased perspiration, constipation, dry mouth, tremors, blurred vision, and asthenia or muscle weakness. Elevations in blood pressure and heart rate have been described, and nurses should monitor these vital sign parameters, especially in patients who have a preexisting history of coronary artery disease. Nurses need to be very familiar with nefazodone (Serzone) and the clinical issues related to its side effects. Nefazodone is a phenylpiperazine antidepressant that is structurally related to trazodone. Its most common side effects include sedation, dizziness, and orthostatic hypotension; less common is increased risk for seizures. Drug–drug interactions between nefazodone and triazolam and alprazolam have been reported, with increased plasma levels of these benzodiazepines, resulting in an enhancement of the psychomotor impairment caused by these agents. Bupropion (Wellbutrin) has a chemical structure unlike any of the other antidepressants. Some of its pharmacologic profile is due to effects on dopamine systems, in addition to effects on serotonin and norepinephrine.

Bupropion's activating effects may be experienced as agitation or anxiety by some patients. Others also experience insomnia and appetite suppression. Rarely, bupropion has produced psychosis, including hallucinations and delusions. Most likely, this is secondary to the stimulation of dopamine systems. Dopamine is also associated with reward and motivated behaviour, which accounts for the increasingly common use of bupropion, under the trade name of Zyban, as a smoking cessation agent. The slightly increased risk for experiencing seizures with bupropion use has received the most attention. Most important, bupropion has not been found to cause sexual dysfunction and often is used in individuals who are experiencing these side effects.

The MAOIs can produce anticholinergic side effects (dizziness, dry mouth, blurred vision, constipation, nausea, peripheral oedema, urinary hesitancy) but at a much-reduced rate compared with the TCAs. Orthostatic hypotension and sexual dysfunction, including decreased libido, impotence, and anorgasmia, can occur with MAOIs. The most serious side effect of the MAOIs is their interaction with tyramine-containing foods and certain medications. The food interaction occurs because MAOIs block the breakdown of tyramine, a trace amine with vasoconstrictor properties. Increased levels of tyramine can cause severe headaches and hypertension, stroke, and, in rare instances, death. Patients who are taking MAOIs are placed on a low-tyramine diet. This diet has been difficult for some individuals to follow, and concerns about the risk for severe hypertension have led many clinicians to rarely use the MAOIs (see Table 13.10).

Table 13.10 Example of a Tyramine-Restricted Diet

Category of Food	Food to Avoid	Food Allowed
Cheese	All matured or aged cheeses. All casseroles made with these cheeses, pizza, lasagna, etc. *Note:* All cheeses are considered matured or aged except those listed under the "Foods Allowed" column	Fresh cottage cheese, cream cheese, ricotta cheese, and processed cheese slices. All fresh milk products that have been stored properly (e.g., sour cream, yogurt, ice cream)
Meat, fish, and poultry	Fermented/dry sausage: pepperoni, salami, mortadella, summer sausage, etc. Improperly stored meat, fish, or poultry. Improperly stored pickled herring	All fresh packaged or processed meat (e.g., chicken loaf, hot dogs), fish, or poultry. Refrigerate immediately and eat as soon as possible
Fruits and vegetables	Fava or broad bean pods (not beans). Banana peel	Banana pulp. All others except those listed in the "Food to Avoid" column
Alcoholic beverages	All tap beers	Alcohol: No more than two domestic bottled or canned beers or 4-fluid-oz glasses of red or white wine per day; this applies to nonalcoholic beer also; please note that red wine may produce a headache unrelated to a rise in blood pressure
Miscellaneous foods	Marmite concentrated yeast extract. Sauerkraut. Soy sauce and other soybean condiments	Other yeast extracts (e.g., brewer's yeast). Soy milk

Adapted from Gardener, D. M., Shulman, K. I., Walker, S. E., & Tailor, S. A. N. (1996). The making of a user-friendly MAOI diet. *Journal of Clinical Psychiatry, 57*, 99–104.

MAOIs in use in Canada include phenelzine (Nardil) and tranylcypromine (Parnate). These are considered irreversible MAOIs because they form unbreakable covalent bonds with MAO. It takes at least 2 weeks to produce replacement enzyme molecules after discontinuation of use of the medication. Moclobemide is an example of a reversible MAOI that is available in Europe and Canada. Although it acts in the same way as the irreversible MAOIs, moclobemide forms weaker bonds that are short lasting. Therefore, a less restrictive diet may be used with moclobemide. In addition to food restrictions, many prescription and nonprescription medications that stimulate the sympathetic nervous system (sympathomimetics) produce the same risk for hypertensive crisis as do foods containing tyramine. The nonprescription medication interactions primarily involve diet pills and cold remedies. Patients should be advised to check the labels of any nonprescription drugs carefully for a warning against use with antidepressants, especially the MAOIs, and then consult their prescriber or pharmacist before consuming these medications. Patients should notify other healthcare providers, including dentists, that they are taking an MAOI before being prescribed or given any other medication.

Suicide is a major concern when working with individuals who are depressed. Systematic suicide risk assessment should be done routinely before initiating antidepressant therapy, in the first 2 to 4 weeks of treatment and for longer if indicated. Some of these medications are more lethal than others. For example, the TCAs pose a significant risk for overdose and are more lethal in children. Symptoms of overdose and treatment are discussed more fully in Chapter 22, but for now, it is important to remember that this potential exists.

Sometimes, the prescriber will provide the patient with only small amounts of the medication, requiring more frequent visits, and will closely monitor use. In general, newer antidepressant medications, such as the SSRIs, are associated with less risk for toxicity and lethality in overdose. Box 13.5 highlights some of the newest antidepressants being tested in clinical trials.

BOX 13.5 Novel Antidepressant Drug Development

Research into the neurobiology of depression has implicated other neurotransmitter and neuroendocrine systems in the aetiology of depression. This has led to the development of new antidepressants, many of which are in clinical trials at this time.

For example, dysregulation of the glutamatergic system is known to cause impaired neurotransmission and neural cell toxicity. It is believed that these synaptic abnormalities may be, at least partially, responsible for mood disorders. Thus, drug agents targeting glutamate and associated receptors may prove to be useful in future treatment of mood disorders (Małgorzata et al., 2020). Ketamine, a specific glutamate receptor antagonist, was shown to attenuate acute suicidal ideation and improve mood (Carreno et al., 2020). The use of ketamine is increasingly being used in the treatment of severe mood disorders.

Phases of Mood Stabilizing and Antidepressant Therapy

Initiation Phase

Overcoming issues such as social stigma, viewing depression and mood disorders as a personal failing, fear about taking a medication, and the decreased energy and motivation associated with depression have made the decision to seek treatment a major hurdle. The nurse plays an important role in helping patient through the phases of drug therapy.

Stabilization Phase

The treatment goal for bipolar disorder is to prevent relapse of the current episode or cycling into the opposite pole. It lasts about 2 to 9 months after acute symptoms resolve. The usual pharmacologic procedure in this phase is to titrate the mood stabilizer while closely monitoring the patient for signs or symptoms of relapse. In depression, patients will experience a lag between starting drug therapy and complete drug effect. Nurses should warn patients about potential side effects, such as nausea and diarrhoea, associated with most antidepressant. Dose increases or the addition of other antidepressant agents occur in this phase.

Maintenance Phase

The goal of treating this phase is to sustain remission and to prevent new episodes or bipolar disorder or depression. The great weight of evidence favours long-term prophylaxis against recurrence after the effective treatment of acute episodes. It is recommended that long-term or lifetime prophylaxis with a mood stabilizer be prescribed after two manic episodes or one severe manic episode or if there is a family history of bipolar disorder. Careful monitoring and follow-up are essential during this phase to assess patient response to medications, adjust dosage if necessary, identify and address side effects, and provide patient support and education.

Discontinuation Phase

Both bipolar I and bipolar II disorders are typically recurrent and progressive; long-term suppressive medication may be indicated. Unlike many psychiatric disorders, depressive disorders may be time limited; thus, medication therapy should be reviewed periodically. The decision to discontinue active treatment is generally based on factors that include the frequency and severity of past episodes, the persistence of dysthymic symptoms after recovery, the presence of comorbid disorders, and patient preference.

Patients may be reluctant to take prescribed antidepressant medications or may self-treat depression.

The continuation of medication, as well as emphasizing potential drug–drug interactions, should be included in the teaching plan.

Antianxiety and Sedative–Hypnotic Medications

Sometimes called anxiolytics, antianxiety medications and sedative–hypnotic medications come from various pharmacologic classifications, including benzodiazepines, nonbenzodiazepines, and nonbarbiturate sedative–hypnotics, such as chloral hydrate. These drugs represent some of the most widely prescribed medications today for the short-term relief of anxiety or anxiety associated with depression.

Benzodiazepines

Commonly prescribed benzodiazepines include chlordiazepoxide (Librium), diazepam (Valium), lorazepam (Ativan), flurazepam (Dalmane), oxazepam (Serax), and clonazepam (Rivotril).

Indications and Mechanisms of Action

Benzodiazepines act as positive modulators at $GABA_A$ ion channels, increasing the ease of GABA binding to its binding site. This enhancement of GABA binding increases both the duration and frequency of channel opening and decreases the firing rate of the nerve cell. This inhibition of nerve cell firing allows this class of drugs to act as anticonvulsants, antianxiety medications, or hypnotics, depending on dose and pharmacokinetic properties. Other neurotransmitter systems are also involved in the effects of benzodiazepines. Of the various benzodiazepines in use to relieve anxiety (and treat insomnia), clonazepam (Rivotril) and lorazepam (Ativan) are often preferred for patients with liver disease and for older adult patients because of their short half-lives.

Pharmacokinetics

The variable rate of absorption of the benzodiazepines determines the speed of onset. Table 13.11 provides relative indications of the speed of onset, from very fast to slow, for some of the commonly prescribed benzodiazepines.

Chlordiazepoxide (Librium) and diazepam (Valium) are slow, erratic, and sometimes incompletely absorbed when given IM, whereas lorazepam (Ativan) and clonazepam (Rivotril) are rapidly and completely absorbed when given IM. Lorazepam is also well absorbed by the sublingual route.

All the benzodiazepines are highly lipid soluble and highly protein bound. They are distributed throughout

Table 13.11 Antianxiety and Sedative–Hypnotic Medications			
Generic (Trade) Drug Name	Usual Dosage Range (mg/day)	Half-Life (Hours)	Speed of Onset After Single Dose
Benzodiazepines			
diazepam (Valium)	4–40	30–100	Very fast
chlordiazepoxide (Librium)	15–100	50–100	Intermediate
clorazepate (Tranxene)	15–60	30–200	Fast
prazepam (Centrax)	20–60	30–200	Very slow
flurazepam (Dalmane)	15–30	47–100	Fast
lorazepam (Ativan)	2–8	10–20	Slow–intermediate
oxazepam (Serax)	30–120	3–21	Slow–intermediate
temazepam (Restoril)	15–30	9.5–20	Moderately fast
triazolam (Halcion)	0.25–0.5	2–4	Fast
alprazolam (Xanax)	0.5–10	12–15	Intermediate
clonazepam (Rivotril)	1.5–20	18–50	Intermediate
Nonbenzodiazepines			
buspirone (BuSpar)	15–30	3–11	Very slow
zolpidem (Sublinox)[a]	5–10	2.6	Fast

[a]5 mg for women and people over 65.

the body and enter the CNS quickly. Other drugs that compete for protein-binding sites may produce drug–drug interactions. The degree to which each of these drugs is lipid soluble affects its duration of action. Most of these drugs have active metabolites, but the degree of activity of each metabolite affects the duration of action and elimination half-life. Most of these drugs vary markedly in the length of half-life. Oxazepam, which is itself an active metabolite of diazepam, and lorazepam have no active metabolites and thus have shorter half-lives. Sustained presence of these drugs after discontinuation may be observed in older adult or obese patients.

Side Effects, Adverse Reactions, and Toxicity

The most commonly reported side effects result from the sedative and CNS depression effects of these medications. Drowsiness, intellectual impairment, anterograde memory impairment, ataxia, and reduced motor coordination are common adverse effects. If used for sleep, then many of these medications, especially long-acting benzodiazepines, produce significant "hangover" effects experienced on awakening. Flunitrazepam (Rohypnol), otherwise known as the "date rape" drug because of its ability to impair anterograde memory, is illegal in Canada. For the older adult, drowsiness mixed with mental confusion can lead to falls and hip fractures. Current clinical guidelines for drug treatments in older adults strongly recommend avoiding benzodiazepine use in this population (Conn et al., 2020). For most patients, the effects subside as tolerance develops; however, alcohol increases all these symptoms and potentiates CNS depression. Indeed, benzodiazepines have a wide therapeutic index but can be lethal when used with alcohol, opioid, or other sedating drugs and substances. Individuals using these medications should be warned to avoid driving or performing other tasks that require

mental alertness. If these tasks are part of the person's work requirements, another medication may be chosen.

Because tolerance develops to most of the CNS depressant effects, individuals who wish to experience the feeling of "intoxication" from these medications may be tempted to increase their own dosage. Psychological dependence is more likely to occur when using these medications for a longer period, which is the reason benzodiazepines are, for the most part, to be used as short-term therapies. Abrupt discontinuation of the use of benzodiazepines may result in a recurrence of the target symptoms, such as rebound insomnia or anxiety. Other withdrawal symptoms appear rapidly, including tremors, increased perspiration, palpitations, increased sensitivity to light, abdominal discomfort or pain, and elevations in systolic blood pressure. These symptoms may be more pronounced with the short-acting benzodiazepines, such as lorazepam. Gradual tapering is recommended for discontinuing the use of benzodiazepines after long-term treatment. When tapering short-acting medications, the prescriber may switch the patient to a long-acting benzodiazepine before discontinuing the use of the short-acting drug.

Individual reactions to the benzodiazepines appear to be associated with sensitivity to their effects. Some patients feel apathy, fatigue, tearfulness, emotional lability, irritability, and nervousness. Benzodiazepines do little for depression symptoms, except for sleep disturbance, and may even exacerbate anhedonia and difficulties concentrating. As such, their use in depression, even with significant comorbid anxiety, should be closely monitored.

Older adults are particularly susceptible to incontinence, memory disturbances, dizziness, and increased risk for falls when using benzodiazepines. Pregnant patients should be aware that these medications cross the placenta and are associated with an increased risk for birth defects, such as cleft palate, intellectual disability, and pyloric stenosis. Infants born addicted to benzodiazepines often exhibit flaccid muscle tone, lethargy, and difficulties sucking. All the benzodiazepines are excreted in breast milk, and breast-feeding women should avoid using these medications. Infants and children metabolize these medications more slowly; therefore, more drug accumulates in their bodies.

Toxicity can develop with liver dysfunction or disease. Symptoms include worsening of the CNS depression, ataxia, confusion, delirium, agitation, hypotension, diminished reflexes, and lethargy. Rarely do the benzodiazepines cause respiratory depression or death. In overdose, these medications have a high therapeutic index and rarely result in death unless combined with another CNS depressant drug, such as alcohol or opioids.

Nonbenzodiazepines: Buspirone and Zolpidem

One of the nonbenzodiazepines, buspirone (BuSpar), was first synthesized in 1968 by Michael Eison who was searching for an improved antipsychotic medication. Later, it was found that buspirone was effective in controlling the symptoms of anxiety but had no effect on panic disorders and little effect on obsessive–compulsive disorder. Another nonbenzodiazepine, zolpidem (Sublinox), is a medication for sleep that acts on the benzodiazepine–GABA receptor complex.

Indications and Mechanisms of Actions

These drugs are effective for treating anxiety disorders without the CNS depressant effects or the potential for abuse and withdrawal syndromes. Canadian treatment guidelines for generalized anxiety disorder caution against long-term use of benzodiazepines and, based on level I evidence, recommend either the SSRI, paroxetine, or the SNRI, venlafaxine (Katzman et al., 2014). Buspirone is also indicated for treating generalized anxiety disorder; therefore, its target symptoms include anxiety and related symptoms, such as difficulty in concentrating, tension, insomnia, restlessness, irritability, and fatigue. Because buspirone does not add to depression symptoms, it has been tried for treating anxiety that coexists with depression. In some instances, it is thought to potentiate the antidepressant actions of other medications. Antipsychotic drugs, and anticonvulsants such as pregabalin, are occasionally used off-label for the treatment of anxiety. Hydroxyzine and propranolol are used as adjunctive agents in treatment refractory anxiety. The use of cannabis to alleviate anxiety symptoms requires further research (Van Ameringen et al., 2020).

Buspirone has no effect on the benzodiazepine–GABA complex but instead appears to control anxiety by blocking the serotonin subtype of receptor, 5-HT_{1a}, at both presynaptic reuptake and postsynaptic receptor sites. It has no sedative, muscle relaxant, or anticonvulsant effects. It also lacks potential for abuse.

Zolpidem (Sublinox), which is indicated for short-term insomnia treatment, appears to increase slow-wave (deep) sleep and to modulate $GABA_A$ receptors, but with less risk for tolerance or withdrawal issues compared with benzodiazepines.

Pharmacokinetics

Buspirone is rapidly absorbed but undergoes extensive first-pass metabolism. Food slows absorption but appears to reduce first-pass metabolism, increasing the bioavailability of the medication. Buspirone is given on a continual dosing schedule of three times a day because of its short half-life of 2 to 3 h. Clinical action depends on reaching steady-state concentrations; taking this medication with food may facilitate this process.

Buspirone is highly protein bound but does not displace most other medications. However, it does displace digoxin and may increase digoxin levels to the point of toxicity. It is metabolized in the liver and excreted predominantly by the kidneys but also through the gastrointestinal tract. Patients with liver or kidney impairment should be given this medication with caution. Buspirone is a major substrate of CYP3A4 and thus demonstrates many drug–drug interactions on this basis.

Buspirone cannot be used on a PRN basis; rather, it takes 2 to 4 weeks of continual use for symptom relief to occur. It is more effective in reducing anxiety in patients who have never taken a benzodiazepine. Buspirone does not block the withdrawal of other benzodiazepines. Therefore, a switch to buspirone must be initiated gradually to avoid withdrawal symptoms. Nurses should closely monitor patients who are undergoing this change of medication for emergence of withdrawal symptoms from the benzodiazepines and report such symptoms to the prescriber.

Zolpidem is metabolized by the liver; it crosses the placenta and enters breast milk. It has a short half-life of 3 h and is excreted in the urine, which makes it an ideal hypnotic.

Side Effects, Adverse Reactions, and Toxicity

Common side effects from higher-dose buspirone include dizziness, drowsiness, nausea, excitement, and headache. Most other side effects occur at an incidence of less than 1%. There have been no reports of death from an overdose of buspirone alone. Older adults, people who are pregnant, and children have not been adequately studied. For now, buspirone can be assumed to cross the placenta and is present in breast milk; therefore, its use should be avoided in people who are pregnant. Individuals taking this medication should not breastfeed.

Rebound effects, such as insomnia and anxiety, from zolpidem are minimal. There are minimal effects on respiratory function and little potential for abuse. Although very rare, there have been cases of sleepwalking, sleep driving, and other complex behaviours while asleep attributed to zolpidem use (Paulke et al., 2015).

Stimulants

Amphetamines were first synthesized in the late 1800s but were not used for psychiatric disorders until the 1930s. Amphetamines were initially prescribed for a variety of symptoms and disorders, but their high abuse potential soon became obvious.

Amphetamines, Methylphenidate, and Modafinil

Methamphetamine, a highly addictive psychoactive substance, is illegal in most countries, including Canada. A prescription form of methamphetamine is available in the United States, but it is highly restricted and seldom prescribed. All stimulants, including cocaine, methamphetamine, and prescription amphetamine (lisdexamfetamine and dextroamphetamine), are all psychoactive substances with the potential for abuse and addiction. For these reasons, amphetamines are now restricted to the treatment of few disorders, including attention deficit hyperactivity disorder (ADHD), narcolepsy, and binge eating. Nonamphetamine drugs are increasingly being used for the treatment of ADHD, narcolepsy, and illness-associated fatigue. These drugs include modafinil, methylphenidate, atomoxetine, and bupropion. Though nonamphetamine drugs are less addictive, they are frequently abused by students and professionals.

Indications and Mechanisms of Action

Among the medications known as stimulants are methylphenidate (Ritalin), dextroamphetamine (Dexedrine), dextroamphetamine and amphetamine (Adderall), and lisdexamfetamine (Vyvanse). They are used for ADHD and narcolepsy, a sleep disorder. Modafinil is a nonamphetamine agent used in the treatment of narcolepsy and illness-associated fatigue, including cancer, depression, and multiple sclerosis. Nonstimulant drugs, such as bupropion (Wellbutrin) and atomoxetine (Strattera), are often used in the treatment of ADHD.

Amphetamine is a racemate or chiral compound, meaning that half of the amphetamine molecules are the mirror image to the other half. Each half of the molecules, dextroamphetamine (D-amphetamine) and levoamphetamine (L-amphetamine), have different pharmacological properties. Dextroamphetamine is typically more potent, has a rapid onset, has more effects on dopamine than norepinephrine, and has been the focus of much research. Lisdexamfetamine is a prodrug converting to dextroamphetamine by hydrolytic activity of the red blood cells. This produces a slower release of dextroamphetamine, a more sustained peak plasma concentration, and lower risk for abuse potential (Heal et al., 2013).

Amphetamines indirectly stimulate the sympathetic nervous system, producing alertness, wakefulness, vasoconstriction, suppressed appetite, and hypothermia. Tolerance develops to some of these effects, such as suppression of appetite, but the CNS stimulation continues. Although the exact mechanism of action is not completely understood, stimulants cause a release of catecholamines, particularly norepinephrine and dopamine, into the synapse from the presynaptic nerve cell. They also block the reuptake of these catecholamines. Methylphenidate is structurally similar to the amphetamines but produces a milder CNS stimulation (Sadek, 2021).

Although the stimulant effects of these medications may seem logically indicated for narcolepsy, a disorder in which the individual frequently and abruptly falls asleep (see Chapter 28), the indications for childhood ADHD seem less obvious. The aetiology and neurobiology of ADHD remain unclear, but psychostimulants produce a paradoxic calming of the increased motor activity characteristic of ADHD. Studies show that medication decreases disruptive activity during school hours, reduces noise and verbal activity, improves attention span and short-term memory, improves ability to follow directions, and decreases distractibility and impulsivity. Although these improvements have been well documented in the literature, the diagnosis of ADHD and subsequent use of psychostimulants with children and adults remain a matter of controversy (see Chapter 30).

Modafinil increases mental alertness by blocking dopamine transporter, thus increasing dopamine levels in the brain. Atomoxetine (Strattera) increases energy by blocking the norepinephrine reuptake transporter. The mechanism of action for bupropion (Wellbutrin) is not well understood, but its metabolites inhibit the reuptake of norepinephrine. It is found to have similar effects to atomoxetine.

Pharmacokinetics

Amphetamines are rapidly absorbed from the gastrointestinal tract and reach peak plasma levels in 1 to 3 h. Considerable individual variations occur between the drugs in terms of bioavailability, plasma levels, and half-life. Table 13.12 compares the primary psychostimulants used in psychiatry. Some of these differences are age dependent because children metabolize these medications more rapidly, producing shorter

Table 13.12 Psychostimulant Medications		
Generic (Trade) Name and Half-Life	Usual Dosage Drug Range (mg/day)	Side Effects
dextroamphetamine (Dexedrine); 6–7 h	5–40	Overstimulation Restlessness Dry mouth Palpitations Cardiomyopathy (with prolonged use or high dosage) Possible growth retardation (greatest risk); risk reduced with drug holidays
methylphenidate (Ritalin); 2–4 h	10–60	Nervousness Insomnia Anorexia Tachycardia Impaired cognition (with high doses) Moderate risk for growth suppression
lisdexamfetamine (Vyvanse); 10–13 h	30–70	Insomnia Tachycardia Decreased appetite Raynaud phenomena Blurred vision

elimination half-lives. Adderall and Ritalin are available in a sustained release form and should not be chewed or crushed.

Amphetamines appear to be unaffected by food in the stomach and should be given after meals to reduce the appetite-suppressant effects when indicated. However, changes in urine pH may affect the rates of excretion. Excessive sodium bicarbonate alkalizes the urine and reduces amphetamine secretion. An increased vitamin C or citric acid intake may acidify the urine and increase its excretion. Starvation from appetite suppression may have a similar effect. All these drugs are highly lipid soluble, crossing easily into the CNS and the placenta. Dextroamphetamine and amphetamine undergo metabolic changes in the liver, where they may affect or be affected by other drugs. Lisdexamfetamine is not metabolized by P450 microsomal enzymes. All amphetamines are primarily excreted through the kidneys; therefore, renal dysfunction may interfere with excretion.

Modafinil is absorbed rapidly and reaches peak plasma concentration in 2 to 4 h. The absorption of modafinil may be delayed by 1 to 2 h if taken with food. Modafinil is eliminated through liver metabolism, with subsequent excretion of metabolites through renal excretion. Modafinil may interact with drugs that inhibit, induce, or are metabolized by P450 enzymes, primarily CYP3A4, including phenytoin, diazepam, and propranolol. Concurrent use of modafinil and other drugs metabolized by CYP3A4 may lead to increased circulating blood levels of the other drugs.

Bupropion and atomoxetine are rapidly absorbed and have a duration of action of 1 to 2 days, allowing for once daily dosing. It may take up to 1 to 2 weeks, particularly for bupropion, for a clinical effect to be observed. Both drugs are extensively metabolized via the CYP 2D6 enzymes and form the basis for many drug–drug interactions, such as increasing serum concentrations of propranolol, tamsulosin, and metoprolol.

All psychostimulants are usually begun at a low dose and increased weekly, depending on improvement of symptoms and occurrence of side effects. With amphetamine-based drugs, children with ADHD are given a morning dose so that their school performance may be compared from morning to afternoon. Rebound symptoms of excitability and talkativeness may occur when use of the medication is withdrawn or after dose reduction. These symptoms also begin about 5 h after the last dose of medication, which may affect the dosing regimen for some individuals. The return of symptoms in the afternoon for children with ADHD may require that a second dose be given at school. Prescribers should work with parents to implement other interventions after school and on weekends when the psychostimulants are not used. Severity of symptoms may require that the medications be continued during these times, but this dosing schedule should be determined after careful evaluation on an individual basis. Use of these medications should not be stopped abruptly, especially with higher doses, because the rebound effects may last for several days.

Side Effects, Adverse Reactions, and Toxicity

The most common side effects of all psychostimulants include appetite suppression, insomnia, irritability, weight loss, nausea, headache, palpitations, blurred vision, dry mouth, constipation, and dizziness. Because there is no compelling reason for an individual who is pregnant to continue to take these medications, patients should be informed and should advise their prescriber immediately if they plan to become pregnant or if pregnancy is a possibility. There are increased risks for congenital malformation with bupropion and modafinil and for low birth weight with amphetamines.

Because amphetamines produce effects on the sympathetic nervous system, some individuals experience blood pressure changes (both hypertension and hypotension), tachycardia, tremors, and irregular heart rates. Blood pressure and pulse should be monitored initially and after each dosage change. Rarely, amphetamines suppress growth and development in children. These effects are a matter of controversy, and research has produced conflicting results. Although the suppression of height seems unlikely to some researchers, others have indicated that amphetamines may have an effect on cartilage. Height and weight should be monitored several times annually for children taking these medications and compared with prior history of growth. Weight should be monitored especially closely during the initial phases of treatment. These effects also may be minimized by drug "holidays," such as during school vacations. Abnormal movements and motor tics may also increase in individuals who have a history of Tourette syndrome. Amphetamines should be avoided by patients with Tourette symptoms or a positive family history of the disorder.

Death is rare from overdose or toxicity of the amphetamines, but a 10-day supply may be lethal, especially in children. Symptoms of overdose include agitation, chest pain, hallucinations, paranoia, confusion, and dysphoria. Seizures may develop, along with fever, tremor, hypertension or hypotension, aggression, headache, palpitations, rashes, difficulty breathing, leg pain, and abdominal pain. Maximum dosage for children is 40 mg per day, with potential death resulting from a 400-mg dose. Parents should be warned regarding the potential lethality of these medications and take preventive measures by keeping the medication in a safe place.

New Medications and Emerging Therapies

Each country has its own approval process for new medications. In Canada, this process is controlled by Health Canada. Through various phases of drug testing, a new drug must be determined to have therapeutic benefit based on known physiologic processes, animal testing, and laboratory models of human disease and its potential toxicity predicted at doses likely to produce clinical improvement in humans (see Box 13.6 for more information). Then, the pharmaceutical company can begin research with human volunteers after filing an *investigational new drug* (IND) application. Many new psychiatric medications, particularly the second-generation antipsychotics and novel antidepressants, are in various phases of clinical testing and are expected to be released in the coming years. Keeping the phases of new drug development in mind will assist the nurse in understanding

BOX 13.6 Phases of New Drug Testing

- *Phase I*: Testing defines the range of dosages tolerated in healthy individuals.
- *Phase II*: Effects of the drug are studied in a limited number of individuals with the target disorder.
- *Phase III*: Extensive clinical trials are conducted at multiple sites throughout the country with larger numbers of patients. Efforts focus on corroborating the efficacy identified in phase II. Phase III concludes with a new drug application (NDA) being submitted to Health Canada.
- *Phase IV*: Postmarketing surveillance continues to detect new or rare adverse reactions and potentially new indications. During this period, adverse reactions from the new medication are required to be reported to Health Canada.

IMPLICATIONS FOR MENTAL HEALTH NURSES

Throughout the phases, side effects and adverse reactions are monitored closely. The studies are tightly controlled, and strict regulations are enforced at each step.

Clinical trials for new drugs usually involve patient populations that have no other health problems but the one under study. This is important to test the drug's effectiveness, but in clinical practice, many patients have other health problems, and postmarketing surveillance helps identify unforeseen benefits or adverse effects in most heterogeneous patient populations.

A newly approved drug is approved only for the indications for which it has been tested. However, there is often a widening of application for other health problems over time (called *off-label* uses).

In Canada, the pharmaceutical companies must follow strict guidelines in terms of product advertising and interaction with health professionals. For example, the companies are not permitted to advertise directly to the public, and there are stringent guidelines regarding any potential sales incentives offered to health professionals. This is to address potential ethical issues around influencing prescriber preferences.

what to expect from drugs newly released to the market. All drugs approved by Health Canada have a Drug Identification Number (DIN).

SEP-856 is a drug currently in clinical trials which may prove to be a useful treatment for schizophrenia, psychosis in Parkinson, and addiction. This drug focuses on modulating the trace amine-associated receptor 1 (TAAR-1) and is a 5HT1A agonist. TAAR-1 may prevent the development of metabolic syndrome and may provide a much-needed pharmacological treatment option for people with amphetamine or cocaine addiction (Dodd et al., 2021).

Tak-831 is a selective inhibitor of D-amino acid oxidase inhibitor prolonging D-serine activity on the NMDA receptor. This drug is early in the investigation and, if effective, may improve negative symptoms of schizophrenia and treat Friedreich ataxia (Correll, 2020).

IV ketamine infusions have been successfully used over the past two decades for the treatment of resistant depression. Building on this knowledge, esketamine, a nasally inhaled ketamine derivative, was approved for use in the United States in 2019. Hydroxynorketamine is believed to provide similar antidepressant effects without dissociative side effects (Bokel et al., 2020).

Cannabis does not have a Drug Identification Number (DIN) nor has it been subject to Health Canada review or phases of drug testing. Research exploring the potential therapeutic benefits of cannabis is in its infancy. The Canadian Pharmaceutical Association produced a drug monograph for Cannabis, outlining potential use of cannabis to treat various conditions. At the current time, there is either insufficient or inconclusive evidence to routinely recommend the use of cannabis for the management of anxiety disorders, post-traumatic stress disorder, schizophrenia, or substance use disorder. There is some promising research to suggest that cannabis use improves the retention of people with opioid use disorder on opioid agonist therapy (Canadian Pharmacists Association, 2018; Okusanya et al., 2020). See phases of new drug testing in Box 13.6.

Other Biologic Treatments

Although the primary intervention remains pharmacologic, some treatments for mental illness are nonpharmacological in nature. Examples of these therapies include electroconvulsive therapy (ECT), phototherapy, and transcranial magnetic stimulation.

Electroconvulsive Therapy

ECT is an effective treatment option for people with severe depression with any or all of the following: psychotic symptoms, psychomotor agitation, and psychomotor retardation (van Diermen et al., 2020). It may also be appropriate to treat moderate severity depression

with ECT, particularly among older adults (Østergaard et al., 2020).

With ECT, a brief electrical current is passed through the brain to produce generalized seizures lasting 25 to 150 seconds. Short-acting anaesthetics and muscle relaxing agents are given before ECT; the patient does not feel the stimulus or recall the procedure. A brief pulse stimulus, administered unilaterally on the nondominant side of the head, is associated with less confusion after ECT. However, some individuals require bilateral treatment for the effective resolution of depressive symptoms. Induction of a seizure is necessary to produce positive treatment outcomes. Individual seizure thresholds vary and increase with age, so the electrical impulse and treatment method also may vary.

Older adults may experience longer postprocedure disorientation; however, it is unclear if changes in electric dose may improve this finding (Magne Bjølseth et al., 2016). Blood pressure and the ECG are monitored during the procedure. This procedure is repeated two or three times a week, usually for a total of 6 to 12 treatments. Because there is no particular difference in treatment efficacy and a twice-weekly regimen produces less accumulative memory loss, this treatment course is often chosen. After symptoms have improved, antidepressant medications are used to prevent relapse. Some patients who cannot take or do not experience response to antidepressant treatment may go on maintenance ECT treatments. Usually, once-weekly treatments are gradually decreased in frequency to once monthly.

Light Therapy (Phototherapy)

Human circadian rhythms are set by time clues (zeitgebers) inside and outside the body. One of the most powerful regulators of these body patterns is the cycle of daylight and darkness. Research findings indicate that some individuals with depressive symptoms that worsen at specific times of the year (have a seasonal pattern) may experience disturbance in these normal body patterns or of circadian rhythms (Kragh et al., 2016). For example, some individuals are more depressed during the winter months, when there is less light, and they improve spontaneously in the spring (see Chapter 22 for a complete description of depression and mood disorders). These individuals usually have symptoms that are somewhat different from classic depression, including fatigue, increased need to sleep, increased appetite and weight gain, irritability, and carbohydrate craving. Administering artificial light to these patients during winter months has reduced these depressive symptoms.

Light therapy, sometimes called **phototherapy**, involves exposing the patient to a specific type of artificial light source to relieve seasonal depression. Artificial light is believed to trigger a shift in the patient's circadian rhythm to an earlier time. Research remains ongoing. The light source must be very bright, full-spectrum light, usually 2,500 lux, which is about 200 times brighter than normal indoor lighting. Harmful ultraviolet light is filtered out.

Transcranial Magnetic Stimulation

Repetitive transcranial magnetic stimulation (rTMS) is an emerging therapy for many psychiatric and neuropsychiatric disorders, including depression, Parkinson, and brain injury resulting from a stroke. Underlying this procedure is the hypothesis that a time-varying magnetic field will induce an electrical field, which, in brain tissue, activates the inhibitory and excitatory neurons, thereby modulating neuroplasticity in the brain. In depression, most treatment protocols apply a high-frequency stimulation at 10 to 20 HZ to the left dorsolateral prefrontal cortex (Lefaucheur et al., 2020). rTMS is an intensive therapy requiring daily sessions lasting approximately 45 minutes each over a period of 6 to 8 weeks. This can be cumbersome and not accessible for people in rural and remote areas of Canada.

Psychosocial Issues in Biologic Treatments

Many factors influence successful medication and other biologic therapies. Of particular importance are issues related to adherence. Adherence refers to following the therapeutic regimen, self-administering medications as prescribed, keeping appointments, and following other treatment suggestions. For instance, as adherence to oral antipsychotic medications is between 40% and 60%, a new tool, the *antipsychotic medication adherence scale*, was developed to assist nurses and other clinicians to better detect potential nonadherence and plan interventions to increase rates of drug adherence (Martins et al., 2016). Box 13.7 lists some of the common reasons for nonadherence. It is also important to not conclude

---

BOX 13.7 Common Reasons for Nonadherence With Medication Regimens

- Uncomfortable side effects and those that interfere with quality of life, such as work performance or intimate relationships
- Lack of awareness of or denial of illness
- Stigma
- Feeling better
- Limited psychoeducation and follow-up
- Difficulties in access to treatment and cost of newer drug therapies
- Substance abuse

---

that the patient is nonadherent until a full assessment is completed.

The most often cited reasons for nonadherence are related to side effects of the medication. Improved functioning may be observed by healthcare professionals but not felt by the patient. Side effects may interfere with work performance or other important aspects of the individual's life. For example, a construction worker cannot afford to be drowsy and sedated while operating a crane at a construction site, or a woman in an intimate relationship may find anorgasmia intolerable. Nurses need to be sensitive to the patient's ability to tolerate side effects and to the impact that side effects have on the patient's life. Medication choice, dosing schedules, and prompt treatment of side effects may be crucial factors in helping patients to continue their treatment, even if the symptoms for which they initially sought help have improved.

Cognitive deficits associated with some psychiatric disorders may make it difficult for the individual to self-monitor, develop insight, make choices, remember to fill prescriptions, or keep appointments. Family members may have beliefs and attitudes that influence the individual not to take the medication as prescribed. Some drug side effects, including decreased sexual libido (SSRI, SNRI) and extrapyramidal side effects (antipsychotics), may impact intimate sexual relationships and cause distress among family members. It is important to discuss these potential side effects with the patient and their loved ones. Patients may also be reluctant to disclose financial constraints, especially in relation to the cost of newer agents and may try to stretch out the prescription or just not fill their prescription. Nurses should have open and frank conversations with patients to identify and address potential barriers to drug adherence.

Adherence concerns must not be dismissed as the patient's or family's problem. Nurses should actively address this issue. A positive therapeutic relationship between the nurse and the patient and family must provide a strong sense of trust that side effects and other difficulties in treatment will be addressed and minimized. When individuals report distressing side effects, the nurse should immediately respond with assessment and interventions to reduce these effects or, at the very least, to validate the patient's concern. It is important to assess adherence often, asking questions in a nonthreatening, nonjudgmental manner.

Adherence can be improved by psychoeducation. This approach is most helpful if it addresses the individual's specific symptoms and concerns. For example, if the patient is having difficulty with understanding the purpose of the medication, then it may be helpful to link taking it to a reduction of specific unwanted symptoms or improved functioning, such as continuing to work.

Furthermore, researchers have noted that antipsychotic drug adherence among persons with severe mental illness and who are experiencing homelessness was associated with connectedness with health services and with a long-acting antipsychotic medication regimen, leading them to conclude that long-acting injectable antipsychotic medication is a reasonable treatment approach to adherence among persons who are experiencing homelessness (Rezansoff et al., 2016).

Other factors that interfere with adherence should also be assessed and plans developed to minimize their effect. For example, an individual who is being considered for clozapine therapy may have missed a number of appointments in the past. On assessment, the nurse may discover that it takes the individual 2 h on three different busses each way to reach the clinic. The nurse can then assist with arranging for a home health nurse to visit the patient's apartment, draw blood samples for analysis, and assess side effects, thus decreasing the number of trips the patient must make to the clinic.

🍁 Summary of Key Points

- Psychopharmacology is the study of medications used to treat psychiatric disorders, including the drug categories of antipsychotics, mood stabilizers, antidepressants, antianxiety medications, and psychostimulants.
- Pharmacokinetics refers to how drugs move through the body. The phases are absorption, distribution, metabolism, and excretion.
- Pharmacodynamics refers to the actions of drugs on living tissue and the human body, with the focus primarily on drug actions at receptor sites, on transporters, and on enzyme activity.
- The importance of receptors is recognized in current psychopharmacology. Biologic action of many drugs depends on how their structure interacts with a specific receptor, functioning either as an agonist, reproducing the same biologic action as a neurotransmitter, or as an antagonist, blocking the response.
- A drug's ability to interact with a given receptor type may be judged on three qualities: (a) selectivity—the ability to interact with specific types of receptors; (b) affinity—the attraction the drug has for the binding site; and (c) intrinsic activity—the ability to produce a certain biologic response.
- Many characteristics of specific drugs affect how well they act and how they affect patients. Nurses must be familiar with characteristics, adverse reactions, and toxicity of certain drugs to administer psychotropic medications safely, educate patients regarding their safe use, and encourage therapeutic adherence.
- Bioavailability describes the amount of the drug that actually reaches the systemic circulation after oral ingestion.
- The wide variations in pharmacokinetic properties across individuals are related to physiologic differences caused by age, genetic makeup, other disease processes, and chemical interactions.
- Antipsychotic medications are drugs used in treating psychotic disorders, such as schizophrenia. They act primarily by blocking dopamine or serotonin postsynaptically. In addition, they have a number of actions on other neurotransmitters. First-generation antipsychotic drugs work on positive symptoms and are inexpensive, but they produce many side effects. Newer second-generation antipsychotic drugs work on positive and negative symptoms; are much more expensive but have far fewer anticholinergic side effects; and are better tolerated by patients, but increase risk for metabolic disorders.
- Medication-related movement disorders are a particularly serious group of side effects that principally occur with the typical antipsychotic medications and that may be acute syndromes, such as dystonia, pseudoparkinsonism, and akathisia, or chronic syndromes, such as tardive dyskinesia.
- The mood stabilizers, or antimania medications, are drugs used to control wide variations in mood related to mania, but these agents may also be used to treat other disorders. Lithium and the anticonvulsants are chemically unrelated and act in different ways to stabilize mood.
- Antidepressant medications are drugs used primarily for treating symptoms of depression but are also used extensively for anxiety disorders and eating disorders. They act by blocking the reuptake of one or more of the monoamines, especially serotonin and norepinephrine. These medications vary considerably in their structure and action. Newer antidepressants, such as the SSRIs, have fewer side effects and are less lethal in overdose than the older TCAs.
- Antianxiety medications also include several subgroups of medications, but SSRIs, NSRIs, benzodiazepines, and nonbenzodiazepines are those principally used in psychiatry. Benzodiazepines act by enhancing the actions of GABA, whereas the nonbenzodiazepine buspirone acts on serotonin. Benzodiazepines can be used on a PRN basis, whereas buspirone must be taken regularly.
- Psychostimulants enhance neurotransmitter activity, acting at a number of different receptor sites. These medications are most often used for treating symptoms related to ADHD and narcolepsy.
- ECT uses the application of an electrical pulsation to induce seizures in the brain. These seizures produce a number of effects on neurotransmission that result in the fairly rapid relief of depressive symptoms.
- Phototherapy involves the application of full-spectrum light in the morning hours, which appears to reset circadian rhythm delays related to seasonal affective disorder and other forms of depression.
- Adherence refers to the ability of an individual to self-administer medications as prescribed and to follow other instructions related to medication treatment. Nonadherence is related to factors such as medication side effects, cost, stigma, and family influences. Nurses play a key role in educating patients and helping them to improve adherence.

Thinking Challenges

Trey is 22 years old and an engineering student at a local university. Trey identifies using the pronouns they/them/their. In their adolescent years, Trey was active in sports and kept fit by swimming nearly each day. Like most busy university students, Trey swam less and less during their first and second year of university due to a heavy academic schedule but remained physically fit. Trey experienced a primary onset of schizophrenia during the summer months between their second and third academic year. They reported that quetiapine helped reduce the terrifying auditory and visual hallucinations but caused tiredness and decreased ability to concentrate in the classroom and while doing homework at home. Trey has since given up swimming to keep on top of their schoolwork. They noticed increased weight gain over

the past 8 months, and, as a result, Trey began to skip many doses of quetiapine. They are now experiencing profound symptoms of schizophrenia again, including poor hygiene, bizarre and erratic behaviour, and poor academic performance. Trey is referred to the university health center for assessment and intervention.

a. How has taking quetiapine impacted Trey's life?
b. What are strategies that can help Trey improve their adherence to antipsychotic medications?

> Visit the Point to view suggested responses. Go to **thePoint.lww.com/activate** and use the activation code found in the front of this text to unlock answers to the "Thinking Challenges" and other online resources.

Web Links

ismp-canada.org This is the site for the Institute for Safe Medication Practices (ISMP), an independent, national, non-profit organization focused on medication safety in healthcare settings. ISMP works with healthcare services, regulatory agencies, patient safety organizations, the pharmaceutical industry, and the public to promote safe practices by analyzing medication incidents, making recommendations for prevention of such incidents, and facilitating quality improvement.

References

Abdel-Baki, A., Thibault, D., Medrano, S., Stip, E., Ladouceur, M., Tahir, R., & Potvin, S. (2020). Long-acting antipsychotic medication as first-line treatment of first-episode psychosis with comorbid substance use disorder. *Early Intervention in Psychiatry, 14*(1), 69–79. https://doi.org/10.1111/eip.12826

Bauer, M., & Gitlin, M. (2016). Treatment of mania with lithium. In *The essential guide to lithium treatment* (pp. 61–70). Springer International Publishing.

Bellivier, F., Belzeaux, R., Scott, J., Courtet, P., Golmard, J.-L., & Azorin, J.-M. (2017). Anticonvulsants and suicide attempts in bipolar I disorders. *Acta Psychiatrica Scandinavica, 135*(5), 470–478. https://doi.org/10.1111/acps.12709

Bokel, A., Rühlmann, A., Hutter, M. C., & Urlacher, V. B. (2020). Enzyme-mediated two-step regio- and stereoselective synthesis of potential rapid-acting antidepressant (2S,6S)-hydroxynorketamine. *ACS Catalysis, 10*(7), 4151–4159. https://doi.org/10.1021/acscatal.9b05384

Brailean, A., Curtis, J., Davis, K., Dregan, A., & Hotopf, M. (2019). Characteristics, comorbidities, and correlates of atypical depression: evidence from the UK Biobank Mental Health Survey. *Psychological Medicine, 50*(7), 1129–1138. https://doi.org/10.1017/s0033291719001004

Brunoni, A. R., Moffa, A. H., Sampaio-Júnior, B., Gálvez, V., & Loo, C. K. (2017). Treatment-emergent mania/hypomania during antidepressant treatment with transcranial direct current stimulation (tDCS): A systematic review and meta-analysis. *Brain Stimulation, 10*(2), 260–262. https://doi.org/10.1016/j.brs.2016.11.005

Canadian Pharmacists Association. (2018). *CPS online: Cannabis.* www.myrxtx.ca. Subscription required.

Carbon, M., Hsieh, C.-H., Kane, J. M., & Correll, C. U. (2017). Tardive dyskinesia prevalence in the period of second-generation antipsychotic use. *The Journal of Clinical Psychiatry, 78*(3), e264–e278. https://doi.org/10.4088/jcp.16r10832

Carreno, F. R., Lodge, D. J., & Frazer, A. (2020). Ketamine: Leading us into the future for development of antidepressants. *Behavioural Brain Research, 383,* 112532. https://doi.org/10.1016/j.bbr.2020.112532

Cendrós, M., Arranz, M. J., Torra, M., Penadés, R., Gonzalez-Rodriguez, A., Brunet, M., Perez-Blanco, J., Ibáñez, L., Serra, A., & Catalán, R. (2020).

The influence of CYP enzymes and ABCB1 on treatment outcomes in schizophrenia: association of CYP1A2 activity with adverse effects. *Journal of Translational Genetics and Genomics, 4,* 210–220. https://doi.org/10.20517/jtgg.2020.21

Chow, C. L., Kadouh, N. K., Bostwick, J. R., & VandenBerg, A. M. (2020). Akathisia and newer second-generation antipsychotic drugs: a review of current evidence. *Pharmacotherapy: The Journal of Human Pharmacology and Drug Therapy, 40*(6), 565–574. https://doi.org/10.1002/phar.2404

Conn, D. K., Hogan, D. B., Amdam, L., Cassidy, K.-L., Cordell, P., Frank, C., Gardner, D., Goldhar, M., Ho, J. M.-W., Kitamura, C., & Vasil, N. (2020). Canadian guidelines on benzodiazepine receptor agonist use disorder among older adults. *Canadian Geriatrics Journal, 23*(1), 116–122. https://doi.org/10.5770/cgj.23.419

Correll, C. U. (2020). Current treatment options and emerging agents for schizophrenia. *The Journal of Clinical Psychiatry, 81*(3). https://doi.org/10.4088/jcp.ms19053br3c

Correll, C. U., & Lauriello, J. (2020). Using long-acting injectable antipsychotics to enhance the potential for recovery in schizophrenia. *The Journal of Clinical Psychiatry, 81*(4). https://doi.org/10.4088/jcp.ms19053ah5c

Davies, J., & Read, J. (2019). A systematic review into the incidence, severity and duration of antidepressant withdrawal effects: Are guidelines evidence-based? *Addictive Behaviors, 97,* 111–121. https://doi.org/10.1016/j.addbeh.2018.08.027

Dodd, S. F., Carvalho, A., Puri, B. K., Maes, M., Bortolasci, C. C., Morris, G., & Berk, M. (2021). Trace Amine-Associated Receptor 1 (TAAR1): A new drug target for psychiatry? *Neuroscience & Biobehavioral Reviews, 120,* 537–541. https://doi.org/10.1016/j.neubiorev.2020.09.028

Egberts, A., Alan, H., Ziere, G., & Mattace-Raso, F. U. S. (2020). Antipsychotics and lorazepam during delirium: are we harming older patients? A real-life data study. *Drugs & Aging, 38*(1), 53–62. https://doi.org/10.1007/s40266-020-00813-7

Fabbri, C., & Serretti, A. (2020). Genetics of treatment outcomes in major depressive disorder: present and future. *Clinical Psychopharmacology and Neuroscience, 18*(1), 1–9. https://doi.org/10.9758/cpn.2020.18.1.1

Fava, G. A., & Cosci, F. (2019). Understanding and managing withdrawal syndromes after discontinuation of antidepressant drugs. *The Journal of Clinical Psychiatry, 80*(6). https://doi.org/10.4088/jcp.19com12794

Fluyau, D., Mitra, P., & Lorthe, K. (2019). Antipsychotics for amphetamine psychosis. A systematic review. *Frontiers in Psychiatry, 10,* 740. https://doi.org/10.3389/fpsyt.2019.00740

Galeotti, N. (2017). Hypericum perforatum (St John's wort) beyond depression: A therapeutic perspective for pain conditions. *Journal of Ethnopharmacology, 200,* 136–146. https://doi.org/10.1016/j.jep.2017.02.016

Gardener, D. M., Shulman, K. I., Walker, S. E., & Tailor, S. A. N. (1996). The making of a user-friendly MAOI diet. *Journal of Clinical Psychiatry, 57,* 99–104.

Giordano, G., Tomassini, L., Cuomo, I., Amici, E., Perrini, F., Callovini, G., Carannante, A., Kotzalidis, G. D., & De Filippis, S. (2020). Aripiprazole long-acting injection during first episode schizophrenia—An exploratory analysis. *Frontiers in Psychiatry, 10,* 935. https://doi.org/10.3389/fpsyt.2019.00935

Goff, D. C., Falkai, P., Fleischhacker, W. W., Girgis, R. R., Kahn, R. M., Uchida, H., Zhao, J., & Lieberman, J. A. (2017). The long-term effects of antipsychotic medication on clinical course in schizophrenia. *American Journal of Psychiatry*, 174(9), 840–849. https://doi.org/10.1176/appi.ajp.2017.16091016

Granger, B. (1999). The discovery of haloperidol. *Encephale*, 25(1), 59–66.

Heal, D. J., Smith, S. L., Gosden, J., & Nutt, D. J. (2013). Amphetamine, past and present—a pharmacological and clinical perspective. *Journal of Psychopharmacology*, 27(6), 479–496. https://doi.org/10.1177/0269881113482532

Kam, H., & Jeong, H. (2020). Pharmacogenomic biomarkers and their applications in psychiatry. *Genes*, 11(12), 1445. https://doi.org/10.3390/genes11121445

Katzman, M. A., Bleau, P., Blier, P., Chokka, P., Kjernisted, K., & Van Ameringen, M. (2014). Canadian clinical practice guidelines for the management of anxiety, posttraumatic stress and obsessive-compulsive disorders. *BMC Psychiatry*, 14(Suppl 1), S1. https://doi.org/10.1186/1471-244x-14-s1-s1

Kennedy, S. H., Lam, R. W., McIntyre, R. S., Tourjman, S. V., Bhat, V., Blier, P., Hasnain, M., Jollant, F., Levitt, A. J., MacQueen, G. M., McInerney, S. J., McIntosh, D., Milev, R. V., Müller, D. J., Parikh, S. V., Pearson, N. L., Ravindran, A. V., & Uher, R. (2016). Canadian network for mood and anxiety treatments (CANMAT) 2016 clinical guidelines for the management of adults with major depressive disorder: Section 3. Pharmacological treatments. *The Canadian Journal of Psychiatry*, 61(9), 540–560. https://doi.org/10.1177/0706743716659417

Kornetova, E. G., Kornetov, A. N., Mednova, I. A., Dubrovskaya, V. V., Boiko, A. S., Bokhan, N. A., Loonen, A. J. M., & Ivanova, S. A. (2019). Changes in body fat and related biochemical parameters associated with atypical antipsychotic drug treatment in schizophrenia patients with or without metabolic syndrome. *Frontiers in Psychiatry*, 10, 803. https://doi.org/10.3389/fpsyt.2019.00803

Kragh, M., Møller, D. N., Wihlborg, C. S., Martiny, K., Larsen, E. R., Videbech, P., & Lindhardt, T. (2016). Experiences of wake and light therapy in patients with depression: A qualitative study. *International Journal of Mental Health Nursing*, 26(2), 170–180. https://doi.org/10.1111/inm.12264

Lefaucheur, J. P., Aleman, A., Baeken, C., Benninger, D. H., Brunelin, J., Di Lazzaro, V., & Ziemann, U. (2020). Evidence-based guidelines on the therapeutic use of repetitive transcranial magnetic stimulation (rTMS): An update (2014–2018). *Clinical Neurophysiology*, 131(2), 474–528. http://doi.org/10.1016/j.clinph.2019.11.002

Łojko, D., & Rybakowski, J. (2017). Atypical depression: current perspectives. *Neuropsychiatric Disease and Treatment*, 13, 2447–2456. https://doi.org/10.2147/ndt.s147317

Magne Bjølset, T., Engedal, K., Šaltytė Benth, J., Bergsholm, P., Strømnes Dybedal, G., Lødøen Gaarden, T., & Tanum, L. (2016). Speed of recovery from disorientation may predict the treatment outcome of electroconvulsive therapy (ECT) in elderly patients with major depression. *Journal of Affective Disorders*, 190, 178–186. https://doi.org/10.1016/j.jad.2015.10.013

Mahmood, I. (2016). Chapter 3: Developmental pharmacology: Impact on pharmacokinetics and pharmacodynamics of drugs. In I. Mahmood & G. Burckart (Eds.), *Fundamentals of pediatric drug dosing* (pp. 23–44). Springer International Publishing.

Małgorzata, P., Paweł, K., Iwona, M. L., Brzostek, T., & Andrzej, P. (2020). Glutamatergic dysregulation in mood disorders: Opportunities for the discovery of novel drug targets. *Expert Opinion on Therapeutic Targets*, 24(12), 1187–1209. https://doi.org/10.1080/14728222.2020.1836160

Martins, M. J., Pereira, A. T., Carvalho, C. B., Castilho, P., Lopes, A. C., Oliveira, A., Roque, C., Mota, D., Tróia, F., Bajouco, M., Madeira, N., Matos, O., Santos, P., Leite, R., Morais, S., Santos, T., Santos, T., Nogueira, V., Santos, V., & Macedo, A. (2016). Antipsychotic Medication Adherence Scale (AMAS): Development and preliminary psychometric properties. *European Psychiatry*, 33(S1), s258–s259. https://doi.org/10.1016/j.eurpsy.2016.01.658

Mentzel, T. Q., van der Snoek, R., Lieverse, R., Oorschot, M., Viechtbauer, W., Bloemen, O., & van Harten, P. N. (2018). Clozapine monotherapy as a treatment for antipsychotic-induced tardive dyskinesia. *The Journal of Clinical Psychiatry*, 79(6). https://doi.org/10.4088/jcp.17r11852

Meyer, J. M. (2007). Antipsychotic safety and efficacy concerns. *Journal of Clinical Psychiatry*, 68(Suppl 14), 20–26.

Mijovic, A., & MacCabe, J. H. (2020). Clozapine-induced agranulocytosis. *Annals of Hematology*, 99(11), 2477–2482. https://doi.org/10.1007/s00277-020-04215-y

Monteleone, P., Cascino, G., Monteleone, A. M., Rocca, P., Rossi, A., Bertolino, A., Aguglia, E., Amore, M., Collantoni, E., Corrivetti, G., Cuomo, A., Bellomo, A., D'Ambrosio, E., Dell'Osso, L., Frascarelli, M., Giordano, G. M., Giuliani, L., Marchesi, C., Montemagni, C., … Maj, M.

(2021). Prevalence of antipsychotic-induced extrapyramidal symptoms and their association with neurocognition and social cognition in outpatients with schizophrenia in the "real-life." *Progress in Neuro-Psychopharmacology and Biological Psychiatry*, 109, 110250. https://doi.org/10.1016/j.pnpbp.2021.110250

Nicolas, J.-M., Bouzom, F., Hugues, C., & Ungell, A.-L. (2017). Oral drug absorption in pediatrics: the intestinal wall, its developmental changes and current tools for predictions. *Biopharmaceutics & Drug Disposition*, 38(3), 209–230. https://doi.org/10.1002/bdd.2052

Nowak, J. K., & Walkowiak, J. (2020). Lithium and coronaviral infections. A scoping review. *F1000Research*, 9, 93. https://doi.org/10.12688/f1000research.22299.2

Nuechterlein, K. H., Ventura, J., Subotnik, K. L., Gretchen-Doorly, D., Turner, L. R., Casaus, L. R., Luo, J., Boucher, M. L., Hayata, J. N., Bell, M. D., & Medalia, A. (2020). A randomized controlled trial of cognitive remediation and long-acting injectable risperidone after a first episode of schizophrenia: Improving cognition and work/school functioning. *Psychological Medicine*, 1–10. Advance online publication. https://doi.org/10.1017/s0033291720003335

Okusanya, B. O., Asaolu, I. O., Ehiri, J. E., Kimaru, L. J., Okechukwu, A., & Rosales, C. (2020). Medical cannabis for the reduction of opioid dosage in the treatment of non-cancer chronic pain: A systematic review. *Systematic Reviews*, 9(1), 1–8. https://doi.org/10.1186/s13643-020-01425-3

Østergaard, S. D., Speed, M. S., Kellner, C. H., Mueller, M., McClintock, S. M., Husain, M. M., Petrides, G., McCall, W. V., & Lisanby, S. H. (2020). Electroconvulsive therapy (ECT) for moderate-severity major depression among the elderly: Data from the pride study. *Journal of Affective Disorders*, 274, 1134–1141. https://doi.org/10.1016/j.jad.2020.05.039

Ott, M., Stegmayr, B., Salander Renberg, E., & Werneke, U. (2016). Lithium intoxication: Incidence, clinical course and renal function—a population-based retrospective cohort study. *Journal of Psychopharmacology*, 30(10), 1008–1019. https://doi.org/10.1177/0269881116652577

Park, L. T., Luckenbaugh, D. A., Pennybaker, S. J., Hopkins, M. A., Henter, I. D., Lener, M. S., Kadriu, B., Ballard, E. D., & Zarate, C. A. (2020). The effects of ketamine on typical and atypical depressive symptoms. *Acta Psychiatrica Scandinavica*, 142(5), 394–401. https://doi.org/10.1111/acps.13216

Paulke, A., Wunder, C., & Toennes, S. W. (2015). Sleep self-intoxication and sleep driving as rare zolpidem-induced complex behaviour. *International Journal of Legal Medicine*, 129(1), 85–88. https://doi.org/10.1007/s00414-014-0997-x

Pluta, M. P., Dziech, M., Czempik, P. F., Szczepańska, A. J., & Krzych, Ł. J. (2020). Antipsychotic Drugs in Prevention of Postoperative Delirium—What Is Known in 2020? *International Journal of Environmental Research and Public Health*, 17(17), 6069. https://doi.org/10.3390/ijerph17176069

Post, R. M. (2016). Treatment of bipolar depression: Evolving recommendations. *Psychiatric Clinics of North America*, 39(1), 11–33. https://doi.org/10.1016/j.psc.2015.09.001

Poyurovsky, M., & Weizman, A. (2020). Treatment of antipsychotic-induced akathisia: Role of serotonin 5-HT2a receptor antagonists. *Drugs*, 80(9), 871–882. https://doi.org/10.1007/s40265-020-01312-0

Preskorn, S. H. (2020). Drug-drug interactions (DDIs) in psychiatric practice, part 9: interactions mediated by drug-metabolizing cytochrome p450 enzymes. *Journal of Psychiatric Practice*, 26(2), 126–134. https://doi.org/10.1097/pra.0000000000000458

Pringsheim, T., Gardner, D., Addington, D., Martino, D., Morgante, F., Ricciardi, L., Poole, N., Remington, G., Edwards, M., Carson, A., & Barnes, T. R. (2018). The assessment and treatment of antipsychotic-induced akathisia. *The Canadian Journal of Psychiatry*, 63(11), 719–729. https://doi.org/10.1177/0706743718760288

Rezansoff, S. N., Moniruzzaman, A., Fazel, S., Procyshyn, R., & Somers, J. M. (2016). Adherence to antipsychotic medication among homeless adults in Vancouver, Canada: A 15-year retrospective cohort study. *Social Psychiatry and Psychiatric Epidemiology*, 51(12), 1623–1632. https://doi.org/10.1007/s00127-016-1259-7

Rieck, K. M., Pagali, S., & Miller, D. M. (2020). Delirium in hospitalized older adults. *Hospital Practice*, 48(Suppl 1), 3–16. https://doi.org/10.1080/21548331.2019.1709359

Rizkalla, M., Kowalkowski, B., & Prozialeck, W. C. (2020). Antidepressant discontinuation syndrome: A common but underappreciated clinical problem. *Journal of Osteopathic Medicine*, 120(3), 174–178. https://doi.org/10.7556/jaoa.2020.030

Sadek, J. (2021). ADHD medications. In *Clinician's guide to psychopharmacology* (pp. 147–189). Springer.

Schou, M. (1978). Lithium treatment. *Western Journal of Medicine*, 128(6), 535–536.

Shnayder, N. A., Bochanova, E. N., Dmitrenko, D. V., & Nasyrova, R. F. (2020). Pharmacogenetics of carbamazepine. *Epilepsy and Paroxysmal Conditions, 11*(4), 364–378. https://doi.org/10.17749/2077-8333.2019.11.4.364-378

Simpson, G. M., & Angus, J. W. S. (1970). A rating scale for extrapyramidal side effects. *Acta Psychiatrica Scandinavica, 212*(Suppl), 11–19. https://doi.org/10.1111/j.1600-0447.1970.tb02066.x

Singh, H., Kaur, S., & Shah, A. (2019). Antidepressant induced bruxism: A literature review. *Journal of Psychiatric Intensive Care, 15*(1), 37–44. https://doi.org/10.20299/jpi.2019.004

Solomon, D. A., Keitner, G. I., Ryan, C. E., & Miller, I. W. (1998). Lithium plus valproate as maintenance polypharmacy for patients with bipolar I disorder. *Journal of Clinical Psychopharmacology, 18*(1), 38–49. https://doi.org/10.1097/00004714-199802000-00007

Spuch, C., López-García, M., Rivera-Baltanás, T., Rodrígues-Amorím, D., & Olivares, J. M. (2020). Does lithium deserve a place in the treatment against COVID-19? A preliminary observational study in six patients, case report. *Frontiers in Pharmacology, 11*, 1347. https://doi.org/10.3389/fphar.2020.557629

Stegmayer, K., Walther, S., & van Harten, P. (2018). Tardive dyskinesia associated with atypical antipsychotics: prevalence, mechanisms and management strategies. *CNS Drugs, 32*(2), 135–147. https://doi.org/10.1007/s40263-018-0494-8

Takeshima, M. (2017). Treating mixed mania/hypomania: A review and synthesis of the evidence. *CNS Spectrums, 22*(2), 177–185. https://doi.org/10.1017/s1092852916000845

Taylor, R. W., Marwood, L., Oprea, E., DeAngel, V., Mather, S., Valentini, B., Zahn, R., Young, A. H., & Cleare, A. J. (2020). Pharmacological augmentation in unipolar depression: A guide to the guidelines. *International Journal of Neuropsychopharmacology, 23*(9), 587–625. https://doi.org/10.1093/ijnp/pyaa033

Van Ameringen, M., Zhang, J., Patterson, B., & Turna, J. (2020). The role of cannabis in treating anxiety. *Current Opinion in Psychiatry, 33*(1), 1–7. https://doi.org/10.1097/yco.0000000000000566

van Diermen, L., Poljac, E., Van der Mast, R., Plasmans, K., Van den Ameele, S., Heijnen, W., Birkenhäger, T., Schrijvers, D., & Kamperman, A. (2020). Toward targeted ECT. *The Journal of Clinical Psychiatry, 82*(1). https://doi.org/10.4088/jcp.20m13287

Won, E., & Kim, Y.-K. (2017). An oldie but goodie: Lithium in the treatment of bipolar disorder through neuroprotective and neurotrophic mechanisms. *International Journal of Molecular Sciences, 18*(12), 2679. https://doi.org/10.3390/ijms18122679

Yatham, L. N., & Kesavan, M. (2017). The treatment of bipolar II disorder. In A. F. Carvalho, & E. Vieta (Eds.), *The treatment of bipolar disorder: Integrative clinical strategies and future directions* (pp. 108–122). Oxford University Press.

Yatham, L. N., Kennedy, S. H., Parikh, S. V., Schaffer, A., Bond, D. J., Frey, B. N., Sharma, V., Goldstein, B. I., Rej, S., Beaulieu, S., Alda, M., MacQueen, G., Milev, R. V., Ravindran, A., O'Donovan, C., McIntosh, D., Lam, R. W., Vazquez, G., Kapc, F., … Berk, M. (2018). Canadian Network for Mood and Anxiety Treatments (CANMAT) and International Society for Bipolar Disorders (ISBD) 2018 guidelines for the management of patients with bipolar disorder. *Bipolar Disorders, 20*(2), 97–170. http://doi.org/10.1111/bdi.12609

Zanardi, R., Prestifilippo, D., Fabbri, C., Colombo, C., Maron, E., & Serretti, A. (2020). Precision psychiatry in clinical practice. *International Journal of Psychiatry in Clinical Practice, 25*, 19–27. https://doi.org/10.1080/13651501.2020.1809680

Zintzaras, E. (2005). Statistical aspects of bioequivalence testing between two medicinal products. *European Journal of Drug Metabolism and Pharmacokinetics, 30*(1–2), 41–46. https://doi.org/10.1007/bf03226406

Cognitive–behavioural therapy (CBT) is a form of psychotherapy that applies the understanding that our thoughts (cognitions) about ourselves, others, and the world influence our emotions and behaviours. When we modify our thoughts, our emotions and behaviours change, too. Knowing this, we are able to identify, analyze, and change, if need be, cognitions that contribute to distressing emotions and problematic behaviours (Beck, 2021). The cognitive interventions in CBT are used to modify maladaptive thinking or beliefs; its behavioural interventions are aimed at decreasing maladaptive responses while increasing adaptive ones, and the learning of new, helpful behavioural practices. Such changes promote more healthy emotional states.

CBT is research-based with its efficacy supported by clinical trials evidence, as well as further understanding achieved through qualitative research findings. It has been shown to be an effective treatment for many mental health problems and disorders, ranging from social phobia and depression to gambling disorder, general anxiety disorder, panic disorder, and posttraumatic stress disorder (PTSD). It is an effective approach to health promotion (see "Research for Best Practice" Box 14.1). Special training is required to become a cognitive–behavioural therapist, but knowledge of CBT principles and interventions is very useful to nurses. It allows nurses to support persons undergoing CBT, but also to help persons change unhealthy behaviours

(e.g., poor eating habits), overcome avoidance behaviours, and deal with stress and anxiety. Knowledge of CBT can help nurses and other healthcare practitioners to better understand and address their own stress and anxiety, common to the demands of care and treatment. In this chapter, examples of research focused on examining CBT's effect on university students' anxieties are featured.

Technology-supported CBT Delivery

CBT can be delivered remotely in real time, similar to in-person therapy situations, via video link (vCBT) or telephone (tCBT), characterized as "high-intensity." Remote CBT can also involve systematic acquisition of information and skills via books (bCBT), computer resources (cCBT), or the internet (iCBT) and are considered "low-intensity" (Wootton, 2016). Both these modalities appear to be similar in acceptability to patients. For instance, the use of technology-delivered (audio- or computer-based) CBT to older adults as intervention in depression was effective in improving mood, acceptable to the older adults, and low-cost (Mortland et al., 2020). Research indicates that both "high-" and "low-intensity" remote treatments can produce significant decrease in symptoms (Wootton). There is some evidence to suggest that digital CBT may produce greater improvements than standard treatment (Felder et al., 2020).

BOX 14.1 Research for Best Practice

NURSING STUDENTS EXPERIENCE CBT STRESS MANAGEMENT INTERVENTION

Terp, U., Bisholt, B., & Hjärthag, F. (2019). Not just tools to handle it: A qualitative study of nursing students' experiences from participating in a cognitive behavioral stress management intervention. *Health Education & Behavior, 46*(6), 922–929. https://doi.org/10.1177/1090198119865319

The Aim: To describe the learning experience of nursing students in a preventive cognitive behavioural therapy–based stress management intervention.

Method: Swedish students (*n* = 14) in their second semester of their nursing education volunteered to participate in a group-delivered intervention that comprised ten sessions for a total of 20 h. Semistructured qualitative interviews were conducted at the completion of the program with participant data interpreted using inductive qualitative content analysis.

Findings: The identified theme was "turning points," defined by the researchers as "a form of learning and development that takes place through experience or insight that in some way reshapes current thoughts, emotions, and behavioral patterns (p. 924)." Participants attributed to the intervention the positive changes to their self-knowledge and deeper insights related to personal patterns and usual reactions, leading to greater self-confidence and belief in their abilities to cope with stress. *Limitations:* As participants are volunteers, there is risk of volunteer bias.

Implications: Research has indicated that stressors associated with nursing education, in addition to those experienced by all university students, include those connected to clinical practice (e.g., perceived inadequate knowledge and skills, fear of making errors). A preventative group CBT-based intervention has the potential to mitigate such stress for nursing students.

KEY CONCEPT

Cognitive–behavioural therapy is a psychotherapy focused on identifying, analyzing, and ultimately changing the habitually inflexible and negative cognitions about oneself, others, and the world that contribute to distress and problematic behaviours.

The ideas underlying CBT can be traced back to ancient times and the Stoic philosopher Epictetus, but it is psychiatrist Aaron Beck and psychologist Albert Ellis who are recognized as separately developing the contemporary therapy of CBT. Each noted that their patients tended to have irrational and inflexible thought patterns that negatively influenced their mood and behaviours. What if these rigid and negative thought patterns could be changed? Would mood improve and behaviour become more functional? By developing interventions that helped individuals change faulty thinking, they discovered that such change did positively affect emotions and behaviours. Albert Ellis termed his therapeutic approach as "Rational Emotive Behavior Therapy." Aaron Beck cofounded *The Beck Institute of Cognitive Behavior Therapy* with his daughter Judith Beck. Although CBT is a mental health treatment, it is based on a cognitive model that is applicable to human experience in all situations. Life skills for problem solving and coping with distress can be learned using this model (see Boxes 14.2 and 14.3).

The Cognitive Model

The cognitive model forms the foundation of CBT, the essence of which is that humans respond primarily to

BOX 14.2 Preparing for the NCLEX: A Cognitive–Behavioural Approach

There is much at stake for nursing students taking credentialing examinations. Writing an examination like the NCLEX can create such anticipatory anxiety that examination performance is diminished. Distorted thinking translates into poor test-taking preparation and behaviour. Recognition of the way thinking impacts performance is an important first step to dealing with the issue. Self-assessment allows for the identification of specific knowledge deficits to be overcome, but negative thinking and problematic behaviours should also be identified. CB techniques such as cognitive restructuring, thought stopping, and visual imagery can then be used to help a student address test anxiety.

BOX 14.3 **Effect of Cognition on Emotion and Behaviour**

In this example, four nursing students in the same clinical group respond to the same situation in four different ways, owing to different patterns of thinking, emotion, and acting.

The Situation: A staff nurse informs the clinical group that they will be responsible for informing the medical team of their assessment of their assigned patient at rounds that day. All the students have been taught, and have clinically used, patient assessment skills.

- **Susanne** thinks, "This is a chance to demonstrate our nursing skills to the medical team. It will be great. We will earn their respect." She tells the staff nurse that she is willing to go first in reporting on her patient.
- **Dylan** thinks, "I know that I can do a thorough assessment on my patient, but I will be so nervous in reporting it at rounds that I will look like an idiot. No one will believe that I know what I am doing." He feels anxious and uncertain and asks himself, "How am I ever going to report to the medical team without embarrassing myself?" He responds behaviourally by checking and rechecking his assessment, much to the consternation of his patient.
- **Jasmine** thinks, "I just know I will miss something important in my patient assessment. If the

team is relying on my information as a basis for her treatment, it may put her at risk. I could do some real harm." Jasmine becomes highly anxious and, behaviourally, when her clinical teacher asks if something is wrong, she responds by saying that she feels ill and asks to leave for the rest of the day.
- **Ella** thinks, "Great. Now we have to perform for the physicians. And medical students! I do not need or value their judgment of my nursing abilities." Ella feels put upon and angry. She responds behaviourally by telling her clinical teacher that the students should not be forced to report to the medical team—they can read the file.

All the students were presented with the identical situation, and all received similar preparation to perform the required skill. The way in which each student *thought about* the situation, however, was very different, consequently leading to emotions as varied as excitement and terror and behaviours as varied as approach and avoidance. It is not the situation itself that influenced the way each of the students responded, but rather each individual's unique interpretation of the situation.

Understanding the way thinking affects emotions and behaviours can be helpful in working with patients who are having difficulty adhering to treatment regimens.

cognitive representations of the environment, and that cognition mediates affect and behaviour (Beck, 2021). In simpler terms, the way we *think* about situations influences our emotions and our behaviour. Our emotions, behaviours, and thoughts all interact in complex and interconnected ways; however, the cognitive model places particular importance on thoughts as the "director" of our experiences (Fig. 14.1). *The* question this model guides us to ask is "What was going through my mind?" (Beck, p. 15).

Cognitive theory proposes that one's perception of situations and events is salient in guiding emotional and behavioural responses (Beck, 2021). Events in and of themselves do not cause us to feel and act in particular ways; rather, it is how we *understand* or think about what happens to us that affects how we *feel* about it and what we *do* about it. Consider, for example, that you are attending a lecture and the professor asks the class if anyone has an opinion about the theory they had just presented. You do have an opinion and when the professor consults the class list and calls your name, would you think, "This is my chance to share my ideas.

I wonder if others will agree?" Or would you think, "Oh no! I don't want to say what I think. It's too risky. What if the class—or worse, the professor—thinks my opinion is stupid?" The way you perceive the situation will determine how you respond.

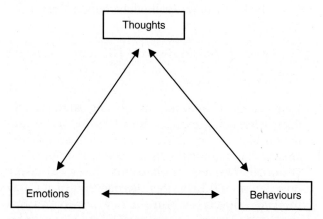

Figure 14.1 Interconnection between thoughts, emotions, and behaviours.

The reasons that individuals perceive, evaluate, and respond to a particular situation or event differently are, in part, accounted for by their core beliefs. See Box 14.3 for an example of students responding differently to the same situation. The cognitive model posits that when an emotion is felt, a thought is behind it, and when behaviour is enacted, a thought is behind it, too.

Levels of Cognition

Cognition has primary importance in CBT, with three levels of cognition being considered: **core beliefs**, **intermediate beliefs**, and **automatic thoughts**.

Core Beliefs

Cognitive theory proposes the existence of core knowledge structures that hold, organize, and interpret all information about one's view of self, others, and the world. These structures are termed core beliefs (or **cognitive schema**) and comprise basic beliefs so fundamental that they tend to be accepted as absolute truths (Beck, 2021). Core beliefs assist in evaluating and assigning meaning to events and thus influence the range of affective and behavioural responses (Beck & Emery, 1985). Core beliefs are so basic that it is challenging to access them or to explicitly identify them and, therefore, are difficult to change. Examples of core beliefs are "I am inadequate," "I am unlovable," "others are not trustworthy," and "the world is an unsafe place."

Core beliefs influence the manner in which we negotiate our way through life. If, for example, individuals hold the belief that they are persons worthy of love then they will likely engage in mutually respectful and fulfilling relationships. Conversely, if the world is believed to be a hostile place in which people are not to be trusted, their outlook may be one of hypervigilance and suspiciousness. They may experience relationships as potentially dangerous. As we go through life, we gather and consider information; our beliefs are processed in a way that is shaped by our view of self, others, and the world. Over time, these beliefs become solidified, rigid, self-confirming, and self-perpetuating in nature (Beck, 2021).

Intermediate Beliefs

Existing at a more accessible level than core beliefs are intermediate beliefs and automatic thoughts. Intermediate beliefs consist of attitudes, rules or expectations, and assumptions that influence one's perceptions, affect, and behaviours (Beck, 2021). They often take the form of "if/then," "should," or "must" statements that are rigid and unrealistic. Our assumptions, rules, and expectations evolve, in part, from the direct teaching or observation of important others early in life. Our cultural background plays a role, too, in creating our understanding and tolerance of what is acceptable. Examples of intermediate beliefs include the following:

- If I'm not liked by everyone, it means I'm no good.
- Assume the worst will happen because it usually does.
- If I show my vulnerability, then I make myself open to attack.
- I must be the best in everything that I do.
- Relationships open you to rejection.

Automatic Thoughts

At an even more superficial level than intermediate beliefs are automatic thoughts. Automatic thoughts are the "knee-jerk" in-the-moment words and images generated in a particular situation. They may not be logical and are often difficult to "shut off." Automatic thoughts are the most accessible of the levels of cognition (Beck, 2021). Although automatic thoughts are accessible, we are not always immediately conscious of their presence. Rather, we may be more aware of the emotion associated with the thought rather than the spontaneous thought itself. In fact, the presence of a strong emotion is often a signal that an important thought is present. For example, when a car cuts you off on the freeway, you might be more likely to respond with anger than to be aware of the thought behind the emotion of anger ("You put the safety of my family at risk!"). In the early phase of therapy, the aim is to bring automatic thoughts into awareness and help us evaluate their impact. As underlying beliefs are revealed, our automatic thoughts begin to make sense (Beck, 2021).

Relationship Between Levels of Cognition

The relationship between automatic thoughts, intermediate beliefs, and core beliefs is illustrated in Figure 14.2. It is demonstrated in two versions of the following situation: A student, Christa, decides to use the library's self-checkout, goes to it, but drops one of the books and bends down to pick it up. At that moment, another student moves to the checkout, piles books on it and begins to scan their library card. Christa thinks, "That person must not have seen me and did not realize that I was here first. I will tell them so they can let me go ahead." This automatic thought spontaneously occurs at the most superficial level of cognition. The deeper intermediate beliefs, rules, and expectations that support this thought might be "People don't intend to be rude." "It's important that we follow social norms." "Being assertive is necessary in social life, especially for women." Under the automatic thoughts and the intermediate rules and expectations is a core belief. "I am worthy of respect." This same situation may be processed very differently by another individual. The three levels still exist; it is the content of the levels that varies. Another student, Sara, may have told herself, "This person saw me drop my book and deliberately used the opportunity to jump into my place at the checkout.

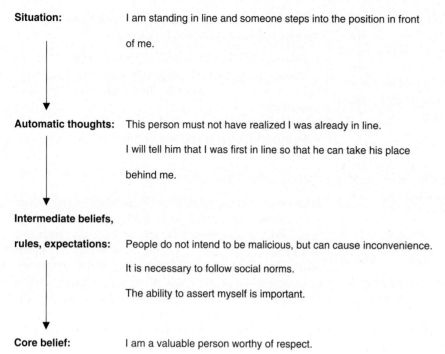

Situation:	I am standing in line and someone steps into the position in front of me.
Automatic thoughts:	This person must not have realized I was already in line.
	I will tell him that I was first in line so that he can take his place behind me.
Intermediate beliefs, rules, expectations:	People do not intend to be malicious, but can cause inconvenience.
	It is necessary to follow social norms.
	The ability to assert myself is important.
Core belief:	I am a valuable person worthy of respect.

Figure 14.2 The relationship between levels of cognition.

They see me as easy to exploit." These automatic thoughts arose from the intermediate beliefs, rules, and expectations that "If you let others exploit you, then it means you are weak and without courage." These thoughts are both driven by a core belief that "My father will not love me if I am not strong." The different thought processes of these two students in this same situation will result in differing emotions and behaviours.

Early experiences, past events, messages from others, and direct observations contribute to the formation of core beliefs and subsequent intermediate beliefs and automatic thoughts. In the individual whose early experiences were primarily nurturing, reliable, and positive, core beliefs are generally an accurate, realistic, and functional reflection of reality. However, the individual who experienced inconsistency, emotional unavailability, and cruelty may develop hypercritical beliefs about the self, others, and the world that are rigid, overgeneralized, and an inaccurate reflection of the current reality. These core beliefs contribute to emotions and behaviours that are intensely negative and harmful.

Principles of Cognitive–Behavioural Therapy

CBT is grounded in a set of specific principles. Treatment strategies employed in CBT are specific to the disorder being treated; however, the basic principles remain common across disorders and are outlined by Judith Beck (2021). A list of these principles appears in Box 14.4.

BOX 14.4 Principles of Treatment

CBT:

1. treatment plans are based on an evolving CB formulation of the patient.
2. requires a sound therapeutic relationship.
3. continuously monitors individual progress.
4. is culturally adapted and tailors treatment to the individual.
5. emphasizes the positive.
6. stresses collaboration and active participation.
7. is aspirational, values based, and goal oriented.
8. initially emphasizes the present.
9. is educative.
10. is time sensitive.
11. sessions are structured.
12. uses guided discovery and teaches individuals to respond to their dysfunctional cognitions.
13. includes Action Plans (therapy homework).
14. uses a variety of techniques to change thinking, mood, and behaviour.

Source: Beck, J. (2021). *Cognitive therapy: Basics and Beyond* (2nd ed., pp. 16–17). Guilford Press.

To provide some understanding of how CBT is enacted, the following is a brief adaptation from the description of CBT principles in action as outlined by Judith Beck (2021).

In CBT, the work with individuals is grounded in a therapeutic relationship, as is care in psychiatric and mental health nursing. Similarly, the formation of an alliance is shaped by the individual's readiness, past experience, strengths, and resources. The culture of the individual may play a role, particularly if the culture of CBT—individual-focused, science-based, rational—is fundamentally different. As with nurses, therapists strive to behave in a culturally respectful way.

The therapist–client relationship needs to be a safe place in which a team of two is formed to set therapeutic goals and develop a treatment plan. CBT is active and educative in nature, as clients learn about the cognitive model and the influence of core and intermediate beliefs on their behaviour. A significant component of therapy is learning what those beliefs are and which are contributing to emotional distress and dysfunctional behaviour. CBT sessions are structured, starting with a renewed connection between client and therapist and a review of the plan of action. Data that the client brings (e.g., mood, automatic thoughts identified, obstacles) sets the session's agenda. Techniques may be used in CBT that are adapted from other therapy approaches, such as gestalt, psychodynamic, or behavioural therapies. There may be integration with mindfulness (see below). Feedback on the treatment strategy and progress is a sessional expectation in CBT, given by both client and therapist.

Treatment Strategies

Both cognitive and behavioural techniques are used to effect change. Some basic CBT strategies are outlined here. Although treatment interventions are described for your understanding, advanced training and clinical supervision are essential to treatment delivery.

Cognitive Techniques

Cognitive techniques revolve primarily around cognitive restructuring, a process that follows a particular path of identifying, analyzing, and modifying the three levels of cognition, beginning with automatic thoughts and working through to core beliefs.

KEY CONCEPT

Cognitive restructuring is a process in which cognitions (automatic thoughts and intermediate and core beliefs) are identified, analyzed, and modified to effect positive change in mood and behaviour.

Identifying Automatic Thoughts

Awareness of one's thinking is the first step toward change. Early in treatment, individuals are often unaware of their internal negative dialogues about themselves, others, and the world. The accompanying emotion may be much more apparent to them than the underlying negative, inflexible thoughts. When introducing individuals to the skill of identifying automatic thoughts, a useful place to begin is to have them attend to shifts in or intensification of their emotions. When a strong emotion is felt or a new emotion is experienced, this is the time that the question "What was going through your mind?" needs to be asked (Beck, 2021). This question often helps individuals to attend to the thinking that drives their emotional experience. For individuals who have difficulty identifying a thought, asking "What image ran through your mind?" may be helpful. Images are another form of cognition (Wenzel, 2017). Another technique to elicit automatic thoughts is to ask the individuals to recount a very recent problematic situation and then encourage them to play back the situation in their mind using all their senses. As the individuals visualize the details of what happened, they are asked questions that will help them identify automatic thoughts and evaluate them for accuracy. Examples of such questions are "What does this situation say about you?" "What does it mean for how others will view you?" "What about this situation is bothering you the most?" (Greenberger & Padesky, 2016).

Evaluating Automatic Thoughts

The goal of evaluating automatic thoughts is to examine thoughts in detail to determine their accuracy. Individuals consider both supporting and unsupported evidence in relation to their automatic thoughts. They need to focus on objective facts rather than interpretations, assumptions, or opinions when generating evidence, although initially this may be difficult. Finding evidence that is unsupportive of automatic thoughts can be aided by key questions such as "What factual evidence supports that automatic thought?" "What are other explanations?" "What are the best-case, worst-case outcomes? The most realistic outcome?" An evaluation of their automatic thoughts often leads individuals to conclude that the evidence for the automatic thought is weaker than that against. This reveals that the thought is not accurate and valid as once considered.

The following case example illustrates the process of evaluating automatic thoughts. A student nurse, Lily, was criticized by a staff nurse for taking too long to complete charting. Lily recognized that the emotions this criticism triggered were shame and fear. Lily then identified related negative automatic thoughts: "They think I'm a bad nurse." "I know they are right. I always mess up." "I am going to fail my practicum." "My parents will be so ashamed." The therapist at health services, whom Lily was seeing, helped Lily determine which automatic thought was the most distressing. It was "I always mess up." Lily was asked to evaluate this thought. What was the evidence of its truth? What factual information did she have? Lily noted this evidence: "I worry so much that I will make a mistake that I take too long to complete tasks." "I am not sleeping well, so being tired slows me down." "My parents were worried about me doing well in the program when I was home last weekend." The therapist then asked Lily to consider evidence that did not support these thoughts. "My midterm clinical evaluation was mostly positive and I was told that some extra lab practice would help me gain more confidence." "My written examination results are above average." "My patient told me yesterday that they appreciated the way I explained aspects of their care as I carried them out."

Evaluating one's automatic thoughts also involves identifying cognitive distortions (thinking errors or problematic thinking styles). These are the characteristic and habitual ways people err in thinking about themselves or others. Thinking errors are problematic as they keep people locked into patterns of negative thinking and behaviour. Burns (2020) has identified types of common cognitive distortions (See Box 14.5). All people engage in distorted thinking; it is not a phenomenon limited to people with mental disorders.

In CBT, the therapist works with the individual to first identify which thinking errors are being used. A handout with a list of cognitive errors and examples may be given to help with identifying and labeling their own thinking distortions. Then the usefulness of such thinking is considered. The aim is to help them respond to their thoughts in a more realistic way. The process of correcting cognitive distortions helps individuals to recognize that their negative automatic thoughts and beliefs about themselves, others, and the world are not valid. They are better prepared to recognize when they are making such errors and to find a clearer way to view an issue or situation. In turn, they will have better options for feeling and responding (Wenzel, 2017).

Returning to our example, Lily recognized having routinely engaged in distorted thinking by jumping to conclusions ("The nurse thinks I'm incompetent." "I am failing.") and overgeneralization ("I always mess up."). Lily worked with a therapist to increase self-awareness of having engaged in this style of thinking and to note how unhelpful and harmful it was.

BOX 14.5 Cognitive Distortions

1. *All-or-nothing thinking*: The tendency to see things in black-and-white, with no shades of grey. There is no middle ground, only extremes, only good or bad. "If I don't receive a 20/20 mark on my lab assignment, it means I will fail this course."

2. *Overgeneralization*: The assumption that one error/problem means a lifetime of the same error/problem. "If I lose this job, I will never succeed in making a living."

3. *Mental filtering*: Filtering out the good things that happen and retaining only the negative. "When I received that award, I could see that Jane didn't think I deserved it."

4. *Discounting the positives*: Refusing to credit the positive aspects of situations. "John said that I looked great today. I guess that I look terrible most days."

5. *Jumping to conclusions*: Concluding things that are not justified based on available evidence. "I saw Peter yawn during my presentation. Everyone was bored." It includes *mind reading*: "My coworker didn't say hello to me today because she's starting to dislike me," and *fortune telling*: "He didn't call me tonight. That's it. He'll never call again."

6. *Labelling*: Putting a negative label on yourself or others as a way to believe that no one can change. "My roommate is a slob. I have to keep everything tidy."

7. *Magnification/minimization*: Over exaggeration of fears, imperfections, or errors. "There is absolutely no way I could have passed that exam. I've totally blown the course."

8. *Personalization and blame*: Feeling responsible for things out of your control. "It is my fault our team lost the game. If only I hadn't dropped the ball in the first half."

9. *Should/must statements*: Thinking in terms of "should" and "must." "I must make no mistakes during the skill laboratory, no matter what."

10. *Emotional reasoning*: Believing something must be true because one "feels" it so strongly, ignoring any evidence to the contrary. "I have friends who say that I'm a good person, but I feel like I'm so bad. They must be wrong."

Adapted from: Burns, D. D. (2020). *Feeling great: The revolutionary new treatment for depression and anxiety.* PESI Publishing and Media.

Modifying Automatic Thoughts

Modification of automatic thoughts is an essential component of CBT. Individuals use what they have learned about identifying and evaluating automatic thoughts to move toward modification. Modifying thoughts involves weighing evidence for and against an automatic thought in an effort to generate a new, more balanced way of thinking. It is not a simple process of changing negative thoughts with positive ones. Not weighing the evidence for automatic positive thoughts is problematic too.

In Lily's case, an examination of the available evidence revealed an alternative understanding of the situation: "I have very high expectations of myself and do not give myself a break when I believe that I have behaved in a less than acceptable way. I screw up at times, but it's relatively infrequent. And I do learn from my mistakes." Making a summary of the evidence regarding an automatic thought is helpful in achieving more balanced thinking. For example, Lily summarized the evidence with "I've jumped to conclusions and acted in negative, unhelpful, and self-harming ways based on those judgments. I am currently doing well on my exams and getting some positive feedback about my clinical practice. I have a strategy now to help me gain confidence: more lab practice." Achieving a more evidence-based viewpoint can relieve the distress triggered by unsupported automatic thoughts.

A *thought record* is a CBT tool to help individuals record their efforts on identifying their automatic thoughts and reactions to them. Three columns can be used to record: (a) a situation with emotional stress; (b) key automatic thoughts; and (c) their emotional reactions and their intensity level. Once the individual gains some experience in working on their cognitive restructuring, other columns may be added, for instance, a column for an adaptive response and another for the outcome of trying out that response.

The *behavioural experiment* is another CBT tool that a therapist may suggest to allow the individual to test their negative automatic thoughts in real life. Does the worst-case scenario that they believed would occur actually happen? If it does, is it as terrible as expected? Did they bear it better than imagined? (Beck, 2021; Wenzel, 2017).

Identifying and Modifying Intermediate Beliefs

The techniques of identifying and modifying automatic thoughts are used with intermediate beliefs or assumptions. Other techniques are also used to get to the deeper level assumptions. Patterns of negative thoughts that emerge in therapy may point to an underlying assumption or core belief. Identifying the rules that individuals live by and expect of others may be useful.

Identifying and Modifying Core Beliefs

Identifying realistic and adaptive core beliefs is an important CBT strategy, as is strengthening them across therapy. Deeply rooted core beliefs may require advanced strategies that include discussing the individual's early life experiences, as core beliefs may be better understood when the context in which they developed is considered. In-depth exploration of painful early experiences, however, is not appropriate in CBT.

Within CBT, individuals identify old, overgeneralized negative beliefs ("I'm scared and all alone in this world."), gather evidence that contradicts them, and form a new adaptive belief ("I have a good friend whom I can count on. We care about and help one another.") The final step is to gather evidence that supports the old belief with the addition of a cognitive reframe ("I find it difficult to trust others so I tend to avoid neighbours and keep co-workers at a distance. This is how I protect myself from getting hurt." "I realize that I am stronger than I imagined. Reaching out to another person does not seem so dangerous after all.")

Behavioural Techniques

Behavioural strategies are primarily utilized in CBT as a way to test and challenge both old maladaptive thinking patterns and newly acquired rational beliefs. Behavioural techniques are employed within the larger scope of CBT and linked back to the cognitive model. *The behavioural experiment*, used as a tool to test negative automatic thoughts, can be used to test and challenge core beliefs. The validity and accuracy of old core beliefs are tested in real-life situations, thus increasing the believability of alternative thoughts. Without this behavioural component, the process of challenging the accuracy and validity of old thoughts and generating new thoughts may be an intellectual exercise and may not lead to meaningful cognitive, emotional, or behavioural change. Behavioural experiments can be challenging for individuals because the prospect of putting new thoughts into action and testing old destructive ways of thinking can be anxiety producing.

Behavioural experiments can be presented to individuals as an opportunity to "test-drive" their new thoughts to see what will really happen as a result. A typical **behavioural experiment** consists of the therapist and the client collaboratively constructing an experiment to test a new belief. For example, the new belief, "I'm a likeable person," could be tested by constructing an experiment in which the client plans to call an acquaintance who also walks their dog at the local dog park and invite them to go together along a path in the river valley. The client makes a prediction about what might happen in the course of the experiment ("They'll agree to go with me, but will find me a bit uninteresting"). Potential obstacles are considered ("I will become nervous and talk only about dogs; therefore, I will be boring"), as well as actions that can be taken to manage the obstacles ("Remind myself that being nervous is okay when you are getting to know people for the first time. Remind myself that even if I only talk about dogs, I can't jump to the conclusion that they will think I'm boring"). The actual result of the experiment is reported: "We walked together with our dogs for an hour and talked about them but about our other interests, too. We have many things in common, including that we are both members of our city's art gallery and we're both shy. They were going to the opening of the exhibit of Picasso's linocut prints and suggested they attend it together. The client takes the next step and rates the support of this new belief. Finally, the client reflects on what has been learned: "If I take the risk of reaching out to others, they can get to know me and we may want to know each other better." Taking action on a new belief as an experiment allows one to experience the change in result. This promotes increased willingness to modify problematic beliefs.

Behavioural Strategies to Modify Symptoms

Numerous types of behavioural strategies for symptom reduction are available, including exposure techniques, relaxation training, and behavioural activation. *Exposure therapy* is utilized in panic disorder, panic disorder with agoraphobia, PTSD, social phobia, and obsessive–compulsive disorder. The common thread among all types of exposure is that they put the individual in contact with feared or avoided thoughts, emotions, behaviours, or situations. To agree to exposure therapy when the idea of being exposed to a highly feared object or situation is terrifying and challenging. The individual's symptoms can be so disruptive to their life, however, that they willingly agree to this strategy. A hoped for outcome to the exposure process is that the individual will discover that an encounter with the feared object or situation will not be as catastrophic as imagined, improving their ability to cope with such an encounter in the future. The most desired outcome is that desensitization to the phobic object or situation will occur. Exposure-based techniques are very specific to the disorder being treated, and the protocols are extensive and comprehensive.

Relaxation strategies, such as controlled breathing and progressive muscle relaxation, may be employed with individuals who have generalized anxiety disorder, panic disorder, and PTSD. These strategies may be useful, as well, to moderate our everyday experiences of anxiety (See Box 14.6, Research for Best Practice). Controlled breathing is the practice of learning how to breathe at an appropriate pace and depth so that this skill can be called on when faced with feared stimuli. The person learns to breathe from the diaphragm rather than the

BOX 14.6 **Research for Best Practice**

WHICH CBT INTERVENTION WORKS BEST FOR TEST ANXIETY: RELAXATION OR IMAGERY RESCRIPTING?

Reiss, N., Warnecke, I., Tolgou, T., Krampen, D., Luks-Krausfrill, U., & Rohrmann, S. (2017). Effects of cognitive behavioural therapy with relaxation vs. imagery rescripting on test anxiety: A randomized controlled trial. *Journal of Affective Disorders, 208,* 483–489.

The Aim: To evaluate the effectiveness of two cognitive behavioural therapy (CBT) group approaches designed to reduce test anxiety.

Method: Students (across faculties; *n* = 138) at two German universities who had a clinical diagnosis of test anxiety were recruited to the study and divided into two treatment groups and a control group, all led by a clinical psychologist. Both treatment groups involved elements of CBT and skill-focused techniques, but relaxation techniques were added to one group; to the other imagery rescripting (i.e., changing the meaning of memories of former aversive experiences) was added. The control was composed of a moderated self-help group (i.e., study and discussion of cases of test anxiety). The groups had weekly 3-hour sessions over 5 weeks. Treatment outcomes were assessed using a test anxiety questionnaire administered prior to and following treatment, and again after 6 months.

Findings: A repeated measures ANOVA for participants with complete data (*n* = 59) indicated a significant reduction of anxiety from baseline to the 6-month follow-up across all three groups.

There was evidence that the image rescripting procedure was helpful in overcoming individual fears.

Limitations: The participants had high levels of test anxiety; the number of participants with complete data was low.

Implications: Group treatments are effective in addressing test anxiety in university settings. While further research is required, the effectiveness of group approaches is important given the high rate of test anxiety at universities.

thorax. Individuals are also educated about the effects of hyperventilation and breath holding, such as increased blood pressure and disturbance of the oxygen–carbon dioxide balance, and how these can worsen anxiety symptoms. Progressive muscle relaxation involves the practice of deliberately tensing and relaxing groups of muscles, beginning with the feet and moving upward to the face. The technique teaches individuals how to relax muscles and induce a sense of physical and mental calmness (see Progressive Muscle Relaxation in Chapter 23). Other relaxation techniques include mindfulness-integrated CBT (MICBT) (see below) and guided imagery (see Chapter 12).

Persons experiencing depression can become immobilized and wait to feel better before engaging in activities. *Behavioural activation* encourages them instead to engage in activity as a way to improve mood. It entails the individual scheduling both necessary and pleasurable activities for the week. The levels of completion and pleasure are rated from 1 to 10. This scheduling is to continue even if the individual has low motivation and rates the pleasure from the activities as low (Sperry & Binensztok, 2019). Experience indicates that as small tasks are accomplished, the person's levels of motivation and pleasure usually increases. For those individuals who resist activity scheduling, discussing current and potential activities within the therapy session can be useful (Beck, 2021).

Mindfulness-Integrated CBT

MICBT is an integration of the mindfulness attitude of acceptance of self, of one's thoughts and emotions, into CBT. CBT is about achieving desired change, but acceptance is a necessary balance to change (Wenzel, 2017). MICBT may be particularly helpful for individuals who worry, who constantly self-criticize, or who concentrate on the negative of life experiences (Beck, 2021).

Grounded in meditation practices, mindfulness is purposefully directing attention on an aspect of the self, such as one's breathing or thoughts or emotions and, most importantly, doing so with openness, nonjudgment, and self-acceptance (Kabat-Zinn, 2013). Its core elements have been identified as attention (receptivity) and awareness (being deeply self-aware and self-monitoring), present-centredness (being in the moment), external events (the outer milieu's impact on the mind and body), and cultivation (the fostering of tranquility and insight); a fifth element, ethical-mindedness (social awareness) links mindfulness to its Buddhist origins as "sati" (Nilsson & Kazemi, 2016).

KEY CONCEPT

Mindfulness is a state achieved by becoming attentive, accepting, and open to the self, to one's thoughts, sensations, and feelings, in the present moment.

Jon Kabat-Zinn (2013) describes an exercise used with those being introduced to mindfulness: eating three raisins. Eating the first raisin is a guided experience as students regard the raisin as if for the time—its colour, shape, feel, smell—allowing any thoughts of raisins to arise (e.g., "I hate raisins" or "I miss Mom's raisin cookies"). Their awareness is moved to the act of eating, the movements of hand, arm, mouth; the experience of salivating, chewing and tasting and swallowing; and, finally, of the body becoming one raisin heavier. The other two raisins are then eaten as the first. Such moment-to-moment attention on our thoughts, body, and emotions is rare for most of us. The "raisin experiment" is in common use today in learning about mindfulness.

Slowing down, achieving calm in our fast-paced world can be highly challenging. Mindfulness can help people to disengage their "automatic pilot" in order to look more carefully at their convictions and thought patterns. The act of pushing away negative thoughts and emotions can actually increase distress. Mindfulness reduces that struggle and allows for calm.

Integrated with CBT, mindfulness promotes a positive approach to obtaining self-understanding of one's thoughts, emotions, and behaviour.

Conclusion

The simple idea that emotion and behaviour are influenced by cognition has generated decades of empirical study, indicating that CBT is a highly effective and cost-efficient treatment for individuals struggling with anxiety, problematic behaviours, and/or mental disorders. The active and collaborative nature of CBT, combined with its orientation toward change, makes it an easy fit with nursing, as is evidenced by the interest and broad appeal of CB interventions among nurses. Psychiatric and mental health nurses are strong advocates of self-reflection and awareness of how one's own experiences influence the therapeutic relationship. With appropriate training, nurses will find CBT to be useful to their therapeutic repertoire. CBT offers an empirically and theoretically sound means to improve, not only the mental health of their individual patients and clients, but their own self-awareness and practice.

🍁 Summary of Key Points

- The cognitive model is based on the idea that the way we think about situations influences our emotion and behaviour.
- CBT is focused on changing negative thought patterns as a means to improve mood and behaviour.
- CBT is a widely researched form of psychotherapy used to treat many mental disorders, including PTSD, bulimia nervosa, panic disorder, and depression.
- The principles of CBT are delineated and act as a fundamental guide to this therapy.
- Cognitive techniques involve cognitive restructuring, a process that follows the steps of identifying, analyzing, and modifying automatic thoughts through to core beliefs.
- Behavioural techniques are used within the cognitive model and are seen as opportunities to test new beliefs.
- Mindfulness is a form of self-awareness training based in meditation and, when integrated with CBT, promotes self-acceptance and awareness and less concentration on self-criticism and negativity.

🧠 Thinking Challenges

1. Toby is a friend in the 2nd year of engineering, who has been feeling "super stressed" about courses and success in the program. Toby has always been a top student, but now is worrying so much that it is interfering with concentration and studying. Toby heard about something called cognitive–behavioural therapy and wonders if it might help. Knowing that you are in your mental health rotation, Toby asks you to explain this therapy. What would you tell Toby about CBT?

2. How do thinking errors contribute to emotional distress?
3. What is the usefulness of behavioural experiments in CBT?
4. What does the integration of mindfulness add to CBT?

> Visit the Point to view suggested responses.
> Go to thePoint.lww.com/activate and use the activation code found in the front of this text to unlock answers to the "Thinking Challenges" and other online resources.

💻 Web Links

https://www.anxietycanada.com/articles/cognitive-behaviour-therapy-cbt/ Anxiety Canada's website has information about CBT, including videos with real stories of individuals' use of CBT and related articles.

http://www.mindfulnessinstitute.ca/ The resources shared at the website of the *mindfulnessinstitute.ca* include information about the emerging research on mindfulness as well as program information.

https://beckinstitute.org/ At this website of *The Beck Institute for Cognitive Behavior Therapy*, there is information about the Institute and, under "Tools and Resources," one can find videos, blogs, and articles freely available.

https://maps.anxietycanada.com/en/ An Anxiety Canada website, *My Anxiety Plans* is a free anxiety management program based on cognitive–behavioural therapy. Taken at one's own pace, there are six units encompassing 45 lessons that take a total of 10 hour to complete.

https://www.anxietycanada.com/resources/mindshift-cbt/ This site has tools for "expanding your comfort zone," creating a "chill zone," a "check-in" tool for keeping track of anxiety and mood over time, and tools and tips for taking better care of yourself, and for goal setting.

References

Beck, J. S. (2021). *Cognitive therapy: Basics and beyond* (3rd ed.). Guilford Press.

Beck, A. T., & Emery, G. (1985). *Anxiety disorders and phobias: A cognitive perspective*. Basic Books.

Burns, D. D. (2020). *Feeling great: The revolutionary new treatment for depression and anxiety*. PESI Publishing and Media.

Felder, J. N., Epel, E. S., Neuhaus, J., Krystal, A. D., & Prather, A. A. (2020). Efficacy of digital cognitive behavioral therapy for the treatment of insomnia symptoms among pregnant women: A randomized clinical trial. *JAMA Psychiatry, 77*, 484–492. https://doi.org/10.1001/jamapsychiatry.2019.4491

Greenberger, D., & Padesky, C. A. (2016). *Mind over mood: Change how you feel by changing the way you think* (2nd ed.). Guilford Press.

Kabat-Zinn, J. (2013). *Full catastrophe living: Using the wisdom of your body and mind to face stress, pain, and illness* (2nd ed.). Random House.

Mortland, M., Shah, A., Meadows, J. T., & Scogin, F. (2020). Development of an audio and computer cognitive behavioral therapy for depression in older adults. *Aging & Mental Health, 24*, 1207–1215. https://doi.org/10.1080/13607863.2019.1609901

Nilsson, H., & Kazemi, A. (2016). Reconciling and thematizing definitions of mindfulness: The big five of mindfulness. *Review of General Psychology, 20*(2), 183–193. https://doi.org/10.1037/gpr0000074

Reiss, N., Warnecke, I., Tolgou, T., Krampen, D., Luks-Krausfrill, U., & Rohrmann, S. (2017). Effects of cognitive behavioral therapy with relaxation vs. imagery rescripting on test anxiety: A randomized controlled trial. *Journal of Affective Disorders, 208*, 483–489. https://doi.org/10.1016/j.jad.2016.10.039

Sperry, L., & Binensztok, V. (2019). *Ultra-brief cognitive behavioral interventions: A new practice model for mental health and integrated care.* Routledge.

Terp, U., Bisholt, B., & Hjärthag, F. (2019). Not just tools to handle it: A qualitative study of nursing students' experiences from participating in a cognitive behavioral stress management intervention. *Health Education & Behavior, 46*(6), 922–929. https://doi.org/ 10.1177/1090198119865319

Wenzel, A. (2017). *Innovations in cognitive behavioral therapy: Strategic interventions for creative practice.* Routledge.

Wootton, B. M. (2016). Remote cognitive-behavior therapy for obsessive-compulsive symptoms: A meta-analysis. *Clinical Psychology Review, 43*, 103–113.

Interventions With Groups

Shelley Marchinko*

Participation in therapeutic groups has powerful treatment effects. Group treatment is effective and efficient for participants to further understand themselves in relation to others through interaction, gain new knowledge and social skills, conquer unwanted thoughts and feelings, and change behaviours. For effective interventions, the nurse must possess leadership skills that can shape, enhance, and monitor group interactions. The decisions regarding which interventions fit best are complex and dependent upon the purpose of the group. Competent group skill development requires the ability to critically select and modify techniques to best accommodate the particular practice conditions. This applies across diverse situations from providing patient and family education or conducting support groups to direct care provision, case management, and program leadership. Understanding group skills and dynamics is also increasingly relevant to contemporary health care education and service delivery with emphasis on effective interprofessional practice collaboration and teamwork (Canadian Interprofessional Health Collaborative, 2010); relationship communication for healthcare professionals (Pagano, 2015); racial and cultural diversity in groups (McRae & Short, 2010); and participatory and transformative pedagogies (Taylor & Cranston, 2012). A challenge in group intervention is the shift from a primarily individual focus to consideration of interpersonal and whole-group interactions. This chapter presents relevant group concepts for psychiatric mental health (PMH) nurses. Group leadership is explored with special emphasis on the groups relevant to PMH nursing practice.

Group: Definitions and Concepts

There are many different definitions of a group. Psychoanalytic tradition draws from the work of Sigmund Freud and considers group interaction as a recapitulation of the family of origin, where unconscious conflicts are interpreted and reexamined. Contemporary psychodynamic theories consider groups a combination of group dynamics and interpersonal and intrapsychic transactions (Rutan et al., 2014). Yalom (1998) and Yalom and Leszcz (2005) suggest that a group is a social microcosm of interpersonal dynamics and advocate a here-and-now, self-reflective approach. The cognitive–behavioural approach considers a group a social arena for corrective change in maladaptive thinking and behaviour patterns, whereas, according to systems theory, a group consists of parts or components that exist to perform some activity or purpose. As group members interact, subsystems form, challenging leaders to understand

---

*Adapted from the chapter "Interventions with Groups" by Carol Ewashen

boundary realignments and the effects of subcomponents on the system and to improve interpersonal communication. A more contemporary development that draws from the rich history of group work and apparent across a wide range of settings is the prevention group that utilizes a full range of group processes, constructive interactions, and positive group cohesion to reduce risk while promoting health and wellness (Harpine, 2013, 2015; Harpine et al., 2010).

A global, but rather simple, definition of a group is two or more people who are in an interdependent relationship with one another (Forsyth & Diederich, 2014). The simplicity of the definition is misleading because interactions within groups, or group dynamics, are anything but simple. Group dynamics influence the group's development and process. In fact, it takes an astute observer to determine the real dynamics of a group and the effects. No matter the type of group, its theoretic orientation, or its purpose, group dynamics influence the effectiveness of a group intervention. Best practice requires that group facilitators understand and articulate the theoretical framework guiding their practice, including the rationale for use of specific techniques and interventions.

In this text, a group is defined as "two or more individuals who are connected to one another by social relationships" (Forsyth, 2006, p. 3). Groups are considered as social microcosms: dynamic living systems of interdependent relations that acquire and expend energy, sustain structure and functionalities, and respond to changing circumstances with capabilities for transformation (Forsyth & Diederich, 2014). As Susan Day states, "at the heart of group is a learning process in a social setting" (2014, p. 25). Groups can be further defined according to the number of people or the relationship of members. A dyad is a group of two people, such as a married couple, siblings, or parent and child. A triad is a group of three people. A family is a special type of group and is discussed in Chapter 16.

KEY CONCEPT

A group is "two or more individuals who are connected to one another by social relationships" (Forsyth, 2006, p. 3). "At the heart of group is a learning process in a social setting" (Day, 2014, p. 25).

Open Versus Closed Groups

A group can be viewed as either an open or a closed system. In an **open group**, new members are welcomed and provided time to learn group norms and expectations. For example, a newly admitted patient may join an anger management group that is part of an ongoing program in an inpatient unit. It is important to help new members engage with the group by inviting member-to-

member interaction. The advantage of an open group is that participants can join at any time. In addition, these groups can function on an ongoing basis and thus can be available to more people.

In a **closed group**, all members begin at the same time, and no new members are admitted. If a member of a closed group leaves, no replacement joins. Advantages of a closed group are that the participants get to know one another over time, the group becomes more cohesive, and members move concurrently through the group process. Closed groups also lend themselves to confidentiality amongst members, as well as a chance to identify with others with similar experiences. For example, a person with an addiction may choose to attend closed-group meetings as part of the closed 12-step program of Alcoholics Anonymous. However, implementing closed-group interventions is often difficult, especially in tertiary settings where the length of stay is short and participant readiness for group work varies greatly.

Group Size

Group size is an important consideration in forming group programs. Many mental health professionals favour small groups, but large groups can also be effective. The age of participants, the group's purpose, the leader's abilities, participant availability, and the resources available impact the decision of whether to form a small or large group.

Small groups (usually a minimum of three and no more than 10 members) become more cohesive, are less likely to form subgroups, and can provide a richer interpersonal experience than large groups. Small groups may function with one group leader, although many small groups are led by two people. An ideal small group is about seven to eight people in addition to the leader or leaders (Corey, 2013; Myers & Anderson, 2020). Small groups often are used for people who are trying to deal with complex emotional issues such as depression, anxiety, eating disorders, substance use disorder, sexual abuse, or trauma. They are also ideal for individuals or families who require more specialized intervention such as families in recovery (Zimmerman & Winek, 2013). These groups work best if they are closed to new members or if new members are gradually introduced. One disadvantage of small groups relates to the loss of members. If places are unfilled, then the group dynamics change, which may alter therapeutic effectiveness.

A large group (more than 10 members) can be therapeutic as well as cost-effective. Some research suggests that large intervention and prevention groups are effective for specific problems, such as smoking, or for settings such as schools and community (Harpine, 2013; McWhirter & McWhirter, 2010). A large group can be ongoing and open-ended. In large group intervention, a challenge for the nurse leader is to include all members in discussion, preventing a sense of alienation with the potential for member dropout.

Leading a group, whether small or large, is complex because of the number of potential interactions, relationships, and conflicts that can form. The leader needs both presentation and group leadership skills. Kottler and Englar-Carlson (2010) suggest that group work requires a different sort of mindset. It is insufficient to be purely a leader—a leader must practice in a therapeutic or facilitative manner while in the midst of a complex interactive event. Practitioners who take on *leadership* of groups require education and supervised training for competent, accountable, and ethical group practices. In large groups, the leader is often both a presenter of educative information and a facilitator of experiential learning among participants. In-depth reflection on participants' feelings and thoughts may not be the focus of group work. Depending on the theoretic orientation and the purpose of the group, leadership style and interventions must change to be effective in meeting the goals of small or large groups.

Group Development

The development of a group is a process much like the development of therapeutic relationships (see Chapter 7). Many researchers view group development as a sequence of phases, particularly in small groups (see Table 15.1). Although models of group development differ, most follow a pattern of a beginning, middle, and ending stage (DeLucia-Waack et al., 2014). These stages should be thought of not as a straight line with one preceding another, but as a dynamic and iterative process with continual revisiting and reexamining of group interactions, changes, and progress toward established goals.

KEY CONCEPT

Group process is "what is happening" in the group. It is how each member and the whole group interacts and relates with each other as a whole group, which involves nonverbal communications, group mood, and group atmosphere, including successes and tensions.

Beginning Stage

Group members get to know one another and the group leader when a group begins. The length of the beginning stage depends on, among other variables, the purpose of the group, the number of members, and the skill of the leader. It may last for only a few sessions or several. "Honeymoon" behaviours characterize the beginning of this stage, and "conflict" emerges at the end. During the initial sessions, members usually are polite and congenial, displaying behaviours typical of those in new social situations. They are "good" and often intellectualize problems; that is, emotional conflict or stress is minimized by excessively using abstract thinking or generalizations. Members are usually anxious and sometimes act in ways that do not truly represent their feelings. In the first few sessions, members test whether they can trust one another. Sometime after the initial sessions, group members experience a period of conflict, either among themselves or with the leader. This conflict is a normal part of group development as members differentiate from each other, and many believe that negotiating conflict and differentiation satisfactorily is necessary to move into a productive working phase. Sometimes, one or more group members become the "scapegoat," or the "one who is blamed or punished for the sins of others" ("scapegoat", n.d., para1). While a scapegoat

Table 15.1 Comparison of Models of Group Development

Tuckman (1965)	Garland et al. (1973)	Corey et al. (2013)
Forming: Get to know one another and form a group	*Theme in all stages: Closeness Pregroup* *Forming*: Preparing for and deciding if this is the right group	*Preaffiliation*: Approach and avoidance; ambivalence around involvement
Storming: Tension and conflict occur; subgroups form and clash with each other	*Power and control*: Testing out and vying for status, authority, autonomy, influence, and connection	*Initial stage*: Orienting; forming relations; establishing group structure and climate of trust
Norming: Develop norms for how to work with each other	*Intimacy*: More intense personal involvement and recognition of others; emergent growth	*Transition*: Emerging differences and potential for conflict
Performing: Reach consensus and develop cooperative relationships	*Differentiation*: Accept uniqueness of each with interdependence; cohesion	*Working*: Involved, interactive, and committed to engaging in productive group work
Adjourning: End of relationships and orientation to the future; sadness and appreciation	*Separation*: Moving apart; review and evaluation	*Final stage*: Consolidation of learning; sadness and anxiety with leaving

often performs a central function for the group, intervening to therapeutically process scapegoating is complex but necessary: a group leader needs to ensure the group is a safe place. The leader may do so by noting the way the scapegoat behaviour relates to other members' issues and may be able to help the scapegoat get beyond such a role, which could be one held in their family of origin (Moreno, 2007).

Middle (Working) Stage

The middle, or working, stage of groups involves a real sharing of ideas and the development of closeness. A group-as-a-whole culture may emerge that is distinct from the individual personalities of its members. The group develops its own rules and rituals and has its own behavioural norms; for example, groups develop regular patterns of seating and interaction. Group norms are formed through the majority of members accepting or rejecting certain behaviour. During this stage, the group realizes its purpose. If the purpose is education, then the participants engage in learning new content or skills. If the aim of the group is to share feelings and experiences, then these activities consume group meetings. The group members take responsibility for starting on time during this stage, and the leader often needs to remind members when it is time to stop.

Ending (Termination) Stage

Ending, or termination, and saying goodbyes can be difficult for a group, especially a successful therapeutic one. During the final stages, members begin to separate and may grieve the loss of the group closeness while transitioning to reestablish themselves as individuals. Individuals terminate and say goodbyes from groups as they do from other relationships (see Chapter 7). One person may not attend the last session, another person may bring up issues that the group has already addressed, and others may demonstrate anger or hostility. During this stage of adjournment, group leaders should recognize these difficult emotional responses and help facilitate the farewell process of saying goodbye to the group and to each other (Pessagno, 2022).

Roles of Group Members

There are two **formal group roles**: the leader and the members. In small groups, however, members often assume **informal group roles** or positions in the group with rights and duties that are directed toward one or more group members. Informal roles can be categorized as task, maintenance, or individual roles. Group roles can be thought of as the different hats members try on and learn from while engaged in a group (Myers & Anderson, 2020). These roles can either facilitate or obstruct the group process and goals.

Task functions involve the business of the group or "keeping things focused." Individuals who assume this function keep the group focused on a main purpose. For any group to be successful, it must have members who assume some of these task roles, such as *information seeker* (asks for clarification), *coordinator* (spells out relationships between ideas), and *recorder* (keeper of the minutes). **Maintenance functions** facilitate the building of group-centred attitudes, behaviours, and processes. Members functioning in maintenance roles help by ensuring a consistent start time, assisting individuals to compromise, and encouraging everyone's participation. These members facilitate maintaining group cohesiveness and may have difficulty with group conflict and differentiation. The *harmonizer* (keeps the peace), *compromiser* (gives and takes), and *standard setter* (sets expectations) are examples of maintenance roles. In a successful group, members take on and learn from both group task and maintenance functions (see Table 15.2). Leader and member responsibilities and functions shift depending upon the group stage and task.

Deviant roles are member roles that detract from group functioning (Myers & Anderson, 2020). These roles are considered dysfunctional to the group, often antagonistic to group building and group maintenance, and they may detract from the group purpose and cohesion. For example, someone who dominates the group conversation inhibits group interaction and interferes with the work of the group and keeping members on task. When deviant roles dominate, the risk is that neither the group task nor group maintenance function is accomplished. Deviant role examples include the aggressor, blocker, recognition seeker, and dominator.

While acknowledged in scholarly and popular literature, member role classification and related functions in contemporary group work have become more controversial. Critiques include the dangers of decontextualizing, generalizing, and categorizing people as well as the potential "colonizing" effects when placing people in pre-existing schemas that may negatively define people (Kottler & Englar-Carlson, 2010). While it is important for the leader to recognize that all groups function through a division of labour, the leader's primary responsibility is to facilitate all members in learning the functions of productive group work in relation to self, others, and group goals. This is especially challenging in contemporary practice where increasingly diverse and multicultural populations are served and where racial and cultural dynamics in group work and member roles cannot be underestimated or silenced (McRae & Short, 2010).

Group Communication

The main responsibilities of group leadership are to *actively listen* and to facilitate both verbal and nonverbal member-to-member communication to meet the

Table 15.2 Leader and Member Responsibilities and Functions

Group Stage	Leader	Member
Pregroup: Formation of a group *Informed decision making:* How does this group fit with this member this purpose?	*Design and plan the group:* Purpose, structure, process, evaluation methods. Solicit group membership. Conduct pregroup screening interviews. Determine the group composition. Provide orientation to members.	*To determine:* Is the group right for me? Do I have enough knowledge to understand the group purpose and process? What do I want from the group experience? How do my expectations fit with the group expectations?
Initial Stage Orientation, exploration, and setting the structure of the group Creating a safe place Sharing information Engaging each other and as a whole group around purpose	Orient group members. Establish ground rules, norms, and expectations. Encourage all members to be involved and express expectations, reactions, and concerns. Clarify understandings. Be open with members' concerns and questions. Provide guidance yet encourage member interaction and initiative.	*To work through:* Will I be accepted? What will the leader think of me? What is expected of me? Establish trust. Form relations with others. Express thoughts, feelings, expectations, and reservations. Become involved. Set goals for self and self-in-relation to others. Be respectful of others. Learn well and share understandings.
Transition Increased anxiety and emergence of differences with potential for conflict Reluctance to voice concerns or frustrations	Teach members the value of recognizing conflict, naming the issue, and negotiating a win–win situation. Practice directness and tactfulness in naming issues in the here and now. Encourage members to share reactions while maintaining a safe environment. Intervene with sensitivity and prevent scapegoating of a particular member. Encourage participatory interaction. Reinforce learning of self in relation to others negotiating difference/conflict in group.	Recognize own defenses and resistances. Recognize and express reactions to the group. Learn to constructively confront issues. Work through conflicts and differences rather than withdraw or form subgroups.
Working High trust High group cohesion High productivity Interactive with willingness to take risks Supportive hopeful climate	Exemplify caring confrontation, disclosure of issues, and support to others. Encourage member risk taking. Interpret meanings of behaviours and interpersonal patterns in group. Explore group themes. Encourage translating insight into action in daily living.	Practice openness with issues. Offer feedback to others. Practice new skills and behaviours in daily life. Initiate constructive challenge and support to others. Initiate active involvement with others.
Final Stage Saying goodbyes Reflection on learning, relations, changes made, and challenges ahead	Encourage saying of goodbyes to each other. Provide opportunity for members to provide feedback to each other. Reinforce changes made. Ensure members have the resources to enable further progress. Reemphasize the importance of confidentiality.	Acknowledge thoughts and feelings with leaving the group. Say goodbye to each member and to the leader. Review gains made and complete unfinished business. Evaluate the impact of the group. Plan for the future.

Adapted from Corey, M., Corey, G., & Corey, C. (2013). *Groups: Process and practice* (8th ed.). Brooks/Cole.

treatment goals of the individual members and the entire group. Developing trusting, working relationships within groups is more complicated than developing a single relationship with another person because of the number of people involved. The communication techniques used in establishing and maintaining individual relationships are similar for groups, but the leader also attends to the communication patterns among the members, the member-to-member communications.

Relational Communication

Group interaction can be viewed as relational communication that is dynamic and variable. It has recognizable phases and interaction patterns oriented to growth and connection. Some patterns of interaction (e.g., sequences of speaking and acting) are more fixed while others are flexible (Clark, 2009). Relational communication posits that human beings yearn for connection, yet paradoxically, patterns of disconnection also occur in developing increasingly complex relational repertoires over time (Comstock et al., 2002; Fedele, 2004).

Interaction Patterns

Asking a colleague to observe and record content and interaction is a useful technique in determining the interaction patterns within a group. The leader may also use an audio or video recorder. In such cases, ethical guidelines must be followed and with the informed consent of group members.

In some groups, one person may always change the subject when another raises a sensitive topic. One person may always speak after another. People who sit next to each other tend to communicate among themselves. By analyzing the group event, content, process, and relational patterns, the leader can determine the existence of communication pathways and form interpretations—who is most liked in the group, who occupies a position of power, what subgroups have formed, where is connection growth-producing, and who is isolated and disconnecting from the group. Burtis and Turman's (2006) network analysis for group discussion provides a way to diagram connections among members, frequency of connections, and interactional patterns. Usually, those who are well liked or display leadership abilities tend to be chosen for interactions more often than do those who are less well liked (see Fig. 15.1). In one study of

communication networks, members who exhibited more dominant behaviours or whom the group perceived as being dominant emerged as more central to the group's communication networks and both sent and received more messages. The study also found that the task at hand affects the communication network. Groups that worked on low-complexity tasks had more centralized communication than when they worked on high-complexity tasks (Brown & Miller, 2000).

Group Themes

Group themes are the collective socioemotional and conceptual underpinnings of a group and express the members' underlying concerns or feelings, regardless of the group purpose. Themes that emerge in groups help members to understand group dynamics. Different groups have different themes. For example, three themes that emerged for a support group for grieving children included vulnerability, the importance of maintaining memories, and the contribution of the group to the process of grieving. Although some predictable themes occur in groups, the obvious or assumed themes at the beginning may actually wind up differing as the process continues. In one hospice support group, the members seemed to be focusing on the memories of their loved ones. However, upon closer examination of the thematic content of group interactions, the discussion was revolving around financial planning for the future (Graham & Sontag, 2011).

Nonverbal Communication

Nonverbal communication is important to understanding group relations. All members, not just the group leader, observe the eye contact, posture, and body gestures of the participants. What is expressed is the result of individual and group, as well as internal and external, processes. For example, if one member is explaining a painful experience and another member looks away and tries to engage still another, then the self-disclosing member may feel devalued and rejected because they interpret the behaviour as disruptive and disinterest. However, if the leader interprets the behaviour as anxiety over the topic, then the leader may intervene and try to engage the other member in sharing reactions to the topic, the anxiety, and the impact on building relations with others.

The leader(s) should remain attuned to the nonverbal behaviour of group members during each session and the effect on group climate and process. Often, one or two people can set the overall mood of the group. Someone who comes to a session very sad or angry can set a tone of sadness or anger for the whole group. An astute group leader recognizes the effects of an individual's mood on the total group. If the purpose of the group is to process emotions, then the group leader may invite

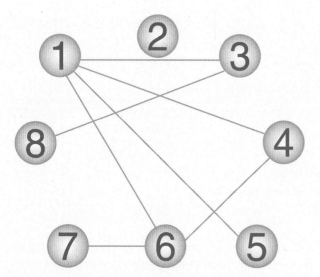

Figure 15.1 Network analysis of group discussion. In this analysis, response pattern was recorded during member interaction. Group members interacted with number *1* the most. Therefore, number *1* is the over-chosen person. Numbers *5* and *7* are under-chosen. Number *2* is never-chosen and is determined to be the isolate.

members to discuss emotional issues at the beginning of the session. The leader thus acknowledges the mood of the person(s) experiencing this and encourages discussion regarding the effect on other group members. If the group's purpose is inconsistent with self-disclosure of personal problems, then the nurse should acknowledge the individual member's distress yet set limits while maintaining the group focus. In this instance, the nurse would limit repeated episodes of self-disclosure from the member(s) or others and redirect discussion to the group task.

Group Norms and Standards

Groups develop norms or rules and standards that establish acceptable group behaviours. Some norms are formalized, such as meeting as a group on time, but others are never really formalized. These standards encourage conformity of behaviour among group members. The group discourages deviations from these established norms. A group member has four options in relation to norms: conform, change the norm, be deviant, or leave the group. Open discussion that encourages healthy interaction while addressing unhelpful or problematic behaviours is one of the most successful ways of renegotiating group norms. *Leadership* is critical in establishing group norms consistent with the group goals to effect desired changes.

Group Cohesion

One of the goals of most group leaders is to foster **group cohesion,** a sense of "we-ness" as a group, where members feel they belong and draw comfort from their peers and where high levels of participation and involvement among members is evident (Pessagno, 2022). Group cohesion through engaging all members in the group process. This involves close monitoring of the group atmosphere to develop a sense of belonging and commitment to the group goals. A particularly effective intervention for enhancing group cohesion is encouraging member-to-member interaction. In supportive and educational groups, leaders can promote social interaction with minimal supervision through organizing refreshment periods and team-building exercises. Cohesiveness is especially important in health education groups that focus on health maintenance behaviours such as exercise and weight control.

Dimock and Kass (2011) state that cohesion is like the glue that holds the group together and that if cohesion decreases, then the group may begin to fall apart. Cohesion is a powerful force that motivates members and correlates with outcomes. In cohesive groups, members are committed to the existence of the group. In large heterogeneous groups, cohesiveness tends to be decreased, with subsequent decreased performance among group

members in completing tasks. Cohesiveness promotes job satisfaction and higher performance when members are strongly committed to completing a task and the leader encourages equal participation (Steinhardt et al., 2003). However, cohesiveness can be a double-edged sword. Members in very cohesive groups are more likely to transgress personal boundaries. Too much cohesiveness can exert powerful social pressure to conform to group standards with low tolerance for difference, while too little cohesiveness can result in mistrust, lack of engagement, and eventual disbanding of the group.

Groupthink and Decision Making

Groups that are strong and healthy encourage creativity, risk taking, differentiation, and change while remaining respectful of all members. Healthy groups encourage aligning with group norms and standards while remaining respectful of each member's unique contributions. However, if feelings of unity become too intense and members are overly invested in maintaining the status quo, then the phenomenon of **groupthink** can occur. Groupthink is the tendency of group members to isolate as a group, avoid conflict, maintain homogeneity, and adopt a closed-mindedness that is often congruent with a lack of impartial group leadership (Janis, 1982; Myers & Anderson, 2020). Such tendencies can lead to poor group decisions. With groupthink, striving for uniformity overrides realistic, fair, and just appraisal of alternative courses of action. Other factors that support groupthink include a charismatic leader whose opinion is known, the interpretation of silence as agreement when members may be afraid of censure, a decision of substantial consequence, and time pressures (Janis, 1972, as cited in Forsyth, 2020; Parks, 2020). Groupthink was demonstrated during the COVID-19 pandemic by groups protesting against public health measures necessary to limiting spread of the virus (Forsyth, 2020).

Nurse leaders are responsible for mobilizing therapeutic and growth fostering factors to support healthy group development and prevent a stagnating groupthink consensus. What factors to mobilize and when depend on the type, purpose, and stage of the group. Supportive factors often emerge spontaneously and include universality, altruism, hope, and acceptance (Pessagno, 2022). **Therapeutic factors** proposed by Yalom and Leszcz (2005), also referred to as principles, can be applied to all groups, regardless of the type or theoretical orientation. There are (Pessagno, 2022)

- the instillation of hope
- universality
- imparting information
- altruism
- the corrective recapitulation of the primary family group
- development of socialization techniques
- imitative behaviour

- interpersonal learning
- group cohesiveness
- catharsis
- existential factors

Growth fostering relations are characterized by relational resilience and include the following dimensions: vitality and energy, capacity and desire for action, awareness of self in relation to others, self-worth, and desire for connection (Miller, 1986), as well as authenticity, empathy, and empowerment (Hartling, 2013).

Group Leadership

In the beginning stage of a group, the group leader establishes the presence of each member; constructs a working environment; builds a working relationship with the group and among participants; and clarifies outcomes, processes, and commitments related to the group purpose (Corey et al., 2013). The leader also considers when and how to participate while attempting to understand the group process. Depending on the purpose of the group and the stage of development, the leader position shifts, for example, from primarily supportive to educative with provision of information to interpretive of **group dynamics**. The leader reflects on, evaluates, and responds to promote effective group work. Leader intervention skills include attention to process while considering timing of interventions, when to clarify and when to interpret, when to intervene with individuals, and when to intervene with the group as a whole. Various techniques and strategies enhance the leader's ability to lead the group effectively and help the group attain its goals (see Table 15.3).

Table 15.3 Techniques in Leading Groups

Technique	Purpose	Example
Support: giving feedback that provides a climate of emotional support	Helps a person or group continue with ongoing activities Informs group about what the leader thinks is important Creates a climate for expressing unpopular ideas Helps the more quiet and fearful members speak up	"We really appreciate your sharing that experience with us. It sounds like it was quite painful."
Confrontation: challenging a participant (needs to be done in a supportive environment)	Helps individuals learn something about themselves Helps reduce some forms of disruptive behaviour Helps members deal more openly and directly with one another	"Tom, this is the third time that you have changed the subject when we have talked about spouse abuse. Is something going on?"
Information and suggestions: sharing expertise and knowledge that the members do not have	Provides information that members can use once they have examined and evaluated it Helps focus group's task and goals	"The medication that you are taking may be causing you to be sleepy."
Summarizing: statements at the end of the session that highlight the session's discussion, any problem resolution, and unresolved problems	Provides continuity from one session to the next Brings to focus still-unresolved issues Organizes past in ways that clarify Brings to focus themes and patterns of interaction	"This session we discussed Sharon's medication problems, and she will be following up with her physicians."
Clarification: restatement of an interaction	Checks on the meanings of the interaction and communication Avoids faulty communication Facilitates focus on substantive issues rather than allowing members to be sidetracked into misunderstandings	"What I heard you say was that you are feeling very sad right now. Is that correct?"
Probing and questioning: a technique for the experienced group leader that asks for more information	Helps members expand on what they were saying (when they are ready to) Gets a more extensive and wider range of information Invites members to explore their ideas in greater detail	"Could you tell us more about your relationship with your parents?"
Repeating, paraphrasing, highlighting: a simple act of repeating what was just said	Facilitates communication among group members Corrects inaccurate communication or emphasizes accurate communication	*Member*: "I forgot about my wife's birthday." *Leader*: "You forgot your wife's birthday."
Reflecting feelings: identifying feelings that are being expressed	Orients members to the feelings that may lie behind what is being said or done Helps members deal with issues they might otherwise avoid or miss	"You sound upset."
Reflecting behaviour: identifying behaviours that are occurring	Gives members an opportunity to see how their behaviour appears to others and to evaluate its consequences Helps members to understand others' perceptions and responses to them	"I notice that when the topic of sex is brought up, you look down and shift in your chair."

Adapted from Sampson, E., & Marthas, M. (1990). *Group process for the health professions* (pp. 222–224). Delmar.

One of the most important **group leadership** skills is *active listening*. A leader who practices active listening provides group members with someone who is responsive to what they say. A group leader who listens also models listening behaviour for others, which helps them improve their skills. Listening enables the leader to process events and track interactions. The leader should be able to listen to the group members and formulate responses based on an understanding of the discussion. Members may need to learn to listen to one another, track discussions without changing the subject, and learn to not speak while others are talking.

The leader tracks the *verbal and nonverbal interactions* throughout the group. Depending on the group purpose, leaders may keep this information private to understand the group process or they may share the observations with the group. For example, if the purpose of the group is psychoeducational, the leader may use the information to facilitate the best learning environment. The leader may point out patterns of interaction if the purpose of the group is to improve the self-awareness and interaction skills of members. The leader needs to be clear about the theoretical orientation and purpose of the group and tailor leadership strategies accordingly.

Additional leadership skills include providing each member with an opportunity to contribute and to demonstrate respect of other's ideas. A leader must also consider the degree of member disclosure warranted in each situation. Leaders tend to be more expressive and interactive in supportive and educative groups. A good rule of thumb in relation to leader self-disclosure is to consider whether the disclosure furthers the purposes of the group. A leader is responsible for understanding the intent and impact of leader self-disclosure on both individual members and the group as a whole. It is also assumed that a leader will engage in continuous learning through ongoing critical reflection with opportunity for regular supervision.

Some generally accepted guidelines in leading groups include establishing group structure and norms by setting start and stop times, arranging for the introduction of new members, and listening while other people talk. Leaders explain these group norms or rules at the first group meeting and continue structuring as an ongoing process. An important group rule is to always begin and end at the scheduled time. This sets a clear and reliable structure that helps reduce initial anxieties, educate members about group process, and encourage members to acquire skills that contribute to a successful group experience.

Understanding different group leadership styles can be useful in deciding which style fits which group situation. Leadership style is influenced by the group leader's personal characteristics and behaviours, theoretic background, and the group structure and purpose. Often leaders have a dominant style that fits more comfortably with who they are; however, developing a repertoire of different styles offers a wider range of interventions. Regardless of style, a leader remains fair and respectful, avoiding favouritism and encouraging participation and involvement of all members with each other (DeLucia-Waack et al., 2014; Pessagno, 2022).

Typology of Leadership Styles

Whatever the leader's theoretic background, leadership styles can be viewed more traditionally as a continuum from direct to indirect or, in keeping with contemporary literature, as transformational, authentic, and/or situational (Benson, 2010; Crowell, 2011). In the *direct leadership style*, the leader is actively authoritarian and controls the interaction by giving directions and information and allowing little discussion. The authoritarian leader literally tells the members what to do. On the other end of the continuum is *indirect leadership*, a form of laissez-faire, where the leader is primarily passive, reflects the group members' discussion, and offers little guidance or information to the group. Leadership is inadequate and lacking.

Effective group leadership is flexible and considers the group task and when to intervene in situations that require attention. The challenge of providing leadership is to know what to do in specific situations so that the group and member goals can be met and group process furthered with enough freedom that members can make mistakes and recover in a supportive, caring learning environment. In *transformational leadership*, both leaders and members gain from one another, energized to perform beyond initial expectations (Grossman & Valiga, 2012), while *authentic leadership* promotes high ethical standards and relational transparency and instills powerful social processes that positively influence members and the group climate as a whole (Forsey, 2019). Finally, leaders emulating a *situational leadership* style demonstrate flexibility in their approach to meet the needs of group members. Nielsen (2013) examined the effect of leadership style on the occurrence of bullying in work groups. Laissez-faire leadership was associated with increased risk of exposure to bullying, while transformational and authentic leadership was associated with less risk.

Selecting the Members

Individuals can self-refer or be referred to groups. The leader is responsible for assessing the individual's suitability to the group. In instances where a new group is forming, the leader preplans, sets criteria for group membership, and invites members with the aim that the group can be well functioning and beneficial for each member. The leader should consider the following criteria when selecting members:

- Does the purpose of the group match the treatment goals of the potential member?
- Does the potential member have the social skills to function comfortably in the group?
- Can the potential member make a commitment to attending group meetings?

Arranging Seating

Spatial seating arrangements contribute to group comfort and interactive group communication. Over time, group members tend to sit in the same places. Where a person sits may offer different insights into group interaction. For example, those who consistently sit close to the group leader may desire power more so than those who sit far away, or those sitting closer to the leader may feel safer. Arranging a group in a circle with chairs comfortably close to one another without a table focuses group work on relations with each other and on communication (see Fig. 15.2). In therapeutic interactive groups, no one should sit outside the group, as this often indicates exclusion and/or resistance. If a table is necessary, then a round table is preferable to a rectangular one as it spatially identifies two distinct positions of power for those who sit at the ends.

Group sessions should ideally be held in a quiet, pleasant room with no distractions, adequate space, and the assurance of privacy and confidentiality. Holding a session in too large or too small a room may inhibit engaged communication and a sense of comfort.

Intervening With Challenging Group Behaviours

Behaviours problematic to the group task can occur in all groups. They can be challenging to the most experienced group leaders and frustrating to new leaders. When intervening with any problematic behaviour or situation, the leader must remember to support the

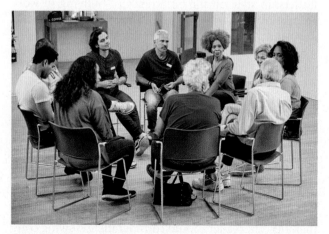

Figure 15.2 Arrangement of Seats. (Shutterstock.com/Monkey Business Images.)

integrity of the individual members and the group as a whole. It is important for the group leader to consider what might be escalating difficult behaviours and to remember that challenging or deviant members may serve a function for the group (American Group Psychotherapy Association, 2007). This could include releasing uncomfortable tension, speaking the unspeakable, or deflecting anger. One of the simpler therapeutic interventions with difficult member behaviour is to describe what is observed and let the member know how it is affecting others (Corey, 2013).

Monopolizing Group Time

Some people tend to monopolize a group by frequent talking or interrupting others. This behaviour is common in the beginning stages of group formation and usually represents anxiety that the member displaying such behaviour is experiencing. This person usually relaxes and spends less time monopolizing the group within a few sessions. However, for some people, monopolizing discussions is an established interpersonal style that will continue. Other group members usually find the behaviour mildly irritating in the beginning and extremely annoying as time passes. Members may drop out of the group to avoid that person. The leader needs to decide if, how, and when to intervene. The best-case scenario is when savvy group members remind the person who is monopolizing to let others speak. The leader can then support the group in reinforcing rules that allow everyone the opportunity to participate. However, the group often waits for the leader to act. There are a couple of ways to manage such situations. The leader can interrupt the person who is monopolizing by acknowledging the member's contribution and redirect the discussion to others, or the leader can become more directive and limit the discussion time per member.

"Yes, But..."

Some people have a patterned response to any suggestions from others. Initially, they agree with suggestions others offer them, but then they add "yes, but..." and give several reasons why the suggestions will not work for them. Leaders and members can easily identify this patterned response. In such situations, it is best to avoid problem solving for the member and encourage the person to develop their own solutions. The leader can role model problem-solving behaviour for the other members and encourage them to let the member develop a solution that would work specifically for them.

Disliked Member

Members clearly dislike one particular member in some groups. This situation can be challenging for the leader because it can result in considerable tension and conflict. This person could become the group scapegoat, a phenomenon that requires therapeutic intervention (Clark, 2009). Often, the group leader intervenes by showing respect for the disliked member and acknowledging their contribution. One solution may be to move the person to a better-matched group depending on the group structure and purpose. Whether the person stays or leaves, the group leader must be willing to accept anger, avoid displaying verbal and nonverbal behaviours that indicate that they too dislike the group member or that they are displeased with the other members for their behaviour, and help the group members learn through processing what is happening in the group. In some instances, getting supervision from a more experienced group leader is useful. Defusing the situation may be possible by using conflict resolution strategies and discussing the underlying issues.

Group Conflict

Most groups experience periods of conflict. It is the avoidance of conflict that is problematic for a group. It is important that conflicts be acknowledged and the leader then decide how best to address the issues. Member-to-member conflict can be negotiated by using the conflict resolution process discussed in Chapter 12. Leader-to-member conflict is more complicated and often difficult for members to express because the leader has the hierarchical position of greater power. In this instance, the leader can use conflict resolution strategies, including encouraging members to directly express concerns, while remaining sensitive to the power differential. Group cohesion often increases as conflictual issues are effectively addressed.

Types of Groups

Different types of groups are identified by the group goals and interactive processes or dynamics. The group leader assumes responsibility for ensuring group processes are in keeping with the group goals. Not every type of group is a therapy group. Types of groups are increasingly responsive to emerging contemporary issues in research, education, and practice; for example, group therapy for women with substance use disorders (Valeri et al., 2018), group play interventions for children (Reddy, 2012), outpatient psychotherapy group treatment for military veterans (Cox et al., 2017), support group for fathers whose partners died from cancer (Yopp & Rosenstein, 2013), effective group work in nurse education (Wong, 2018), and preventing health disparities (Stone & Kwan, 2016). In today's virtual world, web-based groups have become more common, as people seek out supports and connections through social media means and access. Leaders for online groups must also be aware of ethical issues associated with web-based delivery such as privacy and security issues, informed consent, as well as crisis situations where a member might require psychiatric emergency care (Stoll et al., 2020).

The life-threatening COVID-19 pandemic caused increased stress and mental health issues for individuals and families. It necessitated a public health requirement of physical distancing that made remote therapy, including the group modality, an important treatment venue. New, complex challenges arise with online group therapy that are similar to those found in face-to-face groups. Weinberg (2020) reviewed the limited amount of research available to identify useful practice recommendations for group therapists. He found that most online therapy groups during the pandemic crisis were synchronous (i.e., online at the same time) rather than asynchronous (i.e., connect to a group forum at different times). As therapeutic alliance (agreement on the goals of therapy and on the tasks of therapy, as well as the bonds between therapist and client) is likely to be as significant with remote group therapy as with in-person therapy, it was a key area to consider. Weinberg determined that agreement of the goals and tasks was readily achievable for online groups, but the quality of the relationship that could be achieved between therapist and clients remained questionable. Eye-to-eye contact is absent and emotions associated with physical presence are difficult to achieve on screen. Predictably, training in remote group therapy is necessary for therapists transitioning from the traditional face-to-face modality.

Structured Groups

Structured groups have an explicit structure predetermined by the group leader. These groups are often short term, oriented to education, and focus on a specific theme such as smoking prevention, substance abuse prevention, stress management, self-esteem for children, and parenting skills. Group goals focus primarily on education, psychosocial skill development, and task completion. In a mixed method research study, Kidd et al. (2013) investigated the impact of a structured group "mindful eating intervention" on weight loss and depression in urban, underserved, overweight women. The group mindfulness intervention was co-facilitated by a PMH clinical nurse specialist and a dietician. The study illustrated the benefits of social support, the significance of relationships, and the women's increased self-efficacy for weight loss.

Psychoeducational Groups

Psychoeducational groups are directed to specific concepts and teaching–learning aims. The process includes focused teaching with ample opportunity for questions, interactive discussions, and activities related to the topic. The group leader primarily imparts information, promotes discussions, and facilitates experiential learning through structured activities. Psychoeducational groups include task groups that focus on completion of specific activities (e.g., planning a week's menu) and teaching groups that are used to enhance knowledge, improve skills, or solve problems. For example, Petrakis and Laxton (2017) explored the effectiveness of inpatient psychoeducation as delivered by a nurse specializing in early psychosis care that was offered to family members of service users experiencing first-episode psychosis. In this *Journey to Recovery* group, the authors' findings suggested that although the families found the targeted information and materials provided during the session to be helpful, further community psychoeducation groups should be provided to families and care providers of individuals experiencing first-episode psychosis.

Other examples include medication groups, anger management groups, and stress management groups. Psychoeducational groups are formally planned, and members are purposefully selected. Members are asked to join specific groups because of the focus of the group. These groups are time limited and last for only a few sessions (see Box 15.1).

Cognitive–Behavioural Groups

The leader in cognitive groups identifies specific distorted thought patterns as the focus of change; whereas, the leader in behavioural groups targets specific behaviours to be modified. Cognitive and behavioural interventions may be combined to offer cognitive–behavioural (CB) group interventions. Cognitive interventions aim to modify distortions in attitudes and beliefs about self, the situation, and the future. Behavioural interventions modify behavioural excess, such as overly aggressive or sexual behaviour; behavioural deficits, such as social isolation or extreme passivity; and behaviours interfering with living, such as phobias and panic attacks (see Chapter 14). For example, Ahmad et al. (2020), found that a web-based mindfulness virtual community intervention based on CB Therapy constructs was effective in reducing symptoms of anxiety, depression, and stress among undergraduate students attending a Canadian University (see Chapter 14).

Interactive Groups

Interactive groups include counseling and therapy groups. They may be short-term or long-term focused and short-term or long-term focused or experiential. Although some structure is predetermined by the group leader, group work primarily emphasizes dynamic, interactive group processes to allow for personal and

---

BOX 15.1 **Research for Best Practice**

PUBLIC HEALTH NURSES AND A GROUP COGNITIVE BEHAVIOURAL THERAPY INTERVENTION FOR POSTPARTUM DEPRESSION

From Layton, H., Bendo, D., Amani, B., Bieling, P. J., & Van Lieshout, R. J. (2020). Public health nurses' experiences learning and delivering a group cognitive behavioral therapy intervention for postpartum depression. *Public Health Nursing, 37,* 863–870.

Objective: To explore the experience and effects on the professional and personal roles of public health nurses (PHNs) trained to deliver a Cognitive Behavioural Therapy (CBT) group intervention, aimed at providing support to women with post-partum depression (PPD), in a public health setting.

Method: In this phenomenological study, PHNs were selected to participate through purposive sampling. The study included six PHNs who volunteered to complete a CBT group intervention training program for PPD in a public health setting. The program included a 2-day in-class training session, 9-week observation of CBT group intervention sessions, and participation in supervised sessions of delivery of the group CBT intervention in the community setting for women experiencing PPD. In-depth, audio-recorded, semi-structured interviews were conducted with each of the six nurses. Interviews were 40 to 60 min in lengths, employed an interview guide, and included open-ended questions about the PHNs' experiences of completing the training program, as well as delivering the CBT group intervention. Interview

transcripts were analyzed according to thematic derivation procedures for identifiable themes.

Findings: Emergent themes from the interviews with the PHNs included the value and benefits of the training for their roles as PHNs, which involved an ability to build their confidence in foundational knowledge of CBT, as well as the opportunity to become more client-centred in their practice. The PHNs also identified implications for practice and the importance of the CBT program as an essential public health intervention. Finally, the PHNs identified that they were able to gain new knowledge and skillsets into their lives as part of addressing and coping with everyday challenges and circumstances.

Implications for Nursing: The training of nurses in delivery of CBT group therapy can be a valuable facet as part of a nurse's skillset and knowledge. The experience of conducting CBT groups for PPD as an intervention can contribute to a nurse's professional development as a rewarding, enriching, and empowering experience. CBT groups implemented by PHNs have the potential benefit of improving the mental health of women experiencing PPD, through the provision of treatment and services that address an identified gap in the public health system.

interpersonal growth through experiential teaching and learning. With this focus, the group becomes, in a sense, a microcosm of society. Group goals focus on addressing personal and interpersonal problems in living as well as modifying and changing more long-standing maladaptive patterns of behaviour.

Supportive Therapy Groups

Supportive therapy groups are usually less intense than psychotherapy groups, and they focus on helping individuals cope with their illnesses and problems as well as build interpersonal connections. Implementing supportive therapy groups is one of the basic functions of the PMH nurse. In conducting this type of group, the nurse focuses on helping members cope with situations that are common for other group members. Counseling strategies are used. For example, a group of patients with stable bipolar illness may discuss at a monthly meeting how to tell other people about the illness or how to cope with a family member who seems insensitive to the illness. Family caregivers of people with mental illnesses benefit from the support of the group as well as additional information about providing care for an ill family member. An example of an innovation in this form of group work includes a group quilting intervention with older women who are African American and transitioning out of homelessness (Washington et al., 2009).

Psychotherapy Groups

Groups that rely primarily on interpretive interventions are known as group psychotherapies. Psychotherapy groups differ depending on the theoretic perspective, including psychodynamic, interpersonal, and existential. These groups focus primarily on increasing cognitive and emotional insight as well as on improving interpersonal relations to help members face their life situations. In group psychotherapy, "therapeutic change is an enormously complex process" (Yalom, 1998, p. 7). At times, these groups can be extremely intense. Psychotherapy groups provide an opportunity for members to examine and resolve psychological and interpersonal issues within a safe environment. Mental health specialists who have a minimum of a master's degree and are trained in group psychotherapy lead such groups. When providing nursing care, communication with the group therapist is important for continuity and collaboration of care. Coulson and Morfett (2013) adeptly illustrate through qualitative data how group work inspired by Irvin Yalom's client-centred approach fosters healing and recovery for adult survivors of sexual abuse in childhood.

Self-Help Groups

Self-help groups are led by lay people, often mental health consumers, who have experienced a specific prob-

lem or life crisis. These groups are generally structured and involve supportive interaction among members (see Syvertsen, 2020). These groups do not explore psychodynamic issues in depth. Professionals usually do not attend these groups or serve as consultants. Alcoholics Anonymous, Overeaters Anonymous, and One Day at a Time (a grief group) are examples of self-help groups. A variation on self-help groups that are led by lay people is the self-help group led by a professional. Professionally led intervention groups (including those led by mental health nurses) can systematically strengthen group processes, which in turn can contribute to social support and empowerment. This was illustrated in a quantitative study by Longden et al. (2018) to evaluate the effectiveness of the Hearing Voices Network self-help group. Participants found the groups to be helpful in enhancing their self-acceptance, coping skills, and emotional wellbeing.

Common Nursing Intervention Groups

Common intervention groups led by nurses include medication, symptom management, anger management, self-care, and health promotion groups. Nurses lead many other groups, including stress management, relaxation groups, and women's groups. As a nurse, the key to being a good group leader is to critically select and modify group interventions to best accommodate the primary focus of therapeutic change in relation to the unique conditions of the setting and the group membership (Garrick & Ewashen, 2001).

Medication Groups

Medication groups led by nurses are common in psychiatric nursing. Not all medication groups are alike, so the nurse must be clear regarding the purpose of each specific medication group (see Box 15.2). A medication group can be used primarily to transmit information about medications, such as action, dosage, and side effects, or it can focus on issues related to medications, such as adherence, management of side effects, and lifestyle adjustments. Many nurses incorporate both perspectives.

It is important to assess a potential member's medication knowledge before they join the group to determine what an individual would like to learn. People with mental illness may have difficulty remembering new information, so assessment of cognitive abilities is important. Assessing attention span, memory, and problem-solving skills gives valuable information that nurses can use in designing the group. The nurse should determine the members' reading and writing skills to select effective patient education materials.

Group members typically use various medications. The nurse should know which medications each member is taking, but the nurse needs to be careful not to

---

BOX 15.2 Medication Group Protocol

Purpose: Develop strategies that reinforce a self-medication routine.

Description: The medication group is an open, ongoing group that meets once a week to discuss topics germane to self-administration of medication. Members will not be asked to disclose the names of their medications.

Member Selection: The group is open to any person taking medication for a mental illness or emotional problem who would like more information about the medication, side effects, and staying on a regimen. Referrals from mental health providers are encouraged. Each person will meet with the group leader before attending the group to determine if the group will meet the individual's learning needs.

Structure: Format is a small group, with no more than eight members and one PMH nurse group leader facilitating a discussion about the issues. Topics are rotated.

Time and Location: 2 to 3 p.m., every Wednesday at the Mental Health Centre.

Cost: No charge for attending.

Topics:

- How Do I Know if My Medications Are Working?
- Side Effect Management: Is It Worth It?
- Hints for Taking Medications Without Missing Doses!
- Health Problems That Medication Affects
- (Other topics will be developed to meet the needs of group members.)

Evaluation: Short pretest and post-test for the instructor's use only.

---

divulge that information to other patients to avoid violating patient confidentiality. Group members can choose to share the names of their medications with one another. A small-group interactive format works best. Using a lecture method of teaching is less effective than engaging the members in the learning process. The nurse should expose the members to various audio and visual educational materials, including workbooks, videos, podcasts, and handouts. Encouraging members to write down key information and supporting them throughout the various modes of teaching can facilitate retention of the information being shared. Evaluation of the learning outcomes begins with the first class. Nurses can develop and give pretests and post-tests, which in combination can measure learning outcomes.

Symptom Management Groups

Nurses often lead groups that focus on helping patients with severe and persistent mental illnesses. Handling hallucinations, being socially appropriate, and staying motivated to complete activities of daily living are a few common topics. Prevention of relapse is often a focus in symptom management groups. Members learn when a symptom indicates that relapse is imminent and what to do to avoid relapse. Increasingly, the focus on treatment and relapse prevention extends to community settings and to diverse populations. Robinson et al. (2018) examined outcomes of a dialectical behaviour therapy program as implemented by a multidisciplinary team, including nurses, for adult outpatients presenting with acute suicidal and self-harm behaviours. The authors determined that the program, consisting of group skills and individual therapy, was effective in reducing symptoms, increasing adaptability in coping skills, and improving the quality of life of participants.

Communication and Anger Management Groups

Communication and anger management are other common themes for groups led by nurses, often in inpatient settings. An inpatient communications group designed and implemented by Graham Paley, a nurse therapist, and colleagues incorporated supportive therapy, interpersonal learning, and a strengths-based focus. Evaluation based on the Yalom model identified the top four therapeutic factors as group cohesiveness, universality, catharsis, and member-to-member guidance (Paley et al., 2013). The purposes of an anger management group are to discuss the concept of anger, identify antecedents to aggressive behaviour, and develop new strategies to deal with anger other than verbal and physical aggression (see Chapter 19). The treatment team refers individuals with a history of being verbally and physically abusive, usually to family members, to these groups to help them better understand their emotions and behavioural responses. Impulsiveness and emotional lability are problems for many of the group members. Anger management usually includes a discussion of associated stressful situations, events that trigger anger, feelings about the situation, and unmet personal needs.

Self-Care Groups

Another common psychiatric group led by nurses is a self-care group. People with psychiatric illnesses often have difficulties with self care and benefit from the structure that a group provides. These groups are challenging because members usually know how to perform these daily tasks (e.g., bathing, grooming, performing personal hygiene), but their illnesses cause a decrease in the motivation to complete them. The leader not only reinforces the basic self-care skills but also, more importantly, helps identify strategies that maintain motivation and provide structure to their daily lives. Contemporary self-care group interventions are increasingly complex and sophisticated in design. For example, researchers from Norway explored Gambling Addiction Norway, an atheoretical self-help group, and concluded that common therapeutic factors exist across various types of self-help groups. Cespedes-Knadle and Munoz's (2011) *Teen Power*, a group mental health intervention for teens with Type I diabetes (who are at significant risk for depression) and a parallel support group for their caregivers involved a collaborative interdisciplinary team effort with the aim of improving diabetes management and adherence. An information–motivation–behavioural skills (IBM) model provided the theoretical underpinnings with a supportive–psychoeducational therapy format.

Reminiscence Groups

Reminiscence therapy has been shown to be a valuable intervention for community-dwelling older adults without dementia, as well as those with dementia living in long-term care. In this type of group, members are encouraged to share life stories and recall events from past years. Such groups can be developed by PMH nurses and easily implemented. Usually, a simple question about an important family event will spark memories. Reminiscence groups have the potential to increase physical and psychosocial wellbeing and satisfaction by contributing to quality of life, social engagement, cognitive skills, and memory; recalling distant memories can be particularly comforting. Reminiscence groups are typically associated with people who have dementia and are having difficulty with recent memory; however, they can also be used for people experiencing depression. Research has shown that participation in reminiscence groups has contributed to improvements in depressive symptoms. Recalling distant memories is comforting to older adults and improves wellbeing (Shropshire, 2020).

Health Promotion Groups

Mental health promotion groups have been shown to be an effective and valuable intervention resulting in positive outcomes for individuals, families, and communities (Sharma et al., 2017). Mental health promotion groups led by nurses and aimed at addressing the bio/psycho/social/spiritual dimensions of health (see Chapter 12) can include a wide array of topics and issues ranging from encouraging a healthy lifestyle and wellness, building self-esteem and resilience, to preventing child and domestic abuse (Barry et al., 2019; Salberg et al., 2018). For example, in a longitudinal observational study by Bounds et al. (2019), an intervention led by a nurse practitioner for runaway adolescents who had been sexually assaulted or exploited was found to have a positive impact on decreasing trauma responses and emotional distress in participants. As part of the intervention, nurse practitioners who were trained in trauma-informed care provided therapeutic support, intensive case management, and led empowerment groups involving problem- or arts-based activities to youth involved in the study. Health promotion groups led by nurses are often part of the treatment program on acute psychiatric inpatient units. Nursing students during clinical practicum experiences can be involved with inpatient groups and take opportunities to work with clientele on various health promotion, wellness, or arts-based activities ("4th Year Mental Health Students", 2014).

🍁 Summary of Key Points

- The definition of group can vary according to theoretic orientation. A general definition of group is "two or more individuals who are connected to one another by social relationships" (Forsyth, 2006, p. 3) and "at the heart of group is a learning process in a social setting" (Day, 2014, p. 25). Group dynamics are the interactions within a group that constitute group development and process.
- Groups can be *open* with every session available to new membership, or *closed* with membership determined at the first session. Leading a group, whether small or large, is complex because dynamics change depending on different sizes of groups and clinical conditions.
- The group development process occurs in stages: beginning, middle (working), and ending (termination). These stages are not fixed but dynamic. Each stage challenges the leader to intervene in different ways. Success at the beginning stage prepares the group to take responsibility for addressing its purpose during the middle (working) stage.
- Although there are only two formal group roles—leader and member—there are many informal group roles. These roles are usually categorized according to purpose—task functions, maintenance functions, and individual-centred roles. Members who assume task functions encourage the group members to stay focused on the group's task. Those who assume

maintenance functions concern themselves more with the group working together than the task itself. Deviant roles can detract from the work of the group as an individual member may increasingly become the focus of communication. Relational communication includes verbal and nonverbal communication, member-to-member connection and disconnection, and the communication network and group themes. Nonverbal communication is complex, open to misinterpretation, and involves eye contact, body posture, and mood of the group.

- Nurse leaders are responsible for mobilizing therapeutic factors to support healthy group development and prevent a stagnating groupthink. What factors to mobilize and when depend on the type, purpose, and developmental stage of the group.
- Seating arrangements affect group interaction. Fewer physical barriers, such as tables, improve potential for interactive communication. Everyone should be engaged as a member of the group and be invited to join in. Interactive groups should take place in a comfortable space with members facing one another in a circle arrangement.

- Leadership skills involve active listening, tracking verbal and nonverbal behaviours, remaining fair and respectful, avoiding favouritism, and encouraging participation and involvement of all members with each other.
- The leader should address challenges to the leadership, group process, or other members to determine whether to intervene and how. In some instances, the leader redirects a monopolizing member; at other times, the leader supports group members to provide feedback on the effects of the behaviour. Periods of group conflict occur in most groups during the transition from the beginning to the middle (working) phase.
- There are many different types of groups. PMH nurses lead psychoeducational and supportive therapy groups. Mental health specialists trained to provide intensive therapy lead psychotherapy groups and cognitive–behavioural groups. Self-help groups are led by participants themselves, and professionals assist only as requested.
- Medication, symptom management, anger management, self-care, and reminiscence health promotion groups are common groups led by nurses.

 ## Thinking Challenges

The nurse is leading a supportive therapy group for senior citizens whose spouses have passed away. They are learning positive coping strategies to deal with a loss.

a. What is the premise behind supportive therapy groups?
b. How is the role of the nurse different than that of the group members?

c. What are the stages of group development?

> Visit **thePoint** to view suggested responses.
> Go to **thePoint.lww.com/activate** and use the activation code found in the front of this text to unlock answers to the "Thinking Challenges" and other online resources.

 ## Web Links

agpa.org The American Group Psychotherapy Association (AGPA) is an interdisciplinary association for enhancing practice, theory, and research in group therapy. Extensive resources are available for members and nonmembers.

camh.net The Centre for Addiction and Mental Health (CAMH) offers valuable practical, educational, group, and research-based resources for health professionals in the field of addictions and mental health, including resources related to concurrent disorders, trauma, policy research, and health promotion.

cgpa.ca The Canadian Group Psychotherapy Association (CGPA) is a national organization dedicated to promoting

group therapy practice and the enhancement of clinical knowledge and skills through training, continuing education, and research. CGPA is multidisciplinary, which results in a rich and diverse membership. The association is responsible for setting national training standards and for accrediting regional training programs. CGPA has three levels of membership that reflects a broad range of expertise and experience, from internationally acclaimed members to students of the mental health professions.

entalhelp.net/selfhelp The American Self-Help Group Clearinghouse provides online self-help resources containing information on many different self-help groups.

References

4th Year Mental Health Students Making a Difference. (2014, October 27). *UM Today News.* https://news.umanitoba.ca/4th-year-mental-health-students-making-a-difference/

Ahmad, F., El Morr, C., Ritvo, P., Othman, N., & Moineddin, R. (2020). An eight-week mindfulness virtual community intervention for students' mental health: Randomized controlled trial. *Journal of Medical Internet Research Mental Health, 7*(2), e15520. http://doi.org/10.2196/15520

American Group Psychotherapy Association. (2007). *Practice guidelines for group psychotherapy.* Sage.

Barry, M. M., Clarke, A. M., Peterson, I., & Jenkins, R. (Eds.). (2019). *Implementing mental health promotion.* Springer Publishing.

Benson, J. (2010). *Working more creatively with groups* (3rd ed.). Routledge.

Bounds, D. T., Edinburgh, L. D., Fogg, L. F., & Saewyc, E. M. (2019). A nurse practitioner-led intervention for runaway adolescents who have been sexually assaulted or sexually exploited: Effects on trauma symptoms, suicidality, and self-injury. *Child Abuse & Neglect, 90,* 99–107. http://doi.org/10.1016/j.chiabu.2019.01.023

Brown, T., & Miller, C. (2000). Communication networks in task-performing groups: Effects of task complexity, time, pressure, and interpersonal dominance. *Small Group Research, 31*(2), 131–157. https://doi.org/10.1177/104649640003100201

Burtis, J., & Turman, P. (2006). *Group communication pitfalls: Overcoming barriers to an effective group experience.* Sage.

Canadian Interprofessional Health Collaborative. (2010). *A national interprofessional competency framework.* http://www.cihc.ca/files/CIHC_IPCompetencies_Feb1210.pdf

Cespedes-Knadle, Y., & Munoz, C. (2011). Development of a group intervention for teens with Type 1 diabetes. *Journal for Specialists in Group Work, 36,* 278–295. https://doi.org/10.1080/01933922.2011.613898

Clark, C. (2009). *Group leadership skills for nurses and health professionals* (5th ed.). Springer.

Comstock, D., Duffey, T., & St. George, H. (2002). The relational-cultural model: A framework for group process. *Journal for Specialists in Group Work, 27*(3), 254–272. https://doi.org/10.1177/0193392202027003002

Corey, G. (2013). *Theory and practice of group counseling* (8th ed.). Brooks/Cole.

Corey, M., Corey, G., & Corey, C. (2013). *Groups: Process and practice* (8th ed.). Brooks/Cole.

Coulson, L., & Morfett, H. (2013). Group work for adult survivors of sexual abuse in childhood. *Mental Health Practice, 17*(1), 14–21. https://doi.org/10.1177/104973159700700103

Cox, D. W., Owen, J. J., & Ogrodniczuk, J. S. (2017). Group psychotherapeutic factors and perceived social support among veterans with PTSD symptoms. *The Journal of Nervous and Mental Disease, 205,* 127–132. https://doi.org/10.1097/NMD.0000000000000635

Crowell, D. (2011). *Complexity leadership: Nursing's role in health care delivery.* F.A. Davis.

Day, S. (2014). A unifying theory for group counselling and psychotherapy. In J. Delucia-Waack, C. Kalodner, & M. Riva (Eds.), *The handbook of group counseling & psychotherapy* (2nd ed., pp. 24–33). Sage.

Delucia-Waack, J., Kalodner, C., & Riva, M. (2014). *The handbook of group counseling & psychotherapy* (2nd ed.). Sage.

Dimock, H. G., & Kass, R. (2011). *Making workgroups effective* (4th ed.). Captus Press.

Fedele, N. (2004). Relationships in groups: Connection, resonance, and paradox. In J. Jordon, M. Walker, & L. Hartling (Eds.), *The complexity of connection: Writings from the Stone Center's Jean Baker Miller Training Institute* (pp. 195–219). Guilford.

Forsey, C. (2019). *What's authentic leadership, & how do you practice it.* https://blog.hubspot.com/marketing/authentic-leadership

Forsyth, D. R. (2020). Group-level resistance to health mandates during the COVID-19 pandemic: A groupthink approach. *Group Dynamics: Theory, Research, and Practice, 24*(3), 139–152. http://dx.doi.org/10.1037/gdn0000132

Forsyth, D. R. (2006). *Group dynamics.* Thomson Nelson.

Forsyth, D. R., & Diederich, T. (2014). Group dynamics and development. In J. Delucia-Waack, C. Kalodner, & M. Riva (Eds.), *The handbook of group counseling & psychotherapy* (2nd ed., pp. 34–45). Sage.

Garland, J., Jones, H., & Kolodny, R. (1973). A model of stages of development in social work groups. In S. Bernstein (Ed.), *Explorations in group work: Essays in theory and practice* (pp. 17–71). Milford House.

Garrick, D., & Ewashen, C. (2001). An integrated model for adolescent inpatient group therapy. *Journal of Psychiatric and Mental Health Nursing, 8,* 165–171. https://doi.org/10.1046/J.1365-2850.2001.00374.X

Graham, M., & Sontag, M. (2011). Art as an evaluative tool: A pilot study. *Art Therapy, 18*(1), 37–43. https://doi.org/10.1080/07421656.2001.10129451

Grossman, S., & Valiga, T. (2012). *The new leadership challenge: Creating the future of nursing* (4th ed.). F.A. Davis.

Harpine, E. (2013). *Prevention groups.* Sage.

Harpine, E. (2015). *Group-centered prevention in mental health.* Springer.

Harpine, E., Nitza, A., & Conyne, R. (2010). Prevention groups: Today and tomorrow. *Group Dynamics: Theory, Research, and Practice, 14,* 268–280. https://doi.org/10.1037/a0020579

Hartling, L. M. (2013). Strengthening resilience in a risky world: It's all about relationships. In J. V. Jordon (Ed.), *The power of connection: Recent developments in relational-cultural theory* (pp. 49–68). Routledge.

Janis, I. (1982). *Groupthink* (2nd ed.). Houghton-Mifflin.

Kidd, L., Graor, C., & Murrock, C. (2013). A mindful eating group intervention for obese women: a mixed methods feasibility study. *Archives of Psychiatric Nursing, 27,* 211–218. https://doi.org/10.1016/j.apnu.2013.05.004

Kottler, J., & Englar-Carlson, M. (2010). *Learning group leadership: An experiential approach.* Sage.

Layton, H., Bendo, D., Amani, B., Bieling, P. J., & Van Lieshout, R. J. (2020). Public health nurses' experiences learning and delivering a group cognitive behavioral therapy intervention for postpartum depression. *Public Health Nursing, 37,* 863–870. https://doi.org/10.1111/phn.12807

Longden, E., Read, J., & Dillon, J. (2018). Assessing the impact and effectiveness of hearing voices network self-help groups. *Community Mental Health Journal, 54,* 184–188. https://doi.org/10.1007/s10597-017-0148-1

McRae, M. B., & Short, E. L. (2010). *Racial and cultural dynamics in group and organizational life.* Sage.

McWhirter, P., & McWhirter, J. (2010). Community and school violence and risk reduction: Empirical supported prevention. *Group Dynamics: Theory, Research, and Practice, 14,* 242–256. https://doi.org/10.1037/a0020056

Miller, J. B. (1986). *What do we mean by relationships?* (Work in Progress, No. 22). Stone Center Working Paper Series.

Moreno, J. K. (2007). Scapegoating in group psychotherapy. *International Journal of Group Psychotherapy, 57*(1), 93–104. https://doi-org.login.ezproxy.library.ualberta.ca/10.1521/ijgp.2007.57.1.93

Myers, S., & Anderson, C. (2020). *The fundamentals of small group communication.* SAGE Publications Inc.

Nielsen, M. B. (2013). Bullying in work groups: The impact of leadership. *Scandinavian Journal of Psychology, 54,* 127–136. https://doi.org/10.1111/sjop.12011

Pagano, M. (2015). *Communication case studies for health care professionals: An applied approach.* Springer.

Paley, G., Danks, A., Edwards, K., Reid, C., & Rawse, H. (2013). Organizing an inpatient psychotherapy group. *Mental Health Practice, 16*(7), 10–15. https://doi.org/10.7748/mhp2013.04.16.7.10.e815

Parks, C. (2020). Group dynamics when battling a pandemic. *Group Dynamics: Theory, Research, and Practice, 24*(3), 115–121. http://dx.doi.org/10.1037/gdn0000143

Pessagno, R. (2022). Group therapy. In K. Wheeler (Ed.), *Psychotherapy for the advanced practice nurse* (3rd ed., pp. 469–493). Springer Publishing Company.

Petrakis, M., & Laxton, S. (2017). Intervening early with family members during first-episode psychosis: An evaluation of mental health nursing psychoeducation within an inpatient unit. *Archives of Psychiatric Nursing, 31,* 48–54. https://doi.org/10.1016/j.apnu.2016.07.015

Reddy, L. A. (2012). *Group play interventions for children: Strategies for teaching prosocial skills.* American Psychological Association.

Robinson, R., Lang, J. E., Hernandex, A., Holz, T., Cameron, M., & Brannon, B. (2018). Outcomes of dialectical behavior therapy administered by an interdisciplinary team. *Archives of Psychiatric Nursing, 32,* 512–516. https://doi.org/10.1016/j.apnu.2018.02.009

Rutan, J. S., Stone, W. N., & Shay, J. J. (2014). *Psychodynamic group psychotherapy* (5th ed.). Guilford Press.

Salberg, J., Folke, F., Ekselius, L., & Öster, C. (2018). Nursing staff-led behavioral group intervention in psychiatric in-patient care: Patient and staff experiences. *International Journal of Mental Health Nursing, 27,* 1401–1410. https://doi.org/10.1111/inm.12439.

Sampson, E., & Marthas, M. (1990). *Group process for the health professions* (pp. 222–224). Delmar.

scapegoat. (n.d). OED Online. December 2020. Oxford University Press. Retrieved February 21, 2021 from https://www-oed-com.login.ezproxy.library.ualberta.ca/view/Entry/171946?rskey=BfVByp&result=1

Sharma, A., Sharma, S. D., & Manasi, S. (2017). Mental health promotion: A narrative review of emerging trends. *Current Opinion in Psychiatry, 30,* 339–345. https://doi.org/ 10.1097/YCO.0000000000000347

Shropshire, M. (2020). Reminiscence intervention for community-dwelling older adults without dementia: A literature review. *British Journal of Community Nursing, 25*(1), 40–44. https://doi.org/10.12968/bjcn.2020.25.1.40

Steinhardt, M. A., Dolbier, C. L., Gottlieb, N. H., & McCalister, K. T. (2003). The relationship between hardiness, supervisor support, group cohesion, and job stress as predictors of job satisfaction. *American Journal of Health Promotion, 17*(6), 382–389. https://doi.org/10.4278/0890-1171-17.6.382

Stoll, J., Müller, J. A., & Trachsel, M. (2020). Ethical issues in online psychotherapy: A narrative review. *Frontiers in Psychiatry, 10,* Article 993. https://doi.org/10.3389/fpsyt.2019.00993

Stone, J., & Kwan, V. (2016). How group processes influence, maintain, and overcome health disparities. *Group Process & Intergroup Relations, 19,* 411–414. https://doi.org/ 10.1177/1368430216642612

Syvertsen, A., Erevik, E. K., Mentzoni, R. A., & Pallesen, S. (2020). Gambling addiction Norway—experiences among members of a Norwegian self-help group for problem gambling. *International Gaming Studies, 20*(2), 246–261. https://doi.org/10.1080/14459795.2020.1722200

Taylor, E., & Cranston, P. (2012). *The handbook of transformative learning: theory, research, and practice.* Jossey-Bass.

Tuckman, B. W. (1965). Development sequence in small groups. *Psychological Bulletin, 63,* 384–399. https://doi.org/10.1037/h0022100

Valeri, L., Sugarman, D. E., Reilly, M. E., McHugh, R. K., Fitzmaurice, G. M., & Greenfield, S. F. (2018). Group therapy for women with substance use disorders: In-session affiliation predicts women's substance use treatment outcomes. *Journal of Substance Abuse Treatment, 94,* 60–68. https://doi.org/10.1016/j.jsat.2018.08.008

Washington, O., Moxley, D., & Garriott, L. (2009). The telling my story: Quilting workshop. *Journal of Psychosocial Nursing, 47*(11), 42–52. http://doi.org/10.3928/02793695-20090930-01

Wong, F. M. F. (2018). A phenomenological research study: Perspectives of student learning through small group work between undergraduate nursing students and educators. *Nurse Education Today, 68,* 153–158. https://doi.org/10.1016/j.nedt.2018.06.013

Weinberg, H. (2020). Online group psychotherapy: Challenges and possibilities during COVID-19—A practice review. *Group Dynamics: Theory, Research, and Practice, 24*(3), 201–211. http://dx.doi.org/10.1037/gdn0000140

Yalom, I. D. (1998). *The Yalom reader: Selections from the work of a master therapist and storyteller.* Basic Books.

Yalom, I. D., & Leszcz, M. (2005). *The theory and practice of group psychotherapy* (5th ed.). Basic Books.

Yopp, J., & Rosenstein, L. (2013). A support group for fathers whose partners died from cancer. *Clinical Journal of Oncology Nursing, 17,* 169–173. http://doi.org/10.1188/13.CJON.169-173

Zimmerman, J., & Winek, J. (2013). *Group activities for families in recovery.* Sage.

CHAPTER 16

Family Assessment and Interventions*

Cindy Peternelj-Taylor and Patricia M. King

LEARNING OBJECTIVES

After studying this chapter, you will be able to independently and competently:

- Discuss the role families and family caregivers provide in the support, advocacy, and recovery of people living with mental illness.
- Develop an accurate genogram that depicts the family structure and family history, relationships, and health patterns across three generations.
- Develop an ecomap to explore a family's existing network of support that includes strengths and resources.
- Identify current family needs and concerns related to mental illness.
- Collaborate to develop a family-centred care plan to address the identified family needs and concerns.

KEY TERMS

- ecomap • extended family • family development • family life cycle • family structure • genogram • immediate family • nuclear family • respite • transition times

KEY CONCEPTS

- comprehensive family assessment • 15-minute family interview • family

Mental illness affects families across the life span. These effects can occur directly within the family when a family member receives a diagnosis or indirectly through social contacts with friends or community members. Mental illness has a significant impact on morbidity and mortality throughout Canada (Canadian Mental Health Association [CMHA], n.d.). Approximately 11 million Canadians who are 15 years of age and older have at least one family member with a mental illness including addiction (Pearson, 2015). Further, an estimated 1.2 million Canadian children and youth are affected by mental illness, and one in four Canadian seniors lives with a mental health issue or illness (MacCourt, 2013). As a group, Indigenous Peoples in Canada experience a disproportionately higher burden of mental illness when compared to the rest of the country (Kirmayer & Valaskakis, 2009; Nelson & Wilson, 2017).

The unique role that families play in promoting wellbeing, providing care, and facilitating recovery is finally being more recognized. Families are often poorly prepared for the inherent demands required of the primary caregiver role. Serious mental illness changes the lives and relationships of families often with a "disturbing and destructive force" (Buckley & Scott, 2017, p. 55). Family engagement and involvement is vital to successful management and wellbeing of members who experience mental health problems.

Evidence suggests that family-based interventions reduce relapse rates and improve the recovery of patients while increasing family wellbeing. Family-based interventions are useful for the following:

- Patients with first-episode psychosis (Petrakis & Laxton, 2017)
- Bipolar disorder in adults and youth (Reinares et al., 2016)
- Families where parents have a mental illness (Reupert & Mayberry, 2016; Afzelius et al., 2018)
- Diverse consumers experiencing mental illness and their families (Coker et al., 2016)

Family-to-family interventions have also been shown to increase empowerment, knowledge, and coping, and they reduce stress among family caregivers (Toohey et al., 2016). Well-supported family caregivers play an essential role in the recovery journey of their ill relatives (Revell & McCurry, 2021).

---

*Adapted from the chapter "Family Assessment and Interventions" by Cindy Peternelj-Taylor.

In 2013, the Mental Health Commission of Canada (MHCC) published the *National Guidelines for a Comprehensive Service System to Support Family Caregivers of Adults with Mental Health Problems and Illnesses*. These are a first for Canada and provide recommendations for mental health services that recognize and address the needs of family caregivers of adults with mental health problems and illnesses (MacCourt, 2013). The purpose of this chapter is to provide an overview of key concepts from these recommendations and other sources to enable nurses to effectively work with families as they navigate family life within the context of mental illness. This chapter includes ideas on assessing family needs and concerns and enhancing family strengths and resources to support persons experiencing illness and improving their recovery journeys.

Patient- and Family-Centred Care in Canada

Philosophically and pragmatically, nurses embrace patient- and family-centred care with increasing intention in attitude and behavioural skills. This philosophy is rooted in the belief that the family's perspective in their experience within health care has been erroneously omitted or ignored in the planning and delivery of health care. Family- and patient-centred care brings that lived experience perspective to the forefront so that patients and their families feel involved in and in control of the planning, delivery, and evaluation of their health care. The goal is to put the patient first and improve patients' experiences in healthcare systems.

Family-centred care has four concepts around which the philosophy is enacted: (a) dignity and unconditional respect for the client and family; (b) information sharing that is tailored in a complete and unbiased manner; (c) participation of the patient and family as a full partner in the care team and care needs decision-making process; and (d) collaboration for effective care in the system. The benefits of this approach are shared decision-making for care and full engagement of the client and family throughout their healthcare journey (Institute for Patient- and Family-Centered Care, 2017).

In 2015, the Registered Nurses Association of Ontario (2015) (RNAO) published their best practice guidelines on *Person- and Family-Centred Care*, which highlights that the person should be involved in and in control of their care. Person- and family-centred care is defined as an approach to care that recognizes the importance of the family to a patient. It actively involves respectful, compassionate, culturally safe and responsive care with the goals of establishing a therapeutic relationship for true care partnerships, continuity of care for the client, autonomy of the client and family, and shared decision-making and power sharing. The ideas of open communication, active collaborative effort, and engagement of client and family are key behaviors required by

healthcare professionals. (See In-A-Life for a testimonial on the importance of family- and patient-centred care on their mental health and wellbeing.)

Characteristics of Canadian Families

The portrait of Canadian families continues to change. In 2011, Statistics Canada (2011) released *Fifty Years of Families in Canada: 1961 to 2011* that highlights the changing face of Canadian families. There is now more diversity in the way families are configured. Married couples form the predominant **family structure** in Canada, accounting for two thirds of all families. In 2006, there were more common-law couples and lone-parent families. Common-law couples outnumbered lone-parent families between 2006 and 2011. The number of same-sex married couples nearly tripled from 2006 to 2011, which reflected the first full 5-year period for which same-sex marriage was legalized across the country. According to the 2016 census, 26% of Canadian families are represented by a couple with children, 26% by a couple without children, 9% are represented by lone-parent families, and 3% of families are multigenerational. Of note, 21% of Canadians on average were in common-law unions, with the highest percentages noted in Quebec (40%) and Nunavat (50%); 35% of young adults aged 20 to 24 lived with their parents; and more seniors were living as a couple when compared to 2001 (Statistics Canada, 2017).

Understanding the characteristics of families within the Canadian context is an important starting point for tailoring family nursing care. Most children under the age of 14 live with married parents; however, an increasing number live with common-law parents. One in 10 children aged 14 and under lived in stepfamilies, while 0.5% of children in this age group were foster children in private households. Over the past decade, more seniors aged 65 and over lived as part of a couple in a private household. During the same period, the proportion of senior women who lived alone declined while it remained relatively stable for senior men. About one in every 12 seniors lived in a collective dwelling, such as a nursing home or a senior citizens residence.

Definitions of the family suggest that families are unique. Unlike other social organizations, families generally incorporate new members by birth, adoption, or marriage, and members leave only by divorce or death. The **nuclear family** was once considered a "traditional" family and is defined as two or more people living together and related by blood, marriage, or adoption. An **extended family** is defined as several nuclear families whose members may or may not live together but function as one group. McGoldrick et al. (2016) suggest that the term "nuclear family" is limiting and exclusive of diverse family forms. The more inclusive term **"immediate family"** refers to "all household members and other family caretakers or siblings of children,

IN·A·LIFE 🏠

Heather Thiessen—Patient-and Family-Centred Care Advocate

No one thinks they will grow up to become a patient for most of their adult life. I had always dreamed of becoming a nurse. However, at the age of 20, I was diagnosed with multiple sclerosis (MS) and had to withdraw from my nursing studies. My MS did not follow a "typical" presentation, and I often questioned if this was truly what I was experiencing. I was eventually diagnosed with a second neurological disorder, myasthenia gravis (MG).

At this point, I had two little girls at home who needed a mother and a husband who needed a wife. Unfortunately, many Christmases, anniversaries, and birthdays were held in either the ICU or the neurology unit. I am grateful for those who were kind and bent rules to allow my children and husband to spend more time in the ICU to visit with me. Having them involved and close was essential to my recovery.

I longed to be more involved in the decisions about my care. Thankfully, in 2009, the *Patient First Review* occurred: over 4,000 patients, families, and care providers were asked what was working well and not so well in health care. There were three reports and 12 recommendations. The overarching recommendation was to shift from a system-centred approach to one that was more patient and family centred.

This document saved my life as a patient as the focus in health care shifted by ensuring that my and my family's voice was fully integrated in my care decisions. I have also been integrated as a patient partner; being able to work so closely with a healthcare system has brought purpose to my life. Although I did not become a nurse, I am able to influence healthcare experiences and change by sharing my experiences in another way.

The impact of being chronically ill and having to navigate the healthcare system has helped me and my family become closer. My children had to grow up faster dealing with a mother who was in and out of the hospital and so very sick. My journey has helped them to appreciate the time we have together. My relationship with my husband is stronger and since we have been through so much together, we have learned to appreciate every day to the fullest and to take each health issue in stride.

In 2020, the Saskatchewan Registered Nurses Association awarded Heather with an Honorary Membership.

Reference: Thiessen, personal communication with Patricia King, November 7, 2020.
2020 SRNA Awards of Excellence. (2020, October 14). https://www.youtube.com/watch?v=1J2jIEliTiU. 2020. https://www.srna.org/about-us/how-we-operate/awards-of-excellence/

whether in a heterosexual couple, single-parent, unmarried, remarried, gay, or lesbian household" (p. xxiv). It is the commitment to each other that is the bond that defines family, rather than the biologic or legal status (McGoldrick et al., 2016). The term "immediate family" is consistent with Shajani and Snell's (2019) all-encompassing conceptualization of family that focuses on belonging, affection, and durability of the relationships in the context of a person's life. In essence, "the family is who they say they are." Another way of conceptualizing family is a complex process where economics, emotion, context, and experiences are weaved and layered (Doane & Varcoe, 2021). These latter conceptualizations seem to be an appropriate "fit" for the changing portrait of Canadian families.

Nurses interact with families in various ways. Nurses may have frequent and long-term contact with families because of the interpersonal and chronic nature of many mental illnesses. Involvement may range from brief telephone contact to meeting family members face-to-face once or twice to treating the whole family as the unit of care. Families often share a unique history and investment in their relationships, caring for each other, and

promoting family member welfare. When one family member experiences the challenges associated with a serious mental health issue, they are also shared by other family members, often in complex ways. Family members are often thrust into the caregiving role and are frequently ill-prepared or equipped to deal with mental illness and all its ramifications (Grebeldinger & Buckley, 2016). The caregiving role is challenging because of the unpredictable nature of many mental illnesses, the current barriers to family involvement in the mental health system, and the stigma associated with mental illness. Despite such obstacles, family members provide support, advocate for the family member who is ill, and contribute to the recovery process (MacCourt, 2013).

The provision of competent and holistic care to families includes ongoing access to information, guidance, and support so they may effectively achieve their caregiving responsibilities while enhancing their own personal health and wellbeing. Additionally, nurses need to be mindful of issues of patient confidentiality as they respond to the family's need for information. The MHCC's Guidelines recognize that when families are well supported, they can enhance the recovery journey of their relatives who are ill, improve their quality of life, and do so with less caregiving stress than when unsupported. The unpaid care provided by family caregivers contributes vastly to Canada's health and social service systems (MacCourt, 2013).

KEY CONCEPT

A family is a group of people committed to each other and involved relationally in a complex process where economics, emotion, context, and experiences are interwoven and multilayered.

Family Caregivers

In 2018, approximately 7.8 million Canadians aged 15 and older provided care for a family member (or friend) with a physical or mental disability or problems related to aging (Statistics Canada, 2020). An earlier national survey conducted of caregivers indicated that 54% were women, 60% were employed, 28% were sandwiched between caregiving and child-rearing, and 89% had been providing care for at least 1 year. Mental illness (e.g., depression, bipolar disorder, and schizophrenia) was the most common reason for parents caring for a sick child and accounted for 23% of family caregivers (Sinha, 2013). Additionally, over one million young carers in Canada under the age of 25 were referred to as a "hidden army" by Stamatopoulos (2015) and provided unpaid care to family members with chronic illness, disability, mental health issues, problems with substance abuse, and/or health challenges related to aging. Young carers are frequently hidden and underrepresented groups and are often both providers and recipients of care. Therefore, young carers must be identified, supported, and provided with the necessary programming to prevent them from becoming secondary users of the healthcare system (Stamatopoulos, 2016).

As parents age, there is a need for succession planning for changing roles and responsibilities in families. Dodge & Smith (2019) studied the responses of sibling caregivers and how they engage with each other and redefined their relationships over time as their parents aged. A sense of familial duty to care was experienced by sibling caregivers. Using narrative methodologies, three themes emerged about sibling caregiving in this research. The first theme, diagnosis and changing sibling relationships, revealed that the sibling caregiving experience changed over time and necessitated a process of accepting their patient's diagnosis. The second theme, adopting the caregiving role, was a gradual process that required a willingness to be involved. The third theme, the process of sibling caregiving, is not without challenges. These challenges involved burdens that needed to be managed. The stories in these narratives revealed that nurses need to understand that the response of

siblings may vary across families, and ambivalence with embracing primary caregiving roles may be evident in families.

Caregiving is a complex interactional and interpersonal process that involves emotional and social labor throughout a family's life course. It consumes time, energy, finances, and other resources. Families caring for adults living with mental illness frequently assist with activities of daily living such as shopping, banking, paying bills, preparing meals, housekeeping, and childcare. Caregiving also includes monitoring symptoms and scheduling and coordinating appointments. Managing behaviours within situations and crises while preventing relapses is the work of family caregivers. Throughout all interactions and roles, family caregivers provide companionship, emotional support, and financial resources. Many caregivers are involved in providing housing and transportation, personal safety and hygiene, guidance, encouragement, and motivation. Family caregivers often assume an informal case management role advocating on their family member's behalf, navigating the health and social services systems, and facilitating continuity of care (MacCourt, 2013; Young et al., 2019). It is not surprising that families experience high caregiver burden levels given the complex demands of caring for and supporting a family member experiencing mental illness, which Wrosch et al. (2011) have equated with the burden reported by dementia caregivers.

Caregiver Burden

Caregiver burden is a common negative consequence experienced by family members involved in providing care for a family member with mental illness. Caregiver burden is defined as: "a caregiver's subjective perception of hardship in providing necessary direct care to an ill individual which will change over time" (Mulud, 2016, p. 142). In a concept analysis of caregiver burden, Mulud (2016) concluded that caregiver burden represents a comingling of attributes (caregiver's subjective perception, hardship, changes over time), antecedents (unexpected events/illnesses, an imbalance between demands and resources, negative coping), and consequences (psychological and physical morbidity, coping, and adaptation). Caregiver burden includes both objective and subjective burdens. Objective burden is associated with the practical objective aspects of care, including time and finances, which may contribute to financial hardships and limitations on social life. Conversely, subjective burden includes an informal caregiver perception of the burden of care. This may include anxiety, depression, and relational problems related to the extent to which the presence, behaviour, and dependency of the person who is ill are perceived as a source of worry, stress, and strain. In a study examining the experiences of female spousal caregivers, Rahmani et al. (2018) found that the caregiving role had a disruptive influence on the emotional relationships in the family. It led to emotional exhaustion and feelings of being trapped in their various caregiving roles: "trapped like a butterfly in a spider's web" (p. 1512). Subjective burden in caregivers was found to be lower when patients had higher levels of functioning and when caregivers experienced good health (Flyck et al., 2015). When patients are unwell, it is imperative that nurses actively and purposefully screen for caregiver burden.

Caring for a family member with a mental illness can exert both a physical and emotional toll on the caregiver. Analyzing data from the *2012 Canadian Community Health Survey—Mental Health*, Pearson (2015) reported that about 10% of people who had one family member (defined as spouse or partner, children, parents, parents-in-law, grandparents, brothers and sisters, cousins, aunts, uncles, nieces, or nephews) with a mental illness reported having experienced symptoms themselves. The rate almost doubled for those with two or more family members with a mental illness. 35% of those with at least one family member with a mental illness said that their time, energy, emotions, finances, or daily activities had been affected because of their family member's experiences with their mental illness. A total of 19% of those who perceived that their lives had been affected reported that they had experienced symptoms of a mental or substance use disorder themselves in the past 12 months, while two thirds (62%) indicated that their family member's problems had caused them to become worried, anxious, or depressed. Interestingly, Ennis and Buntig (2013) found that people who perceived that their lives had been affected (as opposed to those who did not perceive an impact) were more likely to report that they had their own mental health problems. Revell and McCurry (2021) discuss the cycle of suffering that family unit experiences when individuals and family caregivers are not able to access appropriate resources and treatment. This cycle perpetuates through the individual crisis, crisis stabilization, inpatient stay, community-based partnerships, and discharge to home. PMH nurses are ideally situated to assist families with managing the intricacies of caring for family members with mental illness through interventions directed to the individual, familial and systems level, interprofessional collaborations, and health policy reforms.

Clearly, caregiver burden is relevant to nursing practice in mental health settings. Nurses need to be mindful of the load and distress experienced by caregivers and prevent family caregivers from becoming "collateral casualties" of mental illness (MacCourt, 2013). By identifying antecedents and consequences, nurses assess for the presence of burden in caregivers and implement specific interventions and programs for those at high risk for developing caregiver burden (Mulud, 2016). Flyck and colleagues (2015) concluded that interventions aimed at relieving family caregivers'

burdens should be congruent with the type of burden (objective vs. subjective) primarily experienced by the caregivers. Success in working with families is enhanced when healthcare professionals and nurses comprehend and are oriented to how mental illness impacts families.

Meeting the Needs of Families

Historically, the impact of mental illness on the family has been mostly ignored. The attention that families received primarily focused on their role in the aetiology of the illness. And while more recently, the family is recognized as a partner in the recovery journey of the person who is ill, family members are not consistently acknowledged or supported. At times, families feel blamed for the problems and issues associated with the mental illness. They are confronted with issues that can arise when healthcare professionals must balance the family's need for information and support with the individual family member's right to confidentiality. This can be particularly frustrating for family members who assume a primary caregiver role.

Family caregivers who participated in the development of the *National Guidelines for a Comprehensive Service System to Support Family Caregivers of Adults with Mental Health Problems and Illnesses* identified several ways healthcare providers can address their needs. Families need to

- Know their relatives are receiving adequate care and services that facilitate their ability to maximize their quality of life
- Have their relationships and caregiving roles recognized by mental health service providers
- Be meaningfully involved in the assessment and treatment planning
- Receive information, skills, support and services from knowledgeable mental healthcare providers, so they can effectively provide care to their relative
- Receive family support and services to sustain their health and emotional wellbeing (MacCourt, 2013)

Failure to address family caregivers' needs increases their risk for developing mental health issues, compromises their physical health, reduces the effectiveness of their support of their relative who is ill, and increases costs to health and social service systems. On the other hand, enhancing caregiving capacity is clinically significant in terms of positive outcomes related to the relative's illness, family relationships with the person who is ill, improved medication adherence (El-Mallakh & Findlay, 2015; Farooq & Naeem, 2014; Miklowitz et al., 2003), fewer relapses and fewer hospitalizations (Falloon, 2005), and assisting with relapse prevention and promotion of recovery in their ill family member (Petrakis & Laxton, 2017).

Contextual Issues to Consider When Working With Families

Some important contextual issues to consider when working with families include stigma, access to services and respite, and family diversity.

Stigma

Mental illness is highly stigmatized in society, and the stigma associated with mental health issues and diagnoses often extend to family members. This phenomenon is known as stigma by association (Bos et al., 2013). Thus, mental illness stigma harms persons with mental illness along with their family members (van der Sanden et al., 2016). Families often experience difficulty coming to terms with mental illness in a family member and may simply deny its existence and retreat in shame. Or worse yet, they may experience cognitive dissonance when faced with the realization that they hold some of the negative stigmatizing beliefs commonly held by the general public, too. As a result, stigma may delay help-seeking, which may increase their isolation and decrease their ability to cope. Children of parents with mental illness are often wary of negative reactions of peers and do not discuss their "family secret" (Gladstone et al., 2011, p. 283). Nurses need to initiate early recognition of how stigma has affected patients and their families and offer reassurance and validation that a diagnosis of a mental illness does not change the worth of the person. Dobransky (2019) indicated two ways that nurses can be active teammates in stigma management for patients and families: normalization and brokering/buffering. Normalization is a patient led activity where patients are encouraged to disclose their illness to the degree to which they are comfortable. Brokering and buffering by a healthcare professional involves protecting the patient from negative reactions and may involve creating contacts and resources of support for the client. Dobransky (2019) concluded that "providers also play key roles in common stigma management strategies taken by those with mental illness: secrecy, withdrawal, education, and activism" (p. 239).

Access to Services and Respite

Families identify that access to needed medical and social services as crucial to recovery. Social services include housing, income assistance, and legal and employment support. Information that is tailored to the educational and literacy level of the family is crucial, as it must be understandable to the family members (Mac-Court, 2013).

Family members also need **respite** supports and services to provide relief from everyday caregiving responsibilities (Brighton et al., 2016). In 2005, the Schizophrenia Society of Canada conducted a national survey on the respite needs of people living with schizo-

phrenia. A total of 372 responses were received from individuals across the country who were identified as care providers. Of this group, 80% were female-identified, with an average age of 63. The remaining 20% were male-identified with an average age of 66, and of this group, 61% were not employed, while 41% were just beyond retirement. Conversely, the average age of care recipients was 49 years (Stuart, 2005). In essence, these data paint a picture of aging parents caring for aging adult children. In answering the question, "What does respite mean to you?" one respondent replied, "It means time to take care of my physical and mental needs so that I can be a better caregiver. Time to recharge and reconnect with my husband" (Stuart, 2005, p. 70). Although this study took place in 2005, it remains relevant today, as little has changed for family caregivers, who continue to have limited access to appropriate respite services. More recently, the Schizophrenia Society of Canada (2020) updated its family psychoeducation program entitled *Family Recovery Journey*, designed to meet the needs of families living with schizophrenia.

Three themes emerged in a study that explored the effect of respite services on carers of individuals with severe mental illness (Brighton et al. 2016). In the first theme, respondents discussed the impact of caregiving on their health and wellbeing (experienced stress, depression and anxiety, and physical health problems). In the second theme, respondents discussed the impact of caregiving on their leisure activities, concluding that caregiving was too great a burden to engage in leisure activities. The final theme focused on formal respite benefits (i.e., a 5-day Recovery Camp) for care recipients. One participant remarked, "We went out for dinner, relaxed, put our feet up…didn't engage in other activities, just needed a rest, a break from looking after her" (Brighton et al., 2016, p. 37). Nurses are ideally situated to assess, assist, and advocate for family members who are caregivers. Understanding caregiver burden and the importance of respite for family caregivers is imperative. Being care providers to adult children with schizophrenia is explored further in Box 16.1.

Diversity of Families

Canada is a multicultural and diverse society. Diversity is about difference and complexity. It includes age, ability, ethnicity, culture, faith, gender, education, income, language, and sexual orientation differences. Diversity is not a neutral concept; the social, political, and economic context of family life needs to be considered, and disparities and power imbalances addressed in the plan of care (Doane & Varcoe, 2021). Diversity in how mental illness is expressed is evident across cultures (Brijnath & Antoniades, 2018). Diversity is also apparent in the characteristics of individual family members, including the individual experiencing mental illness. Life cycle stage, gender, age, type and severity of illness, and type of treatments may influence needs.

BOX 16.1 Research for Best Practice

PARENT CAREGIVERS OF ADULT CHILDREN WITH SCHIZOPHRENIA

Young, L. Vandyk, A. D., Jacob, J. D., McPherson, C., & Murata, L. (2019). Being parent caregivers for adult children with Schizophrenia. *Issues in Mental Health Nursing, 40*(4), 297–303. https://doi.org/10.1080/01612840.2018.1524531

Purpose: The aim of this study was to explore parent caregivers' experiences of providing care to adult children with schizophrenia.

Methods: In collaboration with the Schizophrenia Society of Ontario, 12 parents of adult children with schizophrenia were recruited to participate in this qualitative study. Data were collected through the use of semistructured, face-to-face interviews and a sociodemographic questionnaire. Participants were encouraged to share stories, reflections, and anecdotes as they answered open-ended questions such as: "Can you tell me about the time that your child was first diagnosed?" "What are some of the challenges (benefits) you experience as a caregiver?"

Findings: Of the 12 parent participants who took part in the study, eight identified as mothers and four as fathers. Their ages ranged from 52 to 77 years, and the ages of their children ranged from 22 to 40 years. Six participants were employed, one was unemployed, and five were retired.

Two participants had additional caregiving responsibilities including caring for other children and older parents. Caregiving responsibilities for a total of 10 children were discussed, and of this group, 9 of the children were sons.

Two themes emerged from the interview data. The first theme, "uncertainty, change, and challenges," was illustrated by poignant reflections and quotes on the uncertainties they encountered, changes in their parenting practices, and the challenges they faced having an adult child with schizophrenia, including accessing and navigating the mental healthcare system, and interactions with police. The second theme, "the meaning of it all," captured the participants' distress, feelings of guilt and worry, their own mental health challenges, and the impact on their work and careers. They also spoke of some of the positive encounters resulting from their caregiving roles including advocacy, volunteer work, and facilitating family support groups.

Implications for Practice: The authors concluded that strategies are required to help parent caregivers cope with their multiple caregiving roles and to navigate the logistical barriers preventing access to timely and appropriate care.

Family configurations may include immediate, blended, or extended families. When "family" is defined as "who they say they are," then those in the circle of care, specifically those who protect the individual with mental illness and support their autonomy and recovery, may include unrelated individuals.

Determining the needs of families is a vital component of a comprehensive nursing assessment and care. When asked, families will let nurses know what has meaning, significance, and importance for them (Doane & Varcoe, 2021). Inquiring how the mental illness influences all family members helps the nurse understand the reciprocity between the illness and family functioning. In this way, nurses can gain an understanding of the complex dynamics of familial context. They can learn about the way a particular family thinks about and organizes themselves around their member's mental illness, including how the illness is interpreted, symptoms are managed, and mental healthcare resources are accessed and used.

Family Assessment

The Canadian national *Guidelines* for services to support family caregivers of adults with mental illness advocate a recovery-focused process (MacCourt, 2013). This means that both caregivers and individuals with mental illness(es) are supported on their journey toward

recovery and wellbeing. Principles in a recovery-focused approach include building relationships that foster hope, empowerment, self-determination, and responsibility. Five principles and values are outlined that are integral components of services. These include family engagement; respect and dignity; choice, determination, and independence; family caregiver needs; and family caregiver sustainability (MHCC, 2009, 2015). These will be discussed in the context of a family nursing assessment recognizing the value of family, friends, and community.

The MHCC (2015) states in its recovery guidelines, "Recovery-oriented practice and service delivery recognizes the unique role of personal and family relationships in promoting wellbeing, providing care and fostering recovery across the lifespan; as well as recognizing the needs of families and caregivers themselves" (p. 44).

A comprehensive family assessment involves collecting relevant data related to family health, psychological and spiritual wellbeing, and social functioning. In this way, the nurse can identify problems, enhance family strengths, and generate solutions *with* the family to address their needs and concerns. The assessment usually consists of a face-to-face interview with family members (although telephone or videoconferencing may be an alternative) and may be conducted over several sessions. A comprehensive family assessment is appropriate when an individual is admitted to the hospital for psychiatric or mental health treatment. If an individual's admission status is voluntary and they are deemed competent to make treatment decisions, then permission to contact the family is in order (Box 16.2). Providing support to family caregivers does not require patient consent as long as confidentiality of patient information is maintained and respected.

Assessing and exploring the family's use of social media and internet literacy skills may include assessing the family's ability to access, understand, and utilize information that can be accessed on the internet. For example, nurses may need to assess which social media sites that families refer to for information. Knowing which social media sites families use can help maximize

the use of appropriate and helpful information while minimizing the effects of social media and other websites that may be potentially harmful. Assessing family members' use of social media provides opportunities for nurses to support families in making informed choices. Connecting families with reliable information and communication channels can be especially beneficial for those who are separated by distance living in rural and remote areas and may have limited access to other information sources (i.e., libraries). Through social media, families can be provided with education regarding mental illness and information regarding specific family needs, peer support, and other useful family resources

---

BOX 16.2 **Family Mental Health Assessment**

Family Name: _____

Family Members Present At Interview: _____

_____

_____

_____

Nurse Interviewer: _____

1. Referral route and presenting problem (include psychiatric diagnosis and current treatment): _____

_____

_____

2. Family composition (complete and attach a family genogram): _____

3. Family life cycle phase (include stage and any pertinent transitional issues): _____

_____

_____

4. Pertinent history of the problem:
   a. Explore what the family's most urgent concerns or needs are at this point in time
   b. Explore the effects of the mental health concern on all family members
   c. Developmental history (including family of origin, health or medical events)
   d. Communication patterns (for solving day-to-day issues or problems)
   e. Previous solutions
   f. Ethnicity/culture
   g. Ecomap showing social supports (internal and external), including financial, housing, educational, and legal resources

5. Strengths and problems (identify the family strengths, resources, and capabilities): _____

_____

_____

6. Summary (include urgent concerns and needs of family, strengths and resources, degree to which they wish to collaborate in care and discharge planning, any pertinent history, positive or negative relational patterns affecting illness symptoms, and preferred communication): _____

_____

7. Goals/plans (list interventions and family responses): _____

_____

(Risling et al., 2017). Refer further to Web Links at the end of this chapter.

Expanding the modality of access to care is an area in community mental health that is of growing interest for patients and their families. It requires computer literacy skills, and there is increasing recognition that care that is accessed via the internet is facilitating patient improvements and reducing attrition rates for appointments. This modality has been endorsed by Health Quality Ontario (2019) as a supplement to in person cognitive–behavioural therapy. In 2018, Gratzer et al. (2018) explored internet-delivered cognitive–behavioural therapy in community-based mental healthcare services. Internet-based care is newer modality that requires further evaluation; it was shown to increase access to care, decrease attrition, and allowed patients to choose when and where they engaged with their therapist, which in turn increased empowerment effects. Internet-based modalities are likely to only expand in the future with growing access to internet and telemedicine approaches.

Engagement

In preparing for a family assessment, the nurse actively promotes a positive nurse–family relationship by cultivating an atmosphere of trust, respect, dignity, and cooperation. Creating this climate begins with the simple act of an introduction. The nurse provides an introduction by using their name and explaining their role for the meeting and its purpose. The nurse refers to the patient and family by name during the meeting (Shajani & Snell, 2019). Many families do not know what to expect from the nurse, which is the first step in decreasing their anxiety and increasing engagement. It is important to remember that families are unique, and their needs, understanding of the situation, expectations for care, and previous experiences with the healthcare system are just some factors that should be explored at the beginning of a therapeutic relationship. It may take more than the initial meeting to build the relationship and complete the assessment.

KEY CONCEPT

A comprehensive family assessment involves collecting all relevant data related to family health, psychological wellbeing, and social functioning to identify problems for which the nurse can generate solutions with the family and enhance family strengths.

When working with families, the nurse needs to engage the family in a manner that demonstrates understanding, competence, and caring. Listening to family members, valuing their contributions, acknowledging their knowledge and expertise, and addressing their immediate needs will build confidence and trust in the therapeutic relationship. For example, a family that needs shelter or food is not ready to discuss a member's medication regimen until these basic needs are addressed. Families are encouraged to participate in the diagnosis, treatment, and recovery process of their family member who is ill. This approach is balanced with privacy and confidentiality rights of that person.

Genogram

The **genogram** is a structural assessment tool used by the nurse to collect diverse information about family members, their relationships, and health and illness patterns over time. The genogram represents an engagement, assessment, and intervention tool. The tool is simple to use and requires only a pencil and paper. Alternatively, this tool may also be available via an app or other software.

Genograms are schematic diagrams of families that list family members and their relationships to one another. A genogram includes the age, dates of marriage/union and death, and each member's geographic location. A genogram includes a key or legend of symbols to depict individual family members. Squares represent men, and circles represent women. Ages are listed inside the figures. Horizontal lines represent marriages/unions, with the date written on the line. Vertical lines connect parents and children. Genograms can be particularly useful in understanding family history, composition, relationships, and illnesses (Fig. 16.1). As diversity of gender identity, sexual orientation, and sexual communication is highly prevalent in Canadian families today, there is a need to ensure that the genograms are inclusive so that sexual and intimacy components of relationships are included. With increasing diversity, Belous et al. (2012) caution against the construction of heteronormative and discriminatory symbology. Transgender individuals get a symbol that represents their current gender identification. For example, a transgender female (M2F) could be depicted by a circle with the M2F descriptor inside the circle. A transgender male could be depicted using a square with the F2M notation inside the square. The letter Q could be added to any person on the genogram who is queer or questioning.

During the genogram creation, the nurse can discern how clients feel about sexual communication and sexual environments. Clients can be seen as sex positive (sex+) where sexual environment and communication are open and nonjudgmental. Sex negative (sex−) would be used where families are closed about sexuality and indicate the negative consequences of sexual behaviours. Sex neutral (sex∅) would be used where sexual environments and communication are silence or ignored (Belous et al., 2012).

Genograms vary from simple to complex. The needs of the patient and family guide the level of assessment

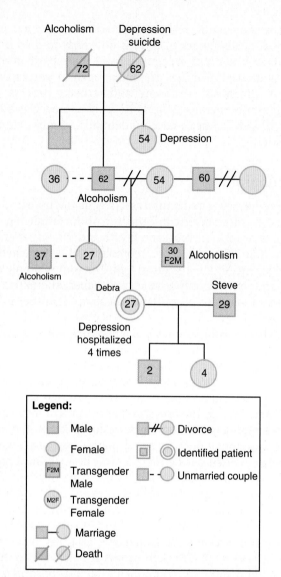

Figure 16.1 Analysis of genogram for Debra. Illness patterns are depressive disorder (maternal aunt and grandmother [suicide]) and alcohol use disorder (brother, father, and grandfather). Relationship patterns show that parents are divorced and neither sibling is married.

a tool that should be explained and an offer should be made to provide family members with a copy should they desire one.

Ecomap

An **ecomap** is a structural assessment tool used to explore the context of family living. The ecomap is a diagram of how the family is linked to the community, culture, and resources (Fig. 16.2). While constructing a family ecomap, the nurse will determine current and past access to mental health inpatient or outpatient/community services, support networks, cultural or religious affiliations, education, employment, and housing. The ecomap can be used as a starting point to identify family needs and family strengths and positive connections in terms of promoting family health. It can be most informative early in the assessment process and can be used to plan for discharge. Family members can actively participate in working on the ecomap during the assessment phase.

The family genogram is placed in a centre circle and labelled family or household. Outer circles represent significant people, organizations, and service providers in the context of living. Lines are drawn from the family to the outside circle and indicate the nature of the relationship. Straight lines indicate a strong connection, dotted lines indicate a tenuous relationship, and slashed or jagged lines indicate stressful or nonexistent relationships.

Analyzing Genogram and Ecomap Data

Genograms and ecomaps can be most useful in a family assessment when the nurse analyzes the data for family composition, mental health patterns in the fam-

detail depicted in the image. The genogram can be simple in a small family with few concerns. In a larger family with multiple concerns, the genogram can reflect these complexities across generations. Nurses can explore important events such as marriages, divorces, deaths, and geographic movements in relation to the presenting concern. Nurses should always include mental health issues and other significant health problems in the genogram.

Questions are more meaningful to the family if they are designed to address the family's particular area of concern rather than a general exploration. The nurse can begin the interview by explaining to family members they will be having a conversation, so the nurse can better understand their situation, their needs and concerns, and their family or support network. The genogram is

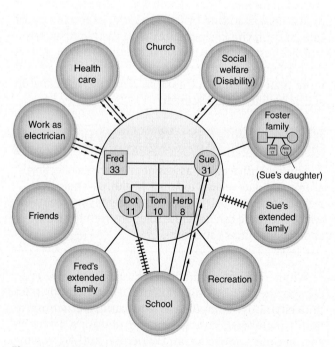

Figure 16.2 Ecomap.

ily, individual family needs, and relationship strengths and problems (particularly related to the mental health concern).

Nurses can begin by exploring family composition. For example: Who is considered to be family? How large is the family? Where do family members live? In what way do the family members show support? A large family whose members live in the same city may have more support than a family in which distance separates members. Of course, this is not always the case. The nurse could also study the genogram for relationship and illness patterns: Who is closer and further apart in the family? How might marriage and divorce influence relationships? What illness patterns might be observed across relationships or generations? For example, depressive or substance use disorders might be evident in past generations and may be risk factors for present and future generations. Exploring the significance and meaning of these health issues with the family is essential to a comprehensive family assessment. This can lead to conversations with the family about family strengths and solution strategies that they have tried. It can improve their understanding of health promotion and illness prevention related to family health risks.

The ecomap may be constructed to explore family connections further. The nurse may ask questions like, "What community agencies are you involved with now?" "Which are most and least helpful?" "How might you describe your work or school relationships?" "Which of your outside connections fosters your sense of wellbeing and gives you the most hope?" "What activities do you do, as a family, find rejuvenating?"

Family Assessment in the Bio/Psycho/ Social/Spiritual Domains

A comprehensive family assessment incorporates information related to the biological, psychological, social, and spiritual domains.

Biologic Domain

Family assessment includes discussing family members' physical and mental health status and how they affect family functioning. A family with multiple physical and mental health problems will be trying to manage the symptoms, their treatments, and obtain needed financial and healthcare resources.

The nurse should ask the family to identify members who have had or have a physical or mental illness using a matter-of-fact and direct approach. The nurse can record family health status information on the genogram. This may include current and past physical or mental illness and disabilities. This is important information to document, as genetic and epigenetic factors contribute to the intergenerational transmission of mental illness (Melchior, 2019). Stresses the family currently experience and their resources may be indicated in the ecomap and in narrative form. It is important for the nurse to explore how physical and mental health problems are affecting family functioning. For example, if a member requires frequent visits to a provider or hospitalizations, then the whole family may feel the effects of focusing more time and financial resources on that member.

In most cultures, mental health problems are associated with stigma and shame (MHCC, 2012). Therefore, exploring a family's history and experience with a mental disorder must be approached with respect and sensitivity. The nurse should be aware that families may experience varied timelines in their readiness to share and disclose details about their lived experience with mental illness. Some families will have closed boundaries that need respect and understanding rather than judgment. Creating a safe space, use of therapeutic silence, and pacing a conversation requires active management by the nurse. How and with whom families share information about the member who is ill can vary greatly, as illustrated in the following quote by a parent: "We went a long time without telling anyone what was going on partly because our son didn't want anyone to know and it would have freaked my family out" (MacCourt, 2013, p. 14).

If family members do not know if there is a family history of mental illness, then the nurse could ask if anyone was treated for "nerves" or had a "nervous breakdown." Overall, a comprehensive family history of mental illness across multiple generations helps the nurse understand the significance of mental illness in the family. The whole family can be affected if one family member has a serious mental illness. Exploring how this is unique to each family is vital to planning, tailoring, and contextualizing care.

Psychological Domain

Assessment of the family's psychological domain focuses on the family's development and life cycle, communication patterns, stress and management abilities, and problem-solving skills. One aim of the assessment is to understand how family members communicate with each other as they negotiate developmental and life transitions, including mental health problems and illnesses. It is essential that nurses explore coping styles and problem-solving abilities of family members relevant to crisis situations, acute episodes, short-term and long-term management of issues associated with their relative's mental illness with an emphasis on hope while planning for a recovery process. Identifying stressful events and assessing family management, strengths, and resources should be a priority to facilitate a family's recovery process.

Family Development

Family development is a broad term that refers to all the processes connected with the family's growth, including changes associated with its economic situation, geographic location, migration, acculturation, and serious illness. In optimal family development, family members are relatively differentiated (capable of autonomous functioning), anxiety is low, and individuals have good emotional relationships with their own families of origin.

Family Life Cycles

It is important for nurses to have a good understanding of the distinction between family life cycles and family development when working with families (McGoldrick et al., 2016). Family development refers to the unique path a family takes shaped by predictable and unpredictable events, such as illness or environmental disasters, and societal trends, such as an economic downturn. The nurse's focus regarding family development is not on categorizing the family but rather on understanding the relational processes that occur as the family evolves and responds to its member's mental illness. Nurses need to "widen their lens" and model inclusivity and respect for the diversity of families encountered in their practice regardless of family structure, family composition, family tasks, or family function. Diversity may also become apparent in how families move through life. Nurses understand the uniqueness of each family's journey.

The **family life cycle** refers to a "typical" path most families go through related to the arrival and departure of family members through birth and death, couple unions and separations, and the raising and launching of children. The family life cycle is a process of expansion, contraction, and realignment of relationship systems to support the entry, exit, and development of family members in a practical way. While there is no single definitive list of stages of a family life cycle that is sufficiently inclusive or representative of diversity, a family's life cycle is conceptualized in terms of stages throughout the years. The family system undergoes changes to move from one stage to the next. Structural and potential structural changes within stages can usually be handled by rearranging the family system (first-order changes), whereas the transition from one stage to the next requires changes in the system itself (second-order changes). In first-order changes, the family system is rearranged, such as when the youngest child enters schooling and the stay-at-home parent returns to work. The system is rearranged, but the structure remains the same. In second-order changes, the family structure changes, such as when a member moves away from the family home to live independently. Families may be transitioning through more than one stage depending

on the family configuration. As suggested, the nurse may use this model to explore potential stress related to family transitions. Multiple transitions can trigger or exacerbate symptoms of mental illness.

Consider the following two situations:

- A family transitioning through various life cycle stages experiences the emotional process and second-order changes when one family member experiences an acute mental illness episode.
- A family is affected when several life cycle changes are interrupted simultaneously, such as a grandparent's death, a job loss, and separation of the parents.

Transition times are any times of addition, subtraction, or change in the status of family members. During transitions, family stresses are more likely to cause symptoms or difficulties. Significant family events, such as the death of a member or the introduction of a new member, also affect the family's ability to function. During these times, families may need help from the mental health system.

Cultural Diversity

It is imperative that nurses consciously attend to cultural diversity given Canada's multicultural climate. In a study conducted in Toronto, Murney et al. (2020) explored stigma utilizing a qualitative methodology and found that stigma can be communicated verbally or nonverbally. The study found that listening effectively is the foundation of all nonstigmatizing communication. This study also revealed that patient encounters where there are cultural misunderstandings leads to exacerbated perceptions of stigma and discrimination. One method for increasing sensitivity to culture has been to identify distinctive characteristics or responses to life cycle transitions or disruptions such as mental illness within specific ethnic communities. Becoming conscious of the characteristics of particular ethnic groups is an important step toward developing an appreciation for cultural diversity, as long as these norms are remembered to be gross generalizations. Labelling and categorizing ethnic groups' behaviours according to general rules can help raise awareness of difference, but it can equally obscure each family's uniqueness. For the nurse, appreciating, acknowledging, and validating ethnic differences, while at the same time acknowledging similarities, can feel like a delicate balancing act. Nurses must be mindful of the personal biases they bring to their practice. In the clinical example provided in Box 16.3, a particular generalization is at play in the description of Judy's rich familial connections and her location in a particular geographic region of Canada. This is an example of a cultural assumption.

Developing sensitivity to one's own beliefs about what constitutes normalcy and functionality in a family

BOX 16.3 John and Judy Jones

John and Judy Jones were married 3 years ago after their graduation from a small university in Eastern Canada. Judy's career choice required that she live on the East Coast, where she would be near her large family. John willingly moved with her and quickly found a satisfying position.

After about 6 months of marriage, John became extremely irritable and depressed. He kept saying that his life was not his own. Judy was very concerned but could not understand his feelings of being overwhelmed. His job was going well, and they had a very busy social life that mostly revolved around her family, whom John loved. They decided to seek counselling and completed the genogram below.

After looking at the genogram, both John and Judy began to realize that part of John's discomfort had to do with the number of family members who were involved in their lives. Judy and John began to redefine their social life and allowed more time with friends and each other.

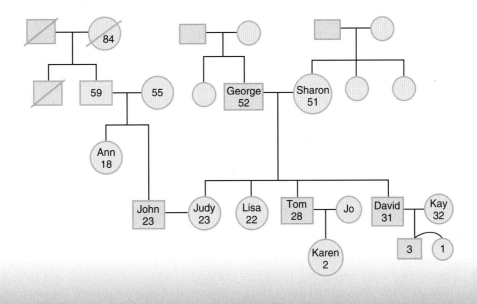

is a challenging and important endeavour for all nurses. It is only in this process of self-reflection that the nurse will develop a rich awareness of the cultural norms and values that are guiding and creating the template against which the nurse is judging and assessing the family life cycle (Doane & Varcoe, 2021). Developing and maintaining sensitivity to ethnicity, culture, and power are important in helping the nurse recognize diversity issues (see Chapters 3 and 4).

Nurses working with Indigenous Peoples must recognize the pervasive and harmful effects colonialism has had on how relationships within healthcare systems and with healthcare providers unfold (Gracey & King, 2009; Nelson & Wilson, 2017; Turpel-Lafond, 2020). In keeping with the Truth and Reconciliation Commission of Canada (TRC) calls to action, acknowledgment of nursing's involvement in past harms to Indigenous Peoples and communities need to be actualized (Symenuk et al., 2020). Active reconciliation should involve the establishment of respectful, equitable, and trusting therapeutic relationships. Nurses need to acknowledge

how family and community stability affect the mental wellbeing of Indigenous Peoples. Family support and community wholeness and connection to culture and the land are of paramount importance to patients who are Indigenous Peoples and must be incorporated into treatment and the delivery of culturally safe, competent care. Nurses must show concern for these social networks and relationships and acknowledge resilience to build trust. "Resilience—what keeps people strong in the face of adversity and stress—has many Indigenous facets: spiritual connections, cultural and historical continuity, and the ties with family, community, and the land" (King et al., 2009, p.82). In a recent study, the concept of complete mental health was explored among Indigenous People in Canada. Researchers found that two thirds of study participants experienced substantial wellbeing, a shift in existing literature. Factors attributed with wellbeing included postsecondary education, having a confidant, and fewer adverse childhood experiences (Fuller-Thomson, et al., 2020). Resiliency of all Indigenous Peoples must be acknowledged and celebrated. Nevertheless, in our relational practice and in our healthcare systems, nurses should work concurrently and tirelessly to reduce systemic structural inequities, barriers to timely care, and disparity in the intersectionality of the social determinants of health.

Families With Low Incomes

Rates of psychological distress and mental disorders, including substance-related disorders and addiction, are higher in populations of people with low incomes. These differences are statistically consistent across the Canadian sociodemographic strata: region/province, gender, age, marital status, immigration, first language, and ethnic origin (Caron & Liu, 2010). People experiencing poverty struggle to make ends meet, and family members may face difficulties meeting their own or other members' basic developmental needs. They may be experiencing homelessness or living in unsafe conditions. To be experiencing poverty does not mean that a family is dysfunctional, but poverty is an important factor that can force even the healthiest families to crumble.

The life cycle may be condensed, such that family members leave their home, mate, have children, and become grandparents at much earlier ages than people from different socioeconomic groups. Consequently, many individuals in such families assume new roles and responsibilities before they are developmentally capable. The condensed life cycle creates adolescents whose educational opportunities are compromised (no time to complete school given the family demands), thereby limiting their employment skills. The cycle of poverty is thus reinforced.

Families experiencing poverty are subject to disruption via abrupt loss of members, loss of unemployment compensation, illness, death, imprisonment, or addiction. Men may die relatively young compared with people from different socioeconomic groups. Everyday problems, such as transportation or a sick child, can become major crises because of a lack of resources.

Reliance on institutional supports is another distinguishing characteristic of families experiencing poverty. Families with low incomes are often forced to seek public assistance, resulting in the additional stress dealing with a governmental agency.

Communication Patterns

Family communication patterns develop over a lifetime. Some family members communicate more openly and freely than others. Family subgroups may have unique communication patterns with one another. During the assessment, the nurse should observe the verbal and nonverbal communication of the family members. The nurse could consider: Who sits next to each other? Who talks to whom? Who answers most questions? Who volunteers information? Who changes the subject? Which subjects seem acceptable to discuss? Which topics are avoided? How are partners intimate with each other? How are family secrets or sensitive topics revealed? Does the nonverbal communication match verbal communication? Nurses can use this information to help identify family problems, strengths, and communication issues.

Nurses should also assess the family for their daily communication patterns. Identifying which family members confide in one another is a place to start examining ongoing communication. Other areas include how often children talk with parents, which child talks to the parents most frequently, and which adult is most likely to discipline the children. Another question considers how family members express positive and negative feelings. In determining how open or closed the family is, the nurse explores the type of information the family shares with nonfamily members. For example, one family may tell others about a member's mental illness, whereas another family may not discuss any illnesses outside the family.

Stress and Coping Abilities

One essential assessment task is to determine how family members deal with major and minor stressful events and their available coping skills. Some families seem to cope with overwhelming stresses, such as the death of a member, major illness, or severe conflict, whereas other families seem to fall apart over relatively minor events. The nurse needs to listen to which situations a family appraises as stressful and help the family identify usual coping responses. The nurse can then evaluate these responses. Taking a strength-based approach can help the nurse identify what the family does well, and acknowledging the family for these strengths is important. If the family's responses are detrimental to health (e.g., substance misuse, physical abuse), then the nurse may discuss the need to develop coping skills that lead to family wellbeing (see Chapter 18). The use of mindfulness within the context of a multifamily support holds promise for families coping with mental illness across the lifespan (Whitehorn et al., 2017). Interestingly, the Schizophrenia Society of Canada (2020) advocated for a change in language to emphasize family management rather than coping when referring to family coping abilities in their psychoeducation document, *Family Recovery Journey*.

Problem-Solving Skills

Nurses assess family problem-solving skills by focusing on the more recent problems the family has experienced and determining how family members solved them. For example, even with the most effective treatment, relapses are likely to occur. When a family member relapses, who is the one to ensure that they seek treatment? Underlying the ability to solve problems is the family's decision-making process. Who makes and implements decisions? How does the family support each other? How does the family handle conflict? All these data provide information regarding the family's problem-solving abilities. Once these abilities are identified, the nurse can build on these strengths in helping families deal with additional problems.

Social Domain

An assessment of the family's social domain provides important data about the operation of the family as a system and its interaction within its environment. Areas of concern include the system itself, perspectives on understanding families, social and financial status, and formal and informal support networks.

Family Systems

A family can be understood as a system with interdependent members. Family system theories view the family as an open system whose members interact with their environment and themselves. One family member's change in thoughts or behaviour can cause a ripple effect and change everyone else's (Shajani & Snell, 2019). For example, a parent of a child with attention deficit hyperactivity disorder (ADHD) who decides to reinforce the child's positive efforts rather than focusing on negative actions may notice a change in the child's behaviour, which may, in turn, result in a reduction of the stress the parent feels when interacting with their child.

One common scenario in the mental health field is the effect of a patient's improvement on the family. Patients are more likely to live independently with new medications and treatments, which subsequently changes the responsibilities and activities of family caregivers. Although family members may be relieved that their caregiving burden is lifted, they will also be adjusting to changes in the demands on their time and energies. This transition may not be easy because it is often less stressful to maintain familiar activities than to venture into uncharted territory. Families may seem as though they want to keep the member who is ill dependent, but, in reality, they are struggling with the change in their family system.

Wright and Leahey's Calgary Family Assessment Model (CFAM) and the Calgary Family Intervention Model (CFIM) are Canadian family nursing models that have been implemented successfully in mental healthcare settings (Leahey & Harper-Jaques, 2010). These relational practice nursing models are based on postmodernism, systems, cybernetics, communication and change theories, and the biology of cognition. These two models are multidimensional frameworks that conceptualize the family into structural, developmental, and functional categories. Each assessment category contains several subcategories. The family structure includes internal (family, gender, sexual orientation, etc.), external (extended family and larger systems), and contextual (ethnicity, race, social class, religion, spirituality, environment) components. Family developmental assessment is organized according to stages, tasks, and attachments. Functional assessment areas include instrumental (activities of daily living) and expressive (communication, problem-solving, roles, beliefs, influence, power, and alliances) (Shajani & Snell, 2019).

When the nurse uses CFAM/CFIM, relational practice develops and evolves during four stages: engagement, assessment, intervention, and termination. The nurse and the family are partners in care as each brings specialized expertise in managing health problems, strengths, and resources to the relationship (Shajani & Snell, 2019).

The *engagement* stage is the initial stage in which the family is greeted and made comfortable. In the *assessment* stage, needs are identified, and relationships develop between family and health providers. The nurse invites the family to tell its story during this stage. The nurse asks exploratory questions and listens to the patient's and family members' expectations, hopes, questions, and ideas. The *intervention* stage is the core of the clinical work and involves providing a context in which recovery is facilitated (see section Family Interventions in this chapter). The nurse communicates regularly with the family to provide cognitive and emotional support. The *termination* phase refers to the process of evaluating the family interviews, recognizing the family efforts in their recovery journey, providing referrals if necessary, and extending an invitation for further interviews depending on the family's needs. The family's role in promoting wellbeing and providing care to their loved one is to be recognized and their needs to be supported (MHCC, 2015).

Perspectives on Understanding Families

Nurses are looking to the ideas of postmodernism and social constructivism to enrich their understanding of families. These ideas support exploring how families make meaning in their lives and construct their reality about their social environment. For instance, the constructivist influence invites nurses to understand that what they see is a product of their assumptions about people, families, and problems and their family's interactions. People are highly influenced by their current relationships and the environments in which they perceive their realities. Therefore, persons with mental illness and their families should be encouraged to express their perspectives (their own "truth") on their situation. Nurses need to be respectful of family stories and viewpoints, within the parameters of values about human safety and rights, including self-determination and protection from interpersonal violence.

Nurses are also using a critical lens derived from feminist, poststructural, and postcolonial theories that support considerations of power, oppression, culture, economic conditions of life, social change, and emancipation. This critical perspective draws the nurse's attention to the sociopolitical, economic, and linguistic contexts within which families are situated and constituted. The focus can then be on exposing underlying sociopolitical structures that are advantaging some people/families and disadvantaging others. The goals are to explore social conditions and revise structures in ways that address inequities (Doane & Varcoe, 2021).

Social and Financial Status

Social status is often linked directly to financial status. Identifying the occupations of family members can be particularly informative. Who works outside the home and inside the home? Who is primarily responsible for the family's financial support? Families of low social status are more likely to have limited financial resources, which can place additional stresses on the family. This information can be recorded on the eco-map and in narrative form. Nurses can use the information on the family's financial status to advocate for appropriate referrals of the family to social service agencies as appropriate.

Formal and Informal Support Networks

Formal and informal networks are important in providing support to individuals and families. These networks are the links among the individual, family, and the community. Assessing the extent of formal support (e.g., hospitals, agencies) and informal support (e.g., extended family, friends, and neighbours) gives a clearer picture of the supports available. In assessing formal support, the nurse could ask about the family's involvement with government institutions and self-help groups such as Alcoholics Anonymous or Strengthening Families Together (refer further to Web Links). Assessing the informal network is particularly valuable in cultural groups with extended family networks or close friends because these individuals can be significant sources of support to patients. This is important information to include in the ecomap. If the nurse does not ask about informal networks, then these influential people may be missed. Nurses can inquire whether family members volunteer at schools, local hospitals, or nursing homes. They can also ask whether the family attends religious services or activities.

There is a growing trend for peer support services to meet the needs of people with mental illness and addictions. It is believed that the formalization of such care relationships can benefit the recipient of care, the giver of the support, and also the healthcare system.

Chronister et al. (2021) explored the meaning of support for persons with serious mental illness from the perspective of family caregivers. They identified five areas where support was needed: person centered (e.g., acceptance and valuing of the person, using concise concrete language); autonomy support (e.g., respecting and encouraging personal choice and decision-making); support for community participation (e.g., engaging in activities aligned with their interests and choices and providing instrumental support); health management support (e.g., assistance with crisis management, medication adherence, promoting healthy living); and day-to-day living support (e.g., support related to housing, finances, appointments etc.).

Peer support can be instrumental in assisting with the five types of support identified by family caregivers. A peer is defined as someone who shares personal, social, or experiential similarities with another. Support includes empathetic and encouraging actions and assistance between two people who are in a reciprocal relationship (Penney, 2018). Peer support defined as "the help and support that people with lived experience of mental illness or a learning disability can give one another" (Shalaby & Agyapong, 2020, p.1). Within supportive networks, peer support can provide hope, increase self-esteem, improve engagement with the healthcare system, and facilitate an improved quality of life of a person with mental illness. Some peer support workers may target families with psychoeductional support and mentoring through the care of family members with mental illness (Gagne et al., 2018). A nurse may work collaboratively within the interprofessional team to assess a family's desire to access such supports, the availability of services, and advocate for an appropriate fit between service worker and family. Collaborative conversation would facilitate an assessment of appetite for such a pairing, the readiness to engage, and the limitations of the caregiving partnership.

Spiritual Domain

Families may find meaning in their experiences by embracing their spiritual or religious beliefs. Religious or faith practices help promote their recovery while strengthening their sense of meaning and purpose. For many families, their religious affiliations will play a key role in their everyday lives. These affiliations can influence the family's understanding of health, illness, healing, and treatment. Religious and spiritual practices can foster family and community support that may be a significant resource to families. It is increasingly recognized in all faith groups that the help and guidance of religious leaders are frequently sought by families who have a member who is mentally ill (Aaron, 2008). Research with Christian clergy suggests that they felt their knowledge regarding mental illness was inadequate (Farrell & Goebert, 2008). Unfortunately, mental health professionals do not tend to view religious leaders collaboratively (Leavey et al., 2007) even though they are frequently seen as conduits to the formal mental health system (Vermaas et al., 2017). However, collaboration can be of significant use to both groups, especially to individuals and families requiring assistance. Religious leaders can provide community-based support and assist health professionals to understand patients' beliefs, which is important to informing treatment planning and improving responses to crises. In turn, nurses and colleagues can assist religious leaders to understand mental disorders and mental health issues and their treatment. Open communication can facilitate the appropriate use of complementary healing practices that can be a part of a group's religious beliefs, and more importantly, it may promote better trust in psychiatric treatment and care.

Collaborating with faith-based nurses (e.g., Christian parish nurses, Jewish congregational nurses, Muslim crescent nurses, etc.) can also be beneficial when working with family caregivers. Four themes emerged in the data of a study that explored the roles Christian parish nurses employed in meeting the family caregivers' needs. Researchers found that parish nurses provided the gift of presence, they were the bearers of blessings, messengers of spiritual care, and they were involved in bridging challenges. In short, they were able to provide family caregivers with emotional, informational, and spiritual support (Grebeldinger & Buckley, 2016).

Finally, in addressing the spiritual domain of family nursing, the nurse needs to recognize that family members may differ widely in their religious beliefs and approach to spirituality. If such variation exists among members' perspectives, then it should inform the family assessment. It may be a source of enrichment, distress, or both for the family. Spirituality helps one look within and the meaning they attribute to events around them, such as the meaning they attribute to the experience of mental illness in the family (Greenstein, 2016).

The Pyramid of Family Care Framework

The pyramid of the Family Care Framework in the MHCC's national guidelines identifies five levels of tasks for meeting the support needs of family caregivers (MacCourt, 2013). As one moves from the bottom to the top of the pyramid, the intensity of family intervention increases while the number of families who require the intervention decreases (Fig.16.3). Nurses have the knowledge, skill, and competency to provide these services based on their education and advanced practice level.

Levels 1 (*connecting and assessment*) and 2 (*general education*) indicate the minimum level of service available to all family caregivers. The need for level 1 and level 2 interventions should be assessed at each point of contact. One of the most important family interventions is

education and health teaching related to mental illness. Families have a central role in the treatment of mental illnesses, and members need to learn about mental disorders, medications, actions, side effects, and overall treatment approaches and outcomes. For example, families are often reluctant to have members take psychiatric medications because they believe the medications will "drug" the patient or become addictive. The family's beliefs about mental illnesses and treatment will often affect how patients manage their illness and recovery.

Level 3 (*psychoeducation*) refers to interventions in which recommendations are made to the family caregivers regarding coping strategies or specific ways to deal with the challenges of the mental illness. Level 4 (*consultation*) may be required by family caregivers with significant challenges supporting an individual living with mental illness. Level 5 (*family therapy*) refers to interventions that work on family relationships and is designed to facilitate change in the family interactional system. Family therapy is useful for families who are having difficulty maintaining family integrity. Various theoretical perspectives are used in family therapy: therapies influenced by postmodernism, hermeneutics, and social constructionism have developed more recently. These focus on collaborative, conversational approaches, and narrative and solution-based therapies. Family therapy can be short term or long term and is conducted by mental health specialists, including advanced practice psychiatric and mental health nurses. Few families require level 4 or 5.

Family Interventions

Each conversation the nurse has with a family member can be meaningful and healing, and it can effect change in the patient's and the family members' bio/psycho/social/spiritual integrity and functioning. Families with loved ones experiencing mental illness have reported that even a short meaningful conversation with a healthcare professional is significant. Therapeutic conversations are the heart of family nursing and are of central importance when working with family caregivers. Developing skill in therapeutic conversations that are sensitive to language, culture, setting, and time available allows nurses to "see" and "do" differently when working with family caregivers (Bell, 2016). In a study addressing a therapeutic conversation intervention with acute psychiatric patients and their families, Sveinbjarnardottir et al. (2013) found that family members receiving this type of intervention by nurses who were educated, trained, and supervised in this approach built on the Calgary Family Assessment and Intervention models perceived significantly higher cognitive and emotional support from nurses, as compared to family members who received standard care. More recently, in a study evaluating the usefulness of family-centred support conversations based upon the Calgary Family

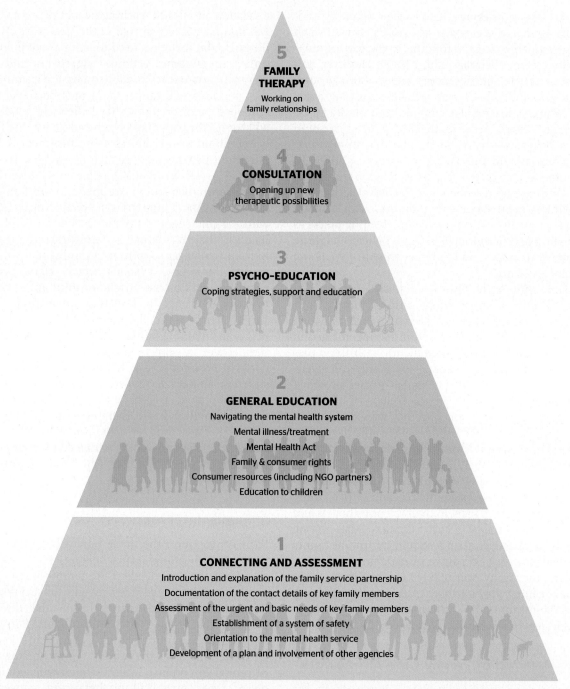

Figure 16.3 Pyramid of Family Care Framework. (Adapted Mottaghipour, Y., & Bickerton, A. (2005). The pyramid of family care: A framework for family involvement with adult mental health services. Australian e-Journal for the Advancement of Mental Health, 4(3), 210–217. https://doi.org/10.5172/jamh.4.3.210)

Assessment Model, researchers found families living with mental illness thought family nursing conversations provided opportunities for the families to "find new meanings and possibilities in everyday life" (Aass et al., 2020, p. 302).

Therapeutic conversation in a brief family interview is purposeful and time-limited. It is an opportunity to acknowledge and affirm the illness experience and patient and family expertise. Listening to the illness story is part of ethical nursing practice. Nurses can focus the conversations using the language of recovery and strength while still addressing the family's needs and concerns. Adopting therapeutic conversations as an intervention strategy, information sharing, emotional support, and patient and family involvement in decision-making can occur. Efforts should be made to enhance the family's choice, determination, and independence.

Wright and Leahey's *15-minute Family Interview* has been used effectively as a framework for family intervention. The following are some specific ideas for conducting a healing, productive, and efficient 15-minute family interview. They are condensed ideas from the CFAM and CFIM that consist of five key components: manners, therapeutic conversations, genogram and eco-map, therapeutic questions, and commending individual and family strengths (Shajani & Snell, 2019):

- Begin the therapeutic conversation with a purpose in mind that can be accomplished in the time period available with the family.
- Use manners to engage with the family by first introducing yourself with your name and your role.
- Provide a brief overview of the purpose of the interview.
- Assess the key areas of internal/external structure, function, and relationships using a genogram and ecomap.
- Identify family needs or concerns by asking key therapeutic questions.
- Commend the family on one or two strengths.
- Evaluate the usefulness of the meeting and conclude the conversation.

KEY CONCEPT

The *15-minute family interview* is an assessment/intervention framework that consists of five key components: manners, therapeutic conversations, genogram and eco-map, therapeutic questions, and commending individual and family strengths.

Therapeutic Questions

Nurses can ask key questions to involve families in care. The questions need to fit with the context in which the nurse encounters the family. The purpose of the questions is to identify the family's imminent needs in supporting their caregiver sustainability. Questions should be built on the responses to the previous question.

Some useful questions include the following:

- What are your main concerns about this hospitalization or illness?
- What information would be most helpful for you at this time?
- How can we be most supportive to you now?

🍁 Summary of Key Points

- Family is a group of people defined as "who they say they are" and involved relationally in a complex process where economics, emotion, context, and experiences are interwoven and multilayered. Families come in various compositions, including immediate, extended, multigenerational, single-parent, same-gender, and blended families. Cultural values and beliefs define family composition and roles.

- Who in the family is most affected by the patient's illness?
- What is the most meaningful way to involve you in the care and treatment plan?

Commending Family and Individual Strengths

It is empowering to enhance the family's sense of worth. One way the nurse can accomplish this is to actively notice and distinguish the family's strengths, courage, resources, and capabilities in the form of a verbal *commendation* (Limacher & Wright, 2003; Shajani & Snell, 2019). A direct, specific comment on their positive actions and solutions can be a powerful intervention for a family that has been challenged, often for many years, with a serious mental health issue. It can be as simple as a nurse telling them, "I am impressed with your strength, your detailed knowledge about the medication regimen, and the way that you have stuck together to support one another by visiting the hospital and attending this family meeting." Families find that participating in strength-based conversation enhances the recovery process.

Implementation

Flexibility is essential in implementing any family intervention, particularly when working with culturally diverse groups. Nurses need to be open to modifying the session's structure and format to implement successful, competent family interventions. Longer sessions are often useful, especially when a translator or an interpreter is used. Nurses also need to respect and work with the changing composition of the family and nonfamily participants (e.g., extended family members, intimate partners, friends and neighbours, community helpers). Nurses may need to hold intervention sessions in community settings (e.g., churches, schools) or at the family's home because of the stigma that some cultural groups associate with seeking help. Finally, ending face-to-face sessions with the family may need to be gradual. The family may need information for further support, consultation, or reengagement should the problems reoccur.

- Families, whether they are relatives of individuals experiencing mental illness or friends who make up a larger circle of support, have a unique role in promoting wellbeing, providing care, and facilitating recovery across the life span.
- Nurses complete a comprehensive family assessment when they care for families for extended periods or if a patient has complex mental health problems.
- Nurses must establish credibility and competence with the family in building relationships with families. The

nurse must first listen and address the family's immediate needs, otherwise the family will have difficulty engaging in the challenges of caring for someone with a mental disorder.

- Families can be engaged and helped through education and programs like parenting and sibling support, financial assistance, peer support, and respite care. Wherever possible, families should be welcomed as partners in care and treatment of their loved ones and should be included in decision-making in a way that respects consent, confidentiality, and privacy.
- The genogram is an assessment and intervention tool that is useful in understanding health, relationships, and social functioning across several generations.
- In assessing the family biologic domain, the nurse determines physical and mental health status and its effects on family functioning.
- Family members are often reluctant to discuss the mental disorders of family members because of the stigma associated with mental illness. In many instances, family members do not know whether mental illnesses were present in other generations.
- The family psychological assessment focuses on family development, the family life cycle, communication patterns, stress and coping abilities, problem-solving skills, strengths, hope, and resourcefulness. Determining how these occur in relationships is key.

- The family life cycle is a process of expansion, contraction, and realignment of the relationship systems to support the entry, exit, and development of family members in a functional way. Families have unique patterns based on their context for living.
- The ecomap is a tool used to assess the family social domain, which includes relationships within formal and informal support networks. The ecomap is particularly useful in care planning and discharge.
- Religious leaders of all faiths may be a significant support to families with a member who is mentally ill in fostering meaning of their situation and in maintaining hope and spiritual strength.
- Family interventions focus on supporting the family's bio/psycho/social/spiritual integrity and functioning as defined by its members. Family nursing interventions include counselling, promotion of self-care activities, eliciting strengths and resources, purposefully commending the family, supportive therapy, education and health teaching, and the use of genograms and ecomaps. Mental health specialists and advanced practice nurses conduct family therapy.
- Education of the family is one of the most useful interventions. Teaching the family about mental disorders, life cycles, family systems, and family interactions can help the family develop a new understanding of family functioning and the effects of mental disorders on the family.

Thinking Challenges

a. Refer to Heather Thiessen's In-A-Life feature presented earlier in the chapter. What might have been different for her, as she navigated her wellness journey, if she had been diagnosed with a major mental illness?

b. When working with families who experience mental illness, it is important for nurses to explore how mental illness influences all family members. Discuss the differences experienced by the various positions that family members hold, for example, parents, spouses/partners, children, siblings, etc. What about the role of the person who experiences mental illness? What

impact does their diagnosis have on their familial responsibilities?

c. How might nurses and the treatment team partner with families embarking on their recovery journey? What challenges might they encounter?

Visit thePoint to view suggested responses.
Go to thePoint.lww.com/activate and use the activation code found in the front of this text to unlock answers to the "Thinking Challenges" and other online resources.

Web Links

www.cmha.ca Founded in 1918, the Canadian Mental Health Association (CMHA) champions mental health for all Canadians through advocacy, education, research, and service. In doing so, CMHA helps people who experience mental illness and their families access the community-based resources they need to build resilience and support recovery in their own communities.

www.heretohelp.bc.ca HeretoHelp represents a group of leading provincial and national mental health and addictions nonprofit agencies, working collaboratively in the prevention and management of mental health and substance

abuse problems. Readers will find here excellent trustworthy resources regarding mental illness and addiction specifically designed for family caregivers.

www.mentalhealthcommission.ca Through this site, readers can access a number of resources including the *National Guidelines for a Comprehensive Service System to Support Family Caregivers of Adults with Mental Health Problems and Illnesses* and a *Caregiver Mobilization Toolkit.*

www.schizophrenia.ca The mission of the Schizophrenia Society of Canada is to improve the quality of life for those affected by schizophrenia and psychosis through education, support programs, public policy, and research. Individuals can access a reference manual here for families and caregivers entitled, *Schizophrenia: Rays of Hope*, and a newly published resource, *Family Recovery Journey.*

References

Aaron, M. (2008). Spirituality, the heart of caring. *A Life in the Day, 12*(4), 23–26.

Aass, L. K., Skunderberg-Kletthagen, H., Schrøder, A., & Moen, O. L. (2020). Young adults and their families living with mental illness: Evaluation of the usefulness of family-centered support conversations in community mental health care settings. *Journal of Family Nursing, 26*(4), 302–314. https://doi.org/10.1177/1074840720964397

Afzelius, M., Plantin, L., & Östman, M. (2018). Families living with parental mental illness and their experiences of family interventions. *Journal of Psychiatric and Mental Health Nursing, 25*, 69–77. https://doi.org/10.1111.jpm.12433

Bell, J. (2016). The central importance of therapeutic conversations in family nursing: Can talking be healing? *Journal of Family Nursing, 22*(4), 439–449. https://doi.org/10.1177/1074840716680837

Belous, C. K., Timm, T. M., Chee, G., & Whitehead, M. R. (2012). Revisiting the sexual genogram. *American Journal of Family Therapy, 40*(4), 281–296. https://doi.org/10.1080/01926187.2011.627317

Bos, A. E. R., Pryor, J. B., Reeder, G. D., & Stutterheim, S. E. (2013). Stigma: Advances in theory and research. *Basic Applied Social Psychology, 35*(1), 1–9. https://doi.org/10.1080/01973533.2012.746147

Brighton, R. M., Patterson, C., Taylor, E., Moxham, L., Perlman, D., Sumskis, S., & Heffernan, T. (2016). The effect of respite services on carers of individuals with severe mental illness. *Journal of Psychosocial Nursing and Mental Health Services, 54*(12), 33–38. https://doi.org/10.3928/02793695-20161208-07

Brijnath, B., & Antoniades, J. (2018). What is at stake? Exploring the moral experience of stigma with Indian-Australians and Anglo-Australians living with depression. *Transcultural Psychiatry, 55*(2), 178–197. https://doi.org/10.1177/1363461518756519

Buckley, M. R., & Scott, S. K. (2017). Relational functioning: Understanding bipolar and related disorders. In J. A. Russo, J. K. Coker, & J. H. King (Eds.), *DSM-5® and family systems* (pp. 55–83). Springer Publishing Company, LLC.

Canadian Mental Health Association. (n.d.). *Fast facts about mental illness.* https://cmha.ca/fast-facts-about-mental-illness

Caron, J., & Liu, A. (2010). A descriptive study of the prevalence of psychological distress and mental disorders in the Canadian population: Comparison between low-income and non-low-income populations. *Chronic Diseases in Canada, 30*(3), 84–94. https://www.canada.ca/content/dam/phac-aspc/migration/phac-aspc/publicat/hpcdp-pspmc/30-3/pdf/cdic-30-3-03-eng.pdf

Chronister, J., Fitzgerald, S., & Chou, C-C. (2021). The meaning of social support for persons with serious mental illness: A family member perspective. *Rehabilitation Psychology, 66*(1), 87–101. https://doi.org/10.1037/rep0000369

Coker, F., Williams, A., Hayes, L., Hamann, J., & Harvey, C. (2016). Exploring the needs of diverse consumers experiencing mental illness and their families through family psychoeducation. *Journal of Mental Health, 25*(3), 197–203. https://doi.org/10.3109/09638237.2015.1057323

Doane, G. H., & Varcoe, C. (2021). *How to nurse: Relational inquiry with individuals and families in changing health care contexts* (2nd ed.). Wolters Kluwer Health.

Dobransky, K. M. (2019). Breaking down walls, building bridges: Professional stigma management in mental health care. *Society and Mental Health, 9*(2), 228–242. https://doi.org/10.1177/2156869317750705

Dodge, C. E., & Smith, A. P. (2019). Caregiving as role transitions: Siblings' experiences and expectations when caring for a brother or sister with Schizophrenia. *Canadian Journal of Community Mental Health, 38*(2), 35–47. https://doi.org.cyber.usask.ca/10.7870/cjcmh-2019-005

El-Mallakh, P., & Findlay, K. (2015). Strategies to improve medication adherence in patients with schizophrenia: The role of support services. *Neuropsychiatric Disease and Treatment, 11*, 1077–1090. https://doi.org/10.2147/NDT.S56107

Ennis, E., & Bunting, B. P. (2013). Family burden, family health, and personal mental health. *BMC Public Health, 13*, 255. https://doi.org/10.1186/1471-2458-13-255

Falloon, I. (2005). Research on family interventions for mental disorders: Problems and perspectives. In N. Sartorius, J. Leff, J. J. López-Ibor, M. Maj, & A. Okasha (Eds.), *Families and mental disorders: From burden to empowerment* (pp. 235–257). Wiley.

Farooq, S., & Naeem, F. (2014). Tackling nonadherence in psychiatric disorders: Current opinion. *Neuropsychiatric Disease and Treatment, 10*, 1069–1077. https://doi.org/10.2147/NDT.S40777

Farrell, J., & Goebert, D. (2008). Collaboration between psychiatrists and clergy in recognizing and treating serious mental illness. *Psychiatric Services, 59*, 437–440.

Flyck, L., Fatouros-Bergman, H., & Koernig, T. (2015). Determinants of subjective and objective burden of informal caregiving of patients with psychotic disorders. *The International Journal of Social Psychiatry, 61*(7), 684–692. https://doi.org/10.1177/0020764015573088

Fuller-Thomson, E., Lee, S., Cameron, R. E., Baiden, P., Agbeyaka, S., & Karamally, T. M. (2020). Aboriginal peoples in complete mental health: A nationally-representative Canadian portrait of resilience and flourishing. *Transcultural Psychiatry, 57*(2), 250–262. https://doi.org/10.1177/1363461519885702

Gagne, C. A., Finch, W. L., Myrick, K. J., & Davis, L. M. (2018). Peer workers in the behavioral and integrated health workforce: Opportunities and future directions. *American Journal of Preventive Medicine, 54*(6), S258–S266. https://doi.org/10.1016/j.amepre.2018.03.010

Gladstone, B. M., Boydell, K. M., Seeman, M. V., & McKeever, P. D. (2011). Children's experiences of parental mental illness: A literature review. *Early Intervention in Psychiatry, 5*, 271–289. https://doi.org/10.1111/j.1751-7893.2011.00287.x

Gracey, M., & King, M. (2009). Indigenous health part 1: Determinants and disease patterns. *The Lancet, 374*, 65–75. https://doi.org/10.1016/S0140-6736(09)60914-4

Gratzer, D., Khalid-Khan, F., Balasingham, S., Yuen, N., & Jayanthinkumar, J. (2018). Internet-delivered cognitive behavioral therapy in a Canadian community hospital: A novel approach to an evidenced based intervention. *Canadian Journal of Community Mental Health, 37*(1), 81–85. https://doi.org/10.7870/cjcmh-2018-001

Grebeldinger, T. A., & Buckley, K. M. (2016). You are not alone: Parish nurses bridge challenges for family caregivers. *Journal of Christian Nursing, 33*(1), 50–56. https://soi.org/10.1097/CNJ.0000000000000252

Greenstein, L. (2016, December 21). *The mental health benefits of religion & spirituality.* National Alliance on Mental Illness. https://www.nami.org/Blogs/NAMI-Blog/December-2016/The-Mental-Health-Benefits-of-Religion-Spiritual

Health Quality Ontario. (2019). *Internet-delivered cognitive behavioural therapy for major depression and anxiety disorders: Health Quality Ontario recommendation.* https://www.hqontario.ca/Portals/0/documents/evidence/reports/recommendation-internet-delivered-cognitive-behavioural-therapy-en.pdf

Institute for Patient- and Family-Centered Care (2017). *Advancing the practice of patient- and family-centered care in hospitals.* https://ipfcc.org/resources/getting_started.pdf

King, M., Smith, A., & Gracey, M. (2009). Indigenous health part 2: The underlying causes of the health gap. *The Lancet, 374*, 76–85. https://doi.org/10.1016/S0140-6736(09)60827-8

Kirmayer, L. J., & Valaskakis, C. G. (2009) *Healing traditions: The mental health of aboriginal peoples in Canada.* University of British Columbia Press.

Leahey, M., & Harper-Jaques, S. (2010). Integrating family nursing into a mental health urgent care practice framework: Ladders for learning. *Journal of Family Nursing, 16*(2) 196–212.

Leavey, G., Lowenthal, K., & King, M. (2007). Challenges to sanctuary. *Social Science and Medicine, 65*(3), 548–559.

Limacher, L. H., & Wright, L. M. (2003). Commendations: Listening to the silent side of a family intervention. *Journal of Family Nursing, 9*(2), 130–150.

MacCourt, P. (2013). *Family Caregivers Advisory Committee, Mental Health Commission of Canada. National guidelines for a comprehensive service system to support family caregivers of adults with mental health problems and illnesses.* Mental Health Commission of Canada. http://www.mentalhealthcommission.ca

McGoldrick, M., GarciaPreto, N., & Carter, B. A. (2016). *The expanding family life cycle: Individual, family and social perspectives* (5th ed.). Pearson.

Melchior, M. (2019). Is children's mental illness "a family affair"? *European Child & Adolescent Psychiatry, 28*, 875–876. https://doi.org/10.1007/s00787-019-01366-w

Mental Health Commission of Canada. (2009). *Toward recovery and well-being: A framework for a mental health strategy for Canada.*

Mental Health Commission of Canada. (2012). *Opening Minds program overview.* https://www.mentalhealthcommission.ca/English/initiatives/11874/opening-minds

Mental Health Commission of Canada. (2015). *Recovery guidelines.*

mdsc.ca The Mood Disorders Society of Canada has evolved to become strong voice for consumers regarding education and advocacy at the national level through partnerships with like-minded public, private, and voluntary sectors.

Miklowitz, D., George, E., Richards, J., Simoneau, T., & Suddath R. (2003). A randomized study of family-focused psycho-education and pharmaco-therapy in the outpatient management of bipolar disorder. *Archives of General Psychiatry, 60*, 904–912. https://doi.org/10.1001/archpsyc.60.9.904

Mottaghipour, Y., & Bickerton, A. (2005). The Pyramid of family care: A framework for family involvement with adult mental health services. *Australian e-Journal for the Advancement of Mental Health, 4*(3), 210–217. https://doi.org/10.5172/jamh.4.3.210

Mulud, Z. A. (2016). Caregiver burden in mental illness. In J. J. Fitzpatrick, & G. M. McCarthy (Eds.), *Nursing concept analysis: Applications to research and practice* (pp. 141–150). Springer Publishing Company LLC.

Murney, M. A., Sapag, J. C., Bobbili, S. J., & Khenti, A. (2020). Stigma and discrimination related to mental health and substance use issues in primary care in Toronto, Canada: A qualitative study. *International Journal of Qualitative Studies on Health and Wellbeing, 15*(1), 1744926, https://doi.org/10.1080/17482631.2020.1744926

Nelson, S. E. & Wilson, K. (2017). The mental health of Indigenous peoples in Canada: A critical review of research. *Social Science & Medicine, 176*, 93–112. https://doi.org/10.1016/j.socscimed.2017.01.021

Pearson, C. (2015, October). *The impact of mental health problems on family members. Health at a Glance.* Statistics Canada. http://www.statcan.gc.ca/pub/82-624-x/2015001/article/14214-eng.htm

Penney, D. (2018). *Defining 'peer support': Implications for policy, practice, and research.* Advocates for human potential. https://www.ahpnet.com/AHPNet/media/AHPNetMediaLibrary/White%20Papers/

Petrakis, M., & Laxton, S. (2017). Intervening early with family members during first-episode psychosis: An evaluation of mental health nursing psychoeducation within an inpatient unit. *Archives of Psychiatric Nursing, 31*, 48–54. https://doi.org/10.1016/j.apnu.2016.07.015

Rahmani, F., Ebrahimi, H., Seyedfatemi, N., Areshtanab, H. N., Ranjbar, F., & Whitehead, B. (2018). Trapped like a butterfly in a spider's web: Experiences of female spousal caregivers in the care of husbands with severe mental illness. *Journal of Clinical Nursing, 27*, 1507–1508. https://doi.org/10.1111/jocn.14286

Registered Nurses Association of Ontario. (2015). *Person- and family-centred care: Best practice guideline.* https://rnao.ca/sites/rnao-ca/files/FINAL_Web_Version_0.pdf

Reinares, M., Bonnin, C. M., Hidalgo-Mazzei, D, Sánchez-Moreno, J., Colm, R., & Vieta, E. (2016). The role of family interventions in bipolar disorder: A systematic review. *Clinical Psychology Review, 43*, 47–57.

Reupert, A., & Mayberry, D. (2016). What do we know about families where parents have a mental illness? A systematic review. *Child & Youth Services, 37*(2), 98–111.

Revell, S. M. H., & McCurry M. K. (2021). Nursing science, mental illness, and the family: A conceptual framework to break the cycle of suffering. *Nursing Science Quarterly, 34*(1), 59–66. https://doi.org/10.1177/0894318420965230

Risling, T., Risling, D., & Holtslander, L. (2017). Creating a social media assessment tool for family nursing. *Journal of Family Nursing, 23*(1), 13–33. https://doi.org/10.1177/1074840716681071

Shajani, Z., & Snell, D. (2019). *Wright and Leahey's nurses and families: A guide to family assessment and intervention* (7th ed). F. A. Davis.

Shalaby, R. A. H., & Agyapong, V. (2020). Peer support in mental health: Literature review. *JMIR Mental Health, 7*(6), e15572. https://doi.org/10.2196/15572

Schizophrenia Society of Canada. (2020). *Family recovery journey.* https://schizophrenia.ca/family-recovery-journey/family-recovery-journey-materials/

Sinha, M. (2013). *Portrait of caregivers, 2012. Spotlight on Canadians: Results for the General Social Survey.* Statistics Canada. Catalogue no. 89-652-x-No. 001. http://www.statcan.gc.ca/pub/89-652-x/89-652-x2013001-eng.htm

Stamatopoulos, V. (2015). One million and counting: The hidden army of young carers in Canada. *Journal of Youth Studies, 18*(6), 809–822. https://doi.org/10.1080/13676261.2014.992329

Stamatopoulos, V. (2016). Supporting young carers: A qualitative review of young carer services in Canada. *International Journal of Adolescence and Youth, 21*(2), 178–194. https://doi.org/10.1080/02673843.2015.1061568

Statistics Canada. (2011). *Fifty years of families in Canada: 1961 to 2011.* http://www12.statcan.gc.ca/census-recensement/2011/as-sa/98-312-x/98-312-x2011003_1-eng.cfm

Statistics Canada (2017). *Families, households and marital status: Key results from the 2016 Census.* https://www150.statcan.gc.ca/n1/daily-quotidien/170802/dq170802a-eng.htm

Statistics Canada. (2020, January 8). *Caregivers in Canada, 2018.* https://www150.statcan.gc.ca/n1/en/daily-quotidien/200108/dq200108a-eng.pdf?st=j69VV2ri

Stuart, H. L. (2005). *Respite needs of people living with schizophrenia: A national survey of schizophrenia society members.* Schizophrenia Society of Canada. http://www.schizophrenia.ca/docs/SSCRespiteReportE.pdf

Sveinbjarnardottir, E., Svararsdottir, E., & Wright, L. (2013). What are the benefits of a short therapeutic conversation intervention with acute psychiatric patients and their families? A controlled before and after study. *International Journal of Nursing Studies, 50*(5), 593–602.

Symenuk, P., Tisdale, D., Bourque Bearskin, D.H. & Munro, T. (2020). In search of the truth: Uncovering nursing's involvement in colonial harms and assimilative policies five years post truth and reconciliation commission. *Witness: The Canadian Journal of Critical Nursing Discourse, 2*(1), 84–96. https://doi.org/10.25071/2291-5796.51

Toohey, M. J., Muralidharan, A., Medoff, D., Lucsted, A., & Dixon, L. (2016). Caregiver positive and negative appraisals. Effects of the National Alliance on Mental Illness Family-to-Family Intervention. *Journal of Nervous and Mental Disease, 204*(2), 156–159. https://doi.org/10.1097/NMD.0000000000000447

Turpel-LaFond, M. E. (2020). *In Plain Sight: Addressing Indigenous-specific racism and discrimination in BC Health Care.* file:///C:/Users/Cindy/Desktop/In-Plain-Sight-Full-Report.pdf

van der Sanden, R. L. M., Pryor, J. B., Stutterheim, S. E., Kok, G., & Bos, A. E. R. (2016). Stigma by association and family burden among family members of people with mental illness: The mediating role of coping. *Social Psychiatry and Psychiatric Epidemiology, 51*, 1233–1245. https://doi.org/10.1007/s00127-016-1256-x

Vermaas, J. D., Green, J., Haley, M., & Haddock, L. (2017). Predicting the mental health literacy of clergy: An informational resource for counselors. *Journal of Mental Health Counseling, 39*(3), 225–241.

Whitehorn, D., Campbell, M. E., Cosgrove, P., Abidi, S., & Tibbo, P. G. (2017). A mindfulness-based support group for families in early psychosis: A pilot qualitative study. *Journal of Mental Health and Addiction Nursing, 1*(1), e30–e34.

Wrosch, C., Amir, E., & Miller, G. E. (2011). Goal adjustment capabilities, coping, and subjective well being: The sample case of caregiving for a family member with mental illness. *Journal of Personality and Social Psychology, 100*(5), 934–946. https://doi.org/10.1037/a0022873

Young, L., Vandyk, A. D., Jacob, J. D., McPherson, C., & Murata, L. (2019). Being parent caregivers for adult children with Schizophrenia. *Issues in Mental Health Nursing, 40*, 297–303. https://doi.org/10.1080/01612840.2018.1524531

Psychological Health and Safety in the Workplace

Diane Kunyk*

The workplace has great potential as a setting in which the health of workers and their families can be promoted, protected, and supported. It offers a venue for health education and healthy workplace policies, for workers to access preventive health services, and for linkages to primary health care. Workplace programs are considered one of the best opportunities to prevent and manage mental health disorders (World Health Organization [WHO], 2020).

These opportunities, however, are far from being optimized. Canadian employees report workplace stress as the primary cause of their mental health problems or illnesses, with depression and anxiety noted as the top two issues (Dewa et al., 2010). Psychological health issues have been estimated to cost the Canadian economy over $50 billion annually and make up about 70% of disability claims among Canadians (Mental Health Commission of Canada [MHCC], 2013a). Mental illness and related claims are approximately two times longer in duration and more costly than the average of all other claim types (Dewa et al., 2010). Further mental health strains amongst Canadian workers have been reported since the onset of the global pandemic. In one example, an April 2021 survey of 3,000 Canadian workers demonstrated significant ongoing and increasing mental stress scores amongst Canadian workers since the beginning of the COVID-19 pandemic (Life-Works, 2021). Clearly, the workplace is an opportune arena for nurses to attend to mental health issues.

Substantive strides have been made in Canada towards improving workplace mental health. The treatment of employees with mental health issues and attitudes towards workplace mental health have improved with time. We are the first country to create national standards for psychological health and safety in the workplace (CSA Group, 2013). Known collectively as the Standard, these standards, although voluntary, are a significant achievement developed from legal and scientific research and through consultation with occupational health and safety experts, industry, unions, professional associations, and government agencies. A growing body of evidence supports this approach. For instance, in a Canadian survey, employees in organizations that implemented the Standard were significantly more likely to describe a workplace where the psychological environment was a relative strength, whereas those who knew that their organization had not implemented the Standard were more likely to describe

---

*Adapted from the chapter "Psychological Health and Safety in the Workplace" by Wendy Austin

workplaces that were psychologically concerning (Ipsos, 2017).

The health and wellbeing of the health workforce is of particular concern: the health of everyone depends upon it. How can safe, compassionate, competent, ethical care be provided by individuals who are unhealthy, fatigued, and burned out? The rationale behind instructing airline passengers to put on their own oxygen masks before helping others can be applied here. Along this line, HealthCare*CAN* and the Mental Health Commission of Canada concluded that although there has been progress in addressing the physical health and safety of healthcare workers and workplaces, there was an urgent need to safeguard their psychological health and safety. For this reason, two additional factors for the Standard were added at that time that are relevant to nurses: protection from moral distress and support for psychological self-care (MHCC, 2021).

This chapter addresses psychological health and safety in the workplace. It considers the relation of work to health and wellbeing and the attributes of a healthy workplace. Outlined are some ways in which workplaces may support and accommodate individuals at risk for, or who have, mental health concerns. Workplace violence, including bullying, is discussed, and healthcare environments are considered as workplaces, particularly from the perspective of nurses.

Work

Work is the term used to signify our paid employment, the job or task we perform to earn a living. As humans, we are meant to work, to contribute and produce in some way, and this very work rewards our psychological health (Table 17.1). Work in its broadest sense is not restricted to places of employment. Some individuals work entirely within their homes, are not employees of any organization, and do not receive any monetary remuneration for their contribution to family, home, and community life.

However, if negative conditions exist, such as high job demands, low job control, low procedural justice, role stress, bullying, and low social support, work can also contribute to mental illness (Harvey et al., 2017). How we perceive our work and workplace is not static,

Table 17.1 Potential Psychological Benefits of Work
1. Income and sense of security
2. Source of identity
3. Sense of purpose in life
4. Source of self-worth and self-esteem
5. Opportunity to develop skills and creativity
6. Autonomy and independence
7. Relationships outside the family
8. Structure
9. Defines leisure time and activities

Source: Gold, L. H., & Shuman, D. W. (2009). *Evaluating mental health disability in the workplace—Model, process, and analysis* (pp. 45–48). Springer.

but rather constantly changing. There are times when we struggle with our work or may exit (temporarily or permanently) the workplace for many reasons. Throughout their workplace life cycle, individuals will shift along the spectrum of mental health in the workplace depending on their circumstances (see Fig. 17.1). This spectrum ranges through seven identified categories:

- Healthy in work
- In work struggling
- In work off sick
- Not in work (less than a year)
- Not in work (more than a year)
- Never worked

Job attitudes, how people think and feel about their job, are important because one's job is important to their identity, health, and satisfaction with life (Judge & Kammeyer-Mueller, 2012). Facets of job satisfaction include satisfaction with work, supervision, coworkers, pay, and promotions. Of these, it is satisfaction with the work itself that is key to overall satisfaction (Herzberg et al., 2009; Judge & Kammeyer-Mueller, 2012). While the quality of workplace environments, particularly potential **hazards** (i.e., sources of physical and/or psychological harm), must be addressed, the quality of the work itself matters, too.

KEY CONCEPT

Work is "the job, occupation, or task one performs as a means of providing a livelihood" (Venes, 2009, p. 2502).

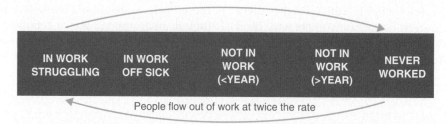

IN WORK STRUGGLING	IN WORK OFF SICK	NOT IN WORK (<YEAR)	NOT IN WORK (>YEAR)	NEVER WORKED

People flow out of work at twice the rate

Figure 17.1 Mental health in the workplace. (Source: Howatt, B., Bradley, L., Adams, J., Mahajan, S., & Kennedy, S. (2017). *Understanding mental health, mental illness, and their impacts in the workplace.* Mental Health Commission of Canada and Morneau Shepell. https://www.morneaushepell.com/permafiles/91248/mental-health-white-paper-2018.pdf)

The Changing Nature of Work

Economic and technologic changes to the workplace, which are aimed at increasing short-term productivity and maximizing profits, continue to shape the nature of contemporary work. These changes include organizational restructuring and downsizing, decreases in job stability, the frantic pace of work and life, and decreases in leisure time. Organizational change is likely to increase given technology advances, new business models, and global economic forces.

This transformation has direct effects on the work life of Canadians. Two thirds of Canadian employees have experienced an organizational change at their current workplace; among them, 40% say it has negatively affected their health and wellbeing. In particular, their position redesign has the strongest correlation with sick leave for physical and mental health reasons (MHCC, 2018). Nurses must be aware that although work has the potential to be a positive factor in sustaining health and wellbeing, work, or the lack of it, can have a negative effect on existing health problems and can contribute to the development of new ones.

Unemployment

Most governments identify an individual as **unemployed** when the person does not have paid employment, wants to be employed, and is actively seeking work. The unemployment rate is often understated and does not include individuals who are **underemployed**: those with insufficient work relative to hours, capabilities, or skills. Nor does this rate include those who want to work but have given up seeking it. When considering a person's employment status, it is more useful to consider employment along a continuum rather than as a dichotomous state of employed or unemployed.

Unemployment places individuals at risk for adverse health effects. An international meta-analysis examining the influence of unemployment on morbidity and mortality found that the unemployed had a significantly higher risk of morbidity and premature mortality compared with their employed counterparts (Hollederer, 2015). When individuals have a strong attachment to the labour market or prior workplace, have high "breadwinning" responsibilities, or are disadvantaged in terms of occupational class, wage, or job quality, there is greater likelihood that unemployment will impair their mental health (Backhans & Hemmingsson, 2011).

Job loss can cause a shift in family roles and power balance and therefore greatly impact family members (McKee-Ryan & Maitoza, 2018). Family members of those who have lost their jobs can also experience hardship and stigma. Insecurity regarding one's job contributes to a sense of insecurity regarding the future. Sharp and/or sustained rises in unemployment negatively impacts a community's wellbeing as people lose jobs, acquire debt, and become unable to maintain their lifestyle. When appropriate measures are not in place, such as adequate unemployment benefits, social services, and community support, the level of stress and mental health problems in a community rises.

Work and Gender

In industrialized nations, women make up nearly half of the paid workforce but remain underrepresented in decision-making positions (the "glass ceiling" continues to exist). In Canada, women are paid 13.3% less than men on average (Statistics Canada, 2019). Although gender stereotypes are less influential in determining job and career choices than they once were, males and females continue to be segregated into different types of work. Registered nurses in Canada, for instance, are overwhelmingly female and despite increases in males entering nursing programs, they represent only 9% of the nursing workforce (Canadian Institute for Health Information, 2020). Attempts are being made to support greater diversity in the workplace. In 2019, a Symposium on Women and the Workplace was held to discuss gender equality and diversity in the workplace. This symposium made suggestions to change workplace culture to provide diversity training, inspire peer support, and prevent gender-based violence and harassment (Government of Canada [GOC], 2019a).

Gender segregation in types of work means that exposure to risk—the likelihood that harm may occur plus the severity of that harm (CSA Group, 2013)—differs between genders. For instance, preliminary findings suggest that female healthcare workers have been at increased risk for stress, burnout, and depression during the COVID-19 pandemic. Triggers for these negative outcomes include personal factors such as lack of social support, organizational factors such as high workload, systems-level factors such as rapidly changing public health guidelines, and a lack of recognition at work (Srihara et al., 2020).

Responses to workplace hazards may also have gender-based variation. Biologically, men and women may be affected differently by such hazards as toxins, due to hormonal differences; psychologically, women report work-related stress more frequently, perhaps due to less power and autonomy or greater vulnerability to harassment (WHO, 2011). Low control over work environment and conditions, however, has been found to correlate with hypertension in male workers but not in female workers (Smith et al., 2013). Biology may shape response to job demands and control, as well. Until rates of work-related injuries and disease are analyzed by gender, our understanding of its influence on workplace health will be insufficient. The dearth of research related to risks and health issues encountered in unpaid work (e.g., cooking, cleaning, care of family members, tending to family business) contributed most often by women also leaves an important knowledge gap (WHO, 2011).

Equity, Diversity, and Inclusion

Equity, diversity, and inclusion (EDI) are at the forefront of many changes in employment policies and practices in institutions across Canada. (Refer to Chapter 3 for further discussion of these concepts.) EDI action plans are being created to recognize and reduce systemic barriers (GOC, 2019b). This movement offers numerous benefits to employers, including, for example, access to a range of experiences, skills, and perspectives, and positively contributes to innovation, creativity, and problem solving (Canadian Centre for Diversity and Inclusion, 2019). No employee should be treated differently, feel stigmatized, or fear going to work. Implementing EDI policies can minimize these feelings by creating an inclusive workplace through practices such as the use of gender-neutral pronouns and name usage, gender-neutral washrooms, parental leaves, and diversity training. Failure to create an inclusive workplace can lead to absenteeism, high turnover, and decreased engagement and productivity (Thoroughgood et al., 2020).

Working From Home

Thanks to technological advances, there are increasing opportunities for employees to work from home. In response to the COVID-19 pandemic, government and organizational policies *required* employees to work from home whenever possible, thereby drawing increased attention to this phenomenon. Although there are direct benefits for employees, such as absence of commuting, flexible work hours, and cost savings, working from home also has challenges (Dockery & Bawa, 2020; Xiao et al., 2021). Some of the negative effects for employees include working long hours, difficulty separating work from home life, exacerbating work–family conflicts, and limited social networking (Dockery & Bawa, 2020). There may be additional strain for those who have housemates, children, or other family members sharing space (Dockery & Bawa, 2020) and can also increase unpaid work if productivity ignores employee care burdens (Craig & Churchill, 2021). This stance did not take into account that care burdens, and childcare/school closures impacted women's paid and unpaid work disproportionately to men's (Craig & Churchill, 2021).

Healthy Workplaces

According to the WHO's framework, a healthy workplace exists when workers and managers continually collaborate to address health and safety concerns in the physical and psychosocial work environment, including the organization of work and workplace culture, and attend to health resources in the workplace and the community (Burton, 2010). The healthy workplace is

an inclusive work culture: open, accessible, and accepting of workers with diverse backgrounds, demographics, and skills. Disparities between groups of workers or difficulties affecting specific workers (e.g., due to gender, ethnicity, or disability) are minimized or eliminated (Burton, 2010).

KEY CONCEPT

Workplace health is the promotion and maintenance of the health and wellbeing of workers through policies, programs, and practices that promote safety, minimize risk, and create a positive, responsive, equitable workplace culture and a supportive workplace climate.

The Psychologically Healthy and Safe Workplace

A psychologically healthy and safe workplace is one where workers understand their roles and believe that they can contribute to decisions about how their work is carried out. There is much evidence that both worker's wellbeing and performance are improved when organizations understand the importance of flexible work design and give their employees as much choice and control as possible (Lowe, 2010). The Mental Health Commission of Canada's recognition of the key contribution that healthy workplaces can make towards the wellbeing of Canadians has informed the development of several resources for employers. Thirteen psychosocial factors for a healthy and safe workplace were identified in 2012 (see Table 17.2) (Samra et al., 2012). The characteristics of psychologically *unsafe* workplaces with increased risks to mental health have similarly been identified (Shain et al., 2013) (see Box 17.1).

The National Standard of Canada for Psychological Health and Safety in the Workplace outlines a systematic framework for employers to use in creating and sustaining healthy, safe workplaces. It includes ways to identify and eliminate environmental hazards and how to assess and control risks associated with hazards that cannot be removed (e.g., inherent job demands and stressors). The standard includes several application annexes with evidence-informed resources including sample implementation models, scenarios, and audit tools (CSA Group, 2013). As mentioned earlier in this chapter, in 2016, HealthCare*CAN* and the Mental Health Commission of Canada concluded that although there has been progress in addressing the physical health and safety of healthcare workers and workplaces, there is an urgent need to safeguard their psychological health and safety. For this reason, two additional factors for the Standard were added at that time that are relevant to nurses (Table 17.3).

Table 17.2 Thirteen Psychosocial Factors in Workplace Health, Safety, and Wellbeing

Factor	Objective for the Workplace	Benefits to Employees
1. Psychological support	Coworkers and supervisors provide support and appropriate responses to employees' psychological and mental health concerns.	Improved psychological health Increased productivity Reduced absenteeism and disability Successful and sustainable return to work
2. Organizational culture	An environment characterized by trust, honesty, and fairness.	Higher job satisfaction and morale Improved teamwork and productivity Enhanced retention and recruitment Positive image in the community
3. Clear leadership and expectations	Effective leadership and support that help employees know what they need to do, how their work contributes, and whether there are impending changes.	Clear expectations for job responsibilities and roles Positive morale and resiliency, particularly in times of stress and change Lessened frustration and conflict Greater trust in the employer
4. Civility and respect	An environment where employees and supervisors are respectful and considerate in their interactions with one another, as well as with clients and the public.	Effective teamwork and positive morale Reduced conflict Fewer grievances and lessened legal risk Improved relationships with clients
5. Psychological competencies and requirements	There is a good fit between employees' interpersonal and emotional competencies and the requirements of the position they hold.	Enhanced performance and overall productivity Greater job satisfaction Increased retention of skilled staff Enhanced recruitment success
6. Growth and development	Employees receive encouragement and support in the development of their interpersonal, emotional, and job skills.	Increased employee competency Retention of skilled staff Effective succession planning/internal promotion Enhanced service quality
7. Recognition and reward	Appropriate, fair, and timely acknowledgement and appreciation of employees' efforts.	Greater employee satisfaction, motivation, and loyalty Improved teamwork and positive employee morale Increased retention and enhanced recruitment of skilled staff Enhanced employee/labour relations
8. Involvement and influence	Employees are included in discussion about how their work is done and how important decisions are made.	Enhanced performance and productivity Greater employee motivation and job satisfaction Employees actively address challenges at work Positive employee/labour relations
9. Workload management	Tasks and responsibilities can be accomplished successfully within the time available.	Enhanced performance and productivity Reduced stress and/or burnout Fewer job-related errors, incidents, accidents, and injuries Increased retention
10. Engagement	Employees feel connected to their work and motivated to do their job well.	Enhanced performance and productivity High morale and motivation Enhanced recruitment and increased retention of skilled staff Improved relationships with clients
11. Balance	An environment where there is recognition of the need for balance between the demands of work, family, and personal life.	Greater job satisfaction and morale Reduced stress and burnout Enhanced performance and productivity Reduced absenteeism and disability
12. Psychological protection	An environment where employees' psychological safety is ensured.	Reduced absenteeism and disability Reduced conflict Fewer job-related errors, incidents, accidents, and injuries Fewer grievances and lessened legal risk
13. Protection of physical safety	Management takes appropriate action to protect the physical safety of employees.	Improved physical and psychological health and safety Fewer job-related errors, incidents, accidents, and injuries Reduced absenteeism and disability Improved labour–management relations Reduced legal and regulatory costs

Adapted from: Standards Council of Canada (2013). Psychological health and safety in the workplace—prevention, promotion, and guidance to staged implementation. (CSA Group and BNQ Publication No. CAN/CSA-Z1003-13/BNQ 9700-803/2013 National Standard of Canada). Retrieved from http://shop.csa.ca/en/canada/occupational-health-and-safety-management/ cancsa-z1003-13bnq-9700-8032013/invt/z10032013

BOX 17.1 The Psychologically Unsafe Workplace

RISKS TO MENTAL HEALTH IN THE WORKPLACE ARE MORE LIKELY TO OCCUR WHEN

* *Job demands and requirements of effort* consistently and chronically exceed worker skill levels or unreasonably exploit them or where work is distributed inequitably.
* *Job control or influence* is deliberately withheld from workers who lack discretion over the means, manner, and methods of their work (including "voice" or the perceived freedom to express views or feelings appropriate to the situation or context).
* *Reward*, such as praise, recognition, acknowledgement, and credit, is withheld from workers without good business reasons.
* *Fairness* is lacking in that there is consistent failure or refusal to recognize and accommodate the legitimate needs, rights, and claims of workers. Workers feel that decisions are made without attention to due process.
* *Support* with regard to advice, direction, planning, and provision of technical and practical resources and information (to the extent that they are available within the organization) is withheld from workers by choice rather than due to systematic organizational constraints.

Adapted from Shain, M., Arnold, I., & GermAnn, K. (2013). *The road to psychological health and safety: Legal, scientific and social foundations for a national standard for psychological safety in the workplace*. A working paper for the Mental Health Commission of Canada. www.mentalhealthcommission.ca

Table 17.3 Healthcare Workers Factors, National Standard of Canada for Psychological Health and Safety in the Workplace

The two additional factors to National Standard of Canada for Psychological Health and Safety in the Workplace for the Standards to address the physical health and safety of health care workers are:
1. Protection from moral distress: A healthcare work environment where staff are able to do their work with a sense of integrity while being supported by their profession, employer, and peers.
2. Support for psychological self-care: A healthcare workplace where staff are encouraged to care for their own psychological health and safety.

Source: Mental Health Commission of Canada. (2021). *Advancing psychological health and safety within healthcare settings.* https://www.mentalhealthcommission.ca/English/what-we-do/workplace/workplace-healthcare

Work–Life Balance

A challenge for many people is to balance the demands of their paid employment with other aspects of their lives, such as family and community. Individuals have many roles beyond that of an employee. Nonwork roles, such as educational, cultural, recreational, and volunteer activities, are important to life satisfaction and contribute to the cohesion of a society (Lero et al., 2009). **Work–life balance** is achieved when individuals find a satisfactory interaction among all the domains of their lives. This balance is not the same for everyone but differs based on personal values, family structure, life situations and expectations, and societal norms. These domains are fluid because they reflect constantly shifting life circumstances.

Work–life conflict occurs when work–life balance is upset, when the demands of work and nonwork roles directly interfere with a person's ability to meet one or more of the roles. Both the number of demands and the control individuals feel over such demands are factors in work–life conflict (Duxbury & Higgins, 2009; Lero et al., 2009). See Box 17.2 for categories of work–life conflict. Job demands (e.g., heavy workload, multiple and/or time-pressured tasks) are a primary antecedent of work–life conflict. In an attempt to meet job demands, workers may stay on the job after regular hours, take work home, or work on days off. These strategies interfere with successful fulfillment of other roles, such as those within the family. Working long hours can keep one from attending family

BOX 17.2 Work–Life Conflict Categories

* **Role overload:** The total demands on time and energy associated with the prescribed activities of multiple roles are too great to perform the roles adequately or comfortably.
* **Role interference:**
  * Work-to-family interference: role conflict when work demands and responsibilities hinder one from fulfilling family-role responsibilities
  * Family-to-work interference: role conflict when family demands and responsibilities make it more difficult to fulfill work role
  * Caregiver strain: strain related to the everyday responsibilities of providing necessary care or assistance to someone, such as a family member

Adapted from Higgins, C., Duxbury, L., & Lyons, S. (2008). *Reducing work-life conflict: What works? What doesn't?* http://www.hc-sc.gc.ca/ewh-semt/pubs/occup-travail/balancing-equilibre/index-eng.php

celebrations and children's school and sports events; pre-occupation with or stress from work can strain family relationships. Family roles and responsibilities, in turn, can interfere with fulfilling one's role at work, as when caring for an ill family member means being absent from the job, or trouble at home impedes work functioning. Technology has further complicated work–life balance. Technological advances, for instance, can make an individual available to work at any time and can make working from home a more viable option. **Role overload** occurs when an individual is unable to satisfy role demands.

The quality and availability of community supports, such as daycare or dependent care, can mitigate pressures on individuals and families, as can flexible working practices, such as varied hours of work, working remotely, opportunity for leave, and "family-friendly" workplaces (Lero et al., 2009; Lowe, 2010). In fact, flexible work design has been identified as the most effective solution for improving employee wellbeing, particularly when it is conceived in a holistic and systemic way (Lowe, 2010). Some employers have recognized the importance of work–life balance and are finding unique strategies to retain their employees. Google, for instance, developed a study, based on the longitudinal Framingham Heart Study, to improve the experience of work. The purpose was to improve wellbeing, cultivate better leaders, keep employees ("Googlers") engaged for long periods of time, and understand how happiness and work impact one another (Block, 2014). In the first round of the study, 69% of participants stated they were unable to draw a line between work and the rest of their life and more than half stated they wanted to achieve a better work–life balance. Google started initiatives to help employees achieve this balance, including having employees drop off their devices at the front desk before leaving work and encouraging employees to use all their vacation days and to ignore off-hours e-mails (Block, 2014). Another company that prioritizes work–life balance is Zoom Video Communications. The business has been ranked one of the top companies for its corporate environment by Glassdoor in 2019 (Howley, 2020). The company provides unlimited vacation, promotes evenings and weekends off, has a "happy crew" that provides employees with monthly experiences, and has a monthly gym membership allowance for all employees. Additionally, the company has virtual celebrations for holidays such as Diwali. They also advocate for mental health and heart disease awareness and have partnered with the American Heart Association (Howley, 2020).

Threats to Workplace Psychological Health and Safety

Stress

Stress at work does not necessarily have a negative effect on employees; it depends upon the nature, intensity,

and duration of the stress and upon the presence of protective factors (e.g., employees feel they have some control regarding their work situation) (Burton, 2010). Indications that an individual's stress is work related include awareness that they function without any difficulty outside of the workplace and that stress is experienced when preparing for work or when thinking primarily about workplace issues (see Chapter 18 for a detailed discussion of stress).

When organizations commit to meeting Canada's voluntary national standard of psychological health and safety, they contribute to creating a less stressful workplace for their employees. There are many freely available resources for them to use, including the Comprehensive Workplace Health and Safety program of the Canadian Centre for Occupational Health and Safety, which addresses psychosocial work environment, workplace health promotion, and organizational community involvement (see Web Links). Proactive initiatives are to an organization's advantage: there are huge costs related to absenteeism, presentism, and voluntary employee turnover (Lowe, 2010; Shain et al., 2013).

Burnout

Burnout is a term that refers specifically to the occupational workplace and not to other areas of everyday life. It has been classified in the 11th Revision of the International Classification of Diseases (ICD-11) as an occupational phenomenon, not a medical condition, and is characterized by three dimensions:

- Feelings of energy depletion or exhaustion
- Increased mental distance from one's job, or feelings of negativism or cynicism related to one's job
- Reduced professional efficacy (WHO, 2019)

However, burnout has been associated with symptoms such as fatigue, anxiety, sleep disorders, headache, reduced concentration, and heart disease (Chuang et al., 2016; Pradas-Hernández et al., 2018). There is some suggestion that the COVID-19 pandemic increased risk for stress, burnout, and depression amongst female healthcare workers. These negative outcomes were triggered by individual-level factors such as lack of social support; family status; organizational factors such as access to personal protective equipment or high workload; and systems-level factors such as prevalence of COVID-19, rapidly changing public health guidelines, and a lack of recognition at work (Sriharan et al., 2020).

Workplace Violence

Workplace violence is gaining attention as a serious global health, safety, and organizational problem rooted in broad cultural and socioeconomic factors. Workplace violence encompasses far more than physical assault; it includes any act in which a person is abused, threatened, intimidated, or assaulted in their place of work (GOC, 2020). Although physical violence is common, psychological violence appears to be more common in the health sector (Mento et al., 2020).

Some workers are at increased risk for violence due to factors related to their work situation. The Canadian Centre for Occupational Health and Safety (2021) identified heightened workplace risk for employees who:

- Work with the public
- Handle money, valuables, or prescription drugs (e.g., cashiers, pharmacists)
- Carry out inspection or enforcement duties (e.g., government employees)
- Provide service, care, advice, or education (e.g., health care staff, teachers)
- Work with unstable or volatile persons (e.g., social services or criminal justice system employees)
- Work in premises where alcohol is served (e.g., food and beverage staff)
- Work alone, in small numbers (e.g., store clerks, real estate agents), or in isolated or low-traffic areas (e.g., isolated reception area, washroom)
- Work in community-based settings (e.g., nurses, social workers, and other home visitors)
- Have a mobile workplace (e.g., taxicab drivers)
- Work during intense organizational change (e.g., during strikes or downsizing)
- Work with third-party workers, such as contractors or subcontractors

KEY CONCEPT

Workplace violence is defined as aggression in which workers are abused, intimidated, or attacked in circumstances related to their work, including commuting to and from work, involving an explicit or implicit challenge to their safety, wellbeing, or health (Mento et al., 2020, p. 1).

Bullying and Incivility

Bullying is usually considered as acts or verbal comments that could hurt or isolate an individual in the workplace (Canadian Centre for Occupational Health and Safety, 2021). Bullying has three defining characteristics: it occurs repeatedly, there is intent to do emotional and/or physical harm, and a power difference exists between the victim and the aggressor (Canadian Council on Learning, 2008). Recognizing these is crucial to eliminating bullying. Labeling every conflict or criticism as bullying diminishes the latter's seriousness, as does dismissing bullying behaviour as "joking" or "roughhousing." Forms of bullying are found in Table 17.4.

Under Canada's Criminal Code, physical bullying, which includes threats of physical aggression or cyberstalking, can constitute as assault. Amongst other offences, sharing intimate images without consent, uttering threats or intimidation, unauthorized use of computer, mischief in relation to data, identity theft, extortion, defamatory libel, and offence against the person and reputation can constitute criminal harassment and make the offender liable for criminal charges (GOC, 2021). The police can be called to investigate such incidents by employees as well as employers.

Persons who are targets of bullying can experience a wide range of reactions, including shock, anger, frustration and/or helplessness, increased sense of vulnerability, loss of confidence, and physical (e.g., loss of appetite and sleeplessness) and psychosomatic (e.g., headaches, panic or anxiety, inability to concentrate) symptoms (Canadian Centre for Occupational Health and Safety, 2021). A wide range of psychosocial and professional support is therefore necessary to address bullying's many potentially traumatic effects. Such support needs to evolve. A Canadian qualitative study of men's experiences of surviving bullying at work found that a central concern of participants was a lack of workplace supports for addressing and resolving bullying; as well, some men believed that healthcare professionals were unwilling or unable to help manage emotional health problems (O'Donnell & MacIntosh, 2016).

Table 17.4 Four Types of Bullying			
Physical	**Relational**	**Verbal**	**Cyber**
Threatening violence	Spreading gossip or rumours	Name-calling	Online verbal or relational bullying
Pushing	Withholding job information	Verbal intimidation	Sending false e-mails under victim's name
Tripping	Overmonitoring of work	Insulting	Forwarding private e-mails and pictures
Punching	Excessive or unjustified criticism	Mocking	Online threats
Kicking	Setting unrealistic goals	Attacking personal attributes	Cyberstalking
Stalking		Attacking private life	
Forcibly confining			

Adapted from Department of Criminal Justice Canada. (2003). *Stalking is a crime called criminal harassment*. http://canada.justice.gc.ca/eng/pi/fv-vf/pub/har/har.html; Canadian Council on Learning. (2008). *Bullying in Canada: How intimidation affects learning*. http://www.ccl-cca.ca/pdfs/LessonsInLearning/Mar-20-08-Bullying-in-Canad.pdf; Public Services Health and Safety Association. (2010). *Bullying in the workplace: A handbook for the workplace.*

Incivility is disrespectful speech or behaviour that involves such actions as making jokes at another person's expense, interrupting or speaking over them, ignoring them or giving them the "silent treatment," or ignoring their input or opinions (Matthews & Ritter, 2016). In a survey study of approximately 1,000 new graduate nurses in Canada, it was found that civility norms (i.e., informal expectations of mutually respectful behaviour) were key to decreasing coworker incivility and to preventing early career burnout of the nurses (Laschinger & Read, 2016).

Emergencies and Disasters

Traumatic events that constitute an emergency or disaster can affect involved workers both physically and emotionally. A traumatic event can be an emergency such as a transportation accident, large chemical spill, nuclear incident, power outage, or terrorist threat, or it can involve a natural disaster such as a disease outbreak, fire, flood, earthquake, or tornado. The workplace may be affected directly by such events, but employees may also bring to the workplace the effect of such events on their personal lives. Health Canada is one employer that has established a psychosocial emergency preparedness and response team to assist their employees exposed to traumatic events such as emergencies and natural disasters (Health Canada, 2012). This team of professionals provides training in "resiliency building" for employees and managers, as well as consultation service to deal with the aftermath of a traumatic event. (See Chapter 18 for further information on disasters.)

The workplace may be a good and familiar place for employees to be after a traumatic event because colleagues can comfort, console, and support one another. Responses to trauma can be planned and enacted together (e.g., holding memorial ceremonies, visiting the injured, attending funerals, setting up a relief fund for families). (See Chapter 18 for more on response to trauma events.)

Mental Health Problems and Disorders in the Workplace

Awareness of the potential for mental health problems and disorders among employees is an essential component of a psychologically healthy and safe workplace. It is important to recognize, for instance, that some employees may be more vulnerable than others, in the short or long term, to stress and other work-related threats to mental health. Such vulnerability may be associated with factors such as gender, age, health status, family situation, life history, or life experiences.

Workplace strategies can be put in place to assist and support specific workers or groups of workers. Examples include workshops for employees nearing retirement, counseling for those exposed to traumatic events, interventions for those with substance-related problems, and support groups for single parents. Individuals with chronic health problems may require individually accommodated support, such as an adaptation of work hours to include rest periods. Strategies can also include educating managers about particular topics (e.g., cross-cultural issues to enable them to assist recently immigrated employees).

Workplace factors can affect the likelihood of mental health problems and disorders, increase the severity of an existing disorder, or impede treatment and rehabilitation (Samra et al., 2012). There is emerging evidence suggesting that the workplace may induce a greater risk of developing common mental health disorders through high job demands, low job control, high effort–reward imbalance, low relational justice, low procedure justice, role stress, bullying, and low social support in the workplace (Harvey et al., 2017). The workplace can also play a more positive role in the prevention and early detection of disorders by improving knowledge of mental health problems and disorders within the organization. For instance, in regard to substance use problems, healthier attitudes and beliefs about the use of tobacco and other psychoactive substances can be promoted, and assistance made available to employees needing to deal with substance use issues. Unfortunately, Canadian survey research ($n = 2,219$) indicates that one third of workers would not tell their managers if they were experiencing a mental health problem, predominately out of fear of damaging their career. Decreasing this form of barrier to disclosure and the discrimination and stigma associated with it would better enable individuals to get the support they need (Dewa, 2014).

The Mental Health Commission of Canada offers Mental Health First Aid programs in which individuals learn how to recognize the signs and symptoms of a mental health problem or illness and how to find appropriate help (see Web Links). Using such a resource is not unlike employers' and employees' accessing training in first aid for physical injuries and illness. See Table 17.5 for work-related symptoms of common mental disorders.

Addressing mental health in the workplace is economically worthwhile. It is estimated that the total annual economic cost from mental illness in Canada in 2021 will be nearly 623 billion dollars (MHCC, 2016). Workplace mental health interventions can positively impact productivity, as well as absenteeism and financial outcomes (Wagner et al., 2016).

Accommodation

Employers in Canada are required to provide reasonable **accommodation** to special needs of current or

Table 17.5 Work-Related Symptoms of Common Mental Disorders		
Depression	**Anxiety Disorders**	**Burnout**
• Trouble concentrating • Trouble remembering • Trouble making decisions • Impairment of performance at work • Sleep problems • Loss of interest in work • Withdrawal: family, friends, and coworkers • Feeling pessimistic and hopeless • Feeling slowed down • Fatigue	• Feeling apprehensive and tense • Difficulty managing daily tasks • Difficulty concentrating	• Becoming cynical, sarcastic, and critical at work • Difficulty coming to work and getting started once at work • More irritable and less patient with coworkers, clients, customers • Lack of energy to be consistently productive at work • Tendency to self-medicate with alcohol or drugs

From Burton, J. (2010). *WHO healthy workplace framework and model: Background and supporting literature and practices.* World Health Organization.

potential employees. Although an employer can show that a discriminatory policy or standard is necessary for a particular job (e.g., good vision for ambulance drivers), accommodation is otherwise a requirement under labour laws and human rights acts and prevents discriminatory employment practices. Accommodation often involves primarily simple, often low-cost strategies. The American Psychiatric Association has identified examples of accommodations that employers can make for people with mental health problems and disorders. These include the following:

• Supportive supervision, such a positive reinforcement and constructive feedback, along with adjustments in level of supervision and additional forms of communication
• Flexible scheduling/remote work, given that flexibility can be valuable during the accommodation process
• Attention to breaks, which can boost attention span and mental ability
• Sick leave for therapy, treatment, recovery, or other mental health-related appointments
• Physical workplace modifications to allow the employee to be more productive
• Providing certain equipment such as recorders for meetings and noise cancelling headsets
• Reasonable modifications to the employee's duties to support their performance of essential tasks such as dividing assignments into smaller components (American Psychiatric Association Foundation Centre for Workplace Mental Health, 2021)

Disability management programs are effective; accommodating employee needs increases productivity and promotes greater trust between workers and employers (Burton, 2010).

Work and Persons Living With a Mental Disorder

Individuals living with mental disorders want, as others do, self-determination and life satisfaction through work. Work can help achieve relief from poverty, diminish reliance on

social assistance, and promote social inclusion. Work can play an important role in recovery from mental illness and is a means to integrate persons with mental disorders back into their community. Nevertheless, finding appropriate employment remains difficult for persons with a mental disorder diagnosis: research has shown that a mental disorder may be a bigger barrier to employment than a physical disability (WISE Employment, 2012). "Unemployed" is the situation for up to 90% of Canadians with serious mental illness, many of whom aspire to be part of the workforce. This situation is sustained by barriers such as stigma and discrimination, income security policies that penalize earned income, and lack of support for getting and holding a job (MHCC, 2013b).

Supported employment is an approach to assisting people with disabilities, such as severe mental illness, in finding appropriate work and supporting them once employed through the services of trained professionals. The Aspiring Workforce research project identified existing and innovative practices in supported employment to help people with serious mental illness achieve meaningful employment and income (MHCC, 2013b). Their findings support that employment should be matched to the client's interests and goals, that family and peer support must be part of the service, and that vocational, social skills, and cognitive training for clients should be provided as needed. Job accommodation needs to be addressed with clients and employers, and ongoing evaluation/support of their adaptation to one another should occur. Further, it is recommended that employment services be integrated with mental health services (MHCC). The reports of the Aspiring Workforce project are an important resource towards accessing the many capabilities of Canadians who live with a mental disorder and support their aspirations for employment.

Nurses and Workplace Psychological Health and Safety

Educating, recruiting, and retaining workers in the health sector continue to be pressing global concerns. Nurses are the largest component of the healthcare workforce, and registered nurses make up 68% of the regulated nursing workforce (Canadian Institute for Health Information, 2020). Nurses' work crosses a wide range of settings, primarily on shift-work schedules, with patients and their families throughout the entire patient experience, and with all other members of the healthcare team (American Nursing Association, n.d.; Canadian Nurses Association, 2021). Nurses' health is a barometer of workplace health in the health sector. See Table 17.6 for recommendations for the workplace health, safety, and wellbeing of the nurse.

Nurses and Burnout

Burnout is considered an occupational phenomenon that results from chronic workplace stress that has not been successfully managed. Burnout is a serious threat to the quality of health care. Its effects reach far beyond the impact on an individual, harming the entire health care system as care standards are not met (Cimiotti et al., 2012). Burnout has been identified as a major concern for nurses in Canada. In a study of the three dimensions of burnout—emotional exhaustion, depersonalization, and personal accomplishment—amongst 7,153 Canadian nurses, participants reported high levels of burnout overall, high levels of emotional exhaustion, and moderate levels of depersonalization and personal

achievement. The researchers noted that their findings correspond with results from other studies confirming that burnout is related to quality of nursing care and job outcomes, including job satisfaction and turnover intention (McGillis Hall & Vasekruna, 2020).

Nurses and Fatigue

Fatigue-related impairment amongst nurses contributes to a multitude of health, safety, and economic consequences (Thompson, 2019). Fatigue was identified as a major negative influence on safe practice in a survey study of 6,312 Canadian nurses. Organizational factors cited as preventing nurses from responding to their fatigue included workload, professional responsibility to be there for patients, feelings of not wanting to let down their colleagues, and the culture of doing more with less. Causes of fatigue reported by the nurses were workload, shift work, patient acuity, lack of time for professional development and mentoring, a decline in organizational leadership and decision-making processes, and inadequate time for "recovery" during and following work shifts (Canadian Nurses Association and Registered Nurses' Association of Ontario, 2010). There are numerous policy recommendations for health care services and standard-setting organizations targeted at reducing nurses' fatigue. The purpose of fatigue risk

Table 17.6   Recommendations for Workplace Health, Safety, and Wellbeing of the Nurse

Organization practice recommendations	Organizations/nursing employers create and design environments and systems that promote safe and healthy workplaces, including strategies.
	Creating a culture, climate, and practices that support, promote, and maintain staff health, safety, and wellbeing.
	Ensuring that the organization's annual budget includes adequate resources (human and fiscal) to implement and evaluate health and safety initiatives.
	Establishing organizational practices that foster mutual responsibility and accountability by individual nurses and organizational leaders to ensure a safe work environment.
	Being aware of the impact of organizational changes (such as restructuring and downsizing) on the health, safety, and wellbeing of nurses, and being responsible and accountable for implementing appropriate supportive measures.
	Implementing and maintaining education and training programs aimed at increasing awareness of health and safety issues for nurses (e.g., safe-lift initiative, employee rights, hazard awareness, etc.).
	Integrating health and safety best practices across all sectors of the healthcare system.
Research recommendations	Researchers actively collaborate with healthcare partners to demonstrate the effectiveness of interventions aimed at improving nurse health, safety, and wellbeing using rigorous research and evaluation methodologies.
	Researchers make full use of existing databases on nurse health, including the National Survey on the Work and Health of Nurses, in order to improve understanding of the key factors contributing to healthy work environments for nurses and to develop and test best practice indicators.
Education recommendations	Nursing education institutions model the integration of health, safety, and wellbeing into their own workplace culture.
	Nursing education institutions incorporate information about the health, safety, and wellbeing of the nurse into the core curriculum of nursing education programs.
System recommendations	Governing/accreditation bodies incorporate the Organization Practice Recommendations from this Healthy Work Environments Best Practice Guideline in their quality health and safety standards for healthcare service and education organizations.

Source: Registered Nurses' Association of Ontario. (2010). *Workplace health, safety and well-being of the nurse.*

management strategies is to promote nurses' health and safety along with patient and public safety. Some examples of these are:

- setting limits on shift length, number of hours and shifts worked per week, and the number of consecutive shifts allowed;
- establishing procedures to protect tasks that are vulnerable to fatigue-related errors;
- promoting education for managers and nurses;
- including fatigue-related factors in incident investigations;
- establishing anonymous near miss and incident reporting systems;
- addressing sleep disorders; and
- striving for continuous improvements (Caruso et al., 2019).

Compassion Fatigue

Compassion fatigue is the term used by caregiving professionals when they experience weariness, numbing of feelings like empathy, and relational disengagement from patients. Although it can appear as burnout, compassion fatigue seems to be rooted in prolonged exposure to others' suffering, coupled with one's own empathic responses. A review of the research literature suggests that the risk of compassion fatigue is increased by factors such as burnout and stress, heightened emotions of patients' families, the inability of the caregiver to maintain self-care, lack of social support, uncontrolled work stressors, lack of defined boundaries, degree of traumatic exposure, and lack of experience (Austin et al., 2013). In a qualitative study of registered nurses and registered psychiatric nurses with compassion fatigue, nurses described feelings of disconnection and disengagement from patients: "I couldn't give or open myself up to interact with the patients and their families … You're going through the motions but there is some disconnection … [you're] not really feeling their suffering" (Austin et al., 2009, p. 204). The nurses tried to overcome compassion fatigue by changing their practice area and schedule and by seeking out new knowledge, but they noted that changes to the healthcare system that improved support for compassionate caregiving were needed. The healthcare workplace has a role in preventing compassion fatigue. An overview of management strategies in a study by Lachman (2016) included recognition of the reality of compassion fatigue and its signs and symptoms, a workplace culture that supports dialogue and debriefing, stress-coping skills, and leaders supportive of a culture of caring.

Violence in the Healthcare Workplace

Healthcare practitioners are at particularly high risk of workplace violence; its high frequency constitutes concern amongst the health system (Mento et al., 2020).

In an early report, Statistics Canada reported that in the course of 1 year of providing direct care in hospitals or long-term care facilities, 34% of nurses were physically assaulted and 47% were emotionally abused by their patients (Shields & Wilkins, 2009).

More recently, in a report by the Canadian Federation of Nursing Unions, McGillis Hall & Vasekruna (2020) noted that workplace violence continues to be a major issue for nurses. About one quarter of the 7,123 nurses surveyed reported that they experienced physical violence from patients or their families "once a month or less" or "a few times a month." About another quarter (26.3%) of the nurses said they experienced physical violence "once a week" (6.8%), "a few times a week," (11.6%) or "every day" (7.9%). Verbal abuse by patients or their families was even more common than physical abuse. About one in five study participants (21.2%) experienced verbal abuse "daily" Another 30% experienced verbal abuse "a few times a week" (20.6%) or "once a week" (9%). About another 30% (28.1%) indicated that verbal abuse occurred a few times during the course of the month or "once a month or less" (McGillis Hall & Vasekruna, 2020).

In their systematic review, Mento and colleagues (2020) determined that workplace violence towards health professionals most frequently occurs in psychiatry, emergency, and geriatric units, and waiting rooms. The psychiatric–mental health nurse is required to utilize safety measures to protect clients, self, and colleagues from potentially abusive situations in the work environment (CFMHN, 2014); the place to start is by identifying the cources of violence, so discussion can begin and strategies be adopted for its prevention. Strategies may be as simple as providing timely information to patients and their friends and family, because to do so effectively lessens the risk of assault in healthcare settings, particularly in cases involving distress and long waiting periods (Chappell & Di Martino, 2006; Mento et al., 2020). Perhaps amongst the most important recommendations to reduce violence in healthcare settings are changes in organizational policies to improve staffing levels during busy periods to reduce wait times, decrease worker turnover, and ensure there is adequate security and mental health personnel on site (Philips, 2016). If there is a violent event, debriefing with those involved in incidents is helpful; counseling by qualified staff or outside specialists may be necessary in more serious cases.

Acceptable behaviours may require definition, systemic recognition, and support, whereas uncivil behaviour should be confronted and addressed in a professional manner.

The Psychological Health of Nurses Working in the COVID-19 Pandemic

The COVID-19 pandemic has placed unprecedented and long-lasting demands on frontline healthcare

BOX 17.3 Research for Best Practice

THE IMPACT OF COVID-19 ON NURSE MENTAL HEALTH

Havaei, F., Smith, P., Oudyk, J., & Potter, G. G. (2021, May 27). The impact of the COVID-19 pandemic on mental health of nurses in British Columbia, Canada using trends analysis across three time points: The impact of COVID-19 on nurse mental health. *Annals of Epidemiology, 62,* 7–12. https://doi.org/10.1016/j.annepidem.2021.05.004

Background: The onset of the COVID-19 pandemic has placed tremendous workplace stressors on health care workers. Some of these include fear of disease exposure or spreading the disease, variable and uncertain pandemic management, and the death of patients and/or their colleagues due to COVID-19.

Purpose: The purpose of this study was to examine the trend of the impact of the COVID-19 pandemic on the prevalence of anxiety and depression symptoms amongst nurses working in long-term settings in British Columbia.

Method: A cross-sectional survey of 48,000 unionized nurses was distributed on three occasions: prepandemic

(September 2020), early pandemic (April 2020), and in June 2020. The survey questions included the Generalized Anxiety Disorder screener and the Patient Health Questionnaire (PHQ-7).

Findings: A total of 10,117 responses were collected across the three surveys. The results determined a significant increase of 10% to 15% on respective indicators of anxiety and depression between the first and second measure. There was also a significant increase between the first and third measure but relative stability between the second and third.

Implications: These findings suggest that the workplace conditions created by the COVID-19 pandemic resulted in a significant and sustained detrimental impact on the mental health of nurses working in long-term settings. The sustained level of symptoms between the second and third measure raises questions regarding adaptability and is worthy of future study.

professionals. During the pandemic, healthcare workers have had to work long hours, sometimes with limited access to supplies, confront emerging ethical dilemmas, maintain currency with rapidly changing policies, and witness high mortality rates (Gavin et al., 2020; Havaei et al., 2021). The working conditions frontline health care staff experience can negatively impact their psychological health, leading to anxiety, depression, burnout, emotional exhaustion, and post-traumatic stress (Giusti et al., 2020). One survey of 18,000 Canadian healthcare workers shows that 70% of respondents reported worsening mental health as a direct result of working through the COVID-19 pandemic. When looking at nurses alone, 37% reported poor mental health (Statistics Canada, 2021). Psychological distress of frontline nurses includes such symptoms as sleep disturbances, anxiety, depression, posttraumatic stress, inability to make decisions, and somatic symptoms (Crowe et al., 2021). Better workplace practices and policies are required to protect the health of frontline healthcare professionals during COVID-19 (Havaei et al., 2021). It is unknown

how these psychological effects will impact healthcare professionals in the long term.

Workers have been providing a range of essential services on the frontlines during the COVID-19 pandemic. It has been reported that nurses, as well as other healthcare workers, may have been particularly vulnerable to negative mental health impacts during the pandemic due to their greater risk of exposure to the virus, concerns about infecting loved ones, intensifying work conditions, and shortages of personal protective equipment. Box 17.3 describes Canadian research on the impact of the pandemic on nurses working in long-term care.

This chapter presented and explored key concepts related to psychological health and safety in the workplace. In particular, examples were provided of the impact of the workplace on nurses' mental health. The increasingly rapid advances in this field reflect better understanding of the importance of a robust and psychologically healthy workforce for all employees along with the ever-shifting dynamics of the workplace.

🍁 Summary of Key Points

- Work influences self-identity, provides income, and plays a significant role in an individual's health and wellbeing. Unemployment and underemployment can cause psychological distress and negatively affect an individual's mental health. There are also adverse effects related to job change that go beyond those who have lost jobs.

- The nature of work has been changing across the globe due to economic and technologic developments; these changes are affecting the mental health of workers.
- Achieving work–life balance can be difficult. Work–life conflict occurs when one role interferes with meeting the demands of another.

- Gender inequality continues to influence the situation of paid workers.
- Nurses need to understand the psychosocial factors that contribute to a healthy and inclusive workplace and the need for flexibility in sustaining a healthy workplace and for accommodating employees with mental health and/or other chronic health problems.
- The Mental Health First Aid and Working Mind programs of the MHCC are educational means of increasing literacy in mental health and decreasing stigma and discrimination.

- Work can help persons with mental disorders in their recovery and in the improvement of their wellbeing. The Supportive Employment approach facilitates acquiring and maintaining employment for persons with severe mental disorders.
- Bullying (physical, relational, verbal, and cyber) involves repeated, intended harm to a person with less power than the aggressor.
- Nurses need to overcome a culture of silence related to workplace violence in healthcare settings.

 ## Thinking Challenges

1. You have nursing experience in intensive care and strived to secure a position in a prestigious hospital. During the orientation into your new position, it was revealed this particular unit has the highest turnover rate and medical leaves of any department in the hospital.

   a. As a staff nurse, what steps would you explore to maintain your wellbeing and success in this position?

   b. As a nursing manager, what strategies you would consider to enhance the psychological health and safety of your staff?

> Visit thePoint to view suggested responses. Go to thePoint.lww.com/activate and use the activation code found in the front of this text to unlock answers to the "Thinking Challenges" and other online resources.

 ## Web Links

https://nursesunions.ca/wp-content/uploads/2019/06/CFNU_EquityToolkit_EN.pdf The Canadian Federation of Nurses Unions (CFNU) has developed a toolkit to assist member organizations to implement procedures and structures that will facilitate EDI. This toolkit includes a section on the power of inclusive language, an environmental scan checklist, a sample accessibility event checklist, and sample workshops to discover gaps or improvements to be made.

https://cmha.ca The Canadian Mental Health Association provides information about their work in workplace mental health, including the employment of persons with mental health problems.

https://www.guardingmindsatwork.ca An excellent comprehensive and research-based resource for the promotion of psychological health and safety in the workplace, developed by the Centre for Applied Research in Mental Health and Addiction (CARMHA).

https://www.ccohs.ca The Canadian Centre for Occupational Health and Safety offers free resources, including podcasts (also at iTunes) such as "Breaking the cycle of workplace bullying" and "Exploring psychosocial issues in the workplace."

https://mhfa.ca Information about the mental health first aid programs can be found here.

https://www.mentalhealthcommission.ca/English/resources/training/working-mind Details about the MHCC's educational program for managers and employees, The Working Mind, are at this site.

https://www.mentalhealthcommission.ca/English/caring-healthcare-workers-assessment-tools This toolkit was created specifically to help healthcare organizations take action on implementing the Standard and its continuous quality improvement cycle.

Acknowledgement

The author thanks Sadie Deschenes, RN, MN, doctoral candidate, for her valuable review, literature search, and other contributions to the chapter.

References

American Nursing Association. (n.d.). *What is nursing?* https://www.nursingworld.org/practice-policy/workforce/what-is-nursing/

American Psychological Association Foundation Centre for Workplace Mental Health. (2021). *Reasonable job accommodations.* https://www.workplacementalhealth.org/mental-health-topics/reasonable-job-accommodations

Austin, W., Brintnell, S., Goble, E., Kagan, L., Kreitzer, L., Larsen, D., & Leier, B. (2013). *Lying down in the ever-falling snow: Canadian health professionals' experience of compassion fatigue.* Wilfrid Laurier University Press.

Austin, W., Goble, E., Leier, B., & Byrne, P. (2009). Compassion fatigue: The experience of nurses. *Ethics and Social Welfare, 3*(2), 195–214.

Backhans, M., & Hemmingsson, T. (2011). Unemployment and mental health—Who is (not) affected? *European Journal of Public Health, 22*(3), 429–433.

Block, L. (2014). *Google's scientific approach to work-life balance (and much more).* Harvard Business Review. https://hbr.org/2014/03/googles-scientific-approach-to-work-life-balance-and-much-more?utm_source=feedburner&utm_medium=feed&utm_campaign=Feed%3A+harvardbusiness+%28HBR.org%29&_ga=1.79658388.1052155481.1390589963

Burton, J. (2010). *WHO healthy workplace framework and model: Background and supporting literature and practices.* World Health Organization.

Canadian Centre for Diversity and Inclusion and Dalhousie University. (2019). *National diversity and inclusion benchmarking study: Senior leaders* and diversity personnel. https://ccdi.ca/media/1979/20190715-research-national-diversity-and-inclusion-benchmarking-study.pdf

Canadian Centre for Occupational Health and Safety. (2021). *Bullying in the workplace*. https://www.ccohs.ca/oshanswers/psychosocial/bullying.html

Canadian Council on Learning. (2008). *Bullying in Canada: How intimidation affects learning*. http://www.ccl-cca.ca/pdfs/LessonsInLearning/Mar-20-08-Bullying-in-Canad.pdf

Canadian Federation of Mental Health Nurses (CFMHN). (2014). *Canadian standards of psychiatric-mental health nursing* (4th ed.).

Canadian Institute for Health Information. (2020). *Nursing in Canada, 2019: A lens on supply and workforce*. https://www.cihi.ca/sites/default/files/document/nursing-report-2019-en-web.pdf

Canadian Nurses Association. (2021). *Role description*. https://www.cna-aiic.ca/en/nursing-practice/tools-for-practice/primary-care-toolkit/role-description

Canadian Nurses Association and Registered Nurses' Association of Ontario. (2010). *Nurse fatigue and patient safety: Research report*. http://www2.cna-aiic.ca/cna/practice/safety/full_report_e/files/fatigue_safety_2010_report_e.pdf

Caruso, C. C., Baldwin, C. M., Berger, A., Chasens, E. R., Cole Edmonson, J., Holmes Gobel, B., Landis, C. A., Patrician, P. A., Redeker, N. S., Scott, L. D., Todero, C., Trinkoff, A., & Tucker, S. (2019). Policy brief: Nurse fatigue, sleep and health, and ensuring patient and public safety. *Nursing Outlook, 67*(5), 615–619. https://doi.org/10.1016/j.outlook.2019.08.004

Chappell, D., & Di Martino, V. (2006). *Violence at work*. International Labour Organization.

Chuang, C. H., Tseng, P. C., Lin, C. Y., Lin, K. H., & Chen, Y. Y. (2016). Burnout in the intensive care unit professionals: A systematic review. *Medicine, 95*(50), e5629. http://dx.doi.org/10.1097/MD.0000000000005629

Cimiotti, J. P., Aiken, L. H., Sloane, D. M., & Wu, E. S. (2012). Nurse staffing, burnout, and health care-associated infection. *American Journal of Infection Control, 40*(6), 486–490.

Craig, L., & Churchill, B. (2021). Working and caring at home: Gender differences in the effects of Covid-19 on paid and unpaid labor in Australia. *Feminist Economics*, 1–17.

Crowe, S., Howard, A. F., Vanderspank-Wright, B., Gillis, P., McLeod, F., Penner, C., Haijan, G. (2021). The effect of COVID-19 pandemic on the mental health of Canadian critical care nurses providing patient care during the early phase pandemic: A mixed method study. *Intensive and Critical Care Nursing, 63*, 102999. doi.org/10.1016/j.iccn.2020.102999

CSA Group. (2013). *National Standard of Canada, CAN/CSA-Z1003-13/BNQ 9700-803/2013: Psychological health and safety in the workplace—Prevention, promotion, and guidance to staged implementation*. http://shop.csa.ca/en/canada/occupational-health-and-safety-management/cancsa-z1003-13bnq-9700-8032013/invt/z10032013

Department of Criminal Justice Canada. (2003). *Stalking is a crime called criminal harassment*. http://canada.justice.gc.ca/eng/pi/fv-vf/pub/har/har.html

Dewa, C. S. (2014). Worker attitudes towards mental health problems and disclosure. *International Journal of Occupational and Environmental Medicine, 5*(15), 175–186.

Dewa, C. S., Chau, N., & Dermer, S. (2010). Examining the comparative incidence and costs of physical and mental health-related disabilities in an employed population. *Journal of Occupational and Environmental Medicine, 52*(7), 758–762. https://doi.org/10.1097/JOM.0b013e3181e8cfb5

Dockery, M., & Bawa, S. (2020). *Working from home in the COVID-19 lockdown*. Bankwest Curtin Economics Centre.

Duxbury, L., & Higgins, C. (2009). *Work-life conflict in Canada in the new millennium: Key findings and recommendations from the 2001 National Work-Life Conflict Study*. Public Health Agency of Canada.

Gavin, B., Hayden, J., Adamis, D., & McNicholas, F. (2020). Caring for the psychological well-being of healthcare professionals in the Covid-19 pandemic crisis. *Irish Medical Journal, 113*(4), 51.

Giusti, E. M., Pedroli, E., D'Aniello, G. E., Badiale, C. S., Pietrabissa, G., Manna, C., Badiale, M. C., Riva, G., Castelnuovo, G., Molinari, E., & Molinari, E. (2020). The psychological impact of the COVID-19 outbreak on health professionals: A cross-sectional study. *Frontiers in Psychology, 11*, 1684.

Gold, L. H., & Shuman, D. W. (2009). *Evaluating mental health disability in the workplace—Model, process, and analysis* (pp. 45–48). Springer.

Government of Canada. (2019a). *Women and the workplace—How employers can advance equality and diversity—Report from the symposium and the workplace*. https://www.canada.ca/en/employment-social-development/corporate/reports/women-symposium.html

Government of Canada. (2019b). *Equity, diversity and inclusion. Tri-agency EDI action plan for 2018-2025*. https://www.nserc-crsng.gc.ca/NSERC-CRSNG/EDI-EDI/Action-Plan_Plan-dAction_eng.asp

Government of Canada. (2020). *Violence and harassment in the workplace: Warning signs*. Canadian Center for Occupational Health and Safety. https://www.ccohs.ca/oshanswers/psychosocial/violence_warning_signs.html

Government of Canada. (2021). *Cyberbullying can have serious consequences*. https://www.canada.ca/en/public-safety-canada/campaigns/cyberbullying/cyberbullying-against-law.html

Harvey, S. B., Modini, M., Joyce, S., Milliigan-Saville, J. S., Tan, L., Mykletun, A., Bryant, R. A., Christensen, H., & Mitchell, P. B. (2017). Can work make you mentally ill? A systematic meta-review of work-related risk factors for common mental health problems. *Occupational and Environmental Medicine, 74*, 301–310. https://doi.org/10.1136/oemed-2016-104015

Havaei, F., & MacPhee, M. (2021). Effect of workplace violence and psychological stress responses on medical-surgical nurses' medication intake. *Canadian Journal of Nursing Research, 53*(2), 133–144. https://doi.org/10.1177/0844562120903914

Health Canada. (2012). *Psychosocial emergency preparedness and response*. http://www.hc-sc.gc.ca/ewh-semt/occup-travail/empl/psychosoc-eng.php

Herzberg, F., Mausner, B., & Bloch Snyderman, B. (2009). *The motivation to work*. Transaction Publishers.

Higgins, C., Duxbury, L., & Lyons, S. (2008). *Reducing work-life conflict: What works? What doesn't?* Health Canada. http://www.hc-sc.gc.ca/ewh-semt/pubs/occup-travail/balancing-equilibre/index-eng.php

Hollederer, A. (2015). Unemployment, health and moderating factors: The need for targeted health promotion. *Journal of Public Health, 23*(6), 319–325. https://doi.org/10.1007/s10389-015-0685-4

Howatt, W., Bradley, L., Adams, J., Mahajan, S., & Kennedy, S. (2017). *Understanding mental health, mental illness, and their impacts in the workplace*. Mental Health Commission of Canada and Morneau Shepell. https://www.morneaushepell.com/permafiles/91248/mental-health-white-paper-2018.pdf

Howley, D. (2020). *A 'happy crew' and unlimited vacation: What it's like working at Zoom*. Yahoo! Finance. https://finance.yahoo.com/news/what-its-like-working-at-zoom-142628732.html

Ipsos. (2017). *Workplaces that are implementing the National Standard of Canada for Psychological Health and Safety in the Workplace described by employees as psychologically-safer environments*. Public release. https://www.ipsos.com/en-ca/news-polls/workplaces-implementing-national-standard-canada-psychological-health-and-safety-workplace

Judge, T. A., & Kammeyer-Mueller, J. D. (2012). Job attitudes. *Annual Review of Psychology, 63*, 341–367.

Lachman, V. D. (2016). Compassion fatigue as a threat to ethical practice: Identification, personal and workplace prevention/management strategies. *MedSurgNursing, 25*(4), 275–278.

Laschinger, H. K. S., & Read, E. A. (2016). The effect of authentic leadership, person-job fit, and civility norms on new graduate nurses: Experiences of coworker incivility and burnout. *Journal of Nursing Administration, 46*(11), 574–580.

Lero, D., Richardson, J., & Korabik, K. (2009). *Cost-benefit review of work-life balance practices—2009*. Canadian Association of Administrators of Labour Legislation.

LifeWorks. (2021). *The Mental Health Index™ Report Canada*. https://lifeworks.com/en/mental-health-index

Lowe, G. (2010). *Creating sustainable organizations: How flexible work improves wellbeing and performance*. http://www.grahamlowe.ca/documents/258/

Matthews, R. A., & Ritter, K. J. (2016). A concise, content valid, gender invariant measure of workplace incivility. *Journal of Occupational Health Psychology, 21*(3), 352–365.

McGillis Hall, L., & Vasekruna, S. (2020). Outlook on Nursing: A snapshot from Canadian nurses on work environments pre-COVID-19. *Canadian Federation of Nurses Unions*. https://nursesunions.ca/research/outlook-on-nursing/

McKee-Ryan, F. M., & Maitoza, R. (2018). Job loss, unemployment, and families. In U.C. Klehe & E. A. van Hooft (Eds.), *The Oxford handbook of job loss and job search* (pp. 87–98). Oxford University Press.

Mental Health Commission of Canada. (2013a). *Making the case for investing in mental health in Canada*. https://www.mentalhealthcommission.ca/sites/default/files/2016-06/Investing_in_Mental_Health_FINAL_Version_ENG.pdf

Mental Health Commission of Canada. (2013b). *The aspiring workforce: Employment and income for people with serious mental illness*. http://www.mentalhealthcommission.ca/sites/default/files/2016-06/Workplace_MHCC_Aspiring_Workforce_Report_ENG_0.pdf

Mental Health Commission of Canada. (2016). *Making the case for investing in mental health in Canada*. https://www.mentalhealthcommission.ca/sites/default/files/2016-06/Investing_in_Mental_Health_FINAL_Version_ENG.pdf

Mental Health Commission of Canada. (2018). *Understanding mental health, mental illness, and their impacts in the workplace*. https://

www.morneaushepell.com/permafiles/91248/mental-health-white-paper-2018.pdf

Mental Health Commission of Canada. (2021). *Advancing psychological health and safety within healthcare settings.* https://www.mentalhealth-commission.ca/English/what-we-do/workplace/workplace-healthcare

Mento, C., Silvestri, M. C., Bruno, A., Muscatello, M. R. A., Cedro, C., Pandolfo, G., & Zoccali, R. A. (2020). Workplace violence against healthcare professionals: A systematic review. *Aggression and Violent Behavior, 51*, 101381. https://doi.org/10.1016/j.avb.2020.101381

O'Donnell, S. M., & MacIntosh, J. A. (2016). Gender and workplace bullying: Men's experience of surviving bullying at work. *Qualitative Health Research, 26*(3), 351–366.

Philips, J. P. (2016). Workplace violence against health care workers in the United States. *The New England Journal of Medicine, 374*(17), 1661–1669. https://doi.org/10.1056/NEJMra1501998

Pradas-Hernández, L., Ariza, T., Gómez-Urquiza, J. L., Albendín-García, L., De la Fuente, E. I., & Canadas-De la Fuente, G. A. (2018). Prevalence of burnout in paediatric nurses: A systematic review and meta-analysis. *PLoS One, 13*(4), e0195039. https://doi.org/10.1371/journal.pone.0195039

Public Services Health and Safety Association. (2010). *Bullying in the workplace: A handbook for the workplace.*

Registered Nurses' Association of Ontario. (2010). *Workplace health, safety and well-being of the nurse.*

Samra, J., Gilbert, M., Shain, M., & Bilsker, D. (2012). *GuardingMinds@ Work.* Centre for Applied Research in Mental Health and Addiction (CARMHA). http://www.guardingmindsatwork.ca

Shain, M., Arnold, I., & GermAnn, K. (2013). *The road to psychological health and safety: Legal, scientific and social foundations for a national standard for psychological safety in the workplace.* A working paper for the Mental Health Commission of Canada. www.mentalhealthcommission.ca

Shields, M., & Wilkins, K. (2009). Factors related to on-the-job abuse of nurses by patients. *Statistics Canada.* http://www.statcan.gc.ca/pub/82-003-x/2009002/article/10835-eng.htm

Smith, P., Mustard, C., Lu, H., & Glazier R. (2013). Comparing the risk associated with psychosocial work conditions and health behaviours on incident hypertension over a nine-year period in Ontario, Canada. *Canadian Journal of Public Health, 104*(1), e82–e86.

Sriharan, A., Ratnapalan, S., Tricco, A. D., Lupea, D., Ayala, A. P., Pang, H., & Lee, D. D. (2020). Stress, burnout and depression in woman in healthcare during COVID-19 pandemic: Rapid scoping review. *Frontiers in Global Women's Health, 1.* https://doi.org/10.3389/fgwh.2020.596690

Statistics Canada. (2019). *The gender age gap in Canada: 1998 to 2018.* https://www150.statcan.gc.ca/n1/pub/75-004-m/75-004-m2019004-eng.htm

Statistics Canada. (2021). *Mental health among health care workers in Canada during the COVID-19 pandemic.* https://www150.statcan.gc.ca/n1/daily-quotidien/210202/dq210202a-eng.htm

Thompson, B. J. (2019). Does work-induced fatigue accumulate across three compressed 12 hour shifts in hospital nurses and aides? *PLoS One, 14*(2), e0211715. https://doi.org/10.1371/journal.pone.0211715

Thoroughgood, C. N., Sawyer, K. B., & Webster, J. R. (2020). Creating a trans-inclusive workplace. *Harvard Business Review.* https://hbr.org/2020/03/creating-a-trans-inclusive-workplace

Venes, D. (Ed.) (2009). *Taber's cyclopedic medical dictionary* (21st ed.). F.A. Davis Company.

Wagner, S. L., Koehn, C., White, M. I., Harder, H. G., Schultz, I. Z., & Williams-Whitt, K. (2016). Mental health intervention in the workplace and work outcomes: A best-evidence synthesis of systematic reviews. *International Journal of Occupational and Environmental Medicine, 7*(1), 1–14.

WISE Employment. (2012). *SMEs attitudes to employing people who have a mental illness.* http://www.wiseemployment.com.au/uploads/publications/Empowermental-McNair_Research.pdf

World Health Organization. (2011). *Gender, work and health.* http://whqlibdoc.who.int/publications/2011/9789241501729_eng.pdf

World Health Organization. (2019). *Burn-out an "occupational phenomenon": International Classification of Diseases.* https://www.who.int/news/item/28-05-2019-burn-out-an-occupational-phenomenon-international-classification-of-diseases

World Health Organization. (2020). *Healthy workplaces: A WHO global model for action.* https://www.who.int/activities/healthy-workplaces-a-who-global-model-for-action

Xiao, Y., Becerik-Gerber, B., Lucas, G., & Roll, S. C. (2021). Impacts of working from home during COVID-19 pandemic on physical and mental well-being of office workstation users. *Journal of Occupational and Environmental Medicine, 63*(3), 181.

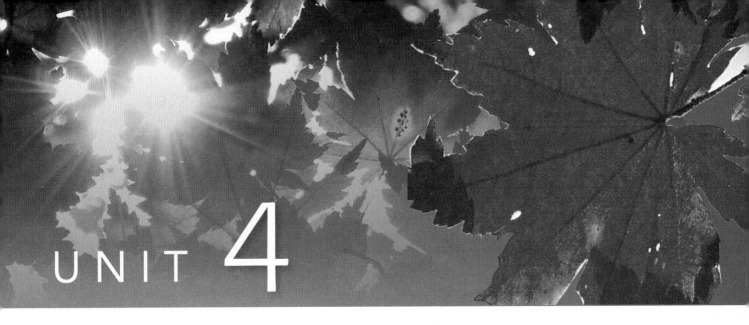

Challenges
to Mental
Health

CHAPTER

18

Stress, Trauma, Crisis, and Disaster

Holly Graham and Wendy Austin*

LEARNING OBJECTIVES

After studying this chapter, you will be able to:

- Discuss the evolution of the concept of stress.
- Use the Transactional Model to assess an individual's stress, adaptation, and coping abilities.
- Differentiate problem-focused and emotion-focused coping.
- Define stress, traumatic stressor, crisis, and disaster and describe human responses to these.
- Define intergenerational trauma, collective trauma, and historical trauma and describe human responses to these.
- Understand the importance of trauma-informed care and differentiate between cultural competence, cultural humility, and cultural safety.
- Explain nursing assessment and interventions of trauma- and stressor-related disorders.
- Identify adaptive and maladaptive responses to disaster and indicators that a survivor may require psychiatric services.

KEY TERMS

- adaptation • allostasis • cognitive appraisal • cultural competence • cultural safety • dissupport • duty to provide care • emotion-focused coping • freeze-hide response • grief • homeostasis • infodemic • psychological first aid • social support

KEY CONCEPTS

- collective trauma • coping • crisis • disaster • historical trauma • psychological resilience • transactional model • trauma-informed care • traumatic stressor

Although stress has been the focus of considerable scientific, clinical, and general interest, most of us would be hard-pressed to explain what it is. As Selye (1980) quipped, "stress, like relativity, is a scientific concept which has suffered the mixed blessing of being too well known, and too little understood" (p. 127). Increasing acknowledgment of the pervasiveness of stressor and trauma experiences has resulted in increasing emphasis on the importance of providing clients with safe and supportive inpatient and care environments that can better serve people who are living with stress and/or who have had traumatic experiences. In this chapter, the concepts of stress, trauma, crisis, and disaster are described and the way that nurses can identify and address the needs of individuals experiencing these events are explained. The system level need for trauma-informed care is also addressed.

Stress

The Evolution of the Concept of Stress

The word stress comes from the Latin word *stringere*, meaning to draw tight (Cooper & Dewe, 2004), and the Middle English word *stresse*, which refers to hardship or distress (Harper, 2001). Throughout the 18th and 19th centuries, the word "stress" was used to denote *force*, *pressure*, or *strain*, which explains why the word "stress" was used almost exclusively by engineers before the beginning of the 20th century.

The early decades of the 20th century saw the rise of *psychosomatic medicine* and a shift away from the prevailing view of the body as a machine (Cooper & Dewe, 2004). Proponents of psychosomatic medicine believed that a mechanistic model was reductionistic and could not explain the role of the mind and spirit in health and

---

*Adapted from the chapter "Trauma- and Stressor-Related Disorders, Crisis, and Response to Disaster" by Gerri Lasiuk, Kathleen Hegadoren, and Wendy Austin

illness. It was in this context that the concept of stress as hardship was taken up by biologic and social scientists as a possible explanation of disease and illness (Bartlett, 1998). Throughout the last century, our understanding of stress evolved through three distinct periods in which it was conceptualized as a physiologic response, as a stimulus, and, finally, as a transaction.

Stress as a Physiologic Response

Walter Cannon and Hans Selye, two pioneers in the study of stress, both conceptualized stress as a response to changing environmental conditions. Cannon (1939), a noted Harvard physiologist, is considered by many to be the father of modern stress research. In his book, *The Wisdom of the Body*, he coined the term **homeostasis** to describe the body's ability to maintain a stable internal environment despite changing environmental conditions. Cannon's thesis was that environmental changes are perceived as threats to personal integrity or safety and signal a compensatory response mediated by the sympathetic branch of the autonomic nervous system (ANS). He also believed that strong emotions like fear and anger are fundamental to the stress response and have evolved because of their high survival value. "Fear," he wrote, "has become associated with the instinct to run, to escape; and anger or aggressive feeling, with the instinct to attack" (p. 227). This notion, later dubbed the *fight or flight* response, remains a key concept in discussions of stress.

Working at McGill University in Montreal, Selye (1956, 1974) developed his general **adaptation** syndrome theory. In this, Selye differentiated stress (a nonspecific response of the body to any demand placed on it) from stressors (events that initiate the response) and argued that stressors can be physical (e.g., infection, intense heat or cold, surgery, debilitating illnesses), psychological (e.g., psychological trauma, interpersonal problems), or social (e.g., lack of social support). Stressors can also be short term (acute) or long term (chronic).

According to Selye, the perception of a stressor triggers an automatic, total-body response. The first stage of this response is the *alarm reaction*, during which virtually all body systems (e.g., sense organs, brain, heart and blood vessels, lungs, digestive system, immune system) respond in a coordinated effort to mediate the stressor. If this effort is successful, the body returns to its normal state. If it is not successful and the stressor remains present for hours or days, the organism moves into the *stage of resistance*, and efforts to adapt continue. In circumstances in which the stressor becomes chronic or is extreme, the body moves into the *stage of exhaustion*, during which the individual's resources deplete, and exhaustion and death ensue.

Although Selye made significant contributions to our understanding of human stress, he was criticized for his notion that stress is a nonspecific response to diverse environmental stimuli. Selye's challengers (e.g., Mason, 1971; Mikhail, 1981) pointed out that many neuroendocrine responses are not general at all but very specific.

Selye's critics argued that all stressors do not necessarily produce the same response in every individual, and what is a stressor for one person may not be a stressor for another (Lazarus & Folkman, 1984). The conceptualization of stress solely as a response was also challenged for its circular reasoning (i.e., an event is stressful because it elicits a stress response).

Stress as a Stimulus

Before the 1960s, the study of stress was a physiologic concept. By the middle of the last century, the disciplines of psychology and psychiatry were on the rise, and researchers and clinicians became interested in the psychological and emotional aspects of stress. With this came the notion that life changes or events were the stimuli (i.e., stressors) that evoked the stress response (e.g., Dohrenwend & Dohrenwend, 1974; Holmes & Rahe, 1967). Within this perspective, stress researchers explored associations between significant life events (e.g., marriage, birth, divorce, relocation, death) and stress. One of the most widely used tools in this type of research is the *Recent Life Changes Questionnaire* (RLCQ) (Holmes & Rahe, 1967; see Table 18.1). A major problem with this conceptualization of stress is that stress-provoking stimuli can be identified only in retrospect, that is, only after a response occurs. Other criticisms are that it does not take into consideration the meaning the individual assigns to an item, the individual's coping abilities, or the implications of chronic or recurrent events (Jones & Kinman, 2001).

Stress as a Person–Environment Transaction

The mid-1970s to the early 1990s was a critical period in stress research. During this period, a debate raged in the literature between two camps of stress researchers. One group favoured the view that critical life events (e.g., the presence of an objective event) mediate the experience of stress. Supporters "urged researchers to measure pure events, uncontaminated by perceptions, appraisals, or reactions" (Dohrenwend & Shrout, 1985, p. 782). On the other side, others maintained that it is the appraisal of an event (e.g., the subjective evaluation of an event or situation) that is critical to the stress experience (Lazarus et al., 1985). Although the debate centred on measurement and other methodologic problems, Lazarus (1999) later wrote that what was at issue was the fundamental nature of stress and the person–environment relationship. In the end, the latter group prevailed, and the view of stress as a relationship between persons and their environment has become the dominant explanatory model.

In their seminal work, *Appraisal and Coping*, Lazarus and Folkman (1984) conceptualized stress as resulting from a perceived imbalance between an individual's resources and the demands placed on them. Within their Transactional Model, stress depends on how a stressor is appraised in relation to the individual's resources for coping with it. The central premise is that stress is "neither

Table 18.1 Recent Life Changes Questionnaire		
Social Area	Life Changes	LCU Values[a]
Family	Death of spouse	105
	Marital separation	65
	Death of close family member	65
	Divorce	62
	Pregnancy	60
	Change in health of family member	52
	Marriage	50
	Gain of new family member	50
	Marital reconciliation	42
	Spouse begins or stops work	37
	Son or daughter leaving home	29
	In-law trouble	29
	Change in number of family get-togethers	26
Personal	Jail term	56
	Sex difficulties	49
	Death of a close friend	46
	Personal injury or illness	42
	Change in living conditions	39
	Outstanding personal achievement	33
	Change in residence	33
	Minor violations of the law	32
	Begin or end school	32
	Change in sleeping habits	31
	Revision of personal habits	31
	Change in eating habits	29
	Change in church activities	29
	Vacation	29
	Change in school	28
	Change in recreation	28
	Christmas	26
Work	Fired at work	64
	Retirement from work	49
	Trouble with boss	39
	Business readjustment	38
	Change to different line of work	38
	Change in work responsibilities	33
	Change in work hours or conditions	30
Financial	Foreclosure of mortgage or loan	57
	Change in financial state	43
	Mortgage (home, car, etc.)	39
	Mortgage or loan less than $10,000 (stereo, etc.)	26

Directions: Total the LCUs for your life change events during the past 12 months.
250 to 400 LCUs per year: Minor life crisis.
More than 400 LCUs per year: Major life crisis.
[a]LCU, Life change unit. The number of LCUs reflects the average degree or intensity of the life change.
From Rahe, R. H. (2000). Recent Life Changes Questionnaire [RLCQ] [1997]. In T. H. Holmes & American Psychiatric Association (Eds.), *Task force for the handbook of psychiatric measures. Handbook of psychiatric measures* (pp. 235–237). American Psychiatric Association.

an environmental stimulus, a characteristic of the person, nor a response, but a relationship between demands and the power to deal with them without unreasonable or destructive costs" (Coyne & Holroyd, 1982, p. 108).

Cognitive Appraisal

Lazarus and Folkman (1984) use the term **cognitive appraisal** to describe the process by which individuals examine the demands and constraints of a situation in relation to their own personal and network resources. Cognitive appraisal has two levels—primary and secondary. In primary appraisal, individuals evaluate the situation and determine whether they are in danger or under threat. If yes, they go on to secondary appraisal, during which the individual considers the options for dealing with the situation. According to Lazarus and Folkman, stress is the perception of threat or harm (primary appraisal) for which an individual has no effective response (secondary appraisal). Figure 18.1 depicts

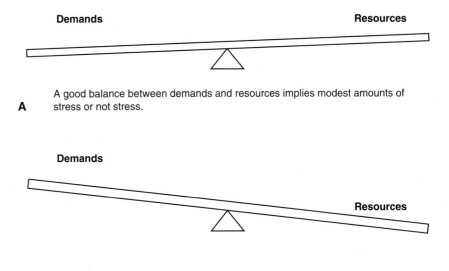

A good balance between demands and resources implies modest amounts of stress or not stress.

A

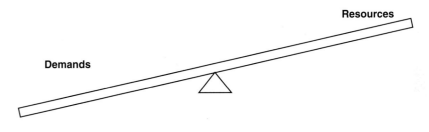

B   High demands with few resources can result in a high stress balance.

Figure 18.1 Lazarus's (1999) seesaw analogy of stress.

C   A low stress balance, which could imply boredom.

Lazarus's (1999, p. 59) seesaw analogy illustrating stress as a balance between environmental demands and personal resources.

KEY CONCEPT

According to the Transactional Model (Lazarus & Folkman, 1984), stress is the relationship between the person and the environment that is appraised as exceeding the person's resources and endangering their wellbeing.

New Understandings of the Stress and the Stress Response

In recent years, the concept of stress has been increasingly criticized for its lack of precision and specificity. Lazarus (1999) argued that while the concept of stress is a useful one, it is not a single, unitary phenomenon. This sentiment is echoed by Woolfolk and colleagues (2007) who contend that stress "is probably best thought of as a generic, nontechnical term, analogous to disease or to addiction" (p. 10). Until the term "stress" is replaced by a more precise label, it is a useful heuristic to aid communication among laypersons, health professionals, and researchers.

Allostasis

A recent refinement in our understanding of stress is the concept of **allostasis**. The word, which literally means *maintaining stability through change*, was coined by Sterling and Eyer (1988) to describe how the cardiovascular system adjusts to resting and active states of the body. Unlike the concept of homeostasis, which posits a single optimum state, allostasis reflects the notion that different environmental circumstances or conditions require different set points. For instance, individuals' ideal blood pressure when asleep is very different from their ideal blood pressure if they are bungee jumping (Sapolsky, 2004). Maintaining an allostatic balance in wide-ranging circumstances calls for continuous systemic adjustments throughout the whole body. For example, the hypothalamus regulates sleep and wakefulness and the production of adrenocortical hormones in response to the light–dark cycle that occurs as the earth rotates on its axis every day. When the light–dark cycle is altered (e.g., long flights across several time zones), the production of adrenocortical hormones is disrupted and alterations occur in the usual patterns of sleep, activity, appetite, and cognitive function (i.e., jet lag).

The term allostatic load (McEwen, 1998) refers to the cumulative negative effects on the body of continually having to adapt to changing environmental conditions and psychosocial challenges. It is mediated by the efficiency of the body's response to these changing conditions and to the number of stressors an individual may experience throughout their lifetime. Allostatic load is more than "chronic stress"; it is the sum total of the "wear and tear" on the body that accumulates from the constant effort required to maintain normal body rhythms in the face of changing environmental conditions, the challenges of daily life, and the adverse physiologic consequences of harmful lifestyle choices (e.g., inactivity, excessive alcohol, smoking).

New Views on Responses to Stress

The Freeze–Hide Response

Although the stress response is typically described in terms of an individual organism defending itself against threat by fighting or fleeing, other responses to stress have also been observed. One of these is the freeze–hide response, which is the tendency to produce a passive response to stress (Korte et al., 2005). Rupia and colleagues (2016), in a study of flatfish, achieved the first experimental evidence that there is a difference in metabolic responses to stressful situations between individuals designated bold or shy according to behavioural assays. During acute stress, those who are designated shy adopted a **freeze–hide response** while the bold adopted a fight-flight response. Although research related to the freeze–hide response has been done with animals, it suggests that the stress response may actually be more differentiated than Cannon predicted.

Tend and Befriend

Another line of research into the human stress response is one proposed by Taylor and colleagues (Taylor et al., 2000, 2002) who argue that women and men respond differently to stress. They theorize that women have the same physiologic response to stress but their resultant behaviours differ. They propose another alternative to fight-or-flight–type behavioural responses—which they call the *tend-and-befriend* behavioural response—characteristic of females of various species. According to these authors, the tend-and-befriend response also has evolutionary advantages and reflects the inclination of females towards affiliation, cooperation, and caretaking.

Tending involves nurturant activities designed to protect the self and offspring that promote safety and reduce distress; befriending is the creation and maintenance of social networks that may aid in this process (Taylor et al., 2000, p. 411).

As Taylor et al. (2000, 2002) explain, the biologic mediators of the tend-and-befriend response appear to involve oxytocin and female reproductive hormones. Oxytocin, dubbed the "love hormone," appears to have a role in a range of social behaviours including social memory, attachment, and bonding; sexual and maternal behaviour; trust; and aggression (Lee et al., 2009). It is also believed that disorders characterized by difficulties with social interactions (e.g., autism and schizophrenia) may also involve oxytocin.

The possibility that the stress response may be gendered opens new horizons for exploring human stress responses.

Flow

With growing attention to the variety of responses to trauma and paths to recovery, including those beyond the reaction to trauma states of "fight or flight" and "freeze or faint," Seng and colleagues (2019) have identified a posttrauma concept to express "anembodied, positive outcome of trauma recovery" (p. 202): *Flow*. This subjective experience in a posttraumatic life is "inviting, positive, dynamic, and responsive to real circumstances: shaped by the stress of trauma but not destroyed; an active state … useful for daily life… and sustainable" (Seng et al., p. 205). This language embeds a strength-based, relational, growth-fostering approach to stress and trauma.

Physiologic Stress Responses

The appraisal of a situation as dangerous or threatening to one's personal integrity triggers an automatic, total-body response. Structures in the brain receive and integrate simultaneous inputs from a number of sources and coordinate a series of physiologic and behavioural responses that enhance an individual's chances of survival.

The physiologic response to stress begins in the central nervous system (CNS) but quickly involves all body systems (refer to Table 18.2). The hypothalamus is

Table 18.2	Stress-Related Symptoms
System	Symptom
Physiologic	Headaches
	Fatigue
	Restlessness
	Sleep difficulties
	Indigestion
Emotional	Crying
	Feeling of pressure
	Easily upset
	Edginess
	Increased anger
	Feeling sick
	Nervousness
	Increased impatience
	Feeling of tension
	Overwhelmed
Cognitive	Memory loss
	Problems with decision-making
	Loss of humour
	Forgetfulness
	Feeling of tension
	Difficulty thinking clearly
Behavioural	Isolation
	Difficulty functioning
	Compulsive eating
	Lack of intimacy
	Intolerance
	Resentment
	Excessive smoking

Adapted with permission from Carpenito-Moyet, L. J. (2017). *Nursing diagnosis: Application to clinical practice* (15th ed.). Wolters-Kluwer.

responsible for maintaining the body's internal environment and for initiating the body's stress response, which it orchestrates through its dense neural connections with the posterior pituitary gland, brainstem, and spinal cord and through its endocrine links with the anterior pituitary gland. The hypothalamus activates the sympathetic branch of the ANS, which stimulates the adrenal medulla to secrete catecholamines and mediates vigilance, arousal, activation, and mobilization (see Fig. 18.2). It also secretes corticotrophin-releasing hormone (CRH) to signal the anterior pituitary gland to release adrenocorticotropic hormone into the systemic circulation, which stimulates the adrenal cortex to secrete cortisol. Also through CRH, the hypothalamus excites firing of the locus coeruleus in the brainstem to increase norepinephrine in the CNS. The hypothalamus also synthesizes arginine vasopressin or antidiuretic hormone (AVP/ADH), which is released by the posterior pituitary gland and increases blood pressure by causing vasoconstriction and water retention.

The activities of the hypothalamic–pituitary–adrenocortical (HPA) axis and the sympathetic–adrenal medullary system operate within different time frames to provide the body with a wide range of defensive responses. Because the neural response of the ANS is instantaneous, it is the body's first line of defense against stressors. The release of AVP/ADH and corticosteroids is slightly slower and augments ANS effects. In the short term, these responses mobilize energy reserves (mainly in the form of glucose to skeletal muscles) and prepare the body to deal with the stressor by running away or fighting it off. If the stressor is prolonged, then the body must make longer-term metabolic adjustments that ensure a sufficient supply of energy. Cortisol is essential to the body's sustained stress response because it

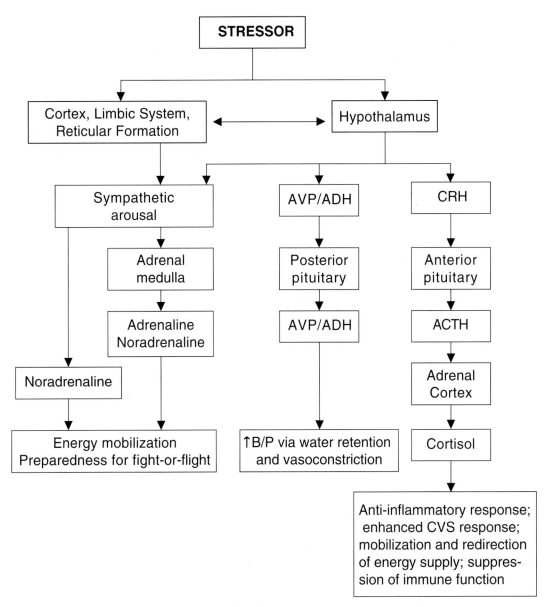

Figure 18.2 Physiologic responses to stress.

mobilizes lipid stores and skeletal protein for energy, which allows the conservation of glucose energy for neural tissue. It also acts on the liver to elevate and stabilize blood glucose levels through gluconeogenesis and lipolysis. As well as having these metabolic effects, cortisol is an anti-inflammatory. By reducing the dilation and permeability of blood vessels, which is part of the inflammatory response, cortisol aids in the maintenance of blood pressure and minimizes fluid loss to the tissue. At the same time, chronically elevated cortisol prolongs healing and leaves the body vulnerable to infection.

Social Support and Stress

Animal and human research consistently demonstrates that **social support** enhances health and wellbeing and, conversely, that a lack of social support increases the risk of morbidity and mortality.

Social Support

Broadly defined as resources provided to us by others, social support has been shown to moderate the adverse effects of stress. Although it takes various forms, social support is broadly categorized as either *functional* or *structural*. Functional support refers to the quality of the relationships and the degree to which an individual believes that help is available; structural support relates to the quantitative characteristics of a social support network (e.g., size, number of interconnections).

Nurses may conclude that social support is a dynamic process that is in constant flux and varies with life events and health status. It is important to keep in mind that not all interpersonal interactions within a network are supportive; an individual can have a large, complex social network but little social support. The concept of **dissupport** (Malone, 1988) derives from the observation that some relationships can be harmful, stressful, and even damaging to an individual's self-esteem. Examples of dissupport include verbal, physical, or emotional abuse; discounting an individual's opinions, feelings, behaviours, or values; blocking access to resources; or consuming an individual's material resources. As one might expect, social dissupport can hinder growth, is emotionally destructive, and depletes resources. Even more complex are those relationships that are both supportive and dissupportive, such as those that provide tangible support (e.g., money) but are also emotionally destructive.

Social Network

We all live within networks of relationships among a defined set of people with whom we have regular face-to-face contact. It is through these relationships that we are socialized and acquire emotional support, material aid, services, and information. An individual's social network can be a resource, enhance the ability to cope with change, and influence the course of illness.

Contacts within a social network are categorized into three levels:

1. *Level I*—6 to 12 people with whom the person has intimate contact (e.g., one's closest family and friends)
2. *Level II*—30 to 40 people whom the person sees regularly (e.g., more distant family and friends, neighbours, coworkers)
3. *Level III*—the several hundred people with whom an individual has direct contact but incidental contact during their day-to-day life (e.g., acquaintances, the grocer, mail carrier). The various levels of an individual's social network often intersect with each other; for example, a friend may be a confidant, a neighbour, and a workout buddy. Generally speaking, the larger and more interconnected a social network is, the more support that is available to its members. An ideal network is dense and interconnected so that each individual within the network relates to the other at various levels. Dense networks are typically better able to respond in times of stress and crisis because they represent a large reservoir of social, emotional, and instrumental resources.

Intensity and reciprocity are two concepts important to understanding social networks. *Intensity* is the degree or closeness of a relationship. Some relationships are naturally more intense than others, and ideally, an individual's social network reflects a balance between intense and less intense relationships. Intense relationships can restrict a person's opportunity to interact with other network members, but a person lacks intimacy without at least a few intense relationships. *Reciprocity* is the extent to which there is balanced give-and-take in a relationship. Network members provide and receive support, aid, services, and information from each other; sometimes, members are on the giving side; at other times, they receive. Reciprocity represents a necessary equilibrium between the two states.

Emotional Responses to Stress

Although it is clear that emotion is key to the human stress response, there is still debate about the relationship between emotion and cognition. On one side, there is the argument that emotions are primary and influence both the form and content of our perceptions, while opponents believe that cognition is primary and gives rise to emotion. Consistent with his transactional view of stress, Lazarus (1991) takes a more integrative approach and contends that cognition and emotion are essentially simultaneous and interdependent. He and his colleagues define emotion as "complex, organized psychophysiologic reactions consisting of cognitive appraisals, action impulses, and patterned somatic reactions" (Folkman & Lazarus, 1991, p. 209).

Cognitive appraisal is fundamental to the experience of emotion because it colours the meaning of a situation or an event. Based on their research, Lazarus and colleagues believe that there are 15 basic emotions, each

Table 18.3	Fifteen Basic Emotions
Emotion	**Relational Meaning**
Anger	A demeaning offense against me and mine
Anxiety	Facing an uncertain, existential threat
Fright	Facing an immediate, concrete, and overwhelming physical danger
Guilt	Having transgressed a moral imperative
Shame	Having failed to live up to an ego ideal
Sadness	Having experienced an irrevocable loss
Envy	Wanting what someone else has
Jealousy	Resenting a third party for the loss of or a threat to another's affection
Disgust	Taking in or being too close to an indigestible object or idea (metaphorically speaking)
Happiness	Making reasonable progress towards the realization of a goal
Pride	Enhancement of one's ego identity by taking credit for a valued object or achievement, either our own or that of someone or a group with whom we identify
Relief	A distressing goal-incongruent condition that has changed for the better or gone away
Hope	Fearing the worst but yearning for better
Love	Desiring or participating in affection, usually but not necessarily reciprocated
Compassion	Being moved by another's suffering and wanting to help

Adapted with permission from Lazarus, R. S. (1999). *Stress and emotion: A new synthesis.* Springer.

of which is elicited in response to a particular perception of what a situation or an event means to the individual (see Table 18.3). Anxiety, for example, is typically associated with the perception of a nonspecific threat or some uncertainty, whereas happiness reflects an appraisal of the person–environment condition that is beneficial. Patterned somatic reactions are the individual's own, unique experience of the physiologic changes associated with an emotion. For one person, a rush of energy is the salient feature of anger, whereas for another person, it is trembling and a feeling of weakness. These physical reactions motivate or inhibit action impulses. For example, the person who feels energized may attack an aggressor, whereas the person who experiences trembling and weakness is likely to withdraw.

Coping

According to Lazarus (1998), the following three principles are vital to an understanding of coping: (a) it continually changes over the course of an encounter; (b) it must be assessed independently of its outcomes; and (c) it consists of what an individual thinks and does in response to the perceived demands of a situation. With those principles in mind, coping is defined as "the efforts we take to manage situations we have appraised as being potentially harmful or stressful" (Kleinke, 2007, pp. 290–291). Coping reflects an individual's continual reappraisal of the person–environment relationship in light of changing conditions, as well as the success of their efforts to mitigate the situation. Those who evaluate their coping responses as effective are likely to feel competent and to repeat those responses in the future. Conversely, individuals who see their efforts as ineffective are likely to feel helpless and overwhelmed. Positive coping leads to adaptation, which is characterized by wellbeing and maximum social functioning. The inability to cope leads to maladaptation and contributes to ill health, a diminished self-concept, and deterioration in social functioning. These ideas are captured in the stress, coping, and adaptation models presented in Figures 18.3 and 18.4.

There are two general approaches to coping: problem-focused and emotion-focused. As Kleinke (2007) explains, problem-focused coping may be inner or outer directed. Outer-directed strategies attempt to eliminate or alter a situation or another's behaviour, while inner-directed strategies aim at altering one's own beliefs, attitudes, skills, responses, and so forth. In **emotion-focused coping**, individuals seek to manage their emotional distress (e.g., through exercise, prayer/meditation, expressing emotions, talking to friends). Table 18.4 contrasts problem-focused and emotion-focused coping.

Coping involves the continuous reevaluation or reappraisal of the changing person–environment relationship. Reappraisal incorporates feedback about the effects of coping and allows for continual processing of new information. No single coping strategy is effective in all situations. Throughout life, a repertoire of coping strategies is developed and adapted to suit different situations, and these strategies become ingrained into patterned responses. Well-adapted individuals are realistic in their appraisal of the demands upon them, are flexible in their use of coping resources, and remain open to learning new coping strategies. Poor reality testing, impaired judgment, inflexibility, limited coping strategies, and an unwillingness to acquire new resources can render individuals vulnerable to stress-related problems and illness.

KEY CONCEPT

Coping is an individual's constantly changing cognitive and behavioural efforts to manage specific external or internal demands that are appraised as taxing or exceeding the individual's resources.

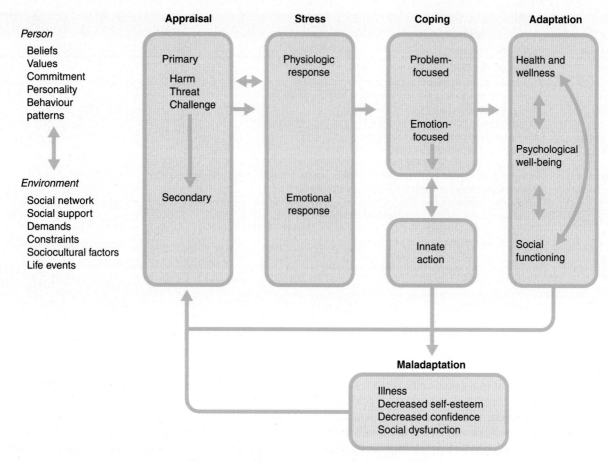

Figure 18.3 Stress, coping, and adaptation model.

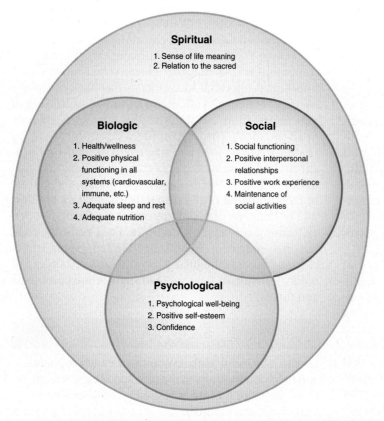

Figure 18.4 Bio/psycho/social/spiritual adaptation.

Table 18.4 Ways of Coping: Problem-Focused Versus Emotion-Focused	
Problem-Focused Coping	Emotion-Focused Coping
Outer-directed When noise from the television in the apartment next door interrupts a student's studying, they experience anxiety about being ready for an important exam the next day. They respond by asking their neighbour to turn the volume down.	A man dislikes visiting his wife's mother because she has two cats that roam her house freely, and the cat fur on all of the furniture irritates him. Rather than refusing to visit his mother-in-law, which causes conflict in his marriage, the man plans strategies that help him manage his distress during visits (e.g., long walks, a good book to distract him, thinking about how pleased his wife is).
Inner-directed When an abused woman feels guilt about leaving her husband, she reminds herself that her children are much happier and doing well in school.	

Stress, Trauma, and Illness

Accumulated research has demonstrated a relationship between stress and illness for more than 50 years. Animal experiments in the 1950s and 1960s demonstrated that a number of stressors (e.g., isolation, crowding, exposure to predators, electrical shock) increased morbidity and mortality from tumours and infections (Sadock et al., 2015).

Between 1995 and 1997, Felitti explored the impact of Adverse Childhood Experiences (ACEs). This is the largest epidemiological study to date in the United States with more than 17,000 middle class adult participants. The ACE study (Felitti et al., 1998) was the first to explore the long-term relationship of abuse in children under 18 years of age and the links to disease, disability, social problems, and early death. Felitti and his colleagues administered a 10-item questionnaire to identify childhood experiences of household dysfunction, abuse, and neglect. The greater the score, then the higher the risk of trauma resulting in compromised health, emotional and cognitive functioning (see Table 18.5).

Inability or ineffective coping negatively impacts health. Some coping strategies actually increase the risk for mortality and morbidity, such as the excessive use of alcohol, drugs, tobacco, or overeating. Although these strategies may provide some short-term stress relief, they often cause long-term secondary stress. The corollary is that healthy coping strategies such as exercising, adequate sleep, leisure activities, and good nutrition reduce the negative effects of stress and promote health and wellbeing. An ideal wellness plan includes physical, emotional, mental, and spiritual components.

Table 18.5 Adverse Childhood Experiences Questionnaire	
ACE Score: Prior to Your 18th Birthday:	Score
1. Did a parent or other adult in the household often or very often … Swear at you, insult you, put you down, or humiliate you? Or Act in a way that made you afraid that you might be physically hurt? If yes, enter 1.	
2. Did a parent or other adult in the household often or very often … Push, grab, slap, or throw something at you? Or Ever hit you so hard that you had marks or were injured? If yes, enter 1.	
3. Did an adult or person at least 5 years older than you ever … Touch or fondle you or have you touch their body in a sexual way? Or Attempt or actually have oral, anal, or vaginal intercourse with you? If yes, enter 1.	
4. Did you often or very often feel that … No one in your family loved you or thought you were important or special? Or your family didn't look out for each other, feel close to each other, or support each other? If yes, enter 1.	
5. Did you often or very often feel that … You didn't have enough to eat, had to wear dirty clothes, and had no one to protect you? Or your parents were too drunk or high to take care of you or take you to the doctor if you needed it? If yes, enter 1.	
6. Were your parents ever separated or divorced? If yes, enter 1.	
7. Was your mother or stepmother: Often or very often pushed, grabbed, slapped, or had something thrown at her? Or sometimes, often, or very often kicked, bitten, hit with a fist, or hit with something hard? Or ever repeatedly hit over at least a few minutes or threatened with a gun or knife? If yes, enter 1.	
8. Did you live with anyone who was a problem drinker or alcoholic, or who used street drugs? If yes, enter 1.	
9. Was a household member depressed or mentally ill, or did a household member attempt suicide? If yes, enter 1.	
10. Did a household member go to prison? If yes, enter 1.	
Total score out of ten	

Source: ACE Response. (2021). *ACE questions and overviews.* http://aceresponse.org/img/uploads/file/ace_score_questionnaire.pdf

Trauma- and Stressor-Related Disorders

Although historical and literary documents dating back to the third-century B.C. describe human responses to extreme stress (e.g., natural disasters, combat, physical/sexual assault; Birmes et al., 2003), modern psychiatry did not officially recognize them until 1980, when posttraumatic stress disorder (PTSD) appeared in the *Diagnostic and Statistical Manual of Mental Disorders (DSM)* (American Psychiatric Association [APA], 1980); 14 years later, acute stress disorder (ASD) was added as a diagnostic label (APA, 1994).

In the fifth and latest version of the *DSM* (APA, 2013), both PTSD and ASD were removed from the list of anxiety disorders and placed in a new category of disorders called *trauma- and stressor-related disorders*. All of the disorders in this category specify exposure to a traumatic or extremely stressful event as a diagnostic criterion. *Trauma* is from the Greek for *wound* and refers to an injury, physical and/or psychic (Oxford English Dictionary Online, 2013, December). A traumatic stressor is considered in the *DSM-5* to be "any event (or events) that may cause or threaten death, serious injury, or sexual violence to an individual, a close family member, or a close friend" (APA, 2013, p. 830). This change in criteria acknowledges that there are wide variations in individuals' responses to a traumatic experience.

KEY CONCEPT

A traumatic stressor is "any event (or events) that may cause or threaten death, serious injury, or sexual violence to an individual, a close family member, or a close friend" (APA, 2013, p. 830).

Acute Stress Disorder

A diagnosis of ASD is made if an individual has experienced, personally or through witnessing others' experience(s), a severe threat in which life or injury is or appears to be at stake. This experience must then continue to affect the individual's mental health status in such areas as arousal, intrusive memories, and changes in behaviour and functioning. Refer to the *DSM-5* (2013) for APA's criteria for the traumatic event and for specific symptoms.

Posttraumatic Stress Disorder

A diagnosis of PTSD is made if an individual experiences or witnesses an authentic, severe threat of death or injury (including sexual injury) to self or others and this experience then affects the individual's mental health in specific ways. Reliving the traumatic experience through intrusive thoughts or images is a key symptom of PTSD. Avoidance of memories of the trauma (emotional avoidance)

or external reminders of it (behavioural avoidance) may occur. Daily functioning can be affected by the inability to concentrate and by alterations in arousal level (e.g., hyperarousal and hypervigilance). PTSD may have negative effects on sleep and relationships, with some individuals experiencing a sense of being isolated and alone. Sareen (2014), in an overview of PTSD, notes that clinicians need to be aware that PTSD symptoms overlap with those of panic disorder, general anxiety disorder, and depression. The physical and mental effects of the trauma event on the individual need ongoing evaluation, as does risk for suicidal behaviour, which is increased with PTSD. Brief, self-report measures (e.g., the PTSD checklist and the Impact of Events Scale) can assist in this evaluation (Sareen, 2014). For symptom criteria for PTSD, please see the *DSM-5* (APA, 2013). Among the most common type of threats related to PTSD include witnessing the killing or injury of others and being in a life-threatening accident (Sareen, 2014). For children and adult refugees, precarious immigration status is associated with PTSD (Kronick, 2017).

Although more than half of individuals will experience a traumatic event at some time in their lives, most people will not develop PTSD (National Collaborating Centre for Mental Health, 2005). A survey study of adults in Ottawa regarding perceived personal threat in response to the terrorist attacks of September 11, 2001, found that the higher the appraisal of personal threat and distress experienced, the more likely it was that positive life changes (e.g., closer to family, refocused priorities) were made; these changes were reported to remain stable nearly a year later (Davis & Macdonald, 2004). For most people, adversity fosters psychological resilience, not psychopathology. Psychological resilience is understood as a dynamic process of effective coping and positive adaptation in the face of adversity (Veer et al., 2021), developed and sustained by bio/psycho/social/spiritual factors (Tay & Lim, 2020). Research suggests that a positive appraisal style (a tendency to "look on the bright side") mediated by the perception that one has social support available are notable resilience factors (Veer et al.). Preferred coping mechanisms tend to: (a) focus on brief time intervals (e.g., think only about the next step); (b) maintain a view of oneself as competent and a view of others as willing and able to provide support; and (c) focus on the current implications of the trauma and avoid regretting past decisions and actions.

KEY CONCEPT

Psychological resilience is effective coping and positive adaptation despite adversity. Developed and sustained by bio/psycho/social/spiritual factors, research indicates that it is promoted by positive appraisal style and perceived social support.

Factors that predict the development of PTSD include being female, type and severity of the trauma, past trauma (including childhood physical, sexual, and emotional abuse), and availability of support at the time of the stressful event (Richardson et al., 2007). Since women are more likely to experience more high-impact trauma, they are also more likely than men to develop PTSD. It is the type of experience, such as interpersonal violence, that accounts for some of this difference (Amstadter et al., 2013; Kelly et al., 2011; Maguen et al., 2012; Rees et al., 2011). Women in the perinatal period have higher rates of PTSD compared with other times across the life span, likely due to exacerbation of preexisting PTSD symptoms (Seng et al., 2010). A study in which structured interviews of 8,441 members of the Canadian Armed Forces (CAF) regarding trauma exposure and PTSD found that PTSD rates were higher among female soldiers. Women had less exposure than men to warlike trauma but greater experience of sexual assault. Although members of the CAF have high exposure to trauma events (85.6% had such exposure), the rate of lifetime PTSD is moderate (6.6%) (Brunet et al., 2015). Children (particularly those under the age of 10 years) are less likely to experience PTSD after trauma than are adults (National Collaborating Centre for Mental Health, 2005), but a systematic review and meta-analysis identified associations between adverse childhood experiences (ACE) and ill health, including mental health, over the life course. Findings support a strong relationship between ACEs and conditions such as depression, anxiety, and illicit drug use (Bellis et al., 2019).

Treatments for PTSD include cognitive–behavioural therapy (CBT), psychotherapy, eye movement desensitization and reprocessing (EMDR), and medication. Treatment may need to be prolonged, and there are many who live with chronic persistent symptoms. Neurobiologic studies related to PTSD first began with Vietnam war veterans who still met criteria for PTSD 20 to 30 years after the war.

Intergenerational Transmission of Stress, Trauma, and Resilience

The processes by which the effects of stress and trauma experienced in one generation can be transmitted to the subsequent generations involve multiple factors and intersecting pathways (Bombay et al., 2009, 2014a; Bowers & Yehuda, 2016; Dekel & Goldblatt, 2008). It is known that adverse experiences in childhood and adulthood may influence the risk for various health and social outcomes in offspring of those who encountered the stressor or trauma directly (Bombay et al., 2009, 2014b; Bowers & Yehuda, 2016; Dekel & Goldblatt, 2008). For example, the experiences of parents have been shown to be linked with the way their children appraise certain situations, including the way they appraise stressful experiences and their ability to contend with these stressors.

These appraisals, in turn, can influence the coping strategies that are endorsed, which will also be influenced by the coping styles or predispositions that individuals bring with them. As a result, these individuals may be at increased risk of further stressor encounters, increased psychological and neurochemical reactivity to stressors, and the promotion of poor mental and physical health outcomes (Bowers & Yehuda, 2016).

This is not only one potential scenario demonstrating how trauma can be transmitted across generations, as other psychological, social, physiologic, cultural, and economic factors have also been shown to be involved in these intergenerational processes. The previous depiction of intergenerational transfer essentially portrays events within a family unit, but it is understood that stressful and traumatic events within this unit do not occur in isolation of other external and indirect factors that might contribute to, or protect against, the intergenerational transfer of stressor effects (e.g., sociocultural environment, physical environment, historical influences, and government policies). These factors, alone or in combination, may result in impaired abilities to provide an adequate early childhood environment for their children, which might result in the recapitulation of the events that occurred in the preceding generation. Of course, not all individuals whose parents face stress and trauma are destined to be at risk for negative outcomes throughout their lifetime, as the transmission of such risk across generations can be mitigated by various protective factors—including internal assets and external resources—that may buffer against the negative experiences faced by their parents (Bowers & Yehuda, 2016; Lee et al., 2012).

Collective Trauma and Historical Trauma

It has been suggested that focusing solely on individual experiences of stress and trauma has resulted in the lack of appropriate consideration of the significant collective experiences and outcomes that can arise when a whole group of people encounter a traumatizing and/or adverse experience (Somasundaram, 2007). Collective trauma refers to instances in which a significant proportion of any given social group—based on political, racial, religious, cultural, or other factors—are collectively exposed to a traumatic event. Such experiences can be as random as a single natural disaster or purposely conducted by one group to another at one time or for an extended period (Bombay et al., 2009, 2014a). Increasing research has demonstrated the potential unique social and psychological outcomes at the collective or community level that can have significant long-term consequences (Somasundaram, 2007, 2014). In addition to the additive effects of individual trauma elicited by such collective experiences, effects at the family and community levels can modify social norms, dynamics, structures, and functioning that are more than the sum of the individual-level effects. For example, community-level changes in the aftermath of mass trauma have included erosion of basic trust; collective silence; deterioration in social norms, morals, and values; and poor leadership (Bombay et al., 2014a, 2014b; Catani et al., 2008; Saul, 2014; Somasundaram, 2007).

In addition to considering the collective nature of some traumatic events, it is also important to consider the traumatic events that the group had previously experienced. Similar to the allostatic overload associated with individual experiences of stress or trauma, the concept of historical trauma highlights the process by which the consequences of multiple collectively experienced adversities experienced by a group over time may be cumulative and be carried forward to subsequent generations if they outweigh contextual and group-level resilience factors (Evans-Campbell, 2008). This perspective allows events occurring across generations to be considered as part of a single traumatic trajectory, expanding the focus from isolated impacts of single events to also considering the interactions and synergies associated with numerous adversities over time (Bombay et al., 2014a, 2014b; Evans-Campbell, 2008).

Many Indigenous Peoples across the world have endured numerous intense collective traumas since first contact that continue in the present day. This was compounded by the suppression of spiritual and traditional practices, which could have otherwise served as a resilience factor (Matheson et al., 2016). Indeed, historic trauma has been suggested and shown to be a contributing factor in relation to the high prevalence of certain psychosocial issues faced by First Nations Peoples and other Indigenous Peoples groups (Braveheart-Jordan & DeBruyn, 1995; Duran et al., 1998; Robin et al., 1996).

Historical trauma can be considered a cumulative emotional and psychological wounding over the life span and across generations that emanates from massive group trauma experiences (Brave Heart, 2003). Duran (2006) describes this as "soul wounding" and is taken from the definition of psychology—the study of the soul. Increasing empirical research supports this concept and intergenerational effects in relation to various mental health outcomes have been observed in the adult offspring of adults who are Indigenous Peoples of the United States and Canada who were affected by forced relocations (Walls & Whitbeck, 2012), or by the forced removal of children who are Indigenous Peoples to residential schools (Native North American boarding schools in the United States), for the purposes of assimilation (Bombay et al., 2014a). For example, it was shown that adults who are Indigenous Peoples of Canada who had a parent or grandparent who attended Native North American residential schools were at greater risk for psychological distress and suicide attempts compared to those whose parents did not attend (Bombay et al., 2014a; McQuaid et al., 2017). Providing evidence for

the cumulative nature of historical trauma events and experiences, it was also found that those with a parent and grandparent who attended—so with two previous familial generations who were directly affected—were at greater risk for these negative outcomes compared to those with only one previous generation who attended (i.e., parent or a grandparent) (McQuaid et al.).

KEY CONCEPT

Collective trauma occurs when a traumatic event is experienced by a significant proportion of a given social group; it can have long-term consequences for the social group beyond its additive effect on individuals such that social norms, dynamics, functioning, and structure of the group may be modified.

KEY CONCEPT

Historical trauma is the process by which a social group is affected by the consequences of multiple, collectively experienced adversities across time that outweigh group resiliency factors, become cumulative, and are carried forward to subsequent generations such that the trauma may be considered as part of a single trajectory.

Responses to Collective and Historical Trauma

For collectivistic societies that place significant value on relationships, healing and recovery from collectively experienced trauma and stress must address the impacts on the collective and do so through integrated multi-level approaches (Somasundaram, 2007, 2014). Though both the *DSM* and World Health Organization (WHO) International Classification of Diseases (ICD) classification systems have traditionally been based on the individual, it has been argued that collective approaches will often have the most benefits from a public health perspective when resources are limited. For example, community-level mental health and psychosocial support interventions have been shown to help communities affected by disasters (Macy et al., 2004; Scholte & Ager, 2014; Somasundaram, 2007, 2014).

Furthermore, community-based approaches enable interventions to reach a larger target population, as well as undertake preventive and promotional public mental health activities at the same time. Individuals and families can be expected to recover and cope when communities become functional, activating healing mechanisms within the community itself (Somasundaram, 2007, 2014). It is important to recognize the manifestations of collective trauma, so that effective interventions at the community level can be used in these complex situations.

Integrated holistic community approaches that were found useful in rebuilding communities include:

* creating public awareness;
* training of grass root workers;
* encouraging traditional practices and rituals;
* promoting positive family and community relationships and processes; and
* rehabilitation and networking with other organizations (Somasundaram, 2007, 2014).

In relation to the historical trauma of Indigenous Peoples of Canada, researchers and scholars who are Indigenous Peoples of Canada have expressed the need for multilevel assessment and intervention strategies to address factors related to health and wellness at individual, family, and community levels (Brave Heart et al., 2011; Evans-Campbell, 2008). A long-term goal of historical trauma intervention research and practice is to reduce inequities faced by Indigenous Peoples by developing culturally responsive interventions driven by communities to improve quality of life and wellbeing. Through individual and community-based initiatives, as well as larger political and cultural processes, Indigenous Peoples of Canada are involved in healing their traditions, repairing the ruptures and discontinuities in the transmission of traditional knowledge and values, and asserting their collective identity and power.

Trauma-Informed Care

Trauma-informed care and practice takes into consideration the prevalence of various types of violence and trauma and the wide range of responses by individuals (British Columbia Provincial Mental Health and Substance Use Planning Council [BCPMH & SUPC], 2013). There are four principles that provide the structure for this practice-informed approach: trauma awareness; emphasis on safety and trustworthiness; opportunity for choice, collaboration, and connection; and strength-based and skill building. Effective trauma-informed care is to equip staff with the knowledge to ensure that they do no further harm or re-traumatize those already exposed to significant trauma (Elliott et al., 2005; Raja et al., 2015). Clients should find those providing their care to be compassionate and trustworthy.

KEY CONCEPT

Trauma-informed care is an approach to all clients takes into consideration the prevalence of various types of violence and trauma and the wide range of responses by individuals (British Columbia Provincial Mental Health and Substance Use Planning Council [BCPMH & SUPC], 2013). There are four principles that provide the structure for this practice-informed approach: trauma awareness; emphasis on safety and trustworthiness; opportunity for choice, collaboration, and connection; and strength-based and skill building.

Health, social, and economic inequities continue to exist across certain racialized and marginalized groups in Canada and the United States, and interpersonal and systemic racism within the healthcare system contributes to these ongoing gaps (Allan & Smylie, 2015; Bombay, 2015; Braveman et al., 2010; Browne et al., 2012; Turpel-Lafond, 2020). In addition to systemic and more blatant forms of discrimination, implicit discrimination in the form of bias, attitudes, and beliefs, even without conscious intent or awareness, can influence provider behaviour in healthcare settings (Dovidio et al., 2008; Johnson et al., 2004; Penner et al., 2010), clinical decision-making, and treatment recommendations, with potential detrimental consequences to the provision of effective and safe care (Green et al., 2007; Turpel-Lafond, 2020).

There is growing attention to the need for **cultural competence** in trauma-informed health care (Ardino, 2014; Huey et al., 2014; Imel et al., 2011). In this conceptions, culture is implied to be indistinguishable from ethnicity (Browne et al., 2009) rather than recognizing that we are all bearers of culture and espouse cultural values. Although it is clearly important to increase knowledge regarding differing culturally embedded world views, experiences and conceptualizations of health (Tervalon & Murray-Garcia, 1998), healthcare practitioners, community members, and researchers have advocated that cultural competence is not enough; we need *cultural safety* and *cultural humility* (Caron, 2017). *Cultural competence* implies a finite skill that can be acquired through training, whereas *cultural humility* is an active and continual engagement in a process of self-critique, reflection, acknowledgment, rectification of imbalances of power, and respectful community partnership in the provision of care (Kumagai & Lypson, 2009; Tervalon & Murray-Garcia, 1998). Approaching cultural competence as a sum of knowledge that can be acquired and implemented, risks reductionism and may result in harm due to stereotyping and cultural assumptions, when this information does not result in changes in practice or in the understanding for the need to adopt a humble stance within cross-cultural interactions (Ben-Ari & Strier, 2010; Tervalon & Murray-Garcia, 1998). A concept compatible with cultural humility is **cultural safety**. Cultural safety was first conceived, developed, and advocated for within health care by nurses who are of Maori origin in Aotearoa/New Zealand and was introduced as a requirement in nursing education in the early 1990s to redress health and healthcare inequalities of Maori people (Papps & Ramsden, 1996; Ramsden & Spoonley, 1993; Richardson, 2004). Central to cultural safety is an examination of colonial, interpersonal, and professional power relationships reflected through racism and discrimination (Allan & Smylie, 2015; Richardson & Carryer, 2005).

It is unlikely for a single paradigm to address the full complexity of intercultural interactions within health care settings, which must be understood in relation to historical contexts and power relations (Kirmayer, 2012). Adding to the complexity, patient's experiences and identities may include a variety of intersections, such as ethnicity, gender, immigrant experiences, sexuality, socioeconomic status, and ability, to name a few, which may interact to influence points of view and care needs (Quiros & Berger, 2015). However, health care provider perceptions and assumptions can and do interfere with care provision (Penner et al., 2010). The concept of cultural safety is potentially useful to improving intercultural care (Tervalon & Murray-Garcia, 1998) and is congruent with, and a core element of, trauma-informed care by creating a respectful and safe environment for all patients (Elliott et al., 2005) and working to reduce health inequities in primary care (Browne et al., 2012).

It is important to consider the impact of repetitive and/or chronic trauma experiences at not only an individual but also a collective or group level. There is growing awareness of repetitive and chronic trauma affecting generations and whole communities, as is the case with historical trauma (Bombay et al., 2014a, 2014b; Brave Heart et al., 2011). In addition to understanding the implications of colonization and other types of collective and historical trauma, it is equally important to adopt a strength-based perspective that respects individual and community resilience and empowerment within marginalized populations (Kirmayer et al., 2009a, 2009b; Million, 2013). Within a Canadian context of colonization, it is imperative for health professionals within mainstream settings to recognize and work towards redressing the intergenerational impacts of the residential school system and other colonizing policies (TRC, 2015) as part of culturally safe trauma-informed care and to "create space for Indigenous healing strategies as part of treatment" (Linklater, 2014, p. 131).

Nursing Care of Individuals Affected by Stress

Nursing assessment of individuals experiencing stress attends to biologic, psychological, emotional, and environmental (physical and social) as well as coping resources. In particular, the nurse should explore recent changes (positive or negative) in the individual's life (e.g., trauma, loss, developmental milestones).

The overall goals of care for those individuals actively experiencing a stress response are to eliminate or moderate the stressor (if possible), to reduce untoward effects of the stress response, and to facilitate the maintenance or development of positive coping skills. The goals of care for individuals who are at high risk for stress (e.g., are experiencing significant life changes, have preexisting vulnerabilities, have limited coping mechanisms) are to recognize the potential for stress and to strengthen

or develop positive coping skills. It is also important to educate clients about human stress responses as a way to help normalize bodily, emotional, and social responses, thereby helping the client to reappraise their own interpretation of these responses.

Biologic Domain

Biologic Assessment

Biologic data are essential for analyzing an individual's physical responses to stress, coping efforts, and adaptation. This information comes from the health history, physical examination, and diagnostic testing (as indicated; see Chapter 10). Nurses should pay particular attention to:

- signs and responses indicating sympathetic and parasympathetic arousal (see Chapter 10);
- alterations in vegetative functions (e.g., appetite and eating patterns, sleep, energy level, sexual activity);
- chronic illness or conditions with a strong stress component (e.g., hypertension, migraine, chronic pain syndromes, irritable bowel syndrome);
- evidence of immune system suppression (e.g., frequent infections);
- physical appearance (e.g., deficits in grooming and hygiene; nonverbal indications of muscle tension, anxiety, or depression); and
- alterations in activity and exercise patterns.

As well, the biologic assessment of stress and coping considers the use of pharmacologic agents, including prescription and nonprescription medications, over-the-counter and herbal preparations, alcohol, tobacco, and illicit drugs. Some individuals begin or increase the frequency of using these agents as a way of coping with stress. At the same time, however, reliance on relaxants or mood-altering substances can become a secondary stressor and contribute to maladaptation. Understanding patterns of use (e.g., frequency, dose, circumstances, and effects) is important to assessing their role in stress management. The more important the substances are to a person's handling of stress, the greater the potential for abuse and addiction.

Interventions for the Biologic Domain

Individuals experiencing or at risk for untoward stress responses may benefit from a number of biologic interventions.

- The importance of (re)establishing regular routines for activities of daily living (e.g., eating, sleeping, self-care, leisure time) cannot be overstated. As well as ensuring adequate nutrition, sleep and rest, and hygiene routines may help to structure an individual's time and give them a sense of personal control or mastery.
- Exercise can reduce the emotional and behavioural responses to stress. In addition to the physical benefits,

Maria Campbell (1940–)

Maria Campbell is a woman of Métis origin and the eldest daughter of seven children. She was born in Park Valley, Saskatchewan, to parents of Scottish, Indigenous Peoples, and French descent. Her autobiography, *Halfbreed* (1973), is considered a foundational work of literature of Indigenous Peoples and has become a Canadian classic. It recounts the first 33 years of her life and tells of how Maria lost her mother when she was only 12 years old, leaving her to care for her younger siblings. In an effort to keep her family together, young Maria married an abusive White man who reported her to child welfare authorities, and her siblings were placed in foster homes. Devastated, Maria moved to Vancouver, where her husband deserted her, and she turned to a life of drugs and prostitution. Alone and desperate, she attempted suicide twice and was hospitalized for psychiatric care. It was in the hospital that Maria joined Alcoholics Anonymous and began a journey of healing. Campbell not only tells her own story but also speaks of the discrimination and racism that affects people who are of Métis origin. In the book's introduction, she writes, "I write this for

all of you, to tell you what it is like to be a half-breed woman in this country. I want to tell you about the joys and sorrows, the oppressing poverty, the frustrations and the dreams" (p. 8). Although Maria's story is one of stress and crises, it is also a story of courage and psychological resilience. She is not a scared little girl but a strong, independent woman full of hope for herself and her people. She is a mother, grandmother, and great-grandmother. Today, Maria is a cultural leader for people who are of Métis origin and an officer of the Order of Canada (awarded in 2008). She continues to write; her translated work, *Stories of the Road Allowance People*, was republished in 2010. In 2012, she retired from the University of Saskatchewan, was awarded a Pierre Elliott Trudeau Fellowship, and joined the Métis Research Group, Institute of Canadian Studies, University of Ottawa. She is the recipient of many writing awards, including the Chalmers Award for best new play, and has four Honorary Doctorate degrees. See Web Links for a brief video with Maria Campbell.

From Campbell, M. (1973). *Halfbreed*. Goodread Biographies.

regular exercise can provide structure to a person's life, enhance self-confidence, and increase feelings of well-being. Under stress, many individuals are not receptive to the idea of exercise, particularly if it has not been a part of their life. Exploration of usual activity patterns, as well as knowledge and beliefs about the value of exercise, will help to identify where the nurse may intervene.

• Activities such as yoga, meditation, deep breathing, and progressive muscle relaxation can help individuals mediate the physical stress response, improve sleep, and reduce pain. Nurses should also consider referring clients for hypnosis, biofeedback, or eye movement desensitization and reprocessing (EMDR) when indicated.

• Health teaching in such areas as nutrition, sleep hygiene, and medication management may also be a part of nursing interventions in this domain.

Psychological Domain

Psychological Assessment

Information about the psychological and emotional dimensions of stress may be forthcoming throughout the assessment process. In particular, the nurse should do the following:

• Observe for behavioural and affective indicators of stress response (e.g., energy level and general presentation; appearance, grooming, and hygiene; psychomotor agitation and retardation; facial expression; speech characteristics).

• Explore reports of recent changes in mood or current emotional distress (e.g., anxiety, fear, irritability, anger, tension, pressure, depression).

• Note alterations or impairment in mental status (e.g., suicidal ideation; self-deprecatory thoughts; impulsivity; ruminations; impaired concentration, problem-solving, or memory).

• Explore the individual's appraisal of significant life events (e.g., losses, physical or sexual abuse or assault, motor vehicle crashes, natural disasters, combat experience), the effect of those experiences, and the commitment to particular outcomes.

• Ask about alterations in day-to-day function or inability to fulfill responsibilities (e.g., family, work, school).

• Explore the individual's current resources and effectiveness of usual coping strategies.

Interventions for the Psychological Domain

Nursing interventions that support psychological functioning and facilitate lifestyle changes for persons coping with stress include cognitive–behavioural interventions (see Chapter 14), psychoeducational (individual or group) interventions (see Chapter 15), relaxation therapy, and assertiveness training.

Social Domain

Social Assessment

Information from a social assessment is invaluable to understanding an individual's coping resources. The ability to make healthy lifestyle changes is strongly influenced by one's social support system. Even the expression of stress is related to social factors, particularly ethnic and cultural expectations and values.

Social assessment also includes identification of the person's social network. The nurse should elicit the following information:

- size and extent of the network, both relatives and non-relatives, and the length and quality of the relationships;
- functions the network serves (e.g., intimacy, social integration, nurturance, reassurance of worth, guidance and advice, access to new contacts);
- degree of reciprocity between the individual and others in the network (i.e., Whom provides support to the client? Whom does the client support?); and
- degree of interconnectedness among network members.

Interventions for the Social Domain

Individuals who are coping with stressful situations often benefit from interventions that facilitate social functioning and promote the health and welfare of social network members. The education of the family regarding the client's disorder and their supportive involvement can be significant. The family and individual members may also require support, including respite. Referral to family therapy may be indicated.

Spiritual Domain

The challenges faced by individuals in times of stress and crisis can lead to an acute questioning about one's life choices and situation, about one's relationships, and about the meaning of one's very existence. Making sense of what is happening to you is fundamental to being human. If we want to believe in a "just world," then one response may be to search for reasons that one deserves to be "punished" (Hafer & Bègue, 2005). In his book, *When Bad Things Happen to Good People*, Kushner (1981) describes how a personal tragedy compelled him to "rethink everything" he had been taught about God and God's ways (p. 1). He could not make sense of what was happening to his family and felt "a deep aching sense of unfairness" (p. 2). Ultimately, Kushner concluded that

suffering happens in our natural world and that there are no exceptions for nice people; God gives humans strength to cope with their misfortunes and does not leave them to suffer alone. While his book reveals the search for meaning that a life crisis can inspire, his conclusions are his own. Others, even those in very similar circumstances, may choose a different resolution. For instance, lasting anger at the sacred power in which one believes may be the response if one feels totally abandoned or one may view the crisis situation as revealing direction for personal growth.

Nurses attending to the spiritual domain of their practice need to recognize the likely occurrence of such searching on the part of clients under duress or in crisis. Nurses need to refrain from providing their own answers to questions of meaning; rather, through listening, they need to provide support. Thoughtful questions may be helpful in understanding the client's perspective: What is sustaining you through this time? Are there spiritual acts, such as prayer or ritual, which you are finding helpful? What, if anything, can you take from this experience to help you in the future?

When a traumatic or crisis event is catastrophic in its scope, entire communities can struggle to understand the cause of what has happened and the meaning of the loss suffered. At one time in Western societies, disasters were understood as evidence of the wrath of the gods or God (Grandjean et al., 2008). The Lisbon earthquake of 1755 is used to mark the beginnings of change in societal attitudes towards disaster: it is called the first modern disaster as it was attributed to "natural" rather than "supernatural" causes. The type of disaster influences this struggle, of course, and can affect the community's recovery (Furedi, 2007). Faith-based support in times of disaster may be absent from organized disaster response, but rituals and sacraments, group prayer, and action on beliefs regarding service and helping others can restore a sense of stability and comfort for those who feel a need to turn to their faith (Clements & Casani, 2016).

Spirituality can positively influence the response to disaster. In a study of psychiatric morbidity following a tsunami in a community with diverse religious beliefs, it was found that altruistic behaviour on the part of community leaders, religious faith, and spirituality (along with family systems and social support) were factors that positively affected the early coping of survivors (Math et al., 2008). In addition to their professional challenges, nurses responding to a disaster in their own community will have to address their personal reaction as members of the community with their own spiritual questions.

Evaluation and Treatment Outcomes

Evaluation is guided by treatment goals established in the plan of care. The goals of individual care relate to improved health, wellbeing, and social function. Depending on the level of intervention, there may also be goals for the family and other members of the client's social network. Family outcomes may relate to improved communication or social support (e.g., reduced caregiver stress). Social network outcomes focus on strengthening the social network and improving its function.

Crisis

Our current understanding of the bio/psycho/social/spiritual implications of a crisis has its roots in Lindeman's (1944) study of bereavement among friends and relatives of the Coconut Grove nightclub fire in Boston in 1942. 439 individuals died in that fire, which at the time was the worst single building fire in U.S. history. In the course of his research, Lindeman learned that family and friends of those who died experienced somatic symptoms, feelings of anger and guilt, and preoccupation with the deceased. From this work, he developed a model that describes *grief as progressing through three stages*: shock and disbelief, acute mourning, and resolution. Lindeman concluded that **grief** is both a natural response to loss and necessary to survivors' mental health. He later extended his ideas about crisis to more common, yet significant, life events (e.g., the birth of a child, marriage, death) and hypothesized that the changes associated with these events cause emotional strain and require individuals to adapt to a new reality (Lindeman, 1956). These adaptive efforts lead to either mastery (psychological growth) or impaired functioning. Lindeman was convinced that by helping individuals through the bereavement process, mental health professionals could prevent later psychological and emotional problems. This thinking reflected two important trends that were germinating in psychiatry around the globe: the recognition of the potential for and the value of early intervention to prevent emotional and psychological problems and the movement from hospital-based to community-based psychiatric treatment.

Although Lindeman did much of the foundational work in the area of crisis, Gerald Caplan is widely acknowledged as the master architect of crisis intervention. A psychiatrist and close colleague of Lindeman's, Caplan (1961) equated mental health with a strong, mature ego, which he defined as (a) the capacity to withstand stress and maintain equilibrium, (b) an accurate perception of reality, and (c) a balanced repertoire of coping strategies based on sound reality testing. Caplan is believed to be the first to apply the term crisis in psychiatry, to relate the concept of homeostasis to crisis intervention, and to describe the stages of a crisis.

Caplan defined crisis as occurring "when a person faces an obstacle to important life goals, that is, for a time, insurmountable through the utilization of customary methods of problem solving" (1961, p. 18). More specifically, a crisis is a response in which psychological equilibrium is disrupted, usual coping methods are ineffective in restoring that equilibrium, and there is evidence of functional impairment (Caplan, 1961; Flannery & Everly, 2000). This disequilibrium causes a rise in inner tension and anxiety that, if it continues, engenders emotional upset and an inability to function (Caplan, 1961). Figure 18.5 summarizes the phases of crisis.

Although crises force individuals into uncharted territory, Caplan (1961) recognized that most individuals achieve resolution without professional help within 4 to 6 weeks. He viewed this time as a period of transition in which the individual, family, or group is more vulnerable to harm and, at the same time, more open to outside intervention. This prompted Caplan to advocate for community-based crisis services aimed at identifying maladaptive responses and intervening early to assist those involved to transform problems into opportunities for personal growth and new learning.

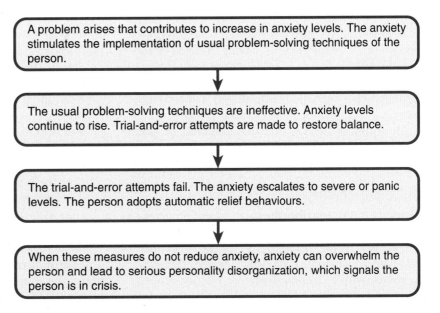

Figure 18.5 Phases of crisis response.

KEY CONCEPT

A crisis response occurs when an individual encounters an obstacle or problem that might affect their life goals and that cannot be solved by customary problem-solving methods. It is acute, is time limited, and may be developmental, situational, or interpersonal in nature.

Types of Crises

Situational Crisis

A situational crisis is any event that overwhelms an individual's coping resources and upsets their equilibrium. The precipitating event may be positive or negative, physiologic, psychological, or social in nature. Examples of situational crises include illness, the death of a loved one, separation or divorce, job loss, school problems, physical or sexual assault, or an unplanned pregnancy. Situational crises also result from less common occurrences such as accidents, natural or human-caused disasters, and acts of terrorism. Box 18.1 discusses the death of a loved one, a situational crisis that each of us will encounter in our lifetime.

Developmental Crisis

Theorists such as Erikson (1959) propose that human development proceeds sequentially through a series of stages, each with a new set of social roles and responsibilities. Stage theorists hold that demands from the social environment exert pressure on an individual to move on to the next developmental stage and that a failure to meet these new expectations precipitates a developmental crisis. Successful resolution of this crisis is necessary for movement into the next stage. Developmental crises are an expected part of maturation and are a time during which individuals acquire new skills and resources.

The concept of developmental crisis assumes that psychosocial development progresses in an orderly, easily identifiable process. Other developmental theories, such as those of Miller (1994) and Gilligan (1994), refute the notion that human development advances in stages (see Chapter 9). That being said, the concept of developmental crisis is useful for describing unfavourable person–environment relationships that relate to maturational events, such as leaving home for the first time, completing school, or the birth of one's first child.

BOX 18.1 Death of a Loved One: A Crisis Event

One of the most common crisis-provoking events is the loss of a loved one through death. Although death is a certainty for all of us, death in contemporary Western societies remains a taboo topic and unaccepted as a normal part of life. Combined with advances in medical science aimed at prolonging life (or postponing death), such attitudes can silence and isolate the bereaved (Lewis et al., 2020).

DEFINITION OF TERMS

Bereavement is typically understood to be the objective event or occurrence of having suffered a loss (Rando, 1993).

Grief is the subjective experience (e.g., thoughts, feelings, behaviours, body sensations) that accompanies the perception of a loss (Rando, 1993).

Mourning is the external manifestation of grief, which is highly influenced by gender, ethnicity, culture, religion, and the cause of death (Wolfelt, 1999).

TASKS OF MOURNING

Worden (2003) describes the four tasks of mourning, which are necessary to the process of adapting to loss and reestablishing equilibrium. Unlike other theorists who conceptualize mourning in terms of *stages* or *phases*, which connote linearity, Worden emphasizes the issues that bereaved individuals must face

and successfully negotiate as they come to terms with their new reality:

1. *Accepting the reality of the loss.* The first task of grieving is to accept the reality and full consequence of the loss. A part of this is recognizing the permanence of death and that life as it was is over forever.

2. *Working through the pain of grief.* It is important for the bereaved individual to experience and acknowledge the pain of grief. Denial or suppression of this pain prolongs grieving.

3. *Adapting to an environment in which the deceased is absent.* This adaptation requires the bereaved individual to adjust to a new reality, which involves developing a new self-identity (e.g., as a widow or single person) and taking on new social roles and responsibilities.

4. *Developing a new relationship with the deceased and reengaging with life.* In coming to terms with the loss, the bereaved individual does not forget the deceased but rather establishes a new relationship with the deceased. This involves healing the wound of the severed attachment so that new attachments can be formed.

Resolution of grief is manifested by the gradual return of feelings of wellbeing and the ability to continue with life. Bereaved persons do not deny their former lives or forget their loved ones but find a way to weave memories of the past into the current reality.

It is important to keep in mind that although the experience of loss is universal, individual responses vary widely, and there is no one clearly defined course or process of bereavement or grieving. Grief is influenced by age, development, gender, history of loss and/or trauma, history of depression, the nature and quality of the relationship with the deceased, and the type of loss (e.g., anticipated, violent, traumatic). Research underscores that the experience and expressions of grief are influenced by such factors as familial relationships and expectations, social and cultural factors, and religion (Center for the Advancement of Health, 2004).

COMPLICATED GRIEF

Complicated grief is also termed abnormal, pathologic, chronic, or exaggerated grief. It refers to grief that does not seem to be advancing the bereaved individual towards acceptance and reorganization. Grief is complicated when an individual does not accomplish one or more of the tasks of mourning. Examples of this include denying the reality of one's loss, prolonged and intense emotions that do not seem to lessen over time, the apparent absence of mourning, and the inability to reinvest in life.

ROLE OF HEALTHCARE TEAMS IN SUPPORTING GRIEF

As members of the healthcare team, nurses participate in supporting bereaved individuals through the process of grieving. The goals of this care are to assist bereaved individuals with the tasks of mourning and to prevent complicated grief. Activities may include sitting in silence with the bereaved, active listening, assistance with practical needs, and referral for ongoing support.

Crisis or Not? The Effects of Balancing Factors

Aguilera (1998) believes that a stressful event developing into a crisis depends on three *balancing factors*: perception of the event, available situational supports, and coping mechanisms. As Figure 18.6 illustrates, the timely and successful resolution of a crisis is more likely if an individual has a realistic view of the situation, adequate supports available, and effective coping mechanisms.

Nursing Care of Individuals Experiencing Crisis

Crisis Intervention

Crisis intervention is the provision of emergency psychological care to assist victims in returning to an adaptive level of functioning and to prevent or moderate the potentially negative effects of psychological trauma. Although there are several models of crisis intervention, virtually all of them incorporate the following principles:

1. **Early intervention.** By their nature, crises are acute and distressing events that overwhelm an individual's coping resources. Inability to resolve a crisis in a timely manner renders those affected at higher risk for long-term health problems. Crisis intervention services are typically community based and operate 24 hours per day. Crisis teams provide telephone triage and counselling but may also travel to the scene of the crisis, where they work closely with other emergency service personnel (e.g., police officers, firefighters, and hospital emergency staff).

2. **Stabilization.** An immediate goal of all crisis intervention efforts is to prevent the situation from worsening. Stabilization involves mobilizing resources and support networks with the aim of minimizing harm and quickly restoring some semblance of order and routine.

3. **Facilitating understanding.** An important part of crisis intervention is helping individuals to develop an accurate understanding of the situation and its potential consequences. This usually involves listening to individuals' accounts of their experience and assisting them to identify and articulate their feelings about what is happening. Facilitating a clear understanding of a situation helps individuals to develop a realistic appraisal of the demands on them and aids the integration of the crisis into their cognitive schema.

4. **Focusing on problem-solving.** A primary task of crisis intervention is the identification and prioritization of immediate problems. Once achieved, interventions focus on assisting those involved to find short-term solutions.

5. **Encouraging self-reliance.** Encouraging and supporting individuals to participate in identifying and solving problems facilitate their return to independent function and the development of a sense of mastery (Flannery & Everly, 2000).

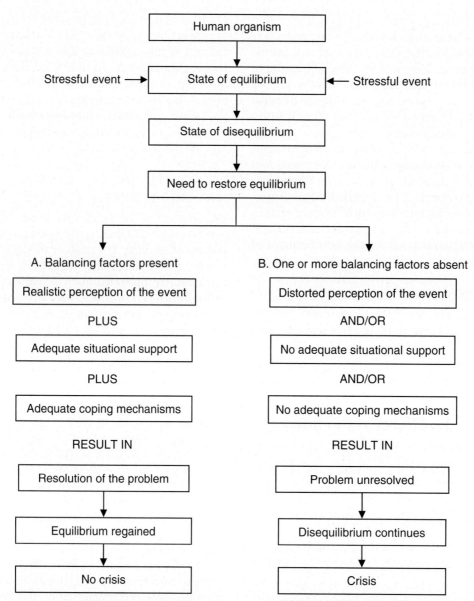

Figure 18.6 The effect of balancing factors in a stressful event. (From Aguilera, D. C. (1998). *Crisis intervention: Theory and methodology* (8th ed.). Mosby.)

The case study in Box 18.2 uses Roberts' Seven-Stage Crisis Intervention Model (Roberts, 1991; Fig. 18.7) to illustrate the application of these principles to a clinical situation.

Telephone Help Lines

Many health authorities now have telephone help lines, typically staffed by mental health professionals or trained volunteers, which offer support for problems such as child abuse, suicide, and family stress. These lines permit immediate access to a spectrum of support and intervention services for individuals who are experiencing a crisis or need help to manage life stressors.

Short-Stay Hospitalization and Community-Based Emergency Housing

Some health authorities also designate a few beds on their psychiatric units for short-stay crisis stabilization. Individuals are admitted to these beds for a brief period of inpatient care (typically 72 hours) when they have no supports in the community, need to have their medications assessed or stabilized, or require some other health service. Community-based emergency housings, such as shelters for children and youth who cannot remain at home, shelters for victims of domestic violence, and short- and long-term accommodations for individuals with serious and persistent mental illness, are also often available. These settings provide users with food, a place

BOX 18.2 Case Study Demonstrating Roberts' Seven-Stage Crisis Intervention Model

The mobile mental health crisis unit in a large Canadian city receives a call from Theresa, the maternal aunt of 19-year-old Billy, an young man who is of Indigenous Peoples origin whose 12-year-old brother died 4 months ago from sniffing gasoline. Upon hearing of his brother's death, Billy quit college and went on a 5-day drinking binge. At the time of the call, he is lying on his bed in the dark. Theresa tells the crisis nurse that Billy has been eating very little for the past several weeks and has been sleeping 12 to 14 hours per day. He rarely leaves his room and speaks only when addressed directly. What little conversation he does offer is preoccupied with his brother and their parents, who died in a car crash a number of years earlier. Theresa has tried everything she can think of to convince Billy to get help; she is worried about leaving him alone for fear he will harm himself.

STAGE 1: Conduct Crisis, Lethality, and Bio/Psycho/Social/Spiritual Assessment. Joanne, the crisis intervention nurse, performs a focused assessment and, using direct questions, ascertains important details about the situation (e.g., caller name, address, and telephone number; nature of emergency; presence of/potential for injury or loss of life; availability of weapons or other potentially dangerous items). Within 2 or 3 minutes, she determines that Billy has experienced major losses (one of them very recently), that his behaviour is suggestive of acute mourning and/or depression, that he is at high risk for self-harm, and that his aunt, who is his primary social support, has exhausted her resources for dealing with the situation. The nurse tells Theresa that she and a colleague are on their way to talk with Billy and that they will be bringing police assistance. The nurse decides to involve the police for two reasons. The first is that by their nature, crises are unpredictable situations and have some potential for violence; a police presence sometimes deters aggressive acting out, and if it does not, it ensures that there are trained personnel to effectively contain it. The second reason is that the police have authority, under provincial mental health legislation, to transport individuals for psychiatric assessment, even against their will. In order to do this, they must have evidence that the individual is in imminent danger to themselves or someone else.

STAGE 2: Establish Rapport and a Working Therapeutic Relationship. Joanne establishes rapport with Theresa on the telephone by listening carefully to her, validating her concerns, and offering concrete and specific assistance. When the nurse and other members of the crisis team arrive at the home, Joanne stays with Theresa while her colleague, Don, begins talking with Billy through his locked bedroom door. Don uses his well-developed interpersonal skills (see Chapter 7) to make a connection with the young man and to convince him to come out of his room and talk face-to-face. When it becomes apparent that Billy is not a danger to himself or others, the police leave.

STAGE 3: Identify Dimensions of Presenting Problem. Fortunately, when the crisis team speaks with Billy, they learn that he has not done anything to harm himself. He is experiencing a great deal of emotional pain for which he has few words, has lost his sense of meaning in life, and has only a vague plan of shooting himself. He does not have immediate access to a firearm. In his conversation with Don, Billy acknowledges that the loss of his parents was devastating, but it is his brother's death that caused his "world to crash apart."

STAGE 4: Explore Feelings and Emotions. Don encourages Billy to talk about his experience and offers him words for the things he is feeling. Eventually, Billy agrees to include his aunt and Joanne in the conversation.

STAGE 5: Generate and Explore Alternatives. Billy, Theresa, Don, and Joanne sit around the kitchen table with cups of tea discussing the supports available to the family.

STAGE 6: Develop a Plan. Theresa states that praying to the creator every day and speaking to a local elder help her to get through many difficult times. Billy says that he will pray with her every day, signs a written safety contract, and agrees to see an intake worker at the mental health centre for an assessment the next day. The safety contract specifies a number of things that Billy will do if he begins to feel overwhelmed again, including praying, talking to Theresa, and calling the crisis line.

STAGE 7: Develop a Follow-Up Plan. Joanne calls Theresa the next afternoon and learns that she and Billy had spent the evening talking and praying together. He had eaten breakfast and showered this morning before attending his appointment at the mental health centre. The intake worker referred Billy to a men's grief support group and was going to speak with the student counselling service at his college to arrange one-to-one counselling.

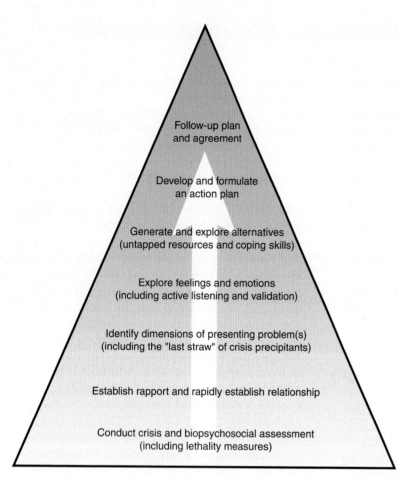

- Follow-up plan and agreement
- Develop and formulate an action plan
- Generate and explore alternatives (untapped resources and coping skills)
- Explore feelings and emotions (including active listening and validation)
- Identify dimensions of presenting problem(s) (including the "last straw" of crisis precipitants)
- Establish rapport and rapidly establish relationship
- Conduct crisis and biopsychosocial assessment (including lethality measures)

Figure 18.7 Roberts' (1991) Seven-Stage Crisis Intervention Model.

to stay, emotional support, and referrals to other community services.

Disaster

Disasters are sudden, severe, and social phenomena. In their framework, Canada's Ministers Responsible for Emergency Management (2016) state: "a disaster occurs when a hazard intersects with a vulnerable community in a way that exceeds or overwhelms the community's ability to cope and may cause serious harm to the safety, health, welfare, property or environment of people; may be triggered by a naturally occurring phenomenon which has its origins within the geophysical or biological environment or by human action or error, whether malicious or unintentional, including technological failures, accidents and terrorist acts." Encompassing such events as floods, wildfires, drought, extreme heat, tropical storms, melting permafrost, coastal erosion, disasters are increasing in frequency and severity across Canada, costing billions of dollars and impacting hundreds of thousands of Canadians (Public Safety Canada, 2019). Disaster events can have far-reaching effects, causing extensive and sustained social and mental health problems, and challenge the resilience of all those affected. The Canada Disaster Database (CDC) contains information on disasters that have occurred since 1900 that directly affected Canadians and tracks significant disas-

ter events (see Web Links). The disasters are categorized in the CDC as natural, conflict, or technology (see Table 18.5 for types of disasters).

KEY CONCEPT

A disaster occurs when a hazard intersects with a vulnerable community which exceeds or overwhelms the community's ability to cope and may cause serious harm to the safety, health, welfare, property, or environment of people. It may be triggered by a naturally occurring phenomenon, originating within the geophysical or biological environment or by malicious or unintentional human action or error, such as technological failures, accidents, and terrorist acts (Ministers Responsible for Emergency Management, 2016).

A Meteorologic-Hydrologic Disaster Example: Fort McMurray Wildfire

When the Fort McMurray wildfire occurred in May 2016, it necessitated the evacuation of all 88,000 residents and became Canada's most expensive natural disaster with recovery costs in billions of dollars (see Fig. 18.8). Although two teenagers died in a vehicle collision while fleeing the city, there were amazingly no deaths directly attributed to the fire. The "safety-first" approach of this

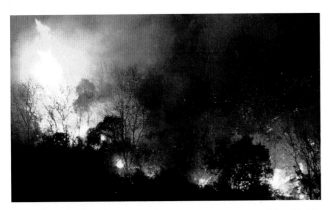

Figure 18.8 A wildfire as occurred in Fort McMurray, May 2016. (shutterstock.com/RoBBQ.)

city, evident its regional Emergency Preparedness Week and the routine fire, evacuation, and lockdown drills at schools and by various businesses, was a significant factor in the successful evacuation (Mamuji & Rozdilsky, 2019). The preparation and response phases of emergency management are over, and the recovery and mitigation phases remain in progress. The psychological and social costs of this disaster were substantial and will likely continue to affect emergency responders and residents of Fort McMurray for some time. Alberta Health Services usually recorded about 1,000 mental health contacts annually in the region, but there were 29,000 between May 2016 and March 2017, with contact numbers remaining high (15,000) the following year. Mitigation efforts are in effect, including creating a Critical Incident Stress Management team for the region and the development of firebreaks around homes (Mamuji & Rozdilsky). Some citizens watched and recorded the wildfire as it moved to their city, uploading their images to YouTube. For a phenomenological analysis of the human experience and examples of the video images, see Slick (2019).

A Biologic Disaster Example: COVID-19 Pandemic

The coronavirus appeared in Canada on January 23, 2020, when the first instance of the COVID-19 virus was presented in a 56-year-old man with mild symptoms of pneumonia who came to the emergency room of Sunnybrook Health Sciences Centre in Toronto. Learning that he had recently returned from China, the staff were altered to the potential for his illness to be a viral disease that was proliferating in Wuhan, China. There were protocols for such a case at the hospital, and the patient was placed in a negative pressure room (Perkel, 2021). This was only the first case of COVID-19 in Canada; the virus was soon rampant across the nation and the world, infecting many millions with the disease (including more than a million Canadians) and causing much sorrow and death.

Pandemics are extraordinary times: chaotic, surreal, transformative. As well as the fear arising due to potential infection and death, the necessary public

health measures changed daily life in significant ways—from physical distancing and mask wearing to closures of schools, workplaces, and nonessential businesses and home confinement—which impacted the mental health of entire communities. Rapid transformation of health care systems was required (e.g., increasing intensive care beds, engaging with patients online or by phone, exclusion of family visitors) (Fig. 18.9).

Recognized as "heroic," healthcare workers faced high workloads affecting work-life balance as well as distress from fears of becoming infected or bringing the virus to their homes. The risks were real. From July 2020 to January 2021, 65,920 healthcare workers were infected by the virus, and 24 lost their lives (Canadian Institute of Health Information, 2021, January 15). Furthermore, a Statistics Canada (2021, February 2) survey (n = 18,000) found 7 in 10 healthcare workers in direct contact with patients who tested positive for COVID-19 reported worsening mental health (Fig. 18.10).

Infodemic is the rapid and large scale spread of health information and disinformation by media and other informational means, including social media, that affects one's ability to differentiate between false and true information. This phenomenon is particularly dangerous to public health if it undermines the receipt of accurate prevention and treatment information, as happened during the COVID-19 pandemic. Disinformation became a worldwide threat to overcoming the spread of the virus, such that the Secretary-General of the United Nations launched the United Nations Communications Response initiative to combat it in April 2020. During the pandemic, 9 out of 10 Canadians sought information related to COVID-19 from online sources: newspapers, news sites, social media posts, etc. In its early months,

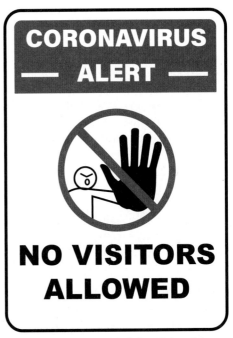

Figure 18.9 Hospital entrance with "No Visitors" sign. (shutterstock.com/TazzyDesigns.)

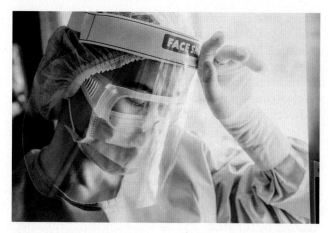

Figure 18.10 An exhausted nurse. (shutterstock.com/Boyloso.)

96% of Canadians using the internet for this purpose stated that they saw information they suspected was false, inaccurate, or misleading and only 4% said they had not seen any (Garneau and Zoosou, 2021, February 2). An example of the misinformation spreading over the internet was to ingest methanol as a preventative measure against COVID-19 (Sell et al., 2021). The spread of disinformation is becoming complex and sophisticated, jeopardizing public health and public trust.

Emergency Preparedness and Response

Role of the United Nations

The United Nations Office for Disaster Risk Reduction's (UNDRR) role is to work with nations to ensure a safer future for our hyperconnected world by reducing disaster risk and losses. The UNDRR is clear about the challenges: the level of risks (new and familiar) is higher than at any time in human history. The systemic nature of risk has become evident with climate change occurring more rapidly than predicted, increasing the frequency and intensity of hazards. Integrated and innovative approaches are required if disasters are to be successfully reduced (UNDRR, 2019).

Disaster risk reduction involves analyzing and decreasing causal factors of disaster by decreasing exposure, reducing vulnerability, increasing resiliency to hazards, improving preparation and early warning abilities regarding adverse events, and identifying wise approaches to sustaining the environment and usage of land and water (UNDRR, 2015).

The UNDRR publishes a global assessment report of disaster risk and management every two years. A global plan for disaster risk reduction is outlined in the Sendai Framework 2015–2030 using four priorities:

- understanding disaster risk;
- strengthening disaster risk governance;
- investing in resilience (economic, social, health, and cultural) of persons, communities, countries, and the environment; and

- improving disaster preparedness in response, recovery, rehabilitation, and reconstruction (using a "build back better" approach) (UNIDRR, 2015).

In Montrèal, in 2017, Canada hosted a meeting of countries and territories in the Americas where a regional disaster risk plan was endorsed that was aligned with the Sendai Framework (Public Safety Canada, 2017). Nurses across the Americas and the globe have a role in enhancing health infrastructure resilience and preparedness, as well as in the promotion of gender equitable and universally accessible (e.g., includes persons with disabilities) disaster preparedness, from response to reconstruction. October 13th is the *International Day for Disaster Risk Reduction.*

Role of Government

Canadians can expect their federal, provincial, and territorial governments to help them and their communities to mitigate and prepare for disaster and to assist them during such an event. When a disaster occurs in Canada, our federal government mobilizes resources, coordinated through Public Safety and Preparedness Canada, for when assistance is requested or when more than one province or territory is involved. Public Safety Canada is responsible for national policy, standards, and response systems related to disaster. The Public Health Agency of Canada's Centre for Emergency Preparedness and Response (CEPR) has information for the public concerning response to chemical, biologic, radiologic, and nuclear threats, as well as scenarios illustrating a natural and a possible bioterrorism threat and CEPR's role (see Web Links).

Indigenous Services Canada, along with First Nations and Inuit health regional offices, including British Columbia's First Nations Health Authority, are responsible for emergency health services to First Nations and Inuit communities, for working to decrease the adverse effects (health, economic) due to disaster, as well as for coordination of the response to a nuclear or radiologic emergency. The Public Health Agency of Canada is the resource for disease information. Environmental and workplace health, including in emergencies and disasters, is also an area of activity (see Chapter 17 for information on emergencies in the workplace). Provincial and territorial governments' responsibilities, policies, and disaster plans can be found on their public websites (see Web Links for an example: British Columbia's Emergency Preparedness, Response & Recovery website).

Canada assists other nations in times of disaster and shares resources and information related to disaster mitigation, responsiveness, and recovery. For instance, Canada is a member of the International Initiative for Mental Health Leadership in which countries (e.g., Australia, New Zealand, England, United States) work together to improve mental health components of disaster planning and response (see Web links).

Role of Nurses

Healthcare professionals play a key role across all phases of disaster: planning, mitigation, response, and recovery. Their society depends upon them to respond responsibly in times of disaster, with skill and expertise; they depend upon their society to reduce the risks they encounter in doing so (e.g., provision of antivirals, protective equipment, risk management protocols) and to plan for recovery and support in the aftermath (e.g., life and disability insurance; practical support). This reciprocal relationship must be evident in the planning phase onward, including the identification of threats to healthcare staff and their families and ways to mitigate them (e.g., child and elder care facilities for responders' family during a disaster).

The Canadian Nurses Association's (CNA, 2017) *Code of Ethics for Registered Nurses* identifies, as an obligation, nurses' **duty to provide care** (with appropriate precautions) during a disaster, communicable disease outbreak or pandemic. It is acknowledged that there may be circumstances when it is acceptable for a nurse to withdraw or refuse to provide care. The concept of unreasonable burden, such as ongoing threats to personal and family well-being, informs this decision. The Code provides examples of ethical decision-making models to assist individual

nurses, and CNA's (2008) *Ethical Considerations for Nurses in a Natural or Human-Made Disaster, Communicable Disease Outbreak or Pandemic*, part of the *Ethics in Practice for Registered Nurses* series, is a further resource.

A relational ethics approach, with its focus on relationship, environmental context, ethical decisions as embodied actions, and the importance of dialogue, may be particularly useful to nurses in preparation for and response to disaster (Austin, 2008). CNA's (2012) position statement on emergency preparation and response supports the International Council of Nurses' (ICN) expectation that nurses are competent and ready to take part in the preparation, response, and recovery involved in responding to disaster events. The ICN's *Core Competencies in Disaster Nursing* Version 2.0 outlines these expectations for both the general professional nurse and the advanced or specialized professional nurse. As the literature on effective disaster response is rapidly evolving, all nurses are encouraged to keep up-to-date with the current literature (International Council of Nurses, 2019).

It is highly problematic that many nurses do not believe that they are sufficiently prepared to respond to disaster events given the expectations of the profession and the reality that nurses are the largest group in the healthcare workforce (see Box 18.3). Nurses who do

BOX **18.3** Research for Best Practice

NURSE PREPAREDNESS FOR DISASTER

McNeill, C., Adams, L., Heagele, T., Swanson, M., & Alfred, D. (2020). Emergency preparedness competencies among nurses: Implications for nurse administrators. *Journal of Nursing Administration, 50*(7), 407–413.

Question: How professionally prepared for emergencies do nurses report themselves to be? What is level of their self-reported personal preparedness, as well as their perceived likelihood of reporting to work in a disaster?

Method: An exploratory, cross-sectional research design was used to survey registered nurses and registered practical nurses across a range of clinical practice areas in three inpatient healthcare facilities and one outpatient facility in the United States. *The Emergency Preparedness Information Questionnaire* was used to measure professional preparedness across eight dimensions: triage and basic first aid; detection; accessing critical resources and reporting; the incident command system; isolation, quarantine, and decontamination; psychological issues; epidemiology and clinical decision-making; and communication and connectivity. Personal preparedness was measured by four items on a five-point Likert scale: general, natural, biological, and terrorist attack disaster readiness. A Likert scale measured likelihood of reporting to work in seven types of disasters: infectious disease pandemic, mass casualty disaster, terrorism event,

natural disaster, chemical disaster, radiologic disaster, and biologic disaster. Completed surveys = 186.

Findings: A positive response to professional preparedness across the disaster response domains was calculated overall at 23%, with 43% providing a positive response to "triage and first aid." Less than 40% gave a positive response for personal preparedness in any scenario, with an overall positive response of 25%. A 55% overall positive response regarding the likelihood of reporting for work was found. Self-reported professional competence correlated more strongly with overall personal preparation ($r = 0.57$) than with likelihood of reporting for work ($r = 0.34$).

Implication for Practice: The researchers found their findings to be "alarming" for all three areas of research interest (p. 410). Given that disasters are increasing worldwide (e.g., natural disaster, terrorism, the spread of new diseases), it is essential that nurses are prepared to respond. A sense of competence can increase the likelihood of reporting to work, as can knowing one's family is prepared. Nursing educators need to ensure that preparation for disaster response is part of curricula. Healthcare services administrators can build upon this foundation through such means as online education, disaster simulations, and drills. Deficits in nurses' readiness to respond in times of public crises and trauma must be overcome.

feel prepared are those with previous participation in a disaster or disaster training (Labrague et al., 2017). Optimally, nurses should have the basic knowledge and skills required in disaster response and public health emergencies, be personally prepared to sustain themselves and their families in a disaster, promote preparedness among their community and within the organization in which they practice, and be proactive at enhancing their professional competence in this area (e.g., participation in drills, disaster exercises). Nurses need to be involved across all aspects of disaster planning if they are to be fully cognizant of their roles and responsibilities when a disaster event occurs (Labrague et al.).

Role of Individuals and Families

Public Safety Canada in collaboration with other government and nongovernment agencies has a *Get Prepared* initiative that assists Canadians and their families to prepare for the first three days following a disaster event. *Get Prepared* has three main components: know the risks and get prepared, make an emergency plan, and get an emergency kit. Guides to doing so, as well as a list of federal–provincial–territorial resources, are available for free (see Web Links); there is an emergency plan guide for persons with disabilities or special needs. A mobile "get prepared" site provides key steps to follow in particular types of emergencies such as floods, wildfires, and so on, as well as how to respond to an evacuation order (see Web Links).

Phases of Disaster

Although the experience of disaster is unique to each individual and community, various phases of disaster can be delineated. It is important to recognize such phases (e.g., preparation, response, recovery, mitigation) as multilayered, complex, and influenced by the interaction of persons–community–environment rather than as discrete and constant categories. Phases of disaster focused on possible psychological and social responses from 1 to 3 days to 1 to 3 years are shown in Figure 18.9.

There are critical factors of disaster that can potentially shape aftermath reactions and postdisaster stress. These include causation (natural or human), degree of personal impact, size and scope, visible impact/low point, and the probability of recurrence (DeWolfe, 2000). When human intent causes a disaster (e.g., bombing), the stress reaction is greater than when the cause is "natural" (an "act of God"). Causes are not always clearly defined, such as when environmental degradation contributes to flooding. If an individual has high exposure to a disaster event or intimate personal loss, the disaster impact will usually be more intense; a disaster that destroys an entire community will have more negative and lasting impact than one of lesser scope. The recovery process is impeded when disasters are neither clearly visible nor defined (i.e., there is no "it's over

and the rebuilding begins" moment), as in the case of toxic spills and nuclear accidents. With such disasters, the devastating consequences continue for years, resulting in chronic stress, fear, and anxiety. When there is a high probability that a disaster will reoccur in a community, the ongoing threat will affect recovery, particularly if disaster mitigation is not occurring (DeWolfe, 2000).

An international review of the effects of disaster on over 60,000 individuals in 102 different events indicates that effects are the greatest when two of the following are present:

- extreme and widespread property damage;
- serious and ongoing finance problems for the community;
- human intent was the cause; and
- high prevalence of trauma: injuries, loss of life (Norris et al., 2002, p. 246).

The spiritual impact that loss of home, possessions, community, and sense of belonging can have difficult to quantify and to address.

Response to Mental Health and Illness in a Disaster

Natural recovery processes and community-based sources of help are foundational to disaster response. Research indicates that social cohesion in a community increases its resilience to disaster and is associated with a significant decrease in psychological distress (Greene et al., 2015). Disaster events can increase social cohesion within a community (Cocking, 2013). The everyday cooperation of community members as survivors are comforted, fed, sheltered, and supported is as important as heroic acts and crucial to recovery. It is helpful to keep people in their normal groups if relocation is necessary and to facilitate their return to normal activities as soon as possible; disaster response should not undermine natural helping networks (Norris et al., 2002).

Key to community-level disaster response is the provision of accurate, timely information that allows informed action in meeting the rapidly changing circumstances inherent to disasters. In Canada, there is mandatory broadcaster participation in the public alerting system regarding disaster. Social networking (e.g., YouTube, Facebook, Twitter) has the potential to facilitate communication in times of disaster: it is broad in reach, user-friendly, and free. Nevertheless, there remain privacy, information accuracy, and trustworthiness concerns related to its use (Trainer & Goel, 2013). Information after disaster should be brief, basic, and focused on promoting coping among survivors. Three components to such information are recommended: reassurance and explanation about normal, to-be-expected reactions; advice to return to daily routines as soon as possible; and guidance regarding where to find help if needed (European Commission, 2008).

Mental Health First Aid

The common model for mental healthcare delivery following an emergency such as a disaster is mental health first aid (MHFA), also known as **psychological first aid** (PFA; WHO, War Trauma Foundation, & World Vision International, 2013). As with medical first aid, MHFA involves intervention with the purpose of immediate relief of distress and the prevention of pathologic sequelae until medical treatment is available or the crisis is resolved. There are three basic steps: recognize a change in behaviour of an individual; respond with confident conversation, and guide to appropriate resources and support.

It can be performed by nonprofessionals with training. Mental Health First Aid Canada, a program of The Mental Health Commission of Canada, offers such training in every province and territory and is included on the Public Health Agency of Canada's Best Practices Portal (see Web Links). MHFA competency domains have been identified as establishing rapport and stabilization at initial contact, performing screening and assessment, intervening in acute distress and fostering coping, triage for immediate or delayed care, referring/advocating for those requiring more intensive care, and being self-aware and self-caring (McCabe et al., 2014).

Much of the distress experienced by individuals at such times will be normative (i.e., grief, anger, and stress related to the trauma of a disaster event) and not require professional treatment. PFA involves promoting five key responses: sense of safety, calming, sense of self, and community efficacy, connectedness, and hope (Hobfoll et al., 2007; Prewitt Diaz, 2013). Hope for recovery can be supported through practical action: the provision of necessary services, housing and relocation, replacement of household goods, and employment help (Prewitt Diaz). See Table 18.6 for public health principles for disaster interventions.

Table 18.6	Types of Disasters With Selected Examples in Canada		
Natural			
	Biologic		
		Epidemic	March–August 2003 SARS outbreak with 44 deaths, most in city of Toronto.
		Infestation	October 2005 *Escherichia coli* bacteria was found in water supply of the Kashechewan reserve. 1,100 people were evacuated, and 74 people hospitalized.
		Pandemic	January 23, 2020 The coronavirus, first appeared in Wuhan, China, in 2019. The first person to test positive for COVID-19 had returned to Canada from China and appeared with respiratory symptoms at a Toronto hospital. The cost in human life and economic repercussions remain open as this textbook is being revised, but vaccines are making a significant difference.
	Meteorologic–hydrologic		
		Avalanche	January–April 2003 Rocky Mountains along the British Columbia–Alberta border experienced the deadliest avalanche season in over 30 years. Thirty people were killed.
		Cold Event	In 1947, temperatures dropped to −63°C in Snag, Yukon—the lowest temperature recorded in North America. It is said that exhaled breath froze, making a hissing sound (The Canadian Encyclopedia, 2013).
		Drought	1990 Parts of the Prairies were stricken by cereal crop drought, and there was an estimated loss of half a billion dollars.
		Flood	June 2013 The worst flood in Alberta's history—4 people were killed, 100,000 people were displaced, and damages were estimated at over $5 billion.
		Hurricane	August 2011 Tropical storm Irene hit Québec and the Maritime provinces. Power outages were experienced throughout the region, and two people were killed.
		Tornado	September 21st, 2018 Six tornadoes touched down in the National Capital Region. The strongest (rated level 3 in intensity on the Enhance Fujita [EF] scale) struck near Ottawa with estimated wind speeds of up to 265 km/h. An EF-2 tornado (138–177 km/h) struck another Ottawa area. Four EF-1 tornadoes (138–177 km/h) touched down near the areas of Calabogie, ON, the Baskatong Reservoir, QC, Val-des-Bois, QC, and Otter Lake, QC. There was estimated $334 million in insured damage.
		Wildfire	May 2016 Wildfire at Fort McMurray, Alberta. An entire community of 88,000 people were evacuated. The fire caused billions of dollars in damages but, incredibly, no person died or was seriously injured.

(Continued)

Table 18.6	Types of Disasters With Selected Examples in Canada (*Continued*)		
	Geologic	Winter storm	March 14–16, 2019 A winter storm produced rain and warm temperatures causing significant flooding in parts of Ontario and Quebec. Moving through Quebec and into the Maritimes, it estimated $124 million in insured losses. brought not only rain but also wind. There was an
		Earthquake	June 2010 5.0-strength earthquake near Val-de-Bois, QC. A bridge collapsed and a highway was closed. 300 houses lost power and a state of emergency was called.
		Landslide	January 2005 A landslide of mud, debris, and snow destroys two homes in North Vancouver. One person was killed and 100 homes were evacuated.
		Tsunami	
Conflict	Arson		January 1980 Arsonists set fire to a social club in Chibougamau, QC, killing 45 people and injuring 55.
	Civil event		June 2011 Hockey fans take to the streets of Vancouver, rioting, burning, and looting. 140 people were taken to the hospital with minor injuries, with four serious injuries.
	Hijacking		May 1984
Technologic	Terrorist		A shooting at the National Assembly of Québec kills three people and injures 13.
	Fire		July 2007 Hundreds of Edmonton residents were affected by "wall of fire" that swept through the neighbourhood, destroying 18 townhomes and damaging 76 more.
	Hazardous chemicals		
	Infrastructure failure		August 2003 Fifty million people throughout Ontario and the eastern United States affected by blackout (with power outages lasting over 48 h) that was caused by sagging transmission lines and untrimmed trees in Ohio.
	Transportation		August 2011 A flight *en route* from Yellowknife, NT, to Resolute Bay, NU, struck a hill and crashed, killing four crewmembers and eight passengers.
	Explosion		July 2013 A train carrying crude oil derails in the town of Lac-Mégantic, QC. Explosions killed 42 people, with 5 missing and presumed dead. Half the town's centre is destroyed.
	Space event		January 1978
	Space launch		Space debris falls upon the Northwest Territories.

References: The Canadian Disaster Database. (2019). *List of event types.* https://www.publicsafety.gc.ca/cnt/rsrcs/cndn-dsstr-dtbs/index-en.aspx; The Canadian Encyclopedia. (2015). *Extreme-weather-in-Canada.* http://www.thecanadianencyclopedia.ca/en/article/extreme-weather-in-canada-feature/

The indications that an individual is not successfully coping with stress following a disaster event and may need assistance with stress management are listed in Box 18.4.

Although it was once believed that PTSD, the mental disorder most often diagnosed in disaster-affected communities, could be prevented by psychological debriefing, the evidence now indicates otherwise. Single-session debriefing may even be harmful (European Commission, 2008). Professional help may be required for those experiencing persistent and complex grieving.

Vulnerable Populations in Disaster

There are persons who are particularly "at risk" in a disaster situation. These include persons with communication difficulties (e.g., those who do not speak the area's dominant language), those who are physically impaired (e.g., visually, hearing, mobility), those who are cognitively or psychologically impaired, those who are geographically or culturally isolated, and those who lack a means of transportation when evacuation becomes necessary (Hagen & Hagen, 2013, p. 582). Issues for some at-risk populations are described below.

Indigenous Peoples and Disaster

As Indigenous communities in Canada may be particularly vulnerable to disaster events as they are often geographically remote, as well as too often marginalized and dealing with poverty and lack of health and social services. Problems that increase vulnerability have been lack of funding for on-reserve mitigation efforts and a

BOX 18.4 Indicators of Need for Assistance With Stress Management After a Traumatic Event

The following signs occurring for more than 2 to 4 weeks indicate that assistance with stress may be necessary:

- Confusion; disorientation
- Problems concentrating; short attention span
- Changes in ability to see or hear
- Becoming easily frustrated; continuous crying; frequent mood swings
- Feelings of hopelessness
- Overwhelming self-doubt and/or feelings of guilt

- Reluctance to leave home
- Fear of crowds, strangers, or being alone
- Increased use of alcohol and/or other drugs, including prescription medication
- Existing medical problems worsening

Adapted from Substance Abuse and Mental Health Services Administration. (2013). *Tips for survivors of a disaster or traumatic event: What to expect in your personal, family, work and financial life.* https://store.samhsa.gov/sites/default/files/d7/priv/sma13-4775.pdf

complicated process for securing the necessary federal financial support after a disaster (Puxley, 2013). Getting the communities the necessary resources in a timely and culturally sensitive way is key to good recovery; the collective wisdom of many Indigenous communities regarding survival in adverse conditions is already strong. Scholars and experts in the field are increasingly recognizing that lessons are to be learned from such traditional knowledge that can inform effective disaster management as a whole (Hagen & Hagen, 2013).

Notions of healing and tradition are central to contemporary efforts to confront the legacy of injustices and suffering brought on by colonization (Kirmayer et al., 2009a, 2009b). Any approach to health services with Indigenous Peoples must consider ongoing uses of tradition in the community and local efforts to assert cultural identity (Kirmayer et al.). Indigenous researchers and scholars have expressed the need for multilevel assessment and intervention strategies to address factors related to health and wellness at individual, family, and community levels (Brave Heart et al., 2011; Evans-Campbell, 2008). A long-term goal of historical trauma intervention research and practice is to reduce inequities faced by Indigenous Peoples by developing culturally responsive interventions driven by communities to improve quality of life and wellbeing. Through individual and community-based initiatives, as well as larger political and cultural processes, Indigenous Peoples in Canada are involved in healing their traditions, repairing the ruptures and discontinuities in the transmission of traditional knowledge and values, and asserting their collective identity and power.

Children and Adolescents

Education of families and teachers on the needs of children in disaster should be part of disaster planning, including age-appropriate inclusion of children and adolescents in such planning. Infants and young children require caregivers who provide care and emotional security. Involving adolescents appropriately in disaster response and recovery tasks can be validating and help mitigate their distress (Masten, 2020).

Children and adolescents will be strongly influenced in their response to disaster by the reactions of the adults around them. Their psychological and behavior responses will be shaped, however, by their developmental stage and their vulnerability increased by separation from significant others, lack of attention from distracted adults, disruptions in routine, and by family strife. Their response behaviours may be misunderstood as being unaffected or as acting out rather than as signs of distress (Morganstein & Ursano, 2020). As with adults, assessment of children's and adolescents' reactions to a disaster event and their resulting mental health needs involves two components: screening and then clinical evaluation for those who are identified during screening as at risk for psychiatric disturbance and for those who (or whose family/close friends) were directly exposed to the disaster.

Persons with an Existing Mental Disorder

Persons living with a mental disorder may be particularly vulnerable during and after a disaster and require access to clinical care, as well as resources to meet basic needs (World Health Organization, 2019). Many individuals living with psychiatric conditions will experience worsening of their symptoms in a disaster. In one international study, self-reported worsening of preexisting psychiatric conditions were experienced by over half of 2,734 psychiatric patients during the pandemic (Gobbi et al., 2020). It was found that factors associated with increased symptoms were female gender, feeling no control of the situation, dissatisfaction with the handling of the pandemic by the state, and reduced interaction with family and friends. Factors associated with less increase of symptoms were optimism, sharing of concerns with family and friends, and use of social media (Gobbi et al.).

During a disaster, mental healthcare infrastructures may be seriously damaged, displacing the resources normally accessed for ongoing care at a time when the need for services increases. It is important that PTSD is not exclusively the focus in disaster management so that persons with other mental disorders, including addictions, will receive assistance.

Disabled Persons

The disruption of infrastructure and support systems during a disaster disproportionally affects persons with disabilities: they are more likely to be left behind in evacuations, and disability can be a discriminating factor in allocation of scarce resources. The needs and perspectives of persons with disabilities must be included across all phases of disaster management if their vulnerability and risk are to be reduced. Article 11 in the United Nations Convention on the Rights of Persons with Disabilities (United Nations, 2006) identifies the obligation of nations to do so. Public Safety Canada's Emergency Preparedness Guide for People with Disabilities/Special Needs provides information about emergency packs, resources, and tips for helping persons with disabilities/special needs and addresses particular types of disability

(e.g., mobility, hearing, vision, nonvisible disabilities like mental illness, heart disease) (see Web Links).

Underrepresented Ethnic Groups

The symptoms of stress, anxiety disorders, and PTSD are identical across cultures (European Commission, 2008). Stress and distress can be reduced if disaster response information to underrepresented ethnic communities is available in their mother tongue and if recovery efforts are culturally appropriate and involve key community figures. When possible, responders should adapt their approach to a person's culture. Things to consider include gender issues, touching, need for certain clothing items, and religious beliefs that will influence the meaning given to the disaster event (WHO et al., 2011).

Disaster Relief Workers

Volunteers are a major source of rescue and recovery assistance in times of disaster. The research on the postdisaster mental health of volunteer responders indicates that volunteers have higher complaint levels when compared with professional workers. The factors that contributed to this were determined as, "identification with victims as a friend, severity of exposure to gruesome events during disaster work, anxiety sensitivity, and lack of post-disaster social support" (Thormar et al., 2010, p. 529).

🍁 Summary

It is important that nurses understand the human experience of stress, crisis, and trauma so that they may respond appropriately to individuals, families, and communities in need. Such knowledge is important to nurses' professional self-development, as well, so that they can be confident and safe as they meet the chal-

lenges of healthcare practice. Being prepared to respond to disaster events is a responsibility that nurses share with other professionals; such preparation requires institutional support. Despite the adversity and challenges that disasters bring, there is also opportunity at such times to positively transform a community's approach to mental health care (WHO, 2013).

🍁 Summary of Key Points

- Many personal factors, such as personality patterns, beliefs, values, and commitment to an outcome, interact with environmental demands and constraints that produce a person–environment relationship.
- Stress occurs when a person–environment relationship is appraised as being unfavourable. Stress responses are simultaneously emotional and physiologic, leading to an innate tendency to act.
- Within the social network, social support can help a person cope with stress.
- The impact of adverse childhood experiences can foster a traumatic response that impacts health, emotional and psychological wellbeing.
- Effective coping can be either problem-focused or emotion-focused. The outcome of successful coping is enhanced health, psychological wellbeing, and social functioning.

- A crisis is a severely stressful situation that causes exaggerated stress responses. The nursing process is similar for the person experiencing a stress response, except that increased attention is paid to safety issues.
- Nurses have an obligation to respond competently across all phases of disasters: planning, mitigation, response, and recovery. Nursing educators and administrators have a responsibility to assist nurses in achieving this competency.
- In a pandemic, the necessary public health measures change daily life in significant way, including the rapid reorganization of healthcare services and the level of demands placed on healthcare workers. An infodemic may occur with disinformation endangering the success of disaster management and response.
- Psychological resilience (i.e., effective coping and positive adaptation to adversity) is developed and sustained by bio/psycho/social/spiritual factors, as well

as facilitated by a positive appraisal style and perceived social support.

• Natural recovery processes and community-based sources of help are foundational to successful disaster

response and need to be supported. Timely information is key.

• Mental Health First Aid (MHFA) is the common model for mental health delivery following a disaster.

 ## Web Links

www.getprepared.gc.ca The Government of Canada's public safety site, where "'72 Hours' Is your family prepared?" and other resources are freely available.

www.publicsafety.gc.ca/cnt/rsrcs/pblctns/2017-mrgnc-mngmnt-frmwrk/2017-mrgnc-mngmnt-frmwrk-en.pdf This is the site of *Canada's National Disaster Mitigation Strategy.*

https://cdd.publicsafety.gc.ca/srchpg-eng.aspx Public Safety's Canadian Disaster Database can be accessed here.

www.undrr.org/youth-voices-childrens-charter *The Children's Charter for Disaster Risk Reduction,* developed for children by children can be found here: preventionweb.net/files/globalplatform/childrencharter.

www.iimhl.com/ International Initiative for Mental Health Leadership

https://www.apa.org/practice/programs/dmhi/research-information/responding-disaster The American Psychological Association's site with resources for coping after disaster.

https://www.health.gov.on.ca/en/pro/programs/emb/pan_flu/pan_flu_plan.aspx An example of a governmental influenza pandemic plan (Ontario's) is available at this site.

https://www2.gov.bc.ca/gov/content/safety/emergency-management British Columbia's *Emergency Preparedness, Response & Recovery* website is at this link.

www.samhsa.gov/nctic/trauma-interventions This site describes six key principles of a trauma-informed approach.

www.trauma-informed.ca The Manitoba Trauma Information Centre is a resource for promoting trauma-informed relationships and practices.

https://www.cna-aiic.ca/-/media/cna/covid-19/cna_covid-19_website.pdf The Canadian Nurses Association's document regarding COVID-19.

www.mhfa.ca/ Mental Health First Aid website.

www.who.int/news-room/fact-sheets/detail/mental-health-in-emergencies World Health Organization's Mental Health in Emergencies can be found here.

https://www.undrr.org/publication/words-action-guidelines-engaging-children-and-youth-disaster-risk-reduction-and *The Words into Action Guidelines: Engaging Children and Youth in Disaster Reduction and Resilience Building* part of the Sendai Framework is available here.

https://www.preventionweb.net/publication/sendai-framework-disaster-risk-reduction-children Sendai Framework for Disaster Risk Reduction for Children.

 ## Thinking Challenges

Drew has been a police constable for nearly 5 years. The supervising staff sergeant has considered Drew as one of their best officers. Recently, Drew has been unusually irritable, looks tired, and seems distracted during report. The sergeant knows Drew had some tough cases to deal with the previous month, including beatings and sexual assaults, but Drew has always been able to stay on top of things. The sergeant spoke with Drew and voiced their concern that Drew didn't seem themself lately. Drew admits to having some trouble sleeping but nothing more. When answering a distress call regarding the rape of a teenage boy later that week, Drew experiences what appears to be an anxiety attack and remains in the patrol car while another officer responds to the situation. The following day, Drew goes to the local Community Mental Health Centre for a health assessment at the sergeant's direction.

1. What elements of a trauma-informed assessment of the psychological domain would you observe or explore in assessing Drew?
2. What is psychological resilience?
3. Are you and your family/friends prepared for an emergency or disaster event?
   a. Identify the elements of such preparation.
   b. What will you do if you are not together and phones and e-mail are unavailable?

Visit thePoint to view suggested responses.
Go to thePoint.lww.com/activate and use the activation code found in the front of this text to unlock answers to the "Thinking Challenges" and other online resources.

References

Aguilera, D. C. (1998). *Crisis intervention: Theory and methodology* (8th ed.). Mosby.

Allan, B., & Smylie, J. (2015). *First Peoples, second class treatment: The role of racism in the health and well-being of Indigenous peoples in Canada*. Wellesley Institute.

American Psychiatric Association. (1980). *Diagnostic and statistical manual of mental disorders* (3rd ed.).

American Psychiatric Association. (1994). *Diagnostic and statistical manual of mental disorders* (4th ed.).

American Psychiatric Association. (2013). *Diagnostic and statistical manual of mental disorders* (5th ed.).

Amstadter, A., Aggen, S., Knudsen, G. P., Reichborn-Kjennerud, T., & Kendler, F. (2013). Potentially traumatic event exposure, posttraumatic stress disorder, and axis I and II comorbidity in a population-based study of Norwegian young adults. *Social Psychiatry and Psychiatric Epidemiology, 48*, 215–223.

Ardino, V. (2014). Trauma-informed care: Is cultural competence a viable solution for efficient policy strategies? *Clinical Neuropsychiatry, 11*, 45–51.

Austin, W. (2008). Relational ethics. In L. Given (Ed.), *The SAGE encyclopedia of qualitative research methods* (pp. 749–750). SAGE Publications, Inc.

Bartlett, D. (1998). *Stress: Perspectives and processes*. Open University Press.

Bellis, M. A., Hughes, K., Ford, K., Rodriguez, G. R., Sethi, D., & Passmore, J. (2019, September 3). Life course health consequences and associated annual costs of adverse childhood experiences across Europe and North America: A systematic review and meta-analysis. *Lancet Public Health, 4*, e517–e528. https://dx.doi.org/10.1016/

Ben-Ari, A., & Strier, R. (2010). Rethinking cultural competence: What can we learn from Levinas? *British Journal of Social Work, 40*, 2155–2167. https://doi:10.1093/bjsw/bcp153

Birmes, P., Hatton, L., Brunet, A., & Schmitt, L. (2003). Early historical literature for post-traumatic symptomatology. *Stress and Health, 19*, 17–26.

Bombay, A. (2015). A call towards eliminating mental health disparities faced by Indigenous Peoples. *The Lancet Psychiatry, 2*, 861–862. https://doi.org/10.1016/S2215-0366(15)00352-1

Bombay, A., Matheson, K., & Anisman, H. (2009). Intergenerational trauma: Convergence of multiple processes among First Nations peoples in Canada. *Journal of Aboriginal Health, 5*, 6–47.

Bombay, A., Matheson, K., & Anisman, H. (2014a). The intergenerational effects of Indian Residential Schools: Implications for the concept of historical trauma. *Transcultural Psychiatry, 51*, 320–338.

Bombay, A., Matheson, K., & Anisman, H. (2014b). *Origins of lateral violence in aboriginal communities: A preliminary study of student-to-student abuse in Indian Residential Schools*. Aboriginal Healing Foundation.

Bowers, M. E., & Yehuda, R. (2016). Intergenerational transmission of stress in humans. *Neuropsychopharmacology, 41*, 232–244.

Brave Heart, M. Y. H. (2003). The historical trauma response among natives and its relationship with substance abuse: A Lakota illustration. *Journal of Psychoactive Drugs, 35*, 7–13.

Brave Heart, M. Y. H., Chase, J., Elkins, J., & Altschul, D. B. (2011). Historical trauma among Indigenous Peoples of the Americas: Concepts, research, and clinical considerations. *Journal of Psychoactive Drugs, 43*, 282–290.

Braveheart-Jordan, M., & DeBruyn, L. (1995). So she may walk in balance: Integrating the impact of historical trauma in the treatment of Native American Indian women. In J. Adleman & G. M. Enguidanos (Eds.), *Racism in the lives of women: Testimony, theory and guides to antiracist practice* (pp. 345–368). Haworth Press.

Braveman, P. A., Cubbin, C., Egerter, S., Williams, D. R., & Pamuk, E. (2010). Socioeconomic disparities in health in the United States: What the patterns tell us. *American Journal of Public Health, 100*(S1), S186–S196.

British Columbia Provincial Mental Health & Substance Use Planning Council. (2013). *Trauma-informed practice guide*. http://bccewh.bc.ca/wp-content/uploads/2012/05/2013_TIP-Guide.pdf

Browne, A. J., Varcoe, C., Smye, V., Reimer-Kirkham, S., Lynam, M. J., & Wong, S. (2009). Cultural safety and the challenges of translating critically oriented knowledge in practice. *Nursing Philosophy, 10*, 167–179. https://doi.org/10.1111/j.1466-769X.2009.00406.x

Browne, A. J., Varcoe, C. M., Wong, S. T., Smye, V. L., Lavoie, J., Littlejohn, D., Tu, D., Godwin, O., Krause, M., Khan, K. B., Fridkin, A., Rodney, P., O'Neil, J., & Lennox, S. (2012). Closing the health equity gap: Evidence-based strategies for primary health care organizations. *International Journal for Equity in Health, 11*, 59.

Brunet, A., Monson, E., Lui, A., & Fikretoglu, D. (2015). Trauma exposure and posttraumatic stress disorder in the Canadian military. *The Canadian Journal of Psychiatry, 60*, 488–496. https:/doi:10.1177/070674371506001104

Campbell, M. (1973). *Halfbreed*. Goodread Biographies.

Canadian Institute of Health Information (2021, January 15). *COVID-19 cases and deaths in health care workers in Canada—Infographic*. https://www.cihi.ca/en/covid-19-cases-and-deaths-in-health-care-workers-in-canada-infographic

Canadian Nurses Association. (2008). *Nurses' ethical considerations in a pandemic or other emergency*. http://www.cna-aiic.ca/~c/media/cna/page%20content/pdf%20en/2013/07/26/10/43/ethics_in_practice_august_2008_e.pdf

Canadian Nurses Association. (2012). *Position statement (PS119): Emergency preparedness and response*.

Canadian Nurses Association. (2017). *Code of ethics for registered nurses*. https://www.cna-aiic.ca/en/on-the-issues/best-nursing/nursing-ethics#toc

Cannon, W. B. (1939). *The wisdom of the body*. WW Norton.

Caplan, G. (1961). *An approach to community mental health*. Grune & Stratton.

Caron, N. (2017, March). *Indigenous Health Interest Group*. Keynote address.

Carpenito-Moyet, L. J. (2017). *Nursing diagnosis: Application to clinical practice* (15th ed.). Wolters Kluwer.

Catani, C., Jacob, N., Schauer, E., Kohila, M., & Neuner, F. (2008). Family violence, war, and natural disasters: A study of the effect of extreme stress on children's mental health in Sri Lanka. *BMC Psychiatry, 8*, 33.

Center for the Advancement of Health. (2004). Report on bereavement and grief research. *Death Studies, 28*, 491–575.

Clements, B., & Casani, J. (2016). *Disasters and public health: Planning and response* (2nd ed.). Butterworth-Heinemann/Elsevier.

Cocking, C. (2013). Collective resilience versus collective vulnerability after disasters: A social psychological perspective. In R. Arora & P. Arora (Eds.), *Disaster management: Medical preparedness, response and homeland security* (pp. 449–463). CABI.

Cooper, G. L., & Dewe, P. (2004). *Stress: A brief history*. Blackwell Publishing.

Coyne, J. C., & Holroyd, K. (1982). Stress, coping and illness: A transactional perspective. In T. Milton, C. Green, & R. Meagher (Eds.), *Handbook of clinical health psychology* (pp. 103–127). Plenum Press.

Davis, C. G., & Macdonald, S. L. (2004). Threat appraisals, distress and the development of positive life changes after September 11th in a Canadian sample. *Cognitive Behaviour Therapy, 33*(2), 68–78.

Dekel, R., & Goldblatt, H. (2008). Is there intergenerational transmission of trauma? The case of combat veterans' children. *American Journal of Orthopsychiatry, 78*, 281–289.

DeWolfe, D. J. (2000). *Training manual for mental health and human service workers in major disasters* (2nd ed.). Abuse and Mental Health Services Administration (DHHS/PHS). http://www.samhsa.gov/dtac/FederalResource/Response/4-Training_Manual_MH_Workers.pdf

Dohrenwend, B. P., & Shrout, P. E. (1985). "Hassles" in the conceptualization and measurement of stress variables. *American Psychologist, 40*, 780–785.

Dohrenwend, B. S., & Dohrenwend, B. P. (1974). *Stressful life events: Their nature and their effects*. Wiley & Sons.

Dovidio, J. F., Penner, L. A., Albrecht, T. L., Norton, W. E., Gaertner, S. L., & Shelton, J. N. (2008). Disparities and distrust: The implications of psychological processes for understanding racial disparities in health and health care. *Social Science & Medicine, 67*, 478–486.

Duran, E. (2006). *Healing the soul wound: Counselling with American Indians and other Native peoples*. Teachers College Press.

Duran, E., Duran, B., Brave Heart, M. Y. H., & Yellow Horse-Davis, S. (1998). Healing the American Indian Soul Wound. In Y. Danieli (Ed.), *International handbook of multigenerational legacies of trauma* (pp. 341–354). Plenum.

Elliott, D., Bjelajac, P., Fallot, R., Markoff, L., & Glover Reed, B. (2005). Trauma-informed or trauma-denied: Principles and implementation of trauma-informed services for women. *Journal of Community Psychology, 33*, 461–477.

Erikson, E. H. (1959). *Identity and the life cycle*. International Universities Press.

European Commission. (2008). *European multidisciplinary guideline: Early psychosocial interventions after disaster, terrorism and other shocking events*. Impact, the Dutch Knowledge & Advice Centre for Post-disaster Psychosocial Care.

Evans-Campbell, T. (2008). Historical trauma in American Indian/Native Alaska communities a multilevel framework for exploring impacts on individuals, families, and communities. *Journal of Interpersonal Violence, 23*, 316–338.

Felitti, V. J., Anda, R. F., Nordenberg, D., Williamson, D. F., Spitz, A. M., Edwards, V., Koss, M. P., & Marks, J. S. (1998). Relationship of childhood abuse and household dysfunction to many of the leading causes of death in adults: The Adverse Childhood Experiences (ACE) Study. *American Journal of Preventive Medicine, 14*(4), 245–258.

Flannery, R. B., & Everly, G. S. (2000). Crisis intervention: A review. *International Journal of Emergency Mental Health, 2*, 119–125.

Folkman, S., & Lazarus, R. S. (1991). The concept of coping. In A. Monat and & R. S. Lazarus (Eds.), *Stress and coping: An anthology* (3rd ed., pp. 209–227). Columbia University Press.

Furedi, F. (2007). The changing meaning of disaster. *Area, 39*, 482–489.

Garneau, K., & Zoosou, C. (2021, February 2). *Misinformation during the COVID-19 pandemic. StatCan COVID-19: Data to Insights for a Better Canada* (Catalogue no. 45280001).

Gilligan, C. (1994). Joining the resistance: Psychology, politics, girls and women. In M. Berger (Ed.), *Women beyond Freud: New concept of feminine psychology* (pp. 99–145). Brunner Mazel.

Gobbi, S., Płomecka, M. B., Ashraf, Z., Radzin, P., Neckels, R., Lazzeri, S., Dedic, A., Bakalovic, A., Hrustic, L., Skórko, S., Es haghi, S., Almazidou, K., Rodríguez-Pino, L., Alp, A. B., Jabeen, H., Waller, V., Shibli, D., Behnam, M. A., Arshad, A. H., … Jawaid, A. (2020, December 16). Worsening of preexisting psychiatric conditions during the COVID-19 pandemic. *Frontiers in Psychiatry, 11*, 581426. https:/doi: 10.3389/fpsyt.2020.581426

Grandjean, D., Rendu, A.-C., MacNamee, T., & Scherer, K. R. (2008). The wrath of the gods: Appraising the meaning of disaster. *Social Science Information, 47*, 187–204.

Green, A. R., Carney, D. R., Pallin, D. J., Ngo, L. H., Raymond, K. L., Iezzoni, L. I., & Banaji, M. R. (2007). Implicit bias among physicians and its prediction of thrombolysis decisions for black and white patients. *Journal of General Internal Medicine, 22*, 1231–1238.

Greene, G., Paranjothy, S., & Palmer, S. R. (2015). Resilience and vulnerability to psychological harm from flooding: The role of social cohesion. *American Journal of Public Health, 105*, 1792–1796.

Hafer, C., & Bègue, L. (2005). Experimental research on just-world theory: Problems, developments, and future challenges. *Psychological Bulletin, 131*(1), 128–167.

Hagen, J., & Hagen, S. (2013). The immediate post-disaster reconstruction phase: Alternative care site settings and vulnerable populations. In R. Arora & P. Arora (Eds.), *Disaster management: Medical preparedness, response and homeland security* (pp. 575–590). CABI.

Harper, D. (2001). *Online etymology dictionary.* http://www.etymonline.com

Hobfoll, S. E., Watson, P., & Bell, C. C. (2007). Five essential elements of immediate and mid-term mass trauma intervention: Empirical evidence. *Psychiatry, 70*, 283–315.

Holmes, T., & Rahe, R. (1967). The social readjustment patient scale. *Journal of Psychosomatic Research, 11*(2), 213–218.

Huey Jr, S. J., Tilley, J. L., Jones, E. O., & Smith, C. A. (2014). The contribution of cultural competence to evidence-based care for ethnically diverse populations. *Annual Review of Clinical Psychology, 10*, 305–338.

Imel, Z. E., Baldwin, S., Atkins, D. C., Owen, J., Baardseth, T., & Wampold, B. E. (2011). Racial/ethnic disparities in therapist effectiveness: A conceptualization and initial study of cultural competence. *Journal of Counseling Psychology, 58*, 290.

International Council of Nurses. (2019). *Core competencies in disaster nursing Version 2.0.* https://www.icn.ch/sites/default/files/inline-files/ICN_Disaster-Comp-Report_WEB.pdf

Johnson, R. L., Saha, S., Arbelaez, J. J., Beach, M. C., & Cooper, L. A. (2004). Racial and ethnic differences in patient perceptions of bias and cultural competence in health care. *Journal of General Internal Medicine, 19*, 101–110.

Jones, F., & Kinman, G. (2001). Approaches to studying stress. In F. Jones & J. Bright (Eds.), *Stress: Myth, theory & research* (pp. 17–44). Prentice Hall.

Kelly, U. A., Skelton, K., Patel, M., & Bradley, B. (2011). More than military sexual trauma: Interpersonal violence, PTSD, and mental health in women veterans. *Research in Nursing and Health, 34*, 457–467.

Kirmayer, L. J. (2012). Rethinking cultural competence. *Transcultural Psychiatry, 49*, 149–164. https://doi.org/10.1177/1363461512444673

Kirmayer, L. J., Brass, G., & Valaskakis, G. G. (2009a). Conclusion: Healing/intervention/tradition. In L. Kirmayer & G. G. Valaskakis (Eds.), *Healing traditions: The mental health of Aboriginal Peoples in Canada* (pp. 440–472). UBC Press.

Kirmayer, L. J., Shedev, M., Whitley, R., Dandeneau, S. F., & Isaac, C. (2009b). Community resilience: Models, metaphors and measures. *Journal of Aboriginal Health, 5*, 62–117.

Kleinke, C. L. (2007). What does it mean to cope? In A. Monat, R. S. Lazarus, & G. Reevy (Eds.), *The Praeger handbook on stress and coping* (pp. 289–308). Praeger.

Korte, S. M., Koolhaas, J. M., Wingfield, J. C., & McEwen, B. S. (2005). The Darwinian concept of stress: Benefits of allostasis and costs of allostatic load and the trade-offs in health and disease. *Neuroscience and Biobehavioral Reviews, 29*, 3–38.

Kronick, R. (2017). Mental health of refugees and asylum seekers: Assessment and intervention. *The Canadian Journal of Psychiatry, 63*, 290–296. https:/doi: 10.1177/0706743717746665

Kumagai, A. K., & Lypson, M. L. (2009). Beyond cultural competence: Critical consciousness, social justice, and multicultural education. *Academic Medicine, 84*, 782–787.

Kushner, H. (1981). *When bad things happen to good people.* Random House Inc.

Labrague, L. J., Hammad, K., Gloe, D. S., McEnroe-Petitte, D. M., Fronda, D. C., Obeidat, A. A., Leocadio, M. C., Cayaban, A. R., & Miranfurentes, E. C. (2017). Disaster preparedness among nurses: A systematic review of literature. *International Nursing Review, 65*, 41–53. https:/doi:10.1111/inr.12369

Lazarus, R. S. (1991). *Emotion and adaptation.* Oxford University Press.

Lazarus, R. S. (1998). *The life and work of an eminent psychologist: An autobiography of Richard S. Lazarus.* Springer.

Lazarus, R. S. (1999). *Stress and emotion: A new synthesis.* Springer.

Lazarus, R. S., DeLongis, A., Folkman, S., & Gruen, R. (1985). Stress and adaptation outcomes: The problem of confounded measures. *American Psychologist, 40*, 770–785.

Lazarus, R. S., & Folkman, S. (1984). *Stress, appraisal and coping.* Springer.

Lee, H. J., Macbeth, A. H., Pagani, J. H., & Young, W. S. (2009). Oxytocin: The great facilitator of life. *Progress in Neurobiology, 88*, 27–51.

Lee, T. Y., Cheung, C. K., & Kwong, W. M. (2012). Resilience as a positive youth development construct: A conceptual review. *Scientific World Journal, 2012*, 390450.

Lewis, L., Tieman, J., Rawlings, D., Parker, D., & Sanderson, C. (2020). Can exposure to online conversations about death and dying influence death competence? An exploratory study within an Australian Massive Open Online Course. *OMEGA, 8*, 242–271. https:/doi/10.1177/0030222818765813

Lindeman, E. (1944). Symptomatology and management of acute grief. *American Journal of Psychiatry, 151*(6 Suppl.), 155–160.

Lindeman, E. (1956). The meaning of crisis in individual and family. *Teachers College Record, 57*, 310.

Linklater, R. (2014). *Decolonizing trauma work: Indigenous stories and strategies.* Fernwood Publishing.

Macy, R. D., Behar, L., Paulson, R., Delman, J., Schmid, L., & Smith, S. F. (2004). Community based, acute posttraumatic stress management: A description and evaluation of a psychosocial intervention continuum. *Harvard Review of Psychiatry, 12*, 217–228.

Maguen, S., Luxton, D., Skopp, N., & Madden, E. (2012). Gender differences in traumatic experiences and mental health in active duty soldiers redeployed from Iraq and Afghanistan. *Journal of Psychiatric Research, 46*, 311–316.

Malone, J. (1988). The social support and dissupport continuum. *Journal of Psychosocial Nursing and Mental Health Services, 26*, 18–22.

Mamuji, A. A., & Rozdilsky, J. L. (2019). Wildfire as an increasingly common natural disaster facing Canada: Understanding the 2016 Fort McMurray wildfire. *Natural Hazards, 98*, 163–180. https://doi.org/10.1007/s11069-018-3488-4

Mason, J. W. (1971). A re-evaluation of the concept of 'non-specificity' in stress theory. *Journal of Psychiatric Research, 8*, 323–333.

Masten, A. (2020). Resilience of children in disasters: A multisystem perspective. *International Journal of Psychology, 56*, 1–10. https:/doi:10.1002/ijop.12737

Math, S. B., John, J. P., Girimaji, S. C., Benegal, V., Sunny, B., Krishnakanth, K., Kumar, U., Hamza, A., Tandon, S., Jangam, K., Meena, K. S., Chandramukhi, B., & Nagaraja, D. (2008). Comparative study of psychiatric morbidity among the displaced and non-displaced populations in the Andaman and Nicobar Islands following the tsunami. *Prehospital and Disaster Medicine, 23*, 29–34.

Matheson, K., Bombay, A., Haslam, A., & Anisman, H. (2016). Indigenous identity transformations: The pivotal role of student-to-student abuse in Indian residential schools. *Transcultural Psychiatry, 53*, 551–573.

McCabe, O. L., Everly Jr, G. S., Brown, L. M., Wendelboe, A. M., Hamid, N. H. A., Tallchief, V. L., & Links, J. M. (2014). Psychological first aid: A consensus-derived, empirically supported, competency-based training model. *American Journal of Public Health, 104*, 621–628.

McEwen, B. S. (1998). Protective and damaging effects of stress mediators. *The New England Journal of Medicine, 338*, 171–179.

McNeill, C., Adams, L., Heagele, T., Swanson, M., & Alfred, D. (2020). Emergency preparedness competencies among nurses: Implications for nurse administrators. *Journal of Nursing Administration, 50*, 407–413.

McQuaid, R. J., Bombay, A., McInnis, O. A., Humeny, C., Matheson, K., & Anisman, H. (2017). Suicide ideation and attempts among First Nations peoples living on-reserve in Canada: The intergenerational and cumulative effects of Indian Residential Schools. *Canadian Journal of Psychiatry, 62*, 422–430.

Mikhail, A. (1981). Stress: A psychophysiological conception. *Journal of Human Stress, 7*, 9–15.

Miller, J. (1994). Women's psychological development: Connections, disconnections, and violations. In M. Berger (Ed.), *Women beyond Freud: New concept of feminine psychology* (pp. 79–97). Brunner Mazel.

Million, D. (2013). Chapter 6: What will our nation be? In *Therapeutic nations: Healing in an age of Indigenous human rights* (pp. 123–145). The University of Arizona Press.

Ministers Responsible for Emergency Management. (2016, June 17). *An emergency management framework for Canada* (2nd ed.). Emergency Management Policy Division, Public Safety Canada. http://www.publicsafety.gc.ca/cnt/rsrcs/pblctns/mrgnc-mngmnt-frmwrk/index-eng.aspx

Morganstein, J. C., & Ursano, R. J. (2020, February 11). Ecological disasters and mental health: Causes, consequences, and interventions. *Frontiers in Psychiatry, 11*, 1–15. https://doi:10.3389/fpsyt.2020.00001

National Collaborating Centre for Mental Health. (2005). *Post-traumatic stress disorder: The management of PTSD in adults and children in primary and secondary care* (NICE Clinical Guidelines, No. 26). Gaskell. http://publications.nice.org.uk/post-traumatic-stress-disorder-ptsd-cg26

Norris, F. H., Friedman, M. J., & Watson, P. J. (2002). 60,000 disaster victims speak: Part II. Summary and implications of the disaster mental health research. *Psychiatry, 65*, 240–260.

Oxford English Dictionary Online. (2013, December). "trauma, n." http://www.oed.com.login.ezproxy.library.ualberta.ca/view/Entry/205242?redirectedFrom=trauma

Papps, E., & Ramsden, I. (1996). Cultural safety in nursing: The New Zealand experience. *International Journal for Quality in Health Care, 8*, 491–497.

Penner, L. A., Dovidio, J. F., West, T. V., Gaertner, S. L., Albrecht, T. L., Dailey, R. K., & Markova, T. (2010). Aversive racism and medical interactions with Black patients: A field study. *Journal of Experimental Social Psychology, 46*, 436–440.

Perkel, C. (2021, January 24). *It wasn't called COVID at the time: One-year since Canada's first COVID-19 case.* The Canadian Press. https://www.ctvnews.ca/health/coronavirus/it-wasn-t-called-covid-at-the-time-one-year-since-canada-s-first-covid-19-case-1.5279999

Prewitt Diaz, J. O. (2013). Community-based psychosocial support: An overview. In R. Arora & P. Arora (Eds.), *Disaster management: Medical preparedness, response and homeland security* (pp. 464–476). CABI.

Public Safety Canada. (2017, March 9). *Fifth regional platform for disaster risk reduction in the Americas endorses action plan demonstrating progress for Canada and Region.* http://www.newswire.ca/news-releases/fifth-regional-platform-for-disaster-risk-reduction-in-the-americas-endorses-action-plan-demonstrating-progress-for-canada-and-region-615822184.html

Puxley, C. (2013, November 19). *First Nations to get disaster relief sooner, Ottawa says.* The Canadian Press. theglobeandmail.com

Quiros, L., & Berger, R. (2015). Responding to the sociopolitical complexity of trauma: An integration of theory and practice. *Journal of Loss and Trauma, 20*, 149–159. https://doi:10.1080/15325024.2013.836353

Rahe, R. H. (2000). Recent Life Changes Questionnaire [RLCQ] [1997]. In T. H. Holmes & American Psychiatric Association (Eds.), *Task force for the handbook of psychiatric measures. Handbook of psychiatric measures* (pp. 235–237). American Psychiatric Association.

Raja, S., Hasnain, M., Hoersch, M., Gove-Yin, S., & Rajagopalan, C. (2015). Trauma informed care in medicine: Current knowledge and future research directions. *Family & Community Health, 38*, 216–226.

Ramsden, I., & Spoonley, P. (1993). The cultural safety debate in nursing education in Aotearoa. *New Zealand Annual Review of Education, 3*, 161–174.

Rando, T. (1993). *Treatment of complicated mourning.* Research Press.

Rees, S., Silove, D., Chey, T., Ivancic, L., Steel, Z., Creamer, M., Teesson, M., Bryant, R., McFarlane, A. C., Mills, K. L., Slade, T., Carragher, N., O'Donnell, M., Forbes, D. (2011). Lifetime prevalence of gender-based violence in women and the relationship with mental disorders and psychosocial function. *Journal of the American Medical Association, 306*, 513–521.

Richardson, F., & Carryer, J. (2005). Teaching cultural safety in a New Zealand nursing education program. *Journal of Nursing Education, 44*, 201.

Richardson, J. D., Naifeh, J. A., & Elhai, J. D. (2007). Posttraumatic stress disorder and associated risk factors in Canadian peacekeeping veterans with health-related disabilities. *Canadian Journal of Psychiatry, 52*, 510–518.

Richardson, S. (2004). Aotearoa/New Zealand nursing: From eugenics to cultural safety. *Nursing Inquiry, 11*, 35–42.

Roberts, A. R. (1991). Conceptualizing crisis theory and the crisis model. In A. R. Roberts (Ed.), *Contemporary perspectives on crisis intervention and prevention* (pp. 3–17). Prentice-Hall.

Robin, R. W., Chester, B., & Goldman, D. (1996). Cumulative trauma and PTSD in American Indian communities. In A. J. Marsella, M. J. Friedman, E. T. Gerrity, & R. M. Scurfield (Eds.), *Ethnocultural aspects of posttraumatic stress disorder: Issues, research, and clinical applications* (pp. 239–253). https://dx.doi.org/10.1037/10555-009

Rupia, E., Binning, S. A., Roche, D. G., & Li, W. (2016). Fight-flight or freeze-hide? Personality and metabolic phenotype mediate physiological defence responses in flatfish. *Journal of Animal Ecology, 85*, 927–937. https://doi:10.1111/1365-2656.12524

Sadock, B. J., Sadock, V. A., & Ruiz, P. (2015). *Kaplan and Saddock's synopsis of psychiatry* (11th ed.). Wolters Kluwer.

Sareen, J. (2014). Posttraumatic stress disorder in adults: Impact, comorbidity, risk factors, and treatment. *The Canadian Journal of Psychiatry, 59*(9), 460–467. https://doi:10.1177/070674371405900902

Sapolsky, R. M. (2004). *Why zebras don't get ulcers* (3rd ed.). Henry Holt.

Saul, J. (2014). *Collective trauma, collective healing: Promoting community resilience in the aftermath of disaster.* Routledge.

Scholte, W. F., & Ager, A. (2014). Social capital and mental health: Connections and complexities in contexts of post conflict recovery. *Intervention, 12*, 210–218.

Sell, T. K., Hosangadi, D., Trotochaud, M., Purnat, T. D., Nguyen, Y., & Briand, S. (2021, February 18). Improving understanding of and response to infodemics during public health emergencies. *Health Security, 19*, 1–2. https://doi.org/10.1089/hs.2021.0044

Selye, H. (1956). *The stress of life.* McGraw-Hill.

Selye, H. (1974). *Stress without distress.* JB Lippincott.

Selye, H. (1980). The stress concept today. In I. L. Kutash, L. B. Schlesinger, & Associates (Eds.), *Handbook on stress and anxiety* (pp. 127–143). Jossey-Bass.

Seng, J., & CAsCAid Group. (2019). From fight or flight, freeze or faint, to flow: Identifying a concept to express a positive embodied outcome of trauma recovery. *Journal of the American Psychiatric Nurses Association, 25*, 200–207. https://doi: 10.1177/1078390318778890

Seng, J., Rauch, S., Resnick, H., Reed, C., King, A., Low, L., McPherson, M., Muzik, M., Abelson, J., & Liberzon, I. (2010). Exploring posttraumatic stress disorder symptom profile among pregnant women. *Journal of Psychosomatic Obstetrics and Gynecology, 31*, 176–187.

Slick, J. (2019). Experiencing fire: A phenomenological study of YouTube videos of the 2016 Fort McMurray fire. *Natural Hazards, 98*, 181–212. https://doi-org.login.ezproxy.library.ualberta.ca/10.1007/s11069-019-03604-5

Somasundaram, D. (2007). Collective trauma in northern Sri Lanka: A qualitative psychosocial-ecological study. *International Journal of Mental Health Systems, 1*, 1–27. https://doi:10.1186/1752-4458-1-5

Somasundaram, D. (2014). Addressing collective trauma: Conceptualisations and interventions. *Intervention, 12*(Suppl 1), 43–60.

Statistics Canada. (2021, February 2). *Mental health among health care workers in Canada during the COVID-19 pandemic.* https://www150.statcan.gc.ca/n1/daily-quotidien/210202/dq210202a-eng.htm

Sterling, P., & Eyer, J. (1988). Allostasis: A new paradigm to explain arousal pathology. In S. Fisher & J. Reason (Eds.), *Handbook of life stress, cognition and health* (pp. 629–649). John Wiley & Sons.

Substance Abuse and Mental Health Services Administration. (2013). *Tips for survivors of a disaster or traumatic event: What to expect in your personal, family, work and financial life.*

Tay, P. K. C., & Lim, K. K. (2020). Psychological resilience as an emergent characteristic for well-being: A pragmatic view. *Gerontology, 66*, 476–483. https://doi:10.1159/000509210

Taylor, S. E., Klein, L. C., Lewis, B. P., Gruenewald, T. L., Gurung, R. A., & Updegraff, J. A. (2000). Biobehavioral responses to stress in females: Tend-and-befriend, not fight-or-flight. *Psychological Review, 107*, 411–429.

Taylor, S. E., Lewis, B. P., Gruenewald, T. L., Gurung, R. A. R., Updegraff, J. A., & Klein, L. C. (2002). Sex differences in biobehavioral responses to threat: Reply to Geary and Flinn. *Psychological Review, 109*, 751–753.

Tervalon, M., & Murray-Garcia, J. (1998). Cultural humility versus cultural competence: A critical distinction in defining physician training outcomes in multicultural education. *Journal of Health Care for the Poor and Underserved, 9*, 117–125.

The Canadian Encyclopedia. (2013). *Extreme-weather-in-Canada.* http://www.thecanadianencyclopedia.ca/en/article/extreme-weather-in-canada-feature/

Thormar, S. B., Gersons, B. P., Juen, B., Marschang, A., Djakababa, M. N., & Olff, M. (2010). The mental health impact of volunteering in a disaster setting: A review. *Journal of Nervous and Mental Disorders, 198*, 529–538.

Trainer, M., & Goel, A. (2013). The role of social networking in disaster management. In R. Arora & P. Arora (Eds.), *Disaster management: Medical preparedness, response and homeland security* (pp. 67–94). CABI.

Truth and Reconciliation Commission of Canada. (2015). *Calls to action.* http://www.trc.ca/websites/trcinstitution/File/2015/Findings/Calls_to_Action_English2.pdf

Turpel-Lafond, M. E. (2020). *In plain sight: Addressing Indigenous-specific racism and discrimination in B.C. health care.* https://engage.gov.bc.ca/app/uploads/sites/613/2020/11/In-Plain-Sight-Full-Report.pdf

United Nations. (2006). *Convention on the rights of persons with disabilities*. http://www.un.org/disabilities/documents/convention/convoptprot-e.pdf

United Nations Office for Disaster Reduction. (2015). *The Sendai framework for disaster reduction 2015–2030*. https://www.undrr.org/publication/sendai-framework-disaster-risk-reduction-2015-2030

United Nations Office for Disaster Risk Reduction. (2019). *Global assessment report on disaster risk reduction*. https://gar.undrr.org/sites/default/files/reports/2019-06/full_report.pdf

Veer, I. A., Riepenhausen, A., Zerban, M., Wackerhagen, C., Puhlmann, L. M. C., Engen, H., Köber, G., Bögemann, S. A., Weermeijer, J., Uściłko, A., Mor, N., Marciniak, M. A., Askelund, A. D., Al-Kamel, A., Ayash, S., Barsuola, G., Bartkute-Norkuniene, V., Battaglia, S., Bobko, Y., … Kalisch, R. (2021). Psycho-social factors associated with mental resilience in the Corona lockdown. *Translational Psychiatry, 11*, 67–78. https://doi.org/10.1038/s41398-020-01150-4

Walls, M. L., & Whitbeck, L. B. (2012). The intergenerational effects of relocation policies on Indigenous families. *Journal of Family Issues, 33*, 1272–1293.

Wolfelt, A. D. (1999). *Dispelling 5 common myths about grief*. http://www.griefwords.com/index.cgi?action=page&page=articles%2Fhelping7.html&site_id=2

Woolfolk, R. L., Lehrer, P. M., & Allen, L. M. (2007). Conceptual issues underlying stress management. In P. M. Lehrer, R. L. Woolfolk, & W. E. Sime (Eds.), *Principles and practice of stress management* (3rd ed., pp. 3–15). Guilford.

Worden, J. W. (2003). *Grief counseling and grief therapy: A handbook for the mental health practitioner*. Brunner-Routledge.

World Health Organization (WHO). (2019, June 11). *Fact Sheet: Mental health in emergencies*. https://www.who.int/news-room/fact-sheets/detail/mental-health-in-emergencies

World Health Organization, War Trauma Foundation and World Vision International. (2013). *Psychological first aid: Guide for field workers*. WHO.

CHAPTER 19

Anger, Aggression, and Violence

Mary-Lou Martin*

LEARNING OBJECTIVES

After studying this chapter, you will be able to:

- Explore feelings about the experience and expression of anger.
- Discuss the bio/psycho/social/spiritual factors that influence anger, aggression, and violence.
- Discuss the theories used to explain anger, aggression, and violence.
- Identify the behaviour or actions that escalate and de-escalate violent behaviour.
- Recognize the risk for aggression and violence towards nurses.
- Generate options for responding to anger, aggression, and violence in nursing practice.
- Apply the nursing process to the management of anger, aggression, and violence in clients.

KEY TERMS

- catharsis • mindfulness • restraint

KEY CONCEPTS

- aggression • anger • assertiveness • structured professional judgment

---

Anger is considered a universal human emotion, identifiable across cultures, by theorists who believe that prototypical emotions exist (DiGiuseppe & Tafrate, 2007). We get our knowledge about emotion in several ways: personal knowledge, knowledge about others' emotions, social norms, and evolving conceptual knowledge (Faucher & Tappolet, 2008). Definitions of anger, aggression, and violence vary and are informed through our experiences, beliefs, culture, and gender. Individuals and groups develop their own views of where the boundaries exist with these: verbally, nonverbally, and behaviourally. Theoretic distinctions can be made between anger, aggression, and violence, but clinically, their expression may be blurred. Each phenomenon may occur alone or in combination.

Most societies develop norms for acceptable and unacceptable behaviour. Today, images and stories about aggressive and violent acts throughout the world appear almost instantaneously in the media. Incidents such as mass killings receive enormous coverage that strongly impacts public perception of the risk for violence, especially that posed by persons with mental illness (Friedman & Michels, 2013), even though most societal violence is caused by individuals who are not mentally ill (Varshney et al., 2016). Or in other words, "the large majority of the perpetrators of violent crimes do not have a diagnosable mental illness, and conversely, most people with psychiatric disorders are never violent" (Swanson, 2021, pp. 1–2).

Healthcare settings are not immune to expressions of anger, aggression, and violence. Aggression and violence reflect the values of the individual, family, community, and society. Many people tend to minimize the frequency and severity of aggressive and violent acts (Freeman et al., 2015). The expression of anger, aggression, and violence by clients, and sometimes families, is a tremendous challenge for nurses, impacting their physical and mental health (Canadian Federation of Nurses Unions [CFNU], 2020). This chapter discusses prominent theories about the nature of these phenomena and offers varying, sometimes controversial, models, theories, and evidence. Clinicians can choose a model as a basis for assessment, nursing care focus, planning, intervention, and evaluation. It is through the application of the nursing process that the nurse identifies strengths and risks; manages angry, aggressive, or violent clients; and prevents or de-escalates situations that may lead to aggression or violence.

---

*Adapted from the chapter "Anger, Aggression, and Violence" by Phillip Woods

Anger

Anger is "a normal human emotion, aroused by frequently occurring violations of our values, beliefs, or rights" (Thomas, 2005, p. 508). Anger is part of the fight-or-flight response of the sympathetic nervous system and is usually described as a temporary state of emotional arousal, in contrast to hostility, which is associated with a more enduring negative attitude. Thomas (2001) asserts that the expression of anger may prevent aggression and help to resolve a situation.

Language pertaining to anger is imprecise and confusing. The word *anger* is used to describe a wide range of feelings, from annoyance at having to wait at a red light when in a hurry, to a severe emotional reaction to the news that a family member has been physically assaulted. Words often used interchangeably with anger include annoyance, irritation, frustration, temper, resentment, hostility, fury, hatred, livid, and rage. In addition, the word *angry* is used to describe both a transient emotional state and a personality trait. Novaco (2007) purports that this imprecision is related to varying beliefs and theories, including the following:

- Anger is a fixed quantity that either dams up or floods the system.
- Anger and aggression are linked. Anger is the feeling, and aggression is the behaviour.
- Anger is the instinctive response to a threat or to the inability to meet goals or desires.
- If the outward expression of anger is blocked, then it turns inward and develops into depression.
- Anger arises out of feelings of hurt or anxiety.

Box 19.1 invites the reader to explore variations in responses to anger using an experiential exercise.

BOX 19.1 Self-Awareness Exercise: Personal Experience of Anger

People's reactions differ when they experience anger. Some people report a sense of power, control, and calmness different from their usual experience; others report feeling shaky, tearful, and on the verge of collapse. Still others describe physical sensations of nausea and dizziness.

Think about the last time that you felt angry. List the body sensations and other emotions that you experienced. Now ask a friend, colleague, or family member to do the same. Compare lists. What are the similarities and differences between you? How will awareness of these differences help you in your clinical practice?

KEY CONCEPT

Anger is an affective state experienced as the motivation to act in ways that warn, intimidate, or attack those who are perceived as challenging or threatening. It occurs when there is a threat, delay, thwarting of a goal, or conflict between goals.

Experience of Anger

The experience of anger is an internal event that involves thoughts, images, and bodily sensations (Kassinove & Tafrate, 2006). The experience of anger can serve as a warning that demands are greater than available resources. Yet, except for anger that arises from specific neurologic damage or biochemical imbalances, angry episodes can also be viewed as social events. The meaning of angry episodes develops from the beliefs held about anger and the interpretation given to the episode, and these are shaped by influences such as culture, language, and gender (Thomas, 2006). Anger is a normal human emotion; it is the dysfunctional expression of anger that may be threatening to the self or others.

Expression of Anger

Verbal (e.g., yelling) and motor behaviours (e.g., stomping one's foot, raising one's fist) are illustrations of the expression of anger (see Fig. 19.1). Difficulties in expressing anger have often been associated with mental health problems. Anger turned inwards has been implicated as a contributor to mood disorders, such as depression and somatic symptom disorder (Koh et al., 2005). Behavioural expressions of anger vary. In the 19th century, anger was viewed as sinful, dangerous, and destructive—an emotion to be contained, controlled, and denied. This negatively viewed emotion was to be dominated and conquered, and an ideal family life was free of anger. Spouses were discouraged from expressing anger towards each other and parenting manuals promoted the suppression of anger in children. This view contributed to the development of a powerful taboo against feeling and expressing anger. People who have accepted this taboo may have difficulty even knowing when they are angry (Thomas, 1993).

Differences in expectations about how men and women should express anger also contribute to the confusion about anger. Varying beliefs about appropriate ways to express anger become apparent when a client and a nurse engage in a therapeutic relationship. Genetic predisposition, emotional development during infancy and childhood, and family environment influence the variations in expression for both the nurse and the client (Thomas, 2009). Previous experiences in

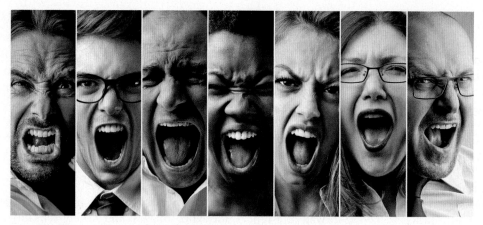

Figure 19.1 Facial expressions of anger.

expressing anger and reactions from others such as parents and peers are also influential. Frequency, duration, intensity, and mode of expression are aspects of anger that can be explored and considered (Novaco, 2007). When the expression of anger has negative outcomes for the person such as personal distress (e.g., shame, guilt, rejection) and consequences (e.g., lost relationships, job loss), it may be considered dysfunctional (Kassinove & Tafrate, 2006). Anger may energize the person to take action that can lead to positive or negative outcomes.

Aggression and Violence

Whereas anger is an emotion, aggression and violence are behaviours. In this chapter, violence and aggression "refer to a range of behaviours or actions that can result in harm, hurt or injury to another person, regardless of whether violence or aggression is physically or verbally expressed, physical harm is sustained, or the intention is clear" (National Institute for Health and Care Excellence, 2015, p. 5). Aggression and violence reflect

a continuum from suspicious behaviour to extreme actions that threaten the safety of others or result in injury or death (see Table 19.1 for examples). The World Health Organization (WHO) (2021a) states that 8% to 38% of healthcare workers experience physical violence during their careers and that most violence towards healthcare workers is due to clients and visitors. WHO also asserts that such violence puts the quality of care and provision of health services at risk.

Research focused on inpatient psychiatric units has found that higher levels of aggression were associated with clients detained under mental health legislation (Bowers et al., 2011), high client turnover, unit doors being locked, and higher patient to staff ratios (Bowers et al., 2009). Furthermore, Bowers and colleagues (2011) found that the imposition of restrictions on clients appeared to be associated with increased aggression. Reasons for aggression in these settings as identified by staff and clients, included client factors (e.g., psychotic symptoms), staff factors (e.g., lack of skill), and environmental factors (e.g., overcrowding, lack of access

Table 19.1	Examples of Behaviours on the Continuum of Aggression and Violence	
Term	Description	Clinical Example
Suspicious behaviour	Hypervigilance to external cues Attends more to cues that fit with current thinking patterns Guarded, nervous, nervous glancing, ill at ease	A female client with a long history of delusional disorder (including the belief that her family wants to "lock her away") questions the motives of a community mental health nurse when she asks the client about her medication regimen. The client misperceives the nurse's inquiry as evidence of a conspiracy against her.
Verbal hostility	Verbal comments that may be loud, sarcastic, and/or blaming and often expressed with the intent to bully, intimidate, or frighten others May be used as a means of getting attention, hurting others, or inviting others to take action	When administration of PRN medication is delayed, a client's mother comes to the care station and starts to yell. She states that the nurses do not care, are lazy, and should work harder. She also demands that someone give her daughter medication. (Family members have been previously reported as using demanding behaviours to have needs met.)
Physical violence	Act of striking out, grabbing, throwing an object, pushing, etc. that appears to be intended to cause harm to a person or object	A young man attending a mental health clinic has missed his appointment with the clinical nurse specialist. When he finds out he cannot be scheduled to see her for another week, he yells at the receptionist, bangs his fist on the desk, and then picks up a chair and throws it at her.

to outside space). A systemic perspective of aggression and violence in mental healthcare has been proposed that identifies four related phenomena: environmental (e.g., layout of the unit, noise level), intrapersonal/client (e.g., age, gender, trauma, diagnosis), clinician (e.g., skills, stress level, attitude towards aggression), and mental healthcare system (e.g., policies, cultural factors, control orientation) (Cutcliffe & Riahi, 2013a, 2013b). A recent literature review found that patient characteristics, management practices, approaches by staff, and the environment of the ward are influencing factors that may give rise to violent behaviour (Asikainen et al., 2020). A recent Norwegian study found that onward violence decreased significantly when changes in practice saw more individualized patient-oriented care, a proportionate increase in female staff, and better-educated nurses (Urheim et al., 2020).

Aggression does not occur in a vacuum. Therefore, a multidimensional framework (Fig. 19.2) is essential for understanding and responding to anger, aggression, and violence.

KEY CONCEPT

Aggression is defined as verbal statements and/or physical actions that are intended to threaten.

Models of Anger, Aggression, and Violence

In this section, some of the dominant theoretical explanations for anger, aggression, and violence are discussed. Because of the complex nature of these emotions and actions, no single model or theory can fully explain anger, aggression, and violence. Instead, the nurse must choose the most useful model(s) for explaining a particular client's experience, for planning interventions, and evaluating outcomes.

Biologic Theories

From a biologic viewpoint, a tendency to have more frequent angry episodes may partially originate from developmental deficits, anoxia, malnutrition, toxins, tumours, or neurodegenerative diseases or trauma affecting the brain. Clients with a history of damage to the cerebral cortex are more likely to exhibit increased impulsivity, decreased inhibition, and decreased judgment. The interaction of neurocognitive impairment and social history of abuse or family violence increases the risk for violent behaviour. The odds of violent behaviour also increase when separate risk factors, such as untreated first-episode psychosis and substance use disorder, coexist in the same person (Latalova, 2014).

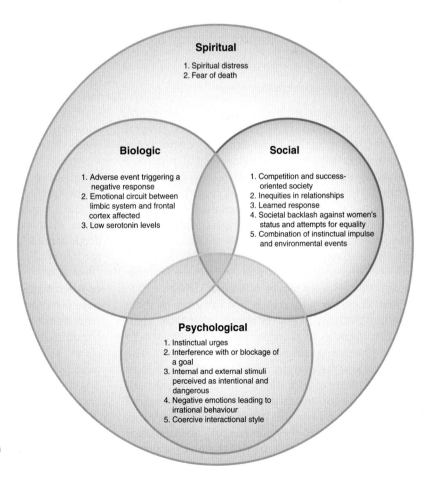

Figure 19.2 Aetiologies for clients with aggression.

BOX 19.2 Self-Awareness Exercise: Intensity of Anger

IMAGINE THIS SCENE

You are coming home after a 12-h shift. You've been at the hospital for your clinical placement and are tired. As you come up the front walk, you trip over a skateboard, probably left by one of the neighbourhood children. Before you know it, you are sprawled across the front sidewalk.

What emotions threaten to overwhelm you at that moment? What contributes to the intensity of the anger that you feel?

- The pain where you scraped your hands and legs across the cement sidewalk?
- Your general state of tiredness?
- The fact that you missed dinner?
- The five cups of caffeinated coffee you had today?
- The careless child who left their skateboard in your way?

If the same thing had happened when you were well rested and feeling good, would the feeling and the intensity of anger be the same?

Before reading additional research evidence, try the anger exercise in Box 19.2.

Cognitive Neuroassociation Model

The cognitive neuroassociation model is one explanation for the interplay of biologic and other internal influences (Berkowitz, 2012). Initially, an adverse event (e.g., pain from tripping over a skateboard) triggers a primitive negative response. Peripheral receptors communicate this response to the spinal cord through the spinothalamic tract to the hypothalamus. The hypothalamus, which synthesizes input from throughout the nervous system, is part of the limbic system. The limbic system mediates primitive emotion and basic drives to produce behaviours for survival, such as the fight-or-flight response (Harper-Jaques & Reimer, 1992).

At first, cognitive appraisal is not involved in these rudimentary feelings of fear or anger, other than identifying the stimulus as aversive; however, higher-order cognitive processing quickly begins to take over. The brain associates the current experience of physiologic sensations with memories, ideas, and previously experienced expressive motor reactions. It then interprets and differentiates the experience. Depending on prior experience and associations, the response may be intensified or suppressed. It is this latter part of the process that is most amenable to modification through psychotherapy.

Neurostructural Model

The brain structures most frequently associated with anger and aggressive behaviour are the amygdala and the hypothalamus (Gouveia et al., 2019). The amygdala processes fear, triggers anger, and motivates action—in essence, it alerts us to danger and activates the fight-or-flight response. It also stimulates the hypothalamus, which plays an important role in the expression of emotions (including pleasure and/or rage). Conversely, the prefrontal cortex of the brain is responsible for reasoning, judgment, and logic and theoretically prepares one to "think before one acts."

Neurochemical Model and Low Serotonin Syndrome

In recent decades, knowledge has exploded about the complex role of neurotransmitters in human behaviour. Serotonin is a major neurotransmitter involved in mood, sleep, and appetite. Low serotonin levels are associated not only with depression but also with irritability, increased pain sensitivity, impulsiveness, aggression, vulnerability to alcoholism, and obsessive–compulsive behaviour.

Serotonin is sensitive to fluctuations in dietary intake of its precursor, tryptophan, which is found in high-carbohydrate foods. Tryptophan intake and the availability of binding sites on the plasma proteins affect the synthesis of serotonin. Thus, assessing overall dietary intake is relevant, particularly of good tryptophan sources, such as wheat, flour, corn, milk, and eggs. In one meta-analysis, a small inverse relationship between tryptophan level and aggression was found, highlighting that the literature continues to have contradictory findings and methodologic limitations (Duke et al., 2013).

People with a history of aggressive behaviour have been found to have a lower than average level of serotonin. Studies of humans with known aggressive tendencies, such as violent offenders, have repeatedly shown lower than average concentrations of 5-hydroxyindole-acetic acid (5-HIAA), the major metabolite for serotonin (Soloff et al., 2000) and prefrontal cortex dysfunction (Best et al., 2002). Similarly, the plasma concentration of tryptophan is lower in people with alcoholism who have a history of aggressive behaviour than in people with alcoholism and no such history. People who have committed impulsive acts of violence have lower levels of 5-HIAA than do people whose acts of violence were premeditated. Impulsivity and difficulty controlling anger are characteristic of people diagnosed with borderline personality disorder, another condition associated with lower than normal serotonin levels (Paris, 2005). Hyperarousal, such as may occur through being constantly vigilant against possible risk to self, may contribute to aggressive behaviour.

This evidence for a biologic component to aggressive behaviour does not mean that only biologic means of treatment can be effective. Feedback between human behaviour and biochemistry is continuous; verbal suggestions and even early life stressors can affect biochemistry, just as biochemistry affects behaviour (Heinz et al., 2001). Environmental and learned behaviours influence the type and degree of aggression expressed, even by those for whom there is a biologic component (da Cunha-Bang & Knudsen, 2021; Soloff et al., 2000).

Psychological Theories

Several psychological explanations exist for aggressive and violent behaviours. This section discusses psychoanalytic, behavioural, and cognitive theories.

Psychoanalytic Theories

Psychoanalytic theorists view emotions as instinctual urges. They view suppression of these urges as unhealthy and as possible contributors to the development of psychosomatic or psychological disorders. Freud struggled to understand the nature and expression of human aggressive behaviour. His ideas were based on his experiences in conducting therapy with clients. In his early works, he linked aggression with libidinal factors; however, this association did not explain destructive actions during wars and armed conflict. In his later writings, Freud identified aggression as a separate instinct, like the sexual instinct. He viewed aggression as an innate human quality that could be expressed when a person is provoked or abused. In doing so, he challenged the commonly held belief that human beings are essentially good.

Freud explained aggressive or violent behaviour as a combination of instinctual impulses and events in the environment that stimulated release of the instinctual urge. Freud's view fostered the use of **catharsis**. Therapeutic approaches, such as primal scream and nursing interventions that direct the client to "let it out" by pounding a pillow, find their origins in this theory (Thomas, 1990). However, results of research studies have been mixed as to if catharsis is helpful in reducing anger (Verona & Sullivan, 2008). Venting can also have negative consequences when the action taken is hurtful to, or blaming of others, or damaging to property.

Erich Fromm (1900–1980), an American psychoanalyst best known for his application of psychoanalytic theory to social and cultural problems, believed that animals and humans share a form of aggression he called *benign*. This genetically programmed response was designed as a defense to protect oneself against a threat. The distinction between humans and animals is that human beings could reason. This capability provided them with options not available to animals.

Thus, unlike animals, human beings can behave aggressively for reasons other than self-preservation. Fromm (1973) defined aggression in humans as any behaviour that causes or intends to cause damage to another person, animal, or object. Humans may foresee both real and perceived threats. Perceived threats that are based on distorted perceptions may lead to aggressive and violent behaviours; for example, the cognitive and information-processing deficits of clients with psychosis or schizophrenia (see Chapter 21) are frequently implicated in episodes of aggression and violence.

Behavioural Theories

The goal of behaviourists is to predict and control behaviour. Introspection has no role in these theories. One behavioural theory, drive theory, suggests that violent behaviour originates externally. A person experiences anger and acts violently in response to interference with or blocking of a goal. Laboratory experiments and the reality of everyday experience have proved the limitations of this theory. Clearly, not all situations in which one's goal is blocked lead to anger or violence.

Another behavioural theory is social learning theory. In his research, Bandura (1973) drew attention to social learning processes whereby the role of learning and rewards in the expression of anger and violence was observed. He studied interactions between mothers and children. The children learned that anger and aggressive behaviour helped them get what they wanted from their mothers. The children learned aggressive behaviour in a context that may have made them understand aggressive behaviour as appropriate. According to this view, people learn to be aggressive by participating in an aggressive environment in which aggression is reinforced. There is some evidence, for instance, that playing violent videogames is associated with aggressive emotions, thoughts, and behaviours, and decreased empathy (Calvert et al., 2017). However, the debate remains ongoing over the significance of the effect of violence in movies, television, and videogames on an individual's propensity for violence (Ontario Ministry of Children, Community and Social Services, 2016).

Cognitive Theories

Cognitive theorists are interested in how people transform internal and external stimuli into useful information. They emphasize understanding how a person takes new information and fits it into an already developed schema. Beck (1976) proposed that cognitive schemas such as judgments, self-esteem, and expectations influence angry responses. In a situation perceived as intentional, dangerous, and unprovoked, the recipient's reaction will be intensified. The person's reaction will be further intensified if they view the offender as undesirable. In psychological disorders, cognitive processing may be compromised (Kornreich et al., 2016; Kurtz et al., 2016).

Rational–emotive theory, a type of cognitive theory, considers cognition, affect, and behaviour to be interrelated psychological processes (Ellis, 1977, 1995). This theory regards anger as an inappropriate negative emotion because it stems from irrational beliefs. Change is directed at altering irrational beliefs by identifying and working to change them and their associated psychological processes. Cognitive theories inform us about how not to get angry in the first place not about what to do when we become angry (Novaco, 2007, 2017). In a systematic review and meta-analysis by David and colleagues (2018) that aimed to summarize the effectiveness and efficacy of 50 years of rational–emotive and behavioural therapy (REBT), only a limited number of studies investigated anger, so it is not possible to draw any strong conclusions.

Sociocultural Theories

Sociocultural theories suggest violent behaviour has multiple determinants, including social experiences in family and peer settings and the social consequences (positive and negative) of physical aggression. These determinants can be influenced by the gender of the individual and the way that gender differences are conceived and enacted within a society (Snyder et al., 2007).

Western society often is characterized by a competitive, success-oriented ideology that values the individual and their accomplishments over collaboration and a sense of community. Self-esteem, particularly for men, may be based on social and economic status and influence over others and the environment (Thomas, 2003). The pursuit of status produces inequities in relationships, whereby one person is superior and the other is subordinate. A hazard inherent in the pursuit of status is the view that a person is entitled to have influence and control and that the "entitled person" has the right to use whatever means necessary to obtain status. These means may include force or disregarding the rights and needs of others. The entitled person may also begin to consider other people responsible for their thoughts, feelings, or actions. Such a belief in entitlement can be used to justify actions such as threatening, hurting, or murdering less powerful individuals (Stosny, 2019)

The World Health Organization (WHO) (n.d.) views violence as a global public health problem and violence against women as being entrenched in gender inequality. The WHO (2021b) acknowledges violence against women as a violation of women's rights and globally (n = 161 countries), one in three women report experiencing violence by sexual partners and/or nonpartners. The WHO asserts that violence is preventable, and economic and sociocultural issues that promote a culture of violence must be tackled. Moreover, WHO (n.d.) indicates prevention must encompass the reduction of risk factors and building capacity in protective factors. This means that individual, interpersonal, community, and societal risk and protective factors must be addressed. The WHO further identifies that issues concerning violence also need to be integrated into undergraduate education and training for healthcare professionals so that they can play an important role in preventing violence and provide comprehensive healthcare to those who experience violence.

Interactional Theory

Morrison (1998) challenged research and theories suggesting that aggression and violence are biologically or psychologically based. She asserted that these views lead to excusing the person's behaviour. She proposed that violence among people in psychiatric settings is the same as violence in other settings. Therefore, the client's behaviour should be considered a social problem and responded to on that basis. This challenge is grounded in several studies that examined the interactional style of the aggressive and violent individual. People with interactional styles that were argumentative or coercive were more likely to engage in aggressive or violent interchanges. Morrison clearly stated her view that the antecedent variables (e.g., history of violence, psychiatric diagnosis, length of hospitalization) and the mediating variable of interactional style are the primary reasons for the behaviour.

A lifespan approach to understanding aggressive behaviour can be taken, one that considers risks factors across the developmental spectrum (Liu et al., 2013). See Table 19.2 for characteristics and risk factors for aggressive behaviour across age groups.

Nursing Management: Human Response to Anger and Aggression

Aggression and violence often arise from a person's belief that their view of a situation is the only correct one and that the other person's view needs to change. Box "Clinical Vignette: Sidney's Anger" illustrates such a scenario in the clinical setting.

Contrary to popular belief, most clients who have mental health problems do not behave aggressively or violently. To develop a means of predicting aggressive and violent behaviours, researchers have examined the relationship between diagnosis and violence. They have also focused on the role of a person's history in predicting violence and examined demographics, client characteristics, and unit climate.

Table 19.2   Characteristics and Risk Factors for Aggressive Behaviour Across Age Groups

Age Group	Characteristics	Underlying and Contextual Risk Factors
Toddlers	Tantrums, crying, screaming, biting, kicking, throwing, and/or breaking objects.	Genetic and biologic factors (e.g., birth complications, nutrition deficit, neglect, abuse/trauma).
School-age children	Aggressive behaviour peaks before age 2. Teasing, irritability, bullying, fighting, cruelty to animals, and fire setting. Nonphysical aggressive behaviour increases (verbal [e.g., insults, taunting] and psychological [e.g., ostracizing]). Symptoms of sexual or physical abuse to the child. It is important to assess for potential abuse in these clients.	Imitation of others' aggression (social learning theory). Neurodevelopment disorders. After repeated exposure to specific social stimuli (social information-processing theory). Psychosocial and environmental factors (such as poor parenting, dysfunctional home environment).
Adolescents	More serious aggressive behaviours and even violence appear. Gang activities including stealing, truancy, etc. Cross-gendered aggressive behaviours, including dating violence, date rape, and sexual assault. Suicide is the third leading cause of death for this group.	Aggressive behaviour that appears in only adolescence and disappears in later life (adolescence-limited antisocial behaviour). Learned aggressive behaviour in childhood that is carried over into adolescence. Depression, family and other relationship difficulties, and a family history of suicide (or personal history of suicide attempts) may place an adolescent at greater risk for suicidal behaviour. Substance abuse.
Adults	Domestic violence, sexual abuse, child abuse, and homicide. Highest homicide rate among age groups.	Drug use. Traumatic brain injury to areas responsible for managing aggression and impulse control.
Older adults	Older adults in nursing homes due to daily interactions with staff and other residents. Aggressive behaviours aimed at caregivers centre on intimate care practices or those that cause pain. Aggressive behaviour aimed at fellow residents in the context of excessive vocalization, territoriality, arguments with roommates, and general loneliness or frustration.	The emergence of dementias such as Alzheimer disease may result in misunderstanding of motives. Aggression may result from this confusion. The annual incidence of homicide–suicide is higher in adults 55 years and older and typically occurs more among couples. Multifactorial aetiology.

Adapted from Liu, J., Lewis, G., & Evans, L. (2013). Understanding aggressive behaviour across the lifespan. *Journal of Psychiatric and Mental Health Nursing, 20*(2), 156–168. Licensed © 2012 Blackwell Publishing.

CLINICAL VIGNETTE

SIDNEY'S ANGER

Sidney, a new client on the unit, appears to be experiencing auditory hallucinations. The nurse calmly approaches Sidney, careful not to invade their personal space, and begins to walk with them. The nurse introduces herself and asks, "How are you?" Sidney responds abruptly with "Fine." To begin developing a therapeutic relationship and assess their current mental status, the nurse points out that they seem tense and restless and asks if the voices have returned. Sidney responds, "They are telling me this place isn't safe." The nurse responds, "This place isn't safe...?" Sidney responds, "The angels in the corner are signaling to me." Nurse responds, "I don't see anyone else here." Sidney responds, "They want me to leave!" Sidney starts to walk towards the door. The nurse attempts to offer an alternative point of view and orient Sidney to the present. The nurse understands that what the client is seeing and hearing are hallucinations. The nurse attempts to increase Sidney's feeling of safety by identifying their perceptions as hallucinations and reassuring them of their safety. Sidney's facial expression changes and they look angry. They shout, "No I won't stay, and you can't make me." Sidney pushes the nurse aside and runs to the door.

What Do You Think?

If you were the nurse in this situation, what would be your next response? How would you acknowledge Sidney's concerns, promote their sense of safety, and encourage them to stay?

Although media attention highlights violence related to mental illness, research shows that "the mentally ill as a group pose little risk of violence" (Friedman & Michels, 2013, p. 455). Persons with severe mental illness, such as schizophrenia or bipolar disorder, may be at a slightly higher risk for violent behaviour (Elbogen & Johnson, 2009; Swanson, 2021; Swanson et al., 2006) but they are overwhelmingly more likely to be victims of violence and violent crime with a prevalence of 6 to 23 times greater than others (Teplin et al., 2005). Research has also shown that factors additional to mental disorder increase the risk of violent behaviour such as historical, clinical, dispositional, and contextual factors (Elbogen & Johnson, 2009). Many possible causes have been identified for aggressive behaviours in individuals experiencing a psychiatric disorder, including the presence of comorbid substance abuse, dependence, and intoxication (Citrome, 2015; DeAngelis, 2021; Elbogen & Johnson, 2009; Swanson, 2021). In addition, individuals experiencing symptom manifestation of hallucinations or delusions or those with neuropsychiatric deficits are identified as posing an increased risk for violence. Individuals with underlying antisocial personality traits may use violent acts to achieve specific goals. Finally, environmental factors that are associated with aggressive behaviours are identified, including a chaotic or unstable home or hospital situation, which may further encourage maladaptive aggressive behaviours (Citrome, 2015; Elbogen & Johnson, 2009; Jensen & Clough, 2016). An important consideration for the nurse is the course of violence related to changes in symptomatology (Bernstein & Saladino, 2007).

Research suggests that some characteristics are predictive of violent behaviours. Low self-esteem that may be further eroded during hospitalization or treatment may influence clients to use force to meet their needs or to experience a sense of empowerment. Many people who have chronic mental health problems "fight" the experience and have difficulty accepting mental health treatment. When admitted to the hospital, they may experience turmoil from both the illness and the anger at the additional loss of control that hospitalization mandates. Clients may resort to violence to force change or to regain or maintain control. Rewards from violence include attention from staff and/or status and prestige among the client group (Harris & Morrison, 1995). For example, the client who behaves violently is observed more frequently and has more opportunities to discuss concerns with nurses. Impaired communication, disorientation, and depression have been found to be consistently associated with aggressive behaviour among nursing home residents with dementia (Talerico et al., 2002).

Nurses bring their own perceptions and reactions to clinical settings. They respond to the behaviours of the clients and families for whom they care. Clients and families, in turn, react to nurses. Nurses' beliefs about themselves as individuals and professionals will influence their responses to aggressive behaviours. For example, the nurse who considers any expression of anger or aggression inappropriate will approach an agitated client in a manner different from that used by the nurse who considers agitated behaviour to be meaningful. In a phenomenological study of client experiences of violent encounters (Carlsson et al., 2006), participants described wanting caregivers who were calm and confident and who did not respond to client anger by disconnecting (e.g., becoming cool and distant). They said that such reactions on the part of caregivers increased their despair and, with it, their aggression. When a caregiver genuinely related to the client as a person and seemed to recognize the suffering being experienced, the client's anger was diffused. The researchers found the clients to be "longing for authentic personal care" (p. 287).

Duxbury and Whittington (2005) studied clients' and nurses' perspectives on inpatient aggression and violence. They found that clients believed poor communication on the part of staff played a significant role, whereas nurses believed it was clients' mental illness that was most significant. Both noted that environmental conditions (e.g., restrictive and underresourced) played a role. Clients advocated for communication training for staff, whereas nurses looked for organizational deficits to be addressed. The nurse's ability to maintain personal control is challenged when faced with angry, provoking clients (see Fig. 19.3). Some clients who are experiencing emotional problems have an uncanny ability to verbally target a nurse's vulnerable characteristics. It is a usual response to become defensive when a person feels vulnerable. However, when nurses lose control of their own responses, the potential for punitive interventions or the use of threats or sarcasm is greater.

Nurses in all areas of clinical practice need to understand angry emotions, know how to prevent aggression and violence, and respond proactively. To better prepare themselves to respond to different types of behaviours, many nurses take assertiveness training courses and workshops. Many nursing schools also teach

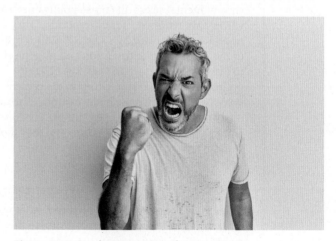

Figure 19.3 Escalating anger and aggression.

assertiveness. Nurses should understand the phenomena of anger, aggression, and violence as meaningful behaviours that warrant attention rather than as disruptive behaviours to control.

KEY CONCEPT

Assertiveness is a set of behaviours and a communication style that is open, honest, direct, and confident. Assertiveness enables the expression of emotions, including anger, in a manner that assumes responsibility. It allows placement of boundaries and prevents acceptance of inappropriate aggression from others.

Predictors of Violence

Prevention of violence requires early identification of risk and the corresponding appropriate intervention. Extensive research has been undertaken to determine variables that are strongly associated with the risk of violence. When assessing a client, their history is probably the most important predictor of potential for violence. Important markers include previous episodes of rage and violent behaviour, escalating irritability, intruding angry thoughts, and fear of losing control. There is reasonable consensus in the literature that actuarial or statistical approaches are not the best for assessing risk of violence and instead the clinician should use a structured professional judgment (SPJ) approach (Hart et al., 2017).

KEY CONCEPT

Structured professional judgment (SPJ) is an analytical method used to understand and mitigate the risk for interpersonal violence posed by individual people that is discretionary in essence but relies on evidence-based guidelines to systematize the exercise of discretion (Hart et al., 2017).

The Historical/Clinical/Risk–20 Version 3 (HCR-20 V3) is one of several prominent instruments to assist predicting long-term violence risk (Douglas et al., 2013). The HCR-20 consists of 10 historical items (violence, other antisocial behaviour, relationships, employment, substance use, major mental disorder, personality disorder, traumatic experiences, violent attitudes, treatment or supervision response); 5 clinical items (insight, violent ideation or intent, symptoms of major mental disorder, instability, treatment or supervision response); and 5 risk items (professional service and plans, living situation, personal support, treatment or supervision response, stress and coping). Extensive research has been published on its predictive accuracy.

The short-term assessment of risk and treatability (START) is an SPJ guide for assessing vulnerabilities, strengths, signature risk signs, and the historical and short-term assessment of seven risk domains including violence to others, suicide, self-harm, self-neglect, unauthorized absence, substance use, and victimization (Webster et al., 2006, 2009). There is also a START version for adolescents. The Structured Assessment of Protective Factors (SAPROF) assesses 17 protective factors with 3 scales for violence risks (de Vries Robbé & de Vogel, 2012).

Two actuarial instruments used to assess imminent violence are the Brøset Violence Checklist (BVC) (Almvik & Woods, 1998; Almvik et al., 2000) and the Dynamic Appraisal of Situational Aggression (DASA) (Ogloff & Daffern, 2002). The BVC consists of six items predictive of violence: confusion, irritability, boisterousness, physical threats, verbal threats, and attacks on objects. The DASA has a version for youth and a version for women. Other risk tools include the Hamilton Anatomy of Risk Management (Chaimowitz & Mamak, 2015); the Fordham Risk Screening Tool (Rosenfeld et al., 2017); the Imminent Risk Rating Scale (Starzomski & Wilson, 2015); and the Violence Risk Screening–10 (Hartvig et al., 2011).

Regardless of the assessment tools utilized, it is important that clients are engaged in the development of their risk management plan. Whether clients understand their own risk for violence informs risk assessment and rehabilitation. For example, if the client lacks insight into their personal risks (e.g., propensity for violence), this needs to be addressed within the risk assessment conducted by staff (Ray & Simson, 2019). There is now acknowledgment that risk assessment can be done by clients as well as by the clinician (Wagstaff, et al., 2018; van den Brink et al., 2015), and research supports that risk assessment can be developed from the perspective of the client (Wagstaff et al., 2018).

Some physiologic and behavioural cues to anger are listed in Table 19.3.

Analysis and Outcome Identification

The nurse analyzes all assessment data across the biologic, psychological, social, and spiritual domains to understand the dangers that the client's behaviour poses for self or others. Angry clients present practical concerns for nurses and other healthcare professionals, and the interplay of their unique biologic, psychological, social, and spiritual experiences must be taken into consideration to ensure the safety of the client and others in the client's environment. The most common nursing care foci for clients experiencing intense aggression include acute anxiety, impulsivity, injury risk, safety, self-harm risk, suicide risk, and violence risk. Outcomes of nursing interventions focus on aggression and violence control.

Table 19.3 Physiologic and Behavioural Cues to Anger

Internal Signs	External Signs
• Increased pulse, respirations, and blood pressure • Chills and shudders • Feeling hot • Prickly sensations • Numbness • Choking sensations • Nausea • Racing thoughts • Headache/pounding in head • Vertigo	• Increased muscle tone • Changes in body posture, finger pointing, clenched fists, hands on hips, arms folded across chest • Changes in facial expression (clenched jaw) • Changes to the eyes: eyebrows lower and drawn together, eyelids tense, eyes assume a "hard" appearance, may have unshed tears • Dilated nostrils • Lips pressed together to form a thin line, or in a square shape • Hands or body shake • Stamping/stomping feet • Pacing • Flushing or pallor • Goose bumps • Twitching • Sweating • Invades another person's personal space • Change in pitch of voice, change in rate of speech • Yelling, arguing, cursing, name-calling, sarcasm, challenging

Planning and Implementing Interventions

This section emphasizes the development of a partnership between the nurse and client, who work together to find solutions to prevent the recurrence of explosive episodes and to de-escalate volatile situations. The plan of care identifies problems, risks, and strengths, and the interventions to address the needs of the client and is revised as the unique needs of the client change. However, sometimes the client's condition (e.g., advanced dementia, psychosis) or the situation prevents the development of a collaborative partnership. In such instances, the nurse must take the lead. The nurse who intervenes from within the context of the therapeutic relationship must be cognizant of the fit of a particular intervention and act accordingly. The nurse's action is based on their response to the client. The client's affective, behavioural, and cognitive response to the intervention provides information about its effects and guides the nurse's next response (Shajani & Snell, 2019). The bio/psycho/social/spiritual interventions for clients with aggression are summarized in Figure 19.4.

The following assumptions are important to consider in planning interventions with this client population:

• Anger is a normal and universal emotion. All people have the right and responsibility to express their

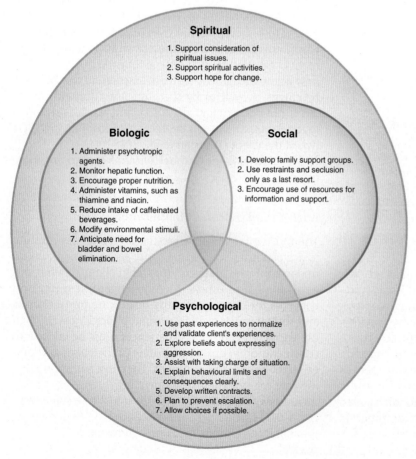

Figure 19.4 Interventions for clients with aggression.

anger in a way that does not, emotionally or physically, threaten or harm others.

- The safety of clients, staff, and others is a priority.
- The nurse and client collaborate to find solutions and alternatives to aggression and violence.
- In most instances, the person who is aggressive or violent can assume responsibility for their behaviour.
- The nurse views the client from the perspective of acknowledging that the client has solved problems before and is only temporarily in need of help.
- The nurse understands that norms for behaviour are created within the context of a particular environment and are influenced by the client's history, capacities, and culture.

Nurses who work collaboratively with potentially violent clients must also keep in mind that they can take certain actions to minimize personal risk:

- Using nonthreatening body language
- Respecting the client's personal space and boundaries

- Positioning themselves so that they have immediate access to the door of the room in case they need to leave
- Choosing to leave the office or examination room door open while talking to a client
- Knowing where colleagues are and making sure those colleagues know where the nurse is
- Removing or not wearing clothing or accessories that could be used to harm them, such as lanyards, scarves, necklaces, or dangling earrings
- Wearing a personal alarm (which is dependent on the clinical setting)
- Informing another staff member you are meeting with a client

When a violent outburst appears imminent or occurs, immediate intervention is required and should be directed by a designated leader. Healthcare facilities will have protocols that outline leader designation and the crisis response process (see Box "Emergency"). It is

EMERGENCY

Guidelines for Crisis Response to Threatening or Violent Client Behaviour

1. Clear the immediate area of other people. Maintain a safe distance from the person in crisis.
2. Call for staff assistance and/or use your personal alarm as designated in unit policy. Avoid engaging with the client until other team members are present. If possible to do so safely, remove objects that may be used as a weapon or may impede movement during a team response.
3. Brief responders and designated team leader on the status of the client, the situation preceding the threatening or violent behaviour, and any action that has been taken.
4. With the team leader, plan intervention, including specific staff roles in the intervention. For example, one staff is designated to communicate with the client during the crisis.
5. Communication should be respectful, precise, and succinct. Speak slowly and calmly.
6. Responders should remove any items from their persons that may cause injury (e.g., watches, pens, pagers, jewelry, mobile phones).
7. The crisis response leader should speak with the client and make the response team's presence evident. The primary goal is to defuse the situation, prevent harm, and promote safety for everyone.
8. The options for intervention depend on the client's mental status, risks, and response. Here are some examples:
   - Calm the client verbally.
   - Direct the client to a safe area (e.g., client's room, the comfort room).
   - Invite the client to talk with a clinician.
   - Prompt the client to use the sensory room.
   - Offer PRN medication.
   - Guide the client in a relaxation exercise or a grounding exercise.
   - Engage the client in diversion activities.
     The client may be offered a choice of these options by the one staff who is the designated communicator with the client. If the client continues to be at risk for harm to others, it may be necessary to consider the use of restraint (physical, mechanical, seclusion, chemical) as a last resort.
9. The team debriefs about the crisis incident. Medical and/or supervisory staff are informed as necessary. A report of the crisis incident is recorded.
10. During the crisis response planning, other staff may be delegated to plan and take action for the safety and wellbeing of other clients and visitors.
11. After the incident, a debriefing is conducted with the client when appropriate.
12. After the incident, a debriefing may be conducted with the client's family/significant other, if appropriate.
13. After the incident, a debriefing is conducted with other select clients, visitors, and learners as appropriate.

each nurse's responsibility to be knowledgeable about the process and policy in their institution so that an informed, coordinated team response can occur.

Nurses who work with potentially aggressive clients do so with respect and concern. The goal is to work collaboratively with clients and cocreate solutions. The nurse approaches these clients calmly, using nonthreatening body language and taking care not to invade the client's personal space boundaries. In dealing with aggression, as in other aspects of nursing practice, the nurse will find that at times the best intervention is silence. It is easy to equate intervention with activity, the sense that "I must do something." But quiet calmness and presence on the nurse's part may be enough to help a client regain control of their behaviour and perspective on the situation.

Trying to clarify what has upset the client is important. The nurse can use therapeutic communication techniques to prevent a crisis or defuse a critical situation (see Box 19.5). During interactions with clients, nurses can intervene in many creative and useful ways. The intervention alone does not serve as the solution; it is the process or art of offering the intervention within the context of the nurse–client relationship that is successful. These interventions will not be successful with all clients all the time. However, it is not the nurse or client's fault when an intervention is ineffective. The intervention simply did not fit the situation at that time.

Biologic Domain

Biologic Assessment

Biologic assessment examines how biologic factors may interact and influence human behaviour. The nurse may encounter clients whose aggressive tendencies have been exacerbated by a biochemical imbalance. However, nurses must recognize that biologic alterations

BOX 19.5 THERAPEUTIC DIALOGUE

The Potentially Aggressive Client

Uli is a 23-year-old client in the high observation area of an inpatient unit. He looks angry and is pacing back and forth. He is pounding one fist into his other hand. In the past 24 h, Uli has been more cooperative and less agitated. The behaviour the nurse observes now is more like the behaviour that he displayed 2 days ago. Yesterday, the psychiatrist told Uli that he would be granted more freedom in the unit if his behaviour improved. The psychiatrist has just seen Uli and refused to change the restrictions on Uli's activities.

Ineffective Approach

Nurse: Uli, I can understand this is frustrating for you.
Uli: How can you understand? Have you ever been held like a prisoner?
Nurse: I do understand Uli. Now you must calm down or more privileges will be removed.
Uli: (voice gets louder, speech is more rapid) But I was told that calm behaviour would mean more privileges. Now you are telling me calm behaviour only gets me what I have got! Can't you talk to the doctor for me?
Nurse: No, Uli. I can't talk to the doctor. The decision is made and you are going to have to work on calming down. (Uli appears more frustrated and angry as the conversation continues.)

Effective Approach

Nurse: Uli, you look upset (observation). I would like to help. What happened in your conversation with the psychiatrist? (seeking information).

Uli: Yesterday, he said calmer behaviour would mean more freedom in the unit. I have tried to be calm and not to swear. You said you noticed the difference. But today, he says "no" to more freedom.
Nurse: Some people might feel disappointed and angry if this happened to them (validation). Is that how you feel?
Uli: Yeah, I feel really cheated. Nothing I do makes a difference. That's the way it is in here and that's the way it is when I am out of the hospital.
Nurse: Sounds like this experience is making you feel powerless (validation).
Uli: I don't have any power, anywhere. Sometimes when I have no power, I get mean. At least then people pay attention to me.
Nurse: In this situation with your doctor, what would help you feel that you had some power? (Inviting client partnership).
Uli: Well, if he would listen to me, if he would read my chart.
Nurse: I am a bit confused by the psychiatrist's decision. I cannot promise that your privileges will change, but would it be okay with you if I talk with him and set up a time for us to meet together?
Uli: That would make me feel like someone is on my side.

CRITICAL THINKING CHALLENGE
- In the first scenario, how did the nurse escalate the situation?
- Compare the first and second scenarios. How are they different? How was the nurse effective in the second scenario?

are neither necessary nor sufficient to account for most aggressive behaviours. In taking the client's history, the nurse listens for evidence of industrial exposure to toxic chemicals, missed doses of medications, alcohol intoxication, substance use withdrawal, or premenstrual dysphoric disorder. Similarly, a history of even minor structural changes, resulting in trauma, haemorrhage, or tumour, may contribute to lowering a client's anger threshold and thus requires investigation.

Sensory Impairment

Communication is an issue for clients who experience sensory impairments because such a disability can negatively affect an individual's physical and mental health. The most common impairments are hearing loss and reduced visual acuity, but sensory impairment can also include loss of smell, taste, and touch. If clients cannot provide information about their hearing and vision, the nurse should ask a family member or friend. If there are any sensory impairments, the nurse should ensure that any sensory augmenting aids, devices, or equipment are accessible and in working order. Impairment of one or more of an individual's senses can be challenging and may interfere with their ability to interact with their environment. Individuals with a diagnosis of autism spectrum disorder may experience challenges with social interaction, speech, and nonverbal communication, which may be experienced as over- or undersensitivity to sensory information, which in turn may influence their emotions or behaviour.

Interventions for the Biologic Domain

Administering and Monitoring Medications

When there is a change in the client's behaviour, such as an increase in aggression, medications should be reviewed and evaluated. Several classes of drugs are used in the management of aggressive behaviour. A common effect of some medications is sedation, which may contribute to risks for falls and disorientation. Important points for the nurse to consider in making decisions about client and family teaching, medication administration, and consultation with physicians and pharmacists are as follows:

* Evidence supports the use of *atypical antipsychotics*, such as clozapine (Clozaril), risperidone (Risperdal), and olanzapine (Zyprexa), in reducing agitation (Caine, 2006; Jensen & Clough, 2016). Extrapyramidal side effects are few, which makes these drugs easier to tolerate than the typical antipsychotics.
* *Benzodiazepines* (e.g., lorazepam [Ativan]) for acute agitation, which can be administered orally, sublingually, intramuscularly, or intravenously (Jensen & Clough, 2016).
* *Selective serotonin reuptake inhibitors* (e.g., fluoxetine [Prozac], paroxetine [Paxil]) are increasingly being used for their antiaggressive effects, as well as for their

antidepressant effects. Their effects on aggressive behaviour usually occur before their effects on depression.
* *β-Adrenergic receptor blockers*, such as propranolol (Inderal), have been reported in one systematic review to have some effect in reducing hostility and aggression (Victoroff et al., 2014).
* *Lithium carbonate* has been effective in treating aggressive behaviour associated with brain injury (Burke et al., 2002).
* *Divalproex sodium* and *carbamazepine, oxcarbazepine, and phenytoin* have been shown to reduce aggressive behaviour in some studies (Huband et al., 2010).
* The liver metabolizes most psychotropic drugs (except lithium). The nurse should be alert to possible hepatic dysfunction in clients with a history of alcohol or drug abuse.

A systematic review and meta-analysis of 53 randomized controlled trials (i.e., whereby groups of subjects instead of individual subjects are randomized) addressing pharmacological interventions for agitated aggressive behaviours found the most effective and safe drugs for rapid tranquilization were olanzapine, haloperidol, and droperidol (Bak et al., 2019).

When there is a change in the client's behaviour, such as an increase in aggression, medications should be reviewed and evaluated as a possible contributing factor.

Managing Nutrition

The interest in the relationship between nutrition and mental health continues to grow because of the significant influence of these factors on a person's health. For example, prolonged use of alcohol can result in thiamine deficiency, which in turn can lead to increased irritability, disorientation, and paranoia (Horton et al., 2015). The complex relationship between the brain, the gut microbiome, and the immune system and how they are connected to human behaviour is an emerging science (Deans, 2016; Firth et al., 2020; Sylvia & Demas, 2018). Current research is investigating the modulating processes between the gut microbiome and the regulation of emotions in the brain. It is known that the gut and the brain are linked through neurotransmitters. For example, serotonin, which affects a person's sleep, appetite, mood, and pain, is largely produced in the gastrointestinal tract. Further research is needed to illuminate the relationships between nutrition, the microbiome, the immune system, the brain, and behaviour before the clinical implications will be known.

Psychological Domain

Psychological Assessment

The nurse interested in working with clients to prevent and manage aggressive and violent behaviours should observe and monitor these clients for disturbances in thought processing. Assessment can be accomplished by listening to the client's story, validating and exploring their beliefs. Clients may have disordered thoughts for various reasons, including associated psychiatric diagnoses. Some common diagnostic categories that the nurse needs to assess for in the client's history are major depressive episode, bipolar disorder, delusional disorders, posttraumatic stress disorder, schizophrenia, and depersonalization. The nurse should also assess for a history or current use of substances because clients who misuse drugs, alcohol, or solvents may also exhibit disordered thought processing. Intoxication can trigger erratic thought processes and unpredicted violence. Some form of thought disorder may remain after a person is detoxified and may become a permanent feature of the person's way of processing ideas. In addition, the nurse must look for acute and chronic medical conditions, such as brain tumour, encephalitis, electrolyte imbalance, and hepatic failure, which may also alter thought processing. The thought processes of greatest interest to the nurse in assessing a client's potential for aggression and violence are perceptions and delusions.

Perception

Perception is awareness of events and sensations and the ability to make distinctions between them. Clients with disordered perceptions may misinterpret objects or events. Such misperception is called an *illusion*. For example, a client may assume that a person walking towards them is going to strike out and thus they act to defend against this illusionary foe. The nurse can explore a client's perception by asking such questions as, "I noticed you were looking overly cautious as I approached you. I wondered what you were thinking."

Delusions

Clients may maintain false or unreasonable beliefs, known as delusions, despite attempts to dissuade them from their point of view. The nurse may not notice any abnormalities in the client's behaviour or appearance until the client begins to discuss delusional ideas. Delusions may cause or contribute to aggressive or violent behaviour. To explore and evaluate these false beliefs, the nurse could, with the client's consent, ask questions respectfully about how these beliefs affect the person's life. The nurse should match the pacing of such questions to the client's responses. Attempts to challenge or dissuade the client from their beliefs are usually ineffective. See Chapters 11 and 21 for further information on delusions and their assessment.

Interventions for the Psychological Domain

Psychological interventions help clients gain control over their expression of anger and aggressive behaviour.

In some instances, these interventions eliminate the need for chemical (medications) or mechanical restraints. De-escalating potential aggression is always preferable to challenging or provoking a client.

Affective Interventions

Affective interventions are designed to reduce or increase intense emotions that may hinder the client from finding alternatives to the use of aggression or violence (Shajani & Snell, 2019). They include using the client's own words, restating feelings, paraphrasing, validating, listening to the client's story, exploring beliefs, and summarizing.

Validating

Clients who experience intense anger and rage can feel isolated. The nurse can reduce the client's feelings of isolation by listening, being present, and acknowledging these intense feelings. By drawing on experience with other clients, the nurse can also reassure the client that others have felt the same way.

Listening to the Client's Illness Experience

Often, clients and their family members are invited to provide details about past medical treatments, medications, hospitalizations, and therapies. The patient and/or family needs to know you are present, you are listening, and you understand their story. Sometimes the experience of the health problem or the experience of interactions with professionals or other clients has involved anger, aggression, or violence. Inviting clients and families to talk about their experience with the healthcare system may highlight their values, concerns, strengths, and recommendations for improvement. A strategy to begin the conversation might be to say to the patient and family, "Tell me what is important to you." See Box "Clinical Vignette: Tracee's Rage" for an example of how a nurse uses this intervention to improve a client's care.

Exploring Beliefs

Exploring the client's beliefs about the expression of angry feelings can be useful. Discussing beliefs that prevent clients from seeking alternate ways of handling distressing emotions and situations may help them to take charge of the situation.

Cognitive Interventions

Cognitive interventions are usually those that provide new ideas, opinions, information, or education about a particular problem. The nurse offers a cognitive intervention with the goal of inviting the client to consider other possibilities (Shajani & Snell, 2019).

CLINICAL VIGNETTE

TRACEE'S RAGE

Tracee, a 22-year-old single woman, was a regular client at the crisis centre. During previous visits, she came alone or with her mother and demanded immediate attention. This time she comes with her mother. The receptionist groans and rolls her eyes as she describes this family to the new intake nurse. "They are so obnoxious. It is best to handle them fast and get them out of here!"

Before the interview, the nurse reviews Tracee's extensive file. She notes that on many occasions Tracee was aggressive and violent while in the centre. The mother has complained to the local health authority about the centre on at least two occasions.

During the interview, the nurse asks the mother and daughter the following questions:

- What was the most useful thing that has happened during previous visits at the centre?
- What was the least useful thing about previous visits at the centre?
- If you are anxious or upset, how would I recognize it? What could I do to help?
- Is there something you would like to talk about when you come to the centre?

The family looks surprised to be asked these questions. They state that previous visits were useful only in providing them with written proof that Tracee could not work. This information was required by the social service agency and ensured continuation of Tracee's disability status (and financial support). Furthermore, Tracee and her mother state that they often left the centre feeling that the nurses were not interested in their concerns and believed that if Tracee tried harder, her auditory hallucinations would decrease. They also said that they often waited 1 to 2 h to be seen, whereas other clients were seen more quickly. Tracee admits that she sometimes made a lot of noise in the waiting room so she would be seen sooner.

The nurse then asks, "What would need to happen during your visit today to make you feel that coming here was worthwhile?" The mother expresses interest in receiving information about hallucinations and how she could help Tracee when she experiences them. Tracee says she wants to know how to handle angry feelings.

After the client and her mother leave the centre, the nurse meets with the receptionist to develop an approach for the next time Tracee comes to the centre.

Examples include giving commendations, offering information, and providing education.

Giving Commendations

A commendation focuses on the client's behaviour pattern over time and highlights their strengths and resources (Limacher & Wright, 2003, 2006). For example, commending a client's decision to request medication or to remove themselves from an overstimulating environment highlights the person's ability to assume responsibility for thoughts and feelings that have previously precipitated aggressive behaviour.

Offering Information

Nurses can offer information or arrange opportunities for clients to receive information from other professionals. Clients may sometimes become anxious, frightened, and overwhelmed with negative emotions and threaten to harm the nurse because they do not know what is expected of them or they do not remember why they need to be in treatment. The nurse can orient them about unit expectations or the reasons for their hospitalization. The nurse can also determine the client's information needs by asking questions. One option in providing information, education, and support is to connect the client to a peer support worker or a family support group, which can provide a forum for responding to general concerns and questions.

In the mental health setting, the nurse must make behavioural limits and consequences clear to the client. When possible, the nurse should match consequences to the client's interests and desires and make sure that the client is aware of and understands these consequences.

Providing Education

Nurses can offer education to clients and families about various topics, including assertive communication, coping strategies for negative emotions, anger management, and strategies to control aggressive behaviours. Greater understanding about mental health problems and altered mental status may help to prevent conflict and aggression by clarifying misunderstandings. Effective use of debriefing techniques after a crisis can give nurses and clients insights into ineffective coping and promote client learning with strategies for future behavioural change.

Behavioural Interventions

Behavioural interventions are designed to assist the client to behave differently (Shajani & Snell, 2019). Examples of such interventions include assigning behavioural tasks, using bibliotherapy, interrupting patterns, and providing choices.

Assigning Behavioural Tasks

Sometimes, the nurse may assign a behavioural task to help the client maintain or regain control over aggressive behaviours. Behavioural tasks might include writing down a list of grievances that the client will discuss with the nurse or observing how other people take charge of anger and aggression. For example, the nurse may ask the client to observe others on the unit, people in the community, or movies or television shows to evaluate how other people in real or fictitious situations manage anger.

Using Bibliotherapy

In bibliotherapy, books, articles, and/or audiovisual materials are used as therapeutic tools. The nurse refers the client to a particular reference and then checks with the client to discuss their impression of the ideas and information provided by it. A client might be referred to an article on anger management and then discuss it with the nurse as they consider whether any of the ideas they read might be used to address their anger.

Interrupting Patterns

Although clients are not usually aware of it, escalation of feelings, thoughts, and behaviour from calmness to violence usually follows a particular pattern. Disruption of the pattern can sometimes be a useful means for preventing escalation and can help the client regain composure and regulate emotions. Nurses can suggest several strategies to interrupt patterns:

- Counting to 10 or using a mantra (sacred name repetition)
- Removing oneself from interactions or stimuli that may contribute to increased distress
- Doing something different (e.g., reading, exercising, gardening, watching television, etc.)

Providing Choices

When possible, the nurse should provide the client with choices, particularly clients who have little control over their situation because of their condition. For example, the client who is experiencing a manic episode and is asked to stay in their room may have few options in their daily schedule. However, they may be allowed to make choices about food, personal hygiene, clothing, and personal activities.

Social Domain

Social Assessment

The nurse should evaluate factors related to the social domain that may be contributing to anger, aggression, or violence in a client. For example, are conditions in the client's home, family, or community leading to aggression or violent episodes? Are school, employment, financial, or legal troubles placing stress on the client that puts them at risk?

Interventions for the Social Domain

Reducing Stimulation

Normally, people adjust their environments to suit their needs: some people seek out the thrill of high-risk sports; others prefer to be spectators.

People whose perceptions or thoughts are disordered from an acquired brain injury, degeneration, or other thought-processing difficulties may be experiencing intense and highly confusing stimulation, even though the environment—from the nurse or family's perspective—is calm and orderly. Considering the environment from the client's viewpoint is essential. Modification of the environment may be one of the main interventions. Introducing more structure into a chaotic environment can enhance the client's sense of safety and decrease the risk for aggressive behaviour (Citrome, 2015). The nurse can make stimuli meaningful or simplify and interpret the environment in many practical ways, such as by identifying people or equipment that may be unfamiliar, providing cues as to what is expected (e.g., using a white board in the patient's room with the assigned nurse's name or photo, and the agenda for the day, posting signs, putting toothbrush and toothpaste by the sink), and removing or silencing unnecessary stimuli (e.g., turning off paging systems, radio, television, etc.).

Anticipating Needs

The nurse can anticipate many needs of clients. In assuming responsibility for clients with cognitive impairment, the nurse needs to know the client's story and information such as when the client last voided and their bowel pattern. Regular toileting routines are not just interventions to prevent incontinence. Similarly, the anticipation of basic needs such as safety, comfort, thirst, hunger, and freedom from pain is important, especially when working with adults or children who cannot readily express their needs. Other needs can arise from situations such as allergic reactions, medication side effects, and adverse drug reactions.

The urge to void can be a powerful stimulus contributing to agitated behaviour. It is not uncommon in a neurologic unit to see a person with a recent head injury become violent just before spontaneously voiding. From a biologic perspective, such a client is probably normally sensitive to a full bladder. They may have sufficient cognitive function to recognize their need to void. Even some level of social inhibition may be operational in that they recognize that voiding while lying on their back in bed, with strangers around, is inappropriate. But if they cannot speak or ask for help, they may become increasingly distressed. Thrashing around in bed, unable to communicate their needs, they may strike out at staff.

Using Restraint and Seclusion

The World Health Organization (2019) is concerned about the use of restraints. The use of any type of physical, mechanical, or chemical **restraint**, including seclusion, is controversial. These coercive interventions must be used judiciously and only when other interventions have failed to safely manage a client's behaviour. Different types of restraints have the potential to cause physical and emotional trauma and contribute to negative health outcomes, even death. The successful use of psychotropic medications since the 1950s has reduced the use of seclusion and physical restraint to interventions of last resort. Reasons cited for using these interventions are to protect the client from injury to self or others, to help the client re-establish behavioural control, and to minimize disruption of unit milieu. The controversy surrounding these interventions and their potential to be applied punitively heightens the need for clear institutional standards for their use. The development and use of clear practice standards can reduce the likelihood that such interventions will be misused (College of Registered Psychiatric Nurses of British Columbia, 2015).

If restraint is used, the nurse must anticipate and be aware of the risks and how to mitigate them.

The Registered Nurses' Association of Ontario (2012) developed best practice guidelines for using restrains. This guideline, "Promoting Safety: Alternative Approaches to the Use of Restraints," highlights the important role of nurses in the prevention, assessment, and application of alternative strategies, safety, de-escalation, debriefing, organizational culture, and quality improvement.

Restraint reduction programs are common. For example, the "Six Core Strategies" program focuses on cultural change at the individual and organizational levels, specifically: (a) leadership towards organizational change; (b) full inclusion of lived experience; (c) using data to inform practice; (d) workforce development; (e) use of seclusion and restraint reduction tools; and (f) debriefing (Huckshorn, 2006). Adoption and implementation of this model across a number of countries and across a number of service sectors has been successful in reducing restraint (Duxbury et al., 2019; Goulet et al., 2017; Hernandez et al., 2017; Huckshorn, 2014; LeBel et al., 2014; Riahi et al., 2016). A study of clients' experiences before, during, and after seclusion and restraint found that client/carer communication was drastically affected and not viewed as therapeutic (Ling et al., 2015). In a modified interpretive phenomenological study, Holmes and colleagues (2015) reported that both patients and nurses indicated that maintaining a good therapeutic relationship was key to seclusion being therapeutic, as a last resort measure. A scoping review by Goulet et al. (2017) indicated that both clients and clinicians need to be involved in a postseclusion and/or restraint review to promote reflection and learning. Fletcher and colleagues (2021) report on patient and staff perspectives on causes of violence and aggression in Box 19.7.

BOX 19.7 Research for Best Practice

COMPARISON OF PATIENTS AND STAFF PERSPECTIVES ON CAUSES OF VIOLENCE AND AGGRESSION

Fletcher, A., Crowe, M., Manuel, J., & Foulds, J. (2021). Comparison of patients' and staff's perspectives on the causes of violence and aggression in psychiatric inpatient settings: An integrative review. *Journal of Psychiatric & Mental Health Nursing, 28,* 924–939. https://doi.org/10.1111/jpm.12758

Proposal: To compare perspectives of inpatients and staff on causes of aggression and violence in a mental health setting because it may contribute to a better understanding of how best to prevent and manage these types of events.

Method: An integrative review of the literature was undertaken and thirty articles met the inclusion criteria. A research synthesis framework was used so that qualitative and quantitative data could be integrated. This method involved data reduction, data display, data comparison, conclusion drawing, and verification.

Results: The perspectives of patients and staff differed on causes of aggression and violence and were influenced by factors within the culture of the inpatient unit. Patients identified disrespect, coercion, boredom, and lack of privacy as part of an inpatient culture that contributed to aggression and violence.

Conclusions and Implications for Practice: Inpatient culture was identified as a contributing cause of aggression and violence. The interpersonal skills of staff were identified as influencing interactions with clients and potentially contributing to aggression and violence. Acknowledging how the culture of the inpatient setting influences collaboration in the interactional dynamics between clients and staff may help to decrease aggression and violence in these settings.

Evaluation is important in the use of seclusion and restraint. The Canadian Institute for Health Information (2011) reported that between 2006 and 2010 nearly one in four patients admitted to the Ontario mental health system had one or more forms of control intervention. Furthermore, within this large group, 21% had physical/mechanical restraint and 20% experienced seclusion. On inpatient units, the monitoring of restraints as part of a primary prevention approach for restraint reduction should also include such strategies as building staff skills and teamwork, promoting relationship-based care, using consultation, and making physical design safer (Johnson, 2010). More recently, Blair and colleagues (2017) found that utilizing evidence-based therapeutic practices for reducing violence and aggression (i.e., routine use of the Brøset Violence Checklist, mandatory education in crisis intervention and trauma-informed care, increased frequency of physician reassessment of need for seclusion and restraint, and formal administrative review of events, and environmental enhancements [e.g., comfort rooms to support sensory modulation]) resulted in statistically significant decreases in both the number of seclusions and the duration of seclusion per admission in an inpatient psychiatric setting.

Spiritual Domain

In addressing the spiritual domain of care for the client who is experiencing anger and aggression, contemplative practices, such as mindfulness, may be valuable to the client and nurse. **Mindfulness** is being fully attentive in the "here and now" moment (Marlatt & Kristeller, 1999). The process of paying attention (without judgment) to what is happening can promote a connection to a person's inner being and spirit. Acknowledging the present moment of reality is the beginning of transforming that reality (Kabat-Zinn, 1993). Mindfulness is like meditation: awareness of breathing and of the body is central to it. It is about acting with attentiveness and concentration as one walks, eats, looks about, and carries out activities of daily living. It is being consciously aware of our body and mind, rather than thinking "about" experience (Sherman & Siporin, 2008). This meditative act can bring a sense of calmness within minutes.

Mindfulness can be found within most religious and spiritual traditions (Sherman & Siporin, 2008). It is a way for a person to recognize a connection with something beyond themselves, to realize that they are not separate nor alone, to experience serenity, and to search for meaning and purpose (Ponte & Koppel, 2015). Shapiro (2008), who researches mindfulness, finds that individuals "often find their faith is deepened as a result of becoming more mindful" (p. 3).

Mindfulness in health literature, however, is most often discussed as a cognitive behavioural technique. This practice tends to utilize a brief, structured format called mindfulness-based stress reduction (MBSR). MBSR programs, initially designed by Kabat-Zinn (1990, 1994), involve three basic techniques: meditation, body scan (involves directing one's attention through the entire body), and yoga. In addition to the resource of healthcare team members trained to teach mindfulness to clients, there are local community programs and scores of educational tools—books, videos, and apps—that are available to learn about this contemplative practice. In a systematic review of mindfulness interventions for clients with psychosis, Aust and Bradshaw (2017) concluded that mindfulness-based therapies can be safely used with clients experiencing psychosis, providing a number of therapeutic benefits with routine care.

Utilizing mindfulness techniques may contribute to client safety by enhancing the nurses' attentiveness and their ability to identify conditions—including their own patterns of thinking and awareness—when addressing anger in the clinician–client/family relationship. Lown (2007) notes that mindfulness in such an encounter allows one to be both a participant and an observer. In taking a moment to assess one's own response to the situation (e.g., anxiety, anger) and to focus on being present in a genuine way to the client/family member, the nurse is better able to respond to the situation (Ponte & Koppel, 2015).

Interactional Processes

When nurses develop collaborative relationships with clients, they can assist the clients to stop exhibiting aggressive behaviour. A review of the research regarding factors affecting violence on psychiatric units showed that violence is influenced by complex interactions among clients, staff, and unit culture (Hamrin et al., 2009). For instance, a qualitative study of experienced mental health nurses found that participants identified workplace stressors (e.g., poor staffing skill mix, inadequate workplace design, and unsupported involuntary admissions) as contributing to increased pressure, fear, and uncertainty on units (Ward, 2013). A positive culture has appropriate levels of stimulation and meaningful client activities, as well as positive staff attitudes and values towards client care. Good assessment of client factors, including history of violence, plays an important role. Therapeutic relationship strategies, including being available, being a client advocate, providing client education, and collaborating with the client in treatment planning, can decrease the potential for violence. "Listening deeply rather than jumping into action is often a more effective way to acknowledge and meet another person's needs" (Ponte & Koppel, 2015, p. 51).

The skills the nurse uses in interactions with the client may invite escalation or de-escalation of a tense situation. When the nurse uses communication skills to draw out the client's experience, together the nurse and client coevolve an alternative view of the problem. Some nursing authors (Leahey & Harper-Jaques, 1996; Shajani & Snell, 2019) have highlighted the importance of attending to notions of reciprocity and circularity when providing nursing care. For example, the nurse explores the meaning of the expression of aggressive behaviours with the client and the client's beliefs about the ability to control aggressive impulses. Or, the nurse and client could discuss the effects of the nurse's behaviours on the client and the effects of the client's behaviours on the nurse. Such an approach facilitates the development of an accepting and collaborative nurse–client relationship. The client is a partner invited to assume responsibility for inappropriate actions. This approach contrasts with the hierarchical nurse–client relationship that emphasizes the nurse's role in controlling the client's behaviours and defining the changes the client must make. In a collaborative approach, the nurse values the client's experience and acknowledges their strengths. The nurse asks the client to use those strengths to either maintain or resume control of behaviour.

In Western cultures, events are typically thought of in a linear fashion (Shajani & Snell, 2019). The nurse who uses a linear causality frame of reference to think about client aggression and violence will view the problem as follows:

PACING → leads to → THREATENING BEHAVIOURS
(Event A)   (Event B)

From this linear perspective, the nurse labels the client as the problem, and all other factors assume secondary importance. The nurse might decide, first, to gain control over the client's behaviour. The nurse may base this decision on their affective response and previous experiences (e.g., that threatening behaviours frighten other clients and disrupt the unit routine). The nurse's response to a client's behaviour could be to ask the client to stop yelling, to inform the client that the behaviour is inappropriate, or to suggest the use of medication if the client does not calm down. When one thinks based on linear causality, they assume that event A (pacing) causes event B (threatening behaviour).

When one thinks using circular causality, there is an attempt to understand the link between behaviours and to determine how the threatening behaviour will influence the continuation or cessation of pacing. The nurse who engages in circular thinking will also know that their responses to the client will influence the situation. The nurse's responses will be in the domains of cognition (ideas, concepts, and beliefs), affect (emotional state), and behaviour. The nurse will be aware of the reciprocal influences of the nurse and client's behaviours (Shajani & Snell, 2019). In viewing the situation from a circular perspective, the nurse is interested in understanding how people are involved, rather than in

discovering who is to blame. This perspective does not ignore individual responsibility for aggressive or violent actions, nor does it blame the victim. It does invite the nurse to consider the multiple influences on the expression of aggressive and violent behaviour.

Responding to Assault

Trauma can be experienced by both clients and clinical staff. They can witness anger, aggression, and violence or they may participate in it. For nurses, trauma can lead to moral distress, burnout, and compassion fatigue. High rates of trauma are found in individuals with mental health issues (Anderson et al., 2016). Trauma can lead to poor health outcomes and potentially people may be re-traumatized. Trauma- and violence-informed care (TVIC) is an approach to care that acknowledges past, recent, and current trauma and violence, and its effects on peoples' physical and mental health and the culture of the organization (Government of Canada, 2018).

In recent years, compelling scientific evidence that violence portrayed in the media is harmful to children has fostered debate about violence and its effects. As a result, television networks have taken voluntary and legislated actions to limit violent programming during hours when children are watching programs. However, these gains in limiting access to violence have been countered by the growing availability of violent videogames and websites, and the increasing influence of social media, which can include a vast array of aggressive and violent content and imagery.

Violence in healthcare settings threatens the safety of staff, clients, family members, and visitors, yet it remains an underreported problem. Proximity to clients by healthcare staff presents a higher risk to experience acts of violence, and nurses are the most frequent victims (Phillips, 2016).

Research shows that the incidence and severity of violence directed towards nurses are on the rise including physical violence (e.g., biting, kicking, slapping, punching) and verbal and psychological violence (e.g., abusive language, rudeness, harassment, intimidation, bullying, threatening behaviours) (CNA, 2019; Luck et al., 2006). Reported violence may be higher in long-term care, emergency departments, and psychiatric facilities (CNA, 2019), but nurses who work in ambulatory care settings or community clinics are not immune to assault (Gerberich et al., 2004). Refer further to Chapter 17.

Variations in statistics can result from differences in definitions of violence, reporting practices, data collection and analysis, and underreporting. Rationale for underreporting is common and includes time constraints, staff attitudes, conflict between the traditional caring role and reporting the violence, belief that an individual will be blamed or perceived as inadequate, minimization of the event by the nurses involved or by their colleagues, lack of visible injuries, and lack of understanding in the importance of data collection (Munro, 2002). The WHO (2014) reported on the status of violence prevention strategies in 133 countries and called for a scaling up of violence prevention programs, stronger legislation, and enforcement of laws relevant for violence prevention, and enhanced services for victims of violence. In 2019, The Canadian Nurses Association prepared a brief for the Standing Committee on Health, with the primary recommendation that the federal government lead a pan-Canadian strategy to determine why workplace violence continues to be an issue, why initiatives continue to have limited success, and to more clearly define the language of workplace violence, to allow for comparisons of data.

Reports of inpatient violence tend to be exclusively from the staff's perspective. Although data indicate one third of incidents are unprovoked, it may be that staff are not recognizing or not recording the antecedents of an incident. Clients' experiences need to be captured if the scope of antecedents is to be better understood (Bowers et al., 2011).

Assaults on nurses by clients can have immediate and long-term consequences. Reported assaults range from verbal threats and minor altercations to severe injuries, rape, and murder. Any assault can produce severe consequences for the victim. Nonphysical violence towards nurses by clients or others can have long-lasting effects on nurses, such as posttraumatic stress disorder (Gerberich et al., 2005).

Lanza's research (Lanza, 1992) indicates that nurses experience a wide range of responses (Table 19.4) like those of victims of any other type of trauma. However,

because of their role as caregivers, nurses may suppress the normal range of feelings after an assault, believing that it is wrong to experience strong feelings of anger and fear in this situation. This belief may relate to the conflict nurses experience in having to care for clients who have hurt them.

Steps can be taken at clinical and management levels to reduce the risk for assaults on nurses by clients. A nursing-based framework that identifies three staff factors that are important to conflict reduction in inpatient psychiatric units is the city model (Björkdahl et al., 2013; Bowers, 2009). These factors are positive appreciation of clients (i.e., psychological understanding of difficult behaviour promoted; humanistic values), self-regulation of emotional responses (i.e., awareness and control of feelings), and effective structure of rules and routine (i.e., teamwork, organizational support, clarity of rules, teamwork). This model aims to use less coercive strategies and to reduce conflict and containment (Bowers et al., 2011). Bowers (2014) introduced the Safewards Model and identified six factors that contribute to conflict (behaviours that potentially result in harm) and containment (e.g., restraint, sedating medication) within mental health wards. This model aims to promote a safer healthcare environment for clients and workers and has at its core staff and patient modifiers, originating domains, flash points, conflict, and containment. Ten interventions were developed: clear mutual expectations; soft words; talk down; positive words; bad news mitigation; know each other; mutual help meeting; calm down methods; reassurance; and discharge messages (Bowers, 2014; Bowers et al., 2014). The Safewards Model is a popular approach globally, and evidence of

Table 19.4	Nurses' Responses to Assault	
Response Type	Personal	Professional
Affective	• Irritability • Depression • Anger • Anxiety • Fear • Helplessness • Apathy	• Erosion of feelings of competence, leading to increased anxiety and fear • Feelings of guilt or self-blame • Fear of potentially violent clients
Cognitive	• Suppressed or intrusive thoughts of assault • Reduced concentration	• Reduced confidence in judgment • Consideration of job change
Behavioural	• Social withdrawal	• Possible hesitation or avoidance in responding to other violent situations • Possible overcontrolling • Possible hesitation to report future assaults • Possible withdrawal from colleagues • Not wanting to work with certain clients • Questioning of capabilities by coworkers
Physiologic	• Changes in sleep • Headaches • Stomach/body aches • Muscle tension • Changes in appetite	• Increased absenteeism because of somatic complaints

its effectiveness continues to emerge, including a study by Bowers et al. (2015) that utilized a cluster randomized controlled trial.

Nurses must be provided with training programs in prevention and management of aggressive behaviour. These programs, akin to courses on cardiopulmonary resuscitation (CPR), impart both knowledge and skill and should be made available to nurses and students so that they have opportunities to practice and regularly update what they have learned. It is assumed that nurses who have participated in preventive training programs are more likely to effectively manage and reduce aggressive or violent situations. A systematic review concluded, however, that there is yet insufficient evidence to determine whether training for interventions such as de-escalation is effective and can improve safety (Price et al., 2015). Training programs need to address the complex interplay of factors related to violent client behaviour. Such training would inform staff about risk assessment, staff interactions, and unit milieu; how to use de-escalation techniques and breakaway techniques; and how to control, manage, and perform postassessment and documentation of an incident of violent patient behaviour (Björkdahl et al., 2013).

Evaluation and Treatment Outcomes

Treatment outcomes can be considered at both individual and aggregate levels. The desired outcome at the individual level is for the client to regain or maintain control over aggressive or potentially aggressive thoughts, feelings, and actions. The nurse may observe that the client shows decreased psychomotor activity, has a more relaxed posture, speaks more directly about feelings of anger and personal needs, requires less sedating medication, shows increased tolerance for frustration and the ability to consider alternatives, and makes effective use of other coping strategies. Evidence of a reduction in risk factors may include decreased noise and confusion in the immediate environment, good communication and calmness on the part of nurses and others, and a climate of clear expectations and mutual acceptance and respect. In units, day hospitals, or group home settings, indicators of positive treatment outcomes might be a reduction in the number and severity of assaults on staff and others, fewer incident reports, and increased staff competency in de-escalating potentially violent situations.

Continuum of Care

Anger and aggression occur in all settings. During periods of extreme aggression, in which people are a risk to themselves or others because of a mental disorder, they may be admitted to an acute psychiatric unit. Removing individuals from their community-based environment and hospitalizing them in a secure psychiatric unit provide safety until the aggressive behaviour dissipates.

Understanding of the phenomena of anger, aggression, and violence in the clinical setting is needed. Research studies that have illuminated this problem from a nursing perspective need to be continued and expanded. Specific areas of study need to examine the links among biology, neurology, and psychology. In addition, further explorations of the reciprocal influence of clients' interactional style and organizational culture will assist in the development and management of humane treatment settings. Research suggests that the very language nurses use may be deemed oppressive and violent (Alex et al., 2013). Finally, and perhaps most importantly, nurses must research the effectiveness of nursing interventions, apply these to practice, and then evaluate the approaches used.

🍁 Summary of Key Points

- Theories used to explain anger, aggression, and violence include the following types:
  - Neurobiologic, including the cognitive neuroassociation model, the neurostructural model, and the neurochemical model
  - Psychological, including psychoanalytic theories, behavioural theories, and cognitive theories
  - Sociocultural theories
  - Interactional theory
- Biologic factors to assess in clients who display aggression and violence, the exposure to toxic chemicals, medications, substance abuse, premenstrual dysphoric disorder, trauma, haemorrhage, and tumour.
- Biologic intervention choices include administering medications and managing nutrition.

- Psychological factors to assess in clients include thought processing and sensory impairment.
- Psychological intervention choices can be affective, cognitive, or behavioural.
- Social intervention choices include reducing stimulation, anticipating needs, and using restraints.
- Clinical judgment and reliable/validated assessment guides should be used to assess risk.
- Mindfulness can be a component of the spiritual domain of care; it is a contemplative practice that may be useful in dealing with anger and aggression.
- Client aggression and violence are serious concerns. Training and policies and procedures for prevention and management of aggression should be available in all clinical settings.

Thinking Challenge

You are supervising clients during mealtime when a client, a new admission to the unit, accuses another client of stealing their dessert. The dining room is noisy and other clients are becoming increasingly agitated. The two clients suddenly start yelling at each other over the dessert issue, and you fear that the interaction will escalate to a physical confrontation.

- How might a nurse intervene in this situation? What approaches should be adopted?

- What interventions could be utilized to de-escalate this situation?
- Could this situation have been prevented? Discuss.

> Visit the**Point** to view suggested responses.
> Go to **thePoint.lww.com/activate** and use the activation code found in the front of this text to unlock answers to the "Thinking Challenges" and other online resources.

Web Links

https://ageinc.ca/ Advanced Gerontological Education (AGE). (2021). Here you will find numerous educational resources including the *Gentle Persuasive Approaches (GPA)* https://ageinc.ca/?s=the+gentle+persuasive+approaches

https://albertaheatlhservices.ca Here you will find the *Restraint as a Last Resort Toolkit, Information for Health Professionals* https://www.albertahealthservices.ca/info/Page15702.aspx

https://cmha.ca/ Here you will find *Feeling angry*. Retrieved from https://cmha.ca/documents/feeling-angry

Canadian Nurses Association & Canadian Federation of Nurses Union. (2015). Workplace Violence. Retrieved from https://cna-aiic.ca/~/media/cna/page-content/pdf-en/workplace-violence-and-bullying_joint-position-statement.pdf?la=en

https://www.patientsafetyinstitute.ca/ Here you will find comprehensive documents on *Mental Health Care: Seclusion and Restraint; Mental Health Care: Diminishing Violence and Aggressive Behaviour; and Mental Health Care: An Introduction to Patient Safety Issues*

https://www.cdc.gov/ Here you will find a free interactive course for nurses—*Online Workplace Violence Prevention Course for Nurses* by the Centers for Disease Control and Prevention, and the National Institute for Occupation Safety and Health. See https://www.cdc.gov/niosh/topics/violence/training.html

https://www.crisisprevention.com/ Here you can access training by the Crisis Prevention Institute including verbal intervention, nonviolent crisis intervention, and nonviolent crisis intervention—advanced physical skills.

https://www.pshsa.ca/ Public Services Health & Safety Association *PSHSA Violence, Aggression & Responsive Behaviour (VARB) Project*. See https://www.pshsa.ca/news/pshsa-violence-aggression-responsive-behaviour-varb-project

https://www.nice.org.uk National Institute for Health and Care Excellence. Here you will find resources/guidelines on Violence and Aggression: Short-Term Management in Mental Health, Health and Community Settings. Retrieved from https://www.ncbi.nlm.nih.gov/books/NBK305020/pdf/Bookshelf_NBK305020.pdf

https://rnao.ca/ Registered Nurses' Association of Ontario. Here you will find a number of resources and best practice guidelines including *Preventing violence, harassment and bullying against health workers* now in its second edition. https://rnao.ca/bpg/guidelines/preventing-violence-harassment-and-bullying-against-health-workers

https://www.safewards.net Here you will find several resources for Safewards implementation.

https://www.who.int/teams/ *Violence Prevention*. Here you will find several documents related to the prevention of interpersonal violence https://www.who.int/teams/social-determinants-of-health/violence-prevention/ and preventing violence against healthcare workers https://www.who.int/activities/preventing-violence-against-health-workers

References

Alex, M., Whitty-Rogers, J., & Panagopoulos, W. (2013). The language of violence in mental health: Shifting the paradigm to the language of peace. *Advances in Nursing Science, 36*(3), 229–242. https://doi.org/10.1097/ANS.0b013e31829edcf3

Almvik, R., & Woods, P. (1998). The Brøset Violence Checklist (BVC) and the prediction of inpatient violence: Some preliminary results. *Psychiatric Care, 5*(6), 208–211.

Almvik, R., Woods, P., & Rasmussen, K. (2000). The Brøset violence checklist: Sensitivity, specificity, and interrater reliability. *Journal of Interpersonal Violence, 15*(12), 1284–1296. https://doi.org/10.1177/088626000015012003

Anderson, F., Howard, L., Dean, K., Moran, P., & Khalifeh, H. (2016). Childhood and treatment and adulthood domestic and sexual violence victimization among people with severe mental illness. *Social Psychiatry and Psychiatric Epidemiology, 51*, 961–970. https://doi.org/10.1007/s00127-016-1244-1

Asikainen, J., Vehviläinen-Julkunen, K., Repo-Tiihonen, E., & Louheranta, O. (2020). Violence factors and debriefing in psychiatric inpatient care: A review. *Journal of Psychosocial Nursing and Mental Health Services, 58*(5), 39–49. https://doi.org/10.3928/02793695-20200306-01

Aust, J., & Bradshaw, T. (2017). Mindfulness interventions for psychosis: A systematic review of the literature. *Journal of Psychiatric and Mental Health Nursing, 24*(1), 69–83. https://doi.org/https://doi.org/10.1111/jpm.12357

Bak, M., Weltens, I., Bervoets, C., DeFruy, J., Samochowiec, J., Fiorillo, A., Sampogna, G., Bienkowski, P., Preuss, W. U., Misiak, B., Frydecka, D., Samochowiec, A., Bak, E., Drukker, M., & Dom, G. (2019). The pharmacological management of agitated behaviour: A systematic review and meta-analysis. *European Psychiatry, 57*, 78–100. https://doi.org/10.1016/j.eurpsy.2019.01.014

Bandura, A. (1973). *Aggression: A social learning analysis*. Prentice-Hall.

Beck, A. T. (1976). *Cognitive therapy and emotional disorders*. International Universities Press.

Berkowitz, L. (2012). A different view of anger: The cognitive-neoassociation conception of the relation of anger to aggression. *Aggressive Behavior, 38*(4), 322–333. https://doi.org/10.1002/ab.21432

Bernstein, K. S., & Saladino, J. P. (2007). Clinical assessment and management of psychiatric patients' violent and aggressive behaviors in general hospital. *Medsurg Nursing, 16*(5), 301–309, 331.

Best, M., Williams, J. M., & Coccaro, E. F. (2002). Evidence for a dysfunctional prefrontal circuit in patients with an impulsive aggressive disorder. *Proceedings of the National Academy of Sciences of the*

United States of America, *99*(12), 8448–8453. https://doi.org/10.1073/pnas.112604099

Björkdahl, A., Hansebo, G., & Palmstierna, T. (2013). The influence of staff training on the violence prevention and management climate in psychiatric inpatient units. *Journal of Psychiatric and Mental Health Nursing*, *20*(5), 396–404. https://doi.org/10.1111/j.1365-2850.2012.01930.x

Blair, E. W., Woolley, S., Szarek, B. L., Mucha, T. F., Dutka, O., Schwartz, H. I., Wisniowski, J., & Goethe, J. W. (2017). Reduction of seclusion and restraint in an inpatient psychiatric setting: A pilot study. *Psychiatric Quarterly*, *88*(1), 1–7. https://doi.org/10.1007/s11126-016-9428-0

Bowers, L. (2009). Association between staff factors and levels of conflict and containment on acute psychiatric wards in England. *Psychiatric Services*, *60*(2), 231–239.

Bowers, L. (2014). Safewards: A new model of conflict and containment on psychiatric wards. *Journal of Psychiatric and Mental Health Nursing*, *21*(6), 499–508. https://doi.org/10.1111/jpm.12129

Bowers, L., Alexander, J., Bilgin, H., Botha, M., Dack, C., James, K., Jarret, M., Jeffery, D., Nijman, H., Owiti, J. A., Papdopulos, C., & Ross, J. (2014). Safewards: The empirical basis of the model and a critical appraisal. *Journal of Psychiatric and Mental Health Nursing*, *21*(4), 354–364.

Bowers, L., Allan, T., Simpson, A., Jones, J., Van Der Merwe, M., & Jeffery, D. (2009). Identifying key factors associated with aggression on acute inpatient psychiatric wards. *Issues in Mental Health Nursing*, *30*(4), 260–271. https://doi.org/10.1080/01612840802710829

Bowers, L., James, K., Quirk, A., Simpson, A., Stewart, D., & Hodsoll, J. (2015). Reducing conflict and containment rates on acute psychiatric wards: The Safewards cluster randomised controlled trial. *International Journal of Nursing Studies*, *52*(9), 1412–1422. https://doi.org/10.1016/j.ijnurstu.2015.05.001

Bowers, L., Stewart, D., Papadopoulos, C., Dack, C., Ross, J., Khanom, H., & Jeffery, D. (2011). *Inpatient violence and aggression: A literature review*. Report from the Conflict and Containment Reeducation Research Programme. Institute of Psychiatry, King's College London. https://www.kcl.ac.uk/ioppn/depts/hspr/archive/mhn/projects/litreview/LitRevAgg.pdf

Burke, J. D., Loeber, R., & Birmaher, B. (2002). Oppositional defiant disorder and conduct disorder: A review of the past 10 years, part II. *Journal of the American Academy of Child and Adolescent Psychiatry*, *41*(11), 1275–1293. https://doi.org/10.1097/00004583-200211000-00009

Caine, E. D. (2006). Clinical perspectives on atypical antipsychotics for treatment of agitation. *Journal of Clinical Psychiatry*, *67*(Suppl 10), 22–31. https://www.psychiatrist.com/read-pdf/2901/

Calvert, S. L., Appelbaum, M., Dodge, K. A., Graham, S., Nagayama Hall, G. C., Hamby, S., Fasig-Caldwell, L. G., Citkowicz, M., Galloway, D. P., & Hedges, L. V. (2017). The American Psychological Association Task Force assessment of violent video games: Science in the service of public interest. *American Psychologist*, *72*(2), 126–143. https://doi.org/10.1037/a0040413

Canadian Federation of Nurses Unions. (2020). *Mental disorder symptoms among nurse in Canada*. https://nursesunions.ca/wp-content/uploads/2020/06/OSI-REPORT_final.pdf

Canadian Nurses Association. (2019). *Violence faced by health-care workers in hospitals, long-term care facilities and in home care settings*. Brief prepared for the Standing Committee on Health. https://www.cna-aiic.ca/-/media/cna/page-content/pdf-en/2019-violence-faced-by-health-care-workers.pdf

Canadian Institute for Health Information. (2011). *Restraint use and other control interventions for mental health inpatients in Ontario*. https://secure.cihi.ca/free_products/Restraint_Use_and_Other_Control_Interventions_AIB_EN.pdf

Carlsson, G., Dahlberg, K., Ekebergh, M., & Dahlberg, H. (2006). Patients longing for authentic personal care: A phenomenological study of violent encounters in psychiatric settings. *Issues in Mental Health Nursing*, *27*(3), 287–305. https://doi.org/10.1080/01612840500502841

Citrome, L. (2015). *Aggression*. https://www.emedicine.com/Med/topic3005.htm

Chaimowitz, G. A., & Mamak, M. (2015). *Companion guide to the AIS and the HARM* (2nd ed.). St. Joseph's Healthcare Hamilton.

College of Registered Psychiatric Nurses of British Columbia. (2015). *Restraint & seclusion*. www.crpnbc.ca/practice-support/topics-in-depth/restraint-and-seclusion/

Cutcliffe, J. R., & Riahi, S. (2013a). Systemic perspective of violence and aggression in mental health care: Towards a more comprehensive understanding and conceptualization: Part 1. *International Journal of Mental Health Nursing*, *22*(6), 558–567. https://doi.org/10.1111/inm.12029

Cutcliffe, J. R., & Riahi, S. (2013b). Systemic perspective of violence and aggression in mental health care: Towards a more comprehensive understanding and conceptualization: Part 2. *International Journal of Mental Health Nursing*, *22*(6), 568–578. https://doi.org/10.1111/inm.12028

da Cunha-Bang, S., & Knudsen, G. M. (2021). The modulatory role of serotonin on human impulsive aggression. *Biological Psychiatry*. Open Access. https://doi.org/10.1016/j.biopsych.2021.05.016

David, D., Cotet, C., Matu, S., Mogoase, C., & Stefan, S. (2018). 50 years of rational-emotive and cognitive-behavioral therapy: A systematic review and meta-analysis. *Journal of Clinical Psychology*, *74*(3), 304–318. https://doi.org/10.1002/jclp.22514

Deans, E. (2016). Microbiome and mental health in the modern environment. *Journal of Physiological Anthropology*, *36*(1), 1. https://doi.org/10.1186/s40101-016-0101-y

DeAngelis, T. (2021). Mental illness and violence: Debunking myths, addressing realities. *Monitor on Psychology*, *52*(3), 31. https://www.apa.org/monitor/2021/04/ce-mental-illness

de Vries Robbé, M., & de Vogel, V. (2012). *SAPROF 2nd edition manual updated Research chapter*. Van der Hoeven Stichting.

DiGiuseppe, R., & Tafrate, R. (2007). *Understanding anger disorders*. Oxford University Press.

Douglas, K. S., Hart, S. D., Webster, C. D., & Belfrage, H. (2013). *HCR-20V3: Assessing risk of violence—User guide*. Mental Health, Law, and Policy Institute, Simon Fraser University.

Duke, A. A., Bègue, L., Bell, R., & Eisenlohr-Moul, T. (2013). Revisiting the serotonin-aggression relation in humans: A meta-analysis. *Psychological Bulletin*, *139*(5), 1148–1172. https://doi.org/10.1037/a0031544

Duxbury, J., Baker, J., Downe, S., Jones, F., Greenwood, P., Thygesen, H., McKeown, M., Price, O., Scholes, A., Thomson, G., Whittington, R. (2019). Minimising the use of physical restraint in acute mental health services: The outcome of a restraint reduction programme ('REsTRAIN YOURSELF'). *International Journal of Nursing Studies*, *95*, 40–48. https://doi.org/10.1016/j.ijnurstu.2019.03.016

Duxbury, J., & Whittington, R. (2005). Causes and management of patient aggression and violence: Staff and patient perspectives. *Journal of Advanced Nursing*, *50*(5), 469–478. https://doi.org/10.1111/j.1365-2648.2005.03426.x

Elbogen, E. B., & Johnson, S. C. (2009). The intricate link between violence and mental disorder: Results from the National Epidemiologic Survey on Alcohol and Related Conditions. *Archives of General Psychiatry*, *66*(2), 152–161. https://doi.org/10.1001/archgenpsychiatry.2008.537

Ellis, A. (1977). *Anger: How to live with and without it*. Citadel Press.

Ellis, A. (1995). Changing rational-emotive therapy (RET) to rational emotive behavior therapy (REBT). *Journal of Rational-Emotive and Cognitive-Behavior Therapy*, *13*(2), 85–89. https://doi.org/10.1007/BF02354453

Faucher, L., & Tappolet, C. (2008). *The modularity of emotions*. University of Calgary Press.

Firth, J., Gangwisch, J. E., Borisini, A., Wootton, R. E., & Mayer, E. A. (2020). Food and mood: How do diet and nutrition affect mental wellbeing? *BMJ*, *369*, m2382. https://doi.org/10.1136/bmj.m2382

Fletcher, A., Crowe, M., Manuel, J., & Foulds, J. (2021). Comparison of patients' and staff's perspectives on the causes of violence and aggression in psychiatric inpatient settings: An integrative review. *Journal of Psychiatric and Mental Health Nursing*, *28*, 924–939. https://doi.org/10.1111/jpm.12758

Freeman, A. J., Schumacher, J. A., & Coffey, S. F. (2015). Social desirability and partner agreement of men's reporting of intimate partner violence in substance abuse treatment settings. *Journal of Interpersonal Violence*, *30*(4), 565–579. https://doi.org/10.1177/0886260514535263

Friedman, R. A., & Michels, R. (2013). How should the psychiatric profession respond to the recent mass killings? *American Journal of Psychiatry*, *170*(5), 455–458. https://doi.org/10.1176/appi.ajp.2013.13010045

Fromm, E. (1973). *The anatomy of human destructiveness*. Holt, Rinehart and Winston.

Gerberich, S. G., Church, T. R., McGovern, P. M., Hansen, H. E., Nachreiner, N. M., Geisser, M. S., Ryan, A. D., Mongin, S. J., & Watt, G. D. (2004). An epidemiological study of the magnitude and consequences of work related violence: The Minnesota Nurses' Study. *Occupational and Environmental Medicine*, *61*(6), 495–503. https://doi.org/10.1136/oem.2003.007294

Gerberich, S. G., Church, T. R., McGovern, P. M., Hansen, H., Nachreiner, N. M., Geisser, M. S., Ryan, A. D., Mongin, S. J., Watt, G. D., & Jurek, A. (2005). Risk factors for work-related assaults on nurses. *Epidemiology*, *16*(5), 704–709. https://doi.org/10.1097/01.ede.0000164556.14509.a3

Goulet, H. H., Larue, C., & Dumais, A. (2017). Evaluation of seclusion and restraint reduction programs in mental health: A systematic review. *Aggression and Violent Behaviour*, *34*, 139–146. https://doi.org/10.1016/j.avb.2017.01.019

Gouveia, F. V., Hamani, C., Fonoff, E. T., Brentani, H., Alho, E. J. L., Borba de Morais, R. M. C., de Souza, A. L., Rigonatti, S. P., & Martinez, R. C. R. (2019). Amygdala and hypothalamus: Historical overview with focus on aggression. *Neurosurgery, 85*(1), 11–30. https://doi.org/10.1093/neuros/nyy635

Government of Canada. (2018). *Trauma and violence-informed approaches to policy and practice.* https://www.canada.ca/en/public-health/services/publications/health-risks-safety/trauma-violence-informed-approaches-policy-practice.html#s1

Hamrin, V., Iennaco, J., & Olsen, D. (2009). A review of ecological factors affecting inpatient psychiatric unit violence: Implications for relational and unit cultural improvements. *Issues in Mental Health Nursing, 30*(4), 214–226. https://doi.org/10.1080/01612840802701083

Harper-Jaques, S., & Reimer, M. (1992). Aggressive behavior and the brain: A different perspective for the mental health nurse. *Archives of Psychiatric Nursing, 6*(5), 312–320. https://doi.org/https://doi.org/10.1016/0883-9417(92)90043-I

Harris, D., & Morrison, E. F. (1995). Managing violence without coercion. *Archives of Psychiatric Nursing, 9*(4), 203–210. https://doi.org/10.1016/s0883-9417(95)80025-5

Hart, S. D., Douglas, K. S., & Guy, L. S. (2017). The structured professional judgement approach to violence risk assessment: Origins, nature, and advances. In D. P. Boer, A. R. Beech, T. Ward, L. A. Craig, M. Rettenberger, L. E. Marshall, & W. L. Marshall (Eds.), *The Wiley handbook on the theories, assessment, and treatment of sexual offending* (pp. 643–666). Wiley Blackwell.

Hartvig, P., Roaldset, J. O., Moger, T. A., Ostberg, V., & Bjorkly, S. (2011). The first step in the validation of a new screen for violence risk in acute psychiatry: The inpatient context. *European Psychiatry, 26*(2), 92–99. https://doi.org/10.1016/j.europsyl29010. 01.003

Hernandez, A., Riahi, S., Stuckey, M. I., Mildon, B. A., & Klassen, P. E. (2017). Multidimensional approach to restraint minimization: The journey of a specialized mental health organization. *International Journal of Mental Health Nursing, 26*(5), 482–490. https://doi.org/10.1111/inm.12379

Holmes, D., Murray, S. J., & Knack, N. (2015). Experiencing seclusion in a forensic psychiatric setting: A phenomenological study. *Journal of Forensic Nursing, 11*(4), 200–213. https://doi.org/10.5172/conu.2006.21.2.251

Horton, L., Duffy, T., Hollins Martin, C., & Martin, C. R. (2015). Comprehensive assessment of alcohol-related brain damage (ARBD): Gap or chasm in the evidence? *Journal of Psychiatric and Mental Health Nursing, 22*(1), 3–14. https://doi.org/https://doi.org/10.1111/jpm.12156

Huband, N., Ferriter, M., Nathan, R., & Jones, H. (2010). Antiepileptics for aggression and associated impulsivity. *Cochrane Database of Systematic Reviews, 2010*(2), CD003499. https://doi.org/10.1002/14651858.CD003499.pub3

Huckshorn, K. A. (2006). *Six core strategies for reducing seclusion and restraint use.* National Association of State Mental Health Program Directors.

Huckshorn, K. A. (2014). Reducing seclusion restraint use in inpatient settings a phenomenological study of state psychiatric hospital leader and staff experiences. *Journal of Psychosocial Nursing and Mental Health Services, 52,* 40–47. https://doi.org/10.3928/02793695-20141006-01

Jensen, L., & Clough, R. (2016). Assessing and treating the patient with acute psychotic disorders. *Nursing Clinics of North America, 51*(2), 185–197. https://doi.org/10.1016/j.cnur.2016.01.004

Johnson, M. E. (2010). Violence and restraint reduction efforts on inpatient psychiatric units. *Issues in Mental Health Nursing, 31*(3), 181–197. https://doi.org/10.3109/01612840903276704

Kabat-Zinn, J. (1990). *Full catastrophe living: Using the wisdom of your body and mind to face stress, pain, and illness.* Dell.

Kabat-Zinn, J. (1993). Mindfulness meditation: Health benefits of an ancient Buddhist practice. In D. Goleman & J. Gurin (Eds.), *Mind/body medicine* (pp. 259–276). Consumer Reports Books.

Kabat-Zinn, J. (1994). *Wherever you go, there you are: Mindfulness meditation in everyday life.* Hyperion.

Kassinove, H., & Tafrate, R. C. (2006). Anger-related disorders: Basic issues, models, and diagnostic considerations. In E. L. Feindler (Ed.), *Anger-related disorders: A Practitioner's guide to comparative treatments* (pp. 1–28). Springer.

Koh, K. B., Kim, D. K., Kim, S. Y., & Park, J. K. (2005). The relation between anger expression, depression, and somatic symptoms in depressive disorders and somatoform disorders. *Journal of Clinical Psychiatry, 66*(4), 485–491. https://doi.org/10.4088/jcp.v66n0411

Kornreich, C., Saeremans, M., Delwarte, J., Noël, X., Campanella, S., Verbanck, P., Ermer, E., & Brevers, D. (2016). Impaired non-verbal emotion processing in Pathological Gamblers. *Psychiatry Research, 236,* 125–129. https://doi.org/https://doi.org/10.1016/j.psychres.2015.12.020

Kurtz, M. M., Gagen, E., Rocha, N. B., Machado, S., & Penn, D. L. (2016). Comprehensive treatments for social cognitive deficits in schizophrenia: A critical review and effect-size analysis of controlled studies. *Clinical Psychology Review, 43,* 80–89. https://doi.org/10.1016/j.cpr.2015.09.003

Lanza, M. L. (1992). Nurses as patient assault victims: An update, synthesis, and recommendations. *Archives of Psychiatric Nursing, 6*(3), 163–171. https://doi.org/10.1016/0883-9417(92)90027-g

Latalova, K. (2014). Violence and duration of untreated psychosis in first-episode patients. *International Journal of Clinical Practice, 68*(3), 330–335. https://doi: 10.1111/ijcp.12327

Leahey, M., & Harper-Jaques, S. (1996). Family–nurse relationship: Core assumptions and clinical implications. *Journal of Family Nursing, 2*(2), 133–151. https://doi.org/10.1177/107484079600200203

Lebel, J., Duxbury, J., Putkonen, A., Sprague, T., Rae, C., & Sharpe, J. (2014). Multinational experiences in reducing and preventing the use of restraint and seclusion. *Journal of Psychosocial Nursing and Mental Health Services, 52*(11), 22–29. https://doi.org/10.3928/02793695-20140915-01

Limacher, L. H., & Wright, L. M. (2003). Commendations: Listening to the silent side of a family intervention. *Journal of Family Nursing, 9*(2), 130–150. https://doi.org/10.1177/1074840703009002002

Limacher, L. H., & Wright, L. M. (2006). Exploring the therapeutic family intervention of commendations: Insights from research. *Journal of Family Nursing, 12*(3), 307–331. https://doi.org/10.1177/1074840706291696

Ling, S., Cleverley, K., & Perivolaris, A. (2015). Understanding mental health service user experiences of restraint through debriefing: A qualitative analysis. *Canadian Journal of Psychiatry, 60*(9), 386–392. https://doi.org/10.1177/070674371506000903

Liu, J., Lewis, G., & Evans, L. (2013). Understanding aggressive behaviour across the lifespan. *Journal of Psychiatric and Mental Health Nursing, 20*(2), 156–168. https://doi.org/10.1111/j.1365-2850.2012.01902.x

Lown, B. A. (2007). Difficult conversations: Anger in the clinician-patient/family relationship. *Southern Medical Journal, 100*(1), 33–39. https://doi.org/10.1097/01.smj.0000223950.96273.61

Luck, L., Jackson, D., & Usher, K. (2006). Survival of the fittest, or socially constructed phenomena? Theoretical understandings of aggression & violence towards nurses. *Contemporary Nurse, 21*(2), 251–263. https://doi.org/10.5172/conu.2006.21.2.251

Marlatt, G. A., & Kristeller, J. L. (1999). Mindfulness and meditation. In W. R. Miller (Ed.), *Integrating spirituality into treatment.* American Psychological Association.

Morrison, E. F. (1998). The culture of caregiving and aggression in psychiatric settings. *Archives of Psychiatric Nursing, 12*(1), 21–31. https://doi.org/https://doi.org/10.1016/S0883-9417(98)80005-8

Munro, V. (2002). Why do nurses neglect to report violent incidents? *Nursing Times, 98*(17), 38–39. https://www.nursingtimes.net/archive/why-do-nurses-neglect-to-report-violent-incidents-23-04-2002/

National Institute for Health and Clinical Excellence. (2015). *Violence and aggression: Short-term management of in mental health, health and community settings* (NG 10). www.nice.org.uk/guidance/ng10

Novaco, R. (2007). Anger dysregulation. In T. Cavell & K. Malcolm (Eds.), *Anger, aggression, and interventions for interpersonal violence* (pp. 3–54). Lawrence Erlbaum Associates.

Novaco, R. W. (2017). Cognitive-behavioral factors and anger in the occurrence of aggression and violence. In P. Sturmey (Ed.), *International handbook of violence and aggression. volume 1. Definition, conception, and development.* John Wiley & Sons.

Ogloff, J., & Daffern, M. (2002). *Dynamic appraisal of situational aggression: In patient version.* Monash University and Forensicare. https://www.swinburne.edu.au/downloads/DASA-Sample.pdf

Ontario Ministry of Children, Community and Social Services. (2016). *Social learning, the media and violence.* http://www.children.gov.on.ca/htdocs/English/professionals/oyap/roots/volume5/chapter10_media_violence.aspx

Paris, J. (2005). Borderline personality disorder. *Canadian Medical Association Journal, 172*(12), 1579–1583. https://doi.org/10.1503/cmaj.045281

Phillips, J. P. (2016, Apr 28). Workplace violence against health care workers in the United States. *New England Journal of Medicine, 374*(17), 1661–1669. https://doi.org/10.1056/NEJMra1501998

Ponte, P. R., & Koppel, P. (2015). Cultivating mindfulness to enhance nursing practice. *American Journal of Nursing, 115*(6), 48–55. https://doi:10.1097/01.NAJ.0000466321.46439.17

Price, O., Baker, J., Bee, P., & Lovell, K. (2015). Learning and performance outcomes of mental health staff training in de-escalation techniques for the management of violence and aggression. *British Journal of Psychiatry, 206*(6), 447–455. https://doi.org/10.1192/bjp.bp.114.144576

Ray, I., & Simson, A. I. F. (2019). Shared risk formulation in forensic psychiatry. *Journal of the American Academy of Psychiatry and the Law, 47*(1). https://doi:10.29158/JAAPL.003813-19

Registered Nurses' Association of Ontario. (2012). *Promoting safety: Alternative approaches to the use of restraints.* https://rnao.ca/sites/rnao-ca/files/Promoting_Safety_-_Alternative_Approaches_to_the_Use_of_Restraints_0.pdf

Riahi, S., Thomson, G., & Duxbury, J. (2016). An integrative review exploring decision-making factors influencing mental health nurses in the use of restraint. *Journal of Psychiatric and Mental Health Nursing, 23*(2), 116–128. https://doi.org/10.1111/jpm.12285

Rosenfeld, B., Foellmi, M., Khadivi, A. Wijetunga, C., Howe, J., Nijdam-Jones, A., & Rotter, M., (2017). Determining when to conduct a violence risk assessment: Development and initial validation of the Fordham risk screening tool (FRST). *Law and Human Behavior, 41*(4), 325–332.

Shajani, Z., & Snell, D. (2019). *Wright and Leahy's nurses and families: A guide to family assessment and intervention* (7th ed.). F. A. Davis.

Shapiro, S. L. (2008). Exploring the effects of mindfulness meditation on health, well-being, and spirituality. *Spirituality in Higher Education, 4*(2), 1–5. https://spirituality.ucla.edu/docs/newsletters/4/Shapiro_Final.pdf

Sherman, E., & Siporin, M. (2008). Contemplative theory and practice for social work. *Journal of Religion & Spirituality in Social Work: Social Thought, 27*(3), 259–274. https://doi.org/10.1080/15426430802202179

Snyder, K., Schrepferman, L., Brooker, M., & Stoolmiller, M. (2007). The roles of anger, conflict with parents and peers, and social reinforcement in the early development of physical aggression. In T. Cavell & K. Malcolm (Eds.), *Anger, aggression, and interventions for interpersonal violence* (pp. 187–214). Lawrence Erlbaum Associates.

Soloff, P. H., Lynch, K. G., & Moss, H. B. (2000). Serotonin, impulsivity, and alcohol use disorders in the older adolescent: A psychobiological study. *Alcoholism, Clinical and Experimental Research, 24*(11), 1609–1619. https://doi.org/10.1111/j.1530-0277.2000.tb01961.x

Starzomski, A., & Wilson, K. (2015). Development of a measure to predict short term violence in psychiatric populations: The imminent risk rating scale. *Psychological Services, 12*(1), 1–8. https://doi.org/10.1037/a0037281

Stosny, S. (2019, February 15). Anger in the age of entitlement: Entitlement and anger go together. *Psychology Today.* https://www.psychologytoday.com/ca/blog/anger-in-the-age-entitlement/201902/anger-in-the-age-entitlement

Swanson, J. W. (2021). Introduction: Violence and mental illness. *Harvard Review of Psychiatry, 29*(1), 1–5. https://doi.org/10.1097/HRP.0000000000000281

Swanson, J. W., Swartz, M. S., Van Dorn, R. A., Elbogen, E. B., Wagner, H. R., Rosenheck, R. A., Stroup, T. S., McEvoy, J. P., & Lieberman, J. A. (2006). A national study of violent behavior in persons with schizophrenia. *Archives of General Psychiatry, 63*(5), 490–499. https://doi.org/10.1001/archpsyc.63.5.490

Sylvia, K. E., & Demas, G. E. (2018). A gut feeling: Microbiome-brain-immune interactions modulate social and affective behaviors. *Hormones and Behavior, 99,* 41–49. https://doi.org/10.1016/j.yhbeh.2018.02.001

Talerico, K. A., Evans, L. K., & Strumpf, N. E. (2002). Mental health correlates of aggression in nursing home residents with dementia. *Gerontologist, 42*(2), 169–177. https://doi.org/10.1093/geront/42.2.169

Teplin, L. A., McClelland, G. M., Abram, K. M., & Weiner, D. A. (2005). Crime victimization in adults with severe mental illness: Comparison with the National Crime Victimization Survey. *Archives of General Psychiatry, 62*(8), 911–921. https://doi.org/10.1001/archpsyc.62.8.911

Thomas, S. P. (1990). Theoretical and empirical perspectives on anger. *Issues in Mental Health Nursing, 11*(3), 203–216. https://doi.org/10.3109/01612849009014555

Thomas, S. P. (1993). *Women and anger.* Springer.

Thomas, S. P. (2001). Teaching healthy anger management. *Perspectives in Psychiatric Care, 37*(2), 41–48. https://doi.org/10.1111/j.1744-6163.2001.tb00617.x

Thomas, S. P. (2003). Men's anger: A phenomenological exploration of its meaning in a middle-class sample of American men. *Psychology of Men & Masculinity, 4*(2), 163–175. https://doi.org/10.1037/1524-9220.4.2.163

Thomas, S. P. (2005). Women's anger, aggression, and violence. *Health Care for Women International, 26*(6), 504–522. https://doi.org/10.1080/07399330590962636

Thomas, S. P. (2006). Culture and gender considerations in the assessment and treatment of anger-related disorders. In E. L. Feindler (Ed.), *Anger-related disorders: A practitioner's guide to comparative treatments* (pp. 71–96). Springer.

Thomas, S. P. (2009). *Transforming nurses' stress and anger: Steps toward healing* (3rd ed.). Springer.

Urheim, R., Palmstierna, T., Rypdal, K., Gjestad, R., Senneseth, M., & Mykletun, A. (2020). Violence rate dropped during a shift to individualized patient-oriented care in a high security forensic psychiatric ward. *BMC Psychiatry, 20*(1), 200. https://doi.org/10.1186/s12888-020-02524-0

Van den Brink, R. H. S., Troquete, N. A. C., Beintema, H., Mulder, T., van Os, T. W. D., Schoevers, R. A., & Wiersma, D. (2015). Risk assessment by client and case manager for shared decision making in outpatient forensic psychiatry. *BMC Psychiatry, 15,* 120. https://doi.org/10.1186/s12888-015-0500-3

Varshney, M., Mahapatra, A., Krishnan, V., Gupta, R., & Deb, K. S. (2016). Violence and mental illness: What is the true story? *Journal of Epidemiology and Community Health, 70*(3), 223–225. https://www.jstor.org/stable/44017698

Verona, E., & Sullivan, E. A. (2008). Emotional catharsis and aggression revisited: Heart rate reduction following aggressive responding. *Emotion, 8*(3), 331–340. https://doi.org/10.1037/1528-3542.8.3.331

Victoroff, J., Coburn, K., Reeve, A., Sampson, S., & Shillcutt, S. (2014). Pharmacological management of persistent hostility and aggression in persons with schizophrenia spectrum disorders: A systematic review. *Journal of Neuropsychiatry and Clinical Neurosciences, 26*(4), 283–312. https://doi.org/10.1176/appi.neuropsych.13110335

Wagstaff, C., Bom, J., Salkeld, R., & Felj, C. M. (2018). Developing risk assessments from the perspective of the patient: Case study report. *International Journal of Mental Health & Psychiatry, 4*(2). https://doi.org/10.4172/2471-4372.1000163

Ward, L. (2013). Ready, aim fire! Mental health nurses under siege in acute inpatient facilities. *Issues in Mental Health Nursing, 34*(4), 281–287. https://doi.org/10.3109/01612840.2012.742603

Webster, C. D., Martin, M. L., Brink, J., Nicholls, T. L., & Desmarais, S. (2009). *Manual for the short-term assessment of risk and treatability (START) (Version 1.1).* Forensic Psychiatric Services Commission and St. Joseph's Healthcare.

Webster, C. D., Nicholls, T. L., Martin, M. L., Desmarais, S. L., & Brink, J. (2006). Short-Term Assessment of Risk and Treatability (START): The case for a new structured professional judgment scheme. *Behavioral Sciences & the Law, 24*(6), 747–766. https://doi.org/10.1002/bsl.737

World Health Organization (n.d.). *Violence—A global public health problem.* Chapter 1. https://www.who.int/violence_injury_prevention/violence/world_report/en/chap1.pdf

World Health Organization. (2014). *Global status report on violence prevention 2014.* WHO Press. http://apps.who.int/iris/bitstream/10665/145086/1/9789241564793_eng.pdf?ua=1&ua=1

World Health Organization. (2019, June 30). *Strategies to end seclusion and restraint.* WHO Quality Rights Specialized training—Course Guide. https://www.who.int/publications/i/item/9789241516754

World Health Organization. (2021a). *Preventing violence against health workers.* https://www.who.int/activities/preventing-violence-against-health-workers

World Health Organization. (2021b). *Violence against women.* https://www.who.int/news-room/fact-sheets/detail/violence-against-women

20 Self-Harm and Suicidal Behaviours

Kristen Jones-Bonofiglio*

LEARNING OBJECTIVES

After studying this chapter, you will be able to:

- Define self-harm, suicidality, and suicide.
- Identify and debunk common myths about suicide.
- Describe specific population groups that are at high risk for self-harm and/or suicidal behaviours.
- Discuss the rights of individuals and other legal issues in the care of patients experiencing suicidality.
- Determine the nurse's role and responsibilities for comprehensive assessment, planning, intervention(s), evaluation, and discharge to the community.
- Identify risk factors, protective factors, and reasons for living (hope) related to suicide.
- Describe factors that increase the risk for suicide completion.
- Describe the nurse's role and responsibilities to promote short- and long-term recovery with patients who are suicidal, and their families, in various health care settings.
- Identify potential impacts on nurses and other health care practitioners when an individual dies by suicide.
- Identify current issues related to self-harm and suicidal behaviours, including compassion fatigue, burnout, moral distress, and moral injury.

KEY TERMS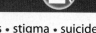

- parasuicide • self-harm behaviours • stigma • suicide attempt • suicidal behaviours • suicidal ideation • suicide intent • suicide plan • suicidality • suicide • survivors of suicide loss

KEY CONCEPTS

- helplessness • hopelessness • lethality • powerlessness • risk/rescue ratio

The spectrum of human behaviours that are understood as self-harm and suicidal occurs along a fluid and complex continuum of intent and self-destructiveness. This chapter provides nurses with evidence-based information, essential assessment skills, and responsive actions for their care of individuals, families, and communities. Studies that privilege knowledge from individuals with lived experiences of self-harm and suicide are highlighted here. Also explored are the effects of this phenomenon on nurses and requirements for self-care.

Common Myths

There are many myths about suicide that interfere with timely and effective care. Findings from an Australian study that surveyed over 3,000 adults showed that individuals most influenced by suicide myths include men

over age 60 and those speaking a language other than English at home (Nicholas et al., 2020). One common myth is that individuals who talk about suicide will not actually "go through with it" and are just seeking attention. Another myth is that there are never warning signs to "see it coming." Other common myths include that individuals exhibiting suicidal behaviours are weak, selfish, attention seeking, manipulative, or crazy. Additionally, there is a misconception that suicide is only an issue among youth. Further, there are beliefs that talking openly to individuals about suicide will cause them to engage in suicidal behaviours; talking about it will put ideas into their head. In fact, none of these myths are true. Suicidality is a symptom of experiencing intolerable distress and not a personal shortcoming. Suicide can be prevented and every conversation about self-harm and suicide is an opportunity. It is a privileged moment

---

*Adapted from the chapter "Self-Harm Behaviour and Suicide" by Elaine Santa Mina

when a nurse is able to engage in a therapeutic dialogue with an individual who is sharing thoughts about ending their life.

Definitions

Self-Harm Behaviours

Self-harm behaviours include self-inflicted, active destruction to body tissues such as cutting, preventing wound healing, head banging, biting, scratching, hitting, poisoning, overdose, burning, inserting objects under the skin, and hair pulling (Gillies et al., 2018). Self-harm is always a sign of psychological distress. Self-harm may also involve indirect, passive behaviours such as self-neglect, refusing food, and not taking prescribed medications (Wand et al., 2018). Some individuals engage in self-harm as a means to cope with suicidal thoughts. These behaviours can be suicidal, but the majority are described by the patient as nonsuicidal acts.

There is little consensus in self-harm terminology. These coping behaviours are also known as self-destructive, self-abuse, automutilation, deliberate self-harm, and nonsuicidal self-injury (NSSI). Individuals who engage in self-harm behaviour are at a higher risk to unintentionally die by suicide; therefore, all acts of self-harm must be taken seriously. **Parasuicide** is self-harm without an expressed intent to die, although death may still occur as an unanticipated outcome (Tzoneva, 2018).

Knowledge about motivations for self-harm behaviours remains incomplete. Thoughts about self-harm can stem from relational difficulties with self/other(s) and may serve as a mechanism to relieve intense negative emotions, such as loneliness, hate, and guilt (Gargiulo & Margherita, 2019). Such acts may produce a tangible, physical pain to substitute for unfamiliar or unbearable psychological suffering (Franklin & Nock, 2017). For some individuals, it can be described as a means of fighting for survival, rather than a wish to die (Roberts, 2018). Individuals may also utilize self-harm as a means of managing experiences of dissociation (Franklin & Nock, 2017; Hoyos et al., 2019). Further, some individuals describe self-harm as an addiction (like a fix with a subsequent high; experimental at first then increasing in frequency), as a release, as a means of control (over pain, to cope with difficult emotions), and as a punishment (Brown & Kimball, 2013). In a comparative study between German and American youth aged 14 to17 years, 25% of teenaged respondents reported that they had participated in NNSI, 9.5% had done so repetitively (more than four times), and 6.5% had made a suicide attempt (Plener et al., 2009). Individuals who self-harm report that they feel misunderstood and isolated due to stigma and the confusion between NSSI and suicidal acts (Brown & Kimball, 2013).

Self-harm behaviours may be an impulsive act or planned in advance. Self-harm may be a single event or repetitive in nature. Individuals may self-harm by one method only, for example, cutting, or multiple methods, for example, cutting and burning. Further, individuals who engage in self-harm may not openly acknowledge their behaviour because it tends to be considered socially unacceptable. Barriers to disclosure to others include shame and fear of judgment (Stirling, 2020). Individuals may not seek help nor come to the attention of health or social service providers; therefore, the prevalence of self-harm is likely to be seriously underestimated. When individuals do seek help, therapeutic responses by nurses can facilitate a positive disclosure experience and influence current as well as future help seeking opportunities (Rosenrot & Lewis, 2020).

Suicidal Ideation and Intent

Suicidal ideation comprises the thoughts, ideas, and feelings that a person experiences that are about wanting to die and/or the wish to permanently end severe emotional pain (Beck et al., 1997). Canada reports that almost 12% (of people surveyed) have thought about suicide in their lifetime, with 2.5% having considered suicide in the past year, and 4% having made actual plans to die (Government of Canada, 2020). **Suicidality** is a symptom and may be experienced in varying degrees of frequency (e.g., intermittent or continuous) and intensity. Suicidal thoughts may be nonintrusive or intrusive and may be related to triggers that can be anticipated. Suicidal thoughts can be expressed directly, indirectly, or not of spoken of at all. **Suicide intent** may be expressed through changes in behaviours, such as suddenly taking care of one's affairs: financial, belongings, and dependents. Sometimes, individuals leave messages about their intent to die by suicide or experiences of serious personal distress in a goodbye note or even a video broadcasting of the suicide event posted to their social media accounts (Behera et al., 2020).

Suicide Plan

An individual who is in enough distress to consider suicide may act impulsively and not plan it out in advance (such as someone under the influence of substances or having a sudden extreme emotional experience). Others may plan the suicide event in detail including the method, location, circumstance, and time. The **suicide plan** may emanate within cogent thought processes and resultant actions may be assessed to be voluntary in nature. Or it may be a component of a psychotic thought process from which the behavioural outcome may be assessed as involuntary, impulsive, and/or compulsive.

Suicidal Behaviours and Suicide

Suicidal behaviours are self-inflicted acts for which the dominant motivation is death. Some individuals describe this motivation as not being able to see a way to continue living while others express the desire to die. These behaviours are described by type (e.g., overdose, gunshot, asphyxiation, hanging), lethality (e.g., low or nonlethal to serious or fatal), and frequency (e.g., number of behaviours by type and how often or under what circumstances). The act of **suicide** is the self-termination of one's own life and was decriminalized in Canada in 1972 (Kellner & Marshall, 2016). In some countries, the act of suicide is still considered a criminal offense that may carry legal penalties for the individual and/or their family members (Shahrour et al., 2018). Suicide is associated with deep despair, overwhelm, and/or extreme distress and death is perceived to be a solution to life's problems.

Suicide Attempt

A **suicide attempt** is a self-destructive behaviour that did not result in death despite the expectation or intention that it would. Though the individual may receive help/support, hospitalization, and/or be grateful for such services, the intent to end one's life was present. This should always be taken seriously. Canada estimates that just over 3% of its population (over 15 years of age) have attempted suicide during their life (Government of Canada, 2020). Further, Canadian data estimate that for every completed suicide by a youth, there were 200 attempts; for every completed suicide among adults, there were 100 attempts; and for every death by suicide among older adults, there were 2 to 4 attempts (Centre for Suicide Prevention, n.d.). There are many complex dimensions associated with suicide that are grounded in an individual's perceptions, experiences of life, and specific factors that are known to put a person at risk to die by suicide.

Effects of Suicide

Stigma

Stigma is often deeply embedded in social and cultural contexts (Dardas & Simmons, 2015). The stigma of suicide can prevent people from openly voicing their suicidal thoughts and seeking help for problems and/or mental health. When a person survives a suicidal act, the visibility of medical intervention can trigger stigmatization by others. Stigma can be addressed in many ways, such as at individual, interpersonal, institutional, and population levels (Tam, 2019). Actions at any and all of these levels contribute to improving access and quality of resources and services. Pathways of stigma prevention include targeting the drivers, types, practices, and experiences (Tam, 2019). Drivers of stigma are stereotypes, colonialism, unfounded fears, inequity, and lack of awareness. Types of stigma are related to a person's identity (e.g., racialized, LGBTQI2SA+, age) and certain health issues

(e.g., HIV/AIDS, mental illness, addiction, obesity). Stigma promoting practices may include policies, behaviours, language, demeaning portrayals, avoidance, exclusion, bullying, and violence. Stigma experiences can be multiple and intersecting and may involve enacted stigma (personal experiences), internalized stigma, anticipated stigma, and secondary stigma (experiences of others). Nurses can demystify suicide and contribute to efforts to prevent the stigmatization of those at risk.

Survivors of Suicide Loss

Stigma may also be experienced by the **survivors of suicide loss**. Suicide affects all ages (e.g., children to older adults), all races and cultures, and all socioeconomic groups. Individuals, families, friends, communities, and cultural groups can be deeply affected by suicide, directly and indirectly. Every year there are approximately 800,000 deaths from suicide worldwide (World Health Organization [WHO], 2019a, 2019b), with each of those deaths having a network of survivors left behind. Prolonged suffering can be caused by the sudden shock, unanswered questions of "why," and potentially the discovery of the body. Nurses must ensure that their postvention responses to survivors of suicide are compassionate and nonjudgmental. Simple explanations, false reassurances, and clichés should be avoided. Survivors of suicide will need time and may require ongoing support to try to understand what has happened. As their personal search for meaning regarding the death transpires, their coping abilities will mediate their grief responses. Survivors may feel personally responsible for their loss, experience a sense of isolation, and may not seek support for their grief and bereavement. Suicide bereavement is different than that experienced by families whose loved one's death is not self-inflicted. Intense experiences of rejection, shame, guilt, anger, and abandonment are reported by loved ones left behind and this can lead to an increased risk of suicidal ideation and other mental health issues among survivors (Berardelli et al., 2020). Such complicated grieving is an individual experience that can be described as a nonlinear and evolving process that can sway from deep grieving to healing and back to grief again over a lifetime (Kaur & Stedmon, 2020).

Settings Where Nurses Work With People With Suicidality

Suicidality includes ideations, plans, high risk behaviours, and attempts of suicide and occurs across diverse healthcare settings. Some people believe that only nurses who work in mental health settings or emergency departments will care for individuals experiencing suicidality. However, human psychological and social distress may be found anywhere in society and hence anywhere in nursing practice. Many people struggle to know what to do when a patient, colleague, friend, loved one, or community experiences suicidality. It is essential that all nurses, regardless of their area of practice and expertise, be knowledgeable about self-harm and suicide, the risk and protective factors, and best practices for assessment and interventions for safety. Caring for individuals demonstrating self-harm and/or suicidal behaviours can be a challenging professional, as well as personal, experience for nurses as well as other health care professionals and first responders.

Economic Costs of Suicide

Suicide remains a significant global public health concern that places heavy demands on healthcare systems around the world despite efforts at both policy and clinical levels (e.g., to identify risk and protective factors, as well as to provide appropriate interventions). There are various economic costs for individuals, communities, provinces/states, and countries. However, accurately estimating the economic cost of suicide is difficult. Data have been gathered to calculate actual medical costs and potential for lost income and lost productivity to attempt to gauge the impact. In an American study that used data from 2013, the average cost of one suicide was estimated at over a million dollars (i.e., $1,329,553); with a total cost for all suicides and attempts during 2013 at $93.5 billion after adjustments were made to account for the underreporting of suicides (Shepard et al., 2016). Authors of this study indicate that there is a 6:1 benefit–cost ratio for investments in services and supports for individuals experiencing suicidality.

Prevention

September is national suicide prevention month in Canada. Nurses play an essential role in suicide prevention because they practice in diverse healthcare settings with individuals, families, and communities. Nurses are among the first frontline healthcare providers who come in contact with an individual experiencing self-harm and/or suicidal behaviours and are pivotal in making a difference in the outcome and preventing death. Due to this unique positioning, nurses are well aligned to contribute to preventive efforts, including raising awareness, early detection, and effective treatment. With knowledge of risk assessment and interventions—understood from a holistic perspective and applied within the context of an individual's family, social world, and broader community—as well as with knowledge of how to engage with and respond to the actively suicidal person, nurses can make a difference by preventing the escalation or chronicity of self-harm and suicidal behaviour. In a systematic review of studies across the past 40 years, Angelakis and colleagues (2020) suggest that suicide prevention therapies should be prioritized for high-risk groups of individuals (namely children and young people) who have experienced trauma in the form of abuse and/or neglect.

Canada's mental health strategy, *Changing Directions, Changing Lives*, contains a comprehensive suicide prevention strategy that cuts across six identified strategic directions (Mental Health Commission of Canada, 2012). These strategic directions include improving frontline practitioner suicide prevention training, supporting suicide awareness and prevention programs in schools and workplaces, decreasing the stigma associated with suicide, supporting the families of persons who are suicidal, improving screening for suicidality, supporting research about suicide and its causes, and addressing social factors like poverty that increase suicide risk for specific groups. In 2016, the Government of Canada released a report titled, *Working Together to Prevent Suicide in Canada: The Federal Framework for Suicide Prevention*. This document highlights three strategic objectives: (a) increasing public awareness/knowledge and decreasing stigma; (b) connecting people, resources, and information about suicide/prevention; and (c) accelerating research and innovation for suicide prevention. Additionally, the World Health Organization (2013) has suicide prevention as an integral component of its mental health action plan. Suicide prevention is possible with evidence-based, timely, and often low-cost options that require a comprehensive and multi-sectoral approach (WHO, 2019a). For example, community pharmacists can be a resource for individuals who are experiencing suicidality (Murphy et al., 2018). Refer to Box 20.1 for information about suicide prevention internationally.

Lived Experiences of Suicidality

Suicidal behaviours tend to be seen as "cries for help" rather than overt expressions of a desire to die. This may

BOX 20.1 Acknowledging Suicide in Our World

World Suicide Prevention Day is September 10th each year. See www.iasp.info to learn about activities for this year. Worldwide, there are an estimated 800,000 deaths by suicide annually; 1 person dies every 40 s (World Health Organization [WHO], 2020). Almost 80% of suicides globally occur in countries with households of low to middle income (WHO, 2019b). International Survivors of Suicide Loss Day is honoured every year on the Saturday before American Thanksgiving. See www.survivorday.org for more details.

be true for some and not for others. Often the lived experiences of past suicide attempt survivors are not fully considered. In an Australian study, 31 adult suicide attempt survivors were interviewed to gain an understanding of their complex experiences of disclosing suicidality before, during, or after attempts (Maple et al., 2020). When and how attempts were disclosed was dependent on both internal and external factors. Internally (within themselves), they described feeling hard to reach (by others) and struggling to find the words to explain their feelings and experiences, with online opportunities to share often being preferred. External factors included how others received their disclosures, such as feeling judged as attention seeking, stigmatized, or positively supported (Maple et al., 2020).

Epidemiology of Suicidal Behaviours

Global Rates of Suicidality

It is generally accepted that global prevalence rates of self-harm and suicide are underestimated and that numbers are not reported consistently. Death by suicide can be difficult to identify as it may be disguised an accident or have an ambiguous cause of death. Even with statistics that may underrepresent the scope of the problem, suicide is one of the leading causes of death worldwide (Ritchie et al., 2015). Further, suicide occurs across all age groups, social classes, and cultures. Approximately 1.4% of deaths in the world are due to suicide, with countries such as South Korea, Qatar, and Sri Lanka having the highest rates (Ritchie et al., 2015). Globally, suicide is a greater cause of death than breast cancer, malaria, or war and homicide combined (WHO, 2019b). It is estimated that for every completed suicide, there are more than 20 nonfatal suicide attempts (WHO, 2016). Every year, it is also estimated that over 160 million people experience suicidal thoughts (Canadian Mental Health Association [CMHA], 2020).

Canadian Data on Suicidality

Although exact statistics are difficult to track, Canada reports a national suicide rate of 11.5 per 100,000 people (Statistics Canada, 2017). Approximately 11 Canadians die by suicide each day; that is, approximately 4,000 deaths per year (Government of Canada, 2020). The age group with the highest rates of suicide in Canada are among those aged 40 to 59 (Statistics Canada, 2017). In 2018, 25,000 Canadians were hospitalized for suicidality, with 30% of those being women and 1 in 9 of those patients having 2 or more hospital stays in 1 year (Canadian Institute for Health Information [CIHI], 2020). In 2019, 2.5 % of Canadians reported that they had experienced suicidal thoughts over the past year with an increase to 6% during the COVID-19 pandemic

in 2020 (CMHA, 2020). The most common means of death by suicide in Canada are hanging, including strangulation and suffocation (44%; more often men), poisoning (25%; more often women), and firearms (16%; more often men) (Statistics Canada, 2017). Although more recent and reliable data are lacking on the full impact of suicide in Canada, it is recognized that self-harm and suicide attempts can result in physical injury and emotional, psychological, and social trauma, acute and lengthy hospitalization, and the need for ongoing community care.

Regional Variations in Canada

Provincial statistics show varied rates of suicide across Canada (see Table 20.1). Urban centres tend to have suicide rates lower than the national average. Northern, rural, and remote areas have some of the highest mortality rates from suicide in Canada. Higher suicide rates may be due to a combination of factors. Many people in these regions live where hunting (and ready access to firearms) is common; social isolation can occur due to geography (low population per square kilometre) and extreme weather conditions; inequities in access to health and social services; and high unemployment rates.

Suicidality and Specific Populations

Suicide is more common among groups with specific risk factors, such as grief and loss, unemployment, transience, recent stressful life events (e.g., financial problems, divorce, moving), family dysfunction, interpersonal distress, mental illness, substance use (e.g., alcohol), and previous attempts. Research indicates

Table 20.1 Canadian Suicide Statistics	
Province/Territory	Suicide Rate[a]
Alberta	15.2 (647 deaths)
British Columbia	11.6 (572 deaths)
Manitoba	16.3 (217 deaths)
New Brunswick	13.0 (100 deaths)
Newfoundland and Labrador	18.5 (98 deaths)
Northwest Territories	30.3 (n/a)
Nova Scotia	14.5 (138 deaths)
Nunavut	66.6 (25 deaths)
Ontario	5.6 (403 deaths)
PEI	16.3 (12 deaths)
Quebec	12.6 (1045 deaths)
Saskatchewan	16.2 (187 deaths)
Yukon	30.3 (12 deaths)
National average	10.4

[a]Per 100,000 people; 2017 data (Canadian Centre for Suicide Prevention, 2020).

Understanding and preventing suicide is a priority within the Canadian Armed Forces (CAF). Retired Lieutenant-General Romeo Dallaire reminds us that, as Canadians, we have a shared responsibility to our veterans: to care for them and not consider mental illness, such as posttraumatic stress disorder (PTSD; see Chapter 18) as simply an individual's problem (Dallaire & Humphreys, 2016). An expert panel on suicide prevention was held in 2016 to address suicide in the CAF (Sareen et al., 2018). Findings include that an average of 16.6 deaths by suicide occur annually, despite having mental health services for service members that exceeds what is available for the general Canadian population. Suicide was acknowledged as a phenomenon that is hard to accurately predict. Eleven recommendations were provided to improve suicide prevention in the CAF, namely: (a) create the role of Canadian Forces Health System Suicide Prevention Quality Improvement Coordinator; (b) conduct a systematic annual review of all CAF suicides since 2010 (approximately 100 deaths); (c) conduct a needs assessment and then targeted training for suicide assessment and safety planning training; (d) conduct a needs assessment and then offer training to CAF clinicians for suicide-specific psychosocial interventions; (e) adopt and implement follow-up communication (e.g., with cell phone) with CAF members after a mental health crisis; (f) screen for mental health issues and suicidality at recruitment/enlistment, pre-deployment, and post-deployment; (g) create a support group and strategies to better support transition to civilian life; (h) offer concurrent treatment options, for mental health and addictions, and train clinicians on this type of integrated approach; (i) improve access to evidence-based treatments for CAF members; (j) work collaboratively with the CPA to encourage safe reporting of suicide in the media; and (k) create a patient and family advisory committee to provide input into assessments, treatments, design of mental health services, and suicide prevention.

that, universally, suicide is strongly associated with mood disorders, mainly depression (Ritchie et al., 2015), and most specifically with a pervasive sense of despair and hopelessness. A strong predictor for suicide is a previous attempt. See Box 20.2 for a discussion of suicide and individuals in the Canadian military.

Age

Children

Suicide is rare among children who are younger than 10 years of age, although it does occur. However, suicides by children may be significantly underestimated, as many question whether children can fully understand the finality of death and therefore unintentionally kill themselves. In an Australian study of over 1,000 children aged 8 to 12 years, predictors of self-harm behaviours included frequent bullying, recent alcohol use, and persistent symptoms of anxiety or depression (Borschmann et al., 2020). Among children aged 10 to 14 years, suicide is actually the leading cause of death (Children First Canada, University of Calgary, & Alberta Children's Hospital, 2020). Children can experience helplessness and hopelessness that leads to suicidality due to experiences such as poverty, food insecurity, abuse/trauma, bullying, mental health issues, and family problems (Carpenter, 2020).

According to recent Canadian statistics of children, 1 in 3 is not experiencing a happy, safe, and healthy childhood; 1 in 3 will experience abuse before turning 15 years of age; and 1 in 5 lives experiencing poverty (Children First Canada, University of Calgary, & Alberta Children's Hospital, 2020).

Adolescents/Youth

Self-harm and suicidal behaviours are a growing concern among youth. More teenagers die from suicide than from cancer, heart disease, birth defects, stroke, pneumonia, influenza, and chronic lung disease combined. In Canada, suicide is the second leading cause of death for youths, age 15 to 24 years (Children First Canada, University of Calgary, & Alberta Children's Hospital, 2020; Stewart et al., 2020). In a recent study conducted in the United Kingdom, 16-year-olds were assessed for suicidality and those most at risk to attempt suicide included individuals who had been exposed to other's self-harm behaviours, had a diagnosed psychiatric disorder, were young women, expressed hopelessness, had a lower IQ, had lower conscientiousness, had higher impulsivity, were high intensity seeking, described body dissatisfaction, and/or were substance involved (Mars et al., 2019).

Adolescents are, generally, at risk for body image concerns, identity issues, and peer pressure. Those with histories of childhood abuse and/or trauma, mental health issues, and those in contact with law enforcement are at an especially high risk for self-destructive behaviours (Nofziger & Callanan, 2016). Further, youth who are presently or formerly engaged with child protective services and child welfare systems are also at greater risk (Brown, 2020). Self-harm and suicide in youth has been linked to personality traits such as impulsivity, aggression, and compulsivity. Prevalence of self-harm behaviours tends to peak in the teen years (current data from a Swedish study suggests 40% of youth participated in NSSI), but many do not continue these behaviours into adulthood (Daukantaité et al., 2021). NSSI is associated with being a stronger predictor for a future suicide attempt than a past suicide attempt (Asarnow et al., 2011). In a prospective cohort study in England, NSSI was correlated with a significantly increased risk for a subsequent suicide (Bergen, Hawton, Waters, et al., 2012; Bergen, Hawton, Ness, et al., 2012).

Midlife Adults

As age increases, suicide rates as a cause of death within the overall age group decline, which is indicative of an increase in pathologic deaths occurring from cancers, heart attacks, and chronic diseases. Canada, however, reports that 1/3 of all deaths by suicide are among people aged 45 to 59 (Government of Canada, 2020). Single people in this age group have double the suicide rates of other age groups. Income is a factor in suicide, as data show that 7% of suicide attempts occurred among the lowest income bracket versus 3% in the highest income bracket (Centre for Suicide Prevention, n.d.).

Older Adults

Although other causes of death are more prominent among older adults, suicide risk is also high. In fact, individuals aged 65 years and older (especially men) have the highest rates of death by suicide (suicide completion) when compared to every other age group in Canada and the United States (Centre for Suicide Prevention, n.d.). Contributing factors to suicide in this age group may include life transitions (grief and loss experiences) and health challenges associated with aging. Substance use is another factor, often under recognized among older adults (Suicide Prevention Resource Center, 2008). Further, suicide risk factors for older adult are associated with less education, widowhood, previous attempts, depressive disorders, financial difficulties, poor physical health and functioning, and loss of autonomy (Heisel & Duberstein, 2017). Finally, many older adults live alone, which makes social isolation another contributing factor as well as a reason that a suicide attempt may result in death because of a reduced possibility of discovery and potential for rescue.

Black Indigenous People of Colour

Black People and People of Colour

Many research studies represent statistics and lived realities of majority populations of non-Hispanic white/ White people in mainly Western contexts. It is important for nurses to educate themselves above and beyond this evidence, as People of Colour (POC) represent more than 1/5 of the Canadian population (Catalyst, 2020). Further, visible underrepresented groups regularly face the added stressors of anticipating and receiving racial and/or ethnic discrimination and bias in their daily encounters. For example, a British study of over 20,000 individuals (aged 16 to 64 years) found the highest rates of self-harm among women who are Black aged 16 to 34 years (Cooper et al., 2010). In this study, minority ethnic groups and people who are Black were less likely to receive proper mental health assessment and less likely return for help with self-harm behaviours. This is an example of structural inequities in care and highlights opportunities for improvement and needed change.

A critical gap in the suicide literature has been identified as the statistically significant increase in rates of suicide among children who are Black, aged 5 to 12 years (Opara et al., 2020). The majority of research has focused on youth who are White, so there are additional, unique risk factors to consider for youth who are Black, as well as culturally appropriate approaches and interventions to explore. However, it is equally important for nurses not to assume that statistics among visible underrepresented groups always have a negative connotation. For example, rates of self-harm behaviours and suicide attempts among people who are Canadian immigrants have been found to be much lower than among the general Canadian population and long-term residents (Centre for Suicide Prevention, n.d.; Saunders et al., 2019).

Indigenous Peoples

"I am here today because my ancestors, starving as they often were, fought to survive. Why did the old people strive to live … and the young people now want to die?" (Nishnawbe Aski Nation Youth, 2004). In Iqaluit, Nunavut, a collaborative workshop was held to share knowledge about suicide and youth who are Inuit and aged 12 to 19 years (Tan et al., 2015). The Inuit word for suicide (*ingminiirniq*) translates to "people who have done it to themselves" and among some groups of Inuit people it is referred to as "cutting off life" (Tan et al., 2015, p. 33). Historically, Inuit people would undertake suicide as an act of self-sacrifice for the greater good of the community if they felt that they were a burden, and this act could be condoned by the collective. However, present-day suicide is very different, and there are generational challenges in understanding and reconciling past and present-day perspectives on suicide. The workshop highlighted cultural norms such as not showing an emotional response as a hallmark of appropriate behaviour for people who are Inuit. Thus, the paradox of allowing youth to express and process their emotions related to suicide and the need to uphold culturally valued behaviour in the community was revealed (Tan et al., 2015).

Suicide disproportionately affects Indigenous Peoples and their communities in Canada. From 2011 to 2016, the reported rate of suicide among First Nations Peoples was approximately 24 deaths per 100,000 persons annually; among people who are Inuit, it was just over 72 deaths per 100,000 annually; and among people who are Métis, it was almost 15 deaths per 100,000 annually (Statistics Canada, 2019). This is in comparison to the rate of suicide for people who are not Indigenous Peoples of 8 deaths per 100,000 annually, which means that the rates of suicide for people who are First Nations are approximately 3 times higher, rates for Inuit people are approximately 9 times higher, and rate for people who are Métis are almost double. Further, it is important to note that suicide rates of Indigenous Peoples may be underreported as data collected by Statistics Canada pertain only to status Aboriginal Peoples, thus excluding nonstatus First Nations, Métis, and Inuit people from the overall Indigenous suicide data. As well, the rate of accidental deaths among Indigenous People is 4 to 5 times higher than in the general population and up to 25% of these deaths may be from suicide (Inuit Tapiriit Kanatami, 2016). Although the rate of suicide is higher, in general and as compared with other Canadians, not every community of Indigenous People in Canada experiences high rates of suicide (Kirmayer et al., 2007). As an example, First Nations People report that 60% of bands have a zero rate of suicide (Statistics Canada, 2019). Therefore, marked differences and

variabilities can be noted between provinces and regions, and even between communities in the same geographic region. A gap in the academic literature can be found with research on suicidality and Indigenous People in Canada. The scope of research needs to be broadened as well as made more inclusive for Métis people, urban/off-reserve populations, and nonstatus individuals that self-identify as Indigenous People. Guidelines have been suggested to develop responsive and respectful research strategies for studying mental health issues among and with Indigenous People (see Box 20.3).

A Canadian study of almost 3,000 First Nation People living off-reserve who have experienced suicidality found factors associated with recovery that included being a woman, speaking an Aboriginal language, being food secure, being older, not having a diagnosis of mental illness or a learning disability, and having a high school degree (Fuller-Thomson et al., 2019). Also, in communities of Indigenous People where there is a high level of autonomy and a strong sense of ownership, culture, and community, there are much lower rates of suicide (Kirmayer et al., 2007). The Truth and Reconciliation Commission (TRC) of Canada (2015) states 94 recommendations to redress the destructive legacy of colonialism, residential schools, and the "sixties scoop." Such strategies aim to mitigate the impacts of abuse, trauma, and marginalization related to the loss of traditions, family and community, political and economic structures, languages, and cultures (Statistics Canada, 2019). Attention to history can help nurses to work "in a good way" with Indigenous People and communities toward a future with less suicide and more hope.

Gender

The reasons for gender differences in suicidality are not entirely understood. Current and past statistics often have a binary approach to gender and exclude individuals

---

BOX 20.3 A Critical Review of the Research on the Mental Health of Indigenous People in Canada

Much of the available literature on the mental health of Indigenous People in Canada is in relation to colonialism and associated processes with an overemphasis on substance abuse and suicide. The following recommendations were raised as a result of a systematic review to address existing gaps in research (Nelson & Wilson, 2017):

- Continue to recognize colonialism as a structural and collective force that impacts health and well-being among populations of Indigenous People.

- Question whether health services and health data adequately respond to the specific mental health needs of Indigenous People.
- Address colonial attitudes, related to the ways in which Indigenous People heal each other, in mainstream mental health services and institutions.
- Address geographic and demographic gaps in mental health research for Indigenous Peoples, especially for people who are Métis, urban, and off-reserve individuals and communities.

who may identify neither as male nor as female (nonbinary). Known factors that affect suicide risk differently by gender include experiences of trauma and violence, family upbringing, economic deprivation, child care responsibilities, having a parent with mental illness, and unemployment. Worldwide, crude suicide death rates from 2016 indicate that men complete suicide at a rate (13.5/100,000) almost double that of women, who are at 7.7/100,000 (WHO, 2018). Canadian data, from 2018, indicate suicide as the ninth leading cause of death with 3,811 deaths by suicide recorded (Statistics Canada, 2020). Within Canada, death by suicide is more than three times higher for men than for women (Government of Canada, 2018). However, suicide attempt rates are highest among young women who tend to choose less lethal methods and are more likely to survive their self-inflicted injuries and to have subsequent attempts.

LGBTQI2SA+

In recent years, sexual orientation has been more openly addressed as a risk factor for suicide. Being part of an underrepresented sexual or gender group can bring experiences of stigma and discrimination. For lesbian, gay, bisexual, transgender, queer, questioning, intersexual, or two-spirit (LGBTQI2SA+) youth, "coming out" can be a risk factor because of the perceived or actual negative reactions of others, particularly from peers and family. In Canada, transgender youth are at increased risk for psychological distress, suicidality, and major depressive episodes when compared with the general population (Veale et al., 2017). Being unable to openly disclose sexual identity because it is unsafe to do and therefore not being able to receive a sense of acceptance, often contributes to a deep sense of isolation. During adolescence in Western countries, generally the major focus of a youth's life is on peers, sexuality, and self-identity. A British study of over 700 university students who identified as gay, lesbian, or bisexual, found that thwarted belongingness was correlated with a higher risk for both NSSI events and suicide attempts (Taylor et al., 2020).

People Who Are Inmates

Suicide in prisons occurs among high-risk populations in environments where concepts of safety and security need an ongoing balance. Many people who are inmates and express suicidality have mental illness and are placed in isolation (e.g., solitary confinement) to prevent self-harm and to protect the prison community. Correction Services Canada (2019) reports that between 2009/2010 and 2016/2017, 70 people who are inmates died by suicide, most by hanging. The majority had life histories with substance misuse (89%) and at least one mental health concern (89%); the majority were on medication for mental illness and were regularly accessing mental health services. A significant number were serving indeterminate sentences and were in custody for homicide-related offences.

People who are inmates experiencing suicidality are placed in isolation (e.g., solitary confinement) to prevent self-harm and to protect the prison community. Since social isolation is a well-known risk factor for suicide (as well as poor mental health in general), placement in isolation can challenge not only an individual's human rights, but also their capacity to cope, and lead to further sequela that do not contribute to recovery. A study done in Italy reviewed this issue in the cases of two people who were inmates who died by suicide, using their underwear to hang themselves (Grassi et al., 2018). These researchers challenge the routine practice of social deprivation (and sometimes clothing deprivation, e.g., allowed underwear only) as being inhumane and as a form of psychosocial torture. They call for the need to establish evidence-informed, standardized practices to manage suicidality in prison settings and to explore alternative forms of detention.

First Responders

First responders (e.g., firefighters, police and correctional services, emergency medical technicians/paramedics, crisis workers, mental health professionals, physicians, nurses, social workers, etc.) can have disproportionate exposure to human violence and trauma when compared to the general population. Heavy workloads, shift work, and high stress environments can contribute to an inability to allocate adequate time and effort for self-care, often resulting in the adoption of unhealthy coping mechanisms. In a study done in America of over 1,000 first responders, routine exposure to suicide was associated with statistically significant impacts on mental health, namely depression, anxiety, and posttraumatic stress disorder (Aldrich & Cerel, 2020).

During the COVID-19 pandemic, such mental health impacts were intensified when first responders experienced stigmatization due to their exposure to the virus. Research focused on understanding their experience found that first responders suffered from "feelings of isolation, lack of support and understanding by family or friends, decreased or forced removal in immediate social interaction (e.g., within family and friend circles), sentiments of being infected or dirty, increased feelings of sadness and anxiety, and reluctance to ask for help or get treatment" (Zolnikov & Furio, 2020, p.375).

These findings speak to the need for nurses to consider that suicidality in their professional work can have (sometimes unexpected) personal impacts that require urgent attention and a strong sense of compassion. Further, first responders need to be aware of the early signs and symptoms of suicidality among their colleagues and be willing to reach out to help others.

KEY CONCEPT

Lethality refers to the likelihood that death will occur as a result of the means used to attempt suicide. Violent suicide attempts (high lethality acts) use the most lethal means to achieve death and serious suicide attempts (moderate lethality acts) use nonviolent means and require intensive-care level hospitalization (Alacreu-Crespo et al., 2020). Measures of lethality are further influenced by the opportunity for rescue and the individual's intent to die (Choo et al., 2019).

KEY CONCEPT

Risk/rescue ratio refers to the potential for death and evaluates lethality, risk factors, and rescue factors. Suicidal risk carries with it a progression of seriousness from suicidal ideation to completed suicide. Risk is lowest when intent is weak and the method used has low lethality. Risk factors include the method, impaired consciousness, required medical treatment, toxicity, and reversibility. Rescue factors include location, rescue person, time and probability for discovery, and accessibility to rescue (Alacreu-Crespo et al., 2020). The likelihood of rescue is dependent on communication of intent and lower lethality of means.

Holistic Risk Factors

The spectrum of suicidal thoughts, feelings, behaviours, and death by suicide occurs in the context of an individual's unique life experiences and is triggered by stressors that are perceived as unmanageable and exceed typical coping efforts. Vulnerabilities are enhanced by engaging in risky behaviours, often used in an effort to deal with stress. Risky behaviours related to suicide include fast, dangerous driving; tempting death; promiscuity; abuse of alcohol or other substances; and acquiring a handgun. A comprehensive assessment identifies the physical, psychological, social, and spiritual factors that contribute to suicidal feelings, thoughts, and behaviours (see Fig. 20.1). The convergence of these dynamic factors can be directly linked to self-harm and suicidal behaviours. Most will agree that suicidality, like many other aspects of humanity, rarely lies within a single sphere of the bio/psycho/social/spiritual model. However, in order to facilitate learning, it will be discussed in relation to each of these spheres separately to establish a baseline understanding of how these factors contribute to self-harm and suicidality across the life span. For example, physical factors include medical illness and substance use; psychological factors include hopelessness, helplessness, psychological distress, mental illness, and low self-esteem; and external social risk factors include lack of social support, family problems, financial hardship, and legal problems. Spiritual risk factors

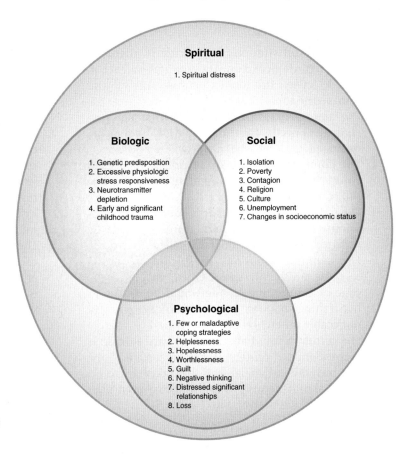

Figure 20.1 Bio/psycho/social/spiritual aetiologies of suicide.

include a loss of meaning or purpose in one's life and may also involve spiritual distress related to religious and/or ethnocultural beliefs and traditions.

Aetiology of Self-Harm Behaviours and Suicidality

Self-harm is more common among adolescent youth than other age groups and is found more often among young women. It is a sign of psychological distress and should always be taken seriously. It should never be stigmatized as simply being attention seeking or manipulative. Researchers in Australia have identified 11 genes associated with self-harm, and further associated some of these genes with a shared genetic susceptibility for suicidal thoughts (Campos et al., 2020). Most individuals who attempt suicide have seen a healthcare professional at least 1 year prior to the attempt (Morrison & Laing, 2011). Therefore, nurses need to be aware that self-harm and suicidality may occur in their practice and have the knowledge to act responsively.

Edwin S. Shneidman (1918–2009) was an American clinical psychologist, thanatologist, suicidologist, founder of the American Association of Suicidology, and founder of the academic journal *Suicide and Life*

Threatening Behavior. Dr. Shneidman became interested in studying suicide in his work with veterans in the 1940s and later described common characteristics of suicide in his famous book *Definition of Suicide* (see Box 20.4). He wrote 20 books on the topic of suicide and suicide prevention over his lifetime.

Biological Theories

Suicide can be understood using biological theories through opportunities to recognize and interpret physiologic, neurologic, and hormonal changes. Theoretical research suggests that behaviours of despair may be driven by early distal risk factors (e.g., mental illness, family history of suicide, childhood adversity) and linked to more proximal failures to produce adaptive, biological responses to acute stress (Miller & Eisenlohr-Moul, 2019). Stress responsiveness ultimately changes an individual's biological functioning. Our current understanding of the role of brain function and various neurotransmitters can be used to explore potential psychopharmacological treatments for suicidality.

Mental illness is the primary reason for the majority of deaths by suicide (Shoib & Kim, 2019), due to the prevalence of major depressive disorders (MDD)

BOX 20.4 Shneidman's Common Characteristics of Suicide

1. **The common stimulus for suicide is unendurable psychological pain.** The core ambivalence in suicide reflects the conflict between survival and unbearable stress.
2. **The common stressor in suicide is frustrated psychological needs.** The clinical rule is to address the frustrated needs and the suicide will not occur.
3. **The common purpose of suicide is to seek a solution.** Suicide is not a random act. It is a way out of a problem or crisis.
4. **The common goal of suicide is "cessation of consciousness."** The main clinical rule is to reduce the suffering and the individual will choose to live.
5. **The common emotions in suicide are hopelessness and helplessness.** Often, people on the edge of committing suicide would be willing to live if things/life were only a little bit better, a just noticeable difference.
6. **The common internal attitude toward suicide is ambivalence.** A prototypical suicidal state is one in which the individual feels that they have to do it and simultaneously yearns and may even plan for rescue and intervention.

7. **The common cognitive state in suicide is "constriction" (tunnel vision).** Suicide is a transient psychological constriction of affect and intellect; a narrowing of the range of options that leads to either/or thinking.
8. **The common interpersonal act in suicide is communication of intention.** Communication of suicidal intent can be a shout, a murmur, or nonverbal. It can be a cry for help; it can be for autonomy or any number of needs. Nonetheless, in most cases of suicide, there is some interpersonal communication related to that intended final act.
9. **The common action in suicide is regression or escape.** It is important to view each suicidal act as an urgently felt effort to answer a question or to resolve an issue or problem.
10. **Suicide is consistent with lifelong coping patterns.** "You can't fire me; I quit." "I'll leave her before she leaves me." Shneidman believes that suicide is sometimes reasonably predictable.

From Shneidman, E. (1985). *Definition of suicide.* John Wiley & Sons.

BOX 20.5 Research for Best Practice

RECOVERY AND THE UNIQUE ROLE OF MENTAL HEALTH NURSES

From Santangelo, P., Procter, N., & Fassett, D. (2018). Mental health nursing: Daring to be different, special and leading recovery-focused care? *International Journal of Mental Health Nursing, 27*(1), 258–266.

Question: How is mental health nursing different from other disciplines and what special contributions can mental health nurses make?

Method: Using a constructivist grounded theory approach, this research involved interviews with 36 Australian mental health nurses. These nurses were asked, "What's special about mental health nursing?" Findings were organized according the 10 P's to describe the professional profile of mental health nurses.

Findings: Mental health nursing was described as being a distinct and special discipline. As providers of quality care, mental health nurses are well placed to have a role that involves being present, personal, professional, phenomenological, pragmatic, psychotherapeutic, proud, and profound. They engage in partnership and power-sharing to fulfill this role.

Implications for Practice: Mental health nurses hold an important role and potential for contributing to positive change and recovery in the lives of individuals, families, and communities. This research offers an opportunity for nurses to more fully engage in contemporary aspects of mental health nursing practice versus more traditional psychiatric approaches to care that closely adhere to the medical model.

that are sometimes comorbid with other psychiatric illnesses. MDD (see Chapter 22) may develop when a person, vulnerable to depression because of genetic or other factors, is subjected to repeated or sustained stress. Psychopathology (e.g., abnormal behaviours, extreme emotional reactions, and distorted thinking) is evident in most suicidal people. The links between poor mental health and suicide are well documented. MDD, generalized anxiety disorders (GAD), personality disorders, bipolar disorders, schizophrenia, and other psychiatric illnesses are frequently present in persons experiencing suicidality. Further, suicidality and substance involvement often co-occur (Agrawal et al., 2017). Moreover, suicide rates tend to be higher in families in which suicide has previously occurred.

Psychological Theories

Suicide can be understood using psychological theories through opportunities to recognize and interpret human development, early childhood experiences, learned responses and defense mechanisms, personality, sexuality, and thoughts, emotions, and behaviours. Our current understanding of the role of psychological aspects of individuals can be used to explore various psychodynamic therapies and interventions.

Coming to understand suicide as it is related to the human psyche is important. According to attachment theory, adult behaviour is shaped by early interactions and relationships with the primary caregiver during infancy. Disturbed attachment results in the individual's inability to form meaningful relationships or constant concern about the viability of a lasting relationship. Isolated individuals lose the resource of co-regulation

that is available through supportive interactions and empathic connections. Therefore, interventions that strengthen an individual's capacity for establishing and maintaining healthy interpersonal bonds and boundaries can be valuable. A psychodynamic theoretical perspective conceptualizes suicidal behaviour as an intra-psychically determined phenomenon. The Interpersonal Theory of Suicide (Van Orden et al., 2010) explores how an individual's sense of hopelessness involves intense experiences of aloneness (thwarted belonging) and feeling like a burden (burdensomeness). However, an individual's capability to carry out suicidal behaviour can be separate from the desire to die. For a small percentage of individuals, there is both the desire and the capability, and thus a suicide attempt occurs.

The widely used cognitive theory of depression espoused by Beck (2011) accounts for how negative thoughts occur, how they tend to be repetitive and intrusive, and how they can lead to suicidal behaviour. Cognitive approaches also attribute suicide to learned helplessness and hopelessness as an automatic and pervasive pathologic scheme for organizing and interpreting experiences. Perhaps due to the sequelae of mental illness, suicidality is also associated with neurocognitive impairments in executive functioning, such as decision-making and inhibition (Allen et al., 2019). For further consideration, the Integrated-Motivational-Volitional (IMV) Model of Suicidal Behaviour posits that suicidal behaviour is largely a cognitive process and is driven by experiences of defeat and entrapment (O'Connor & Kirtley, 2018). The transition from thought to action is influenced by volitional moderators (VMs; e.g., means, past behaviours, exposure, mental imagery, capability, impulsivity, planning). Therefore, it is the combination of vulnerability and stress that initially develops suicidal ideation and intention, and then later leads to suicidal behaviours. Finally, Opara and colleagues (2020) propose the Interpersonal-Psychological Theory of Suicide with Intersectionality Theory to provide a broader context to understand suicide. They use a socioecological model of suicidality that includes consideration for the individual (e.g., hope, belonging, mental health), their immediate environment (e.g., supports), their community (e.g., violence, poverty, discrimination, racism), and their culture and society (e.g., race, sex, class, sexual orientation).

Social Theories

Suicide can be understood using social theories through opportunities to recognize and interpret family dynamics, an individual's roles and responsibilities, gender and cultural norms, and sociocultural experiences. Social factors are particularly important to the aetiology of suicide. As humans, we are inherently a part of the social fabric in which we exist. Humans are wired to live with and connect with others. Suicide, then, is the desire to estrange oneself from the world; to isolate and withdraw permanently. Some individuals with suicidality describe a desire to "feel nothing for a while" that expresses a request for a temporary respite from life and the world. Studying the social factors that contribute to rates of suicide, sociologist Emile Durkheim developed a theoretical framework outlining social causes of suicide and believed that the degree of social integration was a variable affecting rates of suicide. Durkheim (1897/2006) classified suicide under four headings: egoistic suicide, altruistic suicide, anomic suicide, and fatalistic suicide. *Egoistic suicide* occurs among individuals who are not significantly bound to others in society. Conversely, *altruistic suicide* occurs when individuals become overly connected to society; for example, patriotic soldiers who kill themselves after a defeated battle because they are ashamed. A society lacking a sense of purpose, social regulation, or community values experiences *anomic suicide*. For example, this type of suicide occurs during times of financial depression. Contrastingly, in areas of overregulation and oppression, *fatalistic suicides* occur. Although Durkheim discussed little about fatalistic suicide, many use the suicide of people who were slaves as an exemplar.

Spiritual Theories

Increasingly, spirituality is recognized as a key component of holistic care in nursing. Suicide can be understood using spiritual theories through opportunities to recognize and interpret an individual's existential life concerns, sense of purpose, reasons for living and hope, and understanding of love. An American study of 110 military veterans explored links between suicide

symptoms and spiritual struggles and found that a greater degree of perceived burdensomeness was associated with increased symptom severity (Raines et al., 2020). Psychospiritual theories and related interventions extend beyond their boundaries into psychological, cultural, religious, and social arenas (Egargo & Kahambing, 2021).

Suicide and Religion

Current studies that explore the topic of suicide and religion have identified this relationship as complex, with inconsistent findings, although historically an inverse association was noted (Gearing & Alonzo, 2018; Hamdan & Peterseil-Yaul, 2020; Lawrence et al., 2016). Some nurses choose to further specialize in the healing capacities of spirituality and religion. As an example, the Canadian Association of Parish Nursing Ministry (CAPNM, 2020) was established in the late 1990s and supports registered nurses to expand their care of individuals and families in a faith community context. In the United States, this speciality is recognized as Faith Community Nursing (FCN) by the American Nurses Association (Chase & Solari-Twadell, 2020).

Suicide Pact, Contagion, and Cluster

Most suicides occur independently, but some individuals mutually plan and act to die together. This is known as a *suicide pact* (Byard et al., 2019). Some individuals plan to die by the hand of someone else, as is seen in the act of *suicide by cop* (SbC). Suicide by cop is usually found among individuals who are young men and non-Hispanic White or of European origin and who have a history of mental health issues and engagement with the law, are intoxicated, and have experienced a romantic conflict (Patton & Fremouw, 2016).

Another social phenomenon, known as *suicide contagion*, occurs when additional suicidal behaviours follow the death of a peer, fellow student, or even a celebrity (Carmichael & Whitley, 2019). When such a ripple effect occurs in a given timeframe and often specific geographic area, it can be known as a *suicide cluster* (Poland et al., 2019). A *mass cluster* is often associated with media reports related to the suicide of a celebrity or other cases of completed suicide with overwhelming attention generated by media saturation. There is a direct relationship between media coverage of suicide and contagion. This social phenomenon was originally termed the "Werther effect" after the young lover in Goethe (1774–1989) whose suicide inspired copycat suicides among readers how are young men (Scherr & Reinemann, 2011). Some scholars, however, suggest that individuals who are influenced by such stories are already in a vulnerable state as a result of other precipitating factors and may not necessarily be influenced by media exposure of suicide (Westerlund et al., 2009). Nevertheless, media guidelines have been developed to address the potential harm of suicide coverage (Sinyor et al., 2017; Stack, 2020). These guidelines emphasize collaboration between mental health professionals and the media to ensure that reporting is done in a way to reduce subsequent suicidal behaviour.

In contrast to mass clusters, *point clusters* are suicides that occur close in time and space and often occur in specific communities, such as hospitals, schools, or prisons (Poland et al., 2019). For example, risk for the occurrence of point clusters occurs in communities of Indigenous People as individuals on reserves are closely related and share the same social predicaments; therefore, a single suicide affects the entire community (Kirmayer et al., 2007). Such circumstances can also manifest as *echo clusters* that occur over an extended period of time after the original cluster.

Bullying, Victimization, Trauma, and Violence

Traditional bullying has been defined as aggressive intentional "harm doing" by one person or a group, generally carried out repeatedly over time (see Chapter 17, Table 17.4 for examples of the four types of bullying: physical, verbal, relational, and cyber). Trauma, victimization, and violence in childhood is commonly associated with peer and/or sibling bullying (Dantchev et al., 2019). Usually, the impacts are only associated with the victims. However, an Australian study considers the possibility of a link between self-harm and exposure to bullying, both for victims and perpetrators (Heerde & Hemphill, 2018). Many countries, including Canada, have initiated anti-bullying legislation and school policies. However, virtual environments now hold unlimited potential for individuals to be unduly influenced and cyberbullied through social media, video recordings, and chat messaging. Further research is required to explore effective means to keep children and young adults safe in their homes, in public spaces, as well as in e-domains.

Caring for People at Risk for (or Engaging in) Self-Harm and/or Suicidal Behaviours

All Canadians have legal rights that healthcare providers must consider and uphold during self-harm and/or suicide prevention, intervention, and postvention activities. Individuals always maintain their right to self-determination unless they have been assessed and found to be incompetent. Individuals have the right to be free from harm. Physically restraining or hospitalizing a patient against their will has the potential for both physical and emotional harm. Such nonconsensual action should be taken only when the patient is under the threat of imminent harm to self or others or when the patient's status is "not competent" under the relevant mental health act. Nurses must be familiar with their provincial or territorial mental health legislation

(see Chapter 8), understand patients' legal rights, be able to explain them clearly, and advocate to ensure that these fundamental rights are upheld.

Privacy and Confidentiality

Disclosing an individual's health information without the expressed permission of the patient violates their right to privacy and may seriously damage the therapeutic relationship. A loss of trust can occur when the nurse shares a patient's suicidal intent with others unless the nurse has specifically explained the limits of confidentiality to the patient. The concept of confidentiality involves safeguarding information acquired within a professional relationship, except when doing so would cause significant harm (Canadian Nurses Association [CNA], 2017; Canadian Federation of Mental Health Nurses [CFMHN], 2014). When informing the patient of existing limits of confidentiality, the nurse must be very clear and specific. The CNA's (2017) *Code of Ethics* is consistent with all provincial legislations. Namely, patients have the right to confidentiality unless they are at risk for harming themselves or others or disclose any form of abuse. In these situations, the nurse must enlist the help of others to protect the patient's or others' safety.

Protecting an individual's right to confidentiality is a special concern when a minor child has suicidal intent. In a study done in Canada, issues related to confidentiality were explored with physicians in the context of mental health care and adolescent clients (Agostino & Burstein, 2020). Researchers found that the provision of confidentiality during care was influenced by the type of diagnosis, the patient's age, and the timing of the visit. Three quarters of participating physicians expressed the desire for further training to provide better confidentiality in their practice. As with adult patients, the nurse is required to describe the right to confidentiality and its limits to minor patients. The nurse must always consider informing parents or legal guardians of a child who has suicidal intent. The parents of a minor child retain the privilege to determine the right care for their child and they need sufficient information to make good decisions. Before beginning any suicide risk assessment, the nurse must let the child know that disclosure of self-harm may be shared with parents, but the child will be told if/when information will be shared. Involving parents/caregivers in decisions about care for their child experiencing suicidality is important. Honesty about what the nurse can and cannot keep confidential ultimately increases a patient's trust and often results in a more therapeutic relationship.

Informed Consent

Obtaining informed consent from patients protects their right to self-determination. However, nurses must inform suicidal patients about limits to their autonomy and work in collaboration with patients in their care. From the time that the nurse encounters a suicidal patient until a suitable placement is made in consultation with other members of the interprofessional team, the nurse must share with the patient their right to be placed in the least restrictive environment that will ensure safety. The least restrictive environment is the setting that puts the fewest constraints on patients' rights while still ensuring their safety. By informing patients about their choices, the nurse has an opportunity to build trust and decreases the likelihood that involuntary hospitalization will be necessary.

The ethical principles of beneficence (doing the most amount of good) and nonmaleficence (doing the least amount of harm) are critical considerations when holding patients against their will. Caring for patients who are suicidal and determined to carry out self-harm behaviours is difficult without touching and actively restraining them. Still, nurses must do their best to disclose to patients the specifics of planned treatments (including restraints, seclusion, and 1:1 observation) and attempt to obtain their consent to proceed. Respect for the patient needs to be maintained throughout the process and trauma–violence informed approaches must influence decision-making. For further discussion of these issues, see Chapter 12.

▌ Nursing Assessment and Interventions

The foundation of quality nursing practice is the therapeutic relationship. Assessment and care of individuals, who are experiencing changes to affect, behaviour, and cognition on the spectrum of self-harm and suicidality, must be grounded in the core principles of *relational practice* (Doane & Varcoe, 2015). Individuals with suicidality often experience hopelessness, helplessness, and powerlessness which need to be assessed and integrated into their plan of care. All individuals who indicate verbally or nonverbally their intention to engage in any self-harm or suicidal behaviour must be taken seriously and assessed for suicide risk. Self-harm and suicidal behaviours are seriously underreported and often not recognized by healthcare professionals. A patient who is acutely suicidal is in a true psychiatric emergency. Nurses must act immediately and responsibly to prevent the patient's death.

KEY CONCEPT

Hopelessness is a perception of having no hope that one's life situation or circumstance will ever change or improve. It is characterized by feelings of inadequacy and an inability to act on one's own behalf. An individual perceives that their circumstances will never get better or change.

KEY CONCEPT

Helplessness is the perception of a state of being with limited ability, motivation, or ambition to change one's current life situation. It is characterized by a sense of being unable to help oneself and a sense that there is a lack of support or protection from others. An individual perceives that no one (including self) can do anything to help them.

KEY CONCEPT

Powerlessness is the perception of having a state of character without power, influence, or control over one's life circumstance, feeling that the world will never be fair, feeling helpless and totally ineffectual, and/or feeling that one lacks legal or other authority.

Bio/Psycho/Social/Spiritual Domains of Nursing Assessment

Nursing interventions, based on a comprehensive assessment of risk, provide a holistic approach to nursing care of the individual and family. The process of risk assessment will be discussed, followed by a discussion of nursing interventions in relation to the biological, psychological, social, and spiritual aspects of care.

Comprehensive Assessment of Risk

A comprehensive nursing assessment provides insight into self-harm and suicidal behaviour and guides planning for appropriate interventions. A nonblaming, nonjudgmental approach allows further exploration of an individual's experiences and gives a message of interest and concern to the patient. Each interaction is an opportunity to build trust as part of the therapeutic alliance (see Box 20.6 for Questions to Guide a Comprehensive Assessment of Risk; see Box 20.7 for Suicide Assessment Tools). Assessment of the context of both current and prior suicidality from the perspective of the patient assists the nurse to formulate an understanding of the complex motivations that are unique to the individual. Exploration of the patient's motivations helps both the patient and the nurse to understand factors that put that person at risk and work toward interventions that may help them to meet their needs in healthier ways. Assessment includes the collection of adequate data to provide the healthcare team with a snapshot understanding of the individual's life and relevant stressors. This includes gathering information about the person's family, peers, and other social relationships as well as workplace (or school) issues. Changes related to grief and loss experiences need to be explored to identify

---

BOX 20.6 Questions to Guide a Comprehensive Assessment of Risk

Stressors

- What is troubling you most at the moment?
  - Explore with curious questions in terms of all areas of the patient's life.
  - Explore each area, asking the patient to tell you more.
  - The idea is to get a clear picture of the patient's life situation and presenting stressors as the patient perceives them.

Symptoms

- Can you tell me about your sleep patterns?
  - Are you having difficulty sleeping?
  - Do you want to stay in bed and sleep through the day?
- Can you tell me about your eating habits?
  - Have you lost your appetite?
  - Do you eat in an attempt to cope with difficulties?
- What do you do for enjoyment?
  - Do you find you no longer enjoy activities you thought were enjoyable?
  - Do you use drugs or alcohol to cope?

Prior Behaviour

- Have you ever thought of harming yourself?
  - Can you tell me about that (e.g., time, place, situation, feelings, meaning)?
  - What was the self-harm about?
  - What happened?
  - What did you expect to happen?
  - What did you want to happen?

Current Plan

- Do you currently have a plan to harm yourself?
  - What would you do?
- Do you have access to the pills (or other methods)?
- Have you picked a specific day or time? Do you want to die?

Resources and Support

- Do you have someone you recognize as supportive?
- Who can you talk to about your concerns?
- Who can you confide in?
- Offer suggestions of a number of people the patient may not have thought of who could be trusted (e.g., parent's friend, colleague, clergy, coach).

---

possible precipitating or contributing factors. Issues related to trauma and/or violence need to be discussed with thoughtfulness and sensitivity.

The patient should be assessed for symptoms of psychiatric disorders, especially those most commonly associated with suicidal behaviour (e.g., MDD, substance use disorder, panic disorder, anxiety disorder, schizophrenia). The broad spectrum of symptoms related to depression, hopelessness, and helplessness must be explored, such as isolating or withdrawing from friends and family, changes to sleeping and eating patterns, not enjoying or ceasing participation in activities that were previously enjoyed, and having no sense of hope for the future (see Chapter 22 for assessment of depression). Increased severity of MDD is associated with a greater likelihood of suicide completion. For adolescents, a key question is whether any family member has attempted or completed suicide. Nurses must be mindful that an individual may not always report suicidality prior to a suicide attempt. An study done in American by Richards et al. (2019) found three main reasons that patients may not disclose, including fear of overreaction, stigma, and loss of autonomy. Further, the study found that patients may answer "no" if they are not thinking of suicide at that moment, and that the actual attempt was often precipitated by heavy alcohol use.

Having a Current Plan

Suicide requires intent, knowledge of how to carry out the act, and few obstacles to completing it. Individuals who complete suicide are less likely to have young children or other immediate responsibilities and may not be concerned with religious prohibitions concerning the act. The relationship between the availability of a method of suicide, the method's lethality, and suicide completion is strong. It is important for the nurse to ask whether the patient has a *current plan for suicide* and *access to the means* to end their life. Further exploration of the plan gives the nurse a more accurate assessment of risk and guides appropriate interventions. Some individuals will plan the suicide event in detail, possibly leaving a suicide note about the anticipated event, the method, location, circumstance, and time. People who engage in chronic self-harm behaviour may resort to their usual methods (such as cutting) and know when and under what triggers they will do this (see Chapter 27 for further information on self-harm related to personality disorders). Self-harm and suicidal behaviour may also be impulsive. People who are under the influence of alcohol or other substances and people who experience sudden negative feelings (e.g., abandonment and rage) may be at risk to impulsively end their lives. Individuals with psychoses

BOX 20.7 Suicide and Self-Harm Assessment Tools

There are many tools that can assist with assessing risk and evaluating progress. Although these references may seem dated, they are classics in the field and still in use by individuals who have been trained to utilize them in mental health practice.

- *Beck Hopelessness Scale*—assists with assessment of the level of hopelessness, as hopelessness is highly associated with suicide (Beck, Weissman, et al., 1974).
- *Beck Scale for Suicide Ideation (BSS)*—assesses five key factors including suicidal ideation, active and passive desire for suicide, planning, and concealment (Beck et al., 1988; Beck, Schuyler, et al., 1974).
- *Columbia-Suicide Severity Rating Scale (C-SSRS)*—assesses suicide from a number of perspectives, including ideation, intensity, behaviour, and lethality (Posner et al., 2008).
- *Geriatric Suicide Ideation Scale (GSIS)*—assesses suicide risk as well as psychological resilience in late life (Heisel & Flett, 2006).
- *Inventory of Motivation for Suicide Attempts (IMSA)*—has 54 statements that are answered on a five-point Likert scale to assess suicidal intent by identifying two factors: intrapersonal and interpersonal motivations (May & Klonsky, 2013).
  - *Intrapersonal* motivations reveal the need to escape or relieve internal emotions and thoughts.
  - *Interpersonal* motivations reveal the desire to communicate with or influence another individual.
- *Inventory of Statements About Self-Injury (ISAS)*—is used to assess the functions (i.e., interpersonal and intrapersonal) and frequency of NSSI (Klonsky & Glenn, 2009).
- *IS PATH WARM*—is a mnemonic tool to recall the main points for assessment of suicidality, including Ideation, Substance abuse, Purposelessness, Anxiety/agitation, Trapped (no options), Helplessness/hopelessness, Withdrawal (isolation), Anger, Recklessness, and Mood changes (Juhnke et al., 2007).
- *Nurses' Global Assessment of Suicide Risk (NGASR)*—used to assess suicide risk and focus further

discussion with the client and/or members of the healthcare team (Cutcliffe & Barker, 2004). Developed as part of the *Tidal Model* (Barker, 2001; Barker & Buchanan-Barker, 2005).
- *SAD PERSONS Scale*—is a mnemonic tool to recall the main points for assessment of the 10 major risk factors for a suicide attempt (Patterson et al., 1983). Risk factors include: **S**, sex; **A**, age; **D**, depression; **P**, previous attempt; **E**, excess alcohol/substance use; **R**, rationale thinking, lacking; **S**, social supports, lacking; **O**, organized plan; **N**, no spouse; and **S**, sickness.
- *Suicidal Affect Behaviour Cognition Scale (C-SABCS)*—is a public domain tool to assess suicide risk, with an accompanying risk barometer that defines risk from nonsuicidal to high suicidal (Harris et al., 2015).
- *Suicide Intent Scale*—is a short and useful tool to determine an individual's intent to die, which assesses circumstances as well as feelings and thoughts (Beck et al., 1979).
- *Suicide Probability Scale (SPS)*—provides a quick measure of suicide risk for screening in outpatient settings (Cull & Gill, 1989).
- *Suicide Risk Assessment Model*—can be used in any care setting and includes stressors, symptoms, prior behaviour, current plan, and available resources and support (Murray, 2003; Murray & Wright, 2006). It can be integrated as part of the focused suicide risk assessment in the *Tidal Model* (Barker, 2001; Barker & Buchanan-Barker, 2005).
- *Reasons for Living Inventory*—tools to measure beliefs about reasons not to die by suicide, including categories such as survival and coping beliefs, moral objections, responsibilities to family, fear of social disapproval, child-related concerns, and fear of suicide itself (Linehan et al., 1983).

Additional tools available from the *Suicide Risk Assessment Guide* (Perlman et al., 2011).

---

may be responding to "voices" that direct them to kill themselves and are at considerable risk because of their inability to separate psychotic thinking from reality.

Protective Factors, Resources, and Support

There are many reasons that a person who has suicidal thoughts and/or a plan does not act on it. As much as someone may wish to die, that person may also

have many reasons to stay alive. The *state of ambiguity* between wanting to live and wanting to die affords an opportunity to explore reasons for living and opportunities for hope, which are considered protective factors (as they protect a person from acting on thoughts, feelings, and plans). It is important, therefore, to assess an individual's unique reasons for living. For some, it may be a child or parent to care for; for others, it may be against religious beliefs to take one's life; for others still, it may be a purpose in life not yet fulfilled. In a study completed in Manitoba, both the pregnancy and postpartum periods were found to have lower rates of mood disorders, substance use, and suicide attempts, although the postpartum period carried an increased rate of psychotic disorder (Mota et al., 2019). Factors that protect against suicide may include good health practices, social support networks, interests and pleasurable activities, a sense of purpose, and little to no access to lethal methods (e.g., firearms) (Canadian Coalition for Seniors Mental Health, 2008). Protective factors are not a guarantee that a person will not take their life, but they do offer strengths upon which a nurse can build on with the patient to promote and sustain hope in living (Bongar et al., 2016).

Resources and supports are also critical considerations for people at risk for self-harm and suicide. Lack of these may put an individual or community at greatest risk. Individuals contemplating suicide often feel socially isolated and struggle to identify and accept support from people in their immediate environment; therefore, it is important to explore all available supports. Interest in the patient's life and attention received during a thorough assessment are therapeutic and can also provide connectedness and engagement with the patient and family. Resources and supports not available through the patient's personal sphere of friends and family may need to be supplemented through any variety of informal community supports and formal referrals to professional services. Assessment of the patient's previous use of, access to, and benefits from resources and supports helps to plan care post discharge from a hospital, crisis centre, or community agency. Assessment of financial resources, such as drug and benefit plans, is also important in considering the scope of available and accessible resources.

Method and Access

Nursing assessment of method and potential for access to that method is important to ascertain potential lethality of any suicidal ideation and behaviour. The method of a suicide attempt may hold meaning for an individual and understanding that meaning may also provide insight. Understanding access to method is also critical to creating a responsive plan of care to ensure safety, for example, removing pills to prevent overdoses. It is important to assess where all potential methods are kept or stored in the environment that the individual will be in.

Assessment and Reassessment

Self-harm and suicide may be a single event in a person's life and with rapid interventions may safely resolve and never occur again. However, as discussed, the thoughts and feelings underlying self-harm and suicide are complex, typically multifaceted, and dynamic, which may make a very fluid situation for many people who suffer such despair. Hence, a suicidal state is often understood as existing along a continuum of wanting to live and wanting to die. An individual's thoughts and feelings may change rapidly with fluctuating biopsychosocial and spiritual circumstances. That is why it is so important for the nurse to be alert to subtle, as well as overt, changes in the patient's behaviours that may indicate a shift in suicidal thinking that will require further assessment. Ongoing and thorough assessments are key components of the intervention process. If some or many of the risk factors for suicide are present, the nurse must determine the steps that are necessary to ensure the patient's safety as the first priority. Until the nurse has identified a patient's safety needs and implemented a plan to ensure this, the nurse must not leave the acutely suicidal individual alone for any reason, not even briefly. Nursing care of an acutely suicidal patient requires consultation with a team approach.

Documentation

The nurse must thoroughly document assessments, interactions, planning, and interventions with an individual experiencing suicidality. This action is important when evaluating the patient's ongoing treatment and for the legal protection of the nurse's professional license and the workplace. Thorough and accurate documentation must reflect that the nurse took every reasonable action in a timely manner to provide for the patient's safety, inclusive of all stages of the nursing process. If contracting for safety has been instituted, the record must contain specific aspects of the agreement.

Planning and Implementing Nursing Interventions

The nurse's genuine interest, concern, and exploration begins to establish a needed trusting, therapeutic relationship with the individual in their care. The nurse should listen, empathize, acknowledge, and validate patient and family experiences. An understanding of the purpose and meaning of an individual's self-harm or suicidal behaviour guides planning and choices of intervention strategies. It also has an opportunity for the patient and family to gain a sense of hope. Using this approach, the nurse can help the patient to identify what (and sometimes who) needs to change in their environment. This approach uncovers concrete areas for planning to improve or change an individual's circumstances and stressors, and opportunities to develop effective coping strategies. A strategy of empowerment can address feelings of hopelessness, helplessness, and powerlessness.

Contracting for Safety

Contracting for safety—having the patient agree and commit, in writing, to no self-harm or suicide attempt for an agreed upon period of time—is an intervention used extensively in some psychiatric settings (Knesper, 2011). Such contracts can only be negotiated after a thorough assessment of the patient has been completed. The nurse must consider an individual's competency in terms of being able to enter into a contract of this nature. The patient cannot be in a psychotic state or under the influence of substances. An individual who has made a previous suicide attempt or is extremely isolated is not a good candidate for safety contracting.

Advantages and disadvantages of no self-harm contracts and several examples of contracts can be found in a review by Range and colleagues (2002). However, the use of safety contracts is under researched: while their effectiveness depends upon the patient's ability to keep a commitment of this kind, the factors influencing this are not fully known or understood (Knesper, 2011). Legal and professional scholars disagree on the ability of children and adolescents to make decisions of this gravity on their own behalf. More recently, *structured safety plans* in the context of discharge to a community setting have been explored, particularly for individuals who fall into the moderate to high-risk categories (Walters, 2020).

Acute Care Treatment

Historically, patients with suicidality were hospitalized for extended periods to ensure that the suicidal crisis had passed and to provide sufficient time to establish a solid base of treatment for any underlying psychiatric disorder. This is no longer the case. Hospitals are highly restrictive environments that may inhibit the patient's development of the self-reliance needed to return to the community. Objectives of acute care hospitalization are to maintain the patient's safety, reduce or relieve the suicidal crisis, decrease the level of suicidal ideation, initiate treatment for any underlying disorder(s), evaluate for substance involvement, reduce the level of social isolation, and connect the patient and family with ongoing outpatient resources and support. If the patient is assessed as acutely suicidal and is at considerable risk for completing suicide, the decision must be made whether to hospitalize the patient (with or without their consent) for the patient's safety. Safety in such cases is commonly determined by whether an individual may be a threat to self or others. Provincial law also requires that restrictions to an individual's right to autonomous decision-making occurs only when it is intended to provide a necessary therapeutic effect and is needed to ensure safety.

Interventions for the Biologic Domain

Ensuring Safety

Ongoing and effective communication with the patient is key to allowing patients to disclose and discuss their life situation and the resulting emotions and behaviour. Patients often feel shaky in the first hours of psychiatric hospitalization, and it is comforting to know that a caring person is nearby. Observational periods can be used to help the patient express a broad range of feelings and strengthen their belief in their own abilities to keep themselves safe. The nurse can help the individual who is not skilled in self-expression or self-management skills to describe their feelings more effectively and cite ways of managing their safety needs. Then, at the next observation time, the nurse may have the opportunity to reinforce the patient's own safety behaviour. Thus, the observation period can be transformed from something negative (e.g., "The patient can't be trusted" or "I am out of control") to something positive (e.g., "The patient is becoming safer" and "Maybe I can keep myself safe after all"). As the patient becomes more confident in understanding and controlling self-harm behaviour, the frequency of observation periods can be gradually reduced.

During the early part of the hospitalization, the most important way to reduce stress is to help the patient feel more secure and hopeful. Nurses can do so by ensuring the patient's safety with as little intrusion as possible on the person's exercise of free will. Achieving this goal can be difficult. The major deterrent to patients' completing suicide in psychiatric hospitals is their engagement in a therapeutic relationship and regular observation by nurses. Each hospital has its own specific protocol for maintaining patients' safety. In addition to nursing standards of care, hospital staffing and other policies that affect the degree to which a suicidal patient can be restrained may influence the procedures mandated for caring for patients. Maintaining a safe environment includes observing the patient regularly for suicidal behaviour, removing any objects that could be used to self-injure, and providing counselling opportunities for the patient. Part of ensuring patient safety is helping patients to reestablish personal control by including them in decisions about their care as much as possible and restricting their behaviour and choices only as necessary.

Seclusion and restraint are two modalities sometimes used in inpatient settings to maintain safety. However, these highly restrictive interventions are extremely stressful for patients and may interfere with their recovery. Moreover, seclusion and restraint should never be used to compensate for inadequate staffing numbers. Unduly restraining patients to prevent self-harm actually interferes with the development of trusting relationships between patients and healthcare providers. The stress associated with restraints can contribute to the biochemical disarray of any underlying psychiatric disorder(s). Further, restraints prevent patients from managing their own dysphoric and anxiety symptoms and may reinforce their sense of hopelessness and helplessness. Restraints also enhance patients' fears that they are "crazy" and incapable of controlling their impulses. These restrictive methods may reinforce a patient's perception of being out of control and lessen their ability to form a partnership with mental health providers. Further, seclusion and restraints can trigger past experiences of trauma and violence. Thus, the use of seclusion and restraints should be a last resort for a time-limited period and then require reassessment.

Psychopharmacological Therapies

Suicidal patients with MDDs will likely receive antidepressant medications and individual patient's response to these treatments must be monitored. The objective of medications for suicidal behaviour is to ameliorate depression and reduce suicide risk. To that end, classifications of antidepressant medications, such as selective serotonin reuptake inhibitors, should be used for those patients who are in imminent danger of harming themselves. Generally, these medications are nontoxic and cause few side effects, especially after being taken for 1 to 2 weeks. They are often faster acting than the older classifications of antidepressant medications, but the onset of action varies with each type of medication. Patients who take an overdose of these medications are likely to have much better outcomes than patients who overdose with older antidepressants. The older classifications of antidepressants, including tricyclics and monoamine oxidase inhibitors, are also effective for severe depression. However, for patients with suicidal behaviour, these medications may not be the best choice because they can be highly toxic and used as a means to die by suicide. The resuscitation of a patient who has taken large amounts of these older medications can be difficult because of cardiotoxicity, and medical sequelae may be long term if the patient is able to be saved. Also, the side effects of these older antidepressants may result in the patient stopping the use of prescribed medication while still having suicidal thoughts.

Electroconvulsive therapy (ECT) may be useful for selected patients with intractable suicidal ideation and severe depression. ECT is used for people who do not experience a response to medication (treatment resistant) or who cannot tolerate antidepressant medications, such as older adults and those with comorbid medical conditions. Although the decision must be made carefully, ECT can be a lifesaving procedure for the acutely suicidal patient. Nurses need to be able to support patients in accepting and understanding this highly stigmatized treatment (see Chapters 13 and 22). Regardless of the treatment intervention that is prescribed, ongoing assessment of the patient's suicidal ideation and behaviour is required. As a patient's depression is lifting, they may find that they may now have the energy to carry out their plan. This is a critical time and the nurse must monitor and be aware of changes in the patient's symptoms.

Substance-Related and Addictive Disorders

Suicidal behaviour is often associated with substance-related and addictive disorders, especially among men. When substance use is an issue for an individual with suicidality, the use must be addressed or the danger of the patient repeating a suicidal attempt will remain high. The nurse should help the patient understand the role that alcohol and/or other substances play in their life and their suicidal behaviour. Harm reduction strategies for substance use disorders should be part of the treatment plan, as appropriate, including referral to specific inpatient or community-based programs (see Chapter 26). Nurses should provide overdose prevention education to patients who are substance involved (especially those who use opioids), that their tolerance will have decreased during hospitalization and using the same dose after discharge may result in an unintentional overdose.

Interventions for the Psychological Domain

It is important for nurses to use the hospitalization period to find out what may have triggered or contributed to the suicidal crisis. Precipitating factors and how the individual's coping processes were ineffective, often become evident. After identifying extreme stressors experienced by the patient, the nurse and patient can help determine ways to avoid or manage those stressors more effectively in the future. During hospitalization, the nurse should evaluate the patient's ways of thinking about problems, problem solving, and carrying out solutions. Some patients, by virtue of their concurrent illness or social learning, have an unusually negative view of life and/or an external locus of control. They may think such thoughts as, "I am no good," "Everything I do is useless," "I have no future," or "Nobody has ever liked me, and nobody ever will." Often patients are unable to recognize the connection between their stressors and their suicidal behaviour. Many patients have had very difficult and traumatic experiences in their lives, and their ability to cope is threatened. It is important for the nurse to help the individual identify what needs to change in their life and how that change can come about most effectively. The prevention of further suicidal behaviour is dependent on the patient's belief that they can drive meaningful change, with the necessary support and resources, to create hope for the future.

Interventions for the Social Domain

Improving Communication

Some individuals can identify family and friends who are willing to help, but in many cases, they are concerned about burdening these people or do not feel comfortable sharing their concerns with others. Helping the individual express these concerns and arrive at ways of reducing them is important. In other cases, because of trauma and abuse, patients may have difficulty identifying anyone in their lives as supportive. These patients are usually at a high risk for suicide because of their perception of aloneness and lack of connection with any significant other. The nurse needs to assist the individual to identify the potential for people in their life to be supportive and make appropriate referrals to professionals with relevant expertise. Within the confines of therapeutic boundaries, the nurse can be one of the supportive clinicians if the nurse is successful in establishing a professional relationship with the patient.

Support Networks and Discharge Planning

Another concern may be patients' embarrassment, shame, or guilt about the hospitalization and their emotional state. Through education, the nurse can do much to destigmatize the situation for both the patient and significant others. Together, with the patient's permission, the nurse can work with the patient and family (or other supportive individuals) to begin to develop a social network for the patient to rely on to remain safe. It is important for the patient and their designated supports to have a plan to contact another person, either a confidante or a mental healthcare provider, when they have questions, distressing thoughts, or feel unable to cope.

Educating the Patient and Family

The objectives of patient and family education are to increase understanding about plans for post-discharge care and offer an opportunity for questions and concerns to be raised. Key areas to explore include the origins of the patient's suicidal behaviour, effective treatments for comorbid mental health issues and/or substance use, ongoing and seamless outpatient treatment, a plan for managing future suicidal ideation, and identifying additional support and resources in the community. Fully achieving these objectives are demanding for both the nurse and patient during a brief hospitalization. When possible, the nurse should schedule educational sessions to include significant others so that they will better understand the patient's illness and also learn about the detailed plans for outpatient care.

Interventions for the Spiritual Domain

Nurses not only must understand the influences within the bio/psycho/social domains on their patients' experiences but also must understand how a sense of purpose in life encompasses the other three domains. In order to understand suicide from a patient perspective, it is important to be open to patients' concepts of spirituality. The lived experience of suicide contemplation needs to be heard in a caring way. By providing a patient with the time and space to explore their own understanding about meaning in their life, their spirituality, and their concept of death and dying, nurses may gain insight into the factors that precipitated the patient's suicidal thoughts and behaviours. Valued members of the health care team such as chaplains and elders, and community clergy and religious figures (e.g., priests, imams, rabbis) can be important resources.

Evaluation and Treatment Outcomes

The most desirable treatment outcome is the patient's return to the community and to optimize their personal baseline functioning. Because most hospitalizations for suicidal behaviour are brief, discharge planning must begin when the patient is being admitted. The nurse needs to explain to the patient that hospitalization is likely to be short term and should immediately begin to form a partnership with the patient and family to ensure a smooth transition back to the community. Partnering means empowering patients to engage in self-care as soon as possible by helping to provide the support, information, and tools they need for informed decision-making, effective problem solving, and adaptive coping.

Referrals, Resources, and Additional Support

Appropriate referrals to professionals in the community and understanding the resources and support that are available and relevant to each individual patient are important steps for the nurse to contribute to recovery. A nurse or therapist in the community will require information about an individual and their history to continue with effective interventions after discharge. Therefore, the nurse ensures that required information is provided, follows up to make sure it has been received, and relays upcoming appointment information to the patient.

It is helpful for community nurses and mental health workers, in addition to visits, to call periodically during the few first weeks after discharge to assess how the patient is doing. This contact will help the patient to feel valued and connected to others. In addition to engaging family and/or other supportive people in the patient's ongoing care, the nurse also explores other sources of help in the community that may be relevant to the individual, such as church groups, drop-in centres, or other social/peer support groups. A patient's inability to name any significant others or means of social support often signals an increased risk for poor outpatient outcomes.

Establishing an Outpatient Care Plan

At the time of discharge from hospital, the patient who has experienced suicidality is still considered very ill. Most repeat attempts of suicide occur during the first week after discharge, and many happen within the first 24 hr. Before the patient's release, a specific, concrete plan for outpatient care must be in place (see Box 20.8 for considerations for imminent risk of harm). There should be continuity of care between inpatient and outpatient settings. Nurses must tell their patients specifically how to obtain emergency psychiatric care, provide patients with written instructions, and ensure that emergency contact numbers are placed in their phones. Lack of continuity of care is thought to contribute to significant suicide mortality after hospital discharge. The outpatient care plan must include scheduled appointments for follow-up care, providing for continuing medication until the first outpatient treatment visit, ensuring postrelease contact between the patient and significant others, and making arrangements for the patient's home environment to provides both structure and safety. The outpatient environment should be made as safe as possible before discharge. The nurse must share the care plan with family members so that they can assist with removing any items in the patient's environment that could be used for self-harm or suicidal behaviours. The nurse must explain this measure to patients to reinforce their sense of self-control and feelings of being an integral part of planning for their safety. It is important to be reasonable in deciding what to remove from the environment. Patients who are truly determined to kill themselves after discharge may ultimately complete suicide, despite best efforts.

At discharge, the patient should have enough medication on hand to last until the first community nurse visit or follow-up appointment with a healthcare provider. At that time, the doctor or nurse practitioner can assess the individual's level of stability and determine whether a full prescription can be safely provided. Further, the patient and healthcare provider can explore a responsive plan of care that specifies the frequency and intensity of outpatient care, to meet the unique and emerging needs of that person. Individuals who feel very unstable after discharge may need two to three outpatient visits per week in the early days after hospitalization in order to maintain their safety in the community. Patients and significant others must have a plan for ongoing supervision, which is established in such a way that the individual does not feel undermined in their ability to manage self-care and make decisions, but is also reassured that help will be available if and when it is needed. Family members/support people should feel that they are resources for the patient but not responsible for the patient's life or death. In the end, it is each individual, and not their support network, who must bear responsibility for their own safety and their life. Individuals who feel connected to, but not dependent on significant others, will be most likely to maintain health, safety, and wellbeing in the community.

Short-Term Outcomes

Short-term outcomes for the suicidal patient include maintaining the patient's safety, averting suicide, and mobilizing the patient's resources. Whether patients are hospitalized or cared for in the community, their emotional distress must be reduced. Understanding the individual and their unique needs will help the nurse to identify shared goals and the best options for providing sustained emotional support. Nursing diagnoses may focus on risk for injury, ineffective coping, self-care

---

BOX 20.8 Emergency: Imminent Risk of Harm

American researchers Steele and colleagues (2018) performed an extensive literature review to explore suicide risk factors across the life span. In their findings, teens were found to be at highest risk if they had conflict with family or significant other, suffered from insomnia, or felt like a burden. However, adults were at greatest risk if they had experienced a major loss (e.g., loss of marriage or job) and/or were substance involved. Older adults showed more significant risk for suicide if they experienced isolation,

a sense of hopelessness, and/or had medical comorbidities. One recommendation from this study is that all individuals with suicidality should be screened to determine the accessibility of firearms.

From Steele, I. H., Thrower, N., Noroian, P., & Saleh, F. M. (2018). Understanding suicide across the lifespan: A United States perspective of suicide risk factors, assessment & management. *Journal of Forensic Sciences*, 63(1), 162–171. https://doi.org/10.1111/1556-4029.13519

deficit, knowledge deficiency, risk for anxiety or fear, complicated grieving, low self-esteem, social isolation/impaired social interaction, powerlessness, or disturbed thought processes. Treatments during the suicidal crisis should also set the stage for meeting long-term objectives.

Long-Term Outcomes

Long-term outcomes must focus on maintaining the patient's mental and physical health and wellbeing, enabling the patient and their support network to identify and manage stress (including any future suicidal crises), and utilizing effective coping strategies. Long-term goals for the patient should include meaningful accomplishments and connections.

Impact on Nurses

Moral Distress and Moral Injury

Professional work centred on relief of emotional suffering involves empathy as a key tool, which can put providers at risk due to secondary or vicarious trauma. Caring for suicidal patients who are close to one's own age or who have a history of being abused or neglected in childhood can be challenging to process. To care successfully for individuals, families, and/or communities in crisis, nurses must attend to their own wellbeing. Self-care with attention to balancing nutrition, sleep/rest, exercise/activity, positive relationships, and effective coping skills facilitates good management of personal and professional stress. Nurses have knowledge of this information but do not always apply it for themselves. Self-awareness is integral to therapeutic nursing practice, particularly in terms of one's feelings of anxiety, depression, and vulnerability. Debriefing (i.e., sharing experiences and feelings) about stressful situations and one's response to them with a colleague and developing support within the team (so that members do not feel isolated, but rather that care burdens are shared) are helpful strategies.

Over time, the emotional labour of caring work can become exhausting, even when the caregiver is diligently maintaining self-care skills. Compassion fatigue and/or burnout may not be recognized as such by an overwhelmed healthcare provider; it is often caring others who realize their colleague is in trouble (Austin et al., 2013). Also of concern are experiences of moral distress, that is, when a nurse feels the need to act to address an ethical issue, but cannot due to a variety of barriers (Jameton, 1993), and moral injury, that is, betrayal of what's right, by a person in authority, in a high stakes situation (Shay, 2014). These, often recurring, experiences are of genuine concern and may result in diminished capacity to function at work, at home, and within personal and professional relationships. The nurse may begin to avoid further stress through absenteeism or presentism (i.e., being physically present but not truly engaged in one's role). This is a signal that a nurse's health is at risk (Mathieu, 2012). There is very little tracked in terms of statistics about nurses who die by suicide, but it does occur and it occurs in a culture of silence (Davidson et al., 2018). Your clinical work presents an opportunity for you, as nurses of the future, to open the dialogue, mitigate the judgment, end the stigma, and address suicide one caring conversation at a time. And if you (or someone you know) are experiencing suicidality, please reach out for help. Canada Suicide Prevention Service takes crisis calls from anywhere in Canada, 24 hr a day/7 days a week, and offers support in French or English, toll-free **1-833-456-4566** (also see Web Links).

Summary of Key Points

- Self-harm and suicide are major global public health concerns.
- Self-harm and suicidal behaviours are associated with biological, psychological, social, and spiritual factors.
- Self-harm and suicidal behaviours are a means of communicating distress and/or overwhelm in an individual's life.
- People who threaten suicide have individual rights that must be preserved.
- An individual with self-harm or suicidal behaviours is likely to feel a profound sense of hopelessness and/or helplessness, is likely to be experiencing a disturbance in emotional regulation, and likely has symptoms of depression.
- Statistically, individuals who engage in self-harm are likely to do so repeatedly and are at greater risk to die by suicide.
- Statistically, parasuicide and multiple suicide attempts are more common among women; men have higher rates of suicide completion because of the use of more lethal means.
- Contracting for safety is a potential means of increasing the suicidal patient's safety.
- The major objectives of brief hospital care are to maintain the patient's safety, reestablish the patient's biological equilibrium, strengthen the patient's cognitive and emotional coping skills, and develop an outpatient support system.
- The nurse who cares for patients, families, and communities and is exposed to suicidality is vulnerable to experiences of moral distress and moral injury, and therefore must take steps to promote and protect personal resilience and wellbeing.

Thinking Challenge

1. A nurse is caring for a client with a history of suicidal ideations. The client has attempted suicide by ingesting large doses of sedatives and is currently on suicide precautions on the psychiatric behavioural health unit.

   a. What are some factors that increase the risk for suicide completion?

   b. What is a no self-harm contract?

   c. How can the nurse ensure safety of this client while in their care?

> Visit thePoint to view suggested responses.
> Go to **thePoint.lww.com/activate** and use the activation code found in the front of this text to unlock answers to the "Thinking Challenges" and other online resources.

Web Links

https://www.suicideprevention.ca/ Canadian Association for Suicide Prevention intends to reduce the rate and consequences of suicide through providing educational materials and resources.

https://ccsmh.ca/booklet/ Canadian Coalition for Seniors' Mental Health is a federal government initiative that provides information and resources to seniors and their families.

https://www.crisisservicescanada.ca/en/ Canada Suicide Prevention Service has been engaging the public since 2002 and is a collaboration of service centres across the country. They believe in partnerships to improve outcomes for those who are expressing suicidality.

https://crise.ca/ Centre for Research and Intervention on Suicide and Euthanasia is an interdisciplinary research centre, known as CRISE, located at the Université du Québec à Montréal. Their work is focused to reduce suicide, suicidal behaviours, and negative consequences.

http://railwaysuicideprevention.com/ Centre for Research and Intervention on Suicide, Ethical Issues, & End-of-Life Practices, at the Université du Québec à Montréal, includes research on railway suicide prevention and other research projects around the world.

https://www.suicideinfo.ca/ Centre for Suicide Prevention provides information about workshops, resources, and events related to responding to people at risk of suicide in Canada.

http://firstnationssuicideprevention.com/ First Nations Youth Suicide Prevention Program Curriculum provides educational materials and strategies to promote resilience and hope among First Nations' youth.

https://thelifelinecanada.ca/resources/ Lifeline Canada Foundation has a gallery of suicide prevention resources.

https://www.canada.ca/en/department-national-defence/services/benefits-military/military-mental-health.html Military Mental Health offers information about suicide awareness and mental health for members of the Canadian Armed Forces.

https://www.thetrevorproject.org/ Trevor Project, founded in 1998, this American resource provides suicide prevention and crisis intervention services for LBGTQIA2+ youth (under age 25).

https://www.mentalhealthcommission.ca/English/308-conversations #308 Conversations is an initiative by the Mental Health Commission of Canada that provides information, templates, and resources to support a suicide prevention event in your community.

References

Agostino, H., & Burstein, B. (2020). 90 perceived barriers to the provision of adolescent confidential care in the tertiary care setting. *Paediatrics & Child Health, 25*(Suppl 2), e37.

Agrawal, A., Tillman, R., Grucza, R. A., Nelson, E. C., McCutcheon, V. V., Few, L., Conner, K. R., Lynskey, M. T., Dick, D. M., Edenberg, H. J., Hesselbrock, V. M., Kramer, J. R., Kuperman, S., Nurnberger, J. I., Schuckit, M. A., Porjesz, B., & Bucholz, K. K. (2017). Reciprocal relationships between substance use and disorders and suicidal ideation and suicide attempts in the Collaborative Study of the Genetics of Alcoholism. *Journal of Affective Disorders, 213*, 96–104. https://doi.org/10.1016/j.jad.2016.12.060

Alacreu-Crespo, A., Olié, E., Guillaume, S., Girod, C., Cazals, A., Chaudieu, I., & Courtet, P. (2020). Dexamethasone suppression test may predict more severe/violent suicidal behavior. *Frontiers in Psychiatry, 11*, 97. https://doi.org/10.3389/fpsyt.2020.00097

Aldrich, R. S., & Cerel, J. (2020). Occupational suicide exposure and impact on mental health: Examining differences across helping professions. *OMEGA-Journal of Death and Dying, 0*(0), 1–15. https://doi.org/10.1177/0030222820933019

Allen, K. J., Bozzay, M. L., & Edenbaum, E. R. (2019). Neurocognition and suicide risk in adults. *Current Behavioral Neuroscience Reports, 6*(4), 151–165. https://doi.org/10.1007/s40473-019-00189-y

Angelakis, I., Austin, J. L., & Gooding, P. (2020). Association of childhood maltreatment with suicide behaviors among young people: A systematic review and meta-analysis. *JAMA Network Open, 3*(8), e2012563. https://doi.org/10.1001/jamanetworkopen.2020.12563

Asarnow, J. R., Porta, G. M. S., Spirito, A., Emslie, G., Clarke, G., Wagner, K. D., Vitiello, B., Keller, M., Birmaher, B., McCracken, J., Mayes, T., Berk, M., & Brent, D. A. (2011). Suicide attempts and nonsuicidal self-injury in the treatment of resistant depression in adolescents: Findings from the TORDIA study. *Journal of the American Academy of Child & Adolescent Psychiatry, 50*(8), 772–781. https://doi.org/10.1016/j.jaac.2011.04.003

Austin, W., Brintnell, E. S., Goble, E., Kagan, L., Kreitzer, L., Larsen, D. J., & Leier, B. (2013). *Lying down in the ever-falling snow: Canadian health professionals' experience of compassion fatigue.* Wilfrid Laurier Press.

Barker, P. (2001). The Tidal Model: Developing an empowering, person-centred approach to recovery within psychiatric and mental health nursing. *Journal of Psychiatric and Mental Health Nursing, 8*, 233–240.

Barker, P., & Buchanan-Barker, P. (2005). *The Tidal Model: A guide for mental health professionals.* Brunner-Routledge.

Beck, A. T. (2011). *Cognitive behavior therapy: Basics and beyond* (2nd ed.). Guilford.

Beck, A. T., Brown, G. K., & Steer, R. A. (1997). Psychometric characteristics of the scale for suicide ideation with psychiatric outpatients. *Behaviour Research and Therapy, 35*, 1039–1046.

Beck, A. T., Kovacs, M., & Weissman, A. (1979). Assessment of suicidal intention: The scale for suicide ideation. *Journal of Consulting and Clinical Psychology, 47*, 343–352.

Beck, A. T., Schuyler, D., & Herman I. (1974). Development of suicidal intent scales. In A. T. Beck II, L. P. Resnik, & D. J. Lettieri (Eds.), *The prediction of suicide.* Charles Press.

Beck, A. T., Steer, R. A., & Ranieri, W. F. (1988). Scale for suicide ideation: Psychometric properties of a self-report version. *Journal of Clinical Psychology, 44*, 499–505.

Beck, A. T., Weissman, A., Lester, D., & Trexler, L. (1974). The measurement of pessimism: The Hopelessness Scale. *Journal of Consulting and Clinical Psychology, 42*(6), 861–865.

Behera, C., Kishore, S., Kaushik, R., Sikary, A. K., & Satapathy, S. (2020). Suicide announced on Facebook followed by uploading of a handwritten suicide note. *Asian Journal of Psychiatry, 52,* e102061. https://doi.org/10.1016/j.ajp.2020.102061

Berardelli, I., Erbuto, D., Rogante, E., Sarubbi, S., Lester, D., & Pompili, M. (2020). Making sense of the unique pain of survivors: A psychoeducational approach for suicide bereavement. *Frontiers in Psychology, 11,* 1244. https://doi.org/10.3389/fpsyg.2020.01244

Bergen, H., Hawton, K., Ness, J., Cooper, J., Steeg, S., & Kupur, N. (2012). Premature death after self-harm: A multicenter cohort study. *Lancet, 380,* 1568–1574. https://doi.org/10.1016/S0140-6736(12)61141-6

Bergen, H., Hawton, K., Waters, K., Ness, J., Cooper, J., Steeg, S., & Kapur, N. (2012). How do methods of non-fatal self-harm relate to eventual suicide? *Journal of Affective Disorders, 136*(3), 526–533. https://doi.org/10.1016/j.jad.2011.10.036

Bongar, B., Sullivan, G., Kendrick, V., & Tomlins, J. (2017). Evaluating and managing suicide risk with the adult patient. *The Oxford Handbook of Behavioral Emergencies and Crises,* 115–125.

Bongar., B., Sullivan, G., Kendrick, V., & Tiomlins, J. (2016). Evaluating and managing suicide risk with the adult patient. In P. M. Kleespies (Ed.), *The Oxford handbook of behavioral emergencies and crises* (pp. 115–125). Oxford University Press. doi:10.1093/oxfordhb/9780199352722.001.0001

Borschmann, R., Mundy, L. K., Canterford, L., Moreno-Betancur, M., Moran, P. A., Allen, N. B., Viner, R. M., Degenhardt, L., Kosola, S., Fedyszyn, I., & Patton, G. C. (2020). Self-harm in primary school-aged children: Prospective cohort study. *PLoS One, 15*(11), e0242802. https://doi.org/10.1371/journal.pone.0242802

Brown, L. A. (2020). Suicide in foster care: A high-priority safety concern. *Perspectives on Psychological Science, 15*(3), 665–668. https://doi.org/10.1177/1745691619895076

Brown, T. B., & Kimball, T. (2013). Cutting to live: A phenomenology of self-harm. *Journal of Marital and Family Therapy, 39*(2), 195–208. https://doi.org/10.1111/j.1752-0606.2011.00270.x

Byard, R. W., Winskog, C., & Heath, K. (2019). Nitrogen inhalation suicide pacts. *Medicine, Science and the Law, 59*(1), 57–60. https://doi.org/10.1177/0025802419828914

Campos, A. I., Verweij, K. J. H., Statham, D. J., Madden, P. A., Maciejewski, D. F., Davis, K. A., John, A., Hotopf, M., Heath, A. C., Martin, N. G., & Rentería, M. E. (2020). Genetic aetiology of self-harm ideation and behaviour. *Scientific Reports, 10*(1), 1–11. https://doi.org/10.1038/s41598-020-66737-9

Canadian Association for Parish Nursing Ministry. (2020). *Parish nursing.* https://www.capnm.ca/

Canadian Centre for Suicide Prevention. (2020). *Suicide stats for Canada, provinces and territories.* https://www.suicideinfo.ca/resource/suicide-stats-canada-provinces/

Canadian Coalition for Seniors' Mental Health. (2008). *Suicide risk and prevention of suicide.* https://ccsmh.ca/projects/suicide/

Canadian Federation of Mental Health Nurses. (2014). *Canadian standards of psychiatric-mental health nursing* (4th ed.). https://www.cfmhn.ca/professional-practice/

Canadian Institute for Health Information. (2020). *Thousands of Canadians a year are hospitalized or die after intentionally harming themselves.* https://www.cihi.ca/en/thousands-of-canadians-a-year-are-hospitalized-or-die-after-intentionally-harming-themselves

Canadian Mental Health Association. (2020). *Light a candle for world suicide prevention day.* https://cmhahkpr.ca/news/world-suicide-prevention-day-on-thursday-sept-10-2020/

Canadian Nurses Association. (2017). *Code of ethics for registered nurses.* https://cna-aiic.ca/~/media/cna/page-content/pdf-en/code-of-ethics-2017-edition-secure-interactive.pdf?la=en

Carmichael, V., & Whitley, R. (2019). Media coverage of Robin Williams' suicide in the United States: A contributor to contagion? *PLoS One, 14*(5), e0216543. https://doi.org/10.1371/journal.pone.0216543

Carpenter, E. (2020). National study says 'our children are not alright' under mounting stress of pandemic. *CBC Calgary.* https://www.cbc.ca/news/canada/calgary/covid-pandemic-children-mental-health-physical-poverty-calgary-study-canada-1.5707493

Catalyst. (2020). *People of Colour in Canada: Quick take.* https://www.catalyst.org/research/people-of-colour-in-canada/

Centre for Suicide Prevention. (n.d.). *Resources.* Canadian Mental Health Association. https://www.suicideinfo.ca/resources/

Chase, S., & Solari-Twadell, P. A. (2020). Faith community nursing: A professional specialty nursing practice. In P. Solari-Twadell & D. Ziebarth (Eds.), *Faith community nursing: An international speciality practice changing the understanding of health (e-book).* Springer. https://doi.org/10.1007/978-3-030-16126-2_1

Children First Canada, University of Calgary, & Alberta Children's Hospital. (2020). *Raising Canada 2020.* https://childrenfirstcanada.org/raising-canada

Choo, C. C., Harris, K. M., & Ho, R. C. (2019). Prediction of lethality in suicide attempts: Gender matters. *OMEGA-Journal of Death and Dying, 80*(1), 87–103.

Cooper, J., Murphy, E., Webb, R., Hawton, K., Bergen, H., Waters, K., & Kapur, N. (2010). Ethnic differences in self-harm, rates, characteristics and service provision: Three-city cohort study. *The British Journal of Psychiatry, 197*(3), 212–218. https://doi.org/10.1192/bjp.bp.109.072637

Correction Services Canada. (2019). *Annual report on deaths in custody 2016–2017.*

Cull, J. G., & Gill, W. S. (1989). *Suicide probability scale (SPS).* Western Psychological Services.

Cutcliffe, J. R., & Barker, P. (2004). The Nurses' Global Assessment of Suicide Risk (NGASR): Developing a tool for clinical practice. *Journal of Psychiatric and Mental Health Nursing, 11*(4), 393–400. http://works.bepress.com/john_cutcliffe/164/

Dallaire, R., & Humphreys, J. D. (2016). *Waiting for first light: My ongoing battle with PTSD.* Random House Canada.

Dantchev, S., Hickman, M., Heron, J., Zammit, S., & Wolke, D. (2019). The independent and cumulative effects of sibling and peer bullying in childhood on depression, anxiety, suicidal ideation, and self-harm in adulthood. *Frontiers in Psychiatry, 10,* 651. https://doi.org/10.3389/fpsyt.2019.00651

Dardas, L. A., & Simmons, L. A. (2015). The stigma of mental illness in Arab families: A concept analysis. *Journal of Psychiatric and Mental Health Nursing, 22*(9), 668–679. https://doi.org/10.1111/jpm.12237

Daukantaitė, D., Lundh, L. G., Wångby-Lundh, M., Claréus, B., Bjärehed, J., Zhou, Y., & Liljedahl, S. I. (2021). What happens to young adults who have engaged in self-injurious behavior as adolescents? A 10-year follow-up. *European Child and Adolescent Psychiatry, 30,* 475–492. https://doi.org/10.1007/s00787-020-01533-4

Davidson, J., Mendis, J., Stuck, A. R., DeMichele, G., & Zisook, S. (2018). Nurse suicide: Breaking the silence. *NAM Perspectives.* https://www.suicideinfo.ca/wp-content/uploads/gravity_forms/6-191a85f36ce9e20de2e2fa3869197735/2018/01/Nurse-Suicide_oa.pdf

Doane, G. H., & Varcoe, C. (2015). *How to nurse: Relational inquiry with individuals and families in changing health and health care contexts.* Wolters Kluwer Health/Lippincott Williams & Wilkins.

Durkheim, E. (1897/2006). *On suicide.* Penguin Classics.

Egargo, F. J., & Kahambing, J. G. (2021). Existential hope and humanism in COVID-19 suicide interventions. *Journal of Public Health (Oxford, England), 43,* e246–e247. https://doi.org/10.1093/pubmed/fdaa171

Franklin, J. C., & Nock, M. K. (2017). Nonsuicidal self-injury and its relation to suicidal behavior. In P. M. Kleespies (Ed.), *The Oxford handbook of behavioral emergencies and crises* (pp. 401–416). Oxford University Press.

Fuller-Thomson, E., Sellors, A. E., Cameron, R. E., Baiden, P., & Agbeyaka, S. (2020). Factors associated with recovery in Aboriginal people in Canada who had previously been suicidal. *Archives of Suicide Research, 24*(2), 186–203. https://doi.org/10.1080/13811118.2019.1612801

Gargiulo, A., & Margherita, G. (2019). Narratives of self-harm: The experience of young women through the qualitative analysis of blogs. *Mediterranean Journal of Clinical Psychology, 7*(1).

Gearing, R. E., & Alonzo, D. (2018). Religion and suicide: New findings. *Journal of Religion and Health, 57*(6), 2478–2499. https://doi.org/10.1007/s10943-018-0629-8

Gillies, D., Christou, M. A., Dixon, A. C., Featherston, O. J., Rapti, I., Garcia-Anguita, A., Villasis, M., Reebye, P., Christou, E., Al Kabir, N., & Christou, P. A. (2018). Prevalence and characteristics of self-harm in adolescents: Meta-analyses of community-based studies 1990–2015. *Journal of the American Academy of Child & Adolescent Psychiatry, 57*(10), 733–741.

Government of Canada. (2016). *Working together to prevent suicide in Canada: The federal framework for suicide prevention.* https://www.canada.ca/content/dam/canada/public-health/migration/publications/healthy-living-vie-saine/framework-suicide-cadre-suicide/alt/framework-suicide-cadre-suicide-eng.pdf

Government of Canada. (2018). *Inequalities in death by suicide in Canada.* https://www.canada.ca/en/public-health/services/publications/science-research-data/inequalities-death-suicide-canada-infographic.html

Government of Canada. (2020). *Suicide in Canada: Key statistics (infographic).* https://www.canada.ca/en/public-health/services/publications/healthy-living/suicide-canada-key-statistics-infographic.html

Grassi, S., Mandarelli, G., Polacco, M., Vetrugno, G., Spagnolo, A. G., & De-Giorgio, F. (2018). Suicide of isolated inmates suffering from psychiatric disorders: When a preventive measure becomes punitive. *International Journal of Legal Medicine, 132*(4), 1225–1230. https://doi.org/10.1007/s00414-017-1704-5

Hamdan, S., & Peterseil-Yaul, T. (2020). Exploring the psychiatric and social risk factors contributing to suicidal behaviors in religious young adults. *Psychiatry Research, 287*, 112449. https://doi.org/10.1016/j.psychres.2019.06.024

Harris, K. M., Syu, J., Lello, O. D., Chew, Y. L. E., Willcox, C. H., & Ho, R. H. M. (2015). The ABC's of suicide risk assessment: Applying a tripartite approach to individual evaluations. *PLoS One, 10*(6), e0127442. https://doi.org/10.1371/journal.pone.0127442

Heisel, M., & Duberstein, P. (2017). Working sensitively and effectively to reduce suicide risk among older adults: A humanistic approach. In P. M. Kleespies (Ed.), *The Oxford handbook of behavioral emergencies and crises* (pp. 115–125). Oxford University Press. https://doi.org/10.1093/oxfordhb/9780199352722.013.25

Heisel, M. J., & Flett, G. L. (2006). The development and initial validation of the Geriatric Suicide Ideation Scale. *The American Journal of Geriatric Psychiatry, 14*(9), 742–751. https://doi.org/10.1097/01.JGP.0000218699.27899.f9

Heerde, J. A., & Hemphill, S. A. (2018). Are bullying perpetration and victimization associated with adolescent deliberate self-harm? A meta-analysis. *Archives of Suicide Research, 23*, 353–381. https://doi.org/10.1080/13811118.2018.1472690

Hoyos, C., Mancini, V., Furlong, Y., Medford, N., Critchley, H., & Chen, W. (2019). The role of dissociation and abuse among adolescents who self-harm. *Australian & New Zealand Journal of Psychiatry, 53*(10), 989–999. https://doi.org/10.1177/0004867419851869

Inuit Tapiriit Kanatami. (2016). *National Inuit suicide prevention strategy.* www.itk.ca

Jameton, A. (1993). Dilemmas of moral distress: Moral responsibility and nursing practice. *AWHONN's Clinical Issues in Perinatal and Women's Health Nursing, 4*, 542–551.

Juhnke, G. A., Granello, P. F., & Lebron-Striker, M. (2007). Is path warm. A suicide assessment mnemonic for counselors. *Professional Counseling Digest, 3.*

Kaur, R., & Stedmon, J. (2020). A phenomenological enquiry into the impact of bereavement by suicide over the life course. *Mortality*, 1–22. https://doi.org/10.1080/13576275.2020.1823351

Kellner, F., & Marshall, T. (2016). Suicide in Canada. *The Canadian Encyclopedia.* https://www.thecanadianencyclopedia.ca/en/article/suicide

Kirmayer, L. J., Brass, G. M., Holton, T., Paul, K., Simpson, C., & Tait, C. (2007). *Suicide among Aboriginal people in Canada.* Aboriginal Healing Foundation.

Klonsky, E. D., & Glenn, C. R. (2009). Assessing the functions of non-suicidal self-injury: Psychometric properties of the Inventory of Statements about Self-injury (ISAS). *Journal of Psychopathology and Behavioral Assessment, 31*(3), 215–219. https://doi.org/10.1007/s10862-008-9107-z

Knesper, D. J. (2011). *Suicide prevention and research: Suicide attempts and suicide details subsequent to discharge from emergency rooms and psychiatric units.* American Association of Suicidology and Suicide Prevention Research Center, Education Development Centre.

Lawrence, R. E., Oquendo, M. A., & Stanley, B. (2016). Religion and suicide risk: A systematic review. *Archives of Suicide Research, 20*(1), 1–21. https://doi.org/10.1080/13811118.2015.1004494

Linehan, M., Goodstein, J., Nielsen, S., & Chiles, J. (1983). Reasons for staying alive when you are thinking of killing yourself: The Reasons for Living Inventory. *Journal of Consulting and Clinical Psychology, 51*, 276–286.

Maple, M., Frey, L. M., McKay, K., Coker, S., & Grey, S. (2020). "Nobody hears a silent cry for help": Suicide attempt survivors' experiences of disclosing during and after a crisis. *Archives of Suicide Research, 24*, 498–516.

Mars, B., Heron, J., Klonsky, E. D., Moran, P., O'Connor, R. C., Tilling, K., Wilkinson, P., & Gunnell, D. (2019). What distinguishes adolescents with suicidal thoughts from those who have attempted suicide? A population-based birth cohort study. *Journal of Child Psychology and Psychiatry, 60*(1), 91–99. https://doi.org/10.1111/jcpp.12878

Mathieu, F. (2012). *The compassion fatigue handbook.* Taylor & Francis Group, LLC.

May, A. M., & Klonsky, E. D. (2013). Assessing motivations for suicide attempts: Development and psychometric properties of the Inventory of Motivations for Suicide Attempts. *Suicide and Life-Threatening Behavior, 43*(5), 532–546.

Mental Health Commission of Canada. (2012). *Changing directions, changing lives: The mental health strategy for Canada.*

Miller, A. B., & Eisenlohr-Moul, T. A. (2019). Biological responses to acute stress and suicide: A review and opportunities for methodological innovation. *Current Behavioral Neuroscience Reports, 6*, 141–150. https://doi.org/10.1007/s40473-019-00185-2

Morrison, K. L., & Laing, L. (2011). Adults' use of health services in the year before death by suicide. *Health Reports, 22*(3), 1–8.

Mota, N. P., Chartier, M., Ekuma, O., Nie, Y., Hensel, J. M., MacWilliam, L., McDougall, C., Vigod, S. & Bolton, J. M. (2019). Mental disorders and suicide attempts in the pregnancy and postpartum periods compared with non-pregnancy: A population-based study. *The Canadian Journal of Psychiatry, 64*(7), 482–491. https://doi.org/10.1177/0706743719838784

Murray, B. L. (2003). Self-harm among adolescents with developmental disabilities: What are they trying to tell us? *Journal of Psychosocial Nursing, 41*(11), 37–45.

Murray, B. L., & Wright, K. (2006). Integration of a suicide risk assessment and intervention approach: The perspective of youth. *Journal of Psychiatric and Mental Health Nursing, 13*(2), 157–161.

Murphy, A. L., Ataya, R., Himmelman, D., O'Reilly, C., Rosen, A., Salvador-Carulla, L., Martin-Misener, R., Burge, F., Kutcher, S., & Gardner, D. M. (2018). Community pharmacists' experiences and people at risk of suicide in Canada and Australia: A thematic analysis. *Social Psychiatry and Psychiatric Epidemiology, 53*(11), 1173–1184.

Nelson, S. E., & Wilson, K. (2017). The mental health of Indigenous peoples in Canada: A critical review of research. *Social Science and Medicine, 176*, 9–112. https://doi.org/10.1016/j.socscimed.2017.01.021

Nicholas, A., Niederkrotenthaler, T., Reavley, N., Pirkis, J., Jorm, A., & Spittal, M. J. (2020). Belief in suicide prevention myths and its effect on helping: A nationally representative survey of Australian adults. *BMC Psychiatry, 20*(1), 1–12.

Nishnawbe Aski Nation Youth. (2004). *What's wrong? Depression, suicide and Aboriginal teenagers.* https://sites.google.com/site/northernontario-aboriginalyouth/

Nofziger, S., & Callanan, J. (2016). Predicting suicidal tendencies among high risk youth with the general theory of crime. *Deviant Behavior, 37*(2), 167–183.

O'Connor, R. C., & Kirtley, O. J. (2018). The Integrated Motivational–Volitional Model of suicidal behaviour. *Philosophical Transactions of the Royal Society, B: Biological Sciences, 373*(1754), 20170268. https://doi.org/10.1098/rstb.2017.0268

Opara, I., Assan, M. A., Pierre, K., Gunn, J. F., III., Metzger, I., Hamilton, J., & Arugu, E. (2020). Suicide among Black children: An integrated model of the Interpersonal-Psychological Theory of Suicide and Intersectionality Theory for researchers and clinicians. *Journal of Black Studies, 51*(6), 611–631. https://doi.org/10.1177/0021934720935641

Patterson, W. M., Dohn, H. H., Bird, J., & Patterson, G. A. (1983). Evaluation of suicidal patients: The SAD PERSONS scale. *Psychosomatics, 24*(4), 343–349.

Patton, C. L., & Fremouw, W. J. (2016). Examining "suicide by cop": A critical review of the literature. *Aggression and Violent Behavior, 27*, 107–120. https://doi.org/10.1016/j.avb.2016.03.003

Perlman, C. M., Neufeld, E., Martin, L., Goy, M., & Hirdes, J. P. (2011). *Suicide risk assessment inventory: A resource guide for Canadian health care organizations.* Ontario Hospital Association and Canadian Patient Safety Institute. https://www.patientsafetyinstitute.ca/en/toolsResources/SuicideRisk/Documents/Suicide%20Risk%20Assessment%20Guide.pdf#:~:text=The%20Suicide%20Risk%20Assessment%20Guide%3A%20A%20Resource%20for,the%20practice%20of%20high-%20quality%20suicide%20risk%20assessment

Plener, P. L., Libal, G., Keller, F., Fegert, J. M., & Muehlenkamp, J. J. (2009). An international comparison of adolescent non-suicidal self-injury (NSSI) and suicide attempts: Germany and the USA. *Psychological Medicine, 39*(9), 1549–1558. https://doi.org/10.1017/S0033291708005114

Poland, S., Lieberman, R., & Niznik, M. (2019). Suicide contagion and clusters—Part 1: What school psychologists should know. *Communiqué, 47*(5), 1, 21–23.

Posner, K., Brent, D., Lucas, C., Gould, M., Stanley, B., Brown, G., Fisher, P., Zelazny, J., Burke, A., Oquendo, M., & Mann, J. (2008). Columbia-suicide severity rating scale (C-SSRS). *Columbia University Medical Center.* https://depts.washington.edu/ebpa/sites/default/files/C-SSRS-LifetimeRecent-Clinical.pdf

Raines, A. M., Macia, K. S., Currier, J., Compton, S. E., Ennis, C. R., Constans, J. I., & Franklin, C. L. (2020). Spiritual struggles and suicidal ideation in veterans seeking outpatient treatment: The mediating role of perceived burdensomeness. *Psychology of Religion and Spirituality.* Advance online publication. https://doi.org/10.1037/rel0000311

Range, L. M., Campbell, C., Kovac, S. H., Marion-Jones, M., Aldridge, H., Kogos, S., & Crump, Y. (2002). No-suicide contracts: An overview and recommendations. *Death Studies, 26*, 51–74.

Richards, J. E., Whiteside, U., Ludman, E. J., Pabiniak, C., Kirlin, B., Hidalgo, R., & Simon, G. (2019). Understanding why patients may not report suicidal ideation at a health care visit prior to a suicide attempt: A qualitative study. *Psychiatric Services, 70*(1), 40–45. https://doi.org/10.1176/appi.ps.201800342

Ritchie, H., Roser, M., & Ortiz-Ospina, E. (2015). *Suicide.* Our World in Data. https://ourworldindata.org/suicide#:~:text=The%20World%20Health%20Organization%20%28WHO%29%20and%20the%20Global,With%20timely%2C%20evidence-based%20interventions%2C%20suicides%20can%20be%20prevented

Roberts, M. (2018). *Understanding mental health care: Critical issues in practice.* Sage.

Rosenrot, S. A., & Lewis, S. P. (2020). Barriers and responses to the disclosure of non-suicidal self-injury: A thematic analysis. *Counselling Psychology Quarterly, 33*(2), 121–141.

Santangelo, P., Procter, N., & Fassett, D. (2018). Mental health nursing: Daring to be different, special and leading recovery-focused care? *International Journal of Mental Health Nursing, 27*(1), 258–266.

Sareen, J., Holens, P., Turner, S., Jetly, R., Kennedy, S., Heisel, M., Cooper, K., Mota, N., Comtois, K., Stein, M. B., Schaffer, A., Thompson, J., & Heber, A. (2018). Report of the 2016 mental health expert panel on suicide prevention in the Canadian Armed Forces. *Journal of Military, Veteran and Family Health, 4*(1), 70–89. https://doi.org/10.3138/jmvfh.2017-0043

Saunders, N. R., Chiu, M., Lebenbaum, M., Chen, S., Kurdyak, P., Guttmann, A., & Vigod, S. (2019). Suicide and self-harm in recent immigrants in Ontario, Canada: A population-based study. *The Canadian Journal of Psychiatry, 64*(11), 777–788. https://doi.org/10.1177/0706743719856851

Scherr, S., & Reinemann, C. (2011). Belief in a Werther effect: Third-person effects in the perceptions of suicide risk for others and the moderating role of depression. *Suicide and Life-Threatening Behavior, 41*(6), 624–634.

Shahrour, T. M., Mohan, S., Siddiq, M., Hammasi, K. E., & Alsaadi, T. (2018). Suicide attempters in Abu Dhabi: Is criminal prosecution associated with patients' guardedness? *Death Studies, 42*(10), 636–639.

Shay, J. (2014). Moral injury. *Psychoanalytic Psychology, 31*(2), 182.

Shepard, D. S., Gurewich, D., Lwin, A. K., Reed, G. A., & Silverman, M. M. (2016). Suicide and suicidal attempts in the United States: Costs and policy implications. *Suicide and Life-Threatening Behaviour, 46*(3), 352–362. https://doi.org/10.1111/sltb.12225

Shneidman, E. (1985). *Definition of suicide.* John Wiley & Sons.

Shoib, S., & Kim, Y. K. (2019). The frontiers of suicide. In Y. K. Kim (Eds.), *Frontiers in psychiatry. Advances in experimental medicine and biology* (Vol. 1192, pp. 503–517). Springer. https://doi.org/10.1007/978-981-32-9721-0_25

Sinyor, M., Schaffer, A., Heisel, M. J., Picard, A., Adamson, G., Cheung, C. P., Katz, L. Y., Jetly, R., & Sareen, J. (2017). Media guidelines for reporting on suicide: 2017 update of the Canadian Psychiatric Association policy paper. *Canadian Psychiatric Association.* https://www.cpa-apc.org/wp-content/uploads/Media-Guidelines-Suicide-Reporting-EN-2018.pdf

Stack, S. (2020). Media guidelines and suicide: A critical review. *Social Science & Medicine,* 112690. https://doi.org/10.1016/j.socscimed.2019.112690

Statistics Canada. (2017). *Suicide rates: An overview.* https://www150.statcan.gc.ca/n1/pub/82-624-x/2012001/article/11696-eng.htm

Statistics Canada. (2019). *Suicide among First Nations people, Métis and Inuit (2011–2016): Findings from the 2011 Canadian Census Health and Environment Cohort (CanCHEC).* https://www150.statcan.gc.ca/n1/en/daily-quotidien/190628/dq190628c-eng.pdf?st=PEUDtD2o

Statistics Canada. (2020). *Table 13-10-0394-01 Leading causes of death, total population, by age group.* https://doi.org/10.25318/1310039401-eng

Steele, I. H., Thrower, N., Noroian, P., & Saleh, F. M. (2018). Understanding suicide across the lifespan: A United States perspective of suicide risk factors, assessment & management. *Journal of Forensic Sciences, 63*(1), 162–171. https://doi.org/10.1111/1556-4029.13519

Stewart, S. L., Celebre, A., Hirdes, J. P., & Poss, J. W. (2020). Risk of suicide and self-harm in kids: The development of an algorithm to identify high-risk individuals within the children's mental health system. *Child Psychiatry & Human Development, 51,* 913–924. https://doi.org/10.1007/s10578-020-00968-9

Stirling, F. J. (2020). Journeying to visibility: An autoethnography of self-harm scars in the therapy room. *Psychotherapy and Politics International, 18,* e1537. https://doi.org/10.1002/ppi.1537

Suicide Prevention Resource Center. (2008). *It takes a community: Report on the summit on opportunities for mental health promotion and suicide prevention in senior living communities.* Substance Abuse and Mental Health Services Administration. http://www.sprc.org/resources-programs/it-takes-community-report-summit-opportunities-mental-health-promotion-suicide

Tam, T. (2019). *Addressing stigma: Toward a more inclusive health system. The chief public health officer's report on the state of public health in Canada in 2019.* Public Health Agency of Canada. https://www.canada.ca/content/dam/phac-aspc/documents/corporate/publications/chief-public-health-officer-reports-state-public-health-canada/addressing-stigma-what-we-heard/stigma-eng.pdf

Tan, J. C. H., Borg, C., Levy, L., Levy, S., & Tierney, J. (2015). *Report on the workshop on suicide contagion among Inuit youth aged 12–19.*

Taylor, P. J., Dhingra, K., Dickson, J. M., & McDermott, E. (2020). Psychological correlates of self-harm within gay, lesbian and bisexual UK university students. *Archives of Suicide Research, 24,* 41–56. https://doi.org/10.1080/13811118.2018.1515136

Truth and Reconciliation Commission of Canada. (2015). *Calls to action.* http://trc.ca/assets/pdf/Calls_to_Action_English2.pdf

Tzoneva, D. (2018). Parasuicide-the aftermath. *Mental Health Matters, 5*(2), 19–22.

Van Orden, K. A., Witte, T. K., Cukrowicz, K. C., Braithwaite, S. R., Selby, E. A., & Joiner, T. E., Jr. (2010). The interpersonal theory of suicide. *Psychological Review, 117*(2), 575. https://doi.org/10.1037/a0018697

Veale, J. F., Watson, R. J., Peter, T., & Saewyc, E. M. (2017). The mental health of Canadian transgender youth compared with the Canadian population. *The Journal of Adolescent Health, 60*(1), 44–49. https://doi.org/10.1016/j.jadohealth.2016.09.014

Walters, A. S. (2020). Implementing a safety plan intervention as part of suicide risk screening. *The Brown University Child and Adolescent Behavior Letter, 36*(3), 8. https://doi.org/10.1002/cbl.30450

Wand, A. P. F., Peisah, C., Draper, B., & Brodaty, H. (2018). Understanding self-harm in older people: A systematic review of qualitative studies. *Aging & Mental Health, 22*(3), 289–298.

Westerlund, M., Schaller, S., & Schmidtke, A. (2009). The role of mass-media in suicide prevention. In D. Wasserman, & C. Wasserman (Eds.), *Oxford textbook of suicidology and suicide prevention: A global perspective* (pp. 515–525). Oxford University Press.

World Health Organization. (2013). *Mental health action plan 2013–2020.* http://apps.who.int/iris/bitstream/10665/89966/1/9789241506021_eng.pdf?ua=1

World Health Organization. (2016). *Practice manual for establishing and maintaining surveillance systems for suicide attempts and self harm.* https://apps.who.int/iris/bitstream/handle/10665/208895/9789241549578_eng.pdf;jsessionid=7C1ADD3241B7078C7903EDBF89DD7450?sequence=1

World Health Organization. (2018). *World health statistics data visualizations dashboard: Suicide.* https://apps.who.int/gho/data/node.sdg.3-4-viz-2?lang=en

World Health Organization. (2019a). *Suicide.* https://www.who.int/news-room/fact-sheets/detail/suicide

World Health Organization. (2019b). *Suicide in the world: Global health estimates.* https://www.who.int/publications/i/item/suicide-in-the-world

World Health Organization (WHO). (2020). *Suicide data.* https://www.who.int/mental_health/prevention/suicide/suicideprevent/en/

Zolnikov, T. R., & Furio, F. (2020). Stigma on first responders during COVID-19. *Stigma and Health, 5,* 375–379. http://dx.doi.org/10.1037/sah0000270

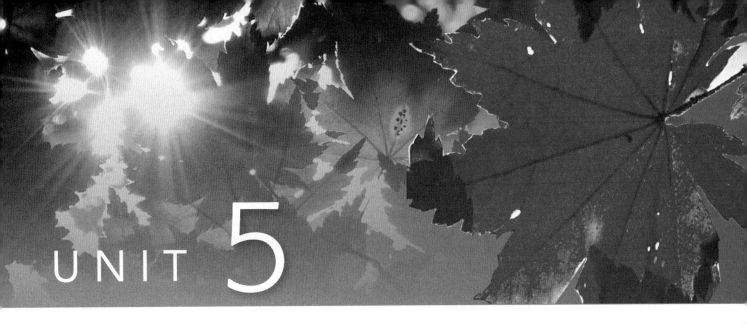

UNIT 5

Care and Recovery for Persons With a Psychiatric Disorder

CHAPTER 21

Schizophrenia Spectrum and Other Psychotic Disorders

Wendy Austin and Tanya Park*

LEARNING OBJECTIVES

After studying this chapter, you will be able to:

- Distinguish and define key features of the schizophrenia spectrum disorders (SSDs) and distinguish the major differences and similarities among them.
- Discuss the theories related to the aetiology of schizophrenia and their relevance to the other SSDs.
- Describe the prevailing epidemiologic findings that form the basis for understanding schizophrenia spectrum and other psychotic disorders.
- Analyze human responses to these disorders, with emphasis on hallucinations, delusions, disorganization, emotional blunting, and social isolation.
- Explain the primary elements involved in assessment, nursing care foci, nursing interventions, and evaluation of individuals with schizophrenia and schizoaffective disorder.
- Formulate a nursing care plan based on a bio/psycho/social/spiritual assessment of persons with schizophrenia and integrate it with the interprofessional care plan.
- Outline the major aspects of nursing care for persons with schizoaffective disorder and identify the aspects of care that differ from care of a person with schizophrenia.
- Discuss special concerns within the nurse–patient relationship common to working with individuals with schizophrenia spectrum disorder.

KEY TERMS

- affective flattening or blunting • affective lability
- akathisia • alogia • ambivalence • anhedonia
- anosognosia • apathy • avolition • bizarre delusions
- delusional disorder • delusions, delusional disorder unspecified type • disorganized behaviour • duration of untreated psychosis • dystonic reactions • echolalia
- echopraxia • erotomanic • extrapyramidal side effects
- first-episode psychosis • grandiose • hallucinations
- hypervigilance • illusions • jealous • metabolic syndrome • neurocognition • nihilistic • persecutory
- shared delusional disorder (folie à deux) • somatic
- stereotypy • tangentiality • tardive dyskinesia • waxy flexibility • word salad

KEY CONCEPTS

- disorganized symptoms • negative (second-rank) symptoms • neurocognitive impairment
- positive (first-rank) symptoms

Classified in the fifth edition of the *Diagnostic and Statistical Manual of Mental Disorders* (DSM-5) under "schizophrenia spectrum and other psychotic disorders [SSDs]" are schizophrenia and schizoaffective, delusional, brief psychotic, and schizophreniform disorders (American Psychiatric Association [APA], 2013). In the *International Classification of Diseases*, 11th Revision, the classification is simply "schizophrenia and other primary psychiatric disorders."

Their common element is the state of psychosis in which an individual can experience these abnormalities: hallucinations, delusions, disorganized thoughts (speech), or behaviour (known as positive symptoms) and/or diminished emotional expression, anhedonia, and avolition (known as negative symptoms). Psychotic disorders may be induced by medications or other substances or may be a symptom of another medical disorder. This chapter introduces the SSDs

---

*Adapted from the chapters, "Schizophrenia" by Tanya Park and "Schizoaffective, Delusional, and Other Psychotic Disorders" by Diana Clarke and Shelley Marchinko

448

and describes the associated nursing care. All nurses need to understand these disorders and advocate to correct stereotyping and misperceptions. Individuals with a serious mental illness may need to access various healthcare services over their lifetime and should expect to receive appropriate, holistic care.

Schizophrenia

Schizophrenia has fascinated and confounded healers, scientists, and philosophers for centuries. It is one of the most severe, complex mental illnesses and is present in all cultures, races, and socioeconomic groups.

Overview of Schizophrenia

The clinical picture of schizophrenia is highly variable and complex. Individual symptoms differ from one another and the experience for a single individual may be different from episode to episode. For some, the illness onset is slow and insidious; for others, it is sudden, seemingly coming from out of the blue. Similarly, the course of schizophrenia is unique and unpredictable. Schizophrenia was once considered a chronic condition, deteriorating over time, but research now indicates that persons

with schizophrenia, living in the community, have significant periods in which symptoms have abated, with fewer hospitalizations and improved functioning over time (Salzer et al., 2018). Recovery is achievable. A study, set in Germany, found that 1 year after discharge, 14% of persons diagnosed with schizophrenia could be viewed as recovered (Spellmann et al., 2017). Schizophrenia remains overall, however, a serious and potentially disabling illness. New advances in our understanding of the aetiology, course, and treatment of schizophrenia spectrum disorders will contribute to further recovery rates.

As is the case with most chronic illnesses, the emphasis in care and treatment must be upon maximizing wellness while minimizing the disability. Recovery does not mean cure. As noted, there is not one predictable outcome for an individual with schizophrenia; rather, it depends on how the illness affects the person, their family, and the kind and type of treatment received. Nurses, in both inpatient and community settings, have an opportunity to help individuals live as well as possible with their illness (Box 21.1).

Acute Illness Period

Initially, the illness behaviours caused by schizophrenia may be confusing and frightening to the person and

BOX 21.1 First Person Accounts of Living With Schizophrenia

Understanding how a disease is experienced by an individual and their family is key to the provision of trustworthy care. It is most meaningful if this insight is achieved directly with them. Learning from first-person accounts shared by others can deepen one's understanding, as well.

Some sources of first-person accounts follow:

- *Schizophrenia Bulletin* offers a series of first-person accounts: https://academic.oup.com/schizophreniabulletin/pages/first_person_accounts
- Daley, T., Jones, N., George, P., & Rosenblatt, A. (2020). First-person accounts of change among young adults enrolled in Coordinated Specialty Care for First-Episode Psychosis. *Psychiatric Services, 71,* 1277–1284. https://doi:10.1176/appi.ps.202000101
- A Canada-wide survey commissioned by the *Schizophrenia Society of Canada* provides insight into the meaning of quality of life. Respondents were people with schizophrenia (*n* = 433) and their families or caregivers (*n* = 570) who shared the importance of hope, optimism, and a belief in recovery. To remain optimistic that recovery is possible when one is unwell and feeling without hope is challenging. To be supportive, nurses and other healthcare professionals need to move beyond a

focus of symptom management to supporting recovery from a body, mind, and spirit perspective. *Schizophrenia Society of Canada* (2009). www.schizophrenia.ca/docs/FINALSSCQOLReport.pdf
- Arndtzén, M., & Sandlund, M. (2020). To live with a schizoaffective disorder. *Journal of Psychiatric and Mental Health Nursing,* 1–5. https://doi:10.1111/jpm.12708
- Demjén, Z., Marszalek, A., Semino, E., & Varese, F. (2019). Metaphor framing and distress in lived-experience accounts of voice-hearing. *Psychosis, 11,* 16–27. https://doi:10.1080/17522439.2018.1563626
- Personal stories by individuals in British Columbia written for *Vision* magazine can be found here: https://www.heretohelp.bc.ca/personal-stories
- Beers, Clifford, W. (1908). The mind that found itself: An autobiography. This is a classic work by a Yale graduate who, in 1900, was placed in an American mental institution for paranoia and depression. Describing his experience and the maltreatment of patients that he witnessed, the book became a best seller. With support from the medical profession and others, reforms to the treatment of the mentally ill began. The book is freely available here: https://www.gutenberg.org/ebooks/11962

the family. At first, the changes (prodromal symptoms) may be subtle and, because they often begin in late adolescence, can even be confused with the anxiety and moodiness of adolescence. However, at some point, the changes in thought and behaviour become so disruptive or bizarre that they can no longer be overlooked. These changes herald the beginning of psychosis. Typically, family and friends become aware that something is not right. Changes might include episodes of staying up all night for several nights, withdrawal from social activities, incoherent conversations, irritability, and/or aggressive acts against self or others. For example, it is not uncommon for parents to report a teenager sneaking around their home for several days, peeking out from behind the curtains, and complaining that their home was under surveillance. Others have noted that their adolescent's first delusional hallucination episode was so convincing that it was frightening—visiting cemeteries and making "mind contact" with the deceased, seeing his deceased grandmother walking around in the home, and certain that there were pipe bombs in objects in his home. Others have reported that their daughter believed that she had been visited by space aliens who wanted to unite their world with Earth and who assured her that she would become the leader of her country.

These experiences are collectively referred to as indicators of **first-episode psychosis (FEP)**, or the initial episode of psychosis, which most often occurs in adolescence or early adult life (see Box "Clinical Vignette"). This early stage of illness, defined as the first 3 to 5 years after the onset of symptoms, is considered a critical period for intervention. Early intervention has been found to lead to more favourable recovery outcomes, and many such programs are offered in Canada and around the world. NAVIGATE, for instance, is a multicomponent treatment program for individuals with FEP and their families that offers individual resiliency training, a family education program, individualized medication treatment and management, and supported employment and education, using a shared decision-making approach (Mueser et al., 2015). The Centre for Addiction and Mental Health (CAMH, 2018) in Toronto has adopted this program. In general, the threefold aim of such programs has been to reduce the **duration of untreated psychosis (DUP)**, intervene appropriately at this early stage of illness, and prevent subsequent relapse, while minimizing the disability. Early intervention efforts have led to new hope for those who develop schizophrenia.

As the DUP increases, affected individuals are less able to care for their basic needs, such as eating, sleeping, and bathing. Substance use is common. Functioning at school or work deteriorates. Dependence on family and friends increases, and those persons recognize the individual's need for treatment. In the acute phase, individuals with schizophrenia are at high risk for suicide and may require hospitalization to protect themselves or others. Initial treatment for schizophrenia focuses upon thorough assessment and the alleviation of symptoms through the initiation of medications, decreasing the risk for suicide through safety measures, normalizing sleep, and reducing substance misuse. Functional deficits may persist during this period, and

CLINICAL VIGNETTE

GRADUATE STUDENT EXPERIENCE

BGW, born in 1985, spent most of his teenage years using drugs and alcohol, behaviour that started when he was 11. He and his small group of friends spent their teenage years outside of school running around on bicycles. He failed 8th grade, repeated it, and made it to 10th grade. He was removed permanently from school at the age of 16. His dress included a dirty denim jacket or Army fatigues, torn tee shirts with rock band logos, and tight-fitting jeans. At age 16, he was hospitalized for a psychotic episode initiated by LSD; it was the scariest moment of his life. His mind had been getting fuzzier every day; he had dabbled with black magic and Satanism. Later, he admitted that for years, he had been trapped in a fantasy land, only partially explained by his drug use.

Years of treatment followed, and even with abstinence from drugs, his mental status fluctuated. Once antipsychotic agents were prescribed, he began to feel like himself. He was motivated to complete his high school diploma and entered college. He kept his mental illness a secret. While in graduate school, his thoughts, feelings, and behaviours began to change. His thinking became delusional, his moods unpredictable, and his behaviours illogical. Finally, he was hospitalized once again, and his condition was stabilized with medications. Currently, he is reapplying to graduate school and this time vowing to keep people close to him aware of his mental status.

Adapted from Oxford University Press and the Maryland Psychiatric Research Center. (2002). Graduate student in peril: A first person account of schizophrenia. *Schizophrenia Bulletin, 28*(4), 745–755.

the individual and family must begin to learn to cope with these. Emotional blunting diminishes the ability and desire to engage in hobbies, vocational activities, and relationships. Limited participation in social activities may spiral into numerous skill deficits, such as difficulty engaging others interpersonally. Similarly, cognitive deficits may lead to problems recognizing patterns in situations and transferring learning and behaviours from one circumstance to another similar one.

Stabilization Period

After the initial diagnosis of psychosis and the initiation of treatment, stabilization of schizophrenia symptoms becomes the focus. Symptoms become less acute but may still be present. Treatment is intense during this period as medication regimens are established and adaptation to various medication side effects occurs. With appropriate assistance and support, adjustment to the situation of living with a serious mental illness takes place for the individual and their family. Ideally, the misuse of substances is eliminated. Socialization with others begins to increase, and rehabilitation begins.

Maintenance and Recovery Period

After the patient's condition is stabilized, there is a focus upon recovery efforts to help them regain a previous level of functioning and improve quality of life. Research indicates that an individual's perception that their treatment is recovery oriented is positively correlated with their subjective quality of life (Sum et al., 2021).

Pharmacologic treatment of schizophrenia has generally contributed to an improvement in symptom remission, but medication is not a cure. Good medication management tends to lessen the severity of impairments in functioning when they do occur and diminishes the extremes individuals might experience. As with any chronic illness, stresses of life and major crises can contribute to exacerbations of acute symptoms.

Clearly, family support and involvement are extremely important at this time. Once the initial diagnosis is made, the individual and their family can be educated regarding early signs of potential relapse and how to cope with it. This is an important theme in nursing those with schizophrenia. A key goal in its treatment is to avoid subsequent relapses after remission of the first episode. This can be challenging. The long-term prognosis for relapse is influenced by the individual's willingness to remain on a maintenance antipsychotic treatment regimen and to access and engage in other therapies and supports as appropriate.

Relapses

Although they are not inevitable, relapse can occur at any time during treatment and recovery and is detrimental

Table 21.1 Fostering Recovery From Schizophrenia
The six key dimensions of recovery-orientated practice
1. Creating a culture and language of hope
2. Recovery is personal
3. Recovery occurs in the context of one's life
4. Responding to the diverse needs
5. Working with First Nations, Inuit, and Métis
6. Métis Transforming services and systems

Mental Health Commission of Canada. (2015). Recovery Guidelines Ottawa, ON: Author. ©2015 Mental Health Commission of Canada

to the successful management of this disorder. With each relapse, rehabilitation is prolonged and recovery takes longer. Medications combined with psychosocial treatments greatly diminish the severity and frequency of relapses (Emsley et al., 2013).

A major reason for relapse is nonadherence to the medication regimen. Side effects of antipsychotic medications are challenging, but discontinuing medications can lead to relapse and, as a stressor, may cause the relapse to be severe and rapid (Freudenreich & Cather, 2012). Lower relapse rates are found among groups whose continuing treatment regimen is effective, so strategies to enhance an individual's recovery are particularly important. Helping the individual derive a realistically hopeful attitude for the future is a worthy goal (see Table 21.1).

Many other factors can trigger a relapse: the degree of impairment in cognition and coping that leaves patients vulnerable to stressors; the accessibility of community resources, such as public transportation, housing, entry-level and low-stress employment, and social services; income supports that buffer the day-to-day stressors of living; the degree of stigmatization that the community holds for mental illness, which undermines the self-concept of patients; and the responsiveness of family members, friends, and supportive others (e.g., peers and professionals) when patients need help.

Diagnostic Criteria

Since the 19th century, schizophrenia has been described as a mixture of positive and negative symptoms (Young et al., 2013). Positive symptoms, or "first-rank" symptoms, reflect an excess or distortion of normal functions, including delusions, **hallucinations**, and thought disturbances. Negative symptoms, or "second-rank" symptoms, reflect a lessening or loss of normal functions, such as restriction or flattening in the range and intensity of emotion (**affective flattening or blunting**), reduced fluency and productivity of thought and speech (**alogia**), withdrawal and inability to initiate and persist in goal-directed activity (**avolition**), and inability to experience pleasure (**anhedonia**).

The DSM-5 criteria for diagnosing schizophrenia include necessary symptomatology, duration of

---

BOX 21.2 DSM-5 Diagnostic Criteria: Schizophrenia

A. Two (or more) of the following, each present for a significant portion of time during a 1-month period (or less if successfully treated). At least one of the symptoms must be (1), (2), or (3):
   1. Delusions
   2. Hallucinations
   3. Disorganized speech (e.g., frequent derailment or incoherence)
   4. Grossly disorganized or catatonic behaviour
   5. Negative symptoms (i.e., diminished emotional expression or avolition)

B. For a significant portion of the time since the onset of the disturbance, level of functioning in one or more major areas, such as work, interpersonal relations, or self-care, is markedly below the level achieved prior to the onset (or when the onset is in childhood or adolescence, there is failure to achieve expected level of interpersonal, academic, or occupational functioning).

C. Continuous signs of the disturbance persist for at least 6 months. This 6-month period must include at least 1 month of symptoms (or less if successfully treated) that meet criterion A (i.e., active-phase symptoms) and may include periods of prodromal or residual symptoms. During these prodromal or residual periods, the signs of

the disturbance may be manifested by only negative symptoms or by two or more symptoms listed in criterion A present in an attenuated form (e.g., odd beliefs, unusual perceptual experiences).

D. Schizoaffective disorder and depressive or bipolar disorder with psychotic features have been ruled out because either (a) no major depressive or manic episodes have occurred concurrently with the active-phase symptoms or (b) if mood episodes have occurred during active-phase symptoms, they have been present for a minority of the total duration of the active and residual periods of the illness.

E. The disturbance is not attributable to the physiologic effects of a substance (e.g., a drug of abuse, a medication) or another medical condition.

F. If there is a history of autism spectrum disorder or a communication disorder of childhood onset, the additional diagnosis of schizophrenia is made only if prominent delusions or hallucinations, in addition to the other required symptoms of schizophrenia, are also present for at least 1 month (or less if successfully treated).

Reprinted with permission from the American Psychiatric Association. (2013). *Diagnostic and statistical manual of mental disorders* (5th ed.).

---

symptoms, evaluation of functional impairment, and elimination of alternate hypotheses that might account for the symptoms (APA, 2013). The diagnostic criteria for schizophrenia are listed in Box 21.2.

KEY CONCEPT

Positive (first-rank) symptoms reflect an excess or distortion of normal functions, including delusions and hallucinations.

KEY CONCEPT

Negative (second-rank) symptoms reflect a lessening or loss of normal functions, such as restriction or flattening in the range and intensity of emotion (affective flattening or blunting), reduced fluency and productivity of thought and speech (alogia), withdrawal (asociality) and inability to initiate and persist in goal-directed activity (avolition), and inability to experience pleasure (anhedonia).

Positive Symptoms of Schizophrenia

Delusions are fixed false beliefs that usually involve a misinterpretation of experience. For example, a person believes someone is reading their thoughts or plotting against them. Types of delusions include the following:

- *Grandiose*: the belief that one has exceptional powers, wealth, skill, influence, or destiny
- *Nihilistic*: the belief that one is dead or a calamity is impending
- *Persecutory*: the belief that one is being watched, ridiculed, harmed, or plotted against
- *Somatic*: beliefs about abnormalities in bodily functions or structures

Hallucinations are perceptual experiences that occur without actual external sensory stimuli. They can involve any of the five senses—auditory, visual, olfactory (smell), gustatory (taste), tactile—and the somatic sense, but *visual* and *auditory* are most common. Auditory hallucinations (e.g., hearing voices commenting on their behaviour) are much more common than visual ones (e.g., seeing a ghostly image that taunts them).

Negative Symptoms of Schizophrenia

Negative symptoms, which affect one in three persons with schizophrenia (Wang et al., 2020), involve the loss of everyday abilities to the extent that long-term functional impairment can occur (Strauss et al., 2018). The losses are complex and related to alterations in brain frontal white matter (FWM), with symptom severity linked to functional connectivity and structural properties of the left FWM (Wang et al., 2020). Negative symptoms comprise the inability to experience pleasure (anhedonia), to self-motivate (avolition), and to socialize (asociality). Facial expressions are diminished or totally lacking (blunted affect) and the ability to converse is significantly diminished (alogia). Thus, while not as dramatic as positive symptoms, negative symptoms are debilitating, interfering greatly with the person's ability to function day to day.

Expression of emotion becomes difficult, so those affected laugh, cry, and get angry less often. They have a flat affect, showing little or no emotion, even when personal loss occurs. They experience ambivalence, which interferes with their ability to make decisions. The avolition may be so profound that simple activities of daily living, such as dressing or combing hair, may not get completed. Speech becomes limited and it becomes difficult to carry on a conversation. Anhedonia prevents them from enjoying life experiences. These symptoms can cause the person to withdraw and experience feelings of severe isolation and loneliness. The pathophysiological mechanisms behind negative symptoms are not well understood, including whether some are primary to schizophrenia while others are secondary to other factors. Fortunately, recognition of their impact on the lives of those living with schizophrenia is driving new investigations in hope of developing treatments for them (Galderisi et al., 2018).

Neurocognitive Impairment

Neurocognition includes short- and long-term memory, vigilance or sustained attention, verbal fluency or the ability to generate new words, and executive functioning, which includes volition, planning, purposive action, and self-monitoring behaviour. Working memory is a concept that includes short-term memory and the ability to store and process information. Neurocognitive impairment exists in schizophrenia and is particularly noted in verbal learning and executive functioning. Impairment is associated primarily more with the disorganized and negative symptoms than with positive symptoms. Long-term memory and intellectual functioning are not necessarily affected. Nevertheless, for many people with this disorder, symptoms interfere with completing educational opportunities and obtaining employment.

It is important that nurses recognize that secondary factors—such medical issues as diabetes or hypertension, or reduced visual acuity—can also contribute to neurocognitive impairment or affect performance on neurocognitive testing. Problems with self-esteem (self-stigma), motivation, and anxiety also influence functioning. It is necessary to take a comprehensive approach when assisting an individual to improve neurocognition, particularly because better functional outcomes are important to quality of life (Moritz et al., 2021).

KEY CONCEPT

Neurocognitive impairment in schizophrenia is noted in memory, vigilance, verbal learning, and executive functioning and can cause poor functional outcome.

KEY CONCEPT

Disorganized symptoms of schizophrenia are those things that make it difficult for the person to understand and respond to the ordinary sights and sounds of daily living. These include disorganized speech and thinking and disorganized behaviour.

Disorganized Thinking

Examples of disturbed speech and thinking patterns can be found in Chapter 11, specifically in Boxes 11.5 and 11.6. Disorganized perceptions often create oversensitivity to colours, shapes, and background activities. **Illusions** occur when the person misperceives or exaggerates stimuli that actually exist in the external environment. This is in contrast to hallucinations, which are perceptions in the absence of environmental stimuli. Ancillary symptoms that may accompany schizophrenia include anxiety, depression, irritability, and hostility.

Disorganized Behaviour

Disorganized behaviour (which may manifest as a very slow, rhythmic, or ritualistic movement), coupled with disorganized speech, makes it difficult for someone with schizophrenia to partake in daily activities. Examples of disorganized behaviour include the following:

- Aggression—behaviours or attitudes that reflect rage, hostility, and the potential for physical or verbal destructiveness (usually occurs when the person believes that someone is going to harm them)
- Agitation—inability to sit still or attend to others, accompanied by heightened emotions and tension
- Catatonic excitement—a hyperactivity characterized by purposeless activities and abnormal movements such as grimacing and posturing

- **Echopraxia**—*involuntary* imitation of another person's movements and gestures
- **Regressed behaviour**—behaving in a manner of a less mature life stage; childlike and immature
- **Stereotypy**—repetitive, purposeless movements that are idiosyncratic to the individual and to some degree outside of the individual's control
- **Hypervigilance**—sustained attention to external stimuli as if expecting something important or frightening to happen
- **Waxy flexibility**—posture held in odd or unusual fixed position for extended periods of time

Schizophrenia in Special Populations

Children

The diagnosis of schizophrenia is rare in children before adolescence. The 2016 incidence ratio in Canada for schizophrenia in persons 10 to 19 years old was 33 per 100,000 (Government of Canada, 2018a). When it does occur in children, the symptoms are essentially the same as in adults. A comprehensive review of clinical studies (1990 to 2014) confirmed that children and adolescents suffering from early-onset schizophrenia experience impairment due to significant positive and negative symptoms, as well as disorganized behaviour. Premorbid and/or comorbid conditions, such as posttraumatic stress disorder and/or attention deficit hyperactivity disorder, tend to be present. While there is usually significant improvement over time, poor pre-illness adjustment and duration of untreated psychosis are associated with less favourable outcomes (Stentebjerg-Olesen et al., 2016). (See Chapter 30, Psychiatric Disorders in Children and Adolescents.)

It is crucial that other medical disorders, including psychiatric disorders, be ruled out before SSD is diagnosed in children and adolescents (APA, 2013; Grover & Avasthi, 2019). For instance, difficulties with speech and language may be related to a developmental disorder, and fantasies, concrete thinking, and social awkwardness indicative of autism spectrum disorder. Even experiences common to these age groups (e.g., imagination, fantasy) may be mistaken as psychopathology (Grover & Avasthi, 2019).

There appears to be a high prevalence of childhood trauma (CT) among adults diagnosed with an SSD, including emotional, physical, and sexual abuse and neglect. In one study of 54 persons with an SSD, more than 75% had experienced CT, all forms of which, except emotional neglect, showed direct correlation with dissociative experiences (disruption in the linkages among self-awareness, feelings, thoughts, and behaviour) in terms of intensity and number of traumas experienced (Álvarez et al., 2021). Experiences of trauma and neglect (as well as substance use) are important epigenetic risk factors for schizophrenia (De Berardis et al., 2021).

It has been proposed within transitional psychiatry that SSDs be reconceived as neurodevelopmental diseases in which interaction of genetics and environment during phases of development leads to neurobiologic vulnerability. Then, in "relatively few cases," emotional dysregulation, basic schizophrenic symptoms, and psychosis may result if there is continuous distress occurring for the individual (De Berardis et al., 2021, p.1).

Older Adults

Older adults with schizophrenia include those who developed the disease as adolescents or young adults, as well as those for whom the onset of schizophrenia occurred between 40 and 60 years of age ("late onset") or after 60 years of age ("very-late onset"). The latter group makes up less than 15% of those with schizophrenia. The clinical presentation is fundamentally similar to early-onset schizophrenia: positive symptoms (particularly paranoid or persecutory delusions), negative symptoms (with less affective blunting), and functional deficits (although social functioning tends to be more intact). Disturbances in sensory functions, primarily hearing and vision losses, may be present (APA, 2013).

In treatment and care of older persons with schizophrenia, a focus on functional recovery is most helpful (Mucci et al., 2021). Approximately half of the older adults who have lived with schizophrenia for many years report a positive quality of life related to remission of symptoms, increased functioning, and recovery (Solomon et al., 2021). Their lifestyle is likely attributable to effectiveness of earlier treatment, the support systems that are in place (including relationships with family members and professionals), and the interaction between environmental stressors and the individual's functional impairments. A 4-year prospective study of more than 600 persons with schizophrenia living in community found that some variables associated with life functioning (i.e., neurocognition, social cognition, avolition, and practical skills) were not a focus of intervention programs. The researchers recommended that personalized, responsive programs, adapted to the needs of the individual, be adopted (Mucci et al., 2021).

Although antipsychotic medication remains a key treatment, often in older adults, dosage can be gradually reduced (Solomon et al., 2021). There is, however, increased susceptibility to this class of drugs' side effects, including increased incidence of tardive dyskinesia. With clozapine, the risk of agranulocytosis is elevated (Galletly et al., 2016). Although older adults with schizophrenia have higher rates of cardiovascular, respiratory, gastrointestinal, neurologic, and endocrine diseases compared with those without schizophrenia, their medical care—beyond the schizophrenia—is less likely to be as good. It is apparent that good medical care and health status monitoring are important to their quality of life and wellbeing, yet these older adults are not as likely as the general population to receive these benefits (Galletly et al., 2016). Loneliness (or perceived social isolation) is common in older adults with schizophrenia, potentially increasing their morbidity and mortality. Depression, too, is common but goes underrecognized and undertreated. Suicidal ideation is higher among these older adults compared with adults without schizophrenia (Solomon et al., 2021).

Older adults with an SSD diagnosis have not been a significant research focus; better understanding of efficacious community-based treatments as well as ways to improve/support cognitive and social functioning need to be achieved. Development of appropriate options for living accommodations can promote enhanced quality of life; attention to end-of-life care for these older adults is also important.

Epidemiology

Schizophrenia occurs in approximately 1% of the population in all cultures and countries. Variations in the incidence and prevalence rates across studies can be explained by the definition of schizophrenia and the sampling method used. Its economic costs are enormous. Direct costs include treatment expenses; indirect costs include lost wages, premature death, and incarceration. In addition, employment among people with schizophrenia is one of the lowest of any group with disabilities (Mental Health Commission of Canada [MHCC], 2013a). In a study of societal factors related to schizophrenia within Norway, a high-income welfare society, it was found that, among working-age individuals with schizophrenia, the employment rate was 10.24%. Although the costs of schizophrenia in terms of individual and family suffering are inestimable, the researchers of this study determined societal costs over a 12-month period were USD 890 million; the average cost per individual with schizophrenia was USD 106 thousand (Evensen et al., 2017).

People with schizophrenia tend to cluster in the lowest social classes in industrialized countries and urban communities. For some, the symptoms of the illness are so pervasive that it is difficult for these individuals to maintain any type of gainful employment. Homelessness is a problem for those with severe and persistent symptoms of schizophrenia. Somewhere between 30% and 40% of people who are homeless are estimated to be suffering from mental illness and of those, 20% to 25% are living with concurrent disorders, that is, with addiction and other health problems (Standing Senate Committee on Social Affairs, Science and Technology, 2006).

Results of a Canadian study that took place over 4 years conducted by the MHCC (2013b), entitled *At Home/Chez Soi*, reinforced the need for secure and safe housing for individuals suffering from serious mental illness. As an example, consider the findings related to mental illness and homelessness among Indigenous People in Vancouver and Winnipeg (Bingham et al., 2019). The participants in the overall study ($N = 1,010$) included 16% ($n = 77$) Indigenous participants of the 497 Vancouver participants and 71% ($n = 362$) of the 513 participants in Winnipeg. Astonishingly high rates of suicidality were found at the time of the study among the Indigenous participants (i.e., 94.7% female and 81.5% male). Further, 65.7% of the female and 66.4% of the male participants were alcohol dependent, with similar rates of other substance dependence for the female participants, but lower (49.1%) for the male participants. Approximately 27% of the female Indigenous participants and 24% of the male Indigenous participants were hospitalized two or more times due to mental illness during the past 5 years. Half of all the Indigenous participants experienced more than over 3 years of homelessness in their lifetime (Bingham et al., 2019).

Risk Factors

Risks for SSDs may be encountered *in utero*, including maternal infection, obstetric complications, preterm birth, or preeclampsia (Stilo & Murray, 2019). Childhood adversity and trauma (i.e., sexual abuse, physical abuse, emotional/psychological abuse, neglect, parental death, and bullying) strongly increases risk. In fact, researchers estimate that if they did not occur, the incidence of psychosis would be reduced by 33% (Varese et al., 2012).

Lower socioeconomic class and social isolation may be factors, given that individuals with FEP are more likely—up to 5 years before diagnosis—to be single, living alone, and unemployed or with a low income. It is known, however, that disability and dependence of those living with schizophrenia are more pronounced in high-income countries, despite availability of health care. The reason why is unclear, but it may be that such an illness inhibits participation in such societies (Stilo & Murray, 2019). Migration (particularly among refugee populations) and urbanicity (particularly if moving from a rural area) create risk, perhaps due to exposure to further risk, such as prenatal influenza, social deprivation, and income inequality. Cannabis use is known to elevate risk of SSDs, especially if use starts early, is frequent, or involves high-potency tetrahydrocannabinol (THC). The risk factors noted here are not necessary or sufficient to cause SSDs. It may be that genetic and environmental risks converge and/or interact to induce brain dysfunction (McCutcheon et al., 2020).

Age of Onset

Schizophrenia is most often diagnosed in late adolescence or early adulthood. When schizophrenia begins before age 25, symptoms seem to develop more gradually and negative symptoms predominate throughout the course of the disease. People with early-onset schizophrenia experience a greater number of neuropsychological problems. Disruptions occur in the achievement of milestone events of early adulthood, such as achieving in education, work, and long-term relationships.

Gender Differences

Men are typically diagnosed with schizophrenia earlier, in their mid-twenties, whereas the average age of onset for women is the late 20s; more women than men experience late-onset schizophrenia (Galletly et al., 2016). Estrogens may play a protective role against the development of schizophrenia that disappears as estrogen levels drop during menopause (Kulkarni et al., 2012), perhaps accounting as well for a more favourable treatment outcome in women. Recent research confirms that estrogens have neuroprotective effects associated with pathways in schizophrenia. Estrogen regulates pathophysiological pathways in schizophrenia, specifically dopamine activity, mitochondrial function, and the stress system. Deficiencies in estrogen in both males and females are associated with increases in psychotic symptoms. Furthermore, estrogen raises the efficacy of antipsychotics (Brand et al., 2021).

Comorbidity and Mortality

Persons with schizophrenia are at significantly higher risk for mortality than those without the disease. Research indicates that with this diagnosis, life expectancy at 20 and 45 years of age may be shortened for males by 11.5 and 8.1 years, respectively; for females, by 13.7 and 9.6 years. The higher risk is chiefly associated with comorbidities, including diabetes mellitus, chronic obstructive pulmonary diseases, and asthma; acute lower respiratory infections; suicide attempts; viral hepatitis; HIV disease and other infections; and epilepsy and other diseases of the nervous system (Bitter et al., 2017). Increases in mortality with SSD may be partly explained by socioeconomic factors, lifestyle, cardiometabolic comorbidities, and inflammation (Keinänen et al., 2018).

Lack of appropriate medical care may play a substantial role, an opinion supported by research that indicates that an SSD diagnosis can bias physicians and increase decision-making mistakes (Yamauchi et al., 2019). In a 5-year Ontario mortality study, of those with a hospital-diagnosed SSD who were 13 times more likely to die compared with controls, it was discovered that 50% of those who died had not seen a physician in the 30 days before the date of death; 17.5% had not seen a physician during the year preceding death (Kurdyak et al., 2021). If individuals diagnosed with an SSD can be engaged and supported in accessing treatment and receive risk monitoring for suicide, mortality can be reduced. Medical focus must go beyond the SSD and address the serious, potential comorbidities that can arise. Better medical education in relation to caring for persons with schizophrenia may be required (Bitter et al., 2017).

During the pandemic, it was learned that a premorbid diagnosis of SSD is a significant risk factor for mortality from COVID-19, ranked only behind the age factor. Mood and anxiety disorders, however, were not associated with COVID-19 mortality (Nemani et al., 2021).

Depression

Depression may occur for individuals with schizophrenia and is an important symptom to recognize. First, depression may be the evidence that the diagnosis of a mood disorder is more appropriate (see Chapter 22). Second, depression is not unusual in all stages of schizophrenia and deserves attention. Third, the suicide rate among individuals with schizophrenia is higher than that of the general population. In a Canadian community-based study, it was found that 32.2% of persons with a diagnosis of schizophrenia had attempted suicide compared with 2.8% of persons without such a diagnosis. After adjusting for sociodemographics, chronic pain, substance use/abuse, childhood adversities, and depression/anxiety, the researchers found that those with schizophrenia were six times more likely to attempt suicide than others (Fuller-Thomson & Hollister, 2016). Further, a 20-year population study in Ontario following 75,989 people with schizophrenia found that 1 out of every 58 died by suicide, usually within the first 4 years of diagnosis. Other predictors in this group included a mood disorder diagnosis, previous suicide attempts, and later age at diagnosis (Zaheer et al., 2020).

Metabolic Syndrome

The incidence of **metabolic syndrome** (MetS), a combination of conditions that put an individual at risk for chronic disease (e.g., heart disease, stroke, type II diabetes), is increasing in persons with schizophrenia worldwide, particularly among the younger age group (Yoca et al., 2020). In the general population of Canada, nearly one in five meet the criteria for this syndrome, having three of the following conditions: high blood pressure, high blood glucose, abnormal cholesterol or triglyceride levels, and excess body fat around the waist (Rao et al., 2014). Large waist circumference (greater than 89 cm for females; greater than 102 cm for males) is the most visible indicator of MetS. Antipsychotic medications, particularly clozapine and olanzapine, play a role in increasing MetS vulnerability. Although haloperidol and perphenazine do not play such a role, their associated risk of extra-pyramidal adverse effects remains a negative factor. These may be the medications of choice, however, for individuals with MetS as well as schizophrenia (Domany & Weiser, 2020).

Nurses need to be very cognizant of this syndrome, given that many individuals in their care will be unaware of its existence. Education regarding the risk and assistance in avoiding or overcoming MetS are appropriate to the nursing role. *Metabolic Syndrome Canada* has developed a research-based CHANGE program to assist healthcare professionals support long-term lifestyle interventions for those with MetS (see Web Links).

Diabetes Mellitus

Research indicates that MetS, diabetes, and hypertension are significantly associated with global cognitive impairment in schizophrenia (Hagi et al., 2021). Diabetic risk appears to be present in individuals at the first episode of schizophrenia because they are at an increased risk of developing diabetes compared with the general population, based on higher levels of fasting blood glucose (Pillinger et al., 2017). The focus on individuals at the onset of their disorder removes the factors of antipsychotic medications and lifestyle (i.e., poor diet and negative symptoms) that have been considered the cause of the 3-fold higher risk for diabetes in those with long-term schizophrenia. Although it is possible that schizophrenia has a direct role in increasing risk of diabetes, other factors may have a role in the development of both diseases, such as shared genetic risk or stress (i.e., increased cortisol levels brought on by receiving such a diagnosis) (Pillinger et al.).

Evidence that supports this view includes a higher rate of type II diabetes in first-degree relatives of people with schizophrenia. However, obesity associated with type II diabetes is complicated in schizophrenia treatment by weight gain that occurs for many taking antipsychotic medications. In addition, some weight gain may be attributed to a return to a healthier lifestyle with treatment (i.e., reduction in symptoms [e.g., delusions] that interfere with appetite and eating). Not surprisingly, weight gain is often cited as a reason for nonadherence to antipsychotic medications.

Substance Use

Prior to Canada's *Cannabis Act* (i.e., the framework for the production, distribution, sale, and possession of cannabis) on October 17, 2018, it was estimated that up to 10% of the Canadian population used cannabis and cannabis-derived substances and up to 25% of people with schizophrenia used cannabis (Imtiaz et al., 2015). Health Canada's *Canadian Cannabis Survey 2020* (Government of Canada, 2020, December) revealed that 14% of Canadians surveyed aged 16 years and older used cannabis for medical purposes, the same rate as in the 2019 survey. The question "Does cannabis use increase the risk of developing psychosis or schizophrenia?" was addressed in an evidence brief of the Canadian government (Government of Canada, 2018b). The answer was "It can." It was noted that cannabinoids change how cells communicate with one another and, in the brain, affect one's perception of the environment, as well as ways of thinking, feeling, and behaving. Risk factors identified for developing a psychosis through cannabis use include the following:

- Initiated before the age of 16
- Use is frequent (i.e., daily or near daily)
- Involves high-potency cannabis

Although the evidence is inconsistent, use of cannabis when one has a family history of schizophrenia may increase one's risk of developing the disorder. It is recommended that those with such a family history refrain from using cannabis. Interestingly, the prevalence of schizophrenia has not increased with increased cannabis use (Government of Canada, 2020).

Tobacco is used by people experiencing their first episode of psychosis at an incidence of over 50% (Grossman et al., 2017). There is uncertainty regarding the effect of nicotine on cognitive alterations in schizophrenia. A systematic review of research literature revealed evidence that one dose of nicotine to persons with schizophrenia improved a range of cognitive functions, such as attention, working memory, executive functions (these effects, however, varied across studies in type of assessment and nicotine intake conditions). Reviewers concluded that, when persons with schizophrenia quit smoking, there could be a potential decrease of cognitive performance (Dondé et al., 2020). Even so, smoking nicotine products is linked to serious disease, diminished health status, and harm to the fetus of people who are pregnant (see Chapter 26).

Aetiology of the Schizophrenia Spectrum Disorders

The search for the causation of schizophrenia is centuries old, but the answer is still to be found. Fortunately, advances in neuroimaging are enabling new research strategies. Structural imaging, specifically computed tomography, magnetic resonance imaging, diffusion tensor imaging (DTI), and functional imaging, including positron emission tomography (PET) and functional magnetic resonance imaging (fMRI), have made viewing the living brain, its form and function, possible. The causes once attributed to

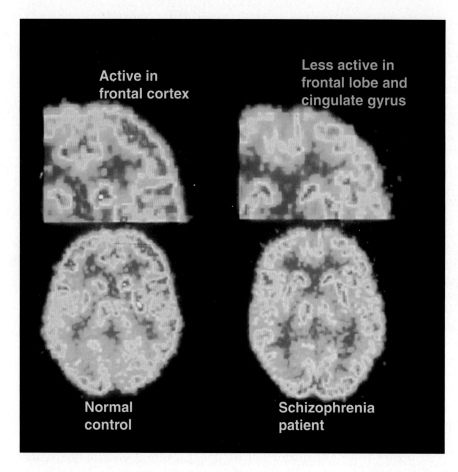

Active in
frontal cortex

Less active in
frontal lobe and
cingulate gyrus

Normal
control

Schizophrenia
patient

Figure 21.1 PET scan with 18F-deoxyglucose shows metabolic activity in a horizontal section of the brain in a control subject (*left*) and in an unmedicated patient with schizophrenia (*right*). *Red* and *yellow* indicate areas of high metabolic activity in the cortex; *green* and *blue* indicate lower activity in the *white* matter areas of the brain. The frontal lobe is magnified to show reduced frontal activity in the prefrontal cortex of the patient with schizophrenia. (Courtesy of Monte S. Buchsbaum, MD, The Mount Sinai Medical Center and School of Medicine, New York, NY.)

schizophrenia, key areas of current interest—genetics, neuroanatomy, neurochemistry—and the dominate hypothesis, dysconnectivity are briefly reviewed here (see Fig. 21.1).

Background

Early on, psychosis was viewed as possession by evil spirits or the devil or as punishment by the gods; later it was physical vapours or pressures that required purging or cutting. By the 1800s, Heinrich Neumann suggested that "insanity" was due to "loosening of the togetherness," a rather poetic interpretation of psychotic symptoms. In 1896, Emil Kraepelin named psychosis as "dementia praecox" (thus denoting a deteriorating trajectory) and identified the clinical symptoms of hallucinations, delusions, and disordered affect. In 1911, Eugen Bleuler described the *group of schizophrenias* and referred to the splitting of thought, behaviour, and emotion that occurs. This is not to be confused with the "split personality" of dissociative identity disorder. Bleuler rejected deterioration as a defining outcome. He viewed schizophrenia as a disease with psychopathologic aspects and categorized symptoms as primary (e.g., disordered affect and volition) and secondary (e.g., hallucinations and delusions) (Lehmann, 1967).

In the mid-twentieth century, those with a psychodynamic orientation understood schizophrenia to be caused by disturbed family relations. Frieda Fromm-Reichman (1948) coined the terrible term "schizophrenogenic mothers," indicating that, through severe rejection and warped interactions, mothers were the source of the disease. Anthropologist Gregory Bateson's et al. (1956) "double-bind" theory of schizophrenia pointed to family interactions that repeatedly involved the individual in "no-win" situations with communications for which no response was appropriate (e.g., "Be spontaneous"). A further example is that of Lyman C. Wynne and colleagues' (1958) "pseudomutuality" in family relationships. Concurrently with these psychodynamic approaches, a "psychiatric revolution" had begun: neuroleptic medications were introduced, replacing drugs like paraldehyde, chloral hydrate, and phenobarbital, which were without antipsychotic effects but used for sedation and chemical restraint (Cancro, 2000).

Influenced by the fact that infectious diseases have single causes, medicine for some time focused on finding *the* cause of a disease. The multicausal nature of noncommunicable diseases (e.g., heart disease, cancer) changed that approach. In psychiatry, however, the search for a single, identifiable cause for disorders continued for some time (Kendler, 2019). Today research consortia and teams around the world find schizophrenia to be a complex neuropsychiatric disorder with a diverse clinical phenotype (Kraguljac & Lahti, 2021).

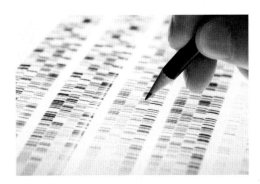

Figure 21.2 A DNA gel sequence. Studies have found more than 100 genetic loci associated with schizophrenia.

Genetic Factors

It is well known that genetic factors play a role in the aetiology of schizophrenia, but a comprehensive understanding of that role remains elusive. The search for such understanding continues, with the schizophrenia genetics knowledge base available as a resource for the research community (Liu et al., 2019) (Fig. 21.2).

Familial Transmission

As far back as Kraepelin, it was noted that heredity was a potential factor in psychosis: in some families, it was present across generations. In familial transmission, the risk of schizophrenia decreases as the number of shared genes decreases. A child born to two parents with schizophrenia has a 40% chance of developing it. In monozygotic twins, there is 45% to 50% chance that if one twin has schizophrenia, the other will; in dizygotic twins, the risk is 12% to 15%. Incidence among first degree relatives is 10% to 12%, among second degree relatives 5% to 6%, and among the general population, 5% (Sadock et al., 2019). Consistent with this hypothesis is that the disorder ranges from very severe to less severe; two parents without the disorder can have a child who develops it, and the risk of schizophrenia decreases as the number of shared genes decreases (Sadock, et al., 2019).

Polygenic Nature of Schizophrenia Spectrum Disorders

There is no longer a search for a schizophrenic gene: the polygenic nature of SSDs is recognized. Genome-wide association studies (GWAS) have found more than 100 genetic loci associated with the disease, with expectations that hundreds more may be found. The research on individual genes continues, but as a means of understanding the clinical and functional relevance of genetic variants identified in GWAS.

A recurrent deletion at chromosome 22q11.2 is one of the strongest risk factors for schizophrenia (Cleyen et al., 2020). Individuals with 22q11.2 deletion syndrome

(DS) (approximately 1 per 3,000 people) (Khan et al., 2020) account for 25% of the adolescents and young adults who have SSDs (Gur et al., 2021). Scientists are pointing to an electrical abnormality among cortical neurons as the cause. Using cortical spheroids (clusters of neurons and other brain cells) from persons carrying 22q11DS and from healthy control subjects, it was determined that neurons of those with 22q11DS were more excitable and had abnormalities in signaling. Antipsychotic medications reversed these defects in the neurons. A gene, DGCR8 (part of chromosomal DNA deleted in 22q11DS), may play a major role. 22q11.2DS offers a window for revealing neurobiologic pathways from genes to psychosis (Gur et al., 2021) with the potential to inform the development of new treatments (see Figure 21.2).

Past investigations into genetic mutations in persons with schizophrenia identified only a fraction in individuals who were studied. New, more advanced techniques, however, have facilitated the discovery of somatic mutations in brain cells. Somatic gene mutations, unlike germline mutations, which occur in egg or sperm cells and are passed onto an embryo, occur *in* the embryo after fertilization and can be present throughout the body. In research using postmortem samples from persons with schizophrenia and those without the disease, mutations were found in genes known to be associated with the disease in brain samples of those with schizophrenia (Kim et al., 2021). The mutations highly affected a protein component of NMDA-type glutamate receptors, GRIN2B, essential to neural signaling. Faults in glutamate receptors have been suspected in schizophrenia neuropathology, suggesting that somatic mutations can contribute to schizophrenia by disrupting neuronal communication. Such mutations, present at even very low levels, can have consequences in an individual's ability to function (Kim et al., 2021).

Interaction of Genes and Environment

Genetics appears to interact with environmental factors to affect a person's susceptibility to SSDs (Marder & Cannon, 2019). It may be that a genetic predisposition to SSD acts in concert with environmental factors during the perinatal to early adulthood periods of life. These factors may include adversity in utero, childhood spent in urban settings, social isolation, traumatic events, living in poverty, and other life-impacting psychosocial stressors.

The Neural Diathesis–Stress Model

The neural diathesis–stress model proposes that early in life, perhaps as early as conception, genetic and environmental factors (acting alone or interacting) increase vulnerability to psychosis by stimulating

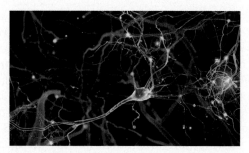

Figure 21.3 Neurons—brain cells—appear to play an important role in the timing of development of schizophrenia. Deficits in *gray* matter volume (and hence fewer neurons) appear to be greater in those with earlier stage of onset of the disease.

degenerative processes that negatively affect neuromaturation and increase risk for psychosis (Pruessner et al., 2017). Such predisposition may involve genes relevant to hypothalamus–pituitary–adrenal (HPA) axis function (i.e., neuroendocrine component of the stress response). Adverse environmental factors include pre-, peri-, and postnatal stress, childhood trauma, negative life events, low socioeconomic or racial–ethnic minority status, and urban setting. Affected individuals respond to stressors in a maladaptive way, contributing further to stress system disruption. Resilience can be promoted through psychosocial support (e.g., strategies that increase self-esteem), stress management strategies, cognitive–behavioural therapy, and other interventions that support mental health (Pruessner et al., 2017) (Fig. 21.3).

Neuroanatomic Factors

In 1976, a landmark study by Johnstone and colleagues reported ventricular dilatation in subjects with chronic schizophrenia, an observation that has been repeatedly confirmed. Dilation is primarily in the third and lateral ventricles. This anatomic ventricular change can be found in other disorders such as Alzheimer disease, so it is not specific to SSDs. Currently, as neuroscience and its neuroimaging tools become increasingly sophisticated, subtle differences in brain structure of persons with SSDs are being identified.

Structural features may contribute to altered physiologic activity and functional connectivity among the prefrontal cortex, temporal cortex, thalamus, hippocampus, and cerebellum (Marder & Cannon, 2019). Better functioning of individuals is associated with integrity of frontolimbic brain regions (e.g., smaller ventricles, greater frontolimbic volumes) (Wojtalik et al., 2017). The brains of individuals with schizophrenia weigh less than the average brain, with earlier age of onset associated with lower weight. Reductions in prefrontal and temporal lobe volumes is also observed in persons at high genetic risk for SSD.

Prefrontal lobe volume deficit (about 3% to 12% smaller than normal controls) has been attributed primarily to gray matter (i.e., neurons, glial cells, and neurophil). In a study that examined brain structural changes in FEP and chronic psychosis stages, individuals in FEP had subtle deficits in volume compared with control subjects, whereas those in the chronic stage of schizophrenia had extensive gray matter decreases, affecting primarily the frontotemporal regions and the insula. On the whole, gray matter volume deficits appeared to be greater in those with earlier stage of onset (Torres et al., 2016). Such a deficit in neuronal connections has consequences in life functioning.

Neuroimaging research has revealed that alterations in FWM of the brain underlie negative symptoms, with functional connectivity and structural properties of the left FWM linked to the severity of symptoms experienced (Wang et al., 2020). Altered sphingosine-1-phosphate (S1P) metabolism may play a role in this. Changes in S1P metabolism may cause deficits in oligodendrocyte differentiation and myelin formation that create structural and molecular abnormalities in FWM (Esaki et al., 2020).

Neurochemical Factors

Psychoses, including the SSDs, involve the dysregulation of multiple neurotransmitters in multiple pathways (Stahl, 2018). Three neurotransmitters—dopamine, glutamate, and serotonin—and their suspected roles in the causation of schizophrenia are briefly reviewed here. There is complex interplay among neurotransmitters, so it is doubtful that a single neurotransmitter theory will evolve to explain schizophrenia. Given that much of the dynamics of this interplay remains obscure, the neurotransmitters will be individually addressed (Fig. 21.4).

Dopamine Hyperactivity Hypothesis

Dopamine (DA) has been of interest in relation to schizophrenia for more than 50 years. Stimulating such

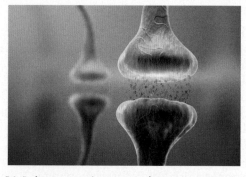

Figure 21.4 A presynaptic neuron releases neurotransmitters that bind to receptors on a postsynaptic cell.

interest was the fact that amphetamine achieves its rewarding effects through elevating extracellular DA, as well as prolonging DA receptor signaling and, in doing so, can cause a paranoid psychotic reaction similar to schizophrenia (Calipari & Ferris, 2013). In addition, antipsychotic medications are effective because of their antagonism to dopamine (primarily to the dopamine D2 receptor), indicating a significant role for dopamine system dysfunction in schizophrenia.

Presynaptic striatal dopaminergic function is elevated in patients with schizophrenia (Howes et al., 2017). So, it is dopamine *hyperactivity* in the mesolimbic dopamine pathway at dopamine D2 receptors that causes the positive symptoms of schizophrenia (i.e., hallucinations, delusions) (Stahl, 2018). Blockade of this heightened transmission, either by decreasing dopamine levels or by blocking dopamine transmission, leads to a resolution of symptoms for most patients. It is the blocking of the D2 receptors in the nigrostriatal pathway that causes the movement disorders that are a significant side effect of most antipsychotic drugs (Stahl, 2018). Sensitization of the dopamine system by the interaction of genetic and environmental factors, such that the system is made vulnerable to acute stress, has been proposed as the cause of progressive dysregulation in an individual's brain functioning, leading to psychosis (Howes et al., 2017).

Glutamate Hypoactivity Hypothesis

Attention focused on glutamate as a potential factor in the aetiology of schizophrenia when it was discovered that antagonists of N-methyl-D-aspartate glutamate (NMDA) receptors, such as phencyclidine (PCP) and ketamine, provoke positive, negative, and cognitive psychotic symptoms in healthy volunteers and worsen such symptoms in persons with schizophrenia. Such *hypofunctioning* of NMDA glutamate receptors on γ-aminobutyric acid (GABA) interneurons in the prefrontal cortex leads to decreased GABAergic inhibition of glutamatergic pyramidal neurons, promoting increased release of synaptic glutamate. This is the basic principle of the NMDA receptor hypofunction/disinhibition model (Egerton et al., 2020).

Measuring the levels of neurochemicals (e.g., neurotransmitters, metabolites) has been made possible by proton magnetic resonance spectroscopy (1H-MRS). Merritt and colleagues (2016) interpret 1H-MRS studies as providing evidence of glutamatergic elevations in schizophrenia, as would be predicted by the model. This conclusion is disputed by other scientists, however, based on the complexity of interpreting differences in glutamate and glutamine MRS signals between individuals with schizophrenia and controls, as well as

competing rationales for this finding (Coyle & Konopaske, 2016). This minor controversy provides us with a glimpse into the sophistication necessary to each small step toward understanding the human brain. The precise nature of glutamate dysfunction continues to be studied, but much remains unknown (McCutcheon et al., 2020).

Serotonin Hyperfunction Hypothesis

Cortical serotonin (5-hydroytryptamine/ 5HT2A) *hyperfunctioning* can result in psychosis.

Hallucinogens like lysergic acid diethylamide (LSD) are primarily 5-HT2A agonists (activators). Release of serotonin-activating 5HT2A receptors causes downstream release of glutamate and the mesolimbic dopamine pathway gets activated. This chain reaction can lead to hallucinations and paranoid delusions. Although this suggests a role for serotonergic dysfunction in the aetiology of schizophrenia, there is no direct evidence that supports this hypothesis (Yang & Tsai, 2017).

Dysconnectivity Hypothesis

In the 1980s, it was first hypothesized (but difficult to test) that schizophrenia could be caused by dysfunctional synapses (Weinberger et al., 1988). Today, brain connectivity patterns in schizophrenia are revealed by fMRIs. Significant functional *hypo*connectivity is consistently found in the brain networks of those with schizophrenia (including within the auditory system, task and cognitive control, self-referential processing, episodic memory and self-projection, and sensory–motor function), supporting the dysregulated brain network hypothesis (Li et al., 2019). Abnormal connectivity—dysconnectivity—in the brain is increasingly viewed as a (*the?*) causal factor in schizophrenia.

Functional dysconnectivity (a "bad" or "abnormal" connection) in subregions of the insula, for instance, affects cognitive, affective, and somatosensory processing. Clinically, the individual experiences worsening cognition and negative symptoms (Sheffield et al., 2020). Dysconnectivity appears to arise through aberrations in brain development (Nath et al., 2021). When the normal evolution of structural and functional brain networks occurs—synaptic connections created during childhood are pruned in adolescence—something goes wrong and excess pruning occurs.

Neuropsychiatry's investigation of the structural and functional etiological processes of schizophrenia may take a new direction. A subfield of artificial intelligence, deep learning (DL), could offer some solutions. DL involves system-modeling algorithms, based on the nervous system, that learn by "training" how to solve problems, which may have some potential in solving the underlying sources of this debilitating disease (Cortes-Briones et al., 2021).

The Eye and Schizophrenia

There is increasing interest in the eye problems (particularly of the retina) of persons with schizophrenia. Notably, research is pointing to the dysfunction in the visual processing regions as an underlying mechanism in schizophrenia (Sendi et al., 2021). For example, results of a study of military conscripts (N = 1,140,710) point to a potential link between poor visual acuity and the later onset of schizophrenia, especially for those whose vision cannot be improved by use of lenses (Hayes et al., 2019). Abnormal visual input may impact schizophrenia, or the altered neurodevelopment seen in schizophrenia may be expressed robustly in the eyes.

What is fortuitous about such findings is that the retina appears to be "a window into the brain" (Silverstein et al., 2021 p. 1): changes in the structure and functioning of the retina, a part the central nervous system, are similar to changes in the brain. There is much potential in having the means to explore the central nervous system that is external to the brain. Imagine: there may be an eye test for psychosis one day (Silverstein et al., 2021).

▌ Interdisciplinary Treatment

The most effective treatment approach for individuals with schizophrenia is interdisciplinary, involving a range of healthcare disciplines: nursing, psychiatry, psychology, social work, occupational and recreational therapies, pharmacy, pastoral counselling, peer support, and others. A team approach is essential given the complex nature of schizophrenia symptoms and the continuum of interventions required to enhance best outcomes. Inpatient teams are often the starting point, but the spectrum of interventions must include outpatient teams and community-based, recovery-oriented programs.

Teams of professionals working in partnership with self-help and peer support programs can shape a favourable recovery environment for stabilizing and enhancing the lives of people who have schizophrenia. However, barriers to this type of treatment abound and include access; inadequate funding; limitations on physician fee reimbursements; staff shortages (in particular, skilled mental health nurses); large caseloads; insufficient inpatient opportunities; and insufficient community supports, facilities, and social services. Despite these barriers, nurses contribute significantly to interdisciplinary care with an emphasis on individuals' and their families' responses to the illness, on functional adaptation, and holistic needs.

▌ Priority Care Issues

There exist priority concerns in the care and treatment of persons with schizophrenia. People who have this disease are at risk for attempted suicide (Hettige et al., 2017). In a Canadian community-based study of a representative sample of persons with schizophrenia (n = 101) and without (n = 21,643), the lifetime prevalence rate of suicide attempts among those with the disease was 39.2% compared with 2.8% of those without it (Fuller-Thomson & Hollister, 2016). After researchers adjusted for sociodemographics, childhood adversities, substance abuse/dependence, depression/anxiety, and chronic pain, individuals with schizophrenia had six times the odds of attempting suicide. Those most vulnerable were individuals who used or were dependent on illicit substances, experienced depression, had undergone childhood physical abuse, and those who were female. Community dwelling persons with schizophrenia appear to be at high risk for suicide attempts (Fuller-Thomson & Hollister). Suicide assessment is an important component of care.

In an inpatient unit, patient safety concerns extend to potential aggressive actions toward self, other patients, and staff during episodes of psychoses. During times of acute illness, treatment with antipsychotic medications is often required. During the recovery phase of schizophrenia, individuals need support in accepting their illness and developing hopeful expectations for their future. A useful framework was developed by Bartram (2019), who identified individual, social, and structural factors that support recovery and wellbeing. Focusing on hope and acceptance and believing that recovery is possible provides much-needed support for people who are struggling with a new or ongoing diagnosis of schizophrenia.

▌ Family Response to Disorder

In 2020, a true story of living with schizophrenia, *Hidden Valley Road: Inside the Mind of an American Family* (Kolker, 2020) examined the many challenges faced by such families. The Galvin family with their 12 children share their story of how six of the ten boys were diagnosed with schizophrenia, their different experiences with treatment, and the health system. The story is, at its core, about family and enduring connections. The manifestations of schizophrenia in a family member are often met with mixed emotions of disbelief, shock, fear, and care and concern. Families initially may seek reasons for the psychotic episode, attributing it to taking illicit drugs or to extraordinary stress or fatigue. Others, particularly parents, may blame themselves. They often do not know how to comfort their ill family member and may find themselves fearful of their behaviours. If the ill person is hostile and aggressive toward family members, the family may respond with anger and hostility, along with fear, confusion, and anxiety. During these episodes, some families may have to seek help from police or a crisis response team to control the situation. Coming to terms with the mental illness of a loved one is often described as an experience of catastrophic proportions (Addington et al., 2005; Wilson, 2012; Young et al., 2019).

The initial period of illness for a patient and family that receive a diagnosis of schizophrenia is extraordinarily challenging. Often, during the initial phase of treatment, families are the primary caregivers for an ill relative. This necessitates that families have opportunities for explanation, education about the illness, and access to timely support. As families acknowledge the meaning of the diagnosis and the potential long-term rehabilitation required, they often feel overwhelmed, angry, and depressed (Schizophrenia Society of Canada, 2021; Wilson, 2012). Diagnostic labels are imbued with history and still resonate with fear and apprehension. During the early moments, when families receive the diagnostic proclamation, they generally hold the same unenlightened notions of schizophrenia as others within our culture. It is imperative then, for nurses and other healthcare providers, to provide families with meaningful explanations of the disease to address any notions of blame or self-reproach. Nurses can help families hold hope for the future of their ill relative.

The issue of family caregiving for a relative with serious mental illness has received attention from the MHCC, and a comprehensive guide for caregivers has been developed. Nurses should familiarize themselves with the recommendations contained in this document, *National Guidelines for a Comprehensive Service System to Support Family Caregivers of Adults with Mental Health Problems and Illnesses* (MHCC, 2013c), and the Schizophrenia Society of Canada's (2021) *Rays of Hope: A Reference Manual for Families & Caregivers*.

Nursing Management: Human Response to Disorder

The nursing management of the person with schizophrenia usually involves a chronic trajectory. Different phases of the illness require various nursing interventions at varying intensity. During exacerbation of symptoms, many patients are hospitalized for stabilization. During periods of relative stability, the nurse helps patients maintain a therapeutic regimen, develop positive mental health strategies, devise strategies to prepare for and cope with the stress, and reclaim their lives as much as possible.

Because of the complexity of this major psychiatric disorder, the nursing management for each domain is discussed separately. In reality, the nursing process steps overlap in all domains. For example, medication management is a direct biologic intervention; however, the effects of medications also are seen in psychological functioning. In the clinical area, effective nursing management requires an integration of the assessment data from all domains into meaningful interventions. Nursing interventions should cover all domains, including biologic, psychological, social (including family functioning), and spiritual. See Box 21.3.

A person with schizophrenia may require several foci of nursing care. This is particularly true given that schizophrenia affects so many aspects of an individual's functioning and that symptoms can be observed in cognitive, emotional, family, social, and physical functioning. It is also important to note that the periods between exacerbations of symptoms are actually very important phases for pursuing recovery goals.

Biologic Domain

Biologic Assessment

The following sections highlight the important assessment areas for people with schizophrenia.

Current and Past Health Status and Physical Examination

It is important to conduct a thorough history and physical examination to rule out medical illness or substance abuse that could cause the psychiatric symptoms. It is also important to screen for comorbid medical illnesses that need to be treated, such as diabetes mellitus, hypertension, and cardiac disease, or a family history of such disorders. People with schizophrenia have a higher mortality rate from physical illness and often have smoking-related illnesses, such as emphysema, and other pulmonary, cardiac, and cancer problems. The nurse should determine whether the patient smokes tobacco, which not only affects the patient's health but also can affect the clearance of medications.

Physical Functioning

The negative symptoms of schizophrenia are often manifested in terms of impairment in physical functioning. Self-care often deteriorates, and sleep may be nonexistent during acute phases. Information regarding physical functioning may best be collected from family members.

Nutritional Assessment

A nutritional history should be completed to determine baseline eating habits and preferences.

Medications can alter normal nutrition, and the patient may need to limit calories or fat consumption.

BOX 21.3   NURSING CARE PLAN

PATIENT WITH PSYCHOSIS: PROBABLE SCHIZOPHRENIA

Jeff Taylor (JT) is a 29-year-old man who was brought to the hospital by his family after they became concerned over the changes in his behaviour. He had stopped going to his job at a museum and had barricaded himself in his apartment. When Sam, his brother, tried to see him, Jeff told him that he knew he was not Sam, that he was an imposter, one of the time travellers from another century who were after him. Jeff began shouting at Sam in a strange language. Sam remembered that Jeff had experienced a psychotic episode when he was 19 years old, shortly after graduation from high school. He had recovered after a few months. Sam called their parents who were able to convince Jeff that he would be safer at the hospital. He agreed it would be a good place to hide temporarily until his allies from the future answered his summons.

Setting: Psychiatric Intensive Care Unit

Baseline Assessment: JT is a 6′1″, 145-lb tired-looking man whose appearance is dishevelled. He has not slept for 4 days and appears frightened. He is hypervigilant, pacing, and mumbling to himself. He is vague about past drug use, but his parents do not believe that he has used drugs. He has delusional ideas about hiding out in the hospital until his protectors from the future arrive. He appears to be hallucinating, conversing as if others are speaking with him. He is confused and has difficulty writing, speaking, or thinking coherently. He is disoriented to time; recognizes that he is in a hospital but views it as a hideout. Lab values are within normal limits except Hgb, 10.2, and Hct, 32.

Associated Psychiatric Diagnosis	Medications
Schizophrenia	Risperidone (Risperdal), 2 mg bid, then titrate to 3 mg if needed
Psychosocial and contextual issues: educational problems (failing), social problems (withdrawn from peers)	

Nursing Focus of Care 1: Hallucinations

Defining Characteristics	Related Factors
Inaccurate interpretation of stimuli (people thinking his thoughts) Cognitive impairment—attention, memory, and executive function impairment Suspiciousness Hallucinations	Uncompensated alterations in brain activity

Outcomes

Initial	Long Term
Decrease or eliminate hallucinations	Use coping strategies to deal with hallucinations or delusions if they reappear
Accurate interpretation of the environment (stop thinking that people are thinking his thoughts)	Communicate clearly with others
Improvement in cognitive functioning (improved attention, memory, and executive functioning)	Maintain cognitive functioning

Interventions	Rationale	Ongoing Assessment
Initiate a nurse–patient relationship by using an accepting, nonjudgmental approach. Be patient.	A therapeutic relationship will provide patient support as JT begins to deal with the realization that he has experienced a psychotic episode that could be the onset of schizophrenia. Be patient and offer information in small, gradual ways. Information processing is likely to be slow at this time.	Determine the extent to which JT is willing to trust and engage in a relationship.

NURSING CARE PLAN (*Continued*)

Interventions	Rationale	Ongoing Assessment
Administer risperidone as prescribed. Observe for effects, side effects, and adverse effects. Begin teaching about the medication and its importance, once symptoms subside.	Risperidone is a D_2 and 5-HT2A antagonist and is indicated for the management of psychotic disorders.	Make sure JT swallows the pills. Monitor for relief of positive symptoms and assess side effects, especially extrapyramidal. Monitor BP for orthostatic hypotension and body temperature increase (neuroleptic malignant syndrome [NMS]).
During hallucinations and delusional thinking, assess significance (are voices telling him that he is in danger or to flee the hospital?) Reassure JT that he is safe in the hospital. (Do not try to convince JT that his delusional ideas are false and hallucinations are not real.) Redirect to the here and now.	It is important to understand the context of the hallucinations and delusions to be able to provide the appropriate interventions. By avoiding arguments about the content, the nurse will enhance communication.	Assess the meaning of the hallucination or delusion to the patient. Determine whether he is a danger to himself or others. Determine whether the patient can be redirected.
Assess the ability for self-care activities.	Disturbed thinking may interfere with JT's ability to carry out activities of daily living (ADLs).	Continue to assess: determine whether the patient can manage self-care.

Evaluation

Outcomes	Revised Outcomes	Interventions
Hallucinations and delusions began to decrease within 5 days.	Participate in unit activities according to interdisciplinary treatment plan.	Encourage attendance at treatment activities.
He is oriented to time, place, and person. Attention and memory are improving.	Agree to continue to take antipsychotic medications as prescribed.	Teach JT about medications. Teach JT about psychosis initially and schizophrenia when diagnosis is confirmed.

Nursing Focus of Care 2: Aggressive Behaviour

Defining Characteristics	Related Factors
Assaultive toward others, self, and environment	Frightened, secondary to auditory hallucinations and delusional thinking
Presence of pathophysiologic risk factors: delusional thinking	Poor impulse control Dysfunctional communication patterns

Outcomes

Initial	Long Term
Avoid acting on fears and fleeing hospital or assaulting others he mistakes for patients or staff. Decrease agitation and aggression.	Control behaviour with assistance from staff and parents.

Continued on following page

NURSING CARE PLAN (*Continued*)

Interventions

Interventions	Rationale	Ongoing Assessment
Acknowledge the patient's fears, hallucinations, and delusions.	Hallucinations and delusions change an individual's perception of environmental stimuli. A patient who is frightened will respond because of his need to stay safe.	Determine whether the patient is able to hear you. Assess his response to your comments and his ability to concentrate on what is being said.
Offer the patient choices of maintaining safety: keeping distance from others; sitting near nurses' station.	By having choices, he will begin to develop a sense of control over his behaviour.	Observe the patient's nonverbal communication for evidence of increased agitation.
Administer prn lorazepam 2 mg for agitation	Lorazepam potentiates the inhibitory neurotransmitter GABA, relieving anxiety, agitation, and produce sedation	Observe for a decrease in agitated behaviour.
JT gradually decreased agitated behaviour. He appeared to feel safer.	Demonstrate control of behaviour by resisting hallucinations and delusions.	Teach JT about the effects of hallucinations and delusions. Problem solve ways of controlling hallucinations if they occur. Emphasize the importance of taking medications.

Fluid Imbalance Assessment

The nurse should remain alert for signs of polydipsia and polyuria to identify disordered water balance, although these signs are quite rare. Patients suspected of having disordered water balance should be assessed for signs and symptoms of hyponatraemia, water intoxication, excessive urination, incontinence, or periodically elevated blood pressure. Signs and symptoms of hypervolaemia that may be evident include puffiness of the face or eyes, abdominal distention, and hypothermia. These patients should be weighed daily, and their urine specific gravity and serum sodium levels should be monitored (Goldman, 2009).

Pharmacologic Assessment

Baseline information about the initial psychological and physical functioning should be obtained before the initiation of medication (or as early as possible). Side effects of medications should be assessed. Patients are often physically awkward and have poor coordination, motor abnormalities, and abnormal eye tracking. Before medication begins, standardized assessment of abnormal motor movements should be conducted using one of several assessment tools designed for that purpose, such as the Abnormal Involuntary Movement Scale (AIMS) (Guy, 1976) (see Web Links), the Dyskinesia

Identification System: Condensed User Scale (Sprague & Kalachnik, 1991) (Fig. 21.5), or the Simpson-Angus Rating Scale (Simpson & Angus, 1970) (see Appendix B), which is designed for Parkinson-like symptoms.

Nursing Focus of Care: Biologic Domain

Typical foci of nursing care for the biologic domain for the person during all phases of schizophrenia include self-care issues and disturbed sleep. During a relapse, the focus of care may be on management of the therapeutic regimen, and on nutrition, fluid intake, and sexual dysfunction. Constipation may occur if the person takes anticholinergic medications.

Interventions: Biologic Domain

Nursing interventions during the initial acute phase of schizophrenia include prompt, safe, and informed administration of antipsychotic medications. During any stage, attention to self-care needs and the patient's ability to maintain hygiene and adequate nutrition are important.

Promotion of Self-Care Activities

For many individuals with schizophrenia, the plan of care will include specific interventions to enhance self-care, nutrition, and overall health knowledge. Negative symptoms commonly leave patients unable to initiate

NAME		I.D.

(HEALTH CARE FACILITY)
Dyskinesia Identification System:
Condensed User Scale (DISCUS)

CURRENT PSYCHOTROPICS/ANTI-
CHOLINERGIC AND TOTAL MG/DAY

_____ ___ mg
_____ ___ mg
_____ ___ mg
_____ ___ mg

See Instructions on the Other Side

EXAM TYPE (check one)
- ☐ 1. Baseline
- ☐ 2. Annual
- ☐ 3. Semi annual
- ☐ 4. D/C—1 month
- ☐ 5. D/C—2 months
- ☐ 6. D/C—3 months
- ☐ 7. Admission
- ☐ 8. Other

COOPERATION (check one)
- ☐ 1. None
- ☐ 2. Partial
- ☐ 3. Full

SCORING
- 0—**Not present** (movements not observed or some movements observed but not considered abnormal)
- 1—**Minimal** (abnormal movements are difficult to detect or movements are easy to detect but occur only once or twice in a short nonrepetitive manner)
- 2—**Mild** (abnormal movements occur infrequently and are easy to detect)
- 3—**Moderate** (abnormal movements occur frequently and are easy to detect)
- 4—**Severe** (abnormal movements occur almost continuously **and** are easy to detect)
- NA—**Not assessed** (an assessment for an item is not able to be made)

ASSESSMENT
DISCUS Item and Score (circle one score for each item)

FACE
1. Tics.. 0 1 2 3 4 NA
2. Grimaces... 0 1 2 3 4 NA

EYES
3. Blinking... 0 1 2 3 4 NA

ORAL
4. Chewing/Lip Smacking......................... 0 1 2 3 4 NA
5. Puckering/Sucking/
   Thrusting Lower Lip.............................. 0 1 2 3 4 NA

LINGUAL
6. Tongue Thrusting/
   Tongue in Cheek.................................. 0 1 2 3 4 NA
7. Tonic Tongue....................................... 0 1 2 3 4 NA
8. Tongue Tremor..................................... 0 1 2 3 4 NA
9. Athetoid/Myokymic/
   Lateral Tongue..................................... 0 1 2 3 4 NA

HEAD/NECK/TRUNK
10. Retrocollis/Torticollis.......................... 0 1 2 3 4 NA
11. Shoulder/Hip Torsion........................... 0 1 2 3 4 NA

UPPER LIMB
12. Athetoid/Myokymic
    Finger–Wrist–Arm............................... 0 1 2 3 4 NA
13. Pill Rolling.. 0 1 2 3 4 NA

LOWER LIMB
14. Ankle Flexion/
    Foot Tapping....................................... 0 1 2 3 4 NA
15. Toe Movement..................................... 0 1 2 3 4 NA

EVALUATION

1. Greater than 90 d neuroleptic exposure?	:	YES NO
2. Scoring/intensity level met?	:	YES NO
3. Other diagnostic conditions?	:	YES NO

(if yes, specify)
_____
_____

4. Last exam date: _____
   Last total score: _____
   Last conclusion: _____

┌─────────────────────────────────┐
│ Preparer signature and title for items 1–4 │
│ (if different from the physician): │
└─────────────────────────────────┘

5. Conclusion (circle one):

A. No TD (if scoring prerequisite met, list other diagnostic conditions or explain in comments)
B. Probable TD
C. Masked TD
D. Withdrawal TD
E. Persistent TD
F. Remitted TD
G. Other (specify in comments)

6. Comments:
_____
_____
_____
_____
_____
_____
_____
_____

COMMENTS/OTHER
_____
_____
_____
_____

TOTAL SCORE
(items 1–15 only)

EXAM DATE

RATER SIGNATURE AND TITLE	NEXT EXAM DATE	CLINICIAN SIGNATURE	DATE

Figure 21.5 The dyskinesia identification system condensed user scale. (From Sprague, R. L., & Kalachnik, J. E. (1991). Reliability, validity, and a total score cutoff for the dyskinesia identification scale system: Condensed user scale (DISCUS) with mentally ill and mentally retarded populations. Psychopharmacology Bulletin, 27, 51–58.)

these seemingly simple activities. Developing a daily schedule of routine activities (e.g., showering and shaving) can help the patient structure the day. Most patients actually know how to perform self-care activities (e.g., hygiene, grooming) but are not motivated (avolition) to carry them out consistently. Interventions include developing a schedule with the patient for various hygiene activities and emphasizing the importance of maintaining appropriate self-care activities.

Activity, Exercise, and Nutritional Interventions

Encouraging activity and exercise is necessary, not only to maintain a healthy lifestyle but also to counteract the side effects of psychiatric medications that cause weight gain. Because the diagnosis of schizophrenia is usually made in late adolescence or early adulthood, it is possible to establish solid exercise patterns early.

During episodes of acute psychosis, individuals are often unable to focus on eating. When patients begin atypical antipsychotic medications, normal satiety and hunger responses change and overeating or weight gain can become a problem. Appetite increases and cravings for food develop when some neuroleptic medications are initiated. Promoting healthy nutrition and caloric monitoring are key interventions. Weight gain is one of the reasons some persons become resistant to taking medication. It also may be a contributing factor to the development of type II diabetes mellitus. As such, this places them at greater risk for several health complications and early death.

Monitoring for diabetes and managing weight are important activities for all care providers to perform. Individuals should be screened for risk factors of diabetes, such as family history, obesity as indicated by a body mass index (BMI) exceeding or equal to 27, and age older than 45 years. Weight should be measured at regular intervals and BMI calculated. Blood pressure readings should be taken regularly. Laboratory findings for triglycerides, HDL cholesterol, and glucose level should be monitored and reviewed regularly as well. All providers should be alert to the development of diabetic ketoacidosis, particularly in individuals known to have diabetes who begin taking new antipsychotic agents. A program to address weight gain should be initiated at the earliest sign of weight gain (probably between 5 and 10 lb over desired body weight). Reduced caloric intake may be accomplished by increasing the patient's access to affordable, healthful, and easy-to-prepare foods. Behavioural management of weight gain includes keeping a food diary, diet teaching, and exercise and weight management support groups.

Thermoregulation Interventions

Individuals with schizophrenia may have disturbed body temperature regulation. In winter, they may seem to be oblivious to cold weather. In the heat of summer, they may dress for winter. Observing patients' responses to temperatures helps identify problems in this area. In those who are taking psychotropic medications, body temperature needs to be monitored, and they need to be protected from extremes in temperature. Sun safety is also important, and regular use of a sunscreen product to avoid skin damage from sunburn should be recommended.

Pharmacologic Interventions

Early in the 20th century, somatic treatment of schizophrenia included hydrotherapy (baths), wet-pack sheets, insulin shock therapy, electroconvulsive therapy, psychosurgery, and occupational and physical therapies. But in the early 1950s, treatment of schizophrenia drastically changed with the recognition that a drug, chlorpromazine, used to induce anaesthesia also calmed patients with schizophrenia. Optimism persists as older medications continue to be used effectively while offering clues into the workings of the brain and as new discoveries about the brain lead to more precise medications for treating schizophrenia.

Antipsychotic drugs have the general effect of blocking dopamine transmission in the brain by blocking D_2 receptors to some degree (see Chapter 13). Some also block other dopamine receptors and receptors of other neurotransmitters to varying degrees. For the most part, the antidopamine effects are not specific to the mesolimbic and mesocortical tracts associated with schizophrenia, but instead travel to all the dopamine receptor sites throughout the brain. This results in desirable antipsychotic effects but also creates some unpleasant and undesirable side effects. The effects of antipsychotic drugs on other neurotransmitter systems may account for additional side effects.

The newer antipsychotic drugs, often referred to as second generation or atypical antipsychotics, such as risperidone (Risperdal; see Box 21.4), olanzapine (Zyprexa), quetiapine (Seroquel), paliperidone (Invega), ziprasidone (Zeldox), and aripiprazole (Abilify), appear to be more efficacious and safer than conventional antipsychotics. They are available in a variety of formulations. Risperidone (Consta) and paliperidone (Invega Sustenna) are both available in a long-acting injectable form. They are effective in treating negative and positive symptoms. These drugs also affect several other neurotransmitter systems, including serotonin. This is believed to contribute to their overall antipsychotic effectiveness.

Monitoring and Administering Medications

Antipsychotic medications are the treatment of choice for patients with psychosis. The use of conventional or

BOX 21.4 DRUG PROFILE ℞

Drug Profile Risperidone (Risperdal; Consta, Long-Acting Injectable)

Drug Class: Atypical antipsychotic.

Receptor Affinity: Antagonist with high affinity for D_2 and $5\text{-}HT_2$, also histamine (H_1) and α_1- and α_2-adrenergic receptors, weak affinity for D_1 and other serotonin receptor subtypes; no affinity for acetylcholine or beta-adrenergic receptors.

Indications: Psychotic disorders such as schizophrenia, schizoaffective illness, bipolar affective disorder, and major depression with psychotic features.

Routes and Dosage: 1-, 2-, 3-, and 4-mg tablets and liquid concentrate (1 mg/mL). 25-, 50-, and 75-mg long-acting IM.

Adult Dosage: Initial dose typically 1 mg bid. Maximal effect at 6 mg/day. Safety not established above 16 mg/day. Use lowest possible dose to alleviate symptoms.

Geriatric: Initial dose, 0.5 mg/day, increase slowly as tolerated.

Children: Safety and efficacy with this age group have not been established.

Injection: Initiate 25 or 50 mg with oral supplementation for 2 to 3 weeks. Then, injections only, every 2 to 3 weeks. Given IM in gluteal area.

Half-Life (Peak Effect): Mean, 20 h (1 h, peak active metabolite = 3 to 17 h).

Select Adverse Reactions: Insomnia, agitation, anxiety, extrapyramidal symptoms, headache, rhinitis, somnolence, dizziness, headache, constipation, nausea, dyspepsia, vomiting, abdominal pain, hypersalivation, tachycardia, orthostatic hypotension, fever, chest pain, coughing, photosensitivity, and weight gain.

Warning: Rare development of NMS. Observe frequently for early signs of tardive dyskinesia. Use caution with individuals who have cardiovascular disease; risperidone can cause ECG changes. Avoid its use during pregnancy or while breast-feeding. Hepatic or renal impairments increase plasma concentration.

Specific Patient/Family Education

- Notify the prescriber if tremor, motor restlessness, abnormal movements, chest pain, or other unusual symptoms develop.
- Avoid alcohol and other CNS depressant drugs.
- Notify the prescriber if pregnancy is possible or planning to become pregnant. Do not breast-feed while taking this medication.
- Notify the prescriber before taking any other prescription or over-the-counter (OTC) medication.
- It may impair judgment, thinking, or motor skills; avoid driving or other hazardous tasks.
- During titration, the individual may experience orthostatic hypotension and should change positions slowly.
- Do not abruptly discontinue.

typical antipsychotics (e.g., haloperidol, chlorpromazine) decreased dramatically with the introduction of the second generation of antipsychotics, commonly referred to as atypical antipsychotics (Dilks et al., 2019). In general, it takes 1 to 2 weeks for antipsychotic drugs to effect a change in symptoms. During the stabilization period, the type of drug selected should be given an adequate trial, generally 6 to 12 weeks, before considering a change in the drug prescription. If treatment effects are not seen, another antipsychotic agent may be tried. Clozapine (Clozaril) use may be initiated when no other atypical antipsychotic is effective. Clozapine is exceptional in that it often works even when other medications have failed; however, because it requires monitoring of white blood cell counts, it is not the first choice for treatment (see Box 21.5).

Adherence to a prescribed medication regimen is the best approach to preventing relapse. Hardeman and Narasimhan (2010) discuss clinical strategies to guide the promotion of adherence, specifically:

- Build a trusting relationship (guard against bias, include the patient in decision-making)
- Positive and respectful communication (clear and concise communication, taking cognitive state into account)
- Explore patients' beliefs (clarifying their beliefs, exploring the meaning/understanding of taking medication)

- Make remission the goal (link to patient's aspirations in life, clearly explain treatment goals)
- Anticipate nonadherence (talk about medication-taking behaviours; acknowledge this problem, facilitate planning *with* the patient)
- Evaluate adherence (explore patient self-report, explore medication adherence questionnaires)
- Simplify medication regimens (utilize long-acting/extended release/depot medications as appropriate)
- Educate patients, families, and caregivers (about the illness, medication regimens, and what to expect from treatment)
- Seek support (family involvement, case management, collaboration with pharmacies)
- Employ technology (handheld devices, cell phones—timer and calendar features)

In these days of spending constraints and funding shortfalls, inpatient facilities are discharging patients before a judgment can be made about the efficacy of a given drug treatment. Nurses and other mental health professionals are charged with ensuring the continuation of these stabilization protocols and to also ensure that outpatient caregivers assume the responsibility for maintaining this stabilization phase of treatment and continue to monitor and manage the patient's symptoms. Outpatient systems should avoid the immediate

BOX 21.5 DRUG PROFILE ℞

Drug Profile Clozapine (Clozaril)

Drug Class: Atypical antipsychotic

Receptor Affinity: D_1 and D_2 blockade, antagonist for 5-HT_2, H_1, α-adrenergic, and acetylcholine. These additional antagonist effects may contribute to some of its therapeutic effects. It produces fewer extrapyramidal effects than standard antipsychotics with lower risk for tardive dyskinesia.

Indications: Severely ill individuals who have schizophrenia and have not responded to standard antipsychotic treatment. Unlabelled use for other psychotic disorders, such as schizoaffective disorder and bipolar affective disorder.

Routes and Dosage: Available only in tablet form, 25- and 100-mg doses.

Adult Dosage: Initial dose of 25 mg PO bid or qid may gradually increase in 25 to 50 mg/day increments, if tolerated, to a dose of 300 to 450 mg/day by the end of the 2nd week. Additional increases should occur no more than once or twice weekly. Do not exceed 900 mg/day. For maintenance, reduce the dosage to the lowest effective level.

Children: Safety and efficacy with children younger than 16 years have not been established.

Half-Life (Peak Effect): 12 h (1 to 6 h).

Select Adverse Reactions: Drowsiness, dizziness, headache, hypersalivation, tachycardia, hypo-/hypertension, constipation, dry mouth, heartburn, nausea/vomiting, blurred vision, diaphoresis, fever, weight gain, hematologic changes, seizures, tremor, and akathisia.

Warning: Agranulocytosis, defined as a granulocyte count of less than 500 mm^3, occurs at about a cumulative 1-year incidence of 1.3%, most often within 4 to 10 weeks of exposure, but it may occur at any time. Required registration with the clozapine. *Patient management system*, a WBC count before initiation, and weekly WBC counts while taking the drug and for 4 weeks after its discontinuation. Rare development of NMS. No confirmed cases of tardive dyskinesia, but it remains a possibility. Increased seizure risk at higher doses. Use caution with individuals who have cardiovascular disease; clozapine can cause ECG changes. Cases of sudden, unexplained death have been reported. Avoid its use during pregnancy or while breast-feeding.

Specific Patient/Family Education

- Need informed consent regarding the risk for agranulocytosis. Weekly blood draws are required. Notify the prescriber immediately if lethargy, weakness, sore throat, malaise, or other flu-like symptoms develop.
- Notify the prescriber if pregnancy is possible or planning to become pregnant. Do not breast-feed while taking this medication.
- Notify the prescriber before taking any other prescription or OTC medication. Avoid alcohol or other CNS depressant drugs.
- It may cause drowsiness and seizures; avoid driving or other hazardous tasks.
- During titration, the individual may experience orthostatic hypotension and should change positions slowly.
- Do not abruptly discontinue.

---

manipulation of dosages and medications during the stabilization phase unless a medical emergency ensues.

Given the nature of a chronic illness like schizophrenia, patients generally face a lifetime of taking antipsychotic medications. Rarely is discontinuation of medications prescribed; however, many patients stop taking medications on their own. Some situations that require the cessation of medication use are neuroleptic malignant syndrome (NMS) (see *Emergency!* later in this chapter) and agranulocytosis (a dangerously low level of circulating neutrophils). Agranulocytosis is most commonly experienced with clozapine (Clozaril) therapy. Discontinuation is an option when tardive dyskinesia develops. Discontinuation of medications, other than in circumstances of a medical emergency, should be achieved by gradually lowering the dose over time. This diminishes the likelihood of withdrawal symptoms, which include withdrawal dyskinesia and withdrawal psychosis.

Monitoring Extrapyramidal Side Effects

Parkinsonism that is caused by antipsychotic drugs is identical in appearance to Parkinson disease and tends to occur in older patients. The symptoms are believed to be caused by the blockade of D_2 receptors in the basal ganglia, which throws off the normal balance between acetylcholine and dopamine in this area of the brain and effectively increases acetylcholine. The symptoms are managed by reestablishing the balance between acetylcholine and dopamine by reducing the dosage of the antipsychotic (increasing dopamine activity) or adding an anticholinergic drug (decreasing acetylcholine activity), such as benztropine (Cogentin) or trihexyphenidyl (Artane). Discontinuation of the use of anticholinergic drugs should never be abrupt, which can cause a cholinergic rebound and result in withdrawal symptoms, such as vomiting, excessive sweating, and altered dreams and nightmares. Thus, the anticholinergic drug dosage should be reduced gradually (tapered) over several days. If a patient experiences akathisia (physical restlessness), an anticholinergic medication may not be particularly helpful. Table 21.2 lists the anticholinergic side effects of anti-Parkinson drugs and several interventions to manage them. Table 21.3 lists the extrapyramidal side effects of antipsychotic drugs.

Dystonic reactions are also believed to result from the imbalance of dopamine and acetylcholine, with the

Table 21.2 Nursing Interventions for Anticholinergic Side Effects

Effect	Intervention
Dry mouth	Sips of water; hard candies and chewing gum (preferably sugar-free)
Blurred vision	Avoid dangerous tasks; teach the patient that this side effect will diminish in a few weeks
Decreased lacrimation	Artificial tears if necessary
Mydriasis	May aggravate glaucoma; teach the patient to report eye pain
Photophobia	Sunglasses
Constipation	High-fibre diet; increased fluid intake; laxatives as prescribed
Urinary hesitancy	Privacy; run water in sink; warm water over perineum
Urinary retention	Regular voiding (at least every 2–3 h) and whenever urge is present; catheterize for residual; record intake and output; evaluate benign prostatic hypertrophy
Tachycardia	Evaluate for preexisting cardiovascular disease; sudden death has occurred with thioridazine (Mellaril)

latter being dominant. Young men seem to be more vulnerable to this particular extrapyramidal side effect. This side effect, which develops rapidly and dramatically, can be very frightening for patients as their muscles tense and their body contorts. The experience often starts with stiffness experienced in the muscles and can rapidly escalate to oculogyric crisis, in which the muscles that control eye movements tense and pull the eyeball so that the patient is looking toward the ceiling. This may be followed rapidly by *torticollis*, in which the neck muscles pull the head to the side, or *retrocollis*, in which the head is pulled back, or *orolaryngeal–pharyngeal hypertonus*, in which the patient has extreme difficulty swallowing. The patient may also experience contorted extremities. These symptoms occur early in antipsychotic drug treatment, when the patient may still be experiencing psychotic symptoms. Experiencing these side effects may compound the patient's fear and anxiety and requires a quick response. The immediate treatment is to administer benztropine (Cogentin), 1 to 2 mg, or diphenhydramine (Benadryl), 25 to 50 mg, intramuscularly or intravenously. This is followed by daily administration of oral anticholinergic drugs and, possibly, by a decrease in antipsychotic medication (Dilks et al., 2019). Refer to Box 21.6 for more information about benztropine).

Akathisia appears to be caused by the same biologic mechanism as other extrapyramidal side effects. Patients are restless and report that they feel driven to keep moving, can't sit still, and exhibit fidgety movements. They are very uncomfortable (Dilks et al., 2019). Frequently, this response is misinterpreted as anxiety or increased psychotic symptoms, and the patient may be inappropriately given increased dosages of the antipsychotic drug, which only perpetuates the side effect. If possible, the dose of the antipsychotic drug should be reduced. A beta-adrenergic blocker such as propranolol (Inderal), 20 to 120 mg, may be required. Failure to manage this side effect is a leading cause of patients ceasing to take antipsychotic medications.

Tardive dyskinesia (impaired voluntary movement, resulting in fragmented or incomplete movements), tardive dystonia, and tardive akathisia are less likely to appear in individuals taking atypical, rather than conventional, antipsychotics. Tardive dyskinesia is late-appearing abnormal involuntary movements (dyskinesia). It can be viewed as the opposite of parkinsonism both in observable movements and in aetiology. Whereas muscle rigidity and the absence of movement characterize parkinsonism, constant movement characterizes tardive dyskinesia. Typical movements involve the mouth, tongue, and jaw and include lip smacking, sucking, puckering, tongue protrusion, the bon-bon sign (where the tongue rolls around in the mouth and protrudes into the cheek as if the patient were sucking

Table 21.3 Extrapyramidal Side Effects of Antipsychotic Drugs

Side Effect	Symptoms
Parkinsonism or pseudoparkinsonism	Resting tremor, rigidity, bradykinesia/akinesia, masklike face, shuffling gait, and decreased arm swing
Acute dystonia	Intermittent or fixed abnormal postures of the eyes, face, tongue, neck, trunk, and extremities
Akathisia	Obvious motor restlessness evidenced by pacing, rocking, and shifting from foot to foot; subjective sense of not being able to sit or be still; these symptoms may occur together or separately
Tardive dyskinesia	Abnormal dyskinetic movements of the face, mouth, and jaw; choreoathetoid movements of the legs, arms, and trunk
Tardive dystonia	Persistent sustained abnormal postures in the face, eyes, tongue, neck, trunk, and limbs
Tardive akathisia	Persisting, unabating sense of subjective and objective restlessness

Adapted from Lilley, L. L., Collins, S. R., Synder, J., & Swart, B. (2017). *Pharmacology for Canadian health care practice* (3rd ed.). Elsevier Canada.

BOX 21.6 DRUG PROFILE ℞

Drug Profile Benztropine Mesylate (Cogentin)

Drug Class: Anti-Parkinson agent

Receptor Affinity: Blocks cholinergic (acetylcholine) activity, which is believed to restore the acetylcholine/dopamine balance in the basal ganglia.

Indications: Used in psychiatry to reduce extrapyramidal symptoms (acute medication–related movement disorders), including pseudoparkinsonism, dystonia, and akathisia (not tardive syndromes), due to neuroleptic drugs such as haloperidol. Most effective with acute dystonia.

Routes and Dosage: Available in tablet form, 0.5-, 1-, and 2-mg doses, also injectable 1 mg/mL.

Adult Dosage: For acute dystonia, 1 to 2 mg IM or IV usually provides rapid relief. No significant difference in the onset of action after IM or IV injection. Treatment of emergent symptoms may be relieved in 1 or 2 days, with 1 to 2 mg orally two to three times per day. Maximum daily dose is 6 mg/day. After 1 to 2 weeks, withdraw the drug to see if continued treatment is needed. Medication-related movement disorders that develop slowly may not respond to this treatment.

Geriatric: Older adults and very thin patients cannot tolerate large doses.

Children: Do not use in children younger than 3 years. Use with caution in older children.

Half-Life: 12 to 24 h, very little pharmacokinetic information is available.

Select Adverse Reactions: Dry mouth, blurred vision, tachycardia, nausea, constipation, flushing or elevated temperature, decreased sweating, muscular weakness or cramping, urinary retention, urinary hesitancy, dizziness, headache, disorientation, confusion, memory loss, hallucinations, psychoses, and agitation in toxic reactions, which are more pronounced in older people and occur at smaller doses.

Warning: Avoid its use during pregnancy or while breastfeeding. Give with caution in hot weather due to a possible heatstroke. Contraindicated with angle-closure glaucoma, pyloric or duodenal obstruction, stenosing peptic ulcers, prostatic hypertrophy or bladder neck obstructions, myasthenia gravis, megacolon, or megaesophagus. It may aggravate the symptoms of tardive dyskinesia or other chronic forms of medication-related movement disorder. Concomitant use of other anticholinergic drugs may increase the side effects and risk for toxicity. Coadministration of haloperidol or phenothiazines may reduce serum levels of these drugs.

Specific Patient/Family Education

- Take with meals to reduce dry mouth and gastric irritation.
- Dry mouth may be alleviated by sucking sugarless candies, adequate fluid intake, or good oral hygiene; increase the intake of fibre and fluids in diet to avoid constipation; stool softeners may be required. Notify the prescriber if urinary hesitancy or constipation persists.
- Notify the prescriber if rapid or pounding heartbeat, confusion, eye pain, rash, or other adverse symptoms develop.
- It may cause drowsiness, dizziness, or blurred vision; use caution while driving or performing other hazardous tasks requiring alertness. Avoid alcohol and other CNS depressants.
- Do not abruptly stop this medication because a flu-like syndrome may develop.
- Use caution in hot weather. Ensure adequate hydration. It may increase the susceptibility to heatstroke.

---

on a piece of hard candy), athetoid (wormlike) movements in the tongue, and chewing. Other facial movements, such as grimacing and eye blinking, also may be present.

Movements in the trunk and limbs are frequently observable. These include rocking from the hips, athetoid movements of the fingers and toes, jerking movements of the fingers and toes, guitar strumming movements of the fingers, and foot tapping. The long-term health problems for people with tardive dyskinesia are choking associated with loss of control of muscles used for swallowing and compromised respiratory function leading to infections and, possibly, respiratory alkalosis.

Because the movements resemble the dyskinetic movements of some patients who have idiopathic Parkinson disease and who have received long-term treatment with L-dopa (a direct-acting dopamine agonist that crosses the blood–brain barrier), the suggested hypothesis for tardive dyskinesia includes the supersensitivity of the dopamine receptor in the basal ganglia.

All patients on antipsychotics should be screened and monitored for movement disorders. However, antipsychotic drugs mask the movements of tardive dyskinesia and have periodically been suggested as a treatment. This is counterintuitive because these are the drugs that cause the disorder. Newer antipsychotic drugs, such as clozapine, may be less likely to cause the disorder. The best management remains prevention through prescription of the lowest possible dose of antipsychotic drug over time that minimizes the symptoms of schizophrenia, prescription of these drugs for psychotic symptoms only, and early case finding by observation of clinical presentation and systematic AIMS screening of everyone receiving these drugs (Dilks et al., 2019). See Chapter 13 for information regarding medication-related movement disorders.

Orthostatic hypotension is another side effect of antipsychotic drugs. The primary antiadrenergic effect is decreased blood pressure, which may be general or orthostatic. Patients may be protected from falls by teaching them to rise slowly and by monitoring blood pressure before doses of the drug. The nurse should monitor and document lying, sitting, and standing blood pressures when any antipsychotic drug therapy begins.

Hyperprolactinaemia can occur and is associated with the use of haloperidol and risperidone. When dopamine is blocked in the tuberoinfundibular tract, it can no longer repress prolactin, the neurohormone that regulates lactation and mammary function. The prolactin level increases and, in some individuals, side effects appear. *Gynaecomastia* (enlarged breasts) can occur among both sexes and is understandably distressing to individuals who may be experiencing delusional or hallucinatory body image disturbances. *Galactorrhoea* (lactation) also may occur. Menstrual irregularities and sexual dysfunction are also possible. If these symptoms appear, the medication should be reduced or changed to another antipsychotic agent. Evidence for long-term consequences of hyperprolactinaemia is still lacking.

Weight gain is related to antipsychotic agents, especially olanzapine and clozapine, which have major antihistaminic properties. Patients may gain as much as 20 or 30 lb within 1 year. Increased appetite and weight gain are often distressing to patients. Diet teaching and monitoring may have some effect on this side effect. Another solution is to increase the accessibility of healthful, easy-to-prepare food. Although nausea and vomiting can occur with the use of these drugs, they most often mask nausea.

Screening for new-onset diabetes in patients taking antipsychotic drugs should be conducted regularly. An association has been made between new-onset diabetes mellitus (type 2 diabetes) and impaired glucose regulation and the administration of atypical antipsychotic agents, especially olanzapine and clozapine (Gough, 2005; Whicher et al., 2018). Patients should be assessed and monitored for clinical symptoms of diabetes. Fasting blood glucose tests are commonly ordered for these individuals (Holt, 2019).

Sedation is another possible side effect of antipsychotic medication. Patients should be monitored for the sedating effects of antipsychotic agents that are antihistaminic. In older patients, sedation can be associated with falls.

Cardiac arrhythmias may also occur. Prolongation of the QT interval is associated with torsade de pointes (polymorphic ventricular tachycardia) or ventricular fibrillation. The potential for drug-induced prolonged QT interval is associated with many drugs, for example, the antipsychotic agent ziprasidone (Zeldox) may be more likely than other drugs to prolong the QT interval and change the heart rhythm. For these patients, baseline electrocardiograms may be ordered. Nurses should observe these patients for cardiac arrhythmias.

Agranulocytosis is a reduction in the number of circulating granulocytes and decreased production of granulocytes in the bone marrow that limits one's ability to fight infection. Agranulocytosis can develop with the use of all antipsychotic drugs, but it is most likely to develop with clozapine use. Although laboratory values below 500 cells/mm^3 are indicative of agranulocytosis, often, granulocyte counts drop to below 200 cells/mm^3 with this syndrome.

Patients taking clozapine must have regular blood tests. White blood cell and granulocyte counts should be measured before the treatment is initiated and at least weekly or twice weekly after the treatment begins. Initial white blood cell counts should be above 3,500 cells/mm^3 before treatment initiation; in patients with counts of 3,500 to 5,000 cells/mm^3, cell counts should be monitored three times a week if clozapine is prescribed. Any time the white blood cell count drops below 3,500 cells/mm^3 or granulocytes drop below 1,500 cells/mm^3, the use of clozapine should be stopped, and the patient should be monitored for fever and infections.

A faithfully implemented program of blood monitoring, however, should not replace careful observation of the patient. It is not unusual for blood cell counts to drop precipitously in a period of 2 to 3 days. This may not be discovered when the patient is on a strict weekly blood monitoring schedule. Any reported symptoms that are reminiscent of a bacterial infection (e.g., fever, pharyngitis, weakness) should be a cause for concern, and immediate evaluation of blood count status should be undertaken. Because patients are frequently discharged before the critical period of risk for agranulocytosis, patient and family education about these symptoms is also essential so that they will report these symptoms and obtain blood monitoring if necessary. In general, granulocytes return to normal within 2 to 4 weeks after discontinuing use of the medication (Box 21.7).

Drug–Drug Interactions

Several potential drug–drug interactions are possible when administering antipsychotic medications. One of the cytochrome P450 enzymes responsible for the metabolism of olanzapine and clozapine is 1A2. If either olanzapine or clozapine is given with another medication that inhibits this enzyme, such as fluvoxamine (Luvox), the antipsychotic blood level would increase and possibly become toxic. On the other hand, cigarette smoking can also induce 1A2 and lower concentration of drugs metabolized by this enzyme, such as olanzapine and clozapine. Individuals that smoke may require a higher dose of these medications than do nonsmokers (Levin & Rezvani, 2007). Similarly, individuals that are unable to smoke (due to smoke-free policies) or have quit smoking are at risk of increased antipsychotic blood levels and possible toxicity. This effect may be of high relevance when an individual is discharged from a nonsmoking institution to a community setting.

Nonadherence to the medication regimen is an important factor in relapse. Patients and their families must be made aware of the importance of consistently taking medications. Medication education should cover the association between medications and the amelioration of symptoms (in general as well as individualized for the patient), side effects and their management, and coaching as to when to report medication effects.

Several atypical antipsychotic agents, including clozapine, quetiapine, and ziprasidone, are metabolized by the 3A4 enzyme. Weak inhibitors of this enzyme include the antidepressants fluvoxamine, nefazodone, and norfluoxetine (an active metabolite of fluoxetine). Potent inhibitors of 3A4 enzyme include ketoconazole (antifungal drug), protease inhibitors, and erythromycin. If these drugs are given with clozapine, quetiapine, or ziprasidone, the antipsychotic level will rise. In addition, the mood stabilizer carbamazepine (Tegretol) is a 3A4 inducer. When this drug is given with clozapine, quetiapine, or ziprasidone, the antipsychotic dose should be increased to compensate for the 3A4 induction. If the use of carbamazepine is discontinued, the dosage of the antipsychotic agent needs to be adjusted.

Risperidone, clozapine, and olanzapine are substrates for the enzyme 2D6. Theoretically, antidepressants (fluoxetine and paroxetine) that inhibit this enzyme could increase these antipsychotics' levels. However, this is not usually clinically significant.

The most important aspects of nursing care for patients with NMS relate to recognizing symptoms early, stopping the administration of any neuroleptic medications, and initiating supportive nursing care. In any patient with fever, fluctuating vital signs, abrupt changes in levels of consciousness, or any of the symptoms presented in Box 21.8, NMS should be suspected. The nurse should be especially alert for early signs and symptoms of NMS in high-risk patients, such as those who are agitated, physically exhausted, or dehydrated, or those who have an existing medical or neurologic illness. Patients receiving parenteral or higher doses of oral neuroleptic drugs or lithium concurrently must also be carefully assessed. The nurse should carefully monitor fluid intake and fluid and electrolyte status.

To prevent NMS from developing in a patient with signs or symptoms of the disorder, the nurse should immediately discontinue the administration of any

EMERGENCY

Neuroleptic Malignant Syndrome

In NMS, severe muscle rigidity develops with elevated temperature and a rapidly accelerating cascade of symptoms (occurring during the next 48 to 72 h), which can include two or more of the following: hypertension, tachycardia, tachypnea, prominent diaphoresis, incontinence, mutism, leukocytosis, changes in the level of consciousness ranging from confusion to coma, and laboratory evidence of muscle injury (e.g., elevated creatinine phosphokinase). NMS occurs in about 1% of those who receive antipsychotic drugs, especially the conventional antipsychotics such as haloperidol and other drugs that block dopamine, such as metoclopramide (Montoya et al., 2003). Up to one third of patients experiencing NMS die as a result of the syndrome. NMS is probably underreported and may account for unexplained emergency room deaths of patients taking these drugs who do not have diagnoses because their symptoms do not seem serious. The presenting symptom is a temperature greater than 37.5°C (usually between 38.3°C and 39.4°C) with no apparent cause.

neuroleptic drugs and notify the physician. In addition, the nurse should hold any anticholinergic drugs that the patient may be taking. A common error made by nurses who fail to analyze the patient's total clinical picture (including vital signs, mental status changes, and laboratory values) is to continue the use of neuroleptic drugs. Figure 21.6 shows how to decide whether to withhold an antipsychotic medication. Medical treatment includes administering several medications. Dopamine agonist drugs, such as bromocriptine (modest success), and muscle relaxants, such as dantrolene or benzodiazepine, have been used. Antiparkinsonism drugs are not particularly useful. While some patients experience improvement with electroconvulsive therapy, Morcos and colleagues (2019) suggest that ECT should be considered in cases of NMS that are unresponsive to pharmacologic intervention.

The vital signs of the patient with symptoms of NMS must be monitored frequently. In addition, it is important to check the results of the patient's laboratory tests for increased creatine phosphokinase, elevated white blood cell count, elevated liver enzymes, or myoglobinuria. The nurse must be prepared to initiate supportive measures or anticipate emergency transfer of the patient to a medical–surgical or an intensive care unit.

BOX 21.8 Diagnostic Criteria for Neuroleptic Malignant Syndrome (NMS)

1. Treatment with neuroleptics within 7 days of onset (2 to 4 weeks for depot neuroleptic medications)
2. Hyperthermia
3. Muscle rigidity
4. Five of the following (concurrently):
   - Change in mental status
   - Tachycardia
   - Hypertension or hypotension
   - Tachypnea or hypoxia
   - Diaphoresis or sialorrhoea
   - Tremor
   - Incontinence
   - Creatinine phosphokinase elevation or myoglobinuria
   - Leukocytosis
   - Metabolic acidosis
5. Exclusion of other drug-induced, systemic, or neuropsychiatric illnesses

Adapted from Lilley, L. L., Collins, S. R., Synder, J., & Swart, B. (2017). *Pharmacology for Canadian health care practice* (3rd ed.). Elsevier Canada.

Treating high temperature (which frequently exceeds 39°C) is an important priority for these patients. High body temperature may be reduced with a cooling blanket and acetaminophen. Because many of these patients experience diaphoresis, temperature elevation, or dysphagia, it is important to monitor fluid hydration. Another important aspect of care for patients with NMS is safety. Joints and extremities that are rigid or spastic must be protected from injury. The treatment of these patients depends on the facility and availability of medical support services.

In general, episodes of anticholinergic crisis are self-limiting, usually subsiding in 3 days. However, if untreated, the associated fever and delirium may progress

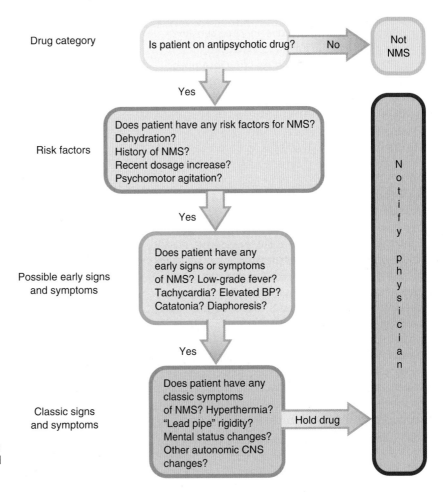

Figure 21.6 Action tree for "holding" a neuroleptic drug because of suspected neuroleptic malignant syndrome.

EMERGENCY

Anticholinergic Crisis

There is also a potential for abuse of anticholinergic drugs. Some patients may find the anticholinergic effects of these drugs on mood, memory, and perception pleasurable. Although at toxic dosages, patients may experience disorientation and hallucinations, lesser doses may cause patients to experience greater sociability and euphoria. Anticholinergic crisis is a potentially life-threatening medical emergency caused by an overdose of or sensitivity to drugs with anticholinergic properties. This syndrome (also called anticholinergic delirium) may result from an accidental or intentional overdose of antimuscarinic drugs, including atropine, scopolamine, or belladonna alkaloids, which are present in numerous prescription drugs and over-the-counter (OTC) medicines. The syndrome may also occur in psychiatric patients who are receiving therapeutic doses of anticholinergic drugs, especially when such agents are combined with other psychotropic drugs that produce anticholinergic side effects. Numerous drugs commonly prescribed in psychiatric settings produce anticholinergic side effects, including tricyclic antidepressants and some antipsychotics. As a result of either drug overdose or drug sensitivity, these anticholinergic substances may produce an acute delirium or a psychotic reaction resembling schizophrenia. More severe anticholinergic effects may occur in older patients, even at therapeutic levels (Ramnarine & Ahmad, 2016).

The signs and symptoms of anticholinergic crisis are dramatic and physically uncomfortable (see Box "Emergency: Signs and Symptoms of Anticholinergic Crisis"). This disorder is characterized by elevated temperature; parched mouth; burning thirst; hot, dry skin; decreased salivation; decreased bronchial and nasal secretions; widely dilated eyes (bright light is painful); decreased ability to accommodate visually; increased heart rate; constipation; difficulty urinating; and hypertension or hypotension. The face, neck, and upper arms may become flushed because of reflex blood vessel dilation. In addition to peripheral symptoms, patients with anticholinergic psychosis may experience neuropsychiatric symptoms of anxiety, agitation, delirium, hyperactivity, confusion, hallucinations (especially visual), speech difficulties, psychotic symptoms, or seizures. The acute psychotic reaction that is produced resembles schizophrenia. The classic description of anticholinergic crisis is summarized in the following mnemonic: "Hot as a hare, blind as a bat, mad as a hatter, dry as a bone."

EMERGENCY

Signs and Symptoms of Anticholinergic Crisis

Neuropsychiatric signs: confusion, recent memory loss, agitation, dysarthria, incoherent speech, pressured speech, delusions, ataxia, and periods of hyperactivity alternating with somnolence, paranoia, anxiety, or coma

Hallucinations: accompanied by "picking," plucking, or grasping motions, delusions, or disorientation

Physical signs: unreactive dilated pupils; blurred vision; hot, dry, flushed skin; facial flushing; dry mucous membranes; difficulty swallowing; fever; tachycardia; hypertension; decreased bowel sounds; urinary retention; nausea; vomiting; seizures; or coma

to coma or cardiac and respiratory depression. Although rare, death is generally due to hyperpyrexia and brainstem depression. Once the use of the offending drug is discontinued, improvement usually occurs within 24 to 36 h.

A specific and effective antidote, physostigmine (an inhibitor of anticholinesterase), is frequently used for treating and diagnosing anticholinergic crisis. Administration of this drug rapidly reduces both the behavioural and the physiologic symptoms. However, the usual adult dose of physostigmine is 1 to 2 mg intravenously, given slowly during a period of 5 min because rapid injection of physostigmine may cause seizures, profound bradycardia, or heart block. Physostigmine is relatively short acting, so it may need to be given several times during the course of treatment. This drug provides relief from symptoms for a period of 2 to 3 h. In addition to receiving physostigmine, patients who intentionally overdose on large amounts of anticholinergic drugs are treated by gastric lavage, administration of charcoal, and catharsis. The dose may be repeated after 20 or 30 min.

It is important for the nurse to be alert for signs and symptoms of anticholinergic crisis, especially in older adults and children, who are much more sensitive to the anticholinergic effects of drugs, and in patients who are receiving multiple medications with anticholinergic effects. If signs and symptoms of the syndrome occur, the nurse should discontinue the use of the offending drug and notify the physician immediately.

Other Somatic Interventions

Electroconvulsive therapy is suggested as a possible alternative when the patient's schizophrenia is not being successfully treated by medication alone. For the most part, this is not indicated unless the patient is experiencing catatonia or has a depression that is not treatable by other means.

Psychological Domain

Although schizophrenia is a brain disorder, the psychological manifestations are the most difficult to assess and treat. Many of these psychological manifestations improve with the use of medications, but they are not necessarily eliminated.

Psychological Assessment

Several assessment scales have been developed and received considerable reliability and validity testing to help evaluate positive and negative symptom clusters in schizophrenia. Box 21.9 lists the standardized instruments used in assessing symptoms of people with schizophrenia. These include the Scale for the Assessment of Positive Symptoms (SAPS) the Scale for the Assessment of Negative Symptoms (SANS), and the Positive and Negative Syndrome Scale (PANSS) (Kay et al., 1987), which assesses both symptom clusters in the same instrument (see Web Links). Tools that list symptoms, such as the

Brief Psychiatric Rating Scale (BPRS) (Overall & Gorham, 1988) (see Web Links), SANS, or SAPS, can also be used to help patients self-monitor their symptoms.

Information about prediagnosis experiences usually requires retrospective reporting by the patient or the family. This reporting is generally reliable for the frankly psychotic symptoms of delusions and hallucinations; however, negative symptoms are more difficult to date. In fact, negative symptoms vary from an imperceptive deviation from normal to a clear impairment. Negative symptoms probably occur earlier than do positive symptoms and are less easily noted by the patient and significant others.

Responses to Mental Health Problems

Schizophrenia robs people of mental health and imposes social stigma. People with schizophrenia struggle to maintain control of their symptoms, which affects every aspect of their life. The person with schizophrenia displays a variety of interrelated symptoms and experiences deficits in several areas. Most patients report the following

---

BOX 21.9 Standardized Scales and Resources Used in Assessing Symptoms of People With Schizophrenia

SCALE FOR THE ASSESSMENT OF POSITIVE SYMPTOMS (SAPS)

From Nancy C. Andreasen, MD, PhD, Department of Psychiatry, College of Medicine, The University of Iowa, Iowa City, IA 52242. Copyright 1984 Nancy C. Andreasen.

SCALE FOR THE ASSESSMENT OF NEGATIVE SYMPTOMS (SANS)

From Nancy C. Andreasen, MD, PhD, Department of Psychiatry, College of Medicine, The University of Iowa, Iowa City, IA 52242. Copyright 1984 Nancy C. Andreasen.

ABNORMAL INVOLUNTARY MOVEMENT SCALE (AIMS)

Guy, W. (1976). *ECDEU: Assessment manual for psychopharmacology* (DHEW Publication No. 76-338). Washington, DC: Department of Health Education and Welfare, Psychopharmacology Branch.

BRIEF PSYCHIATRIC RATING SCALE (BPRS)

Overall, J. E., & Gorham, D. R. (1988). The brief psychiatric rating scale (BPRS): Recent developments in ascertainment and scaling. *Psychopharmacology Bulletin, 24*, 97–99.

DYSKINESIA IDENTIFICATION SYSTEM: CONDENSED USER SCALE (DISCUS)

Sprague, R. L., & Kalachnik, J. E. (1991). Reliability, validity, and a total score cutoff for the dyskinesia

identification scale system: Condensed user scale (DISCUS) with mentally ill and mentally retarded populations. *Psychopharmacology Bulletin, 27*(1), 51–58.

SIMPSON-ANGUS RATING SCALE

Simpson, G. M., & Angus, J. W. (1970). A rating scale for extrapyramidal side effects. *Acta Psychiatrica Scandinavica, 212*, 11–19. Copyright 1970, Munksgaard International Publishers, Ltd.

ADDITIONAL RESOURCES

Blanchard, J. J., & Cohen, A. S. (2006). The structure of negative symptoms within schizophrenia: Implications for assessment. *Schizophrenia Bulletin, 32*(2), 238–235.

Correll, C. U., & Schooler, N. R. (2020). Negative symptoms in schizophrenia: A review and clinical guide for recognition, assessment, and treatment. *Neuropsychiatric Disease and Treatment, 16*, 519–534. https://doi.org/10.2147/NDT.S225643

Kay, S. R., Fiszbein, A., & Opler, L. A. (1987). The positive and negative syndrome scale (PANSS) for schizophrenia. *Schizophrenia Bulletin, 13*(2), 261–276. https://doi.org/10.1093/schbul/13.2.261

Kumari, S., Malik, M., Florival, C., Manalai, P., & Sonje, S. (2017). An assessment of five (PANSS, SAPS, SANS, NSA-16, CGI-SCH) commonly used symptoms rating scales in schizophrenia and comparison to newer scales (CAINS, BNSS). *Journal of Addiction Research & Therapy, 8*(3), 324. https://doi.org/10.4172/2155-6105.1000324

Rege, S., Castle, D., Pai, N., & Dark, F. (2022, January 20). *Negative symptoms in schizophrenia –A review of neurobiology, diagnosis and management.* https://psychscenehub.com/psychinsights/negative-symptoms-in-schizophrenia/

prodromal symptoms (in order of frequency): tension and nervousness, lack of interest in eating, difficulty concentrating, disturbed sleep, decreased enjoyment and loss of interest, restlessness, forgetfulness, depression, social withdrawal from friends, feeling laughed at, more religious thinking, feeling bad for no reason, feeling too excited, and hearing voices or seeing things.

Mental Status and Appearance

The patient with schizophrenia may look eccentric or dishevelled or have poor hygiene and bizarre dress. The patient's posture may suggest lethargy or stupor.

Mood and Affect

Patients with schizophrenia often display altered mood states. In some cases, they may show heightened emotional activity; others may display severely limited emotional responses. Affect, the outward expression of mood, is categorized on a continuum: flat (emotional expression entirely absent), blunted (expression of emotions present but greatly diminished), and full range. Inappropriate affect is marked by incongruence between the emotional expression and the thoughts expressed. Other common emotional symptoms include the following:

- **Affective lability**—abrupt, dramatic, unprovoked changes in the type of emotions expressed
- **Ambivalence**—the presence and expression of two opposing feelings, leading to inaction
- **Apathy**—reactions to stimuli are decreased; diminished interest and desire

Speech

Speech patterns may reflect obsessions, delusions, pressured thinking, loose associations, or flight of ideas and neologisms. Speech is an indicator of thought content and other mental processes and is usually altered. An assessment of speech should note any difficulty articulating words (dysarthria) and difficulty swallowing (dysphagia) as indicators of medication side effects. In many instances, what an individual says is as important as how it is said. Both content and speech patterns should be noted.

Thought Processes and Delusions

Delusions can be distinguished from strongly held ideas by the degree of conviction with which the belief is held despite clear contradictory evidence (APA, 2013). Culture must be considered when evaluating delusions. Delusional beliefs are those not sanctioned or held by a cultural or religious subgroup.

Bizarre delusions alone are sufficient to diagnose schizophrenia. It can often be difficult to distinguish between bizarre and nonbizarre delusions. Nonbizarre delusions generally have themes of jealousy and persecution and are derived from ordinary life experiences. For example, a woman believes that her husband, from whom she has recently separated, is trying

to poison her, or a man believes that members of the Mafia are trying to kill him because, when he was in high school, he reported to the principal that several of his classmates were selling drugs at school.

Bizarre delusions are those that are implausible, not understandable, and not derived from ordinary life experiences. Bizarre delusions often include delusions of control (that some outside force controls thoughts and actions), thought broadcasting (that others can read or hear one's thoughts), thought insertion (that someone has placed thoughts into one's mind), and thought withdrawal (that someone is removing thoughts from one's mind) (APA, 2013). For example, a patient who has been with a hypnotist for 2 months reports that the hypnotist continued to read his mind and was "picking his brain away piece by piece." Another patient was convinced that a computer chip was placed in her vagina during a gynaecologic examination and that this somehow directly influenced her physical movements and her thoughts.

Assessing and judging the content of the delusion and exploring other aspects of the delusional experience are helpful in understanding the significance of these false beliefs. The underlying feeling that accompanies the delusion should be identified. Other aspects to consider include the conviction with which the delusion is held; the extent to which other aspects of the individual's life are incorporated into or affected by the delusion; the degree of internal consistency, organization, and logic evident in the delusion; and the amount of pressure (in terms of preoccupation and concern) individuals feel in their lives as a result of the delusion (see Box 21.10).

Hallucinations

Hallucinations are the most common example of disturbed sensory perception observed in patients with schizophrenia. Hallucinations can be experienced in all sensory modalities; however, auditory hallucinations are the most common in schizophrenia. Some specific hallucinations may be sufficient to diagnose schizophrenia, such as hearing voices conversing with each other, or carrying on a discussion with someone who is not there. Because most individuals will not spontaneously share their hallucinatory experiences with an interviewer, the nurse may need to rely on indirect evidence in the patient's behaviour, such as (a) pauses during conversations in which the individual seems preoccupied or appears to be listening to someone other than the interviewer; (b) looking toward the perceived source of a voice; or (c) responding to the voices in some manner. Although patients may not spontaneously share their hallucinations, many validate observations of the examiner or admit to a history of hallucinations when asked (see Box 21.11).

Disorganized Communication

The other aspect of thought content and processes that may be altered in schizophrenia is the organization of expressed thoughts. Impaired verbal fluency (ability to

BOX 21.10 THERAPEUTIC DIALOGUE

The Patient With Delusions
John joined the nurse in a game of pool. The following conversation occurred as they played.

Ineffective Approach

John: The RCMP put a transmitter in my molar, here (points to his right cheek).
Nurse: No one would put a transmitter in your tooth; come on, the RCMP isn't looking for you.
John: You get the striped balls. Yeah, they want to monitor me while I'm here. I know that they have the real Governor General here in the hospital. They are trying to get the Prime Minister to intervene with the Ontario Provincial Police. Mark from Ottawa told me that.
Nurse: The Governor General can't possibly be here; I saw him on television this morning.
John: Maybe—he does have lighter hair and has different-coloured contacts to disguise his eyes, but they're just trying to keep people from knowing what they're doing.
Nurse: John, he isn't in the hospital; if he were, I would know it because I work here.
John: (With anger) You don't know anything! You are probably from the RCMP also. I have nothing else to say to you.

Effective Approach

John: The RCMP put a transmitter in my molar, here (points to his right cheek).
Nurse: Oh. Which balls are mine?
John: You get the striped ones. Yeah, they want to monitor me while I'm here. I know that they have the real Governor General here in the hospital. They are trying to get the Prime Minister to intervene with the Ontario Provincial Police. Mark from Ottawa told me that.

Nurse: Do you suppose that you saw someone who looks like the Governor General?
John: Maybe—he does have lighter hair and has different-coloured contacts to disguise his eyes. But they're just trying to keep people from knowing what they're doing.
Nurse: You sound a little overwhelmed with all the information you have.
John: No, no. I can handle it. The RCMP can't do anything to me, I'll never talk. They are trying to confuse me so that I stay away from the Governor General. They all think they can keep me from my mission.
Nurse: Who is it that worries you, John?
John: Everyone in the government. The RCMP, CSIS, CRA—all those alphabets.
Nurse: It must be rather frightening to feel all these people are looking for you. You must be scared a lot of the time.
John: It's scary but I can handle it. I've handled it all my life.
Nurse: You've been in scary situations all your life?
John: Yeah. I don't know. Maybe not scary, just hard. I never seemed to be able to do as well as my parents wanted—or as I wanted.

CRITICAL THINKING CHALLENGE

- How did the nurse's argumentative responses cause the patient to react in the first scenario?
- What effective communication techniques did the nurse use in the second scenario?

produce spontaneous speech) is commonly present. Abrupt shifts in the focus of conversation are a typical symptom of disorganized thinking. The most severe shifts in focus may occur after only one or two words (**word salad**), after one or two phrases or sentences (flight of ideas or loose associations), or somewhat less severely as a shift that occurs when a new topic is repeatedly suggested and pursued from the current topic (**tangentiality**). In some individuals, speech may be a simple repetition of words or phrases spoken by others (**echolalia**).

Cognitive Impairments

Although cognitive impairments in schizophrenia vary widely from patient to patient, several primary problems have been identified:

- Attention may be increased and sustained on external stimuli over a period of time (hypervigilance).
- The ability to distinguish and focus on relevant stimuli may be diminished.

- Familiar cues may go unrecognized or be improperly encoded.
- Information processing may be diminished, leading to inappropriate or illogical conclusions from available observations and information (Sheffield et al., 2014).

Cognitive impairments are not easy to recognize. By relying only on clinical assessment, the nurse can miss the extent of the impairment. Using a standardized instrument such as the Mini-Mental Status Examination (MMSE), the Cognitive Assessment Screening Instrument (CASI), or the 7-Minute Screen can provide a screening measurement of cognitive function (see Chapter 11). If impairment is suspected, neuropsychological testing by a qualified psychologist may be necessary.

Memory and Orientation

Impairments in orientation, memory, and abstract thinking may be observed. Orientation to time, place, and person may remain relatively intact unless the

BOX 21.11 THERAPEUTIC DIALOGUE

The Patient With Hallucinations

The following conversation took place in a dayroom with several staff members present. The patient was potentially very violent. Although it is a good example of dealing with someone who is hallucinating, it is not a situation that should be taken lightly. Always make certain that you have a means to leave a situation (i.e., you are not in the corner of a room) and that you have sufficient staff members close by to ensure safety. Take careful note of whether the patient has a potential weapon near at hand.

Jason approached the nurse and asked to play pool. The nurse debated about playing but chose to play because Jason appeared distracted and the game might give him something to focus on.

Ineffective Approach

Nurse: Shall I break?

Jason: (Had been looking off to his right, but turns and looks directly at the nurse.) Yeah, go ahead. (Looks at the table briefly and then turns to look out the door and down the hallway.)

Nurse: (Breaking the pool balls without putting any in a pocket.) It's your turn. You can hit any ball that you'd like.

Jason: (Turning back to the table.) Huh? (Shaking his head as he stared at the table.) What?

Nurse: You know, Jason, you really should pay attention.

Jason: (Hits a ball in and moves to the other side of the table. Stops in line with the next shot but doesn't bend down to take aim. Stands very still and then shakes his head slightly and quickly. Leans down to take aim and then stands up again.)

Nurse: Jason. (Looks at the nurse.) Jason! Are you going to play or not? I don't have all day.

Jason: Oh yeah. (Leans down, takes aim, and misses.)

Nurse: (Moves to where the next shot is. Position is near where Jason is standing. The nurse watches him carefully, moving closer to him.) Please move over, Jason.

Jason: No. (Doesn't move. In peripheral vision, the nurse sees Jason's lips move and he again looks to his right and shakes his head in a staccato motion, as if trying to shake something out of his head.)

Effective Approach

Nurse: Shall I break?

Jason: (Had been looking off to his right, but turns and looks directly at the nurse.) Yeah, go ahead. (Looks at the table briefly and then turns to look out the door and down the hallway.)

Nurse: (Breaking the pool balls without putting any in a pocket.) Your turn; you can hit any ball that you'd like.

Jason: (Turning back to the table.) Huh? (Shakes his head as he stares at the table.) What?

Nurse: You can hit any ball you like. I didn't get any.

Jason: (Hits a ball in and moves to the other side of the table. Stops in line with the next shot but doesn't bend down to take aim. Stands very still and then shakes his head slightly and quickly. Leans down to take aim and then stands up again.)

Nurse: Jason. (He looks at nurse.) Are you aiming at the 10 ball?

Jason: Oh yeah. (Leans down, takes aim, and misses.)

Nurse: (Moving to where her next shot is. The position is very close to where Jason is standing. The nurse watches him carefully while moving closer to him.) Here, let me take this shot.

Jason: Oh. (Moves back. In peripheral vision, the nurse sees Jason's lips move and again he looks to his right and shakes his head in a staccato motion, as if trying to shake something out of his head.)

Nurse: I missed again. (Moves away from the table and turns to Jason, who moves up to the table. He leans down and then stands up again. His lips move again as he turns his head to the right and then looks over his back toward the doorway.) Jason. Jason. (He looks at the nurse.) You have the striped ones.

Jason: (Nods and leans down to take a shot, which he makes. He then misses the next shot. He stands up and moves back from the table, again looking back toward the doorway. He shakes his head.)

Nurse: (Watches him closely and moves to the opposite side of the table, making the next shot. Lining up the next shot, Jason leans the pool cue against the table, looks past the nurse, and turns and walks away toward the door. Looks down the hallway, takes a few steps, stops for a minute or so, turns back into the room, and again looks past the nurse. Sits down and shakes his head again. Holds his head in his hands, with his hands covering his ears. The nurse picks up his pool cue and places both against the wall, out of the way. The nurse, recognizing that Jason is likely experiencing auditory hallucinations, remains where she can observe him, noting, as well, that another staff member is near at hand.)

CRITICAL THINKING CHALLENGE

- How did the nurse's impatience translate into Jason's behaviour in the first scenario?
- What effective communicating techniques did the nurse use in the second scenario?

patient is particularly preoccupied with delusions and hallucinations. Although all aspects of memory may be affected in schizophrenia, registration or the recall within seconds of newly learned information may be particularly diminished. This affects the individual's short- and long-term memories. The ability to engage in abstract thinking may be impaired.

Insight and Judgment

Individuals display insight when they display evidence of knowing their own thoughts, the reality of external objects, and their relationship to these. Judgment is the ability to decide or act on a situation. Insight and judgment are closely related and depend on cognitive functions that are frequently impaired in people with schizophrenia.

In schizophrenia, however, it is estimated that 57% to 98% of persons with the disease exhibit signs of lack of insight or **anosognosia,** from Greek "without disease knowledge" (Lehrer & Lorenz, 2014). There is evidence that anosognosia in schizophrenia is due to a neurologic deficit (involving the prefrontal cortex, the inferior parietal, and anterior cingulate cortices) that deprives the individual from recognizing that some of their ideas, perceptions, and/or behaviour are indicative of an illness requiring treatment (Little & Bell, 2021). This denial can have serious consequences for the person's wellbeing because they do not seek medical help when ill, which can lead to requiring emergency services. Amador (2012), author of *I Am Not Sick. I Don't Need Help! How To Help Someone With Mental Illness Accept Treatment,* uses his experience with a family member living with schizophrenia to offer a strategy to address this lack of insight: LEAP. LEAP stands for listening (reflectively), empathizing, agreeing (on some areas; agree to disagree on others) and partnering. The person may believe they do not need medication but, wanting to stay out of hospital or to stop loved ones worrying, may agree to accept it.

Behavioural Responses

During periods of psychosis, unusual or bizarre behaviour often occurs. These behaviours can usually be understood within the context of the patient's disturbed thinking. The nurse needs to understand the significance of the behaviour to the individual. For example, one patient moved the family furniture into the yard because he thought that evil spirits were hiding in the furniture. His bizarre behaviour was an attempt to protect his family. Another patient painted a sequence of numbers on his bedroom walls. He said that the numbers were the language of the angels. His bizarre thoughts were at the basis of his behaviour.

Because of the negative symptoms, specifically avolition, patients may not seem interested or organized to complete their normal daily activities. They may stay in bed most of the day or refuse to take a shower. Many times, they will agree to get up in the morning and go to

school or work, but they never get around to it. Several specific behaviours are associated with schizophrenia, including stereotypy (idiosyncratic repetitive, purposeless movements), echopraxia (involuntary imitation of others' movements), and waxy flexibility (posture held in odd or unusual fixed position for extended periods). In some cases, certain behaviours need to be evaluated carefully to distinguish them from movements that are associated with medication side effects, such as grimacing, stereotypic behaviour, or agitation.

Self-Concept

Self-concept is usually poor for people with schizophrenia. Patients often are aware that they are hearing voices others do not hear. They recognize that they are different from others and are often afraid of "going crazy." Many are aware of the loss of expectations for their future achievements. The pervasive stigma associated with having a mental illness contributes to poor self-concept. Body image can be disturbed, especially during periods of hallucinations or delusions. One patient believed that her body was infected with germs and she could feel them eating away her insides.

Stress and Coping Patterns

Stressful events are often linked to psychiatric symptoms. It is important to determine stresses from the patient's perspective because a stressful event for one may not be stressful for another (see Chapter 18). It is also important to determine typical coping patterns, especially negative coping strategies, such as the use of substances or aggressive behaviour.

Risk Assessment

Because of high suicide and attempted suicide rates among patients with schizophrenia, the nurse needs to assess patients risk for self-injury: Do patients speak of suicide, have delusional thinking that could lead to dangerous behaviour, and have command hallucinations telling them to harm themselves or others? Do patients have homicidal ideations? Do patients have access to weapons? Do patients lack social support and the skills to be engaged with other people or a vocation? Substance-related disorders are also common among patients with schizophrenia, and nurses should assess for substance misuse or abuse.

Nursing Focus of Care: Psychological Domain

Many nursing care foci can be generated from data collected assessing the psychological domain. Disturbed thought processes can be used for delusions, confusion, and disorganized thinking. Disturbed sensory perception is appropriate for hallucinations or illusions. Other examples of foci include distortion of body image, low self-esteem, personal identity issue, at risk for violence, and knowledge deficits.

Interventions for Psychological Domain

All the psychological interventions, such as counselling, conflict resolution, behaviour therapy, and cognitive interventions, are appropriate for patients with schizophrenia. The following discussion focuses on applying these interventions.

Special Issues in the Nurse–Patient Relationship

The development of the nurse–patient relationship with patients with schizophrenia centres on developing trust and accepting the person as a worthy human being. People with schizophrenia are often reluctant to engage in any relationship because of previous rejection and, in some instances, an underlying suspicion that is a part of the illness. If they are having hallucinations, their images of other people may be distorted and frightening. They struggle to trust their own thoughts and perceptions, and engaging in an interaction with another human being may prove too overwhelming.

The nurse should approach the patient in a calm and caring manner. Engaging the patient in a relationship may take time. Brief interactions are best for a patient who is experiencing psychosis. Being consistent in interactions and following through on promises will help establish trust within the relationship.

Establishing a therapeutic relationship is crucial, especially with patients who deny that they are ill. Patients are more likely to agree to treatment if these recommendations are made within the context of a safe, trusting relationship. Even if some patients deny having mental illness, they may take medication and attend treatment activities because they trust the nurse.

Management of Disturbed Thoughts and Sensory Perceptions

Although antipsychotic medications may relieve positive symptoms, they do not always eliminate hallucinations and delusions. The nurse must continue helping the patient develop creative strategies for dealing with these sensory and thought disturbances. Information about the content of the hallucinations and delusions is needed, not only to determine whether the medications are effective but also to assess safety and the meaning of these thoughts and perceptions to the patient. In caring for a patient who is experiencing hallucinations or delusions, nursing actions should be guided by three general patient outcomes:

- Decrease the frequency and intensity of hallucinations and delusions.
- Recognize that hallucinations and delusions are symptoms of a brain disorder.
- Develop strategies to manage the recurrence of hallucinations or delusions.

When interacting with a patient who is experiencing hallucinations or delusions, the nurse must remember that these experiences are real to the patient. The

BOX 21.12 TEACHING POINTS

Teaching patients that hallucinations and delusions are part of the disorder becomes easier after the medication begins working and a therapeutic relationship is established. Once patients believe and acknowledge that they have a mental illness and that some of their thoughts are delusions and some of their perceptions are hallucinations, they can develop strategies to manage their symptoms.

nurse should never tell a patient that these experiences are not real. Discounting the experiences blocks communication. It also is dishonest to tell the patient that you are having the same hallucinatory experience. It is best to validate the patient's experiences and identify the meaning of these thoughts and feelings to the patient. For example, a patient who believes that they are under surveillance by the police probably feels frightened and suspicious of everyone. By acknowledging how frightening it must be to always feel like you are being watched, the nurse focuses on the feelings that are generated by the delusion, not the delusion itself. The nurse can then offer to help the patient feel safe within this environment. The patient, in turn, begins to feel that someone understands them (Box 21.12).

Self-Monitoring and Relapse Prevention

Patients benefit greatly by learning techniques of self-regulation, symptom monitoring, and relapse prevention. By monitoring events, time, place, and stimuli surrounding the appearance of symptoms, the patient can begin to predict high-risk times for symptom recurrence. Cognitive–behavioural therapy is often used in helping patients monitor and identify their emerging symptoms in order to prevent relapse (see Chapter 14).

Another important nursing intervention is to help the patient identify who and where to talk about delusional or hallucinatory material. Unfortunately, because self-disclosure of these symptoms immediately labels someone as having a mental illness, patients should be encouraged to evaluate the environment for negative consequences of disclosing these symptoms. It may be fine to talk about it at home but not at the grocery store.

Enhancement of Cognitive Functioning

After identifying deficits in cognitive functioning, the nurse and the individual can develop interventions that target specific deficits. If the ability to focus or attend is an issue, activities that improve attention, such as computer games, can be encouraged. For memory problems, making lists and writing down important information can be helpful. Executive functioning problems are the most challenging for persons with a schizophrenia spectrum disorder. For planning and problem-solving impairments, coaching the individual using interventions that closely simulate real-world problems is most helpful and supports the development of problem-solving skills. Cognitive remediation interventions can assist individuals to improve both their cognition and functioning. Researchers evaluating such training advocate for its inclusion in clinical guidelines and its implementation in clinical practice (Vita et al., 2021). *Computerized* cognitive remediation therapy has proven efficacious for improvements in both cognition and negative symptoms, with age not being a factor in overall benefits (Tan et al., 2020). Participants' sense of mental wellbeing and competence can be positively affected, as well (Siu et al., 2021).

Solution-focused therapy is another approach to helping individuals learn new strategies for dealing with problems. It focuses on the perspectives, strengths, and positive attributes that of that person. For example, the person is asked to identify their most important problem. This focuses on the situation from their perspective and allows nurses and the team to respond to the problem the person finds most pressing. Once that issue is successfully addressed, the next issue can be examined together for solutions (Good Therapy, 2018).

Behavioural Interventions

Behavioural interventions can be very effective in helping patients improve motivation and organize routines and daily activities, such as maintaining a regular schedule and completing activities. Reinforcement of positive behaviours (e.g., getting up on time, completing hygiene, going to treatment activities) can easily be included in a treatment plan. In hospital, individuals and the team can identify rewards for following the agreed-upon treatment plan.

Stress and Coping Skills

Developing skills to cope with personal, social, and environmental stresses are important to everyone, but particularly to those with a severe mental illness. Stresses can easily trigger symptoms that the individual is trying to avoid. Learning better coping skills through education or counselling can improve wellbeing. Nursing research indicates, for instance, that a program of relaxation exercises and music therapy significantly can decrease psychological symptoms and feelings of depression in persons living with schizophrenia (Kavak et al., 2016).

Digital mobile apps are evolving as means to provide healthcare support. In a review of apps identified as relevant to "schizophrenia" and "psychosis," Lagan and colleagues (2021) found only six out of hundreds were evidence based and clinically relevant. Many were games, including stigmatizing ones like *schizophrenia*, a ping pong game that will "make you lose your mind!… "(p. 98). Nevertheless, apps have high potential as a mental health resource if quality and access are substantially addressed.

Patient Education

Cognitive deficits (difficulty in processing complex information, maintaining steady focus of attention, distinguishing between relevant and irrelevant stimuli, and forming abstractions) may challenge the nurse planning educational activities. Evidence indicates that people with schizophrenia may learn best in an errorless learning environment; that is, they are directly given correct information and then encouraged to write it down. Asking questions that encourage guessing is not as effective in helping them retain information. Trial-and-error learning is avoided.

Education sessions should occur in an environment with minimal distractions. Terminology should be clear and unambiguous. Visual aids can supplement verbal information, but these materials should have simple information stated in simple language. The nurse takes care not to overcrowd the visual material or incorporate images that draw attention away from the important content. Teaching should occur in small segments with frequent reinforcement. Most important of all, teaching should occur when the patient is ready. Regular assessments of cognitive abilities with standardized instruments can help determine this readiness. These suggestions can be adapted for teaching during any phase of the illness.

Skill-training interventions should be designed to compensate for cognitive deficits. To help patients learn to process complex activities, such as catching a bus, preparing a meal, or shopping for food or clothing, nurses should break the activity into small parts or steps and list them for the patient's reference. For example:

- Check that you have the correct bus fare in your pocket.
- Leave your apartment with your keys in your hand.
- Close the door.
- Walk to the corner.
- Turn right and walk three blocks to the bus stop.

Family Education

Because having a family member with schizophrenia is a life-changing event for the family and friends who provide care and support, educating patients and their families or significant others is crucial. It is a primary concern for the mental health nurse. Family support and education are crucial to help patients maintain their treatment. Education should include information about the disease course, treatment regimens, support systems, and life management skills. The most important factor to reinforce during patient and family education is the consistent taking of medication. Ensure

> ### BOX 21.13 Psychoeducation Checklist: Schizophrenia
>
> When working with the person with schizophrenia and their family or caregiver, be sure to include the following topic areas in the education plans:
>
> ✓ Psychopharmacologic agents, including drug action, dosage, frequency, and possible adverse effects. Stress the importance of adherence to the prescribed regimen
> ✓ Management of hallucinations
> ✓ Coping strategies such as self-talk, getting busy
> ✓ Management of the environment
> ✓ Use of contracts that detail the expected behaviours, with goals and consequences
> ✓ Community resources
> ✓ Community educational opportunities for families
> ✓ Family peer supports/family navigator contacts in the community

that there is opportunity to discuss their concerns about side effects and that patient and family are cognizant of reporting significant changes in side effects or worrisome new ones (e.g., symptoms of tardive dyskinesia). See Box 21.13 for a psychoeducation checklist.

Social Domain

Social Assessment

Several difficulties with social functioning occur in schizophrenia. As the disorder progresses, individuals can become increasingly socially isolated. On a one-to-one basis, this occurs because the individual seems unable to connect with people in their environment. Several aspects of the symptoms already discussed can contribute to this, for example, emotional blunting and anhedonia (the inability to form emotional attachment and experience pleasure). Cognitive deficits that contribute to difficult social functioning include problems with the face and affect recognition, deficiencies in recall of past interactions, problems with decision-making and judgment in conflictual interactions, and poverty of speech and language. Poor functioning and the inability to complete activities of daily living are manifested in poor hygiene, malnutrition, and social isolation.

Social Systems

In schizophrenia, support systems become very important in maintaining the patient in the community. The individual may become socially isolated if the treatment and management occur in long-term care facilities and group homes away from family and friends. One challenge in treating schizophrenia is to identify and maintain the patient's links with family and significant others. Assessment of the patient's formal support (e.g., family caregivers, healthcare providers) and informal support (e.g., neighbours, friends) should be conducted.

Quality of Life

People with schizophrenia often have a poor quality of life, especially older people who may have spent many years in a long-term hospital. The nurse should assess the patient's quality of life and how it could be improved. Simple changes, such as arranging for a different roommate or improving access to social activities by meeting transportation needs, can greatly improve a patient's quality of life. Stable housing is key to making any improvements to the patient's quality of life (MHCC, 2013b).

Family Assessment

The assessment of the family can take many forms, and the family assessment guide presented in Chapter 16 can be used. In many instances, the patient will be young and living with their parents. This is most often the case when a young person experiences the first episode of psychosis. Often, the nurse's first contact with the patient and family is in the initial phases of the disorder. The family is dealing with the shock and disbelief of seeing a child with a mental illness that may have lifelong consequences. Ideally, in this instance, the assessment process may be extended over several sessions to provide the family with support and education about the disorder. Certainly, the emergence of psychotic illness is a distressing and confusing time, not only for young persons experiencing these perplexing changes but also for their parents.

The family, and in particular the parents, play a critical role in early intervention for psychosis, both as a vehicle for early identification and treatment, and as a supportive context for recovery. Understanding of this caregiving experience was gleaned from a qualitative study that employed a phenomenological approach to uncover four distinct stories: *a story of Protection, a story of Loss, a story of Stigma*, and a final story of *Enduring Love* (Wilson, 2012). The experiences of parent caregivers suggest that healthcare providers, and nurses in particular, can have more discretion, insight, and discernment in clinical approaches and might also serve to shape future policies, which will recognize and affirm the strengths and resilient capacities of families (Smith, 2020) (see Box 21.14).

Because women with schizophrenia generally have better treatment outcomes than do men, many will marry and have children. These women experience the same life stresses as other women and may find themselves single parents, raising children in poverty-stricken conditions. Managing a psychiatric illness and trying to be an effective parent in a socially stigmatizing society are exceedingly challenging because of the lack of financial resources and social support. This family will need an extensive assessment of financial need and social support.

BOX 21.14 Research for Best Practice

BEING A HEALTH PROFESSIONAL AND MOTHER OF AN ADULT CHILD WITH SCHIZOPHRENIA

Klages, D., East, L., Usher, K., & Jackson, D. (2020). Health professionals as mothers of adult children with schizophrenia. *Qualitative Health Research*, *30*(12), 1807–1820. https://doi.org/10.1177/1049732320936990

Question: This study aimed to understand the complex interplay between being a health professional and being a mother of a child with schizophrenia. The research question was: What are the stories that mothers, who are health professionals, tell of their experiences of negotiating care with the mental health system for their children diagnosed with schizophrenia?

Methods: In this qualitative narrative study, 13 mothers from Canada, Australia, Scotland, and the United States of America were recruited to participate in interviews. The participants shared their stories of accessing the mental healthcare system for support for their child.

Findings: There was one overarching theme, *mothering in the context of uncertainty: unbalancing and rebalancing*

as mothers, and three major themes: *disrupted mothering* (living with fear and distress; navigating the unknown alone, creating tentative hope); *reconfigured mothering* (fighting for their right to be heard; using their professional knowledge, transforming their mothering practices); and *resolute mothering* (bearing the weight of caring; reflecting on their dual experience; finding meaning in their disrupted lives).

Implications for Practice: The experience of feeling ignored, unheard, and excluded is an experience that nurses can and must change for mothers and all family members. This study clearly demonstrates the importance of listening to mothers, involving them in the care of their child, and supporting the family as an integral component of mental health care. Healthcare professionals with a dual role as family member have expertise that can inform the delivery of services for those who live schizophrenia and their families.

Nursing Focus of Care: Social Domain

The nursing care foci based on an assessment of the social domain are typically related to social interaction, role performance, and family coping and processes. Outcomes will depend on areas of focus.

Interventions for Social Domain

Promoting Patient Safety

Although violence is not a consistent behaviour of people with schizophrenia, it is always a concern during the initial phase when hallucinations or delusions may put patients at risk for harming themselves or others. Nonviolent patients who are experiencing hallucinations and delusions can also be at risk for victimization by more aggressive patients. The patient who is hallucinating needs to be protected. This protection may include increased staff monitoring and, if necessary, a safer environment in a secluded area.

The nurse's best approach to avoiding violence or aggression is to demonstrate respect for the patient and the patient's personal space, assess and monitor for signs of fear and agitation, and use preventive interventions before the patient loses control. Medications should be administered as ordered. Because most antipsychotic and antidepressant medications take 1 to 2 weeks to begin moderating the patient's behaviour, the nurse must be vigilant during the acute illness.

Reducing environmental stimulation is particularly important for individuals who are experiencing

hallucinations but can be helpful for all patients when signs of fear and agitation are observed. Allowing patients to use private rooms or seclusion for brief periods can be an important preventive method.

Other techniques of managing the environment (milieu management) have been found to be helpful in inpatient settings. One researcher who examined aggression and violence in psychiatric hospitals found violent behaviour to be associated with the following predictors: a history of violence, a coercive interaction style of using violence to obtain what is desired, and an environment in which violence is inadvertently rewarded, for example, by gaining staff attention (Morrison & Love, 2003). In 1992, Morrison proposed the following methods to help avoid acts of violence or aggression— these approaches remain relevant today:

- Take a thorough history that includes information about the patient's past use of violence.
- Help the patient to talk directly and constructively with those with whom they are angry, rather than venting anger to staff about a third person.
- Set limits with consistent and justly applied consequences.
- Involve the patient in formulating a contract that outlines patient and staff behaviours, goals, and consequences.
- Schedule brief but regular time-outs to allow the patient some privacy without the attention of staff either before or after the time-out (these time-outs may be patient activated).

Staff members need to have planned sessions after all incidents of violence or physical management in which the event is analyzed. These sessions allow staff members to learn how to better manage these situations and evaluate patients' cues. With sensitive leadership, these sessions can help staff to learn more about the interaction of patient and staff characteristics that can contribute to these incidents.

Convening Support Groups

People with mental illness benefit from support groups that focus on daily problems and the stress of dealing with a mental illness. These groups are useful throughout the continuum of care and help reduce the risk for suicide. In the hospital setting, the focus of the group can be simply sharing the experience of living with a mental illness. In the community, a regular support group can provide interaction with people with similar problems and issues and the opportunity to share stories of recovery. Friendships often develop from these groups.

Implementing Milieu Therapy

Individuals with schizophrenia can be hospitalized or live in group homes for a long period of time. It is unrealistic to expect people who have an illness that interferes with their ability to live with family members to live in peace and harmony with complete strangers. Arranging the treatment environment to maximize recovery is crucial to the rehabilitation of the patient.

Developing Psychiatric Rehabilitation Strategies

Rehabilitation strategies are used to support the individual's recovery and integration into the community. Community-based psychosocial rehabilitation programs usually offer long-term intensive case management services to adults with schizophrenia. Programs provide a continuum of services to meet the changing needs of people with psychiatric disabilities. Patients set rehabilitation goals, and services are then provided to help "clients" (most programs do not use the term "patients") reach their goals. Services range from daily home visits to providing transportation, occupational training, and group support. Social skills training shows much promise for patients with schizophrenia, both individually and in groups. This is a method for teaching patients specific behaviours needed for social interactions. The skills are taught by lecture, demonstration, role-playing, and homework assignments (see Chapters 12 and 15). Nurses may be team members and involved in case management or provision of services. These and other psychological treatment approaches, combined with breakthroughs in biologic therapy, continue to help improve the functioning and quality of life for patients with schizophrenia.

Family Interventions

When schizophrenia first becomes apparent, the patient and family must negotiate the mental health system for the first time (in most cases)—a challenge that almost equals that of confronting the family member's illness. In most provincial jurisdictions, the mental health system is complex and is usually ignored unless a family member becomes seriously mentally ill. The system includes inpatient and outpatient clinics supported by provincial health insurance and publicly funded community mental health clinics and hospitals.

Family members should be encouraged to participate in educational and support groups that help family members deal with the realities of living with a loved one with a mental illness. Family members should be given information about local community and provincial resources and organizations such as mental health associations and those that can help families negotiate the complex system.

See Box 21.15 for care of a patient with a more persistent form of schizophrenia.

Spiritual Domain

Many people living with schizophrenia find comfort in their spirituality, as well as the strength to deal with life events that interfere with their recovery journeys. Religious or spiritual beliefs can be a resource for both patients and their families. Such beliefs may help, for instance, to reappraise difficult events into a positive light (e.g., God gives us only difficulties that we are able to handle). A relationship with the sacred through ritual, prayer, worship, meditation, or other spiritual activities may offer solace, peace, and serenity. These activities may also help to structure the daily lives of individuals with schizophrenia, an important rehabilitation goal. The experience of living with a serious and chronic illness, however, can also cause a crisis of faith or lead one to question the purpose and meaning of one's life. This may be especially true if one's illness brings stigma and rejection by the members of one's community. The sense of connection and hope that supports spiritual growth may be diminished if one is labelled "crazy" by others.

Spiritual nursing care actively supports patients in their efforts to sustain and enhance their spirituality. This support can take many forms, from safeguarding the dignity of the patient to understanding the potential impact of hallucinations on spiritual needs to ensuring spiritual activities can occur. In psychiatric and mental health settings, there may be reluctance on the part of staff to consider the spirituality of a patient who is experiencing the psychotic symptoms of delusions and hallucinations, especially if there are religious overtones to the "voices" and/or fixed beliefs. Knowledge of the patient and of the disease, along with a broad, rich understanding of spirituality, should nevertheless enable the nurse and other staff to address the spiritual

BOX 21.15 NURSING CARE PLAN

PATIENT WITH SCHIZOPHRENIA

MP is a 53-year-old woman who was brought to the crisis support clinic by her community nurse case manager. MP had made a number of telephone calls to her case manager and to the police in rapid succession in the previous 24 h to report that her next-door neighbour was spying on her. When the nurse case manager arrived, MP was very agitated and distrusting. The case manager also received a call from MP's landlord to report that MP has been making threatening hand gestures to neighbours from her apartment window. MP disclosed to her nurse case manager that her neighbours had tampered with her medications and that she had not been taking them for several days. MP was acutely paranoid and agreed to a hospitalization to keep her safe. She had been attending the Community Clubhouse Program but had not been there for 2 weeks. She failed to attend her follow-up appointment at the mental health clinic to pick up her biweekly dosette of pills.

Setting: Crisis Support Team: Psychosocial Rehabilitation Unit

Baseline Assessment: MP is a 5′4″, 155-lb woman whose appearance is dishevelled. She has not slept for 2 days and appears frightened. She is hypervigilant, suspicious, irritable, and wringing her hands. She is vague about when she last took her treatment medications. She is oriented to time and place and person. Lab values are within normal limits. She has a history of at least 12 former admissions to the psychiatric ward for self-discontinuation of treatment medications.

Associated Psychiatric Diagnosis	Medications
Schizophrenia	Olanzapine, 5 mg bid
Social problems/context: landlord threatening to evict MP from her apartment	
Estranged from her two adult sons	
Support system limited to a few acquaintances at the clubhouse	

Nursing Focus of Care 1: Self-Care Challenges

Defining Characteristics	Related Factors
MP does not remember when she last took her medications. Two weeks of pills are still in the dosette box. MP has not taken the pills for at least 2 weeks, possibly more. MP has not attended the Clubhouse program for 2 weeks. MP did not attend her appointment at the clinic to get a refill of pills in her dosette. MP has been calling the police and the case manager several times in the past 24 h.	Paranoid delusions are contributing to her thought disturbance. Suspiciousness is contributing to her reluctance to leave her apartment. Inability to make thoughtful judgments. Ineffective individual coping.

Outcomes

Initial	Long Term
Restarts medications in the hospital. Agreement from MP to a referral to the ACT team. Increased ability to self-administer medications. Demonstrates willingness to take her medications independently while in hospital using a blister pack dosette.	MP will communicate her understanding of and demonstrate follow-through with the mutually agreed on health maintenance plan. MP will show the ability to perform health maintenance activities needed to function in her apartment independently with ACT team assistance.

Continued on following page

NURSING CARE PLAN (*Continued*)

Interventions

Interventions	Rationale	Ongoing Assessment
Take initial steps to help MP feel safe in the hospital setting.	When a person feels safe, trust is more likely to develop.	Determine when MP's suspiciousness is diminishing. Assess when she is ready to discuss plans for discharge.
Listen carefully, making eye contact. Make efforts to clarify what MP is thinking and feeling.	Listening attentively will help MP to feel safe and cared for.	
Contact all community care providers and convene an interdisciplinary meeting to discuss possible changes to the current community care plan.	A meeting of all care providers will provide a forum to explore alternative support/treatment solutions to improve MP's health maintenance once discharged.	Assess MP's readiness for discharge and transition to the ACT team in addition to returning to the community clubhouse.
	ACT team will be able to increase visitation to MP's home at more frequent intervals. ACT team will provide a more intense level of support.	

Evaluation

Outcomes	Revised Outcomes	Interventions
MP's delusions begin to decrease.	MP meets with the ACT team and agrees to include this team in her follow-up health maintenance plan.	Problem solve ways for MP to respond to ongoing worries and suspicions.
MP uses some distraction techniques to draw her away from focusing upon the neighbours.		Develop a written, mutually agreed-upon relapse prevention and crisis action plan and send to all community care partners.

Nursing Focus of Care 2: Disturbed Thinking

Defining Characteristics	Related Factors
Inaccurate interpretation of stimuli (neighbours tampering with her medications) Cognitive impairment—attention, memory, and executive function impairment Suspiciousness Hallucinations (hears voices telling her that her sons are in danger)	Uncompensated alterations in brain activity

Outcomes

Initial	Long Term
Decrease or eliminate hallucinations.	Use coping strategies to deal with hallucinations or delusions if they reappear.
Have accurate interpretation of the environment.	
Exhibits some reality-based thinking.	
Demonstrates improvement in cognitive functioning (improved attention, memory, and executive functioning).	Communicate clearly with others. Maintain cognitive functioning.
Interacts appropriately with others.	

NURSING CARE PLAN (*Continued*)

Interventions

Interventions	Rationale	Ongoing Assessment
Initiate a nurse–patient relationship by using an accepting, nonjudgmental approach. Be patient.	A therapeutic relationship will provide patient support as she begins to deal with the realization that she is in hospital once again. Be patient and offer reassurance as required until MP feels safe. Do not argue with the false beliefs.	Determine the extent to which MP is willing to trust and engage in a relationship. Make every effort to help MP attend to real rather than internal stimuli, orient her to the real situation, and encourage MP to focus upon distracting concrete activities. Make determined efforts to steer thinking in alternate directions.
Administer olanzapine as prescribed. Observe for effects, side effects, and adverse effects. Begin teaching about the potential switch to an injectable form of antipsychotic medication.	Olanzapine is a D_2 and $5\text{-}HT_{2A}$ antagonist and is indicated for the management of psychotic disorders.	Make sure MP swallows the pills. Monitor for relief of positive symptoms and assess side effects, especially extrapyramidal. Monitor BP for orthostatic hypotension and body temperature increase (NMS).
Assess the ability for self-care activities.	Disturbed thinking may interfere with MP's ability to carry out ADLs.	Continue to assess: determine whether the patient can manage self-care.

Evaluation

Outcomes	Revised Outcomes	Interventions
Delusions began to decrease within 6 days.	Participate in Community Clubhouse activities as soon as possible to bridge the transition from hospital back to the community.	Encourage attendance at the Clubhouse while in hospital to reconnect with the activity/recreational group, which MP enjoys.

Nursing Focus of Care 3: Anxiety Related to Delusional Ideas

Defining Characteristics	Related Factors
Constantly asking nurses for reassurance that her neighbours are not on the unit. Presence of pathophysiologic risk factors: delusional thinking.	Frightened, secondary to *paranoia* (feelings of being unsafe), and delusional thinking.

Outcomes

Initial	Long Term
MP is able to describe a reduction in anxiety.	MP will demonstrate decreased anxiety while at home.
Decreased agitation, gesturing, and pacing.	MP will refrain from gesturing at neighbours.

Interventions

Interventions	Rationale	Ongoing Assessment
Acknowledge MP's fear and paranoid delusions. Be genuine and empathetic.	Anxiety and delusions change an individual's perception of environmental stimuli. A patient who is frightened will respond because of her need to stay safe.	Assess her response to your comments and her ability to concentrate on what is being said.

Continued on following page

NURSING CARE PLAN (*Continued*)

Interventions	Rationale	Ongoing Assessment
Reassure MP verbally at frequent intervals. Make frequent brief supportive contacts. Acknowledge MP's distress.	It is helpful to validate the anxious feelings MP is experiencing.	Observe MP's nonverbal communication for evidence of increased anxiety and agitation.
Administer lorazepam, 2 mg, for agitation. Oral route is preferable over injection.	Exact mechanisms of action are not understood, but this medication is believed to potentiate the inhibitory neurotransmitter GABA, relieving anxiety and producing sedation.	Observe for a decrease in anxiety.

Evaluation

Outcomes	Revised Outcomes	Interventions
MP gradually decreased anxious behavior. Lorazepam was given regularly for the first 4 days.	Demonstrate control of behaviour by resisting delusions.	Teach MP about the effects of delusions. Problem solve ways of controlling hallucinations if they occur. Emphasize the importance of taking medications.

domain of care. Employing a relational ethics approach can move the nurse to consider the context and environment of the patient's situation to safeguard dignity (Wilson, 2009) (see Chapter 8).

Evaluation and Treatment Outcomes

Schizophrenia was once considered to have a progressively long-term and downward course, but it is now known that schizophrenia can be successfully treated and managed. In one older but significant study, the researchers interviewed patients 20 to 25 years after diagnosis and found that 50% to 66% experienced significant improvement or recovery (Harding et al., 1987). This study is important because it occurred before the development of atypical antipsychotic agents. Ways to support recovery are currently being developed. Research indicates, for instance, that persons with a severe mental illness, such as schizophrenia, can recover and maintain daily functioning through cognitive adaptive training. This approach involves individual assessment (e.g., functional skills, specific strengths/weaknesses) as a foundation for environmental support interventions, embedded in daily routine care provided by nurses, thereby assisting the person to achieve their goals. This approach leads to improvements in daily functioning and has the potential to improve executive functioning (Stiekema et al., 2020).

Inpatient-Focused Care

Persons with schizophrenia may be hospitalized many times, often involuntarily, for a short period. During the stabilization period, the status is changed to voluntary admission, whereby the patient agrees to treatment.

Community Care

Most of the care of patients with schizophrenia in Canada will be in the community through publicly

EMERGENCY

Emergency care ideally takes place in a hospital emergency room, but the crisis often occurs in the home. Patients are usually relapsing and do not recognize their bizarre or aggressive behaviours as symptoms. In many urban communities, a specially trained crisis team is sent to assess the emergency and recommend further treatment. Patients are brought to the emergency room not only because of relapse but also because of medication side effects. Nurses should refer to the previous discussion for nursing management.

supported mental health delivery systems. Community services include assertive community treatment, outpatient therapy, case management, and psychosocial rehabilitation, including clubhouse programs. For a very small number of patients with a community treatment order in effect that delineates the conditions required to live in the community, services must be congruent with those conditions (see Chapter 8). For all patients in the community, health care should be integrated in a holistic manner with physical health care. Nurses should be especially vigilant that patients with mental illnesses receive proper primary and medical health care.

Mental Health Promotion

The stresses of seeking care and services may be such that they affect the wellbeing of the person with schizophrenia. Healthcare systems are complex and mental health care may not be well resourced as other areas. Development of assertiveness and conflict resolution skills can help the person in negotiating access to services. Developing a positive support system for stressful periods will help promote a positive outcome.

A summary of the bio/psycho/social/spiritual interventions is presented in Figure 21.7.

Schizoaffective Disorder

Schizoaffective disorder was recognized in 1933 by Kasanin, who described varying degrees of symptoms of both schizophrenia and mood disorders beginning in youth. Since then, there has been debate about the status of this disorder (Malhi & Bell, 2019), including challenges in diagnosing schizoaffective disorder when it must be determined that symptoms are not more consistent with a mood disorder (Peterson et al., 2019; WHO, 2020). Despite the debate, schizoaffective disorder remains a separate disorder in the *Diagnostic and Statistical Manual of Mental Disorders, 5th ed. (DSM-5)* (APA, 2013) and in the *ICD-11* (WHO, 2020). In a study of 5581 admissions, schizoaffective disorder accounted for 5% compared to 17% for schizophrenia (Feeney et al., 2020). A systematic review of the neuropsychological and neuroimaging underpinnings of this disorder concluded that the abnormalities associated with it resemble schizophrenia more than bipolar disorder (Madre et al., 2016).

Clinical Course

This disorder is episodic in nature and characterized by intervals of intense symptoms alternating with quiescent periods, during which psychosocial functioning is adequate. At times, there are symptoms of schizophrenia; at other times, it appears to be a depressive disorder or

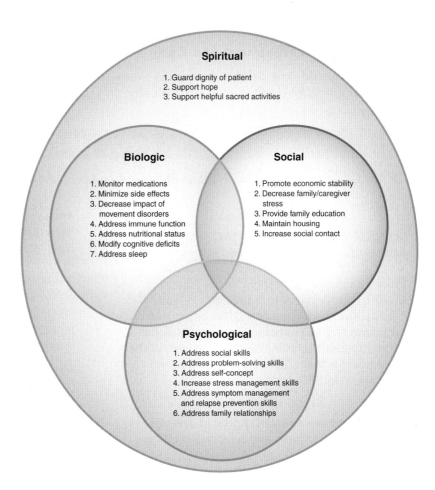

Figure 21.7 Bio/psycho/social/spiritual interventions for people with schizophrenia.

bipolar disorder. Psychosis and pervasive mood changes can occur concurrently. Individuals may feel that they are on a "chronic roller-coaster ride" of symptoms, often more difficult to cope with than those of schizophrenia or an affective disorder.

To receive a diagnosis of schizoaffective disorder, a person must have an uninterrupted period of illness when there is a major depressive, manic, or mixed episode along with some symptoms of schizophrenia, such as delusions, hallucinations, or other indicative symptoms. In addition, although the person's problems with mood are present much of the time, the positive symptoms of schizophrenia must be experienced without the mood symptoms at some time. To clarify this disorder further, two related subtypes of schizoaffective disorder have been identified (APA, 2013); see the DSM-5 for specific diagnostic criteria and subtypes.

Epidemiology and Risk Factors

The lifetime prevalence of schizoaffective disorder is estimated to be around 0.3% (APA, 2013) but is very difficult to track. There is a greater incidence of women with this disorder (APA, 2013). It is not yet clear if this is related to biologic differences or to a diagnostic bias. Women are reported to have better outcomes than men in terms of symptom control and sometimes employment. Twenty-five percent of individuals with this diagnosis experience postpsychotic depression and panic attacks.

Interprofessional Treatment and Care

Persons with schizoaffective disorder benefit from a comprehensive treatment plan and a cohesive interprofessional treatment team that includes the individual (and, when possible, their family). Pharmacologic intervention is needed to stabilize the symptoms, and it presents specific challenges. Long-term atypical antipsychotic agents are as effective as the traditional combination of a standard antipsychotic agent and an antidepressant drug. Mood stabilizers, such as lithium or valproic acid, may also be used. A combination of antipsychotic and antidepressant agents is sometimes used (see Chapter 13). After the patient's condition has stabilized (i.e., the patient exhibits a decrease in positive and negative symptoms), the treatment that led to remission of symptoms should be continued. Titrating antipsychotic agents to the lowest dose that provides suitable protection may enable optimal psychosocial functioning while slowing recurrence of new episodes. Electroconvulsive therapy (see Chapter 13) is considered when symptoms are refractory to other interventions or when the patient's life is at risk and a rapid improvement is required (Pompili et al., 2013). Psychotherapy may help manage interpersonal relationships and mood changes. Social services are often needed to obtain disability benefits or services.

A priority care issue is that of suicide; comorbidity with substance abuse may increase the risk.

Nursing Care

Assessment of these patients is similar to that required for persons with schizophrenia and mood disorders, including the range and duration of symptoms and any physiologic problems experienced, such as sleep pattern disturbances, difficulties with self-care, or poor nutritional habits. Common foci of nursing care are *disturbed thought process*, *disturbed sensory perception*, and *disturbed sleep*

IN-A-LIFE 🏠

Louis Riel Métis Leader (1844–1885)

Public Persona

Louis Riel, leader of the Métis in Manitoba and Saskatchewan, has been remembered as the man who negotiated for the establishment of Manitoba as a province and who led the fight for the protection of Métis and Aboriginal land and rights in Western Canada. Arrested for treason in 1884, he showed symptoms of grandiosity and paranoid delusions. He was declared "sane" by the superintendent of the Asylum for the Insane in Toronto, stood trial, and was hanged in 1885.

Personal Realities

Riel had numerous episodes of profound depression, apparent psychosis, and delusional thinking throughout his life. At times, he believed he had been substituted for the real Louis Riel who had died. At other times, he talked about his "mission" to form a new religion and replace the Pope. He was hospitalized and committed to insane asylums on numerous occasions. In retrospect, he has been "diagnosed" variably in the literature with paranoid schizophrenia, schizoaffective disorder, and bipolar disorder.

From Perr, I. N. (1992). Religion, political leadership, charisma and mental illness: The strange story of Louis Riel. *Journal of Forensic Science, 37*(2), 574–584; Waite, P. (1987). Between three oceans: Challenges of a continental destiny. In C. Brown (Ed.), *The illustrated history of Canada* (pp. 279–373). Lester & Orpen Dennys.

patterns. Interventions are based on the needs identified in the bio/psycho/social/spiritual assessment. Self-care deficits are often related to lack of motivation. For deficits created by severe mood symptoms, establishing a routine and setting goals can be useful. Helping the individual to establish a regular sleep pattern by using a routine can promote or reestablish normal rest patterns. Focusing on the principles of good nutrition and identifying any barriers to healthy eating can improve nutritional status.

Pharmacologic Interventions

An in-depth history of the patient's medication allows an evaluation of response to past medications and any issues related to medication management. Clozapine can reduce hospitalizations and risk for suicide in treatment-refractory patients although it carries with it significant side effect risk. A study of individuals diagnosed with schizoaffective disorder in Finland (*n* = 7,655) and Sweden (*n* = 7,525), with a follow-up time averaging over 11 years, found that clozapine and long-acting injectable antipsychotics were consistently associated with decreased risk of psychosis hospitalization but also of treatment failure (indicated by psychiatric hospitalization, medication change, death) (Lintunen et al., 2021). Atypical antipsychotic agents (e.g., quetiapine) appear to have thymoleptic (mood stabilizing), as well as antipsychotic, effects (see Chapter 13). If depressive symptoms persist, adjunctive use of an antidepressant agent may be helpful (see Chapter 22).

Side effects such as weight gain and sexual dysfunction can be very distressing to the individual and may lead to unilateral discontinuation of the medications. They need to be made particularly aware of extrapyramidal symptoms and the possibility of developing metabolic syndrome—a triad of diabetes, dyslipidemia, and hypertension with associated obesity. Regular monitoring of abdominal obesity and fasting blood glucose is effective in detecting risk for cardiovascular morbidity, and counselling regarding nutrition and healthy lifestyle choices (e.g., smoking cessation, physical exercise) is a supportive response (refer to Teaching points in Box 21.16).

Although using lithium alongside antipsychotic medications is common practice, particularly in cases of acute mania or hypomania, caution must be used: it has occurred that haloperidol and lithium taken together has resulted in an encephalopathic syndrome and irreversible brain damage (Boora et al., 2008). Lithium may interact similarly with other antipsychotic agents. It may also prolong the effects of neuromuscular blocking agents. Use of nonsteroidal anti-inflammatory drugs may increase plasma lithium levels. Diuretics and angiotensin-converting enzyme inhibitors should be prescribed cautiously with lithium, which is excreted through the kidney.

In schizoaffective disorder, individuals vacillate between mood dysregulation and disturbed thinking. Typical nursing foci of care for this domain include

BOX 21.16 TEACHING POINTS

- Ensure the individual knows the target symptoms of their medications and the times of administration.
- Encourage individuals to discuss the side effect profiles of their medications, seeking input on their level of tolerance for them. If necessary, negotiate for a medication with a different side effect profile but comparable efficacy. Medication tolerance and effectiveness should be reevaluated regularly.
- Advise patients taking olanzapine and clozapine to monitor body weight and report any rapid weight gain.
- Explain orthostatic hypotension to the individual and provide instruction for getting up slowly from a lying or sitting position and advice re: maintaining adequate fluid intake.
- Advise individuals and, if possible, their families to contact case coordinator/healthcare provider immediately if there is a dramatic change in body temperature (neuroleptic malignant syndrome), inability to control motor movement (dystonia), or dizziness.
- Advise against use of over-the-counter medications without consultation with their primary healthcare provider.
- Advise patients to report symptoms of diabetes mellitus (frequent urination, excessive thirst, etc.).
- Determine whether the person has sufficient resources to obtain medications. Explore coverage in provincial medication plans for those on social assistance.

hopelessness, powerlessness, coping, and self-esteem issues. Structured, integrated, and problem-solving psychotherapeutic interventions should be used to develop or increase the patient's insight. Psychoeducational interventions can help to decrease symptoms, enhance recognition of early regression, and hone psychosocial skills. The collaborative development of a crisis plan can help individuals to identify triggers and prodromal symptoms of decompensation and preplan coping mechanisms, including ways to engage supports. With the patient's permission, family members can be valuable resources for strengthening the patient's ability and willingness to follow treatment, monitor symptoms, and continue with rehabilitation and recovery. Families should be encouraged to seek out self-help support groups in the community; early interventions focused on those in a caregiving role can improve quality of life and reduce distress (Yesufu-Udechuku et al., 2015). (See Chapter 16 for guidance in working with families.)

Social dysfunction is common in this illness so a thoughtful assessment of social skill deficits and issues with interpersonal conflicts should be made. Typical nursing foci of care include *assisting the family with healthy functioning, personal and environment self-care*, and *difficulties managing social expectations*. The person may use fantasy and fighting as a means of coping and those who report the most severe peer rejection may present with the angriest dispositions and display antisocial behaviours. Social skills training is useful and may foster social adjustment. Education focusing on conflict-resolution skills, promoting compromise, negotiation, and expression of negative feelings can promote positive social adjustment. Social skills can be improved through role-playing and assertiveness training. Cognitive–behavioural therapy (CBT) can be useful.

Spiritual concerns may focus on finding meaningful ways to cope with such a serious illness, one that can bring social rejection and isolation. A relationship with the sacred through ritual, prayer, or other activities may offer daily comfort. Mindfulness-based strategies may also be of significant benefit (see Chapter 14).

Delusional Disorder

Delusional disorder (DD) has not been studied in a systematic manner and is more likely to be encountered in a medical–surgical rather than a psychiatric setting. Thus, nurses practicing in nonpsychiatric settings need to be able to recognize and understand it if meaningful care is to be given. Delusional disorder is a psychotic disorder characterized by nonbizarre, logical, stable, and well-systemized delusions that occur in the absence of other psychiatric symptoms. The delusions are typically nonbizarre delusions and plausible in the context of the person's background and life. Rarer are bizarre delusions that are clearly implausible and are not derived from ordinary life experiences (APA, 2013). Examples of real-life situations include being followed, poisoned, infected, loved at a distance, or deceived by a spouse or lover. Diagnosis is based on the presence of one or more nonbizarre delusions for at least 1 month, nor attributed to other psychiatric disorders (Sadock et al., 2015). Other psychotic features are not typically seen. Research indicates that global functioning may be affected (i.e., in the cognitive symptom domain and verbal memory performance) beyond the severity of the delusion (Díaz-Caneja et al., 2020). In general, however, behaviour is not odd or bizarre, but normal, except when the patient focuses on the delusion (APA, 2013).

The subtypes of delusional disorders involve beliefs that one is:

* loved intensely by a public figure or a stranger (**erotomanic**)
* a great, unrecognized talent or actually a prominent person (**grandiose**)
* being betrayed by an unfaithful spouse or lover (**jealous**)
* the victim of treachery (**persecutory**).

There is a **delusional disorder unspecified type** in which the person's delusional beliefs cannot be clearly determined. This category includes *illusions of doubles* or *Capgras syndrome* in which a familiar person seems to be replaced by an impostor (Salvatore et al., 2014). There is a **shared delusional disorder** (or **folie à deux**), in which the delusional ideas of one person (the primary) are transferred to another person (the secondary) living in close proximity, often adult siblings. This diagnosis does not appear in the *DSM-5*; rather, *delusional symptoms in partner of individual with delusional disorder* is noted in the "other specified" category (APA, 2013).

Other Psychotic Disorders

Schizophreniform Disorder

The essential features of this disorder are those of criteria A for schizophrenia but with less duration of the illness. Altered social or occupational functioning may occur but is not necessary. Most patients experience interruption in one or more areas of daily functioning (APA, 2013).

Brief Psychotic Disorder

Sudden in onset, there appears at least one of the positive symptoms of schizophrenia in a brief episode. Impairment, however, can be severe with suicide is a risk. An uncommon disorder, it usually appears in early adulthood (Sadock et al., 2015).

Substance-/Medication-Induced Psychotic Disorder

A psychotic disorder with prominent hallucinations or delusions that are the direct physiologic effects of medication or a substance. The symptoms cause clinically significant distress or impairment of functioning (APA, 2013).

Psychotic Disorder Due to Another Medical Condition

Evidence shows that the hallucinations and/or delusions causing clinically significant distress or impairment in functioning are the direct pathophysiologic consequence of another medical condition and are not better explained by another mental disorder or delirium (APA, 2013).

Other Specified Presentations

Symptoms, characteristic of psychotic disorders, cause clinically significant distress or impairment of functioning occur but do not meet the full criteria of a diagnostic class.

🍁 Summary of Key Points

- The person with schizophrenia displays a complex constellation of symptoms typically categorized as positive symptoms (those that exist but should not), such as delusions or hallucinations and disorganized thinking and behaviour, and negative symptoms (characteristics that should be there but are lacking), such as alogia, avolition, anhedonia, and affective blunting.

- In the past, the diagnosis and treatment of schizophrenia focused on the more observable and dramatic positive symptoms (i.e., delusions and hallucinations), but scientists and researchers have shifted their focus to the disorganizing symptoms of cognition.

- The clinical presentation of schizophrenia occurs in three phases: phase 1, first-episode psychosis, entails the initial diagnosis and first treatment; phase 2 includes periods of stabilization between episodes of overt signs and symptoms but during which the patient needs sustained treatment; phase 3 includes periods of exacerbation or relapse that require hospitalization or more frequent contacts with mental health professionals and increased use of resources.

- The etiological theories of schizophrenia include genetic, neuroanatomic, neurochemical (dopamine, glutamate and serotonin), and the dominant hypothesis of dysconnectivity. Advances in structural and functional neuroimaging are enabling increased understanding of schizophrenia.

- Biologic assessment of the patient with schizophrenia must include a thorough history and physical examination to rule out any medical illness or substance abuse problem that might be the cause of the patient's symptoms, assessment of risk for self-injury or injury to others, and documentation of baseline health information before medications are administered. Several standardized assessment tools are available to help assess characteristic abnormal motor movements.

- Several nursing interventions address the biologic domain: promotion of self-care activities (activity, exercise, and nutritional), thermoregulation, and fluid balance interventions. In general, the antipsychotic drugs used to treat schizophrenia block dopamine transmission in the brain but also cause some troublesome and sometimes serious side effects, primarily anticholinergic side effects and extrapyramidal side effects (motor abnormalities). Newer antipsychotic agents block serotonin as well as dopamine. The nurse should be familiar with these drugs, their possible side effects, and the interventions required to manage side effects.

- The **extrapyramidal side effects** of antipsychotic drugs can appear early in drug treatment and include acute parkinsonism or pseudoparkinsonism, acute dystonia, and akathisia, or they can appear late in treatment after months or years. The primary example of late-appearing extrapyramidal side effects is tardive dyskinesia, which is a severe syndrome of abnormal motor movements of the mouth, tongue, and jaw.

- Psychological assessment must include equal attention to manifestations of both positive and negative symptoms and a concentrated focus on the cognitive impairments that make it so difficult for patients to manage their disorder. Several standardized assessment tools assess for positive and negative symptoms. Developing the nurse–patient relationship is essential in helping patients manage disturbed thoughts and sensory perceptions. Interventions should be designed to enhance cognitive functioning. Patient and family education are critical interventions for the person with schizophrenia.

- Because schizophrenia is a lifetime disorder and patients require the continued support and care of mental health professionals and family or friends, one of the primary nursing interventions is ensuring that patients and families are properly educated about the course of the disorder, the importance of medication adherence, and the need for consistent care and support. Research is demonstrating that interaction between patients and their families is key to the success of long-term treatments and outcomes.

- Schizoaffective disorder has symptoms typical of both schizophrenia and depressive disorders and/or bipolar disorders but is a separate disorder. Although these patients experience mood problems most of the time, the diagnosis of schizoaffective disorder depends on the presence of positive symptoms (i.e., delusions or hallucinations) without mood symptoms at some time during the uninterrupted period of illness.

- Patients with schizoaffective disorder have fewer awareness deficits and appear to have more insight than do patients with schizophrenia, a fact that can be used in teaching patients to control symptoms, recognize early regression, and develop psychosocial skills. Nursing care for patients with schizoaffective disorder is focused on minimizing psychiatric symptoms through promoting medication maintenance and on helping patients maintain optimal levels of functioning and self-care.

- Delusional disorder is characterized by stable, well-systematized, and logical nonbizarre delusions that could occur in reality and are plausible in the context of the patient's ethnic and cultural background. These delusions may or may not interfere with an individual's ability to function socially.

- Other psychotic disorders, distinguished particularly by duration of symptoms or specifically identified cause, include schizophreniform disorder, brief psychotic disorder, substance-/medication-induced disorder, and psychotic disorder due to another medical condition.

- The therapeutic relationship is crucial to the successful treatment of the patient with any psychotic disorder. Nurses must be aware of the patient's fragile self-esteem and unusual vulnerabilities and try to establish a trusting relationship through a flexible, nonjudgmental approach that promotes empathy, trust, and support.

Thinking Challenges

a. Sharon has a diagnosis of schizophrenia. She was admitted to hospital via the mental health act after neighbours became concerned when she barricaded herself in her home and could be seen sitting near a window, looking afraid and holding a knife. Periodically, she would open the window and scream, "Leave me alone or I'll kill you!" In hospital, Sharon initially seemed relieved to be there. Today, the second day of her admission, you notice that she appears hypervigilant, regarding other patients and some staff members with suspicion. She refused to eat breakfast in the cafeteria and is sitting near the unit door, intent on watching who comes and goes. You surmise that Sharon is responding to her delusional beliefs. What nursing actions are appropriate at this time?

b. James has been newly diagnosed with schizophrenia and has been placed on antipsychotic medication. He is very concerned about the potential for developing tardive dyskinesia. What can you tell James about the steps that can be taken to lessen the risk of this serious side effect happening?

c. Self-stigma occurs for many individuals living with schizophrenia. Describe three interventions that may be useful in diminishing this sense of shame and despair for an individual.

> Visit the Point to view suggested responses. Go to thePoint.lww.com/activate and use the activation code found in the front of this text to unlock answers to the "Thinking Challenges" and other online resources.

 Web Links

https://www.waombudsman.org/files/2013/09/AIMS-Test-Abnormal-Involuntary-Movement-Test.pdf The Abnormal Involuntary Movement Scales (AIMS) and directions of its use are at this site. The scale is in public domain.

artbeatstudio.ca Art Beat is a Winnipeg-based art studio established by a mental health consumer and his family. The website provides examples of the studio's stated vision to "enable consumers of mental health services to engage in artistic expression that promotes recovery, empowerment, and community."

https://www.psychdb.com/_media/psychosis/bprs.pdf The Brief Psychiatric Rating Scale (BPRS) can be found here.

https://www.bbrfoundation.org/ This is the site of the Brain & Behavior Research Foundation.

https://www.camh.ca/en/health-info/mental-illness-and-addiction-index/antipsychotic-medication This site of the Centre for Addiction and Mental Health provides plain language information re: antipsychotic medication, suitable for those individuals prescribed it.

https://www.camh.ca/-/media/files/guides-and-publications/first-episode-psychosis-guide-en.pdf Here you will find First Episode Psychosis: An Information Guide that provides information regarding a first episode of schizophrenia, its treatment and recovery.

https://www.cna-aiic.ca/en/nursing-practice/tools-for-practice/learning-module-de-stigmatizing-practices-and-mental-illness A national training program for nurses and other healthcare professionals that specifically confront mental health stigma and discrimination in the healthcare environment: the module is made available from the Canadian Nurses Association in partnership with the Mental Health Commission of Canada and the Mood Disorders Association of Canada.

https://cmha.ca/ This is the site of the Canadian Mental Health Association, a charitable organization that promotes mental health and supports the resilience and recovery of those with mental illness.

https://www.lifetimeresources.net/assets/discus.pdf

https://www.earlypsychosis.ca/resources-and-downloads/ Early Psychosis Program of the Fraser Health Authority in BC with downloadable resources is at this site.

www.metabolicsyndromecanada.ca/about-metabolic-syndrome Information about metabolic syndrome can be found here.

https://mentalhealth.com/home/ Internet Mental Health provides extensive information on schizophrenia and schizoaffective disorder and their treatments.

https://mentalhealthcommission.ca/English The Mental Health Commission of Canada (MHCC) website contains all the reports of the commission and the National Strategy for Mental Health. It also offers access to Collaborative Spaces, an electronic repository of recovery-oriented mental health resources and discussions.

https://www.mentalhealthcommission.ca/English/media/3150 Readers will find the Mental Health First Aid Canada Psychosis First Aid Guidelines. These were developed to help members of the Canadian public assist someone who may be experiencing a psychotic episode until professional help becomes available.

https://www.mentalhealthcommission.ca/English/initiatives/11869/guidelines-recovery-oriented-practice Guidelines for recovery-oriented care from the Mental Health Commission of Canada.

https://www.nami.org/Home "You are not alone." This is the site of the National Alliance on Mental Illness, which is the largest grassroots organization for people with mental illness and their families in the United States.

https://www.sciencedirect.com/topics/medicine-and-dentistry/positive-and-negative-syndrome-scale Positive and Negative Syndrome Scale (PANSS)

https://psychcentral.com/ Tips, stories, and resources about mental health are here.

https://www.psychosissucks.ca/ This is a British Columbia early psychosis intervention site with links to other excellent resources.

https://schizophrenia.ca/ Site of the Schizophrenia Society of Canada, an organization committed to alleviating suffering caused by the disease.

https://www.schizophrenia.ca/docs/FINALSSCQOLReport. pdf A report on Quality of Life: As defined by people living with schizophrenia and their families is available here. FINALSSCQOLReport.pdf. Schizophrenia Society of Canada.

https://www.signnow.com/fill-and-sign-pdf-form/63822-simpson-angus-scale-pdf The Simpson-Angus Rating Scale is available at this site.

References

Addington, J., McCleery, A., & Addington, D. (2005). Three-year outcome of family work in an early psychosis program. *Schizophrenia Research, 79*(1), 107–116.

Álvarez, M. J., Masramom, H., Foguet-Boreu, Q., Tasa-Vinyals, E., García-Eslava, J. S., Roura-Poch, P., Escoté-Llobet, S., & Gonzalez, A. (2021). Childhood trauma in schizophrenia spectrum disorders: Dissociative, psychotic symptoms, and suicide behavior. *The Journal of Nervous and Mental Disease, 209*, 40-48. https://doi.org/10.1097/NMD.0000000000001253

Amador, X. (2012). *I am not sick I don't need help! How to help someone with mental illness accept treatment.* Vida Press.

American Psychiatric Association. (2013). *Diagnostic and statistical manual of mental disorders* (5th ed.).

Bartram, M. (2019). Toward a shared vision for mental health and addiction recovery and well-being: An integrated two-continuum model. *Journal of Recovery in Mental Health, 2*(2-3), 55–72. https://jps.library.utoronto.ca/index.php/rmh/article/view/32749

Bateson, G., Jackson, D. D., Haley, J., & Weakland, J. (1956). Toward a theory of schizophrenia. *Behavioral Science, 1*(4), 251–264.

Bingham, B., Moniruzzaman, A., Patterson, M., Sareen, J., Distasio, J., O'Neil, J., & Somers, J. M. (2019). Gender differences among Indigenous Canadians experiencing homelessness and mental illness. *BMC Psychology, 7*, 1–12. https://doi.org/10.1186/s40359-019-0331-y

Bitter, I., Czobor, P., Borsi, A., Fehé, L., Nagy, B. Z., Bacskai, M., Rakonczai, P., Hegyi, R., Németh, T., Varga, P., Gimesi-Országh, J., Fadgyas-Freyler, P., Sermon, J., & Takács, P. (2017). Mortality and the relationship of somatic comorbidities to mortality in schizophrenia. A nationwide matched-cohort study. *European Psychiatry, 45*, 97–103. http://dx.doi.org/10.1016/j.eurpsy.2017.05.022

Boora, K., Xu, J., & Hyatt, J. (2008). Encephalopathy with combined lithium-risperidone administration. *Acta Psychiatrica Scandinavica, 117*, 394–395. https://doi.org/10.1111/j.1600-0447.2008.01165.x

Brand, S. A., de Boer, J. N., & Sommer, I. E. C. (2021). Estrogens in schizophrenia: Progress, current challenges and opportunities. *Current Opinion in Psychiatry, 34*(3), 228–337. https://doi.org/10.1097/YCO.0000000000000699

Calipari, E. S., & Ferris, M. J. (2013). Amphetamine mechanisms and actions at the dopamine terminal revisited. *Journal of Neuroscience, 33*, 8923–8925. https://doi.org/10.1523/JNEUROSCI.1033-13.2013

Cancro, R. (2000). The introduction of neuroleptics: A psychiatric revolution. *Psychiatric Services, 51*, 333–335.

Centre for Addiction and Mental Health. (2018, July 24). *CAMH-led collaboration will introduce a new model of early psychosis care across Ontario.* https://www.camh.ca/en/camh-news-and-stories/camh-led-collaboration-will-introduce-a-new-model-of-early-psychosis-care-across-ontario

Cleynen, I., Engchuan, W., Hestand, M. S., Heung, T., Holleman, A. M., Johnston, H. R., Monfeuga, T., Epstein, M. P., Williams, N. M., & Bassett, A. S. (2020, February). Genetic contributors to risk of schizophrenia in the presence of a 22q11.2 deletion. *Molecular Psychiatry, 26*, 4496–4510. https://doi.org/10.1038/s41380-020-0654-3

Cortes-Briones, J. A., Tapia-Rivas, N. I., D'Souza, D. C., & Estevez, P. A. (2021, June 5). Going deep into schizophrenia with artificial intelligence. *Schizophrenia Research.* S0920-9964(21)00179-1. https://doi.org/10.1016/j.schres.2021.05.018. Online ahead of print.

Coyle, J. T., & Konopaske, G. (2016, June 15). Opinion: Glutamatergic dysfunction in schizophrenia evaluated with magnetic resonance spectroscopy. *JAMA Psychiatry, 73*, 649–650. https://doi.org/10.1001/jamapsychiatry.2016.0575

De Berardis, D., De Filippis, S., Masi, G., Vicari, S. & Zuddas, A. (2021). A neurodevelopment approach for a transitional model of early onset schizophrenia. *Brain Sciences, 11*, 1–16. https://doi.org/10.3390/brainsci11020275

Díaz-Caneja, C., Cervilla, J., Haro, J., Arango, C. & Portugal, E. (2020). Cognition and functionality indelusional disorder. *European Psychiatry, 55*, 52–60. https://doi.org/10.101/j.eurpsy.2018.09.010

Dilks, S., Xavier, R. M., Kelly, C., & Johnson, J. (2019). Implications of antipsychotic use: Antipsychotic-induced movement disorders, with a focus on tardive dyskinesia. *Nursing Clinics of North America, 54*, 595–608. https://doi.org/10.1016/j.cnur.2019.08.004

Domany, Y., & Weiser, M. (2020). Insights into metabolic dysregulations associated with antipsychotics. *Lancet Psychiatry, 7*, 6–7. https://doi.org/10.1016/ S2215-0366(19)30473-0

Dondé, C., Brunelin, J., Mondino, M., Cellard, C., Rolland, B., & Haesebaert, F. (2020). The effects of acute nicotine administration on cognitive and early sensory processes in schizophrenia: A systematic review. *Neuroscience & Biobehavioral Reviews, 118*, 121–133. https://doi.org/10.1016/j.neubiorev.2020.07.035

Egerton, A., Grace, A. A., Stone, J., Bossong, M. G., Sand, M., & McGuire, P. (2020). Glutamate in schizophrenia: Neurodevelopmental perspectives and drug development. *Schizophrenia Research, 223*, 59–70. https://doi.org/10.1016/j.schres.2020.09.013

Emsley, R., Chiliza, B., Asmal, L., & Harvey, B. (2013). The nature of relapse in schizophrenia. *BioMedCentral Psychiatry, 13*, 50. http://www.biomedcentral.com/1471-244X/13/50

Esaki, K., Balan, S., Iwayama, Y., Shimamoto-Mitsuyama, C., Hirabayashi, Y., Dean, B., & Yoshikawa, T. (2020). Evidence for altered metabolism of sphingosine-1-phosphate in the corpus callosum of patients with schizophrenia. *Schizophrenia Bulletin, 46*, 1172–1181. https://doi.org/10.1093/schbul/sbaa052

Evensen, S., Wisløff, T., Ullevoldsæter Lystad, J., Bull, H., Ueland, T., & Falkum, E. (2017). Prevalence, employment rate, and cost of schizophrenia in a high-income welfare society: A population-based study using comprehensive health and welfare registers. *Schizophrenia Bulletin, 42*, 476–483. https://doi.org/10.1093/schbul/sbv141

Feeney, A., Umama-Agada, E., Curley, A., Anamdi, C., Asghar, M., & Kelly, B. D. (2020, December 4). Voluntary and involuntary admissions with schizoaffective disorder: Do they differ from schizophrenia? *Irish Journal of Psychological Medicine*, 1–8. https://doi.org/10.1017/ipm.2020.123

Freudenreich, O., & Cather, C. (2012). Antipsychotic medication nonadherence: Risk factors and remedies. *Focus, 10*(2), 124–129.

Fromm-Reichman, F. (1948). Notes on the development of treatment of schizophrenics by psychoanalytic psychotherapy. *Psychiatry, 11*(3), 263–273.

Fuller-Thomson, E., & Hollister, B. (2016). Schizophrenia and suicide attempts: Findings from a representative community-based Canadian sample. *Schizophrenia Research and Treatment, 2016*, 3165243. http://dx.doi.org/10.1155/2016/3165243

Galderisi, S., Mucci, A., Buchanan, R. W., & Arango, C. (2018). Negative symptoms of schizophrenia: New developments and unanswered research questions. *Lancet Psychiatry, 5*, 664–677. http://dx.doi.org/10.1016/S2215-0366(18)30050-6

Galletly, C., Castle, D., Dark, F., Humberstone, V., Jablensky, A., Killackey, E., Kulkarni, J., McGorry, P., Nielssen, O., & Tran, N. (2016). Royal Australian and New Zealand College of Psychiatrists clinical practice guidelines for the management of schizophrenia and related disorders. *Australian & New Zealand Journal of Psychiatry, 50*, 410–472. https://doi.org/10.1177/0004867416641195

Goldman, M. B. (2009). The mechanism of life-threatening water imbalance in schizophrenia and its relationship to the underlying psychiatric illness. *Brain Research Review, 61*(2), 210–220.

Good Therapy. (2018). *Solution focused brief therapy (SFBT).* https://www.goodtherapy.org/learn-about-therapy/types/solution-focused-therapy

Government of Canada. (2018a). *Canadian chronic disease surveillance system 2018: Schizophrenia.* https://health-infobase.canada.ca/ccdss/data-tool/Age?G=00&V=5&M=1

Government of Canada. (2018b). *Cannabis Evidence Brief: Does cannabis use increase the risk of developing psychosis or schizophrenia?.*

Government of Canada. (2020, December). *Canadian cannabis survey 2020: Summary.* https://www.canada.ca/en/health-canada/services/drugs-medication/cannabis/research-data/canadian-cannabis-survey-2020-summary.html

Grossman, M., Bowi, R., Lepage, M., Malla, A. K., Joober, R., & Iyer, S. N. (2017). Smoking status and its relationship to demographic and clinical characteristics in first episode psychosis. *Journal of Psychiatric Research, 85*, 83–90.

Grover, S., & Avasthi, A. (2019). Clinical practice guidelines for the management of schizophrenia in children and adolescents. *Indian Journal of Psychiatry, 61*, 277–93. https://doi.org/10.4103/psychiatry.IndianJPsychiatry_556_18

Gough, E. (2005). Diabetes and schizophrenia. *Practical Diabetes, 22*(1), 23–26.

Gur, R. E., Roalf, D. R., Alexander-Bloch, A., McDonald-McGinn, M., & Gur, R. C. (2021). Pathways to understanding psychosis through rare— 22q11.2DS - and common variants. *Current Opinion in Genetics and Development, 68*, 35–40. https://doi.org/10.1016/j.gde.2021.01.007

Guy, W. (1976). *ECDEU: Assessment manual for psychopharmacology* (DHEW Publication No. 76-338). Department of Health Education and Welfare, Psychopharmacology Branch.

Hagi, K., Nosaka, T., Dickinson, D., Lindenmayer, J. P., Lee, J., Friedman, J., Boyer, L., Han, M., Abdul-Rashid, N. A., & Correll, C. U. (2021, March 3). Association between cardiovascular risk factors and cognitive impairment in people with schizophrenia: A systematic review and meta-analysis. *JAMA Psychiatry, 78*, 510–518. https://doi.org/10.1001/jamapsychiatry.2021.0015

Hardeman, S. M., & Narasimhan, M. (2010). Adherence according to Mary Poppins: strategies to make the medicine go down. *Perspectives in Psychiatric Care, 46*(1), 3–13.

Harding, C., Zubin, J., & Strauss, J. (1987). Chronicity in schizophrenia: Fact, partial fact or artifact? *Hospital and Community Psychiatry, 38*(5), 477–486.

Hayes, J. F., Picot, S., Osborn, D. J. P., Lewis, G., Dalman, C., & Lundin, A. (2019). Visual acuity in late adolescence and future psychosis risk in a cohort of 1 million Men. *Schizophrenia Bulletin, 45*, 571–578. https://doi.org/10.1093/schbul/sby084

Hettige, N. C., Bani-Fatemi, A., Kennedy, J. J., & De Luca, V. (2017). Assessing the risk for suicide in schizophrenia according to migration, ethnicity and geographical ancestry. *BMC Psychiatry, 17*, 63.

Howes, O. D., McCutcheon, R., Owen, M. J., & Murray, R. (2017). The role of genes, stress, and dopamine in the development of schizophrenia. *Biological Psychiatry, 81*, 9–20. http://dx.doi.org/10.1016/j.biopsych.2016.07.014

Holt R. (2019). Association between antipsychotic medication use and diabetes. *Current Diabetes Reports, 19*(10), 96. https://doi.org/10.1007/s11892-019-1220-8

Imtiaz, S., Shield, K. D., Roerecke, M., Cheng, J., Popova, S., Kurdyak, P., Fischer, B., & Rehm, J. (2015). The burden of disease attributable to cannabis use in Canada in 2012. *Addiction, 111*, 653–662.

Johnstone, E. C., Crow, T. J., Frith, C. D., Husband, J., & Kreel, L. (1976). Cerebral ventricular size and cognitive impairment in chronic schizophrenia. *Lancet, 2*, 924–926.

Kasanin, J. (1933). The acute schizo-affective psychoses. *American Journal of Psychiatry, 13*, 97–126.

Kavak, F., Ünal, S., & Yılmaz, E. (2016). Effects of relaxation exercises and music therapy on the psychological symptoms and depression levels of patients with schizophrenia. *Archives of Psychiatric Nursing, 30*(5), 508–512. https://doi:10.1016/j.apnu.2016.05.003

Kay, S. R., Fiszbein, A., & Opler, L. A. (1987). The positive and negative syndrome scale (PANSS) for schizophrenia. *Schizophrenia Bulletin, 13*, 261–276.

Keinänen, J., Mantere, O., Markkula, N., Partti, K., Perälä, J., Saarni, S. I., Härkänen, T. & Suvisaari, J. (2018). Mortality in people with psychotic disorders in Finland: A population-based 13-year follow-up study. *Schizophrenia Research, 192*, 113–118. https://doi.org/10.1016/j.schres.2017.04.048

Kendler, K. S. (2019). From many to one to many—The search for causes of psychiatric illness. *JAMA Psychiatry, 76*, 1085–1091. https://doi.org/10.1001/jamapsychiatry.2019.1200

Khan, T. A., Revah, O., Gordon, A., Yoon, S-J., Krawisz, A. K., Goold, C., Sun, Y., Kim, C. H., Tian, Y., Li, M-Y., Schaepel, J. M., Ikeda, K., Amin, N. D., Kakail, N., Yazawa, M., Kushan, L., Nishino, S., Porteus, M. H., Papoport, J. L. … Pasca, S. P. (2020). Neuronal defects in a human cellular model of 22q11.2 deletion syndrome. *Nature Medicine, 26*, 1888–1898. https://doi.org/10.1038/s41591-020-1043-9

Kim, M-H., Kim, I. B., Lee, J., Cha, D. H., Park, S. M., Kim, J. H., Kim, R., Park, J. S., An, Y., Kim, K., Kim, S., Webster, M. J., Kim, S., & Lee, J. H. (2021). Low-level brain somatic mutations are implicated in schizophrenia. *Biological Psychiatry, 90*, 35–46. https://doi.org/10.1016/j.biopsych.2021.01.014

Klages, D., East, L., Usher, K., & Jackson, D. (2020). Health Professionals as mothers of adult children with schizophrenia. *Qualitative Health Research, 30*(12), 1807–1820.

Kolker, R. (2020). *Hidden Valley Road: inside the mind of an American family.* Anchor Books, A division of Penguin Random House LLC.

Kraguljac, N. V., & Lahti, A. C. (2021, March 11). Neuroimaging as a window into the pathophysiological mechanisms of schizophrenia. *Frontiers of Psychiatry, 12*, 1–16. https://doi.org/10.3389/fpsyt.2021.613764

Kulkarni, J., Hayes, E., & Gavrilidis, E. (2012). Hormones and schizophrenia. *Current Opinions in Psychiatry, 25*(2), 89–95.

Kurdyak, P., Mallia, E., de Oliveira, C., Carvalho, A. F., Kozloff, N., Zaheer, J., Tempelaar, W. A., Anderson, K. K., Correll, C. U., & Voineskos, A.

N. (2021). Mortality after the first diagnosis of schizophrenia-spectrum disorders: A population-based retrospective cohort study. *Schizophrenia Bulletin, 47*, 864–874. https://doi.org/10.1093/schbul/sbaa180

Lagan, S., Camacho, E., & Torous, J. (2021). Is there a clinically relevant, publicly accessible app for that? Exploring the clinical relevance and availability of mobile apps for schizophrenia and psychosis. *Schizophrenia Research, 230*, 98–99. https://doi.org/10.1016/j.schres.2020.11.007

Lehmann, H. E. (1967). Psychotic disorders. I: Schizophrenic reactions. In A. M. Freedman & H. I. Kaplan (Eds.), *Comprehensive textbook of psychiatry* (pp. 593–598). Williams & Wilkins Co.

Lehrer, D. S., & Lorenz, J. (2014). Anosognosia in schizophrenia: Hidden in plain sight. *Innovations in Clinical Neurosciences, 11*, 10–17.

Levin, E., & Rezvani, A. (2007). Nicotinic interactions with antipsychotic drugs, models of schizophrenia and impacts on cognitive function. *Biochemical Pharmacology, 74*(8), 1182–1191.

Li, S., Hu, N., Zhang, W., Tao, B., Dai, J., Gong, Y., Tan, Y., Cai, D., & Lui, S. (2019, July). Dysconnectivity of multiple brain networks in schizophrenia: A meta- analysis of resting-state functional connectivity. *Frontiers in Psychiatry, 10*, 1–8. https://doi.org/10.3389/fpsyt.2019.00482

Lilley, L. L., Collins, S. R., Synder, J. S., & Swart, B. (2017). *Pharmacology for Canadian health care practice* (3rd ed.). Elsevier Canada.

Lintunen, J., Taipale, H., Tanskanen, A., Mittendorfer-Ruz, E. Tihonen, J., & Lähteenvuo, M. (2021, February). Long-Term real-world effectiveness of pharmacotherapies for schizoaffective disorder. *Schizophrenia Bulletin, 47*, 1099–1107. https://doi-org.login.ezproxy.library.ualberta.ca/10.1093/schbul/sbab004

Little, J. D., & Bell, E. (2021). Anosognosia and schizophrenia— a reminder. *Australasian Psychiatry, 29*, 344–345. https://doi.org/10.1177/1039856220928866

Liu, C., Kanazawa, T., Tian, Y., Saini, S. M., Mancuso, S., Mostaid, M. S., Takahashi, A., Zhang, D., Zhang, F., Yu, H., Shin, H. D., Cheong, H. S., Ikeda, M., Kubo, M., Iwata, N., Woo, S-I., Yue, W., Kamatani, Y., Shi, Y., … Bousman, C. (2019). The schizophrenia genetics knowledgebase: A comprehensive update of findings from candidate gene studies. *Translational Psychiatry, 9*, 1–7. https://doi.org/10.1038/s41398-019-0532-4

Madre, M., Canales-Rodriguez, E. J., Ortiz-Gil, J., Murru, A., Torrent, C., Bramon, E., Perez, V., Orth, M., Brambilla, P., Vieta, E., & Amann, B. L. (2016). Neuropsychological and neuroimaging underpinnings of schizoaffective disorder: A systematic review. *Acta Psychiatrica Scandinavica, 134*(1), 16–30. https://doi.org/10:1111/acps.12564

Malhi, G. S., & Bell, E. (2019). Schizoaffective disorder: Time to refine our thinking not the criteria? *Schizophrenia Research, 208*, 34–35. https://doi.org/10.1016/j.schres.2019.04.019

Marder, S. R., & Cannon, T. D. (2019). Schizophrenia. *New England Journal of Medicine, 381*, 1753–1761. https://doi.org/10.1056/NEJMra1808803

McCutcheon, R. A., Krystal, J. H., & Howes, O. D. (2020). Dopamine and glutamate in schizophrenia: Biology, symptoms, and treatment. *World Psychiatry, 19*, 15–33. https://onlinelibrary.wiley.com/doi/epdf/10.1002/wps.20693

Mental Health Commission of Canada (MHCC). (2013a). *Aspiring workforce: Employment and income for people with serious mental illness.* http://www.mentalhealthcommission.ca/English/node/7606

Mental Health Commission of Canada (MHCC). (2013b). *At home/Chez soi.* http://www.mentalhealthcommission.ca/English/initiatives-and-projects/home?routetoken=ff8ead4644148979334f1198d0bb826f&terminitial=38

Mental Health Commission of Canada (MHCC). (2013c). *National guidelines for a comprehensive service system to support family caregivers of adults with mental health problems and illnesses.* http://www.mentalhealthcommission.ca/English/node/8601/#sthash.FZdfsot1.dpuf

Merritt, K., Egerton, A., Kempton, M. J., Taylor, M. J., & McGuire, P. K. (2016). Nature of glutamate alterations in schizophrenia: A meta-analysis of proton magnetic resonance spectroscopy studies. *JAMA Psychiatry, 73*, 665–674. https://doi.org/10.1001/jamapsychiatry.2016.0442

Montoya, A., Ocampo, M., & Torres-Ruiz, A. (2003). Neuroleptic malignant syndrome in Mexico. *Canadian Journal of Clinical Pharmacology, 10*(3), 111–113.

Morcos, N., Rosinski, A., Maixner, D. F. (2019). Electroconvulsive therapy for neuroleptic malignant syndrome: A case series. *The Journal of ECT, 35*(4), 225–230. https://doi: 10.1097/YCT.0000000000000600

Moritz, S., Silverstein, S. M., Beblo, T., Özaslan, Z., Zink, M., & Gallinat, J. (2021). Much of the neurocognitive impairment in schizophrenia is due to factors other than schizophrenia itself: Implications for research and treatment. *Schizophrenia Bulletin Open, 2*, 1–11. https://doi.org/10.1093/schizbullopen/sgaa034

Morrison, E. F. (1992). A coercive interactional style as an antecedent to aggression in psychiatric patients. *Research in Nursing and Health, 15*, 421–431.

Morrison, E. F., & Love, C. C. (2003). An evaluation of four programs for the management of aggression in psychiatric settings. *Archives in Psychiatric Nursing, 17*(4), 146–155.

Mucci, A., Galderisi, S., Gibertoni, D., Rossi, A., Rocca, P., Bertolino, A., Aguglia, E., Amore, M., Bellomo, A., Biondi, M., Blasi, G., Brasso, C.,

Bucci, P., Carpiniello, B., Cuomo, A., Dell'Osso, L., Maria Giordano, G., Marchesi, C., Monteleone, P., ... Maj, M.; Italian Network for Research on Psychoses. (2021, February). Factors associated with real-life functioning in persons with schizophrenia in a 4-year follow-up study of the Italian Network for Research on Psychoses [Online]. *JAMA Psychiatry, 78,* 550–559. https://doi.org/10.1001/jamapsychiatry.2020.4614

Mueser, K. T., Penn, D. L., Addington, J., Brunette, M. F., Gingerich, S., Glynn, S. M., Lynde, D. W., Gottlieb, J. D., Meyer-Kalos, P., McGurk, S. R., Cather, C., Saade, S., Robinson, D. G., Schooler, N. R., Rosenheck, R. A., & Kane, J. M. (2015). The NAVIGATE program for first-episode psychosis: Rationale, overview, and description of psychosocial components. *Psychiatric Services, 66,* 680–690. https://doi.org/10.1176/appi.ps.201400413

Nath, M., Wong, T. P., & Srivastava, L. K. (2021). Neurodevelopmental insights into circuit dysconnectivity in schizophrenia. *Progress in Neuro-Psychopharmacology and Biological Psychiatry, 104,* 1–7. https://doi.org/10.1016/j.pnpbp.2020.110047

Nemani, K., Li, C., Olfson, M., Blessing, E. M., Razavian, N., Chen, J., Petkova, E., & Goff, D. C. (2021). Association of psychiatric disorders with mortality among patients with COVID-19. *JAMA Psychiatry, 78*(4), 380–386. https://doi.org/10.1001/jamapsychiatry.2020.4442

Overall, J. E., & Gorham, D. R. (1988). The Brief Psychiatric Rating Scale (BPRS): Recent developments in ascertainment and scaling. *Psychopharmacology Bulletin, 24,* 97–99.

Oxford University Press and the Maryland Psychiatric Research Center. (2002). Graduate student in peril: A first person account of schizophrenia. *Schizophrenia Bulletin, 28*(4), 745–755.

Perr, I. N. (1992). Religion, political leadership, charisma, and mental illness: The strange story of Louis Riel. *Journal of Forensic Sciences, 37*(2), 574–884.

Peterson, D. L., Webb, C. A., Keeley, J. W., Gaebel, W., Zielasek, J., Rebello, T. J., Robles, R., Matsumoto, C., Kogan, C. S., Kulygina, M., Farooq, S., Green, M. F., Falkai, P., Hasan, I., Galderisi, S., Larach, V., Krasnov, V., & Reed, G. M. (2019). The reliability and clinical utility of ICD-11 schizoaffective disorder: A field trial. *Schizophrenia Research, 208,* 235–241. https://doi.org/10.1016/j.schres.2019.02.011

Pillinger, T., Beck, K., Gobjila, C., Donocik, J. G., Jauhar, S., & Howes, O. D. (2017). Impaired glucose homeostasis in first-episode schizophrenia: A systematic review and meta-analysis. *JAMA Psychiatry, 74,* 261–269. https://doi.org/10.1001/jamapsychiatry.2016.3803

Pompili, M., Lester, D., Dominici, G., Longo, L., Marconi, G., Forte, A., Serafini, G., Amore, M., & Girardi, P. (2013). Indications for electroconvulsive treatment in schizophrenia: A systematic review. *Schizophrenia Research, 146*(1–3), 1–9. http://dx.doi.org/10.1016/j.schres.2013.02.005

Pruessner, M., Cullen, A. E., Aas, M., Walkerd, E. F. (2017). The neural diathesis-stress model of schizophrenia revisited: An update on recent findings considering illness stage and neurobiological and methodological complexities. *Neuroscience and Biobehavioral Reviews, 73,* 191–218. http://dx.doi.org/10.1016/j.neubiorev.2016.12.013

Ramnarine, M., & Ahmad, D. A. (2016, July 28). Anticholinergic toxicity clinical presentation. *Medscape.* http://emedicine.medscape.com/article/812644-clinical

Rao, D. P., Dai, S., Lagacé, C., & Krewski, D. (2014). Metabolic syndrome and chronic disease. *Chronic Diseases and Injuries in Canada, 34,* 36–45.

Sadock, B. J., Ahmad, S., & Sadock, V. A. (2019). *Kaplan & Sadock's pocket handbook of clinical psychiatry* (6th ed.). Lippincott Williams & Wilkins.

Sadock, B. J., Sadock, V. A., & Ruiz, P. (2015). *Kaplan and Sadock's synopsis of psychiatry* (11th ed.). Wolters Kluwer Health/Lippincott Williams & Wilkins.

Salvatore, P., Bhuvaneswar, C., Tohen, M., Khalsa, H. M., Maggini, C., & Baldessarini, R. J. (2014). Capgras' syndrome in first episode psychotic disorders. *Psychopathology, 47*(4), 261–269. https://doi.org/10.1159/000357813

Salzer, M. S., Brusilovskiy, E., & Townley, G. (2018). National estimates of recovery-remission from serious mental illness. *Psychiatric Services, 69,* 523–528. https://doi.org/10.1176/appi.ps.201700401

Schizophrenia Society of Canada. (2021). *Rays of hope: A reference manual for families & caregivers* (5th ed.). https://schizophrenia.ca/wp-content/uploads/2021/06/SSC-Rays-of-Hope-2021-WEB.pdf

Sendi, M. S. E., Pearlson, G. D., Mathalon, D. H., Ford, J. M., Preda, A., van Erp, T. G. M., & Calhoun, V. D. (2021). Multiple overlapping dynamic patterns of the visual sensory network in schizophrenia. *Schizophrenia Research, 228,* 103–111. https://doi.org/10.1016/j.schres.2020.11.055

Sheffield, J. M., Gold, J. M., Strauss, M. E., Carter, C. S., Macdonald, A. W., III, Ragland, J. D., Silverstein, S. M., & Barch, D. M. (2014). Common and specific cognitive deficits in schizophrenia: Relationships to function. *Cognitive, Affective, & Behavioral Neuroscience, 14*(1), 161–174.

Sheffield, J. M., Rogers, B. P., Blackford, J. U., Heckers, S., & Woodward, N. P. (2020). Insula functional connectivity in schizophrenia. *Schizophrenia Research, 220,* 69–77. https://doi.org/10.1016/j.schres.2020.03.068

Silverstein, S. M., Keane, B. P., & Corlett, P. R. (2021, February). Oculomics in schizophrenia research [Editorial]. *Schizophrenia Bulletin, 47,* 577–579. https://doi.org/10.1093/schbul/sbab011

Simpson, G. M., & Angus, J. W. S. L. (1970). A rating scale for extrapyramidal side effects. *Acta Psychiatrica Scandinavica, 212,* 11–19.

Siu, A. M. H., Ng, R. S. H., Poon, M. Y. C., Catherine, S. Y., Chong, C. S. Y., Siu, C. M. W., & Lau, S. P. K. (2021). Cognition evaluation of a computer-assisted cognitive remediation program for young people with psychosis: A pilot study. *Schizophrenia Research: Cognition, 23,* 1–8. https://doi.org/10.1016/j.scog.2020.100188

Smith, E. M. (2020). A first episode of psychosis. Helping loved ones cope and care for patients who have a lack of insight. *Nursing Made Incredibly Easy, 18,* 23–26. https://doi.org/10.1097/01.NME.0000668368.84427.77

Solomon, H. V., Sinopoli, M., & DeLisi, L. E. (2021). Ageing with schizophrenia: An update. *Current Opinion in Psychiatry, 34,* 266–274. https://doi.org/10.1097/YCO.0000000000000694

Spellmann, I., Schennach, R., Seemüller, F., Meyer, S., Musil, R., Jäger, M., Schmauß, M., Laux, G., Pfeiffer, H., Naber, D., Schmidt, L. G., Gaebel, W., Klosterkötter, J., Heuser, I., Bauer, M., Adli, A., Zeiler, J., Bender, W., Kronmüller, K-T., ... Möller, H-J. (2017). Validity of remission and recovery criteria for schizophrenia and major depression: Comparison of the results of two one-year follow-up naturalistic studies. *European Archives of Psychiatry Clinical Neuroscience, 267,* 303–313. https://doi.org/10.1007/s00406-016-0741-2

Sprague, R. L., & Kalachnik, J. E. (1991). Reliability, validity, and a total score cutoff for the Dyskinesia Identification Scale System: Condensed User Scale (DISCUS) with mentally ill and mentally retarded populations. *Psychopharmacology Bulletin, 27,* 51–58.

Stahl, S. M. (2018). Beyond the dopamine hypothesis of schizophrenia to three neural networks of psychosis: Dopamine, serotonin, and glutamate. *CNS Spectrums, 23,* 187–191. https://doi.org/10.1017/S1092852918001013

Standing Senate Committee on Social Affairs, Science and Technology. (2006). *Out of the shadows at last: Transforming mental health, mental illness and addiction services in Canada.* http://www.parl.gc.ca/39/1/parlbus/commbus/senate/Com-e/SOCI-E/rep-e/rep02may06-e.htm

Stentebjerg-Olesen, M., Pagsberg, A. K., Fink-Jensen, A., Correll, C. U., & Jeppesen, P. (2016). Clinical characteristics and predictors of schizophrenia-spectrum psychosis in children and adolescents: A systematic review. *Journal of Child and Adolescent Psychopharmacology, 26,* 410–427. https://doi.org/10.1089/cap.2015.0097

Stiekema, A. P. M., van Dam, M. T., Bruggeman, R., Redmeijer, J. E., Swart, M., Dethmers, M., Rietberg, K., Wekking, E. M., Velligan, D. I., Timmerman, M. E., Aleman, A., Castelein, S., van Weeghel, J., Pijnenborg, G. M. H., & van der Meer, L. (2020). Facilitating recovery of daily functioning in people with a severe mental illness who need longer-term intensive psychiatric services: Results from a cluster randomized controlled trial on cognitive adaptation training delivered by nurses. *Schizophrenia Bulletin, 46*(5), 1259–1268. https://doi.org/10.1093/schbul/sbz135

Stilo, S. A., & Murray, R. M. (2019). Non-genetic factors in schizophrenia. *Current Psychiatry Reports, 21*(100), 1–10. https://doi.org/10.1007/s11920-019-1091-3

Strauss, G. P., Nuñez, A., Ahmed, A. O., Barchard, K. A., Granholm, E., Kirkpatrick, B., Gold, J. M., & Allen, D. N. (2018). The latent structure of negative symptoms in schizophrenia. *JAMA Psychiatry, 75,* 1271–1279. https://doi.org/10.1001/jamapsychiatry.2018.2475

Sum, M. Y., Chan, S. K. W., Tse, S., Bola, J. R., Ng, R. M. K., Hui, C. L. M., Lee, E. H. M., Chang, W. C., & Chen, E. Y. H. (2021). Relationship between subjective quality of life and perceptions of recovery orientation of treatment service in patients with schizophrenia and major depressive disorder. *Asian Journal of Psychiatry, 57,* 1–6. https://doi.org/10.1016/j.ajp.2021.102578

Tan, S., Zhu, X., Fan, H., Tan, Y., Yang, F., Wang, Z., Zhao, Y., Fan, F., Guo, J., Li, Z., Quan, W., Wang, X., Reeder, C., Zhou, D., Zou, Y., & Wykes, T. (2020). Who will benefit from computerized cognitive remediation therapy? Evidence from a multisite randomized controlled study in schizophrenia. *Psychological Medicine, 50,* 1633–1643. https://doi.org/10.1017/S0033291719001594

Torres, U. S., Duran, F. L. S., Schaufelberger, M. S., Crippa, J. A. S., Louzã, M. R., Sallet, P. C., Kanegusuku, C. Y. O., Elkis, H., Gattaz, W. G., Bassitt, D. P., Zuardi, A. W., Hallak, J. A. C., Leite, C. C., Castro, C. C., Santos, A. C., Murray, R. M., & Busatto, G. F. (2016). Patterns of regional gray matter loss at different stages of schizophrenia: A multisite, cross-sectional VBM study in first-episode and chronic illness. *NeuroImage Clinical, 12,* 1–15. http://dx.doi.org/10.1016/j.nicl.2016.06.002

Varese, F., Smeets, F., Drukker, M., Lieverse, R., Lataster, T., Viechtbauer, W., Read, J., van Os, J., & Benta, R. P. (2012). Childhood adversities increase the risk of psychosis: A meta-analysis of patient-control, prospective- and cross-sectional cohort studies. *Schizophrenia Bulletin, 4,* 661–671. https://doi.org/10.1093/schbul/sbs050

Vita, A., Barlati, S., Ceraso, A., Nibbio, G., Ariu, C., Deste, G., & Wykes, T. (2021, April). Effectiveness, core elements, and moderators of response of cognitive remediation for schizophrenia: A systematic review and meta-analysis of randomized clinical trials. *JAMA Psychiatry, 78,* 848– 858. https://doi.org/10.1001/jamapsychiatry.2021.0620

Waite, P. (1987). Between three oceans: Challenges of a continental destiny. In C. Brown (Ed.), *The illustrated history of Canada* (pp. 279–373). Lester & Orpen Dennys.

Wang, X., Lu, F., Duan, X., Han, S., Guo, X., Yang, M., Zhang, Y., Xiao, J., Sheng, W., Zhao, J., & Chen, H. (2020). Frontal white matter abnormalities reveal the pathological basis underlying negative symptoms in antipsychotic-naïve, first-episode patients with adolescent-onset schizophrenia: Evidence from multimodal brain imaging. *Schizophrenia Research, 222,* 258–266. https://doi.org/10.1016/j.schres.2020.05.039

Weinberger, D. R., Berman, K. P., & Illowsky, B. P. (1988). Physiological dysfunction of dorsolateral prefrontal cortex in schizophrenia. III. A new cohort and evidence for a monoaminergic mechanism. *Archives of General Psychiatry, 45,* 609–615. https://doi.org/10.1001/archpsyc.1988.01800310013001

Whicher, C. A., Price, H. C., & Holt, R. G. (2018). Antipsychotic medication and type 2 diabetes and impaired glucose regulation. *European Journal of Endocrinology, 178,* R245–R258. https://doi.org/10.1530/EJE-18-0022

Wilson, J. H. (2009). Moving beyond policy rhetoric: Building a moral community for early psychosis intervention. *Journal of Psychiatric and Mental Health Nursing, 16*(7), 621–628.

Wilson, J. H. (2012). *First episode psychosis: The experience of parent caregivers.* Doctoral dissertation, University of Alberta, Edmonton, AB.

Wojtalik, A., Smith, M. J., Keshavan, M. S., & Eack, S. M. (2017). A systematic and meta-analytic review of neural correlates of functional outcome in schizophrenia. *Schizophrenia Bulletin, 43,* 1329–1347. https://doi.org/10.1093/schbul/sbx008

World Health Organization. (2020). *International statistical classification of diseases (ICD) related health problems* (11th ed.). https://icd.who.int/

Wynne, L. C., Ryckoff, I. M., Day, J., & Hirsch, S. I. (1958). Pseudo-mutuality in the family relations of schizophrenics. *Psychiatry, 21*(2), 205–220. https://doi.org/10.1080/00332747.1958.11023128

Yamauchi, Y., Shiga, T., Shikino, K., Uechi, T., Koyama, Y., Shimozawa, N., Hiraoka, E., Funakoshi, H., Mizobe, M., Imaizumi, T., & Ikusaka, M. (2019). Influence of psychiatric or social backgrounds on clinical decision making: A randomized, controlled multi-centre study. *BMC Medical Education, 19,* 1–10. https://doi.org/10.1186/s12909-019-1897-z

Yang, A. C., & Tsai, S-J. (2017). New targets for schizophrenia treatment beyond the dopamine hypothesis. *International Journal of Molecular Sciences, 18,* 1–14. https://doi.org/10.3390/ijms18081689

Yesufu-Udechuku, A., Harrison, B., Mayo-Wilson, E., Young, N., Woodhams, P., Shiers, D., Kuipers, E., & Kendall, T. (2015). Interventions to improve the experience of caring for people with severe mental illness: Systematic review and meta-analysis. *British Journal of Psychiatry, 206,* 2268–2274. https://doi.org/10.1192/bjp.bp.114.147561

Yoca, G., Yağcıoğlu, A. E. A., Eni, N., Karahan, S., Türkoğlu, I., Yıldız, E. A., Mercanlıgil, S. M., & Yazıcı, M. K. (2020). A follow-up study of metabolic syndrome in schizophrenia. *European Archives of Psychiatry and Clinical Neuroscience, 270,* 611–618. https://doi.org/10.1007/s00406-019-01016-x

Young, A., Halari, R., & Gray, R. (2013). Negative symptoms in schizophrenia: Meeting the challenge. *Progress in Neurology and Psychiatry, 17*(5), 33–36.

Young, L., Murata, L., McPherson, C., Jacob, J. D., & Vandyk, A. D. (2019). Exploring the experiences of parent caregivers of adult children with schizophrenia: A systematic review. *Archives of Psychiatric Nursing, 33,* 93–103. https://doi.org/10.1016/j.apnu.2018.08.005

Zaheer, J., Olfson, M., Mallia, E., Lamb, J. S. H., de Oliveira, C., Rudoler, D., Carvalho, A. F., Jacob, B. J., Juda, A., & Kurdyak, P. (2020). Predictors of suicide at time of diagnosis in schizophrenia spectrum disorder: A 20-year total population study in Ontario, Canada. *Schizophrenia Research, 222,* 382–388. https://doi.org/10.1016/j.schres.2020.04.025

Depressive, Bipolar, and Related Disorders

Katherine S. Bright*

The World Health Organization (WHO) (2020) identifies major depression as one of the most common and costly public health concerns worldwide. The economic burden is a result of its high prevalence rates and the debilitating nature of the illness (Greenberg et al., 2015). In their report from 2009, WHO estimated that by the year 2030, depression will be the leading cause of disease burden globally. Depression not only directly affects a person's quality of life but also impacts the family relationships and functioning of women at work (Hofmann et al., 2017). A study using mental health data from the 2019 Canadian Community Health Survey (Statistics Canada, 2020) indicated that approximately 4.4 million Canadians (14%) aged 12 years and older reported having a diagnosed mood or anxiety disorder, up from 3.7 million (12%) in 2015. The prevalence of mood disorders in Canada was greatest in the group 18 to 34

years of age (up from 13% to 17%) with females (17%) reflecting significantly higher levels of mood or anxiety disorders than males (11%). Of note, of those 18 to 34 years of age, 17% reported a diagnosed mood or anxiety disorder, up from 12% in 2015. Females (17%) in 2019 were more likely than males (11%) to report a diagnosed mood or anxiety disorder, also up from 2015, when 15% of females and 9% of males reported a mood or anxiety disorder. Indeed, studies show that the lifetime rate of major depression is 1.98 to 2.02 times greater in females than in males, with risk increasing especially between adolescence and mid-50s, perhaps triggered by fluctuations in female hormones and more sensitivity to interpersonal relationships (Findlay, 2017). Reflecting this higher prevalence rate of depression in women, using cross-sectional data from the National Population Health Survey (NPHS), general health cycles of the

---

*Adapted from the chapter "Depressive, Bipolar, and Related Disorders" by Carol Rupcich

Canadian Community Health Survey (CCHS), and two mental health-focused iterations of the CCHS called the CCHS 1.2 and CCHS-MH in Canada between 2002 and 2012, women were twice as likely to meet criteria for major depression (Patten et al., 2016a) and prescribed antidepressants twice as often as were men (Rotermann et al., 2014).

Studies show the connection of depressive disorders with the incidence of chronic conditions such as hypertension, arthritis, pain, heart disease, diabetes, and chronic obstructive pulmonary disorder (Bhattacharya et al., 2014; Canadian Mental Health Association, 2013). A major concern is the extent that untreated mood disorders are concurrent with elevated suicide rates. Suicide accounts for 1.4% of all premature deaths worldwide, and chronic physical and mental diseases account for numbers that are 10 times as high when compared with the general population (Bachmann, 2018). These "premature and preventable" deaths prompted the WHO to declare the necessity of building awareness, developing prevention strategies, and improving crisis intervention treatments to stop such dire consequences (WHO, 2017). Caring, connecting, and a holistic perspective, primary tenets of nursing foster a unique therapeutic context that places the nurse in an essential position to prevent suicide through the identification, treatment, and referral of individuals experiencing a mood disorder.

Common features of depressive disorders, and bipolar and related disorders, as described in the fifth edition of the American Psychiatric Association's *Diagnostic and Statistical Manual of Mental Disorders* (*DSM-5*) (APA, 2013) "include the presence of sad, empty, or irritable mood, accompanied by somatic and cognitive changes that significantly affect the individual's capacity to function" (p. 155). In depressive and bipolar-related disorders, mood is the primary alteration rather than thought or perceptual disturbances. Several terms describe **affect**, or the observable expression of mood (APA, 2013), such as the following:

- *Blunted*: Significantly reduced intensity of emotional expression
- *Flat*: Absent or nearly absent affective expression
- *Inappropriate*: Discordant affective expression accompanying speech content or ideation
- *Labile*: Varied, rapid, and abrupt shifts in affective expression
- *Restricted or constricted*: Mildly reduced in range and intensity of emotional expression

Primary mood disorders include depressive (**unipolar**) and **bipolar** (manic–depressive) disorders. Although the *DSM-5* has separated its discussion of depressive disorders from bipolar and related disorders, what endure related to both groupings are the common features noted above. Specific criteria differentiating the diagnostic classification of these disorders are detailed according to "issues of duration, timing, or presumed etiology"

(APA, 2013, p. 155). Although several mood categories are described in the *DSM-5*, this chapter focuses primarily on the nurse's role in caring for persons who have these disorders:

- *Depressive disorders*: Major depressive disorder, single or recurrent; and dysthymic disorder
- *Bipolar disorders*: Bipolar I disorder, bipolar II disorder, and cyclothymic disorder
- *Mood disorder* caused by a general medical condition
- *Substance-induced mood disorder*

Additional specifiers for depression further classify these diagnoses:

- Severity specifier: mild, moderate, or severe
- With mixed features: allows for the presence of manic symptoms in depressed patients who do not meet the full criteria for a manic episode
- With anxious distress: allows for the presence of anxiety because the addition of anxiety may affect prognosis, treatment, and patient response to treatment
- Seasonal depression: recognized, recurrent, annual pattern with a specific onset related to seasonal light deprivation, typically occurring during the fall and winter months, followed by symptom reprieve during the spring and summer. Seasonal variations in mood occur most commonly in northern latitudes (APA, 2013)
- Peripartum onset: recognized onset of an episode during pregnancy or within the first 4 weeks postpartum (National Institute for Health and Care Excellence, 2020)

The advantages of diagnosing a mood disorder early (e.g., early intervention, community nursing support) can be constrained by the adverse effect of a psychiatric diagnosis as a negative social label. Early diagnosis can influence the chronicity and secondary risks associated with mood disorders such as suicidal ideation and substance misuse (Iorfino et al., 2019). Accessing effective care can be inhibited by the need to keep the diagnosis hidden, even from oneself through self-stigma (Corrigan & Nieweglowski, 2021). Increased awareness is a principal "weapon against stigma" and fundamental to combating misperceptions. Awareness would lead to clarity in detection, to acceptance by patients and their families, and ultimately to the required support and treatment (Nihayati et al., 2020).

KEY CONCEPT

Mood is the predominant, pervasive, and sustained emotion colouring the patient's perception of the world and ability to function in it. Normal variations in mood, such as sadness, euphoria, and anxiety, occur as responses to specific life experiences and are time limited, not associated with significant or chronic functional impairment.

Depressive Disorders

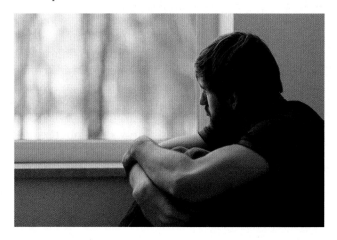

Clinical Course

The criteria in the *DSM-5* indicate that a major depressive disorder can occur as a single episode, although episodes often recur. To constitute a **major depressive**

episode (MDE), either a depressed mood or a loss of interest or pleasure in nearly all activities must be present for at least 2 weeks. Additionally, four of the following seven symptoms are usually present: disruption in sleep, appetite (or weight), concentration, or energy; psychomotor agitation or retardation; excessive guilt or feelings of worthlessness; and suicidal ideation (see Box 22.1 for the APA's DSM-5 criteria). Individuals often report feeling depressed, hopeless, or discouraged. If a person complains of feeling sad and empty, a depressed mood may be inferred from their facial expression and demeanour. Depression may also be demonstrated by other behaviours such as withdrawal and excessive ruminations, typically with the themes of guilt and/or shame (Gambin & Sharp, 2018).

The course of major depression is variable, but increasingly this illness is considered persistent and recurrent. Over time, depressive episodes can increase in frequency, severity, and duration. The severity, number of episodes, and the amount of time that major depression is left untreated influences the long-term prognosis

---

BOX 22.1 DSM-5 Diagnostic Criteria: Major Depressive Disorder

A. Five (or more) of the following symptoms have been present during the same 2-week period and represent a change from previous functioning; at least one of the symptoms is either (a) depressed mood or (b) loss of interest or pleasure.

   1. Depressed mood most of the day, nearly every day, as indicated by either subjective report (e.g., feels sad, empty, hopeless) or observation made by others (e.g., appears tearful). (*Note:* In children and adolescents, can be irritable mood.)

   2. Markedly diminished interest or pleasure in all, or almost all, activities most of the day, nearly every day (as indicated by either subjective account or observation).

   3. Significant weight loss when not dieting or weight gain (e.g., a change of more than 5% of body weight in a month) or decrease or increase in appetite nearly every day. (*Note:* In children, consider failure to make expected weight gain.)

   4. Insomnia or hypersomnia nearly every day.

   5. Psychomotor agitation or retardation nearly every day (observable by others, not merely subjective feelings of restlessness or being slowed down).

   6. Fatigue or loss of energy nearly every day.

   7. Feelings of worthlessness or excessive or inappropriate guilt (which may be delusional)

nearly every day (not merely self-reproach or guilt about being sick).

   8. Diminished ability to think or concentrate, or indecisiveness, nearly every day (either by subjective account or as observed by others).

   9. Recurrent thoughts of death (not just fear of dying), recurrent suicidal ideation without a specific path, or a suicide attempt, or a specific plan for committing suicide.

B. The symptoms cause clinically significant distress or impairment in social, occupational, or other important areas of functioning.

C. The episode is not attributable to the physiologic effects of a substance or to another medical condition.

D. The occurrence of the major depressive disorder is not better explained by schizoaffective disorder, schizophrenia, schizophreniform disorder, delusional disorder, or other specified and unspecified schizophrenia spectrum and other psychotic disorders.

E. There has never been a manic episode or a hypomanic episode.

Reprinted with permission from the *Diagnostic and statistical manual of mental disorders* (5th ed.). (Copyright 2013). American Psychiatric Association.

(Dohm et al., 2017). Complicating the course of major depression may be the frequently occurring bidirectional link between alcohol dependence and depression. Research suggests that problematic alcohol use is associated with more severe levels of MDE (Pavkovic et al., 2018). Further, suicide as a result of major depression underscores the serious and lethal progression this disorder can take. Yet despite the potentially problematic course of major depression, it is important to note that many of those who experience a depressive episode are likely to recover fully from it (Oluboka et al., 2018).

Dysthymic disorder is a persistent yet less severe form of major depressive disorder (Carta et al., 2019). Dysthymic disorder, along with a depressed mood, includes two or more of the following symptoms: eating and sleeping behaviour changes (eating or sleeping too little or too much), loss of energy, difficulty concentrating and making decisions, low self-esteem, and feelings of hopelessness (Patel & Rose, 2020). MDE superimposed on dysthymia is often referred to as "double depression" (Case et al., 2018).

Depressive Disorders in Special Populations

Children and Adolescents

The rates of anxiety and depression among children and adolescents are increasing (Caldwell et al., 2019). Depressive disorders in children have similar presentations to those seen in adults, with some exceptions in presentation and developmental expression. In major depressive disorder, children are less likely to present with psychosis, but when they do, auditory hallucinations are more common than are delusions. They are also less likely to express subjectively, hopelessness and dysphoria, and more likely to have anxiety symptoms characterized as internalizing disorders, which are often expressed somatically in the form of stomach aches and headaches. Externalizing behavioural abnormalities, such as fear of separation, aggression, hyperactivity, and rule-breaking behaviours, are often demonstrated in young children (Rodas et al., 2017). Psychiatric visits to the emergency department among children and youth are increasing across Canada, and the greatest rise is in those ages 14 to 21 years, high-acuity cases, and those with symptoms of anxiety and mood disorders (Chiu et al., 2020). In adolescence, major depressive disorder is twice as common in female as in male populations, whereas prepubertal boys and girls are noted to be equally affected. Insomnia, hypersomnia, and irritability instead of sad mood may predominate in a depressed adolescent. Adolescent boys are more likely than girls to present with disruptive behaviour disorders and attention deficit hyperactivity disorders (ADHDs) (Georgiades et al., 2019). Hickie and colleagues (2019) discuss the importance of "right care, first time" when working with adolescents with onset mood disorders. Recognizing that long-term consequences of such disorders can prevail, they discuss the importance of utilizing a personalized measurement-based early intervention model that includes "social and occupational function; self-harm, suicidal thoughts, and behaviour; alcohol or other substance misuse; physical health; and illness trajectory" (p. S4). The risk for suicide is real in children and adolescents and peaks around age 13 to 15 years in girls and after age 15 in boys (Steinhoff et al., 2021). Transgender boys/men and nonbinary youth are at higher risk of suicide (Veale et al., 2017). See Chapter 20 regarding suicidal behaviour.

Older Adults

The aging demographic in Canada necessitates that nurses take a leadership role in ensuring that the health care needs of the older adult are met (Canadian Nurses Association, 2016), especially depression in this population. Older patients experiencing depressive symptoms do not always meet the full criteria for major depression, and this disorder can manifest comorbidly with dementia, complicating the presentation of both conditions. It is estimated that 8% to 20% of older adults in the community, and as many as 33% in primary care settings, experience depressive symptoms (Neufeld et al., 2021). Treatment is successful in 60% to 80%, but response to treatment is slower than in younger adults. Depression in older adults often is associated with chronic illnesses, such as heart disease, diabetes, stroke, and cancer; symptoms may be somatically focused (Liu et al., 2019). Suicide is a very serious risk for older adults, especially men. In Canada, significant mortality rates due to suicide are reported in people older than 80 years of age. Statistics also reflect more deaths by suicide in adults aged 80 to 90+ years. Between 1979 and 2012, a rate of 20 to 24 suicides per 100,000 was reported (Statistics Canada, 2012). Rates were substantially higher among men than among women in individuals older than 85 years; rates for men are 6 to 10 times as high as those for women (Skinner et al., 2016).

Indigenous and First Nations Populations

Limited and variable data exist regarding the prevalence rates of major depression in Canada's Indigenous and First Nations populations. When compared with the general population, however, there are significantly elevated rates of suicide in Indigenous Peoples, which may reflect a high incidence of depression that is twice that of the general population (Chahar Mahali et al., 2021). In addition to cultural engagement and structural determinants of health, depression in Indigenous Peoples is tied to social circumstances related to colonialism, assimilationist policies, cultural destruction, discrimination, stereotyping, and transgenerational trauma

(Hackett et al., 2016; Wilk et al., 2017). Pertinent is that depressive symptoms evidenced among Indigenous Peoples may be quite distinct with respect to their own unique cultural practices (Fiedeldey-Van Dijk et al., 2017). The spiritual beliefs of this population play a vital part in their mental health, and the use of a term such as "spirit" to connote mood does not fit with Western descriptions of depression (Bellamy & Hardy, 2015). Thus, it is critical that nurses possess a clear understanding of how each Indigenous person conceptualizes their depression to ensure accurate assessment and intervention.

COVID-19

COVID-19 emerged in China in December 2019 and quickly became a global pandemic. As of January 2022, more than 364 million people have contracted COVID-19, and there have been more than 5.6 million deaths from COVID-19 (World Health Organization, n.d.); these include more than 3 million cases in Canada, including more than 33,000 deaths (World Health Organization, n.d.), as of January 2022, with more expected during the fifth wave of the pandemic. Beyond the enormous global threat to physical health and life, there are significant concerns over the international impact on mental health (Gruber et al., 2021; Pfefferbaum & North, 2020). COVID-19 has affected the health, safety, and wellbeing of individuals and communities causing insecurity, emotional isolation, stigma, financial loss, work and school closures, and inadequate resources for medical and mental health response (Pfefferbaum & North, 2020). As a result, individuals may develop a range of emotional reactions (depression, anxiety, loneliness, suicide) and substance misuse behaviours (Gruber et al., 2021). Findlay and colleagues (2020) reported that 54% of Canadians aged 15 and older reported "excellent or very good mental health" during the COVID-19 pandemic; however, they concluded that those experiencing physical health concerns, socioeconomic stressors, and family stress from confinement were at risk of lower perceived mental health. Anecdotally, nurses know that the pandemic has had (and continues to have) a significant impact on the mental health of Canadians. Telehealth modalities are already effective interventions for mental health. Individuals may benefit from increased access to such telemedicine, which helps nurses reach those who are most vulnerable to the mental health impact of the pandemic.

Epidemiology

In Canada, to evaluate national trends in the prevalence of major depression during the past two decades, data were examined from a series of representative Canadian surveys, conducted from 1994 to 2012. No increase in the yearly prevalence of major depression over time was noted and stability was evident in a 4.7% annual

IN-A-LIFE

James Eugene Carrey (1962–)

CANADIAN-BORN ACTOR AND COMEDIAN

Public Persona

Jim Carrey grew up in Toronto. His fame as a comedian began on *The Carol Burnett Show* at the age of 10. His stage talents ripened through the comedy routines he performed for classmates throughout his school years. Carrey, a high school dropout, began his acting career in comedy clubs and with bit-part television and movie performances. His unique on-screen characteristics were recognized quickly, and he became a box-office success. Jim Carrey is well known for his performances in such films as *The Mask, Ace Ventura: Pet Detective, Dumb and Dumber,* and more recently, *Me, Myself & Irene, Bruce Almighty, Dumb and Dumber To, Eternal Sunshine of the Spotless Mind, A Christmas Carol, Sonic the Hedgehog,* and played Joe Biden on *Saturday Night Live.* He was inducted into Canada's Walk of Fame in 2004.

Personal Reality

In 2004, Carrey publicly discussed his struggle with depression on the U.S. news programme, *60 Minutes*, exposing a serious, complicated side of himself as a person who was continually questioning himself and the world. Carrey was candid about periods of desperation in his life: the poverty, deprivation, and anger that marked some of his early childhood and adolescence; the struggles through two failed marriages; the highs and the lows bordering on despair; and the extended use of Prozac that helped him "out of a jam." Through it all, Jim, using the mask of *comedy* as a shield, maintains "life is beautiful" and that he is committed to giving full expression to the "realness" of his being.

Source: Leung, R. (2004, November). Carrey: Life is too beautiful. *60 Minutes, CBS NEWS.* http://www.cbsnews.com/stories/2004/11/18/60minutes/main656547.shtml

prevalence rate in 2012 and a 4.8% annual prevalence rate in 2002 (Patten et al., 2016b). Specific factors associated with this stability are unclear, but it may be that heightened public recognition of depression, increased mental health literacy, improved diagnosis, and increased access to treatment as well as increased antidepressant use have exerted an effect (Patten et al., 2016a). Dobson and colleagues (2020) reviewed trends in the prevalence of depression among working age Canadians between 2000 and 2016 and noted that the prevalence of a major depressive disorder was 5.4%; these estimates were slightly higher among those who were unemployed. Moreover, the authors concluded that a gap exists in the study of depression among the Canadian labour force.

Despite some evidence that major depression in Canada may be stabilizing, it remains a serious public health concern because it occurs so commonly and has a chronic–recurrent trajectory (Carta et al., 2017). Moreover, this illness presents comorbidly with other medical disorders, and particularly endocrine disorders, cardiovascular disease, neurologic disorders, autoimmune conditions, infectious diseases, and cancer (Kim & Jeon, 2018), as well as nutritional deficiencies, and as a direct physiologic effect of a substance such as corticosteroid treatment (Joëls, 2018). Further, major depression usually coexists with other mental illnesses, particularly anxiety and substance-use disorders. Importantly, major depression predicts serious role performance impairments, which have significant personal and social economic ramifications (Leach & Butterworth, 2020). Thus, the magnitude of major depression as a significant public health problem occurring throughout the life span must register with nurses practicing in all healthcare contexts.

Ethnic and Cultural Differences

Although prevalence rates in Canada are said to be unrelated to race, culture can influence the experience and communication of depressive symptoms. Culture is a complex concept and the context in which all human emotions, experiences, and actions are understood. Canada is a country of vast regional differences and numerous "microidentities" populated by a variety of cultures. Many groups of inhabitants, such as those of Ukrainian and Asian cultures, maintain "homeland" beliefs and ideologies that may influence how individual patients experience and express emotional disturbances. Culture may dictate an iron resolve to keep feelings in check or unexpressed. In some cultures, somatic symptoms, rather than sadness or guilt, may predominate. Complaints of "nerves" and headaches (in Ukrainian cultures); weakness, tiredness, or "imbalance" (in Chinese and other Asian cultures); or problems of the "heart" (in Middle Eastern cultures) may be ways of expressing experience of depression. Although

culturally distinctive experiences must be distinguished from symptoms, it is imperative that a symptom not be dismissed merely because it may be viewed as a culture-specific norm. It is important for the nurse to be cognizant of emergent Canadian immigration trends; Syrian, Latin American, South Asian, Indian, and African populations may have their own ways of characterizing a depressive disorder. Nurses must be equipped to care for an increasingly diverse population. To achieve this aim, culturally competent mental health nursing care must value different beliefs and multiple ways of knowing, engaging, and expressing so that proper assessments may be conducted in a culturally and linguistically sensitive manner (International Council of Nurses, 2013).

Risk Factors

Depression is so common that it is sometimes difficult to identify risk factors. The Adverse Childhood Experiences study indicates devastating risk links between childhood emotional, physical, and sexual abuses and subsequent life experiences of depression (Felitti et al., 1998; Petruccelli et al., 2019). Other generally acknowledged risk factors include the following:

- Prior episode of depression
- Family history of depressive disorder
- Lack of social support
- Stressful life events
- Current substance use
- Medical comorbidity
- Economic difficulties

Aetiology

The aetiology of major depression is undoubtedly understood from a biopsychosocial model with the spiritual component increasingly recognized. In the biologic domain, a proliferation of research over the past 50 years has led to a clear understanding that multifactorial biologic disturbances are involved in the aetiology of major depression. Box 22.2 explores research into differences in the level of depressive symptoms of men and women.

Genetics

Family, twin, and adoption studies conducted to determine a heritable aetiology for major depression suggest a genetic liability for this disorder. Twin studies offer compelling data that major depressive disorder is demonstrated more commonly among first-degree biologic relatives of people with this illness than among the general population (Ormel et al., 2019). New understandings about genetics and major depression continue to

BOX 22.2 Research for Best Practice

GENDERED DEPRESSION: VULNERABILITY OR EXPOSURE TO WORK AND FAMILY STRESSORS?

Marchand, A., Bilodeau, J., Demers, A., Beauregard, N., Durand, P., & Haines, V. (2016). Gendered depression: Vulnerability or exposure to work and family stressors? *Social Science and Medicine, 166*, 160–168. http://dx.doi.org/10.1016/j.socscimed.2016.08.021

Question: Are differences in the level of depressive symptoms of men and women explained by differentials in their vulnerability and exposure to work and family circumstances, as well as the mediating effects of work-to-family conflict (WFC) and family-to-work conflict (FWC)? Two hypotheses were advanced: the vulnerability hypothesis (women react more intensely than do men to stressful conditions) and the exposure hypothesis (the distribution of psychosocial risks and resources in the workplace and in the family are gendered).

Method: Data in this study were derived from the Salveo Study, which occurred from 2009 to 2012. It included a random sample of 1,935 employees (women constituted 48.9% of the sample) working in Quebec, Canada. Multilevel path analysis models were used to test the differential exposure hypothesis; gender stratification of the data was used to test for a differential vulnerability hypothesis.

Results: Both hypotheses were supported. Differences in vulnerability and exposure risks did impact depressive symptoms in men and women, with exposure risks having the most empirical support. Overall, it was the WFC that had a mediating effect between work–family stressors and depression (i.e., increased depression levels in women). In terms of the vulnerability hypothesis, results indicated only one gendered pathway, and it pertains to the relationship between WFC and depression. For men, lower skill utilization and higher job security were associated with higher depressive symptoms; psychological

demands and abusive supervisors were the only work factors associated with women's higher symptoms. Couple-related problems and WFC were associated with higher depressive symptoms in both genders, with child-related problems associated with increased symptoms for women. The importance of the relationship between family income and WFC was greatest in women. When work, family, and WFC factors were accounted for, differences in symptoms of depression between women and men were not significant because variables such as working hours, irregular work schedules, and skill acted as mediators for both genders. Increased working hours and irregular work schedules were also associated with WFC. More women than men reported higher WFC, but fewer working hours, a more regular work schedule, and lower skill use.

Nursing Implications: Nurses must be cognizant that the higher rate of depression in women compared with men may be related to differential social experiences that are formed by gendered social structures and gendered organizations. Despite increased gender equity in home life, women typically take on and juggle more family responsibilities while simultaneously working in occupational environments that do not afford them the same possibilities as men. Gendered role meanings for women are fundamentally linked to work–family conflict, and significant role strain may occur in women in the domains of work and family. Nurses need to integrate into their assessments how work and family domains are influencing depressive symptoms in men and women so more effective nursing interventions can be implemented. As well, assessing women for gendered role strain, promoting individual self-care, and offering family support in the context of gendered work–family conflict may decrease a vulnerability to depression.

emerge through research in linkage studies examining coinheritance of genetic markers for major depression. However, the extent to which shared gene–environment factors influence familial MDE risk remains unclear. Advances in epigenetics are enhancing the understanding of how early life experiences can trigger changes in the association between gene and environment expression, which results in mood disorders (Peña & Nestler, 2018).

Neurobiologic Hypotheses

The evolution of early neurobiologic theories has resulted in new paradigms regarding the cause of depression in which it is attributed to a wide range

of complex and intertwining neurobiologic abnormalities. Advances in the neurobiology of depression are seen in the areas of increased phasic rapid eye movement sleep, poor sleep maintenance, elevated cortisol levels, impaired cellular immunity, and decreased activity in the dorsolateral prefrontal cortex, low levels of the serotonin metabolite 5-hydroxyindoleacetic acid (5-HIAA), and increases in limbic responses (Ferrari & Villa, 2017). Depression is also linked to abnormalities in either the excretion of the neurotransmitters norepinephrine (NE), dopamine (DA), and serotonin (5-HT) or their receptor functions (Wang et al., 2020). The homeostasis of these neurotransmitters, and their cellular responses to stress, can be disrupted so that an increase or decrease results depending on how stressful events are cognitively processed and encoded. Other notable developments in the neurobiology of clinical depression are related to newer neuroimaging capabilities that have identified brain regions and structures integral to the expression of depressive symptoms such as decreased hippocampal volume (Dean & Keshavan, 2017).

Neuroendocrine and Neuropeptide Hypotheses

Major depressive disorder is associated with multiple endocrine alterations, specifically of the hypothalamic–pituitary–adrenal axis (HPA), the hypothalamic–pituitary–thyroid axis, the hypothalamic–growth hormone axis, and the hypothalamic–pituitary–gonadal axis (Xu et al., 2017). Increased HPA activity is considered the trademark of the human stress response. Sustained hypercortisolism damages the integrity of HPA axis regulation and in doing so plays an important role in the pathophysiology of depression (Zhong et al., 2020). Hyperactivity of the HPA and increased levels of glucocorticoid hormones, features seen in depressed people, are attributed to a disrupted feedback regulation possibly due to altered glucocorticoid receptor functioning. Glucocorticoid receptor involvement in depression is evident in recent research evidence concerning the role of the amygdala in the aetiology of major depression (Farrell et al., 2018). Results obtained from studying post-mortem brain tissue of people diagnosed with major depression showed increased expression of glucocorticoid protein levels in amygdala tissue (Enache et al., 2019). There is mounting evidence that components of neuroendocrine axes (e.g., neuromodulatory peptides such as corticotropin-releasing factor) may contribute to depressive symptoms. Evidence also suggests that the secretion of these hypothalamic and growth hormones is controlled by many of the neurotransmitters implicated in the pathophysiology of depression (Liu et al., 2018).

Psychoneuroimmunology

Psychoneuroimmunology is a recent area of research into a diverse group of proteins known as *chemical messengers* between immune cells. These messengers, called cytokines, signal the brain and serve as mediators between immune and nerve cells. The connection between brain–immune interactions and susceptibility to major depression is a complex and ongoing study (Dean & Keshavan, 2017).

Psychological Theories

Psychodynamic Factors

Most psychodynamic theorists acknowledge some debt to Freud's drive theory, which ascribes the aetiology of depression to an early lack of love, care, warmth, and protection, with resultant anger, guilt, and helplessness turned inward (Fulmer, 2018). A more modern hypothesis about the onset of depression rests on four major presuppositions: (a) Forces behind the scenes are influential. This includes biologic impulses, psychological motives, and cultural pressures. (b) Personality shapes experience. A person's development, preferred defensive processes, and the manifestation of psychological health affect personal experience. (c) The past is powerful. Past relationships shape the lens through which people see future relationships and feelings. (d) Psychic determinism is real. Unawareness and hidden forces impact people's lives (Fulmer, 2018).

Behavioural Factors

Behaviourists hold that depression occurs primarily as the result of a severe reduction in rewarding activities or an increase in unpleasant events in one's life. The resultant depression then leads to further restriction of activity, thereby decreasing the likelihood of experiencing pleasurable activities, which in turn intensifies the mood disturbance.

Developmental Factors

Developmental theorists pose that depression results from early adverse life events that become formed and progressively evolve into core dysfunctional attitudinal patterns, activated in later life by stressful events that lead to depression. Early experiences such as child maltreatment, parental loss possibly through death or emotionally inadequate parenting, as well as other factors such as a disrupted attachment system, and negative familial interactional influences can lead to a vulnerability for major depression (Kuhlman et al., 2020).

Social Theories

Family Factors

Family theorists Wright and Leahey contend that the family is who they say they are (Shajan & Snell, 2019). Wright and Leahey have ascribed maladaptive "circular" patterns in family interactions as contributing to the onset of depression in family members. Disruption to family dynamics deriving from multiple causes can manifest as depression experienced by an individual single family member. Nurses must be vigilant in identifying whether the individual's depressive experience is symptomatic of family distress. In such cases, a "family unit" assessment and assistance may be warranted and, indeed, possibly the best predictor of a positive outcome for the individual (see Chapter 16).

Social Factors

Social isolation, lack of connectedness, diminished sense of belonging, loneliness, and financial distress are all risk factors for ensuing depression (Kok et al., 2018). Depression may also follow loss and adverse or traumatic life events, especially those involving the loss of an important human relationship or role in life. Grieving after the loss of a loved one has been regarded as a normal process unless it endures for inordinate and extensive time periods and ultimately results in the symptoms equated with major depression. The dawn of the *DSM-5* has generated debate related to *grief* and whether or not it warrants labeling as a diagnostic mental disorder. For many, this topic became a contentious issue instigating debate about what "should" be considered normal, and/or normal variations of grieving, and why that should earn entry and be labeled within the rubric of mental disorder. Grief is said to be "an inescapable part" of the human condition and medicalizing what is regarded as normal bereavement has several consequences for the ways that people understand their grief and themselves (Granek, 2017). Pathologizing grief places an unrealistic expectation for how people grieve and how long they grieve. As a result, grief is treated with medications such as antidepressants, antianxiety drugs, and sleeping medications. However, both grief and depression may follow a major loss and possess overlapping features, introducing a complexity to each experience. Thus, the *grief diagnosis* may be thought of as a way to identify any harmful extremes of a grief response in order to facilitate treatment of an associated depression (Bonanno & Malgaroli, 2020). Helping patients process their feelings about a loss gives them the opportunity to understand this experience in a meaningful way and could prevent progression into a depressive episode.

Interdisciplinary Treatment

Although depressive disorders are the most commonly occurring mental disorders, they are usually treated within the primary care setting, not the psychiatric setting. Patients with depression enter mental health settings when their symptoms become so severe that hospitalization is needed, usually for suicide attempts or if they self-refer because of incapacitation. Interprofessional treatment of these disorders, which are often lifelong, needs to include a wide array of health professionals in all areas. The specific goals of treatment are to:

- Reduce/control symptoms and, if possible, eliminate signs and symptoms of the depressive syndrome;
- Improve occupational and psychosocial functioning as much as possible; and
- Reduce the likelihood of relapse and recurrence.

Priority Care Issues

The overriding concern for people with mood disorders is safety. In depressive disorders, suicide risk must be evaluated and suicide assessments should be done frequently to protect the patient (see Chapter 20).

Family Response to Disorder

Depression in one family member has a far-reaching impact and affects the whole family. Spouses, children, parents, siblings, and friends experience frustration, guilt, anger, and even their own mental health issues when the functional ability of a family member is compromised by depression. It is often difficult for others to understand the depth of the low mood and how disabling it can be. Financial hardship can occur when the family member cannot work and spends days in bed. The lack of understanding and challenges of living with a person with depression can lead to family estrangement. Nurses can be facilitators in three key areas for families: recognizing and ensuring appropriate distance among family members so adequate reflection about the illness can occur, encouraging daily stability and structure, and fostering transparent communication among family members (Zhang, 2018).

Nursing Management: Human Response to Depressive Disorder

The diagnosis of major depressive disorder is made when *DSM-5* criteria are met. An awareness of the risk factors for depression, a comprehensive bio/psycho/social/spiritual assessment, and a history of the patient's illness and any past treatment are key to formulating a treatment plan and evaluating outcomes. Interviewing a family member or close friend about the patient's day-to-day functioning and specific symptoms may be helpful in determining the course of the illness, current symptoms, and level of functioning.

Depression during pregnancy and the postpartum period warrants special consideration. A mood disorder in these contexts is particularly important to identify and treat because it has the potential to disrupt the maternal–foetal bond as well as the postpartum maternal–infant bond. Such outcomes also have negative ramifications for infant attachment, which in turn can affect the infant's mental health and developmental trajectory (Apter et al., 2017; Flowers et al., 2018). Infants need an environment that supports and nurtures their capabilities for emotional regulation, one that is protective and fosters a positive developmental trajectory. Symptoms of depression can inhibit the mother's ability to respond sensitively to the infant (Dau et al., 2019). However, treating women who are pregnant and women in the postpartum phase with antidepressant medications presents a unique challenge due to the potential effects of these medications on the foetus and breast-feeding infants. When decisional conflict arises about this topic, a risk and benefit discussion about both the impact of the medications and untreated maternal depression is always necessary (Barker et al., 2020). It is important that nurses not express judgment toward people who choose to take antidepressants during pregnancy (Schmied, 2020).

Biologic Domain

Assessment

Symptoms of depression can be similar to some medical problems or side effects of medication therapies; therefore, a biologic assessment must include a physical systems review and thorough history of medical problems, with special attention to central nervous system function, endocrine function, anaemia, chronic pain, autoimmune illness, diabetes, or menopause. Additional medical history includes surgeries, medical hospitalizations, head injuries, episodes of loss of consciousness, and pregnancies, childbirths, miscarriages, and abortions. Also, a complete list of prescribed, over-the-counter (OTC) medications and herbal supplements should be compiled, including the reason for taking them. Information about the frequency and dosage of prescribed OTC medications and supplements should be obtained, and any abrupt discontinuation of medications warrants further assessment. With depressive disorders, the nurse must always assess the lethality of the medication being taken. For example, if a patient has sleep medications at home, the patient should be questioned about the number of pills in the bottle. The use of alcohol, marijuana, other mood-altering medications, as well as herbal substances must be assessed as they can cause drug–drug interactions (see Chapter 13).

Physical examination is recommended with baseline vital signs and laboratory tests, which include a comprehensive blood chemistry panel, complete blood count, liver function tests, thyroid function tests, urinalysis, and electrocardiogram. Biologic assessment also includes evaluating the patient for the characteristic neurovegetative symptoms listed below.

- *Appetite and weight changes* are a set criterion in major depression (APA, 2013): Changes from baseline can include decrease or increase in appetite with or without significant weight loss or gain (i.e., a change of more than 5% of body weight in 1 month). Weight loss occurs when not dieting, and weight gain presents more as an atypical feature of depression. Older adults with moderate to severe depression need to be assessed for dehydration as well as weight changes.
- *Sleep disturbance*: The most common sleep disturbance associated with major depression is insomnia. *DSM-5* (APA, 2013) addresses varied forms of insomnia, such as initial insomnia (difficulty falling asleep), middle insomnia (waking up during the night and having difficulty returning to sleep), or terminal insomnia (waking too early and being unable to return to sleep). Additionally, there can be hypersomnia (prolonged sleep episodes at night or increased daytime sleep). The patient, with either insomnia or hypersomnia, complains of not feeling rested upon awakening (see Chapter 28).
- *Decreased energy, tiredness, and fatigue*: Fatigue associated with depression is a subjective experience of feeling tired regardless of how much sleep or physical activity a person has had. Even the smallest tasks require substantial effort (APA, 2013).
- *Loss of interest or pleasure* is to some degree always present (APA, 2013): Activities that brought pleasure in the past (e.g., hobbies, golfing, etc.) hold no interest in periods of depression.
- *Difficulty thinking, concentrating, or making decisions*: Problems associated with memory, focus, and decision-making can contribute to difficulties with concentration and the completion of tasks. As a result of difficulties with decision-making, individuals may actively avoid having to make decisions as a coping strategy.

Physical assessment should also include current weight, noting any changes, and assessment of loss of appetite, sleep habits and related disturbances, fatigue factors, and loss of interest.

Nursing Care Foci for the Biologic Domain

Nursing care foci within the biologic domain are formulated based upon assessment data and include sleep (insomnia and hypersomnia), nutrition imbalances, fatigue, nausea, activity intolerance, treatment nonadherence, and loss of libido.

Interventions for Biologic Domain

Prolonged periods of disturbed sleep patterns and nutritional imbalances worsen the progression of depressive disorders. Counseling and education should be aimed at establishing normal sleep patterns and healthy nutrition to help patients move toward remission or recovery. Health teaching about physical care should focus on encouraging patients to practice positive sleep hygiene measures such as avoiding any caffeine intake prior to sleep and avoiding the use of electronics in bed (see Chapter 28). Patients should be encouraged to regularly eat well-balanced meals. Regular activity and exercise are also critical for improving depressed mood state. Most people find that regular exercise is hard to maintain, and people who are depressed may find it impossible. When teaching about exercise, it is important to start with the patient's current activity level and increase it slowly. For example, if the patient is spending most of the time in bed, encouraging the patient to get dressed every day and walk for 5 or 10 min may be all that the patient can tolerate. Gradually, patients should be encouraged to have a regular exercise programme.

Pharmacologic Interventions

A cornerstone of treatment for mood disorders is pharmacologic intervention with antidepressants and mood stabilizers. Patients may be reluctant to take prescribed medications or may self-treat with medications, substances, and/or alcohol. Adherence with medication regimens, emphasizing any potential drug–drug interactions should always be included in the patient teaching plan. A complete discussion of antidepressants and mood stabilizers as well as the nurse's role related to them is found in Chapter 13.

Other Biologic Interventions

*Biologic treatment*s, the term applied to treatments working at a somatic or physical level, are nonpharmacologic in nature. Historically, somatic therapies were developed and used as treatments to change the physiologic mechanisms thought to be the prevailing cause of psychiatric disorders. Early somatic treatments believed to relieve mania, psychosis, and depressive symptoms included insulin or atropine coma, hemodialysis, hyperbaric oxygen therapy, continuous sleep therapy, lobotomies, as well as ether and carbon dioxide inhalation therapies. Seizures were also noted to improve some psychiatric symptoms, and this effect led to seizure induction as a treatment modality. Camphor-induced seizures, prevalent in the 16th century, were used to reduce psychosis and mania symptoms. Other chemicals administered as inhalants were also used to induce a seizure, but difficulty controlling their adverse reactions and sometimes fatal results rendered them prohibitive. The advent of pharmacologic therapies replaced these somatic treatments apart from electroconvulsive therapy (ECT), which has remained an efficacious and safely used treatment for depression. ECT is one of several neuromodulatory approaches (i.e., modulates the activity of neural networks implicated in the pathophysiology of depression) to treat depression. In the past 10 years, new neuromodulatory modalities have emerged such as repetitive transcranial magnetic stimulation (rTMS) (Brunoni et al., 2019) and vagus nerve stimulation (VNS) (Kong et al., 2018). These modalities developed in conjunction with advances in engineering and neuro-

imaging, and they show some promise as research continues to investigate their efficacy as future treatments for depression (Brunoni et al., 2019). Other biologic interventions such as phototherapy and nutritional therapy are gaining some acceptance too but remain under inquiry.

Electroconvulsive Therapy

ECT was formally introduced in Italy in 1938 to treat mental illness. Each year, over one million people in the world receive ECT as treatment (Read et al., 2019). ECT, however, is not a first-line treatment for depression but rather used to treat patients whose disorder is refractory, patients who are intolerant to initial drug treatments, and patients who are so severely ill that rapid treatment is required (e.g., patients with malnutrition, catatonia, or suicidality). ECT is also used in other disorders, such as mania and schizophrenia, when other treatments have failed. Although patients with a severe form of depression, with psychosis present, are considered the best candidates for ECT, reliable predictors of a person's response to this modality remain unclear.

The ECT procedure involves the administration of a muscle relaxant followed by an anaesthetic. An electrical current is then passed through the brain to produce generalized seizures lasting 25 to 150 s. A brief pulse stimulus, administered unilaterally on the nondominant side of the head, is associated with less confusion post ECT. However, some individual patients require bilateral treatment for effective resolution of depressive symptoms. Bilateral lead placement, with increased voltage, is associated with more negative cognitive outcomes (Li et al., 2020b; Vasavada et al., 2017). Seizure induction appears to be necessary to produce positive treatment outcomes. Individual seizure thresholds vary and increase with age; therefore, the electrical impulse and treatment method also may differ. Typically, the lowest possible electrical stimulus necessary to produce seizure activity is used. Blood pressure and ECG monitoring occur during the procedure. The ECT procedure is repeated two or three times weekly, usually for 6 to 12 treatments in total. Twice-weekly regimes are favoured because they produce less accumulative memory loss. After symptoms have improved, an aggressive trial of antidepressant medications is used for relapse prevention. Some patients who cannot tolerate or do not respond to antidepressant treatment may go on maintenance ECT treatments where once-weekly treatments are gradually decreased to once monthly. ECT can be administered to inpatients and outpatients.

The exact antidepressant action of ECT is unclear. Positron emission tomography (PET) scans show an increase in glucose and blood flow followed by a marked decrease, particularly in the frontal lobes. This decreased blood flow is a mechanism thought to have antidepressant effects. ECT also affects all neurotransmitters, but it particularly downregulates β-adrenergic receptors in much the same way as do antidepressant medications. However, unlike antidepressant therapy, ECT produces an upregulation in serotonin, especially 5-HT$_2$. Additionally, ECT also exerts other effects on neurochemistry, including increased influx of calcium and effects on second messenger systems (Ostroff et al., 2019).

Brief, usually transient episodes of hypotension or hypertension, bradycardia or tachycardia, and minor arrhythmias are among the adverse effects that may occur during and immediately after the procedure. Cognitive side effects include *transient postictal* ("after seizure") *disorientation* that clears in minutes to hours (Porter et al., 2020). Common aftereffects from ECT include headache, nausea, and muscle pain. Memory loss or disturbance is the most troublesome effect of ECT with *anterograde amnesia* (amnesia for events occurring during and soon after a course of ECT) that varies in severity. In this context, a patient might find a diary helpful. Other possible cognitive effects are *short-term retrograde amnesia* (gaps in memory about things occurring a few weeks or months before the ECT) that usually clears within weeks and *retrograde memory loss* (persistent, severe memory deficits) that rarely occurs (Porter et al., 2020). Many patients experience no amnesia at all. Since memory loss is a symptom of untreated depression, it can present as a confounding factor in determining the extent of memory deficits related to ECT.

ECT is contraindicated in patients with an increased intracranial pressure. Risk also increases in patients with recent myocardial infarction, recent cerebrovascular accident, retinal detachment, or pheochromocytoma (an adrenal cortex tumour) and in patients at high risk for complications from anaesthesia. The nursing care for patients undergoing ECT is to provide educational and emotional support for the patient and family, assess baseline or pretreatment levels of functioning, prepare the patient for the ECT process, and monitor and evaluate the patient's response to the treatment and communicate it to the ECT team so treatment modifications can occur if necessary.

New Somatic (Neuromodulatory) Therapies

Repetitive transcranial magnetic stimulation (rTMS) and VNS are two recognized somatic treatments for depression. Both directly affect brain activity by stimulating nerve cell firing rates. Transcranial magnetic stimulation was introduced in 1985 as a noninvasive, painless method to stimulate the cerebral cortex. Rapidly alternating magnetic fields are applied to the scalp at subconvulsive levels. Underlying this procedure is the hypothesis that a time-varying magnetic field will induce an electrical field, which, in brain tissue, activates the inhibitory and excitatory neurons thereby modulating

neuroplasticity in the brain (Lefaucheur et al., 2020). The low-frequency electrical stimulation from rTMS triggers lasting anticonvulsant effects in rats, and the therapeutic benefits of rTMS in humans are considered related to action like that produced by anticonvulsant medication. rTMS relies on the cumulative effects of intermittent application that may occur four to five times a week for 40 min while the patient is awake (Lefaucheur et al., 2020). rTMS stimulation of the brain's prefrontal cortex may help some depressed patients in much the same way as ECT but without the cognitive side effects. Thus, it has been proposed as an alternative to ECT in managing symptoms of depression. Research is mixed about the efficacy of this procedure, and more investigation about it as a treatment modality is necessary. Side effects of rTMS include scalp pain, mild headaches, and dizziness (Hett et al., 2020).

VNS is a new somatic treatment that requires the surgical implantation of a pulse generator that delivers chronic intermittent electrical signals at low frequency to the vagus nerve (Lv et al., 2019). VNS was initially used for treatment refractory epilepsy, and mood improvement was noted in patients with epilepsy that received this treatment (Lv et al., 2019). For years, scientists have been interested in identifying how autonomic functions modulate activity in the limbic system and higher cortex. The vagus nerve has traditionally been considered a parasympathetic efferent nerve responsible only for regulating autonomic functions, such as heart rate and gastric tone. However, the vagus nerve (cranial nerve X) also carries sensory information to the brain from the head, neck, thorax, and abdomen. Research identified that the vagus nerve has extensive projections of its sensory afferent connections to many brain areas. Although the basic mechanism of action of VNS is unknown, incoming sensory, or afferent, connections of the left vagus nerve directly project into many of the very same brain regions implicated in depressive disorders. It is also thought that VNS changes levels of several neurotransmitters implicated in the development of major depression, including serotonin, norepinephrine, GABA, and glutamate. Chronic VNS may cause side effects such as voice alteration, cough, pharyngitis, throat discomfort, dyspnea, headache, nausea, and vomiting (Müller et al., 2018). Presently, it is used as a supplemental treatment for chronic refractory depression (Johnson & Wilson, 2018).

Other Somatic Treatments

Light Therapy (Phototherapy)

Another somatic therapy is phototherapy, used in seasonal affective disorder. Human circadian rhythms are set by time clues (zeitgebers) inside and outside the body (Nussbaumer-Streit et al., 2019). One of the most powerful regulators of these body patterns is the cycle of daylight and darkness. Individuals vulnerable to seasonal depression may experience disturbances either in these normal body patterns or in circadian rhythms. They usually have symptoms that are somewhat different from classic depression, such as irritability, fatigue, and increased need to sleep, increased appetite and weight gain, and carbohydrate craving. Administering artificial light to such patients during winter months has reduced these depressive symptoms (Maruani & Geoffroy, 2019).

Phototherapy involves exposing the patient to a specific type of artificial light source to relieve seasonal depression. Artificial light is believed to trigger a shift in the patient's circadian rhythm to an earlier time. The light source must be very bright, full-spectrum light, usually 2,500 lux, which is about 200 times brighter than normal indoor lighting. Harmful ultraviolet light is filtered out. Exposure to this light source has produced improvement and relief of depressive symptoms for significant numbers of seasonally depressed individuals. It does not produce change for individuals who are not seasonally depressed. Morning phototherapy is thought to produce a better response than either evening or morning and evening timing of the phototherapy session (Nussbaumer-Streit et al., 2019). Light banks with full-spectrum light are readily available. Light visors, visors containing small, full-spectrum light bulbs that shine on the eyelids, have also been developed. The patient is instructed to sit in front of light banks at about 3 ft, engaging in a variety of other activities, but glancing directly into the light every few minutes. This action should be done immediately on rising and is most effective before 8 a.m. The duration of administration may begin with as little as 30 min and increase to 2 to 5 h. One to two hours is usually sufficient, and the antidepressant response begins in 1 to 4 days, with the full effect usually complete after 2 weeks. Full antidepressant effect is usually maintained with daily sessions of 30 min.

Side effects of phototherapy are rare, but eyestrain, headache, and insomnia are possible. An ophthalmologist should be consulted if the patient has a preexisting eye disorder. In rare instances, phototherapy has been reported to produce mania. Melatonin may also be used in conjunction with phototherapy to treat seasonal affective disorder (Nussbaumer-Streit et al., 2019). Follow-up visits with the phototherapy prescriber are necessary to help manage side effects and assess positive results.

Nutritional Therapies

The neurotransmitters necessary for normal healthy functioning are produced from amino acids absorbed from the foods we eat. Nutritional deficiencies, such as deficits in iron, folic acid, pantothenic acid, magnesium, vitamin C, or biotin, may produce symptoms of psychiatric disorders such as fatigue, apathy, and depression.

Logically, treating these deficiencies with nutritional supplements should improve the psychiatric symptoms. In 1967, Linus Pauling espoused this idea as a theory and posited psychiatric disorders were caused by an ascorbic acid deficiency. He implemented *megavitamin therapy* or *orthomolecular therapy* as a treatment for schizophrenia that included administering large doses of ascorbic acid and other vitamins. Initial interest in Pauling's hypothesis resulted in scepticism when his research and claims could not be proven. Research about the role of vitamins as a treatment for depression continues. Some moderate, short-term improvement in depressive symptoms and quality of life noted when methylated vitamin B complex was administered to patients diagnosed with an MDE or a related depressive disorder (Mikkelsen et al., 2016). Others have speculated that depression may be caused by oxidative stress, and they suggest that treatment to reduce this process with antioxidants, such as vitamin E and curcumin, may be effective in mitigating depression (Li et al., 2017; Zhang et al., 2020).

Previous theories purported that diets and specific foods control behaviour. High sugar intake was thought to produce hyperactivity in children, and Benjamin Feingold developed a diet to eliminate food additives he believed increased hyperactivity. Recent advances in technology led researchers to identify dietary precursors for the bioamines. As an example, tryptophan (5-HTP), a dietary precursor of serotonin, has been extensively investigated in relation to low serotonin levels. Some patients with mild depression and insomnia respond to tryptophan (100 mg to 2 g daily), which has been used as an adjunct to antidepressant drugs (Samad et al., 2019).

Many patients are turning to dietary herbal preparations to address psychiatric symptoms. More than 17% of the adult population has used herbal preparations to address their mood or emotions. Dietary herbal preparations such as St. John's wort are used to treat depression. Ng et al. (2017) conducted a meta-analysis of the effectiveness and safety of St John's wort extract and found this herbal remedy had comparable efficacy as SSRIs for mild to moderate depression. However, more research in this area is needed. Unlike pharmaceutical supplements, however, herbal preparations are often unregulated; therefore, the bioactive compounds available may vary significantly. Nurses, using a nonjudgmental approach, must assess phytomedicinal use by the patient during the initial assessment to determine any drug interactions and to understand the patient's treatment preferences.

Medications may also influence the development of nutritional deficiencies that may worsen psychiatric symptoms. For example, drugs with strong anticholinergic actions (i.e., tricyclic antidepressants, antipsychotics, and antiepileptics) often produce impaired or enhanced gastric motility, which may lead to the generalized malabsorption of vitamins and minerals. Additionally, many nutritional supplements have toxicities of their own when given in excess. For example, daily ingestion of more than 100 mg pyridoxine (vitamin B_6) can produce neurotoxic symptoms, photosensitivity, and ataxia (Hemmiger & Wills, 2021). Robust research is needed to identify how the underlying mechanisms of supplements and dietary precursors of the bioamines are related to mood, behaviour, and psychopharmacologic medications. It is important for nurses to recognize that diet can affect mood and behaviour, and dietary supplements have the potential to cause drug–drug interaction.

Psychosocial Issues in all Biologic Treatments

Many factors influence the success of medication and other biologic therapies and notably adherence. Adherence refers to following the therapeutic regimen, self-administering medications as prescribed, keeping appointments, and following other treatment suggestions. It exists on a continuum and can be conceived of as full, partial, or absent.

Psychological Domain

Assessment

The mental status examination is an effective clinical tool to evaluate the psychological aspects of major depression, which causes disturbances in mood, affect, thought processes and content, cognition, memory, and attention. The comprehensive mental status examination is described in detail in Chapter 11.

Mood

The person with depression has a sustained period of feeling depressed, sad, or hopeless and may experience anhedonia (loss of interest or pleasure). The patient may report "not caring anymore" or not feeling any enjoyment in activities that were previously considered pleasurable. In some individuals, this may include a decrease in or loss of libido and sexual function. Depressed mood may be severe enough to provoke thoughts of suicide.

Numerous assessment scales are available for assessing depression. Easily administered self-report questionnaires can be valuable detection tools. These questionnaires cannot be the sole basis for making a diagnosis of MDE, but they are sensitive to depressive symptoms. A commonly used self-report scale questionnaire is the Beck Depression Inventory (BDI). The Hamilton Rating Scale for Depression (HAM-D; see Appendix E) is a clinician-completed rating scale often used and may be somewhat more precise than self-report questionnaires in detecting depression (Hamilton, 1986).

Thought Content

Individuals with depression often have an unrealistic, negative evaluation of their worth or have guilty preoccupations or ruminations about minor past failings. Neutral or trivial day-to-day events are interpreted as evidence of personal defects and contain an exaggerated sense of responsibility for untoward events. As a result, feelings of being helplessness, hopelessness, worthlessness, and powerlessness may ensue. Thus, an exploration of the patient's perspective on self, the world, and the future should be included in the overall assessment, as should the possible occurrence of disorganized thought processes (e.g., tangential or circumstantial thinking) and perceptual disturbances (e.g., hallucinations, delusions).

Suicidal Behaviour

Patients with major depressive disorder are high risk for suicide. Suicide risk is dynamic and should be assessed initially and throughout the course of treatment. It is important for the nurse to distinguish between thoughts, planning, and intent. Suicidal ideation can be passive in nature with thoughts that range from a belief that others would be better off if the person were dead, to active thoughts of death with an organized plan for committing suicide. The frequency, intensity, and lethality of these thoughts may vary and can help determine the seriousness of intent. The more specific the plan and the more accessible the means, the more serious is the intent. Risk factors that must be carefully considered are the availability and adequacy of social supports, history of suicidal ideation or behaviour, presence of psychosis or substance abuse, and decreased ability to control suicidal impulses. Importantly, behavioural indicators toward suicide, such as hoarding medications to overdose, need to be determined and immediately addressed. Questioning to verify behavioural indicators determines whether the person has a plan and is acting on it. Such questions should be interfaced with a deliberate suicide risk assessment (see Chapter 20).

Cognition and Memory

Many individuals with depression report an impaired ability to think, concentrate, or make decisions. They may appear easily distracted or complain of memory difficulties. In older adults with major depressive disorder, memory difficulties may be the chief complaint and may be mistaken for early signs of a dementia. When the depression is fully treated, the memory problem often improves or fully resolves.

Nursing Care Foci for the Psychological Domain

Nursing care foci in the psychological domain with patients with depression are numerous. They include loss of self-worth, loss of self-identity, and loss of self-esteem; hopelessness; grief; coping impairment; and safety. Assessment data of patients with depression may reveal that they are at risk for self-harm and/or suicide, which requires a thorough suicide risk assessment.

Interventions for Psychological Domain

Often pharmacotherapy is used in conjunction with psychosocial and psychoeducational treatments. The most effective therapies for patients with severe or recurrent major depressive disorder are combinations of psychotherapy (including interpersonal therapy [IPT], cognitive–behavioural therapy [CBT], behaviour therapy) and pharmacotherapy. Adding a course of CBT may be an adjunct strategy for preventing relapse in patients who have had only a partial response to pharmacotherapy alone (see Chapter 13). Moreover, a combination of medication and psychotherapy may be particularly useful in more complex situations (e.g., depression in the context of concurrent, chronic general medical or other psychiatric disorders or in patients who fail to respond completely to either treatment alone). Further, depressive symptomatology can be complicated by stressful lifestyle circumstances, perhaps presenting as work related or located in social aspects of an individual's life. CBT and other psychotherapies (individual, marital, or group) can be helpful in addressing such situational life complexities. Mindfulness-based cognitive therapy is increasingly valued as a supportive intervention modality that can be implemented in community health programmes by nurse therapists (Williams et al., 2015).

Therapeutic Relationship

One of the most effective therapeutic tools for treating any psychiatric disorder is the therapeutic alliance, a helpful and trusting relationship between clinician and patient. The alliance is built from several activities, including the following:

- Establishment and maintenance of a supportive relationship
- Availability in times of crisis
- Vigilance regarding dangerousness to self and/or others
- Education about the illness and treatment goals
- Encouragement and feedback concerning progress
- Guidance regarding the patient's interactions with the personal and work environment
- Realistic goal setting and monitoring

Interacting with patients with depression can be challenging because they tend to be withdrawn and have difficulty expressing feelings and engaging in interpersonal interactions. The therapeutic alliance partly depends on winning the patient's trust through a warm and empathic stance within the context of professional

boundaries (see Chapter 7). Understanding the individual's personal experience of receiving a psychiatric diagnosis enables the nurse to respond more effectively.

Cognitive Therapy

Cognitive therapy is successful in reducing depressive symptoms during the acute phase of major depression (APA, 2013). Techniques such as monitoring thoughts, emotions, and actions are used to identify irrational, distorted thinking and beliefs (see Chapter 14). The use of cognitive therapy in the acute phase of treatment, combined with medication, has grown in the past few years. Cognitive therapy is also considered first-line treatment for outpatients with mild to moderate depression. Varied modalities for implementing cognitive therapy have been made convenient through computer-assisted technology, with some early promise in this area and more research needed. For example, a meta-analysis of the research in computerized CBT demonstrated short-term reduction in depression but no significant long-term clinical and functional outcomes for patients with mood disorders (Chiang et al., 2017).

Behaviour Therapy

Behaviour therapy for depression encompasses behavioural activation techniques, which are effective in the treatment of patients with depression and particularly when they are combined with pharmacotherapy (Bot et al., 2019). Therapeutic techniques include activity scheduling, self-control therapy, social skills training, and problem solving.

Interpersonal Therapy

IPT is a form of brief therapy that is used to recognize, explore, and resolve any current interpersonal losses, role confusion and transitions, social isolation, and deficits in social skills that may precipitate depressive states (Stuart & Robertson, 2012). It is based on a biopsychosocial stress-diathesis model. In IPT, losses must be mourned and related affects appreciated, role confusion and transitions must be recognized and resolved, and social skills deficits must be overcome to acquire social supports (Zhou et al., 2017).

Family and Marital Therapy

Patients who experience high family stress are at risk for greater future severity of illness, increased utilization of health services, and higher healthcare expenses. Family and marital problems may be an outcome of major depressive disorders but can also increase susceptibility to the disorder and, in some instances, inhibit recovery. Assisting the adjustment of the partner, and of all family members, may be invaluable in averting a relapse of depression for the recovering patient. Since marital and family problems are common among patients with mood disorders; comprehensive treatment requires that these problems be assessed and interventions suggested to ensure the family is part of the therapeutic system. Many family–nursing interventions (see Chapter 16) may be used by the nurse in providing targeted family-centred care. These include

- Monitoring patient and family for indicators of stress
- Teaching stress management techniques
- Counseling family members on coping skills for their own use
- Providing necessary knowledge of options and support services
- Facilitating family routines and rituals
- Assisting family to resolve feelings of guilt
- Assisting family with conflict resolution
- Identifying family strengths and resources with family members
- Facilitating communication among family members

Group Therapy

The role of group therapy in treating depression is based on clinical experience rather than on systematic, controlled studies. It may be particularly useful for depression associated with bereavement or chronic medical illness (Maass et al., 2020). Patients may benefit from the example of others who have dealt successfully with similar losses or challenges. Survivors can gain self-esteem as successful role models for new group members. Medication support groups can provide information to the patient and to family members regarding prognosis and medication issues, thereby providing a psychoeducational forum (see Chapter 15).

Teaching Patients and Families

Patients with depression and their close family members often incorrectly believe that their illness is their own fault and that they should be able to "pull themselves up by their bootstraps" or "snap out of it." It is vital to educate patients and their families about the nature, prognosis, and treatment of depression to dispel these false beliefs and unnecessary associated guilt (Gautam et al., 2017).

Patients need to know the full range of suitable treatment options before consenting to participate in treatment. Nurses can provide opportunities for patients to question, discuss, and explore their feelings about past, current, and planned use of medications and other treatments. Developing strategies to enhance adherence and to raise awareness of early signs of relapse can be important aids to making treatment more effective.

Social Domain

Assessment

Social assessment focuses on the patient's developmental history, family psychiatric history, patterns of relationship, education and work history, the quality of their support system, and the impact of physical or sexual abuse on their interpersonal functioning (see Chapter 11). Depression can colour a patient's perception of the quality of their relationships; therefore, including a family member or close friend in the assessment process can be helpful. Changes in patterns of relating (especially social withdrawal) and changes in occupational functioning are commonly reported and may represent a significant deterioration from baseline behaviour. Increased use of "sick days" may occur. The family's level of support and understanding of the disorder also need to be assessed.

Nursing Care Foci for the Social Domain

The focus of nursing care in the social domain may include impairment in role performance and family coping, challenges with activities of daily living, and caregiver fatigue (if the patient is also a caregiver).

Interventions for Social Domain

Patients experiencing depression often withdraw from daily activities such as engaging in family routines, attending work, and participating in community events. During hospitalization, patients often withdraw to their rooms and refuse to participate in unit activities. Nurses are challenged to help the patient balance the need for privacy with the need to return to normal social functioning. Patients with depression should never be approached in an overly enthusiastic manner; this approach may be irritating and block communication. On the other hand, patients should be encouraged to set realistic goals to reconnect with family and community. Explaining to patients the importance of attending social activities, however, much they may not feel like doing so, will promote the recovery process.

Milieu Therapy

While hospitalized, milieu therapy (see Chapter 12) helps patients with depression maintain socialization skills and continue to interact with others. When depressed, people are often unaware of their environment and withdraw into themselves. On a psychiatric unit, patients with depression should be encouraged to attend and participate in unit activities. These individuals have a decreased energy level and thus may be moving more slowly than others; however, their efforts should be acknowledged.

Safety

In many cases, patients are admitted to an acute mental health unit because of a suicide attempt. Suicide risk is dynamic and should continually be evaluated, especially at transition points in the patient's care such as when there is a change in the care level, prior to anticipated leaves from hospital, and at discharge. During the depths of depression, patients may not have the energy to complete a suicide, but as they begin to feel better, and their energy increases, they may be at a greater risk. If a previously depressed patient appears to have become energized overnight, they may have decided to commit suicide and thus may be relieved the decision is finally made. The nurse may misinterpret the mood improvement as a positive move toward recovery; however, this patient may be very intent on suicide. Emphasis is always on protecting the patient and ensuring the development of a strong therapeutic alliance, which fosters a hopeful milieu. Ongoing, careful monitoring must take place to maintain safety. It is imperative to collaborate with the patient in the development of a written suicide safety plan to help the patient stay safe in the hospital and community (see Chapter 20).

Consumer-Oriented Interventions

Nurses are exceptionally well positioned to engage patients and their families in the active process of improving daily functioning, increasing knowledge and skill acquisition, and increasing independent living. Consumer-oriented support groups can help to enhance the self-esteem and the support network of participating patients and their families. Advice, encouragement, and the sense of group camaraderie may make an important contribution to recovery. Organizations providing support and information about depression (and bipolar disorder) include the Canadian Mental Health Association (CMHA), Canadian Alliance on Mental Illness and Mental Health, the Mood Disorders Society of Canada (MDSC), the Native Mental Health Association of Canada (NMHAC), and the Organization for Bipolar Affective Disorders (OBAD). Many other internet resources are available that can provide patients and families with education and support for mood disorders (see Web Links section below).

Interventions for Family Members

The family needs education and support during and after the treatment of a family member with depression. Nurses should be attentive to family distress and caregiver burden and provide appropriate support and education. Because major depressive disorder can recur, the family needs information about specific antecedents to a family member's depression and what steps to take should decompensation occur. For example, one patient may routinely become depressed during the fall of each

year, with the initial symptom manifesting as excessive sleepiness. For another patient, a major loss, such as a child going to college or the death of a pet, may precipitate a depressive episode. Families of older patients need to be aware of the possibility of depression and related symptoms, which may occur after such triggering events as the death of a friend or relative. Families of children who are depressed often misinterpret depression as behaviour problems.

Spiritual Domain

Understanding the relevance of spirituality in today's varied arenas of "pluralistic" health care can be daunting and even problematic, particularly given the varied interpretations of spirituality as a concept. Paine and Sandage (2017) recognizes that aspects of spirituality and religion overlap and correlate with less stress, decreased depression, decreased suicide, as well as better coping. Moreover, essential constructs associated with spirituality such as forgiveness, flourishing, and resilience may serve as protective factors in mental health recovery (Pandey et al., 2020). However, religion can also increase guilt and despair in some people who view themselves as failures when they are unable to live up to the high standards of their faith. Therefore, health care providers must consider the religious and spiritual activities of their patients and recognize the potential of spirituality as both an important mental health resource and possible stressor (Oxhandler & Parrish, 2018).

Assessment

Spirituality involves thoughts and feelings that contribute meaning, purpose, connectedness, and hope about one's existence (Ransome, 2020). Spirituality is an important social determinant that drives holistic health care (Ransome, 2020). When a person experiences depression, they may have despairing thoughts and express a lack of spiritual wellbeing. Conducting a spiritual assessment facilitates exploration of how this integral component is related to the patient's mental health recovery (Milner et al., 2020). The intensely personal and intimate nature of this domain justifies a cautionary and tentative approach. Patients with mood disorders may feel especially guarded in discussing their spirituality, fearing that clinicians may belittle or "pathologize" their experience. In attending to the spiritual domain, Timmins and Caldeira (2017) have endorsed an initial basic spiritual screening, and then if deemed advisable, this screening should be followed by an in-depth spiritual assessment.

Spiritual Screening and In-depth Assessment

An initial spiritual screening can determine the persons' basic needs related to their religious affiliation and if they desire additional attention in this domain.

Queries posed tentatively and with sensitivity are more likely to have the desired effect of eliciting concerns, should they exist. This initial assessment gives an indication of whether spirituality is an organizing principle in the depressed person's life and if further assessment is appropriate (Timmins & Caldeira, 2017). Spiritual screening questions may include those developed from the collective feedback of a focus group composed of mental health providers and consumers tasked to delineate spiritual assessment questions: Is spirituality, religion, or faith important to you? Has your spirituality, religion, or faith been in your past? Is it something that you would like to explore as part of your mental health recovery? (Timmins & Caldeira, 2017). The predominant focus in a spiritual assessment is directly on the patient's understanding of spirituality and its importance in their lives. The intent of the assessment is an exploration of the person's religious history and/or spiritual practice and how they might wish to have spiritual concerns included in their recovery work (Timmins & Caldeira, 2017). Within an interprofessional context, this exploration may also default to (or be done in consultation with) pastoral counsellors or clinicians deemed most proficient in addressing the spiritual dimension of a patient's experience. The spiritual assessment can also help to determine if more support for the patient is necessary, such as ensuring contact with a religious representative (e.g., minister, priest, chaplain, elder, imam, rabbi). If indicated, a spiritual assessment can be followed by an in-depth spiritual history using a tool that identifies themes in the patient's spiritual concerns and recognizes the impact of those concerns on the patient's condition (Borneman et al., 2010). A broadly used and researched model of spiritual history taking, implemented to help establish relevant care, is based on the acronym FICA: "**F**—faith, presence of faith and specific beliefs that give the person's life meaning. **I**—importance; what is the importance and influence of faith and beliefs on the person's life? **C**—community, is there any spiritual or religious community involvement? **A**—address in care, how can healthcare providers use the information about spirituality in the person's care? (Borneman et al., 2010, p. 166).

Nursing Care Foci for the Spiritual Domain

Nursing care within the spiritual domain focuses on distress of the spirit. Very often these are situation specific. Within the realm of mood disorders, these are often expressed as disturbances in one's belief system related to loss of hope, uncertainty about the meaning of life, suffering, discouragement, and despair.

Interventions for Spiritual Domain

Spiritual interventions can have positive outcomes for patients suffering depression and other mood disorders.

Where need presents, appropriate people can intervene with patients by way of guided conversations, personal life storytelling, and ritual experiences. Spiritual activities can be encouraged, including prayer, the reading of religious texts, and attendance at devotional services or ceremonies. Such care modalities may serve to relieve distress, make meaning of suffering, nurture hope, promote spiritual resolution, and foster wellness.

Evaluation and Treatment Outcomes

The major goals of treatment are to help the patient to be as independent as possible and to achieve stability, remission, and recovery from major depression. It is often a lifelong struggle for the individual. An ongoing evaluation of the patient's symptoms, functioning, and quality of life should be carefully documented in the patient's record to monitor treatment outcomes.

Continuum of Care

If the prevalence of major depressive disorders in Western countries escalates, it is not unrealistic to speculate that demands for services will increasingly threaten the capacity for service delivery (Bickman, 2020). Nurses can expect to encounter individuals with depressive disorders in all areas of practice. Initially, they may present in inpatient and outpatient medical and primary care settings, emergency departments (EDs), and inpatient and outpatient mental health settings (see Chapter 5). Thus nurses must be able to recognize depression in their patients and make appropriate interventions or referrals. The continuum of care, however, goes beyond these settings and may include partial hospitalization or day treatment programmes; individual, family, or group psychotherapy; home visits; and psychopharmacotherapy. Although most patients with major depression are treated in outpatient settings, brief hospitalization may be required if the patient is suicidal or psychotic.

Nurses working on inpatient units provide a wide range of direct services, including administering and monitoring medications and monitoring target symptoms, conducting psychoeducational groups, and, more generally, structuring and maintaining a therapeutic environment. Community nurses are well situated to detect undiagnosed depressive disorders and make appropriate referrals. Nurses providing home care, by virtue of their in-home role, can be particularly helpful in helping both patients living with a mood disorder and their families to address the everyday challenges this illness brings.

Nursing practice requires a coordinated, ongoing interaction among patients, families, and providers to deliver comprehensive services. This includes using the complementary skills of other disciplines for forming overall goals, plans, and decisions and for providing continuity of care as needed. Integrated multidisciplinary

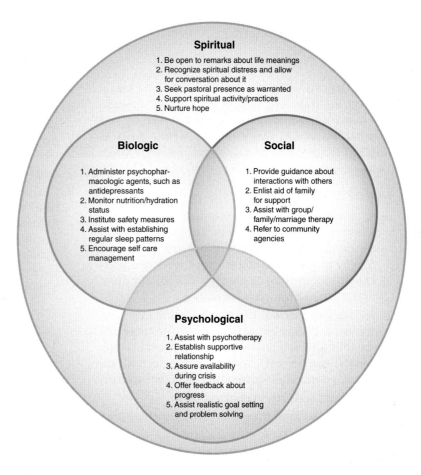

Spiritual
1. Be open to remarks about life meanings
2. Recognize spiritual distress and allow for conversation about it
3. Seek pastoral presence as warranted
4. Support spiritual activity/practices
5. Nurture hope

Biologic
1. Administer psychopharmacologic agents, such as antidepressants
2. Monitor nutrition/hydration status
3. Institute safety measures
4. Assist with establishing regular sleep patterns
5. Encourage self care management

Social
1. Provide guidance about interactions with others
2. Enlist aid of family for support
3. Assist with group/family/marriage therapy
4. Refer to community agencies

Psychological
1. Assist with psychotherapy
2. Establish supportive relationship
3. Assure availability during crisis
4. Offer feedback about progress
5. Assist realistic goal setting and problem solving

Figure 22.1 Holistic interventions for patients with major depressive disorder.

care aimed at holistic interventions is key to achieving the remission of symptoms and physical wellbeing, restoring baseline occupational and psychosocial functioning, and reducing the likelihood of relapse or recurrence (Fig. 22.1).

Bipolar Disorders

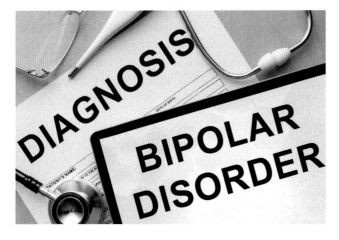

Diagnostic Criteria

Bipolar disorders are distinguished from depressive disorders by the occurrence of manic or hypomanic (i.e., mildly manic) episodes in addition to depressive episodes. The *DSM-5* divides bipolar disorders into bipolar I (characterized by one or more manic episodes generally with a major depressive occurrence), bipolar II (periods of major depression accompanied by at least one incidence of hypomania), and **cyclothymic disorder** (periods of hypomanic episodes and depressive episodes that do not meet full criteria for an MDE) (see Box 22.3 for the APA's DSM-5 criteria) (Fig. 22.2).

A manic episode is characterized by **euphoria**, a state of elation experienced as a heightened sense of wellbeing. During a manic episode, patients often manifest an expansive mood, in which they show an inappropriate lack of restraint in expressing feelings, and they frequently overvalue their own importance. Expansive qualities include an unceasing and indiscriminate enthusiasm for interpersonal, sexual, or occupational interactions and involve behaviours the patient later regrets and that have a high potential for painful consequences. It is important to note that an irritable rather than euphoric mood is often the first sign of mania. This irritability manifests as easy annoyance and anger, particularly when the patient's wishes are challenged or thwarted. Additionally, in manic episodes, the mood can be labile, altering between euphoria, depression, and irritability within minutes or hours. Other symptoms include inflated self-esteem or grandiosity, which

BOX 22.3 DSM-5 Diagnostic Criteria: Bipolar I Disorder

For a diagnosis of bipolar I disorder, it is necessary to meet the following criteria for a manic episode. The manic episode may have been preceded by and may be followed by hypomanic or MDEs. (Refer to Box 22.1 for the DSM-5 Diagnostic Criteria for Major Depressive Episodes.)

MANIC EPISODE

A. A distinct period of abnormally and persistently elevated, expansive, or irritable mood and abnormally and persistently increased goal-directed activity or energy, lasting at least 1 week and present most of the day, nearly every day (or any duration if hospitalization is necessary).

B. During the period of mood disturbance and increased energy or activity, three (or more) of the following symptoms (four if the mood is only irritable) are present to a significant degree and represent a noticeable change from usual behaviour:

1. Inflated self-esteem or grandiosity
2. Decreased need for sleep (e.g., feels rested after only 3 h of sleep)
3. More talkative than usual or pressure to keep talking
4. Flight of ideas or subjective experience that thoughts are racing
5. Distractibility (i.e., attention too easily drawn to unimportant or irrelevant external stimuli), as reported or observed
6. Increase in goal-directed activity (either socially, at work or school, or sexually) or psychomotor agitation (i.e., purposeless non–goal-directed activity)
7. Excessive involvement in activities that have a high potential for painful consequences (e.g., engaging in unrestrained buying sprees, sexual indiscretions, or foolish business investments)

C. The mood disturbance is sufficiently severe to cause marked impairment in social or occupational functioning or to necessitate hospitalization to prevent harm to self or others, or there are psychotic features.

D. The episode is not attributable to the physiologic effects of a substance (e.g., a drug of abuse, a medication, or other treatment) or to another medical condition.

HYPOMANIC EPISODE

A. A distinct period of abnormally and persistently elevated, expansive, or irritable mood and abnormally and persistently increased activity or energy, lasting at least 4 consecutive days and present most of the day, nearly every day.

B. During the period of mood disturbance and increased energy or activity, three (or more) of the following symptoms (four if the mood is only irritable) have persisted, represent a noticeable change from usual behaviour, and have been present to a significant degree:

1. Inflated self-esteem or grandiosity
2. Decreased need for sleep (e.g., feels rested after only 3 h of sleep)
3. More talkative than usual or pressure to keep talking
4. Flight of ideas or subjective experience that thoughts are racing
5. Distractibility (i.e., attention too easily drawn to unimportant or irrelevant external stimuli), as reported or observed
6. Increase in goal-directed activity (either socially, at work or school, or sexually) or psychomotor agitation (i.e., purposeless non–goal-directed activity)
7. Excessive involvement in activities that have a high potential for painful consequences (e.g., engaging in unrestrained buying sprees, sexual indiscretions, or foolish business investments)

C. The episode is associated with an unequivocal change in functioning that is uncharacteristic of the individual when not symptomatic.

D. The disturbance in mood and the change in functioning are observable by others.

E. The episode is not severe enough to cause marked impairment in social or occupational functioning or to necessitate hospitalization. If there are psychotic features, the episode is, by definition, manic.

F. The episode is not attributable to the physiologic effects of a substance (e.g., a drug of abuse, a medication, or other treatment).

Reprinted with permission from the *Diagnostic and statistical manual of mental disorders* (5th ed.). (Copyright 2013). American Psychiatric Association.

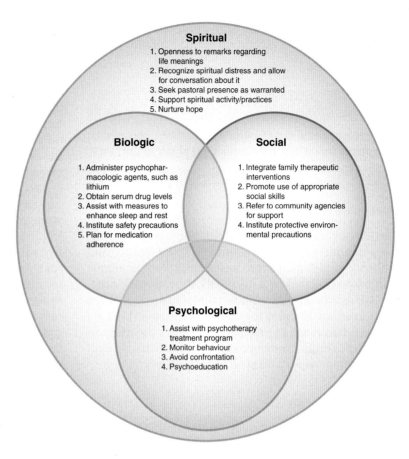

Figure 22.2 Holistic interventions for patients with bipolar I disorder.

may range from unusual self-confidence to delusions about possessing special powers or abilities. Delusions occur in 77.8% of patients experiencing mania, and they can be either congruent or incongruent with the mood state (Parker et al., 2020). As well in a manic episode, there is frequently a decreased need for sleep, pressured speech (excessive talkativeness), racing thoughts, distractibility, and a decrease in goal-directed activity or psychomotor agitation. As the mania increases, the patient feels more pressured to speak and at times is difficult to interrupt. Speech can become incoherent and associations in thought become quite loose and even disorganized. When thoughts skip rapidly among seemingly unrelated topics with a decreased logical connection between them, it is termed flight of ideas. Further, decreased inhibition, impulsivity, and distractibility in bipolar disorder can negatively affect cognition in diffuse areas such as *attention* and *concentration* (Morsel et al., 2018). During a manic episode, patients experience an increase in energy that manifests as pressure of activity, often with less sleep to feel rested. The patient often remains awake for long periods at night or wakes up several times a night, full of energy. Increased motor activity and agitation, which may be purposeful at first (e.g., cleaning the house), may deteriorate into inappropriate or disorganized actions. The patient may get involved unrealistically in several new endeavours, such as overspending sprees, or in reckless sexual encounters, drug or alcohol use, or other high-risk activities such as driving too fast or taking up dangerous sports. Frequently, hospitalization may be required to prevent self-harm.

Other psychiatric disorders have symptoms resembling a manic episode. Borderline personality disorder, attention deficit disorder, and substance abuse involving stimulants should be ruled out when assessing for mania. When considering any symptoms of bipolar disorder, it must be noted that the *DSM-5* criteria indicate that the presenting disturbances must be severe enough to cause marked impairment in social activities, occupational functioning, and interpersonal relationships (APA, 2013).

The criteria describing a **hypomanic episode** are the same as those detailed in a manic episode, apart from a longer duration of time noted in the expression of symptoms during the latter. An important feature, in hypomania, is that generally no marked impairment in social or occupational functioning occurs. Moreover, should there be fluctuations in the way the patient presents throughout the duration of an acute illness episode, for example, demonstrating high anxiety, agitation, and irritability alternating with the occurrence of depressive symptoms, the patient may be described as having **mixed features**. Such presentations can occur when the criteria for a manic or hypomanic episode are present. Mixed symptoms can also be associated with an MDE. If a patient presents with symptoms that meet full episode criteria for both mania and depression simultaneously, the diagnosis would rightfully be "manic episode, with mixed features" (*DSM-5*), (APA, 2013, p. 150). Hypomanic episodes can be considered less intense manic episodes.

KEY CONCEPT

Central features of mania include overactivity, elevated or irritable mood, and grandiose ideas of self-importance (Parker et al., 2020).

Secondary Mania

Underlying medical disorders such as certain metabolic abnormalities, neurologic disorders, CNS tumours, and particular medications can cause mania. Further, mania can be precipitated by some medical treatments, notably steroid therapy. As well, certain substances of abuse such as stimulants and cocaine induce mania (Li et al., 2020a). This range of precipitants requires the nurse to consider them as distinct possibilities for mania onset if there is no previous history of bipolar disorder.

Clinical Course

Bipolar disorder is a chronic, multicomponent, cyclic disorder (Rowland & Marwaha, 2018). With mixed states of mania, extreme turmoil can occur with possible suicidal ideation presenting especially high risk. Bipolar disorders can lead to severe functional impairments, resulting in job losses and financial duress and culminating in alienation from family, friends, and coworkers.

Epidemiology

Distribution and Onset

Bipolar disorder affects approximately 2.4% of the world's population globally irrespective of ethnicity and socioeconomic status, and it is a leading cause of disability in the younger population (Alonso et al., 2011; Dong et al., 2019). The results of a Canadian epidemiologic study conducted by McDonald et al. (2015) estimated the prevalence of bipolar I and bipolar II disorders at 0.87% and 0.57%, respectively.

The mode of onset for bipolar disorder can be variable, manifesting as a mild form of depression, hypersomnia, or as an episode of overt psychosis. Onset may also be characterized by several depressive episodes preceding the first manic occurrence (O'Donovan & Alda, 2020). Bipolar onset often occurs in adolescence; paediatric bipolar disorder (PBD) is rare, and must be distinguished from ADHD, which has a much earlier onset (Meier et al., 2018). Depression may be the initial presentation in children, though the hallmark of PBD is demonstrations of intense rage. Children may display seemingly unprovoked rage episodes for as long as 2 to 3 h. The symptoms of bipolar disorder reflect the devel-opmental level of the child. Whereas children younger than 9 years exhibit more irritability and emotional lability, older children exhibit more classic symptoms, such as euphoria and grandiosity. The first contact with the mental health system often occurs when the behaviour becomes disruptive and these children may have comorbid psychiatric disorders such as ADHD and conduct disorder (Meier et al., 2018). Noteworthy is that, on average, the delay between onset of bipolar disorder and diagnosis can range from 5 to 10 years (Mistry et al., 2019).

Recognizing bipolar disorder in the older adult can be challenging as it occurs less frequently than in younger populations and the symptoms are often atypical. Mood changes are likely to manifest as irritability rather than euphoria and anger instead of excessive spending may dominate the clinical presentation. Moreover, geriatric patients with mania often demonstrate more neurophysiologic abnormalities and cognitive disturbances such as confusion and disorientation, which can be confused with dementia or delirium (Omer et al., 2021). Therefore, a careful history must be obtained where mood symptoms duration and presentation and a previous history are identified. The use of new medications must also be identified. When possible, collaborative sources should be included in the assessment of bipolar problems in an older adult patient.

Gender, Ethnic, and Cultural Differences

Although no significant gender differences have been found in the lifetime prevalence of bipolar I disorder, the incidence of bipolar II disorder is reportedly greater in females than in males (Rowland & Marwaha, 2018). In addition, some data indicate that female patients with bipolar disorder are at greater risk for depression, whereas male patients are prone to manic episodes (Rowland & Marwaha, 2018).

While prevalence rates in Canada are said to be unrelated to race and ethnicity, data from research studies suggest immigration is a risk factor for mood disorders, including bipolar disorder, particularly if migration occurs during early childhood. Specifically, those from infancy to 5 years of age had the highest prevalence rates and risk for mood disorders when compared to their migration generation cohorts and especially adults (Villatoro et al., 2018). These data invite speculation about how those subject to mood-related disorders are affected by social factors including the process of transitioning and their situational circumstances dispose new migrants to affective reactivity. Factors that could give the young this vulnerability include the sense of being remote from one's homeland, feeling situationally isolated in a land where language and local customs are experienced as "strange," and living where they experience transgenerational distress related to their parents' social status loss and precarious employment prospects. The need exists for studies to identify contextual circumstances that may dispose to possible "immigration risk." At this time, no significant differences in prevalence have been found based on race or ethnicity.

Comorbidity

Medical comorbidity in patients with bipolar disorder is a significant issue as it complicates diagnosis and management of the illness and may have a negative impact on patient outcomes (APA, 2013). Rao et al. (2019) analyzed data from a clinical research study regarding medical burden in bipolar patients and found high rates of cardiovascular, metabolic, and alcohol disorders. Cardiovascular comorbidities, and associated problems, such as low HDL and high triglycerides, were suggested to be related to weight gain during depression as well as the medications prescribed. Noteworthy in this data analysis is that mania was negatively related to cardiac and metabolic problems but positively correlated to alcohol problems (Sylvia et al., 2015). Substantial evidence exists suggesting that bipolar disorder in and of itself is an independent risk factor for weight gain, diabetes mellitus, hypertension, dyslipidaemia, cardiovascular disease, and metabolic syndrome (Rao et al., 2019). How these medical problems, specifically rates of obesity, in bipolar disorder interact is difficult to determine due the confounding variables of medication side effects and unhealthy lifestyle choices. Preventing and treating obesity in patients with bipolar disorder could decrease the morbidity and mortality related to physical illness, enhance psychological wellbeing, and possibly improve the course of the disorder (Kittel-Schneider et al., 2020).

Other comorbid psychiatric conditions are anxiety disorders (most prevalent: panic disorder and social phobia) and substance use, notably alcohol and marijuana. In individuals with bipolar disorder and a comorbid anxiety disorder, 60% to 80% of them are more likely to experience a more severe course (McIntyre et al., 2020). The 2012 CCHS—Mental Health data suggested that a history of substance use is associated with increased symptomatology and complicates the prognosis of bipolar illness by decreasing treatment adherence and chances for remission (Đào et al., 2019)

Aetiology

Current theories of the aetiology of bipolar disorders are associated with chronic abnormalities of neurotransmission, which are thought to result in compensatory but maladaptive changes in brain regulation. In addition, the use of controlled structural and functional imaging studies of patients with mood disorders have generated hypotheses that CNS dysfunction is associated with specific structural brain abnormalities and functional CNS alterations (Giridharan et al., 2020).

Chronobiologic Theories

Sleep and schedule disturbances are important aspects of depression and can predict mania. Sleep patterns appear to be regulated by an internal biologic clock centred in the hypothalamus (see Chapter 10). Events that cause sleep deprivation such as time zone changes and childbirth may trigger symptoms. Several neurotransmitter and hormone levels follow circadian patterns; therefore, sleep disruption may lead to biochemical abnormalities that affect mood. Preliminary research evidence suggests that bipolar disorder can be characterized by biologic and behavioural disturbances in the individual's circadian rhythm and sleep deprivation as well as life events that disrupt schedules can trigger manic symptoms (Gold & Sylvia, 2016).

Sensitization and Kindling Theory

Sensitization (increase in response to a drug with repetition of the same dosage) and the related phenomenon of kindling (subthreshold stimulation of a neuron generates an action potential; see Chapter 13) refer to animal models. Repeated chemical or electrical stimulation of certain regions of the brain produces stereotypical behavioural responses or seizures. The amount of the chemical or electricity required to evoke the response or seizure decreases with each experience. These phenomena have been used as models to explain why, over time, affective episodes, particularly those seen in patients with bipolar disorder, recur in shorter and shorter cycles and with less relation to environmental precipitants. It is hypothesized that repeated affective episodes might be accompanied by the progressive alteration of brain synapses that lower the threshold for future episodes and increase the likelihood of illness. The kindling theory also helps explain the value of using antiseizure medication, such as carbamazepine and valproic acid, for mood stabilization (Carvalho et al., 2020).

Genetic Factors

A risk factor for bipolar disorder is having a first-degree relative, and particularly a parent, with this illness. The genetic basis for the development of bipolar disorder is increasingly seen in results from family, adoption, and twin studies that indicate a bipolar disorder familial pattern can be seen (Boland et al., 2021). Heritability for bipolar disorder is estimated to range from 70% to 90% (Gordovez & McMahon, 2020). There is a 2.4% incidence rate in the general population, compared with a 10% incidence rate for first-degree relatives of a patient with bipolar disorder, and 70% for a monozygotic twin of a bipolar patient (Gordovez & McMahon, 2020). Modes of genetic transmission and the cumulative effects of multiple genes interacting with environmental influences have yet to be definitively identified. A compelling Canadian longitudinal study, (Duffy et al., 2019) conducted over two decades, addressed the genetic associations between parents with bipolar disorder and the risks posed to their offspring. Researchers found that bipolar disorder in individuals at familial risk, typically appeared in a progressive clinical sequence, with symptoms of childhood sleep and anxiety disorders noted to be important predictors to the illness trajectory. As evidence mounts, an increase in our understanding as to the nature of possible neurodevelopmental correlates may occur. Likely a vulnerability to bipolar disorder is related to many genetic risk factors interacting with family and environment specific influences. Genomic studies support this model and research continues to identify candidate genes, structural genomic variations, and protein damaging mutations in individual genes possibly implicated in transmitting bipolar disorder (Kerner, 2014).

Psychological and Social Theories

Bipolar disorder encompasses two extremes of a continuum; depression locates at one end and mania at the other. Regarding depression, most psychological and social theories of mood disorders focus on loss as its cause in genetically vulnerable individuals. Mania is considered to be a biologically rooted condition, but when viewed from a psychological perspective, it is usually regarded as a state that arises from an attempt to overcompensate for depressed feelings rather than a disorder in its own right.

Interdisciplinary Treatment of Disorder

Patients with bipolar disorder struggle with the complexity of their illness and must be treated by an interdisciplinary team. Nurses, physicians, social workers, psychologists, occupational, and recreation therapists all have valuable expertise for bipolar patients. For children with bipolar disorder, schoolteachers and counsellors are included in the team. In older adults, the primary care physician is an integral part of the team. An important treatment goal is to minimize and prevent either manic or depressive episodes as the fewer the episodes, the more likely the person can live a normal, productive life. Another important goal is to provide psychoeducation and support for the client and family about the disorder so to assist them in managing it.

Priority Care Issues

During a manic episode, protecting the patient is a priority. Poor judgment and impulsivity result in risk-taking behaviours that can have dire consequences for the patient and family. For example, the person suddenly begins excessively spending money and partying. As well, during a manic episode, the patient may believe that they have supernatural powers, such as the ability to fly, and then may act on them. During a manic phase, suicidality as the result of poor judgment and poor impulse control may increase. When patients recover from a manic episode, they may be devastated by the consequences of poor judgment and impulsivity so

that suicide is considered as a way to deal with shame. Nurses play an important role in promoting improved self-esteem after patients experience a manic episode.

Family Response to Disorder

Bipolar disorder can devastate families, who often feel that they are on an emotional roller coaster, especially if they have difficulty understanding the mood shifts. They can be burdened by their family member's problematic behaviours (e.g., impulsive behaviour during manic episodes, such as excessive debt, assault charges, and sexual infidelities) and the disruption of household routine.Qualitative nursing research, concerned with close family members who have a relative with bipolar disorder, highlights the need for nurses to provide holistic support to both the individual affected by this illness and their family to affect the unpredictability it causes in their life and to make life more liveable for them (Lekoadi et al., 2019). Family members can also experience emotional distress and become significant users of mental health resources themselves. It is important to understand, however, that families do report developing coping strategies that make life more liveable for them such as finding respite from caring for ill relatives and ensuring appropriate boundaries (Doody et al., 2017). Nurses must recognize that families can feel strained to the limit when a family member has bipolar disorder and that they too need support, education, and assistance navigating the mental health system.

Nursing Management: Human Response to Bipolar Disorder

The nursing care of patients with bipolar disorder can be one of the greatest challenges in psychiatric nursing. In general, the behaviour of patients with bipolar disorder is often symptom free between episodes. Nursing care of a patient experiencing bipolar disorder should be approached in a multifaceted and compassionate manner during periods of acute illness and during states of remission.

Biologic Domain

Assessment

In the biologic domain, the assessment emphasis is on evaluating symptoms of mania and, most particularly, changes in sleep patterns. In the manic phase of bipolar disorder, the patient often experiences sleeplessness, resulting in irritability and physical exhaustion. Eating habits usually change during a manic or depressive episode, and the nurse should, therefore, assess changes in diet and body weight. Patients with mania may experience malnutrition and fluid imbalance. The nurse must monitor laboratory studies, such as electrolytes and thyroid functioning. Abnormal thyroid function can be responsible for the mood and behavioural disturbances. Excessive use of alcohol and other substances may also occur, and therefore, the individual must also be assessed for these behaviours. Usually, a drug screen is ordered to determine current use of substances. A further concern during a manic phase is that patients often become hypersexual and engage in risky sexual practices. Changes in sexual practices should be explored.

Pharmacologic Assessment

When a patient is in a manic state, previous use of antidepressants should be assessed as they can precipitate such an episode. In such cases, antidepressant use should be discontinued. Often, manic or depressive episodes occur after patients stop taking their mood stabilizer, at which time the reason for stopping the medication should be explored. Patients may stop taking their medications because of side effects or because they no longer believe they have a mental disorder. As well, patients with known bipolar disorder who take antidepressants without attendant mood stabilizers could be at risk for a manic episode.

Nursing Care Foci for the Biologic Domain

Nursing care within the biologic domain focuses on sleep disturbances (i.e., sleep deprivation leading to exhaustion), rest, inadequate nutrition, self-care, and treatment nonadherence (i.e., medication). If patients are in the depressive phase of illness, the previously discussed nursing care foci for depression should also be considered.

Interventions for Biologic Domain

Physical Care

In a state of mania, the patient's primary physical needs are rest, adequate hydration and nutrition, and reestablishment of physical wellbeing. Self-care has usually deteriorated. For a patient who is unable to sit long enough to eat, snacks and high-energy and finger foods that can be eaten while moving should be provided. Alcohol should be avoided. Sleep hygiene is a priority but may not be realistic until medications take effect. Limiting stimuli is important in decreasing agitation and promoting sleep.

Teaching Points

Once the patient's mood stabilizes, the nurse should focus on monitoring changes in physical functioning in sleep or eating behaviour and teaching patients to identify antecedents to mood episodes. A regular sleep routine should be maintained if possible. High-risk times for manic episodes, such as changes in work schedule (day to night), should be avoided if possible. The postpartum period is a particularly high-risk period for exacerbation of bipolar illness as women are very sleep deprived. They should be encouraged to sleep when the baby sleeps and advised to obtain childcare respite if possible. Patients with a bipolar disorder should be taught to monitor the amount of their sleep each night and report a pattern of decreased sleep and sleeplessness as this may indicate a shift toward a manic episode.

Lithium Carbonate and Related Nursing Interventions

Pharmacotherapy is essential in treating bipolar disorder to achieve two goals: the rapid control of symptoms and the prevention of future episodes—or, at least, reduction in their severity and frequency. Pharmacotherapy continues through the various phases of bipolar disorder; see Chapter 13.

The mainstay of therapy for bipolar disorder is mood-stabilizing drugs and notably lithium carbonate (lithium), which has an impressive efficacy profile in the treatment of this disorder. Other medications used in the treatment of bipolar disorder include anticonvulsants such as divalproex for acute manic episodes; carbamazepine for acute mania and mixed states often when lithium has been ineffective; and lamotrigine, an effective mood stabilizer for depressive episodes but less effective for manic episodes. Lithium, however, is the most widely used mood stabilizer in bipolar disorder (see Box 22.4). It is a very effective treatment for euphoric mania but less so in mania with mixed features, **rapid cycling** bipolar disorder, and secondary manias in the presence of comorbid substance abuse. The supplemental use of antipsychotics is often a beneficial adjunct to treatment with lithium. Due to its significant side-effect burden (Table 22.1), lithium can be poorly tolerated, and small differences in dose or blood levels can cause adverse and even life-threatening outcomes because of its narrow therapeutic index (Day et al., 2017).

Lithium is a salt, and the interaction between lithium levels and sodium levels in the body and the relationship between lithium levels and fluid volume in the body remain crucial issues in its safe, effective use. High sodium levels in the body lower the lithium level and vice versa. Thus, changes in dietary sodium intake can affect lithium blood levels that, in turn, may affect therapeutic results or increase the incidence of side effects. The same applies to fluid volume. If body fluid decreases significantly because of a hot climate, strenuous exercise, vomiting, diarrhoea, fever, a drastic reduction in fluid intake, or diuretic use, then lithium levels can rise sharply, causing an increase in side effects, progressing to lethal lithium toxicity (Hedya et al., 2019). Before lithium administration, a physical assessment that includes laboratory tests to determine electrolytes, thyroid and renal functioning, an electrocardiogram, a baseline pregnancy test, weight status, and concomitant medications is necessary. The nurse must also be cognizant

BOX 22.4 DRUG PROFILE ℞

Lithium (Eskalith)

Drug Class: Mood stabilizer

Generic Name: Lithium carbonate lithiu **(Trade) Name:** (Eskalith, Lithane)

Receptor Affinity: Alters sodium transport in nerve and muscle cells, increases norepinephrine uptake and serotonin receptor sensitivity, slightly increases intra-neuronal stores of catecholamines, and delays some second messenger systems. Exact mechanism of action is unknown.

Indications: Treatment and prevention of manic episodes in bipolar affective disorder. Used successfully in a number of off-label uses such as prophylaxis of cluster headaches, bulimia, etc.

Routes and Dosage: Dosing is done according to clinical response, side effects, and serum levels. Targeted dosages are between 900 and 1,800 mg/daily by mouth. 150-, 300-, and 600-mg capsules. Lithobid, 300-mg slow-release tablets; Eskalith CR, 450-mg controlled-release tablets.

Adult: In acute mania, optimal response is usually 600 mg tid or 900 mg bid. Obtain serum levels twice weekly in acute phase. Maintenance: Use lowest possible dose to alleviate symptoms and maintain serum level of 0.6 to 1.2 mEq/L. In uncomplicated maintenance, obtain serum levels every 2 to 3 months. Do not rely on serum levels alone. Monitor patient side effects.

Geriatric: An increased risk for toxic effects; use lower doses, and monitor frequently.

Children: Safety and efficacy in children younger than 12 years has not been established.

Half-Life (Peak Effect): Mean, 24 h (peak serum levels in 1 to 4 h). Steady state reached in 5 to 7 days.

Select Adverse Reactions: Weight gain. A common side effect of lithium is hand tremors and dosage needs to be monitored.

Warning: Avoid use during pregnancy or while breast-feeding. Hepatic or renal impairments increase plasma concentration.

There is a fine line between therapeutic levels and toxicity levels. Mindfulness is required in use of lithium as a treatment agent.

Specific Patient/Family Education:

- Avoid alcohol or other CNS depressant drugs.
- Notify the prescriber if pregnancy is possible or planned. Do not breast-feed while taking this medication.
- Notify the prescriber before taking any other prescription, OTC medication, or herbal supplements.
- May impair judgment, thinking, or motor skills; avoid driving or other hazardous tasks.
- Do not abruptly discontinue use.

Table 22.1 Serum Lithium Concentration and Associated Side Effects

Mild Toxicity 1.5-2 mmol/L	Metallic taste
	Ataxia
	Nausea
	Vomiting
	Diarrhea
	Dry mouth
	Polydipsia
	Polyuria
	Fine hand tremor
	Fasciculation
	Lethargy
	Fatigue
	Muscle weakness
	Edema
	Weight gain
Moderate Toxicity 2-3.5 mmol/L	Severe diarrhea
	Nausea and vomiting
	Moderate ataxia
	Slurred speech
	Tinnitus
	Blurred vision
	Confusion
	Agitation
	Acute delirium
	Disorientation
	Tachycardia
	Hypertonia (increased muscle tone)
Severe Toxicity > 3.5 mmol/L	Cardiac arrhythmias
	Blackouts
	Course or severe tremor
	Fasciculations
	Visual or tactile hallucinations
	Extrapyramidal symptoms
	Neuroleptic malignant syndrome
	Oliguria
	Renal failure
	Nystagmus
	Hyperthermia
	Hypotension
	Confusion
	Seizures
	Coma
	Death

Adapted from: Hedya, S. A.; Avula, A., & Swoboda, H. D. (2021) Lithium Toxicity. *StatPearls.* National Library of Medicine. https://www.ncbi.nlm.nih.gov/books/NBK499992/ and Procyshyn, R, M., Bezchilibnyk-Butler, K. Z., & Jeffires, J. J. (2019). *Clinical Handbook of Psychotropic Drugs* (23rd ed.). Hogrefe Publishing.

that lithium has serious interactions with medications and other substances as seen in Table 22.2. Table 22.3 describes nursing interventions for lithium side effects.

Psychological Domain

Assessment

The assessment of the psychological domain should follow the process explained in Chapter 11. Individuals with bipolar disorder can usually participate in many parts of the assessment.

Table 22.2   Lithium Interactions With Medications and Other Substances

Substance	Effect of Interaction
Angiotensin-converting enzyme inhibitors, such as • Captopril • Lisinopril • Quinapril	Increases serum lithium; may cause toxicity and impaired kidney function
Acetazolamide	Increases the renal excretion of lithium, decreases lithium levels
Alcohol	May increase serum lithium level
Caffeine	Increases lithium excretion, increases lithium tremor
Carbamazepine	Increases neurotoxicity, despite normal serum levels and dosage
Fluoxetine	Increases serum lithium levels
Haloperidol	Increases neurotoxicity, despite normal serum levels and dosage
Loop diuretics, such as furosemide	Increases lithium serum levels but may be safer than thiazide diuretics; potassium-sparing diuretics (amiloride, spironolactone) are safest
Methyldopa	Increases neurotoxicity without increasing serum lithium levels
Nonsteroidal anti-inflammatory drugs, such as • Diclofenac • Ibuprofen • Indomethacin • Piroxicam	Decreases renal clearance of lithium Increases serum lithium levels by 30%–60% in 3–10 days Aspirin and sulindac do not appear to have the same effect
Osmotic diuretics, such as • Urea • Mannitol • Isosorbide	Increases renal excretion of lithium and decreases lithium levels
Sodium chloride	High sodium intake decreases lithium levels; low sodium diets may increase lithium levels and lead to toxicity Caution warranted regarding salt intake
Thiazide diuretics, such as • Chlorothiazide • Hydrochlorothiazide	Promotes sodium and potassium excretion; increases lithium serum levels; may produce cardiotoxicity and neurotoxicity
TCAs	Increases tremor; potentiates pharmacologic effects of TCAs

Table 22.3   Interventions for Lithium Side Effects

Side Effect	Intervention
Oedema of the feet or hands	Monitor intake and output; check for possible decreased urinary output. Monitor sodium intake. The patient should elevate the legs when sitting or lying. Monitor weight.
Fine hand tremor	Provide support and reassurance if it does not interfere with daily activities. Tremor worsens with anxiety and intentional movements; minimize stressors. Notify the prescriber if it interferes with the patient's work and compliance will be an issue. More frequent smaller doses of lithium may also help.
Mild diarrhoea	Take lithium with meals. Provide for fluid replacement. Notify the prescriber if becomes severe; may need a change in medication preparation or may be early sign of toxicity.
Muscle weakness, fatigue, or memory and concentration difficulties	Provide support and reassurance; this side effect will usually pass after a few weeks of treatment. Short-term memory aids such as lists or reminder calls may be helpful. Notify the prescriber if becomes severe or interferes with the patient's desire to continue treatment.
Metallic taste	Suggest sugarless candies or throat lozenges. Encourage frequent oral hygiene.
Nausea or abdominal discomfort	Consider dividing the medication into smaller doses or give it at more frequent intervals. Give medication with meals.
Polydipsia	Reassure the patient that this is a normal mechanism to cope with polyuria.
Polyuria	Monitor intake and output. Provide reassurance and explain nature of side effect. Also explain that this causes no physical damage to the kidneys. Withhold medication.
Toxicity	Notify the prescriber. Use symptomatic treatments.

Mood

By definition, bipolar disorder is a disturbance of mood. If the patient is depressed, using an assessment tool for depression may help determine the severity of depression. If mania predominates, evaluating the quality of the mood (elated, grandiose, irritated, or agitated) becomes important. Usually, mania is determined by clinical observation.

Cognition

In a depressive episode, the patient may not be able to concentrate enough to complete cognitive tasks, such as those called for in the Mini-Mental State Exam. During the acute phase of a manic or depressive episode, mental status may be abnormal, and in a **manic episode**, insight and judgment is impaired by extremely rapid, disjointed, and distorted thinking. Moreover, feelings such as grandiosity can interfere with normal executive functioning.

It is not uncommon for patients with bipolar disorder to experience deterioration in their cognitive function, including memory, and the ability to plan, attend, and learn, which has a negative impact on their ability to engage in activities of daily living. Further deterioration in executive functioning has been associated with the frequency of manic episodes requiring hospitalization. Sawalha and colleagues (2021) discuss the importance of identifying first-episode bipolar disorder as a way of ensuring appropriate early intervention, thereby reducing the burden of disease. Utilizing machine learning techniques, patients with chronic bipolar disorder and patients with a first episode of bipolar disorder (and matched healthy controls) were subjected to a battery of neurocognitive tests. The machine learning model was able to differentiate patients with chronic bipolar disorder with 77% accuracy, and those with first-episode bipolar disorder with 76% accuracy. The authors concluded that machine models have the potential to contribute to more informed and accurate diagnoses, which may lead to early intervention strategies, and a more positive prognosis for those living with bipolar disorder (Sawalha et al., 2021).

Thought Disturbances

Psychosis commonly occurs in patients with bipolar disorder, especially during acute manic episodes. Auditory hallucinations and delusional thinking may constitute the clinical picture. In children and adolescents, psychosis may not be easily detected, due to possible differential disorders such as ADHD.

Stress and Coping Factors

Stress and coping are critical assessment areas for a patient with bipolar disorder. A stressful event often triggers a manic or depressive episode. In some instances, there may be no apparent stress precipitating the episode, regardless it is important to discuss the possibility of a specific trigger. Determining the patient's usual coping skills for managing stresses lays the groundwork for developing interventional strategies. Negative coping skills, such as substance use or aggression, should be identified because these skills need to be replaced with more appropriate and functional coping.

Risk Assessment

Patients with bipolar disorder are at high risk for suicide. A complex interplay between the illness, environment, and person is considered the likely cause of suicide (Dome et al., 2019). Violent behaviours may occur during severe manic episodes, particularly when irritability, poor insight, limited judgment, as well substance abuse and personality disorder problems, are present; thus, patients should be assessed promptly for suicidal or homicidal risk. Behavioural control of violence is often achieved through medicating the patient to prevent harm (Gaynes et al., 2017).

Nursing Care Foci for the Psychological Domain

Nursing care associated with the psychological domain of bipolar disorder includes attention to hallucinations and delusions, exaggerated self-esteem, risky health behaviours, impulsivity, poor judgment, impairment in coping, which may lead to safety issues, self-harm risks, risk for suicide, and violence risk.

Interventions for Psychological Domain

Although pharmacotherapy is the primary treatment for bipolar disorder, structured psychotherapies and adjunctive therapies for bipolar disorder have notable benefits. Research about psychotherapy for bipolar disorder has focused predominantly on patients with a chronic illness course. However, researchers are exploring the feasibility of implementing a new therapy for patients. Family-focused therapy has also been shown to have primary benefit in preventing relapse. Other modalities such as psychoeducation, IPT, and social rhythm therapy are adjunct therapies for reducing relapses (Goldstein et al., 2018). Integration of these therapies is fundamental to reducing manic episodes and/or depression and preventing possible relapses. Through early intervention, these therapies can be effective in promoting appropriate lifestyle management, improving medication adherence, and ultimately preempting intense symptom reoccurrence (Chia et al., 2019).

Other risk factors for illness reoccurrence include obesity, high rates of nonadherence to medication therapy, marital conflict, separation, divorce, unemployment, and underemployment. The goals of psychosocial interventions aim to address these risk factors and associated features, which are difficult to address with pharmacotherapy alone. Of particular importance to the intents of interventions in this domain are improving medication adherence, decreasing the number and length of hospitalizations and relapses, enhancing social and occupational functioning, improving quality of life, increasing the patient's and family's acceptance of the disorder, and reducing the suicide risk (Chen et al., 2019).

Psychoeducation

Psychoeducation is designed to provide information on bipolar disorder, treatment, and recovery, and it usually focuses on medication adherence. Research suggests that psychoeducation, particularly in a group context, that specifically includes information about the importance of adherence to medications in addition to relapse prevention is effective in averting relapses and decreasing mania (Jawad et al., 2018). Nurses can provide psychoeducational information and identify any obstacles to recovery. Other important psychoeducational interventions nurses can implement include teaching patients to recognize warning signs and symptoms of relapse and offering strategies to help cope with residual symptoms and functional impairments (Chen et al., 2019). As well, resistance to accepting the illness and to taking medication, the symbolic meaning of taking medication, and worries about the future should be discussed openly. In the interest of improved medication adherence, it is helpful to listen carefully to patients' concerns about the medication, the dosing schedules, any changes in dosage, and side effects. Health teaching and weight management should be a component of any psychoeducation programme. In addition to individual variations in body weight, many of the antipsychotic and mood stabilizing medications are associated with weight gain. Monitoring weight and developing individual weight management plans that include exercise can reduce the relapse risk that is related to medication cessation, which is related to these concerns. Nurses must also be cognizant of the fact that poverty can negatively impact the patient's ability to maintain a healthy diet. Overall, the plan to support adherence should be made to fit the attitude, knowledge, and skills of the individual patient.

Psychotherapy

Psychotherapy is an integral aspect of bipolar disorder treatment. Often treatment is overlooked due to a focus on medication adherence. In addition to addressing the the symptoms experienced by the patient, psychotherapy can temper the stressors that trigger episodes and increase the patient's acceptance of the need for medication. Patients should be encouraged to keep their appointments with their therapist, communicate their needs, and provide feedback on the efficacy of their treatment. Kay Redfield Jamison offers important qualitative support for the benefits of psychotherapy and medications in treating bipolar disorder in her book *An Unquiet Mind* (1995).

Social Domain

Assessment

One of the tragedies of bipolar disorder is its effect on social and occupational functioning. Cultural views of mental illness profoundly influence the patient's acceptance of the disorder (Davis, 2014). During illness episodes, patients often behave in ways that jeopardize their social relationships. Losing a job or going through a divorce are common events. When performing an assessment of social function, the nurse should identify changes resulting from a manic or depressive episode.

Nursing Care Foci for the Social Domain

Nursing care within the social domain focuses on patients' role performance within social situations and within their families, the impact of the illness on family members, caregiver fatigue, and caregiver role strain.

Interventions for Social Domain

Interventions focusing on the social domain are integral to nursing care for all ages. During mania, patients usually violate others' boundaries. Roommate selection for patients requiring hospital admittance needs to be carefully considered. If possible, a private room is ideal because patients with bipolar disorder tend to irritate others, who quickly tire of the intrusiveness. These patients may miss the cues indicating anger and aggression from others. The nurse should protect the patient experiencing mania from self-harm, as well as harm from other patients.

Support groups are helpful for people with this disorder. Participating in groups allows the person to meet others with the disorder and learn management and preventive strategies. Support groups also are helpful in dealing with the stigma associated with mental illnesses (see Box 22.5).

Family Interventions

Marital and family interventions are often needed at different periods and multiple time points in the life of a person with bipolar disorder. For the family with a child with this disorder, additional parenting support and skills may be needed to manage the child's behaviours. The goals of family interventions are to help the family understand and cope with the disorder. Interventions may range from occasional counseling sessions to intensive family therapy. Research indicates family

BOX 22.5 **Stigma**

Receiving a diagnosis of bipolar disorder can be a stigmatizing experience that affects the lives and self-esteem of individuals with this disorder (Au et al., 2019).

In a phenomenological study, Hayne (2003) examined the response to receiving a psychiatric diagnosis, as differentiated from experiencing the illness itself. Emphasized in the lived description of psychiatric diagnosis was the notion that the diagnosis places the individual in a context of reflective self-knowledge. Below are excerpts of the experiences of two participants, Matt and Jeff, as well as before and after drawings that exemplified their perceptions of a "legitimized/delegitimized self."

Matt desperately wanted to avoid being "abnormal." A diagnosis spelled "insanity" and he shuddered at the prospect of it. Why not "bizarre experience" or something less caustic? The diagnosis threatened to reveal "a secret he held to himself about himself," confronting him with, "I am flawed! Not, I have a flaw, but, I am flawed!" He sketches "diagnosis" in "Before" and "After" self-profiles. Prediagnosis self has a halo to arc dark (blue) hair (he interprets this as ominous). With diagnosis, there is no evading the ill-fated knowledge and Matt accommodates the diagnosis, colouring his hair bright (green) to represent hope and "self-acceptance."

Jeff viewed embracing the diagnosis as central to his mental illness experience in that it supplied him "a battleground for living." Before diagnosis, he felt empty, forlorn, immobilized ("a scarecrow, suspended in a field"). Diagnosis resulted in "knowledge made knowledgeable" to him. With that he was able to reformulate (pictured as a snowman). Someone "cared" enough to assist this reconstituting (the therapeutic encounter). Therefore, he is not cold as a snowman (scarf); he wears a smile. Rediscovery of his personal significance (top hat) equips him to take up his future (hands outstretched).

The nursing implications from this research are that it fosters a greater understanding of the significance of receiving a psychiatric diagnosis and this knowledge may better prepare nurses to help patients sustain hope and self-acceptance. As well, it encourages nurses to implement early intervention strategies that address shame and stigma. It is also knowledge that may be transferred to understanding the potential life-changing ramifications of any medical diagnosis.

Diagnosis: Matt Before and After.
Diagnosis: Jeff Before and After.

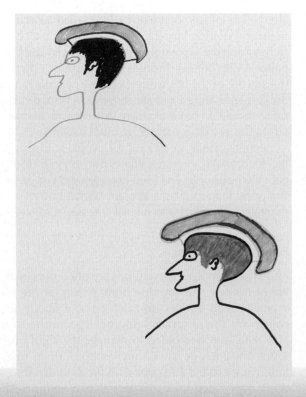

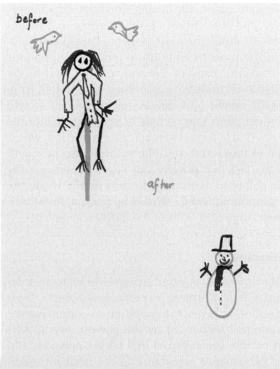

Box 22.6 Psychoeducation Checklist: Bipolar I Disorder

When caring for the family and their family member who has a bipolar I disorder, be sure to include the following topic areas in the teaching plan:

- ✓ Psychopharmacologic agents, including drug action, dosage, frequency, and possible adverse effects
- ✓ Medication and treatment regimen adherence
- ✓ Strategies to decrease agitation and restlessness
- ✓ Safety measures
- ✓ Recognizing and responding to early warning signs and triggers
- ✓ Self-care management
- ✓ Preventing relapse and promoting wellness
- ✓ Follow-up laboratory testing
- ✓ Support services

psychoeducation, as an adjunct treatment to pharmacotherapy, is effective in assisting families to cope, in decreasing the risk for relapse and hospitalization, and in improving outcomes at 6 months postintervention (Kolostoumpis et al., 2015) (see Box 22.6).

Spiritual Domain

The nursing approach to the spiritual domain in the care of the person with a bipolar disorder is the same as for the person with a major depressive disorder.

Evaluation and Treatment Outcomes

Desired treatment outcomes are mood stabilization and enhanced quality of life. Primary tools for evaluating outcomes are nursing observation and patient self-report (see Box 22.7).

BOX 22.7 NURSING CARE PLAN

THE PATIENT WITH BIPOLAR DISORDER

Steven was a young businessman in the oil sector. He was married with three young children and lived in a large metropolitan city. When his business began to fail, he lost millions of dollars within weeks. He describes feeling desperate and going into "overdrive" trying to save the company, spare his employees from being laid off, and evade an inevitable bankruptcy. "I just wouldn't quit," he says. "Because I wouldn't quit, my mind quit. And it just literally went into la-la-land. My mind just shut down. I kind of lost contact with everything." Steven unwittingly stepped in front of a car and was hit. "I jumped up and just carried on," he says. Bystanders, however, mobilized his transport to a hospital ED. "The doctor looked at me for 8 s and said 'manic depressive!'"

Steven sees his condition as a gift: "I'm very likable … and creative…. With mania you think faster and when you

think faster you process more. So I just process more information quicker…. I have the energy that most people can only dream of … I mean incredible energy … I can do anything, anytime, anywhere…. And everything seems in its right space. And it can be you have no money, no house, no job, no family, no friends, no food, and you feel incredible. None of that matters! It's like the ultimate high!"

The first hospitalization established a medical regimen for Steven, and his health stabilized for a time. An initial manic episode very often involves treatment with lithium carbonate resulting in mood stabilization. Recurring mania with episodes of depression may benefit from treatment with TCAs and MAOIs, though this course of action was not necessary for Steven.

Steven found his psychiatric diagnosis was "a destructive (gift) of difference!" "I went from 1 day being gifted to

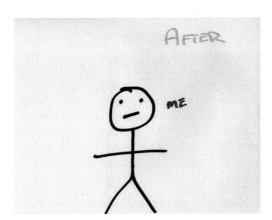

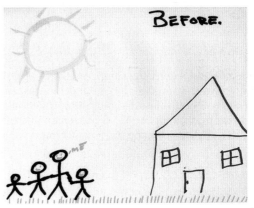

Continued on following page

NURSING CARE PLAN (*Continued*)

the next day being mentally ill. That's a very large step." He depicts his experience in a before-diagnosis drawing, stating, "I had everything before: a wife, three children, a home! The sun shone in my world." This state is contrasted in an after-diagnosis portrayal, where "the sun is gone." "I lost it all. There is just me! No job, no friends, no home, no family! My wife thought she married a gifted person. When she realized the mental illness, she took the kids and left." Within months of his discharge from the hospital, Steven became confused and disorganized. A restaurant owner reported him for causing a disturbance. When police arrived, he was incoherent and behaving erratically. He was transported to the psychiatric ED.

Setting: Acute Care Psychiatric Unit in a General Hospital

Baseline Assessment: From the ED, Steven is admitted to acute care inpatient services where he presents with symptoms of mixed bipolar mood disorder. His mood is quite labile and he is easily irritated. His speech is pressured. He is unable to account for his behaviour and is exhibiting flight of ideas. Historical records indicate his prior admission and discharge on lithium, which he admits he did not take. When asked why he stopped his medication he states, "I completely disagreed with it. I didn't think that my gift needed treatment."

Diagnostic Features	Medications
Bipolar I disorder	L-Thyroxine 0.1 mg q a.m. × 1 day
Hypothyroidism	Clonazepam 0.5 mg bid for sleep and agitation
Social problems (Divorce finalized 18 months ago. Ex-wife has full custody of three children. Patient has supervised visitations.)	Carbamazepine added on transfer to be titrated up to 400 mg tid

Setting: Acute Care Psychiatric Unit in a General Hospital

Associated Features	Related Factors
Potential for life-threatening injury	Elation and expansive feelings
Poor judgment and impulse control	Excitement vacillating with desolation
Lack of support system	Loss secondary to finances/job, divorce

Goals of Care

Initial	Discharge
1. Will seek out appropriate support	5. Will discuss the complexity of his illness
2. Will adhere to unit regulations	6. Will express antecedents of treatment related to mania and depression
3. Will participate in programme activities	7. Will discuss need for adherence to meds
4. Will achieve balance in activities of daily living (e.g., rest, hydration, nutrition)	8. Will identify antecedents and indicators of impending illness exacerbation

Interventions	Rationale	Ongoing Assessment
Initiate a nurse–patient relationship; demonstrate acceptance of the patient as a worthwhile human being through the use of nonjudgmental statements and behaviour.	A sense of worthlessness often underlies despair. A positive therapeutic relationship can maintain the patient's dignity and foster improved self-esteem.	Assess the stages of the relationship and determine whether a therapeutic relationship is actually being formed. Identify indicators of trust.

NURSING CARE PLAN (*Continued*)

Interventions	Rationale	Ongoing Assessment
Initiate suicide precautions per hospital policy. Apply vigilant observation routines. Implement individual suicide safety plan with patient.	Safety of the individual is a priority with people who have poor impulse control.	Determine risk of self-harm.
Help the client to develop a relapse prevention plan that includes seeking professional mental health support when they feel suicidal.	A relapse prevention plan can help the patient maintain wellness and safety by encouraging the resistance of impulses and providing a stepwise plan to address any exacerbation of symptoms.	Determine the patient's ability to commit to the relapse plan.
	A relapse prevention plan requires an understanding of *denial* as an expected coping mechanism. This coping mechanism should be connected with the client's underlying emotional struggle with their illness.	

Evaluation

Outcomes	Revised Outcomes	Interventions
Has not harmed self; denies self-harm thoughts/intent. Identifies people and resources to assist when suicidality heightens	Absence of risk or self-harm intent will continue	Discontinue precautions incrementally; maintain ongoing assessment for safety
Made a suicide safety plan with nurse, agrees to keep it after discharge	Maintains suicide safety plan and reviews it regularly with outpatient mental health provider	Support and reinforce this suicide safety plan, updating it regularly

Associated Impairment—Sense of Self and Self-Esteem

Defining Characteristics	Related Factors
Expressions of grandiosity vacillating with expressions of shame and guilt Lack of success in business endeavours and relationships	Labile mood (elation and despair noted) Feelings of abandonment secondary to separation from significant others Feelings of failure secondary to bankruptcy and relationship problems Unrealistic expectations of self

Goals of Care

Initial	Discharge
1. Realistic self-appraisal	3. Verbalize acceptance of personal limitations
2. Modify excessive and unrealistic self-expectations	4. Report freedom from untoward symptoms
	5. Avoid behavioural risks

Continued on following page

NURSING CARE PLAN (*Continued*)

Interventions	Rationale	Ongoing Assessment
Enhance the patient's sense of self by being attentive; validate interpretation of what is being said or experienced; help to make consistent, realistic verbalizations.	By showing respect and helping the patient frame happenings realistically, the nurse can support and help build the patient's sense of self.	Determine whether the patient confirms realistic interpretation of situations and verbalizes with moderation in rate and volume.
Assist to reframe and redefine negative statements ("not a failure, but a setback").	Reframing an event positively can help the patient view the situation in an alternative way and it directs dialogue toward enhancing change.	Assess whether the patient can actually view the world in a different way.
Problem-solve with the patient about how to approach finding satisfying employment.	Work is very important to adults. Bankruptcy can decrease self-esteem. Focusing on the possibility of a future job can provide hope.	Assess the patient's problem-solving ability. Note indicators of realistic plans.
Encourage positive physical habits (healthy eating patterns, exercise, adequate sleep).	A healthy lifestyle promotes wellbeing, increasing self-esteem.	Determine willingness to consider making lifestyle changes.
Teach the patient to validate consensually with others.	Low self-esteem is generated by negative interpretations of the world. Through consensual validation, the patient can determine whether others view situations in the same way.	Assess the patient's ability to participate in this process.
Teach constructive self-appraisal. Helpful exercises might include self-affirmations, imagery, use of humour, meditation/prayer, and relaxation.	There are many different approaches that can be practiced to increase self-esteem.	Assess the patient's energy level and ability to focus on learning new skills.
Assist in establishing appropriate personal boundaries.	In an attempt to meet their own needs, people with a compromised sense of self often violate other people's boundaries and/or allow others to take advantage of them. Helping patients establish their own boundaries will improve the likelihood of needs being met in an appropriate manner.	Assess the patient's ability to understand the concept of boundary violation and its significance.
Provide an opportunity within the therapeutic relationship to express thoughts and feelings. Use open-ended statements and questions. Encourage expression of both positive and negative statements.	The individual with compromised self-esteem may have difficulty expressing thoughts and feelings. Varied outlets for expression may help improve how thoughts and feelings are expressed.	Monitor thoughts and feelings that are expressed in order to help the patient examine them.
Explore opportunities for positive socialization.	Individuals with insecurity issues may be in social situations that reinforce artificial self-evaluation. Helping the patient identify new positive situations will present other options.	Assess whether the new situations are potentially positive or are a re-creation of other negative (self-aggrandizing) situations.
Steven began to modify excessive and unrealistic expectations of self.	Strengthen ability to affirm realistic aspects and examine expectations related to work and relationships.	Refer to mental health clinic for cognitive–behavioural psychotherapy.

NURSING CARE PLAN (*Continued*)

Interventions	Rationale	Ongoing Assessment
Verbalized defeatist thinking related to finding worthwhile employment	Identify important aspects of tentative employment so that he can begin looking for a job that has those characteristics.	Attend a support group that focuses on job interviewing skills.
As Steven's mood stabilized, he was able to sleep through the night, and he began eating again. He also expressed positive thoughts about his future.	Maintain a stable mood to promote a positive and realistic self-concept.	Monitor mood and identify antecedents to mood escalation and/or depression.

Associated Coping Impairment

Defining Characteristics	Related Factors
Verbalization in inability to cope or ask for help Reported difficulty with life stressors Compromised ability to problem-solve Alteration in social participation Disinhibited behaviour resulting in self-risk Distorted thoughts and self-control Substance abuse	Altered mood (alternating mania and depression) caused by changes secondary to body chemistry (bipolar disorder) Altered mood caused by changes secondary to intake of mood-altering substance (alcohol) Unsatisfactory support system Sensory overload secondary to excessive activity Unreliable psychological resources for consistency of employment

Goals of Care

Initial	Discharge
1. Accept support through the nurse–patient relationship. 2. Identify areas of ineffective coping. 3. Examine current efforts at coping. 4. Identify realistic areas of strength. 5. Learn new coping skills.	6. Practice new coping skills. 7. Focus on realistic strengths.

Interventions	Rationale	Ongoing Assessment
Identify current stresses in Steven's life, including the acceptance of bipolar disorder.	When the patient verbalizes areas of concern, he will be able to focus on one issue at a time. If he identifies the mental disorder as a stressor, he will more likely be able to develop strategies to deal with it.	Determine whether Steven is able to identify problem areas realistically. Continue to assess for self-risk behaviours.
Identify Steven's strengths in dealing with past stressors.	By focusing on past successes, he can identify strengths and build on them in the future.	Assess if Steven can identify any previous successes in his life.
Assist Steven in discussing, selecting, and practicing positive coping skills (jogging, yoga, volunteer work).	New coping skills take a conscious effort to learn and will at first seem strange and unnatural. Practicing these skills will help build a repertoire of coping strategies.	Assess whether Steven follows through on learning new skills.

Continued on following page

NURSING CARE PLAN (*Continued*)

Interventions	Rationale	Ongoing Assessment
Educate the patient on the use of alcohol and its relationship to bipolar disorder.	Alcohol is an ineffective coping strategy that can exacerbate the symptoms of bipolar disorder.	Assess for the patient's willingness to control drinking.
Assist the patient in coping with bipolar disorder, beginning with education about it.	A mood disorder is a major stressor in a patient's life. To manage the stress, the patient needs a knowledge base.	Determine Steven's knowledge about bipolar disorder.
Administer lithium as ordered (give with food or milk). Reinforce the action, dosage, and side effects. Review laboratory results to determine whether lithium is within therapeutic limits. Assess for toxicity. Recommend a normal diet with normal salt intake; maintenance of adequate fluid intake.	Lithium carbonate is effective in the treatment of bipolar disorder, but it must be managed. The patient should have a thorough knowledge of the medication and side effects.	Assess for target action, side effects, and toxicity.

Goals of Care

Hypothyroidism Interventions	Rationale	Ongoing Assessment
Administer thyroid supplement as ordered. Review thyroid functioning laboratory results. Discuss the symptoms of hypothyroidism and how they are similar to depression. Emphasize the importance of taking lithium and L-thyroxine. Explain about the long-term effects of lithium on thyroid functioning.	Hypothyroidism can be a side effect of lithium carbonate and also mimics symptoms of depression.	Determine whether the patient understands the relationship between thyroid dysfunction and lithium carbonate.

Evaluation

Outcomes	Revised Outcomes	Interventions
Clonazepam 0.5 mg bid for sleep and agitation		
Steven is easily engaged in a therapeutic relationship. He examined the areas in his life where he coped ineffectively.	Establish a therapeutic relationship with a therapist at the mental health clinic.	Refer to mental health clinic.
He identified his strengths and how he coped with stressors, especially his illness, in the past.	Continue to view illness as a potential stressor that can disrupt life.	Seek advice immediately if there are any problems with medications.
He learned new problem-solving skills and reported that he learned a lot about his medication. He plans to adhere to medication regimen.	Continue to practice new coping skills as stressful situations arise.	Discuss with the therapist the outcomes of using new coping skills.

Continuum of Care

Inpatient Management

Inpatient admission is the treatment setting necessary when patients are severely psychotic or are an immediate threat to themselves or others. In acute mania, nursing interventions focus on patient safety, because patients in this state are prone to injury due to hyperactivity and are often unaware of injuries they sustain. Patients are often impulsive, disinhibited, and interpersonally inappropriate during acute mania. Redirecting conversation as well as behaviour and implementing boundaries is required when a patient is talking or acting inappropriately. Removal to a quieter environment may be necessary if other interventions have not been successful, but the patient should be carefully monitored. The nurse should avoid a confrontational approach and instead, respectfully implement limits.

Medication management including control of side effects is a major nursing responsibility during inpatient hospitalization. Nurses should be familiar with drug–drug interactions (Chapter 13) and with interventions to help control side effects.

Intensive Outpatient Programmes

When hospitalization is not necessary, or in order to prevent or shorten hospitalization, intensive outpatient programs for several weeks of acute-phase care during a manic or depressive episode are used. These programs are usually called *partial hospitalization* or *day hospitalization*. Close medication monitoring and milieu therapies that foster the restoration of a patient's previous adaptive abilities are the major nursing responsibilities in these settings. Setting up frequent office visits and crisis telephone calls are additional nursing interventions that can help to shorten or prevent hospitalization. Psychoeducation that includes the patient and significant others are alternatives. Severely and persistently ill patients may need ongoing intensive treatment, but the frequency of visits can be decreased for patients whose conditions stabilize and who enter the continuation or the maintenance phase of treatment.

Spectrum of Care

In today's healthcare climate, with efforts to reduce hospitalization, most patients with bipolar disorder are treated as outpatients. Hospitalizations are usually brief, and treatment focuses on restabilization. Patients with mood disorders are likely to need long-term medication regimens and supportive psychotherapy to function in the community. Therefore, medication regimens and additional treatment planning need to be tailored to individual needs. Patients need extended and continued follow-up to monitor medication trials and side effects, reinforce self-care management, and provide continued psychosocial support (see Chapter 5).

Mental Health Promotion

Mental health promotion activities should be the focus during remissions. During this period, patients have an opportunity to learn new coping skills that promote positive mental health. Stress management and relaxation techniques can be practiced for use when needed. A plan for managing emerging symptoms can also be developed during this period.

🍁 Summary of Key Points

- Mood disorders are characterized by persistent or recurring disturbances in mood that cause significant psychological distress and functional impairment. Mood disturbances can be broadly categorized as manic or dysphoric (typified by exaggerated feelings of elation or irritability) or depressive or dysthymic (typified by feelings of sadness, hopelessness, loss of interest, and fatigue).
- Primary mood disorders include both depressive disorders (unipolar depression) and manic–depressive disorders (bipolar disorders).
- Genetics undoubtedly play a role in the aetiology of mood disorders. Risk factors include family history of mood disorders; prior mood episodes; lack of social support; stressful life events; substance abuse; and medical problems, particularly chronic or terminal illnesses.
- The recommended depression treatment guidelines include antidepressant medication, alone or with psychotherapeutic management or psychotherapy; ECT for severe depression; or phototherapy for patients with seasonal depressive symptoms.
- Nurses must be knowledgeable about antidepressant medications: their therapeutic effects and associated side effects, toxicity, dosage ranges, and contraindications. Nurses must also be familiar with ECT protocols and associated interventions. Patient education and the provision of emotional support during and after the course of treatment are also nursing responsibilities.
- Many symptoms of depression, such as weight and appetite changes, sleep disturbance, decreased energy, and fatigue, are similar to those of medical illnesses. Assessment includes a thorough medical history and physical examination to detect or rule out medical or psychiatric comorbidity.
- Bio/psycho/social/spiritual assessment includes assessing medical and health status; mood; speech patterns; thought content and processes; suicidal, filicidal, or

homicidal thoughts; cognition and memory; social factors such as patterns of relationship, quality of support systems, and changes in occupational functioning; and spiritual beliefs and practices. Several self-report scales, such as the BDI and the Hamilton Rating Scale, are helpful in evaluating depressive symptoms.

- Establishing and maintaining a therapeutic nurse–patient relationship is key to successful outcomes. Nursing interventions that foster the therapeutic relationship include being available in times of crisis, providing understanding and education to patients and their families regarding goals of treatment, providing encouragement and feedback concerning the patient's progress, providing guidance in the patient's interpersonal interactions (within the work environment, the community), and helping to set and monitor realistic goals.

- Psychosocial interventions for mood disorders include self-care management, cognitive therapy, behaviour therapy, IPT, patient and family psychoeducation regarding the nature of the disorder and treatment goals, marital and family therapy, and group therapy that includes medication maintenance support groups and other consumer-oriented support groups.

- Bipolar disorders are characterized by one or more manic episodes or mixed mania (co-occurrence of manic and depressive states) that cause marked impairment in social activities, occupational functioning, and interpersonal relationships and may require hospitalization to prevent self-harm.

- Manic episodes are periods in which the patient experiences abnormally and persistently elevated, expansive, or irritable mood characterized by inflated self-esteem, decreased need to sleep, excessive energy or hyperactivity, racing thoughts, easy distractibility, and inability to stay focused. Other symptoms can include hypersexuality and impulsivity.

- Similar to treatment of major depressive disorder, pharmacotherapy is the cornerstone of treatment of bipolar illness, but adjunctive psychosocial interventions are also needed. Pharmacologic therapy includes treatment with mood stabilizers alone or in combination with antipsychotics or benzodiazepines if psychosis, agitation, or insomnia is present and antidepressants for unremitted depression.

- ECT is a valuable alternative for patients with severe mania that do not respond to other treatment.

- Recent major advances in bipolar disorder treatment research validate the efficacy of integrated psychosocial and pharmacologic treatment involving family or couples therapies, psychoeducational programmes, and individual cognitive–behavioural or interpersonal therapies.

Thinking Challenges

A nurse is caring for Violet, a 65-year-old woman who has a diagnosis of major depression. In reviewing the chart, the nurse learns that Violet was first diagnosed with depression in her early 20s, and over the years has taken several different antidepressants, each offering limited effectiveness, as well as side effects that she finds disconcerting. She recently lost her husband, her adult children live in another province, and she no longer is employed due to her ongoing challenges associated with her diagnosis. Her psychiatrist is recommending a course of ECT.

1. What are the common features of a major depressive disorder?

2. What are the bio/psycho/social and spiritual factors that the nurse should consider in working with Violet?

3. In which populations is ECT treatment contraindicated or noted to have high risk of complications?

4. What other forms of short-term and long-term treatment should the nurse consider in working with Violet?

Visit thePoint to view suggested responses.
Go to thePoint.lww.com/activate and use the activation code found in the front of this text to unlock answers to the "Thinking Challenges" and other online resources.

Web Links

ccsa.ca Canadian Centre on Substance Use and Addiction website where information exists issues related to alcohol, other substances, and mood disorders.

canmat.org The site of the Canadian Network for Mood and Anxiety Treatment has information for health professionals, patients and families, and the public, including guidelines for management and treatment of mood disorders.

camimh.ca The Canadian Alliance on Mental Illness and Mental Health (CAMIMH) offers information on services of member mental health organizations for healthcare practitioners, consumers, and their families. The organization is committed to raising mental health awareness and making accessibility to care and support for the mentally ill and their families a priority for government and communities.

cmha.ca This is the site of the Canadian Mental Health Association, which uses a wellness model to approach such topics as mental fitness and how it is defined, acquired, and maintained across the life span.

cpa.ca The Canadian Psychological Association takes an advisory role for people wanting to know about issues and care alternatives. Areas of focus include mental health problems related to mood disorders and the psychological factors necessary to maintain wellness in the context of such mood-related disorders.

cdrin.org Canadian Depression Research and Intervention website. It discusses the coalitions participating in an endeavour to promote research by collaborating with provincial and national organizations about depression and PTSD.

https://www.suicideinfo.ca/ Centre for Suicide Prevention. Here you will find a Senior's Suicide Prevention Toolkit, a Toolkit on Indigenous People, trauma, and suicide prevention, and other relevant resources and events.

internationalbipolarfoundation.org International bipolar foundation (IBPF) organization (nonprofit) that offers information in 60 languages about bipolar disorder and its treatment. There are videos and webinars available as well as resources for families and caregivers.

isbd.org International Society for Bipolar Disorder Professional international organization publishing the journal Bipolar Disorder. It supports research about bipolar treatment and has sections for patients and families.

mdsc.ca The Mood Disorders Society of Canada (MDSC) is a volunteer organization with a commitment to optimizing the quality of life for people with mood disorders. The MDSC gives a voice to consumers by establishing a national research agenda and developing strategies of care.

nccah-ccnsa.ca National Collaborating Centre for Aboriginal Health website containing information, webinars, and publications about the health and mental health of Indigenous populations.

nimh.nih.gov The site of the U.S. National Institute of Mental Health (NIMH) provides a forum for worldwide research into mental illness. In addition to offering a wealth of information on the latest research, the site offers education information pamphlets on depression, bipolar disorder, and other

mental illnesses that can be ordered or printed free of charge. These publications are in the public domain and can be reproduced without copyright infringement, as long as authorship is acknowledged.

nmhac.ca This site is the Native Mental Health Association of Canada which developed from the Canadian Psychiatric Association of Mental Health. NMHAC offers educational information and understanding to promote culturally relevant mental health care for Indigenous Peoples.

https://nnmh.ca/ This is the site of the National Network for Mental Health, which functions as an advocate and educational resource for Canadian mental health consumers and their families and friends. The organization's goal is to unite and empower individuals.

obad.ca This is the site of the Organization for Bipolar Affective Disorders (OBADs). This organization offers peer support for anyone affected by mood disorders, aiming to assist them to be active in their recovery and gain a sense of resolution in their lives.

suicideprevention.ca This is the site of the Canadian Association for Suicide Prevention, which provides information on suicide and resources related to its prevention—the location of crisis centres, survivor support groups, and related library materials. Guidelines to minimize the suicide risk of loved ones are available here.

statcan.gc.ca Statistics Canada website contains statistical information about depression and bipolar disorder.

https://www.who.int/news-room/fact-sheets/detail/depression The World Health Organization, information on depression can be found here, including handouts and videos on depression.

who.int/mental_health/management/depression/who_paper_depression_wfmh_2012.pdf The World Health Organization (2012) report titled *Depression: A Global Crisis* is available here.

References

Alonso, J., Petukhova, M., Vilagut, G., Chatterji, S., Heeringa, S., Üstün, T. B., Alhamzawi, A. O., Viana, M. C., Angermeyer, M., Bromet, E., Bruffaerts, R., de Girolamo, G., Florescu, S., Gureje, O., Haro, J. M., Hinkov, H., Hu, C. Y., Karam, E. G., Kovess, V., … Kessler, R. C. (2011). Days out of role due to common physical and mental conditions: results from the WHO World Mental Health surveys. *Molecular psychiatry, 16*(12), 1234–1246. https://doi.org/10.1038/mp.2010.10

American Psychiatric Association. (2013). *Diagnostic and statistical manual of mental disorders* (5th ed.).

Apter, G., Bobin, A., Genet, M. C., Gratier, M., & Devouche, E. (2017). Update on mental health of infants and children of parents affected with mental health issues. *Current Psychiatry Reports, 19*(10), 72. https://doe.org/10.1007/s11920-017-0820-8/

Au, C. H., Wong, C. S. M., Law, C. W., Wong, M. C., & Chung, K. F. (2019). Self-stigma, stigma coping and functioning in remitted bipolar disorder. *General Hospital Psychiatry, 57*, 7–12. https://doi.org/10.1016/j.genhosppsych.2018.12.007

Bachmann, S. (2018). Epidemiology of suicide and the psychiatric perspective. *International Journal of Environmental Research and Public Health, 15*(7), 1425. https://doi.org/10.3390/ijerph15071425

Barker, L. C., Dennis, C. L., Hussain-Shamsy, N., Stewart, D. E., Grigoriadis, S., Metcalfe, K., Oberlander, T. F., Schram, C., Taylor, V. H., & Vigod, S. N. (2020). Decision-making about antidepressant medication use in pregnancy: A comparison between women making the decision in the preconception period versus in pregnancy. *BMC Psychiatry, 20*(1), 54. https://doi.org/10.1186/s12888-020-2478-8

Bellamy, S., & Hardy, C. (2015). *Understanding depression in Aboriginal communities and families*. National Collaborating Centre for Aboriginal Health. http://www.nccah-ccnsa.ca/Publications/Lists/Publications/Attachments/150/2015-10-07-RPT-MentalHealth03-Depression-BellamyHardy-EN-Web.pdf

Bhattacharya, R., Shen, C., & Sambamoorthi, U. (2014). Excess risk of chronic physical conditions associated with depression and anxiety. *BMC Psychiatry 14*, 10. https://doi.org/10.1186/1471-244X-14-10

Bickman, L. (2020). Improving mental health services: A 50-year journey from randomized experiments to artificial intelligence and precision mental health. *Administration and Policy in Mental Health and Mental Health Services Research, 47*(5), 795–843. https://doi.org/10.1007/s10488-020-01065-8

Boland, R., Verduin, M. L., & Ruiz, P. (2021). *Kaplan and Sadock's synopsis of psychiatry* (12th ed.). Wolters Kluwer.

Bonanno, G. A., & Malgaroli, M. (2020). Trajectories of grief: Comparing symptoms from the DSM-5 and ICD-11 diagnoses. *Depression and Anxiety, 37*(1), 17–25. https://doi.org/10.1002/da.22902

Borneman, T., Ferrell, B., & Puchalski, C. (2010). Evaluation of the FICA tool for spiritual assessment. *Journal of Pain and Symptom Management, 40*(2), 163–173. https://doi.org/10.1016/j.jpainsymman.2009.12.019

Bot, M., Brouwer, I. A., Roca, M., Kohls, E., Penninx, B., Watkins, E., van Grooteheest, G., Cabout, M., Hegerl, U., Gili, M., Owens, M., Visser, M., & MooDFOOD Prevention Trial Investigators. (2019). Effect of multinutrient supplementation and food-related behavioral activation therapy on prevention of major depressive disorder among overweight or obese adults with subsyndromal depressive symptoms: The MooDFOOD randomized clinical trial. *JAMA, 321*(9), 858–868. https://doi.org/10.1001/jama.2019.0556

Brunoni, A. R., Sampaio-Junior, B., Moffa, A. H., Aparício, L. V., Gordon, P., Klein, I., Rios, R. M., Razza, L. B., Loo, C., Padberg, F., & Valiengo, L. (2019). Noninvasive brain stimulation in psychiatric disorders: A primer. *Revista brasileira de psiquiatria (Sao Paulo, Brazil: 1999), 41*(1), 70–81. https://doi.org/10.1590/1516-4446-2017-0018

Caldwell, D., Davies, S., Hetrick, S., Palmer, J., Caro, P., López-López, J., Gunnell, D., Kidger, J., Thomas, J., French, C., Stockings, E., Campbell, R., & Welton, N. (2019). School-based interventions to prevent anxiety and depression in children and young people: A systematic review and network meta-analysis. *The Lancet Psychiatry*, 6, 1011–1020.

Canadian Mental Health Association. (2013). *Connection between mental and physical health.* http://ontario.cmha.ca/mental-health/connection-between-mental-and-physical-health/

Canadian Nurses Association. (2016). *Dementia in Canada: Recommendations to support care for Canada's aging population.* https://cna-aiic.ca/~/media/cna/page-content/pdf-en/dementia-in-canada_recommendations-to-support-care-for-canadas-aging-population.pdf?la=en

Carta, M. G., Paribello, P., Nardi, A. E., & Preti, A. (2019). Current pharmacotherapeutic approaches for dysthymic disorder and persistent depressive disorder. *Expert Opinion on Pharmacotherapy*, 20(14), 1743–1754. https://doi.org/10.1080/14656566.2019.1637419.

Carta, M. G., Patten, S., Nardi, A. E., & Bhugra, D. (2017). Mental health and chronic diseases: A challenge to be faced from a new perspective. *International Review of Psychiatry*, 29(5), 373–376. https://doi.org/10.1080/09540261.2017.1364885

Carvalho, A. F., Firth, J., & Vieta, E. (2020). Bipolar disorder. *New England Journal of Medicine*, 383, 58–66. https://doi.org/10.1056/NEJMra1906193

Case, S. M., Sawhney, M., & Stewart, J. C. (2018). Atypical depression and double depression predict new-onset cardiovascular disease in US adults. *Depression and Anxiety*, 35(1), 10–17. https://doi.org/10.1002/da.22666

Chahar Mahali, S., Beshai, S., & Wolfe, W. L. (2021). The associations of dispositional mindfulness, self-compassion, and reappraisal with symptoms of depression and anxiety among a sample of Indigenous students in Canada. *Journal of American College Health*, 69, 872–880. https://doi.org/10.1080/07448481.2020.1711764.

Chen, R., Zhu, X., Capitão, L. P., Zhang, H., Luo, J., Wang, X., Xi, Y., Song, X., Feng, Y., Cao, L., & Malhi, G. S. (2019). Psychoeducation for psychiatric inpatients following remission of a manic episode in bipolar I disorder: A randomized controlled trial. *Bipolar Disorders*, 21(1), 76–85. https://doi.org/10.1111/bdi.12642

Chia, M. F., Cotton, S., Filia, K., Phelan, M., Conus, P., Jauhar, S., Marwaha, S., McGorry, P. D., Davey, C., Berk, M., & Ratheesh, A. (2019). Early intervention for bipolar disorder—Do current treatment guidelines provide recommendations for the early stages of the disorder? *Journal of Affective Disorders*, 257, 669–677. https://doi.org/10.1016/j.jad.2019.07.062

Chiang, K. J., Tsai, J. C., Liu, D., Lin, C. H., Chiu, H. L., & Chou, K. R. (2017). Efficacy of cognitive-behavioral therapy in patients with bipolar disorder: A meta-analysis of randomized controlled trials. *PLoS One*, 12(5), e0176849. https://doi.org/10.1371/journal.pone.0176849

Chiu, M., Gatov, E., Fung, K., Kurdyak, P., & Guttmann, A. (2020). Deconstructing the rise in mental health–related ED visits among children and youth in Ontario, Canada: Study examines the rise in mental health-related emergency department visits among children and youth in Ontario. *Health Affairs*, 39(10), 1728–1736. https://doi.org/10.1377/hlthaff.2020.00232

Corrigan, P. W., & Nieweglowski, K. (2021). Difference as an indicator of the self-stigma of mental illness. *Journal of Mental Health*, 30, 417–423. https://doi.org/10.1080/09638237.2019.1581351

Đào, G. J., Brunelle, C., & Speed, D. (2019). Impact of substance use and mental health comorbidity on health care access in Canada. *Journal of Dual Diagnosis*, 15(4), 260–269. https://doi.org/10.1080/15504263.2019.1634856

Dau, A. L. B., Callinan, L. S., & Smith, M. V. (2019). An examination of the impact of maternal fetal attachment, postpartum depressive symptoms and parenting stress on maternal sensitivity. *Infant Behavior and Development*, 54, 99–107. https://doi.org/10.1016/j.infbeh.2019.01.001

Davis, S. (2014). *Community mental health in Canada: theory, policy, and practice.* UBC Press.

Day, R. O., Snowden, L., & McLachlan, A. J. (2017). Life-threatening drug interactions: What the physician needs to know. *Internal Medicine Journal*, 47(5), 501–512. https://doi.org/10.1111/imj.13404

Dean, J., & Keshavan, M. (2017). The neurobiology of depression: An integrated view. *Asian Journal of Psychiatry*, 27, 101–111. https://doi.org/10.1016/j.ajp.2017.01.025

Dobson, K. G., Vigor, S. N., Mustard, C., & Smith, P. M. (2020). Trends in the prevalence of depression and anxiety disorders among working-age Canadian adults between 2000 and 2016. *Health Reports*, 31(12), 12–23. https://www.doi.org/10.25318/82-003-x202001200002-eng

Dohm, K., Redlich, R., Zwitserlood, P., & Dannlowski, U. (2017). Trajectories of major depression disorders: A systematic review of longitudinal neuroimaging findings. *Australian & New Zealand Journal of Psychiatry*, 51(5), 441–454. https://doi.org/10.1177/0004867416661426

Dome, P., Rihmer, Z., & Gonda, X. (2019). Suicide risk in bipolar disorder: A brief review. *Medicina*, 55(8), 403. https://doi.org/10.3390/medicina55080403

Dong, M., Lu, L., Zhang, L., Zhang, Q., Ungvari, G. S., Ng, C. H., Yuan, Z., Xiang, Y., Wang, G., & Xiang, Y. T. (2019). Prevalence of suicide attempts in bipolar disorder: A systematic review and meta-analysis of observational studies. *Epidemiology and Psychiatric Sciences*, 29, e63. https://doi.org/10.1017/S2045796019000593

Doody, O., Butler, M. P., Lyons, R., & Newman, D. (2017). Families' experiences of involvement in care planning in mental health services: An integrative literature review. *Journal of Psychiatric and Mental Health Nursing*, 24(6), 412–430. https://doi.org/10.1111/jpm.12369

Duffy, A., Goodday, S., Keown-Stoneman, C., & Grof, P. (2019). The emergent course of bipolar disorder: observations over two decades from the Canadian high-risk offspring cohort. *American Journal of Psychiatry*, 176(9), 720–729. https://doi.org/10.1176/appi.ajp.2018.18040461

Enache, D., Pariante, C. M., & Mondelli, V. (2019). Markers of central inflammation in major depressive disorder: A systematic review and meta-analysis of studies examining cerebrospinal fluid, positron emission tomography and post-mortem brain tissue. *Brain, Behavior, and Immunity*, 81, 24–40. https://doi.org/10.1016/j.bbi.2019.06.015

Farrell, C., Doolin, K., O' Leary, N., Jairaj, C., Roddy, D., Tozzi, L., Morris, D., Harkin, A., Frodl, T., Nemoda, Z., Szyf, M., Booij, L., & O'Keane, V. (2018). DNA methylation differences at the glucocorticoid receptor gene in depression are related to functional alterations in hypothalamic-pituitary-adrenal axis activity and to early life emotional abuse. *Psychiatry Research*, 265, 341–348. https://doi.org/10.1016/j.psychres.2018.04.064

Felitti, V. J., Anda, R. F., Nordenberg, D., Williamson, D. F., Spitz, A. M., Edwards, V., Koss, M. P., & Marks, J. S. (1998). Relationship of childhood abuse and household dysfunction to many of the leading causes of death in adults. The Adverse Childhood Experiences (ACE) Study. *American Journal of Preventive Medicine*, 14(4), 245–258. https://doi.org/10.1016/s0749-3797(98)00017-8

Ferrari, F., & Villa, R. F. (2017). The neurobiology of depression: An integrated overview from biological theories to clinical evidence. *Molecular Neurobiology*, 54(7), 4847–4865. https://doi.org/10.1007/s12035-016-0032-y

Fiedeldey-Van Dijk, C., Rowan, M., Dell, C., Mushquash, C., Hopkins, C., Fornssler, B., Hall, L., Mykota, D., Farag, M., & Shea, B. (2017). Honoring Indigenous culture-as-intervention: Development and validity of the Native Wellness AssessmentTM. *Journal of Ethnicity in Substance Abuse*, 16(2), 181–218. https://doi.org/10.1080/15332640.2015.1119774

Findlay, L. (2017). *Depression and suicidal ideation among Canadians aged 15 to 24.* https://www150.statcan.gc.ca/n1/pub/82-003-x/2017001/article/14697-eng.htm

Findlay, L. C., Arin, R., & Kohen, D. (2020). Understanding the perceived mental health of Canadians during the COVID-19 pandemic. *Health Reports*, 30(1), 22–27. https://www.doi.org/10.25318/82-003-x202000400003-eng

Flowers, A. G., McGillivray, J. A., Galbally, M., & Lewis, A. J. (2018). Perinatal maternal mental health and disorganised attachment: A critical systematic review. *Clinical Psychologist*, 22(3), 300–316. https://doi.org/10.1111/cp.12145

Fulmer, R. (2018). The evolution of the psychodynamic approach and system. *International Journal of Psychological Studies*, 10(1). https://doi.org/10.5539/ijps.v10n3p1

Gambin, M., & Sharp, C. (2018). The relations between empathy, guilt, shame and depression in inpatient adolescents. *Journal of Affective Disorders*, 241, 381–387. https://doi.org/10.1016/j.jad.2018.08.068

Gautam, S., Jain, A., Gautam, M., Vahia, V. N., & Grover, S. (2017). Clinical practice guidelines for the management of depression. *Indian Journal of Psychiatry*, 59(Suppl 1), S34. https://doi.org/10.4103/0019-5545.196973

Gaynes, B. N., Brown, C. L., Lux, L. J., Brownley, K. A., Van Dorn, R. A., Edlund, M. J., Coker-Schwimmer, E., Weber, R. P., Sheitman, B., Zarzar, T., Viswanathan, M., & Lohr, K. N. (2017). Preventing and de-escalating aggressive behavior among adult psychiatric patients: A systematic review of the evidence. *Psychiatric Services (Washington, D.C.)*, 68(8), 819–831. https://doi.org/10.1176/appi.ps.201600314

Georgiades, K., Duncan, L., Wang, L., Comeau, J., Boyle, M. H., & 2014 Ontario Child Health Study Team. (2019). Six-month prevalence of mental disorders and service contacts among children and youth in Ontario: Evidence from the 2014 Ontario Child Health Study. *The Canadian Journal of Psychiatry*, 64(4), 246–255. https://doi.org/10.1177/0706743719830024

Giridharan, V. V., Sayana, P., Pinjari, O. F., Ahmad, N., da Rosa, M. I., Quevedo, J., & Barichello, T. (2020). Postmortem evidence of brain inflammatory markers in bipolar disorder: A systematic review. *Molecular Psychiatry, 25*(1), 94–113. https://doi.org/10.1038/s41380-019-0448-7

Gold, A. K., & Sylvia, L. G. (2016). The role of sleep in bipolar disorder. *Nature and Science of Sleep, 8*, 207. https://doi.org/10.2147/NSS.S85754

Goldstein, T. R., Merranko, J., Krantz, M., Garcia, M., Franzen, P., Levenson, J., Axelson, D., Birmaher, B., & Frank, E. (2018). Early intervention for adolescents at-risk for bipolar disorder: A pilot randomized trial of Interpersonal and Social Rhythm Therapy (IPSRT). *Journal of Affective Disorders, 235*, 348–356. https://doi.org/10.1016/j.jad.2018.04.049

Gordovez, F. J. A., & McMahon, F. J. (2020). The genetics of bipolar disorder. *Molecular Psychiatry, 25*, 544–559. https://doi.org/10.1038/s41380-019-0634-7

Government of Canada. (2021, August 31). *COVID-19 daily epidemiology update.* https://health-infobase.canada.ca/covid-19/epidemiological-summary-covid-19-cases.html

Granek, L. (2017). Is grief a disease? The medicalization of grief by the psy-disciplines in the twenty-first century. In N. Thompson & G. R. Cox (Eds.), *Handbook of the sociology of death, grief, and bereavement: A guide to theory and practice.* Routelage.

Greenberg, P. E., Fournier, A. A., Sisitsky, T., Pike, C. T., & Kessler, R. C. (2015). The economic burden of adults with major depressive disorder in the United States (2005 and 2010). *The Journal of Clinical Psychiatry, 76*(2), 155–162. https:doi.org/10.4088/JCP.14m09298

Gruber, J., Prinstein, M. J., Clark, L. A., Rottenberg, J., Abramowitz, J. S., Albano, A. M., Aldao, A., Borelli, J. L., Chung, T., Davila, J., Forbes, E. E., Gee, D. G., Hall, G., Hallion, L. S., Hinshaw, S. P., Hofmann, S. G., Hollon, S. D., Joormann, J., Kazdin, A. E., … Weinstock, L. M. (2021). Mental health and clinical psychological science in the time of COVID-19: Challenges, opportunities, and a call to action. *The American Psychologist, 76*(3), 409–426. https://doi.org/10.1037/amp0000707

Hackett, C., Feeny, D., & Tompa, E. (2016). Canada's residential school system: Measuring the intergenerational impact of familial attendance on health and mental health outcomes. *Journal of Epidemiology and Community Health, 70*(11), 1096–1105. https://doi.org/10.1136/jech-2016-207380

Hamilton, M. (1986). The Hamilton rating scale for depression. In *Assessment of depression* (pp. 143–152). Springer.

Hayne, Y. (2003). Experiencing psychiatric diagnosis: Client perspectives on being named mentally ill. *Journal of Psychiatric and Mental Health Nursing, 10*(6), 722–729. https://doi.org/10.1046/j.1365-2850.2003.00666.x

Hedya, S. A., Avula, A., & Swoboda, H. D. (2019). Lithium toxicity. In *StatPearls* https://www.ncbi.nlm.nih.gov/books/NBK499992/

Hemmiger, A., & Wills, B. L. (2021). Vitamin B6 toxicity. *StatPearls* https://www.ncbi.nlm.nih.gov/books/NBK554500/

Hett, D., Rogers, J., Humpston, C., & Marwaha, S. (2020). Repetitive transcranial magnetic stimulation (rTMS) for the treatment of depression in adolescence: A systematic review. *Journal of Affective Disorders, 278*, 460–469. https://doi.org/10.1016/j.jad.2020.09.058

Hickie, I. B., Scott, E. M., Cross, S. P., Iorfino, F., Davenport, T. A., Guastella, A. J., Naismith, S. L., Carpenter, J. S., Rohleder, C., Crouse, J. J., Hermens, D. F., Koethe, D., Markus Leweke, F., Tickell, A. M., Sawrikar, V., & Scott, J. (2019). Right care, first time: A highly personalised and measurement-based care model to manage youth mental health. *The Medical Journal of Australia, 211*(Suppl 9), S3–S46. https://doi.org/10.5694/mja2.50383

Hofmann, S. G., Curtiss, J., Carpenter, J. K., & Kind, S. (2017). Effect of treatments for depression on quality of life: A meta-analysis. *Cognitive Behaviour Therapy, 46*(4), 265–286. https://doi.org/10.1080/16506073.2017.1304445

International Council of Nurses. (2013). *ICN code of ethics for nurses. Cultural and linguistic competence.* http://www.icn.ch/images/stories/documents/publications/position_statements/B03_Cultural_Linguistic_Competence.pdf

Iorfino, F., Scott, E. M., Carpenter, J. S., Cross, S. P., Hermens, D. F., Killedar, M., Nichles, A., Zmicerevska, N., White, D., Guastella, A. J., Scott, J., McGorry, P. D., & Hiclie, I. B. (2019). Clinical stage transitions in persons aged 12 to 25 years presenting to early intervention mental health services with anxiety, mood, and psychotic disorders. *JAMA Psychiatry, 76*(11), 1167–1175. https://doi:10.1001/jamapsychiatry.

Jawad, I., Watson, S., Haddad, P. M., Talbot, P. S., & McAllister-Williams, R. H. (2018). Medication nonadherence in bipolar disorder: A narrative review. *Therapeutic Advances in Psychopharmacology, 8*(12), 349–363. https://doi.org/10.1177/2045125318804364

Joëls, M. (2018). Corticosteroids and the brain. *Journal of Endocrinology, 238*(3), R121–R130. https://doi.org/10.1530/JOE-18-0226

Johnson, R. L., & Wilson, C. G. (2018). A review of vagus nerve stimulation as a therapeutic intervention. *Journal of Inflammation Research, 11*, 203–213. https://doi.org/10.2147/JIR.S163248

Kerner, B. (2014). Genetics of bipolar disorder. *The Application of Clinical Genetics, 7*, 33–42. https://doi.org/10.2147/TACG.S39297

Kim, K., & Jeon, H. J. (2018). Clinical, biological, and therapeutic characteristics between depression with and without medical illness. In Y. K. Kim (Ed.), *Understanding depression* (pp. 175–186). Springer. https://doi.org/10.1007/978-981-10-6577-4_13

Kittel-Schneider, S., Bury, D., Leopold, K., Haack, S., Bauer, M., Pfeiffer, S., Sauer, C., Pfennig, A., Völzke, H., Grabe, H. J., & Reif, A. (2020). Prevalence of prediabetes and diabetes mellitus type II in bipolar disorder. *Frontiers in Psychiatry, 11*, 314. https://doi.org/10.3389/fpsyt.2020.00314

Kok, J. K., Pheh, K. S., & Hor, G. L. (2018). Psychological and social factors of depression recovery: A narrative review. *Pertanika Journal of Social Science Humanities, 26*(1), 41–58.

Kolostoumpis, D., Bergiannaki, J., Peppou, L., Louki, E., Fousketaki, S., Patelakis, A., & Economou, M. (2015). Effectiveness of relatives' psychoeducation on family outcomes in bipolar disorder. *International Journal of Mental Health, 44*(4), 290–302. https://doi.org/10.1080/00207411.2015.1076292

Kong, J., Fang, J., Park, J., Li, S., & Rong, P. (2018). Treating depression with transcutaneous auricular vagus nerve stimulation: State of the art and future perspectives. *Frontiers in Psychiatry, 9*, 20. https://doi.org/10.3389/fpsyt.2018.00020

Kuhlman, K. R., Chiang, J. J., Bower, J. E., Irwin, M. R., Cole, S. W., Dahl, R. E., Almeida, D. M., & Fuligni, A. J. (2020). Persistent low positive affect and sleep disturbance across adolescence moderate link between stress and depressive symptoms in early adulthood. *Journal of Abnormal Child Psychology, 48*(1), 109–121. https://doi.org/10.1007/s10802-019-00581-y

Leach, L. S., & Butterworth, P. (2020). Depression and anxiety in early adulthood: Consequences for finding a partner, and relationship support and conflict. *Epidemiology and Psychiatric Sciences, 29*, E141. https://doi.org/10.1017/S2045796020000530

Lefaucheur, J. P., Aleman, A., Baeken, C., Benninger, D. H., Brunelin, J., Di Lazzaro, V., Filipović, S. R., Grefkes, C., Hasan, A., Hummel, F. C., Jääskeläinen, S. K., Langguth, B., Leocani, L., Londero, A., Nardone, R., Nguyen, J. P., Nyffeler, T., Oliveira-Maia, A. J., Oliviero, A., … Ziemann, U. (2020). Evidence-based guidelines on the therapeutic use of repetitive transcranial magnetic stimulation (rTMS): an update (2014-2018). *Clinical neurophysiology: official journal of the International Federation of Clinical Neurophysiology, 131*(2), 474–528. https://doi.org/10.1016/j.clinph.2019.11.002

Lekoadi, R. G., Poggenpoel, M., Temane, M. A., & Myburgh, C. P. (2019). Lived experiences of family members caring for individuals living with Bipolar disorder. *Africa Journal of Nursing and Midwifery, 21*(1), 1–19. https://doi.org/10.25159/2520-5293/5819

Li, C., Palka, J. M., & Brown, E. S. (2020a). Cognitive impairment in individuals with bipolar disorder with and without comorbid alcohol and/or cocaine use disorders. *Journal of Affective Disorders, 272*, 355–362. https://doi.org/10.1016/j.jad.2020.03.179

Li, M., Yao, X., Sun, L., Zhao, L., Xu, W., Zhao, H., Zhao, F., Zou, X., Cheng, Z., Li, B., Yang, W., & Cui, R. (2020b). Effects of electroconvulsive therapy on depression and its potential mechanism. *Frontiers in Psychology, 11*, 80. https://doi.org/10.3389/fpsyg.2020.00080

Li, Y., Lv, M. R., Wei, Y. J., Sun, L., Zhang, J. X., Zhang, H. G., & Li, B. (2017). Dietary patterns and depression risk: A meta-analysis. *Psychiatry Research, 253*, 373–382. https://doi.org/10.1016/j.psychres.2017.04.020

Liu, J., Son, S., McIntyre, J., & Narushima, M. (2019). Depression and cardiovascular diseases among Canadian older adults: A cross-sectional analysis of baseline data from the CLSA Comprehensive Cohort. *Journal of Geriatric Cardiology: JGC, 16*(12), 847. https://doi.org/10.11909/j.issn.1671-5411.2019.12.001

Liu, Y., Zhao, J., & Guo, W. (2018). Emotional roles of mono-aminergic neurotransmitters in major depressive disorder and anxiety disorders. *Frontiers in Psychology, 9*, 2201. https://doi.org/10.3389/fpsyg.2018.02201

Lv, H., Zhao, Y. H., Chen, J. G., Wang, D. Y., & Chen, H. (2019). Vagus nerve stimulation for depression: A systematic review. *Frontiers in Psychology, 10*, 64. https://doi.org/10.3389/fpsyg.2019.00064

Maass, U., Hofmann, L., Perlinger, J., & Wagner, B. (2020). Effects of bereavement groups–a systematic review and meta-analysis. *Death Studies*, 1–11. https://doi.org/10.1080/07481187.2020.1772410

Maruani, J., & Geoffroy, P. A. (2019). Bright light as a personalized precision treatment of mood disorders. *Frontiers in Psychiatry, 10*, 85. https://doi.org/10.3389/fpsyt.2019.00085

McDonald, K., Bulloch, A., Duffy, A., Bresee, L., Williams, J., Lavorato, D., & Patten, S. (2015). Prevalence of bipolar I and II disorder in Canada. *Canadian Journal of Psychiatry, 60*(3), 151–156. http://doi.org/10.1177/070674371506000310

McIntyre, R. S., Rodrigues, N. B., Lipsitz, O., Nasri, F., Gill, H., Lui, L. M., Subramaniapillai, M., Kratiuk, K., Teopiz, K., Ho, R., Lee, Y., Mansur, R. B., & Rosenblat, J. D. (2020). The effectiveness of intravenous ketamine in adults with treatment-resistant major depressive disorder and bipolar disorder presenting with prominent anxiety: Results from the Canadian Rapid Treatment Center of Excellence. *Journal of Psychopharmacology, 35*(2), 128–136. https://doi.org/10.1177/0269881120954048

Meier, S. M., Pavlova, B., Dalsgaard, S., Nordentoft, M., Mors, O., Mortensen, P. B., & Uher, R. (2018). Attention-deficit hyperactivity disorder and anxiety disorders as precursors of bipolar disorder onset in adulthood. *The British Journal of Psychiatry: the Journal of Mental Science, 213*(3), 555–560. https://doi.org/10.1192/bjp.2018.111

Mikkelsen, K., Stojanovska, L., & Apostolopoulos, V. (2016). The effects of vitamin B in depression. *Current Medicinal Chemistry, 23*(38), 4317–4337. https://doi.org/10.2174/0929867323666160920110810

Milner, K., Crawford, P., Edgley, A., Hare-Duke, L., & Slade, M. (2020). The experiences of spirituality among adults with mental health difficulties: A qualitative systematic review. *Epidemiology and Psychiatric Sciences, 29*, e34. https://doi.org/10.1017/S2045796019000234

Mistry, S., Escott-Price, V., Florio, A. D., Smith, D. J., & Zammit, S. (2019). Genetic risk for bipolar disorder and psychopathology from childhood to early adulthood. *Journal of Affective Disorders, 246*, 633–639. https://doi.org/10.1016/j.jad.2018.12.091

Morsel, A. M., Morrens, M., Dhar, M., & Sabbe, B. (2018). Systematic review of cognitive event related potentials in euthymic bipolar disorder. *Clinical Neurophysiology, 129*(9), 1854–1865. https://doi.org/10.1016/j.clinph.2018.05.025

Müller, H., Moeller, S., Lücke, C., Lam, A. P., Braun, N., & Philipsen, A. (2018). Vagus nerve stimulation (VNS) and other augmentation strategies for therapy-resistant depression (TRD): Review of the evidence and clinical advice for use. *Frontiers in Neuroscience, 12*, 239. https://doi.org/10.3389/fnins.2018.00239

National Institute for Health and Care Excellence. (2020). *Antenatal and postnatal mental health: Clinical management and service guidance.* Clinical Guideline. https://www.nice.org.uk/guidance/cg192

Neufeld, E., Freeman, S., Spirgiene, L., & Horwath, U. (2021). A cross-sectoral comparison of prevalence and predictors of symptoms of depression over time among older adults in Ontario, Canada. *Journal of Geriatric Psychiatry and Neurology, 34*(1), 11–20. https://doi.org/10.1177/0891988720901790

Ng, Q. X., Venkatanarayanan, N., & Ho, C. Y. X. (2017). Clinical use of *Hypericum perforatum* (St John's wort) in depression: A meta-analysis. *Journal of Affective Disorders, 210*, 211–221. https://doi.org/10.1016/j.jad.2016.12.048

Nihayati, H. E., Istizabana, E. S., & Nastiti, A. A. (2020). The influence of family psychoeducation to self-awareness family in caring for family members who have mental disorders. *EurAsian Journal of BioSciences, 14*(1), 1589–1595.

Nussbaumer-Streit, B., Forneris, C. A., Morgan, L. C., Van Noord, M. G., Gaynes, B. N., Greenblatt, A., Wipplinger, J., Lux, L. J., Winkler, D., & Gartlehner, G. (2019). Light therapy for preventing seasonal affective disorder. *The Cochrane Database of Systematic Reviews, 3*(3), CD011269. https://doi.org/10.1002/14651858.CD011269.pub3

O'Donovan, C., & Alda, M. (2020). Depression preceding diagnosis of bipolar disorder. *Frontiers in Psychiatry, 11*, 500. https://doi.org/10.3389/fpsyt.2020.00500

Oluboka, O. J., Katzman, M. A., Habert, J., McIntosh, D., MacQueen, G. M., Milev, R. V., McIntyre, R. S., & Blier, P. (2018). Functional recovery in major depressive disorder: Providing early optimal treatment for the individual patient. *The International Journal of Neuropsychopharmacology, 21*(2), 128–144. https://doi.org/10.1093/ijnp/pyx081

Omer, E., Braw, Y., Amiaz, R., & Ravona-Springer, R. (2021). Executive functioning of older adults with bipolar disorder. *International Journal of Geriatric Psychiatry, 36*, 106–115. https://doi.org/10.1002/gps.5402

Ormel, J., Hartman, C. A., & Snieder, H. (2019). The genetics of depression: successful genome-wide association studies introduce new challenges. *Translational Psychiatry, 9*(1), 1–10. https://doi.org/10.1038/s41398-019-0450-5

Ostroff, R., Kitay, B., Wilkinson, S., & Taylor, J. (2019). Interventional psychiatry, a new competency for 21st century psychiatry residents. *Brain Stimulation: Basic, Translational, and Clinical Research in Neuromodulation, 12*(2), 475. https://doi.org/10.1016/j.brs.2018.12.547

Oxhandler, H. K., & Parrish, D. E. (2018). Integrating clients' religion/spirituality in clinical practice: A comparison among social workers, psychologists, counselors, marriage and family therapists, and nurses. *Journal of Clinical Psychology, 74*(4), 680–694. https://doi.org/10.1002/jclp.22539

Paine, D. R., & Sandage, S. J. (2017). Religious involvement and depression: The mediating effect of relational spirituality. *Journal of Religion and Health, 56*(1), 269–283. https://doi.org/10.1007/s10943-016-0282-z

Pandey, R., Tiwari, G. K., Parihar, P., & Rai, P. K. (2020). The relationship between self-forgiveness and human flourishing: Inferring the underlying psychological mechanisms. *Polish Psychological Bulletin, 51*, 23–36. https://doi.org/10.24425/ppb.2020.132649

Parker, G., Spoelma, M. J., Tavella, G., Alda, M., Hajek, T., Dunner, D. L., O'Donovan, C., Rybakowski, J. K., Goldberg, J. F., Bayes, A., Sharma,

V., Boyce, P., & Manicavasagar, V. (2020). The bipolar disorders: A case for their categorically distinct status based on symptom profiles. *Journal of Affective Disorders, 277*, 225–231. https://doi.org/10.1016/j.jad.2020.08.014

Patel, R. K., & Rose, G. M. (2020). Persistent depressive disorder (Dysthymia). *StatPearls [Internet].* https://www.ncbi.nlm.nih.gov/books/NBK541052/

Patten, S. B., Williams, J. V., Lavorato, D. H., Wang, J. L., Bulloch, A. G., & Sajobi, T. (2016a). The association between major depression prevalence and sex becomes weaker with age. *Social Psychiatry and Psychiatric Epidemiology, 51*(2), 203–210. https://doi.org/10.1007/s00127-015-1166-3

Patten, S. B., Williams, J. V., Lavorato, D. H., Wang, J. L., McDonald, K., & Bulloch, A. G. (2016b). Major depression in Canada: What has changed over the past 10 years? *The Canadian Journal of Psychiatry, 61*(2), 80–85. https://doi.org/10.1177/0706743715625940

Pavkovic, B., Zaric, M., Markovic, M., Klacar, M., Huljic, A., & Caricic, A. (2018). Double screening for dual disorder, alcoholism and depression. *Psychiatry Research, 270*, 483–489. https://doi.org/10.1016/j.psychres.2018.10.013

Peña, C. J., & Nestler, E. J. (2018). Progress in epigenetics of depression. In *Progress in Molecular Biology and Translational Science* (Vol. 157, pp. 41–66). Academic Press.

Petruccelli, K., Davis, J., & Berman, T. (2019). Adverse childhood experiences and associated health outcomes: A systematic review and meta-analysis. *Child Abuse & Neglect, 97*, 104127. https://doi.org/10.1016/j.chiabu.2019.104127

Pfefferbaum, B., & North, C. S. (2020). Mental health and the Covid-19 pandemic. *New England Journal of Medicine, 383*, 510–512. https://doi.org/10.1056/NEJMp2008017

Porter, R. J., Baune, B. T., Morris, G., Hamilton, A., Bassett, D., Boyce, P., Hopwood, M. J., Mulder, R., Parker, G., Singh, A. B., Outhred, T., Das, P., & Malhi, G. S. (2020). Cognitive side-effects of electroconvulsive therapy: What are they, how to monitor them and what to tell patients. *BJPsych Open, 6*(3), e40. https://doi.org/10.1192/bjo.2020.17

Procyshyn, R. M., Bezchilibnyk-Butler, K. Z., & Jeffries, J. J. (2019). *Clinical Handbook of Psychotropic Drugs* (23rd ed.). Hogrefe Publishing.

Ransome, Y. (2020). Religion spirituality and health: new considerations for epidemiology. *American Journal of Epidemiology, 189*(8), 755–758. https://doi.org/10.1093/aje/kwaa022

Rao, P. P., Rebello, P., Safeekh, A. T., & Mathai, P. J. (2019). Medical comorbidity in inpatients with psychiatric disorders. *International Journal of Research Review, 6*(8), 222–233.

Read, J., Kirsch, I., & McGrath, L. (2019). Electroconvulsive therapy for depression: A review of the quality of ECT versus Sham ECT trials and meta-analyses. *Ethical Human Psychology and Psychiatry, 21*(2), 64–103. https://doi.org/10.1891/EHPP-D-19-00014

Rodas, N. V., Eisenhower, A., & Blacher, J. (2017). Structural and pragmatic language in children with ASD: Longitudinal impact on anxiety and externalizing behaviors. *Journal of Autism and Developmental Disorders, 47*(11), 3479–3488. https://doi.org/10.1007/s10803-017-3265-3

Rotermann, M., Sanmartin, C., Hennessy, D., & Arthur, M. (2014). Prescription medication use by Canadians aged 6 to 79. *Health Reports.* No. 82-003-x, 1–9. http://www.statcan.gc.ca/pub/82-003-x/2014006/article/14032-eng.pdf

Rowland, T. A., & Marwaha, S. (2018). Epidemiology and risk factors for bipolar disorder. *Therapeutic Advances in Psychopharmacology, 8*(9), 251–269. https://doi.org/10.1177/2045125318769235

Samad, N., Yasmin, F., & Manzoor, N. (2019). Biomarkers in drug free subjects with depression: correlation with tryptophan. *Psychiatry investigation, 16*(12), 948–953. https://doi.org/10.30773/pi.2019.0110

Sawalha, J., Cao, L., Chen, J., Selvitella, A., Liu, Y., Yang, C., Li, X., Zhang, X., Sun, J., Zhang, Y., Zhao, L., Cui, L., Zhang, Y., Sui, J., Greiner, R., Li, X. M., Greenshaw, A., Li, T., & Cao, B. (2021). Individualized identification of first-episode bipolar disorder using machine learning and cognitive tests. *Journal of Affective Disorders, 282*, 662–668. https://doi.org/10.1016/j.jad.2020.12.046

Schmied, V. (2020). Understanding perinatal mental health problems. In J. M. Ussher, J. C. Chrisler, & J. Perz (Eds.), *Routledge International handbook of women's sexual and reproductive health* (pp. 360–377). Routledge.

Shajan, Z., & Snell, D. (2019). *Wright & Leahey's nurses and families: A guide to family assessment and intervention* (7th ed.). FA Davis.

Skinner, R., McFaull, S., Draca, J., Frechette, M., Kaur, J., Pearson, C., & Thompson, W. (2016). Suicide and self-inflicted injury hospitalizations in Canada (1979 to 2014/15). *Health Promotion and Chronic Disease Prevention in CANADA: Research, Policy and Practice, 36*(11), 243. https://doi.org/10.24095/hpcdp.36.11.02

Statistics Canada. (2020). *Canadian Community Health Survey, 2019.* https://www150.statcan.gc.ca/n1/daily-quotidien/200806/dq200806a-eng.htm

Statistics Canada. (2012). *Suicides and suicide rate, by sex and by age group.* http://www.statcan.gc.ca/tables-tableaux/sum-som/l01/cst01/hlth66a-eng.htm

Steinhoff, A., Ribeaud, D., Kupferschmid, S., Raible-Destan, N., Quednow, B. B., Hepp, U., Eisner, M., & Shanahan, L. (2021). Self-injury from early adolescence to early adulthood: Age-related course, recurrence, and services use in males and females from the community. *European Child & Adolescent Psychiatry, 30,* 937–951. https://doi.org/10.1007/s00787-020-01573-w

Stuart, S., & Robertson, M. (2012). *Interpersonal psychotherapy: A clinician's guide.* CRC Press.

Sylvia, L. G., Shelton, R. C., Kemp, D. E., Bernstein, E. E., Friedman, E. S., Brody, B. D., McElroy, S. L., Singh, V., Tohen, M., Bowden, C. L., Ketter, T. A., Deckersbach, T., Thase, M. E., Reilly-Harrington, N. A., Nierenberg, A. A., Rabideau, D. J., Kinrys, G., Kocsis, J. H., Bobo, W. V., … Calabrese, J. R. (2015). Medical burden in bipolar disorder: Findings from the clinical and health outcomes initiative in comparative effectiveness for bipolar disorder study (Bipolar CHOICE). *Bipolar Disorder, 17,* 212–223. https://doi.org/10.1111/bdi.12243

Timmins, F., & Caldeira, S. (2017). Assessing the spiritual needs of patients. *Nursing Standard, 31*(29), 47–53. https://doi.org/10.7748/ns.2017.e10312

Vasavada, M. M., Leaver, A. M., Njau, S., Joshi, S. H., Ercoli, L., Hellemann, G., Narr, K. L., & Espinoza, R. (2017). Short- and long-term cognitive outcomes in patients with major depression treated with electroconvulsive therapy. *The Journal of ECT, 33*(4), 278–285. https://doi.org/10.1097/YCT.0000000000000426

Veale, J. F., Watson, R. J., Peter, T., & Saewyc, E. M. (2017). Mental health disparities among Canadian transgender youth. *Journal of Adolescent Health, 60*(1), 44–49. https://doi.org/10.1016/j.jadohealth.2016.09.014

Villatoro, A. P., Mays, V. M., Ponce, N. A., & Aneshensel, C. S. (2018). Perceived need for mental health care: The intersection of race, ethnicity, gender, and socioeconomic status. *Society and Mental Health, 8*(1), 1–24. https://doi.org/10.1177/2156869317718889

Wang, F., Yang, J., Pan, F., Ho, R. C., & Huang, J. H. (2020). Neurotransmitters and emotions. *Frontiers in Psychology, 11.* https://doi.org/10.3389/fpsyg.2020.00021

Wilk, P., Maltby, A., & Cooke, M. (2017). Residential schools and the effects on Indigenous health and well-being in Canada—a scoping review. *Public Health Reviews, 38.* https://doi.org/10.1186/s40985-017-0055-6

Williams, H., Simmons, L. A., & Tanabe, P. (2015). Mindfulness-based stress reduction in advanced nursing practice: A nonpharmacologic approach to health promotion, chronic disease management, and symptom control. *Journal of Holistic Nursing, 33*(3), 247–259. https://doi.org/10.1177/0898010115569349

World Health Organization. (n.d.). *WHO Coronovirus (COVID-19) Dashboard.* https://covid19.who.int/

World Health Organization. (2012). *Depression: a global crisis.* https://www.who.int/mental_health/management/depression/who_paper_depression_wfmh_2012.pdf

World Health Organization. (2017). WHO Methods and Data Sources for Country-Level Causes of Death 2000–2015; Global Health Estimates Technical Paper WHO/HIS/IER/GHE/2016.3; World Health Organization.

World Health Organization. (2020, November 4). *Depression.* https://www.who.int/newsroom/fact-sheets/detail/depression

Xu, Y. Y., Liang, J., Cao, Y., Shan, F., Liu, Y., & Xia, Q. R. (2017). High levels of Nesfatin-1 in relation to the dysfunction of the hypothalamic–pituitary–adrenal and hypothalamus–pituitary–thyroid axes in depressed patients with subclinical hypothyroidism. *Neuropsychiatric Disease and Treatment, 13,* 1647–1653. https://doi.org/10.2147/NDT.S138954

Zhang, Y. (2018). Family functioning in the context of an adult family member with illness: A concept analysis. *Journal of Clinical Nursing, 27*(15–16), 3205–3224. https://doi.org/10.1111/jocn.14500

Zhang, Y., Li, L., & Zhang, J. (2020). Curcumin in antidepressant treatments: An overview of potential mechanisms, pre-clinical/clinical trials and ongoing challenges. *Basic & Clinical Pharmacology & Toxicology, 127*(4), 243–253. https://doi.org/10.1111/bcpt.13455

Zhong, X., Ming, Q., Dong, D., Sun, X., Cheng, C., Xiong, G., Li, C., Zhang, X., & Yao, S. (2020). Childhood maltreatment experience influences neural response to psychosocial stress in adults: An fMRI study. *Frontiers in Psychology, 10,* 2961. https://doi.org/10.3389/fpsyg.2019.02961

Zhou, S. G., Hou, Y. F., Liu, D., & Zhang, X. Y. (2017). Effect of cognitive behavioral therapy versus interpersonal psychotherapy in patients with major depressive disorder: A meta-analysis of randomized controlled trials. *Chinese Medical Journal, 130*(23), 2844–2851. https://doi.org/10.4103/0366-6999.219149

23

Anxiety, Obsessive–Compulsive, and Related Disorders*

Emily Jenkins and Lynn C. Musto

LEARNING OBJECTIVES

After studying this chapter, you will be able to:

- Discuss anxiety as an adaptive human response to a perceived threat.
- Identify the physical, cognitive, and social manifestations of anxiety.
- Describe the neurobiologic correlates of anxiety.
- Differentiate "normal" anxiety, worry, and anxiety disorder.
- Identify the shared and unique features of specific anxiety disorders.
- Describe the treatments available for anxiety.

KEY TERMS

- allostasis • cognitive–behavioural therapy
- depersonalization • derealization • distraction
- existential anxiety • exposure therapy • fear • fear conditioning • generalized anxiety disorder • hoarding disorder • obsessive–compulsive disorder • panic disorder (PD) • paresthesia • phobias • positive self-talk
- systematic desensitization • worry

KEY CONCEPTS

- anxiety • compulsions • obsessions • panic

In recent decades, we have gained considerable insight into the mechanisms and processes that influence the experience of anxiety. Importantly, researchers have started to clarify the physiologic mechanisms that underpin the mind–body–brain connection. Clearer understanding of the integrated nature of physiologic and mental processes has highlighted the bidirectional relationship between mind and body. While physiologic responses can shape behaviour, the opposite is also true; thoughts can change behaviour and influence physiologic processes (Mallorquí-Bagué et al., 2016; Van Cappellen et al., 2018). This knowledge has been used to inform treatment of anxiety disorders to the extent that a range of modalities is being used to intervene with people diagnosed with anxiety disorders, such as mind–body techniques, cognitive–behavioural therapies, or a combination of mindfulness and cognitive therapies and pharmaceutical interventions.

Although fear and anxiety are common human experiences, they are complex ones that involve both physiologic and psychological processes (LeDoux, 2015). Most of us would be challenged to define them precisely or explain how they are similar and different. In the literature, a few authors do argue that fear and anxiety are indistinguishable; however, most experts claim that they are distinct phenomena (Toh & Yang, 2020) with different aetiologies, response patterns, intensity, and time courses.

In this chapter, the position that fear and anxiety are distinct but related emotions that function "to signal danger, threat, or motivational conflict and to trigger appropriate adaptive responses" is endorsed (Steimer, 2002, p. 233). **Fear** is an emotional response to a specific and proximal threat to an organism's life or integrity—for example, being held at gunpoint or encountering a snarling dog (Mobbs, 2018). Anxiety, on the other hand, is an emotion characterized by the apprehension or dread of a potentially threatening or uncertain outcome (Xi, 2020). Stated differently, fear is a "primitive alarm in response to present danger" (Barlow, 2002, p. 104), whereas anxiety is a "future-oriented" state (Barlow, 2002, p. 64) that helps one prepare for *potentially aversive* situations. Based on these definitions, the key differences between anxiety and fear relate to characteristics of the trigger (stimulus). Characteristics of the trigger include its immediacy or temporal orientation (i.e., whether it exists in the present or future) and its ambiguity or specificity (Nebel-Schwalm & Davis, 2013).

---

*Adapted from the chapter "Anxiety and Obsessive-Compulsive Disorders" by Kathleen Hegadoren and Gerri Lasiuk

A related concept is **worry**, which has been defined as thoughts and images centring on adverse outcomes that engender negative affect and are relatively uncontrollable (Borkovec et al., 1983; Kircanski et al., 2018). Fear and anxiety are emotions, and worry involves negative thoughts and images; worry is considered a symptom of fear and anxiety.

The anxiety disorders are a family of disorders that all share excessive fear or anxiety as their core symptom; specific anxiety disorders differ from one another based on their key feature(s) (e.g., panic attacks, phobias) (American Psychiatric Association [APA], 2013). The anxiety disorders discussed in this chapter include **generalized anxiety disorder** (GAD), social anxiety disorder (social phobia, SAD), **panic disorder (PD)**, and specific **phobias** (grouped as anxiety disorders in the *Diagnostic and Statistical Manual of Mental Disorders*, 5th edition (*DSM-5*)) (APA, 2013). In earlier versions of the *DSM*, **obsessive–compulsive disorder** (OCD) was categorized as an anxiety disorder and while it will be discussed in this chapter, in the *DSM-5*, it is grouped under obsessive–compulsive and related disorders (which includes body dysmorphic disorder, **hoarding disorder**, trichotillomania, and excoriation disorder). Acute stress disorder (ASD) and posttraumatic stress disorder were also previously considered to be anxiety disorders but now appear in the newly created category Trauma- and Stressor-Related Disorders (discussed in Chapter 18).

Significant anxiety and anxiety disorders are not restricted to mental health practice; they are seen across all practice settings and continua of care. Indeed, inpatient psychiatric care is rare in instances where an anxiety disorder is the primary diagnosis. More common to inpatient settings are anxiety disorders that are comorbid with disorders such as severe depression or schizophrenia. Outpatient psychiatric clinics, primary care services, general practice settings, chronic disease management clinics, and private practitioners all provide various types of treatment for individuals experiencing an anxiety disorder. Anxiety disorders are often difficult to treat and symptoms often persist over many years. These disorders are thus frequently chronic in their longitudinal course, with acute episodes occurring in response to stressors or other health problems (Bandelow et al., 2017).

Normal Versus Abnormal Anxiety Response

From an evolutionary perspective, an emotion is a transient response to a specific stimulus that produces an arousal reaction characterized by changes in subjective feelings and behaviour (Pessoa & McMenamin, 2017). At low to moderate intensities, acute anxiety is an adaptive response to a perceived threat and can motivate one to act. On the other hand, when anxiety is extreme or chronic, it can produce paralysis and inaction. An anxiety disorder differs from adaptive ("normal") anxiety in that it is greater than expected in intensity and/or duration for one's age and the situation, and it interferes with one's quality of life and ability to function (APA, 2013).

McEwen (2005) conceptualizes normal responses to stress as **allostasis**, the adaptive processes that maintain homeostasis through the production of various brain and peripheral stress-related chemicals. These mediators of the stress responses promote adaptation to perceived threat or stress. However, they also contribute to allostatic load, the cumulative wear and tear on biologic systems that over time that can increase the risk for stress-related disorders and physical health problems like cardiovascular and metabolic disorders.

The perception of a threat triggers physical and emotional changes in all individuals. A normal emotional response to anxiety consists of three parts: physiologic arousal, cognitive processes, and coping strategies. Physiologic arousal is the signal that an individual is facing a threat. During this part of the anxiety process, sensory input is increasing. Next, cognitive processes in the brain decipher the various inputs and yield judgments about the extent of danger and whether the perceived threat should be approached or avoided. Behaviours include "fight" or "flight" (i.e., escape) as described by Selye (1956) and later updated to include "freeze" (i.e., immobilization) (Porges, 2007). Finally, coping strategies can be used to resolve the threat. Table 23.1 summarizes many physical, affective, cognitive, and behavioural symptoms associated with anxiety.

KEY CONCEPT

Anxiety is an emotion characterized by apprehension or dread of a potentially threatening or uncertain outcome. It is triggered by the perception of a threat and is manifested in physical, emotional, cognitive, and/or behavioural ways.

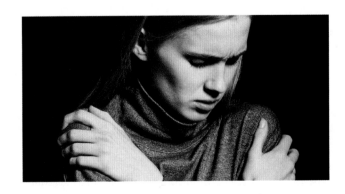

Overview of Anxiety Disorders

As a group, anxiety disorders represent the most common of all mental illnesses in Canada and around the globe. Research informing Canadian clinical practice

Table 23.1	Symptoms of Anxiety	
Physical		
Cardiovascular	**Neuromuscular**	**Gastrointestinal**
Sympathetic	Increased reflexes	Loss of appetite
Palpitations	Startle reaction	Revulsion towards food
Heart racing	Eyelid twitching	Abdominal discomfort
Increased blood pressure	Insomnia	Diarrhoea and vomiting
	Unsteadiness	
Respiratory		**Eyes**
Rapid breathing	**Skin**	Dilated pupils
Difficulty getting air	Face flushed or pale	
Shortness of breath	Sweating	**Urinary Tract**
Pressure of chest	Feeling hot or cold	Pressure to urinate
Shallow breathing		
Lump in throat		
Choking sensations		
Gasping		
Affective	**Cognitive**	**Behavioural**
Edgy	**Sensory–Perceptual**	Inhibited
Impatient	Feeling dazed	Tonic immobility
Uneasy	Objects seem blurred/distant	Flight
Nervous	Environment seems different/unreal,	Avoidance
Wound up	feelings of depersonalization	Impaired coordination
Anxious	Self-consciousness	Restlessness
Fearful	Hypervigilance	Postural collapse
Apprehensive		Hyperventilation
Scared	**Thinking Difficulties**	Jumpy
Frightened	Cannot recall important things	Jittery
Alarmed	Confused	
Terrified	Difficulty focusing attention	
	Difficulty concentrating	
	Fear of losing control or not being able to cope	
	Fear of physical injury or death	
	Fear of going crazy	
	Fear of negative evaluation	
	Frightening visual images	
	Repetitive fearful ideation	

Adapted from Beck, A. T., Emery, C., & Greenberg, R. L. (1985). *Anxiety disorders and phobias: A cognitive perspective* (pp. 23–27). Basic Books.

guidelines for the management of anxiety disorders and OCD reports the lifetime prevalence of anxiety disorders to be "as high as 31% higher than the lifetime prevalence of mood disorders and substance use disorders" (Katzman et al., 2014, p. 1). They are the most treated psychiatric disorders in childhood and adolescence (Essau et al., 2018). In fact, symptoms of anxiety disorder often begin in adolescence (de Lijster et al., 2017). Multiple factors contribute to the development of anxiety disorders in childhood, including genetic inheritance, as well as parental behaviours and modelling and stressful life events at key developmental stages (Schiele & Domschke, 2018). Children and adolescents with anxiety disorders are more likely to demonstrate suicidal behaviour and educational underachievement later in life (Collie et al., 2019; Doering et al., 2019). Further, researchers have found that individuals diagnosed with childhood anxiety disorders are more likely to be diagnosed with substance misuse disorders later in life (Groenman et al., 2017).

Anxiety disorders remain common in adulthood. Statistics Canada's (2013) *Community Health Survey of Mental Health* found that 2.6% of Canadians 15 years and older reported symptoms meeting the diagnostic criteria for GAD in the previous 12 months. Like many mental disorders, there appear to be differences in prevalence across gender, with girls and women more likely than boys and men to be diagnosed with any anxiety disorder during their lifetime (Watterson et al., 2017). For example, lifetime prevalence of anxiety disorders was found to be 10.4% in men and 16.0% in women in a Canadian-based community sample (Meng & D'Arcy, 2015). In terms of aetiology, specific anxiety disorders show more evidence of genetic vulnerability, particularly PD, OCD, and phobias, while environmental factors have also been identified as contributing to the development of anxiety disorders (Meier & Deckert, 2019).

Anxiety may exist as a primary disorder, but as noted earlier, it often co-occurs with other health conditions (Osland et al., 2018). In fact, this comorbidity can contribute to challenges in distinguishing between symptoms of anxiety and symptoms of physical conditions that share similar features (e.g., shortness of breath, racing heart). Evidence from community-based samples indicates that persons diagnosed with an anxiety disorder will likely have at least one comorbid psychiatric disorder, either concomitantly or in their lifetime (for a full discussion, see Merikangas et al., 2010). Individuals who live with chronic anxiety report more functional impairment, increased use of both psychiatric and non-psychiatric healthcare services, and decreased productivity than those in the general population (Edlund et al., 2018; Simo et al., 2018). After adjusting for sociodemographic factors and other mental disorders, the presence of any anxiety disorder is significantly associated with suicidal ideation and suicide attempts (Adhikari et al., 2020).

Generalized Anxiety Disorder

GAD is characterized by unwarranted, enduring anxiety across life situations, especially those in which the individual feels a lack of control. These anxiety symptoms significantly impact the person's functioning and bring with it associated physical symptoms. Thus, the amount of time spent worrying; the degree of control one has over one's worrying; and the impact on personal, social, and occupational functioning are key components of the assessment of GAD. GAD can be a debilitating disorder with serious impact on quality of life (Zhou et al., 2017). For the APA criteria for GAD, please see the DSM-5.

GAD is a common anxiety disorder. Most community-based population studies report lifetime prevalence rates of GAD ranging between 2% and 8%, depending on the country and the definitional and measurement criteria employed (Ruscio et al., 2017). In a Canadian sample, the prevalence estimates of GAD were reported at 2.6% (Public Health Agency of Canada, 2016). Onset of GAD is often early in life and often follows a chronic course with more severe symptoms being triggered by acute stressors. Persons living with GAD often feel powerless to change, frustrated with life, demoralized, and hopeless, and comorbid depression is very common (Price et al., 2019). In fact, less than one third of those with GAD are without a comorbid disorder (Lamers et al., 2011). Rovira and colleagues (2012) reported that 7.9% of those attending a primary care setting had GAD, highlighting the importance of comprehensive mental and physical health assessment in these settings. Assessment of persons with GAD must include the assessment of mood, somatic symptoms, specific worries, and worry management strategies employed. A standardized questionnaire, such as the Generalized Anxiety Disorder Scale (GAD-7), may help assess the severity of the symptoms and health impacts (Spitzer et al., 2006).

Social Anxiety Disorder

Social anxiety disorder (social phobia; SAD) involves a marked or intense fear of social situations in which the individual feels scrutinized and negatively evaluated by others. People with SAD appear to be highly sensitive to disapproval or criticism, tend to evaluate themselves negatively, and have poor self-esteem and a distorted view of personal strengths and weaknesses. These individuals magnify personal flaws and underrate any talents, and the resulting fear or anxiety is out of proportion to the actual risk of being negatively evaluated. Generalized SAD brings with it reduced quality of life (Dryman et al., 2016) and in children is associated with significant decreases in school performance (Vilaplana-Pérez et al., 2020). Despite substantial functional impairment, treatment seeking usually results from a comorbid mental disorder (Koyuncu et al., 2019). For APA criteria of SAD, please see the DSM-5.

The onset of SAD usually occurs in early adolescence. There are two subtypes of this disorder: generalized social phobia and specific social phobia. Generalized social phobia is diagnosed when an individual experiences fears related to most social situations, including public performances and social interactions. These individuals are likely to demonstrate deficiencies in social skills, and their phobias interfere with their ability to function. Individuals with specific social phobias fear and avoid only one or two specific social situations. Classic examples of the latter are eating, writing, or speaking in public or using public bathrooms.

Although there seems to be some genetic vulnerability to SAD, research indicates that negative familial relationships and/or environment (e.g., abuse, insecure child–parent relationships, sibling bullying) increase children's and adolescents' susceptibility to the disorder. Environmental factors, however, appear to be protective against the development of SAD, including close family relationships, peer support and acceptance, and supportive teachers in adolescence, with a cumulative effect of emotional support across family, peers, and school (Olson, 2021).

Data from the World Mental Health Survey Initiative indicate that SAD has a lifetime prevalence of 4% in the general population (Stein et al., 2017). People who experience both social phobia and depression have more severe symptoms and greater functional impairment than those with social phobia alone. Individuals who experience these two disorders in tandem tend to be younger and have an earlier diagnosis of major depression (Adams et al., 2016).

Panic Disorder

Panic disorder (PD) is characterized by repeated episodes of panic. These panic "attacks" are abrupt surges of intense fear or discomfort that peak within minutes and are associated with multiple key physical and cognitive symptoms (see "Clinical Vignette: Panic Disor-

BOX 23.1 DSM-5 Diagnostic Criteria: Panic Disorder

A. Recurrent unexpected panic attacks. A panic attack is an abrupt surge of intense fear or intense discomfort that reaches a peak within minutes, and during with time four (or more) of the following symptoms occur:

Note: The abrupt surge can occur from a calm state or an anxious state.

1. Palpitations, pounding heart, or accelerated heart rate
2. Sweating
3. Trembling or shaking
4. Sensations of shortness of breath or smothering
5. Feelings of choking
6. Chest pain or discomfort
7. Nausea or abdominal distress
8. Feeling dizzy, unsteady, light-headed, or faint
9. Chills or heat sensations
10. **Paresthesias** (numbness or tingling sensations)
11. **Derealization** (feelings of unreality) or **depersonalization** (being detached from oneself)
12. Fear of losing control or "going crazy"
13. Fear of dying

Note: Culture-specific symptoms (e.g., tinnitus, neck soreness, headaches, uncontrollable screaming or crying) may be seen. Such symptoms should not count as one of the four required symptoms.

B. At least one of the attacks has been followed by 1 month (or more) of one or both of the following:

1. Persistent concern or worry about additional panic attacks or their consequences (e.g., losing control, having a heart attack, "going crazy").
2. A significant maladaptive change in behaviour related to the attacks (e.g., behaviours designed to avoid having panic attacks, such as avoidance of exercise or unfamiliar situations).

C. The disturbance is not attributable to the physiologic effects of a substance (e.g., a drug of abuse, a medication) or another medical condition (e.g., hyperthyroidism, cardiopulmonary disorders).

D. The disturbance is not better explained by another mental disorder (e.g., the panic attacks do not occur only in response to feared social situations, as in social anxiety disorder; in response to circumscribed phobic objects or situations, as in specific phobia; in response to obsessions, as in obsessive–compulsive disorder; in response to reminders of traumatic events, as in posttraumatic stress disorder; or in response to separate from attachment figures, as in separation anxiety disorder).

CLINICAL VIGNETTE

PANIC DISORDER

Matt, a 22-year-old man, has experienced several life changes, including a recent engagement, loss of his father to cancer and heart disease, graduation from college, and entrance to the workforce as a computer engineer in a large inner-city company. Because of his active lifestyle, his sleep habits have been poor. He frequently uses sleeping aids at night and now drinks a full pot of coffee to start each day. He has started smoking to "relieve the stress." While sitting in heavy traffic on the way to work, he suddenly experienced chest tightness, sweating, shortness of breath, feelings of being "trapped," and foreboding that he was going to die. Fearing a heart attack, he went to an emergency room, where his discomfort subsided within a half hour. After several hours of testing, the doctor informed him that his heart was healthy. During the next few weeks, he experienced several episodes of feeling trapped and slight chest discomfort on his drive to work. He fears future "attacks" while sitting in traffic and while in his crowded office cubicle.

WHAT DO YOU THINK?

- What risk factors does Matt have that might contribute to the development of panic attacks?
- What lifestyle changes do you think would help Matt reduce stress?

der" and Box 23.1). Panic attacks can occur in response to a serious threat but can also occur "out of the blue" with no apparent triggering environmental stimulus or stressor. PD is characterized by recurrent unexpected panic attacks and fear of prompting another attack, which limits the individual's ability to function socially, occupationally, and interpersonally.

PD is a chronic condition with exacerbations and remissions. Lifetime prevalence estimates vary widely (1.4% to 20.5%), depending on the age of the sampled population and the methodologic approaches used to study it. In Canada, the lifetime prevalence of PD is estimated at 3.7% (Government of Canada, 2006). Recent longitudinal data suggest that having panic attacks increases the risk of developing a mood and/or anxiety disorder in the future (De Jonge et al., 2018). Higher rates of PD occur in women and among those 40 to 49 years old, the average age of onset is in the mid- to late-20s (Olaya et al., 2018). Several risk factors have been implicated in the development of PD, including previous triggered panic attacks, a family history of psychological difficulties, childhood trauma, being female, and history of mood disorder (Asselmann et al., 2018; Tibi et al., 2013). Adolescents with PD may be at higher risk for suicidal thoughts or attempt suicide more often than their peers (Miché et al., 2018).

In addition to comorbid psychiatric disorders, certain physical health problems are also common among individuals with PD, including vertigo, cardiac disease, gastrointestinal disorders, and asthma. One might ponder whether these medical conditions produce similar somatic sensations to anxiety and over time increase the risk of development of PD. The population with both physical health problems and panic symptoms reports poorer quality of life than do those without such comorbidity.

PD can occur with and without agoraphobia. Those who experience PD with agoraphobia tend to have more coexisting anxiety disorders, anxiety attacks, and anticipatory anxiety than do those who have PD without agoraphobia. Women appear more likely to experience PD with agoraphobia (Inoue et al., 2016) and to have poorer outcomes manifesting as missed work time and more frequent visits to healthcare providers (e.g., family doctor, emergency department visits) (Shin et al., 2020).

Panic attacks are typically accompanied by fear of death because their symptoms often mimic those of a heart attack, which are both physically taxing and psychologically frightening to the individual. Affected individuals often seek emergency medical care because they feel as if they are dying, but most have normal results upon cardiac workup. People experiencing panic attacks may also believe that the attacks stem from an underlying major medical illness. Even with sound medical testing and assurance of no underlying disease, it can be difficult for individuals with PD to feel reassured. Recognition of the seriousness of the panic attacks should be communicated to the person. However, individuals with PD continue to experience panic attacks with or without predisposing conditions (see "Clinical Vignette: Panic Disorder").

KEY CONCEPT

Panic can be a normal but extreme, overwhelming form of anxiety often initiated when an individual is placed in a real or perceived life-threatening situation.

Agoraphobia and Other Specific Phobias

Panic attacks can lead to the development of phobias or persistent, unrealistic fears of situations, objects, or

BOX 23.2 Common Phobias

Acrophobia (fear of heights)
Agoraphobia (fear of open spaces)
Ailurophobia (fear of cats)
Algophobia (fear of pain)
Arachnophobia (fear of spiders)
Brontophobia (fear of thunder)
Claustrophobia (fear of closed spaces)
Cynophobia (fear of dogs)
Entomophobia (fear of insects)
Haematophobia (fear of blood)

Microphobia (fear of germs)
Nyctophobia (fear of night or dark places)
Ophidiophobia (fear of snakes)
Phonophobia (fear of loud noises)
Photophobia (fear of light)
Pyrophobia (fear of fire)
Topophobia (stage fright)
Xenophobia (fear of strangers)
Zoophobia (fear of animal or animals)

activities. People with phobias will go to great lengths to avoid the feared objects or situations to deter panic attacks. Box 23.2 presents examples of common phobias. Agoraphobia, fear of certain environments such as open spaces (including shopping malls), travelling on public transportation (buses, subways), or being in closed and crowded spaces (elevators, theatres) often co-occurs with PD, leading to avoidance behaviours. Fear arising in places with limited opportunity to escape or when outside alone is characteristic of agoraphobia (APA, 2013).

The process often begins with an intense, irrational fear of being in an open space, being alone, or being in a public place where escape might be difficult or embarrassing (e.g., a movie theatre). The person fears that if a panic attack occurred, help would not be available, so they begin to avoid such situations. Such avoidance interferes with routine functioning and eventually renders the person afraid to leave the safety of home. Some affected individuals continue to face feared situations but with significant trepidation (i.e., going in public only to take children to school or attend a medical appointment).

Specific phobia (i.e., simple phobia) is a disorder marked by an irrational fear of a specific object or situation that the person realizes is unreasonable. The lifetime prevalence varies by subtype, with highest occurrence among those with natural environment phobias (8.9% to 11.6%), followed by situational phobias (5.2% to 8.4%), animal phobias (3.3% to 7%), and blood injection injury phobias (3.2% to 4.5%) (LeBeau et al., 2010).

Exposure to the stimulus object or situation engenders anxiety; the intensity of anxiety is usually related to both the proximity of the object and the degree to which escape is possible. For example, anxiety heightens as a cat approaches a person who fears cats and lessens when the cat moves away. At times, the level of anxiety can escalate to a full panic attack, particularly when the person must remain in a situation from which escape is deemed impossible. Fear of specific objects is fairly common, and the diagnosis of specific phobia is not made unless the fear significantly interferes with functioning or causes marked distress.

Careful assessment differentiates simple phobia from other diagnoses with overlapping symptoms. Blood injection injury–type phobia merits special consideration here because the phobia is fairly common across all healthcare settings. Before beginning a procedure, nurses should routinely ask whether the person has had any prior difficulty and should continue to monitor the person closely during and afterwards. The physiologic processes exhibited during phobic exposure to a procedure or treatment (e.g., needle poke, suturing) includes a strong vasovagal response, which significantly increases blood pressure and pulse, followed by the deceleration of the pulse and lowering of blood pressure resulting in fainting. Factors that predispose individuals to specific phobias include prior traumatic events; unexpected panic attacks in the presence of the phobic object or situation; observation of others experiencing a trauma; or repeated exposure to information warning of dangers, such as parents' repeatedly warning young children that dogs bite.

IN-A-LIFE 🏠

Ryan Reynolds (born October 23, 1976)

CANADIAN ACTOR

Public Persona

Ryan Reynolds is a well-known Canadian actor. He began acting in his mid-teens in television and transitioned to leading roles in highly popular feature films. Most recently he played the lead in *Deadpool*, a movie that received critical praise, had financial success, and was nominated for numerous awards.

Personal Realities

In a 2018 interview with the *New York Times*, Reynolds opened up about his lifelong struggle with anxiety, which he attributes to growing up in a volatile household and a tumultuous relationship with his father. Reynolds relayed that during his 20s, he was, at times, paralyzed by anxiety. To cope, he tended to self-medicate. As he has got older, he has developed healthier strategies to manage his anxiety, including the use of a meditation app called *Headspace*. Reynolds also uses humour to alleviate his anxiety and identifies his relationship with his wife, Blake Lively, as a strong source of support.

Source: A story in the *New York Times*, May 2, 2018 by Cara Buckley: *This story has already stressed Ryan Reynolds out.* https://www.nytimes.com/2018/05/02/movies/ryan-reynolds-deadpool-2.html

Obsessive–Compulsive and Related Disorders

This cluster of disorders includes OCD, body dysmorphic disorder, hoarding disorder, trichotillomania (also known as hair-pulling disorder), and excoriation disorder (skin-picking disorder) (APA, 2013). OCD and hoarding disorder are being discussed in this chapter.

OCD is a psychiatric disorder characterized by severe obsessions (repetitive, intrusive, thoughts), compulsions (repetitive, ritualistic behaviours), or both. A key feature of OCD is the relationship between obsessions and compulsions; the obsessions cause anxiety, and the compulsions are an attempt to reduce or eliminate it. Obsessive thinking and/or compulsive behaviours are not necessarily signs of a psychiatric disorder if they are not persistent and do not significantly interfere with the person's ability to function. However, when they are severe and persistent, obsessions can interfere with a person's reality testing and judgment to the degree that most of their day is spent performing actions in an attempt to minimize severe anxiety. Affected individuals feel chronically anxious and powerless to control the obsessions and compulsions.

Commons patterns seen in OCD are that of fear of contamination (e.g., from dirt, germs), pathologic doubt (e.g., requiring repeated checking that an action was carried out, such as windows closed), and need of symmetry (e.g., table settings, desktop) (Olatunji et al., 2019). Common compulsions include hand washing, checking and arranging things, and counting. Individuals who perform checking rituals repeatedly check locks, stoves, and/or switches; check for errors; or check that they have not harmed someone or themselves. For example, after hitting a bump in the road, an individual may obsess for hours over whether they hit someone. Some individuals with OCD have somatic fears and frequently seek medical treatment for physical symptoms, often just to get reassurance. Other compulsions include arranging things in perfect symmetry, counting rituals, or doing-and-undoing rituals (e.g., repeatedly turning on and off the alarm clock).

Persons with religious obsessions ruminate over the meaning of sins and whether they have followed the letter of the law. In the case of religious obsessions and compulsions, a diagnosis of OCD is not made unless the thoughts or rituals clearly exceed cultural or religious norms, occur at inappropriate times as described by members of the same religion or culture, or interfere with social obligations. (For the APA criteria for Obsessive–Compulsive Disorder, please see the DSM-5.)

The prevalence of OCD is similar across community samples drawn from different countries. For example, lifetime prevalence estimates of OCD in a mixed South Asian population were reported as 1.6% (Naveed et al., 2020), 0.9% in a Canadian sample (Osland et al., 2018), and 3.5% in a Swiss population (Fineberg et al.,

2013). Each of these studies reported men as having a younger age of onset than women. The typical age of onset of OCD is in the early 20s to mid-30s, although symptoms of OCD can begin in childhood. Despite this early onset, it takes an average of 8 years after the onset of symptoms before individuals access professional help (Stengler et al., 2013).

The most common reasons that individuals with OCD seek professional help include higher symptom severity, poor quality of life, and concurrent mental disorder (Robinson et al., 2017). For instance, researchers have estimated that 78% of individuals with OCD will experience a comorbid mental disorder, with depression, GAD, social anxiety disorder, and PD commonly co-occurring (Brakoulias et al., 2017; Lochner et al., 2014). Because children subscribe to myths, superstition, and magical thinking and enjoy obsessive and ritualistic behaviours, OCD may go unnoticed in younger persons. It is increasing concerns about social, academic, and personal impairments that differentiate common childhood behaviours from OCD. Predictors of poorer treatment outcomes for adults include earlier age of onset; longer duration of symptoms; high symptom severity; comorbidity with other mental disorders, especially depression; a family history of OCD or other anxiety disorders; personality disorders; sexual obsessions; and hoarding and compulsions (Fullana et al., 2020). In children, the predictors of poorer outcomes also include severity and family history of OCD, but family accommodation of OCD behaviours has been demonstrated to predict poorer outcomes (Kagan et al., 2017).

KEY CONCEPT

Obsessions are unwanted, intrusive, and persistent thoughts, impulses, or images that are incongruent with the person's usual thought patterns and cause significant anxiety and distress. The person tries to ignore, suppress, or neutralize the thoughts by some other thought or action but is unable to do so.

KEY CONCEPT

Compulsions are behaviours performed repeatedly, in a ritualistic fashion, with the goal of preventing or relieving anxiety and distress caused by obsessions.

Hoarding Disorder

Sometimes people who have OCD may exhibit hoarding behaviours; in fact, hoarding was originally considered as a symptom or subtype of OCD. As per the DSM-5, hoarding is now recognized as a discreet diagnostic syndrome (APA, 2013). Hoarding disorder is characterized by the excessive acquisition of inability or unwillingness to discard material possessions. Accumulated possessions clutter active living areas and become barriers to their use for daily living. There is impairment in social, occupational, and family functioning. Individuals who hoard may feel compelled to check their belongings repeatedly to see that all is accounted for and they may check the garbage to ensure that nothing of value has been discarded. Hoarding is a "debilitating psychiatric disorder that can lead to considerable health risks, functional impairment, family conflict, and substantial financial burden for sufferers, family members, and the community" (Stekettee et al., 2015, p. 728).

Individuals who hoard may collect items that appear to have no apparent value. Some hoarders collect newspapers, decorations, and other collectables; others hoard animals. Excessive accumulation of objects creates fire hazards, insect and rodent infestations, food contamination, unsanitary living conditions, and associated health hazards (Elsenhauer, 2017). The clutter can be so severe that individuals with hoarding disorder have been found dead in their homes after being trapped in a "clutter avalanche" (Brakoulias & Milicevic, 2015). (For APA criteria for Hoarding Disorder, please see the DSM-5.)

Hoarding disorder is a chronic progressive disorder affecting approximately 2% to 6% of the population. Similar to anxiety disorders, females tend to be overrepresented in clinical samples. Symptoms often are present during adolescence and become increasingly severe as individuals age. The disorder is most prevalent in older adults, with 50 being the average age of those seeking treatment. Hoarding behaviours can be seen in approximately 20% of persons with dementia and 14% of those with brain injury (Sadock et al., 2015). Individuals with hoarding disorder frequently present with a co-occurring mood or anxiety disorder, with high rates of comorbid OCD or attention deficit hyperactivity disorder (ADHD).

Individuals with hoarding disorder rarely voluntarily seek treatment, given that greater than 50% of those with the disorder experience poor insight (Kress et al., 2016).

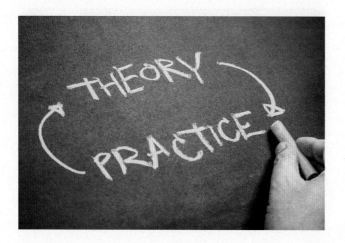

Instead, they may be pressured to seek treatment by family members, public health officials, and/or mental health professionals. It is not uncommon for a number of community services to be involved, including the fire department, public health, animal control, law enforcement, mental health services, and public works (Elsenhauer, 2017; Kress et al., 2016). Cognitive–behavioural therapy that includes a focus on decision-making skills can be an effective treatment approach, with aspects of the therapy occurring in home (Muroff & Otte, 2019).

Aetiologic Theories of Anxiety Disorders

There are many similarities and overlaps among aetiologic theories of the various anxiety disorders and the various theories are not mutually exclusive. Such commonalities may indicate that the current classification of the anxiety disorders will change as the research evolves.

Genetic Theories

The foremost aetiologic theory of anxiety disorders is the diathesis–stress model in which genetic and environmental stressors are viewed, individually and together, as heightening an individual's vulnerability to the disorders (Ask et al., 2021). The inheritability of anxiety disorders, estimated from twin studies, is low to moderate (20% to 60%) and appears to involve an interaction of multiple genes with only small effects on susceptibility that interact with environmental influences, such as low socioeconomic status and early adversity (e.g., parental discord, maltreatment, death of a parent or other significant losses, exposure to threats and trauma) (Ask et al., 2021; Beesdo et al., 2009; Schiele & Domschke, 2018). Yet researchers have found that, even with an interaction of childhood adversity and a genotype that appears to confer vulnerability to SAD and PD (e.g., the 5-HTTLPR variant of the serotonin transporter gene), high levels of general self-efficacy can act as a protective factor. This discovery indicates that adaptive coping may compensate for effects of genetic and environmental risk (Schiele et al., 2016).

Neurobiology of Anxiety

The concept of learned associations provides a useful framework to understand the nature of emotional responsiveness and how anxiety can be manifested in our emotions, thoughts, and behaviour. Advances in research methods and neuroimaging techniques have increased our understanding of the roles of different neurotransmitters and the regions of the brain involved in anxiety and specific anxiety disorders.

Fear conditioning is a type of learning during which an organism is conditioned to associate a neutral stimulus with an aversive one. Over time, the neutral stimulus elicits an automatic emotional response previously associated with the aversive one, and the individual is conditioned to respond with fear to what was once a neutral stimulus. The anxiety and fear response can further generalize to similar stimuli and become a pattern of response to stimuli that are tangentially similar to the original (e.g., a fear of dogs can generalize to all furry animals). This has led to the belief that anxiety disorders reflect an exaggeration of the normal fear response. Extinction (the gradual decrease in a conditioned fear response) can occur when repeated exposure to the conditioned stimulus does not elicit an anxiety or fear response, although the memory is still there and can be re-established to produce the fear response in the face of a similar threat. These dynamics partially explain the chronicity of anxiety disorders and have shaped many of the current interventions and treatments for anxiety and anxiety disorders.

The major structures of the brain involved in fear conditioning are the hippocampus and the amygdala. The hippocampus is involved with memory acquisition and storage. Short-term memory is believed to be related to enhancement of glutamate neurotransmission, whereas longer-term memory is considered to be the result of long-term synaptic potentiation, a process whereby synaptic activity is enhanced by increased gene expression and protein synthesis. The amygdala is a crucial area for encoding and storing fearful memories. Studies using functional magnetic resonance imaging have shown increased amygdalar activity during associative learning (i.e., pairing stimuli with previously experienced stimuli and the prior emotional responses).

The Role of Neurotransmitters and Neuropeptides

Serotonin (5-hydroxytryptamine [5-HT]) is indirectly implicated in the aetiology of anxiety disorders in that drugs that facilitate serotonergic neurotransmission are effective in treating anxiety and panic symptoms. Indeed, selective serotonin reuptake inhibitors (SSRIs) are considered first-line pharmacotherapy for those with anxiety. Norepinephrine is implicated in anxiety disorders because of its effects on the systems associated with the physical sensations of anxiety—the cardiovascular, respiratory, and gastrointestinal systems via stimulation of the sympathetic arm of the autonomic nervous system. Cell bodies of norepinephrine neurons in the brain are located in the locus coeruleus, which is one of the internal regulators of sleep and alertness. Electrical stimulation of the locus coeruleus in monkeys increases fear and anxiety, and studies indicate that norepinephrine-based medications (i.e., serotonin–norepinephrine reuptake inhibitors—SNRIs) are also effective in treating anxiety (Jakubovski et al., 2019).

Gamma-aminobutyric acid (GABA) is the most abundant inhibitory neurotransmitter in the brain. Very small GABAergic neurons (interneurons) affect the firing rates of neurons distributed throughout the brain, which explains why GABA has such pervasive effects within the brain. Although a direct role of GABA in fear conditioning or anxiety disorders has yet to be clearly demonstrated, drugs that enhance GABA neurotransmission are commonly used to treat anxiety symptoms during the day and to help with sleep disturbance that often accompanies significant anxiety.

Corticotropin-releasing hormone (CRH) is a neuropeptide and hormone found in many areas of the brain; it is the initial hormone released from the hypothalamus that activates one of the major stress response systems, the hypothalamic–pituitary–adrenal (HPA) axis. CRH receptors are widely distributed in the hypothalamus, as well as brain regions associated with fear and fear conditioning. Activation of the HPA axis results from many stimuli, including perception of threat, and increases arousal, attention to environmental cues, and glucose availability to skeletal muscles to promote survival responses like "fight or flight." Cortisol, the final output of the HPA axis in humans, is significantly elevated during panic attacks (Bandelow et al., 2000) and appears to decrease or become blunted among those experiencing persistent stress or panic states, such as PD (Wintermann et al., 2016). Increasing levels of cortisol act as negative feedback to decrease further release of CRH; however, many other neurotransmitters and neuropeptides help regulate the HPA axis. CRH receptor antagonists have been suggested as a mechanism to treat anxiety, but no drugs based on this mechanism are currently on the market.

Cholecystokinin (CCK) became a neuropeptide of interest when administered in challenge tests; CCK induces panic attacks in persons with PD and, to a much lesser degree, in people without PD (Ruland et al., 2015). High concentrations of CCK are found in the cerebral cortex, amygdala, and hippocampus—areas implicated in fear and stress responses. Although specific CCK_B receptor antagonists would be a potential treatment mechanism, these compounds did not show sufficient efficacy to be marketed.

Other neurochemicals have been associated with anxiety, including growth hormone (GH), female sex hormones, arginine vasopressin (AVP), and oxytocin (OT). OT has been strongly associated with social behaviours, particularly those related to bonding (e.g., mother–infant; couples). Environmental events early in life can change the OT system and behaviours and thus affect changes in adult social behaviours (Russell et al., 2018).

In healthy subjects, stimulating α-adrenergic receptors elevates GH. This process is blunted in individuals with PD (Sallee et al., 2000). Neuroactive steroids, including the various metabolites of progesterone, have been implicated in the development of panic attacks, which may help to explain why women show an increased susceptibility to PD (Lovick, 2014). AVP and OT help regulate the activity of the HPA axis in a gender-specific fashion, with AVP being able to stimulate the axis independent of CRH and OT decreasing further release of CRH, thus dampening down HPA axis activity.

Neuroimaging Data Related to Specific Anxiety Disorders

The increasing sophistication of neuroimaging techniques has enabled researchers to better understand the physiology of anxiety and the involved neural network or circuits. Most neuroimaging work related to anxiety disorders has focused on PD, with magnetic resonance imaging (MRI) studies demonstrating significant volumetric reductions in grey matter in the frontolimbic regions, thalamus, brainstem, and cerebellum and decreased white matter volume in the frontolimbic, thalamocortical, and cerebellar pathways (Konishi et al., 2014). Studies have also demonstrated consistent increases in blood supply or glucose uptake (indicators of increased neuronal activity) in the amygdala of those with PD, GAD, or SAD (Demenescu et al., 2013; Makovac et al., 2016; Sladky et al., 2015). In individuals with SAD, resting state functional MRI scans indicate that there is abnormal regional and network level functioning of the precuneus (an area of the brain involved in self-consciousness) that correlates with pathologic fear and avoidance (Yuan et al., 2018).

Functional MRI studies also identify abnormal activation patterns in response to provocation paradigms. Consistent findings across neuroimaging studies have led to a consensus that there is a close relationship between the prefrontal cortex and amygdala. Altered connectivity between the amygdala and the ventrolateral prefrontal cortex, as well as other structures within the prefrontal arousal networks, has been found in youth with anxiety disorders (Strawn et al., 2018). The amygdala is activated when an individual is confronted with a novel or fearful situation. Learning from experience that a stressor can be coped with, is under control, or no longer requires attention is termed "emotional processing" and is associated with specific regions of the prefrontal cortex (Sánchez-Navarro et al., 2014). However, cumulative data suggest a distinction between two classes of anxiety disorders. Those disorders involving intense fear and panic (i.e., PD and specific phobias) seem to be characterized by hypoactivity of distinct prefrontal cortex areas, thus disinhibiting the amygdala. Disorders that involve worry and rumination, such as GAD or cognitions of negative consequences in social anxiety disorder, seem to be more associated with hyperactivity of the prefrontal cortex (Greenberg et al., 2012; Kawashima et al., 2016).

Psychodynamic Theories

Psychodynamic theories focus on the psychological influences on human behaviour, feelings, and emotions, and explore how these relate to early life experience. Early life experiences lay a template in the brain and body that shapes the response to stressors across the lifespan (Schore, 2014). A particular contribution of psychodynamic theories to the understanding of anxiety disorders is their emphasis on the important role of separation and loss on the development of anxiety. Individuals with anxiety disorders report greater numbers and severity of recent personal losses at symptom onset than do healthy controls. This statistic is recognized in the diathesis–stress model, which regards both genetic and environmental stressors and their interaction as increasing vulnerability to anxiety disorders. That psychological factors, such as positive coping behaviours, can decrease such vulnerability needs to be recognized as well.

Nursing Management of Significant Anxiety Symptoms and Specific Anxiety Disorders

Primary anxiety disorders are usually treated in primary care settings, in outpatient clinics, or by private practitioners. Hospitalization is limited to acute exacerbation of anxiety or panic symptoms or comorbid mental disorders such as depressive disorder or schizophrenia. Given the comorbidity of significant anxiety and GAD among individuals with chronic physical health conditions such as cardiovascular problems, assessment of anxiety should be part of the overall approach to chronic disease management.

Assessment within a bio/psycho/social/spiritual framework is the foundation of holistic care. Physiologic symptoms tend to be the impetus for individuals to seek health care. Often, persons with PD are initially seen in emergency rooms as they seek treatment for their panic attack. Biologic, psychological, social, and spiritual assessments unveil potential contributing factors and identify sources of strength that can guide the nurse to develop an individual action plan.

Biologic Domain

Assessment

Once it is determined that anxiety symptoms have led to significant impairment in occupational, social, and interpersonal functioning, the nurse should assess for any potential environmental triggers and obtain a detailed history of any previous similar experiences. Questions to ask the person might include the following:

- What did you experience preceding and during times of increased anxiety or a panic attack, including physical symptoms, feelings, and thoughts?

- Have you ever experienced some of these symptoms before? If so, under what circumstances?
- Has anyone in your family ever had similar experiences?
- What do you do when you have these experiences that help you to feel less anxious?
- What has helped you in the past to manage your symptoms?

Substance Use

Assessment for panicogenic substance use, such as sources of caffeine intake, pseudoephedrine, amphetamine, cocaine, or other stimulant use, may rule out contributory issues either related or unrelated to PD. Individuals with anxiety disorders may use alcohol to self-treat their symptoms. Details of typical alcohol and other substance use are an important part of the assessment.

Sleep Patterns

Sleep is often disturbed in those with anxiety disorders. Panic attacks can occur during sleep and the person may fear sleep for this reason. Nurses should closely assess the impact of sleep disturbance as it can increase the risk of further panic attacks and the development of major depressive disorder.

Interventions for Biologic Domain

These interventions can assist individuals with either severe anxiety or panic symptoms.

Physical Activity

Interventions that focus on the physical aspects of anxiety and panic are particularly helpful in reducing the number and severity of the attacks, giving the individual an increasing sense of accomplishment and control. Routine leisure walking can create time for reappraisal and reflection of triggering stimuli. Active participation in an exercise program may help individuals reassess automatic thinking that relates increased heart rate and shortness of breath with a physical crisis. Physical activity can also improve sleep.

Breathing Control

Hyperventilation is common for people with anxiety disorders. Often, people are unaware that they take rapid, shallow breaths when they become anxious. Other common sensations are choking and pressure on the chest, restricting normal breathing. Teaching breathing control is a simple intervention that has immediate results. Begin by encouraging the person to simply observe the rate, pattern, and depth of their breathing. Next, invite the person to perform the following abdominal or diaphragmatic breathing exercise:

- Sit in an upright position, feet flat on the floor, and arms supported on the side-arms of a chair or on your lap. (Rationale: This position increases the capacity of the lungs to fill with air and for the limbs to be comfortably supported.)
- Place your hand on your abdomen, slightly above your umbilicus (bellybutton).
- Inhale slowly through the nose to the count of four and feel your abdomen rise.
- Exhale slowly through the mouth to the count of six and feel your abdomen fall.
- As you exhale, feel all of your muscles relax and let go.
- Repeat a series of 10 slow abdominal breaths, followed by normal breathing.

Abdominal breathing may also be used to interrupt an episode of panic as it begins. Once individuals have learned to identify their own early signs of panic, they can use abdominal breathing to divert or decrease the severity of the attack.

Nutrition Planning

Persons with an anxiety disorder need to work towards reducing and eventually eliminating stimulants such as caffeine from their diet. Many over-the-counter remedies, especially "energy drinks" used to boost energy or increase mental performance, have high levels of caffeine. Individuals need to be informed regarding other potential sources of stimulants, such as those found in some cold remedies and herbal products. The nurse should provide information about caffeine-free substitutes for these substances.

Relaxation Techniques

Teaching relaxation techniques is another way to help with anxiety and anxiety disorders. Many individuals are unaware of the tension they carry in their bodies and first need to learn to monitor their own tension. Isometric exercises and progressive muscle relaxation are helpful methods to learn to differentiate muscle tension from muscle relaxation. This method of relaxation is also helpful for those who have difficulty clearing the mind, focusing, or visualizing a scene, which are often required in other forms of relaxation such as meditation. Box 23.3 provides one method of progressive muscle relaxation.

Pharmacotherapy for Anxiety and Anxiety Disorders

As mentioned previously, there are known neurotransmitter systems associated with anxiety and anxiety disorders, but not all of these associations have led to specific drug therapies. For example, drugs such as propranolol

BOX 23.3 Progressive Muscle Relaxation

Choose a quiet, comfortable location where you will not be disturbed for 20 to 30 min. Your position may be lying or sitting, but all parts of your body should be supported, including your head. Wear loose clothing and remove restrictive items such as glasses and shoes.

Begin by closing your eyes and clearing your mind. Moving from head to toe, focus on each part of your body and assess the level of tension. Visualize each group of muscles as heavy and relaxed.

Take two or three slow abdominal breaths, pausing briefly between each breath. Imagine the tension flowing from your body.

Each muscle group listed below should be tightened (or tensed isometrically) for 5 to 10 s and then abruptly released; visualize this group of muscles as heavy, limp, and relaxed for 15 to 20 s before tightening the next group of muscles. There are several methods to tighten each muscle group, and suggestions are provided below. Each muscle group may be tightened two to three times until relaxed. Do not over tighten or strain. You should not experience pain.

- Hands (tighten by making fists)

- Biceps (tighten by drawing forearms up and "making a muscle")
- Triceps (extend forearms straight, locking elbows)
- Face (grimace, tightly shutting mouth and eyes; open mouth wide and raise eyebrows)
- Neck (pull head forward to chest and tighten neck muscles)
- Shoulders (raise shoulders towards ears; push shoulders back as if touching them together)
- Chest (take a deep breath and hold for 10 s)
- Stomach (suck in your abdominal muscles)
- Buttocks (pull buttocks together)
- Thighs (straighten your legs and squeeze the muscles in thighs and hips)
- Leg calves (pull toes carefully towards you, avoid cramps)
- Feet (curl toes downwards and point toes away from your body)

Finally, repeat several deep abdominal breaths and mentally check your body for tension. Rest comfortably for several minutes, breathing normally, and visualize your body as warm and relaxed. Get up slowly when you are finished.

act primarily on b-adrenergic receptors and reduce the peripheral symptoms of anxiety, but they have limited effectiveness against panic symptoms.

Selective Serotonin and Serotonin–Norepinephrine Reuptake Inhibitors

The SSRIs and SNRIs are generally considered the first-line pharmacotherapy long-term treatment for most anxiety disorders (Bandelow et al., 2015; Strawn et al., 2018). Overall, SSRIs and SNRIs produce fewer side effects than do other drugs used to treat anxiety, are safer to use, and are not lethal in the event of overdose. Details regarding these two classes of antidepressants can be found in Chapter 13.

Tricyclic Antidepressant Therapy

Like the SSRIs and the SNRIs, the tricyclic antidepressants imipramine (Tofranil), nortriptyline (Pamelor), and clomipramine (Anafranil) reduce anxiety and panic symptoms by inhibiting serotonin and norepinephrine reuptake. However, this class of drugs also interacts with many more neurotransmitter systems and brings with them significant side effects. Thus,

they are usually only considered in the event that SSRIs or SNRIs have failed to produce symptom remission. Details regarding this class of antidepressants can be found in Chapter 13.

Benzodiazepine Therapy

All benzodiazepines produce anxiolytic action, and their therapeutic onset is much faster (hours, not weeks) than that of antidepressants. Therefore, benzodiazepines are very useful in treating intensely distressed patients. However, evidence to support their use in long-term treatment of anxiety disorder is limited; they should only be used for short periods of time for acute anxiety and sleep disturbance (Rickels & Moeller, 2019). Alprazolam (Xanax), lorazepam (Ativan), and clonazepam (Rivotril) are widely used for anxiety disorders. They are well tolerated but carry the risk for withdrawal symptoms, like rebound anxiety and sleep disturbance, upon discontinuation of use.

Administering and Monitoring Benzodiazepines

Treatment may include administering benzodiazepines concurrently with antidepressants for the first 4 weeks and then tapering the benzodiazepine. This strategy provides rapid symptom relief but avoids the complications of long-term benzodiazepine use. Details regarding this class of drugs can be found in Chapter 13. Short-acting benzodiazepines, such as alprazolam and lorazepam, are associated with rebound anxiety or anxiety that increases after the peak effects of the medication have decreased.

Medications with short half-lives should be given in three or four small doses spaced throughout the day, with a higher dose at bedtime to allay anxiety-related insomnia. Clonazepam, a longer-acting benzodiazepine, requires less frequent dosing and has a lower risk for rebound anxiety. Rebound anxiety and insomnia are also common with higher dosing regimens and the abrupt cessation of benzodiazepine treatment. Benzodiazepines should be used with extreme caution to treat anxiety in the older adults due to significantly increasing the risk of falls and anterograde memory difficulties, which can be misinterpreted as signs of dementia (Gerlach et al., 2018).

Psychological Domain

Assessment

A complete psychological assessment is necessary to determine patterns of anxiety, characteristic symptoms, and the person's emotional, cognitive, and behavioural responses (see Chapter 11). A comprehensive assessment includes overall mental status, suicidal tendencies and thoughts, cognitive thought patterns, avoidance behaviour patterns, and any comorbid depression symptoms. The individual's perceptions regarding their symptoms should be discussed, as well as present and past coping strategies.

Self-Report Scales

Self-evaluation can be difficult in anxiety disorders. Specific triggers are often no longer present or have generalized so that it is difficult to be aware of subtle associations that increase symptoms. Several tools are available to characterize and rate the individual's state of anxiety and to differentiate between different anxiety disorders. Examples of these symptom and behavioural rating scales are provided in Box 23.4. The majority of these tools are self-report measures and, as such, are limited by the individual's self-awareness and openness. However, the Hamilton Rating Scale for Anxiety (HAM-A), provided in Table 23.2, is an example of a scale rated by the clinician (Hamilton, 1959). This 14-item scale reflects both psychological and somatic aspects of anxiety.

Assessment of Thought Patterns

Catastrophic misinterpretations of trivial physical symptoms can trigger intense anxiety and panic symptoms. Once identified, these sensations and associated thoughts should serve as a basis for individualizing patient education to address the resulting fear. Table 23.3 presents an example of a scale to assess catastrophic misinterpretations of the symptoms of panic. Several studies have found that individuals who have strategies for coping with uncomfortable sensations and feel a sense of control have fewer severe panic attacks. Individuals who fear loss of control during a panic attack often make the following types of statements:

- "I feel trapped."
- "I think I might die."
- "I'm afraid others will know, or I'll hurt someone."
- "I feel alone. I can't help myself."
- "I'm losing control."

BOX 23.4 Rating Scales for Assessment of Panic Disorder and Anxiety Disorder

PANIC SYMPTOMS

Panic-Associated Symptom Scale (PASS; Argyle et al., 1991)

Acute Panic Inventory (Dillon et al., 1987)

National Institute of Mental Health Panic Questionnaire (NIMH PQ; Scupi et al., 1992)

COGNITIONS

Anxiety Sensitivity Index (Reiss et al., 1986)

Agoraphobia Cognitions Questionnaire (Chambless et al., 1984)

Body Sensations Questionnaire (Chambless et al., 1984)

PHOBIAS

Mobility Inventory for Agoraphobia (Chambless et al., 1985)

Fear Questionnaire (Marks & Matthews, 1979)

ANXIETY

State-Trait Anxiety Inventory (STAI; Spielberger et al., 1976)

Penn State Worry Questionnaire (PSWQ; Meyer et al., 1990)

Beck Anxiety Inventory (Beck et al., 1988)

Table 23.2	Hamilton Rating Scale for Anxiety	

Hamilton (1959) designed this scale to help clinicians gather information about states of anxiety. The symptom inventory provides scaled information that classifies anxiety behaviour and assists the clinician in targeting behaviours and achieving outcome measures. Provide a rating for each indicator based on the following scale:

0 = None	**1 =** Mild	**2 =** Moderate
3 = Severe	**4 =** Severe, grossly disabling	

Item	Symptoms	Rating
Anxious mood	Worries, anticipation of the worst, fearful anticipation, irritability	
Tension	Feelings of tension, fatigability, startle response, moved to tears easily, trembling, feelings of restlessness, inability to relax	
Fear	Fear of dark, strangers, being left alone, animals, traffic, crowds	
Insomnia	Difficulty falling asleep, broken sleep, unsatisfying sleep and fatigue on waking, dreams, nightmares, night terrors	
Intellectual (cognitive)	Difficulty concentrating, poor memory	
Depressed mood	Loss of interest, lack of pleasure in hobbies, depression, early waking, diurnal swings	
Somatic (sensory)	Tinnitus, blurred vision, hot and cold flushes, feelings of weakness, picking sensation	
Somatic (muscular)	Aches and pains, twitching, stiffness, myoclonic jerks, grinding of teeth, unsteady voice, increased muscular tone	
Cardiovascular symptoms	Tachycardia, palpitations, chest pain, throbbing of vessels, fainting feelings, heart missing beat	
Respiratory symptoms	Pressure or constriction in chest, choking feelings, sighing, dyspnea	
Gastrointestinal symptoms	Difficulty swallowing, wind, abdominal pain, burning sensation, abdominal fullness, nausea, vomiting, borborygmi (stomach rumbling), looseness of bowels, loss of weight, constipation	
Genitourinary symptoms	Frequent micturition, urgent micturition, amenorrhea, menorrhagic, development of frigidity, premature ejaculation, loss of libido, impotence	
Autonomic symptoms	Dry mouth, flushing, pallor, tendency to sweat, giddiness, tension headache, raising of hair	
Behaviour at interview	Fidgeting, restlessness or pacing, tremor of hands, furrowed brow, strained face, sighing or rapid respiration, facial pallor, swallowing, belching, brisk tendon jerks, dilated pupils, exophthalmos	

From Hamilton, M. (1959). The assessment of anxiety states by rating. *British Journal of Medical Psychology, 32*(1), 54.

Such individuals also tend to show low self-esteem, feelings of helplessness, demoralization, and overwhelming fears of experiencing panic attacks. They may have difficulty with assertiveness or expressing feelings.

Interventions and Therapies Within the Psychological Domain

Current clinical guidelines for the treatment of anxiety disorders suggest that either pharmacotherapy or specific psychotherapies can be efficacious and, in the short term, a combination of both modes of therapy can be superior to using only one or the other in isolation (Cuijpers et al., 2014; Ströhle et al., 2018). Nurses can assist individuals to identify triggers and eventually learn to manage their responses.

Peplau (1989) was one of the first to develop guidelines for nursing interventions for treating individuals experiencing problems with anxiety. These interventions help the person attend to and react to input other than the subjective experience of anxiety. Although Peplau's work is over 30 years old, many of the interventions she described are still relevant today (see Table 23.4).

Box 23.5 offers a comparison of effective and ineffective dialogue with a person with an anxiety disorder.

Distraction

Once individuals can identify the early symptoms of panic, they can learn to use **distraction** behaviours to shift their attention away from the uncomfortable physical sensations. Distraction activities include initiating a conversation with a nearby person or engaging in a physical activity (e.g., walking, gardening, house cleaning). Performing simple, repetitive activities such as snapping a rubber band against the wrist, counting backwards from 100 by threes, and counting objects along the roadway are other strategies for deterring an attack.

Positive Self-Talk

During states of increased anxiety and panic, individuals can learn to counter frightening or negative thoughts with positive coping statements, also called **positive self-talk**. Examples of positive self-talk include "This is only anxiety and it will pass," "I can handle these symptoms,"

Table 23.3 Panic Attack Cognition Questionnaire

Rate each of the following thoughts according to the degree to which you believe each thought contributes to your panic attack.

1 = Not at all   **2** = Somewhat
3 = Quite a lot   **4** = Very much

Thought	Rating
I'm going to die.	
I'm going insane.	
I'm losing control.	
This will never end.	
I'm really scared.	
I'm having a heart attack.	
I'm going to pass out.	
I don't know what people will think.	
I won't be able to get out of here.	
I don't understand what is happening to me.	
People will think I'm crazy.	
I'll always be this way.	
I am going to throw up.	
I must have a brain tumour.	
I'll choke to death.	
I'm going to act foolish.	
I'm going blind.	
I'll hurt someone.	
I'm going to have a stroke.	
I'm going to scream.	
I'm going to babble or talk funny.	
I'll be paralyzed by fear.	
Something is physically wrong with me.	
I won't be able to breathe.	
Something terrible will happen.	
I'm going to make a scene.	

Adapted from Panic attack cognitions questionnaire in Clum, G. A. (1990). *Coping with panic: A drug-free approach to dealing with anxiety attacks.* Brooks/Cole.

and "I'll get through this." These positive statements are most effective when they are grounded in truth, because they offer the individual a focal point and challenge

fear-provoking thoughts (e.g., "I am going to die," or "I can't handle this"). Some individuals carry positive statements written on a small card in their purse or wallet or on a handheld device. These messages can quickly be retrieved and read at the onset of panic symptoms.

Cognitive–Behavioural Therapy and Other Psychotherapeutic Approaches to Anxiety

Cognitive–behavioural therapy (CBT), individual or group, is a primary treatment of choice for anxiety and obsessive–compulsive–related disorders (Cuijpers et al., 2016; Reddy et al., 2020), including for individuals who have not responded well to medications. [There are, of course, disorders, such as a specific phobia, for which behavioural strategies may be more beneficial.] New self-help therapy approaches, such as virtual reality exposure, are potential ways to augment CBT (Reddy et al., 2020). Self-help manuals based on CBT principles and online structured modules have also been shown to be effective (Cuijpers et al., 2016).

CBT is also an effective treatment for depression, sleep problems, chronic pain, and eating disorders and tends to have fewer side effects and better treatment retention as compared with pharmacotherapy (Leichsenring & Steinert, 2017). There is evidence that individuals prefer psychological interventions such as CBT to medication, and psychosocial interventions are first-line treatment for children, adolescents, and people who are pregnant or breastfeeding (Bandelow et al., 2017). Although CBT principles are applied in many different situations, the basic principles are simple and remain constant (Burns, 1999):

1. Thoughts, feelings, behaviours (actions, choices), and body sensations affect each other.
2. Because thoughts, feelings, behaviours (actions, choices), and body sensations are connected, even small changes in one area can affect the others.

Table 23.4 Nursing Interventions Based on Degrees of Anxiety

Degree of Anxiety	Nursing Interventions
Mild	Learning is possible. The nurse assists the patient to use the energy that anxiety provides to encourage learning.
Moderate	The nurse needs to check his or her own anxiety so that the patient does not empathize with it. Encourage the patient to talk: to focus on one experience, to describe it fully, then to formulate the patient's generalizations about that experience.
Severe	Learning is less possible. Allow relief behaviours to be used but do not ask about them. Encourage the patient to talk: ventilation of random ideas is likely to reduce anxiety to a moderate level. When this is observed by the nurse, proceed as above.
Panic	Learning is impossible. The nurse needs to stay with the patient. Allow pacing and walk with the patient. No content inputs to the patient's thinking should be made by the nurse. (They burden the patient, who will distort them.) Pick up on what the patient says, for example, Pt: "What's happening to me—how did I get here?" N: "Say what you notice." Short phrases by the nurse—direct, to the point of the patient's comment, and investigative—match the current attention span of the patient in panic and, therefore, are more likely to be heard, grasped, and acted on, with the patient's responses gradually reducing the anxiety in a helpful way. Do not touch the patient; patients experiencing panic are very concerned about survival, are experiencing grave threat to self, and usually distort intentions of all invasions of their personal space.

Adapted from Peplau, H. (1989). Theoretical constructs: Anxiety, self, and hallucinations. In A. O'Toole & S. Welt (Eds.), *Interpersonal theory in nursing practice: Selected works of Hildegard E. Peplau.* Springer.

BOX 23.5 THERAPEUTIC DIALOGUE

Panic Disorder With Agoraphobia

Matt, a 55-year-old man, was admitted 4 days ago to the psychiatric unit with exacerbation of anxiety symptoms and panic attacks during the last 3 weeks. He has a 30-year history of uncontrolled anxiety that is refractory to medications and psychotherapies. On admission, he stated that he feels suicidal at times because he thinks that his life is not within his control. He feels embarrassed, angry, and "trapped" by his disorder. During the past 24 h, Matt is seen crying at times; he also isolates himself in his room. Michelle, Matt's nurse, enters his room to make a supportive contact and to assess his current mental status.

Ineffective Approach

Nurse: Oh.... Why are you crying?

Patient: (Looks up, gives a nervous chuckle) Obviously, because I'm upset. I am tired of living this way. I just want to be normal again. I can't even remember what that feels like.

Nurse: You look normal to me. Everyone has bad days. It'll pass.

Patient: I've felt this way longer than you've been alive. I've tried everything and nothing works.

Nurse: You're not the first depressed person that I've taken care of. You just need to go to groups and stay out of your room more. You'll start feeling better.

Patient: (Angrily) Oh, it's just that easy. You have no idea what I'm going through! You don't know me! You're just a kid.

Nurse: I can help you if you help yourself. A group starts in 5 min, and I'd like to see you there.

Patient: I'm not going to no damn group! I want to be alone so I can think!

Nurse: (Looks about anxiously) Maybe I should come back after you've calmed down a little.

Effective Approach

Nurse: Matt, I noticed that you are staying in your room more today. What's troubling you?

Patient: (Looks up) I feel like I've lost complete control of my life. I'm so anxious and nothing helps. I'm tired of it.

Nurse: I see. That must be difficult. Can you tell me more about what you are feeling right now?

Patient: I feel like I'm going crazy. I worry all the time about having panic attacks. They make me scared I'm going to die. Sometimes I think I'd be better off dead.

Nurse: (Remains silent, continues to give eye contact)

Patient: Do you know what it's like to be a prisoner to your emotions? I can't even go out of the house sometimes, and when I do, it's terrifying. I don't know what to think anymore.

Nurse: Matt, you have lived with this disorder for a long time. You say that the medications do not work to your liking, but what has helped you in the past?

Patient: Well, I learned in relaxation group that panic symptoms are probably caused by chemicals in my brain that are not working correctly. I learned that medications can help, but they don't work well for me. I tried an exposure plan and relaxation techniques to deal with my fears of leaving the house and my chronic anxiety. That did help some, but it's scary to do.

Nurse: It sounds like you have learned much about your illness, one that can be treated, so that you don't always have to feel this way.

Patient: This is easier to say right now when I'm here and can get help if I need it. It's hard to remember this when I'm in the middle of a panic attack and think I'm dying.

Nurse: It's harder when you're alone?

Patient: Much harder! And I'm alone so much of the time.

Nurse: Let's talk about some ways you can manage your panics when you're alone. Tell me some of the techniques you've learned.

CRITICAL THINKING CHALLENGE

- What tone is established by the nurse's opening question in the first scenario?
- Which therapeutic communication techniques did the nurse use in the second scenario to avoid the pitfalls encountered in the first scenario?
- What information was uncovered in the second scenario that was not touched on in the first?
- What predictions can you make about the interpersonal relationship likely to develop between the nurse and the patient in each scenario?

---

3. CBT focuses on events and situations in the "here and now" and does not try to understand how or where they began.
4. CBT encourages self-awareness.
5. CBT emphasizes learning and practising new skills (homework).

CBT strategies include psychoeducation, self-monitoring, cognitive restructuring, and somatic exercises. CBT is offered to individuals and groups and over a 12- to 20-week period, although longer treatment may be necessary to maintain an initial response. (See Chapter 14, *Cognitive–Behavioural Interventions*.)

CBT has proven to be efficacious in treating hoarding disorder (with maintenance over the long term possible), but having only small to moderate effects on the depressive symptoms that are often comorbid to the disorder. Usually, many CBT sessions are involved (20+) and include tasks to resist acquiring behaviours, cognitive restructuring of hoarding-related beliefs, and training to improve problem-solving skills. There may be home visits involving assistance with sorting and discarding (Rodgers et al., 2021).

Clinicians may combine the principles of CBT with other treatment modalities, such as mindfulness, to achieve better outcomes with patients who have challenging anxiety disorders and/or OCD (Kladnitski et al., 2020; Külz et al., 2019). Research scientist Jeffrey Schwartz (2016) developed a four-step self-treatment method for patients struggling with OCD that combines aspects of mindful awareness with the principles of CBT (see Box 23.6). Components of mindfulness that seem to be effective in helping people shift their thoughts are mindful awareness or dispositional mindfulness, being aware of one's present-moment experiences, thoughts, and sensations in a nonjudgmental way, and the selective focusing of attention (Blanck et al., 2018).

Importantly, built into each of the steps is a *fifteen-minute rule* whereby the intent is for the person to delay their response to the obsessive thought or compulsion by 15 min. During this time, the individual is encouraged to be mindfully aware that they are relabelling, reattributing, or refocusing their attention. These four steps integrate mindful awareness to support cognitive restructuring.

BOX 23.6 A Four-Step Self-Treatment Method.

1. Relabel—whereby the patient learns to recognize the thought for what it is, an obsessive thought or a compulsive urge.
2. Reattribute—when the person recognizes that the messages they are receiving are false and a result of a medical condition.
3. Refocus—is when the person intentionally engages in a different activity, thereby focusing their attention on different, more pleasurable, activity.
4. Revalue—as the person becomes more adept at recognizing OCD symptoms, they recognize the symptoms as distractions and devalue the thoughts and compulsions. At the same time, the person can begin to revalue their lives.

From Schwartz, J. M. (2016). *Brain lock.* Harper Collins.

Exposure therapy is the treatment of choice for agoraphobia, specific phobias, and OCD. Patients are repeatedly exposed to increasingly complex and real or simulated anxiety-provoking situations until they become desensitized and anxiety subsides. **Systematic desensitization**, another exposure method used to desensitize patients, exposes the patient to a hierarchy of feared situations that the patient has rated from least to most feared. The patient is taught to use muscle relaxation as levels of anxiety increase through multisituational exposure. Planning and implementing exposure therapy require special training. Because of the multitude of outpatients in treatment for agoraphobia, exposure therapy would be a useful tool for home health psychiatric nurses. Outcomes of home-based exposure treatment are similar to clinic-based treatment outcomes.

Psychoeducation programs help to educate individuals and families about the symptoms of anxiety and panic. Individuals with PD legitimately fear "going crazy," losing control, or dying because of their physical symptoms. Attempting to convince a person that such fears are groundless only heightens anxiety and impedes communication. Information and physical evidence, such as electrocardiogram results and laboratory test results, should be presented in a caring and open manner that demonstrates acceptance and understanding of the person's situation. Box 23.7 suggests psychoeducation topics for individual or small group discussion. It is especially important to cover such topics as the differences between panic attacks and heart attacks, the difference between PD and other psychiatric disorders, and the effectiveness of various treatment methods.

Social and Occupational Domains

Individuals with anxiety disorders often deteriorate socially as the disorder takes its toll on relationships with family and friends. Occupational success and work satisfaction are often compromised. If the disorder becomes severe enough, the person may experience extreme isolation. Therefore, it is an important area for assessment and active intervention if necessary.

Assessment

During the assessment, the nurse needs to assess the patient's understanding of how anxiety or panic symptoms and associated avoidance behaviours have affected their social and work life along with that of the family. Pertinent questions include the following:

- How has the disorder affected your family's social life?
- How has the disorder affected your work and work–life balance?

BOX 23.7 Psychoeducation Checklist

When caring for the patient with anxiety disorders, be sure to include the following topic areas in the teaching plan:

✓ Psychopharmacologic agents (anxiolytics or antidepressants) if ordered, including drug action, dosage, frequency, and possible adverse effects
✓ Breathing control measures
✓ Potential dietary triggers
✓ Exercise
✓ Progressive muscle relaxation
✓ Distraction behaviours
✓ Relevant psychotherapies and where they are available
✓ Time and specific stress management strategies
✓ Positive coping strategies

- What limitations related to travel has the disorder placed on you or your family?
- What coping strategies have you used to manage the symptoms?
- How has the disorder affected your family members or others?

Cultural Factors

Cultural competence calls for the understanding of cultural knowledge, cultural awareness, cultural assessment skills, and cultural practice (see Chapter 4). Therefore, cultural differences must be considered in the assessment of anxiety disorders. Different cultures interpret anxiety-related sensations, feelings, or understandings differently. "Nervousness" may be more accepted by some cultural groups, and several cultures do not have a word to describe "anxiety" or to denote "anxiousness" but instead may use words or meanings to suggest somatic complaints. Showing anxiety may be a sign of weakness in some cultures (Curcio & Corboy, 2020).

Interventions for Social and Occupational Domains

Individuals with anxiety disorders, especially those with significant anxiety sensitivity, may need assistance in re-evaluating their lifestyles. Casual comments by friends or coworkers can be misinterpreted or overinterpreted and be triggers for intense anxiety or panic symptoms. Time management can be a useful tool. In the workplace or at home, underestimating the time needed to complete a chore or being overly involved in several activities at once increases stress and anxiety. Procrastination, lack

of assertiveness, and difficulties with prioritizing or delegating tasks intensify these problems.

Writing a list of tasks to be completed and estimating the time needed to complete them provides concrete feedback to the individual. Crossing-out each activity as it is completed helps the patient to regain a sense of control and accomplishment. Large tasks should be broken into a series of smaller tasks to minimize stress and maximize a sense of achievement. Rest, relaxation, and family time—frequently omitted from the daily schedule—must be included.

Family Response to Anxiety Disorders

Affected families often have difficulty with overall communication. Parents with agoraphobia may become discouraged and self-critical regarding their child-rearing abilities, which may cause their children to be overly dependent. Parents with PD may inadvertently cause excessive fears, phobias, or excessive worry in their children. Family members may get frustrated with the chronic nature of anxiety disorders and show irritation when anxiety symptoms are exacerbated by acute stressors.

Pregnancy can increase anxiety symptoms for women who have preexisting anxiety disorders. Assessment of mood and anxiety symptoms both in the antepartum and the postpartum period, as well as available resources to manage such symptoms, should be part of routine maternity care.

Spiritual Domain

Anxiety can be understood as basic to the human condition. Existentialist thinkers (see Box 23.8) argue that, because we humans are aware of our own mortality, the apprehension that death will end our existence fills us with foreboding. This **existential anxiety** must be accepted and faced, or it can subvert our everyday life. We can feel alienated and estranged (not at home) in the world. We look to find meaning in our lives, a *raison d'être*. Existentialists note that, as neither nature nor culture can do this for us, individual humans are, in a sense, self-making. Frankl (1992), in *Man's Search for Meaning*, wrote about how it is every human's wish to have a meaningful life (see Chapter 9 for a brief discussion of logotherapy).

Tillich (1952), the author of *The Courage to Be* and a theistic existentialist, finds that existential anxiety involves three areas of apprehension: fate and death (the absolute threat to self), emptiness and meaninglessness (worry that there is no ultimate meaning), and guilt and condemnation (perceived threats to one's identity). Being human involves confronting and reconciling such anxiety.

BOX 23.8 Some Existentialist Thinkers and an Example of Their Work

Søren Kierkegaard   *Either/Or: A Fragment of a Life* (1843/1944)
Friedrich Nietzsche   *Thus Spoke Zarathustra* (1883/1985)
Martin Heidegger   *Being and Time* (1927/1962)
Karl Jaspers   *On My Philosophy* (1941/1955)
Gabriel Marcel   *The Mystery of Being* (1951)
Jean-Paul Sartre   *Being and Nothingness* (1943/1956)
Simone de Beauvoir   *The Second Sex* (1949/1953)
Henrik Ibsen   *A Doll's House* (1879/1889)
Albert Camus   *The Myth of Sisyphus* (1942/1955)
Fyodor Dostoevsky   *Notes from the Underground* (1864/1918)
Samuel Beckett   *Waiting for Godot* (1953/1955)
Eugène Ionesco   *The Chairs* (1952/1958)

Researchers are exploring the importance of understanding the relation between existential anxiety and clinical anxiety. The existential anxiety scale (EAS) has been developed, for instance, based on Tillich's theory. Early results suggest that existential anxiety, as measured by the EAS, is common and associated with symptoms of anxiety and depression (Weems et al., 2004). In a critical review of the literature, Koslande and colleagues (2009) concluded that "it is evident that addressing patients' existential and spiritual needs helps them improve mentally" (p. 40). They argue that an existential perspective should be an element of mental health care. See Irving Yalom's (1980) classic work, *Existential Psychotherapy,* for an in-depth understanding of this form of therapy.

Evaluation and Treatment Outcomes

Patients can be assisted to keep a daily log of the severity of anxiety and the frequency, duration, and severity of anxiety symptoms and panic episodes. This log will be a basic tool for monitoring progress as symptoms decrease. A number of self-help books can provide a rich source of reinforcement of simple interventions that can attenuate the intensity and frequency of panic symptoms. Rating scales may also be helpful to monitor changes in misinterpretations or other symptoms related to panic. Figures 23.1 and 23.2 illustrate a number of examples of bio/psycho/social/spiritual interventions and treatment outcomes for individuals with PD.

Continuum of Care

As with any disorder, the continuum of patient care across multiple settings is crucial. Individuals are treated in the least restrictive environment that will meet their safety needs.

Inpatient Care

Inpatient settings provide care and treatment for individuals experiencing severe anxiety with comorbid depression, increased risk of suicide, or poor treatment response to typical treatment strategies.

Family Interventions

The entire family needs support in adjusting to the disorder. A referral for family therapy may be indicated. Children with OCD living in families who are highly accepting of obsessive thoughts and compulsive behaviours have poorer treatment outcomes and a more chronic course (Monzani et al., 2020). Involving the entire family in the therapy process is imperative. Families experience the symptoms, treatments, clinical setbacks, and recovery from chronic anxiety and panic as a unit. Misunderstandings, misconceptions, false information, and stigma of mental illness, singly or collectively, impede recovery efforts.

Community Treatment

Most individuals with anxiety disorders will be treated on an outpatient basis, and it is important that nurses who work in these settings have access to up-to-date lists of community resources and support groups. In outpatient or primary care settings, nurses are directly involved in treatment, collaborative care management (van der Feltz-Cornelis et al., 2017), conducting psychoeducation groups on relaxation and breathing techniques, and teaching symptom management. Advanced practice nurses conduct CBT and individual and family psychotherapies.

Recovery from anxiety disorders involves the engagement of individuals in self-management of their anxiety disorder. Self-management of anxiety disorders is explored by Coulombe and colleagues in Box 23.9.

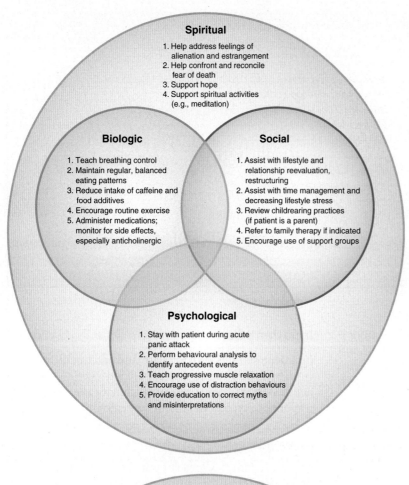

Figure 23.1 Bio/psycho/social/spiritual interventions for patients with panic disorder.

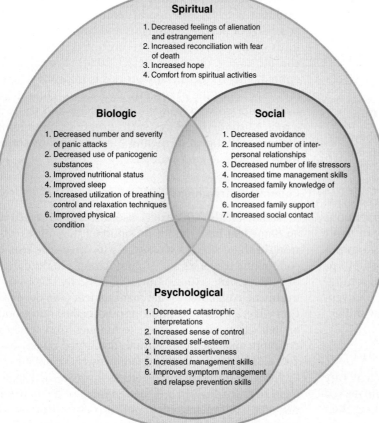

Figure 23.2 Bio/psycho/social/spiritual outcomes for patients with PD.

EMERGENCY CARE

Because individuals with PD are likely to first present for treatment in an emergency room or primary care setting, nurses and nurse practitioners working in these settings should be involved in early recognition and referral. Consultation with a psychiatrist or mental health professional by the primary care provider can decrease both anxiety symptoms and costs to the healthcare system (Kroenke & Unutzer, 2017). Several interventions may be useful in reducing the number of emergency room visits related to panic symptoms. Psychiatric consultation and patient teaching can be provided in the emergency department, including the following:

- Stay with the person and maintain a calm demeanour. (Rationale: Anxiety often produces more anxiety, and a calm presence will help calm the patient.)
- Reassure the patient that you will not leave, that this episode will pass, and that they are in a safe place.

(Rationale: A person experiencing a panic episode often fears dying and cannot see beyond the panic attack.)

- Give clear, concise directions, using short sentences. Do not use medical jargon. (Rationale: A person in the throes of panic is in crisis and has difficulty shifting focus away from his or her internal experience.)
- Walk or pace with the patient to an environment with minimal stimulation. (Rationale: Activity can help an individual focus excessive energy.)
- Administer PRN anxiolytic medications as ordered and appropriate. (Rationale: Benzodiazepines are effective in treating acute panic.)

After the panic attack has resolved, allow the patient to express their feelings. Using a shared decision-making process, ensure a plan for follow-up is in place.

BOX 23.9 Research for Best Practice

PROFILES OF RECOVERY FROM MOOD AND ANXIETY DISORDERS

Coulombe, S., Radziszewski, S., Meunier, S., Provencher, H., Hudon, C., Roberge, P., Provencher, M. D., & Houle, J. (2016). Profiles of recovery from mood and anxiety disorders: A person-centred exploration of people's engagement in self-management. *Frontiers in Psychology, 7*, 584. https://doi.org/10.3389/fpsyg.2016.00584

Purpose: The purpose of this study was to identify profiles underlying mental health recovery including participant characteristics and associations with specific criterion variables.

Methods: One hundred and forty-nine participants with diagnoses of anxiety disorder depression or bipolar disorder were recruited from community organizations located in Quebec and France. In this quantitative study, participants completed a number of questionnaires addressing self-management, clinical recovery, personal recovery, as well as specific criterion variables (including personal goal appraisal, social participation, self-care, and coping strategies).

Findings: Utilizing a latent profile analysis, three profiles emerged: the *Floundering* profile, the *Flourishing* profile, and the *Struggling* profile. Those in the *Floundering* profile rarely engaged in self-management strategies,

experienced moderately severe symptoms, and reported the lowest positive mental health. Individuals in this group were more likely to be male, single, and with a low income. Those in the *Flourishing* profile frequently used self-empowerment strategies, experienced the least severe symptoms, and reported the highest mental health. Participants in this group had the most favourable scores on personal goal appraisal, social participation, self-care, and coping. Participants in the *Struggling* profile actively engaged in self-management strategies focused on symptom reduction and a healthy lifestyle, despite the fact that they reported high symptom severity and moderately high positive mental health.

Implications for Nursing: Recovery is a multifaceted process and individuals in this study used a variety of approaches to promote their mental health and recovery (and not solely focused on symptom reduction strategies). The importance of individualized person-centred care is critical. Nurses should work *with* their patients by exploring recovery-oriented strategies being utilized, utilizing teachable moments to encourage diversity in self-care management and recovery strategies, and to offer patients positive feedback to assist them with building confidence.

Assessment and Treatment Issues Specific to Obsessive–Compulsive Disorder

Symptoms of OCD can be difficult to treat because of the pathology of the disorder, and individuals diagnosed with OCD are treated in specific outpatient programs. Short-term hospitalization may be necessary for treatment of comorbid depression and for treatment refractory symptoms. When this occurs, it is important to have a clear plan of care and to ensure that all staff members follow it consistently (see "Clinical Vignette: Obsessive–Compulsive Disorder").

Individuals with OCD do not consider their compulsions pleasurable. Often, they recognize them as odd and may initially try to resist them. Resistance eventually fails, and the individual incorporates repetitive behaviours into daily routines, performing activities in a specific, ritual order. If this sequence is disturbed, the person experiences extreme anxiety until the process can be repeated in the correct sequence. Interpersonal relationships suffer, and the person may actively isolate themselves. Indeed, individuals with OCD are more likely to be young, separated or divorced, and unemployed.

Assessment

The nurse should assess the type and severity of the patient's obsessions and compulsions. Most individuals will appear neatly dressed and groomed, cooperative, and eager to answer questions. Orientation and memory are not usually impaired, but these individuals may be distracted by obsessive thoughts. Individuals with severe symptoms may be preoccupied with fears or with

discussing their obsessions, but in most instances, direct questions must be asked to reveal symptoms. For example, the nurse may begin indirectly by asking how long it takes the individual to dress in the morning or leave the house, but usually follow-up questions are needed, such as "Do you find yourself frequently returning to the house to make sure that you have turned off the lights or the stove, even when you know that you have already checked this?" "Does this happen every day?" "Are you ever late for work or for important appointments?"

Although individuals with OCD do not have a higher prevalence of physical disease, some may report multiple physical symptoms. In individuals with late-onset OCD (after 35 years of age) or in children who develop symptoms after a febrile illness, cerebral pathology should be excluded. Those whose compulsions involve washing should be checked for dermatologic lesions caused by repetitive hand washing, excessive cleaning with caustic agents, or bathing. Osteoarthritis joint damage secondary to cleaning rituals may also be observed.

Identifying the degree to which the OCD symptoms interfere with the person's daily functioning is important. Several rating scales can be used to identify symptoms and monitor improvement. Examples of these scales are provided in Box 23.10. The Yale-Brown Obsessive–Compulsive Scale (Y-BOCS) is a popular, clinician-rated 16-item scale that obtains separate subtotals for the severity of obsessions and compulsions. The Maudsley Obsessive–Compulsive Inventory is a 30-item, true-false, self-assessment tool that may help the individual to recognize individual symptoms.

Nurses must consider sociocultural factors when evaluating OCD. At times, cultural or religious beliefs may be misunderstood and mistaken for obsessions

CLINICAL VIGNETTE

OBSESSIVE–COMPULSIVE DISORDER

Robert, a 32-year-old man, is a new patient at a psychiatric unit. He admitted himself to have his medicines evaluated because his obsessive thoughts and depression have worsened since his recent divorce. While in the hospital, he has quickly become viewed as a "problem patient" because he hoards linens and demands a new bar of soap for each of his five daily showers. He is compelled to open and close his door five times when he leaves or enters his room but does not know why. This behaviour has led to arguments with his roommate. In an effort to "help him," the staff locked his bathroom door to prevent him from showering so frequently. He tried to enter his bathroom to shower and panicked when the staff refused to allow him to shower, telling him "You can live without it." After receiving PRN medication for extreme anxiety, Robert signed out of the hospital against medical advice because of embarrassment and anger towards the nursing staff.

WHAT DO YOU THINK?

- How could the staff have handled the situation differently in order not to disrupt Robert's or the unit's clinical care?
- What nursing interventions might be appropriate in providing Robert's care?

BOX 23.10 Rating Scales for Assessing Obsessive–Compulsive Symptoms

Yale-Brown Obsessive–Compulsive Scale (Y-BOCS; Goodman et al., 1989)

The Maudsley Obsessional–Compulsive Inventory (MOC; Rachman & Hodgson, 1980)

The Leyton Obsessional Inventory (Cooper, 1970)

---

or compulsions. Shame and embarrassment over the irrational thoughts and behaviours often lead to social isolation and relational difficulties. The time demands related to the compulsions often lead to decreased occupational success. Assessment of current level of functioning in social, occupational, and personal spheres is, therefore, important.

Family Response to Disorder

Individuals whose OCD symptoms are severe are more likely to demonstrate social skill deficits and have more difficulties with intimacy; consequently, they are less likely to marry. Some studies have also shown higher divorce rates for individuals with OCD, particularly when comorbid with other mental disorders (Muhlbauer et al., 2020). They also have higher rates of celibacy, possibly because they fear becoming contaminated.

OCD often diminishes the quality of family relationships. Individuals with this disorder may ask family members to become involved in their rituals of checking or providing repeated reassurance (Albert et al., 2017). Those with OCD can become very angry and frustrated with family members for failing to comply with their requests for help with rituals. This can result in verbal and even physical altercations. Many family members find themselves modifying routines to suit the person's symptoms and report this to be at least moderately distressing for them (Walseth et al., 2019). The most troublesome symptoms of OCD for families to cope with include the family member's ruminations, long-standing unemployment, rituals, noncompliance with medication, depression, withdrawal from social and family contact, lack of motivation, and excessive arguing (Stewart et al., 2017).

Spouses report a variety of issues such as sexual difficulties, overwhelming feelings of frustration, anger, guilt, and fatigue, and disrupted family and social life. Other relatives report moderate to severe burden in coping with an individual with OCD. They state that they have poor social relationships and neglect their hobbies due to their relative's illness (Stewart et al., 2020).

Family education regarding OCD may be helpful to support genuine understanding of the strength of an obsession and a compulsion for a person with this disorder and the degree of fear and anxiety that can be involved.

Treatment

Specific clinical pharmacotherapy reviews for OCD support that long-term SSRIs are the first-line treatment of choice (Jakubovski et al., 2019). Modern stereotactic surgical techniques that produce lesions of the cingulum (a bundle of connective pathways between the two hemispheres) or the anterior limb of the internal capsule (a region near the thalamus and part of the circuit connecting to the cortex) may bring about substantial clinical benefit in some persons without causing significant morbidity (Brown et al., 2016; Kim et al., 2003). Other treatment options include radiotherapy and deep brain stimulation in which electrical current is applied through an electrode inserted into the brain (Vicheva et al., 2020).

For the individual with cleaning or hand washing compulsions, attention to skin condition is necessary. Encourage them to use tepid water when washing and hand cream after washing. Remove harsh, abrasive soaps and replace with moisturizing soaps. The treatment team should work with the person to decrease the frequency of washing by structuring time schedules and time-limited washing.

Specific Psychotherapeutic Interventions for OCD

The front-line psychotherapeutic treatments for OCD are exposure with response prevention (ERP) and CBT. During ERP, the person is exposed to situations or objects that are known to induce anxiety but is asked to refrain from performing the ritualistic behaviours. One goal of this procedure is to help the patient understand that resisting the rituals while exposed to the object of anxiety is less stressful and time consuming than performing the rituals. Another goal is to confound the expectation of distressing outcomes and eventually extinguish the compulsive behaviours. Cognitive restructuring is another intervention to teach the patient to restructure dysfunctional thought processes by defining and testing them (Beck et al., 1985). Its goal is to alter the patient's immediate, dysfunctional appraisal of a situation and perception of long-term consequences.

Community Treatment

Partial hospitalization programs and day treatment programs care for most patients with OCD. They allow patients to maintain significant independence while beginning medications and behavioural therapies. Specific day treatment psychotherapy programs for OCD are available in some larger urban centres. Specific outpatient clinics may also be available. Self-help groups and self-help books can also help individuals keep their symptoms under control.

Assessment and Treatment Issues Specific to Hoarding Disorder

Assessment

Individuals experiencing hoarding disorder often also experience physical health conditions such as fibromyalgia, chronic fatigue syndrome, and obesity; thus, a compressive physical and mental status assessment should be completed. When assessing patients, multiple sources of information are included in the overall assessment including police reports, public health reports, and reports from family members (with the patient's consent). Objective measures such as the Saving Inventory—Revised (Frost et al., 2004) or the Hoarding Rating Scale—Interview (Tolin et al., 2010) are also useful formal measures for assessment.

Family Response

Hoarding disorder can have a negative impact on the health and wellbeing of family members and significant others. Those who live with a person with hoarding disorder frequently experience embarrassment because of the cluttered living environment and frustration with the individual's unwillingness or inability to change. Family

members may not be aware of the individuals hoarding and as a result experience shock and disbelief, while others may be aware, but fear judgment and shame, for not being able to assist the person (Neziroglu et al., 2020).

Treatment

Treatment for hoarding disorder is complex and consists of a combination of treatment approaches including cognitive–behaviour therapy, psychopharmacological treatment, family assistance, and multidisciplinary community-based care. Traumatic life events have been associated with the onset of hoarding; thus, trauma-informed approach to working with individuals is warranted. CBT, however, is the gold standard treatment for hoarding disorder, focusing specifically on three areas of hoarding: disorganization, difficulty discarding items, and excessive acquisition. Antidepressants such as paroxetine (Paxil) and extended-release venlafaxine (Effexor XR) have been effective in improving symptoms of hoarding disorder and comorbid symptoms of depression and anxiety (Brakoulias & Milicevic, 2015; Kress et al., 2016).

The importance of the nurse–patient relationship cannot be overemphasized. Individuals with hoarding disorder need to be treated with respect. Nurses need to exercise self-awareness, be careful not to judge patients (or their families), and mitigate their treatment expectations. Community-based approaches that include mental health services and the inclusion of professional organizations that can assist with home clean out can be very helpful (Kysow et al., 2020).

🍁 Summary of Key Points

- Anxiety-related disorders are the most common of all psychiatric disorders and significantly impair individuals' social and occupational functioning.
- The anxiety disorders are a family of disorders that share excessive fear or anxiety as their core symptom; specific anxiety disorders differ from one another according their key feature(s).
- Significant anxiety and anxiety disorders are seen across all practice settings and along the continuum of care.
- Although anxiety can be a primary diagnosis, it is more often comorbid with other psychiatric disorders (e.g., depression, schizophrenia) and/or physical illnesses (e.g., coronary artery disease, irritable bowel disease).
- Those experiencing anxiety disorders have high levels of physical and emotional symptoms and often experience comorbid or concurrent diagnoses with other anxiety disorders, substance use disorder, or depression. These disorders often significantly impair individuals' abilities to function socially, occupationally, and personally.
- Treatment approaches for all anxiety-related disorders include pharmacotherapies, psychological treatments, or often a combination of both.

- Current research points to a combination of biologic, psychological, social, and spiritual factors that cause persistent anxiety. Other research demonstrates that there are also personality traits that predispose individuals to anxiety disorders, including low self-esteem, external locus of control, some negative family influences, and some traumatic or stressful precipitating event. These components combine to yield a true bio/psycho/social/spiritual theory of causation.
- Nurses employ interventions from each of the dimensions—biologic, psychological, social, and spiritual—in the care of persons experiencing anxiety. Approaching these individuals with knowledge of the disorders, understanding, and with a calm demeanour is key. Nurses can be instrumental in crisis intervention, medication management, and psychoeducation. Psychoeducation is crucial in the management of anxiety disorders and includes methods to help individuals understand and manage anxiety symptoms (e.g., diaphragmatic breathing, stress reduction, relaxation techniques), education regarding medication side effects and management, and education of family members to understand these disorders.

Thinking Challenges

a. A nursing student, Julie, began her first clinical rotation in an active treatment hospital this morning. She was so excited about starting this phase of her education that she barely got any sleep last night. During report, however, Julie begins to feel dizzy and short of breath and starts trembling. She becomes pale and looks as if she might faint. When asked if she feels ill, Julie shakes her head and flees from the unit. What is your assessment of what was happening to Julie? Based on your assessment, describe the information and/or interventions that may be offered to Julie when she seeks assistance at a health centre to prevent such

an episode from happening again or to better deal with one if it does.

b. What would you tell a family member of a person with a hoarding disorder who asks you to explain the disorder?

c. Nurses need to consider sociocultural factors when evaluating an individual's OCD. Describe how this can be accomplished.

> Visit thePoint to view suggested responses. Go to **thePoint.lww.com/activate** and use the activation code found in the front of this text to unlock answers to the "Thinking Challenges" and other online resources.

 Web Links

www.cmha.ca/documents/anxiety-disorders . The Canadian Mental Health Association (CMHA) is one of the most recognized mental health organizations in Canada. With a presence in every province and territory across the nation, CMHA contributes advocacy on mental health issues as well as resources to support those struggling with mental health challenges, including anxiety, and to facilitate recovery and resilience.

www.anxietycanada.ca/ Anxiety Disorders Association of Canada is dedicated to the awareness, prevention, and treatment of anxiety disorders in Canada and to improve the lives of Canadians who experience anxiety disorders.

www.canmat.org/ The Canadian Network for Mood and Anxiety Treatments (CANMAT) is a federally incorporated, academically based, not-for-profit research organization linking healthcare professionals from across Canada who have a special interest in mood and anxiety disorders.

References

Adams, G. C., Balbuena, L., Meng, X., & Asmudson, G. J. G. (2016). When social anxiety and depression go together: A population study of comorbidity and associated consequences. *Journal of Affective Disorders, 206,* 48–54.

Adhikari, K., Metcalfe, A., Bulloch, A. G., Williams, J. V., & Patten, S. B. (2020). Mental disorders and subsequent suicide events in a representative community population. *Journal of Affective Disorders, 277,* 456–462. https://doi.org/10.1016/j.jad.2020.08.053

Albert, U., Baffa, A., & Maina, G. (2017). Family accommodation in adult obsessive–compulsive disorder: Clinical perspectives. *Psychology Research and Behavior Management, 10,* 293–304. https://doi.org/10.2147/PRBM.S124359

American Psychiatric Association (APA). (2013). *Diagnostic and statistical manual of mental disorders* (5th ed.).

Argyle, N., Deltito, J., Allerup, P., Maier, W., Albus, M., Nutzinger, D., Rasmussen, S., Ayuso, J. L., & Bech, P. (1991). The panic-associated symptom scale: Measuring the severity of panic disorder. *Acta Psychiatrica Scandinavica, 83,* 20–26.

Ask, H., Cheesman, R., Jami, E. S., Levey, D. F., Purves, K. L., & Weber, H. (2021, February). Genetic contributions to anxiety disorders: Where we are and where we are heading. *Psychological Medicine, 51,* 1–16. https://doi.org/10.1017/S0033291720005486

Asselmann, E., Stender, J., Grabe, H. J., König, J., Schmidt, C. O., Hamm, A. O., & Pané-Farré, C. A. (2018). Assessing the interplay of childhood adversities with more recent stressful life events and conditions in predicting panic pathology among adults from the general population. *Journal of Affective Disorders, 225,* 715–722. https://doi.org/10.1016/j.jad.2017.08.050

Bandelow, B., Michaelis, S., & Wedekind, D. (2017). Treatment of anxiety disorders. *Dialogues in Clinical Neuroscience, 19*(2), 93–107. https://doi.org/10.31887/DCNS.2017.19.2/bbandelow

Bandelow, B., Reitt, M., Röver, C., Michaelis, S., Görlich, Y., & Wedekind, D. (2015). Efficacy of treatments for anxiety disorders: A meta-analysis. *International Clinical Psychopharmacology, 30*(4), 183–192.

Bandelow, B., Wedekind, D., Pauls, J., Brooks, A., Hajak, G., & Ruther, E. (2000). Salivary cortisol in panic attacks. *American Journal of Psychiatry, 157,* 454–456.

Barlow, D. H. (2002). *Anxiety and its disorders: The nature and treatment of anxiety and panic.* Guilford Press.

Beck, A. T., Emery, C., & Greenberg, R. L. (1985). *Anxiety disorders and phobias: A cognitive perspective.* Basic Books.

Beck, A. T., Epstein, N., Brown, G., & Steer, R. (1988). An inventory for measuring clinical anxiety: The Beck Anxiety Inventory. *Journal of Consulting and Clinical Psychology, 56,* 893–897.

Beesdo, K., Knappe, S., & Pine, D. S. (2009). Anxiety and anxiety disorders in children and adolescents: Developmental issues and implications for DSM-V. *The Psychiatric Clinics of North America, 32*(3), 483–524. https://doi.org/10.1016/j.psc.2009.06.002

Blanck, P., Perleth, S., Heidenreich, T., Kröger, P., Ditzen, B., Bents, H., & Mander, J. (2018). Effects of mindfulness exercises as stand-alone intervention on symptoms of anxiety and depression: Systematic review and meta-analysis. *Behaviour Research and Therapy, 102,* 25–35. https://doi.org/10.1016/j.brat.2017.12.002

Borkovec, T. D., Robinson, E., Pruzinsky, T., & DePree, J. A. (1983). Preliminary exploration of worry: Some characteristics and processes. *Behaviour Research and Therapy, 21*(1), 9–16.

Brakoulias, V., & Milicevic, D. (2015). Assessment and treatment of hoarding disorder. *Australian Psychiatry, 23*(4), 358–360.

Brakoulias, V., Starcevic, V., Belloch, A., Brown, C., Ferrao, Y. A., Fontenelle, L. F., Lochner, C., Marazziti, D., Matsunaga, H., Miguel, E. C., & Reddy, Y. C. J., do Rosario, M. C., Shavitt, R. G., Shyam Sundar, A., Stein, D. J., Torres, A. R., & Viswasam, K. (2017). Comorbidity, age of onset and suicidality in obsessive–compulsive disorder (OCD): An international collaboration. *Comprehensive Psychiatry, 76,* 79–86. https://doi.org/10.1016/j.comppsych.2017.04.002

Brown, L. T., Mikell, C. B., Youngerman, B. E., Zhang, Y., McKhann, G. II., & Sheth, S. A. (2016). Dorsal anterior cingulotomy and anterior capsulotomy for severe, refractory obsessive-compulsive disorder: A systematic review of observational studies. *Journal of Neurosurgery, 124*(1), 77–89.

Burns, D. (1999). *Feeling good: The new mood therapy.* Plume.

Chambless, D. L., Caputo, G. C., Bright, P., & Gallagher, R. (1984). Assessment of fear in agoraphobics: The body sensations questionnaire and the agoraphobic cognitions questionnaire. *Journal of Consulting and Clinical Psychology, 52,* 1090–1097.

Chambless, D. L., Caputo, G. C., Jasin, S. E., Gracely, E. J., & Williams, C. (1985). The mobility inventory for agoraphobia. *Behaviour Research and Therapy, 23,* 35–44.

Clum, G. A. (1990). *Coping with panic: A drug-free approach to dealing with anxiety attacks.* Brooks/Cole.

Collie, R. J., Martin, A. J., Nassar, N., & Roberts, C. L. (2019). Social and emotional behavioral profiles in kindergarten: A population-based latent profile analysis of links to socio-educational characteristics and later achievement. *Journal of Educational Psychology, 111*(1), 170–187. https://doi.org/10.1037/edu0000262

Cooper, J. (1970). The leyton obsessional inventory. *Psychiatric Medicine, 1*, 48.

Coulombe, S., Radziszewski, S., Meunier, S., Provencher, H., Hudon, C., Roberge, P., Provencher, M. D., & Houle, J. (2016). Profiles of recovery from mood and anxiety disorders: A person-centered exploration of people's engagement in self-management. *Frontiers in Psychology, 7*, 584. https://doi.org/10.3389/fpsyg.2016.00584

Cuijpers, P., Cristea, I. A., Karyotaki, E., Reijnders, M., & Huibers, M. J. (2016). How effective are cognitive behavior therapies for major depression and anxiety disorders? A meta-analytic update of the evidence. *World Psychiatry, 15*(3), 245–258. https://doi.org/10.1002/wps.20346

Cuijpers, P., Sijbrandij, M., Koole, S. L., Andersson, G., Beekman, A. T., & Reynolds, C. F. III. (2014). Adding psychotherapy to antidepressant medication in depression and anxiety disorders: A meta-analysis. *World Psychiatry, 13*(1), 56–67.

Curcio, C., & Corboy, D. (2020). Stigma and anxiety disorders: A systematic review. *Stigma and Health, 5*(2), 125–137. https://doi.org/10.1037/sah0000183

De Jonge, P., Roest, A., Lim, C., Levinson, D., & Scott, K. (2018). Panic disorder and panic attacks. In K. Scott, P. De Jonge, D. Stein, & R. Kessler (Eds.), *Mental disorders around the world: Facts and figures from the WHO World Mental Health Surveys* (pp. 93–105). Cambridge University Press.

de Lijster, J. M., Dierckx, B., Utens, E. M. W. J., Verhulst, F. C., Zieldorff, C., Dieleman, G. C., & Legerstee, J. S. (2017). The age of onset of anxiety disorders: A meta-analysis. *The Canadian Journal of Psychiatry, 62*(4), 237–246. https://doi.org/10.1177/0706743716640757

Demenescu, L. R., Kortekass, R., Cremers, H. R., Renken, R. J., van Tol, R. M. J., van der Wee, N. J. A., Veltman, D. J., den Boer, J. A., Roelofs, K., & Aleman, A. (2013). Amygdala activation and its functional connectivity during perception of emotional faces in social phobia and panic disorder. *Journal of Psychiatric Research, 47*(8), 1024–1031.

Dillon, D. J., Gorman, J. M., Liebowitz, M. R., Fyer, A. J., & Klein, D. F. (1987). Measurement of lactate-induced panic and anxiety. *Psychiatry Research, 20*, 97–105.

Doering, S., Lichtenstein, P., Gillberg, C., Middeldorp, C. M., Bartels, M., Kuja-Halkola, R., & Lundström, S. (2019). Anxiety at age 15 predicts psychiatric diagnoses and suicidal ideation in late adolescence and young adulthood: Results from two longitudinal studies. *BMC Psychiatry, 19*, 363. https://doi.org/10.1186/s12888-019-2349-3

Dryman, M. T., Gardner, S., Weeks, J. W., & Heimberg, R. G. (2016). Social anxiety disorder and quality of life: How fears of negative and positive evaluation relate to specific domains of life satisfaction. *Journal of Anxiety Disorders, 38*, 1–8. https://doi.org/10.1016/j.janxdis.2015.12.003

Edlund, M. J., Wang, J., Brown, K. G., Forman-Hoffman, V. L., Calvin, S. L., Hedden, S. L., & Bose, J. (2018). Which mental disorders are associated with the greatest impairment in functioning? *Social Psychiatry and Psychiatric Epidemiology, 53*(11), 1265–1276. https://doi.org/10.1007/s00127-018-1554-6

Elsenhauer, A. (2017, February). Preparing for patients with hording disorder. *EMSWorld*, 45–47.

Essau, C. A., Lewinsohn, P. M., Lim, J. X., Moon-Ho, R. H., & Rohde, P. (2018). Incidence, recurrence and comorbidity of anxiety disorders in four major developmental stages. *Journal of Affective Disorders, 228*, 248–253. https://doi.org/10.1016/j.jad.2017.12.014

Fineberg, N. A., Hengartner, M. P., Bergbaum, C., Gale, T., Rössler, W., & Angst, J. (2013). Lifetime comorbidity of obsessive-compulsive disorder and sub-threshold obsessive-compulsive symptomatology in the community: Impact, prevalence, socio-demographic and clinical characteristics. *International Journal of Psychiatry in Clinical Practice, 17*(3), 188–196. https://doi.org/10.3109/13651501.2013.777745

Frankl, V. (1992). *Man's search for meaning: An introduction to logotherapy* (4th ed.). Beacon Press.

Frost, R. O., Steketee, G., & Grisham, J. (2004). Measurement of compulsive hoarding: Saving Inventory-Revised. *Behaviour Research and Therapy, 42*, 1163–1182.

Fullana, M. A., Tortella Feliu, M., Fernández de la Cruz, L., Chamorro, J., Pérez-Vigil, A., Ioannidis, J., Solanes, A., Guardiola, M., Almodóvar, C., Miranda-Olivos, R., Ramella-Cravaro, V., Vilar, A., Reichenberg, A., Mataix-Cols, D., Vieta, E., Fusar-Poli, P., Fatjó-Vilas, M., & Radua, J. (2020). Risk and protective factors for anxiety and obsessive-compulsive disorders: An umbrella review of systematic reviews and meta-analyses. *Psychological Medicine, 50*(8), 1300–1315. https://doi.org/10.1017/S0033291719001247

Gerlach, L. B., Wiechers, I. R., & Maust, D. T. (2018). Prescription benzodiazepine use among older adults: A critical review. *Harvard Review of Psychiatry, 26*(5), 264–273. https://doi.org/10.1097/HRP.0000000000000190

Goodman, W., Price, L., Rasmussen, S., Mazure, C., Fleischmann, R. L., & Hill, C. L. (1989). The Yale-Brown Obsessive Compulsive Scale (Y-BOCS): Part 1. Development, use and reliability. *Archives of General Psychiatry, 46*, 1006–1011.

Government of Canada. (2006). *The human face of mental health and mental illness in Canada, 2006*. Minister of Public Works and Government Services Canada. Catalogue no.: HP5-19/2006E.

Greenberg, T., Carlson, J. M., Cha, J., Hajcak, G., & Mujica-Parodi, L. (2012). Ventromedial prefrontal cortex reactivity is altered in generalized anxiety disorder during fear generalization. *Depression and Anxiety, 30*(3), 242–250.

Groenman, A. P., Janssen, T. W. P., & Oosterlaan, J. (2017). Childhood psychiatric disorders as risk factor for subsequent substance abuse: A meta-analysis. *Journal of the American Academy of Child & Adolescent Psychiatry, 56*(7), 556–569. https://doi.org/10.1016/j.jaac.2017.05.004

Hamilton, M. (1959). The assessment of anxiety states by rating. *British Journal of Medical Psychology, 32*, 54.

Inoue, K., Kaiya, H., Hara, N., & Okazaki, Y. (2016). A discussion of various aspects of panic disorder depending on presence or absence of agoraphobia. *Comprehensive Psychiatry, 69*, 132–135.

Jakubovski, E., Johnson, J. A., Nasir, M., Müller-Vahl, K., & Bloch, M. H. (2019). Systematic review and meta-analysis: Dose–response curve of SSRIs and SNRIs in anxiety disorders. *Depression and Anxiety, 36*(3), 198–212. https://doi.org/10.1002/da.22854

Kagan, E. R., Frank, H. E., & Kendall, P. C. (2017). Accommodation in youth with OCD and anxiety. *Clinical Psychology: Science and Practice, 24*(1), 78–98. https://doi.org/10.1111/cpsp.12186

Katzman, M. A., Bleau, P., Blier, P., Chokka, P., Kjernisted, K., & Van Ameringen, M. (2014). Canadian clinical practice guidelines for the management of anxiety, posttraumatic stress and obsessive-compulsive disorders. *BMC Psychiatry, 14*(Suppl. 1), S1.

Kawashima, C., Tanaka, Y., Inoue, A., Nakanishi, M., Okamoto, K., Maruyama, Y, Oshita, H., Ishitobi, Y., Aizawa, S., Masuda, K., Higuma, H, Kanehisa, M., Ninomiya, T., & Akiyoshi, J. (2016). Hyperfunction of left lateral prefrontal cortex and automatic thoughts in social anxiety disorder: A near-infrared spectroscopy study. *Journal of Affective Disorders, 206*, 256–260.

Kim, C. H., Chang, J. W., Koo, M. S., Kim, J. W., Suh, H. S., Park, I. H., & Lee, H. S. (2003). Anterior cingulotomy for refractory obsessive-compulsive disorder. *Acta Psychiatrica Scandinavica, 107*(4), 241–243.

Kircanski, K., Thompson, R. J., Sorenson, J., Sherdell, L., & Gotlib, I. H. (2018). The everyday dynamics of rumination and worry: Precipitant events and affective consequences. *Cognition & Emotion, 32*(7), 1424–1436. https://doi.org/10.1080/02699931.2017.1278679

Kladnitski, N., Smith, J., Uppal, S., James, M. A., Allen, A. R., Andrews, G., & Newby, J. M. (2020). Transdiagnostic internet-delivered CBT and mindfulness-based treatment for depression and anxiety: A randomised controlled trial. *Internet Interventions, 20*, 100310. https://doi.org/10.1016/j.invent.2020.100310

Konishi, J., Asami, T., Hayano, F., Yoshimi, A., Hayasaka, S., Fukushima, H., Whitford, T. J., Inoue, T., & Hirayasu, Y. (2014). Multiple white matter volume reductions in patients with panic disorder: Relationships between orbitofrontal gyrus volume and symptom severity and social dysfunction. *PLoS One, 9*(3), e92862. https://doi.org/10.1371/journal.pone.0092862

Koslander, T., Barbosa da Silva, A., & Roxberg, A. (2009). Existential and spiritual needs in mental health care: An ethical and holistic perspective. *Journal of Holistic Nursing, 27*(1), 34–42.

Koyuncu, A., İnce, E., Ertekin, E., & Tükel, R. (2019). Comorbidity in social anxiety disorder: Diagnostic and therapeutic challenges. *Drugs in Context, 8*, 212573. https://doi.org/10.7573/dic.212573

Kress, V. E., Stargell, N. A., Zoldan, C. A., & Paylo, M. J. (2016). Hoarding disorder: Diagnosis, assessment and treatment. *Journal of Counseling & Development, 94*, 83–90.

Kroenke, K., & Unutzer, J. (2017). Closing the false divide: Sustainable approaches to integrating mental health services into primary care. *Journal of General Internal Medicine, 32*, 404–410. https://doi.org/10.1007/s11606-016-3967-9

Külz, A. K., Landmann, S., Cludius, B., Rose, N., Heidenreich, T., Jelinek, L., Alsleben, H., Wahl, K., Philipsen, A., Voderholzer, U., Maier, J. G., & Moritz, S. (2019). Mindfulness-based cognitive therapy (MBCT) in patients with obsessive–compulsive disorder (OCD) and residual symptoms after cognitive behavioral therapy (CBT): A randomized controlled trial. *European Archives of Psychiatry and Clinical Neuroscience, 269*(2), 223–233. https://doi.org/10.1007/s00406-018-0957-4

Kysow, K., Bratiotis, C., Lauster, N., & Woody, S. R. (2020). How can cities tackle hoarding? Examining an intervention program bringing together fire and health authorities in Vancouver. *Health & Social Care in the Community, 28*(4), 1160–1169. https://doi.org/10.1111/hsc.12948

Lamers, F., van Oppen, P., Comijs, H. C., Smit, J. H., Spinhoven, P., Anton, J. L. M., Nolen, W. A., Zitman, F. G., Beekman, A. T. F., & Penninx, B. W. J. H. (2011). Comorbidity patterns of anxiety and depressive disorders in a large cohort study: The Netherlands Study of Depression and Anxiety (NESDA). *Journal of Clinical Psychiatry, 72*(3), 341–348.

LeBeau, R. T., Glenn, D., Liao, B., Wittchen, H. U., Beesdo-Baum, K., Ollendick, T., & Craske, M. G. (2010). Specific phobia: A review of DSM-IV specific phobia and preliminary recommendations for DSM-V. *Depression and Anxiety, 27*(2), 148–167.

LeDoux, J. (2015). *Anxious: Using the brain to understand and treat fear and anxiety.* Penguin Books.

Leichsenring, F., & Steinert, C. (2017). Is cognitive behavioral therapy the gold standard for psychotherapy?: The need for plurality in treatment and research. *JAMA, 318*(14), 1323–1324. https://doi.org/10.1001/jama.2017.13737

Lochner, C., Fineberg, N. A., Zohar, J., Van Ameringen, M., Juven-Wetzler, A., Alfredo Carlo Altamura, A. C., Cuzen, N. L., Hollander, E., Denys, D., Nicolini, H., Dell'Osso, B., Pallanti, S., & Stein, D. J. (2014). Comorbidity in obsessive–compulsive disorder (OCD): A report from the International College of Obsessive–Compulsive Spectrum Disorders (ICOCS). *Comprehensive Psychiatry, 55*(7), 1513–1519.

Lovick, T. A. (2014). Sex determinants of experimental panic attacks. *Neuroscience & Biobehavioural Reviews, 46*(3), 465–471.

Makovac, E., Meeten, F., Watson, D. R., Herman, A., Garfinkel, S. N., Critchley, H. D., & Ottaviana, C. (2016). Alterations in amygdala-prefrontal functional connectivity account for excessive worry and autonomic dysregulation in generalized anxiety disorder. *Biological Psychiatry, 80*(10), 786–795.

Mallorquí-Bagué, N., Bulbena, A., Pailhez, G., Garfinkel, S. N., & Critchley, H. D. (2016). Mind-body interactions in anxiety and somatic symptoms. *Harvard Review of Psychiatry, 24*(1), 53–60.

Marks, I. M., & Matthews, A. M. (1979). Brief standard self-rating for phobic patients. *Behaviour Research and Therapy, 17*, 263–267.

McEwen, B. (2005). Stressed or stressed out: What is the difference? *Journal of Psychiatry and Neuroscience, 30*, 315–318.

Meier, S. M., & Deckert, J. (2019). Genetics of anxiety disorders. *Current Psychiatry Reports, 21*, 16. https://doi.org/10.1007/s11920-019-1002-7

Meng, X., & D'Arcy, C. (2015). Comorbidity between lifetime eating problems and mood and anxiety disorders: Results from the Canadian Community Health Survey of Mental Health and Well-being. *European Eating Disorders Review, 23*(2), 156–162. https://doi.org/10.1002/erv.2347

Merikangas, K. R., He, J. P., Burstein, M., Swanson, S. A., Avenevoli, S., Cui, L., Benjet, C., Georgiades, K., & Swendsen, J. (2010). Lifetime prevalence of mental disorders in U.S. adolescents: Results from the National Comorbidity Survey Replication—Adolescent Supplement (NCS-A). *Journal of the American Academy of Child and Adolescent Psychiatry, 49*(10), 980–989.

Meyer, T., Miller, M., Metzger, R., & Borkovec, T. (1990). Development and validation of the Penn State Worry Questionnaire. *Behaviour Research and Therapy, 28*(6), 487–495.

Miché, M., Hofer, P. D., Voss, C., Meyer, A. H., Gloster, A. T., Beesdo-Baum, K., & Lieb, R. (2018). Mental disorders and the risk for the subsequent first suicide attempt: Results of a community study on adolescents and young adults. *European Child & Adolescent Psychiatry, 27*(7), 839–848. https://doi.org/10.1007/s00787-017-1060-5

Mobbs, D. (2018). The ethological deconstruction of fear(s). *Current Opinion in Behavioral Sciences, 24*, 32–37. https://doi.org/10.1016/j.cobeha.2018.02.008

Monzani, B., Vidal-Ribas, P., Turner, C., Krebs, G., Stokes, C., Heyman, I., Mataix-Cols, D., & Stringaris, A. (2020). The role of paternal accommodation of paediatric OCD symptoms: Patterns and implications for treatment outcomes. *Journal of Abnormal Child Psychology, 48*, 1313–1323. https://doi.org/10.1007/s10802-020-00678-9

Muhlbauer, J. E., Ferrão, Y. A., Eppingstall, J., Albertella, L., do Rosário, M. C., Miguel, E. C., & Fontenelle, L. F. (2020). Predicting marriage and divorce in obsessive-compulsive disorder. *Journal of Sex & Marital Therapy, 47*(1), 90–98. https://doi.org/10.1080/0092623X.2020.1804021

Muroff, J., & Otte, S. (2019). Innovations in CBT treatment for hoarding: Transcending office walls. *Journal of Obsessive-Compulsive and Related Disorders, 23*, 100471. https://doi.org/10.1016/j.jocrd.2019.100471

Naveed, S., Waqas, A., Chaudhary, A. M. D., Kumar, S., Abbas, N., Amin, R., Jamil, N., & Saleem, S. (2020). Prevalence of common mental disorders in South Asia: A systematic review and meta-regression analysis. *Frontiers in Psychiatry, 11*, 899. https://doi.org/10.3389/fpsyt.2020.573150

Nebel-Schwalm, M., & Davis, T. E. (2013). Nature and etiological models of anxiety disorders. In E. Storch & D. McKay (Eds.), *Handbook of treating variants and complications in anxiety disorders* (pp. 3–21). Springer.

Neziroglu, F., Upston, M., & Khemlani-Patel, S. (2020). The psychological, relational and social impact in adult offspring of parents with hoarding disorder. *Children Australia, 45*(3), 153–158. https://doi.org/10.1017/cha.2020.42

Olatunji, B. O., Christian, C., Brosof, L., Tolin, D. F., & Levinson, C. A. (2019). What is at the core of OCD? A network analysis of selected obsessive-compulsive symptoms and beliefs. *Journal of Affective Disorders, 257*, 45–54. https://doi.org/10.1016/j.jad.2019.06.064

Olaya, B., Moneta, M. V., Miret, M., Ayuso-Mateos, J. L., & Haro, J. M. (2018). Epidemiology of panic attacks, panic disorder and the moderating role of age: Results from a population-based study. *Journal of Affective Disorders, 241*, 627–633. https://doi.org/10.1016/j.jad.2018.08.069

Olson, C. M. (2021). Familial factors in the development of social anxiety disorder. *Journal of Psychosocial Nursing, 59*, 23–34. https://doi.org/10.3928/02793695-20210219-01

Osland, S., Arnold, P. D., & Pringsheim, T. (2018). The prevalence of diagnosed obsessive compulsive disorder and associated comorbidities: A population-based Canadian study. *Psychiatry Research, 268*, 137–142. https://doi.org/10.1016/j.psychres.2018.07.018

Peplau, H. (1989). Theoretic constructs: Anxiety, self, and hallucinations. In A. O'Toole & S. Welt (Eds.), *Interpersonal theory in nursing practice: Selected works of Hildegard E. Peplau.* Springer.

Pessoa, L., & McMenamin, B. (2017). Dynamic networks in the emotional brain. *The Neuroscientist, 23*(4), 383–396. https://doi.org/10.1177/1073858416671936

Porges, S. W. (2007). The Polyvagal perspective. *Biological Psychology, 74*(2), 116–143. https://doi.org/10.1016/j.biopsycho.2006.06.009

Price, M., Legrand, A. C., Brier, Z. M., & Hébert-Dufresne, L. (2019). The symptoms at the center: Examining the comorbidity of posttraumatic stress disorder, generalized anxiety disorder, and depression with network analysis. *Journal of Psychiatric Research, 109*, 52–58. https://doi.org/10.1016/j.jpsychires.2018.11.016

Public Health Agency of Canada. (2016). Report from the Canadian chronic disease surveillance system: Mood and anxiety disorders in Canada, 2016. http://healthycanadians.gc.ca/publications/diseases-conditions-maladies-affections/mood-anxiety-disorders-2016-troubles-anxieux-humeur/alt/mood-anxiety-disorders-2016-troubles-anxieux-humeur-eng.pdf

Rachman, S., & Hodgson, R. (1980). *Obsessions and compulsions.* Prentice-Hall.

Reddy, Y. C. J., Sudhir, P. M., Manjula, M., Arumugham, S. S., & Narayanaswamy, J. C. (2020). Clinical practice guidelines for cognitive-behavioral therapies in anxiety disorders and obsessive-compulsive and related disorders. *Indian Journal of Psychiatry, 62*, s230–s250. https://doi.org/10.4103/psychiatry.IndianJPsychiatry_773_19

Reiss, S., Peterson, R. A., & Gursky, D. M. (1986). Anxiety sensitivity, anxiety frequency, and the prediction of fearfulness. *Behaviour Research and Therapy, 24*, 1–8.

Rickels, K., & Moeller, H. J. (2019). Benzodiazepines in anxiety disorders: Reassessment of usefulness and safety. *The World Journal of Biological Psychiatry, 20*(7), 514–518. https://doi.org/10.1080/15622975.2018.1500031

Robinson, K. J., Rose, D., & Salkovskis, P. M. (2017). Seeking help for obsessive compulsive disorder (OCD): A qualitative study of the enablers and barriers conducted by a researcher with personal experience of OCD. *Psychology and Psychotherapy: Theory, Research and Practice, 90*(2), 193–211. https://doi.org/10.1111/papt.12090

Rodgers, N., McDonald, S., & Wootton, B. M. (2021). Cognitive behavioral therapy for hoarding disorder: An updated meta-analysis. *Journal of Affective Disorders, 290*, 128–135. https://doi.org/10.1016/j.jad.2021.04.067

Rovira, J., Albarracin, G., Salvador, L., Rejas, J., Sánchez-Iriso, E., & Cabasés, J. M. (2012). The cost of generalized anxiety disorder in primary care settings: Results of the ANCORA study. *Community Mental Health Journal, 48*(3), 372–383.

Ruland, T., Domschke, K., Schütte, V., Zavorotnyy, M., Kugel, H., Notzon, S., Vennewald, N., Ohrmann, P., Arolt, V., Pfleiderer, B., & Zwanzger, P. (2015). Neuropeptide S receptor gene variation modulates glutamatergic anterior cingulate cortex activity during CCK-4 induced panic. *Pharmacopsychiatry, 25*(10), 1677–1682.

Ruscio, A. M., Hallion, L. S., Lim, C. C., Aguilar-Gaxiola, S., Al-Hamzawi, A., Alonso, J., Andrade, L. H., Borges, G., Bromet, E. J., Bunting, B., de Almeida, J. M. C., Demyttenaere, K., Florescu, S., de Girolamo, G., Gureje, O., Haro, J. M., He, Y., Hinkov, H., Hu, C., … Scott, K. M. (2017). Cross-sectional comparison of the epidemiology of DSM-5 generalized anxiety disorder across the globe. *JAMA Psychiatry, 74*(5), 465–475. https://doi.org/10.1001/jamapsychiatry.2017.0056

Russell, A. L., Tasker, J. G., Lucion, A. B., Fiedler, J., Munhoz, C. D., Wu, T-y. J., & Deak, T. (2018). Factors promoting vulnerability to dysregulated stress reactivity and stress-related disease. *Journal of Neuroendocrinology, 30*, 1–13. https://doi.org/10.1111/jne.1264

Sadock, B. J., Sadock, V. A., & Ruiz, P. (2015). *Kaplan & Sadock's synopsis of psychiatry: Behavioral sciences/clinical psychiatry* (11th ed.). Wolters Kluwer.

Sallee, F., Sethuraman, G., Sine, L., & Liu, H. (2000). Yohimbine challenge in children with anxiety disorders. *American Journal of Psychiatry, 157,* 1236–1242.

Sánchez-Navarro, J. P., Driscoll, D., Anderson, S. W., Tranel, D., Bechara, A., & Buchanan, T. W. (2014). Alterations of attention and emotional processing following childhood-onset damage to the prefrontal cortex. *Behavioral Neuroscience, 128*(1), 1–11.

Schiele, M. A., & Domschke, K. (2018). Epigenetics at the crossroads between genes, environment and resilience in anxiety disorders. *Genes, Brain and Behavior, 17,* 1–15. https://doi.org/10.1111/gbb.12423

Schiele, M. A., Ziegler, C., Holitschke, K., Schartner, C., Schmidt, B., Weber, H., Reif, A., Romanos, M., Pauli, P., Zwanzger, P., Deckert, J. & Domschke, K. (2016). Influence of 5-HTT variation, childhood trauma and self-efficacy on anxiety traits: A gene-environment-coping interaction study. *Journal of Neural Transmission, 123,* 895–904. https://doi.org/10.1007/s00702-016-1564-z

Schore, A. N. (2014). The right brain is dominant in psychotherapy. *Psychotherapy, 51*(3), 388–397. https://doi.org/10.1037/a0037083

Schwartz, J. M. (2016). *Brain lock.* Harper Collins.

Scupi, B. S., Maser, J. D., & Uhde, T. W. (1992). The National Institute of Mental Health Panic Questionnaire: An instrument for assessing clinical characteristics of panic disorder. *Journal of Nervous and Mental Disease, 180,* 566–572.

Selye, H. (1956). *The stress of life.* McGraw-Hill.

Shin, J., Park, D. H., Ryu, S. H., Ha, J. H., Kim, S. M., & Jeon, H. J. (2020). Clinical implications of agoraphobia in patients with panic disorder. *Medicine, 99*(30), e21414. https://doi.org/10.1097/MD.0000000000021414

Simo, B., Bamvita, J. M., Caron, J., & Fleury, M. J. (2018). Patterns of health care service utilization by individuals with mental health problems: A predictive cluster analysis. *Psychiatric Quarterly, 89,* 675–690. https://doi.org/10.1007/s11126-018-9568-5

Sladky, R., Höflich, A., Küblböck, M., Kraus, C., Baldinger, P., Moser, E., Lanzenberger, R., & Windischberger, C. (2015). Disrupted effective connectivity between the amygdala and orbitofrontal cortex in social anxiety disorder during emotion discrimination revealed by dynamic causal modeling for fMRI. *Cerebral Cortex, 25*(4), 895–903.

Spielberger, C. D., Gorsuch, R. L., & Luchene, R. E. (1976). *Manual for the state-trait anxiety inventory.* Consulting Psychologists Press.

Spitzer, R. L., Kroenke, K., Williams, J. B. W., & Löwe, B. (2006). A brief measure for assessing generalized anxiety disorder: The GAD-7. *Archives of Internal Medicine, 166,* 1092–1097.

Statistics Canada. (2013). Canadian community health survey: Mental health, 2012. http://www.statcan.gc.ca/daily-quotidien/130918/dq130918a-eng.pdf

Steimer, T. (2002). The biology of fear- and anxiety-related behaviors. *Dialogues in Clinical Neuroscience, 4*(3), 231–249.

Stein, D. J., Lim, C. C., Roest, A. M., de Jonge, P., Aguilar-Gaxiola, S., Al-Hamzawi, A., Alonso, J., Benjet, C., Bromet, E. J., Bruffaerts, R., de Girolamo, G., Florescu, S., Gureje, O., Haro, J. M., Harris, M. G., He, Y., Hinkov, H., Horiguchi, I., Hu, C., … & WHO World Mental Health Survey Collaborators. (2017). The cross-national epidemiology of social anxiety disorder: Data from the World Mental Health Survey Initiative. *BMC Medicine, 15*(1), 143. https://doi.org/10.1186/s12916-017-0889-2

Stekettee, G., Kelley, A. A., Wernick, J. A., Muroff, J., Frost, R. O., & Tolin, D. F. (2015). Family patterns of hording symptoms. *Depression and Anxiety, 32,* 728–736.

Stengler, K., Olbrich, S., Heider, D., Dietrich, S., Riedel-Heller, S., & Jahn, I. (2013). Mental health treatment seeking among patients with OCD: Impact of age of onset. *Social Psychiatry and Psychiatric Epidemiology, 48*(5), 813–819.

Stewart, S. E., Hu, Y. P., Leung, A., Chan, E., Hezel, D. M., Lin, S. Y., Belschner, L., Walsh, C., Geller, D. A., & & Pauls, D. L. (2017). A multisite study of family functioning impairment in pediatric obsessive-compulsive disorder. *Journal of the American Academy of Child & Adolescent Psychiatry, 56*(3), 241–249. https://doi.org/10.1016/j.jaac.2016.12.012

Stewart, K. E., Sumantry, D., & Malivoire, B. L. (2020). Family and couple integrated cognitive-behavioural therapy for adults with OCD: A meta-analysis. *Journal of Affective Disorders, 277,* 159–168. https://doi.org/10.1016/j.jad.2020.07.140

Strawn, J. R., Mills, J. A., Sauley, B. A., & Welge, J. A. (2018). The impact of antidepressant dose and class on treatment response in pediatric anxiety disorders: A meta-analysis. *Journal of the American Academy of Child & Adolescent Psychiatry, 57*(4), 235–244. https://doi.org/10.1016/j.jaac.2018.01.015

Ströhle, A., Gensichen, J., & Domschke, K. (2018). The diagnosis and treatment of anxiety disorders. *Deutsches Ärzteblatt International, 115*(37), 611. https://doi.org/10.3238/arztebl.2018.0611

Tibi, L., van Oppen, P., Aderka, I. M., van Balkom, A. J. L. M., Batelaan, N. M., Spinhoven, P., Penninx, B. W., & Anholt, G. E. (2013). Examining determinants of early and late age at onset in panic disorder: An admixture analysis. *Journal of Psychiatric Research, 47*(12), 1870–1875.

Tillich, P. (1952). *The courage to be.* Yale University Press.

Toh, W. X., & Yang, H. (2020). Similar but not quite the same: Differential unique associations of trait fear and trait anxiety with inhibitory control. *Personality and Individual Differences, 155,* 109718. https://doi.org/10.1016/j.paid.2019.109718

Tolin, D. F., Frost, R., & Steketee, G. (2010). A brief interview for assessing compulsive hoarding: The Hoarding Rating Scale—Interview. *Psychiatric Research, 178,* 147–152.

Van Cappellen, P., Rice, E. L., Catalino, L. I., & Frederickson, B. L. (2018). Positive affective processes underlie positive health behavior change. *Psychology and Health, 33*(1), 77–97. https://doi.org/10.1080/08870446.2017.1320798

van der Feltz-Cornelis, C., van Marwijk, H., & Hakkaart-van Roijen, L. (2017). Collaborative care models for the management of mental disorders in primary care. In A. F. Carvalho & R. S. McIntyre (Eds.), *Mental disorders in primary care: A guide to their evaluation and management* (pp. 34–44). Oxford University Press.

Vicheva, P., Butler, M., & Shotbolt, P. (2020). Deep brain stimulation for obsessive-compulsive disorder: A systematic review of randomised controlled trials. *Neuroscience & Biobehavioral Reviews, 109,* 129–138. https://doi.org/10.1016/j.neubiorev.2020.01.007

Vilaplana-Pérez, A., Pérez-Vigil, A., Sidorchuk, A., Brander, G., Isomura, K., Hesselmark, E., Kuja-Halkola, R., Larsson, H., Mataix-Cols, D., & de la Cruz, L. F. (2020). Much more than just shyness: The impact of social anxiety disorder on educational performance across the lifespan. *Psychological Medicine, 51*(5), 861–869. https://doi.org/10.1017/S0033291719003908

Walseth, L. T., Launes, G., Sunde, T., Klovning, I., Himle, J., Haaland, V. Ø., & Håland, Å. T. (2019). Present in daily life: Obsessive compulsive disorder and its impact on family life from the partner's perspective. A Focus Group Study. *Journal of Family Psychotherapy, 30*(3), 185–203. https://doi.org/10.1080/08975353.2019.1631027

Watterson, R. A., Williams, J. V. A., Lavorato, D. H., & Patten, S. B. (2017). Descriptive epidemiology of generalized anxiety disorder in Canada. *The Canadian Journal of Psychiatry, 62*(1), 24–29. https://doi.org/10.1177/0706743716645304

Weems, C., Costa, N., Dehon, C., & Berman, S. (2004). Paul Tillich's theory of existential anxiety: A preliminary conceptual and empirical examination. *Anxiety, Stress, and Coping, 17*(4), 383–399.

Wintermann, G.-B., Kirschbaum, C., & Petrowski, K. (2016). Predisposition or side effect of the duration: The reactivity of the HPA-axis under psychosocial stress in panic disorder. *International Journal of Psychophysiology, 107,* 9–15.

Xi, Y. (2020). Anxiety: A concept analysis. *Frontiers of Nursing, 7*(1), 9–12. https://doi.org/10.2478/fon-2020-0008

Yalom, I. (1980). *Existential psychotherapy.* Basic Books.

Yuan, C., Zhua, H., Rena, Z., Yuan, M., Gao, M., Zhang, Y., Li, Y., Meng, Y., Gong, Q., Lui, S., Qiu, C., & Zhang, W. (2018). Precuneus-related regional and network functional deficits in social anxiety disorder: A resting-state functional MRI study. *Comprehensive Psychiatry, 82,* 22–29. https://doi.org/10.1016/j.comppsych.2017.12.002

Zhou, Y., Cao, Z., Yang, M., Xi, X., Guo, Y., Fang, M., Cheng, L., & Du, Y. (2017). Comorbid generalized anxiety disorder and its association with quality of life in patients with major depressive disorder. *Scientific Reports, 7,* 40511. https://doi.org/10.1038/srep40511

24

Somatic Symptom and Related Disorders

Duncan Stewart MacLennan

LEARNING OBJECTIVES

After studying this chapter, you will be able to:

- Explain the concept of somatization and its presentation in people with mental health problems.
- Discuss epidemiologic factors related to somatic symptom and related disorders.
- Compare the etiologic theories of somatic symptom and related disorders from a bio/psycho/social/ spiritual perspective.
- Contrast the major differences between somatic symptom disorders and factitious disorders.
- Discuss human responses to somatic symptom and related disorders.
- Apply the elements of nursing management to a client with somatic symptom and related disorders.

KEY TERMS

- factitious disorder • illness anxiety disorder
- malingering • pseudoneurologic symptoms • somatic symptom disorder

KEY CONCEPT

- somatization

The connection between the mind and the body has been described for centuries. For example, "broken heart syndrome" or Takotsubo cardiomyopathy causes the heart to enlarge and pump poorly in response to very stressful situations (such as the death of a loved one). In contrast, the term somatization is used when unexplained physical symptoms occur in the presence of psychological distress or psychiatric illness. Somatic symptom and related disorders describes conditions in which a psychological state contributes to the development or experience of physical symptoms or illness. This chapter explores the concept of somatization and explains the care of clients experiencing somatic symptom disorders.

Although somatization occurs commonly in many psychiatric disorders, including depression, anxiety, and psychosis, it is the *primary* symptom of somatic symptom disorders. Somatic symptom and related disorders occur when a person experiences physical symptoms causing psychological distress and/or abnormal patterns of thought and behaviour (Henningsen, 2018). The prevalence of somatic symptoms and related disorders in the general population is approximately 5% to 7% (D'Souza & Hooten, 2021). There may or may not be an organic cause for the symptom. A factitious disorder is one in which clients simulate or inflict injury on themselves or others to receive medical treatment or for another secondary purpose. Unlike other somatic

symptom disorders, the physical symptoms in a factitious disorder are deliberately produced by the client.

Historically, people with "medically unexplained symptoms" were said to have a somatic symptom disorder. This diagnostic approach relied on the assumption that all other likely or possible diagnoses were fully explored *and* excluded. Practitioners were reluctant to diagnose somatic symptom or related disorders, in part, due to the impossible task of excluding other alternative diagnoses. This reluctance frequently contributed to treatment delays.

In 2013, the American Psychiatric Association responded to the complexity contributing to the seemingly underdiagnoses of somatic symptom and related disorders by significantly revising earlier diagnostic criteria in the fifth edition of the *Diagnostic and Statistical Manual of Mental Disorders* (DSM-5). These newer criteria have been criticized primarily because of the shifted focus on treating clients' distress to a symptom, whether arising from a physical cause or not. Since 2013, there has been much debate on the usefulness of the changes in diagnostic criteria for somatic symptom and related disorders. Refer to the DSM-5 for full diagnostic criteria.

More recently, there have been calls to reclassify nonspecified somatic symptoms as functional somatic disorders (Burton et al., 2020). Functional somatic disorders would include disorders such as fibromyalgia and irritable bowel syndrome. The call to reclassify somatic symptom disorders reflect the ongoing challenges clinicians have in diagnosing somatic symptom disorders and clients acceptance of such diagnoses.

There are fears that clinicians might inappropriately mislabel people with mental illness by failing to clearly distinguish mental illness from normal variants in human expression, or missing legitimate diagnoses altogether. A case report, for instance, describes anterior cutaneous nerve entrapment syndrome (ACNES) being misdiagnosed as a somatic symptom disorder. The client subsequently endured many months of chronic pain and developed depressive symptoms. After months of inappropriate psychotherapy for a misdiagnosed somatic symptom disorder, the client underwent surgery to remove the source of the painful stimuli. The symptoms (including depression) subsequently disappeared (Arts et al., 2016; Longstreth, 2015). Of note, up to 8% of people referred for specialist evaluation of a medically unexplained symptom did have previously overlooked physical causes to explain the symptoms (Henningsen, 2018).

This chapter presents the nursing care of clients experiencing somatic symptoms and related disorders. Somatization is explained in detail because it is the core symptom of all somatic symptom and related disorders.

KEY CONCEPT

Somatization is the term used when unexplained physical symptoms are present that are related to psychological distress.

▌ Somatization

Anyone who feels the pain of a sore throat or the ache of influenza has a somatic symptom (from *soma*, meaning body). **Somatization**, however, occurs when a person has disturbed ways of feeling, thinking, and behaving when experiencing a distressing somatic symptom. With the current understanding of somatization, the focus is on how an individual reacts to a somatic symptom rather than focusing solely on the lack of an explanatory medical diagnosis. This contemporary understanding is intended to produce the following: (a) fewer inappropriate mental illness diagnoses in people coping well with unexplained somatic symptoms and (b) increased diagnosis and treatment of somatic symptom and related disorders among those responding abnormally to a medically explained somatic symptom.

With somatization, individuals typically develop a preoccupation, amplify, and seek medical care for the somatic symptoms. People with somatization disorders often view their personal problems in physical rather than psychosocial terms. For example, a person quits her job because she is chronically tired instead of recognizing that she is emotionally distressed from a coworker's constant harassment.

▌ Somatic Symptom Disorder

Somatic symptom disorder is a condition characterized by emotional distress and a disruption of daily living caused by one or more physical symptoms. Somatic symptom disorder may lead to a disproportionate focus on bothersome symptoms, cause anxiety, and interfere with work, school, and activities of daily life. Recurrent visits to the emergency department, extensive diagnostic investigations, repeated hospitalizations, and multiple specialist consultations are common (Henningsen, 2018).

Clinical Course

In somatic symptom disorder, clients have one or more clinically significant somatic concerns that may involve several body systems. Physical symptoms in somatic symptom disorder occur in all body systems, such as gastrointestinal (nausea, vomiting, diarrhoea), neurologic (headache, backache), or musculoskeletal (aching legs). The physical symptom, which may be present all the time or may come and go, typically lasts 6 months or longer. These individuals perceive themselves as being "sicker than sick" and report all aspects of their health as poor. They often cannot work or take part in routine activities of daily living. Since no medical explanation of the symptom can be identified, these individuals often become frustrated with primary healthcare providers. Consequently, they seek opinions from many healthcare providers until they find one who will give them new medication, hospitalize them, or perform surgery. People with somatic symptom disorder sometimes cause frustration among healthcare providers. Nurses need to recognize their own feelings toward such clients and deal with these feelings constructively. This may include discussing their feelings with the colleague who is their mentor or clinical supervisor.

Because a psychiatric diagnosis of somatic symptom disorder is made only after numerous unexplained physical problems, psychiatric and mental health nurses do not usually care for these individuals early in the disorder; rather, these clients are more likely to have been encountered initially by nurses in primary care and medical–surgical settings. This is one of the reasons for nurses in all practice areas to have some foundational knowledge in mental health and psychiatry.

Diagnostic Criteria

The diagnosis is made when there is an *abnormal* response to a somatic symptom. It is important to remember that not all people experiencing an "unexplained symptom" have a somatic symptom disorder. Like many other disorders, a diagnosis may only be considered if the symptom is found to be interfering with the client's quality of life, social interactions, or other areas of functioning (American Psychiatric Association, 2013). For the diagnostic criteria for somatic symptom disorders, see the DSM-5.

The Somatic Symptom Disorder–B Criteria Scale (SSD-12) is the first tool developed to assess the psychological features after the 2013 DSM-5 revisions (Toussaint et al., 2016, 2017a). The SSD-12 is a reliable and valid self-report measure used in diagnosing somatic symptom disorders and has been tested in different populations and languages (Hüsing et al., 2018; Kop et al., 2019; Li et al., 2020; Toussaint et al., 2017b). The Patient Health Questionnaire 15 (PHQ-15) and the shortened Somatic Symptom Scale-8 (SSS-8) are valid and reliable tools to measure somatic symptom disease burden (Gierk et al., 2015) and can be used with the SSD-12 when screening for somatic symptom disorder (Toussaint et al., 2019).

Somatic Symptom Disorder in Special Populations

Evidence suggests that this disorder occurs in all populations and cultures. However, the type and frequency of somatic symptoms may differ across cultures.

Children

Although many children experience unexplained symptoms, somatic symptom disorder is not usually diagnosed until adolescence. Although some degree of somatization may be a normal element of childhood development and coping, early detection and treatment may impact longer-term outcomes by decreasing functional disability and healthcare utilization later in life (Saunders et al., 2020). Children at increased risk for somatic symptom disorder use fewer and less effective coping strategies. Further, children who are insecure, who internalize their emotions, or who tend toward perfectionism experience somatic symptom disorder more frequently (Malas et al., 2017).

In children, the protective instincts of the parent may falsely attribute ineffective drug therapy and inability to find a pathologic cause for the symptom to disease severity. This may introduce distrust between client and healthcare provider and further distance the child from receiving proper care. Clinicians must not delay diagnosing somatic symptom disorder in children (Morabito et al., 2020). Pain symptoms, particularly widespread pain in children and teens without a physical cause, is associated with depression, abuse and neglect, family psychiatric history, parental substance use disorder, trauma, and stress-related disorders (Ibeziako et al., 2021; LaVigne et al., 2020). Further, fewer than 10% of paediatric clients have normal school attendance. A potential indicator for somatic symptom disorder severity may be proportional to number of days missed at school (Vassilopoulos et al., 2020).

About 6% of hospitalized children have somatic symptom disorder, and healthcare costs are increased due to increased long hospital stays, multiple specialist involvement, and expensive diagnostic tests (Kullgren et al., 2020). Few of these clients receive mental healthcare

hospitalization (Saunders et al., 2020). The development of multidisciplinary somatization care pathways may yield healthcare savings and increase health outcomes for children and adolescents with somatic symptom disorder (Kullgren et al., 2020; Morabito et al., 2020).

Older Adults

Somatic symptom disorder occurs in the older adult but less prevalently than in other age groups. This may in part be related to increased prevalence of symptoms more easily attributable to other chronic health issues. For the same reasons, traditional somatization questionnaires may not be effective tools to reliably identify somatic symptom disorder in this population (van Driel et al., 2018). However, somatization may correlate with disease severity of illnesses such as Parkinson disease. This is relevant because interventions targeting people with Parkinson disease and somatic symptom disorder may improve coping with motor and nonmotor symptoms and quality of life (Polo-Morales et al., 2020). Regardless, new onset of somatic symptoms in later life warrants a thorough investigation for hidden medical or psychiatric disorders. In the older adult, somatic symptoms can represent many things, such as depression, grief or bereavement, and difficulty coping with symptoms of chronic diseases.

Epidemiology

Although a new definition for somatic symptom disorder was introduced in 2013 by the American Psychiatric Association, the definition remains controversial. Unexplained symptoms are often labelled differently in various medical specialties. For example, "functional abdominal pain" is used in gastroenterology and "pelvic pain syndrome" is used in urology and gynaecology. Terms such as "functional somatic symptoms" and "bodily distress syndrome" are sometimes seen as less associated with mental illness and less prone to stigmatization (Henningsen, 2018). As a result, it is very difficult to measure the true prevalence of somatic symptom disorder in the general population.

However, it is generally believed that somatic symptom disorder occurs in 5% to 7% of individuals younger than 65 years compared with older adults (1.5% to 13%) (Henningsen, 2018; Hilderink et al., 2013). This difference may reflect a biased approach to attribute somatic complaints by older clients to mere aging.

Gender, Ethnic, and Cultural Differences

It was initially believed that females experienced somatic symptom disorder more frequently than did males; however, Karkhanis and Winsler (2016) demonstrated no significant gender differences. There is no research using the contemporary definition of somatic symptom disorder describing differences between people of different genders.

Norms, values, perceptions, and expectations about illness and wellness are culturally based. In cultures in which great stigma toward mental illness exists, the expression of psychological distress can occur through physical symptoms. Cultural differences also influence how nurses recognize and manage somatization. Despite cultural and ethnic differences, the comorbidity of depression and somatic symptoms is consistent around the world (American Psychiatric Association, 2013). In many areas, however, sets of somatic symptoms hold cultural meaning to describe feelings of distress.

People who are refugees, however, do exhibit more somatic symptoms than the general population (Jongedijk et al., 2020). It is believed that this increase in somatic symptoms among refugee populations is related to lifetime trauma and worsened by forced migration (Tarsitani et al., 2020). Nurses should look for subtle cues of somatization and pay careful attention to how clients describe their symptoms. For instance, stomach or head pain may be idioms referring to stress (Lanzara et al., 2019). Given the global rise in refugees fleeing war, terrorism, and climate crises around the world, identifying and addressing somatic symptoms among the refugee population is increasingly relevant.

Comorbidity

Somatic symptom disorder frequently coexists with other psychiatric disorders, most commonly depression and anxiety. Somatic symptom disorder may also become more pronounced when coupled with existing impairment from other medical conditions. Somatic symptom disorder can be manifested as psychological distress in people who experience chronic diseases (e.g., inflammatory bowel disease) and can influence quality of life (Regev et al., 2021).

A disproportionately high number of people who eventually receive diagnoses of somatic symptom disorder have been treated for irritable bowel syndrome, polycystic ovary disease, fibromyalgia, and other functional somatic syndromes. Many of these clients have had prior investigations or treatments associated with a functional somatic syndrome. For instance, women with chronic pelvic pain have undergone hysterectomies, whereas those with irritable bowel syndrome have experienced many invasive diagnostic tests such as endoscopy or colonoscopy or both.

Aetiology

The cause of somatic symptom disorder is unknown. The following are theories regarding the development of the disorder.

Biologic Theories

Neuropathologic Theory

The neuropathology of somatic symptom disorder is unknown. Evidence suggests decreased activity in certain brain areas, such as the caudate nuclei, left putamen, and right precentral gyrus (Garcia-Campayo et al., 2001; Hakala et al., 2002). These findings indicate that hypometabolism may be associated with somatization. More recently, autopsy studies of people with semantic dementia (who are prone to somatic symptom disorder) found increased prevalence of frontotemporal degeneration (Gan et al., 2016). This finding supports a theory that somatic symptom disorder may be a perceptual disorder of how one interprets and constructs meaning of a symptom within their brain.

Genetic

Although somatization disorder has been shown to run in families, the exact transmission mechanism is unclear. Because many people with somatization disorder live in chaotic families, environmental influence could explain the high prevalence in first-degree relatives.

There is research that suggests that genetic variability within the serotoninergic and hypothalamic–pituitary–adrenal axis (HPA) may contribute to somatization (Holliday et al., 2010). This has led to early drug trials using serotonergic agents to evaluate for clinical effect in treating somatic symptom disorders. While these agents may improve symptoms of depressive and anxiety disorders, they have not demonstrated significant efficacy in reducing somatic disorder symptoms (Holster et al., 2017).

Biochemical Changes

Research thus far is insufficient to identify specific biochemical changes that would lead to somatization disorder. However, because these clients experience other psychiatric symptoms, such as depression or panic, clearly many neurobiologic changes occur. The HPA axis is currently being studied for potential links between proinflammatory cytokines and somatization (Iob et al., 2019; Miyauchi et al., 2019). This research is important to determine if antidepressant medications might be useful in the management of somatic symptom disorder. A clearer link between HPA axis and expression of somatic symptoms seems to be emerging.

Psychological Theories

Somatization has been explained as a form of social or emotional communication, meaning the bodily symptoms express an emotion that cannot be verbalized. The adolescent who experiences severe abdominal pain when witnessing their parents fighting or the spouse who receives nurturing from their significant other only when they have back pain are two examples of how the body expresses emotions. From this perspective, somatization may be a way of maintaining relationships. With time, physical symptoms develop automatically in response to perceived threats. Finally, somatic symptom disorder develops when somatizing begins to interfere with daily life or pervades thought. Research is indicating that lack of social support, perceived violence within the community, and external stressors can contribute to somatization (Hart et al., 2012; Karkhanis & Winsler, 2016).

Social Theories

While somatic symptom disorder occurs everywhere, the symptoms may vary between cultures. The stigmatization of mental illness, particularly when this becomes the social norm, discourages emotional expression associated with depression, anxiety, and even grief and bereavement. The expression of physical symptoms, in this context, seems to be more socially acceptable. Although there is worldwide progress in recognizing and supporting people with mental illness, stigmatization persists across the globe.

Previously, somatization was viewed as a primary product of Western culture and that nonwestern cultures did not adequately make a distinction between mind and body. Although this may be true in some contexts, this belief is misleading and produces unnecessary cultural stereotypes. In fact, the diversity of opinions and tendency toward stigmatization vary considerably within each culture and population of people across the globe.

In situations where an individual fears stigmatization of mental illness, euphemisms and somatic symptoms often become prevalent. For example, complaints of headache, stomach pain, back pain, or "nerve" issues may be reported rather than using terms like sadness or hopelessness associated with major depression.

Risk Factors

Somatic symptom disorder tends to "run in families," and children of mothers with multiple unexplained somatic complaints are themselves more likely to have somatic problems. Substance use and depressive and anxiety disorders seem to be risk factors, and women with somatic symptom disorder appear more likely to have been sexually abused as children than do those with other psychiatric conditions, such as mood disorders (Steine et al., 2017). Individuals with depression are especially likely to experience somatization (Aksu, 2020).

Interdisciplinary Treatment

The care of clients with somatic symptom disorder involves three approaches:

- Providing long-term general management of the chronic condition
- Conservatively treating symptoms of comorbid psychiatric and physical problems
- Providing care in special settings, including group treatment

The cornerstone of management is trust. Ideally, the client sees only one healthcare provider at regularly

scheduled visits. During each primary care visit, the provider should conduct a partial physical examination of the organ system in which the client has complaints. Physical symptoms are to be treated conservatively using the least intrusive approach. In the mental health setting, the use of cognitive–behaviour therapy (CBT; see Chapter 14) has produced significant clinical benefits beyond other current treatment methods such as antidepressants or supportive psychotherapy (Cooper et al., 2017). In a review of 31 clinical trials, clients treated with CBT showed more improvement than control subjects did in 71% of the studies. Benefits were observed irrespective of the amelioration of psychological distress (Kroenke & Swindle, 2000). Increasingly, exposure-based CBT via the internet has demonstrated effect in treating somatic symptom disorders (Hedman et al., 2016). Acceptance commitment therapy may be useful in somatization among people with a history of trauma (Kroska et al., 2018).

Nursing Management: Human Response to Disorder

Somatization is the primary response to this disorder. The defining characteristics, depicted in the bio/psycho/social/spiritual model (Fig. 24.1), are so well integrated that separating the psychological and social dimensions is difficult. The most common characteristics include the following:

- Reporting the same symptoms repeatedly
- Receiving support from the environment that otherwise might not be forthcoming (e.g., gaining a spouse's attention because of severe back pain)
- Expressing concern about the physical problems inconsistent with the severity of the illness

Biologic Domain

During the assessment interview, allow enough time for the client to explain all medical problems; a hurried assessment interview blocks communication.

Assessment

Previous medical treatment may have been ineffective because it did not address the underlying psychiatric disorder. However, nurses typically see these clients for coexistent problems related to the psychiatric disorder, such as depression, rather than for the somatic symptom disorder itself. While taking the client's history, the nurse will discover that the individual has had medical problems or multiple surgeries and realize that somatic symptom disorder is a strong possibility. If the client has not already received a diagnosis of somatic symptom disorder, the nurse should screen for it by determining the presence of the most commonly reported

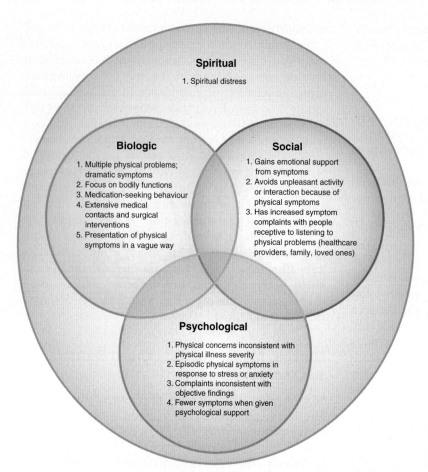

Spiritual

1. Spiritual distress

Biologic

1. Multiple physical problems; dramatic symptoms
2. Focus on bodily functions
3. Medication-seeking behaviour
4. Extensive medical contacts and surgical interventions
5. Presentation of physical symptoms in a vague way

Social

1. Gains emotional support from symptoms
2. Avoids unpleasant activity or interaction because of physical symptoms
3. Has increased symptom complaints with people receptive to listening to physical problems (healthcare providers, family, loved ones)

Psychological

1. Physical concerns inconsistent with physical illness severity
2. Episodic physical symptoms in response to stress or anxiety
3. Complaints inconsistent with objective findings
4. Fewer symptoms when given psychological support

Figure 24.1 Bio/psycho/social/spiritual characteristics of clients with somatic symptom disorder.

problems associated with this disorder, which include dysmenorrhoea, lump in throat, vomiting, shortness of breath, burning in sex organs, painful extremities, and amnesia. If the client has these symptoms, they should be seen by a mental health provider qualified to make the diagnosis.

Review of Systems

Although these clients' symptoms have usually received considerable attention from the medical community, a careful review of systems is important to ensure that nothing is overlooked. Even as the nurse continues to see the client for mental health reasons, an ongoing awareness of biologic symptoms is important, particularly because these symptoms are deemphasized in the overall management.

Pain is the most common problem in people with this disorder. Because it is usually related to symptoms of all the major body systems, it is unlikely that a somatic intervention such as an analgesic will be effective on a long-term basis. The nurse must remember that although there is potentially no medical explanation for the pain, the client's pain is real and has serious psychosocial implications. A careful assessment should include the following questions:

- What is the pain like?
- What is the extent of the pain?
- When is the pain at its best? Worst?
- What has worked in the past to relieve the pain?

Physical Functioning

The actual physical functioning of these individuals is often limited. They usually have problems with sleep, fatigue, activity, and sexual functioning. Assessment of these areas will generate data to be used in establishing nursing care foci. The amount and quality of sleep are important, as are the times when the individual sleeps. For example, an individual may sleep a total of 6 h each diurnal cycle, but only from 2 to 6 a.m., plus a 2-h afternoon nap.

Fatigue is a constant problem, and a variety of physical problems, such as pain, interferes with normal activity. These clients report overwhelming lack of energy, which makes maintaining usual routines or accomplishing daily tasks difficult. Fatigue is accompanied by the inability to concentrate on simple functions, leading to decreased performance and disinterest in social activities. Clients tend to be apathetic and often have little energy (see Clinical Vignette).

CLINICAL VIGNETTE ✚

SOMATIC SYMPTOM DISORDER AND STRESS

Ms. J, age 42 years, has been coming to the mental health clinic for 2 years for her "nerves." She has only seen her primary healthcare provider for prescription medication. The care provider referred her to the nurse's new "Stress Management Group" because she is experiencing side effects of all the medications that have been tried. The psychiatrist has diagnosed somatic symptom disorder and wants her to learn to manage her "nerves" without medication.

At the first meeting with the nurse, Ms. J was preoccupied with chest pain and bloating that had been ongoing for the past 6 months. Her chest pain is constant and sharp at times. The pain does not prevent her from going to her job but does interfere with meal preparation at night for her family and her ability to have sexual intercourse. She has numerous other physical problems, including allergies to certain perfumes, dysmenorrhoea, ovarian polycystic disease, chronic urinary tract infections, and rashes. She is constantly fatigued and has frequent leg cramps. She states that she is too tired to prepare dinner for her family. On days off from work, she takes a nap in the afternoon, sleeping until evening. She is unable to fall asleep at night.

She believes that she will soon have to have her gallbladder removed because of occasional referred pain to her back and nausea that occurs several hours after eating. She is not enthusiastic about a stress management group and does not believe that it will help her, but she has agreed to consider it, while insisting that the psychiatrist continue prescribing her diazepam (Valium).

What Do You Think?

- How would you prioritize Ms. J's physical symptoms?
- What strategies would you use in the group to help Ms. J explore the roots of her stress and fatigue?

Female clients with this disorder usually have had multiple gynaecologic problems. The reason is not known, but symptoms of dysmenorrhoea, painful intercourse, and pain in the sex organs suggest involvement of the hypothalamic–pituitary–gonadal axis. Physiologic indicators, such as those produced by laboratory tests, are not available. However, a careful assessment of the client's menstrual history, gynaecologic problems, and sexual functioning is important. The physical manifestations of somatic symptom disorder often lead to altered sexual behaviour.

Pharmacologic Assessment

A psychopharmacologic assessment of these clients is challenging. Clients with somatic symptom disorder frequently see many different healthcare providers, perhaps seeing seven or eight different providers within a year. Because they often receive prescriptions from each provider, they are usually taking a large number of medications. They tend to protect their sources and may not truthfully identify the actual number of medications they are ingesting. A thorough pharmacologic best possible medication history (BPMH) and assessment of all current home medications, herbal supplements, over-the-counter vitamins, and medications is needed not only because of the number of medications but also because these individuals frequently may have multiple drug–drug interactions and unusual side effects. Moreover, because of their somatic sensitivity, they often report side effects to many medications.

Clients with somatic symptom disorder spend much of their life trying to find out what is wrong with them. When one provider after another finds little or no explanation for their symptoms, the client may become anxious. To alleviate their anxiety, they either self-medicate with over-the-counter medications and substances of abuse (e.g., alcohol, marijuana) or find a provider who prescribes anxiolytics or other narcotics. Because the anxiety of their disorder cannot be treated within a few weeks with an anxiolytic agent, they may become dependent on medication that should not have been prescribed in the first place.

Although anxiolytics have a place in therapeutics, most are addictive and therefore not recommended for long-term use. They also tend to complicate the treatment of somatic symptom disorders. Unfortunately, by the time a client with a somatic symptom disorder sees a mental health provider, they have often already begun taking one or more benzodiazepine agents. Often, the reason a client agrees to see a mental health provider is that the primary health provider has refused to continue prescribing an anxiolytic until the client has undergone psychiatric evaluation.

Nursing Care Focus for the Biologic Domain

Because somatic symptom disorder is a chronic illness, a client could experience any number of concerns requiring a nursing care focus at some point in their life. At least one likely will be related to the individual's physical state. Fatigue, pain, and disturbed sleep patterns are usually supported by the assessment data. The challenge in devising outcomes for these problems is to avoid focusing on the biologic aspects and instead help the client overcome the fatigue, pain, or sleep problem through bio/psycho/social/spiritual approaches.

Nursing Care Focus for the Biologic Domain

Nursing care focus of the biologic dimension becomes especially important because medical treatment must be conservative, and aggressive pharmacologic treatment must be avoided. Each time a nurse sees the client, time spent on the physical complaints should be limited. The goal is to help the person better understand the meaning behind the physical manifestations of the somatic symptom disorder. Several biologic interventions, including pain management, activity enhancement, nutrition regulation, relaxation, and pharmacologic interventions, may also be useful in caring for clients with somatic symptom disorder.

Pain Management

Pain is a primary issue, but a single approach to its management rarely works. After a careful pain assessment, the nurse should encourage nonpharmacologic management strategies. If gastrointestinal pain is frequent, for example, eating and bowel habits should be explored and modified where possible. For back pain, exercises and consultation from a physical therapist may be useful. While headaches are particularly challenging, self-monitoring and tracking, engage the client in the therapeutic process and may help to identify psychosocial triggers.

Activity Enhancement

Helping the client establish a daily activity routine, especially during times when the client does not work, may alleviate some of the difficulty with sleeping. Encouraging good sleep hygiene with established patterns and times for sleeping and waking is especially helpful. Although clients typically use various reasons to avoid activity, regular exercise is important to improve the overall physical state. The nurse needs to work with the client to foster adequate movement for healthier living.

Nutrition Regulation

Clients with somatic symptom disorder often have gastrointestinal problems including special nutritional needs. The nurse should discuss with the client the nutritional value of foods. Because these individuals often take medications that lead to weight gain, weight control strategies may be discussed (see Chapter 12). Clients who are overweight should be given suggestions for healthy, low-calorie foods. To increase their awareness of food choices, clients should be taught about balancing dietary intake with activity levels.

Relaxation

Clients taking anxiolytic medication for stress reduction can also be taught relaxation techniques. The challenge is to help a client develop strategies for routine practice and evaluation of effect. The nurse may consider a variety of techniques, including simple relaxation techniques, distraction, and guided imagery (see Chapter 12).

Psychopharmacologic Interventions

No particular medication is recommended for somatic symptom disorder. However, psychiatric symptoms of comorbid disorders, such as depression and anxiety, may be treated pharmacologically as appropriate. Clients with this disorder often suffer from depression and anxiety. While depressed mood itself is not an indication to initiate antidepressant treatment, when a depressive disorder is present, aggressive psychopharmacologic management is indicated. A wide variety of drugs are available, including the selective serotonin reuptake inhibitors (SSRIs), tricyclic antidepressants (TCAs), and monoamine oxidase inhibitors (MAOIs; see Chapter 13). Clients with somatic symptom disorder usually take several different antidepressants throughout the course of the disorder. Evidence should be sought that the depressive symptoms are cleared before discontinuing use of the medication.

Amitriptyline is one of the TCAs found effective in treating not just depression (see Chapter 13) but also the chronic pain and headaches common in people with somatic symptom disorder. Increasingly, drugs such as tramadol (an analgesic agent) are being used to treat comorbid pain syndromes. Both drugs have an effect on serotonin, and caution is required to prevent the development of serotonin syndrome.

Anxiety associated with a somatic symptom disorder is more difficult than is depression to treat pharmacologically. Nonpharmacologic approaches such as biofeedback or relaxation are preferred. Benzodiazepines should be avoided because of the high potential for abuse and physiologic dependence associated with these medications. Buspirone (BuSpar), a nonbenzodiazepine, does not lead to tolerance or withdrawal and, although not as potent as benzodiazepines, may be useful for relief of anxiety. Other agents, such as the SSRIs, are effective in the management of generalized anxiety and panic disorders and may be effective in the management of anxiety associated with somatic symptom disorder.

The film *Medicating Normal* has won multiple awards for its in-depth look at how over-prescribing medication is impacting society. The premise focuses on the medicalization of normal expressions or normal variants of human expression. The result of doing so has caused a belief in society that any uncomfortable emotion of sensation should be treated with a pharmacologic substance. There is an overlap here with the use of prescription or over-the-counter drugs for the treatment of somatic symptom disorder. Many medications, some which cause significant changes to a person's life, should not be used without a clear pathoanatomic diagnosis.

Monitoring Medications, Interactions, and Side Effects

In somatic symptom disorder, clients are usually treated in the community, where they often use multiple over-the-counter and prescription medications. Once the nurse completes a BPMH of all current home medicinal substances, including self-prescribed and over-the-counter remedies, vitamins and herbal supplements, etc., the information should be documented and reported to the rest of the interdisciplinary team. The nurse questions and listens carefully to determine the full scope of medications, how they are used, and effects that the client attributes to each substance. Using the BPMH, an evaluation of possible drug–drug interactions needs to be completed by the prescriber through a medication reconciliation process. The nurse needs to work with the client, pharmacist, nurse practitioner, and physician to support the client in maintaining a safe and effective pharmacotherapeutic regimen. Individuals with somatic symptom disorder often have idiosyncratic reactions to their medications. Side effects should be assessed, but the client should be encouraged to compare the benefits of the medication with any problems related to side effects.

In working with clients with somatization disorder, the nurse must always monitor for drug–drug interactions. Medications clients are taking for physical problems could interact with psychiatric medications. Clients may be taking alternative medicines, such as herbal supplements (e.g., Valerian for management of anxiety), and these also need to be evaluated for possible adverse interactions. The client should be encouraged to use the same pharmacy to fill all prescriptions so that possible reactions can be checked.

Psychological Domain

The cognitive functioning of individuals with somatic symptom disorder is usually within normal limits. However, these individuals seem preoccupied with personal illnesses and often keep a record of symptoms and illnesses. They constantly focus on bodily functions, and "living with diseases" truly becomes a way of life.

Individuals with somatic symptom disorder usually have intense emotional reactions to life stressors. They often have a series of personal crises beginning at an early age. Typically, a new symptom or medical problem develops during times of emotional stress. It is critical that the physical assessment data be linked to psychological and social events. A history of major psychological events should be compared with the chronology of physical problems. Special attention should be paid to any history of sexual abuse or trauma in the client's younger years. Early sexual abuse also may interfere with self-esteem, belonging, and sexual fulfillment in adulthood.

Response to physical symptoms is often exaggerated, such as interpreting a simple cold as pneumonia or a brief chest pain as a heart attack. Family members may not believe the physical symptoms are real, instead viewing them as attention-seeking behaviour, given that the symptoms often do improve when the client receives attention. For example, a person who has been in bed for 3 weeks with severe back pain may suddenly feel much better once their children visit them—paying them attention.

Assessment

While gathering information from the biologic domain, the nurse concurrently assesses mental status in the psychological domain. Components include appearance, psychomotor behaviour, mood, affect, perception, thought content and process, sensorium, insight, and judgment (see Chapter 11).

Nursing Care Focus for the Psychological Domain

Nursing care focus related to the psychological domain and typical of people with somatic symptom disorder includes anxiety, compromised interpersonal relationships, therapeutic self-care management, coping, and sexual intimacy.

Interventions for the Psychological Domain

The choice of psychological intervention depends on the specific problem the client is experiencing. Cognitive–

BOX 24.1 THERAPEUTIC DIALOGUE

Establishing a Relationship

Ineffective Approach

Nurse: Good morning, CM.
Client: I'm in so much pain. Take that breakfast away.
Nurse: You don't want your breakfast?
Client: Can't you see? I hurt! When I hurt, I can't eat!
Nurse: If you don't eat now, you probably won't be able to have anything until lunch.
Client: Who cares. I have no intention of being here at lunchtime. I don't belong here.
Nurse: CM, I don't think that your physician would have admitted you unless there is a problem. I would like to talk to you about why you are here.
Client: Nurse, I'm just here. It's none of your business.
Nurse: Oh.
Client: Please leave me alone.
Nurse: Sure, I will see you later.

Effective Approach

Nurse: Good morning, CM
Client: I'm in so much pain. Take that breakfast away.
Nurse: (Silently removes the tray, pulls up a chair, and sits down.)
Client: My back hurts.
Nurse: Oh, when did the back pain start?
Client: Last night. It's this bed. I couldn't get comfortable.

Nurse: These beds can be pretty uncomfortable.
Client: My back pain is shooting down my leg.
Nurse: Does anything help it?
Client: Sometimes if I straighten out my leg it helps.
Nurse: Can I help you straighten out your leg?
Client: Oh, it's OK. The pain is going away. What did you say your name is?
Nurse: I'm Susan Miller, your nurse while you are here.
Client: I won't be here long. I don't belong in a psychiatric unit.
Nurse: While you are here, I would like to spend time with you.
Client: OK, but you understand I do not have any psychiatric problems.
Nurse: We can talk about whatever you want. But, since you want to get out of here, we might want to focus on what it will take to get you ready for discharge.

CRITICAL THINKING CHALLENGE

- What communication mistakes did the nurse in the first scenario make?
- What communication strategies helped the client feel comfortable with the nurse in the second scenario? How is the second scenario different from the first?

---

behavioural therapy, which helps the client identify, connect, and change feelings, thoughts, and behaviour, is the most effective treatment for somatic symptom disorder (Cooper et al., 2017). Supportive psychotherapy, counselling, and client education are also useful strategies. The most important and ongoing intervention is the development and maintenance of a therapeutic relationship.

Developing a Therapeutic Relationship

The most difficult yet crucial aspect of nursing care is developing a sound, person-centred, positive, and supportive nurse–client relationship. Without it, the nurse is just one more provider who fails to meet the client's needs and expectations. Developing this relationship requires time and patience. Therapeutic communication techniques are used to help the client explore underlying psychosocial and spiritual problems related to the physical manifestations of the disorder (Box 24.1).

During periods when symptoms of other psychiatric disorders surface, additional therapeutic interventions may be needed (see Chapter 7). For example, the onset of depression requires additional supportive or cognitive approaches.

Counselling

Counselling, with a focus on problem-solving, is needed from time to time. Clients with somatic symptom disorder frequently have chaotic lives and need support through a multitude of crises. Although they sometimes appear confident and self-assured, their constant complaints may irritate others. The consequences of their impaired social interactions must be examined within a counselling framework. The nurse helps the client identify stressors, explore related thoughts and feelings, and develop positive coping responses.

Patient Education: Health Teaching

Health teaching is useful throughout the nurse–patient relationship. Clients who experience somatic symptom disorder have many questions about illnesses, symptoms, and treatments. Emphasis should be upon positive healthcare practices rather than the effects of serious illness. Because of problems in managing medications and treatment, the therapeutic regimen needs constant monitoring; this provides ample opportunity for teaching. One area that might require special health teaching is impaired sexuality. Because clients with this diagnosis often have a history

BOX 24.2 Psychoeducation Checklist: Somatic Symptom Disorder

When caring for the client with somatic symptom disorder, be sure to include the following topic areas in the teaching plan:

✓ Psychopharmacologic agents if prescribed, including drug, action, dosage, frequency, and possible adverse effects
✓ Nonpharmacologic approaches to pain relief
✓ Exercise
✓ Nutrition
✓ Social interaction
✓ Appropriate health maintenance practices
✓ Problem-solving
✓ Relaxation and anxiety-reduction techniques
✓ Sexual functioning

of physical problems related to sexual activity (frequently pain), clients may have difficulty carrying out normal sexual activity, such as masturbation, intercourse, or reaching orgasm. Basic teaching about sexual function is often needed. Refer to Box 24.2 for a psychoeducation checklist.

Social Domain

People with somatic symptom disorder spend excessive time seeking medical care and attending to their multiple illnesses. Because they believe themselves to be very sick, they also often believe that they are disabled and cannot work; their unemployment rate is therefore high. Although these individuals are rarely satisfied with healthcare providers who can find no basis for a medical diagnosis, their social network may consist more of these providers than of their peers. Identifying a support network requires sorting out healthcare providers from their family and friends.

Assessment

It is important to identify both beneficial and harmful relationships within the client's family. Family members may become weary of the client's constant physical complaints. In assessing relations, however, it is important that other members with social problems and psychiatric disorders are identified, as the individual suffering from somatic symptom disorder may live in a chaotic family with multiple challenges.

Symptoms of somatic symptom disorder may disrupt the family's social life. A change in routine or a major life event often precipitates a symptom's appearance. For example, a client planning a vacation with the family may decide at the last minute that they cannot go because their back pain has returned, and they will be unable to sit in the car. Such family disruptions are common.

Nursing Care Focus in the Social Domain

Clients with somatic symptom disorder typically experience social isolation, strained and chaotic family relationships, and impaired coping within their families and communities; family members may experience caregiver role strain.

Interventions for the Social Domain

Clients with somatic symptom disorders may be isolated from family and community. Strengthening relationships and encouraging social activity often become the focus of nursing care. The nurse should help clients identify individuals with whom contact is desired, encourage them to reinitiate a relationship, and ask for a commitment to contact them. The nurse should counsel clients about talking too much about their symptoms with these individuals and emphasize that medical information should be shared with the nurse.

Group Interventions

Although individuals with somatic symptom disorder may not be good candidates for insight oriented group psychotherapy, they do benefit from cognitive–behavioural groups that focus on developing coping skills for everyday life (Hedman et al., 2016). Participation in gender-specific groups that use gender theories, such as queer theory or feminism, should be encouraged; this may help to strengthen their assertiveness skills and improve self-esteem (Fig. 24.2).

When leading a group that has members with somatic symptom disorder, redirection can keep the group from giving too much attention to a person's illness. However, persons experiencing this disorder need reassurance and support while in a group. The client may report feeling as though they do not fit in with or belong in the group; in reality, they are likely feeling insecure and threatened in the situation. The group leader needs to show patience and understanding to engage the individual effectively in meaningful group interaction (refer to Chapter 15).

Family Interventions

The results of a family assessment often reveal a need for education about the disorder, helpful strategies for dealing with the client's symptoms, and, usually, help in developing more effective communication and problem-solving strategies. Many people with somatic symptom disorder have experienced a chaotic family life and often experienced physical and/or sexual abuse. The nurse must assess and offer interventions such as those identified using a thorough family assessment (see Chapter 16).

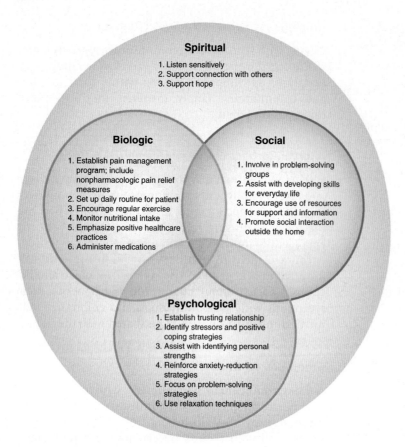

Spiritual
1. Listen sensitively
2. Support connection with others
3. Support hope

Biologic
1. Establish pain management program; include nonpharmacologic pain relief measures
2. Set up daily routine for patient
3. Encourage regular exercise
4. Monitor nutritional intake
5. Emphasize positive healthcare practices
6. Administer medications

Social
1. Involve in problem-solving groups
2. Assist with developing skills for everyday life
3. Encourage use of resources for support and information
4. Promote social interaction outside the home

Psychological
1. Establish trusting relationship
2. Identify stressors and positive coping strategies
3. Assist with identifying personal strengths
4. Reinforce anxiety-reduction strategies
5. Focus on problem-solving strategies
6. Use relaxation techniques

Figure 24.2 Bio/psycho/social/spiritual interventions for clients with somatic symptom disorder.

Spiritual Domain

The spiritual domain assesses how people with a somatic symptom disorder connect experiences, make meaning of their disorder, and find purpose in life. Somatic symptom disorder produces a continuous physical awareness of the body's pain or distress. Over time, clients may begin to resent their bodies, become bitter by living in a world of ongoing challenges, and experience conflict with their religious beliefs. A spiritual assessment provides important information needed to help clients regain spiritual health.

Assessment

To assess spiritual health, nurses enquire about topics such as meaning, ambiguity, and hope using open-ended questions such as *What is "being ill" like for you? What does "being ill" mean in your life?* Personal strengths are assessed with such questions as *What brings joy and peace to you? How has your illness changed the way you understand the world? Do you have spiritual beliefs that have been affected by your illness experience?* Questions to elicit information about connections with self, others, and a higher power may be phrased as *How are you right now? What sustains or heals your spirit? Who is significant to you?*

How do you feel connected to the world and events around you? Are there spiritual acts, such as prayer, that you find helpful?

Nursing Care Focus for the Spiritual Domain

Nursing care foci related to the spiritual domain and typical of people with somatic symptom disorder include addressing feelings of hopelessness and spiritual angst, and exploring opportunities for spiritual wellbeing.

Interventions for the Spiritual Domain

Individuals with somatic symptom disorders sometimes feel estranged from others. For those who belong to a religious group, this can include estrangement from their faith communities. Nurses intervene by creating a safe and caring environment to help the person explore deep questions related to connection, meaning, and purpose. Trust, rapport, and a mutual plan for care are developed using presence, empathy, and sensitivity. Based on the person's assessed needs, nurses may also facilitate religious practices, assist with life review or reminiscence therapy, or make a referral to spiritual care experts (Chida et al., 2016).

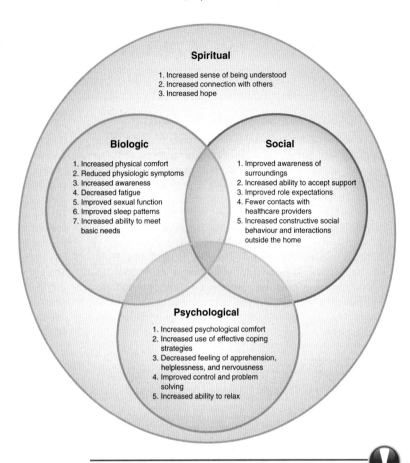

Figure 24.3 Bio/psycho/social/spiritual outcomes for clients with somatic symptom disorder.

Evaluation and Treatment Outcomes

The outcomes for clients with somatic symptom disorder must be realistic and formulated with the client. Because this is a lifelong disorder, small successes should be expected. Specific outcomes should be identified. Over time, there should be a gradual reduction in the number of healthcare providers the individual contacts and gradual improvement in the ability to cope with stresses (Fig. 24.3).

Continuum of Care

For individuals experiencing somatic symptom disorder, mental health services ranging from hospital-based care to health promotion may occur in various healthcare settings over the course of their lives.

Hospital-Based Care

Ideally, individuals with somatic symptom disorder will spend minimal time in the hospital. Such stays occur when the client's comorbid psychiatric disorders become symptomatic. To provide consistent care during hospitalization, the client should be the responsibility of one primary nurse who provides or oversees all the nursing care. The primary nurse must establish a relationship with the client (and family) and consult other nursing staff members about this disorder.

EMERGENCY CARE

The emergencies these individuals experience may be physical (e.g., chest pain, back pain, gastrointestinal symptoms) or stress responses related to a psychosocial crisis. Careful assessment must be used so as not to overlook the symptoms of acute and/or potentially fatal illness.

Community Treatment

Individuals with somatic symptom disorder can spend a lifetime in the healthcare system and still have little continuity of care. Switching from provider to provider is detrimental to their long-term care. Most clients are treated in the community. When they are hospitalized, it is usually for evaluation of physical problems. When their comorbid psychiatric disorders, such as depression, become symptomatic, these clients may require brief hospitalization (see Box 24.3).

Mental Health Promotion

Clients with somatic symptom disorder are encouraged to focus on staying healthy rather than on the symptoms of their illness. For these individuals, approaching the topic of health promotion usually has to be within the

BOX 24.3 NURSING CARE PLAN

The Client With Somatization Disorder

SC is a 48-year-old person making a weekly visit to their primary care nurse practitioner for unexplained multiple somatic problems. This week, the concern is recurring abdominal pain that fits no symptom pattern. Upon physical examination, no cause of the abdominal pain could be found. SC is requesting a refill of lorazepam (Ativan), which is the only medication that "relieves my pain." SC is also in the process of applying for disability income because of being completely disabled by neck and shoulder pain. The nurse practitioner and office staff avoid this client whenever possible. The nurse practitioner will not refill the prescription until SC is evaluated by the consulting mental health team that provides weekly evaluations and services.

Setting: Primary Care Office

Baseline Assessment: SC is a 48-year-old client who presents as frustrated and angry. The client resents being forced to see a psychiatric clinician for "the only medication that works to alleviate my pain." SC denies any psychiatric problems or emotional distress. SC's hair is in disarray because "its too much trouble to comb my hair." Cognitive aspects of mental status appear normal, but SC admits to being slightly depressed and takes the lorazepam for "nerves." SC says she has nothing to live for but denies any thoughts of suicide. The client is dependent on family for everything and feels very guilty about it. SC spends most of their waking hours going to various clinicians, searching the internet for alternative treatments, and taking combinations of medications and supplements. SC has no friends or nonfamily social contacts.

Associated Psychiatric Diagnosis and Other Conditions That May Be a Focus of Clinical Attention	Medications
R/O depression Somatic symptom disorder S/P gastric bypass S/P carpel tunnel release Chronic shoulder, neck pain, vertigo Social problems (father died 6 months ago, divorced 9 months) Economic problems (depends on social assistance) Occupational problems (potential disability)	Lorazepam (Ativan), 1 mg three times daily Ranitidine HCl (Zantac), 150 mg twice daily Simethicone 125 mg four times daily with meals Calcium carbonate, 1,000 mg daily Multiple vitamin, daily Zopiclone (Imovane), 7.5 mg at night as needed Ibuprofen, 600 mg every 6 h, as needed, for pain

Nursing Care Focus 1: Chronic Low Self-Esteem

Defining Characteristics	Related Factors
Self-negating verbalizations (long standing) Hesitant to try new things Expresses feelings of guilt Evaluates self as being unable to cope with events	Feeling unimportant to family Feeling rejected by ex-spouse Constant physical problems interfering with normal social activities

Outcomes

Initial	Long-term
Identify need to increase self-esteem.	Participate in individual or group therapy for self-esteem building.

NURSING CARE PLAN (*Continued*)

Interventions

Interventions	Rationale	Ongoing Assessment
Establish rapport with the client.	Individuals with low self-esteem feel vulnerable and may be reluctant to discuss true feelings.	Ask the client for their perceptions of care and the helping relationship.
Encourage the client to spend time dressing and grooming appropriately.	Confidence and self-esteem improve when a person looks well groomed.	Monitor responses.
Encourage the client to discuss various somatic problems, as well as psychological and interpersonal issues.	Clients with somatic symptom disorder need time to express their physical problems. It helps them feel valued. The best way to build a relationship is to acknowledge physical symptoms.	Monitor time that the client spends explaining physical symptoms.
Explore opportunities for SC to meet other people with similar, nonmedical interests.	Focusing SC on meeting others will improve the possibilities of increasing contacts.	Observe willingness to identify other interests besides physical problems.

Evaluation

Outcomes	Revised Outcomes	Interventions
SC admitted to having low self-esteem but was very reluctant to consider meeting new people.	Focus on building self-esteem.	Identify activities that will enhance self-esteem.

Nursing Care Focus 2: Problems With Therapeutic Self-Care Management

Defining Characteristics	Related Factors
Choices of daily living ineffective for meeting healthcare goal Verbalizes difficulty with prescribed regimens	Inappropriate use of benzodiazepine agents

Outcomes

Initial	Long-term
Openly discuss the use of medications.	Use nonpharmacologic means for stress reduction.

Continued on following page

NURSING CARE PLAN (Continued)

Interventions

Interventions	Rationale	Ongoing Assessment
Clarify the frequency and purpose of taking lorazepam.	Unsupervised polypharmacy is common.	Carefully track self-report of medication use; assess drug adherence and safety.
Educate the client about the effects of combining medications.	Education about combining medication is the beginning of helping the client become independent in medication management.	Observe the client's ability and willingness to consider potential adverse effects.
Explore ways to gradually reduce the number of medications, including other means of managing physical symptoms.	Help the client to identify appropriate ways and means to manage healthcare regimens.	Evaluate the client's ability to solve problems.

Evaluation

Outcomes	Revised Outcomes	Interventions
Client disclosed the use of medications but was unwilling to consider changing ineffective use of medication.	Identify next step if the nurse practitioner or physician does not refill prescription.	Discuss the possibility of not being able to obtain lorazepam. Refer the client to mental health clinic for further evaluation.

context of preventing further problems. Setting aside time for themselves and identifying activities that meet their psychological and spiritual needs, such as connecting with their faith group, are important in maintaining a healthy balance.

Other Somatic Symptom and Related Disorders

The following discussion summarizes other somatic symptom and related disorders and highlights the primary focus of nursing management.

Illness Anxiety Disorder

The exclusion of hypochondriasis from the *DSM-5* has brought about the emergence of illness anxiety as a new *DSM* disorder. The majority of individuals previously diagnosed with hypochondriasis seemingly fit well into the criteria for somatic symptom disorder. With **illness anxiety disorder**, clients experience excessive anxiety and preoccupation with having or acquiring a serious illness. Physical symptoms, if present, are a minor aspect of this diagnosis. Persistent worry regarding illness invades multiple aspects of an individual's life. For instance, illness becomes a frequent topic of discussion as they repeatedly discuss illness within their social circle and seek reassurance from family and friends. They will spend hours researching suspected illnesses and

continuously examine their body for signs of illness. This impacts their quality of life, potentially limiting activities of daily living (looking after family, going to work) and, in extreme cases, results in the inability to go to work or school.

The estimated prevalence of illness anxiety disorder in the general population is approximately 0.1% though the true rate remains unclear (French & Hammed, 2021; Scarella et al., 2019). The aetiology is also unknown, but it is proposed that a serious childhood illness or abuse may be a precursor (Berens et al., 2020; Hovens et al., 2015). Careful evaluation of illness anxiety disorder must be carried out and other psychiatric illnesses, such as obsessive–compulsive disorder, delusional disorder, and generalized anxiety, excluded.

Several interventions have been effective in reducing client's fears of experiencing serious illnesses. Cognitive–behavioural therapy, stress management, and group interventions lead to a decrease in intensity and increase in control of symptoms (Axelsson & Hedman-Lagerlöf, 2019). It is unknown whether the positive outcomes result from the intervention itself or from the symptom validation and increased attention given to the client. Nursing management should include listening to the client's report of symptoms and fears, validating it by acknowledging that the fears may be real, asking the client to monitor symptoms in a journal, and encouraging the client to bring the journal to clinical visits. By seeing the symptom pattern, the nurse can continue assessment and help the client better understand the significance and implications of symptoms. The outcome of this approach should be to decrease fear and achieve better symptom control.

Conversion Disorder

Conversion disorder, also known as functional neurologic symptom disorder, is the somatization of neurologic conditions such as paralysis. Symptoms associated with conversion disorder are called **pseudoneurologic symptoms**. Clients with conversion disorder present with symptoms of impaired coordination or balance, paralysis, aphonia (inability to produce sound), difficulty swallowing or a sensation of a lump in the throat, and urinary retention. They also may have loss of sensation, vision problems, blindness, deafness, seizures, and hallucinations. Females experience conversion disorder two to three times more frequently than do males (Baizabal-Carvallo & Jankovic, 2019). Clients with conversion disorder are said to experience "la belle indifférence" a French term meaning "beautiful ignorance" because they have an absence of psychological distress despite being paralyzed, or experiencing blindness (Gokarakonda & Kumar, 2020). These symptoms do not follow neurologic pathways but rather the individual's conceptualization of the problem. The nurse must understand that the physical sensation is real for the client. There is evidence of a relationship between childhood trauma (e.g., sexual abuse) or other stressful life events and conversion disorder (Diez et al., 2021; Van der Feltz-Cornelis et al., 2020). In approaching this client, the nurse treats the conversion symptom as a real symptom that may have distressing psychological aspects. The nurse intervenes by acknowledging the pain and helps the client deal with it. As trust develops within the nurse–client relationship, the nurse can help the client develop approaches to solving everyday problems.

IN-A-LIFE

Emily Carr (1871–1945)

CANADIAN PAINTER AND WRITER
Public Persona

Emily Carr was an accomplished artist and writer best known for her vivid depictions of Indigenous culture and Canadian West Coast nature. Influenced by early educational sojourns in San Francisco, England, and France and later encouraged by the important artists known as the Group of Seven, Carr developed her unique impressionistic style in both painting and writing. Embellished with dramatizations and idealism, works like *Growing Pains* autobiographically depict the struggle of her life. Raised in a strict Victorian home, Carr has been described as rebellious, irritable, and socially insecure.

Personal Realities

Carr's career was interrupted many times with bouts of poor health. Not much more than a century ago, Carr was treated in an English sanatorium. Many of the symptoms she described were representatives of what today is called illness anxiety disorder, clinical depression, and/or conversion disorder.

Psychological Factors Affecting Other Medical Conditions

Within this category, clients engage in behaviours that negatively impact the outcome of an existing medical condition. In mild cases, clients may, for instance, not take their antidiabetic medication appropriately and intentionally increase their risk for diabetic complications. In more severe cases, the client's behaviour may lead to life-threatening complications and risk of death. For example, a client may ignore a life-threatening infection rather than seek help. This diagnosis can only be established in the absence of other diagnoses that may better characterize or explain such risky behaviour, such as major depressive disorder, delusion disorder, or posttraumatic stress disorder (American Psychiatric Association, 2013).

Factitious Disorders

The other type of psychiatric disorder characterized by somatization is **factitious disorder**. There are two classes of factitious disorders: factitious disorder imposed on self and factitious disorder imposed on another. Clients with this disorder intentionally cause, fabricate, or exaggerate physical or psychiatric symptoms, illness, or injury for primary gain, often the attention of healthcare workers (Carnahan & Jha, 2021). These individuals are motivated solely by the desire to become a client, or have those in their care become clients, just so they themselves can develop a dependent relationship with a healthcare provider. See the DSM-5 for more specific details on diagnostic criteria of factitious disorders.

Factitious Disorder, Imposed on Self

Although feigned illnesses have been described for centuries, it was not until 1951 that the term *Munchausen syndrome* was used to describe the most severe form of this disorder, which is characterized by fabricating a physical illness, having recurrent hospitalizations, and going from one healthcare provider to another (Asher, 1951). Today, this disorder is called factitious disorder and is differentiated from **malingering**, in which the individual who intentionally produces illness symptoms is motivated by another specific self-serving *secondary* gain, such as being classified as disabled or avoiding work, seeking drugs, incarceration, or even military service (Carnahan & Jha, 2021). They generally show poor adherence to treatment, and once the secondary gain is achieved, they no longer express concern about the assumed illness (Alozai & McPherson, 2021).

Clients with factitious disorder injure themselves covertly. The illnesses are produced in such a manner that the healthcare provider is tricked into believing that a true physical or psychiatric disorder is present. The self-produced physical symptoms appear as medical illnesses such as seizure disorders, wound-healing disorders, the abscess processes (introduction of infectious material below the skin surface), and feigned fever (rubbing the thermometer). Unlike malingering, the *primary* gain for those with factitious disorder is the creation of physical and/or psychological symptoms in order to assume a sick role (Alozai & McPherson, 2021).

Epidemiology

The estimated prevalence of factitious disorders is between 0.5% and 2% (Fischer et al., 2016). However, the true prevalence of factitious disorder is difficult to determine because its secretive nature interferes with traditional epidemiologic research methods. Recovery from this condition is seldom addressed in academic literature and effective treatment approaches are not well known.

Nursing Management: Human Response to Disorder

The overall goal of treatment is for the client to replace the dysfunctional, attention-seeking behaviours with positive behaviours. To begin treatment, the client must acknowledge the deception, but confrontation does not appear to lead to acknowledgement. Nonetheless, a supportive, nonpunitive approach may be beneficial in order to establish a therapeutic relationship and encourage psychotherapy (Fischer et al., 2016). The mental health team has to accept and value the client as a human being who needs help. As the pattern of self-injury is well established, giving up the behaviours is difficult.

Assessment

Early childhood experiences, particularly instances of abuse, neglect, or abandonment, should be identified to understand the underlying psychological dynamics of the individual and the role of self-injury. Family assessment is important; relationships become strained as family members become aware of this disorder's self-inflicted nature. Factitious disorder is a secretive disorder. Even though clients are known to cause self-injury

and undergo risky procedures, many clients are undiagnosed and untreated, and when confronted, many are lost to treatment (Carnahan & Jha, 2021).

Nursing Interventions

The fabrications and deceits may provoke anger and a sense of betrayal in the nurse. To be effective, the nurse must be aware of these feelings and resolve them by developing a better understanding of the underlying psychodynamic issues. Therapeutic confrontation in the context of a helping relationship can be effective if the client feels supported and accepted and if there is clear communication between the client, the mental healthcare team, and family members. All care should be centralized within one facility, and the client should see providers regularly, even when not in active crisis. Clients with this disorder generally have a poor prognosis; the treatment goal is recovery, not confession.

Factitious Disorder, Imposed on Another

Within the category of factitious disorder, the *DSM-5* includes a rare but dramatic disorder, factitious disorder imposed on another, once called *Munchausen by proxy*, also known as caregiver-fabricated illness in a child (Koetting, 2015). It involves a person's inflicting injury on another—often a parent and usually the mother—on their own child—hoping thereby to gain the attention of a healthcare provider and extra support and caring. These actions include inducing seizures, poisoning, or smothering. This most severe form of child abuse is usually identified in the emergency department of hospitals or by critical care nurses. The parent rarely admits to injuring the child and thus is not amenable to treatment; if this is the case, the child is removed from the offending parent's care. This form of child abuse is distinguished from other forms by the routine, unwitting involvement of healthcare workers, who subject the child to physical risk and emotional distress through tests, procedures, and medication trials.

🍁 Summary of Key Points

- Somatic symptom and related disorders manifest psychological distress and abnormal thought patterns in relation to physical symptoms, independent of whether the symptom may be medically explained.
- Somatization is affected by sociocultural and traumatic childhood experiences and generally occurs less frequently in older adults.
- Clients with somatic symptom disorder are often seen on the medical–surgical units of hospitals and can go years without receiving a correct diagnosis. In most cases, they eventually receive mental health treatment because of comorbid conditions such as depression and panic.

- The development of the nurse–client relationship is crucial to assessing these clients and identifying appropriate nursing diagnoses and interventions. Because these clients deny any psychiatric basis for their problem and continue to focus on their symptoms having a medical basis, the nurse must take a nonjudgmental, open approach that acknowledges the symptoms while helping the client explore and understand his or her behaviour and focus on new ways of coping with stress.
- Health teaching is important in helping the individual develop positive lifestyle changes in place of somatization responses. Identifying personal strengths and supporting the development of positive skills improve self-esteem and personal confidence. Teaching the use of biofeedback and relaxation provides the client with positive coping skills.
- Illness anxiety disorder occurs when an individual's preoccupation with having or acquiring an illness causes excessive distress.
- Conversion disorder manifests as one or more somatic symptoms involving altered voluntary motor or sensory function.
- Factitious disorders are manifested by individuals intentionally inflicting or feigning injury or illness on themselves or others to gain medical attention.

 ## Thinking Challenges

A nurse is caring for a client diagnosed with factitious disorder. The client has been trying to injure herself at work to get the affection of the factory manager, to no avail. She is now being seen in the neurologic clinical because she is having seizures that have no medical foundation.

a. What are the characteristics of this somatic disorder?
b. What is the overall goal of the treatment of this client population?
c. How is factitious disorder different from malingering?
d. How is it different from factitious disorder imposed on another?

> Visit thePoint to view suggested responses.
> Go to **thePoint.lww.com/activate** and use the activation code found in the front of this text to unlock answers to the "Thinking Challenges" and other online resources.

Web Links

Medicatingnormal.com This is a webpage that host the film Medicating Normal and provides resources and information about the negative consequences of using prescription medications inappropriately.

dsm.psychiatryonline.org This website holds the "DSM Library." You can search the website for information regarding somatic symptom and other disorders.

heretohelp.bc.ca/infosheet/health-anxiety This is a Mental Health and Substance Use information source based in British Columbia. It offers information and resources on a variety of health topics.

https://www.psychiatry.org/patients-families/somatic-symptom-disorder This is an excellent site for patients and families wanting to learn more about somatic symptom disorder, including diagnosis, and treatment.

References

Aksu, M. H. (2020). Relationship between somatization and psychiatric symptoms, especially anxiety, depression, alexithymia, and severity of addiction in male patients with alcohol and heroin addiction. *Dusunen Adam: The Journal of Psychiatry and Neurological Sciences*, 33, 120–129. https://doi.org/10.14744/dajpns.2020.00071

Alozai, U. U., & McPherson, P. K. (2021, June 26). Malingering. *Stat Pearls*. https://www.ncbi.nlm.nih.gov/books/NBK507837/

American Psychiatric Association. (2013). *Diagnostic and statistical manual of mental disorders, 5th Edition: DSM-5* (5th ed.).

Arts, M., Buis, J., & de Jonge, L. (2016). Misdiagnosis of anterior cutaneous nerve entrapment syndrome as a somatization disorder. *European Psychiatry*, 33(S1), S387–S388. https://doi.org/10.1016/j.eurpsy.2016.01.1392

Asher, R. (1951). Munchausen's syndrome. *The Lancet*, 257(6650), 339–341. https://doi.org/10.1016/s0140-6736(51)92313-6

Axelsson, E., & Hedman-Lagerlöf, E. (2019). Cognitive behavior therapy for health anxiety: Systematic review and meta-analysis of clinical efficacy and health economic outcomes. *Expert Review of Pharmacoeconomics & Outcomes Research*, 19(6), 663–676. https://doi.org/10.1080/14737167.2019.1703182

Baizabal-Carvallo, J. F., & Jankovic, J. (2019). Gender differences in functional movement disorders. *Movement Disorders Clinical Practice*, 7(2), 182–187. https://doi.org/10.1002/mdc3.12864

Berens, S., Banzhaf, P., Baumeister, D., Gauss, A., Eich, W., Schaefert, R., & Tesarz, J. (2020). Relationship between adverse childhood experiences and illness anxiety in irritable bowel syndrome—The impact of gender. *Journal of Psychosomatic Research*, 128, 109846. https://doi.org/10.1016/j.jpsychores.2019.109846

Burton, C., Fink, P., Henningsen, P., Löwe, B., & Rief, W. (2020). Functional somatic disorders: Discussion paper for a new common classification for research and clinical use. *BMC Medicine*, 18(1), 34. https://doi.org/10.1186/s12916-020-1505-4

Carnahan, K. T., & Jha, A. (2021, January 9). Factitious disorder. *StatPearls*. StatPearls Publishing. https://www.ncbi.nlm.nih.gov/books/NBK557547/

Chida, Y., Schrempft, S., & Steptoe, A. (2016). A novel religious/spiritual group psychotherapy reduces depressive symptoms in a randomized clinical trial. *Journal of Religion and Health*, 55(5), 1495–1506. https://doi.org/ 10.1007/s10943-015-0113-7

Cooper, K., Gregory, J. D., Walker, I., Lambe, S., & Salkovskis, P. M. (2017). Cognitive behaviour therapy for health anxiety: A systematic review and meta-analysis. *Behavioural and Cognitive Psychotherapy*, 45(2), 110–123. https://doi.org/10.1017/s1352465816000527

D'Souza, R. S., & Hooten, W. M. (2021, March 21). Somatic syndrome disorders. *StatPearls*. StatPearls Publishing. https://www.ncbi.nlm.nih.gov/books/NBK532253/

Diez, I., Larson, A. G., Nakhate, V., Dunn, E. C., Fricchione, G. L., Nicholson, T. R., Sepulcre, J., & Perez, D. L. (2021). Early-life trauma endophenotypes and brain circuit–gene expression relationships in functional neurological (conversion) disorder. *Molecular Psychiatry*, 26, 3817–3828. https://doi.org/10.1038/s41380-020-0665-0

Fischer, C. A., Beckson, M., & Dietz, P. (2016). Factitious disorder in a patient claiming to be a sexually sadistic serial killer. *Journal of Forensic Sciences*, 62(3), 822–826. https://doi.org/10.1111/1556-4029.13340

French, J. H., & Hammed, S. (2021, February 7). StatPearls. StatPearls Publishing. https://www.ncbi.nlm.nih.gov/books/NBK554399/

Gan, J. J., Lin, A., Samimi, M. S., & Mendez, M. F. (2016). Somatic symptom disorder in semantic dementia: The role of alexisomia. *Psychosomatics, 57*(6), 598–604. https://doi.org/10.1016/j.psym.2016.08.002

Garcia-Campayo, J., Sanz-Carrillo, C., Baringo, T., & Ceballos, C. (2001). SPECT scan in somatization disorder patients: An exploratory study of eleven cases. *Australian & New Zealand Journal of Psychiatry, 35*(3), 359–363. https://doi.org/10.1046/j.1440-1614.2001.00909.x

Gierk, B., Kohlmann, S., Toussaint, A., Wahl, I., Brünahl, C. A., Murray, A. M., & Löwe, B. (2015). Assessing somatic symptom burden: A psychometric comparison of the Patient Health Questionnaire—15 (PHQ-15) and the Somatic Symptom Scale—8 (SSS-8). *Journal of Psychosomatic Research, 78*(4), 352–355. https://doi.org/10.1016/j.jpsychores.2014.11.006

Gokarakonda, S. B., & Kumar, N. (2020, July 15). La Belle indifférence. *StatPearls.* StatPearls Publishing. www.ncbi.nlm.nih.gov/books/NBK560842/

Hakala, M., Karlsson, H., Routsalainen, U., Koponen, S., Bergman, J., Stenman, H., Kelavuori, J. P., Aalto, S., Kurki, T., & Niemi, P. (2002). Severe somatization in women is associated with altered cerebral glucose metabolism. *Psychological Medicine, 32*(8), 1379–1385. https://doi.org/10.1017/s0033291702006578

Hart, S. L., Hodgkinson, S. C., Belcher, H. M. E., Hyman, C., & Cooley-Strickland, M. (2012). Somatic symptoms, peer and school stress, and family and community violence exposure among urban elementary school children. *Journal of Behavioral Medicine, 36*(5), 454–465. https://doi.org/10.1007/s10865-012-9440-2

Hedman, E., Axelsson, E., Andersson, E., Lekander, M., & Ljótsson, B. (2016). Exposure-based cognitive–behavioural therapy via the internet and as bibliotherapy for somatic symptom disorder and illness anxiety disorder: Randomised controlled trial. *British Journal of Psychiatry, 209*(5), 407–413. https://doi.org/10.1192/bjp.bp.116.181396

Henningsen, P. (2018). Management of somatic symptom disorder. *Body-Mind Interaction in Psychiatry, 20*(1), 23–31. https://doi.org/10.31887/dcns.2018.20.1/phenningsen

Hilderink, P., Collard, R., Rosmalen, J., & Oude Voshaar, R. (2013). Prevalence of somatoform disorders and medically unexplained symptoms in old age populations in comparison with younger age groups: A systematic review. *Ageing Research Reviews, 12*(1), 151–156. https://doi.org/10.1016/j.arr.2012.04.004

Holliday, K. L., Macfarlane, G. J., Nicholl, B. I., Creed, F., Thomson, W., & McBeth, J. (2010). Genetic variation in neuroendocrine genes associates with somatic symptoms in the general population: Results from the EPIFUND study. *Journal of Psychosomatic Research, 68*(5), 469–474. https://doi.org/10.1016/j.jpsychores.2010.01.024

Holster, J., Hawks, E. M., & Ostermeyer, B. (2017). Somatic symptom and related disorders. *Psychiatric Annals, 47*(4), 184–191. https://doi.org/10.3928/00485713-20170308-03

Hovens, J. G. F. M., Giltay, E. J., van Hemert, A. M., & Penninx, B. W. J. H. (2015). Childhood maltreatment and the course of depressive and anxiety disorders: The contribution of personality characteristics. *Depression and Anxiety, 33*(1), 27–34. https://doi.org/10.1002/da.22429

Hüsing, P., Bassler, M., Löwe, B., Koch, S., & Toussaint, A. (2018). Validity and sensitivity to change of the Somatic Symptom Disorder–B Criteria Scale (SSD-12) in a clinical population. *General Hospital Psychiatry, 55,* 20–26. https://doi.org/10.1016/j.genhosppsych.2018.08.006

Ibeziako, P., Randall, E., Vassilopoulos, A., Choi, C., Thomson, K., Ribeiro, M., Fernandes, S., Thom, R., & Bujoreanu, S. (2021). Prevalence, patterns, and correlates of pain in medically hospitalized pediatric patients with somatic symptom and related disorders. *Journal of the Academy of Consultation-Liaison Psychiatry, 62*(1), 46–55. https://doi.org/10.1016/j.psym.2020.05.008

Iob, E., Kirschbaum, C., & Steptoe, A. (2019). Persistent depressive symptoms, HPA-axis hyperactivity, and inflammation: The role of cognitive-affective and somatic symptoms. *Molecular Psychiatry, 25*(5), 1130–1140. https://doi.org/10.1038/s41380-019-0501-6

Jongedijk, R. A., Eising, D. D., van der Aa, N., Kleber, R. J., & Boelen, P. A. (2020). Severity profiles of posttraumatic stress, depression, anxiety, and somatization symptoms in treatment seeking traumatized refugees. *Journal of Affective Disorders, 266,* 71–81. https://doi.org/10.1016/j.jad.2020.01.077

Karkhanis, D. G., & Winsler, A. (2016). Temperament, gender, and cultural differences in maternal emotion socialization of anxiety, somatization, and anger. *Psychological Studies, 61*(3), 137–158. https://doi.org/10.1007/s12646-016-0360-z

Koetting, C. (2015). Caregiver-fabricated illness in a child. *Journal of Forensic Nursing, 11*(2), 114–117. https://doi.org/10.1097/JFN.0000000000000066

Kop, W. J., Toussaint, A., Mols, F., & Löwe, B. (2019). Somatic symptom disorder in the general population: Associations with medical status and health care utilization using the SSD-12. *General Hospital Psychiatry, 56,* 36–41. https://doi.org/10.1016/j.genhosppsych.2018.10.004

Kroenke, K., & Swindle, R. (2000). Cognitive-behavioral therapy for somatization and symptom syndromes: A critical review of controlled clinical trials. *Psychotherapy and Psychosomatics, 69*(4), 205–215. https://doi.org/10.1159/000012395

Kroska, E. B., Roche, A. I., & O'Hara, M. W. (2018). Childhood trauma and somatization: Identifying mechanisms for targeted intervention. *Mindfulness, 9*(6), 1845–1856. https://doi.org/10.1007/s12671-018-0927-y

Kullgren, K. A., Klein, E. J., Sturza, J., Hutton, D., Monroe, K., Pardon, A., Sroufe, N., & Malas, N. (2020). Standardizing pediatric somatic symptom and related disorders care: Clinical pathway reduces health care cost and use. *Hospital Pediatrics, 10*(10), 867–876. https://doi.org/10.1542/hpeds.2020-0004

Lanzara, R., Scipioni, M., & Conti, C. (2019). A clinical-psychological perspective on somatization among immigrants: A systematic review. *Frontiers in Psychology, 9,* 2792. https://doi.org/10.3389/fpsyg.2018.02792

LaVigne, T. W., Laake, L. M., & Ibeziako, P. (2020). Somatic symptom and related disorders in pediatric patients: Associations with parent psychiatric and substance use histories. *Clinical Child Psychology and Psychiatry, 25*(4), 932–944. https://doi.org/10.1177/1359104520931579

Li, T., Wei, J., Fritzsche, K., Toussaint, A. C., Jiang, Y., Cao, J., Zhang, L., Zhang, Y., Chen, H., Wu, H., Ma, X., Li, W., Ren, J., Lu, W., Müller, A. M., & Leonhart, R. (2020). Validation of the Chinese version of the somatic symptom disorder–B criteria scale for detecting DSM-5 somatic symptom disorders: A multicenter study. *Psychosomatic Medicine, 82*(3), 337–344. https://doi.org/10.1097/psy.0000000000000786

Longstreth, G. F. (2015). Carnett's legacy: Raising legs and raising awareness of an often misdiagnosed syndrome. *Digestive Diseases and Sciences, 61*(2), 337–339. https://doi.org/10.1007/s10620-015-3885-4

Malas, N., Ortiz-Aguayo, R., Giles, L., & Ibeziako, P. (2017). Pediatric somatic symptom disorders. *Current Psychiatry Reports, 19*(2), 11. https://doi.org/10.1007/s11920-017-0760-3

Miyauchi, T., Tokura, T., Kimura, H., Ito, M., Umemura, E., Sato (Boku), A., Nagashima, W., Tonoike, T., Yamamoto, Y., Saito, K., Kurita, K., & Ozaki, N. (2019). Effect of antidepressant treatment on plasma levels of neuroinflammation-associated molecules in patients with somatic symptom disorder with predominant pain around the orofacial region. *Human Psychopharmacology: Clinical and Experimental, 34,* e2698. https://doi.org/10.1002/hup.2698

Morabito, G., Barbi, E., & Cozzi, G. (2020). The unaware physician's role in perpetuating somatic symptom disorder. *JAMA Pediatrics, 174*(1), 9–11. https://doi.org/10.1001/jamapediatrics.2019.4381

Polo-Morales, A., Alcocer-Salas, N., Rodríguez-Violante, M., Pinto-Solís, D., Solís-Vivanco, R., & Cervantes-Arriaga, A. (2020). Association between somatization and nonmotor symptoms severity in people with Parkinson disease. *Journal of Geriatric Psychiatry and Neurology, 34*(1), 60–65. https://doi.org/10.1177/0891988720901787

Regev, S., Odes, S., Slonim-Nevo, V., Friger, M., Schwartz, D., Sergienko, R., Eliakim, R., & Sarid, O. (2021). Differential relationships of somatization, depression, and anxiety to severity of Crohn's disease. *Journal of Health Psychology, 26,* 2390–2401. https://doi.org/10.1177/1359105320909879

Saunders, N. R., Gandhi, S., Chen, S., Vigod, S., Fung, K., De Souza, C., Saab, H., & Kurdyak, P. (2020). Health care use and costs of children, adolescents, and young adults with somatic symptom and related disorders. *JAMA Network Open, 3*(7), e2011295. https://doi.org/10.1001/jamanetworkopen.2020.11295

Scarella, T. M., Boland, R. J., & Barsky, A. J. (2019). Illness anxiety disorder: Psychopathology, epidemiology, clinical characteristics, and treatment. *Psychosomatic Medicine, 81*(5), 398–407. https://doi.org/10.1097/psy.0000000000000691

Steine, I. M., Winje, D., Krystal, J. H., Bjorvatn, B., Milde, A. M., Grønli, J., Nordhus, I. H., & Pallesen, S. (2017). Cumulative childhood maltreatment and its dose-response relation with adult symptomatology: Findings in a sample of adult survivors of sexual abuse. *Child Abuse & Neglect, 65,* 99–111. https://doi.org/10.1016/j.chiabu.2017.01.008

Tarsitani, L., Todini, L., Roselli, V., Serra, R., Magliocchetti, V., D'Amore, D., … & Biondi, M. (2020). Somatization and traumatic events in asylum seekers and refugees resettled in Italy. *Trauma: Psychopathology, Boundaries An Treatment, 26,* 41. https://doi.org/10.36148/2284-0249-374

Toussaint, A., Hüsing, P., Kohlmann, S., & Löwe, B. (2019). Detecting DSM-5 somatic symptom disorder: Criterion validity of the Patient Health Questionnaire-15 (PHQ-15) and the Somatic Symptom Scale-8 (SSS-8) in combination with the Somatic Symptom Disorder—B Criteria Scale (SSD-12). *Psychological Medicine, 50*(2), 324–333. https://doi.org/10.1017/s003329171900014x

Toussaint, A., Löwe, B., Brähler, E., & Jordan, P. (2017a). The Somatic Symptom Disorder - B Criteria Scale (SSD-12): Factorial structure, validity and population-based norms. *Journal of Psychosomatic Research, 97,* 9–17. https://doi.org/10.1016/j.jpsychores.2017.03.017

Toussaint, A., Murray, A. M., Voigt, K., Herzog, A., Gierk, B., Kroenke, K., Rief, W., Henningsen, P., & Löwe, B. (2016). Development and validation of the somatic symptom disorder–B criteria scale (SSD-12). *Psychosomatic Medicine, 78*(1), 5–12. https://doi.org/10.1097/psy.0000000000000240

Toussaint, A., Riedl, B., Kehrer, S., Schneider, A., Löwe, B., & Linde, K. (2017b). Validity of the somatic symptom disorder–B criteria scale (SSD-12) in primary care. *Family Practice, 35*(3), 342–347. https://doi.org/10.1093/fampra/cmx116

Van der Feltz-Cornelis, C. M., Allen, S. F., & Van Eck van der Sluijs, J. F. (2020). Childhood sexual abuse predicts treatment outcome in conversion disorder/functional neurological disorder. An observational longitudinal study. *Brain and Behavior, 10*(3), e01558. https://doi.org/10.1002/brb3.1558

van Driel, T. J. W., Hilderink, P. H., Hanssen, D. J. C., de Boer, P., Rosmalen, J. G. M., & Oude Voshaar, R. C. (2018). Assessment of somatization and medically unexplained symptoms in later life. *Assessment, 25*(3), 374–393. https://doi.org/10.1177/1073191117721740

Vassilopoulos, A., Poulopoulos, N. L., & Ibeziako, P. (2020). School absenteeism as a potential proxy of functionality in pediatric patients with somatic symptom and related disorders. *Clinical Child Psychology and Psychiatry, 26*(2), 342–354. https://doi.org/10.1177/1359104520978462

25

Eating Disorders

Kathryn Weaver

LEARNING OBJECTIVES

After studying this chapter, you will be able to:

- Distinguish the characteristics of eating disorders.
- Describe biologic, psychological, and social aetiologic theories of anorexia nervosa, bulimia nervosa, and binge-eating disorder within the broader spiritual dimension.
- Explain the importance of body image, body dissatisfaction, and gender identity in developmental theories that explain aetiology of anorexia nervosa, bulimia nervosa, and binge-eating disorder. Appreciate the role obesity plays in the development of anorexia nervosa and bulimia nervosa and as a consequence of binge-eating disorder.
- Describe the neurobiology, neurochemistry, and physiologic consequences associated with anorexia nervosa, bulimia nervosa, and binge-eating disorder.
- Explain the impact of sociocultural norms on the development of eating disorders.
- Describe the risk factors and protective factors associated with the development of eating disorders.
- Formulate nursing care problems for individuals living with eating disorders.
- Develop nursing interventions for individuals experiencing anorexia nervosa, bulimia nervosa, and binge-eating disorder.
- Analyze special concerns within the nurse–client relationship for the nursing care of individuals struggling with eating disorders.
- Identify strategies for the prevention and early detection of eating disorders.

KEY TERMS

- anorexia nervosa • binge-eating disorder • body image • body mass index • bulimia nervosa • cue elimination • self-monitoring

KEY CONCEPTS

- body dissatisfaction • body image distortion • dietary restraint • drive for thinness • enmeshment • interoceptive awareness • maturity fears • social comparison

---

Parallels between religious practices and eating disorders have been traced to the history of religious fasting in the Judeo-Christian religious tradition. To illustrate, the story of Saint Catherine of Siena (1347–1380) provides a medieval example of self-starvation honoured by the Catholic Church. Fasting in response to the death of her sister and opposing her parents' demand that she be married, Catherine starved herself and tirelessly cared for the sick, denying her own needs until she died from

malnutrition at 33 (Sukkar et al., 2017). Saint Catherine became a model of virtue through starvation to deny physical desires and atone for sin. However, support of the church's endorsement of fasting ended in the late Middle Ages reformation when asceticism was condemned. Eventually, religious fasting became less common and self-starvation became associated with mental illness (Dell'Osso et al., 2016). In 1694, English physician Richard Morton described a woman who suffered a "nervous consumption" that caused her wasting. "Anorexia nervosa" was coined in 1873 by Sir William Withey Gull and "hysterical anorexia" by Ernest Charles Lasègue the same year (Valente, 2016). The first Canadian publication on anorexia nervosa was by New Brunswick physician Peter Inches (1895) who reported a 17-year-old's low weight, loss of menses, and "almost complete refusal of food of any kind" (p. 74).

This chapter focuses on **anorexia nervosa** (AN), **bulimia nervosa** (BN), and **binge-eating disorder** (BED) with other eating issues that do not fully meet clinical criteria for AN, BN, or BED. The role of obesity in the development of eating disorders and as a specific consequence of BED is considered. Drawing on the transdiagnostic model (Fairburn et al., 2015), the various eating disorders are understood as having comparable characteristics and underlying core psychopathology that are reflected in similar attitudes, behaviours, and dysfunctional self-worth beliefs. For persons living with eating disorders, their sense of self-esteem is primarily determined by their ability to control weight and shape. Consequently, they attempt to follow various dieting regimes, often extremely restrictive or irrational, such as complete avoidance of carbohydrates or eating only 400 kcal a day. Breaking these restrictive regimes usually prompts a binge-eating episode, which leads to even stricter dietary restrictions and a sense of guilt. When a binge-eating episode is followed by compensatory behaviour (e.g., induced vomiting, strenuous physical exercise, or intake of laxatives), the risk of another binge is increased through a dysfunctional belief that compensatory behaviour helps control weight. Some persons who do not use compensation use binge eating to cope with stressful life events or regulate negative emotions and mood may experience overweight and obesity over time. For individuals who rarely or never engage in binge eating, dietary restrictions cause gradual loss of body mass, leaving them underweight.

Manifestations of eating disorders (e.g., dieting, binge eating, weight fluctuations, and preoccupation with weight and shape) overlap, so they may be viewed holistically within a continuum of eating experiences (Fig. 25.1). On one end is *unrestricted eating*, whereupon eating and appearance are not at issue for the individual. For most, this is a time of healthy eating, exercise, weight, and **body image**; however, unrestricted eating can include binge eating. *Watchful eating* includes paying attention to food composition and calories, tracking calories, and physical activity for the purpose of modifying daily energy balance. At this stage of watchful eating, the individual is becoming dissatisfied with body appearance and may weigh self more than usual, relating weight changes to calories ingested or expended. The individual's identity is shifting to one of a dieter and/or body sculptor. Watchful eating is not the same as mindful eating, an emerging healthy weight regulation

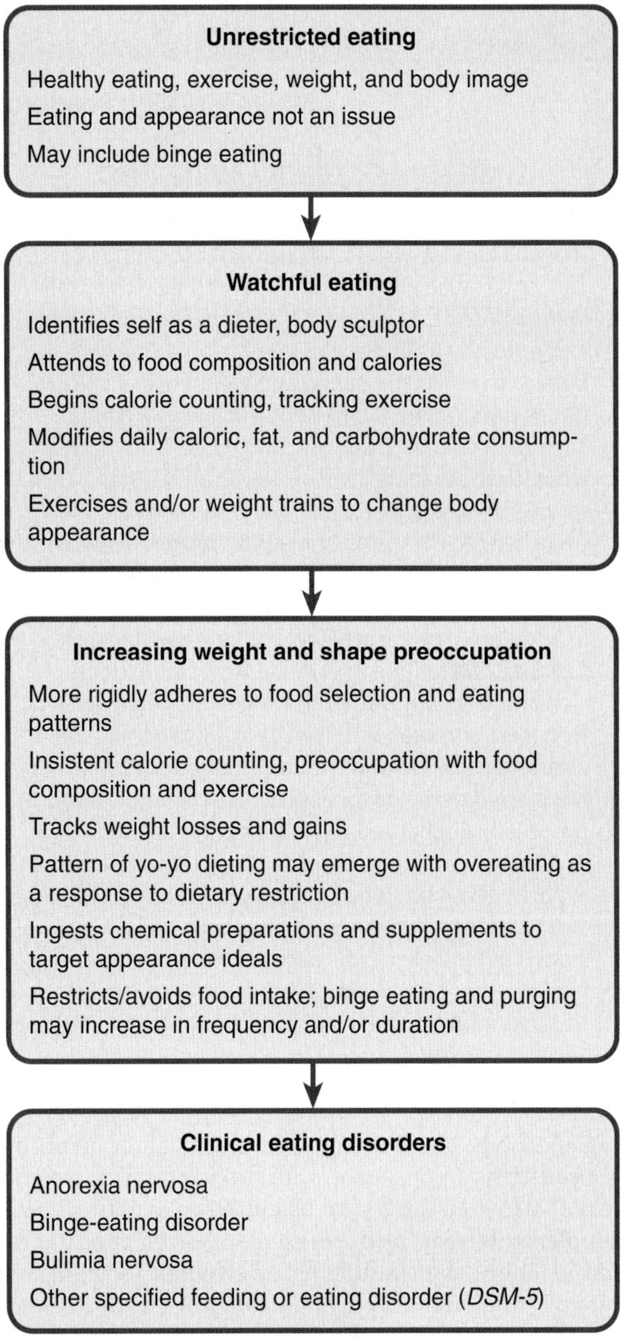

Figure 25.1 Continuum of eating experiences.

approach for maintaining a nonjudgmental awareness of physical feelings, thoughts, and perceptions in the present moment. Next on the continuum of eating experiences is *increasing weight and shape preoccupation*. The individual more rigidly adheres to food selection and eating patterns, insistently comparing energy expended to energy ingested and tracking weight losses and gains. A pattern of dietary restriction in response to weight gain may follow. *Orthorexia* is a term that describes a dietary pattern in which an individual restricts intake to include only "healthy" foods such as vegetables or

IN-A-LIFE 🏠

Melanie Mallet: Roadblocks in the Struggle to Recover

LIMITED ACCESS TO CARE AND SUPPORT

"I would almost wish that I just had something like cancer because it would be less embarrassing to tell someone and you would feel a lot more sympathy and empathy from people," said Melanie. She first began to restrict her eating and weigh herself every day as a young adult. She kept track of everything she put in her body, and she calculated it no matter what it was. Melanie lived in New Brunswick and attended university in Halifax, NS. When she sought treatment, her first stay at the Halifax treatment centre was successful. Yet upon returning to university and her part time job, she relapsed within 6 weeks. In addition to physical ailments like nerve damage, hair loss, and fatigue, Melanie suffered from depression and felt shame about having eating disorders. By her second year of university in Nova Scotia, she attempted suicide and was hospitalized. She was transferred to the hospital in her NB hometown and eventually discharged but had not recovered.

Melanie could not afford to attend a private clinic in NB because her insurance only covered up to $500 a year, the equivalent of just four private sessions. For Melanie, it was necessary to travel to Halifax (a distance of 461 km or a 5-h drive) to receive treatment for anorexia and bulimia, while working part time in New Brunswick. Halifax was the closest city east of Quebec with a public treatment centre. The NB government paid Melanie's clinical fees, but did not cover gas, lodging, and meal expenses. She could, therefore, attend the clinic only 1 day a week.

At the Halifax eating disorder clinic, Melanie was able to meet with people who suffered from similar illnesses. She would eat breakfast at the clinic and attend a check-in afterwards to dispel anxiety around the meal. She and other patients talked in a group about goals, nutrition, and strategies to deal with negative thoughts and behaviours. The group was helpful because few people understood her struggle. "You can't quite understand it or grasp it unless you're suffering from it. But then you don't wish for anybody to actually suffer through this… You don't want to talk to people about how you make yourself throw up seven times a day," Melanie disclosed.

Although the therapy was beneficial, Melanie said the financial stress of travelling took its toll on her. She likened this to facing a wall and bashing her head against it.

Source: Yard, B. (2016). Bathurst woman faces barriers to eating disorder treatment: Province covers treatment costs but not expenses for travel, meal or lodging. *CBC News.* https://www.cbc.ca/news/canada/new-brunswick/bathurst-barrier-eating-disorder-1.3441747

---

organic foods, but in doing so develops significant problems, such as an obsession with food and severe weight loss (Valente et al., 2020). Chemical preparations and supplements may also be used to target appearance ideals. Episodes of restricting or avoiding food intake, binge eating, and purging may develop. At the far end of the continuum, as the eating disturbance increases in frequency and/or duration, *clinical eating disorders* emerge as AN, BN, BED, or as partial clinical disorders that meet some but not all criteria of full clinical eating disorders. Individuals may cycle back and forth among these disorders. Definitions, clinical course, aetiologies, and interventions for the different eating disorders are considered separately in this chapter. Yet, because their risk factors and prevention strategies are similar, these are discussed under one heading.

Anorexia Nervosa

The term "anorexia nervosa" is deceptive as its literal meaning is lack or absence of appetite of nervous origin. Persons with AN suffer, rather, from a deep fear of "becoming fat" that is accompanied by a disturbance in the way in which they perceive and experience their body. This fear motivates them to strictly limit food intake.

Clinical Course

Although the risk of eating disorders occurs across the lifespan, the onset of AN is usually in adolescence or early adulthood (Statistics Canada, 2015). This onset is often associated with a stressful transition (e.g., leaving home) and can be slow with serious dieting present long before an emaciated body is noticed. In a longitudinal study of Canadian adolescents in Quebec, 57.1% of girls desired a thinner body at age 14 years, with prevalence increasing to 65.8% at age 18 years; this was compared with 44.0% among adolescent boys at age 14, which remained unchanged 4 years later (Dion et al., 2015). The prevalence of body dissatisfaction was found to be lower than desire for thinness. As well, 25- to 29-year-old

Canadian women were more likely to be dissatisfied than 12- to 14-year-olds (20.76% vs. 6.34%). The level of body dissatisfaction increased across increasing levels of internet use (Carter et al., 2017). Eating disorders in later life are frequently unrecognized or masked behind medical conditions, depression, or the natural changes of aging. Approximately 50% of 67- to 84-year-old Quebec men and women were dissatisfied with their bodies and misperceived their current body sizes (Roy et al., 2015). Among those dissatisfied with their body weight, 90.7% perceived themselves as being "too fat," and only 9.3% perceived themselves as being too thin; the prevalence of body weight dissatisfaction was higher among women as compared with men. Although the importance given to body image as it relates to physical appearance was lower in comparison with younger populations, tensions regarding the aging body (e.g., appearance vs. health) as well as a double standard of aging were reported. Further, results of an internet survey of women aged 60 to 90 years (n = 245) indicated that eating pathology factors of perfectionism, depression, and sociocultural pressure to be thin matched those reported for younger women (Midlarsky et al., 2017).

The long-term outcome of AN has improved during the past 20 years because awareness has increased early detection. Still, prognosis is variable, and less than 50% recover (Fichter et al., 2017). Currently, AN is regarded as a chronic condition, with relapses characterized by significant weight loss. Treatment drop-out was predicted by having reduced motivation measured by motivational questions or the Anorexia Stages of Change Questionnaire, lower presenting BMI, and binge–purge subtype of AN; greater eating disorder pathology and reduced motivation predicted poorer outcome (Gregertsen et al., 2019). The presence and persistence of binge eating and purging behaviours alongside comorbid depression is particularly devastating (Franko et al., 2018). Findings from a 22-year longitudinal study reported that most women living with AN and BN who achieved full recovery were two times less likely to be depressed or five times less likely to engage in a substance use disorder than those actively ill with the eating disorder (Keshishian et al., 2019). Other positive prognostic factors for AN include shorter duration of illness, shorter duration of first inpatient treatment, and insight (Errichiello et al., 2016).

AN has a higher all-cause mortality than do all other psychiatric disorders with the exception of substance misuse and postpartum admission. AN comorbid with alcohol dependence or insulin-dependent diabetes mellitus is associated with up to 50 times and 10 times higher (respectively) than each of these illnesses alone (Sharan & Sundar, 2015). Poorer health-related quality of life and increased healthcare utilization and healthcare costs were associated with AN compared with the healthy population (Ágh et al., 2016). Moreover, premature death in the young client population leads to significant indirect costs to society, mainly due to the loss of production.

Diagnostic Criteria

The diagnostic criteria for full clinical AN are shown in the *DSM-5* (see Box 25.1). Changes from the previous *DSM-IV* criteria include revision of the weight-loss criterion, clarification that fear of weight gain does not need to be verbalized if behaviours interfering with weight gain can be observed, and elimination of the criterion of amenorrhoea. Using these revised criteria, the lifetime prevalence estimate of *DSM-5*–defined AN (0.8%) slightly increased from that of *DSM-IV*–defined AN at 0.6% (Udo & Grilo, 2018). Among community-based young adult women, Mustelin et al. (2016) found an increase of 60%. The *DSM-5* uses **body mass index** (BMI) cutoffs to denote severity. BMI, calculated as weight in kilograms per height in metres squared, defines limits of body weight as agreed upon by the Centers for Disease Control and Prevention and the World Health Organization. For example, a BMI below 16.5 kg/m^2 for an adult is considered to indicate severe underweight.

AN is categorized as (a) restricting or (b) binge–purge type. The purging associated with the binge–purge type may occur through self-induced vomiting or misuse of laxatives, diuretics, or enemas even after eating a normal or small-sized meal or snack. Many of the clinical features associated with AN result from malnutrition or semistarvation. Classic research with volunteers who semistarved, and observations of prisoners of war and conscientious objectors, have demonstrated that these states of starvation are characterized by food preoccupation, binge eating, depression, obsession, and apathy.

A central feature of AN is a distortion in body image, the mental picture of one's own body (Dalhoff et al., 2019). Body image constructs include dissatisfaction, overvaluation, and preoccupation with weight and/or shape. Overvaluation is the assignment of excessive importance to body weight and/or shape in evaluating one's self-worth, whereas dissatisfaction with weight/shape is the negative evaluation of one's body weight and/or shape. Preoccupation is excessive thinking about weight and/or shape. Body dissatisfaction is a strong predictor of disordered eating in a range of populations from children through to young adults (Rosewall et al., 2018; Turel et al., 2018). Preoccupation with weight and shape predicted increased odds of beginning to use unhealthy weight control behaviours, as well as beginning to diet in both adolescent men and women participants (Sharpe et al., 2018). Dissatisfaction predicted increased odds or severity for a range of outcomes in adolescent women (e.g., unhealthy weight control behaviours, binge eating, and depressive symptoms)

BOX 25.1 Diagnostic Characteristics for Anorexia Nervosa

DSM-5: Feeding and Eating Disorders
Anorexia Nervosa: 307.1 (F50.01 or F50.02)
A. Restriction of energy intake relative to requirements leading to a significantly low body weight in the context of age, sex, developmental trajectory, and physical health. *Significantly low weight* is defined as a weight that is less than minimally normal or, for children and adolescents, less than that minimally expected.
B. Intense fear of gaining weight or "becoming fat," or persistent behaviour that interferes with weight gain, even though at a significantly low weight.
C. Disturbance in the way in which one's body weight or shape is experienced, undue influence of body weight or shape on self-evaluation, or persistent lack of recognition of the seriousness of the current low body weight.

Specify if:
• In partial remission:
  • After full criteria for anorexia nervosa were previously met, criterion A has not been met for a sustained period, but either criterion B or C is still met.

• In full remission:
  • After full criteria for anorexia nervosa were previously met, none of the criteria have been met for a sustained period of time.

Specify current severity:
The minimum level of severity is based, for adults, on current BMI (see below) or for children and adolescents, on BMI percentile. The ranges below are derived from World Health Organization categories for thinness in adults; for children and adolescents, corresponding BMI percentiles should be used. The level of severity may be increased to reflect clinical symptoms, the degree of functional disability, and the need for supervision.

• Mild: BMI > 17 kg/m^2
• Moderate: BMI = 16 to 16.99 kg/m^2
• Severe: BMI = 15 to 15.99 kg/m^2
• Extreme: BMI < 15 kg/m

Reprinted with permission from American Psychiatric Association. (2013). *Diagnostic and Statistical Manual of Mental Disorders* (5th ed.). https://doi.org/10.1176/appi.books.9780890425596

---

that persisted into adulthood; for adolescent men participants, dissatisfaction predicted increases in depressive symptoms over the follow-up adult period. Overvaluation in adolescence predicted increased odds of starting to experience binge eating over the 15-year follow-up.

KEY CONCEPT

Body image distortion occurs when the individual perceives his or her body disparately from how the world or society views it.

Neurobiology, Neurochemistry, and Physiologic Consequences of Anorexia Nervosa

Essential to the diagnosis of AN are semistarvation behaviours, relentless drive for thinness (women) or for muscularity (men) or a morbid fear of "becoming fat," and signs and symptoms resulting from the starvation. Individuals living with AN ignore body signals or cues, such as hunger and weakness, and concentrate all efforts on controlling food intake. Their entire mental focus narrows to one goal: weight loss. Typical thought

patterns are "If I gain half of a kilo, then I'll keep gaining. I'll never stop until I am huge!" Such all-or-nothing thinking keeps these individuals on rigid regimens for weight loss. Their behaviours become organized around food-related activities, such as preparing food, counting calories, and reading cookbooks. Much behaviour concerning what, when, and how they eat is ritualistic; for example, they may cut food into tiny pieces, refuse to eat in the presence of others, or fix elaborate meals for others that they themselves do not eat. Box 25.2 lists common psychological characteristics.

Individuals with AN feel inadequate, so many fear emotional maturation and the unknown challenges the next developmental stages will bring. For some, remaining physically small symbolizes remaining childlike; weight loss becomes a way to experience control and combat feelings of inadequacy and ineffectiveness. Every lost kilogram is viewed as a success, and weight loss often confers a feeling of virtuousness. Perfectionism is an important characteristic found in both adult and adolescent women (Petersson et al., 2017) and athletes (Abbott et al., 2021) experiencing AN.

Arising from a "lost sense of emotional self" (p. 1), individuals living with AN may avoid conflict and may suppress or have difficulty expressing negative emotions

BOX 25.2 Psychological Characteristics Related to Eating Disorders

Anorexia Nervosa
- Decreased interoceptive awareness
- Sexuality conflict/fears
- Maturity fears
- Ritualistic behaviours
- Perfectionism
- Dietary restraint

Bulimia Nervosa
- Impulsivity
- Boundary problems
- Limit-setting difficulties
- Dietary restraint

Binge-Eating Disorder
- Negative mood
- Self-deprecation
- Social insecurity

Anorexia, Bulimia Nervosa, and Binge-Eating Disorder
- Difficulty expressing anger
- Low self-esteem
- Body dissatisfaction
- Powerlessness
- Ineffectiveness
- Obsessiveness
- Compulsiveness
- Nonassertiveness
- Cognitive distortions

(e.g., amenorrhoea, decreased libido). Table 25.1 presents the medical complications, signs, and symptoms of AN and the other eating disorders that result from starving or binge eating and purging. For instance, purging behaviours may cause electrolyte disturbances. It has been identified that individuals with AN who have diabetes mellitus may "purge" through decreasing insulin doses to subsequently decrease carbohydrate metabolism (Goebel-Fabbri et al., 2019).

KEY CONCEPT

Drive for thinness is an intense physical and emotional process that overrides all physiologic body cues.

KEY CONCEPT

Interoceptive awareness is a term used to describe the sensory response to emotional and visceral cues, such as hunger.

Epidemiology

The prevalence of AN in Canada is 0.3% to 1% (Statistics Canada, 2015), similar to the global weighted ranges of lifetime prevalence of 1.4% (0.1% to 3.6%) for women and 0.2% (0% to 0.3%) for men (Galmiche et al., 2019). AN appears to be more prevalent within underrepresented ethnic group and in other countries than previously recognized or reported. Cultural change may be associated with increased vulnerability to eating disorders, and newcomers to Canada experience dietary acculturation that includes increased consumption of foods high in sugar, salt, and fat (Lane et al., 2019).

Age of Onset

The age of onset is typically between 14 and 16 years, with the highest incidence rates for adolescent women aged 15 to 19 years. Adolescents are vulnerable because of stressors associated with their development, especially concerns about body image, autonomy, and peer pressure, and their susceptibility to such influences as the media, which extols an ideal body type and discusses dieting and exercise as ways to achieve success, popularity, and power. Recently, 874 Quebec children aged 8 to 12 years old reported body dissatisfaction with girls significantly more dissatisfied than boys (Côté et al., 2020). It was suggested that (a) girls present a higher risk of being exposed to media and beauty pressure, resulting in higher preoccupation with their weight and

(Oldershaw et al., 2019). They may have difficulty defining feelings because they are confused about or unsure of emotions and visceral cues, such as hunger; therefore, their responses to cues are inaccurate and inappropriate. Often, they cannot name the feelings they are experiencing. This uncertainty and confusion in interpreting signals from the body is called a lack of interoceptive awareness, and it is thought to be partially responsible for developing and maintaining the eating disorder.

Because of the ritualistic behaviours, all-encompassing focus on food and weight, and feelings of inadequacy that accompany AN, social contacts are gradually reduced and the person becomes isolated. With more severe weight loss comes other symptoms, such as apathy, depression, and even mistrust of others.

The nutritional compromise associated with AN may affect most organs and can produce physiologic disturbances that include cardiac arrhythmias, loss of bone density, neuronal deficits, and hormonal changes

Table 25.1	Complications of Eating Disorders
Body System	**Symptoms**
From Starvation to Weight Loss	
Musculoskeletal	Loss of muscle mass and loss of fat (emaciation)
	Osteopenia (*bone mineral* deficiency) and less frequently, osteoporosis
Metabolic	Hypothyroidism (symptoms include lack of energy, weakness, intolerance to cold, and bradycardia)
Cardiac	Hypoglycaemia and decreased insulin sensitivity
Gastrointestinal	Bradycardia, hypotension, loss of cardiac muscle, small heart, cardiac arrhythmias including atrial and ventricular premature contractions, prolonged QT interval, ventricular tachycardia, and sudden death
	Delayed gastric emptying, bloating, constipation, abdominal pain, gas, and diarrhoea
Reproductive	Amenorrhoea, low levels of luteinizing hormone and follicle-stimulating hormone, and irregular periods
Dermatologic	Dry, cracking skin and brittle nails due to dehydration, lanugo (fine baby-like hair over body), oedema, and acrocyanosis (bluish hands and feet); hair thinning
Hematologic	Leucopenia, anaemia, thrombocytopaenia, hypercholesterolaemia, and hypercarotenaemia
	Abnormal taste sensation (possible zinc deficiency)
Neuropsychiatric	Neurologic deficits in cognitive processing of new information; decreased total brain volume; increased brain ventricular size
	Apathetic depression, mild organic mental symptoms, sleep disturbances, and fatigue
Related to Purging (Vomiting and Laxative Abuse)	
Metabolic	Electrolyte abnormalities, particularly hypokalaemia and hypochloremic alkalosis; hypomagnesaemia; increased blood urea nitrogen
Gastrointestinal	Salivary gland and pancreatic inflammation and enlargement with increase in serum amylase; oesophageal and gastric erosion (oesophagitis); dysfunctional bowel with haustral dilation; superior mesenteric artery syndrome
Dental	Erosion of dental enamel (perimylolysis), particularly frontal teeth with decreased decay
Neuropsychiatric	Seizures (related to large fluid shifts and electrolyte disturbances), mild neuropathies, fatigue, weakness, and mild organic mental symptoms
Cardiac	Ipecac cardiomyopathy arrhythmias
Binge Eating to Weight Gain	
Gastrointestinal	Heartburn; abdominal discomfort; bloating; gastric rupture; symptoms of fullness may interrupt sleep
Metabolic	Gall bladder disease; type 2 diabetes
Cardiac	Hypertension and hypercholesterolaemia
Musculoskeletal	Arthritis
Respiratory	Shortness of breath; asthma; sleep apnoea; snoring

body shape and (b) boys' body dissatisfaction occurs later or boys want to look fit and muscular rather than thin. Nationally, a significant proportion of Canadian students with overweight (21%) and obesity (27%) reported they were "doing something" to lose weight (Public Health Agency of Canada, 2015). At the international level, the prevalence of adolescent binge eating and purging has almost doubled from age 14 to age 16 (Bartholdy et al., 2017). According to Moore et al. (2016), recollections of disliking the physical changes of puberty and feeling underprepared relate to disordered eating symptoms, feelings of ineffectiveness, and difficulties with interpersonal relationships in the postpubertal period.

Differences Among People Diagnosed With AN

Anorexia nervosa occurs predominantly in women and is one of the most common psychiatric conditions in young women (Statistics Canada, 2015). This disparity may be attributed to society's influence on women to achieve an ideal body type and to men's reluctance to seek help for what is widely perceived as a women's issue. Box 25.3 highlights findings about eating disorders in men, while Box 25.4 summarizes current research promoting positive change and sustaining positive developmental assets in girls.

Ethnic and Cultural Differences

Contextual variables that may influence eating disorders include level of acculturation, socioeconomic status, peer socialization, family structure, and immigration. In Canada, nearly 2.2 million children under the age of 15, or 37.5% of the total population of children, are in a family of people who have immigrated (Statistics Canada, 2017). Greater exposure to fast food outlets and less exposure to supermarkets selling familiar nutritious foods and to opportunities for physical activity such as walking or cycling contribute to new Canadians who have adopted unhealthy eating and exercise habits, which may increase the likelihood of developing higher BMI (Vitale & Doherty, 2016). Results from a scoping review focusing on body image dissatisfaction among children and adolescents who are from an underrepresented ethnic group within Canada and the United States suggest these individuals experience higher levels of body image dissatisfaction

BOX 25.3 Boys and Men With Eating Disorders

Eating disorders have been present in men for as long as in women. Indeed, the first English-language publication of symptoms in the absence of medical disease was reported in a 16-year-old boy (Morton, 1694, as cited in Robinson et al., 2013). Men get eating disorders with increasing prevalence now than in years past. Research suggests that men make up to "33% of cases of anorexia and bulimia diagnoses" (Griffiths et al., 2015, p. 108).

Boys and men involved in an occupation or a sport with a greater emphasis on weight classes and aesthetic ideals such as wrestling, weightlifting, dancing, jockeying, and body building exhibit high rates of weight and shape preoccupation, intensive body modification practices, binge eating, and BN (National Eating Disorders Collaboration, 2017). However, eating disorders in men and boys are often underdiagnosed, undertreated, and misunderstood. Despite the development of the Eating Disorder Assessment for Men by Stanford and Lemberg in 2012, symptomatology in men is not adequately captured with currently available measures such as the Eating Disorder Examination Questionnaire that were designed primarily for women (Arnow et al., 2017). Compared to women, adolescent men were found more likely to present with diagnoses other than AN or BN, to exhibit similar rates of anxiety, and to less likely present with a mood disorder (Kinasz et al., 2016). Men attribute the symptoms in the context of fitness, sport, and concerns of body images, whereas women mention family tension as a causative factor (Arnow et al., 2017).

Commonly, men only seek treatment or receive a correct medical diagnosis when symptoms become severe. The stigma associated with having a "woman's disease" may contribute to a delay in seeking help. Despite this, men matched to women by age and percent of ideal body weight who present at eating disorder clinics were found to be more aware of the consequences of the illness in their lives and more likely to describe their symptoms as arising in the context of factors external to them (e.g., sports, getting healthy, performance, or personal transitions) while women internalized the disorder as part of their identity (Arnow et al., 2017). Because the men tended to view the eating disorder as separate from their personality, they may feel unhappy with or ashamed of their behaviour, and more willing to engage in therapy.

Most of the risk factors for developing for eating disorders are a shared experience (e.g., perfectionism, bullying, dieting, trauma, childhood obesity). For men, the social construct of "drive for muscularity," a preoccupation with increasing musculature rather than a lower body weight, has been identified as a counterpart to the woman "drive for thinness" (Arnow et al., 2017). Eating disorders among men concern the need for muscle expansion instead of body mass reduction (Jaworski et al., 2019). Anabolic steroid use may indicate body preoccupation. The images of perfect body for men coming from pop culture, sports figures, and the media can lead to feelings of low self-esteem in young men, which contribute to the body image disturbance associated with AN and BN. The unique cultural messages men are exposed to can increase their vulnerability toward developing an eating disorder. These messages extol the ideal physical body shape for men as lean and muscular to the exclusion of other male body types, as well as the notion that men need to be in control. Thus, when coping with particular issues beyond their control, men can sometimes displace these anxieties onto their bodies to manifest control through excessive exercise and dieting.

Men who recovered from eating disorders experienced psychosocial wellbeing in terms of diminished preoccupations with food or disordered eating behaviours and growth of self-confidence, insight, inner peace, empathy, and interpersonal relationships (Lewke-Bandara et al., 2020). These men emphasised the importance of support systems and improved resilience to deflect triggers that would otherwise cause relapse.

Preventive methods include maintaining a healthy body image and healthy self-esteem. The masculine body shape portrayed in society is often not realistic. Teaching young men that there is not one "right way" to be/look like a man is essential in preventing eating disorders (Cottrell & Williams, 2016). A strength-based approach that emphasizes affirming emotional strengths, virtues, and capacities can enable men and boys to flourish (Sangha et al., 2019). Such approach will aid men in acknowledging their problems and accepting professional help as a conduit to healthy self-management.

BOX 25.4 Research for Best Practice

IMPROVING POSITIVE SELF-IDENTITY IN GIRLS

Gilham, C., Thompson, K., & Ruckstuhl, S. (2020). Improving girls' developmental assets using a mentor-led approach in Atlantic Canada. *Gender Issues*, *37*(4), 340–354. https://doi.org/10.1007/s12147-020-09251-6

Background: Adolescent girls' positive self-identity drops by 35% through the middle school years. Social pressures and cultural messages have an eroding effect on the wellbeing of girls and affect their capacity to participate fully and equally in society. Media, parents, and peers play a role, intentionally and/or unintentionally, in imposing girl-stifling conditions, such as when parents convey messages to their daughters about the importance of physical attractiveness, and girls police each other through conformity to thinness and sexiness. Girl-specific empowerment programs support girls in skill-building enhancing social connections, and building self-esteem through culturally safe/appropriate group activities that are asset-based, empowerment-oriented/voice-centred, gender specific, and participatory-driven to build protective factors and reduce the impacts of objectification in their lives.

Purpose: To explore the positive impact of the Amplify program on key developmental assets for girls in a rural Atlantic Canadian community.

Methods: The Developmental Assets Profile Survey was used to assess the developmental assets (e.g., the skills, relationships, and behaviours that help young people thrive and include support, empowerment, boundaries and expectations, constructive use of time, commitment to learning, positive values, social competencies, and positive identity) of 115 middle-school girls who are from households with low incomes prior to, and after, the Amplify intervention program. The program was delivered by first-year nursing students who are women and trained as mentors through the local college's Nurse Practitioner program to facilitate the girls' groups. The Amplify program was chosen because of its Canadian background and content, the breadth of activities facilitators and girls could choose from, its alignment with

best practice recommendations, and its social justice, participatory foundations.

Findings: The Amplify program had a positive impact on rural girls' developmental assets, particularly for those girls who initially scored as vulnerable on one or more developmental assets. Findings showed statistically significant increases in the external assets of boundaries and constructive use of time, and the internal assets of positive identity, positive values, and commitment to learning. Girls who initially scored as not vulnerable on any of the assets maintained their relative scores across all developmental assets. Thus, the findings show that this type of approach can improve developmental assets that are protective among rural girls who are vulnerable for developing negative mental, physical, and social health outcomes. Given the high percentage (70%) of girls who initially scored as vulnerable on one or more of the assets, the findings suggest that this work at this age range is timely. The more assets young people develop, the better off they tend to be across a range of academic, psychological, social–emotional, and behavioural indicators of wellbeing.

Implications for Nursing: This study contributes to the growing body of evidence pursuing mentoring as part of a comprehensive approach to eating disorder prevention. Prevention is crucial given the limited therapeutic intervention and support available in many Canadian provinces (identified in the *Canadian Eating Disorders Strategy 2019–2029*). The increase in girls' positive identity is a hopeful outcome, and the cumulative effect of assets can potentially help overcome risk factors for anxiety, depression, and substance abuse for this important population. School-based prevention programs permit easy student access and participation, addressing rural challenges such as transportation and intense parent work schedules. Having nursing student mentors external to the school facilitated open and honest discourse with program participants and enabled the nurses to gain invaluable practical experience with children in a group-based format that provided project training and mentor support as part of their required course work.

compared to their white counterparts (Kimber, Couturier et al., 2015). Kimber, Georgiades, et al. (2015) reported that a 19-year-old woman who immigrated to Ontario actively changed her eating habits after seeing her cousin in a bathing suit and feeling like she could not wear the same swimwear:

> "I was bigger, and I didn't think that it would be nice looking. I was like, okay, I can't wear that and I want to. So, then I started just not eating, I think I was worse than her even, she would actually eat kind of normally, but I just went overboard. (p. 126)"

Familial Predisposition

There is increased risk among first-degree biologic relatives of individuals with AN (Statistics Canada, 2015). Relatives who are women also have high rates of depression, leading researchers to hypothesize that a shared genetic factor may influence the development of both disorders.

Comorbidity

Data from the Canadian Community Health Survey of Mental Health and Wellbeing indicate that the lifetime

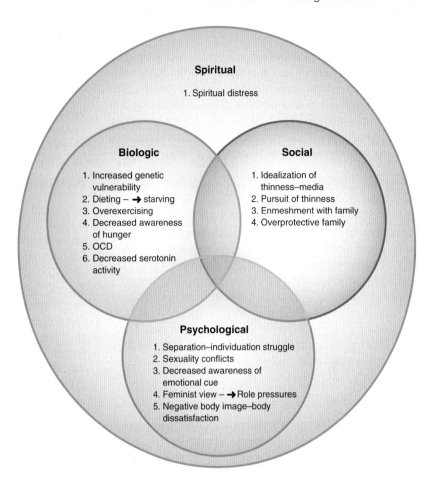

Figure 25.2 Bio/psycho/social/spiritual aetiologies for clients with AN.

prevalence of eating problems is 1.7% among Canadians; almost half of those with eating problems also had mood or anxiety disorders and reported more unmet needs (Meng & D'Arcy, 2015). Comorbid major depression and substance abuse disorders are common in AN (Keshishian et al., 2019), as are obsessive–compulsive disorder or OCD, anxiety disorders such as posttraumatic stress, and avoidant personality disorder. AN is associated with high risk of a suicide attempt; the risk is significantly increased with comorbid diagnoses of personality disorder, depression, bipolar affective disorder, and substance misuse (Cliffe et al., 2020). Substance use can begin before, at the same time as, or after the onset of an eating disorder. Some women seek substances (e.g., methamphetamines or diet pills) to try to reduce their weight, while others turn to substances to dampen urges to binge eat (Muhlhein, 2019). Increased severity from combined psychological disturbance could interfere with treatment and decrease the likelihood of recovery. Comorbid conditions may resolve when AN has been treated successfully. At other times, symptoms of a premorbid condition, such as OCD, remain even though an individual has recovered, leading many to believe that anxiety may actually influence the development of the disorder.

Aetiology

Some risk factors and aetiologic factors for eating disorders overlap. For example, dieting is a risk factor for the development of AN, but it is also a biologic aetiologic factor, and in its most serious form—starving—it is also a symptom. Most experts agree that eating disorders are multidimensional and multidetermined. Figure 25.2 depicts the aetiologic factors for AN within their larger spiritual dimension.

Biologic Theories

The many comorbid conditions associated with the diagnosis, such as depression and OCD, of AN may have a shared aetiology. Although the relationship between these clinical manifestations and the biologic changes caused by starvation is not well understood, many of the biologic changes noted in AN are determined to be the result of starvation and thus are state, rather than trait or causative, factors. Little evidence exists to substantiate that dysregulations in appetite–satiety systems cause AN. Appetite dysregulation is best viewed as the end product or result of an interaction between the environment and physiology. The bio/psycho/social/spiritual model of this interaction explains the aetiology (see Fig. 25.2).

Neuropathologic Theories

Magnetic resonance imaging and computed tomography disclose changes in the brain of individuals with AN who have significant weight loss. The most common findings are increased activation of the amygdala (coordinates with the prefrontal cortex during encoding of emotion-based learning, and with memory structures such as the hippocampus in retaining that learning), altered activation of the cingulate cortex (involved in perception and integration of body stimuli), and gray and white matter reduction correlating with the extent of malnourishment and mostly reversible with recovery (Scharner & Stengel, 2019). The amygdala was found to be more activated in persons experiencing AN when feeling hungry compared to healthy controls, pointing towards a more fearful emotional response. Reduced activation in the attention network was found after women diagnosed with AN viewed images of their own bodies; a finding interpreted as avoidance of perceiving their body. Gray matter changes, however, may not fully return to normal after months of weight restoration.

Genetic Theories

The field of genetics in AN and other eating disorders is still in an early stage. Twin-based heritability estimates are at 50% to 60% (Watson et al., 2017). A genome-wide association study identified significant genetic correlations between AN and psychiatric disorders, physical activity, and metabolic, lipid, and anthropometric traits. These results may be key to improving outcomes as they direct attention to both psychiatric and metabolic components (Watson et al., 2017). Shih and Woodside (2016) call for a focused effort to understand gene–diet interactions in AN as this will lead to a more personalized treatment approach and promote discovery of novel nutritional and pharmacologic interventions.

Biochemical Theories

Undernutrition and weight regulatory behaviours such as vomiting and laxative abuse can lead to a range of biochemical problems in AN, most commonly hypokalaemia and hypophosphatemia in persons who engage in vomiting, laxative abuse, or diuretic use. Hypochloremic metabolic alkalosis may develop in clients who vomit, and hyperchloremic metabolic acidosis may develop in those who abuse laxatives (Kardalas et al., 2018). Hyponatraemia may result from excessive water ingestion and chronic energy deprivation or diuretic misuse; low urea and creatinine concentrations may mask dehydration or renal dysfunction (Boyd & Durant, 2018). Hypoglycaemia is common (Rosen et al., 2016). Most persons admitted with AN have altered regulation of the hypothalamic–pituitary–thyroid axis during starvation with low T3 and low-normal free T4 and thyroid-stimulating hormone (Hoermann et al., 2015).

Neurotransmitter and neuroendocrine abnormalities, such as blunted serotonergic function in clients with low weight, must be viewed with caution as causative factors because these disturbances are considered state related and tend to normalize after symptom remission and weight gain.

Psychological Theories

The most widely accepted theory of AN is psychodynamic. In this theory, key tasks of separation–individuation and autonomy are interrupted. Struggles around identity and role, body image formation, sexuality, and maturity fears predominate (Treasure & Cardi, 2017). During early adolescence, when individuals begin to establish their independence and autonomy, some may feel inadequate or ineffective. Dieting and weight control may be viewed as a means to defend against these feelings. In later adolescence, when separation–individuation is a developmental task, similar conflicts arise when an adolescent is ill prepared for this stage and feels inadequate and ineffective in going forward emotionally. Because AN is usually diagnosed between 14 and 18 years of age, developmental struggles of adolescence are one acceptable theory of causation (Rohde et al., 2015).

Girls and boys begin to differ dramatically in self-esteem just before adolescence. At the time self-doubt increases in girls, pubertal weight gain can also occur, resulting in a more rounded, mature shape. These normal developmental occurrences can add to confusion about identity. Such confusion and self-doubt are further promoted by conflicting messages that girls receive from society about their roles in life. Girls may interpret expectations about how they should look, what roles they should perform, and what they should achieve in society as pressures to achieve "all." They often try to please others to avoid conflicts around perceived expectations. Compared to adolescent and young adult women, adolescent and young adult men are less likely to report eating in response to negative emotion, experience a sense of loss of control when binge eating, and restrict their food intake in response to body dissatisfaction. One adolescent described the difficulty of others recognizing his eating disorder amid pubertal development:

> My friends, for the most part, didn't notice ... This seems incredible to me—when I look at photos from that time, I'm so obviously sick. But at 12, everyone's body is transforming. Furthermore, from my experience, boys generally spend a lot less time scrutinising each other's bodies than girls. It was easier for me to slip under the radar (Pollen, 2019).

Adolescent and young adult men who are gay or bisexual exhibit higher rates of eating disorder pathology. Young men developing eating disorders are more likely than young women to engage in excessive exercise (Limbers et al., 2018). Feminists have focused on role pressure to partly explain the increase in eating disorders and the greater prevalence in women. Box 25.5 outlines some feminist perspectives regarding role, feminisms, eating disorder development, and applicability to both women and men.

BOX 25.5 Feminist Ideology and Eating Disorders

Feminist scholars claim that women are socialized to avoid self-expression in the face of conflict, seek attachment through putting others first, judge self by external standards, and present an outward compliant self. These societal factors and gender beliefs specific to Westernized cultures foster a view of one's self as the way an outside observer would see one; this may fuel constant body monitoring and comparison to societal standards, shame, and disordered eating (Borowsky et al., 2016). Body size and weight are aspects of identity upon which difference is identified. Women are consistently scrutinized for their weight, clothing choices, and other aspects of their everyday life. This even more disproportionately affects women of colour and LGBTQI2SA+ women, who find themselves facing various forms of institutional prejudice that are noticeable in the ways in which women who are of Black Canadian or African origin are chastised for their natural hairstyles, or transgender students have to fight to wear the clothing of their preference for school prom (Carlo, 2018).

Social and health discourses have co-constructed a body hierarchy that positions people who are slender as the norm and people who are overweight as the "other." In doing so, the ideal slender body type is conferred with implicit and explicit advantages and privileges that include greater likelihood for employment, romantic relationships, popularity, and protection from peer victimization. In contrast, people who are obese or overweight are marginalized as individuals to be laughed at, presumed as lazy and ugly, and in need of health advice. Feminism is part of belonging to a group of people who all want to see improvements in the world and see its citizens value themselves. Understanding the extent to which ideals and discourses about body weight and shape act to delimit social and class status can help address the influence of the internalization of such ideals. Taking a step back to look at the inequalities and injustices of restricted gender roles and widely accepted ideas of femininity that society subjects people to, both politically and even mentally, gives a better understanding of how to get past the setbacks experienced personally and gives something larger to be a part of and fight for (Reichmann, 2018).

Feminists take issue with the biomedical explanation of eating disorders, seeing it as limiting and patriarchal. In a culture that rewards thinness and toned bodies but simultaneously peddles consumer products encouraging excess, it can be difficult to decipher how to attain a body identified as healthy and ideal (LaMarre & Rice, 2016). The everyday sexism and historically lower social status experienced by women as well as sexual abuse and violence are seen as pathways that expose women to risk for body disturbances (Borowsky et al., 2016). The recovery of society must occur to decrease the prevalence of eating disorders. For this to occur, women must be supported to speak out and challenge the eating disorder.

The core belief behind feminist philosophy is that all human beings are equal to one another despite gender, appearance, and insecurities. The characterization of eating disorders as body image problems may miss the wider experiences of "restricted agency" that are structurally gendered (Holmes et al., 2017).

> Dieting keeps us focused on our bodies and the mirror, rather than our minds and our sense of purpose. And it is hard to change the world when 80% of your time is sucked up by changing your weight. Ergo, dieting keeps femmes and females from gaining political power, freedom, and choice (Reichmann, 2018, para. 2).

Principles of the feminist relational model apply to men with eating disorders. A feminist relational approach proposes that, in growing up, boys may long for connection but are pushed to become autonomous before they have developed the ability to identify their feelings and needs. The increase in eating disorders among males reveals a need to explore their gender roles and expectations, globalized exposure to media images of idealized men's bodies, and the possibility that men express distress through their bodies. This approach focuses less on pathology and more on responses to pressures, expectations, roles, or environment. According to Carlo (2018), as long as men who develop eating disorders are scorned as "weak" or "feminine," or are prevented from opening up about mental health issues which are often at the root of AN, BN, and BED, "we will continue to allow the oppression of women while simultaneously letting these illnesses eat men up from the inside" (Carlo, 2018, para. 14).

KEY CONCEPT

Maturity fears or feeling overwhelmed by adult responsibilities are often underlying issues for individuals with AN. Starvation is viewed as a response to these fears.

Social Theories

The media, the fashion industry, and peer pressure are significant social influences in the development of eating disorders. Magazines and television shows depict young girls and adolescents with thin and often emaciated bodies as glamorous to young women. In a study with 179 youth aged 10 to 17 years, media influence to lose weight was found a significant predictor of engagement in unhealthy weight control behaviours for girls with average to low self-esteem, while media influence to lose weight was related to frequency of engaging in unhealthy weight control behaviours for boys with higher BMIs (Mayer-Brown et al., 2016). Among girls, media exposure and appearance conversations (talking about clothes, looks, and hairstyles) with peers were the strongest predictors of dietary restraint (Damiano et al., 2015). The mere presence of advertising reinforced rather than directly caused disorder for 15- to 35-year-old women inpatients of an eating disorders unit in Spain who were already dissatisfied with their body (Moral-Agúndez & Carrillo-Durán, 2020).

Body dissatisfaction resulting from perceiving one's own body as falling short of an ideal may include dissatisfaction about one's weight, shape, size, or even a certain body part. In a study that investigated relationships between body weight perception, BMI, physical activity, and food choices among 1,212 adolescent girls and boys from California (Gaylis et al., 2020), more girls (39.3%) perceived themselves as overweight compared to their boy counterparts (26.0%), and weight control practices were more prevalent among girls. Adolescents who perceived themselves to be thin tended to consume unhealthier foods, such as hamburgers and regular soda daily, where those who perceived themselves as fit and overweight made healthier food choices by eating more salad and vegetables. Dietary behaviours initiated in adolescence are likely to carry over into adulthood and may have long-term impacts on health. The perception of body weight is not exclusive to adolescents. Blackburn et al. (2016) compared anthropometric data from 428 men and women from Quebec aged 18 to 35 years with their actual 3D image to evaluate the relationship between women and men's perception of their "real" body, ideal body image, and levels of self-esteem. For both women and men, the most important factor explaining higher level of self-esteem was higher satisfaction with aspects of their bodies. In men, a distorted body image, either by seeing themselves as thinner than

the reality or by not having a good perception of their body shape, improved self-esteem. Media pressure was not significant. However, women who had a higher level of internalized media ideals as personal standards of attractiveness were found to have a lower level of self-esteem. Women who claimed to never expect a change in their silhouette before buying new clothes, as well as those who attempted to control their weight in the last year, showed better self-esteem.

Social comparison theory helps explain how sociocultural pressure may influence the development of eating disorders. The central premise of social comparison theory is that people have an innate drive to evaluate their own standing on a wide range of characteristics, and in the absence of objective standards, people compare themselves with others in the social environment to obtain information about their own qualities or performance (Homan & Lemmon, 2016). Appearance comparisons with those considered more attractive are referred to as upward appearance comparisons, whereas comparisons made with those considered less attractive are called downward appearance comparisons. Women who engaged in upward or downward appearance comparisons were more likely to exhibit higher levels of drive for thinness and dietary restraint (Lin & Soby, 2016). In addition to this, Ntoumanis et al. (2020) found that body image discrepancy from upward appearance comparisons was negatively influenced by the appreciation of one's appearance. The indirect effect of upward appearance evaluation on body image discrepancy via appearance evaluation was significant only when need frustration (basic psychological needs thwarted within social contexts) was high. Ntoumanis et al. recommended that potential opportunities for intervention work are needed to foster appearance self-compassion, feelings of body competence, and positive body image.

KEY CONCEPT

Body dissatisfaction is the belief that one's current body size differs from a highly valued ideal body size and that this difference deserves negative appraisal and may be expressed through comments including "I feel too fat/too gross." Body dissatisfaction has been related to low self-esteem, depression, dieting, binge eating, and purging.

KEY CONCEPT

Social comparison—evaluating oneself against idealized others, such as models or attractive peers—is a major factor in body dissatisfaction, weight anxiety, and disturbed eating.

Family Responses

Early family theories and observations classically labelled the family of the individual experiencing AN as *enmeshed*, overprotective, rigid, and unable to resolve conflicts. In an enmeshed family, boundaries that define individual autonomy are weak: One member may relay communication from another to a third, and excessive togetherness may intrude on privacy. An enmeshed, overprotective, and rigid family engenders and maintains the eating disorder, whereas a highly cohesive and flexible family style is considered more favourable for the children's wellbeing as they move into maturation and independence. In their narrative review of contemporary studies of families with members with eating disorders, Erriu et al. (2020) found a trend in that most persons and their families now living with eating disorders represented their families as connected and flexible, with low levels of entanglement, rigidity, and chaos and moderate levels of communication. This trend points toward high family unity as protecting adolescents from the risk of developing disordered eating behaviours. It is appropriate to (a) consider families as trying to function with different styles and levels of adaptation in relation to their internal organization and coping strategies and (b) take into consideration the different views of family members, as such information may represent an essential resource in healthcare settings.

KEY CONCEPT

Enmeshment refers to an extreme form of intensity in family interactions.

Spiritual Theories

Spirituality involves developing a personal quest for understanding answers to ultimate questions about life, meaning, and a relationship with the transcendent even if one does believe in God, but also encompassing strong personal beliefs. One woman identified "the SOLE REASON I did not commit suicide when I was deep into my eating disorder … [was that] my religious beliefs literally saved my life" (Scott Richards et al., 2018, p. 97). Women's struggles in the formation of their body image, sense of self, relationship building, and connection with the world often reflect an underlying intergenerational journey to achieve a stable authentic self-identity (Richey et al., 2020). Meaning in life is a protective factor against eating disorder symptoms. Women may turn to disordered eating as a method of acquiring meaning to meet their deep-seated needs for purpose and value, as illustrated in a young woman's question of identity and values:

> Finding out who I was, what makes me, me and what I value, what I want to stand for, what I don't want to stand for, those type of things. What, what's life? … It

gave me something to move on with because if I was to let go of my AN, well, what'll I do? Who am I? And that gave me something to develop and explore, … something that was purposeful (Conti, 2018, p. 83).

Historically, the example of Catherine of Sienna (1347–1380), who fasted as part of extreme asceticism, demonstrated profound preoccupation with eating. Weinberger-Litman et al. (2016) have suggested that individuals who are intrinsically motivated toward religion are more internally motivated in general and are less likely to make decisions based on appearance or externalities. Intrinsic religious orientation may serve as a buffer to the development of disordered eating and body dissatisfaction via lower levels of thin-ideal internalization.

Risk Factors

Similar risk factors may put individuals at risk for AN, BN, and BED. The risk factors are classified in the same way as are the aetiologic categories: biologic, psychological, social, and spiritual (Fig. 25.3).

Biologic

Biologic risk factors include dieting, altered metabolic rate, and a history of overweight or obesity. Dieting despite weight loss and an increase in basal metabolic rate are the most studied biologic risk factors. Individuals diet because of body dissatisfaction, a need for control, an actual weight gain, and the fear of weight gain. Girls at risk for developing AN may begin to diet in response to a prepubertal weight increase. The starvation of AN may lead to binge eating followed by purging as a compensatory behaviour when restricting food intake is no longer effective or not possible to maintain. The less socially desirable symptoms (e.g., binge eating) and increasing compulsivity of existing symptoms are troubling (Potterton et al., 2020). For individuals at risk for BN, purging ensues because of fear of "becoming fat," and further dieting occurs in response to the binge eating and its associated negative effect. Those who develop obesity as a consequence of BED may have a history of "yo-yo" dieting also known as weight cycling, which has impaired their metabolic response so that over time their dieting efforts become ineffective as the cycle of gaining weight back and attempting to lose the weight recurs (Contreras et al., 2019).

High-level exercise and compulsive physical activity have been associated with eating disorder symptoms of dietary restraint, weight and shape concerns, obsession with food, poor concentration, drive for thinness, body dissatisfaction, and binge eating (Rizk et al., 2015). Youth with a history of overweight or obesity represent a substantial portion of treatment-seeking adolescents and adults with restrictive eating disorders (Rastogi & Rome, 2020) and BED (McCuen-Wurst

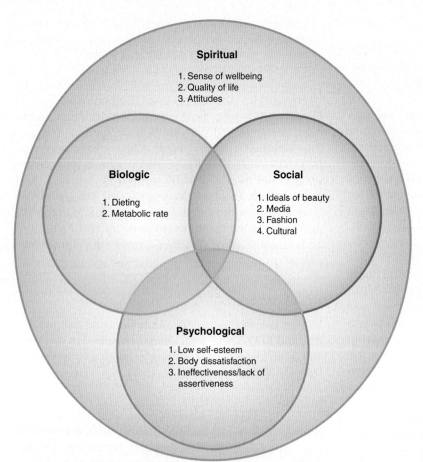

Spiritual

1. Sense of wellbeing
2. Quality of life
3. Attitudes

Biologic

1. Dieting
2. Metabolic rate

Social

1. Ideals of beauty
2. Media
3. Fashion
4. Cultural

Psychological

1. Low self-esteem
2. Body dissatisfaction
3. Ineffectiveness/lack of assertiveness

Figure 25.3 Bio/psycho/social/spiritual risk factors for eating disorders.

et al., 2018). Body dissatisfaction also predicted depressive symptoms for adolescents with low and median BMI, while adolescents with high BMI presented with higher body dissatisfaction but similar levels of depressive symptoms as adolescents with lower BMI (Carapeto et al., 2020). Adolescent girls are more likely to use disordered eating behaviours to relieve depressive symptoms, and reciprocally, disordered eating gives rise to negative self-evaluations and depressed affect (Evans et al., 2017). Early-appearing hyperactivity/inattention is a risk factor for adolescent binge eating (Sonneville et al., 2015).

Pubertal growth puts girls at increased risk relative to boys given that the pubertal physical changes (e.g., increased adiposity) move them away from society's ideal body shape for women, while physical changes in boys (i.e., increased muscle mass and shoulder width) move them closer to the sociocultural valued changes for men's body shape and size, such as athletic ability. Boys who are late maturing are more likely to have higher levels of body dissatisfaction, be less popular with their peers, have more conflict with parents, and show more depressive symptoms. Early maturation for girls is associated with more depressive symptoms and higher BMI (Hoyt et al., 2020) both of which may contribute to greater risk of body dissatisfaction.

Psychological

Depressive symptoms and low self-esteem are two psychological risk factors associated with restrictive eating (Haynos et al., 2016). In writing of their experiences with AN, women expressed constant performance anxiety, low self-esteem, depressed state of mind, and self-destructive behaviours and engaged in self-harm practices of cutting, vomiting, or extreme physical training stating "Nothing cures pain as effectively as pain" (Dahlborg Lyckhage et al., 2015, p. 4). Adolescent girls who experience low body esteem and high social appearance anxiety were more at risk to develop disturbed eating behaviours (Li, 2020). Low body esteem is a negative experience, usually accompanied with body shame, rumination, and negative social appearance evaluation fears and anxiety. This can, in turn, direct individuals to lose weight to maintain what they consider to be a "good" body shape and may result in problematic eating behaviours. Instead of seeing their eating problems as a problematic set of behaviours and cognitions that are separate from the self, they view them as reflections of their self-worth. Women with restricting AN report higher scores on perceived physical appearance and global self-worth than do those with the binge-eating–purging subtype or BN as illustrated by "I think I was worth more as a person when I was anorexic than when I'm bulimic, I sort of think of it as a very hierarchical thing" (Mortimer, 2019, p. 369).

Self-compassion, the tendency to respond to one's own suffering by adopting an attitude of caring and kindness rather than judgment and by viewing personal pain as common within humanity rather than as isolating, influences body satisfaction and eating pathology. Pullmer et al. (2019) found self-compassion was positively related to body satisfaction and negatively related to eating pathology in Canadian boys and girls, and higher self-compassion protected girls against declines in body satisfaction and increases in eating pathology. Fears that self-compassion will result in a failure to meet personal and interpersonal standards and will give rise to difficult emotions such as grief and unworthiness (emotional vulnerability) lower self-compassion and readiness to self improve and recover (Geller et al., 2020).

Experiencing negative life events during childhood is a risk factor for eating disorder development or worsening. Childhood sexual abuse is associated with binge–purging behaviours (AN binge–purge [AN-BP]), BN, BED, and subclinical forms of BN and BED (Micali et al., 2017). Sexual abuse perpetrated by a nonstranger was twice as prevalent among women with AN-BP, but as prevalent as sexual abuse by a stranger for BN and BED. Childhood unhappiness was associated with higher odds of developing restricting AN, BN, BED, and subclinical purging. Childhood life events of parental separation or divorce were positively associated with all but subclinical eating disorders. Reporting low maternal warmth was also associated with increased BN, BED, and subclinical binge-eating and purging disorders. Women who reported a more oppressive relationship with parents had higher odds of developing AN-BP, BED, subclinical BN, AN, and purging.

An external locus of control was associated with BED and interpersonal sensitivity with all eating disorders (Micali et al., 2017). Perceived criticism and parental expectations of perfectionism were associated with bulimic behaviours, while more positive maternal care was protective for BN (La Mela et al., 2015). In addition to perfectionism, the trait of impulsivity has been associated with the presence of binge eating, laxative misuse, fasting, and frequency of vomiting (Schaumberg et al., 2020). In contrast, anxiety was associated with exercise, fasting, concern over mistakes, high standards, and parental expectations.

The prevalence of disordered eating behaviours for most sexual orientation groups decreased between 1999–2001 and 2011–2013; however, the odds of fasting, using diet pills, and purging to control weight remained mostly unchanged for women who are bisexual and increased among women who are lesbians (Watson et al., 2017). LGBTQI2SA+ students report a significantly higher prevalence of disordered eating than heterosexual students.

Women report higher levels of binge-eating symptoms, anxiety, and stress than men; women have higher rates of BED. Further study of the idea that binge eating may serve to decrease one domain (i.e., anxiety) but increase another (i.e., depression) is recommended (Rosenbaum & White, 2015). In a review of the associations between men of colour and eating disorder, Stewardson et al. (2020) found that being a member of a racial group having experiences of discrimination, racism, and acculturative stress, and regular exposure to idealized media images of bodies of White men that do not affirm one's own body, may increase risk for body dissatisfaction. A history of obesity has also been shown to be linked to eating disorders and body image dissatisfaction in men of colour (Stewardson et al., 2020).

Social

In families, weight teasing and parental under involvement are correlates of childhood BED (Saltzman & Liechty, 2016). Although family meals protect against dieting for girls whose families engaged in no or low-level weight-related teasing, exposure to family meals became a risk factor for engaging in dieting when weight teasing was present (Loth et al., 2015). Appearance-related teasing by mothers, fathers, siblings, and peers was associated with higher body dissatisfaction among girls and appearance-related teasing by fathers was associated with a greater drive for muscularity among boys (Schaefer & Salafia, 2014). Sibling teasing was reported more frequently than teasing from mothers or fathers, and the odds of being teased by siblings increased dramatically if adolescents were teased by either parent. Beyond adolescence, men who receive negative commentary (compared to positive commentary) are more likely to experience eating pathology and body dissatisfaction and report more dieting behaviours (Schuster et al., 2013).

The media, the fashion industry, and society's focus on the ideal body type are social risk factors for eating disorders. In addition, peer pressure and attitudes reinforce societal messages regarding the importance of thinness or popularity. Some adolescents reported that dieting, binge eating, and purging were learned behaviours that resulted from peer pressure and a perceived need to conform. As demonstrated by their scores on eating behaviour scales, young women who experienced weight-related teasing by peers during childhood and adolescence were more likely to develop disturbed eating behaviours and eating disorders than were their non–weight-teased peers. Bullying predicts eating disorder symptoms for both bullies and victims, with victims displaying increases in anorexic, bulimic, and binge-eating symptoms and bullies having high prevalence of both binge eating and vomiting. In a longitudinal study across a 4-year interval of 10- to 14-year-olds who lived in households of middle incomes in Canada, girls reported significantly higher bullying victimization at every time point except grade 6, higher symptoms of anxiety at every time point, and higher levels of disordered eating behaviour in grade 8. Both girls and boys with disordered eating behaviour were at elevated risk of being bullied by their peers (Lee & Vaillancourt, 2019). Being victimized increased the risk of perpetrating future bullying, which in turn catalyzed disordered eating behaviour. The experience of criticizing/teasing others may sensitize bullies to their own physical attributes and shortcomings; bullies may experience regret or guilt following bullying incidents, and this contributes to impulsive eating behaviours (Copeland et al., 2015).

Although peers increase in importance throughout adolescence, romantic partners become primary sources of personal feedback and satisfaction during adulthood. In a community-based study, women reported the onset of eating disorder symptoms were triggered by abusive intimate relationships, weight-related teasing from a partner, and coping with neglect or overcontrolling by a partner (Mitchison et al., 2016).

The ways in which individuals cope with weight stigma from the public can be seen as risk factors for promoting or prolonging adverse eating behaviours. For example, exposure to weight-stigmatizing stimuli in individuals with obesity and BED reinforces binge-eating intentions and behaviour and leads to increased calorie consumption. Negative stereotypes toward individuals with BN and AN promote social rejection and limit help seeking. People were found to have more blame, distrust, and desire for social distance with a person experiencing AN, BN, and BED compared to a person living with major depressive episodes; moreover, persons experiencing BED and obesity elicited more blame and were held most responsible for their situation (Thörel et al., 2020).

Athletes are at greater risk for developing disorders. The actual performance demands of a sport and the sports environment itself can intensify body- and weight-related concerns because of such factors as pressure from coaches and parents, social comparisons with teammates, team weigh-ins, physique-revealing uniforms, and judging criteria. Elite athletes are particularly at risk (Stoyel et al., 2020). Ballet dancers are at high risk because of the need to maintain a particular appearance and performance, and athletes for other sports are at risk for developing eating disorders. In particular, boys and men involved in weight-classed sports that necessitate weight restrictions, such as wrestling, bodybuilding, rowing, ski jumping, and swimming, are more likely to engage in pathogenic eating and weight control behaviours than are endurance athletes.

Spiritual

Research into the relationship of spirituality and eating pathology is emerging and findings conflictive. Some research suggests that specific aspects of religious involvement are protective against the development of body dissatisfaction and dysfunctional eating. For example, attendance and prayer buffer the relationship between binge eating and self-esteem. Also seeing one's body as having sacred qualities is associated with more body satisfaction and less body objectification (Tiggemann & Hage, 2019). Spirituality's general emphasis on greater purpose and connectedness may encourage individuals to define themselves more by their contributions to society or relationships than by their appearance, perhaps promoting self-acceptance regardless of their discrepancy or similarity to a cultural ideal. In other research, the importance of religion in one's life has been recently correlated with greater eating pathology. Goulet et al. (2017) suggest that women who place greater importance on religion may be more attentive to religious teachings about fasting for religious purposes or reconciliation for sins (e.g., gluttony). As well, worrying about being deserted by God/Higher Power or seeking to avoid attachment to God/Higher Power (Buser & Gibson, 2016) are associated with increased levels of bulimic symptoms.

Interdisciplinary Treatment

Treatment of the client who experiences AN focuses on initiating nutritional rehabilitation, resolving conflicts around body image disturbance, increasing effective coping, addressing the underlying conflicts related to maturity fears and role conflict, and assisting the family with healthy functioning and communication. The preferred method of treatment is outpatient care that includes family-based interventions if the client is a child or adolescent (Couturier et al., 2020). The acuity of the eating disorder is carefully monitored. Inpatient hospital admission is warranted if health deteriorates and the client meets the criteria outlined in Table 25.2. Clients are often ambivalent about being admitted for weight restoration. Considering the difficulty clients experience in consenting to relinquish the AN, Woodside et al. (2016) recommend the adult client and clinician mutually negotiate a set of goals and plan with no preconceived notions, aside from goals that are realistic for the setting and consistent with the maintenance or improvement of health.

Treatment goals are developed around medical stabilization, nutritional rehabilitation to achieve weight restoration, management of refeeding and its potential complications, and interruption of purging/compensatory behaviours. For full recovery from an eating disorder, weight restoration alone is not a sufficient end goal. It is important that distorted body image and

Table 25.2	Criteria for Hospitalization of Children, Adolescents, and Adults With Eating Disorders

Presence of One or More of the Following:

Medical	Psychiatric
<ul><li>Weight loss that is</li><li>≤75% below median BMI for age, sex, and height</li><li>Rapid, for example, >15% in 1 mo</li><li>Associated with physiologic instability unexplained by another medical condition</li><li>Rapidly approaching weight at which physiologic instability occurred in the past</li><li>BMI < 16 for adults</li><li>Heart rate for children, adolescents, and adults (resting daytime) <40 bpm</li><li>ECG abnormalities (e.g., bradycardia, other cardiac arrhythmias, prolonged QT)</li><li>Cardiac oedema</li><li>Hemodynamic compromise (bradycardia, hypotension, hypothermia)</li><li>Orthostasis</li><li>Hypoglycaemia</li><li>Electrolyte disturbance (hypokalaemia, hyponatraemia, hypophosphataemia, and/or metabolic acidosis or alkalosis)</li><li>Acute medical complications due to starvation (e.g., syncope, seizures, cardiac failure, pancreatitis)</li><li>Comorbid medical or psychiatric condition that hinders appropriate outpatient treatment (e.g., severe depression, suicide ideation, obsessive–compulsive disorder, type 1 diabetes)</li><li>Uncertainty of the diagnosis of an eating disorder</li></ul>	<ul><li>Acute food refusal</li><li>Suicidal thoughts or actions</li><li>Significant comorbid diagnosis that interferes with the treatment of an eating disorder (e.g., severe depression, OCD, anxiety)</li><li>Failure of outpatient treatment</li><li>Uncontrollable binge eating and/or purging</li><li>Inadequate social support and/or follow-up medical or psychiatric care</li></ul>

Source: Academy for Eating Disorders' Medical Care Standards Committee. (2016). Eating disorders: A guide to medical care: Critical points for early recognition & medical risk management in the care of individuals with eating disorders. In *AED REPORT* (3rd ed.). [Endorsed by the Canadian Paediatric Society]. https://www.aedweb.org/publications/medical-care-standards

other disordered thoughts/behaviours, psychological comorbidities, and social or functional impairments be addressed. Treatment requires an interdisciplinary approach of professionals who together strive to meet the multidisciplinary needs of the client (Lock et al., 2015). Dieticians plan a weight-increasing program; physicians, nurses, psychologists, and social workers monitor the refeeding process and its effects and establish the intensive therapies that must be instituted after the refeeding phase. Team members may include a consulting psychiatrist, occupational therapist, and dentist. Family must be considered members of the team.

Individuals may not present as emaciated. They may not be convinced that they have a condition that needs treatment, or they are ashamed to volunteer personal information to a health professional (Davies, 2017). It is, therefore, important to remember the high rates of mortality and medical complications among individuals with eating disorders. If they are severely malnourished and their somatic systems are seriously compromised, then a medical unit might be the choice for the initial intensive refeeding phase that requires close monitoring (see Table 25.1). The intensive therapies needed to help clients with their underlying issues (e.g., body dissatisfaction and low self-esteem) and families with

communication typically begin after refeeding because concentration is usually impaired in the severely undernourished individual. During this phase of treatment, a privilege-earning program is often implemented in which positive reinforcers, such as having visitors and receiving passes to go outside the hospital, are earned based on weight gain. After an acceptable weight (at least 85% of ideal) is established, the client may be discharged to a partial hospitalization program or an intensive outpatient program. Art therapy and psychodrama may be more effective than traditional group therapy for adolescents during the acute phases, when the concentration required for verbal therapy may be impaired. Art therapy can provide access to feelings and emotions that have long been repressed or suppressed, and this increases bodily awareness, helping to clarify central problems such as identity (Kramer, 2015). Family therapy typically begins while the individual is still hospitalized. The first Canadian Practice Guidelines developed to evaluate the evidence on treatments focused specifically on children and adolescents diagnosed with eating disorders strongly recommends family-based treatment (FBT) and the least intensive treatment environment for AN or BN, especially for those who have been ill less than 3 years (Couturier et al., 2020).

Pharmacologic Interventions

Many experts claim that the symptoms of AN, such as body distortion and hyperactivity, are primarily the result of starvation, which causes changes in brain chemistry. Therefore, restoring weight influences symptom remission more than psychopharmacology. It is generally held that the core symptoms of AN are unresponsive to psychotropic medications; however, these medications may be useful in treating comorbid psychiatric conditions and preventing relapses (Garner et al., 2016). For safety, tricyclic antidepressants and monoamine oxidase inhibitors are not recommended (Marvanova & Gramith, 2018). Use of selective serotonin reuptake inhibitors (SSRIs) are not efficacious for the early treatment of AN, possibly because low body weights cause low protein stores and protein is needed for SSRI metabolism. However, SSRIs can be effective later, during outpatient treatment and after weight restoration, to address symptoms such as obsessiveness, ritualistic behaviours, and perfectionism. SSRIs must be used with caution, and the client's weight must be constantly monitored because, during the initiation phase, some SSRIs may cause weight loss. Bupropion is contraindicated because of increased risk of seizures (Valeant Canada, 2017). Attia et al. (2019) documented a modest therapeutic effect of olanzapine compared with placebo on weight in adult outpatients being treated for AN but found no evidence that olanzapine had a significant impact on obsessionality and overconcern with gaining weight. In fact, shape concerns increased more among clients in the olanzapine group than among those in the placebo group. Marzola et al. (2015) found promising results on the effectiveness of aripiprazole augmentation in reducing eating-related obsessions and compulsions, although caution is needed when interpreting these findings as those clients who were started with an augmentation agent were characterized by greater clinical severity upon admission than those who received SSRIs as monotherapy.

There is no evidence to support the efficacy of mood stabilizers (e.g., lithium) for treating AN (Couturier et al., 2020). These medications should be used if comorbid bipolar disorders are identified (Tseng et al., 2017) and with extreme caution in clients with dehydration and compromised renal function. Investigation of prokinetic agents to alleviate gastrointestinal complaints associated with refeeding (e.g., bloating, early satiety) resulted in removal of cisapride (Prepulsid) from the market because of potentially fatal cardiac effects (Kerr, 2016). Oestrogen replacement therapy in the form of oral contraceptive pills has not been found effective in preventing osteopenia/osteoporosis in AN (Steinman & Shibli-Rahhal, 2019). A practical reason to refrain from using hormonal therapy is that it may cause resumption of menses, which in turn may give a false sense of being cured and reinforce denial in women who are still at a low weight. The use of bisphosphonates has shown a trend toward improved bone mass density in women living with AN, but the evidence is still insufficient at this point (Steinman & Shibli-Rahhal, 2019). No significant improvement was found in adolescents living with AN. These differing results in adults versus adolescents may reflect differences in bone turnover in the two age groups. Because bisphosphonates with their extremely long half-life can persist in the body for many years after the discontinuation of treatment and possibly affect foetal bone development, their use is cautioned in adolescents and young women of reproductive age. Body weight is the most important determinant of bone density; optimal intervention promotes weight restoration. Therefore, standard treatment for AN consists of nutritional rehabilitation and psychotherapy. There is little evidence supporting the use of medications (Walsh, 2017).

Priority Care Issues

Age at first hospital admission, percentage of ideal body weight, comorbidities, and hypotension were significantly associated with increased mortality risk. Predictors of clinical recovery include short duration of inpatient treatment, short duration of disorder, early age at first inpatient treatment, and insight (Errichiello et al., 2016). In Canada, the limited number of specialized, publicly funded ED clinics or treatment centres are mainly concentrated in urban areas in British Columbia, Alberta, Ontario, Quebec, and Nova Scotia. Most provinces have private clinics and practitioners, while there exist little to no services in the territories (Canadian Eating Disorders Alliance, 2019). A milestone document, the *Canadian Eating Disorders Strategy: 2019–2029*, developed through direct conversations and surveys targeted at the general public, professionals, caregivers, and people with lived experience recommends prevention, public education and awareness, treatment, caregiver support, training, and research. The focus of prevention is on early identification and identification of people at risk of developing eating disorders, appropriate messaging in specific settings (e.g., schools), and timely referral to either information resources or appropriate care. Public education to mitigate stigmatization, low mental health literacy, and the barriers to treatment and detection is needed (Canadian Eating Disorders Alliance, 2019).

Consistent with principles in the Canada Health Act, all Canadians living with eating disorders must have equitable access to medically necessary services no matter where they live and without discrimination. Varying levels of care available across the country include (a) short-term residential facilities with meal support and around-the-clock care for individuals who are medically stable but require intensive levels of service; (b) inpatient units within specialized eating disorder units or medical units of general hospitals for those who are medically unstable or require intensive 24-h care and support to interrupt their symptoms and/or initiate weight restoration; (c) day treatment group-based programs housed in tertiary care facilities for those who are medically stable but who require intensive 6 to 10 h of support every day for 4 to 5 days per week; (d) intensive outpatient programs for those who require less intensive treatment than a day treatment program but more services than one treatment contact per week; (e) outpatient programs usually housed in hospitals providing group-based and individual therapy by an interdisciplinary team; (f) step-down outpatient services for inpatient and day treatment programs that offer once/week individual psychological therapy and medical/dietetic monitoring; and (g) transitional/supportive housing for individuals who have completed more intensive training to reside until they are able to return to their home communities. General, paediatric, and adult eating disorder programs differ in availability of interprofessional teams, services offered, and treatment inclusion and exclusion criteria.

This fragmented system results in Canadians having unequal access to care as there are some provinces that have no treatment centres available, or it results in care not matched to the client's developmental or symptom level needs. Early treatment of eating disorders has been shown to lead to better recovery outcomes, particularly in the length of illness and likelihood of recovery. *Canadian Eating Disorders Strategy 2019–2029* recommends funding and implementing specialized services to address eating disorders across all levels of treatment intensity. It recommends that networks in provinces and territories where they do not exist be established and linked to pan-Canadian networks to coordinate resources and collaborative care. The experiences of Melanie, the woman from New Brunswick who traveled weekly to another province to obtain help for eating disorders (see In-A-Life box, Roadblocks in the Struggle to Recover), illustrate provincial health inequities. Clients fall through the cracks when their symptoms or demographics (e.g., rural, LGBTQI2SA+ community, men, communities of Indigenous Peoples, Northern communities, cultural and ethnic underrepresented groups) do not match the available services in their geographical region. As well, the delivery of bilingual, culturally appropriate, and gender-sensitive training for health professionals is recommended to help those in situations similar to Melanie's receive appropriate care and services.

Opportunities to help health professionals develop skills in providing care and services to persons experiencing eating disorders include workshops, conferences, and online learning modules offered by eating disorder specialists or provincial discipline-based associations. Other recommendations for training health professionals are job shadowing, clinical supervision by another professional in a specialized eating disorder program, developing a learning credit-based continuing professional development webinar series by Canadian eating disorder specialists, and creating a task force to identify minimum standards for graduate education in eating disorders within all health disciplines. Advanced research training will further innovation in the field and help clinical research findings reach clinicians across the country, benefiting individuals who experience eating disorders. Also recommended is more help for family caregivers through better financial supports, improved access to resources and respite care, more flexible workplaces, and appropriate engagement as part of the care team.

The importance of a co-ordinated continuum of care from outpatient to residential care is emphasized. This need is particularly apparent for those who require intensive inpatient and residential services, those who are medically stable but have psychiatric comorbidities, and those who need longer term treatment in a highly structured environment.

In 2017, over 3.3 million healthy life years worldwide were lost because of eating disorders. A standardized mortality ratio of 5.2 was reported for AN (van Hoeken & Hoek, 2020). According to the Canadian Eating Disorders Alliance (2019), the overall mortality rate for eating disorders is between 10% and 15%, and together, AN and BN kill approximately 1,000 to 1,500 Canadians per year. The true lethality of eating disorders is hidden when death certificates do not record eating disorders as the cause of death but instead record the medical complication that killed the person or, if applicable, suicide, as the cause of death.

Most recently, the COVID-19 pandemic has triggered those who have eating disorders. Because eating disorder behaviours are constructed around anxiety and unpredictability, turning to food or eating rituals gives people the illusion that they have a sense of control and predictability (Hensley, 2020). Therefore, the idea of certain items being unavailable in grocery stores during the COVID-19 pandemic can escalate anxiety. Pairing that with self-isolation and global anxiety and unpredictability is a dangerous combination for those dealing with an eating disorder. These clients are at high physical risk (e.g., frailty in AN, electrolyte disturbances in BN, and cardiovascular risk in BED) and psychological stress due to confinement, distress caused by uncertainty, and decreased usual treatment (Dalle Grave, 2020).

Stigma, discussed previously as a risk factor for promoting or prolonging adverse eating behaviours, is an issue that may impede seeking treatment. Because eating disorders are perceived as trivial and self-inflicted, affected individuals believe they are not ill enough to seek help and personally responsible for their condition. When the aetiology of AN was conceptualized as biologic rather than sociocultural, Bannatyne and Abel (2015) found lower levels of reported blame-based stigma among university students.

Nursing Management: Human Response to Anorexia Nervosa Disorder

Establishing therapeutic alliance with individuals who live with AN may be difficult initially because they may be suspicious and mistrustful. They often express fear of adults, especially healthcare professionals, whom they believe want to "make them fat." They are often impatient and irritable because of low body weight and

starvation. A matter of fact, accepting approach is important. Providing a rationale for all interventions helps build trust. Power struggles regarding eating are common; remaining nonreactive is a challenge. In avoiding such power struggles, the nurse monitors and reduces personal feelings of frustration and need for control (see Box 25.6).

Nursing management involves bio/psycho/social/spiritual assessment and interventions (see Box 25.7).

Biologic Domain

Assessment

A thorough evaluation of the client's body systems is important because many systems can be compromised by starvation. A detailed history from both the individual with AN and the family, including the length and duration of symptoms, such as avoiding meals and over exercising, is necessary to assess altered nutrition. The longer the duration of these behaviours typically means more difficult and prolonged recovery.

BOX 25.6 THERAPEUTIC DIALOGUE

The Client With an Eating Disorder

Ineffective Approach

Nurse: You haven't eaten your lunch yet.
Client: I can't. I'm already fat.
Nurse: Look at you, you're skin and bones.
Client: I'll eat when I go out this afternoon on pass.
Nurse: You can't go on pass. You have to start realizing that you are sick. Because you can't take care of yourself, we are in charge.
Client: You're trying to control me.
Nurse: We are trying to be responsible.
Client: I won't eat!
Nurse: Then you will also lose the next pass.
Client: Well I won't go out! At least I won't get fatter.

Effective Approach

Nurse: You haven't eaten your lunch.
Client: I can't. I'm already fat.
Nurse: You're uncomfortable with how you see yourself and with eating?
Client: I'll eat when I go out on pass.
Nurse: You and I and the other members of your treatment team wrote your behavioural plan together.

You know then that you will not be able to go out because your pass is dependent on you eating both breakfast and lunch.
Client: You're trying to control me.
Nurse: The plan is to help you learn to take control over the eating disorder. It sure does mean a lot of hard work for you. How can I help you right now with this meal?
Client: What if I eat half?
Nurse: You are to eat all of it. Why don't I sit here while you eat? Eating is scary for you. We can talk about other choices you have on the unit; tonight, you can choose the movie or board games.
Client: Okay, at least I have some choices.

CRITICAL THINKING CHALLENGE

• What effect did the first interaction have on the client's behaviour? Why?
• In the second interaction, what theories and interventions regarding eating disorders did the nurse use in her approach to the client?

BOX 25.7 NURSING CARE PLAN

NURSING CARE PLAN FOR A CLIENT WITH AN, BINGE–PURGE TYPE

Maddison is a 19-year-old university student who is 163 cm (5′4″) tall and weighs 44.4 kg (98 lb). A 2nd year Arts student, she initially sought treatment at the University of Calgary Medical Clinic for diarrhoea, cramps, gas, and bloating, saying "I think I have a nervous stomach." She tells the nurse that she is having difficulty sleeping, is stressed out to the point of wanting to stay in bed all day, and states "I feel like such a waste of a university education. I have been trying so hard to be my best and do well. But I can't seem to function. It might be best if I took enough sleeping pills to never wake up!"

Maddison believes that her eating is out of control. Unwanted eating binges as often as once or twice a day have provoked her to try to avoid the feared weight gain through taking laxatives in addition to self-inducing vomiting after eating what she perceives as too much. "I force myself to vomit when I eat regular salad dressing instead of fat-free. I shouldn't be eating so much and it takes so long to get it all back out of my stomach! But I can't let myself get fat again like I was in high school. I felt sad all the time then, as I do now. But never again will I let others call me 'Fatty Maddy' or take advantage of me." She added "I'm so on my own. I can't go out with my friends because they always want me to go and eat or drink with them. I don't want them to find me puking in the restaurant or bar toilet. They say I am lucky to have such a fast metabolism. Little do they know that inside I am falling apart! Right now, I can't handle the 25-minute train ride home from the university without bingeing and purging. I even developed the insane habit of bingeing on chips in the back of the train and throwing up into my empty Red Bull can. I pray to God that nobody ever saw it!"

Maddison was hospitalized for suicidality and assessment of anorexia nervosa, binge–purge type.

Setting: Inpatient Psychiatric Unit

Baseline Assessment: Maddison appears dishevelled and tearful. She discloses she has been watching her diet since high school and began using laxatives to help prevent her from gaining as she sometimes binges on potato chips and energy drinks. Her symptoms of binge eating and purging worsened over the past month as a result of realizing past sexual abuse by an older relative. She is depressed and angry and has not told anyone about the abuse.

History: Maddison lives alone in an apartment just outside city limits. She weighs herself before and after every meal or snack. She lost 12 kg since graduating from high school 2 years ago, by skipping meals and restricting the quantity of food consumed. She had tried using diet tea and slimming pills on a few occasions. Despite being underweight, she perceives herself as being "too fat." She acknowledges the frequency of self-induced vomiting as 7 to 10 times per week; she takes 6 Ex-Lax tablets daily "to hurry the food out of my system." Maddison has occasionally experienced heart palpations, weakness, dizziness, and fatigue. She feels ashamed and guilty about binge eating, self-induced vomiting, and laxative use. She perceives her weight to be much higher than she wishes and desires a slimmer face and thinner legs. She feels that she deserves punishment for her eating behaviour and is contemplating suicide.

Physical findings include dehydration and swollen parotid glands. BMI = 16.7. Laboratory results are all within normal range except for slightly elevated amylase level (116 μ/L suggesting she has been vomiting) and slight metabolic alkalosis (elevated serum bicarbonate level = 33 mmol/L). The only slightly elevated serum bicarbonate level despite vomiting may relate to her misuse of laxatives, which decreases serum bicarbonate levels due to loss of alkaline fluid from the bowel. Her electrocardiogram shows sinus bradycardia. Her menstruation is irregular, 3 to 4 days duration every 30 to 45 days. Her scores on the drive for thinness, bulimia, interoceptive awareness, and perfectionism subscales of the Eating Disorder Inventory (EDI) are significantly increased when compared with the scores of normal undergraduates who are women in North America.

Upon admission, Maddison's fluoxetine hydrochloride dose was increased from 20 to 40 mg. She is encouraged to participate in the psychiatric unit milieu by normalizing her mealtime frequency to three times daily with an evening snack to reduce the binge-eating and purging episodes. She is also expected to start interpersonal therapy (IPT) and attend the unit's stress management group that aims to improve coping strategies.

Associated Psychiatric Diagnosis	Medications
Anorexia nervosa Binge-eating/purging type	

Continued on following page

NURSING CARE PLAN (*Continued*)

Nursing Care Focus 1: Suicide Risk

Defining Characteristics	Related Factors
Feelings of worthlessness	History of sexual trauma
Difficulty sleeping, wanting to stay in bed all day	History of obesity and weight discrimination
Feels hurt, sad, deserving of punishment, angry	She wants to never again be victimized
"I feel like such a waste of a university education … It might be best if I took enough sleeping pills to never wake up!"	

Outcomes

Initial	Long Term
Agrees to seek out nurse if feeling suicidal	Develops self-compassion, self-acceptance
Remains safe from self-harm	Develops alternative and positive ways of coping

Interventions

Interventions	Rationale	Ongoing Assessment
Initiate a nurse–client relationship, convey acceptance of Maddison as a deserving, worthwhile person.	The nurse–client relationship builds trust and acceptance.	Assess the development of trust.
Initiate suicide precautions as per institution policy. Frequent regular round-the-clock observations.	Maddison's safety is the priority of care.	Determine risk of self-harm.
Support Maddison to contact sexual assault centre for information, self-care skills training, therapeutic/social support, and assistance with reconciliation measures as wanted.	Coping strategies and support can facilitate moving past the trauma, rebuilding sense of control and self-worth, and developing resilience.	Evaluate self-care capacity.
Help promote sleep hygiene.	Attention to environment, limiting consumption of caffeine, and establishing a regular bedtime routine improves sleep.	Assess quality of sleep by asking if Maddison feels rested upon awakening.

Evaluation

Outcomes	Revised Outcomes	Interventions
Entered a no-harm contract with the nurse	Has not harmed self; denies self-harm ideas/intentions. Agrees to continue the contract with outpatient clinic nurse after discharge	
Connects with others via participation in the unit milieu and community supports		

Nursing Care Focus 2: Altered Nutrition: Malnutrition Risk

Defining Characteristics	Related Factors
Underweight; BMI below healthy range	Purging (self-induced vomiting and laxative misuse)
Electrolyte and metabolic disturbances	Decreased potassium level from vomiting and laxative use
Weakness, dizziness, and fatigue	Dehydrated

NURSING CARE PLAN (*Continued*)

Outcomes

Initial	Long Term
Adhere to meal and snack schedule of hospital. This decreases the incidence of binge eating, which is often precipitated by starvation and fasting	Eats three nondieting meals and at least one snack per day. Maintains healthy BMI
Ceases purging for 1 week	Develops positive ways of managing emotions and stress rather than binging and purging

Interventions

Interventions	Rationale	Ongoing Assessment
Continue to develop a therapeutic relationship with Maddison. Encourage her to verbalize feelings such as anxiety related to food, weight, and situations associated with or that trigger binge eating.	Through relationship with the nurse and examining her feelings, Maddison may be more likely to cooperate with the nutritional regimen.	Determine anxiety level when discussing food, body image, and weight. Support Maddison in following her nutritional regimen.
Monitor meals and snacks; record the amount eaten.	Skipping meals triggers hunger, which may precipitate an episode of binge eating. Binge eating triggers the compulsion to purge.	Assess Maddison's ability to complete regularly scheduled meals.
Teach to incorporate adequate daily fibre intake.	To restore normal peristalsis without laxatives.	Monitor BM pattern.
Encourage making a journal of incidents and feelings before, during, and after binge episode.	To increase understanding and responsibility taking.	Assist Maddison in identifying triggers to binge eating.
Monitor Maddison's behaviour after meals and snacks for purging. Monitor vital signs daily, electrolytes regularly.	Physical signs of impending complications include evidence of purging, hypotension, and hypokalaemia. Reduce potential for cardiac arrhythmia associated with hypokalaemia from purging.	Monitor vital signs, weight, and electrolytes, especially potassium.
Assist Maddison to identify activities to try if she feels compelled to purge. Contract with Maddison to approach the nurse when she feels the urge to binge or purge so that feelings and alternative ways of coping can be explored.	Positive coping skills will enable her to build capacity to hold and mitigate distress.	Monitor restless behaviour. Evaluate her practice of activities to delay a binge or purge.
Provide psychoeducational intervention. Teach risks of laxative dependency, foods to meet potassium needs, dangers of caffeine-laced energy drinks and slimming pills, importance of adequate water intake, ineffectiveness and risks of purging to prevent weight gain, and role of potassium in heart and muscle function.	Increase awareness of health needs and risks.	Observe comprehension of material.

Continued on following page

NURSING CARE PLAN (*Continued*)

Evaluation

Outcomes	Revised Outcomes	Interventions
Maddison cooperates with meal regimen.	Ceases purging episodes for 1 week. Approaches nurse if she feels driven to binge or purge.	Regular blood work. Praise her successes. Arrange for discharge to outpatient or community clinic.
She has begun to acknowledge the seriousness of her illness and the life-threatening aspects of dieting and purging.	Establish and maintain regular, adequate nutritional eating habits.	Participation in relapse prevention classes.

Nursing Care Focus 3: Distorted Perception in Body Size and Shape

Defining Characteristics	Related Factors
Verbalizes that she is too fat	Inaccurate perceptions of physical appearance secondary to anorexia nervosa Desires a slimmer face and thinner legs
"I have been trying so hard to be my best and do well" but not able to function at this level	Believes that she is failing to measure up to an internalized desired ideal
Hides body in baggy, loose fitting clothing	History of depression, sexual trauma, weight loss, and dieting

Outcomes

Initial	Long Term
Verbalizes feelings related to changing body shape and weight	Acknowledges negative consequences of too little fat on body
Identifies beliefs about controlling body size	Identifies positive aspects of her body and its ability to function

Interventions

Interventions	Rationale	Ongoing Assessment
Explore Maddison's beliefs and feelings about body. Maintain a nonjudgmental approach. Provide opportunities to talk about her experiences of being teased about body changes or sexual abuse.	The past experiences of sexual trauma and weight-related teasing may lead to negativity toward her body. To help Maddison gain a more positive body image, an understanding of her own views is important.	Monitor for statements that identify perceptions of her body. Is her view *distorted* or *dissatisfied*? Monitor for PTSD symptom and need for trauma-oriented psychotherapy and referral.
Assist Maddison in identifying positive and realistic physical characteristics.	In AN, the body is viewed negatively. By focusing on parts of the body that are positive, such as the eyes or hands, or that enhance function, such as strong legs for running, Maddison can begin to experience a positive image of her body.	Observe for her reaction to her body. Which areas are viewed positively? Observe for negative statements related to body size and self-esteem.
Clarify Maddison's views about an ideal body.	Many societal cues idealize an unrealistically thin woman body.	Monitor for statements indicating external pressures to lose weight.
Provide education related to normal growth of women's bodies and the protective role of fat.	Providing education will help in reinforcing a broader view of the importance of a healthy body.	Assess willingness to learn information.

NURSING CARE PLAN (*Continued*)

Evaluation

Outcomes	Revised Outcomes	Interventions
Maddison revealed her belief that she is too fat. She has difficulty identifying aspects of herself and body she likes. She believes that those who are overweight have lost control of their lives.	Maddison accepts alternative beliefs related to her own abilities and body.	Gradually, focus on other positive aspects of Maddison's whole self and body. Challenge her beliefs about loss of personal control and overweight.
Willing to read information about normal body functioning.	Maddison accepts a new view of body functioning as a complex phenomenon.	Discuss the biologic aspect of the development of body weight. Emphasize multiple factors that determine body weight.

Nursing Care Focus 4: Impaired Ability to Experience Meaning and Purpose in Life Through Connectedness With Self and Others

Defining Characteristics	Related Factors
Questions or expresses inner conflict about herself, the meaning or purpose of her life	"I'm so on my own. I can't go out with my friends."
Evinces guilt, hopelessness, despair, and/or abandonment	Tearful, depressed, and angry
Withdrawal from, or absence of, relationships	Believes others would treat her negatively if they knew she binges and purges
Guilt and shame about disordered eating behaviours and abuse	Secretive vomiting. Has not disclosed past sexual abuse to anyone

Outcomes

Initial	Long Term
Begins to express inner distress in acceptable ways (e.g., talking, journaling, art work)	Spiritual health as evidenced by using a type of spiritual experience/expression that provides her comfort. Connecting with others to share thoughts, feelings, and beliefs

Continued on following page

NURSING CARE PLAN (*Continued*)

Interventions

Interventions	Rationale	Ongoing Assessment
Model self-awareness and acceptance without harsh self-judgment.	Maddison will not trust a nurse who does not demonstrate self-comfort.	Ask, "How do you feel about the changes in your life that have come about because of the eating disorder?" "The abuse?"
Create an accepting, nonjudgmental atmosphere.	Providing ongoing, unconditional support establishes rapport and therapeutic relationship, which promotes communication, open expression, and opportunity to explore inner world of meaning and experience.	Assess her ability to see and affirm her self-worth and identity. What does she see as her strengths? Does she define herself as *the eating disorder*? The younger victim *(Fatty Maddy)*?
Spend nontask time with Maddison.	Being with the person who is suffering gives meaning to their experience. It confirms to Maddison that she is important and of value. The nurse's presence helps alleviate the client's sense of isolation, anxiety, and abandonment.	Is she feeling distant and disconnected from others? What are her relations with family? Does she know what she does and does not have control over? Does she accept her human limitations within the context of her traumatic experiences?
Encourage Maddison to experience and verbalize feelings, perceptions, and fears.	Helps her access potential healing resources to wellbeing. Releasing emotions can provide energy and freedom.	Assess her ability to name and identify her feelings.
Encourage her to identify values that guide her everyday behaviour and her actions in times of crisis, loss, and tragedy.	Helps her clarify values and beliefs by reflecting on past behaviours. Experience is a major source for values development.	Assess her ability to challenge counterproductive beliefs.
Observe and listen empathetically to her communication, offering patience, repetition, and reassurance over an extended period of time.	Listening to the "unacceptable" helps the process of finding meaning, healing, growth, and re-entering life with a renewed sense of purpose and connection to others and self.	Assess her growth beyond the prior traumatic experiences. Does she accept herself and her past? What, if anything, would she change now?
Help Maddison tell her story about the eating disorder and any painful traumatic experiences in descriptive rather than evaluative terms.	Storytelling minimizes self-judgment and allows emergence of patterns that aid understanding.	Monitor her capacity for informed understanding.
Help Maddison develop a healthy, positive outlook through such things as letter writing, meditation, and/or imagery.	Helps her access potential healing resources to enhance wellbeing and reduce negative affectivity.	Assess her ability to care for self.

Evaluation

Outcomes	Revised Outcomes	Interventions
She has begun to acknowledge the meaning of the eating disorder in her life but has not developed a non–self-blaming understanding of the abuse.	Establish and maintain appropriate self-care strategies that include adequate nutrition and eating practices and self-development.	Participation in comprehensive and individualized treatment program.

Nursing Care Focus for Biologic Domain

A primary nursing care focus is inadequate nutritional status.

Interventions for Biologic Domain

Weight restoration is the chief intervention during the hospital or initial stage of treatment for AN (Fig. 25.4). The nurse will encounter resistance to eating and weight gain and carefully monitors and records all intake as part of the weight gain protocol. For instance, an adult with an eating disorder who is significantly malnourished and has had very low intake prior to hospitalization might be safely started at approximately 1,600 kcal per day and increased by 300 kcal per day every 2 to 3 days until consistent weight gain of at least 1 to 2 kg (2 to 4 lb) per week is achieved. Children and adolescents are in a state of growth and development. Their treatment goal weights and nutritional needs will change as they continue to grow and develop. Supplemental enteral feeds may be indicated when rates of weight gain are low less than 1 kg (2 lb) per week.

Methods of refeeding that "start low and go slow" have been replaced by more rapid refeeding with close medical monitoring during inpatient treatment. The risk of refeeding syndrome is related to the degree of malnutrition at presentation (i.e., less than 70% median BMI in adolescents, BMI less than 15 in adults). Refeeding syndrome is a rare but potentially fatal condition that can occur during refeeding of severely malnourished individuals. After prolonged starvation, the body begins to use fat and protein to produce energy because there are not enough carbohydrates. Upon refeeding, there is a surge of insulin (because of the ingested carbohydrates) and a sudden shift from fat to carbohydrate metabolism. One of the key features of refeeding syndrome is hypophosphatemia (abnormally low levels of phosphate in the blood), which occurs primarily because the insulin surge during food ingestion leads to a cellular uptake of phosphate. Phosphate dysregulation affects almost every system in the body and can lead to leucocyte dysfunction, respiratory failure, cardiac failure, hypotension, arrhythmias, seizures, coma, and sudden death (Støving, 2019).

Weight-increasing protocols usually take the form of a behavioural plan, using positive reinforcements (e.g., outings or passes) and negative reinforcements (e.g., returning to bed rest). The reinforcements are incremental, informed by client preferences, and based on progress. For example, phone calls, walks around the unit, and walks outside the hospital occur before the day passes and then weekend passes. These protocols provide consistent responses to food avoidance behaviours and are carried out in a caring and supportive context. However, activity restrictions may be perceived negatively by clients (Moola et al., 2015). During the implementation of negative reinforcements, the client is helped to see that these actions are not punitive. On

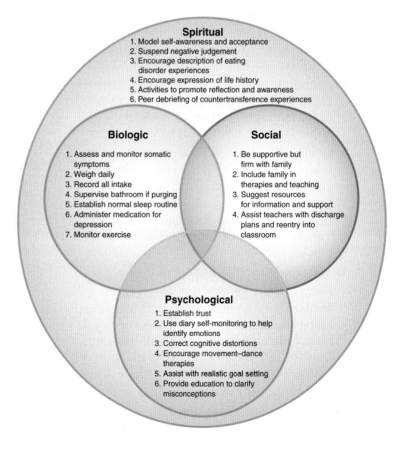

Figure 25.4 Bio/psycho/social/spiritual interventions for individuals with AN.

rare occasions when the client is unable to recognize or accept the eating disorder as harmful, nasogastric tube feedings may be necessary to enable weight restoration.

Menses history also is assessed. Most young women with AN have reached menarche but may have experienced amenorrhoea for some months because of starvation. A return to regular menses signifies substantial body fat restoration. Sleep disturbance is also common, and individuals may sleep little but usually awaken in an energized state. A structured, healthy sleep routine is established to conserve energy and calorie expenditure. To further conserve energy, clients are often relegated to bed rest until a certain amount of weight is regained. Exercise is generally not permitted during refeeding and only with caution after this phase. Inpatient clients are closely supervised because they are often found exercising in their rooms (or while on bed rest).

Psychological Domain

Assessment

The psychological symptoms that individuals with AN experience are listed in Box 25.2. The classic symptoms—low weight, unrealistic expectations and thinking, and ritualistic behaviours—may be noted during a clinical interview. Conflicts that underlie this disorder, such as maturity or independence fears and feelings of ineffectiveness, may not be apparent during the interview. Assessing individuals with low self-esteem and high social anxiety may be particularly difficult, as clients may believe the clinician is negatively evaluating them, whereas their low self-worth may make them feel that they are not worth the effort of referral or therapy.

A variety of instruments are available to clinicians and researchers for determining the presence and severity of symptoms. Box 25.8 lists well-known instruments used to assess psychological symptoms associated with eating disorders. The Eating Attitude Test is frequently used with community and clinical populations. The abbreviated 26-item version of this test, EAT-26 for adolescents and adults, is readily available online (www.eat-26.com/) and is particularly useful in screening for eating disorder risk in high school students, in university students, and in other groups such as athletes. The results can help identify the most significant symptoms and indicate if an individual should be referred for evaluation of an eating disorder.

BOX 25.8 Assessment Tools for Eating Disorder Symptoms

1. **Screening Tools**
   a. *SCOFF*

      www.ceed.org.au/sites/default/files/resources/documents/SCOFF%20Questionnaire%20August%202016.pdf

      Morgan, J. F., Reid, F., & Lacey, J. H. (1999). The SCOFF questionnaire: Assessment of a new screening tool for eating disorders. *British Medical Journal, 319*, 1467–1468.

   b. Eating Attitude Test (EAT)

      www.drshepp.com/wp-content/uploads/2015/06/eatingattitudestest.pdf

      Garner, D. M., & Garfinkel, P. E. (1979). The Eating Attitude Test: An index of the symptoms of anorexia nervosa. *Psychosomatic Medicine, 10*, 647–656.

2. **Assessment/Diagnostic Measures**
   a. *Eating Disorder Assessment for Men (EDAM)*

      Stanford, S. C., & Lemberg, R. (2012). Measuring eating disorders in men: development of the eating disorder assessment for men (EDAM). *Eating Disorders, 20*(5), 427–436. https://doi.org/10.1080/10640266.2012.715522

   b. Eating Disorder Examination

      rcpsych.ac.uk/pdf/EDE_16.0.pdf

      Cooper, Z., & Fairburn, C. G. (1987). The Eating Disorder Examination: A semi-structured interview for the assessment of the specific psychopathology of eating disorders. *International Journal of Eating Disorders, 6*, 1–8.

   c. Eating Disorder Examination Questionnaire (EDE-Q) www.phenxtoolkit.org/toolkit_content/PDF/PX230104.pdf

      Carter, J. C., Stewart, D. A., & Fairburn, C. G. (2001). Eating Disorder Examination Questionnaire: Norms for adolescent girls. *Behaviour Research and Therapy, 39*, 625–632.

   d. Eating Disorder Inventory-3 (EDI-3) and EDI-3 Symptom Checklist (EDI-3-SC)

      river-centre.org/wp-content/uploads/2015/10/EDI-3-Scale.pdf

      Garner, D. M. (2011). *Eating disorder inventory-3: Professional manual.* Psychological Assessment Resources.

   e. Yale-Brown-Cornell Eating Disorder Scale (YBC-EDS)

      www.phenxtoolkit.org/toolkit_content/PDF/PX650501.pdf

      Mazure, C. M., Halmi, K. A., Sunday, S. R., Romano, S. J., & Einhorn, A. M. (1994). Yale-Brown-Cornell Eating Disorder Scale:

BOX 25.8 Assessment Tools for Eating Disorder Symptoms *(Continued)*

Development, use, reliability, and validity. *Journal of Psychiatric Research, 28,* 425–445.

f. Three-Factor Eating Questionnaire-R18

www.med.umich.edu/pdf/weight-management/TFEQ-r18.pdf

de Lauzon, B., Romon, M., Deschamps, V., Lafay, L., Borys, J-M., Karlsson, J., … Fleurbaix Laventie Ville Sante Study Group. (2004). The Three-Factor Eating Questionnaire-R18 is able to distinguish among different eating patterns in a general population. *Journal of Nutrition, 134*(9), 2372–2380.

3. **Tests of Body Dissatisfaction/Body Image**

a. *Body Shape Questionnaire (BSQ)*

www.psyctc.org/tools/bsq/

Cooper, P., Taylor, M., Cooper, Z., & Fairburn, C. (1987). The development and validation of the BSQ. *International Journal of Eating Disorders, 6,* 485–494.

b. Colour-a-Person Test

Wooley, S. C., & Kearney-Cooke, A. (1986). Intensive treatment of bulimia and body image disturbance. In K. D. Brownell & J. P. Foreyt (Eds.), *Handbook of eating disorders: Physiology, psychology and treatment of obesity, anorexia, and bulimia* (pp. 476–502). Basic Books.

c. Body Parts Dissatisfaction Scale

http://www.midss.org/sites/default/files/body_parts_dissatisfaction_scale.pdf

Corning, A. F., Gondoli, D. M., Bucchianeri, M. M., & Blodgett-Salafia, E. H. (2010). Preventing the development of body issues in adolescent girls through intervention with their mothers. *Body Image, 7,* 289–295.

d. Body Dissatisfaction Scale

www.nspb.net/index.php/nspb/article/view/249

Mutale, G. T., Dunn, A., Stiller, J., & Larkin, R. (1996). Development of a body dissatisfaction scale assessment tool. *The New School Psychology Bulletin, 13*(2), 47–57.

4. **Tests of Emotional and Cognitive Components**

a. *Cognitive–Behavioural Dieting Scale*

Martz, D. M., Sturgis, E. T., & Gustafson, S. B. (1996). Development and preliminary validation of the Cognitive Behavioral Dieting Scale. *International Journal of Eating Disorders, 19,* 297–309.

b. Emotional Eating Scale

Arrow, B., Kenardy, J., & Agras, W. S. (1995). The Emotional Eating Scale: The development of a measure to assess coping with negative affect by eating. *International Journal of Eating Disorders, 18,* 79–90.

c. Compulsive Eating Scale

www.moray.gov.uk/downloads/file93345.doc

Kagan, D. M., & Squires, R. L. (1984). Compulsive eating, dieting, stress, and hostility among college students. *Journal of College Student Personnel, 25*(3), 213–220.

d. The Restraint Scale (RS)

Herman, C. P., & Polivy, J. (1975). Anxiety, restraint, and eating behavior. *Journal of Abnormal Psychology, 84,* 66–72.

e. Three-Factor Eating Questionnaire Cognitive Restraint Scale (TFEQ-R)

www.med.umich.edu/pdf/weight-anagement/TFEQ-r18.pdf

Stunkard, A. J., & Messick, S. (1985). The Three-Factor Eating Questionnaire to measure dietary restraint, disinhibition, and hunger. *Journal of Psychosomatic Research, 29,* 71–83.

5. **Behavioural Tests**

a. *Test Meals*

Andersen, A. E. (1995). A standard test meal to assess treatment response in anorexia nervosa patients. *Eating Disorders, 3,* 47–55.

6. **Risk Factors Identification**

a. *The McKnight Risk Factor Survey*

bml.stanford.edu/resources/documents/MRFS_6-12_WEB.pdf

Shisslak, C. M., Renger, R., Sharpe, T., Crago, M., McKnight, K. M., Gray, N., … Taylor, C. B. (1999). Development and evaluation of the McKnight Risk Factor Survey for assessing potential risk and protective factors for disordered eating in preadolescent and adolescent girls. *International Journal of Eating Disorders, 25*(2), 195–214.

(Versions are available for younger and older children.)

Nursing Care Focus for Psychological Domain

Two common nursing care foci in AN are anxiety and altered body image perception.

Interventions for Psychological Domain

Most individuals with AN experience interoceptive awareness problems (inability to experience visceral cues and emotions) and use a somatic complaint such as "I feel bloated" or "I'm fat" to replace a negative emotion such as guilt or anger. Although these complaints may be related to refeeding, they often are part of body dissatisfaction. Research into the experiences of women with eating disorders has demonstrated body shame as a major theme influencing self-criticism (Zelkowitz & Cole, 2019), nondisclosure (Dimitropoulos et al., 2016), and social rank perceptions (Matos et al., 2015). To make it possible for women to speak about such feelings, the nurse can normalize the shame experience in conversation with the client and can encourage clients to keep a journal, help them to identify feelings by having them write a description of the "fat feeling," and list possible underlying emotions and troublesome situations next to this description.

In preparing to interact with an individual struggling with AN, first make meaning of personal experiences with eating issues and self-preservation strategies. Self-awareness and acceptance cannot be effectively modelled without having engaged in this critical self-development. A student nurse who reflected on their belief that young people with eating disorders are manipulative could identify their own fear of being manipulated, which led to their feeling suspicious about interactions with the individual:

> There can be a lot of manipulation around eating disorders … I think that sits at the back of my mind, that I fear that I could be easily manipulated … and I don't want to let the young person down; I don't want to let them away with something (Farrington et al., 2020, p.684).

In order for the student nurse to develop their practice, a process of exploration of such personal knowledge is needed.

Box 25.9 outlines a research project to gain knowledge of health, ideal body image, healthy eating, and eating disorders from the perspective of First Nations Elders to better understand how these concepts may relate to the wellbeing of Indigenous Peoples youth.

Understanding Feelings

Identifying feelings, such as anxiety and fear, and especially negative emotions, such as anger, helps individuals decrease conflict avoidance and develop effective strategies for managing these feelings. It is unhelpful to attempt to change distorted body image by pointing out that the individual is actually too thin. This characteristic is often the last to resolve itself, and it may take years for individuals to see their bodies realistically. Body tracing, mirror exposure, and teaching techniques to facilitate body-acceptance and nonjudgmental attitude towards one's body may help individuals face the fear of hypothetical fatness in breaking the avoidance–anxiety cycle (Kostecka et al., 2019). Individuals may continue to fear "becoming fat" but no longer be driven to act on the distortion by starving. The fear of "becoming fat" eventually lessens with time.

Nurses may contribute to productive physical outcomes and a positive client experience by relying on positive and well-timed interactions. Clients have indicated that their motivation to adhere to care was derived from strong therapeutic alliance where an interest was expressed in the client as a person and not just the eating disorder and understanding of the client's feelings was demonstrated. According to an adolescent with AN-BP, "You really need to see the person and… relate to that person and then… say somebody's buried in there, it is just, you have to help pull that person out" (Zaitsoff et al., 2016, p. 253). The nurse can help individuals restructure the way they view the world, especially relative to food, eating, weight, and shape. Faulty ways of viewing these situations result in ineffective coping. Table 25.3 lists some cognitive distortions commonly experienced by individuals with eating disorders and some typical restructuring responses that challenge the distortion, which the nurse can present as more realistic ways of perceiving situations. Other therapies, such as movement and dance therapy, can help individuals experience pleasure from their bodies, although dance should be used cautiously during refeeding because of energy-expenditure concerns. Imagery and relaxation are often used to overcome distortions and decrease anxiety.

Psychotherapy

Interpersonal psychotherapy (IPT) is a type of treatment that focuses on uncovering and resolving developmental and psychological issues underlying the disorder. Role transitions, conflicts, and interpersonal deficits leading to social isolation or chronically unsatisfactory relationships typically are the focus (Melville, 2016). Cognitive–behavioural therapy (CBT) or enhanced cognitive–behaviour therapy (CBT-E) may address faulty beliefs about food and social interactions; CBT-E has been shown to be effective in eradicating the eating disorder psychopathology (i.e., disturbed way of eating and low weight, extreme weight-control behaviours, and concerns about eating, shape and weight), correcting the mechanisms that maintain the psychopathology specified in the client's formulation, and ensuring

BOX 25.9 Research for Best Practice

Alani-Verjee, T., Braunberger, P., Bobinski, T., & Mushquash, C. (2017). First Nations Elders in Northwestern Ontario's perspectives of health, body image and eating disorders. *Journal of Indigenous Wellbeing, 2*(1), 76–96. https://journalindigenouswellbeing.com/journal_articles/first-nations-elders-in-northwestern-ontarios-perspectives-of-health-body-image-and-eating-disorders/

Background: Health, healthy eating, and ideal body image often are conceptualised from a Eurocentric perspective. Indigenous Peoples' perspectives may differ and are needed to better understand eating disorders among Indigenous Peoples.

Purpose: This study sought knowledge of health, ideal body image, healthy eating, and eating disorders from the perspective of First Nations Elders to gain a better understanding of these concepts, and how they may relate to the wellbeing of Indigenous youth.

Methods: Five Elders living in Northwestern Ontario were interviewed and each transcript was thematically analyzed. Elders were chosen as participants because they are considered the holders of knowledge, and their wisdom and stories are valued by others. Ongoing consultation with these Elders entailed sharing and discussing the themes with them to ensure their perspectives were appropriately captured.

Findings: First Nations belief systems affirm health as balance in all parts of the Medicine Wheel and that health and illness can exist simultaneously as long as this balance is maintained. Physical attractiveness is having "balance" and being "strong" and able-bodied; beauty is in one's definition of self-worth, not about conforming to external standards. Prior to contact with Europeans, Indigenous Peoples' ideal bodies were healthy bodies. The process of colonization forced many children to move away from their families and into boarding school-type facilities with high rates of physical, emotional, and sexual abuse. Connections with family and Indigenous identity were lost. Consequences also included increased consumption of store-bought food high in sugar, salt, or fat, and lower levels of activity related to food procurement. Food consumption was further related to emotion regulation and coping with negative feelings. Choosing to eat salt, sugar, and foods high in fat that are often the most pleasurable and cheapest foods to access may relate to engaging in overeating, and similarly to drugs and addictions. Society creates an environment detrimental to achieving health where Indigenous Peoples are more likely to experience jealousy, fear, and shame through representations in the media. Colonization and current messages in the media negatively affect Indigenous people's body image, creating a shift away from understanding beauty as health and balance. Disordered eating emanates from not feeling good about oneself and using food as a coping mechanism.

Implications for Nursing: Current expectations of health, body image, and healthy eating do not necessarily align with First Nations understandings of these concepts. Conceptualizations of eating disorder etiology, symptom presentations, and consequences need to be understood via culturally relevant explanatory models of health. Otherwise, having to conform to Western models of illness and wellbeing is oppressive, as it does not recognise or allow for other ways of feeling, experiencing, and being. Working with Elders and youth to gain these understandings is essential to increase wellness for youth, and to resist discourses of Indigenous Peoples as weak, sick, and in need of saving. The nursing duty to help clients from a highly stigmatized group make positive behaviour changes requires opportunities to learn about client issues and use of available resources, and the importance of striking a balance between communicating acceptance towards their clients' current state, and facilitating forward movement in formal treatment. To avoid continued colonization and marginalization, Indigenous Peoples must lead initiatives in making accessible information about physical health and nutrition and positive ways of coping with stress, so that people can understand the effect of the food they eat.

the changes are long-lasting by helping clients respond promptly to any setbacks (Frostad et al., 2018). Refer further to Chapter 14. A third treatment option, specialist supportive clinical management (SSCM), includes education, care, support, and therapeutic alliance that promotes adherence to treatment through use of praise, reassurance, and advice. Supportive clinical management emphasizes the resumption of normal eating and the restoration of weight; verbal and written information are provided on weight maintenance strategies, energy requirements, and relearning to eat normally (McIntosh, 2015). Family-based therapy (FBT) is currently the only treatment for adolescents living with AN that is supported by scientific evidence. In particular, behaviourally based family therapy is superior to individual therapy (Couturier et al., 2020). No one specialist treatment has been shown to be best for treatment of adults with AN. However, a significant therapy effect was found using each—CBT, IPT, and SSCM (McIntosh et al., 2016).

Table 25.3	Cognitive Distortions Typical of Patients With Eating Disorders, With Restructuring Statements
Distortion	**Clarification or Restructuring**
Dichotomous or all-or-nothing thinking "I've gained 1 kilo (2 pounds), so I'll be up by 50 kilos (100 pounds) soon."	"You have not ever gained 50 kilos (100 pounds), but I understand that gaining 1 kilo (2 pounds) is scary."
Magnification "I binged last night, so I can't go out with anyone."	"Feeling bad and guilty about a binge are difficult feelings, but you are in treatment and you have been monitoring and changing your eating."
Selective abstraction "I can only be happy 5 kilos (10 pounds) lighter." or "People will only love me if I am thin."	"When you were 5 kilos (10 pounds) lighter, you were hospitalized. You can choose to be happy about many things in your life." "People love you for being you—your kindness, sense of humour, and so on. Let's talk about qualities that make you a good friend/sister."
Overgeneralization "I didn't eat anything yesterday and did okay, so I don't think *not* eating for a week or two will harm me."	"Any starvation harms the body, whether or not outward signs are apparent to you. The more you starve, the more problems your body will encounter."
Catastrophizing "I purged last night for the first time in 4 months—I'll never recover." or "I am so evil—if I have whipped cream on my latte, my stomach will be over my jeans like a muffin in the tin."	"Recovery includes ups and downs, and it is expected you will still have some mild but infrequent symptoms." "No, that's not true. You are working hard to ensure you take in enough to meet your body's needs, such as the extra energy it takes you to walk all the way to the coffee shop."

Client Education

As weight is restored and concentration improved, individuals with AN can maximally benefit from psychoeducation. Although these individuals have much knowledge about food and calories, they also have misinformation that needs clarifying. For example, they are often unclear about the role of "fats" in a healthy diet and try to be as "fat-free" as possible. A thorough assessment of their knowledge is important because they may need information on the importance of including all nutrients in a healthy diet. Furthermore, individuals with AN are often perfectionistic; they may set unrealistic goals and end up frustrated. Teaching them to set smaller, progressive, attainable eating goals is one of the most helpful interventions. To help these clients learn to develop appropriate goals around food and other activities, the nurse can help them consider essential topic areas pertinent to their recovery (see Box 25.10) and patiently support them to gain skill in formulating realistic, attainable goals.

Social Domain

Nursing Care Focus for Social Domain

Difficulty managing social roles, responsibilities, and social expectations.

Interventions for Social Domain

Younger individuals with AN who may have lost some time at school because of hospitalization may find integrating back into a school and classroom setting difficult. Shame and guilt about having an eating disorder and being hospitalized need to be addressed. These clients typically have isolated themselves before hospitalization and treatment, so renewing friendships and relationships with peers may provoke anxiety. Involving school nurses and teachers in the reentry process may help.

When parents learn their child has a diagnosis of AN, tension begins:

> The atmosphere in the house was horrendous, you know because it takes over, actually the whole house really, because you trying to get her to eat and she's sitting there in tears and its horrendous and it's the worst thing ever and it's happening under your nose and you know it's dreadful (McCormack & McCann, 2015, p. 144).

BOX 25.10 Psychoeducation Checklist: Anorexia Nervosa

When caring for the client with AN, be sure to include the following topic areas in the teaching plan:

✓ Psychopharmacologic agents, if used (rarely), including drug, action, dosage, frequency, and possible adverse effects
✓ Nutrition and eating patterns
✓ Effect of restrictive eating or dieting
✓ Weight monitoring
✓ Safety and comfort measures
✓ Avoidance of triggers
✓ Self-monitoring techniques
✓ Trust
✓ Realistic goal setting
✓ Resources

BOX 25.11 What Family and Friends Can Do to Help Those Living With Eating Disorders

- Tell the person you are concerned, you care, and you would like to help. Suggest that the person seek professional help from a physician or therapist.
- If the person refuses to seek professional help, then encourage reaching out to an adult, such as a teacher, school nurse, or counsellor.
- Do not discuss weight, the number of calories being consumed, or particular eating habits. Do try to talk about things other than food, weight, counting calories, and exercise.
- Avoid making comments about a person's appearance. Concern about weight loss may be interpreted as a compliment; comments regarding weight gain may be felt as criticism.
- It will not help to become involved in a power struggle. You cannot force the person to eat.
- You can offer support. Ultimately, however, the responsibility and the decision to accept help and to change rest with the person.
- Read and educate yourself regarding these disorders.
- Care for yourself (e.g., have periods of rest as a way to regain energy).

Parents may feel lost alongside their child who is ill and in need of information, support, and inclusion in treatment decisions (Weaver et al., 2016). They want treatment for their child to shift from weight-focused to a more holistic, individualised, consistent care approach with better balance in targeting psychological and physical problems from an early stage; improved professionals' knowledge and attitudes towards clients and their families at all levels of care from primary to specialist; and enhanced peer and family support (Mitrofan et al., 2019). Box 25.11 provides a list of general strategies that may assist families and friends.

Nurses help family members manage feelings, increase effective communication and capacity to provide helpful nonintrusive support, decrease protectiveness, and resolve guilt. Successful family treatment addresses underlying issues such as negative body image, intergenerational coalitions between parents and children, fear of separation, and undeveloped marital relationships. Goals in the therapy include helping the parents work together, strengthening silenced voices, bringing out repressed emotions, and keeping conversations going between family members. Family are helped to focus on issues of separation–individuation, autonomy, ineffective communication, symptom interruption, and on practical issues, such as how to effectively monitor food intake. A major focus is to help family members see each other's strengths and begin to work together to address the eating issue.

Siblings require support as they report a decrease in quality of life brought about by the eating disorder, such as having decreased motivation for social activities and feeling helpless and afraid about the future. Siblings may also experience guilt due to their past remarks or actions. In-depth interviews with siblings revealed a sense of grief and sacrifice, as well as feeling they lost their family, normal childhood, and individual identity (Maon et al., 2020). It is helpful to have siblings attend family sessions with parents to discuss these feelings and the effect the eating disorder has had on them.

Spiritual Domain

Overcoming eating disorders requires attention to the individual's physical, psychological, social, and spiritual fullness. Core components of recovery include having input into one's own recovery and sense of empowerment (Fogarty & Ramjan, 2016). Empowerment can be experienced through regaining some control by learning new coping strategies and skills such as increasing self-worth and respect. Spiritual interventions entail establishing trust, rapport, consistency, and support while enabling clients to voice and make meaning of their eating disorder experiences. The nurse helps clients recognize patterns and identify and clarify values. Encouraging activities that promote reflection and self-awareness helps clients access potential solutions to wellbeing and reduce depression, anxiety, relationship distress, social role conflict, and eating disorder symptoms. Some important skills during treatment are learning to resist comparing self with others and to impart self-kindness; a client attributed their recovery to developing a deeper sense of their own identity, connecting to what they love, and being able to be present in a relationship despite having imperfections (Lea et al., 2015).

The need for ongoing self-awareness on the part of the nurse is critical when interacting with an individual whose body has served as a container for pain, suffering, and disgust and has subsequently been starved, stuffed, or purged. The nurse therapist may encounter body countertransference or the phenomenon of experiencing a similar type of discomfort in the nurse's own body (Verbeek, 2018).

The nurse's particular physical characteristics, shape, size, and weight are likely to play a part in the unconscious dynamics of the therapeutic process with a client who experiences eating and body image problems, so the nurse needs to attune to these body sensations and anticipate this phenomenon throughout the working relationship. If the nurse therapist has also recovered from an eating disorder, then it is important they have explored their own embodied experiences and/or eating issues in personal therapy to feel "recovered enough" to work safely and ethically with the individual presenting with an eating disorder. In working with clients, it is necessary to process countertransference issues concerning relationships with one's own weight, eating patterns, and body image as well as with the clients' tendencies to scrutinize and comment about the nurse/therapist's body and the degree of self-disclosure in the therapeutic relationship (Seah et al., 2017). Clients having therapy for eating disorders report wanting their service provider to be genuinely curious, elicit trust, have eating disorder expertise to inform the therapy, engage by listening and sharing in conversations, and establish a safe and comfortable environment that reflects the therapist's caring. Nurses have to be able to express interest in clients when they say they binged, threw up, or ate without hunger. Nurses need to investigate, in great detail, instances of clients hating their bodies or shaming themselves because of their bodies. Without awareness and self-monitoring, the nurse may communicate any personal body discomfort to the client. Individual or group peer debriefing sessions are helpful to manage such countertransference.

Evaluation and Treatment Outcomes

Among the varied factors influencing therapeutic outcomes, higher entry BMI and early weight gain predict positive treatment outcome in individuals receiving specialist AN inpatient treatment (Wales et al., 2016). Intensive ongoing outpatient treatment, including nutritional counselling and support, can prevent relapse and facilitate full recovery. Many of the instruments used to assess eating disorder symptoms (see Box 25.9) can be used throughout the individual's treatment to evaluate attitudes and thinking processes.

Continuum of Care

Hospitalization

AN in its acute stage requires hospitalization.

EMERGENCY CARE

Death may result from cardiac problems associated with starvation and suicide. However, emergency care is not usually needed for individuals with AN. Family members and peers usually notice the weight loss and emaciation before the individual's systems are compromised to the degree that they require emergency treatment. The individual is admitted immediately for inpatient care if systems are compromised or if the individual is suicidal. In hospital, individuals are evaluated for discharge to day hospitalization or outpatient therapy, depending on the resources available, the extent of family support, and comorbidity. In both instances, the individual and family participate in a combination of individual and family therapy. Family therapy, initiated in the hospital, is continued more intensively after discharge (see Chapter 16).

Outpatient Treatment

After weight restoration, treatment of AN may take place on an outpatient basis and involve continued individual and family therapy, nutrition counselling to reinforce healthy eating patterns and attitudes, and physician visits to monitor weight and evaluate somatic recovery. Support groups that respect the views and needs of each participant and provide a continuous feedback cycle can help participants develop a sense of empowerment, allow their voices to be heard, and foster a belief they could begin new relationships and friendships (Nicholls et al., 2016). However, support groups are not a substitute for therapy. This is because some self-directed support groups that lack professional leadership can actually delay or prevent needed professional treatment. In particular, online communities may validate the pro-anorexic identity in the cycle of disclosure–response exchanges (Chang & Bazarova, 2016). The role of support groups to maintain recovery requires further study.

Bulimia Nervosa

Until about 35 years ago, BN was thought to be a subtype of AN. However, findings from extensive investigations identified BN as a separate entity. Individuals with BN are usually older at onset than are those with AN. The usual treatment is outpatient therapy. Outcomes are better for BN than for AN, and mortality rates are lower. From a 22-year longitudinal study with women who met diagnostic criteria for BN, the only predictor that increased the likelihood of having a diagnosis of BN at the 22-year assessment was having more weeks during the study when the diagnostic criteria for BN were met (Franko et al., 2018).

Clinical Course

There are few outward signs associated with BN. Individuals binge and purge in secret and are typically of normal weight; therefore, BN does not come to the attention of parents and peers as quickly as AN. Consequently, treatment can be delayed for years as individuals attempt on their own to get their eating under control. Once treatment is undertaken and completed, they are capable of full recovery, except when personality disorders and comorbid serious depression are also present.

Individuals with BN may present as overwhelmed and overly committed and have difficulty with setting limits and establishing appropriate boundaries. They have many rules regarding food and food restriction, and they feel ashamed, guilty, and disgusted about binge eating and purging. They may also be impulsive in other areas of their lives, such as spending.

BN Symptomatology

According to Mayo Clinic Staff (2018), persons struggling with BN may purge through self-induced vomiting; misusing laxatives, diuretics, or enemas; or fasting, strict dieting, or excessive exercise after eating only a small snack or a normal-size meal. BN can be hard to overcome when individuals are preoccupied with their weight and body shape and severely judge self-perceived flaws.

Dietary restriction serves to regulate painful feelings. It may also alter one's perceptual reactivation to food cues, making them more irresistible. Restriction may make persons who diet more prone to feel distress over their dietary "failures," especially if dieting has become a way to overcome body dissatisfaction and to compensate for distress through binge eating. Pearson et al. (2015) identified both state-based and trait-based ways in which women increase their risk to begin engaging in the impulsive behaviour of binge eating and purging. With state-based ways, the experience of negative mood in women attempting to restrain eating leads to the depletion of self-control and thus increased risk for loss of control of eating. With trait-based ways, increased negative urgency, or the tendency to act rashly when distressed, increases risk for loss of control. These behaviours, when reinforced, put women at further risk for developing BN. Consequently, whether the eating is influenced by hunger, the attraction of forbidden foods, or internal needs to assuage perceived failure, restraining one's intake may instigate a drive toward repletion and subsequent overeating. State and trait factors transact to increase risk. Women who are high in negative urgency and experience distress from the environment (e.g., relationship stress) or eating disorder behaviour (e.g., food restriction) have a harder time engaging in self-regulation and experience self-control depletion

quickly. Expecting that eating behaviour will alleviate their distress, they are at increased risk for binge eating. If expecting that thinness will lead to life improvement, then they are at increased risk to then purge. In this way, the state of self-control depletion mediates the influence of the trait of negative urgency on BN behaviour.

As shown in Figure 25.5, dietary restraint leads to hunger. Hunger may occur in response to inadequate intake or as hedonic hunger, the drive to eat to obtain pleasure in the absence of an energy deficit. Individuals high in hedonic hunger exhibit heightened responsivity to food cues, which exist independently of hunger state. Hedonic hunger appears to be closely related to loss of control and binge eating and serves to distinguish among individuals with eating problems that include loss of control eating (i.e., BN or BED) versus those which do not (non-BED obesity and AN-restricting type) (Espel-Huynh et al., 2018). Rapid ingestion of food during a short period of time (binge eating) is followed by feelings of guilt, remorse, and often self-contempt, leading to purging. To assuage the out-of-control feeling, severe dieting referred to as dietary restraint is instituted. Restrictions are viewed as "rules," such as no sweets or fats. Each binge seems to influence stricter rules about what cannot be consumed, leading to more frequent binge eating, subsequent guilt, and self-loathing. Purging or dietary restraint may follow (Fig. 25.5). Accurso et al. (2016) found adolescents over age 16 who practiced weight suppression while having a higher BMI engaged in more frequent binge eating, while those with a low current BMI engaged in less frequent binge eating. The binge–purge cycle prompts clinicians to focus on

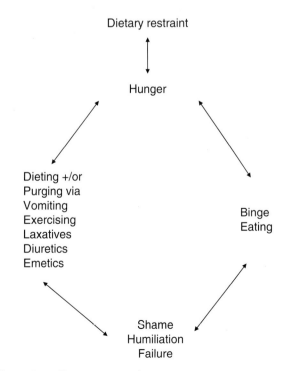

Figure 25.5 Binge–purge cycle.

interventions related to weight suppression and dietary restraint as well as purging behaviours.

KEY CONCEPT

Dietary restraint, a cognitive effort to restrict food intake for the purpose of weight loss or the prevention of weight gain, was originally described to explain the differences between the eating patterns of people who are obese and those of people who are of healthy weight. Restraint is often initiated as a response to weight gain, and the sustained effort to monitor and control food intake characterizes successful long-term weight maintenance.

Epidemiology

Approximately 1% to 3% of young women develop BN in their lifetime (Statistics Canada, 2015). Using symptom frequency of once a week criteria, the lifetime prevalence (proportion of a population who, at some point in life up to the time of assessment, ever had the characteristic) of BN was reported as 2.15% in a large UK sample of women in midlife (Micali et al., 2017), while the period prevalences (proportion of a population who has the characteristic at any point during a given time period) of AN and BED were reported as 3.64% and 1.96%, respectively.

Age of Onset

Typically, the onset of BN begins in adolescence or early adulthood and may coincide with a developmental transition (e.g., leaving home to attend university) or psychosocial stress such as from unexpected loss of a close relative (Su et al., 2016).

Differences Among People Diagnosed With BN

In the community setting, one case in four cases of BN is a man (Dr. Blake Woodside, Director of the Program for Eating Disorders at Toronto General Hospital). Approximately 1.1% of Canadian adolescent young men exhibit a subthreshold eating disorder associated with impairments in psychosocial functioning (Flament et al., 2015).

Ethnic and Cultural Differences

BN is related to culture in the same way as AN. In Western cultures and those becoming westernized in their norms, the focus on achieving an idealized thin body underlies the dieting and dietary restraint that set up the trajectory toward an eating disorder. Women who are of Hispanic or Latinx ethnicity and women who are of non-Hispanic White or European origin have higher reported rates than women who are of Asian origin and

women who are Black American or African origin. A cross-cultural comparison of BMI and waist circumference of 126 university students from Mexico and Canada having disordered eating behaviours, thin-ideal internalization, and body image dissatisfaction found students from Mexico at 4.6 times greater risk than the students from New Brunswick to have values of overweight, obesity, abdominal obesity, and disordered eating behaviour (Saucedo-Molina et al., 2017). The presence of thin-ideal internalization and body image dissatisfaction was similar between samples. There is still a paucity of research exploring ethnic and culture differences among Canadian women.

Familial Differences

Individuals with family members diagnosed with BN have an increased risk of developing eating disorders, BN in particular. The heritability of BN is estimated at approximately 0.60 (Bulik et al., 2019).

Comorbidity

Common comorbid conditions are substance misuse, depression, and anxiety disorders. Higher occurrence of substance use, depression, and anxiety in BN may be characteristics such as a history of sexual or physical abuse (Patel et al., 2018). Anxiety disorders are the most common comorbidity for each person experiencing BN. Anxiety disorders may start in the childhood period before the diagnosis of the eating disorder, leading to the question: Are anxiety disorders also risk factors for the development of BN? PTSD was found to be approximately three times more frequent in individuals living with BN and AN-BP as opposed to those with AN-R (Hocaoglu, 2017). Men had the highest levels of general anxiety syndrome comorbidity with BN (Ulfvebrand et al., 2015). There is a higher occurrence of BN in clients with attention deficit hyperactivity disorder (Svedlund et al., 2017). Cluster B disorders, such as borderline personality disorder (BPD), are also identified frequently with BN. The presence of a comorbid diagnosis of BN among women with BPD is significantly and uniquely associated with recent suicidal ideation, self-harm behaviour, and suicide attempts during treatment (Reas et al., 2015). Women with premenstrual syndrome and premenstrual dysphoric disorder have higher odds of having BN, independent of comorbid mental health conditions (Nobles et al., 2016).

Aetiology

Some of the predisposing or risk factors for BN overlap with theories of causality (see Fig. 25.2). For example, dieting may put an individual at risk for developing BN. The dieting can turn into dietary restraint, which can lead to binge eating and purging in vulnerable individuals.

The interplay of other risk factors (e.g., body dissatisfaction and separation–individuation issues) also helps explain the development of this disorder.

Biologic Theories

Dieting may occur in girls as young as 9 years of age. At 12 years, girls have significantly higher depressive symptom and body dissatisfaction scores than boys. Higher eating disorder symptoms at 9 years have significantly predicted higher eating disorder symptoms at 12 years for both boys and girls, while greater dietary restraint at 7 years was a significant predictor for boys (Evans et al., 2017). In a large sample of junior and high school students aged 12 to 18 years, Haynos et al. (2016) found that nearly half reported dieting and that, after 5 years, roughly half of those dieters had initiated disordered restrictive eating. Factors that predicted the restrictive eating were elevated depression, lower self-esteem, weight concerns, lower body satisfaction, weight-related teasing, and peer dieting. Dieting is believed to affect the neurotransmitters, including serotonin, which are involved in appetite, satiety, and eating patterns of BN. Levels of cholecystokinin (CCK), a hormone associated with satiation, is decreased in individuals diagnosed with BN. Decreased CCK functioning may contribute to impaired satiety and thus binge eating (Culbert et al., 2016). Depending on the macronutrient composition of food choices, CCK release can be influenced. For instance, protein is a potent stimulator of a CCK response. Eating more protein-rich meals increases the release of CCK, increasing satiety and ending a meal.

Neuropathologic

The changes in the brain are the result rather than the cause of eating dysregulation. As with AN, these changes resolve when symptoms such as dietary restraint, binge eating, and purging remit.

Genetic

A specific gene responsible for BN has not been identified. However, genes acting within serotonin and dopamine systems may influence both eating- and personality-related psychopathology either directly or indirectly (i.e., in interaction with traumatic childhood experiences). This is believed to contribute to variations in the presentation of comorbid traits and to increased psychopathology and body mass in bulimia disorders.

Biochemical

As with genetics, the most frequently studied biochemical theories in BN relate to lowered serotonin and dopamine neurotransmission. People experiencing BN are believed to have altered modulation of central serotonin neuronal systems (Mayhew et al., 2018). Even following recovery from BN, findings of altered serotonin levels persist that potentially contribute to BN symptomatology and responses to medication. Dopamine is considered the primary neurotransmitter involved in the reinforcing effects of food. Low levels of dopamine can increase hunger; increased dopamine concentration can decrease appetite. These differences in dopamine levels may help explain why those with BN are more attentive to food stimuli.

Psychological and Social Theories

Psychological factors in the aetiology of BN have been studied extensively, and most experts believe that these factors converge with environmental or sociocultural factors within individuals who have a biologic predisposition, which causes symptoms to develop. Stress precedes the occurrence of bulimic behaviours and increases in negative affect following stressful events may maintain bulimic behaviours. Investigating the neural reactions to food cues following a stressful event in women diagnosed with BN, Collins et al. (2017) found decreased blood flow in a part of the brain associated with self-reflection, compared with increased blood flow in women not having BN. This suggests that women living with BN shift away from self awareness because of negative thoughts regarding performance or social comparisons in order to focus on more concrete stimuli, such as food. As with AN, psychoanalytic developmental theories that explain separation–individuation and sociocultural factors regarding societal focus on the ideal body type are important in causality. Because the age of onset for BN is late adolescence/early adulthood, leaving home (e.g., for employment or educational opportunities) may represent the first physical separation for adolescents unprepared for the emotional separation. A young woman receiving therapy to help with BN revealed the life–historical development of BN as stemming from low self-esteem, poor self-concept, and a negative view of the future. She spoke of feeling inferior and resorting to BN to feel in control:

I felt that I was fat and ugly and when those feelings would come up, they were overwhelming, and I didn't know what to do. So one night that I went to bed hungry and I was so hungry I couldn't sleep, so … I got up and ate so much … and felt full for the first time in months, but my stomach hurt so much after that, umm, I went to the bathroom and I didn't even have to try, everything just came out, and then I was able to sleep peacefully for the first time in a long time. I had found the way to stay slim and eat anything at the same time. I started feeling better about myself, and guys started hitting on me and I started, like, dating just like everyone else (Stavrou, 2018, p. 504).

Cognitive Theory

Within the view of BN as a disorder of thinking, distortions are the basis of behaviours such as binge eating and purging. Core low self-esteem is exacerbated by dependence on perfectionist standards toward weight, shape, and eating control. Interpersonal problems maintain the binge-eating and purging symptoms of BN, and repeated experience and heightened perception of these interpersonal problems further exacerbate and contribute to the core low self-esteem (Lampard & Sharbanee, 2015). For instance, cues such as stress related to interpersonal difficulties (e.g., an argument with a loved one), negative emotions, physiologic state (e.g., hunger, fullness), and environment (e.g., the presence of attractive food, a remark about the person's weight or amount being eaten, or catching sight of self in a mirror) may activate personal negative self-beliefs of "I'm unlikeable" or "I'm a failure." This activation generates considerable emotional distress. Eating provides a distraction and is commonly associated with a decreased intensity of emotional states. In this way, eating is initially interpreted positively and linked to positive beliefs (e.g., "Eating will take away my painful feelings"). However, eating can also be closely linked with negative beliefs about the potential consequences (e.g., "I'll gain weight"). The person experiencing BN is caught in a state of conflict in which positive and negative beliefs about eating coexist. The binge provides only temporary relief from the original distress and is subject to negative interpretation (e.g., as a sign of failure) that, in turn, reinforces the negative self-beliefs in the first place. In contrast, purging may result when negative beliefs about eating dominate positive beliefs and the person switches from eating to vomiting or other compensatory behaviour. Once the compensatory behaviour has ceased, any initial sense of relief at having gotten rid of the food starts to dissipate and the negative consequences of yet another episode of binge eating, purging, negative mood, and arousal start to increase again. These cognitive and emotional regulation explanations account for maintaining the binge eating once it has been established (Burton & Abbott, 2019).

Family

As with AN, the convergence of many factors at a vulnerable stage of individual development contribute to the development of BN. Originating with work at the Maudsley Hospital in London in the late 1970s, a paradigm shift directed attention away from presuming an aetiologic role for family dynamics and toward regarding the family as a resource in therapy to collaboratively help interrupt the pattern of binge eating and purging and reduce the surrounding shame and secrecy.

Spirituality and Attachment Theory

BN is symbolic of a difficulty in finding other more satiating ways to deal with important needs and emotional issues, some of which may not be accessible to awareness. BN may thus be connected to one's identity and purpose in life, covering a true hunger for meaning about where one belongs. It can be frightening for individuals to accept and acknowledge their spirituality because it means confronting greater issues about death, life, and one's place in the world. Churruca et al. (2017) identified conflicting constructions of food in participants' accounts of making sense of the range of bulimic behaviours they engaged in; for example, binge eating was explained through the construction of "comfort food," and restrictive eating through an understanding that certain foods were "bad" while others were "good." Constructing food as both comfort and forbidden pleasure allowed participants to rationalize their binge eating as a form of self-care, or as a disruption to their self-control. In offering participants opportunities to constitute themselves as "virtuous, as morally corrupt, as spiritually cleansed, or as loved" (p. 1502), these constructions provided motivation for binge eating and purging behaviours.

Attachment theory describes one's relationship with a main early caregiver and the subsequent development of internal working models, which may guide one's view of self and the nature of relationships with others. Attachment can be conceptualized as being either secure or insecure. Investigating the link between attachment to God/Higher Power and BN with college students, Buser and Gibson (2016) found significant links between insecure attachments to God/Higher Power and bulimic symptoms. It may be that an individual who fears being abandoned by God/Higher Power and questions God's/Higher Power's love is more vulnerable to accepting sociocultural messages and pressures about body image. Also, an individual who places little value on having a relationship with God/Higher Power may feel upset about this lack of a personal spiritual connection, experience unpleasant emotions, and then use bulimic behaviours to alleviate the negative emotions.

Risk Factors

The risk or predisposing factors for BN are included in Figure 25.3.

Interdisciplinary Treatment

Individuals experiencing BN benefit from a comprehensive multifaceted treatment approach that usually takes place in an outpatient setting, except when the client is suicidal or when past outpatient treatment has failed (see Table 25.2). Therapy for BN focuses on psychological issues, including boundary setting and separation–individuation conflicts, and on changing problematic behaviours and dysfunctional thought patterns and attitudes, especially about eating, constructions of food, weight, and shape. Intensive psychotherapy and pharmacologic interventions are necessary. Nutrition counselling helps stabilize and normalize eating, which means stopping the binge–purge cycle. Support groups may also be involved. Family therapy is not usually a part of the treatment for affected people living away from home and on their own. Usually, the treatment becomes less intensive as symptoms remit. In short, therapeutic relationships, nutrition counselling, and cognitive interventions are priorities in the nursing care of individuals with eating disorders.

Priority Care Issues

Some individuals struggling with BN may become suicidal and engage in self-harm, given the comorbid conditions of depression, anxiety, substance misuse, and BPD. Financial and legal difficulties have been associated with high impulsivity (e.g., shoplifting, overspending).

Nursing Management: Human Response to Bulimia Nervosa Disorder

The primary nursing care foci for clients with BN are inadequate nutrition, malnourishment, inability to exercise personal control, anxiety, and difficulties managing social expectations.

Therapeutic Relationship

Individuals with BN experience shame and guilt and have an intense need to please and be liked. They are too ashamed to discuss their symptoms but do not want to disappoint others, so they may discuss more superficial social or unrelated issues in an attempt to engage the nurse. A nonjudgmental approach stressing the importance of the relationship and outlining its purpose is important from the outset. Explaining the nature of the relationship and the goals of therapy will help clarify the boundaries (see Chapter 7).

Biologic Domain

Most individuals with BN maintain normal weights. Those who purge risk fluid and electrolyte abnormalities, particularly hypokalaemia, that contribute to muscle weakness and fatigability, cardiac arrhythmias, palpitations, and cardiac conduction defects. Neuropsychiatric disturbances, such as poor concentration and attention, and sleep disturbances are common.

Assessment

The nurse assesses current eating patterns, determines the number of times a day the individual binges and purges, and notes dietary restraint practices. Sleep patterns, oral health, and exercise habits are also important.

Nursing Care Foci for the Biologic Domain

Poor nutritional status and sleep disturbances are typical concerns requiring nursing care foci.

Interventions for Biologic Domain

If the client is admitted to the hospital, then all food intake is strictly monitored to normalize eating. Bathroom visits are also supervised to prevent purging. Outpatients are asked to record their intake, binges, and purges to establish a foundation for changing behaviours with psychotherapy. Individuals living with BN often have chaotic lifestyles, and often overcommit themselves, so sleep may be a low priority. Sleep-deprived individuals may assume that food would be helpful, and they begin to eat which triggers a binge. To encourage regular sleep patterns, individuals are encouraged to go to bed and rise at about the same time every day. Clients who purge by inducing vomiting are instructed in proper oral care practices to mitigate enamel erosion and caries.

Pharmacologic Interventions

Pharmacotherapy is effective for symptom remission in BN. Antidepressant treatment may additionally benefit comorbid affective symptoms. Fluoxetine (Prozac) has been the most studied medication for BN in clinical trials (see Box 25.12). It is approved by the U.S. Food and Drug Administration for treatment of an eating disorder; however, in Canada, it is not indicated for use in clients below the age of 18 years (Eli Lilly Canada Inc., 2016). Effective doses are usually 60 mg per day, a higher dosage than that used to treat depression. Weight is monitored as decreased appetite and weight loss are common during the first few weeks of administration. It is also important to monitor the intake of medication for possible purging after administration. The effect of the medication depends on the time taken for its absorption. As with AN, bupropion (Wellbutrin) is contraindicated for the treatment of BN due to its seizure risk.

TEACHING POINTS

Individuals should be instructed to take medication as prescribed. SSRIs should be taken in the morning because they can cause insomnia. Individuals should be informed that any weight loss they initially experience is temporary and is usually regained after a few weeks, when the medication dosage has stabilized. Treatment dropout is high (Furukawa et al., 2019); monitoring adverse effects and eliciting the client's understanding of the reasons why the clinician recommended the pharmacotherapy may help direct interventions.

BOX 25.12 DRUG PROFILE ℞

Fluoxetine Hydrochloride (Prozac)

Drug Class: Selective serotonin reuptake inhibitor

Receptor Affinity: Inhibits central nervous system neuronal uptake of serotonin with little effect on norepinephrine; thought to antagonize muscarinic, histaminergic, and alpha-adrenergic receptors

Indications: Treatment of depressive disorders, most effective in major depression, obesity, bulimia, and OCD

Routes and Dosage: Available in 10- and 20-mg Pulvules and 20 mg per 5 mL oral solution

Adults: 20 mg per day in the morning, not to exceed 80 mg per day. Full antidepressant effect may not be seen for up to 4 weeks. If no improvement, dosage is increased after several weeks. Dosages above 20 mg per day may be administered on a once-a-day (morning) or BID schedule (i.e., morning and noon). For eating disorders, typically, 60 mg per day, administered in the morning, is recommended for reducing the frequency of binge eating and vomiting.

Geriatric: Administer at lower or less frequent doses; monitor responses to guide dosage.

Children: Safety and efficacy have not been established.

Half-Life (Peak Effect): 2 to 3 days (6 to 8 h)

Selected Adverse Reactions: Headache, nervousness, insomnia, drowsiness, anxiety, tremors, dizziness, light-headedness, nausea, vomiting, diarrhoea, dry mouth, anorexia, dyspepsia, constipation, taste changes, upper respiratory infections, pharyngitis, painful menstruation, sexual dysfunction, urinary frequency, sweating, rash, pruritus, weight loss, asthenia, and fever

Warnings: Avoid use in pregnancy and while breast-feeding. Use with caution in clients with impaired hepatic or renal function and diabetes mellitus. Possible risk for toxicity if taken with tricyclic antidepressants.

Special Client and Family Education

- Be aware that the drug may take up to 4 weeks to get full antidepressant effect.
- Take the drug in the morning or in divided doses, if necessary.
- Report any adverse reactions.
- Avoid driving a car or performing hazardous activities because the drug may cause drowsiness or dizziness.
- Eat small, frequent meals to help with complaints of nausea and vomiting.

Psychosocial Domain

Assessment

Psychological assessment focuses on cognitive distortions—cues or stimuli that lead to dysfunctional behaviour affecting symptom development—and knowledge deficits. The psychological characteristics typical of individuals with BN are presented in Box 25.2. Examples of cognitive distortions present in BN are given in Table 25.3. These thought patterns form the basis for "rules" and lead the way to destructive eating patterns. During routine history taking, individuals may relate many of these distortions. Situations that produce feelings of being overwhelmed and powerless need to be explored, as does the individual's ability to set boundaries, control impulsivity, and maintain quality relationships. These underlying issues may precipitate binge eating. Several assessment tools are available to gauge such characteristics as body dissatisfaction and impulsivity (see Box 25.9). Body dissatisfaction should be openly explored. Mood is evaluated because many people having BN also have depression.

Nursing Care Focus for the Psychosocial Domain

Limited understanding of one's illness and cognitive distortions feature prominently in the nursing management in the psychosocial domain.

Interventions for Psychosocial Domain

CBT is the most empirically supported treatment for BN. In a recent clinical trial, the majority (95.7%) of persons participating in CBT exhibited fewer binge and/or vomit and/or laxative use behaviours compared to persons treated using a different treatment (71.4%) (MacDonald et al., 2017). CBT is usually conducted in a group with one or two sessions a week. CBT has also been effectively delivered in guided self-help format. IPT has had positive outcomes but may take longer to change binge eating and purging symptoms. Behavioural therapy alone has not been as effective as CBT. While binge eating may persist, little work can be done on underlying interpersonal issues, such as boundary setting, because the client feels out of control with eating. Therefore, cognitive therapy is begun first, to address the distorted thinking processes influencing dietary restraint, binge eating, and purging. Decreasing these symptoms will help eliminate the out-of-control feelings.

Behavioural Techniques

The behavioural techniques, such as **cue elimination** and response prevention, require **self-monitoring** to individualize the therapy. Self-monitoring is accomplished using a diary, in which the individual records binges, purges, precipitating emotions, and environmental cues including physiologic/nutritional and psychological pressures to eat, as well as individuals and situations that may be associated with negative feelings such as depression, anger, or anxiety. Self-monitoring allows the nurse and client to jointly evaluate problematic behavioural patterns, identifies progress, helps clients develop awareness of what is happening in the moment so that they can begin to change behaviours that may have seemed automatic or beyond their control, and is considered the best predictor of short- and long-term treatment outcomes for BN (Barakat et al., 2017). The client's records are jointly reviewed at each session, and any difficulties are addressed in the session. Emotional and environmental cues are identified, and alternative responses are formulated, tried, and reinforced. When a cue or stimulus leads to a dysfunctional or unhealthy response, the response can be eliminated, or an alternate, healthier response to the cue can be substituted, tried, and then reinforced. The client is encouraged to focus on longer-term consequences (e.g., social isolation) rather than shorter-term relief of uncomfortable feelings. The proliferation of health-related apps with self-monitoring of eating habits as a major feature may be helpful for people with eating disorders and for eating disorder professionals. There is a need to evaluate the added workload and potential harm to the client–nurse/clinician collaboration as well as the clinical utility of such apps (Lindgreen et al., 2018). Figure 25.6 gives two examples of behavioural interventions. In example 1, for AN, the response is modified or altered to a healthier one; in example 2, for the context of BN, the cue is changed to produce a different, healthier response. Other techniques, such as postponing binges and purges through distraction to interrupt the cycle, are also effective.

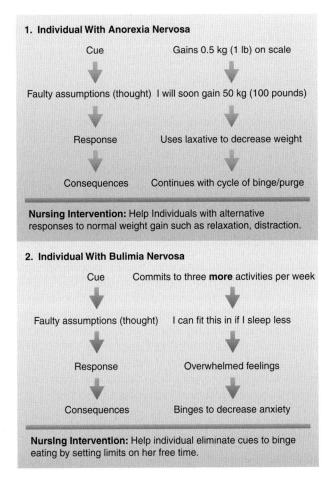

Figure 25.6 Examples of the relationship of cues, thoughts, and responses: behavioural interventions.

Psychoeducation

The nurse can assist clients to understand the binge–purge cycle and the role of rigid rules in contributing to this cycle. The value of eating meals regularly to ward off hunger and reduce the possibility of a binge is important. Individuals who misuse laxatives are taught that although these drugs produce water weight loss, they are ineffective for true, lasting weight loss. Moreover, individuals also need information about potassium depletion, electrolyte imbalances, dehydration, and the medical consequences of purging. Other topics for psychoeducation are included in Box 25.13. Psychoeducation equips participants with concrete scientific evidence to recognize the severity of their illness, challenge disordered thoughts, improve motivation for eating behaviour change, and work towards treatment goals (Belak et al., 2017).

TEACHING POINTS

Psychoeducation for BN focuses on setting boundaries and healthy limits, developing assertiveness, learning nutritional concepts related to healthy eating, discussing societal definitions of beauty, and clarifying misconceptions about food. Research findings related to semistarvation, weight regulation, dieting, obesity, and the sociocultural milieu that influences the development and perpetuation of eating disorders are discussed. Cognitive distortions are addressed because of their role in dietary restraint and resultant binge eating. Measures such as Garner's abbreviated Eating Attitudes Test (EAT-26; see Box 25.9) can be used to assess clients' eating concerns before, during, and after psychoeducation.

Family Assessment and Intervention

For parents, their children's purging behaviours elicit stronger emotional reactions than binge eating (Hoste et al., 2015). The *Canadian Eating Disorders Strategy 2019–2029* recommends that caregivers/families are connected with evidence-informed resources and information to help them better navigate healthcare system and social services and support their own health.

Group Therapy

Group therapy is cost-effective and effectively increases learning because individuals learn from each other as well as from the nurse or other therapist. Some experts have recommended 12-step programs for treating BN. However, many clinicians who work in this specialty have noted that these programs, with their strict rules, can be counterproductive for individuals struggling with BN, who already have stringent rules (e.g., dietary restraint) and are "abstinent" in many ways that lead to binge eating. Broad parameters regarding food choices (e.g., allowing all foods in moderation), together with knowledge about healthy eating, are encouraged instead. As symptoms subside, individuals can concentrate on underlying interpersonal issues in therapy, such as feelings of inadequacy and low self-esteem, and can work with other group members to develop assertiveness.

Spiritual Domain

Assessment

The role of spirituality in the lives of individuals with BN can be assessed through their expressions of loss and powerlessness, self-care capacity, quality of relationships, history of conflicts and painful traumatic experiences, attitudes about food and overeating, harm avoidance strategies, self-directedness, and self-judgments. The nurse must strive to see the person beyond the dieting, binge-eating, and purging behaviours. Women with a diagnosis of BN who experience depression are at greater risk of suicide (Udo et al., 2019). This suggests the need to monitor depression severity as the most important target of treatment and suicide prevention.

Nursing Care Focus in the Spiritual Domain

Loss and powerlessness are among the common concerns requiring nursing management in the spiritual domain.

Interventions for the Spiritual Domain

The nurse encourages clients to express feelings of loss and powerlessness without negative self-judgment. Clients will benefit from exploring what they do and do not have control over and to accept their human limitations. Those who binge eat and purge can learn to delay these behaviours through engaging in activities such as journal writing, affirming positive self-worth, meditation, and imagery. These strategies may help clients living with BN to build support from self and to help deal with comorbid depression and anxiety. Nurses can further help create the context for clients with BN to enlist support from others.

Evaluation and Treatment Outcomes

Individuals experiencing BN may have better recovery outcomes than do those with AN. Outcomes have improved since the early 1990s, partially because of earlier detection, research on treatments that are most effective, and neuropharmacologic research and advances. Recovery from BN has been described by women as a process of beginning with renewed self-esteem. There is progress from feeling stuck in BN, getting ready to change, breaking free of bulimia symptomatology, and grasping a new reality of self-acceptance. The process goes back and forth between progress and relapse, and women express strong ambivalence about leaving the illness behind. Essential for their recovery is developing a unique explanation of the cause of their illness. These findings indicate a need for care that bolsters women's self-efficacy through strengthening beliefs in their own abilities and instilling hope for recovery (Lindgren et al., 2015).

Continuum of Care

Individuals living with BN are less likely than those with AN to require hospitalization. However, those with extreme dehydration, electrolyte imbalance, depression, suicidality, or symptoms that have not remitted with outpatient treatment need hospitalization. After treatment, referrals to recovery groups and support groups are important to prevent relapse.

Binge-Eating Disorder

BED was introduced into the *DSM-IV* as a provisional diagnosis in 2004 and included in the *DSM-5* (APA, 2013) as its own category of eating disorders (refer to *DSM-5* for full diagnostic criteria). BED is more prevalent than either AN or BN and is not uncommon in men. Lifetime prevalence for BED in Canada is 3.19% (Gill & Kaplan, 2021). It is associated with overweight and has high comorbidity comparable to that of BN. When diagnosed, the usual treatment is outpatient therapy.

Clinical Course

Investigators have shown that individuals diagnosed with BED, when compared to those with BN, have lower dietary restraint and are higher in weight, even though many are not obese. It has been estimated that 10% to 30% of people who are obese have BED. In a community study that completed annual diagnostic interviews during the entire adolescent period, the peak age for onset of BED was between 16 and 17 years (Marzilli et al., 2018). Binge eating episodes in adolescence are difficult to differentiate from nonclinical behaviours, as youths may indulge in large food consumption due to developmentally specific growth spurts, which may include rapid neurobiological and body modifications. The criterion of loss of control (LOC) eating is considered the most salient marker of BED. Adolescent young women report less overeating than adolescent men, but more severe indicators of LOC and distress during binge eating episodes. In a separate study by Kelly-Weeder et al. (2019), women with BED expressed, "I need to keep eating to fill up some hole. I'm not fulfilled until I feel sick from eating so much" (p. 174). They further said, "There is no control. I see my hands reaching for the food and bringing it to my mouth without consciously choosing to do so or willing to do so" (p. 175). Participants referred to feeling removed from themselves, as if someone else was taking over their bodies. "It's like you are not even conscious of what you are doing and you don't feel like yourself or like it was your conscious decision to eat" (p. 176). Attributing the binge eating to an unconscious compulsion provides the means to deny personal responsibility for the binge eating.

Outward signs associated with BED may include overweight, obesity, and consequences such as gallbladder disease and arthritis. Through these manifestations, BED may come to the attention of family and peers. Treatment can be delayed for years as individuals attempt on their own or with commercial weight-loss programs to control their eating. Outcomes have not been extensively studied; poor prognosis is expected given the difficulty of attempting to achieve and maintain weight loss, and in cases where mood and anxiety disorders are present.

Individuals living with BED may miss work, school, or social activities to binge eat. Those who become obese often are extremely distressed by their binge eating, feel bad about themselves, and are preoccupied with their appearance. Most feel ashamed, may avoid social gatherings, and try to hide their problem. Often, they are so successful that close family members and friends do not know that they binge eat.

Diagnostic Criteria

BED shares with the other major eating disorders of AN and BN a high body dissatisfaction (Schmitz et al., 2016). BED differs from AN and BN in terms of dietary restraint and drive for thinness. In AN, for example, an excessively strong drive for thinness and fear of weight gain may trigger restriction, refusal of normal food amounts, and subsequently lead to underweight. In contrast, in BN and BED, excessive food intake related to loss of control while eating may trigger fear of weight gain, but in the case of BN, inappropriate compensatory behaviours (e.g., self-induced vomiting or misuse of laxatives) arise. Women who have been diagnosed with BED neither compensate for binge eating directly nor counter regulate its effect indirectly by restrictive eating between the episodes of binge eating. As a consequence, weight differs between the diagnostic groups, from underweight in AN to possible overweight in BED (Schmitz et al., 2016). Persons experiencing BED are typically ashamed of their eating and try to conceal symptoms from others.

Binge-Eating Disorder in Special Populations

BED is more prevalent among those seeking weight-loss approaches, with 9% to 29% of those reporting binge eating episodes (McCuen-Wurst et al., 2018). However, only 1% to 2% of those seeking weight loss treatment meet full *DSM* criteria for BED. BED is also prevalent in persons living with diabetes (Gagnon et al., 2017).

Epidemiology

BED is more common than AN or BN. Those under the age of 30 are at a higher risk compared to older individuals (McCuen-Wurst et al., 2018). The lifetime occurrence of BED is higher for adults who are overweight and obese. Similarly, the prevalence of BED is elevated in those waiting for bariatric surgery. Between 25% and 50% of clients seeking surgical treatment for obesity meet the diagnostic criteria for BED (Davis, 2015).

Age of Onset

Onset of binge eating typically begins in late adolescence or early adulthood, often after a period of significant dieting or weight loss (Lock et al., 2015). The Public Health Agency of Canada reported that in 2017, 64% of Canadians over the age of 18 are overweight or obese, and 30% of children aged 5 to 17 are overweight or obese. The majority of Canadian youth report being unhappy with their appearance or weight. In fact, children begin reporting body dissatisfaction between the ages of 6 and 9, which increases into middle and high school years, and may continue throughout life. These results begin to inform an understanding of body dissatisfaction among Canadians that requires further study to determine if persons affected are initiating dietary restraint or engaging in unhealthy weight practices to modify shape, weight, and appearance.

Differences Among People Diagnosed With BED

A ratio of two to six adult women to one adult man experience BED (Davis, 2015).

Ethnic and Cultural Differences

Western culture may be necessary for the emergence of BED given that there is no evidence of this disorder in individuals not exposed to Western culture. As well, Western ideals may be accompanied by other cultural shifts crucial for the emergence of BED, including increased industrialization and urbanization that influence food availability. In many regions around the world, the availability of large quantities of readily edible food may be insufficient for binge-eating episodes to occur (Keel, 2017). Underrepresentation of ethnic or racial groups among individuals suffering with eating disorders that include BED seems to relate more to biases in treatment seeking than to any protective factors afforded by underrepresented ethnic or racial group status.

Familial Differences

BED aggregates in families and is heritable. Twin-based heritability estimates are between 0.39 and 0.45. First-degree relatives report significantly higher lifetime rates of anxiety disorders, mood disorders (in particular, bipolar I or II disorder and any depressive disorder), and eating disorders than the first-degree relatives of those without BED. Significant genetic correlations exist between binge-eating and bulimia symptoms, as well as between binge-eating and alcohol dependence. Obesity and BED are also moderately genetically correlated (Bulik et al., 2019).

Comorbidity

BED is associated with medical conditions related to obesity, including diabetes, hypertension, dyslipidaemias, sleep problems/disorders, and pain conditions. Specifically, BED may be associated with type 2 diabetes and with metabolic syndrome in adults and children (Mitchell, 2016). Adolescents struggling with severe obesity experience the most common comorbid conditions of dyslipidaemia (74.4%), chronic back or joint pain (58.3%), obstructive sleep apnea (56.6%), and hypertension (45.0%) (Zeller et al., 2015). Besides obesity, BED in adolescence was predictive of social impairment and other psychological difficulties including depressive symptoms, anxiety, emotional distress, substance use, propensity to suicide, and deliberate self-harm (Marzilli et al., 2018). BED is also associated with asthma and GI symptoms and disorders and, among women, with menstrual dysfunction, pregnancy complications, intracranial hypertension, and polycystic ovary syndrome (Olguin et al., 2017).

Mood and substance use disorders co-occur frequently among adult clients experiencing BED. Nearly 80% of those with lifetime BED have suffered from another lifetime psychiatric disorder of mood, anxiety, or substance use (McCuen-Wurst et al., 2018). In persons diagnosed with BED, depression scores were significantly high (Çelik et al., 2015).

Complications

Medical complications of BED include the above comorbidities of obesity, diabetes, hypertension, high cholesterol, gallbladder disease, kidney disease and/or failure, heart disease, arthritis, certain types of cancer, bone deterioration, menstrual irregularities, ovarian abnormalities, complications of pregnancy, depression, anxiety, and suicidal thoughts. BED is also associated with impaired quality of life and increased healthcare utilization. Individuals who are obese living with BED may also experience the consequences of stigma; for example, increased risk of depression, economic hardship, isolation, and social withdrawal. These stigmatized individuals have negative body image, poorer psychosocial functioning, and higher incidence of binge eating. They have reported feelings of discouragement and social inadequacy, which in turn have generated insecurity, social escape, and relationship difficulties. When BED has led to obesity, these persons are blamed more for their condition than those living with AN and BN, even though people who are obese who struggle with BED are held less personally responsible for their condition than people who are obese without BED (Thörel et al., 2020). A further finding that individuals presenting with BED were more likely to be treated for a weight problem than for the eating disorder suggests trivialization of BED with a reduced likelihood of being appropriately referred to treatment.

As a stigmatized condition, obesity negatively affects the relationship between clients and healthcare providers. Clients living with obesity have reported that healthcare professionals' ambivalence toward their health needs amplified the extent to which these clients felt personally responsible for their condition. This contributed to their hesitancy in accessing and using services. For example, they cancelled medical appointments if they believed they would be weighed (Phelan et al., 2015) and were less probable to attend clinical breast examination (Hellmann et al., 2015) and gynaecologic examination or Papanicolaou smear testing (Mignot et al., 2019).

Aetiology

It is postulated that binge eating functions to modulate negative emotional states. Examining the association between coping strategies and emotion regulation in adults who report binge-eating symptoms, Mac

Vie (2016) found a positive association between self-reported binge-eating behaviour and self-reported difficulties regulating emotions and a negative association between self-reported binge-eating behaviour and self-reported positive coping strategies. With BED, individuals may lack effective strategies for managing negative emotions or their typically functional strategies for coping with negative emotions do not work. Binge-eating episodes are triggered by and provide relief from negative effect. Neuroimaging studies show hyperactivity of the medial orbitofrontal cortex and hypoactivity in the prefrontal network in these individuals. Regions in the frontal brain are responsible for processing basic sensory information about food, while areas in the prefrontal cortex control food-related responses. Clients who experience BED demonstrate low impulse control activity (Iqbal & Rehman, 2020). As adolescents, they may be able to anticipate long-term negative consequences but do not chose more advantageous behaviours given their impulsive nature. Coffino and colleagues (2016) found dietary restraint mediated the relationship between impulsivity and binge-eating severity in their under- and normal-weight sample. However, they found impulsivity had a direct effect on binge-eating severity in their overweight and obese sample.

Biologic Theories

While AN and BN tend to be characterized by high levels of most forms of dietary restraint, including extreme restrictive behaviours, BED tends to be associated with low levels of dietary restraint. The peculiar food choice (e.g., fats, sweets, and snacks) that clients make during binge-eating episodes has been related to a hypothesis of "hedonic deprivation," where eating impulsiveness can be triggered by everyday food restrictions (Amianto et al., 2015).

Genetic

Significantly increased rates of BED were reported in first-degree family members of individuals with BED, a finding corroborated by twin studies (Bulik et al., 2019). Candidate gene association studies of binge eating have examined neurotransmitter systems or genetic variants implicated in appetite and obesity, including the serotonin and dopamine systems. Research suggests that a predisposing risk factor for BED may be a heightened sensitivity to reward, which could manifest as a strong dopamine signal in the brain's striatal region (Davis, 2015). Candidate gene studies, however, have not clearly confirmed the involvement of any one gene or genetic pathway. In other research, individuals with a specific mutation in the location of the FTO (fat mass and obesity-associated protein) gene were found to have higher circulating levels of the "hunger hormone," ghrelin, in their blood, which means they start to feel hungry again soon after eating a meal. Individuals with the FTO gene variation were 20% more likely to binge eat; girls specifically were 30% more likely to binge eat (Micali et al., 2015). Significant genetic correlations also exist between binge-eating and alcohol dependence.

Psychological and Social Theories

Woman living with BED show higher harm avoidance scores than women who do not binge eat (Buelens et al., 2020). Harm avoidance manifests as pessimistic worry, fear of uncertainty, social inhibition, shyness, and passivity in situations when self-assertiveness/advocacy is needed. Guillaume et al. (2016) found clients who are women living with BED in an outpatient eating disorders unit of a European hospital reported moderate/severe childhood emotional abuse (30.77%), childhood sexual abuse (19.23%), and moderate/severe childhood emotional neglect (34.62%). Beyond childhood abuse, women have attributed the development of their eating disorder to their relationship with an abusive partner. The abuse was most commonly reported as weight-related teasing, overcontrol, or neglect. One woman described the daily experience of this abuse and the impact on her self-esteem and behaviour as follows:

> …a vicious cycle—the more I ate, the more I became overweight. The more overweight I became, the more cruel he became… It sort of started with the fat jokes, like 'oh you're getting podgy'… He'd go: 'You just worked out for an hour, so you can't eat such and such'… And then he'd go and do something and I'd quickly go to the fridge and just shove whatever I could in my mouth 'cause I'd be starving. And then quickly finish before he got back because heaven forbid he see that I was eating something… And I think I would be like halfway through and feel 'oh well I might as well keep eating because what's the point? And I'm doing this exercise and I'm not losing weight and he still calls me fat and I'm still fat' (Mitchison et al., 2016, p. 7–8 of 13).

People who are obese and struggling with BED are more likely to request professional psychological help than obese non–binge-eating individuals. Their greater sense of social insecurity and the impairment in interpersonal relationships associated with being overweight may contribute to this issue, and the intrinsic feeling of ineffectiveness and self-deprecation maintained by social stigmatization promotes the vicious circle leading to binge eating through negative feedback on self-esteem.

Cognitive Theory

Overvaluation of shape and weight and rumination are central in interpreting BED because overvaluation contributes to preoccupation with thoughts about food and eating, weight, and shape; repeated body checking or avoidance (e.g., avoiding looking at their body or reflections in mirrors); and attempts at dietary restraint (Wang et al., 2017). Rumination is associated with severity of the eating-disorder psychopathology and weight-bias internalization beyond the influence of overvaluation of shape/weight. Individuals with greater rumination might be more likely to dwell on and internalize negative attitudes from weight-based discrimination experiences. Through a cognitive theory lens, overvaluation could be interpreted as a cognitive distortion deriving from (a) how individuals filter, process, organize, and assign meanings to internal and environmental stimuli and (b) the schemas, or core beliefs, that individuals hold about themselves. For example, an individual may have a negative self schema related to being overweight ("I am ugly") or many negative self schemas that are interrelated ("I am worthless because I am ugly") and easily activated by various events or stimuli. Binge eating is associated with a number of early maladaptive schemas including emotional inhibition, abandonment, vulnerability to harm, emotional deprivation, defectiveness/shame, failure to achieve, insufficient self-control, mistrust/abuse, social undesirability, and social isolation (Pugh, 2015). An individual who is overweight would likely regularly encounter events or stimuli that could be interpreted as demeaning, embarrassing, or discriminating. With a negative core schema of ugliness activated, individuals would interpret and filter the information they receive to confirm their ugliness and worthlessness because they connect their body/appearance with their worth.

The cognitive profile of BED is characterized by a poorer performance in decision-making, poorer cognitive flexibility, lower accuracy, a lack of attention, and difficulty adapting to changes in a new situation compared to clients with AN and healthy controls. With BED, longer average time in providing answers could be explained by slowed thinking as a characteristic symptom of depression (Aloi et al., 2015). Because of the inflexibility of the eating schemes, any minor transgression can lead to an all-or-nothing reaction whereby attempts to control eating are abandoned and result in a binge. In reviewing the most prominent theoretical models including the schema theory of binge eating, Burton and Abbott (2017) concluded there may be maintaining factors not being addressed in treatment and that further research should aim to improve understanding of the cognitive factors thought to maintain binge-eating behaviour.

Spiritual Theories

Underlying reasons for eating without being hungry include subjective experiences of distress and disconnection that do not encourage trust in others and prior relationships characterized by insecurity. Individuals who

come to regard food as a kind of substitute attachment object may use it to fill the emptiness, often hiding their food and eating from others and thus increasing their sense of disconnection from self and others. "Because I used my eating disorder to numb my feelings, I was no longer able to feel a spiritual connection with God and most of the time I felt utterly alone" (Scott Richards et al., 2018, p. 92). Examining the relationship between religion and obesity using data from a large nationally representative sample, Krause and Hayward (2016) found the odds of being obese higher for those who received the least amount of spiritual support from religious others, and lowest for those with higher spiritual support and/or emotional support. Some people experience significant personal growth when confronted by a stressful life event; having a sympathetic, understanding religious other available to assist in working through ambiguous feelings about God/Higher Power may go a long way toward alleviating the psychological distress. Higher rate of exposure to stress has been associated with a greater risk of becoming obese (Kiecolt-Glaser et al., 2015). Having a secure relationship with God/Higher Power may provide benefits that are not unlike the benefits that arise from close relationships with human beings.

Risk Factors

The risk or predisposing factors for BED are included in Figure 25.3.

Interdisciplinary Treatment

Women presenting with BED have self-identified their issues as concerns about mood, weight loss, and body image/food issues. Among those with obesity, a greater proportion of these women indicated body image/food issues were their top treatment priorities, suggesting that these persons may be more apt to seek treatment beyond weight management for their problematic eating patterns (Rosenbaum et al., 2016). The treatment methods for BED in current use include CBT, interpersonal psychotherapy, medications, self-help support groups, and commercial weight-loss and exercise programs. Surgical interventions are recommended for morbid obesity (BMI > 40) when other weight-loss attempts have failed. However, in a 2-year RCT, Burguera et al. (2015) found that an intense lifestyle intervention obtained an average weight loss (10%) significantly better compared to bariatric surgery (1% to 2%). Participants who followed the supervised lifestyle intervention incorporated healthy lifestyles and exercise in their daily routine. In other studies, adult clients receiving bariatric surgery for obesity reported lower scores for quality of life compared with individuals who are obese and without BED (Costa & Pinto, 2015). General practitioners may not refer for surgery due to uncertainty about long-term efficacy and safety in addition to their opinion that surgery is not appropriate because it only treats symptoms (Roebroek et al., 2019). As with the treatment of AN and BN, a comprehensive interdisciplinary approach is needed. Treatment goals in outpatient settings focus on reducing binge eating, effecting and maintaining weight loss if overweight or obese, restructuring dysfunctional thinking about food and appearance, alleviating comorbid depression and anxiety, and addressing harassment.

Nutrition counselling for BED targets portion size and control, the role of emotions on eating behaviours, healthy food and nutrient choices, self-monitoring, and strategies to delay binge eating. Greater reductions in binge frequency and improved glycemic control was found in those treated with chromium (Sala et al., 2017), an essential mineral that affects insulin and serotonin functioning and has the potential to also influence dopamine functioning. Any role for chromium supplementation within treatment guidelines requires further research. Commercial weight-loss and fitness programs may also be accessed. Alternative therapies monitored by holistic health professionals may also be helpful, such as relaxation and yoga.

Priority Care Issues

Comorbid obesity, overweight, depression, and anxiety can contribute to cardiac and other health crises. The risk of type 2 diabetes is significant in the presence of obesity.

Nursing Management: Human Response to Binge-Eating Disorder

The primary nursing care focus for clients living with BED may include excessive caloric intake, inability to independently engage in personal care activities, insufficient energy to complete personal care activities, decreased energy, difficulties managing social expectations, and inability to engage and sustain actions to meet health needs. The nurse establishes a therapeutic relationship and through this connection helps the client monitor self-care abilities including dietary intake and activity, teaches and models effective problem solving, and suggests nutritional recommendations that take into account the client's individual needs.

Therapeutic Relationship

Individuals who have BED may experience a great deal of shame and guilt in response to negative judgments of their eating behaviours and any resulting obesity. They often are reluctant to participate in formal fitness programs for fear of being ridiculed. They may opt out of such programs when they believe they have nothing in common with other group members. Often, they suffer with BED for years, feeling very lonely. The nurse builds a relationship of trust through modelling a self-accepting, nonjudgmental approach, and discussing the role of the nurse–client relationship with respect to the goals of therapy (see Chapter 7). The hallmarks of BED are low self-esteem experiences, weak therapeutic alliance, and low mastery experiences, which, in turn, predict treatment dissatisfaction and early discontinuation of care (Amianto et al., 2015). Previous session alliance is significantly associated with lower subsequent session binge eating (Tasca et al., 2016). Thus, by attending to the quality of the therapeutic relationship, nurses may help clients reduce binge eating.

Biologic Domain

Most individuals with BED become overweight or obese. The medical consequences of cardiovascular disease, diabetes, and arthritis as well as other health threats are considered in all aspects of the nursing process.

Assessment

The nurse assesses current binge-eating patterns and associated symptoms of gastric distress (e.g., acid regurgitation, heartburn, dysphagia, bloating, upper abdominal pain, diarrhoea, urgency, and constipation). Physical mobility, activity, and sleep patterns are also evaluated.

Nursing Care Foci for Biologic Domain

Altered nutrition: risk for overweight BMI, altered mobility, and activity intolerance are examples of nursing care foci for the biologic domain.

Interventions for Biologic Domain

Clients are asked to record their intake, binges, and feelings associated with food and eating to form a foundation for changing behaviours. Clients are monitored for complications such as diabetes, cardiovascular disease, and arthritis.

Pharmacologic Interventions

Lisdexamfetamine dimesylate (Vyvanse), a prescription medicine used for the treatment of attention deficit hyperactivity disorder (ADHD) in clients 6 years and above, is the first medication with an approved indication for the treatment of moderate to severe BED in adults in Canada (Shire US Inc, 2015). It is not known if Vyvanse is safe and effective for weight loss in the treatment of obesity. Topiramate and orlistat are currently used in the long-term treatment of obesity. Investigations have shown that topiramate (an antiepileptic agent) has been effective in decreasing binge eating and appetite. Topiramate has demonstrated efficacy in the treatment of BED-related obesity (Guerdjikova et al., 2018). Orlistat inhibits GI lipase, an enzyme that breaks down triglycerides in the intestine so that triglycerides from the diet are prevented from being hydrolyzed into absorbable free fatty acids and are excreted undigested, thus preventing approximately 30% of dietary fat from being absorbed. In a double-blind trial, orlistat was compared with polyglucosamine (a low molecular weight substance that binds fats to make them nonbioavailable yet partially eliminated or used by colonic bacteria as a fuel). Both medications yielded weight loss; however, BMI and waist circumference reduction were more consistent with polyglucosamine than with orlistat (Stoll et al., 2017). Polyglucosamine side effects of stomachache, bloating, nausea, vomiting, constipation, palpitations, and mood swings were reasons participants gave for withdrawing from the study. The side effects resulting from orlistat's mode of action (e.g., oily spotting, liquid stools, faecal urgency or incontinence, flatulence, and abdominal cramping) were not cited by participants. Further research will confirm polyglucosamine's feasibility in the treatment of obesity associated with BED. Other medications, usually SSRIs, may treat anxiety and depression symptomatology. Fluoxetine (Prozac) is often used to reduce binge eating (see Box 25.13).

TEACHING POINTS

Individuals taking the above weight-loss agents should be informed that weight will be regained if the medication is stopped unless lifestyle interventions that include physical activity and stress management are incorporated. Those taking antiobesity drugs should be instructed in what side effects to expect. The instructions for SSRI use are contained in Chapter 13.

Psychosocial Domain

Assessment

Psychological assessment for the individual with BED is similar to that for the individual with BN, requiring identification of cognitive distortions and knowledge deficits. Dissociation is evaluated given that binge eating may be a means to escape negative emotion (Vanderlinden et al., 2015). Symptoms of mood and anxiety disorders are explored in-depth in Chapters 22 and 23, respectively.

Nursing Care Focus for Psychosocial Domain

Common nursing concerns requiring nursing management include anxiety, knowledge deficit, and limited sense of connection with others and society.

Interventions for Psychosocial Domain

Psychotherapy and structured self-help, both based on cognitive–behavioural interventions, are recommended as the first-line treatments for BED (Amianto et al., 2015; Hilbert et al., 2019). When BED is an aspect of complex trauma-related disorders, it must be treated in sequenced stages consisting of (a) establishing safety, stabilization, and symptom reduction; (b) confronting, working through, and integrating traumatic memories; and (c) supporting identity integration and rehabilitation (Vanderlinden et al., 2015). Treatment must also educate clients (and families) about dissociation and related impulsive behaviours. Compared to eating disorders without complex trauma and dissociation, the nurse must be aware that both weight-loss and/or binge-eating behaviours may function to avoid confrontation with painful emotions and memories. The nurse must try to motivate and help clients normalize eating habits and weight through teaching techniques to monitor and change eating habits, as well as to change the way they respond to difficult and stressful situations. CBT is the psychotherapy of choice for BED (Iqbal & Rehman, 2020). In addition to clinician-led CBT, self-help–based CBT is effective for treating BED.

Family

There is little research into family needs; families of individuals with BED may need support themselves.

Psychoeducation

The nurse can assist the individual with BED to eat appropriately portioned meals at regular intervals to reduce hunger and binge eating. Individuals also need information about the medical consequences of binge eating. Other topics for psychoeducation are included in Box 25.14.

BOX 25.14 Psychoeducation Checklist: Binge-Eating Disorder

When caring for the individual with BED, consider the following topics:

✓ Health and lifestyle
✓ How weight reduction can be attained
✓ Applied knowledge about food and healthy eating
✓ Principles of dieting
✓ The importance of being present of one's body and choices
✓ Relaxation techniques
✓ Stress management
✓ The importance of physical activity
✓ Strength training: instruction and practical exercises
✓ Accessing resources: computers as an aid in eating well and achieving nutritional goals
✓ Planning for holidays

Spiritual Domain

Assessment

The nurse assesses the client's reported satisfaction with relationships and lifestyle choices, is watchful of client expressions of self-judgment and self-acceptance, and enables the client to describe any painful traumatic experiences with harassment and discrimination. The nurse listens to client stories of social exclusion, developmental interruption, and denied extracurricular opportunities such as shopping for clothing, attending parties, and participating in recreational/sporting events.

Nursing Care Focus in the Spiritual Domain

Potential nursing care foci for the spiritual domain include dissatisfaction with life, loss of self-identity, and loss of self-worth. Individuals with BED who binge eat in response to various biopsychosocial experiences, environmental cues, trauma, and nonevents may struggle to protect themselves from such underlying issues as isolation and discrimination, filling themselves with food without awareness of deeper unmet needs.

Interventions for Spiritual Domain

Provide clients living with BED opportunities to discuss any experiences of stress, relationship conflict, and trauma. Support them to narrate themes of disappointment and pain in response to stigma. Through the safety of the nurse–client relationship, they can develop their capacity to reconnect with self, others, and, when appropriate, the larger universal life force. The nurse may offer anticipatory guidance to individuals who need to catch up with developmental milestones such as dating and intimacy that were missed due to the overarching presence of eating disorder symptoms of social withdrawal and low self-esteem.

Evaluation and Treatment Outcomes

In a trial comparing effectiveness of CBT with IPT, longer duration of the eating disorder (equal to or greater than 8 years) and higher levels of the importance of shape were associated with the severity of eating disorder features at 60-week follow-up (Cooper et al., 2016). Those with low self-esteem at baseline who received CBT had lower scores on the severity of eating disorder features than those who received IPT. For those whose baseline self-esteem scores were higher, there was no relative advantage for either treatment. As also used to treat BN, CBT-E (enhanced cognitive–behaviour therapy) addresses overvaluation of shape and weight, low self-esteem, perfectionism, and interpersonal problems.

TEACHING POINTS

Keeping in mind that many BED clients are overweight or obese and may have experienced harassment, psychoeducation focuses on principles of dieting, lifestyle changes to maintain weight loss, the importance of being self-aware, relaxation techniques, strength training, and stress management. High attrition rate is reported for psychoeducational programs (Amianto et al., 2015). Therefore, it is important that nurses attend to client emotional comfort, briefing, and debriefing.

Long-term outcome studies indicate that BED may have a more favourable remission rate than other eating disorders. The majority of RCTs for CBT have reported remission rates greater than 50%. CBT has generally not produced meaningful weight loss but has demonstrated improvements in eating disordered psychopathology, depression, social adjustment, and self-esteem that are generally well maintained at 1- to 4-year follow-up. Individual and group treatments appear to produce similar results. Poor treatment outcomes have been associated with a history of weight problems during childhood, high levels of emotional eating at baseline, overvaluation of weight and shape, interpersonal dysfunction, and low group cohesion during group CBT. The presence of a cluster B personality disorder (e.g., borderline, histrionic, antisocial, and narcissistic personality disorders) predicts higher levels of binge eating at 1-year follow-up (Saules et al., 2015). Positive treatment outcomes have been associated with low levels of emotional eating at baseline, older age of onset, weight-loss history that is negative for amphetamine use, and decreases in depressive symptoms during treatment. Early response to treatment (defined as a 65% to 70% reduction in binge eating within 4 weeks of starting treatment) is associated with greater long-term (1 to 2 year) remission from BED and lower eating disorder psychopathology (Saules et al., 2015).

Continuum of Care

Although individuals typically do not require hospitalization for BED, the consequence of obesity may involve hospitalization for surgical intervention such as gastric bypass or gastric banding surgery. Ongoing assessment of maladaptive eating following surgery is important as LOC eating and binge eating may impede weight loss.

Prevention of Eating Disorders

Eating disorders are among the most preventable mental disorders. *Canada's Eating Disorders Strategy 2019–2029* recommends prevention efforts target the time period before an eating disorder develops. Adolescence and young adulthood are critical periods for the initial development of eating disorders, with nearly all (95%) first-time cases occurring by age 25 years (Ward et al., 2019). This finding suggests that prevention efforts may best be targeted to adolescent or younger individuals. However, diagnosis and treatment of eating disorders at older ages should also be prioritized given the risk of relapse and continued eating disorder prevalence throughout the lifespan. National eating disorder awareness and advocacy groups work toward educating the general public, those at risk, and those who work with those at risk, such as teachers, coaches, and college student health centre staff. The awareness and advocacy groups promote greater awareness of early signs of eating disorders and available resources to those at risk for developing eating disorders. They also monitor the media, striving to remove unhealthy advertisements and articles in magazines appealing to vulnerable individuals. A list of online resources is found in the Web Links.

Prevention and early detection strategies for parents and schoolteachers are often the focus of school nurses and community mental health nurses. There is growing evidence for the importance of positive body image in terms of body appreciation and body acceptance (Sharpe et al., 2018). Specific strategies to promote positive body image have included The Body Project, based on the principal of cognitive dissonance, and designed to encourage high school and college students to explore the costs of pursuing the thin ideal. The Body Project was found to reduce risk for onset of eating disorders, reaching 3.5 million girls and young women in 125 countries (Becker & Stice, 2017). The Body Project Canada is currently offered in Newfoundland and Labrador (edfnl.ca/body-project-canada), at the Universities of Manitoba and Waterloo, and by Registered Provisional Psychologists in Calgary. The National Eating Disorder Information Centre (NEDIC) offers *Beyond Images* (nedic.ca/health-promotion-prevention), a free downloadable body image and self-esteem curriculum for grades 4 to 8 that includes activities to combat appearance-based bullying and negative stereotypes. NEDIC's **Body Pride** program provides additional ideas for educators. Another prevention resource is a children's picture book called *Shapesville* that is designed to increase the appearance satisfaction and awareness of healthy eating in 5- to 9-year-old girls (www.edcatalogue.com/small-book-fills-big-need-for-children). National and provincial eating disorder associations also contain information about available prevention programs. Successful overweight and obesity prevention programs are delivered in school settings with program leaders having access to specialist support.

Other strategies for parents and children appear in Table 25.4 and are based on research of risk factors and protective factors. These protective factors mainly concern the quality of family relationships (Langdon-Daly

Table 25.4	Prevention Strategies for Parents and Children	
Education for Parents	**Education for Children**
Real versus ideal weight	Peer pressure regarding eating and weight
Influence of attitudes, behaviours, and teasing	Menses, puberty, and normal weight gain
Ways to increase self-esteem	Strategies for obesity
Role of media: TV and magazines	Ways to develop or improve self-esteem
Signs and symptoms	Body image traps: media and retail clothing
Interventions for obesity	Adapting and coping with problems
Boys at risk also	Reporting friends with signs of eating disorders
Observe for rituals	**Screening:** for risk factors
Supervision of eating and exercise	**Assessment:** for treatment
	Follow-up: monitor for relapse

& Serpell, 2017). They include family composition (living in a two parent household, having siblings to "dilute" parental expectations and pressure), satisfaction with family life (greater family connectedness, positive family communication, and clear family boundaries), social support (feeling loved/supported by family and friends), and healthy family environment around eating and weight (positive atmosphere at family meals, frequent family meals, and avoiding comments about weight). Dieting, low self-esteem, and body dissatisfaction are examples of risk factors underlying eating disorder development that can be reversed with early identification and intervention.

Future Directions in Eating Disorder Knowledge

The classification of eating disorders underwent significant revision in 2013 with the *DSM-5*. Refer to the *DSM-5* (2013) for comprehensive detailing of AN, BN, and BED as well as other feeding and eating disorders that require ongoing research and development. As described earlier, the first Canadian practice guidelines to evaluate the evidence on psychotherapeutic and psychopharmacological treatments for children and adolescents diagnosed with eating disorders was developed by a team of diverse expert stakeholders from across the country (Couturier et al., 2020). A critical finding of both these practice guidelines and of *Canada's Eating Disorder Strategy 2019–2029* is the need for peer support (client and parent) in times of transition between different levels of care and from the paediatric to adult system of care.

Society has begun to engage in an effort to help young individuals resist developing eating disorders. Many of the Web Links have online help and resources for young individuals, families, teachers, and healthcare professionals.

Summary of Key Points

- AN, BN, and BED have some common symptoms, risk factors, and aetiologic factors, and individuals may migrate between the different diagnostic entities, which are discrete disorders.
- Eating disorders are best viewed along a continuum that includes normal unrestricted eating, mild disturbed eating, increasing weight and shape preoccupation, and clinical eating disorders. These symptomologic patterns occur more frequently than full eating disorders, and they may be overlooked; however, once identified, they can be prevented from worsening.
- Similar factors predispose individuals to the development of AN, BN, and BED, and these factors represent a bio/psycho/social/spiritual model of risk that threatens health and wellbeing. Identifying risk factors assists with prevention strategies.
- Combined aetiologic factors contribute to the development of eating disorders; no one factor provides a complete explanation.

- Mood and anxiety disorders are significantly more frequent in individuals with eating disorders than the general community.
- All of the eating disorders have physical, emotional, social, and spiritual consequences that influence health, wellbeing, and even life.
- Treatment of AN almost always includes hospitalization for refeeding; BN and BED are treated primarily on an outpatient basis.
- For individuals with BN, CBT improves symptoms sooner than does IPT. For individuals with AN, family therapy plus individual IPT are the most effective. Research on best practice for BED is still accumulating; CBT and pharmacological interventions (both alone and in combination) foster remission.
- Pharmacotherapy can be effective for BN and BED but less so for AN, especially during acute malnourishment.
- Individuals with eating disorders require responsive treatment addressing both specific (e.g., eating behaviour) and nonspecific (e.g., underlying) vulnerabilities.
- The outcomes for BN are better than those for AN and BED. The type and severity of comorbid conditions and the length of the illness influence outcomes.

Thinking Challenges

Laura, 15 years old, is a high school student diagnosed with anorexia nervosa—restricting subtype. She is the youngest of four children and lives at home alone with her parents since her siblings moved away to attend college. Laura is a competitive swimmer and plays the piano in addition to being involved in the school's student council. Laura recalls reducing her eating at the start of the COVID-19 pandemic because "I wanted to improve myself since school and sports activities were closed." When her weight loss was noticed by her parents who are well-educated health professionals, Laura began individual weekly visits with a paediatrician, a community health clinic, and a nurse psychotherapist. Within several weeks, Laura complied with eating three nondieting meals and a bedtime snack every day. She continued to swim twice a week, play the piano, and attend school in-person or online as COVID-19 restrictions permitted. Laura's parents, while pleased that Laura was eating, noted that Laura did not sit still, paced a lot, and spent most of her time either in her room with the door closed or in the bathroom taking hour-long baths. On several

occasions, Laura appeared flushed when she exited her room. Her weight began to decline again. "I am not exercising," she told her concerned parents. "Please leave me alone!" The parents asked to meet with the clinic nurse. They believed Laura was exercising in her room and sought the clinic's help with how to best approach Laura's request to be left alone.

a. You are the clinic nurse. How do you respond to the parents request for help in approaching Laura about her level of physical activity?
b. What strategies would you consider to help Laura reduce her physical exertion?
c. How would you discuss these strategies with Laura?

> Visit thePoint to view suggested responses.
> Go to **thePoint.lww.com/activate** and use the activation code found in the front of this text to unlock answers to the "Thinking Challenges" and other online resources.

Web Links

bana.ca This site of the Bulimia Anorexia Nervosa Association (BANA) at the University of Windsor has information on specialized treatment education, support services for individuals affected directly and indirectly by eating disorders, and prevention of eating disorders, negative body image, and low self-esteem.

Daniellesplace.org Danielle's Place, Burlington, ON, became a part of ROCK (Reach Out Centre for Kids) in April 2015. Programming includes groups for children and youth up to age 17—body image and self-esteem group for girls through grades 4 to 8, *Boy Zone* for boy's body issues, an eating disorder workshop series, anxiety management group, yoga, meditation, and an active parenting group.

Edac-atac.ca Eating Disorders Association of Canada–Association des Troubles Alimentaires du Canada (EDAC/ARAC) is a Canadian organization of professionals in the field of eating disorders and related areas. The mandate is to promote a reflective, responsive approach in the provision of services among providers.

edfc.ca The Eating Disorder Foundation of Canada supports local community awareness campaigns, education in the schools, and fundraising toward establishing treatment programs, transition housing, and ongoing research.

edoyr.com Eating Disorders of York Region (EDOYR), a grassroots, community-based, registered nonprofit organization provides eating disorder and substance addiction help/support through an expressive, therapeutic art program funded by the Ontario Trillium Foundation.

feast-ed.org Families Empowered and Supporting Treatment of Eating Disorders (F.E.A.S.T) is an international organization providing information on evidence-based treatment and mutual support to caregivers of eating disorder clients with over 6,000 members on four continents.

www.hopeseds.org Hope's Eating Disorders Support provides education, resource support and advocacy services free of charge for all individuals, as well as for their family and friends, who struggle with disordered eating or have been affected by an eating disorder.

kidshelpphone.ca This Kids Help Phone site offers a toll-free (1-800-668-6868) national telephone counselling service for Canadian children and youth experiencing violence, alcohol or drug abuse, or issues related to suicide or who are suffering from an eating disorder. It features tips for parents and others.

www.killingussoftly4.org Using a wide range of contemporary print and television ads, Kilbourne examines these images against the real-world backdrop of eating disorders, men's violence against women, and the political backlash directed at feminism. Kilbourne challenges young people to question traditional gender norms and think critically about the fundamental relationship between representation and power.

www.lookingglassbc.com Residential care, Summer Camp, online peer support group, educational scholarships, and family support to those affected by eating disorders.

Nedic.ca The National Eating Disorder Information Centre (NEDIC) provides information and resources for individuals, families, friends, and teachers on eating disorders and weight preoccupation.

nied.ca The National Initiative for Eating Disorders aims to increase awareness and education of the chronic situation facing persons living with eating disorders and their families in Canada and to ensure eating disorders are included in mental health discussions, policies, mental health organizations, programs, decisions, campaigns, and agendas.

sheenasplace.org This site describes Sheena's Place, Canada's first community-based centre to offer services at no cost to people affected by severe eating and body image issues. The site provides information and support to parents, siblings, friends, spouses, partners, teachers, and other care providers.

something-fishy.org A website (available in English and French) about eating disorders that is dedicated to raising awareness. It emphasizes that eating disorders are *not* about food and weight but are symptoms of something deeper going on, inside.

References

Abbott, W., Brett, A., Brownlee, T. E., Hammond, K. M., Harper, L. D., Naughton, R. J., Anderson, L., Munson, E. H., Sharkey, J. V., Randell, R. K., & Clifford, T. (2021). The prevalence of disordered eating in elite male and female soccer players. *Eating and Weight Disorders, 26*(2), 491–498. https://doi.org/10.1007/s40519-020-00872-0

Accurso, E. C., Lebow, J., Murray, S. B., Kass, A. E., & Le Grange, D. (2016). The relation of weight suppression and BMI to bulimic symptoms in youth with bulimia nervosa. *Journal of Eating Disorders, 4*, 1–6. https://doi.org/10.1186/s40337-016-0111-5

Ágh, T., Kovács, G., Supina, D., Pawaskar, M., Herman, B. K., Vokó, Z., & Sheehan, D. V. (2016). A systematic review of the health-related quality of life and economic burdens of anorexia nervosa, bulimia nervosa, and binge eating disorder. *Eating and Weight Disorders, 21*(3), 353–364. https://doi.org/10.1007/s40519-016-0264-x

Aloi, M., Rania, M., Caroleo, M., Bruni, A., Palmieri, A., Cauteruccio, M. A., De Fazio, P., & Segura-García, C. (2015). Decision making, central coherence and set-shifting: A comparison between Binge Eating Disorder, Anorexia Nervosa and Healthy Controls. *BMC Psychiatry, 15*, 6. https://doi.org/10.1186/s12888-015-0395-z

American Psychiatric Association. (2000). *Diagnostic and statistical manual of mental disorders* (4th ed., Text revision).

American Psychiatric Association. (2013). *Diagnostic and statistical manual of mental disorders* (5th ed.).

Amianto, F., Ottone, L., Daga, G. A., & Fassino, S. (2015). Binge-eating disorder diagnosis and treatment: A recap in front of DSM-5. *BMC Psychiatry, 15*, 70. https://doi.org/10.1186/s12888-015-0445-6

Arnow, K. D., Feldman, T., Fichtel, E., Lin, I. H.-J., Egan, A., Lock, J., Westerman, M., & Darcy, A. M. (2017). A qualitative analysis of male eating disorder symptoms. *Eating Disorders, 25*(4), 297–309. https://doi.org/10.1080/10640266.2017.1308729

Arrow, B., Kenardy, J., & Agras, W. S. (1995). The Emotional Eating Scale: The development of a measure to assess coping with negative affect by eating. *International Journal of Eating Disorders, 18*, 79–90.

Attia, E., Steinglass, J. E., Walsh, B. T., Wang, Y., Wu, P., Schreyer, C., Wildes, J., Yilmaz, Z., Guarda, A. S., Kaplan, A. S., & Marcus, M. D. (2019). Olanzapine versus placebo in adult outpatients with anorexia nervosa: A randomized clinical trial. *American Journal of Psychiatry, 176*(6), 449–456. https://doi.org/10.1176/appi.ajp.2018.18101125

Bannatyne, A. J., & Abel, L. M. (2015). Can we fight stigma with science? The effect of aetiological framing on attitudes towards anorexia nervosa and the impact on volitional stigma. *Australian Journal of Psychology, 67*(1), 38–46. https://doi.org/10.1111/ajpy.12062

Barakat, S., Maguire, S., Surgenor, L., Donnelly, B., Miceska, B., Fromholtz, K., Russell, J., Hay, P., & Touyz, S. (2017). The role of regular eating and self-monitoring in the treatment of bulimia nervosa: A pilot study of an online guided self-help CBT program. *Behavioral Sciences (Basel, Switzerland), 7*(3), 39. https://doi.org/10.3390/bs7030039

Bartholdy, S., Allen, K., Hodsoll, J., O'Daly, O. G., Campbell, I. C., Banaschewski, T., Bokde, A. L. W., Bromberg, U., Büchel, C., Quinlan, E. B., Conrod, P. J., Desrivières, S., Flor, H., Frouin, V., Gallinat, J., Garavan, H., Heinz, A., Ittermann, B., Martinot, J. L., et al. (2017). Identifying disordered eating behaviours in adolescents: How do parent and adolescent reports differ by sex and age? *European Child & Adolescent Psychiatry, 26*(6), 691–701. https://doi.org/10.1007/s00787-016-0935-1

Becker, C. B., & Stice, E. (2017). From efficacy to effectiveness to broad implementation: Evolution of the Body Project. *Journal of Consulting and Clinical Psychology, 85*(8), 767–782. https://doi.org/10.1037/ccp0000204

Belak, L., Deliberto, T., Shear, M., Kerrigan, S., & Attia, E. (2017). Inviting eating disorder patients to discuss the academic literature: A model program for psychoeducation. *Journal of Eating Disorders, 5*(1), 49. https://doi.org/10.1186/s40337-017-0178-7

Blackburn, M.-E., Auclair, J., Dion, J., Lessard, I., Bellemare, J., & Lapalme, L. (2016). Body dissatisfaction and self-esteem: Perception vs reality. Appearance Matters 7, London. http://ecobes.cegepjonquiere.ca/media/tinymce/Publication-Sante/AfficheMEBlack_30Juin16_3.pdf

Borowsky, H. M., Eisenberg, M. E., Bucchianeri, M. M., Piran, N., & Neumark-Sztainer, D. (2016). Feminist identity, body image, and disordered eating. *Eating Disorders, 24*(4), 297–311. https://doi.org/10.1080/10640266.2015.1123986

Boyd, E. D., & Durant, N. H. (2018). Recurrent hyponatremia in a young adult woman with anorexia nervosa and the effects of insufficient communication. *International Journal of Eating Disorders, 51*(12), 1378–1381. https://doi.org/10.1002/eat.22973

Buelens, T., Luyckx, K., Verschueren, M., Schoevaerts, K., Dierckx, E., Depestele, L., & Claes, L. (2020). Temperament and character traits of female eating disorder patients with(out) non-suicidal self-Injury. *Journal of Clinical Medicine, 9*(4). https://doi.org/10.3390/jcm9041207

Bulik, C. M., Blake, L., & Austin, J. (2019). Genetics of eating disorders: What the clinician needs to know. *Psychiatric Clinics of North America, 42*(1), 59–73. https://doi.org/10.1016/j.psc.2018.10.007

Burguera, B., Jesús Tur, J., Escudero, A. J., Alos, M., Pagán, A., Cortés, B., González, X. F., & Soriano, J. B. (2015). An intensive lifestyle intervention is an effective treatment of morbid obesity: The TRA-MOMTANA study—A two-year randomized controlled clinical trial. *International Journal of Endocrinology, 2015*, 194696. https://doi.org/10.1155/2015/194696

Burton, A. L., & Abbott, M. J. (2017). Conceptualising binge eating: A review of the theoretical and empirical literature. *Behaviour Change, 34*(3), 168–198. https://doi.org/10.1017/bec.2017.12

Burton, A. L., & Abbott, M. J. (2019). Processes and pathways to binge eating: Development of an integrated cognitive and behavioural model of binge eating. *Journal of Eating Disorders, 7*(1), 18. https://doi.org/10.1186/s40337-019-0248-0

Buser, J. K., & Gibson, S. (2016). Attachment to God/higher power and bulimic symptoms Among College Women. *Journal of College Counseling, 19*(2), 124–137. https://doi.org/10.1002/jocc.12036

Canadian Eating Disorders Alliance. (2019). *The Canadian eating disorders strategy: 2019–2029.* https://nied.ca/wp-content/uploads/2019/11/NIED_Strategy_Eng_CR_MedRes_SinglePages_REV.pdf

Carapeto, M. J., Domingos, R., & Veiga, G. (2020). Is the effect of body dissatisfaction on depressive symptoms dependent on weight status? A study with early-to-middle adolescents. *European Journal of Investigation in Health, Psychology and Education, 10*(4), 1020–1034. https://www.mdpi.com/2254-9625/10/4/72

Carlo, A. (2018, 30 September). Why feminism can help resolve the unspoken issue of eating disorders among men. *The Independent.* https://www.independent.co.uk/voices/eating-disorders-men-anorexia-feminism-male-bulimia-binge-food-a8561821.html

Carter, A., Forrest, J. I., & Kaida, A. (2017). Association between internet use and body dissatisfaction among young females: Cross-sectional analysis of the Canadian Community Health Survey. *Journal of Medical Internet Research, 19*(2), e39. https://doi.org/10.2196/jmir.5636

Çelik, S., Kayar, Y., Önem Akçakaya, R., Türkyılmaz Uyar, E., Kalkan, K., Yazısız, V., Aydın, Ç., & Yücel, B. (2015). Correlation of binge eating disorder with level of depression and glycemic control in type 2 diabetes mellitus patients. *General Hospital Psychiatry, 37*(2), 116–119. https://doi.org/10.1016/j.genhosppsych.2014.11.012

Chang, P. F., & Bazarova, N. N. (2016). Managing stigma: Disclosure-response communication patterns in pro-anorexic websites. *Health Communication, 31*(2), 217–229. https://doi.org/10.1080/10410236.2014.946218

Churruca, K., Ussher, J. M., & Perz, J. (2017). Just desserts? Exploring constructions of food in women's experiences of bulimia. *Qualitative Health Research, 27*(10), 1491–1506. https://doi.org/10.1177/1049732316672644

Cliffe, C., Shetty, H., Himmerich, H., Schmidt, U., Stewart, R., & Dutta, R. (2020). Suicide attempts requiring hospitalization in patients with eating disorders: A retrospective cohort study. *International Journal of Eating Disorders, 53*(5), 728–735. https://doi.org/10.1002/eat.23240

Coffino, J. A., Orloff, N. C., & Hormes, J. M. (2016). Dietary restraint partially mediates the relationship between impulsivity and binge eating only in lean individuals: The importance of accounting for body mass in studies of restraint. *Frontiers in Psychology, 7*, 1499. https://doi.org/10.3389/fpsyg.2016.0149

Collins, B., Breithaupt, L., McDowell, J. E., Miller, L. S., Thompson, J., & Fischer, S. (2017). The impact of acute stress on the neural processing of food cues in bulimia nervosa: Replication in two samples. *Journal of Abnormal Psychology, 126*(5), 540–551. https://doi.org/10.1037/abn0000242

Cooper, Z., Allen, E., Bailey-Straebler, S., Basden, S., Murphy, R., O'Connor, M. E., & Fairburn, C. G. (2016). Predictors and moderators of response to enhanced cognitive behaviour therapy and interpersonal psychotherapy for the treatment of eating disorders. *Behaviour Research and Therapy, 84*, 9–13. https://doi.org/10.1016/j.brat.2016.07.002

Conti, J. E. (2018). Recovering identity from anorexia nervosa: Women's constructions of their experiences of recovery from Anorexia Nervosa Over 10 Years. *Journal of Constructivist Psychology, 31*(1), 72–94. https://doi.org/10.1080/10720537.2016.1251366

Contreras, R. E., Schriever, S. C., & Pfluger, P. T. (2019). Physiological and epigenetic features of yoyo dieting and weight control. *Frontiers in Genetics, 10*, 1015. https://doi.org/10.3389/fgene.2019.01015

Copeland, W. E., Bulik, C. M., Zucker, N., Wolke, D., Lereya, S. T., & Costello, E. J. (2015). Does childhood bullying predict eating disorder

symptoms? A prospective, longitudinal analysis. *International Journal of Eating Disorders, 48*(8), 1141–1149. https://doi.org/10.1002/eat.22459

Costa, A. J. R. B., & Pinto, S. L. (2015). Binge eating disorder and quality of life of candidates to bariatric surgery. *Arquivos Brasileiros de Cirurgia Digestiva: ABCD = Brazilian Archives of Digestive Surgery, 28*(Suppl. 1), 52–55. https://dx.doi.org/10.1590/S0102-6720201500S100015

Côté, M., Legendrea, M., Aiméb, A., Braultc, M.-C., Dionc, J., & Bégin, C. (2020). The paths to children's disordered eating: The implications of BMI, weight-related victimization, body dissatisfaction and parents' disordered eating. *Clinical Psychology in Europe, 2*(1). https://doi.org/https://doi.org/10.32872/cpe.v2i1.2689

Cottrell, D. B., & Williams, J. (2016). Eating disorders in men. *Nurse Practitioner, 41*(9), 49–55.

Couturier, J., Isserlin, L., Norris, M., Spettigue, W., Brouwers, M., Kimber, M., McVey, G., Webb, C., Findlay, S., Bhatnagar, N., Snelgrove, N., Ritsma, A., Preskow, W., Miller, C., Coelho, J., Boachie, A., Steinegger, C., Loewen, R., Loewen, T., et al. (2020). Canadian practice guidelines for the treatment of children and adolescents with eating disorders. *Journal of Eating Disorders, 8*(1), 4. https://doi.org/10.1186/s40337-020-0277-8

Culbert, K. M., Racine, S. E., & Klump, K. L. (2016). Hormonal factors and disturbances in eating disorders. *Current Psychiatry Reports, 18*, 65. https://doi.org/10.1007/s11920-016-0701-6

Dahlborg Lyckhage, E., Gardvik, A., Karlsson, H., Törner, J. M., & Berndtsson, I. (2015). Young women with anorexia nervosa. *SAGE Open, 5*(1), 1–8. https://doi.org/10.1177/215824401557654

Dalhoff, A. W., Romero Frausto, H., Romer, G., & Wessing, I. (2019). Perceptive body image distortion in adolescent anorexia nervosa: Changes after treatment. *Frontiers in Psychiatry, 10*, 748. https://doi.org/10.3389/fpsyt.2019.00748

Dalle Grave, R. (2020). *Coronavirus disease 2019 and eating disorders. Eating disorders: the facts.* https://www.psychologytoday.com/us/blog/eating-disorders-the-facts/202003/coronavirus-disease-2019-and-eating-disorders

Damiano, S. R., Paxton, S. J., Wertheim, E. H., McLean, S. A., & Gregg, K. J. (2015). Dietary restraint of 5-year-old girls: Associations with internalization of the thin ideal and maternal, media, and peer influences. *International Journal of Eating Disorders, 48*(8), 1166–1169. https://doi.org/10.1002/eat.22432

Davies, N. (2017). The role of the nurse in eating disorder recovery. *Independent Nurse.* https://www.independentnurse.co.uk/clinical-article/the-role-of-the-nurse-in-eating-disorder-recovery/152976/

Davis, C. (2015). The epidemiology and genetics of binge eating disorder (BED). *CNS Spectrums, 20*(6), 522–529. https://doi.org/10.1017/s1092852915000462

Dell'Osso, L., Abelli, M., Carpita, B., Pini, S., Castellini, G., Carmassi, C., & Ricca, V. (2016). Historical evolution of the concept of anorexia nervosa and relationships with orthorexia nervosa, autism, and obsessive-compulsive spectrum. *Neuropsychiatric Disease and Treatment, 12*, 1651–1660. https://doi.org/10.2147/NDT.S108912

Dimitropoulos, G., Freeman, V. E., Muskat, S., Domingo, A., & McCallum, L. (2016). "You don't have anorexia, you just want to look like a celebrity": Perceived stigma in individuals with anorexia nervosa. *Journal of Mental Health, 25*(1), 47–54. http://dx.doi.org.proxy.hil.unb.ca/10.3109/09638237.2015.1101422

Dion, J., Blackburn, M.-E., Auclair, J., Laberge, L., Veillette, S., Gaudreault, M., Vachon, P., Perron, M., & Touchette, É. (2015). Development and aetiology of body dissatisfaction in adolescent boys and girls. *International Journal of Adolescence and Youth, 20*(2), 151–166. https://doi.org/10.1080/02673843.2014.985320

Eli Lilly Canada Inc. (2016). *Product monograph: Prozac.* Date of revision: July 7, 2016. http://pi.lilly.com/ca/rozac-ca-pmi.pdf

Errichiello, L., Iodice, D., Bruzzese, D., Gherghi, M., & Senatore, I. (2016). Prognostic factors and outcome in anorexia nervosa: A follow-up study. *Eating and Weight Disorders, 21*(1), 73–82. https://doi.org/10.1007/s40519-015-0211-2

Erriu, M., Cimino, S., & Cerniglia, L. (2020). The role of family relationships in eating disorders in adolescents: A narrative review. *Behavioral Sciences (Basel, Switzerland), 10*(4), 71. https://doi.org/10.3390/bs10040071

Espel-Huynh, H. M., Muratore, A. F., & Lowe, M. R. (2018). A narrative review of the construct of hedonic hunger and its measurement by the Power of Food Scale. *Obesity Science & Practice, 4*(3), 238–249. https://doi.org/10.1002/osp4.161

Evans, E. H., Adamson, A. J., Basterfield, L., Le Couteur, A., Reilly, J., Reilly, J., & Parkinson, K. N. (2017). Risk factors for eating disorder symptoms at 12 years of age: A 6-year longitudinal cohort study. *Appetite, 108*, 12–20. https://doi.org/10.1016/j.appet.2016.09.005

Fairburn, C. G., Bailey-Straebler, S., Basden, S., Doll, H. A., Jones, R., Murphy, R., O'Connor, M. E., & Cooper, Z. (2015). A transdiagnostic comparison of enhanced cognitive behaviour therapy (CBT-E) and interpersonal psychotherapy in the treatment of eating disorders. *Behaviour Research and Therapy, 70,* 64–71. https://doi.org/10.1016/j.brat.2015.04.010

Farrington, A., Huntley, M. S., & Donohue, G. (2020). "I found it daunting": An exploration of educational needs and experiences of mental health student nurses working with children and adolescents with eating disorders. *Journal of Psychiatric and Mental Health Nursing, 7*(6), 678–688. https://doi-org.proxy.hil.unb.ca/10.1111/jpm.12619

Fichter, M. M., Quadflieg, N., Crosby, R. D., & Koch, S. (2017). Long-term outcome of anorexia nervosa: Results from a large clinical longitudinal study. *International Journal of Eating Disorders, 50*(9), 1018–1030. https://doi.org/10.1002/eat.22736

Flament, M. F., Henderson, K., Buchholz, A., Obeid, N., Nguyen, H. N. T., Birmingham, M., & Goldfield, G. (2015). Weight status and DSM-5 diagnoses of eating disorders in adolescents from the community. *Journal of the American Academy of Child & Adolescent Psychiatry, 54*(5), 403–413. https://doi.org/10.1016/j.jaac.2015.01.020

Fogarty, S., & Ramjan, L. M. (2016). Factors impacting treatment and recovery in Anorexia Nervosa: Qualitative findings from an online questionnaire. *Journal of Eating Disorders, 64,* 1–9. https://doi.org/10.1186/s40337-016-0107-1

Franko, D. L., Tabri, N., Keshaviah, A., Murray, H. B., Herzog, D. B., Thomas, J. J., Coniglio, K., Keel, P. K., & Eddy, K. T. (2018). Predictors of long-term recovery in anorexia nervosa and bulimia nervosa: Data from a 22-year longitudinal study. *Journal of Psychiatric Research, 96,* 183–188. https://doi.org/10.1016/j.jpsychires.2017.10.008

Frostad, S., Danielsen, Y. S., Rekkedal, G. Å., Jevne, C., Dalle Grave, R., Rø, Ø., & Kessler, U. (2018). Implementation of enhanced cognitive behaviour therapy (CBT-E) for adults with anorexia nervosa in an outpatient eating-disorder unit at a public hospital. *Journal of Eating Disorders, 6*(1), 12. https://doi.org/10.1186/s40337-018-0198-y

Furukawa, T. A., Cipriani, A., Cowen, P. J., Leucht, S., Egger, M., & Salanti, G. (2019). Optimal dose of selective serotonin reuptake inhibitors, venlafaxine, and mirtazapine in major depression: A systematic review and dose-response meta-analysis. *The Lancet, 6*(7), 601–609. https://doi.org/10.1016/S2215-0366(19)30217-2

Gagnon, C., Aimé, A., & Bélanger, C. (2017). Predictors of comorbid eating disorders and diabetes in people with type 1 and type 2 diabetes. *Canadian Journal of Diabetes, 41*(1), 52–57. https://doi.org/10.1016/j.jcjd.2016.06.005

Galmiche, M., Déchelotte, P., Lambert, G., & Tavolacci, M. P. (2019). Prevalence of eating disorders over the 2000–2018 period: A systematic literature review. *American Journal of Clinical Nutrition, 109*(5), 1402–1413. https://doi.org/10.1093/ajcn/nqy342

Garner, D. M. (2011). *Eating disorder inventory-3: Professional manual.* Psychological Assessment Resources.

Garner, D. M., Anderson, M. L., Keiper, C. D. Whynott, R., & Parker, L. (2016). Psychotropic medications in adult and adolescent eating disorders: Clinical practice versus evidence-based recommendations. *Eating and Weight Disorders, 21,* 395–402. https://doi.org/10.1007/s40519-016-0253-0

Garner, D. M., & Garfinkel, P. E. (1979). The Eating Attitude Test: An index of the symptoms of anorexia nervosa. *Psychosomatic Medicine, 10,* 647–656.

Gaylis, J. B., Levy, S. S., & Hong, M. Y. (2020). Relationships between body weight perception, body mass index, physical activity, and food choices in Southern California male and female adolescents. *International Journal of Adolescence and Youth, 25*(1), 264–275. https://doi.org/10.1080/02673843.2019.1614465

Geller, J., Kelly, A. C., Samson, L., Iyar, M. M., & Srikameswaran, S. (2020). The relation between two barriers to self-compassion and clinical characteristics in individuals with eating disorders. *European Eating Disorders Review, 28*(6), 766–772. https://doi.org/10.1002/erv.2764

Gilham, C., Thompson, K., & Ruckstuhl, S. (2020). Improving girls' developmental assets using a mentor-led approach in Atlantic Canada. *Gender Issues, 37*(4), 340–354. https://doi.org/10.1007/s12147-020-09251-6

Gill, S. K., & Kaplan, A. S. (2021). A retrospective chart review study of symptom onset, diagnosis, comorbidities, and treatment in patients with binge eating disorder in Canadian clinical practice. *Eating and Weight Disorders, 26*(4), 1233–1242. https://doi.org/10.1007/s40519-020-01026-y

Goebel-Fabbri, A., Copeland, P., Touyz, S., & Hay, P. (2019). EDITORIAL: Eating disorders in diabetes: Discussion on issues relevant to type 1 diabetes and an overview of the Journal's special issue. *Journal of Eating Disorders, 7*(1), 27. https://doi.org/10.1186/s40337-019-0256-0

Goulet, C., Henrie, J., & Szymanski, L. (2017). An exploration of the associations among multiple aspects of religiousness, body image, eating pathology, and appearance investment. *Journal of Religion and Health, 56,* 493–506. https://doi.org/10.1007/s10943-016-0229-4

Gregertsen, E. C., Mandy, W., Kanakam, N., Armstrong, S., & Serpell, L. (2019). Pre-treatment patient characteristics as predictors of drop-out and treatment outcome in individual and family therapy for adolescents and adults with anorexia nervosa: A systematic review and meta-analysis. *Psychiatry Research, 271,* 484–501. https://doi.org/10.1016/j.psychres.2018.11.068

Griffiths, S., Murray, S. B., & Touyz, S. (2015). Extending the masculinity hypothesis: An investigation of gender role conformity, body dissatisfaction, and disordered eating in young heterosexual men. *Psychology of Men & Masculinity, 16*(1), 108–114. https://doi.org/10.1037/a0035958

Guerdjikova, A. I., Williams, S., Blom, T. J., Mori, N., & McElroy, S. L. (2018). Combination phentermine-topiramate extended release for the treatment of binge eating disorder: An open-label, prospective study. *Innovations in Clinical Neuroscience, 15*(5–6), 17–21.

Guillaume, S., Jaussent, I., Maimoun, L., Ryst, A., Seneque, M., Villain, L., Hamroun, D., Haynos, A. F., Watts, A. W., Loth, K. A., Pearson, C. M., & Neumark-Stzainer, D. (2016). Factors predicting an escalation of restrictive eating during adolescence. *Journal of Adolescent Health, 59*(4), 391–396. https://doi.org/https://doi.org/10.1016/j.jadohealth.2016.03.011

Haynos, A. F., Watts, A. W., Loth, K. A., Pearson, C. M., & Neumark-Stzainer, D. (2016). Factors predicting an escalation of restrictive eating during adolescence. *Journal of Adolescent Health, 59*(4), 391–396. https://doi.org/10.1016/j.jadohealth.2016.03.011

Hellmann, S. S., Njor, S. H., Lynge, E., von Euler-Chelpin, M., Olsen, A., Tjønneland, A., Vejborg, I., & Andersen, Z. J. (2015). Body mass index and participation in organized mammographic screening: A prospective cohort study. *BMC Cancer, 15*(1), 294. https://doi.org/10.1186/s12885-015-1296-8

Hensley, L. (2020, March 28). Why the coronavirus pandemic is triggering those with eating disorders. *Global News.* https://globalnews.ca/news/6735525/eating-disorder-coronavirus/

Hilbert, A., Petroff, D., Herpertz, S., Pietrowsky, R., Tuschen-Caffier, B., Vocks, S., & Schmidt, R. (2019). Meta-analysis of the efficacy of psychological and medical treatments for binge-eating disorder. *Journal of Consulting and Clinical Psychology, 87*(1), 91–105. https://doi.org/10.1037/ccp000035810.1037/ccp0000358.supp (Supplemental)

Hocaoglu, C. (2017). Eating disorders with comorbid anxiety disorders. In Ignacio Jáuregui-Lobera (Ed.). *Eating disorders—A paradigm of the biopsychosocial model of illness* (pp. 99–122). Retrieved from http://www.intechopen.com/books/eating-disorders-a-paradigm-of-the-biopsychosocial-model-of-illness

Hoermann, R., Midgley, J. E. M., Larisch, R., & Dietrich, J. W. (2015). Homeostatic control of the thyroid–pituitary axis: Perspectives for diagnosis and treatment. *Frontiers in Endocrinology, 6,* 177. https://doi.org/10.3389/fendo.2015.00177

Holmes, S., Drake, S., Odgers, K., & Wilson, J. (2017). Feminist approaches to Anorexia Nervosa: A qualitative study of a treatment group. *Journal of Eating Disorders, 5*(1), 36. https://doi.org/10.1186/s40337-017-0166-y

Homan, K. J., & Lemmon, V. A. (2016). Perceived relationship with God moderates the relationship between social comparison and body appreciation. *Mental Health, Religion and Culture, 19*(1), 37–51, https://doi.org/10.1080/13674676.2016.1140372

Hoste, R. R., Lebow, J., & Le Grange, D. (2015). A bidirectional examination of expressed emotion among families of adolescents with bulimia nervosa. *The International Journal of Eating Disorders, 48*(2), 249–252. http://doi.org/10.1002/eat.22306

Hoyt, L. T., Niu, L., Pachucki, M. C., & Chaku, N. (2020). Timing of puberty in boys and girls: Implications for population health. *SSM - Population Health, 10,* 100549. https://doi.org/https://doi.org/10.1016/j.ssmph.2020.100549

Inches, P. R. (1895). Anorexia nervosa. *Maritime Medical News, 7,* 73–75.

Iqbal, A., & Rehman, A. (2020). Binge eating disorder. In *StatPearls [Internet].* StatPearls Publishing. https://www.ncbi.nlm.nih.gov/books/NBK551700/

Jaworski, M., Panczyk, M., Śliwczyński, A., Brzozowska, M., Janaszek, K., Małkowski, P., & Gotlib, J. (2019). Eating disorders in males: An 8-year population-based observational study. *American Journal of Men's Health, 13*(4), 1557988319860970. https://doi.org/10.1177/1557988319860970

Kardalas, E., Paschou, S. A., Anagnostis, P., Muscogiuri, G., Siasos, G., & Vryonidou, A. (2018). Hypokalemia: A clinical update. *Endocrine Connections, 7*(4), R135–R146. https://doi.org/10.1530/ec-18-0109

Keel, P. K. (2017). Who suffers from eating disorders? In *Eating disorders* (2nd ed., pp. 27–53). Oxford University Press. https://cpncampus.com/biblioteca/files/original/0d99816f9022c2fb6f4ba9550bd06187.pdf

Kelly-Weeder, S., Willis, D. G., Mata Lopez, L., Sacco, B., & Wolfe, B. E. (2019). Binge eating and loss of control in college-age women. *Journal of the American Psychiatric Nurses Association, 25*(3), 172–180. https://doi.org/10.1177/1078390319829814

Keshishian, A. C., Tabri, N., Becker, K. R., Franko, D. L., Herzog, D. B., Thomas, J. J., & Eddy, K. T. (2019). Eating disorder recovery is associated with absence of major depressive disorder and substance use disorders at 22-year longitudinal follow-up. *Comprehensive Psychiatry, 90,* 49–51. https://doi.org/10.1016/j.comppsych.2019.01.002

Kerr, M. (2016). Prokinetic agents: Cisapride. *Healthline.* http://www.healthline.com/health/gerd/prokinetics#1

Kiecolt-Glaser, J. K., Habash, D. L., Fagundes, C. P., Andridge, R., Peng, J., Malarkey, W. B., & Belury, M. A. (2015). Daily stressors, past depression, and metabolic responses to high-fat meals: A novel path to obesity. *Biological Psychiatry, 77*(7), 653–660.

Kimber, M., Couturier, J., Georgiades, K., Wahoush, O., & Jack, S. M. (2015). Ethnic minority status and body image dissatisfaction: A scoping review of the child and adolescent literature. *Journal of Immigrant and Minority Health, 17*(5), 1567–1579. http://dx.doi.org.proxy.hil.unb.ca/10.1007/s10903-014-0082-z

Kimber, M., Georgiades, K., Jack, S. M., Couturier, J., & Wahoush, O. (2015). Body image and appearance perceptions from immigrant adolescents in Canada: An interpretive description. *Body Image, 15,* 120–131. https://doi.org/10.1016/j.bodyim.2015.08.002

Kinasz, K., Accurso, E. C., Kass, A. E., & Le Grange, D. (2016). Does Sex Matter in the Clinical Presentation of Eating Disorders in Youth? *The Journal of Adolescent Health, 58*(4), 410–416. https://doi.org/10.1016/j.jadohealth.2015.11.005

Kostecka, B., Kordynska, K., Murawiec, S., & Kucharska, K. (2019). Distorted body image in women and men suffering from anorexia nervosa: A literature review. *Archives of Psychiatry and Psychotherapy, 21*(12), 13–21. https://doi.org/10.12740/APP/102833

Kramer, J. L. (2015). *Art therapy in the treatment of eating disorders. Salucore.* https://www.edcatalogue.com/art-therapy-in-the-treatment-of-eating-disorders/

Krause, N., & Hayward, R. D. (2016), Anxious attachment to God, spiritual support, and obesity: Findings from a recent nationwide survey. *Journal for the Scientific Study of Religion, 55,* 485–497. https://doi.org/10.1111/jssr.12284

La Mela, C., Maglietta, M., Caini, S., Casu, G. P., Lucarelli, S., Mori, S., & Ruggiero, G. M. (2015). Perfectionism, weight and shape concerns, and low self-esteem: Testing a model to predict bulimic symptoms. *Eating Behaviors, 19,* 155–158. doi:10.1016/j.eatbeh.2015.09.002.

LaMarre, A., & Rice, C. (2016). Normal eating is counter-cultural: Embodied experiences of eating disorder recovery. *Journal of Community and Applied Social Psychology, 26*(2), 136–149. https://doi.org/10.1002/casp.2240

Lampard, A. M., & Sharbanee, J. M. (2015). The cognitive-behavioural theory and treatment of bulimia nervosa: An examination of treatment mechanisms and future directions. *Australian Psychologist, 50,* 6–13. https://doi.org/10.1111/ap.12078

Lane, G., Nisbet, C., & Vatanparast, H. (2019). Dietary habits of newcomer children in Canada. *Public Health Nutrition, 22*(17), 3151–3162. https://doi.org/10.1017/S1368980019001964

Langdon-Daly, J., & Serpell, L. (2017). Protective factors against disordered eating in family systems: A systematic review of research. *Journal of Eating Disorders, 5,* 1–15. https://doi.org/10.1186/s40337-017-0141-7

Lea, T., Richards, P. S., Sanders, P. W., McBride, J. A., & Allen, G. K. (2015). Spiritual pathways to healing and recovery: An intensive single-N study of an eating disorder patient. *Spirituality in Clinical Practice, 2*(3), 191–201. https://doi.org/10.1037/scp0000085

Lee, K. S., & Vaillancourt, T. (2019). A four-year prospective study of bullying, anxiety, and disordered eating behavior across early adolescence. *Child Psychiatry & Human Development, 50*(5), 815–825. https://doi.org/10.1007/s10578-019-00884-7

Lewke-Bandara, R. S., Thapliyal, P., Conti, J., & Hay, P. (2020). "It also taught me a lot about myself": A qualitative exploration of how men understand eating disorder recovery. *Journal of Eating Disorders, 8*(1), 3. https://doi.org/10.1186/s40337-020-0279-6

Li, Y. (2020). Linking body esteem to eating disorders among adolescents: A moderated mediation model. *Journal of Health Psychology, 25*(10/11), 1755–1770. https://doi.org/10.1177/1359105319886048

Limbers, C. A., Cohen, L. A., & Gray, B. A. (2018). Eating disorders in adolescent and young adult males: Prevalence, diagnosis, and treatment strategies. *Adolescent Health, Medicine and Therapeutics, 9,* 111–116. https://doi.org/10.2147/AHMT.S147480

Lin, L., & Soby, M. (2016). Appearance comparisons styles and eating disordered symptoms in women. *Eating Behaviors, 23,* 7–12. https://doi.org/10.1016/j.eatbeh.2016.06.006

Lindgren, B., Enmark, A., Bohman, A., & Lundström, M. (2015). A qualitative study of young women's experiences of recovery from bulimia nervosa. *Journal of Advanced Nursing, 71*(4), 860–869. https://doi.org/10.1111/jan.12554

Lindgreen, P., Clausen, L., & Lomborg, K. (2018). Clinicians' perspective on an app for patient self-monitoring in eating disorder treatment. *International Journal of Eating Disorders, 51*(4), 314–321. https://doi.org/10.1002/eat.22833

Lock, J., LaVia, M., & American Academy of Child and Adolescent Psychiatry Committee on Quality Issues. (2015). Practice parameter for the assessment and treatment of children and adolescents with eating disorders. *Journal of American Academy of Child and Adolescent Psychiatry, 54*(5), 412–425.

Loth, K., Wall, M., Choi, C., Bucchianeri, M., Quick, V., Larson, N., & Neumark-Sztainer, D. (2015). Family meals and disordered eating in adolescents: Are the benefits the same for everyone? *International Journal of Eating Disorders, 48*(1), 100–110. https://doi.org/10.1002/eat.22339

Mac Vie, J. D. (2016). The association between emotion regulation strategies and symptoms of binge eating disorder (Order No. 10146447). Available from ProQuest Dissertations & Theses A&I; ProQuest Dissertations & Theses Global (1829545297). ttps://login.proxy.hil.unb.ca/login?url=http://search.proquest.com.proxy.hil.unb.ca/docview/1829545297?accountid=14611

MacDonald, D. E., McFarlane, T. L., Dionne, M. M., David, L., & Olmsted, M. P. (2017). Rapid response to intensive treatment for bulimia nervosa and purging disorder: A randomized controlled trial of a CBT intervention to facilitate early behavior change. *Journal of Consulting and Clinical Psychology, 85*(9), 896–908. doi: 10.1037/ccp0000221

Maon, I., Horesh, D., & Gvion, Y. (2020). Siblings of individuals with eating disorders: A review of the literature. *Frontiers in Psychiatry, 11,* 604. https://doi.org/10.3389/fpsyt.2020.00604

Marvanova, M., & Gramith, K. (2018). Role of antidepressants in the treatment of adults with anorexia nervosa. *The Mental Health Clinician, 8*(3), 127–137. https://doi.org/10.9740/mhc.2018.05.127

Marzilli, E., Cerniglia, L., & Cimino, S. (2018). A narrative review of binge eating disorder in adolescence: Prevalence, impact, and psychological treatment strategies. *Adolescent Health, Medicine and Therapeutics 9,* 17–30. https://doi.org/https://doi.org/10.2147/AHMT.S148050

Marzola, E., Desedime, N., Giovannone, C., Amianto, F., Fassino, S., & Abbate-Daga, G. (2015). Atypical antipsychotics as augmentation therapy in anorexia nervosa. *PLoS One, 10*(4), e0125569. http://doi.org/10.1371/journal.pone.0125569

Matos, M., Ferreira, C., Duarte, C., & Pinto-Gouveia, J. (2015). Eating disorders: When social rank perceptions are shaped by early shame experiences. *Psychology and Psychotherapy: Theory, Research and Practice, 88*(1), 38–53. https://doi.org/10.1111/papt.12027

Mayer-Brown, S., Lawless, C., Fedele, D., Dumont-Driscoll, M., & Janicke, D. M. (2016). The effects of media, self-esteem, and BMI on youth's unhealthy weight control behaviors. *Eating Behaviors, 21,* 59–65. https://doi.org/10.1016/j.eatbeh.2015.11.010

Mayhew, A. J., Pigeyre, M., Couturier, J., & Meyre, D. (2018). An evolutionary genetic perspective of eating disorders. *Neuroendocrinology, 106*(3), 292–306. https://doi.org/10.1159/000484525

Mayo Clinic Staff. (2018). *Bulimia nervosa.* https://www.mayoclinic.org/diseases-conditions/bulimia/symptoms-causes/syc-20353615

McCormack, C., & McCann, E. (2015). Caring for an adolescent with anorexia nervosa: Parent's views and experiences. *Archives of Psychiatric Nursing, 29*(3), 143–147. https://doi.org/10.1016/j.apnu.2015.01.003

McCuen-Wurst, C., Ruggieri, M., & Allison, K. C. (2018). Disordered eating and obesity: Associations between binge-eating disorder, night-eating syndrome, and weight-related comorbidities. Annals of the New York Academy of Sciences, 1411(1), 96–105. https://doi.org/10.1111/nyas.13467

McIntosh, V. (2015). Specialist supportive clinical management (SSCM) for anorexia nervosa: Content analysis, change over course of therapy, and relation to outcome. *Journal of Eating Disorders, 3*(1), O1. https://doi.org/10.1186/2050-2974-3-S1-O1

McIntosh, V. V., Jordan, J., Carter, J. D., Luty, S. E., Carter, F. A., McKenzie, J. M., Frampton, C. M., & Joyce, P. R. (2016). Assessing the distinctiveness of psychotherapies and examining change over treatment for anorexia nervosa with cognitive-behavior therapy, interpersonal psychotherapy, and specialist supportive clinical management. *The International Journal of Eating Disorders, 49*(10), 958–962. https://doi.org/10.1002/eat.22555

Melville, N. A. (2016). IPT effective for depression, anxiety, eating disorders. *Medscape.* http://www.medscape.com/viewarticle/861812#vp_2

Meng, X., & D'Arcy, C. (2015). Comorbidity between lifetime eating problems and mood and anxiety disorders: Results from the Canadian Community Health Survey of Mental Health and Well-being. *European Eating Disorders Review, 23*(2), 156–162. https://doi.org/10.1002/erv.2347

Micali, N., Field, A. E., Treasure, J. L., & Evans, D. M. (2015). Are obesity risk genes associated with binge eating in adolescence? *Obesity, 23*(8), 1729–1736. https://doi.org/10.1002/oby.21147

Micali, N., Martini, M. G., Thomas, J. J., Eddy, K. T., Kothari, R., Russell, E., Bulik, C. M., & Treasure, J. (2017). Lifetime and 12-month prevalence of eating disorders amongst women in mid-life: A population-based study of diagnoses and risk factors. *BMC Medicine, 15*(1), 12. https://doi.org/10.1186/s12916-016-0766-4

Midlarsky, E., Marotta, A. K., Pirutinsky, S., Morin, R. T., & McGowan, J. C. (2017). Psychological predictors of eating pathology in older adult women. *Journal of Women & Aging, 3*, 1–15. doi:10.1080/08952841.2017.1295665

Mignot, S., Ringa, V., Vigoureux, S., Zins, M., Panjo, H., Saulnier, P.-J., & Fritel, X. (2019). Pap tests for cervical cancer screening test and contraception: analysis of data from the CONSTANCES cohort study. *BMC Cancer, 19*(1), 317. https://doi.org/10.1186/s12885-019-5477-8

Mitchell, J. E. (2016). Medical comorbidity and medical complications associated with binge-eating disorder. *International Journal of Eating Disorders, 49*(3), 319–323. https://doi.org/10.1002/eat.22452

Mitchison, D., Dawson, L., Hand, L. Mond, J., & Hay, P. (2016). Quality of life as a vulnerability and recovery factor in eating disorders: A community-based study. *BMC Psychiatry, 16*, 328. https://doi.org/10.1186/s12888-016-1033-0

Mitrofan, O., Petkova, H., Janssens, A., Kelly, J., Edwards, E., Nicholls, D., McNicholas, F., Simic, M., Eisler, I., Ford, T., & Byford, S. (2019). Care experiences of young people with eating disorders and their parents: Qualitative study. *BJPsych Open, 5*(1), e6. https://doi.org/10.1192/bjo.2018.78

Moola, F. J., Gairdner, S., & Amara, C. (2015). Speaking on behalf of the body and activity. Investigating the activity experiences of Canadian women living with anorexia nervosa. *Mental Health and Physical Activity, 8*, 44–55. https://doi.org/10.1016/j.mhpa.2015.02.002

Moore, S. R., McKone, K. M. P., & Mendle, J. (2016). Recollections of puberty and disordered eating in young women. *Journal of Adolescence, 53*, 180–188. https://doi.org/10.1016/j.adolescence.2016.10.011

Moral-Agúndez, A. D., & Carillo-Dúan, M. V. (2020). Body-cult television advertisement recall among young women suffering from anorexia nervosa or bulimia nervosa. *Saúde e Sociedade, 29*(1), e170418. https://doi.org10.1590/s0104-12902020170418

Mortimer, R. (2019). Pride before a fall: Shame, diagnostic crossover, and eating disorders. *Journal of Bioethical Inquiry, 16*(3), 365–374. https://doi.org/10.1007/s11673-019-09923-3

Muhlhein, L. (2019). *Eating disorders and substance abuse: How are they related and how are they treated?* https://www.verywellmind.com/eating-disorders-and-substance-abuse-4585199

Mustelin, L., Silen, Y., Raevuori, A., Hoek, H. W., Kaprio, J., & Keski-Rahkonen, A. (2016). The DSM-5 diagnostic criteria for anorexia nervosa may change its population prevalence and prognostic value. *Journal of Psychiatric Research, 77*, 85–91. https://doi.org/10.1016/j.jpsychires.2016.03.003

National Eating Disorders Collaboration. (2017). *NEDC fact sheet— Eating disorders in males.* http://www.nedc.com.au/eating-disorders-in-males

Nicholls, D., Fogarty, S., Hay, P., & Ramjan, L. M. (2016). Participatory action research for women with anorexia nervosa. *Nurse Researcher, 23*(5), 26–30.

Nobles, C. J., Thomas, J. J., Valentine, S. E., Gerber, M. W., Vaewsorn, A. S., & Marques, L. (2016). Association of premenstrual syndrome and premenstrual dysphoric disorder with bulimia nervosa and binge-eating disorder in a nationally representative epidemiological sample. *International Journal of Eating Disorders, 49*(7), 641–650. https://doi.org/10.1002/eat.22539

Ntoumanis, N., Stenling, A., Quested, E., Nikitaras, N., Olson, J., & Thøgersen-Ntoumani, C. (2020). Self-compassion and need frustration moderate the effects of upward appearance comparisons on body image discrepancies. *The Journal of Psychology, 154*(4), 292–308. https://doi.org/10.1080/00223980.2020.1716669

Oldershaw, A., Startup, H., & Lavender, T. (2019). Anorexia nervosa and a lost emotional self: A psychological formulation of the development, maintenance, and treatment of anorexia nervosa. *Frontiers in Psychology, 10*, 219. https://doi.org/10.3389/fpsyg.2019.00219

Olguin, P., Fuentes, M., Gabler, G., Guerdjikova, A. I., Keck, P. E., & McElroy, S. L. (2017). Medical comorbidity of binge eating disorder. *Eating and Weight Disorders, 22*(1), 13–26. https://doi.org/10.1007/s40519-016-0313-5

Patel, R. S., Olten, B., Patel, P., Shah, K., & Mansuri, Z. (2018). Hospitalization outcomes and comorbidities of bulimia nervosa: A nationwide inpatient study. *Cureus, 10*(5), e2583. https://doi.org/10.7759/cureus.2583

Pearson, C. M., Wonderlich, S. A., & Smith, G. T. (2015). A risk and maintenance model for bulimia nervosa: From impulsive action to compulsive behavior. *Psychological Review, 122*(3), 516–535. https://doi.org/10.1037/a0039268

Petersson, S., Johnsson, P., & Perseius, K. (2017). A Sisyphean task: Experiences of perfectionism in patients with eating disorders. *Journal of Eating Disorders, 5*, 1–11. https://doi.org/10.1186/s40337-017-0136-4

Phelan, S., Burgess, D., Yeazel, M., Hellerstedt, W., Griffin, J., & van Ryn, M. (2015). Impact of weight bias and stigma on quality of care 2266 and outcomes for patients with obesity. *Obesity Reviews, 16*(4), 319–326. http://doi.org/10.1111/obr.1

Pollen, S. (2019, 28 March). 'Male eating disorders tend to fly under the radar': How it feels to suffer from anorexia as a teenage boy. *The Independent.* https://www.independent.co.uk/life-style/eating-disorder-awareness-week-anorexia-boys-men-what-its-samuel-pollen-not-eating-a8796416.html

Potterton, R., Austin, A., Allen, K., Lawrence, V., & Schmidt, U. (2020). "I'm not a teenager, I'm 22. Why can't I snap out of it?": A qualitative exploration of seeking help for a first-episode eating disorder during emerging adulthood. *Journal of Eating Disorders, 8*(1), 46. https://doi.org/10.1186/s40337-020-00320-5

Public Health Agency of Canada. (2015, February 24). *Health behaviour in school-aged children in Canada: Focus on relationships.* http://healthy-canadians.gc.ca/publications/science-research-sciences-recherches/health-behaviour-children-canada-2015-comportements-sante-jeunes/index-eng.php#c9a6

Pugh, M. (2015). A narrative review of schemas and schema therapy outcomes in the eating disorders. *Clinical Psychology Review, 39*, 30–41. https://doi.org/10.1016/j.cpr.2015.04.003

Pullmer, R., Coelho, J. S., & Zaitsoff, S. L. (2019). Kindness begins with yourself: The role of self-compassion in adolescent body satisfaction and eating pathology. *International Journal of Eating Disorders, 52*(7), 809–816. https://doi.org/10.1002/eat.23081

Rastogi, R., & Rome, E. S. (2020). Restrictive eating disorders in previously overweight adolescents and young adults. *Cleveland Clinic Journal of Medicine, 87*(3), 165–171. https://doi.org/https://doi.org/10.3949/ccjm.87a.19034

Reas, D. L., Pedersen, G., Karterud, S., & Rø, Ø. (2015). Self-harm and suicidal behavior in borderline personality disorder with and without bulimia nervosa. *Journal of Consulting and Clinical Psychology, 83*(3), 643–648. https://doi.org/10.1037/ccp0000014

Reichmann, C. (2018, June 4). Feminist and eating disordered: The ultimate conundrum. *Wildflower Therapy.* https://www.colleenreichmann.com/2018/06/04/feminist-and-eating-disordered-the-ultimate-conundrum/

Richey, M., Bilodeau, C., & Martin, M. (2020). Women, identity development and spirituality in the Anglican Church of Canada: A qualitative study. *Journal of Spirituality in Mental Health, 22*(4), 330–354. https://doi.org/10.1080/19349637.2019.1593917

Rizk, M., Lalanne, C., Berthoz, S., Kern, L., EVHAN Group, & Godart, N. (2015). Problematic exercise in anorexia nervosa: Testing potential risk factors against different definitions. *PLoS One, 10*(11), e0143352. http://doi.org/10.1371/journal.pone.0143352

Robinson, K. J., Mountford, V. A., & Sperlinger, D. J. (2013). Being men with eating disorders: Perspectives of male eating disorder service users. *Journal of Health Psychology, 18*, 176–186.

Roebroek, Y. G. M., Talib, A., Muris, J. W. M., van Dielen, F. M. H., Bouvy, N. D., & van Heurn, L. W. E. (2019). Hurdles to take for adequate treatment of morbidly obese children and adolescents: Attitudes of general practitioners towards conservative and surgical treatment of paediatric morbid obesity. *World Journal of Surgery, 43*(4), 1173–1181. https://doi.org/10.1007/s00268-018-4874-5

Rohde, P., Stice, E., & Marti, C. N. (2015). Development and predictive effects of eating disorder risk factors during adolescence: Implications for prevention efforts. *International Journal of Eating Disorders, 48*(2), 187–198. https://doi.org/10.1002/eat.22270

Rosen, E., Sabel, A. L., Brinton, J. T., Catanach, B., Gaudiani, J. L., & Mehler, P. S. (2016). Liver dysfunction in patients with severe anorexia nervosa. *International Journal of Eating Disorders, 49*(2), 153–160. https://doi.org/10.1002/eat.22436

Rosenbaum, D. L., Kimerling, R., Pomernacki, A., Goldstein, K. M., Yano, E. M., Sadler, A. G., Carney, D., Bastian, L. A., Bean-Mayberry, B. A., & Frayne, S. M. (2016). Binge eating among women veterans in primary care: Comorbidities and treatment priorities. *Women's Health Issues, 26*(4), 420–428. https://doi.org/10.1016/j.whi.2016.02.004

Rosenbaum, D. L., & White, K. S. (2015). The relation of anxiety, depression, and stress to binge eating behavior. *Journal of Health Psychology, 20*(6), 887–898. https://doi.org/10.1177/1359105315580212

Rosewall, J. K., Gleaves, D. H., & Latner, J. D. (2018). An examination of risk factors that moderate the body dissatisfaction-eating pathology relationship among New Zealand adolescent girls. *Journal of Eating Disorders, 6*(1), 38. https://doi.org/10.1186/s40337-018-0225-z

Roy, M., Shatenstein, B., Gaudreau, P., Morais, J. A., & Payette, H. (2015). Seniors' body weight dissatisfaction and longitudinal associations with weight changes, anorexia of aging, and obesity: Results from the NuAge Study. *Journal of Aging and Health, 27*(2), 220–238. https://doi.org/10.1177/0898264314546715

Sala, M., Breithaupt, L., Bulik, C. M., Hamer, R. M., La Via, M. C., & Brownley, K. A. (2017). A double-blind, randomized pilot trial of chromium picolinate for overweight individuals with binge-eating disorder: Effects on glucose regulation. *Journal of Dietary Supplements, 14*(2), 191–199. https://doi.org/10.1080/19390211.2016.1207124

Saltzman, J. A., & Liechty, J. M. (2016). Family correlates of childhood binge eating: A systematic review. *Eating Behaviors, 22*, 62–71. https://doi.org/10.1016/j.eatbeh.2016.03.027

Sangha, S., Oliffe, J. L., Kelly, M. T., & McCuaig, F. (2019). Eating disorders in males: How primary care providers can improve recognition, diagnosis, and treatment. *American Journal of Men's Health, 13*(3), 1557988319857424. https://doi.org/10.1177/1557988319857424

Saucedo-Molina, T. d. J., Zaragoza Cortés, J., & Villalón, L. (2017). Eating disorder symptomatology: Comparative study between Mexican and Canadian university women. *Revista Mexicana de Trastornos Alimentarios, 8*(2), 97–104. https://doi.org/https://doi.org/10.1016/j.rmta.2017.05.002

Saules, K. S., Carey, J., Carr, M. M., & Sienko, R. M. (2015). Binge-eating disorder: Prevalence, predictors, and management in the primary care setting. *Journal of Clinical Outcomes Management, 22*(11), 512–528. http://www.turner-white.com/pdf/jcom_nov15_binge.pdf

Schaefer, M. K., & Salafia, E. H. B. (2014). The connection of teasing by parents, siblings, and peers with girls' body dissatisfaction and boys' drive for muscularity: The role of social comparison as a mediator. *Eating Behaviors, 15*(4), 599–608. https://doi.org/10.1016/j.eatbeh.2014.08.018

Scharner, S., & Stengel, A. (2019). Alterations of brain structure and functions in anorexia nervosa. *Clinical Nutrition Experimental, 28*, 22–32. https://doi.org/https://doi.org/10.1016/j.yclnex.2019.02.001

Schaumberg, K., Wonderlich, S., Crosby, R., Peterson, C., Le Grange, D., Mitchell, J. E., Crow, S., Joiner, T., & Bardone-Cone, A. M. (2020). Impulsivity and anxiety-related dimensions in adults with bulimic-spectrum disorders differentially relate to eating disordered behaviors. *Eating Behaviors, 37*, 101382. https://doi.org/10.1016/j.eatbeh.2020.101382

Schmitz, C., Schnicker, K., & Legenbauer, T. (2016). Influence of weight on shared core symptoms in eating disorders. *Behavior Modification, 40*(5), 777–796. https://doi.org/10.1177/0145445516643487

Schuster, E., Negy, C., & Tantleff-Dunn, S. (2013). The effects of appearance-related commentary on body dissatisfaction, eating pathology, and body change behaviors in men. *Psychology of Men and Masculinity, 14*(1), 76–87. https://doi.org/10.1037/a0025625

Scott Richards, P. S., Caoili, C. L., Crowton, S. A., Berrett, M. E., Hardman, R. K., Jackson, R. N., & Sanders, P. W. (2018). An exploration of the role of religion and spirituality in the treatment and recovery of patients with eating disorders. *Spirituality in Clinical Practice, 5*(2), 88–103. https://doi.org/10.1037/scp0000159

Seah, X. Y., Tham, X. C., Kamaruzaman, N. R., & Yobas, P. K. (2017). Knowledge, attitudes and challenges of healthcare professionals managing people with eating disorders: A literature review. *Archives of Psychiatric Nursing, 31*(1), 125–136. https://doi.org/10.1016/j.apnu.2016.09.002

Sharan, P., & Sundar, A. S. (2015). Eating disorders in women. *Indian Journal of Psychiatry, 57*(Suppl 2), S286–S295. https://doi.org/10.4103/0019-5545.161493

Sharpe, H., Griffiths, S., Choo, T.-H., Eisenberg, M. E., Mitchison, D., Wall, M., & Neumark-Sztainer, D. (2018). The relative importance of dissatisfaction, overvaluation and preoccupation with weight and shape for predicting onset of disordered eating behaviors and depressive symptoms over 15 years. *The International Journal of Eating Disorders, 51*(10), 1168–1175. https://doi.org/10.1002/eat.22936

Shih, P. B., & Woodside, D. B. (2016). Contemporary views on the genetics of anorexia nervosa. *European Neuropsychopharmacology, 26*(4), 663–673. https://doi.org/10.1016/j.euroneuro.2016.02.008

Shire US Inc. (2015). *Vyvanse® for adults with moderate to severe binge eating disorder.* http://www.vyvanse.com/binge-eating-disorder-treatment

Sonneville, K. R., Calzo, J. P., Horton, N. J., Field, A. E., Crosby, R. D., Solmi, F., & Micali, N. (2015). Childhood hyperactivity/inattention and eating disturbances predict binge eating in adolescence. *Psychological Medicine, 45*(12), 2511–2520. https://doi.org/ 10.1017/S0033291715000148

Stavrou, P. (2018). How does a woman experience bulimia nervosa? the link between bulimia nervosa, low self-esteem and insecure attachment: A phenomenological approach *Journal of Psychology & Clinical Psychiatry, 9*(5), 502–508. https://doi.org/10.15406/jpcpy.2018.09.00580

Statistics Canada. (2015). *Section D—Eating disorders.* http://www.statcan.gc.ca/pub/82-619-m/2012004/sections/sectiond-eng.htm

Statistics Canada. (2017). *Census in Brief: Children with an immigrant background: Bridging cultures.* Minister of Industry. https://www12.statcan.gc.ca/census-recensement/2016/as-sa/98-200-x/2016015/98-200-x2016015-eng.cfm

Steinman, J., & Shibli-Rahhal, A. (2019). Anorexia nervosa and osteoporosis: Pathophysiology and treatment. *Journal of Bone Metabolism, 26*(3), 133–143. https://doi.org/10.11005/jbm.2019.26.3.133

Stewardson, L., Nolan, J., & Talleyrand, R. (2020). Eating disorders and body image concerns in men of color: Cultural considerations. *Journal of Mental Health Counseling, 42*(2), 110–123. https://doi.org/10.17744/mehc.42.2.02

Stoll, M., Bitterlich, N., & Cornelli, U. (2017). Randomised, double-blind, clinical investigation to compare orlistat 60 milligram and a customized polyglucosamine, two treatment methods for the management of

overweight and obesity. *BMC Obesity, 4*, 1–9. https://doi.org/10.1186/s40608-016-0130-4

Støving, R. K. (2019). Mechanisms in endocrinology: Anorexia nervosa and endocrinology: A clinical update. *European Journal of Endocrinology, 180*(1), R9. https://doi.org/10.1530/eje-18-0596

Stoyel, H., Shanmuganathan-Felton, V., Meyer, C., & Serpell, L. (2020). Psychological risk indicators of disordered eating in athletes. *PLoS One, 15*(5), e0232979. https://doi.org/10.1371/journal.pone.0232979

Stunkard, A. J., & Messick, S. (1985). The three-factor eating questionnaire to measure dietary restraint and hunger. *Journal of Psychosomatic Research, 29*, 71–83.

Su, X., Liang, H., Yuan, W., Olsen, J., Cnattingius, S., & Li, J. (2016). Prenatal and early life stress and risk of eating disorders in adolescent girls and young women. *European Child and Adolescent Psychiatry, 25*(11), 1245–1253. https://doi.org/10.1007/s00787-016-0848-z

Sukkar, I., Gagan, M., & Kealy-Bateman, W. (2017). The 14th century religious women Margery Kempe and Catherine of Siena can still teach us lessons about eating disorders today. *Journal of Eating Disorders, 5*(1), 23. https://doi.org/10.1186/s40337-017-0151-5

Svedlund, N. E., Norring, C., Ginsberg, Y., & von Hausswolff-Juhlin, Y. (2017). Symptoms of attention deficit hyperactivity disorder (ADHD) among adult eating disorder patients. *BMC Psychiatry, 17*(1), 19. https://doi.org/10.1186/s12888-016-1093-1

Tasca, G. A., Compare, A., Zarbo, C., & Brugnera, A. (2016). Therapeutic alliance and binge-eating outcomes in a group therapy context. *Journal of Counseling Psychology, 63*(4), 443–451. https://doi.org/10.1037/cou0000159

Thörel, N., Thörel, E., & Tuschen-Caffier, B. (2020). Differential stigmatization in the context of eating disorders: Less blame might come at the price of greater social rejection. *Journal of Stigma and Health, 6*(1), 100–112. https://doi.org/10.1037/sah0000274.supp (Supplemental)

Tiggemann, M., & Hage, K. (2019). Religion and spirituality: Pathways to positive body image. *Body Image, 28*, 135–141. https://doi.org/10.1016/j.bodyim.2019.01.004

Treasure, J., & Cardi, V. (2017). Anorexia nervosa, theory and treatment: Where are we 35 years on from Hilde Bruch's foundation lecture? *European Eating Disorders Review, 25*(3), 139–147. https://doi.org/10.1002/erv.2511

Tseng, M.-C. M., Chang, C.-H., Liao, S.-C., & Chen, H.-C. (2017). Comparison of associated features and drug treatment between co-occurring unipolar and bipolar disorders in depressed eating disorder patients. *BMC Psychiatry, 17*, 81. https://doi.org/10.1186/s12888-017-1243-0

Turel, T., Jameson, M., Gitimu, P., Rowlands, Z., Mincher, J., & Pohle-Krauza, R. (2018). Disordered eating: Influence of body image, sociocultural attitudes, appearance anxiety and depression—A focus on college males and a gender comparison. *Cogent Psychology, 5*(1), 1483062. https://doi.org/10.1080/23311908.2018.1483062

Udo, T., Bitley, S., & Grilo, C. M. (2019). Suicide attempts in US adults with lifetime DSM-5 eating disorders. *BMC Medicine, 17*(1), 120. https://doi.org/10.1186/s12916-019-1352-3

Udo, T., & Grilo, C. M. (2018). Prevalence and correlates of DSM-5-defined eating disorders in a nationally representative sample of U.S. adults. *Biological Psychiatry, 84*(5), 345–354. https://doi.org/10.1016/j.biopsych.2018.03.014

Ulfvebrand, S., Birgegård, A., Norring, C., Högdahl, L., & von Hausswolff-Juhlin, Y. (2015). Psychiatric comorbidity in women and men with eating disorders results from a large clinical database. *Psychiatry Research, 230*(2), 294–299. https://doi.org/10.1016/j.psychres.2015.09.008

Valeant Canada. (2017). *WELLBUTRIN SR (bupropion hydrochloride) sustained-release tablets. Manufacturer's standard.* Retrieved March 20, 2017, from https://pdf.hres.ca/dpd_pm/00038603.PDF

Valente, S. (2016). The hysterical anorexia epidemic in the French nineteenth-century. *Dialogues in Philosophy, Mental and Neuro Sciences, 9*(1), 22–23. Crossing Dialogues Association 20160601

Valente, M., Syurina, E. V., Muftugil-Yalcin, S., & Cesuroglu, T. (2020). "Keep Yourself Alive": From healthy eating to progression to orthorexia nervosa a mixed methods study among young women in the Netherlands. *Ecology of Food and Nutrition, 59*(6), 578–597. https://doi.org/10.1080/03670244.2020.1755279

Vanderlinden, J., Claes, L., De Cuyper, K., & Vrieze, E. (2015). Dissociation and dissociative disorders. In T. Wade (Ed.), *Encyclopedia of feeding and eating disorders.* Springer Science & Business Media Singapore. 10.1007/978-981-287-087-2_33-1. https://lirias.kuleuven.be/bitstream/123456789/530325/1/Dissociation+and+dissociative+disorders+encyclopedia+of+feeding+and+eating+disorders+(002).pdf

van Hoeken, D., & Hoek, H. W. (2020). Review of the burden of eating disorders: Mortality, disability, costs, quality of life, and family burden. *Current Opinion in Psychiatry, 33*(6), 521–527. https://journals.lww.com/co-psychiatry/Fulltext/2020/11000/Review_of_the_burden_of_eating_disorders_.3.aspx

Verbeek, L. (2018). 'The recovered therapist': Working with body image disturbance and eating disorders—Researching the countertransference. In P. Valerio (Ed.), *Introduction to countertransference in therapeutic practice: A myriad of mirrors* (pp. 185–199). Routledge. https://doi.org/10.4324/9781315462097

Vitale, M., & Doherty, S. (2016). Acculturation and post-immigration changes in obesity, physical activity, and nutrition: Comparing Hispanics and Asians in the Waterloo region, Ontario, Canada." Theses and Dissertations (Comprehensive). https://scholars.wlu.ca/cgi/viewcontent.cgi?referer=https://www.google.com/&httpsredir=1&article=2988&context=etd

Wales, J., Brewin, N., Cashmore, R., Haycraft, E., Baggott, J., Cooper, A., & Arcelus, J. (2016). Predictors of positive treatment outcome in people with anorexia nervosa treated in a specialized inpatient unit: The role of early response to treatment. *European Eating Disorders Review, 24*(5), 417–424. https://doi.org/10.1002/erv.2443

Walsh, T. (2017). *Anorexia nervosa in adults: Pharmacotherapy.* Retrieved from http://www.uptodate.com/contents/anorexia-nervosa-in-adults-pharmacotherapy

Wang, S. B., Lydecker, J. A., & Grilo, C. M. (2017). Rumination in patients with binge-eating disorder and obesity: Associations with eating-disorder psychopathology and weight-bias internalization. *European Eating Disorders Review, 25*(2), 98–103. https://doi.org/10.1002/erv.2499

Ward, Z. J., Rodriguez, P., Wright, D. R., Austin, S. B., & Long, M. W. (2019). Estimation of eating disorders prevalence by age and associations with mortality in a simulated nationally representative US cohort. *JAMA Network Open, 2*(10), e1912925. https://doi.org/10.1001/jamanetworkopen.2019.12925

Watson, R. J., Adjei, J., Saewyc, E., Homma, Y., & Goodenow, C. (2017). Trends and disparities in disordered eating among heterosexual and sexual minority adolescents. *International Journal of Eating Disorders, 50*, 22–31. https://doi.org/10.1002/eat.22576

Weaver, K., Martin-McDonald, K., & Spiers, J. (2016). Lost alongside my daughter living with an eating disorder. *GSTF Journal of Nursing and Health Care (JNHC), 3*(2). https://doi.org/10.5176/2345-718X_3.2.122.

Weinberger-Litman, S. L., Rabin, L. A., Fogel, J., Mensinger, J. L., & Litman, L. (2016). Psychosocial mediators of the relationship between religious orientation and eating disorder risk factors in young Jewish women. *Psychology of Religion and Spirituality, 8*(4), 265–276. https://doi.org/10.1037/a0040293

Woodside, B., Twose, R. M., Olteanu, A., & Sathi, C. (2016). Hospital admissions in severe and enduring anorexia nervosa: When to admit, when not to admit, and when to stop admitting. In S. Touyz, D. Le Grange, J. Hubert Lacey, & P. Hay (Eds.), *Managing severe and enduring anorexia nervosa: A clinician's guide* (pp. 171–184). Routledge.

Zaitsoff, S., Pullmer, R., Menna, R., & Geller, J. (2016). A qualitative analysis of aspects of treatment that adolescents with anorexia identify as helpful. *Psychiatry Research, 238*, 251–256. https://doi.org/10.1016/j.psychres.2016.02.045

Zelkowitz, R. L., & Cole, D. A. (2019). Self-criticism as a transdiagnostic process in nonsuicidal self-injury and disordered eating: Systematic review and meta-analysis. *Suicide & Life-Threatening Behavior, 49*(1), 310–327. https://doi.org/10.1111/sltb.12436

Zeller, M. H., Inge, T. H., Modi, A. C., Jenkins, T. M., Michalsky, M. P., Helmrath, M., … Buncher, R. (2015). Severe obesity and comorbid condition impact on the weight-related quality of life of the adolescent patient. *Journal of Pediatrics, 166*(3), 651–659.e4. https://doi.org/10.1016/j.jpeds.2014.11.022

CHAPTER 26

Substance-Related and Addictive Disorders*

Diane Kunyk

LEARNING OBJECTIVES

After studying this chapter, you will be able to:

- Conceptualize addiction as a prevalent, chronic, relapsing, and treatable medical disorder.
- Describe the features of the bio/psycho/social/spiritual theories for understanding addiction in Canadian settings.
- Describe the principles of safe and effective treatment of substance-related and addictive disorders.
- Outline essential components of screening, comprehensive assessment, matching individuals with appropriate multimodal treatment interventions, as well as monitoring progress and effectiveness of treatment.
- Formulate an individualized nursing care plan.
- Contemplate the role of the nurse in advocating for individuals with addiction.

KEY TERMS

- addiction • addictive substances • alcohol
- ambivalence • brief intervention • caffeine
- cannabinoids • cannabis • contemporaneous use
- craving • delirium tremens • detoxification • gambling disorder • hallucinogens • harm reduction • inhalants
- intoxication • motivational interviewing • opioids
- relapse • screening • therapeutic alliance • withdrawal

KEY CONCEPT

- addiction

Addiction is recognized by both major disease classification systems as a bona fide, chronic, and relapsing medical condition (American Psychiatric Association [APA], 2013; World Health Organization, 2021a, 2021b). Advances in brain imaging and other research methods have demonstrated that repeated exposure to alcohol, tobacco, and/or other psychoactive substances over time may alter brain structure, chemistry, and function in susceptible individuals, leading to potential loss of control over the use of one or more substances and continued use despite harm or the knowledge of risk of harm. This conceptualization, along with emerging theories and understandings, has made advances in safe and effective treatment possible and provides increasingly optimistic outcomes for individuals and families affected by addiction.

Addiction may be expressed in individuals regardless of their age, gender identity, socioeconomic status, education, culture, occupation, or other characteristics. Because addiction is the leading preventable cause of death and disease globally, amongst the most prevalent of all mental disorders, and the single greatest contributor to excess healthcare spending, it has been argued that addiction continues to be the most important illness of our time (Els, 2007). The future burden of addiction on Canadian society is uncertain given the current unparalleled opioid epidemic and the potential increase in cannabis use given legalization in October 2018.

Despite its importance and prevalence, addiction is often unrecognized, neglected, and undertreated in Canadian society. Conceptualizations of addiction as resulting from moral failure continue to be expressed in our public policies and popular media (Kunyk et al., 2016a, 2016b). Individuals affected with addiction are often alienated and isolated from their families, workplaces, and communities. There are significant barriers, particularly stigma and lack of resources, for persons with addiction to overcome to access the treatment they need, and these systemic barriers may be as intractable as the disease of addiction itself.

Nurses encounter individuals and their families who are struggling with addiction in their everyday practices and are favourably situated to help. With the necessary knowledge, skills, and attitudes conducive to health promotion and disease intervention, nurses are able to safely and effectively work with individuals, families, and communities experiencing the effects of addiction and thereby effectively reduce this healthcare deficit.

---

*Adapted from the chapter "Substance-Related and Addictive Disorders" by Diane Kunyk and Charl Els

This chapter reviews the categories of substance-related and addictive disorders, current theories regarding the aetiology of substance use disorders (SUDs), and evidence-based treatment interventions. The role of the nurse is discussed in terms of early identification, assessment, and intervention planning with the purpose of helping to meet the needs of individuals, their families, and our broader society, and to consider nurses' ethical duty for advocacy.

KEY CONCEPT

Addiction, a chronic, relapsing, and treatable medical condition, is the leading preventable cause of death, disability, and disease globally. It is a disease of the brain and not an expression of moral character.

IN-A-LIFE

Robert Munsch (June 11, 1945)

CANADIAN AUTHOR
Public Persona

Robert Munsch is a well-known and highly revered author of children's literature. One of his books, *Love You Forever*, was written after Munsch and his wife lost two stillborn babies. This story chronicles the unconditional love between a mother and son throughout the cycle of life. It has sold more than 30 million copies and has been translated into French and Spanish. In 1999, Munsch was made a Member of the Order of Canada for his body of work. Amongst many accomplishments, Munsch is proud to be the most popular author whose books are borrowed but never returned from the Toronto Public Library saying, "I am happy to see thieves like my books and will continue to try to serve the needs of the reading underworld" (Robinson, 2015, p. 7).

Personal Realities

Robert Munsch studied for 7 years to become a Jesuit priest, only to decide that he was "lousy priest material." He subsequently earned a Master of Education in Child Studies from Tufts University. In a note to parents on his website, Munsch writes that he has struggled with addiction and has attended 12-step recovery meetings for more than 25 years. He also revealed that he has been diagnosed with obsessive–compulsive and manic-depressive disorders.

Sources: www.robertmunsch.com; Robinson, M. (July 15, 2015). Gone but not forgotten: 100,000 Toronto library books outstanding. *The Star*. Retrieved from https://www.thestar.com/news/gta/2015/07/15/gone-but-not-forgotten-100000-toronto-library-books-outstanding.html

Definition

The American Society of Addiction Medicine (ASAM, 2019, para. 1) provides the following definition:

Addiction is a "treatable, chronic medical disease involving complex interactions among brain circuits, genetics, the environment, and the individual's life experiences. People with addiction use substances or engage in behaviours that become compulsive and often continue despite harmful consequences."

Addiction is characterized by inability to consistently abstain, impairment in behavioural control, **craving**, diminished recognition of significant problems with one's behaviours and interpersonal relationships, and a dysfunctional emotional response. Like other chronic diseases, addiction often involves cycles of relapse and remission. Without treatment or engagement in recovery activities, addiction is progressive and can result in disability or premature death (ASAM, 2019, para. 1 and 2).

Neurobiology

Addictive substances, regardless of their legal classifications of licit and illicit, are used and misused for many reasons. These may include for their pleasurable effects, to alter mental status, to improve performance, to relieve boredom, or to self-medicate. These substances, when taken in excess, have in common the direct activation of the brain reward system. Stimulation of the reward pathway occurs, in part, through increasing extracellular dopamine concentrations in the limbic regions of the brain. Dopamine, a neurotransmitter, is involved in many aspects of reward and pleasure and is involved in the production of memories and behavioural reinforcement. Given their activation of the reward pathways of the brain, taking substances can be considered a reinforced behaviour. Chronic exposure to addictive substances may lead to pervasive changes in brain function at structural (molecular and cellular) and neurophysiologic levels, thereby undermining the individual's voluntary control over its use. These underlying changes in brain circuits may persist beyond withdrawal, and the behavioural effects of these changes may be exhibited in the repeated experiences of craving and relapse of individuals exposed to drug-related stimuli. From a neurobiologic perspective, addiction is conceptualized as a *chronic, relapsing disease* of the brain, and the associated abnormal behaviour is the result of dysfunction of brain tissue.

Given equal exposure to psychoactive substances, not all individuals who are exposed to addictive substances will develop addiction. Addiction comes to expression in individuals who may be considered potentially susceptible on any one or more of the following levels: biologic, psychological, social, or spiritual. For example, individuals who start using substances in adolescence are at higher risk of developing addiction than are those who start later in life. It has also been estimated that 40% to 60% of the vulnerability to addiction is attributable to genetic factors (Volkow & Warren, 2014). Gender differences have been established, with the prevalence among males consistently demonstrating higher rates of addiction (Crum, 2014). Women, however, are considered more vulnerable for developing addiction and at higher risk of health consequences from their use (Agabio et al., 2016). Regardless of putative vulnerabilities, the manifestation of addiction has been described as "a cluster of cognitive, behavioural, and physiologic symptoms indicating that the individual continues using the substance despite significant substance-related problems" (APA, 2013, p. 483).

Diagnostic Criteria

The APA's (2013) *Diagnostic and Statistical Manual of Mental Disorders*, 5th ed. (*DSM-5*) classification refers to disorders related to taking of substances of abuse and includes two categories: SUDs and substance-induced disorders (substance intoxication, substance withdrawal, and other substance/medication-induced mental disorders).

The diagnosis of SUD is substance specific (e.g., alcohol, opioid, or cannabis use disorder). It is based on a pathologic pattern of 11 behaviours (criteria) grouped into (1) impaired control, (2) social impairment, (3) risky use, and (4) pharmacologic categories. The number of criteria met determines the severity of the SUD (mild,

moderate, or severe). Changes in severity may be observed across time (APA, 2013). (See Box 26.1 for Alcohol Use Disorder Criteria as an example). For specific details of the 11 criteria for each SUD, please consult the *DSM-5*.

The substance-induced disorder of **intoxication** is described as the development of a reversible substance-specific syndrome due to the recent ingestion of (or exposure to) a substance. The maladaptive behaviours associated with intoxication (e.g., belligerence, mood lability, cognitive impairment, impaired judgment, impaired social or occupational functioning) are due to the direct physiologic effects of the substance on the central nervous system (APA, 2013). These behaviours place the individual at significant risk for adverse effects (e.g., accidents, general medical complications, disruption in social and family relationships, vocational or financial difficulties, and legal problems).

Substance **withdrawal** is the development of a substance-specific maladaptive behavioural change that is due to the cessation, or reduction, of heavy and prolonged substance use. This may cause clinically significant distress or impairment in social, occupational, or other important areas of functioning, and as a result, most individuals experience craving to readminister the substance to reduce the discomforting symptoms (APA, 2013). Some withdrawal syndromes are life threatening, others are uncomfortable, and some are less pronounced.

BOX 26.1 Key Diagnostic Criteria for Substance Use Disorders

Alcohol Use Disorder Diagnostic Criteria

1. Alcohol is often taken in larger amounts or over a longer period than was intended.

2. There is a persistent desire or unsuccessful efforts to cut down or control alcohol use.

3. A great deal of time is spent in activities necessary to obtain alcohol, use alcohol, or recover from its effects.

4. Craving, or a strong desire or urge to use alcohol.

5. Recurrent alcohol use resulting in a failure to fulfill major role obligations at work, school, or home.

6. Continued alcohol use despite having persistent or recurrent social or interpersonal problems caused or exacerbated by the effects of alcohol.

7. Important social, occupational, or recreational activities are given up or reduced because of alcohol use.

8. Recurrent alcohol use in situations in which it is physically hazardous.

9. Alcohol use is continued despite knowledge of having a persistent or recurrent physical or

psychological problem that is likely to have been caused or exacerbated by alcohol.

10. Tolerance, as defined by either of the following:
   a. A need for markedly increased amounts of alcohol to achieve intoxication or desired effect.
   b. A markedly diminished effect with continued use of the same amount of alcohol.

11. Withdrawal, as manifested by either of the following:
   a. The characteristic withdrawal syndrome for alcohol.
   b. Alcohol (or a closely related substance, such as a benzodiazepine) is taken to relieve or avoid withdrawal symptoms.

Specify current severity:
   Mild: Presence of 2 to 3 symptoms
   Moderate: Presence of 4 to 5 symptoms
   Severe: Presence of 6 or more symptoms

Classes of Substances

Although not fully distinct, there are 10 described classes of substances referred to in the *DSM-5*. The classification system includes **alcohol**; **caffeine**; **cannabis** (marijuana); **hallucinogens** (with separate categories for phencyclidine [PCP] or similarly acting arylcyclohexylamines, and other hallucinogens); **inhalants**; **opioids**; sedatives, hypnotics, and anxiolytics; stimulants; tobacco (nicotine); and other (or unknown) substances (APA, 2013, p. 481). This last classification is for newer designer drugs entering the market. The diagnosis of SUD can be applied to all 10 classes of substances except for caffeine. The pharmacologic mechanisms by which each of these drugs produces reward to the brain are different, but what is common to these classes of drugs is that when they are taken in excess, the brain reward system is intensely activated (APA, 2013).

Clinical Course

Addiction is best described as a *chronic disease*, more specifically a chronic mental disorder, one that potentially threatens the health and wellbeing of individuals with the disorder as well as their family, friends, colleagues, community, and economy. There is considerable heterogeneity among people with SUD, but it is often observed that there are periods of sustained substance use that are interrupted by periods of partial or complete remission (a period when symptoms have abated). In some individuals, addiction to a single substance may lead to the **contemporaneous use** of (and possible addiction to) other psychoactive substances. Of particular note in this regard is the use of tobacco and caffeine, as these are often contemporaneously encountered with other substances.

It is well acknowledged that when addiction is neglected and untreated, the course of the disease often typically progresses in severity and may result in premature death. SUDs are widely considered to be amenable to evidence-based treatment, as with other chronic disease conditions, such as diabetes, asthma, or hypertension. Most persons with SUDs will have one or more **relapses** (a return to substance use after a drug-free period) during their process of recovery. Some of the most commonly cited precursors to relapse include substance-related reminder cues (e.g., sights, sounds, smells, or thoughts), negative or positive mood states, and sampling the drug itself (even in small doses). Current craving (the experience of a strong desire or urge to take the substance) is assessed because it may be a signal of impending relapse (APA, 2013).

Non–Substance-Related Disorders

Other repetitive behaviours have been postulated to form part of the addiction-related disorder spectrum. These include such behaviours as internet gaming addiction, sex addiction, exercise addiction, shopping addiction, food addictions, mobile phone addiction, and others. More research is needed for these non–substance-related disorders (SRDs) and related conditions to reach the necessary internal consistency of criteria or the diagnostic stability for inclusion in the *DSM-5* classification system.

The *DSM-5* (APA, 2013) does include **gambling disorder** in its classification system due to the body of evidence indicating that gambling behaviours activate reward systems similar to those activated by substances of abuse and appear to produce some behavioural symptoms comparable with those of SUD. Please refer to the *DSM-5* for diagnostic criteria.

Epidemiology

Nurses should be open to the possibility that individuals are unlikely ever too young or old, too healthy or ill, or too educated or wealthy to have problems with substance use. In their practices, nurses are well positioned to detect areas of potential or actual need for individuals and their families in regard to substance use in all of the settings in which nursing is practised (e.g., home, community, ambulatory, inpatient, and long-term settings). The following section addresses the most commonly used substances in Canadian society.

Alcohol

In most instances, alcohol is used in moderation but, in general, the frequency of drinking alcohol *increases* with age, income, and education just as smoking and other substance use *decreases* across these variables. Alcohol is the most used substance in Canada. In 2018, more than 78% of Canadians older than 15 years report drinking in the last 12 months (Canadian Centre on Substance Use and Addiction [CCSA], 2019). Almost 20% of Canadians over the age of 12 were classified as heavy drinkers in that year (Statistics Canada, 2019a). Among many Canadians, alcohol use has increased during the COVID-19 pandemic. However, 22% overall and 33% of those between the ages of 15 and 29 years reported a decrease in alcohol consumption during that time (Statistics Canada, 2021a). The prevalence rate of 12-month and lifetime alcohol use disorders (AUDs) are 13.9% and 29.1%, respectively, with only 19.8% with lifetime AUD ever treated (Grant et al., 2015). Globally, AUDs are the most prevalent of all SUDs and have a standardized prevalence rate of 1,320.8 cases per 100,000 people (GBD 2016 Alcohol and Drug Use Collaborators, 2018).

Caffeine

Caffeine is the most widely used substance globally. Coffee, tea, and soft drinks are the major dietary sources of caffeine, and energy drink consumption continues to sharply increase each year. Approximately one in six energy drink consumers in Canada exceeds the guidance for maximum daily caffeine consumption (400 mg of caffeine daily), potentially increasing their risk of experiencing adverse effects (Reid et al., 2017). Caffeine is generally considered a functional or beneficial drug because it can improve mood and alertness at low doses. However, caffeine use can become disordered or problematic; among caffeine consumers who attempt to permanently stop using caffeine, more than 70% report withdrawal symptoms and 24% report headache plus other symptoms that interfered with functioning (APA, 2013).

Cannabis

Cannabis production, distribution, sales, and nonmedical use became legal in Canada on October 17, 2018 (Statistics Canada, 2021b). The *Cannabis Act* serves to protect the health and safety of Canadians by preventing youth from accessing cannabis, minimize the illegal cannabis market by creating a regulated supply chain, and implementing rules surrounding access to cannabis (Government of Canada, 2021a).

Almost half of all Canadians older than 15 years have tried cannabis (Statistics Canada, 2019b). According to the Canadian Cannabis Survey 2020, 27% of Canadians used cannabis in the previous 12 months, an increase from 25% in the previous year (Government of Canada, 2021b). Canadians between the ages of 16 and 24 years reported using cannabis at almost twice the rate of those older than 25 years. During the COVID-19 pandemic, 56% of people reported using the same amount of cannabis as before the pandemic, 22% reported using more, and the same percentage reported using less (Government of Canada, 2021b).

Before its legalization, cannabis was the fourth most used substance in Canada after caffeine, alcohol, and tobacco. The prevalence of 12-month and lifetime cannabis use disorder are 2.5% and 6.3%, respectively. Only 13.2% with lifetime cannabis use disorder have participated in professional treatment or 12-step programs (Hasin et al., 2016). Globally, cannabis dependence is the third most prevalent of all SUDs and have a standardized prevalence rate of 289.7 cases per 100,000 people (GBD 2016 Alcohol and Drug Use Collaborators, 2018).

Opioids

It has been established that Canada has the world's second highest per capita levels of prescription **opioid** consumption globally, second in usage only to the United States. Their widespread use has resulted in a national epidemic of opioid addiction, overdose, suicide, and deaths. The cause of the epidemic has been attributed to a confluence of efforts to improve pain management by doctors, aggressive, fraudulent marketing by some phar-

maceutical manufacturers, and the emergence of highly potent illegally manufactured opioids such a street fentanyl. Between January 2016 and December 2020, there were 21,174 opioid toxicity deaths in Canada. In 2020 alone, there were 6,214 opioid toxicity deaths, 96% of which were accidental (Government of Canada, 2021c). In Canada, the past-year prevalence of prescription opioid use in the general population was 11.8% and nonmedical opioid use was 2.9% (CCSA, 2020a). Given its increasing and high consumption levels, it has been estimated that prescription opioids now constitute the third highest level of substance use burden of disease (after alcohol and tobacco) in Canada (CCSA, 2020a). Globally, opioid dependence is the second most prevalent of all SUDs and have a standardized prevalence rate of 353.0 cases per 100,000 people (GBD 2016 Alcohol and Drug Use Collaborators, 2018).

Tobacco

The use of tobacco products remains the most important preventable cause of death and disease globally. With around 8 million lives lost annually, tobacco-related diseases claim more lives than do HIV, AIDS, malaria, and tuberculosis combined (WHO, 2021a, 2021b). The deaths of 28% of males and 23% of females in Canada are attributable to the use of tobacco products (Manuel et al., 2016). Tobacco is a risk factor for six of the eight leading causes of mortality, and tobacco smoking remains the dominant risk factor for cancer in Canada (Kruegar et al., 2016). Given that 15.8% of the population smoked daily or occasionally in 2018 (Statistics Canada, 2019c), in an average use of 13.9 cigarettes per day, tobacco continues to have the highest rates of addiction of any substance in Canada (Reid et al., 2017). While e-cigarettes do not contain tobacco, they are harmful to one's health and increase the risk of heart and lung disease. Long-term effects of e-cigarettes are still unknown but are particularly risky when used by children, adolescents, and women who are pregnant (WHO, 2021a, 2021b).

Societal Costs

Alcohol, tobacco, and other substance use exact a heavy toll on the health of individuals, their families, and communities. It is estimated that substance use costs Canadian society almost $46 billion a year or almost $1,258 for every person in Canada (CCSA, 2020b). When substance use costs are analyzed by key sectors, lost productivity accounted for 44%, healthcare costs 28%, criminal justice 20%, and other direct costs contributed 8%. Alcohol and tobacco use cost the Canadian economy and public health more than all of other substances combined and were responsible for 76% of the 751,356 years of life lost due to substance use in 2017.

▊ Aetiologic Theories

Addiction (used synonymously with the *DSM-5* designation of SUD) can be conceptualized as a disorder with a multifactorial pathogenesis and predisposing, precipitating, and modulating factors that encompass the body, the mind (psyche), and the spirit. It is further shaped and affected by social, environmental, cultural, economic, and political influences in the development and expression of the disease, which may affect conceptualizing and formulating safe and effective treatment. Addiction is not all-or-none but rather a matter of degree (West, 2006, p. 3). This disease typically develops, and comes to expression, in behavioural ways with varying degrees of embedded biologic, psychological, social, and spiritual aspects that cannot be explained in isolation or with any reductive theory. Environmental or conditioned cues—of which there may be tens of thousands that individuals associate with their substance use or addictive disorder—also become a part of the addiction, and these are experienced within a complex environment where a range of dynamic factors likely influence the course of the disease.

Biologic Theories

When considering processes that increase the risk for addiction, the interplay between stressors in the environment and genes (the field of epigenetics) is a burgeoning field. Factors such as trauma, prenatal and postnatal stress, and adverse childhood experiences have the potential to change gene expression. These alternations may dysregulate the hypothalamic–pituitary axis (HPA), which may result in an increased sensitivity to stress. In turn, this may increase the risk of the individual in using substances to relieve this stress. At the same time, the use of substances can dysregulate the HPA, leading to a vicious cycle of worsening sensitivity to stress and substance use (Simkin, 2014).

There is large body of evidence examining the influence of addictive substances on the brain, including sophisticated brain imaging techniques that demonstrate structural and functional changes. The addicted brain has been demonstrated to be fundamentally different from the nonaddicted brain, and this is manifested by changes in gene expression, receptor availability, metabolic activity, and responsiveness to environmental cues (Volkow & Warren, 2014). These pervasive changes in brain function may persist on molecular, cellular, structural, and functional levels long after the individual stops consuming the substance. The demonstrated changes to brain structure and function form the foundation and evidence for addiction to be classified as a disease of the brain and a mental disorder.

The use of addictive substances has been found to increase extracellular levels of dopamine. The dopamine-related "high" (euphoria) becomes a reinforcement mechanism in the brain. The brain, in essence, remembers this pleasure and wants it repeated. But the neurochemical status in the brain readjusts to these increased levels of dopamine as being the "normal" neurochemical state; the individual then requires increased amounts of substances to produce the same dopamine-related effects (Volkow & Warren, 2014). Just as food is linked to daily survival, once the brain has become addicted to a substance, it attaches the same level of salience or significance to consuming the substance as it does to the level of life-sustaining functions or behaviours. The substance is no longer sought only for pleasure but for the need to relieve distress or withdrawal; on a subconscious level, it may be enjoyed at the same level of salience as life-sustaining elements of behaviour. Eventually, the drive to obtain and use the substance becomes one of the most important priorities despite adverse (and at times devastating) consequences.

Psychological Theories

The psychological theories on addiction refer to the relative contribution of psychological and psychiatric factors that reflect the individual's preferences, experiences, or problems. It is postulated that these factors influence the likelihood that addictive substances or behaviours will be used initially or that the individual will develop an addiction. These theories suggest that some individuals are born with certain temperaments and subsequently develop particular personality traits or vulnerabilities that may make them more susceptible to addiction. From this theoretical perspective, addiction is considered a behavioural disorder occurring in a vulnerable phenotype, in which an intrinsic predisposed state determines the neuroplasticity that is induced (Swendsen & Le Moal, 2011).

Research increasingly focuses on the possibility that vulnerabilities acquired early in life may predispose individuals to psychiatric conditions (including addiction). Children of mothers who experience stress during pregnancy, or children who have experienced disrupted maternal care during infancy and other early adverse experiences, are considered important factors associated with substance initiation and addiction. It is postulated that the disrupted development and stress from such adverse childhood events (often defined by social and economic disadvantages) contribute to subsequent vulnerability to addiction (Swendsen & Le Moal, 2011).

There is a large body of literature demonstrating that SUDs are strongly associated with other mental disorders. Individuals with SUD often have mood, anxiety, or other psychiatric conditions (Chapter 33 provides more detail on the concurrence of SUD with other mental disorders). Self-medication, whereby substances are used (at least in part) as a means for reducing anxiety, depression, or other symptoms, is one explanation for this finding. The reverse causal association has also been proposed, whereby the use of substances may induce anxiety or other psychiatric conditions. By contrast, shared aetiologic models suggest that there may be specific factors that increase the risk of individuals developing more than one condition (Swendsen & Le Moal, 2011).

Social Theories

The WHO has determined that there are significant differences between some countries in their prevalence of alcohol, tobacco, and other substance addictions (WHO, 2009). These differences exist even between countries of similar income and geographic region. These findings may be attributable, in part, to differences in substance availability, legislation, and other health policies.

Migration studies have compared rates of addiction for homogeneous ethnic groups in the country of origin with those of the host country possessing a different culture.

Stigmatisation is a social phenomenon that is highly relevant to addiction. Labels—"addict" and "drug abuser" are commonly used, even within health care—perpetuate stigma. Stigmatisation is a barrier to seeking help across the continuum of care, with many individuals not receiving the necessary treatment to avoid being stigmatised (Wogen & Restrepo, 2020). Many public (e.g., criminalization) and professional policies are punitive, focusing on the behaviour, rather than restorative for the disease condition. Stigma is so pervasive that even healthcare professionals themselves are often reluctant to seek help for the disease of addiction (Kunyk et al., 2016a, 2016b).

Spiritual Theories

Spirituality has a close relationship with the field of addiction treatment; individuals who have recovered from addiction often mention spiritual experiences or motivation as a major contributory factor in their recovery. Spirituality can be defined as the relationship between an individual and the sacred (numinous), perhaps represented by a transcendent higher being (or higher power) or force (or mind of the universe). This relationship is personal to the individual and does not require affiliation with any organized religion; religion is *not* necessary for an individual to develop his or her spirituality or, for that matter, to recover from addiction. Spirituality is an integral dimension of the 12-step tradition of Alcoholics Anonymous (AA). The 12 steps, formulated by William Wilson or "Bill W.," were derived from his experiences of living with alcohol addiction. These reference "a power greater than us," "God," "Higher Power," and "a spiritual experience" (refer to Box 26.2).

Prevention

Epidemiologic research has demonstrated that the onset of substance use typically begins during the adolescent years. Given this pattern, and the potential progression from experimental use to addiction, prevention initiatives often target children and adolescents. Knowledge-based programs in schools have *not* been shown to be

BOX 26.2 The 12 Steps of Alcoholics Anonymous

1. We admitted we were powerless over alcohol—that our lives had become unmanageable
2. Came to believe that a Power greater than ourselves could restore us to sanity
3. Made a decision to turn our will and our lives over to the care of God *as we understood Him*
4. Made a searching and fearless moral inventory of ourselves
5. Admitted to God, to ourselves, and to another human being the exact nature of our wrongs
6. Were entirely ready to have God remove all these defects of character
7. Humbly asked Him to remove our shortcomings
8. Made a list of all persons we had harmed and became willing to make amends to them all
9. Made direct amends to such people wherever possible, except when to do so would injure them or others
10. Continued to take personal inventory and, when we were wrong, promptly admitted it
11. Sought through prayer and meditation to improve our conscious contact with God as we understood Him, praying only for knowledge of His will for us and the power to carry that out
12. Having had a spiritual awakening as a result of these steps, we tried to carry this message to alcoholics and to practise these principles in all our affairs

Source: The Twelve Steps are reprinted with permission of Alcoholics Anonymous World Services, Inc. ("A.A.W.S."). Permission to reprint the Twelve Steps does not mean that the A.A.W.S. has reviewed or approved the contents of this publication or that A.A. necessarily agrees with the views expressed herein. A.A. is a program of recovery from alcoholism *only*—use of the Twelve Steps in connection with programs and activities, which are patterned after A.A., but which address other problems, or in any other non-A.A., does not imply otherwise.

effective, and those that target social competence and social influence have shown a *small* effect (Faggiano et al., 2014). The evidence for behavioural counselling interventions to prevent the initiation of drug use is inconsistent with some interventions showing a reduction (O'Connor et al., 2020). Effective interventions imbed school programs within a comprehensive approach that includes programs that teach parents and other ways to monitor their children and the skills to communicate with them effectively; community-based programs, such as mass media campaigns; and public policies, such as minimum purchasing age for tobacco (Griffin & Brown, 2014). Future research is needed to find ways to effectively disseminate the most promising prevention programs into our schools, families, and communities.

Interdisciplinary Treatment

The adaptation in the brain that results from chronic substance exposure is long lasting; therefore, addiction interventions must also reflect its chronic (and relapsing) nature. This model is similar to those for other chronic conditions (such as asthma, diabetes, and hypertension). Not surprisingly, the rates of recovery for addiction are comparable to those chronic conditions, and discontinuation of treatment is likely to result in similar rates of relapse (McLellan et al., 2000). As with other chronic diseases, effective addiction interventions require the involvement of multiple brain circuits (reward, motivation, learning, inhibitory control, and executive function), and their associated disruption of behaviour indicates the need for a multimodal approach in its treatment. Within this paradigm, relapse is not interpreted as failure but rather as a temporary setback, and recovery is conceptualized as a "process" and not as an event.

To reflect treatment concepts and recommendations, the National Institute on Drug Abuse (NIDA) updated their seminal document *Principles of Drug Addiction Treatment* in 2020. These principles are intended to address addiction to alcohol, tobacco, and other drugs and are based on the existing body of scientific evidence. They provide a critical starting point for any discussion about the treatment of addiction (Box 26.3).

BOX 26.3 Principles of Addiction Treatment

1. Addiction is a complex but treatable disease that affects brain function and behaviour. Drugs of abuse alter the brain's structure and function, resulting in changes that persist long after drug use has ceased. This may explain why drug abusers are at risk for relapse even after long periods of abstinence and despite the potentially devastating consequences.

2. No single treatment is appropriate for everyone. Treatment varies depending on the type of drug and the characteristics of the patients. Matching treatment settings, interventions, and services to an individual's particular problems and needs is critical to his or her ultimate success in returning to productive functioning in the family, workplace, and society.

3. Treatment needs to be readily available. Because drug-addicted individuals may be uncertain about entering treatment, taking advantage of available services the moment people are ready for treatment is critical. Potential patients can be lost if treatment is not immediately available or readily accessible. As with other chronic diseases, the earlier treatment is offered in the disease process, the greater the likelihood of positive outcomes.

4. Effective treatment attends to multiple needs of the individual, not just his or her drug abuse. To be effective, treatment must address the individual's drug abuse and any associated medical, psychological, social, vocational, and legal problems. It is also important that treatment be appropriate to the individual's age, gender, ethnicity, and culture.

5. Remaining in treatment for an adequate period of time is critical. The appropriate duration for an individual depends on the type and degree of his or her problems and needs. Research indicates that most addicted individuals need at least 3 months in treatment to significantly reduce or stop their drug use and that the best outcomes occur with longer durations of treatment. Recovery from drug addiction is a long-term process and frequently requires multiple episodes of treatment. As with other chronic illnesses, relapses to drug abuse can occur and should signal a need for treatment to be reinstated or adjusted. Because individuals often leave treatment prematurely, programs should include strategies to engage and keep patients in treatment.

6. Behavioural therapies—including individual, family, or group counselling—are the most commonly used forms of drug abuse treatment. Behavioural therapies vary in their focus and may involve addressing a patient's motivation to change, providing incentives for abstinence,

BOX 26.3 Principles of Addiction Treatment *(Continued)*

building skills to resist drug use, replacing drug-using activities with constructive and rewarding activities, improving problem-solving skills, and facilitating better interpersonal relationships. Also, participation in group therapy and other peer support programs during and following treatment can help maintain abstinence.

7. Medications are an important element of treatment for many patients, especially when combined with counselling and other behavioural therapies. For example, methadone, buprenorphine, and naltrexone (including a new long-acting formulation) are effective in helping individuals addicted to heroin or other opioids stabilize their lives and reduce their illicit drug use. Acamprosate, disulfiram, and naltrexone are medications approved for treating alcohol dependence. For persons addicted to nicotine, a nicotine replacement product (available as patches, gum, lozenges, or nasal spray) or an oral medication (such as bupropion or varenicline) can be an effective component of treatment when part of a comprehensive behavioural treatment program.

8. An individual's treatment and services plan must be assessed continually and modified as necessary, to ensure that it meets his or her changing needs. A patient may require varying combinations of services and treatment components during the course of treatment and recovery. In addition to counselling or psychotherapy, a patient may require medication, medical services, family therapy, parenting instruction, vocational rehabilitation, and/or social and legal services. For many patients, a continuing care approach provides the best results, with the treatment intensity varying according to a person's changing needs.

9. Many drug-addicted individuals also have other mental disorders. Because drug abuse and addiction—both of which are mental disorders—often co-occur with other mental illnesses, patients presenting with one condition should be assessed for the other(s), and when these problems co-occur, treatment should address both (or all), including the use of medications as appropriate.

10. Medically assisted detoxification is only the first stage of addiction treatment and by itself does little to change long-term drug abuse. Although medically assisted detoxification can safely manage the acute physical symptoms of withdrawal and, for some, can pave the way for effective long-term addiction treatment, detoxification alone is rarely sufficient to help addicted individuals achieve long-term abstinence. Thus, patients should be encouraged to continue drug treatment following detoxification. Motivational enhancement and incentive strategies, begun at initial patient intake, can improve treatment engagement.

11. Treatment does not need to be voluntary to be effective. Sanctions or enticements from family, employment settings, and/or the criminal justice system can significantly increase treatment entry, retention rates, and the ultimate success of drug treatment interventions.

12. Drug use during treatment must be monitored continuously, as lapses during treatment do occur. Knowing their drug use is being monitored can be a powerful incentive for patients and can help them withstand urges to use drugs. Monitoring also provides an early indication of a return to drug use, signalling a possible need to adjust an individual's treatment plan to better meet his or her needs.

13. Treatment programs should assess patients for the presence of HIV/AIDS, hepatitis B and C, tuberculosis, and other infectious diseases as well as provide targeted risk reduction counselling, linking patients to treatment if necessary. Typically, drug abuse treatment addresses some of the drug-related behaviours that put people at risk of infectious diseases. Targeted counselling specifically focused on reducing infectious disease risk can help patients further reduce or avoid substance-related and other high-risk behaviours. Counselling can also help those who are already infected to manage their illness. Moreover, engaging in substance abuse treatment can facilitate adherence to other medical treatments. Substance abuse treatment facilities should provide on-site, rapid HIV testing rather than referrals to off-site testing as research shows that doing so increases the likelihood that patients will be tested and receive their test results. Those providing treatment should also inform patients that highly active antiretroviral therapy (HAART) has proven effective in combating HIV, including among drug-abusing populations, and link them to HIV treatment if they test positive.

NIDA. (2020, September 18). *Principles of effective treatment.* Retrieved August 6, 2021, from https://www.drugabuse.gov/publications/principles-drug-addiction-treatment-research-based-guide-third-edition/principles-effective-treatment

Goals of Addiction Treatment

Addiction treatment programs have as their goal not simply stabilizing the individual's condition but altering the course of the SUD as well as their overall functioning. Safe and effective treatment for individuals with SUD requires the completion of screening, a comprehensive assessment, matching treatment to include the evidence-based modalities available for the particular disorder and comorbidities, monitoring of outcomes, and follow-up on a longitudinal basis. Treatment ought to be culturally sensitive and appropriate, taking into account the specific needs and preferences of the individual. Issues related to gender identity and expression, pregnancy and lactation, culture, spirituality, age, and other medical needs are to be considered as well in the treatment provision. Box 26.4 outlines specific goals of addiction treatment.

The multimodal treatment of addiction typically involves a combination of psychosocial interventions as well as pharmacotherapy where (and if) available for a particular condition. A longitudinal approach for management of this chronic disease is ideal, and in general, the iterative approach to treatment is first to screen, engage, assess, motivate, and help to retain the patient in a safe and effective evidence-based treatment setting. Treatment retention and adherence to mutually agreed-upon goals generally maximize the potential benefits of treatment and improve outcomes.

Treatment further seeks to help educate individuals, family members, caregivers, and significant others about addiction as a bona fide disease including its causes, consequences, longitudinal approaches to, and the options for, interdisciplinary treatment. For some individuals, **harm reduction** may be an interim step towards recovery, and these philosophies are not considered to

be mutually exclusive or incompatible. Understanding the complementary nature of these approaches is vital.

The **therapeutic alliance** (or the "helping alliance") between the nurse and the individual is a key ingredient for treatment success. This therapeutic alliance ideally builds a foundation of empathy, mutual respect, and trust; provides hope for recovery; and begins at the very first meeting with the patient. Nurses should aim to establish rapport and create a positive alliance with the individual. This rapport is the foundation for establishing the trusting relationship within which change can be negotiated. A healthy treatment relationship generally facilitates treatment, improves adherence with treatment, and ultimately improves outcomes.

To establish a therapeutic alliance, the nurse should aim to minimize or avoid premature and inappropriate confrontations, judgment, negative interactions, advice without permission, and other approaches not congruent with motivation-based techniques. Some health professionals may experience an element of negative bias or stereotyping of people, perhaps stemming from their own particular background, psychodynamics, or their own losses or experiences with addiction. For the ethical professional, it is important to make the effort of processing any unresolved conflicts and losses in their own life and to successfully work through any related issues.

The evidence clearly suggests that a confrontational interpersonal style is generally not helpful for achieving goals in addiction treatment and can lead to the individual being more defensive, displaying increased levels of denial, decreased levels of treatment acceptance, and even disengagement in treatment. Among the most important and valuable skills and attitudes translating into treatment success are the nurse's appropriate empathy, boundary setting, confidence, instillation of hope, and the provision of support and encouragement to the individual.

Principles of Matching Treatment

As an overarching principle, treatment should be offered on the least restrictive level of care that is proven to be safe and likely to be effective. Patients are matched to the most appropriate level of care based on availability along with the assessment of their condition and comorbidities and with respect to the individuals' preferences. The American Society of Addiction Medicine (ASAM) recommends six dimensions of multidimensional assessment to create a holistic, biopsychosocial assessment of an individual for planning services and treatments. Following the assessment, there are detailed descriptions of the most appropriate level of care for the individual, which range from early intervention (0.5), outpatient (1), intensive outpatient services (2.1), partial hospitalization services (2.5), clinically managed low-intensity residential services (3.1), clinically managed population-specific high-intensity residential services (3.3), clinically managed medium-intensity for adolescents and high-intensity

---

BOX 26.4 Goals of Addiction Treatment

The goals of addiction treatment include the following:

- Treatment retention
- Reduction in severity and frequency of substance use episodes
- Reducing harm caused by substances, with the ultimate goal of total abstinence
- Management of comorbid psychiatric and medical conditions
- Improving the patient's quality of life
- Improving all areas of life affected by addiction (e.g., employment, interpersonal relationships, interface with the law/criminal justice system, physical health)
- Improving all levels of adaptive functioning
- Preventing relapse to substance use

BOX 26.5 The Six Dimensions of Multidimensional Assessment

The six dimensions of multidimensional assessment are as follows:

1. Acute intoxication and/or withdrawal potential
2. Biomedical conditions and complications
3. Emotional, behavioral, or cognitive conditions and complications
4. Readiness to change
5. Relapse, continued use, or continued problem potential
6. Recovery or living situation

Adapted from the American Society of Addiction Medicine. (2015). *What are the ASAM levels of care?* Retrieved from http://asamcontinuum.org/knowledgebase/what-are-the-asam-levels-of-care

---

BOX 26.6 The CAGE Questionnaire

Higher scores indicate alcohol problems. A total score of 2 or greater is considered clinically significant.

Question	Yes	No
C: Have you ever felt you should **C**ut down on your drinking?	1	0
A: Have people **A**nnoyed you by criticizing your drinking?	1	0
G: Have you ever felt bad or **G**uilty about your drinking?	1	0
E: Have you ever had a drink first thing in the morning to steady your nerves or get rid of a hangover (**E**ye opener)?	1	0

Ewing, J. A. (1984). Detecting alcoholism. The CAGE questionnaire. *JAMA, 252*(14), 1905–1907. https://doi.org/10.1001/jama.1984.03350140051025

---

residential services for adults (3.5), medically monitored high-intensity inpatient services for adolescents and medically monitored intensive inpatient services withdrawal management for adults (3.7), and medically managed intensive inpatient services for adolescents and adults (4.00) (Box 26.5; ASAM, 2015).

Screening, Brief Intervention, and Referral

It has been estimated that about one in five adults accessing any primary care services reports problems related to substance use. The high number reinforces the need for early identification and intervention. Screening (*Ask*), brief intervention (*Advice and Assess*) and, when appropriate, referral (*Assist*) and follow-up (*Arrange*) for substance-related and addictive disorders are evidence-based and key nursing interventions. Yet, SUD identification is often missed because of a lack of screening. A number of valid and reliable screening tools exist and are readily accessible. Screening for alcohol and drug use disorders, brief intervention, and referral for treatment are feasible and effective strategies when brief interventions and treatment facilities are available for referral.

Screening is used to identify individuals who are likely to have a substance use problem as determined by their responses to certain key questions. An example of a preliminary question about alcohol use is, "Do you sometimes drink beer, wine, or other alcoholic beverages?" If a positive response, screening would occur with options. The CAGE tool is one example of such a screening tool (Box 26.6). If the screen is negative, what should follow is individually tailored advice to maintain consumption below the "at-risk" drinking limits (Box 26.7). Concentration of alcohol in a standard drink can be found in Box 26.8. If the screen is positive, the patient may be advised to undergo more

---

BOX 26.7 Canada's Low-Risk Alcohol Drinking Guidelines

Reduction of long-term health risks can be achieved by drinking no more than:
- 10 drinks a week for women, with no more than 2 drinks a day most days
- 15 drinks a week for men, with no more than 3 drinks a day most days.
- Plan nondrinking days every week to avoid developing a habit.

Drinking is not advised when:
- Driving a vehicle or using machinery and tools
- Taking medicine or other drugs that interact with alcohol
- Doing any kind of dangerous physical activity
- Living with mental or physical health problems
- Living with alcohol dependence
- Responsible for the safety of others (including work)
- Pregnant or planning to get pregnant or about to breastfeed

Source: *Canada's low-risk alcohol drinking guidelines.* Canadian Centre on Substance Use and Addiction. https://www.ccsa.ca/sites/default/files/2020-07/2012-Canada-Low-Risk-Alcohol-Drinking-Guidelines-Brochure-en_0.pdf

BOX 26.8 Conversion Into a Standard Drink

Alcohol consumption is measured in terms of the number of "standard drinks," each of which contains 17.05 mL or 13.45 g of alcohol. Different beverages contain different alcohol concentrations, and conversion into a "standard drink" is shown below.

- A glass of wine (142 mL, 5 oz, 12% alcohol)
- A bottle of beer (341 mL, 12 oz, 5% alcohol)
- A bottle of beer (341 mL, 12 oz, 5% alcohol)
- A glass of wine (142 mL, 5 oz, 12% alcohol)
- A shot glass of spirits (43 mL, 1.5 oz, 40% alcohol)

detailed diagnostic testing to confirm or rule out the disorder and/or to arrange for clinical follow-up.

Screening must also include identifying women who are pregnant or considering pregnancy to provide advice on substance abstention. Alcohol, tobacco, and other substances can have harmful effects on the foetus and may be responsible for lifelong consequences such as foetal alcohol spectrum disorder (FASD). Substances may also be transmitted into breast milk, and the nursing mother can expose the breastfed baby to harmful chemicals, with a range of adverse outcomes and risks. It is important for nurses to note that due to stigma and fear, women in these circumstances may underreport their consumption of alcohol and other substances (Zgierska & Fleming, 2011).

Brief interventions can be defined as time-limited (i.e., 1 to 20 minutes), individual-centred counselling designed to reduce substance use. There is good evidence, for example, that individuals who do not meet the diagnostic criteria for AUDs but are exceeding safe drinking limits can be supported and helped through brief intervention. Similarly, the *Canadian Best Practice Guidelines for Smoking Cessation* recommend that the assessment of tobacco use status should be updated for all individuals by health providers on a regular basis (CAN-ADAPTT, 2011). The Canadian Nurses Association (2011) agrees that nurses ought to be involved in tobacco cessation through assessing and documenting all forms of tobacco use, willingness to quit, and risk of exposure to second-hand smoke.

Screening and brief interventions are promising interventions, but further evidence is required regarding their use.

Multidimensional Assessment

Assessment serves as an early mechanism to engage, motivate, and retain the individual in treatment and to assess for any imminent risk of harm. It further aims to guide ongoing management while allowing for the measurement of progress and outcomes. This assessment process aims to gather information from many different sources that are relevant to the life of the patient affected by substance use. Such assessment involves evaluation of the following domains:

A comprehensive *substance use* assessment, including

- Onset of use or change of pattern of use
- Quantity per day or per week
- Frequency of use and periods of abstinence
- Route of use (e.g., oral, inhalation, ingestion, snort, injection)
- Prior treatment received (e.g., 12 steps, residential care)
- Sources of substances (e.g., retailer, double doctoring, black market)

A comprehensive *psychiatric assessment*, including

- Obtaining a family and social history
- Details of any emotional and behavioural condition or complications (psychiatric, emotional, behavioural status, including any potential for imminent and substantial risk of harm to self or to others; e.g., risk of suicide or risk of aggression, including homicide)

A comprehensive *physical assessment*, including

- Screening for infectious diseases (e.g., HIV, STDs, hepatitis)
- The assessment of biomedical conditions and complications associated with substance use
- Focus on the risk for acute intoxication and/or withdrawal potential
- Laboratory testing (e.g., liver function testing)

Collateral information from others (with necessary consent):

- Assessment of the individual's level of *treatment acceptance* and elements of resistance
- Assessment of risk for relapse (relapse potential) and recovery environment
- Use of structured rating scales to help quantify clinical features and provide baseline for serial monitoring of progress

Management of Intoxication and Withdrawal

Intoxication is the result of being under the influence of, and responding to, the acute effects of alcohol and/or other substances. In the clinical setting, it is important to determine the substance(s) involved, the quantity of the ingested substance(s), and the individual's level of consciousness. Life-threatening intoxication is of immediate concern, and the first priority is for supportive care. Symptoms of intoxication and withdrawal specific to each class of substances are identified in the *DSM-5*.

In general, the signs and symptoms of withdrawal are the opposite of a substance's direct pharmacologic effects. **Detoxification** is a process by which, under care of a health provider, individuals are systematically withdrawn from addictive substances in either an inpatient or outpatient setting. The goal of detoxification is to provide withdrawal from substance use in a way that is compassionate and protects the individual's dignity and to prepare them for ongoing treatment of their SUD. It is important to recognize that detoxification is not SUD treatment. It is simply the management of withdrawal symptoms.

Harm Reduction

Harm reduction is a community health intervention designed to the consequences of substance use to the individual, their family, and society, and differs from moral or criminal approaches to substance abuse and addiction. This approach acknowledges that substance use is a part of society and works to minimize its harmful effects. Respecting the rights of people who use drugs, evidence-based approaches, stigma reduction, and a commitment to social justice are key elements to harm reduction.

Harm reduction forms a part of the continuum of care and places more focus on reducing stigma, decriminalization, and safe supply rather than abstinence. The purpose of harm reduction is to *reduce the risk* for adverse consequences arising from substance use, and this approach works with the individual using substances regardless of their commitment to treatment. Fischer (2005, p. 13) suggests five general principles of harm reduction that continue to be foundational:

- Harm reduction focuses on the consequences of substance use, not on the use itself, requiring decisions about which harms to be targeted and in what order based on what is known about patient's welfare, public health, and the severity of the problem.
- Harm reduction focuses on the pragmatic and effective minimization of use-related harms.
- Meaningful and realistic efforts must be made to actively understand and consider the social and environmental context in which substance use occurs.
- Education, knowledge, and informed decision-making by substance users and potential users are key pillars of harm reduction.
- Misinformed or ineffective interventions or policy can be considered sources of substance-related harms and must also be targeted for harm reduction interventions.

Harm reduction refers to a range of policies, programs, and practices that aim to reduce the negative consequences of substance use, to reduce harms and promote wellness, and to address the determinants of health without requiring abstinence (Schmidt et al., 2019). As examples, alcohol-related harm reduction interventions include providing food where alcohol is served to reduce the incidence of rapid intoxication, encouraging the use of a "designated driver," and "wet" shelters. (Box 26.9 addresses impaired driving.) Some examples of interventions for drug-related harm

---

BOX 26.9 Impaired Driving

Operating a motor vehicle while impaired by alcohol, cannabis, or other substance is the largest cause of criminal death and one of the leading criminal causes of injury in Canada. The level of impairment resulting from the use of *alcohol* is determined by measuring breath or blood alcohol levels (BALs), and the level at which a person is considered to be legally impaired varies with jurisdiction. Under the Criminal Code of Canada, the operator of a vehicle could be charged for driving with a BAL over 0.08%. Some provinces have passed legislation allowing for progressive administrative penalties for drivers with lower BALs (i.e., between 0.03% and 0.08%). These penalties do not include criminal charges; rather, they may include vehicle seizure, licence suspension, and fines.

The standard to determine impairment by *cannabis* has not yet been established. The presence of THC, the major psychoactive component in the plant, can be detected by roadside saliva testing. There is an emerging body of evidence that suggests oral fluid testing can rule out impairment, depending on the time the test is done. The level of THC must be measured through a blood test. Determining the level of THC by which someone is impaired by cannabis is complex. The individual's tolerance to THC can affect the degree of impairment. Furthermore, as it dissipates rapidly, the THC level may have dropped by the time the blood is collected from the suspected driver. In addition, frequent users can exhibit persistent levels long after use, while THC levels can decline more rapidly among occasional users. Resolving this issue is a pressing problem given the increased use of cannabis for medical treatment and recreation.

reduction include naloxone distribution, supervised consumption sites, and needle exchange programs.

Psychosocial Interventions

Effective psychosocial treatment exists for addictive disorders and includes motivational interviewing (MI); cognitive–behavioural therapy (CBT); other behavioural therapies (e.g., contingency management, community reinforcement, cue exposure and relaxation training, and aversion therapy); self-help groups and 12-step facilitation; relapse prevention; psychodynamic and interpersonal therapy; group therapy and family therapy; brief therapies; self-guided therapies; and hypnotherapy. The more common interventions are discussed in the following narrative.

Motivational Interviewing

Motivational interviewing (MI) is a directive, patient-centred style of counselling that helps patients to explore and resolve their **ambivalence** (the presence of both positive and negative feelings) about changing (Miller & Rollnick, 2002). Although it has wide application in practice for behavioural change, MI enjoys substantive uptake within the field of addiction. Some of the techniques in MI involve listening reflectively, eliciting motivational statements, and examining ambivalence. Those using this form of counselling avoid nontherapeutic responses such as directing and giving advice without patient permission, threatening with consequences, being coercive, and inappropriately raising concern without permission because these place the patient in an unhelpful, passive role. This model allows for the process of change to be viewed along a continuum where concrete steps can be taken to help individuals increase readiness for changing behaviour (see Chapter 7 for further discussion of MI).

Cognitive–Behavioural Therapy

Cognitive approaches to addiction hypothesize that if an individual can change the way he or she thinks about a situation, both the emotional reaction to it and the behavioural response will change. Psychoeducational materials, groups, and one-on-one interactions with nurses also impart information to reduce knowledge deficits related to alcohol, tobacco, and other substance dependence. For additional discussion on CBT, refer to Chapter 14.

Twelve-Step Programs

Twelve-step programs emphasize the conceptualization of addiction as an incurable, progressive disease that has spiritual, cognitive, and behavioural components.

AA was the first 12-step self-help group and has become a worldwide fellowship of people with problems (current or past) related to alcohol, which provide support, individually and at meetings, to others who seek help. The only criterion for entry into AA is the "desire to quit drinking." Many treatment programs discuss concepts from AA, hold meetings at treatment facilities, and encourage patients to attend community meetings when appropriate. They also encourage continue use of AA and other self-help groups as part of an ongoing plan for continued abstinence.

Twelve-step programs firmly endorse the need for abstinence and are considered by followers as lifelong programs of recovery with success attained "one day at a time." The importance of recognizing and relying on a "higher power," or a power greater than the individual, is a central element of these programs. Members of 12-step groups can attend meetings on a self-determined or prescribed schedule that, if necessary, may be every day or even twice a day. Periods associated with high risk of relapse (e.g., holidays, weekends, family functions) are considered particularly appropriate times for attending meetings. A sponsor who is compatible with the individual can be particularly supportive and offer guidance, particularly during periods of high stress or increased craving. There are now many kinds of 12-step fellowships available worldwide, including Alcoholics Anonymous, Cocaine Anonymous, Narcotics Anonymous, and Dual Recovery Anonymous.

Inclusion in 12-step groups is considered a routine part of addiction treatment in most settings. In a Cochrane review, 12-step interventions were found to be more effective than other established treatments, such as CBT, for increasing abstinence with AUDs (Kelly et al., 2020). Self-help groups are not beneficial for all people, and some persons may not embrace the spiritual dimension of the program. The evidence is mixed about the relative importance of spiritual/religious changes for explaining increased abstinence (Cavacuiti et al., 2011). An individual's refusal to participate in a self-help group should not be considered synonymous with their resistance to treatment in general.

Group Therapy

An integral and valuable component of the treatment regimen for many with an SUD is group therapy, and advantages of this approach include the following:

- The presence of others with an addiction may provide comfort.
- Other group members who are further along in their recovery may act as role models.
- Group members may offer a wide menu of coping strategies.

- The public nature of group settings can act as a deterrent for relapse. It has been noted that individuals recovering from SUDs may be highly skilled at detecting each other's concealed substance use or early relapse.

The efficacy of group therapy is similar to individual therapy, and it can be a successful component of a combined treatment program. For more detailed information about group therapy, refer to Chapter 15.

Family Therapy

Long-term family therapy is often beneficial following the initial stages of detoxification and stabilization. Families can often unwittingly enable addiction by, for instance, continuing to supply money to the individual, allowing adult children to live at home while continuing their substance use, and rescuing individuals from legal and other difficulties that result from substance use. Family therapy can bring these behaviours to light and assist family members to adopt alternative, more helpful ways of support. More detailed information is available in Chapter 16.

Pharmacotherapy

Pharmacotherapy, when available and appropriate, is routinely combined with psychosocial treatment and is not recommended for use in isolation from psychosocial interventions. Medications for SRD are generally utilized to treat intoxication and withdrawal, to reduce the reinforcing effects of drugs, to prevent relapse, and to treat comorbid medical or psychiatric conditions. For most of the SRDs, there is insufficient evidence for the use of pharmacotherapy. However, for the disorders related to alcohol, opioids, and tobacco, the empirical evidence supports the use of pharmacotherapy, and these will be specifically addressed by substance in the following section on nursing interventions for specific SRDs.

Relapse Prevention

Recovery from SUD can, for some, be defined as a long-term and ongoing process rather than a singular event. Ten interventions have been identified for the purposes of reducing relapse risk (Douaihy et al., 2011) and continue to be salient. These include helping individuals to

- Understand relapse as a possible part of the recovery process and to learn how to identify warning signs
- Identify high-risk situations for relapse and develop effective cognitive and behavioural coping
- Enhance communication skills and interpersonal relationships and to develop a recovery social network

- Reduce, identify, and manage negative emotional states (i.e., the acronym **HALT** warns not to become too Hungry, too Angry, too Lonely, or too Tired)
- Identify and manage cravings and any cues that may precede cravings
- Identify and challenge cognitive distortions
- Work towards a more balanced lifestyle
- Consider the use of medications in combination with psychosocial treatments
- Facilitate the transition between the levels of care between residential or hospital-based treatment programs and structured partial hospital or intensive outpatient programs
- Incorporate strategies to improve adherence to treatment and medications

Mindfulness-based relapse prevention (MBRP) is being investigated as a promising strategy for relapse prevention, with mixed results. There is some evidence that mindfulness is a useful and appropriate intervention for marginalized young adults and that this may be related to reduced stress (Davis et al., 2018). Another study indicated that MBRP as an adjunct to usual care with individual in early recovery did not improve outcomes but postulated that greater adherence to MBRP may improve long-term drinking outcomes (Zgierska et al., 2019).

Toxicology Testing/Drug Screening

Toxicology testing/drug screening can be a critical tool in the multimodal approach to addiction treatment. These tests can detect the presence of a substance (or its metabolite) in the body for a specified window period. These may be done to contribute to the confirmation of a diagnosis of SUD; to support recovery through frequent, random testing; and (more increasingly) are used in the workplace (i.e., pre-employment, periodic, or postaccident testing). The most commonly used matrices for drug testing are urine and serum, but other body fluids may be utilized under certain circumstances. Specific protocols (e.g., chain of custody) are followed to ensure integrity of the specimens, and a medical review officer typically interprets results. With the exception of alcohol, the level of the substance detectable does not provide any reliable indication of the amount used or the level of impairment at the time of use or the time of testing. Drug testing does not have the technologic sophistication to distinguish between recreational use, drug abuse, drug misuse, accidental exposure, or addiction.

Nursing Interventions for Specific Substance-Related Disorders

There is no standardized intervention that will work for all individuals with an SRD because they may differ greatly with respect to severity, substance of abuse, and their own unique biologic, psychological, social, and spiritual considerations. Often, several approaches can work together; others may be deemed inappropriate. Treatment programs usually combine psychosocial interventions with other approaches to provide a comprehensive plan based on the individual's needs. Nursing interventions vary depending on the nature of the current problems, the status and severity of the illness, and the individual's situation. For an individual who is being detoxified, physical interventions (e.g., monitoring vital signs and neurologic functioning) are necessary. When the SUD is secondary to other physical or psychiatric problems, it may be a priority to address these concurrently rather than sequentially.

The following section is organized by the classes of substances and addresses some of their unique features. Greater level of detail has been provided to the substances most frequently abused in Canadian society: alcohol, cannabis, caffeine, opioids, and tobacco. These are the ones nurses are more likely to encounter in everyday practice including mental health and other settings (i.e., community health, hospital, and primary care).

Alcohol-Related Disorders

The effects of alcohol depend on a multitude of physiologic factors that include, among many others, dose, genetic factors, level of tolerance, gender, body mass, body fat, liver mass, and metabolic rate. The acute effects of alcohol are usually characterized by feelings of warmth, relaxation, mild sedation, and a sense of social disinhibition. In alcohol-naive individuals, a blood alcohol concentration of 160 mg% is associated with obvious intoxication symptoms and signs, which may not be evident in persons who have developed tolerance on physiologic or behavioural levels. In progressively higher concentrations, there is a greater depressant effect on inhibition and behavioural control, producing heightened emotions, emotional lability (or mood swings), impulsivity, and impaired motor and cognitive functioning (including impairment in memory, concentration, attention span, and judgment). In increasingly higher concentrations, it also leads to more severe impairment of motor functions and speech, blackouts, confusion, delirium, respiratory failure, stupor, coma (at about 400 to 560 mg%), and death. Although sedating, alcohol impairs the quality of sleep by disturbing the normal sleep architecture.

Alcohol use is associated with worsening of certain psychiatric conditions and their symptoms, may increase the risk of depression, and may increase the risk of harm to self or others. Alcohol induces the liver enzyme system, which in turn leads to more rapid metabolism of therapeutic (and other) compounds, with an anticipated potential for lower therapeutic effects. Excessive or long-term use of alcohol can adversely affect any or all body systems, some of which could be serious, disabling, and irreversible even if alcohol use is discontinued. These include varying degrees of cognitive impairment, amnestic disorder, dementia, and other neurologic complications (e.g., neuropathies, cerebellar degeneration, and brain atrophy). In the category of alcohol-induced cognitive disorders, there are the conditions of Wernicke syndrome and Korsakoff syndrome. The former develops as a result of thiamine deficiency and manifests with oculomotor dysfunction, ataxia, and confusion, whereas the latter is characterized by retrograde and anterograde amnesia with confabulation (fabricated, distorted, or misinterpreted memories without any intention to deceive) as a key feature.

Alcohol contributes to an increased risk of developing such chronic conditions as diabetes, heart disease, and liver cirrhosis. It is also one of the top leading risk factors for death from cancer worldwide and causal link is noted between alcohol consumption and cancers of the oral cavity, pharynx, esophagus, colon, rectum, liver, and breast (CCSA, 2019). In 2017, the rate of hospitalizations caused entirely by alcohol (249 per 100,000) was more than those for heart attacks (243 per 100,000) and 13 times more than for opioids (227 hospitalizations/day for alcohol and 17 hospitalizations/day for opioids) (CCSA, 2019).

Alcohol Withdrawal

Reduction of consumption, or abstinence, may lead to withdrawal symptoms from alcohol that may even progress into life-threatening complications. Symptoms of withdrawal typically start hours after the last consumption of alcohol and may include nausea and vomiting, tactile disturbances, tremor, auditory disturbances, paroxysmal sweats, visual disturbances, anxiety, headaches (or sensations of fullness in the head), agitation, and disturbances in orientation and clouding of the sensorium. It may also include autonomic disturbances, for example, blood pressure increases, tachycardia, and diaphoresis, and in severe cases, withdrawal may progress to seizures (tonic–clonic), delirium (**delirium tremens**), or death. (Box 26.10 discusses the clinical features of alcohol withdrawal.)

Alcohol detoxification treatment consists of achieving safe withdrawal from alcohol followed by psychosocial interventions and the option of pharmacotherapy. Management of intoxication and withdrawal requires a safe environment, and hospitalization may be indicated if there is a history of seizures, delirium, or comorbid medical or psychiatric conditions. The level of withdrawal is used to determine the most appropriate dose of pharmacotherapy-assisted symptom-triggered

BOX 26.10 Clinical Features of Alcohol Withdrawal

Minor Withdrawal: Patients are anxious and may experience nausea and vomiting, coarse tremor, sweating, tachycardia, and hypertension. Symptoms typically appear 6 to 12 hours after the last drink, or shortly after the BAL reaches 0, and are usually resolved within 48 to 72 hours.

Intermediate Withdrawal: Patients experience the symptoms of minor withdrawal in addition to seizures, dysrhythmias, and/or hallucinosis. Within 12 to 72 hours after cessation of drinking, grand mal and nonfocal seizures typically occur. Dysrhythmias range in severity from occasional ectopic beats to atrial fibrillation and supraventricular or ventricular tachycardia. Patients are aware of the unreal nature of their auditory or visual hallucinations and remain oriented and alert.

Major Withdrawal (Delirium Tremens): Patients experience severe agitation, gross tremulousness, marked psychomotor and autonomic hyperactivity, global confusion, disorientation, and auditory, visual, or tactile hallucinations. They tend to occur 5 or 6 days after severe, untreated withdrawal. Symptoms fluctuate and are often more severe at night. These may include severe diaphoresis and vomiting, tachycardia, hypertension, and fever. Sudden death can occur.

Adapted from Brands, B., Kahan, M., Selby, P., & Wilson, L. (2000). *Medical management of alcohol and drug-related problems: A physician's manual* (2nd ed.). Centre for Addiction and Mental Health.

detoxification management and is measured by conducting a brief rating scale, the Clinical Institute Withdrawal Assessment for Alcohol (CIWA-Ar), which is available in Box 26.11.

Medication (e.g., benzodiazepines) administered early in the course of withdrawal (and in sufficient dosages) can prevent the development of delirium tremens. A nursing care plan in this chapter provides an example of patient at risk for symptoms of alcohol withdrawal and medication management (Box 26.12).

Poor nutrition and vitamin deficiencies are often symptoms of alcohol addiction. Thiamine (vitamin B_1) may be needed when a patient is in withdrawal to decrease ataxia (loss of control of body movements) and other symptoms of deficiency. It is usually given orally, 100 mg daily, but can be given intramuscularly or by intravenous infusion with glucose. Folic acid deficiency is corrected with administration of 1 mg orally, four times daily (Muncie et al., 2013). The use of benzodiazepines, multivitamins, and thiamine, as well as fluid balance, should be monitored and supportive treatment provided.

Alcohol Use Disorder

The goal of treatment depends on the nature, extent, and severity of the AUD. Coexisting conditions are also important determinants of the therapeutic approach and methods used. Psychosocial interventions, as described earlier, should be offered at all stages of treatment in combination with pharmacotherapy and at the appropriate level of care. The suggestion to include attendance at AA is routinely offered. The outcome monitoring for AUD treatment includes reporting on sobriety and abstinence. Serial monitoring of liver function tests, ethyl glucuronide, ethyl sulfate, carbohydrate-deficient transferrin, and early detection of alcohol consumption (EDAC) testing can provide valuable information on the course of the condition, success of treatment, and supplement the self-reported abstinence and sobriety.

Following detoxification (when necessary), there are several medication options to support the treatment of alcohol addiction. These include the following:

- *Naltrexone*, originally used as a treatment for opioid-related disorders, targets alcohol's effects on the brain and requires relatively normal liver functions. The use of this opioid antagonist medication cannot be in conjunction with any opioid medication as it will trigger an opioid withdrawal syndrome. It is further contraindicated in pregnancy and suicidal patients. Naltrexone may be particularly useful in patients who continue to drink heavily. Targeted use of naltrexone also may be effective for decreasing alcohol consumption levels among problem drinkers who do not suffer from addiction.
- *Acamprosate* has the ability to curb cravings for alcohol and may be an effective adjunct treatment in motivated persons who are also receiving psychosocial interventions.
- *Topiramate*, not yet approved for this use, may represent a useful first-line treatment option for the management of AUD. It has been shown to have a greater beneficial effect in patients with a typology of craving characterized by drinking obsessions and automaticity of drinking (Guglielmo et al., 2015).
- *Gabapentin*, although not yet approve for this use, has shown promise in managing mild to moderate alcohol withdrawal. Gabapentin can be considered a safer outpatient option for the management of withdrawal if there are concerns of benzodiazepine misuse. It can be considered a long-term option when withdrawal has subsided (British Columbia Centre on Substance Use, 2019).

BOX 26.11 Assessing Alcohol Withdrawal

The Clinical Institute Withdrawal Assessment of Alcohol Scale, Revised (CIWA-Ar), used to determine levels of alcohol withdrawal.

Clinical Institute Withdrawal Assessment of Alcohol Scale, Revised (CIWA-Ar)

Patient:_____ Date: _____ Time: _____ (24 hour clock, midnight = 00:00)

Pulse or heart rate, taken for one minute:_____ Blood pressure:_____

NAUSEA AND VOMITING -- Ask "Do you feel sick to your stomach? Have you vomited?" Observation.
0 no nausea and no vomiting
1 mild nausea with no vomiting
2
3
4 intermittent nausea with dry heaves
5
6
7 constant nausea, frequent dry heaves and vomiting

TREMOR -- Arms extended and fingers spread apart. Observation.
0 no tremor
1 not visible, but can be felt fingertip to fingertip
2
3
4 moderate, with patient's arms extended
5
6
7 severe, even with arms not extended

PAROXYSMAL SWEATS -- Observation.
0 no sweat visible
1 barely perceptible sweating, palms moist
2
3
4 beads of sweat obvious on forehead
5
6
7 drenching sweats

ANXIETY -- Ask "Do you feel nervous?" Observation.
0 no anxiety, at ease
1 mild anxious
2
3
4 moderately anxious, or guarded, so anxiety is inferred
5
6
7 equivalent to acute panic states as seen in severe delirium or acute schizophrenic reactions

TACTILE DISTURBANCES -- Ask "Have you any itching, pins and needles sensations, any burning, any numbness, or do you feel bugs crawling on or under your skin?" Observation.
0 none
1 very mild itching, pins and needles, burning or numbness
2 mild itching, pins and needles, burning or numbness
3 moderate itching, pins and needles, burning or numbness
4 moderately severe hallucinations
5 severe hallucinations
6 extremely severe hallucinations
7 continuous hallucinations

AUDITORY DISTURBANCES -- Ask "Are you more aware of sounds around you? Are they harsh? Do they frighten you? Are you hearing anything that is disturbing to you? Are you hearing things you know are not there?" Observation.
0 not present
1 very mild harshness or ability to frighten
2 mild harshness or ability to frighten
3 moderate harshness or ability to frighten
4 moderately severe hallucinations
5 severe hallucinations
6 extremely severe hallucinations
7 continuous hallucinations

VISUAL DISTURBANCES -- Ask "Does the light appear to be too bright? Is its color different? Does it hurt your eyes? Are you seeing anything that is disturbing to you? Are you seeing things you know are not there?" Observation.
0 not present
1 very mild sensitivity
2 mild sensitivity
3 moderate sensitivity
4 moderately severe hallucinations
5 severe hallucinations
6 extremely severe hallucinations
7 continuous hallucinations

HEADACHE, FULLNESS IN HEAD -- Ask "Does your head feel different? Does it feel like there is a band around your head?" Do not rate for dizziness or lightheadedness. Otherwise, rate severity.
0 not present
1 very mild
2 mild
3 moderate
4 moderately severe
5 severe
6 very severe
7 extremely severe

BOX 26.11 Assessing Alcohol Withdrawal *(Continued)*

AGITATION -- Observation.
0 normal activity
1 somewhat more than normal activity
2
3
4 moderately fidgety and restless
5
6
7 paces back and forth during most of the interview, or constantly thrashes about

ORIENTATION AND CLOUDING OF SENSORIUM -- Ask "What day is this? Where are you? Who am I?"
0 oriented and can do serial additions
1 cannot do serial additions or is uncertain about date
2 disoriented for date by no more than 2 calendar days
3 disoriented for date by more than 2 calendar days
4 disoriented for place/or person

Total **CIWA-Ar** Score _____
Rater's Initials _____
Maximum Possible Score 67

*The **CIWA-Ar** is not* copyrighted and may be reproduced freely. This assessment for monitoring withdrawal symptoms requires approximately 5 minutes to administer. The maximum score is 67 (see instrument). Patients scoring less than 10 do not usually need additional medication for withdrawal.

Sullivan, J. T., Sykora, K., Schneiderman, J., Naranjo, C. A., Sellers, E. M. (1989). Assessment of alcohol withdrawal: The revised Clinical Institute Withdrawal Assessment for Alcohol scale (**CIWA-Ar**). *British Journal of Addiction, 84,* 1353–1357.

BOX 26.12 NURSING CARE PLAN

PATIENT WITH ALCOHOL USE DISORDER

Kenneth W. is a 55-year-old lawyer with a 25-year history of alcohol use disorder. He is the youngest of three children born and raised on a farm. His mother is still living with his older sister, but his father died of cirrhosis, a complication of years of alcohol use. Kenneth is married and has two children who he rarely sees. Kenneth started binge drinking on weekends when he was in university, and this developed into a regular pattern once he started his law practice. His drinking has escalated after he started having difficulties with his partners at work, and he reports consuming up to 2 L of vodka a day and one package of cigarettes.

Recently, Kenneth was involved in a car accident and has been charged with operating a vehicle with a BAC over 0.08%. He was admitted to the hospital through the emergency department following the collision, with a gash above his right eye. Kenneth began to have symptoms of alcohol withdrawal and became anxious shortly after admission. He requested hospital admission for alcohol detoxification and was transferred to a detoxification and brief treatment unit.

Setting: Inpatient Detoxification Unit, Psychiatric Hospital

Baseline Assessment: First admission, last drink and cigarette at 7 PM. Admission vital signs: T 37.3°C, HR 98, R 20, and BP 140/88 on admission to the ER. He has a history of withdrawal seizures and hallucinations (likely delirium tremens during past withdrawal). He had a BAL of 0.15 mg%, became increasingly anxious and restless over the next hour. His CIWA score was 17, and he was given diazepam, 20 mg PO, as ordered, at that time. Decision to conduct CIWA assessments hourly.

Five hours after admission, vital signs were T 37.8°C, HR 110, R 22, and BP 152/100. He continued to be anxious and was tremulous, diaphoretic, and nauseous. CIWA score had increased to 22, and diazepam 20 mg PO stat was given. The next CIWA score was 15, and 4 hours later, it was 10.

Continued on following page

BOX 26.12 NURSING CARE PLAN (*Continued*)

Associated Psychiatric Diagnosis	Medications
Alcohol use disorder (severe)	Deferred until detoxification is complete, after which consideration will be given to acamprosate, naltrexone, or disulfiram
Alcohol withdrawal	Thiamine, 300 mg IV QD Diazepam, 10–20 mg stat, followed by CIWA score, based on elevated BP, HR, and tremors Haloperidol, 5.0 mg IM PRN, for hallucinations or agitation Folic acid 1 mg orally, QID
Tobacco withdrawal	Transdermal nicotine patch 21 mg QD PRN Nicotine inhaler 10 mg, puff on cartridge for 45 minutes, as directed PRN
Tobacco use disorder	Deferred, but continuation of nicotine replacement is offered post detoxification

Nursing Care Focus 1: Associated Risks of Alcohol Withdrawal

Defining Characteristics	Related Factors
Altered vital signs Altered cerebral function secondary to alcohol withdrawal Altered mood states	Withdrawal is common among patients consuming more than 40 drinks per week or in those with other risk factors. Symptoms of detoxification include fever, high blood pressure, tachycardia, tremor or sweating, confusion, and dehydration. Level of consciousness, orientation, perceptual disturbances (hallucinations or illusions), mood, and thought processes including suicide ideation and cognitive deficits

Goals of Care

Initial	Discharge
1. Detoxification from alcohol will be monitored, based on CIWA score, and management implemented to treat symptoms and to prevent complications	2. Bridging from inpatient from level IV care for detoxification to a regimen that is acceptable to Kenneth and keeps him engaged in ongoing treatment

Interventions

Interventions	Rationale	Ongoing Assessment
Welcome to treatment and assure Kenneth that he is in a safe place. Inform of what he may expect during withdrawal. Start with engagement for treatment.	Begin to establish relationship, a therapeutic alliance, with the patient.	See Boxes 26.10 and 26.11.
Monitor vital signs, orientation, and identify stage of alcohol withdrawal and severity of symptoms.	The more severe the reactions, the more likely that anxiety, disorientation, confusion, and restlessness increase.	Administer (symptom triggered, CIWA) diazepam (for elevated BP, HR, and tremors) and haloperidol (for hallucinations or tremors) PRN and report symptoms.
Institute seizure precautions (bed in low position, padded side rails).	Withdrawal seizures usually occur within 48 hours after last drink.	Monitor for seizure activity.
Orient the patient to surroundings and call light, and maintain consistent physical environment.	Disorientation often occurs as BAL drops. These symptoms can last several days.	Determine Kenneth's level of orientation to surroundings and whether he can use call light.
Avoid sudden moves, loud noises, bright lights, discussion of the patient at bedside, and lighting that casts shadows downward.	Decreased environmental stimulation helps calm the patient, which in turn promotes optimal CNS responses.	Observe reactions to loud noises and monitor room environment.
Monitor for respiratory depression and minimize risk of aspiration (elevate head of the bed) related to side effects of diazepam.	Side effects from medications such as diazepam can alter breathing patterns and lead to an increased risk of pneumonia or a medical emergency.	Monitor respiratory rate.

BOX 26.12 NURSING CARE PLAN (*Continued*)

Outcomes

Outcomes (at 3 days)	Revised Goals of Outcomes	Interventions
Oriented, hydrated, and no seizure activity	Engage in the development of a recovery plan and motivational interviewing to gauge motivation to quit.	Continue to monitor for any signs of disorientation. Engage with MI techniques to gauge motivation to quit.

Nursing Care Focus 2: Discomfort Related to Tobacco Withdrawal

Defining Characteristics	Related Factors
Symptoms of tobacco withdrawal include irritability, restlessness, anxiety, insomnia, and fatigue.	Discomfort related to tobacco withdrawal may be difficult to distinguish from alcohol withdrawal.

Outcomes

Initial	Discharge
Will be comfortable without smoking during hospitalization period	Will be provided additional resources and supports to extend tobacco abstinence into a cessation attempt, if desired

Intervention	Rationale	Ongoing Assessment
Discuss prevention of discomfort related to tobacco withdrawal.	The blood level of nicotine begins to drop immediately after smoking a cigarette.	Monitor Kenneth's level of comfort.
Offer a 21-mg transdermal nicotine patch QD to prevent tobacco withdrawal. Offer nicotine inhaler for breakthrough cravings.	The higher dose 21-mg nicotine patch recommended for those smoking one pack per day; may not be of sufficient dosage to prevent breakthrough cravings. Side effects may include sleep disruption.	Assess for sleep disruption; if present, may remove patch at bedtime.

Evaluation

Outcomes (Day 2)	Revised Outcomes	Interventions
Continues to use nicotine patch and has nicotine gum available for breakthrough cravings.	Avoidance of withdrawal symptoms is a strong motivator for quit attempts.	Continue to monitor for any signs of withdrawal. Engage with MI techniques to gauge motivation to cut down or quit smoking.

Caffeine-Related Disorders

Caffeine is a mild CNS stimulant that is found in many drinks (e.g., coffee, tea, cocoa, soft drinks, and energy drinks), chocolate, and many over-the-counter medications (e.g., analgesics, stimulants, appetite suppressants, and cold relief preparations). A typical cup of brewed coffee contains 100 mg caffeine, but the content may vary greatly depending on the type of product or beverage.

Caffeine is not associated with any life-threatening illnesses, and typical daily dietary doses can be consumed under many circumstances. Caffeine has valuable therapeutic effects; it curbs fatigue and increases mental acuity, exerts stimulating effects on both mental and motor performance, and is subjectively viewed as beneficial by some in alleviating mood. It may, however, cause or exacerbate tremors; impair or improve motor performance; and lead to anxiety, dysphoria, and insomnia. Higher doses increase the heart rate; stimulate respiratory, vasomotor, and vagal centres and cardiac muscles, resulting in increased heart contractibility; dilate pulmonary and coronary blood vessels; and constrict blood flow to the cerebral vascular system. The pervasive use of caffeine, and its integration into daily customs and routines, makes the recognition and treatment of caffeine-associated problems challenging.

Caffeine Intoxication

Symptoms of caffeine intoxication include restlessness, nervousness, excitement, insomnia, flushed face, diuresis, and gastrointestinal complaints. Symptoms that generally appear at levels of more than 1 g per day include muscle twitching, rambling flow of thought and speech, tachycardia or cardiac arrhythmia, periods of inexhaustibility, and psychomotor agitation (APA, 2013). The symptoms usually remit within the first day or so and do not have any known long-lasting consequences. Caffeine intoxication has been observed after consumption of highly caffeinated products, including energy drinks. Individuals who have consumed very high doses of caffeine may require immediate medical attention because such doses may be lethal (APA, 2013).

Caffeine Withdrawal

When used in high doses over the course of time, caffeine can be associated with unpleasant withdrawal symptoms when abruptly tapered or discontinued. Withdrawal symptoms may include headache, insomnia, abnormal dreams, drowsiness, fatigue, impaired psychomotor performance, difficulty concentrating, craving, yawning, and nausea. Preferentially, caffeine should be reduced gradually in those considered to be consuming in excess, and this may occur over the course of days or weeks. Psychoeducation can help individuals learn about the caffeine contents of beverages and medication, providing the ability to gradually switch to decaffeinated beverages.

Cannabis-Related Disorders

There are more than 100 cannabinoids in cannabis. Although occasionally classified as a hallucinogenic drug, the effects of **cannabinoids** are less intense than those of other hallucinogens. Depending on the dose and route of administration, the effects of cannabis begin shortly after administration (when smoked) and typically last from 1 to 3 hours (longer when ingested). Cannabis' effects include relaxation, euphoria, at times dyscoria (abnormal pupillary reaction or shape), distortion of senses, conjunctival injection, spatial misperception, time distortion (time standing still), tachycardia, hypotension, and increased appetite/food cravings ("the munchies"). Cannabis use and cannabis use disorders are associated with adverse consequences including impaired driving ability, cognitive decline, impaired education or occupational attainment, emergency department visits, psychiatric symptoms, stroke, testicular cancer, and other drug use (Hasin et al., 2016; Sohn,

2019). Adolescents, women who are pregnant, and people with an increased risk of mental illness have the highest risk for developing adverse effects (Sohn, 2019).

Cannabinoids are also synthetically produced and commercially available for the treatment of selected medical conditions/symptoms (e.g., appetite stimulation related to medical illness in HIV/AIDS, to remedy pain in some conditions, and for the treatment of nausea).

In the short term, cannabis can result in motor impairment, loss of coordination and balance, and slowed reaction time. These responses translate into the potential for significant impairment in the ability to work in safety-sensitive positions (such as nursing) and safely operate machinery or a vehicle. When smoked, cannabis delivers to the body toxic chemicals similar to tobacco, and exposure during pregnancy may result in cognitive problems in offspring. Long-term use may impair consolidation of memory, recall ability, and cognition, hence interfering with academic functioning. Weight gain can also occur as a result of chronic appetite stimulation. Persons consuming high-potency cannabis, or heavy doses, may develop psychotic symptoms, and the use of cannabis is recognized as an independent risk factor in the development of schizophrenia and psychosis. The developing brain is especially vulnerable to cannabis, and its use among adolescents has long-term effects. Early use can affect the organization of white matter in the brain and lead to an increase in impulsivity, accelerated memory loss, and impaired executive functioning (Sohn, 2019). Early use and high frequency of use in adolescence has been particularly linked to an increased risk of depression in adulthood (Hengartner et al., 2020).

The mainstay for the treatment of cannabis use disorders is psychosocial treatment. This includes motivational enhancement, psychodynamic and interpersonal therapy, and relapse prevention. There is no medication proven to be superior to placebo in the treatment of this condition.

Hallucinogen-Related Disorders

The hallucinogens (the psychedelic drugs) represent a broad classification encompassing agents with varied chemical structures that can elicit varied pharmacologic effects but produce similar alterations of perception, mood, and cognition in users. Some of these include a class of drugs, termed "entheogens," that are ingested to produce a nonordinary state of consciousness for religious or spiritual purposes. Emerging research explores whether some drugs within this classification, particularly LSD, may have potential therapeutic properties for psychiatric symptomatology (Fuentes et al., 2020).

There are more than 100 different hallucinogens, with substantially different molecular structures and unique features. They fall into two different chemical groups: serotonin or tryptamine related and phenylethylamine or amphetamine related. In addition, miscellaneous ethnobotanical compounds are within this classification (e.g., *Salvia divinorum*), but cannabis is not. Some of these substances (i.e., LSD) have a long half-life and extended duration to the extent that the user may spend a day using and/or recovering from their effects, and others are short acting (APA, 2013). This classification also includes the "designer drugs" that sometime emerge on the market.

The hallucinogens have salient effects in changing the senses (e.g., visual, auditory, gustatory, tactile, and olfactory) and may induce euphoria or dysphoria, altered body image, distorted sensory perceptions, confusion, incoordination, and impaired judgment and memory. Hallucinogens typically affect the autonomic and regulatory nervous systems first, increasing heart rate and body temperature, and slightly elevating blood pressure. The individual may experience dry mouth, dizziness, and subjective feelings of being hot or cold. Intense mood and sexual behaviour changes may occur, and the subject may feel unusually close to others or distant and isolated. In severe cases, individuals have reported paranoia, depersonalization, illusions, delusions, and hallucinations.

Inhalant-Related Disorders

Inhalants refer to a group of chemical vapours or gasses, including organic solvents or *volatile substances*, that are inhaled, causing a high. These substances are not intended for human consumption, and although the effects may vary, several are considered CNS depressants. Inhalants typically are used by younger individuals in lower socioeconomic settings where they are often available, accessible, and generally affordable. The inhalants are divided into four classes, but there are hundreds of different chemicals belonging to each class:

1. Volatile solvents (benzene, toluene, xylene, acetone, hexane, felt-tip markers, hobby glue, airplane glue, polyvinyl chloride cement, rubber cement, dry cleaning fluid, spot removers, degreasers, computer cleaners, paint and nail polish removers, paint thinners, correction fluids, lighter fluid)
2. Aerosols or spray cans (whipped cream and cooking oil sprays, hair spray, fluorocarbon, butane [pressurized liquids or gasses], asthma sprays, deodorants, air fresheners)
3. Gasses (oxide [laughing gas], chloroform, halothane, ether, butane, propane, enflurane, isoflurane, ethyl chloride)
4. Nitrates (amyl, butyl, isopropyl nitrate)

As a class, the inhalants are known to cause euphoria, sedation, emotional lability, and/or impaired judgment. In some cases, intoxication can result in respiratory depression, stupor, and coma. The chemical structure of the various types of inhalants is diverse, making it difficult to generalize about their effects. However, serious health consequences may ensue, including hearing loss, damage to the liver, kidney, lungs, and heart, as well as bone marrow suppression.

Opioid-Related Disorders

The opioids represent a broad category of psychoactive substances that act by attaching to the endogenous opioid receptors in the brain. The opioid family of substances include the following:

1. Pure opioid agonists:
   a. Naturally occurring alkaloids: opium, morphine, and codeine
   b. Semisynthetic substances (e.g., heroin [diacetylmorphine])
   c. Synthetic substances (e.g., oxycodone, methadone, fentanyl, meperidine, hydrocodone, propoxyphene, tramadol)
4. Mixed agonist–antagonists (e.g., pentazocine, butorphanol)
5. Partial agonists: buprenorphine (combined with naloxone)

Opioids cause CNS depression, sleep or stupor, and analgesia and possess strong reinforcing properties that can quickly trigger addiction when used improperly. Opiates elicit their effects by binding to opioid receptors that are widely distributed throughout the brain and body. Two important effects produced by opioids are pleasure (or reward) and pain relief (analgesia). The brain itself also produces substances known as endorphins that activate the opiate receptors. Endorphins are involved in many functions, including respiration, nausea, vomiting, pain modulation, and hormonal regulation (Canadian Research Initiative on Substance Misuse [CRISM], 2018).

Opioids may cause tolerance and physical dependence (sometimes rapidly) that appear to be specific for each receptor subtype. In the early stages, the use of opioids may be associated with euphoria in some cases. Tolerance develops particularly to the analgesic, respiratory depression, and sedative actions of the opioids. The common physical effects associated with the use of the opioids include sweating, nausea, constipation (which can progress to narcotic bowel syndrome), and dose-dependent sedation, fatigue, confusion, cognitive impairment, respiratory depression, as well as reproductive and endocrine effects (e.g., suppression of testosterone in men and menstrual irregularities in women). In some cases, opioids are used concurrently with other sedative substances (e.g., benzodiazepines, alcohol, barbiturates, or sedating antidepressants). In these cases, the risk of CNS and respiratory depression may be especially salient, thus warranting an even higher level of vigilance in their assessment and management. There is further a phenomenon called medication-induced headaches, for example, with the chronic use of analgesics, where the analgesic drug is causally linked to the exacerbation of the headache, and improvement is noticed when the analgesic is discontinued.

The demonstrated effectiveness of opioid analgesics for the management of acute pain and the limited therapeutic alternatives for chronic pain have combined to produce an overreliance on opioid medications (Els et al., 2017a, 2017b). The resultant increased usage of opioid prescribing has resulted in alarming increases in diversion, overdose, and addiction in Canada. It was first believed that pain protected against the development of addiction to opioid medications. However, the *iatrogenic* (caused by medical treatment) introduction of opioid addiction has now been well established, and rates are estimated to be from 15% to 24% (Volkow & McLellan, 2016), and contributory to the existing and escalating opioid epidemic.

Opioid Intoxication

Signs of opioid intoxication include miosis (pinpoint pupils), dysarthria (slurred speech), lethargic appearance, and slower movements. The individual may also have hypotension (low blood pressure), decreased heart rate, lower body temperature, and experience less physical pain. Other more critical symptomatology may include cyanosis and decreased level of consciousness.

Opioid intoxication typically does not require treatment except in cases where CNS or respiratory depression is a risk or where it is combined with other depressants (e.g., alcohol, barbiturates, or benzodiazepines). The use of an opioid receptor blocker, for example, naloxone or naltrexone, may be indicated in such cases, along with supportive treatment and monitoring of vital signs.

High doses of opioids, especially potent opioids such as fentanyl, can cause breathing to stop completely, which can lead to death (NIDA, 2021). This is because opioid receptors are also found in the areas of the brain that control breathing rate. Fentanyl has emerged as a drug of misuse and is increasingly being reported as an accidental cause of death in Canada. Pharmaceutical-grade fentanyl is 50 to 100 times more potent than morphine, and street versions of the drug are often mixed with heroin and can be even more potent. As fentanyl is such a strong opiate, the chances of overdose occurring are greater than in the less-potent opioid medications. A fentanyl overdose can cause serious short-term and long-term health consequences, and in many cases, fentanyl misuse can be fatal. It is important that people understand the symptoms of overdose so that action can be taken as soon as possible to reduce the likelihood of a negative and potentially fatal outcome. (Box 26.13 discusses fentanyl overdose in the community setting.)

BOX 26.13 Fentanyl Overdose Management in Community Settings

Background: The increased recreational use of fentanyl and accidental fentanyl ingestion has seen a corresponding increase in fatal and nonfatal opioid poisonings in Canada. Severe opioid intoxication and overdose is a medical emergency that may cause preventable deaths and thus requires immediate attention.

Symptoms: The characteristic signs of opioid toxicity may include the following: varying degrees of clouded consciousness (e.g., confusion, drowsiness, unresponsive coma); respiratory problems (e.g., severe respiratory depression, respiratory arrest); markedly constricted (pinpoint) pupils; seizures, bradycardia; and hypotension.

Immediate Management: Once fentanyl overdose symptoms begin, it is important to get the individual help as soon as possible to reduce long-term or even fatal consequences. Calls to 911 or seeking emergency services as soon as possible are critical first steps. Starting CPR if the person stops breathing or has no pulse is fundamental. Another step is to take any remaining pills from the person's mouth or patches from his or her skin so the person does not absorb more of the opioid.

Pharmacologic Therapy: Naloxone is given for acute opioid overdose. It works by binding to opioid receptors blocking the effects of any opioid drug. Naloxone is available as a nasal spray and in injectable form. Naloxone kits can be obtained from any pharmacy without a prescription and can be used for accidental overdose. There are very few contraindications to administering naloxone in an emergency setting.

Follow-up: The effects of naloxone last only a few minutes. Anyone who has received naloxone should be seen in the emergency department to ensure their breathing is not compromised and for overdose monitoring. Depending on opiate concentrations, the individual may require ongoing infusion and/or management programs. This may be an entry point to gauge interest in Opioid Agonist Treatment (OAT) for long-term management.

Adapted from National Institute on Drug Abuse. (2021). *Drug-Facts—Fentanyl.* https://www.drugabuse.gov/publications/drug-facts/fentanyl

Opioid Withdrawal

When opioid use is discontinued or rapidly tapered after a period of continuous use, a rebound hyperexcitability withdrawal syndrome may occur. Withdrawal may be associated with severe cravings and mimics a "bad case of the flu," involving both the respiratory and GI systems. It may include symptoms of anxiety, dysphoria, nausea, vomiting, muscle aches, lacrimation or rhinorrhoea, papillary dilation, piloerection, sweating, diarrhea, yawning, fever, and insomnia. These withdrawal symptoms are not typically life threatening but can be particularly uncomfortable and may lead to significant distress. Medically ill, pregnant, very young, and very old individuals at risk of opioid withdrawal may be more prone to developing medical complications during withdrawal from opioids or combination substances. The Clinical Opiate Withdrawal Scale (COWS), a validated 11-item scale, is used for monitoring withdrawal symptoms. This scale is integrated into many electronic records and is also available for smartphones.

General supportive measure for managing withdrawal includes providing a safe and supportive environment with close monitoring. Detoxification management is usually not associated with medical complications and serves only as the first stage of ongoing treatment for addiction to opioids. Detoxification is conducted with the use of short-acting opioids such as morphine or hydromorphone with considerations to transition to a medication for opioid use disorder such as buprenorphine/naloxone or methadone. Clonidine is also useful in curbing withdrawal symptoms during abrupt discontinuation of opioids and can be combined with naltrexone. Care must be taken to avoid the development of orthostatic hypotension during detoxification using clonidine (Tetrault & O'Connor, 2014).

Individuals who have completed inpatient withdrawal management alone are at increased risk of death from opioid overdose. This is attributed to decreased tolerance to opioids that occurs after withdrawal. Because of these risks, "withdrawal management is not recommended unless it is integrated into ongoing addiction treatment" (Canadian Research Initiative in Substance Misuse [CRISM], 2018, p. 36).

Opioid Use Disorder

For the treatment of opioid use disorders, there may be the option of opioid maintenance treatment (OMT, e.g., methadone maintenance treatment [MMT]) along with psychosocial interventions. The pharmacologic options available in Canada include methadone, buprenorphine (Suboxone, i.e., with naloxone), methadone, and naltrexone (CRISM, 2018). The prescribing physician or nurse practitioner is required to have completed special training and to have been granted exemption and be registered at the provincial professional regulatory body.

In persons with opioid use disorder, discontinuation of the opioid rapidly reverses tolerance and dependence within days or weeks. However, the underlying clinical changes persist for months or longer, leaving the person particularly vulnerable to overdose. The intense drive to take the drug persists, but the tolerance that previously protected the individual from overdosing is no longer present. This risk of relapse can potentially be fatal and must draw nurses' attention to the increased vulnerability of individuals to overdose in their postrehabilitation period.

Sedative, Hypnotic, and Anxiolytic-Related Disorders

Sedative, hypnotic, and anxiolytic-related (antianxiety) agents are synthetic medications that are sedating, induce sleep, and reduce anxiety. Barbiturates were the first class of drugs used to treat sleep disturbances and anxiety and have largely been replaced by benzodiazepines because of their comparative safety with regard to potential toxicity and addictive qualities. Benzodiazepines are often used to sedate individuals preoperatively, to treat seizures and alcohol withdrawal, and as muscle relaxants. The effects of benzodiazepines and other sedative–hypnotics include decreased anxiety, increased sedation, muscle relaxation, and increase seizure threshold.

The abuse of sedative, hypnotic, and anxiolytic-related agents is common and complex, especially among people who abuse other drugs to enhance their effects (e.g., opioids and alcohol) or to ease the agitation of drugs that have stimulant effects, such as ecstasy or cocaine. This is extremely dangerous and can put individuals at risk for overdose, causing coma or death. The combination of benzodiazepines and alcohol also complicates withdrawal treatment because the individual may seem to improve after the alcohol withdrawal symptoms subsides, only to have similar symptoms emerge as the benzodiazepine withdrawal syndrome appears. The severity of symptoms during benzodiazepine withdrawal depends on the duration and dosage of regular use as well as host factors such as psychiatric comorbidity, concurrent use of other substances, concurrent medical conditions, age, and gender (Dickinson & Eickelberg, 2014).

Stimulant-Related Disorders

This category of substances includes amphetamine and amphetamine-type stimulants, substances that are structurally different but have similar effects, such as methylphenidate and cocaine. Amphetamines and other stimulants may be obtained by prescription for the treatment of obesity, attention deficit hyperactivity disorder, and narcolepsy. These prescribed stimulants may be diverted to the black market.

Cocaine is a powerful and addictive stimulant that is snorted (powder), smoked (crack), or injected. Cocaine is highly addictive and is often coadministered with other addictive substances like alcohol or tobacco. When snorted, injected, or smoked, cocaine rapidly crosses the blood–brain barrier and peak intoxication occurs within seconds after intravenous injection or crack smoking. Injecting releases the substance directly into the bloodstream and heightens the intensity of its effects. Smoking entails the inhalation of cocaine vapour or smoke into the lungs, where absorption into the bloodstream is as rapid as by injection. Cocaine use causes tachycardia, hypertension, dilated pupils, and rises in body temperature. It may contribute to seizures, myocardial infarcts, and cerebrovascular accidents and crosses the placenta.

When cocaine is used concomitantly with alcohol, a potentially dangerous interaction may develop. Taken in combination, the two drugs are converted by the body to cocaethylene, which has a longer duration of action in the brain and is more cardiotoxic than is either drug alone.

Shortly after cocaine is snorted, smoked, or injected, the individual experiences a sudden burst of alertness and energy ("cocaine rush"), euphoria, and increased feelings of self-confidence, being in control, and sociability. There is an increase in sense awareness (e.g., sexuality is heightened, and sound, touch, and sight are more acute). There is also a decreased need for sleep and a lowering of appetite. Along with this, anxiety and restlessness as well as agitation may occur. With the use of higher doses, there may also occur panic, mania, psychosis (hallucinations, disorganization, and delusions), and erratic and bizarre behaviours, potentially leading up to violence and potential risk of harm. In an individual with a vulnerability to depression, mania, or psychosis, the use of cocaine may experience exacerbation of symptoms of related psychiatric conditions.

The high is followed by a significant and intense depressive phase (letdown effect or "cocaine crash") in which the subject feels irritable, depressed, and tired and displays increased appetite and powerful cravings for the drug. The individual may desperately seek cocaine or even other drugs, to self-medicate some of the unpleasant side effects of the crash phase. Similar to the severe anxiety, restlessness, and agitation of intoxication, these symptoms may also appear during withdrawal. These, along with drug-seeking behaviour, may last for weeks, contributing to the extremely high relapse rates observed in these persons.

Long-term cocaine use depletes norepinephrine and, when the drug is discontinued, results in a "crash" causing the user to sleep 12 to 18 hours. Upon awakening, withdrawal symptoms may occur that are characterized by sleep disturbances with rebound rapid eye movement (REM) sleep, anergia (lack of energy), decreased libido, depression with possible suicidality, anhedonia, poor concentration, and cocaine craving. Depression typically resolves, and unless an underlying major depressive disorder is demonstrated, the use of antidepressants is not indicated.

Stimulant Withdrawal

Withdrawal from cocaine is usually relatively uncomplicated. There is a high risk of relapse, and the challenge is often to establish a recovery environment in which this risk is minimized. Cocaine detoxification is not typically associated with medical complications and usually requires only supportive care. However, if a patient develops psychotic symptoms (e.g., hallucinations, delusions, or paranoia) during intoxication phases, specific treatments to remedy them may be required, such as the use of atypical antipsychotics. Amphetamine withdrawal symptoms are not as pronounced as those of cocaine withdrawal and are treated similarly. Evidence in support of treatment for addiction using pharmacologic agents is limited and is similar to that used for cocaine.

Stimulant Use Disorder

Treatment is complex and involves assessing the psychobiologic, social, and pharmacologic aspects of abuse. Psychosocial interventions form the mainstay of treatment for cocaine addiction treatment, and residential care may be required in cases where relapse risk cannot be adequately managed on an outpatient basis. Stabilization of the patient's recovery environment is pivotal in achieving lasting abstinence from cocaine, and inclusion in a 12-step program is recommended (e.g., Narcotics Anonymous). Patients using cocaine should be advised to abstain from alcohol as well and, if applicable, offered opportunities to quit smoking.

Tobacco-Related Disorders

If tobacco were introduced to the market today, it could not become a legal product because of its high lethality index. Tobacco smoke contains over 7,000 chemicals, of which there are at least 172 toxic substances, 33 hazardous air pollutants, 47 chemicals restricted as hazardous waste, and 67 known human or animal carcinogens (U.S. Department of Health and Human Services, 2010). These exist whether tobacco smoke is inhaled in the act of smoking or by nonsmokers out of the air indoors or outdoors. Nicotine is an addictive substance found within the tobacco plant, has both stimulant and depressant effects, and is considered as the fundamental chemical "driver" of the process of addiction in the brain. The use of tobacco products without nicotine would not be addictive, but paradoxically, nicotine is not the harmful chemical found within tobacco products, and pharmaceutical-grade (and dosage) nicotine is generally considered to be safe. It is the tar and other substances and additives in tobacco products that threaten health.

A cigarette provides approximately 10 puffs, and a person who smokes 20 cigarettes per day (one pack) is taking 200 doses of nicotine daily. No other drug—not even cocaine—is dosed that frequently, and conditioned cues to smoke become established. As a result, desiring a cigarette becomes associated with everyday events such as getting up in the morning, drinking coffee or alcohol, taking a break, and having a conversation. The quantity and power of this conditioning are unique to cigarette smoking, and it is one of the reasons that smoking is so difficult to quit. Most Canadians initiate the use of tobacco between the ages of 11 and 15; for this reason, tobacco addiction is described as a paediatric disease that in most cases continues into adulthood unless successfully managed in childhood and adolescence. Signs of tobacco use disorder include the urge to smoke within minutes of waking, smoking at regular intervals throughout the day, and continuing to smoke despite wanting to quit. People who are addicted may become tolerant to the desired effects and may no longer experience pleasure from smoking but continue to smoke in order to avoid nicotine withdrawal. Quitting smoking improves wellbeing and health status, reduces mortality, and increases life span (U.S. Department of Health and Human Services, 2020).

Tobacco Withdrawal

Symptoms of tobacco withdrawal vary but may include cravings, irritability, restlessness, difficulty concentrating, depression, frustration, anxiety, insomnia, fatigue, and increased appetite. Most symptoms reach maximum intensity at 24 to 48 hours and are relieved within a few weeks, but some individuals may be unable to concentrate and have strong cravings to smoke for weeks or months after quitting smoking. In recognition of the harmful effects of second-hand smoke for the patients, staff, visitors, and others, most hospitals and healthcare facilities are smoke free. Some patients are placed into involuntary tobacco withdrawal as a result of protections from second-hand smoke policies.

Detoxification interventions are safe and reliable and minimize the suffering from tobacco withdrawal. Detoxification is not considered cessation intervention and, by itself, does not contribute to long-term abstinence. Detoxification is achieved through identifying patients who smoke, offering nicotine replacement therapy (NRT) at sufficient doses, and not expecting a commitment to quit smoking. Effective detoxification requires repeated opportunities to receive NRT and provision of a supportive environment that includes omission of cues to smoke. Systematic measures that are required to ensure rapid treatment delivery include standing orders for NRT, ward stock for quick access, and supplies of a broad spectrum of NRT on hospital formulary (Els & Kunyk, 2017).

Tobacco Use Disorder

There are individuals who are able to stop using tobacco independently (unassisted cessation), but others require formal assistance to achieve long-term abstinence. For some, quitting can be a complex process spanning months and/or years that requires support, medication, and multiple attempts. The optimal treatment design for tobacco use disorder treatment requires a comprehensive and multimodal approach that may include psychosocial and pharmacologic interventions. Canadian clinical practice guidelines that can serve as a suitable template for the delivery of smoking cessation treatments by nurses can be found in Box 26.14.

There are many opportunities for nurses to positively intervene with patients who smoke, given that more than 70% of smokers want to quit, almost half have tried to quit at least once in the past year, and fully one third report that they want to quit in the next month (Reid et al., 2017). In a Cochrane review of nursing interventions, Rice et al. (2017) concluded that smoking cessation and/or counselling given by nurses is effective. One nursing challenge is the incorporation of smoking behavioural monitoring and smoking cessation interventions as part of their daily practice. All patients should be asked about their tobacco use and provided with information and/or counselling to quit along with reinforcement and follow-up. To enhance the likelihood of a successful quit attempt, clinical findings support the offer, and provision, of simple and strategic behavioural counselling and pharmacotherapy to every person interested in quitting. Those who are not ready to make an attempt at cessation should be offered empathetic counselling designed to permit a reassessment of their reasons for continued smoking and an invitation to seek assistance with at any time. Several levels of evidence support the use of the following modalities.

Psychosocial Interventions

Psychosocial interventions, such as group, individual, telephone, office, or web-based counselling, should be routinely offered in combination with medication for increased successful cessation rates (Dragonetti & Zhang, 2017). The provision of simple advice regarding the avoidance of high-risk relapse situations, recognition of settings or circumstances where smoking has been particularly common, management of acute cravings, and development of smoke-free guidelines for home and vehicles are all important in accentuating the likelihood of cessation success. Although the evidence suggests that interventions are effective across a broad range of populations, tailored interventions may be advised for selected subpopulations (e.g., individuals with mental illness, women who are pregnant, and smokeless tobacco users).

BOX 26.14 CAN-ADAPTT Summary Statements for Counselling and Psychosocial Approaches

Ask: Tobacco use status should be updated for all patients/clients, by all healthcare providers on a regular basis.

Advise: Healthcare providers should clearly advise patients/clients to quit.

Assess: Healthcare providers should assess the willingness of patients/clients to begin treatment to achieve abstinence (quitting).

Assist: Every tobacco user who expresses the willingness to begin treatment to quit should be offered assistance.

a. Minimal intervention, of 1 to 3 minutes, is effective and should be offered to every tobacco user. However, there is a strong dose–response relationship between the session length and successful treatment, and so intensive interventions should be used whenever possible.

b. Counselling by a variety or combination of delivery formats (self-help, individual, group, helpline, web-based) is effective and should be used to assist patients/clients who express a willingness to quit.

c. Because multiple counselling sessions increase the chances of prolonged abstinence, healthcare providers should provide four or more counselling sessions where possible.

d. Combining counselling and smoking cessation medication is more effective than either alone; therefore, both should be provided to patients/clients trying to stop smoking where feasible.

e. Motivational interviewing is encouraged to support patients/clients willingness to engage in treatment now and in the future.

f. Two types of counselling and behavioural therapies yield significantly higher abstinence rates and should be included in smoking cessation treatment: (1) providing practical counselling on problem-solving skills or skill training and (2) providing support as a part of treatment.

Arrange Follow-up: Healthcare providers:

a. Should conduct regular follow-up to assess response, provide support, and modify treatment as necessary.

b. Are encouraged to refer patients/clients to relevant resources as part of the provision of treatment, where appropriate.

Reprinted with permission from CAN-ADAPTT. (2011). *Canadian smoking cessation clinical practice guideline.* www.nicotinedependenceclinic.com

Pharmacologic Interventions

Nicotine replacement therapy (NRT) is available in five forms: transdermal patch, chewing "gum," inhaler/vapouriser, lozenge, and spray. Individuals who smoke seek to maintain a certain individualized level of nicotine, and when their nicotine levels fall, distinct and significant discomfort usually occurs (withdrawal symptoms). NRT stimulates nicotine receptors and relieves withdrawal symptoms, and its appropriate use roughly doubles success rates of quit attempts. Combinations of NRT (e.g., patch and a short-acting version concurrently) have the advantage of allowing patients to titrate their nicotine intake to meet their unique needs and are associated with increased levels of success.

Bupropion is an antidepressant that was serendipitously found to be effective in tobacco cessation. Bupropion inhibits the reuptake of dopamine in the reward centres of the brain, as well as norepinephrine, a chemical associated with withdrawal symptoms. Its use has been shown to double success rates in those attempting to quit smoking.

Varenicline, a third-generation smoking cessation pharmacotherapy, directly and distinctly binds to $\alpha_4\beta_2$ nicotinic receptors. These receptor sites are completely blocked but only partially stimulated reducing the transmission of neurologic impulses and causing a reduced amount of dopamine to be released in the reward centres of the brain. Consequently, the patient experiences little to no withdrawal symptoms and no pleasurable sensation if a cigarette is smoked. Varenicline has been shown to more than double the chances of quitting when compared with placebo and helps about 50% more people to quit when compared to NRT. Combining two types of NRT has been shown to be as effective as varenicline.

Gambling Disorder

Gambling is the activity of risk taking for the purposes of gaining an advantage or benefit and produces vast revenue for investors as well as for government. Gambling disorder typically develops over the course of years, and most individuals with the disorder gradually increase their frequency of gambling and amount of wagering. The prevalence of gambling disorder is estimated at 0.2% to 0.3% in the general population. Males are more likely to have a gambling disorder (although this gap appears to be narrowing); the lifetime prevalence for males is about 0.6% (APA, 2013). The internet has expanded the range and accessibility of gambling. There is blurring between the industries of gambling and gaming, for example, raising concerns of gamers being "exposed to gambling content, sometimes in the form of predatory monetization schemes" (Puiras et al., 2021, p. 183).

The mainstay of treatment for gambling disorder is psychotherapy, specifically cognitive and behavioural modalities. Brief interventions and motivational enhancement have also shown to have benefit in improving outcomes. There are no registered pharmacotherapeutic options, although some benefits have been demonstrated with the use of opioid antagonists (e.g., naltrexone), bupropion, lithium, and selective serotonin reuptake inhibitors (e.g., paroxetine and fluvoxamine). Individuals report benefit from attendance at Gamblers Anonymous (12-step based), and in some situations, voluntary self-exclusion programs may offer some degree of protection. Due to the high rates of co-occurrence of other psychiatric conditions, assessment and treatment of comorbid symptoms and syndromes are deemed prudent. The high rates of suicide in gambling addiction warrant special attention to prevention.

Special Populations and Situations

Youth

Adolescence constitutes the life stage with the greatest vulnerability to developing SUDs. Adolescence is a transition period that is characterized by considerable neurobiologic changes and an associated increased propensity for substance use, and it is also a time of increased sensitivity to stress. It is a time of life when self-regulatory executive functions are still maturing, associated with the enhanced neuroplasticity of their brains and their underdeveloped frontal cortex. This period is characterized by pronounced changes in behaviour, including loss of self-control, increased risk taking, novelty and sensation seeking, social interactions, and high activity. At the same time, there may be low levels of anxiety regarding the risk of harm, strong emotional states, and mood instability. During this age, the prefrontal cortex and limbic systems are undergoing prominent reorganization in myelination, neuronal plasticity, and structural rearrangements, and drug exposure might result in different neuroadaptations than those that occur during adulthood. Substance use during this critical period of cortical development may lead to increased vulnerability

to addiction and to lifelong changes of executive function. In general, the younger individuals start using substances, the more likely they are to progress and exceed occasional experimentation and to move into frequent abuse, with a higher chance of developing addiction.

Not all young people who experiment with substances proceed to levels that bring health problems. The serious risks of substances to youth are physical (e.g., liver and heart damage, impaired brain function, impaired reproductive organ development), psychological (e.g., depression, sleep disorders, conduct disorders), and social (e.g., academic performance, relationships with family/friends, and increased exposure to risk situations). It is important to address a developing substance problem in young people as early as possible, with a recognition that they are different from adults in many ways: their unique developmental (e.g., difficulty comprehending future consequences) and psychiatric issues, differences in values and belief systems, and environmental considerations (such as strong peer influence). Family involvement plays a critical role in an adolescent's treatment and recovery.

Postsecondary Education Students

Peak lifetime alcohol use generally occurs in an individual's late teens and early 20s. The prevalence of heavy episodic (or binge) drinking (defined as reaching a BAL of 0.08 or higher, usually by consuming five or more drinks for males, four or more for females, in a 24-hour period) and the detrimental consequences resulting from this type of drinking have led to the classification of college binge drinking as a major public health problem. One promising approach to identify students at risk for dangerous drinking behaviour is perceptions of peer alcohol use. Students who binge drink have significantly higher perceptions of peer alcohol use than their non–binge-drinking and abstaining peers (Lee et al., 2021).

Advances are being made in identifying effective strategies to reduce alcohol (and other substance) consumption and its consequences among this population. Environmental interventions are emerging as important components of an overall prevention strategy. They include such strategies as promoting alcohol-free options, creating an environment that supports health-promoting norms, limiting alcohol availability, restricting alcohol promotion, and developing policies/laws about consumption. More targeted interventions include developing CBT skills (such as identifying and planning for or avoiding risky situations using protective strategies such as drink spacing, counting drinks, and limit setting), norm clarification (correcting misperceptions about drinking norms), using MI to reduce resistance and promote change, and challenging expectations.

Pregnancy and Lactation

Alcohol, tobacco, and other drug use during pregnancy can have serious detrimental effects on the course of pregnancy, as well as on the physiologic status of the foetus and newborn. Pregnancy may result in increased motivation to seek treatment for SUD. Some individuals are able to stop during the pregnancy, but others may have difficulty stopping due to the severity of the addiction or withdrawal. Nurses should be aware that the use of substances is more stigmatized in pregnancy, so that women may minimize or deny their use, its harmful effects, and the need to seek care. The nurse should be aware of special social, emotional, and legal issues involving the treatment of pregnant women and be sensitive to their special needs. For example, women may fear that, by seeking prenatal care, their drug use will be detected by urine toxicology tests and cause them to lose custody of their children. Screening for intimate partner violence should be routine in this population because 34% of substance-abusing pregnant women report physical abuse (Wunsch & Weaver, 2011) (see Chapter 34).

In most cases, providing information alone is insufficient to achieve sobriety/abstinence in the woman who is pregnant, as with other populations. A comprehensive approach to treatment in the perinatal period, including prenatal and perinatal care; pharmacologic interventions, such as methadone maintenance programs; life skills training, such as relapse prevention and social skills training; mother–infant development assessment; and early childhood development programs and social work services, as required, is recommended. The newborn will require evaluation for neonatal intoxication and abstinence syndromes, as well as for foetal effects of psychoactive substance use. Substances are transmitted into breast milk, and the nursing mother can expose the breastfed baby to harmful chemicals, with a range of adverse outcomes and risks. However, women actively engaged in addiction treatment should be encouraged to breastfeed as long as drug screens are clear.

Concurrent Substance Use and Other Mental Disorders

The risk for addiction in individuals with mental illness is significantly higher than for the general population, and many individuals with addiction also have concurrent mental disorders. Also known as dual diagnosis, comorbid substance use mental disorders, or concurrent mental disorders, these can be defined as the coexistence of at least one mental disorder and at least one other SUD as defined by the *DSM-5*. Some mental disorders are in part a by-product of long-term SUDs; some mental disorders predispose the individual to alcohol, tobacco, or other drug use. Nurses need to remember that individuals do not compartmentalize their problems, so health professionals should not either. Concurrent disorders are discussed in detail in Chapter 33.

Nurses With Substance Use Disorders

Nurses, similar to other health professionals, may also develop SUD. Rather than being protected by any special knowledge, skills, or insights they may have due to our education or professional experiences, there is research indicating that nurses may be at particular risk for SUD because of high job strain, disruption, and fatigue related to shift work, ease of access to medications in the workplace, and their knowledge of the benefits of medications. The evidence suggests that the prevalence of SUD among nurses is similar to, or greater than, the general population (Kunyk, 2015). When nurses abuse or become addicted to substances, more than their own health and welfare are placed at risk. There are also patient safety concerns due to the risk associated of impaired nursing practice, and when drugs are accessed from the workplace, patients may suffer from undermedication. To reduce these risks, and improve the recovery of the impaired nurse, the focus must be on prevention, early identification, multimodal treatment, and return to practice with long-term supports.

The issue of SUDs among nurses is sensitive and challenging to address. Nurses with SUD may not be able to recognize their illness or be constrained from seeking help because of stigma, risk of professional discipline or job loss, and loss of status (Kunyk et al., 2016a, 2016b). This inability places some responsibility on others to intervene. Nurses have a responsibility in this situation to ensure patient safety and to assist their nurse colleague in accessing appropriate care and supports (e.g., confidential employee assistance programs are available in many workplaces throughout Canada), with the goal of successful return to practice. Evidence does not support the use of discipline as an effective remedy in reducing the risks of nurses practising while impaired by the use of substances (Kunyk, 2015). Box 26.15 describes research on an alternative-to-discipline approach for nurses with addiction.

Aftercare programs for healthcare professionals have been established as an effective mechanism for early intervention, supporting long-term recovery and detecting a relapse upon return to work. These monitor for continued engagement in evidence-based treatment programs that include random drug testing. This Canadian study followed physicians in these programs and demonstrated outcomes of approximately 80% practising after 5 years (Brewster et al., 2008). The recognition of addiction as a treatable medical illness (as opposed to a moral weakness or lifestyle choice) places a "duty to accommodate" on the employer, and this is increasingly being reflected in employee wellness programs. For further information, see Chapter 17.

BOX 26.15 Research for Best Practice

THE BUSINESS OF MANAGING NURSES' SUBSTANCE-USE PROBLEMS

From Ross, C. A., Jakubec, S. L., Berry, N. S., & Smye, V. (2020). The business of managing nurses' substance-use problems. *Nursing Inquiry, 27*(1), e12324. doi: 10.1111/nin.12324

Background: Nurses' substance use problems, when active and not treated, may place their own health and nursing care at risk. Alternative-to-discipline (ATD) programs have been designed to provide supervised, standardized, and mandated treat and recovery programs to reduce these risks.

Purpose: To investigate nurses experiences in an ATD treatment program, and its institutional organization, in a Canadian context.

Method: Data for this institutional ethnography study included semi-structured interviews with 12 nurses who were enrolled in this ATD program and three of its program administrators. Institutional texts such as reports and contracts were also obtained and analyzed to determine how power relations and current practices affected nurses' experiences.

Findings: There was a disconnect between the texts and the nurse participants' experiences in the program. Power imbalances, potential and actual conflicts of interest, and prevailing corporate interests were uncovered. Nurses in the program were not afforded the same rights to quality ethical health care. Nurses' knowledge was deemed subordinate to that of physicians.

Conclusion: Major deficiencies in this ATD program were uncovered. Individualized treatment alternatives that reflect evidence-based practice, that include nurses in the decision-making process, are recommended instead.

Nurses as Health Advocates

The Code of Ethics for Registered Nurses (Canadian Nurses Association [CNA], 2017) serves as a foundation for nurses' ethical practice, and this includes endeavours that nurses may undertake to address social inequities. Nurses are expected to uphold principles of justice by safeguarding human rights, equity, and fairness and by promoting the public good. Individuals with addiction are among the more marginalized and impoverished members of Canadian society. The challenges associated with their illness are often exacerbated by the experience of stigma, placing an additional burden for overcoming barriers to accessing care. Stigma includes having fixed ideas and judgments—such as thinking that people with substance use and mental health problems are not normal, that they caused their own problems, or that they could simply get over their problems if they wanted to do so. The stigma and shame associated with SUD can, in effect, isolate those with addiction from the rest of society.

The use of substances threatens the overall welfare of our nation and our healthcare system and poses a massive economic burden. Nurses are well positioned on the frontlines of the healthcare system to be provided opportunities to understand the needs and vulnerabilities of those with SUDs, to be aware of available services and resources, and to advocate to improve existing deficits. It is well within the role of the nurse to seek opportunities to reduce the stigma and misunderstanding associated with addiction, as well as to collaborate and advocate for broader societal changes through policy, legislation, and other mechanisms to improve conditions for preventing and treating addiction at a population level. In these times of healthcare reform, nurses may have to proactively advocate for healthcare systems that ensure accessibility, universality, and comprehensiveness of services in order to meet the needs of individuals with addictions and their families.

Summary of Key Points

- Addiction is recognized by the major global disease classification systems as a chronic medical disorder characterized by periods of remission and relapse. Substances of abuse alter the brain's structure and function, resulting in changes that persist long after their use has discontinued. Addiction is amenable to evidence-based treatment, yet it remains largely untreated.
- The *DSM-5* classification of substance-related and addictive disorders includes SUDs (ranging in severity from mild to severe) and substance-induced disorders (including substance intoxication and substance withdrawal). These are classified according to the class of substance: alcohol; caffeine; cannabis (marijuana); hallucinogens; inhalants; opioids; sedatives, hypnotics, and anxiolytics; stimulants; tobacco (nicotine); and other (or unknown) substances.
- The bio/psycho/social/spiritual model conceptualizes addiction as a disorder with multifactorial pathogenesis, including predisposing, precipitating, and modulating factors, that encompasses the body, the mind (psyche), and the spirit, as well as social and environmental influences.
- Accurate and comprehensive assessment is crucial in planning addiction treatment interventions. Assessment should consider all substances for pattern of use,

including factors of tolerance; withdrawal symptoms; consequences of use; loss of control over amount, frequency, or duration of use; desire or efforts to cease or control use; social, vocational, and recreational activities affected by use; and history of previous addiction treatment. It also includes investigating family and social support systems. Treatment plans must be assessed continually and modified as necessary to ensure that they meet the changing needs of the patient.

- In some individuals, reducing consumption or abstaining from substances may lead to withdrawal symptoms that may progress into life-threatening complications. Of note, returning to opioid use after abstinence can be life threatening due to decreased tolerance.

- Substance withdrawal can be assisted through symptom-triggered detoxification. It is important to recognize that detoxification is not SUD treatment. Rather, it is the management of withdrawal symptoms.

- The use of tobacco products remains the leading preventable cause of death and disease globally. Tobacco addiction is vastly undertreated; most individuals who smoke want to quit, but few are helped in doing so. Nurses can effectively intervene and, as a minimum, should incorporate the 5As (Ask, Advise, Assess, Assist, and Arrange follow-up) into their daily practice.

- The purpose of harm reduction is to reduce the risk for adverse consequences arising from substance use and works with the individual to achieve this goal regardless of their commitment to reduce use. Harm reduction forms one part of a continuum of care.

- Many individuals with SUDs have other mental disorders, and individual presenting with one condition should be assessed for others. When these conditions co-occur, treatment should address both (or all) at the same time (integrated or parallel treatment).

- Stigma can be a massive barrier for individuals with SUDs, and nurses are well placed to reduce this stigma and misunderstanding. It is within the nursing role to collaborate and advocate for broader societal changes through policy, legislation, and other mechanisms to improve conditions for preventing and treating addiction.

 ## Thinking Challenge

1. A nurse is caring for an individual diagnosed with opioid use disorder.
   a. What are the four criteria of opioid use disorder (SUD) according to the *DSM-5*?
   b. Create a nursing care plan to monitor and care for an individual experiencing opioid use withdrawal.

> Visit the **Point** to view suggested responses.
> Go to **thePoint.lww.com/activate** and use the activation code found in the front of this text to unlock answers to the "Thinking Challenges" and other online resources.

 ## Web Links

www.aa.org This is the official site for the program of AA. Information about this program, access to resources, and locations are available.

www.al-anon.org The purpose of Al-Anon is to help families and friends recover from the effects of living with the problem drinking of a relative or friend.

https://www.camh.ca The Centre for Addiction and Mental Health (CAMH) is Canada's largest addiction and mental health teaching hospital, as well as one of the world's leading research centres in the area of addiction and mental health.

https://www.canada.ca/en/health-canada/services/substance-use/get-help-problematic-substance-use.html#s2

This is the Government of Canada website to guide Canadians to get help with substance use.

https://www.ccsa.ca The Canadian Centre on Substance Use and Addiction is a national agency that promotes informed debate on substance abuse; disseminates information on the nature, extent, and consequences of substance abuse; and supports and assists organizations involved in substance abuse treatment, prevention, and educational programming.

https://crism.ca The Canadian Research Initiative in Substance Misuse facilitates communication and collaboration across the pillars of addiction service providers, researchers, policy-makers, patients, and individuals who use substances.

https://www.drugabuse.gov The National Institute on Drug Abuse website has research and treatment reports, news, and educational materials.

Acknowledgment

The author thanks Michael Lee, NP, MN, for his valuable review and clinical perspective and Sadie Deschenes, RN, MN, and doctoral candidate, for her literature search and other contributions to the chapter.

References

Agabio, R., Campesi, I., Pisanu, C., Gessa, G., & Franconi, F. (2016). Sex differences in substance use disorders: Focus on side effects. *Addiction Biology, 21,* 1030–1042.

American Psychiatric Association. (2013). *Diagnostic and statistical manual of mental disorders* (5th ed.).

American Society of Addiction Medicine. (2014). *What is the ASAM criteria?* https://www.asam.org/asam-criteria/about

American Society of Addiction Medicine. (2015). *What are the ASAM levels of care?* http://asamcontinuum.org/knowledgebase/what-are-the-asam-levels-of-care

American Society of Addiction Medicine. (2019). *Definition of addiction.* https://www.asam.org/Quality-Science/definition-of-addiction

Brands, B., Kahan, M., Selby, P., & Wilson, L. (2000). *Medical management of alcohol and drug-related problems: A physician's manual* (2nd ed.). Centre for Addiction and Mental Health.

Brewster, J., Kaufmann, M., Hutchinson, S., & MacWilliam, C. (2008). Characteristics and outcomes of a dependence monitoring programme in Canada: Prospective descriptive study. *BMJ, 337,* a2098.

British Columbia Centre on Substance Use. (2019). *Provincial guidelines for the clinical management of high-risk drinking and alcohol use disorder.* https://www.bccsu.ca/wp-content/uploads/2021/01/AUD-Guideline.pdf

CAN-ADAPTT. (2011). *Canadian smoking cessation clinical practice guideline.* https://www.nicotinedependenceclinic.com/en/canadaptt/Pages/CAN-ADAPTT-Guidelines.aspx

Canadian Centre of Substance Use and Addiction. (2019). *Canadian drug summary: Alcohol.* https://www.ccsa.ca/sites/default/files/2020-10/CCSA-Canadian-Drug-Summary-Alcohol-2019-en.pdf

Canadian Centre on Substance Use and Addiction. (2020a). *Canadian drug summary: Prescription opioids.* https://www.ccsa.ca/sites/default/files/2020-07/CCSA-Canadian-Drug-Summary-Prescription-Opioids-2020-en.pdf

Canadian Centre on Substance Use and Addiction. (2020b). *Substance use in Canada costs almost $46 billion a year according to latest data.* https://www.ccsa.ca/substance-use-canada-costs-almost-46-billion-year-according-latest-data

Canadian Nurses Association. (*2017*). *Code of ethics for registered nurses.* Ottawa, ON: Author.

Canadian Nurses Association. (2011). *Joint position statement: The role of health professionals in tobacco cessation.* http://www2.cna-aiic.ca/CNA/documents/pdf/publications/JPS_Tobacco_Cessation_2011_e.pdf

Canadian Research Initiative on Substance Misuse. (2018). *CRISM national guideline for the clinical management of opioid use disorder.* https://crism.ca/wp-content/uploads/2018/03/CRISM_NationalGuideline_OUD-ENG.pdf

Cavacuiti, C. A., Vasic, A., McCrady, B. S., & Tonigan, J. S. (2011). Recent research into twelve-step programs. In C. Cavacuiti (Ed.), *Principles of addiction medicine: The essentials* (pp. 355–361). Lippincott Williams & Wilkins.

Crum, R. M. (2014). The epidemiology of substance use disorders. In R. K. Ries, D. A. Fiellin, S. C. Miller, & R. Saitz (Eds.), *The ASAM principles of addiction medicine* (5th ed., pp. 19–35). Wolters Kluwer.

Davis, J. P., Berry, D., Dumas, T. M., Ritter, E., Smith, D. C., Menard, C., & Roberts, B. W. (2018). Substance use outcomes for mindfulness based relapse prevention are partially mediated by reductions in stress: Results from a randomized trial. *Journal of Substance Abuse Treatment, 91,* 37–48.

Dickinson, W. E., & Eickelberg, S. J. (2014). Management of sedative-hypnotic intoxication and withdrawal. In R. K. Ries, D. A. Fiellin, S. C. Miller, & R. Saitz (Eds.), *The ASAM principles of addiction medicine* (5th ed., pp. 652–684). Wolters Kluwer.

Douaihy, A., Daley, D. C., Marlatt, G. A., & Spotts, C. E. (2011). Relapse prevention: Clinical models and intervention strategies. In C. Cavacuiti (Ed.), *Principles of addiction medicine: The essentials* (pp. 340–344). Lippincott Williams & Wilkins.

Dragonetti, R., & Zhang, V. (2017). Intensive psychosocial interventions for tobacco cessation. Managing tobacco withdrawal in hospital settings. In C. Els, D. Kunyk, & P. Selby (Eds.). *Disease interrupted: A clinical guide to tobacco reduction and cession* (Chapter 9, pp. 141–156). Centre for Addiction and Mental Health, Toronto.

Els, C. (2007). Addiction is a mental disorder, best managed in a (public) mental health setting—But our system is failing us. *Canadian Journal of Psychiatry, 52*(3), 167–169.

Els, C., & Kunyk, D. (2017). Managing tobacco withdrawal in hospital settings. In C. Els, D. Kunyk, & P. Selby (Eds.), *Disease interrupted: A clinical guide to tobacco reduction and cession* (pp. 317–328). Centre for Addiction and Mental Health, Toronto.

Els, C., Jackson, T., Hagtvedt, R., Kunyk, D., Sonnenberg, B., Lappi, V. G., & Straube, S. (2017a). High-dose opioids for chronic non-cancer pain: An overview of Cochrane reviews. *Cochrane Database of Systematic Reviews,* (7), CD012299. https://doi:10.1002/14651858.CD012299

Els, C., Jackson, T., Kunyk, D., Lappi, V. G., Sonnenberg, B., Hagtvedt, R., Sharma, S., Kolahdooz, R., & Straube, S. (2017b). Adverse events associated with medium and long term use of opioids for chronic non-cancer pain: An overview of Cochrane reviews. *Cochrane Database of Systematic Reviews, 10,* CD012509. https://doi:10.1002/14651858.CD012509

Ewing, J. A. (1984). Detecting alcoholism: The CAGE questionnaire. *Journal of the American Medical Association, 252,* 1905–1907.

Faggiano, F., Minozzi, S., Versino, E., & Buscemi, D. (2014). Universal school-based prevention for illicit drug use. *Cochrane Database of Systematic Reviews, 12,* CD003020.

Fischer, B. (2005). Harm reduction. In Canadian Centre on Substance Abuse (Ed.), *Substance abuse in Canada: Current challenges and choices* (pp. 11–15). Canadian Centre on Substance Abuse.

Fuentes, J. J., Fonseca, F., Elices, M., Farré, M., & Torrens, M. (2020). Therapeutic use of LSD in psychiatry: A systematic review of randomized-controlled clinical trials. *Frontiers in Psychiatry, 10,* 943. https://doi./10.3389/fpsyt.2019.00943

GBD 2016 Alcohol and Drug Use Collaborators. (2018). The global burden of disease attributable to alcohol and drug use in 195 countries and territories, 1990–2016: A systematic analysis for the Global Burden of Disease Study 2016. *The Lancet Psychiatry, 5*(12), 987–1012. https://doi.org/10.1016/S2215-0366(18)30337-7

Government of Canada. (2021a). *What you need to know about cannabis.* https://www.canada.ca/en/services/health/campaigns/cannabis/canadians.html#a3

Government of Canada. (2021b). *Canadian Cannabis Survey 2020: Summary.* https://www.canada.ca/en/health-canada/services/drugs-medication/cannabis/research-data/canadian-cannabis-survey-2020-summary.html#a2

Government of Canada. (2021c). *Opioid- and stimulant-related harms in Canada.* https://health-infobase.canada.ca/substance-related-harms/opioids-stimulants/

Grant, B. F., Goldstein, R. B., Saha, T. D., Chou, P., Jung, J., Zhang, H., Pickering, R. P., June Ruan, W., Smith, S. M., Huang, B., & Hasin, D. S. (2015). Epidemiology of DSM-5 alcohol use disorder results from the national epidemiologic survey on alcohol and related conditions III. *JAMA Psychiatry, 72,* 757–766. https://doi.org/10.1001/jamapsychiatry.2015.0584

Griffin, K. W., & Brown, G. J. (2014). Preventing substance use among children and adolescents. In R. K. Ries, D. A. Fiellin, S. C. Miller, & R. Saitz (Eds.), *The ASAM principles of addiction medicine* (5th ed., pp. 1572–1579). Wolters Kluwer.

Guglielmo, R., Martinotti, G., Quatrale, M., Ioime, L., Kadilli, I., Di Nicola, M., & Janiri, L. (2015). Topiramate in alcohol use disorders: Review and update. *CNS Drugs, 29*(5), 385–395. https://doi.org/10.1007/s40263-015-0244-0

Hasin, D. S., Kerridge, B. T., Saha, T. D., Huang, B., Pickering, R., Smith, S. M., Jung, J., Zhang, H., & Grant, B. G. (2016). Prevalence and correlates of DSM-5 cannabis use disorders, 2012–2013: Finding from the national epidemiologic survey on alcohol and related conditions—III. *American Journal of Psychiatry, 173*(6), 588–599. doi:10.1176/appi.jp.2015.15070907

Hengartner, M. P., Angst, J., Ajdacic-Gross, V., & Rössler, W. (2020). Cannabis use during adolescence and the occurrence of depression, suicidality and anxiety disorder across adulthood: Findings from a longitudinal cohort study over 30 years. *Journal of Affective Disorders, 272,* 98–103. https://doi.org/10.1016/j.jad.2020.03.126

Kelly, J. F., Humphreys, K., & Ferri, M. (2020). Alcoholics Anonymous and other 12-step programs for alcohol use disorder. *Cochrane Database of Systematic Reviews, 3,* CD012880. doi:10.1002/14651858.CD012880.pub2

Kruegar, H., Andres, E. N., Doot, J. M., & Resilly, B. S. (2016). The economic burden of cancers attributable to tobacco smoking, excess weight, alcohol use, and physical inactivity in Canada. *Current Oncology, 23*(4), 241–249. https://doi.org/10.3747/co.23.2942

Kunyk, D. (2015). Substance use disorders among registered nurses: Prevalence, risks and perceptions in a disciplinary jurisdiction. *Journal of Nursing Management, 23,* 54–64. https://doi.org/10.1016/j.inurstu.2016.05.001

Kunyk, D., Inness, M., Reisdorfere, E., Morris, H., & Chambers, T. (2016a). Help seeking by health professionals for addiction: A mixed studies review. *International Journal of Nursing Studies, 60,* 200–215. https://doi.org/10.1111/nin.121444

Kunyk, D., Milner, M., & Overend, A. (2016b). Disciplining virtue: Investigating the discourses of opioid addiction in nursing. *Nursing Inquiry, 23*(4), 315–326. doi:10.1111/nin.121444

Lee, M. J., Schick-Makaroff, K. & Kunyk, D. (2021). Frequency of binge drinking and perception of peer alcohol use—A survey of university students in a Western Canadian province. *Journal of Addictions Nursing, 32*(2), 132–140. https://doi.org/10.1097/JAN.0000000000000400

Manuel, D. G., Perez, R., Sanmartin, C., Taljaard, M., Hennessy, D., Wilson, K., Tanuseputro, P., Manson, H., Bennett, C., Tuna, M., Fisher, S., & Rosella, L. C. (2016). Measuring burden of unhealthy behaviours using a multivariable predictive approach: Life expectancy lost in Canada attributable to smoking, alcohol, physical inactivity, and diet. *PLoS Medicine, 13*(8), 31002082. https://doi.org/10.1371/journal.ped.1002082

McLellan, A. T., Lewis, D., O'Brien, C., & Kleber, H. (2000). Drug dependence, a chronic medical illness: Implications for treatment, insurance, and outcomes evaluation. *Journal of the American Medical Association, 284*(13), 1689–1695.

Miller, W. R., & Rollnick, S. (2002). *Motivational interviewing: Preparing people for change*. Guilford Press.

Muncie, H. L., Jr., Yasinian, Y., & Oge', L. (2013). Outpatient management of alcohol withdrawal syndrome. *American Family Physician, 88*(9), 590–595.

National Institute on Drug Abuse (NIDA). (2020). *Principles of drug addiction treatment: A research-based guide* (3rd ed.).

National Institute on Drug Abuse (NIDA). (2021). *Drug facts—Fentanyl.* https://www.drugabuse.gov/publications/drugfacts/fentanyl

O'Connor, E., Thomas, R., Senger, C. A., Perdue, L., Robalino, S., & Patnode, C. (2020). Interventions to prevent illicit and nonmedical drug use in children, adolescents, and young adults: Updated evidence report and systematic review for the US Preventive Services Task Force. *JAMA, 323*(20), 2067–2079. https://doi.org/10.1001/jama.2020.1432

Puiras, E., Cummings, S., & Mazmanian, D. (2021). Playing to escape: Examining escapism in gamblers and gamers. *Journal of Gambling Issues, 46*, 182–198. http://igi.camh.net/doi/pdf/10.4309/jgi.2021.46.10

Reid, J., McCrory, C., White, C. M., Martineau, C., Vanderkooy, P., Fenton, N., & Hammond, D. (2017). Consumption of caffeinated energy drinks among youth and young adults in Canada. *Preventive Medicine Reports, 5*, 65–60. https://doi.org/10.1016/j.pmedr.2016.11.012

Rice, V. H., Heath, L., Livingstone-Banks, J., & Hartmann-Boyce, J. (2017). Nursing interventions for smoking cessation. *Cochrane Database of Systematic Reviews, 12*. https://doi.org/10.1002/14651858.CD001188.pub5

Robinson, M. (July 15, 2015). Gone but not forgotten: 100,000 Toronto library books outstanding. *The Star.* https://www.thestar.com/news/gta/2015/07/15/gone-but-not-forgotten-100000-toronto-library-books-outstanding.html

Ross, C. A., Jakubec, S. L., Berry, N. S., & Smye, V. (2020). The business of managing nurses' substance-use problems. *Nursing Inquiry, 27*(1), e12324. https://doi.org/10.1111/nin.12324

Schmidt, R., Wolfson, L., Stinson, J., Poole, N., & Greaves, L. (2019). *Mothering and opioids: Addressing stigma and acting collaboratively*. Centre of Excellence for Women's Health. https://bccewh.bc.ca/wp-content/uploads/2019/11/CEWH-01-MO-Toolkit-WEB2.pdf

Simkin, D. R. (2014). Neurobiology of addiction from a developmental perspective. In R. K. Ries, D. A. Fiellin, S. C. Miller, & R. Saitz (Eds.), *The ASAM principles of addiction medicine* (5th ed., pp. 1580–1600). Wolters Kluwer.

Sohn, E. (2019). Weighing the dangers of cannabis. *Nature, 572*(7771), S16–S18. https://www.nature.com/articles/d41586-019-02530-7

Statistics Canada. (2019a). *Health fact sheets: Heavy drinking, 2018.* https://www150.statcan.gc.ca/n1/pub/82-625-x/2019001/article/00007-eng.htm

Statistics Canada. (2019b). *Analysis of trends in the prevalence of cannabis use and related metrics in Canada.* https://www150.statcan.gc.ca/n1/pub/82-003-x/2019006/article/00001-eng.htm

Statistics Canada. (2019c). *Health Fact Sheets: Smoking, 2018.* https://www150.statcan.gc.ca/n1/pub/82-625-x/2019001/article/00006-eng.htm

Statistics Canada. (2021a). *Alcohol and cannabis use during the pandemic: Canadian perspectives survey series 6.* https://www150.statcan.gc.ca/n1/daily-quotidien/210304/dq210304a-eng.htm

Statistics Canada. (2021b). *Looking back from 2020, how cannabis use and related behaviours changed in Canada.* https://www150.statcan.gc.ca/n1/pub/82-003-x/2021004/article/00001-eng.htm

Swendsen, J., & Le Moal, M. (2011). Individual vulnerability to addiction. *Annals of the New York Academy of Sciences, 1216*, 73–85.

Tetrault, J. M., & O'Connor, P. G. (2014). Management of opioids intoxication and withdrawal. In R. K. Ries, D. A. Fiellin, S. C. Miller, & R. Saitz (Eds.), *The ASAM principles of addiction medicine* (5th ed., pp. 668–684). Wolters Kluwer.

U.S. Department of Health and Human Services. (2010). *How tobacco smoke causes disease: The biology and behavioral basis for smoking-attributable disease: A report of the Surgeon General.* U.S. Department of Health and Human Services, Centers for Disease Control and Prevention, National Center for Chronic Disease Prevention and Health Promotions, Office on Smoking and Health.

U.S. Department of Health and Human Services. (2020). *Smoking cessation: A report of the Surgeon General.* U.S. Department of Health and Human Services, Centers for Disease Control and Prevention, National Center for Chronic Disease Prevention and Health Promotions, Office on Smoking and Health. https://www.hhs.gov/sites/default/files/2020-cessation-sgr-full-report.pdf

Volkow, N., & McLellan, T. (2016). Opioid abuse in chronic pain—Misconceptions and mitigation strategies. *New England Journal of Medicine, 374*(13), 1253–1264. doi:10.1056/NEJMra1507771

Volkow, N. D., & Warren, K. R. (2014). Drug addiction: The neurobiology of behavior gone awry. In R. K. Ries, D. A. Fiellin, S. C. Miller, & R. Saitz (Eds.), *The ASAM principles of addiction medicine* (5th ed., pp. 3–18). Wolters Kluwer.

West, R. (2006). *Theory of addiction*. Blackwell Publishing/Addiction Press.

Wogen, J., & Restrepo, M. (2020). Human rights, stigma, and substance use. *Health and Human Rights Journal, 22*(1), 51–60.

World Health Organization. (2009). *Global health risks. Morality and burden of diseases attributable to selected major risks*. WHO Press.

World Health Organization. (2021a). *International statistical classification of disease and related health problems* (11th ed.). WHO Press.

World Health Organization. (2021b). *Tobacco.* https://www.who.int/news-room/fact-sheets/detail/tobacco

Wunsch, M. J., & Weaver, M. F. (2011). Alcohol and other drug use during pregnancy: Management of mother and child. In C. Cavacuiti (Ed.), *Principles of addiction medicine: The essentials* (pp. 448–453). Lippincott Williams & Wilkins.

Zgierska, A. E., Burzinski, C. A., Mundt, M. P., McClintock, A. S., Cox, J., Coe, C. L., Miller, M. M., & Fleming, M. F. (2019). Mindfulness-based relapse prevention for alcohol dependence: Findings from a randomized controlled trial. *Journal of Substance Abuse Treatment, 100*, 8–17.

Zgierska, A., & Fleming, M. F. (2011). Screening and brief intervention. In C. Cavacuiti (Ed.), *Principles of addiction medicine: The essentials* (pp. 81–86). Lippincott Williams & Wilkins.

CHAPTER 27

Personality Disorders and Disruptive, Impulse Control, and Conduct Disorders*

Jean Daniel Jacob and Amanda Vandyk

LEARNING OBJECTIVES

After studying this chapter, you will be able to:

- Discuss the concepts of personality and personality trait.
- Describe what is known about the aetiology of personality disorders.
- Identify the common features of personality disorders.
- Name components of maladaptive personality functioning that can be used to describe the severity of a personality disorder.
- Distinguish among the three clusters of personality disorders.
- Formulate nursing assessment and interventions for clients with a personality disorder.
- Plan the nursing care of clients with borderline personality disorder.
- Identify concerns within the nurse–client relationship common to caring for clients with a personality disorder.
- Name the disruptive, impulse control, and conduct disorders and describe intermittent explosive disorder, pyromania, and kleptomania.

KEY TERMS

- affective instability • attachment • communication triad • dialectical behaviour therapy • dichotomous thinking • dissociation • emotional dysregulation • emotional vulnerability • emotions • identity diffusion • impulsivity • invalidating environment • kleptomania • metacognition • parasuicidal behaviour • projective identification • pyromania • reframing • self-identity • separation–individuation • skills groups • temperament • thought-stopping • traits • trichotillomania

KEY CONCEPTS

- personality • personality disorder • personality traits

Historically, the term personality was derived from the Greek *persona*, the theatrical mask used by dramatic players. With time, the connotation changed from being an external surface representation to the internal traits of an individual. Today, personality is conceptualized as a complex pattern of psychological characteristics that, while not easily altered, can change and evolve across the lifespan, as both learned and inherited attributes interact with environmental factors and experiences (Newton-Howes et al., 2015). These characteristics, known as **traits**, are largely outside the person's awareness and include the individual's specific ways of perceiving, thinking, and feeling about self, others, and the environment. These traits are similar and coherent across many different social or personal situations and are expressed in almost every facet of functioning. Intrinsic and pervasive, they emerge from a complicated interaction of genetics, neurobiologic dispositions, psychosocial experiences, and environmental situations that ultimately make up the individual's distinctive personality (Widiger, 2012).

Although various theories about personality have evolved, the approach to understanding human personality through analysis of traits, as attributes that consistently shape an individual's ideas and actions, has been used since Hippocrates' description of **temperament**. Hippocrates defined four types of temperament, each due to the dominance of one of four bodily humours: sanguine (blood), melancholic (black bile), choleric (yellow bile), and phlegmatic (phlegm) (Friedman & Schustack, 2012). In contemporary times, temperament is considered as the recognizable, distinctive, and relatively stable pattern of individual differences that are evident early in life.

---

*Adapted from chapter "Personality Disorders and Disruptive, Impulse Control, and Conduct Disorders" by Wendy Austin

Personality is a complex pattern of characteristics, largely outside the person's awareness, that creates their distinctive and enduring pattern of perceiving, feeling, thinking, coping, and behaving. The personality emerges from a complicated interaction of biologic dispositions, psychological experiences, and environmental situations.

Personality traits are persistent patterns of perceiving, thinking, feeling, and behaving that shape the way a person responds to the world. Key traits have been identified as openness to experience, conscientiousness, extraversion, agreeableness, and neuroticism.

Personality Disorders

No sharp division exists between normal and abnormal personality functioning. Instead, personalities may be viewed on a continuum from normal at one end to abnormal at the other. Many of the same processes involved in the development of a "normal" personality are responsible for the development of a personality disorder (PD). "Normality" involves being able to function autonomously and with competence, to be adaptive in relation to one's social environment, as well as being able to self-develop and experience contentment. Deficits in these dimensions may manifest as core features of personality disorders: adaptive inflexibility, self-defeating pattern of behaviour, and lack of resilience under subjective stress (Millon, 2016). To receive a DSM-5 diagnosis of a PD, an individual must demonstrate these behaviours persistently and to such an extent that they impair their ability to function socially and occupationally (American Psychiatric Association [APA], 2013). In some people, the underlying thoughts, feelings, and behaviours may be intermittent and interfere interpersonally without obvious distress or impairment. Instead of having a PD, these individuals are said to have traits of a personality disorder.

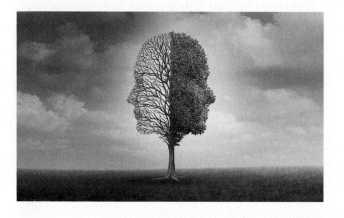

A **personality disorder** is diagnosed when the perceptions, emotion, cognition, and behaviour of an individual substantially deviate from cultural expectations in a persistent and inflexible way, causing distress or impairment (APA, 2013).

A significant shift in the approach to PDs occurred with the 11th revision of the World Health Organization's *International Classification of Disease* (ICD-11). The ICD-11 adopted a new dimensional approach to categorizing PDs based on core personality dysfunction (of self and/or interpersonal) ranging from nonpathological ("personality difficulty"; Watts, 2019) to mild, moderate, or severe. Clinicians have the option of specifying one or more trait domain qualifiers: negative affectivity, detachment, disinhibition, dissociality, and anankastia (obsession–compulsion) (Gamache et al., 2021). There is a qualifier for borderline pattern, as well, but psychoticism is excluded. The ICD-11 classification is congruent with the Alternative Model for Personality Disorders (AMPD) offered in the DSM-5. As the classifications were independently developed, this congruence offers validity to both (Gutiérrez et al., 2021).

Diagnosis of Personality Disorders

Personality disorders are delineated in the American Psychiatric Association's (APA) *Diagnostic and Statistical Manual of Mental Disorders* (*DSM-5*) (APA, 2013). There are 10 PDs recognized as psychiatric diagnoses in the *DSM-5*, organized into three clusters (APA):

- Cluster A: paranoid (PPD), schizoid (SZPD), and schizotypal (STPD)
- Cluster B: borderline (BPD), antisocial (ASPD), histrionic (HPD), and narcissistic (NPD)
- Cluster C: avoidant (AVPD), dependent (DPD), and obsessive–compulsive (OCPD)

These PDs are discussed in this chapter. The disorders within a cluster have some similarities. Cluster A disorders, for instance, have social aversion in common; those in cluster B, dysregulation in emotion and behaviour; and in cluster C, fearfulness. BPD is highlighted in the chapter because persons with this disorder are often seen within the healthcare context and their care requires the development of specific nursing knowledge, skills, and judgment. Disruptive, impulse control, and conduct disorders, which commonly coexist with other mental disorders, are summarized at the end of the chapter. For the official APA diagnostic criteria of disorders in this chapter, which are most commonly used to define personality disorders, please refer to the DSM-5. Interestingly, an alternative approach for the diagnosis of personality disorders was being developed during the work for the *DSM-5*. This alternative approach is designed to be dimensional, characterizing PDs by impairments in personality functioning (self [i.e., identity, self-direction] and interpersonal [i.e., empathy and intimacy]), as well as by pathologic traits (negative affectivity, detachment, antagonism, disinhibition, psychoticism). This alternative model for PDs is regarded by many as innovative and is being explored through research studies (Waugh et al., 2017); however, it was not adopted as the official diagnostic approach for the DSM-5. For more information, refer to Section III of the *DSM-5*.

Epidemiology

Although Canadian prevalence data are lacking for PDs, the reported prevalence of PDs is very similar across studies. In Statistics Canada's *Health State Descriptions for Canadians* (Langlois et al., 2012, modified 2013), it is estimated that 6% to 15% of the population are affected by PDs. Among the most common PDs are OCPD (7.7%), AVPD (6.6%), PPD (5.6%), BPD (5.4%), and STPD (5.2%). Comorbidity between PDs is common. There is some consensus across studies that BPD is the most frequent PD seen in clinical populations. Further, among persons in substance use clinics, prisons, and/or forensic settings, up to 70% are reported to have ASPD (APA, 2013). Interestingly, despite some variability when considering specific PDs (presented later in the chapter), gender does not appear to influence the development of a PD.

Aetiology

The exact aetiology of PDs is unclear. What enables the development of a normal or disordered personality might be genetic, epigenetic, neurobiologic, trauma and stress induced, environmental, or an interaction of said factors. Research findings indicate that personality traits, evident in childhood, are about 50% inherited (genotype), and about 50% dependent on the person's interaction with their environment and unique life experiences (phenotype). At one time, it was believed that personality traits were mostly fixed; however, personality traits are now believed to be more plastic (i.e., changeable), which supports the potential effectiveness of clinical interventions (Newton-Howes et al., 2015).

As highlighted earlier, temperament is said to be a core feature of personality, shaped by physiologic, neurobehavioural, genetic, epigenetic, and cultural influences. As such, the influence of temperament and environment on the development of PDs is currently being explored. Researchers interested in this domain primarily utilize the five-factor model of personality (Putnam & Gartstein, 2017), also known as the Big Five: Openness (to experience), Conscientiousness, Extraversion,

Agreeableness, and Neuroticism (emotional instability) (Friedman & Schustack, 2012). (Hint: Use the mnemonic **OCEAN** to remember them.) A person who rates high in openness, for instance, is curious, actively seeks experiences, and is open to new ideas; one who is high in conscientiousness is organized, self-directed, and persevering. Extraversion is about the amount and intensity of an individual's need for activity, stimulation, and social interaction, while agreeableness is about levels of helpfulness, altruism, and empathy. Neuroticism refers to the level of emotional adjustment; someone with a high level of neuroticism is vulnerable to stress and shows instability in emotional responses, such as anger or depressiveness (Widiger & Costa, 2013).

A prospective, longitudinal study with adolescents explored temperament and maltreatment in predicting the emergence of BPD and ASPD. Measures of temperament, maltreatment, BPD, and ASPD symptoms were completed by 11- to 13-year-old participants (*n* = 245), most of whom (*n* = 206) were assessed again in 2 years. Childhood neglect was found to be a significant predictor of an increase in BPD symptoms, while childhood abuse predicted an increase in ASPD symptoms. Findings also suggested that high capacity for interpersonal affiliation and self-regulation may protect children from developing such disorders in the presence of an adverse environment (Jovev et al., 2013). A challenge in determining the aetiology of PDs is their potential overlap with other mental disorders. For example, AVPD can overlap with social anxiety disorder (social phobia), and clients with diagnoses of social phobia may also met the criteria for AVPD.

Common Features of Personality Disorders

The PD diagnosis is based on pervasive, maladaptive perceiving, thinking, feeling, and behaviour that have manifested in an individual's functioning across situations since adolescence or early adulthood (APA, 2013). Common features of PDs include impaired cognition, maladaptive emotional responses, impaired self-identity and interpersonal functioning, as well as impulsivity and destructive behaviour. Each of these features is described below.

Impaired Metacognition

A significant, defining ability of the human mind is the capacity to take account of one's own—and other's—mental states in order to understand and predict behaviour (Fonagy, 1991). When a person has a PD, there is evidence that this capacity, termed **metacognition**, is impaired (Dimaggio & Brüne, 2016; Fonagy, 1991). Metacognition (also known as "mentalizing" or "mindreading") is the ability to consider and identify one's own state of mind, as well as the state of mind of others, reflect upon these mental states, deliberate upon their accuracy, and then apply this knowledge to problem solving. It allows us to form coherent and stable understandings of ourselves and others, to separate facts from fiction, to consider other persons' points of view, and to question our own. When a person has difficulty with these mental tasks, they may respond to others and events in dysfunctional ways. In different PDs, different aspects of metacognition can be impaired (Moroni et al., 2016).

Maladaptive Emotional Response

Emotions are psychophysiologic reactions that define a person's mood. They can be categorized as negative (e.g., anger, fright, anxiety, guilt, shame, sadness, envy, jealousy, disgust), positive (e.g., happiness, pride, relief, love), and neutral (e.g., hope, compassion, empathy, sympathy, contentment). Emotions can affect one's ability to learn and function by affecting memory, as well as access and storage of information. Emotions can also affect one's ability to accurately perceive the environment. Dysfunction in emotional regulation (over- or underemotional arousal or both) is characteristic of some PDs. For instance, individuals with BPD are said to react to social rejection with greater than normal emotional intensity (McMain et al., 2015), whereas individuals with AVPD appear to be emotionally inhibited, because they have difficulty recognizing and communicating their feelings (Moroni et al., 2016). Emotional responses may also vary depending on the individual as well as their diagnosis. For example, people who have NPD may appear unaffected by losses that would cause deep grief in others. If said loss affects their self-esteem, however, then intense emotional distress may occur (Ronningstam, 2017).

Impaired Self-Identity and Interpersonal Functioning

Self-identity is central to the normal development of personality. Self-identity includes an integration of social and occupational roles and affiliations, self-attributed personality traits, attitudes about gender roles, beliefs about sexuality and intimacy, long-term goals, political ideologies, and religious beliefs. Without an adequately formed identity, an individual's goal-directed behaviour may be impaired, and interpersonal relationships might equally be disrupted. Abilities, limitations, and goals are shaped by one's identity. In personality disorders, self-identity is often impaired or incomplete.

Impulsivity and Destructive Behaviour

Individuals with PDs may come to the attention of mental health clinicians because their impulsive behaviour results in negative consequences to others or themselves. They have difficulty recognizing or appreciating the consequences of their actions, and thus tend to act abruptly on their impulses.

Severity of Disorder

Five reliable, clinically relevant components of maladaptive personality functioning have been identified in a series of research studies (Verheul et al., 2008). These components and their facets are as follows:

- Self-control (stable self-image, self-reflective, emotional and aggressive regulation)
- Identity integration (enjoyment, purposefulness, self-respect, frustration tolerance)
- Relational capacities (intimacy, enduring relationships, feeling recognized)
- Responsibility (trustworthiness, responsible industry)
- Social concordance (respect, cooperation)

These components are associated with the severity of the PD, and long-term changes in the functioning of a client can be determined using the measure that evolved from the research, the Severity Indices of Personality Problems (SIPP-118) (Verheul et al., 2008).

Contextual Considerations

As with other psychiatric disorders, diagnosis of a PD relies heavily on the assessment of social functioning in relation to some form of societal expectations and related perceived maladaptive patterns of thinking and interacting. As a result, there is a need to exercise caution when attributing such labels, and one must ensure that contextual considerations are taken into account when forming an overall clinical picture. For example, emigrating to a new country may prove to be challenging for people who must adapt to new cultural norms. In these instances, the diagnosis of a PD is often delayed in the attempt to differentiate challenges encountered as part of an expected adjustment period versus the manifestations of a PD.

Developmental Stage Across the Lifespan

Another contextual and increasingly necessary consideration in the diagnosis of a PD relates to a person's development stage across the lifespan. For example, it is highly unusual for children to be diagnosed with a PD, and this was previously true for adolescents, as well. However, with growing evidence that certain PDs, such as BPD, may develop during adolescence and benefit from early intervention, in some cases, a PD diagnosis may be given during adolescence (Ronningstam et al., 2014). Recognition of PDs across the lifespan, including in older adults, is important for improving the health of individuals of all ages.

Gender

Although gender does not appear to affect the prevalence of PDs as a whole, we do observe differences in diagnosis patterns when looking at specific PDs, differences that need to be reviewed from a critical standpoint. For example, males are much more likely to be diagnosed with ASPD than females (Oltmanns & Powers, 2012). Yet, ASPD may be underdiagnosed in females because the manifestation of the illness may be different. Specifically, evidence of conduct disorder before the age of 15 is required for an ASPD diagnosis. With conduct disorder, there is an emphasis on aggression against people or animals, behaviours not stereotypically assigned to girls and female adolescents. In contrast, females appear to be more likely to receive diagnoses of somatization (see Chapter 24) or histrionic disorders (discussed later in this chapter). Further, it has been commonly assumed that BPD is more common in females, but higher prevalence rates among females are considered an artifact of sampling in clinical settings because females, especially adult women, are more likely to seek treatment.

Stigma and Personality Disorders

Understanding PDs is necessary for safe and ethical client-centred nursing practice. The term PD itself is highly stigmatized and is sometimes used to describe clients exhibiting challenging symptoms, regardless of whether these symptoms meet the diagnostic criteria for a PD. The term might also be used in a disparaging way, as "more a term of abuse than a diagnosis" (Tyrer et al., 2015, p. 717). Too often clients with PDs report stigmatization because of their disorder and past negative experiences with healthcare providers, which contribute to their avoidance of certain facilities (Lohman et al., 2017).

In practice, healthcare professionals can become impatient with persons who have a PD or traits of a PD, expecting them to have control over their behaviour and change a way of being in the world that is less than optimal. Lack of knowledge about PDs, as well as their associated stigma, can affect both treatment-seeking behaviour and referrals for help (Sheehan et al., 2016). In other words, the manifestations of the disorders, as well as the negative and stereotypical views associated with the labels, may provoke negative reactions from clinicians that interfere with the ability to provide effective care.

As a subset of clients with PDs, persons with BPD may seek care for suicidal ideation, self-harm, safety, situational crises, depression, anxiety, and substance use. These clients may be received negatively by hospital staff and treated differently than other psychiatric clients if labelled as difficult, manipulative, attention seeking, and self-destructive (Mack & Nesbitt, 2016). Rogers and Dunne (2011) found that clients with BPD both perceive these negative staff attitudes and receive suboptimal care because of them. Specifically, the participants in their study encountered healthcare providers who made them feel guilty for being unable to control their behaviours, undeserving of hospital beds, and as though they were less of a priority compared with clients with other diagnoses. Solutions to nurses' issues

regarding caring for individuals with BPD need to be developed and implemented. Promising solutions are theoretical and skill-related education regarding BPD for nurses, as well as an interdisciplinary team approach that includes an evidence-based therapeutic framework, clinical supervision, and peer support (Dickens et al., 2016). McKenzie and colleagues (2021) conducted a systematic literature review that aimed to identify and review existing literature regarding mental health workers attitudes toward clients with a diagnosis of BPD. Not unlike previous research, the researchers concluded that their findings suggested that mental health workers have more negative attitudes toward clients labelled as having BPD, when compared to other mental health diagnoses such as depression. Factors associated with the label BPD, workers perceptions of BPD symptoms, and past experiences providing care for this group need to be considered when addressing negative responses toward clients with BPD.

In a recent study, set within the Canadian context, Vandyk et al. (2019) found that, although persons with BPD most often seek health care for reasons related to their mental illness, they are routinely discharged without proper or targeted community follow-up. Thus their healthcare-seeking patterns are cyclical: this unstable community management re-initiates self- or crisis presentation to hospital (see Box 27.1, Research for Best Practice). In fact, persons with BPD tend to be frequent users of all health services, including inpatient, outpatient, and primary care. Despite this reliance on the healthcare system, the work of Jacob and colleagues (2021) highlights the ways in which processes, structures, and rules within the healthcare system create a context of care where the very symptoms leading to a BPD diagnosis are used to label the client as difficult and undeserving of care. The combined effect of complex and challenging BPD symptoms, healthcare provider preconceptions, and structural processes that are incompatible with the needs of clients with BPD means that often these clients are excluded from the treatments and therapeutic interventions needed to manage their disorder.

Comorbidities and Personality Disorders

Comorbidities are important to consider when caring for a client with PDs. Comorbid mood disorders, substance use disorders, eating disorders, and anxiety disorders are prevalent in this population (Hong, 2016; Moran et al., 2016). For instance, in a review study, Parmar and Kaloiya (2018) reported that between 35% and 73% of clients treated for addictions are also diagnosed with a PD. Although comorbid alcohol use disorder is shown to be highest in persons with BPD and ASPD, all of the PDs are associated with an elevated risk for alcohol use disorder compared with the general population (Rosenström et al., 2018). Of note, clients with comorbid PDs and substance use disorders have a poorer prognosis in

BOX 27.1 Research for Best Practice

EXPLORING THE PERSPECTIVES OF PERSONS WITH BORDERLINE PERSONALITY DISORDER REGARDING THEIR EXPERIENCE IN THE EMERGENCY DEPARTMENT

Vandyk, A., Bentz, A. Bissonette, S., & Cater, C. (2019). Why go to the emergency department? Perspectives from persons with borderline personality disorder. *International Journal of Mental Health Nursing, 28*, 757–765. https://doi.org/10.1111/inm.12580

Aim: To advance clinical knowledge through gaining understanding of the use of emergency services by persons seeking treatment related to their primary diagnosis of borderline personality disorder.

Method: Interpretive inquiry, an inductive approach to clinical phenomena in healthcare delivery that is based on the constructivist paradigm (i.e., each individual constructs their own understanding of the world through experience; multiple realities exist) was used. There were six participants (22 to 66 years old); all had a family physician, three had a psychiatrist. The number of emergency department (ED) visits over a 1-year period ranged from 13 to 27 each. Researchers had psychiatric and mental health expertise and emergency services experience.

Findings: Three pathways to ED visits were noted: aggressive or disorganized behaviour (brought to ED by police), medication seeking (self-referral), and intense emotions often triggered by loss (e.g., loneliness; negative self-perception). The latter pathway was taken after community crisis services or self-management strategies (often maladaptive such as substance use, suicide attempts) were insufficient or failed. Feeling connected to others prevented need of ED care, whereas lost relationships triggered intense ED use. Stigmatizing reactions from ED staff perpetuated participants' negative self-image. Participants used coping methods to reduce ED visits when possible (adaptive [e.g., seeking connection with others], self-destructive [e.g., self-cutting]). The study captured the cyclic nature of participants' ED use.

Implications: There are key patterns in ED use of persons diagnosed with BPD that could inform tailoring community care to be more effective. There is a need to change the perceptions of and actions toward persons with BPD by healthcare staff to ensure their equitable access to good care.

terms of treatment response and outcome (Parmar & Kaloiya, 2018; see Chapter 33 on care of persons with concurrent disorders). From a physical health perspective, recent study findings reveal strong associations between several physical ailments and PDs (Dokucu & Cloninger, 2019). As with many clients with psychiatric illness, the physical health of persons with PDs is often overlooked. Completing a thorough health assessment is always important, regardless of primary diagnosis.

Recovery and Treatment for Personality Disorders

Recovery involves having hope, understanding one's capabilities and challenges, achieving a positive sense of self, connecting meaningfully with others, and engaging in life (see Chapter 2). Research exploring the experiences of recovery for persons with a PD indicates that facilitators of recovery are also core vulnerabilities: interpersonal relationships and social interaction. Participants in this research describe tensions between an alienating outside world and an isolating, but safe, inner world (Gillard et al., 2015). Gillard and colleagues conclude that the process of recovering involves discovering a sense of self that can exist in both worlds.

Psychological and psychosocial interventions are the primary approaches to the treatment of PDs, with psychopharmacology used adjunctively and usually on

a short-term basis for specific symptoms. The overall goal is not to change an individual's fundamental personality, but to help them build on their strengths and minimize problematic effects of their disorder (Lyness, 2016). The aims of treatment can include the reduction of life-threatening symptoms, the improvement of distressing mental state symptoms, greater social and interpersonal adjustment, and the acquisition of life skills (Bateman et al., 2015). Factors outside of therapy, such as the person's circumstances, resources, life events, and cultural background, can have strong effects on recovery; it is important for therapists to recognize and ally with such factors (Pederson, 2015; Stone, 2016). There is no all encompassing approach to the care and treatment of persons with a PD. Further, accessing required therapies can be difficult and expensive. Selected approaches to psychotherapy used in the treatment of PDs are described below.

Dialectical Behaviour Therapy

Dialectical behaviour therapy (DBT), developed by Marsha Linehan (1993a) to treat individuals experiencing suicidality and self-injury, uses cognitive–behavioural therapy (CBT) strategies but also draws on Zen principles, dialectical philosophy, and behavioural science. DBT consists of four treatment components: individual therapy, group skills training, telephone coaching, and therapist consultation teams (i.e., therapy for the therapist). A variety of interventions including "mindfulness practice, skills training, relationship strategies, cognitive and behavioural techniques, and environmental interventions" are used (Pederson, 2015, p. 2). (See Chapter 14 for information on cognitive–behavioural techniques and mindfulness.)

For DBT to be effective, therapists and coaches must work with clients as partners and be willing to focus on interconnected behaviours (e.g., parasuicidal and substance abuse) and not a single diagnosis. Clients actively participate in treatment by collecting information about their own behaviours to recognize patterns and identify behaviours to change. Problem-solving, exposure techniques (i.e., gradual exposure to cues that set off aversive emotions), skills training, contingency management (i.e., reinforcement of positive behaviour), and cognitive modification are core components of this therapeutic approach.

Skills groups are an integral part of DBT in which members practice emotional regulation, interpersonal effectiveness, mindfulness, and distress tolerance. Skills taught to manage intense, labile moods involve helping the client to name and analyze the context of the emotion, and to use strategies to reduce **emotional vulnerability**. Learning to observe and describe emotions, without judging or blocking them, allows the individual to experience emotions without stimulating secondary feelings that cause more distress. For example, describing the emotion of anger without judging it as being "bad" can eliminate feelings of guilt that lead to self-injury.

Interpersonal effectiveness skills include the development of assertiveness and problem-solving skills within an interpersonal context. Clients are given strategies to meet their goals in a particular situation, while at the same time maintaining relationships with others and sustaining their self-respect. Distress tolerance skills involve learning to tolerate and accept distress as a part of normal life. Self-management skills focus on learning how to control, manage, or change behaviours, thoughts, or emotional responses to events.

Cognitive–Behavioural Therapy

The principles and techniques of CBT are addressed in Chapter 14 of this textbook. When applied to the treatment of PDs, CBT focuses on "clinical assessment," "cognitive conceptualization," "technical interventions," and the "therapeutic relationship" (David & Freeman, 2015, p. 16). For some PDs, such as ASPD, clinical assessment involves not only a clinical interview and self-report psychological tests but also psychological tests based on clinicians' or relevant others' assessments and data. The relationship with the client is a key component that includes modelling for change, as well as collaboration and empathy (David & Freeman, 2015).

Mentalization-Based Treatment

Mentalization-based treatment (MBT) was originally developed to treat clients with BPD in day hospital settings, but MBT is now used to treat a range of PDs, including ASPD. Mentalization is the necessary, everyday human ability to recognize and interpret one's own and others' thoughts, feelings, and intensions. It influences how one acts and reacts in the world. The importance of our ability to infer the meaning of our own and others' mental states needs to be recognized, as is the reality that it is not difficult to be mistaken. This ability requires a capacity to be inquisitive, to separate fact from fiction, and to learn from others' perspectives and behaviour. The capacity to mentalize evolves within one's early childhood relationships and is affected by caregivers' ability to validate the child's mental states and to convey understanding, as well as by the quality of the child's social environment (Bateman & Fonagy, 2016). An experimental study of the mentalization ability of individuals with BPD found that while they were equal to control group members on simple mentalization tasks, deficits became apparent as the complexity of the tasks increased. Childhood experiences of punishment were negatively correlated to mentalization ability (i.e., as the level of trauma increased, mentalization skills decreased) for both the BPD and control groups (Petersen et al., 2016). The term "mentalization" is sometimes used interchangeably with "metacognition"; there is a difference, however, because the work on mentalization emphasizes the role of early attachments (Dimaggio & Brüne, 2016; Fonagy, 1991).

The focus of MBT is assisting clients through a therapeutic process to learn about their mental states and then to explore how errors may lead to difficulties. Treatment involves engaging the client in the treatment process from assessment and diagnosis to treatment termination. It includes the identification of problems that might affect treatment, formulation of a hierarchy of therapeutic aims, the addressing of social and behavioural problems, planning for crisis, and monitoring of outcomes. Psychoeducation is important to the MBT process, as is the combination of individual and group therapy (Bateman & Fonagy, 2016).

Metacognitive Interpersonal Therapy

In this approach, as in most other psychotherapies, the therapeutic relationship is seen as the ground for validating clients' experiences and facilitating positive change. Initially, the therapist will assess clients' capacity for sharing a narrative of their life experience and their metacognitive abilities and then use the assessment to modulate each client's metacognitive interpersonal therapy (MIT) experience. Autobiographical details from clients focuses therapy on their specific problems in emotional and cognitive awareness, revealing the way beliefs triggered in specific life episodes have led to particular responses. Maladaptive interpersonal schema can then be explored and changed. Clients practice new behaviours and gain a sense of control over their actions (Dimaggio et al., 2017). There is some nongeneralizable evidence that MIT can be effective. For example, a case study of three non-BPD, non-ASPD clients who completed 2 years of weekly MIT found that at 3 months posttherapy, each showed overall improvement in symptoms and emotional regulation (Dimaggio et al., 2017).

Specific Personality Disorders

Cluster A Disorders

Paranoid Personality Disorder

The most prominent features of paranoid personality disorder (PPD) are mistrust of others and the desire to avoid relationships in which one is not in control. Individuals with PPD are suspicious and guarded. They are consistently mistrustful of others' motives, even those of relatives and close friends. Actions of others are often misinterpreted as deception, deprecation, and betrayal, especially regarding fidelity or trustworthiness of a spouse or friend (Millon et al., 2004). Minor innocuous incidents are often misinterpreted as having sinister or hidden meaning, and suspicions are magnified into major distortions of reality. People with paranoid personalities distance themselves from others and can be outwardly argumentative and abrasive; internally, they may hold private hopes of being understood and feel powerless, fearful, and vulnerable (Hayward, 2007). Imagine living with the belief that you can trust no one and that there are some persons or organizations actively "out to get you?" (Note: the PPD diagnosis excludes psychotic symptoms, like paranoid delusions and hallucinations.)

Other hallmark features of PPD are persistent ideas of self-importance (i.e., important enough to be the target of the harmful intentions of others) and the tendency to be rigid and in control. The individual wants to appear in control and objective, yet often reacts emotionally, displaying signs of nervousness, anger, envy, and jealousy. Fearful, the person will be hypervigilant to any environmental changes. Essentially, PPD is "a stable pattern of nonpsychotic paranoid behaviour" (Hopwood & Thomas, 2012, p. 582). If help is sought, it is unlikely that it will be from mental health professionals but rather from a resource, such as the police, that the person with PPD believes could stop the harm others are doing.

Demographically, PPD is most often associated with low income and disadvantaged populations; stress, trauma, and neglect appear to be causative factors. In clinical populations, PPD is a predictor of aggressive behaviour. In the forensic field, it is associated with excessive litigation, stalking, and violent behaviour.

Paranoid ideas can develop after sustaining a brain injury and in Alzheimer dementia (Lee, 2017).

PPD is difficult to treat; it is primarily psychotherapy, but the ongoing suspicion and mistrust experienced by the client can severely hamper therapeutic alliance and process. Research involving a general population (n = 2,137) with a 15-year follow-up found that PPD was associated with temperament dimensions of high novelty-seeking, high harm aversion, low reward dependence, and explosive temperament. This finding was sustained over age, gender, and socioeconomic factors (Saarinena et al., 2018). These results support psychotherapeutic interventions that focus on the development of self-regulation of temperamental vulnerabilities.

There remains controversy regarding PPD as a distinct diagnostic construct. It is questioned whether or not paranoid symptoms are uniquely attributed to the PPD diagnosis; they may be fully explained by personality traits or psychotic disorders (Hopwood & Thomas, 2012). Mistrust encountered in persons whose experiences may have created mistrust (e.g., people who are refugees or immigrants, migrant workers) should not be confused with that seen in PPD.

Nursing Care

Nurses are most likely to see these clients for other health problems but will need to formulate their foci of nursing care based on the client's underlying suspiciousness. An assessment of individuals with PPD reveals disturbed or illogical thoughts that demonstrate the misinterpretation of environmental stimuli. For example, an individual with PPD might become convinced that their partner was having an affair with a neighbour based on the observation that they both left for work at the same time each morning. Even if following them never revealed any sign of them together, the person may continue to believe, without question, that they were having an affair.

Because of their difficulty with developing relationships, individuals with PPD are often socially isolated and lack social support systems. Although they do not usually demonstrate the loneliness of those desiring connection with others, they are disadvantaged by their insecurity in social situations.

Nursing interventions based on the establishment of a nurse–client relationship are difficult to implement because of the person's mistrust. A professional, matter-of-fact approach and the creation of a nonthreatening environment in which the client can feel as secure as possible are helpful. Nurses must ensure that their own response to a client who does not readily accept them as trustworthy does not further impede relationship building. (This will require professional self-awareness because a negative response to another who assesses one as untrustworthy is a common human response.) If a trusting relationship is established, the nurse helps the individual identify specific problematic areas, such as getting along with particular others or improving workplace behaviour. Through therapeutic techniques such as acceptance and reflection, as well as recognition by the nurse of the ramifications of the client's view of the world (e.g., what it feels like to believe one's spouse is having an affair), the nurse and the client can examine a problematic area to gain another view of the situation. Changing thought patterns takes time. Client outcomes are evaluated in terms of small changes in thinking and behaviour. Although antipsychotics might be considered in its treatment, such as when there is escalating paranoia (Lyness, 2016), no medications have been found to be specifically effective in treating PPD (Silk & Feurino, 2012).

Schizoid Personality Disorder

Individuals with schizoid personality disorder (SZPD) are expressively impassive and interpersonally unengaged (Millon et al., 2004). They tend to be unable to experience the joyful and pleasurable aspects of life. They are introverted and reclusive, and clinically they appear distant, aloof, apathetic, and emotionally detached. They have difficulties making friends, seem uninterested in social activities, and appear to gain little satisfaction in personal relationships. In fact, they appear to be incapable of forming social relationships. Interests are directed at objects, things, and abstractions. As children, they engaged primarily in solitary activities, such as stamp collecting, computer games, electronic equipment, or academic pursuits such as mathematics or engineering. In addition, there seems to be a cognitive deficit characterized by obscure thought processes, particularly about social matters. Communication with others is confused and lacks focus. These individuals reveal minimum introspection and self-awareness, and interpersonal experiences are described in a very mechanical way. The low incidence of SZPD diagnoses without a comorbid diagnosis of another PD has raised questions about the usefulness of SZPD as a PD diagnostic category; it is argued that it should be omitted from future classifications of PDs (Hummelen et al., 2015).

Nursing Care

Impaired social interactions and chronic low self-esteem are typical diagnoses of individuals with SZPD. Major treatment goals are to enhance the experience of pleasure, prevent social isolation, and increase emotional responsiveness to others. Because these individuals often lack customary social skills, social skills training is useful in enhancing their ability to relate in interpersonal situations. The primary focus is to increase the person's ability to experience enjoyment. The nurse balances interventions between encouraging enough social activity that prevents the individual from retreating to a fantasy world and too much social activity that becomes intolerable. Because persons with SZPD typically shy away from interactions, establishing a therapeutic relationship can be challenging; patience in achieving a sense of relatedness is required (Hess, 2016). The evaluation of early outcomes may simply be in terms of increasing the client's feelings of satisfaction with solitary activities.

Schizotypal Personality Disorder

People with the schizotypal personality disorder (STPD) are characterized by a pattern of social and interpersonal deficits. They do not form friendships easily and may be close only to first-degree relatives. Their beliefs about their world are often inconsistent with their cultural norms and appear odd to others. Ideas of reference (i.e., incorrect interpretations of events as having special, personal meaning) are often present, as are unusual perceptual delusions and odd, circumstantial, and metaphorical thinking and speech. Mood is constricted or inappropriate, and there are excessive social anxieties of a paranoid character that do not diminish with familiarity. Appearance and behaviour can be characterized as eccentric, or peculiar. An avoidant behaviour pattern is usually exhibited. The requirement that five of nine *DSM* criteria need to be met for an STPD diagnosis means that two individuals with STPD may share only one diagnostic feature (Kwapil & Barrantes-Vidal, 2012).

In the ICD-11, the schizotypal category is not classified as a PD, but as part of the spectrum of schizophrenia (Bach & First, 2018). A study of individuals with SZPD and STPD using structural magnetic resonance imaging found that, when compared with healthy individuals in a control group, persons with either SZPD or STPD had greater white matter volume in the superior area of the corona radiata, which may relate to the cognitive and motor changes seen in these schizophrenia-related PDs (Via et al., 2016; Waldeck & Miller, 2000). If an individual with STPD becomes psychotic, they will seem highly disoriented and confused and may exhibit posturing, grimacing, inappropriate giggling, rambling speech, and peculiar mannerisms. Fantasy, hallucinations, and bizarre, fragmented delusions may be present. Regressive acts such as enuresis and encopresis may occur. These individuals may consume food in an infantile or ravenous manner. Symptoms mirror but fall short of features that would justify the diagnosis of schizophrenia. Individuals with STPD may be unable to engage in social interaction that can keep them functional.

Nursing Care

Depending on the amount of decompensation (i.e., deterioration of functioning and exacerbation of symptoms), the assessment of a client with an STPD can generate a range of concerns requiring nursing attention. If a person has severe symptoms, such as delusional thinking or perceptual disturbances, the nursing care foci are similar to those for a person with schizophrenia (see Chapter 21). If symptoms are mild, the typical nursing care foci include social isolation, ineffective coping, low self-esteem, and impaired social interactions.

People with STPD need help in increasing their sense of self-worth and recognizing their positive attributes. Limiting dependency and supporting self-directed activities appropriately are focuses of care. Individuals with this PD can benefit from interventions (e.g., social skills training; environmental management) that increase psychosocial functioning. As eccentric thoughts and behaviours alienate others, reinforcing and modelling socially appropriate dress and behaviour for a person with STPD can help to improve overall appearance and ability to relate (Hayward, 2007). A challenge for the person with STPD will be to generalize from one situation to another, so attention to cognitive skills is important (Waldeck & Miller, 2000).

Continuum of Care for Cluster A Personality Disorders

Persons with cluster A personality disorders are rarely seen in mental health treatment unless their daily activities are seriously affected, or symptoms of depression or anxiety appear. Improvement in quality of life for persons with these PDs is possible through psychotherapy, although symptoms such as suspiciousness, lack of trust, and impaired social interactions can make it difficult to establish a therapeutic relationship (Hayward, 2007). Engaging therapeutically with individuals with cluster A disorders can be at variance with the standard approach used with other clients, given the difficulty these clients have in forming emotional connections. In order to reduce the extreme anxiety that interpersonal engagement can cause, nurses will need to carefully judge appropriate therapeutic distance (Hayward, 2007). Brief interventions, including self-care assistance, reality orientation, and role enhancement, can be helpful (Bulechek et al., 2008).

▌ Cluster B Disorders

Borderline Personality Disorder

Clinical Course of Disorder

In 1938, the term *borderline* was first used to refer to a group of disorders that did not quite fit the definition of either neurosis or psychosis (Stern, 1938). The term evolved from the psychoanalytic conceptualization of the disorder as a dysfunctional personality structure. In 1980, BPD was formally recognized as a distinct disorder in the *DSM-III*. Today, in the *DSM-5*, the essential feature of BPD is "a pervasive pattern of instability

of interpersonal relationships, self-image, and affects, and marked impulsivity that begins by early adulthood and is present in a variety of contexts" (APA, 2013, p. 663). Instability is a core component of this disorder, as exemplified by instability in mood, self-image, identity, and interpersonal relationships, as well as impulse and behavioural control (Santangelo et al., 2020). A meta-analysis of the prevalence of BPD in university students, across 43 studies with a total of 26,343 participants from six countries, indicated a range from 0.5% to 32.1% with a lifetime prevalence of 9.7% (Meaney et al., 2016). More recently, Winsper and colleagues (2020) conducted a global systematic review and meta-analysis of personality disorder prevalence in the community and found that a global lifetime prevalence of cluster B diagnoses to be 2.8%.

Individuals with BPD have difficulty with interpersonal relationships in that they experience them as intensive, alternately idealize and devalue others, and become frantic if they feel that they may be abandoned. They have problems with unstable, highly reactive moods, with developing a sense of self, with feelings of emptiness, and with maintaining reality-based cognitive processes. Intense, inappropriate anger and its control can be a problem for them. Impulsive or destructive behaviour, such as suicidal or self-mutilating acts, is an ongoing possibility (Sadock et al., 2019). Persons with BPD may appear more competent than they actually are and often set unrealistically high expectations for themselves. When these expectations are not met, they experience intense shame, self-hate, and self-directed anger. They seem to live from one crisis to another. Some of the crises are caused by the individual's dysfunctional lifestyle or inadequate social milieu, but many are simply challenging human experiences, like the death of a spouse or diagnosis of an illness, to which they react emotionally with minimal coping skills. The intensity of their dysregulation often frightens themselves and others. Friends, family members, and coworkers may come to limit their contact with them, which furthers their sense of aloneness, abandonment, and self-hatred. It also diminishes opportunities for learning self-corrective measures.

Affective Instability

Affective instability (i.e., rapid and extreme shift in mood) is a core characteristic of BPD and is evidenced by erratic emotional responses to situations and intense sensitivity to criticism or perceived slights. For example, a person may greet a casual acquaintance with intense affection, yet later be aloof with the same acquaintance. Friends describe individuals with BPD as moody, irresponsible, or intense. These individuals fail to recognize their own emotional responses, thoughts, beliefs, and behaviours. Clinically, when a stressful situation is encountered, the person with BPD reacts with shifts in emotions, appearing to have limited success in developing emotional buffers to stressful situations. Regulating anger, anxiety, and sadness is particularly problematic. Difficulty with the intensity and regulation of emotion negatively affects social behaviours and relationships, including relations with health professionals. These affective symptoms are a central component of the disorder (Sadock et al., 2019).

Research does suggest that **emotional dysregulation** may play a central role in the development and maintenance of BPD (Stepp et al., 2014). When individuals with innate biologic propensity for intense emotional reactivity develop in an environment that is unsupportive of learning ways to regulate one's emotions, such a deficit will contribute to increased affective instability and dysregulated cognitions, behaviours, and interpersonal relationships. If this is so, helping the individual with BPD to develop emotional awareness and clarity and to improve their ability to cope with negative emotions may be effective in improving other BPD symptoms, as well (Stepp et al., 2014).

Identity Disturbances

Identity diffusion occurs when a person lacks aspects of personal identity or when personal identity is poorly developed (Erikson, 1968). Four factors of identity are most commonly disturbed: role absorption (i.e., narrowly defining self within a single role), painful incoherence (i.e., distressed sense of internal disharmony), inconsistency (i.e., lack of coherence in thoughts, feelings, and actions), and lack of normative commitment (Weston et al., 2011). Other factors of personality identity (e.g., religious ideologies, moral value systems, and sexual attitudes) appear to be less important in identity diffusion. Clinically, these clients appear to have little sense of their own identity and direction; this becomes a source of great distress to them and is often manifested by chronic feelings of emptiness and boredom. It is not unusual for persons with BPD to direct their actions in accord with the wishes of other people.

Unstable Interpersonal Relationships

Individuals with BPD have an extreme fear of abandonment as well as a history of unstable, insecure attachments. Such a history is significant as attachment has been considered within psychology (since the time of Freud) to be an essential aspect in early human development. From this perspective, an infant needs to experience a secure physical and emotional bond to at least one primary caregiver to successfully develop a coherent sense of self and the ability to connect with others. Contemporary theorists, such as Schore (2017), propose that **attachment** is a psychobiologic mechanism that supports early development of abilities to regulate the emotional self. A fear of abandonment may stem from difficulties in early childhood attachment with the primary caregiver. Although there are variations in individual histories, many persons with BPD have never experienced a consistently secure, nurturing relationship and thus are constantly seeking reassurance and validation. In an attempt to meet their interpersonal needs, they idealize others and establish intense relationships that violate others' interpersonal boundaries, which ultimately lead to rejection (Bartholomew & Horowitz, 1991). When these relationships do not live up to their expectations, the person with BPD tends to devalue the other person. Continually disappointed in relationships, this individual can feel estranged from others and inadequate in the face of perceived social standards. Intense shame and self-hate will follow. These feelings often result in self-injurious behaviours, such as cutting the wrist, self-inflicted burns, or head banging.

In social situations, persons with BPD can use elaborate strategies to structure interactions. That is, they restrict their relationships to ones in which they feel in control. They distance themselves from groups when feeling anxious (which is most of the time) and rarely use their social support system. Even if they are married or have a supportive extended family, they can be reluctant to share their feelings (Krause et al., 2003). They do not want to burden anyone, fear rejection, and assume that others are tired of hearing them repeat the same issues.

Cognitive Dysfunctions

An aspect of BPD is **dichotomous thinking**. Individuals with BPD will evaluate experiences, people, and objects in terms of mutually exclusive categories (e.g., good or bad, success or failure, trustworthy or deceitful); this informs extreme interpretations of events that would normally be viewed as including both positive and negative aspects. There are also times when thinking becomes disorganized. Irrelevant, bizarre notions and vague or scattered thought connections can be present, as well as delusions and hallucinations.

Another cognitive dysfunction common in BPD is **dissociation**, in which thoughts and ideas can be split off from consciousness. Dissociation can be conceptualized as lying on a continuum from minor dissociations of daily life, such as daydreaming, to a breakdown in the usually integrated functions of consciousness, memory, perception of self or the environment, and sensorimotor behaviours. For example, in driving familiar roads, people often get lost in their thoughts or dissociate and suddenly do not remember what happened during that part of the trip. Environmental stimuli are ignored, and there are changes in the perception of reality. The individual is physically present but mentally in another place. Dissociation can be a coping strategy for avoiding disturbing events. In dissociating, the person does not have to be aware of or remember traumatic events.

There is a strong correlation between dissociation and self-injurious behaviour (Zanarini et al., 2000).

Dysfunctional Behaviours

Impaired Problem-Solving

In BPD, there is often a failure to engage in active problem-solving. Instead, problem-solving is attempted by soliciting help from others in a helpless, hopeless manner (Linehan, 1993a). Suggestions are rarely taken.

Impulsivity

Impulsivity is also characteristic of the individual living with BPD. When impulse driven, individuals have difficulty delaying gratification or thinking through the consequences before acting on their feelings; their actions are often unpredictable. They literally act in the moment and then must face the consequences afterwards. Thus they are particularly vulnerable in situations where there may be direct impacts on their health and/or social trajectory, such as money management (e.g., gambling), eating habits (e.g., binge eating), safe sex practices (unprotected sex), etc. Job losses, interrupted education, and unsuccessful relationships are common to the history of persons with BPD.

Self-Injurious Behaviours

Unsuccessful interpersonal relationships and turmoil in social experiences may lead the person with BPD to undermine them when a goal is about to be reached. The most serious consequences are suicide attempts or **parasuicidal behaviours** (i.e., deliberate self-injury with intent to harm oneself; see Chapter 20). Individuals who self-injure show a higher threshold and greater tolerance for pain and report less pain intensity compared with healthy control subjects with no history of self-injury. It remains unknown whether this is a risk factor in the development of such behaviour or a consequence of repeated episodes of self-injury (Koenig et al., 2016). In a systematic review and meta-analysis, the prevalence of nonsuicidal self-injury behaviour was determined as 17.2% for adolescents, 13.4% for young adults, and 5.5% for adults (Swannell et al., 2014).

Prevalence rates of nonsuicidal self-injury (NSSI) within the general population are estimated to be approximately 17% in adolescents and 6% in adults. However, in those diagnosed with BPD, the prevalence rates of 95% for adolescents and 90% for adults have been noted in the literature. Additionally, researchers have also found that 75% of individuals with BPD have also attempted suicide (Reichl & Kaess, 2021). In an earlier study of adults with NSSI, with and without BPD, it was found that the self-injury of those with BPD was more frequent and severe than of those without a BPD

diagnosis. Those with BPD had higher rates of skin carving, head banging, self-punching, and self-scratching and reported more severe symptoms, suicidal ideation, and emotional dysregulation. They did not differ from the non-BPD individuals in rates of mood, substance use, nor psychotic disorders, but had greater incidence of anxiety disorders (Turner et al., 2015).

Self-injurious behaviour can be compulsive, episodic, or repetitive and is more likely to occur when the individual with BPD is depressed; has highly unstable interpersonal relationships, especially problems with intimacy and sociability; and is hypervigilant (i.e., alert, watchful) and resentful (Paris, 2005). Self-injurious behaviours associated with BPD are listed below.

- *Compulsive self-injurious behaviours* that may occur many times daily and are repetitive and ritualistic. For example, hair pulling, which can be a separate disorder (**trichotillomania**) or behaviour associated with other personality disorders, involves pulling out hair, especially from the scalp, eyebrows, and eyelashes. Hair is plucked, examined, and sometimes eaten. Hair-pulling sessions may take several hours. Most of those afflicted do not seek help unless the symptoms are severe and then they usually consult dermatologists or family practitioners.
- *Episodic self-injurious behaviours* are especially common in people with BPD and develop into habitual coping behavioural patterns during periods when stress (i.e., progressive tension manifested by feelings of anger, depression, or anxiety) rises to an intolerable level. The individual reports being numb or empty and ends this dissociated state with a self-injurious behaviour that elicits feeling. As noted previously, some individuals with BPD who self-injure experience little or no associated pain (Koenig et al., 2016); rather, tension is relieved and a sense of calmness or even pleasure may follow. These feelings are believed to be reinforcing, and the person learns to relieve stress and anxiety by self-mutilation. The individuals harm themselves to feel better, get rapid relief from distressing thoughts and emotions, and gain a sense of control.
- *Repetitive self-mutilation* occurs when occasional self-injury turns into an overwhelming preoccupation. Persons can be labelled as "cutters" or "burners," for example, and describe themselves as being addicted to self-harm. In a now classic interpretive phenomenologic study of people with BPD, Nehls (1999) described the emotional conflict when efforts to comfort oneself are interpreted by others as manipulation, resulting in care being denied.

Risk for Suicide

All self-injurious behaviours should be considered potentially life threatening and taken seriously. Indicators of increased suicide risk for persons with BPD include changes in the type or pattern of self-harm, increases in the use of substances, significant changes in the individual's mental state, recent adverse life events, and recent discharge from hospital or treatment (National Health and Medical Research Council, 2012). Differentiating acute suicide risk from the long-term risk experienced by some persons with BPD for whom suicidal thoughts are an enduring symptom is challenging but informs the appropriate intervention. The focus for long-term risk is on helping the client develop a sense of control over their behaviour, whereas safety must be prioritized for acute risk (Warrender, 2018). For individuals with BPD who attempt suicide, the mortality rate is 8% to 10%, much higher than in the general population (Leichsenring et al., 2011).

Aetiology

The answer to what causes BPD is becoming clearer but remains undetermined. BPD appears to be caused by the interaction between genetic, neurobiologic, and psychosocial influences that affect brain development (Kulacaoglu & Kose, 2018).

This is a "highly individualized disorder" so the diagnosis of BPD likely reflects many "unique influences and developmental trajectories" (Hooley et al., 2012, p. 415). A brief overview of the existing knowledge related to the aetiology of BPD follows.

Neurobiologic and Genetic Factors

Connections between genetic factors and neurobiology may increase the risk of BPD. There is evidence that genetic factors are involved in the development of BPD: it is five times more common among "first-degree biologic relatives" of individuals with BPD than among the general population (APA, 2013, p. 665). Empirical studies of the neurobiology of BPD have involved neuroendocrinology and biologic specimens, and structural and functional neuroimaging (Ruocco & Carcone, 2016). A systematic and integrative review of these studies found that endogenous stress hormones, neurometabolism, and brain structure and circuits (white matter pathways, grey matter volume) appear to be involved but that the casual interconnections among them and their association with emotion, cognition, and sense of self in persons with BPD need to be clarified, as does the role of the amygdala in coordinating the relevance of emotional stimuli for the individual (Ruocco & Carcone, 2016). There has been speculation that individuals with BPD have reduced volume in the amygdala, but the evidence for this remains inconsistent. Persons with BPD appear to have abnormal serotonergic function, associated with impulsive aggressive symptoms, and such a defect might be related to genetic factors (Leichsenring et al., 2011).

BPD may be related to "stress-induced compromises" in the neural circuits underlying regulatory processes (Hooley et al., 2012, p. 428). Genetic and environmental factors (e.g., childhood trauma) may together be affecting the response of the hypothalamus–pituitary–adrenal (HPA) axis, which plays a main role in the stress response, in persons with BPD. The genetic variants in the HPA axis were found to be a contributor to the pathogenesis of BPD with childhood trauma having a modulating effect when investigated in a large sample of individuals with BPD and healthy controls (Martin-Blanco et al., 2016). PET studies support the hypothesis that persons with BPD have abnormalities in the prefrontal brain regions (associated with emotion control); functional MRI studies add support to the hypothesis that persons with BPD have a dysfunctional frontolimbic network.

Psychosocial Risk Factors

Various studies show that childhood maltreatment appears to be a significant risk factor for BPD: 55% to 80% of individuals with BPD have reported a history of childhood sexual abuse and/or physical abuse (Jordan, 2004). Childhood neglect has been correlated with increase in BPD symptoms (Jovev et al., 2013). Clearly, more studies are needed to identify risk factors for the development of BPD.

Psychological Theories

Psychoanalytic Theories

The psychoanalytic views of BPD focus on two important psychoanalytic concepts: **separation–individuation** and **projective identification**. According to this theory, a person with BPD has not achieved the normal and healthy developmental stage of separation–individuation, during which a child develops a sense of self, a permanent sense of significant others (object constancy), and integration of seeing both bad and good components of self (Mahler et al., 1975). Object relations theory explains how "objects" (i.e., real and internalized relationships with significant people) contribute to personality and are expressed through defences and interpersonal interactions (Clarkin et al., 2006; Magnavita, 2004). Within this theory, individuals with BPD are viewed as lacking the ability to separate from the primary caregiver and develop a separate and distinct personality or self-identity. Psychoanalytic theory suggests that these separation difficulties occur because the primary caregivers' behaviours have been inconsistent or insensitive to the needs of the child. The child develops ambivalent feelings regarding interpersonal relationships and, therefore, has no basis for establishing trusting and secure relationships in the future. Children experience feelings of intense fear and anger in separating themselves from others. This problem continues into adulthood, and they continue to experience difficulties in maintaining personal boundaries and in interpersonal interactions and relationships. These individuals may falsely attribute to others their own unacceptable feelings, impulses, or thoughts, termed projective identification. In this theory, projective identification is believed to play an important role in the development of BPD and is a defence mechanism by which people with BPD protect their fragile self-image. For example, when overwhelmed by anxiety or anger at being disregarded by another, they defend against the intensity of these feelings by unconsciously blaming others for what happens to them. They project their feelings onto a significant other with the unconscious hope that the other knows how to deal with it. Projective identification becomes a defensive way of interacting with the world, which leads to more rejection.

Maladaptive Cognitive Processes

Individuals with personality disorders develop maladaptive cognitive schemas leading them to misinterpret environmental stimuli continuously, which in turn lead to rigid and inflexible behaviour patterns in response to new situations and people. Because those with BPD have been conditioned to anticipate rejection and disappointment in the past, they become entrenched in a pattern of fear and anxiety regarding encountering new people or situations. They have fears that a disaster is going to strike any minute. Early in life, individuals with BPD and other personality disorders develop maladaptive schemas or dysfunctional ways of interpreting people and events. Table 27.1 explains 18 major maladaptive schemas at work in those with personality disorders. The work of cognitive therapists is to challenge these distortions in thinking patterns and replace them with realistic ones. Therapists, too, have personal schemas regarding themselves and others; they need to identify their own schemas and ensure that therapeutic progress is not impeded by an unrecognized conflict with the schema of their clients (Leahy & McGinn, 2012).

Table 27.1 Maladaptive Schemas	
Domain	Schemas With Definitions
I. Disconnection and rejection	1. *Abandonment/instability* Important people will not be there 2. *Mistrust/abuse* Other people will use the client for own selfish ends 3. *Emotional deprivation* Emotional connection will not be fulfilled 4. *Defectiveness/scheme* One is flawed, bad, or worthless 5. *Social isolation/alienation* Being different from or not fitting in
II. Impaired autonomy and performance	1. *Dependence/incompetence* Belief that one is unable to function on one's own 2. *Vulnerability to harm and illness* Fear that disaster is about to strike 3. *Enmeshment/undeveloped self* Excessive emotional involvement at the expense of normal social development 4. *Failure* Belief that one has failed
III. Impaired limits	1. *Entitlement/grandiosity* Belief that one is superior to other; entitled to special rights 2. *Insufficient self-control/self-discipline* Difficulty or refusal to exercise sufficient self-control
IV. Other directedness	1. *Subjugation* Excessive surrendering of control to others because of feeling coerced 2. *Self-sacrifice* Excessive focus on voluntarily meeting the needs of others at the expense of one's own gratification 3. *Approval seeking/recognition seeking* Excessive emphasis on gaining approval, recognition, or attention
V. Overvigilance and inhibition	1. *Negativity/pessimism* Lifelong focus on the negative aspects of life 2. *Emotional inhibition* Excessive inhibition of spontaneous action, feeling, or communication 3. *Unrelenting standard/hypercriticalness* Belief that one must meet very high standards; perfectionistic, rigid 4. *Punitiveness* Belief that people should be harshly punished

Young, J. E. (1999). *Cognitive therapy for personality disorders: A schema-focused approach.* Sarasota, FL: Professional Resource Press. Used with permission.

Biosocial Theories

The biosocial learning theory was developed by Theodore Millon, who viewed BPD as a distinct disorder that develops as a result of both biologic and psychological factors (Millon & Davis, 1999). While he supported the biologic determination of personality, he believed that a child's interaction with the environment and learning and experience could greatly affect their biologic predisposition. He argued that individuals possess biologically based patterns of sensitivities and behavioural dispositions that shape their experiences, including active–passive behaviour or a tendency to take initiative versus reacting to events, sensitivity to pleasure or pain, and sensitivity behaviour to self and others. Millon believed that BPD is a particular cycloid personality pattern representing a moderately dysfunctional dependent or ambivalent orientation, often expressed in intense endogenous moods, described as patterns of recurring dejection and apathy interspersed with spells of anger, anxiety, or euphoria.

A further elaboration of Millon's multidimensional model incorporates biologic explanations into the behaviour. Cloninger and colleagues (1998) described personality disorder behaviours based on temperament and character dimensions derived from a factor analysis design. Cluster A disorders are associated with low-reward dependence and social attachment mediated by norepinephrine and serotonin. Cluster B disorders are associated with high novelty-seeking mediated by dopamine. Novelty-seeking behaviour includes exhilaration, exploration, impulsivity, extravagance, and irritability. Cluster C

disorders are associated with high harm avoidance mediated by γ-aminobutyric acid (GABA) and serotonin.

A biosocial theory of BPD proposed by Marsha Linehan and colleagues is similar to Millon's theory, with a focus on the interaction of both biologic and social learning influences. Their primary focus is on the particular behavioural patterns observed in BPD, including emotional vulnerability, self-invalidation, unrelenting crises, inhibited grieving, active passivity, and apparent competence (Linehan, 1993a; Box 27.2).

This biosocial viewpoint presents BPD as a multifaceted problem, a combination of a person's innate emotional vulnerability and their inability to control that emotion in social interactions (emotional dysregulation) and the environment (Linehan, 1993a). The emotional dysregulation and aggressive impulsivity entail both social learning and biologic regulation. Much of the neurobiologic research is directed at neurotransmitter functions (Silk, 2000) and neural firing between the limbic system and the frontal and prefrontal cortex. When these pathways are functional, the person has a greater capacity to think about their emotions and modulate behaviours more responsibly.

The biosocial viewpoint supports the notion that the ability to control one's emotion is in part a learning process, learned from one's private experiences and encounters with the social environment. A risk factor associated with BPD is believed to develop when emotionally vulnerable individuals interact with an invalidating environment, a social situation that negates the individual's private emotional responses and communication. That

---

BOX 27.2 Behavioural Patterns in BPD

1. *Emotional vulnerability.* Person experiences a pattern of pervasive difficulties in regulating negative emotions, including a high sensitivity to negative emotional stimuli, high emotional intensity, and slow return to emotional baseline.

2. *Self-invalidation.* Person fails to recognize one's own emotional responses, thoughts, beliefs, and behaviours and sets unrealistically high standards and expectations for self. This may include intense shame, self-hate, and self-directed anger. Person has no personal awareness and tends to blame social environment for unrealistic expectations and demands.

3. *Unrelenting crises.* Person experiences a pattern of frequent, stressful, negative environmental events, disruptions, and roadblocks—some caused by the individual's dysfunctional lifestyle, others by an inadequate social milieu, and many by fate or chance.

4. *Inhibited grieving.* Person tries to inhibit and overcontrol negative emotional responses, especially those associated with grief and loss, including sadness, anger, guilt, shame, anxiety, and panic.

5. *Active passivity.* Person fails to engage actively in solving own life problems but will actively seek problem-solving from others in the environment; learned helplessness and hopelessness.

6. *Apparent competence.* Tendency for individuals to appear deceptively more competent than they actually are; it is usually due to failure of competencies to generalize across expected moods, situations, and time and failure to display adequate nonverbal cues of emotional distress.

From Linehan, M. (1993a). *Cognitive-behavioral treatment of borderline personality disorder* (p. 10). Guilford Press.

is, when others whom the person respects or values are continuously insensitive to the person's core emotional responses, respond irrationally and inappropriately, or trivialize their painful experiences, the person receives confused messages about expressing feelings. Further, the message from significant others may be that negative emotions, in particular, are not to be expressed. Invalidation occurs as the individual's emotions are continuously dismissed, trivialized, devalued, punished, and discredited.

The most severe form of invalidation occurs in situations of child sexual abuse. Often, the abusing adult has told the child that this is a "special secret" between them, that the child should feel guilty if they tell anyone, and that telling someone would end their trust and special relationship. The child experiences feelings of fear, pain, and sadness, yet this trusted adult continuously dismisses the child's true feelings and tells the child what they should feel. Children often learn to endure sexual abuse for years, suppressing their true feelings. In disclosing the secret to a nonoffending adult, the child risks not being believed or attended to and possible punishment.

All children, not just those who are emotionally vulnerable, must learn to trust their own feelings and learn when and how to express them by interacting with their environments, including parents, families, friends, and social situations. If they constantly meet with an **invalidating environment**, they cannot learn to trust their own feelings—when to be angry, sad, or happy—they become emotionally dysregulated. This emotional dysregulation leads to further difficulties in identity disturbances, interpersonal relationships, and the development of impulsive, parasuicidal behaviours.

Interdisciplinary Treatment

BPD is a very complex disorder that requires the involvement of the entire healthcare team in its treatment. BPD often involves not only ongoing treatment but also urgent intervention for self-harm and suicidal behaviours. Although psychotherapy has not been shown to lead to remission of BPD (i.e., the diagnostic criteria are no longer met), it can help the individual better manage symptoms of the disorder (Leichsenring et al., 2011), such as dysfunctional moods, impulsive behaviours, and self-injurious behaviours. Evidence-based psychotherapy has been found to be more effective and less expensive to healthcare systems than other approaches (Meuldijk et al., 2017). Characteristics of evidence-based treatment for BPD include manual-directed (structured) approach, encouragement of a sense of agency (i.e., self-control), and therapists who are active, are validating, and assist with the connection of emotion to actions and events (Bateman et al., 2015). Specially trained therapists, representing a variety of mental health disciplines, including psychology, social work, and advanced practice nursing, are often involved. This can be a lifelong

disorder requiring ongoing treatment as the individual copes with multiple interpersonal crises.

Dialectical behaviour therapy is used to treat BPD as it has demonstrated effectiveness in decreasing self-harm behaviour and suicidality in BPD (Lyness, 2016). (See the DBT entry in the section on treatment of PDs in this chapter.) Behaviour patterns of BPD are perceived in this treatment approach as based in a dysfunctional emotional regulation system that evolved from biologic vulnerabilities and an invalidating environment. There are three facets: sensitivity to both positive and negative emotional stimuli, emotional intensity, and slow return to emotion baseline (Lynch & Cuper, 2012, p. 786).

When used on an inpatient basis, DBT requires staff commitment and reinforcement; significant improvement in depression, anxiety, and dissociation symptoms and a highly significant decrease in parasuicidal behaviour have been shown (Bohus et al., 2000). DBT is more often incorporated into a long-term outpatient treatment approach because the greatest effectiveness occurs when skills are learned over time and practised in a variety of daily living settings (Feigenbaum, 2007). Members of the treatment team maintain a positive skills-coaching role with clients.

Psychopharmacotherapy

Although individuals with BPD are treated with medication, the efficacy of such treatments appears to be symptomatic at best. There is evidence that BPD symptoms can be alleviated in the short term by mood stabilizers (e.g., topiramate, for emotional dysregulation and impulsive–aggressive symptoms) and some second-generation antipsychotics (e.g., olanzapine, for cognitive–perceptual and impulsive–aggressive symptoms) (Bateman et al., 2015). Evidence does not support medication as treatment for overall reduction of severity of the disorder (National Health and Medical Research Council [Australia], 2012). Some medications used to treat BPD symptoms have side effects that are potentially harmful (e.g., valproate semisodium for females of child-bearing age) or are neurologic or metabolic in nature (e.g., antipsychotics) (Leichsenring et al., 2011). Risks/benefits must be carefully considered in the symptomatic treatment of BPD.

Family Response to Disorder

The family of clients with BPD may feel captive to the symptoms of the disorder. Family members can be afraid to disagree with them or refuse to meet their multiple needs, fearing that self-destructive behaviours will follow. During the course of the disorder, family members can get "burned out" and withdraw from the individual, only adding to the person's fear of abandonment (Hoffman et al., 2007). They can experience stress, distress, and hopelessness, as well as the significant burden and the loss of their own social support. Psychoeducation for family members and friends can be effective in offering them knowledge regarding the disorder, problem-solving skills, family relationship skills, and a social network (Pearce et al., 2017). When a psychoeducation group intervention for family and friends of youth with BPD was evaluated, participants reported subjective burden was significantly decreased and knowledge of BPD increased; objective burden and distress, however, were unchanged. Longer follow-up after the conclusion of such groups may be required for behavioural change to be practised and established (Pearce et al., 2017). DBT treatment that includes the involvement of family and friends has been developed (Van Wel et al., 2006). Refer further to Chapter 16.

Nursing Care

It is important to recognize that BPD is a devastating disorder that involves much emotional pain and distress and, too often, it is stigmatized (Hooley et al., 2012). Individuals living with BPD experience instability in a variety of areas, including mood, interpersonal relationships, self-esteem, and self-identity, and they can exhibit behavioural and cognitive dysregulations. These manifest in a number of ways, the most prominent of which are listed in Box 27.3. Due to their patterns of response, clients may have problems in daily living: maintaining

---

BOX 27.3 Response Patterns of Individuals With BPD

Affective (mood) dysregulation
Mood lability
Problems with anger
Interpersonal dysregulation
Chaotic relationships
Fears of abandonment
Self-dysregulation
Identity disturbance or difficulties with sense of self
Sense of emptiness
Behavioural dysregulation
Parasuicidal behaviour or threats
Impulsive behaviour
Cognitive dysregulation
Dissociative responses
Paranoid ideation

Courtesy of M. Linehan, Department of Psychology, Box 351525, University of Washington, Seattle, WA 98195–1525.

---

intimate relationships, keeping a job, and living within the law (see Clinical Vignette).

Individuals with BPD may enter the mental health system early (young adulthood or before), but because of their chaotic lifestyle, they typically do not receive consistent treatment. They drop in and out of treatment and usually do not remain with one clinician for long-term treatment. Persons with BPD usually seek help from healthcare workers because of consequences of life crises, medical conditions, or other psychiatric disorders (e.g., depression) or for physical treatment of self-injury. Thus, other problems may need attention before the client's underlying personality disorder can be addressed; at times, the nurse will not know that the person has BPD. During an assessment, however, it usually becomes clear that the client is affected by things more intensely than the average person or has an inflexible view of the world. The great difficulty the client has in changing behaviour, no matter the consequences, will also become apparent. Clients face difficulty in successfully relating to other people and struggle to live a satisfying life.

Nurses often struggle to provide care to clients with a diagnosis of BPD. In a recent study, the perspective of individuals diagnosed with BPD was sought regarding their perceptions of nurses they believed facilitated positive therapeutic relationships. Utilizing a qualitative methodology, 12 participants were interviewed by researchers. The participants identified five overarching attitudes demonstrated by nurses that they believed contributed to their recovery: confidence in their ability to recover, nonjudgmental, used humour, were available, and demonstrated humanity. Clearly, nurses' attitudes are key to the therapeutic relationship; exploring ways to gain a better understanding of this disorder, and subsequent emotional reactions may assist nurses in adopting more positive attitudes when working with this population (Romeu-Labayen et al., 2022).

Biologic Domain

Biologic Assessment

The client with BPD is usually able to maintain personal hygiene and physical functioning. Because of the comorbidity of BPD and eating disorders and substance abuse, a nutritional assessment may be needed. The assessment should also include the use of caffeinated beverages (e.g., coffee, tea, soft drinks) and alcohol. With individuals who engage in bingeing or purging, an assessment should include examining the teeth for pitting and discoloration, as well as the hands and fingers for redness and calluses caused by inducing vomiting. The client should be queried about physiologic responses of emotion. Sleep patterns also should be assessed because sleep alterations may suggest coexisting depression or mania.

CLINICAL VIGNETTE ✚

BORDERLINE PERSONALITY DISORDER

JS is a 22-year-old single woman who was recently fired from her job as a data entry clerk. She is living with her mother and stepfather, who brought her to the emergency room after finding her crouched in a foetal position in the bathroom, her wrists bleeding. She seemed to be in a daze. This is her first psychiatric admission, although her mother and stepfather have suspected that she has "needed help" for a long time. In high school, she received brief treatment for a potential eating disorder. She remains very thin but is able to eat at least one meal per day. During periods of stress, however, she will go for days without eating.

JS is the second of three children. Her parents divorced when she was 3 years old. She has not seen her father since he left. Although she has pleasant memories of her father, her mother has told her that he beat JS and her sisters when he was drinking. When JS was 6 years old, her older sister died following an automobile accident. JS was in the car but was uninjured. As a child, JS was seen as a potential singing star. Her natural musical talent attracted her teachers' support, which encouraged her to develop her talent. She received singing lessons and entered provincial competitions in high school. Although she enjoyed the attention, she was never really comfortable in the limelight and felt "guilty" about having a talent that she sometimes resented. She was able to make friends but found that she was unable to keep them. They described her as "too intense" and emotional. She had one boyfriend in high school, but she was very uncomfortable with any physical closeness. After ending the relationship with the boyfriend, she concentrated on dieting to have a "perfect body." When her dieting attracted her parents' attention, she vowed to eat just enough to keep them "off her back about it." She spent much of her leisure time with her grandmother. She attended university briefly but was unable to concentrate. It was during her time at university and after her grandmother's death that JS began cutting her wrists during periods of stress. It seemed to calm her.

After leaving university, JS returned home. She had several jobs and short-lived friendships. She was usually fired from her job because of "moodiness," and it would take her several months before she would again find another. She would spend days in her room listening to music. Her recent episode followed being fired from work and spending 3 days in her bedroom.

What Do You Think?

- How would you describe JS's mood?
- Are JS's losses (father, sister, grandmother) really severe enough to affect her ability to relate to others now? Do the losses seem to relate to the self-injury?
- What behaviours indicate that there are problems with self-esteem and self-identity?

Physical Indicators of Self-Injurious Behaviours

Clients with BPD should be assessed for self-injurious behaviours or suicide attempts. It is important to ask the individual about specific self-abusive behaviours, such as cutting, scratching, or overdosing. Clients frequently wear long sleeves to hide an injury on the arms. Specifically asking about thoughts of hurting oneself when experiencing a major upset provides an opportunity for prevention and for coaching the client towards alternative self-soothing measures.

Pharmacologic Assessment

The medications that clients with BPD are taking need to be identified and assessed. Initially, individuals may

be reluctant to disclose all their medications as they may be concerned that some or all of their medication may be stopped. The development of rapport with special attention to a nonjudgmental approach is especially important when eliciting current medication practices. The client will play an important role in determining the efficacy of a medication in relieving targeted symptoms. The use of alcohol and street drugs should also be carefully assessed to determine drug interactions.

Nursing Care Foci for the Biologic Domain

Nursing foci of care in the biologic domain can include sleep disturbance, nutritional problem, self-harm or risk for self-harm, and therapeutic regimen issue(s).

Interventions for the Biologic Domain

The interventions for the biologic domain may address a whole spectrum of care issues. Usually, clients are effectively managing hydration, self-care, and pain. The focus here is on the more common care concerns.

Sleep Enhancement

The facilitation of regular sleep–wake cycles may be needed because of disturbed sleep patterns. Conservative approaches should be exhausted before recommending medication (see Chapter 28). Establishing a regular bedtime routine, monitoring bedtime snacks and drinks, and avoiding foods and drinks that interfere with sleep should be tried. If relaxation exercises are used, they should be adapted to the tolerance of the individual. Moderate exercises (e.g., brisk walking) 3 to 4 hours before bedtime activate both serotonin and endorphins, thereby enhancing calmness and a sense of wellbeing before bedtime. For individuals who have difficulty falling asleep and experience interrupted sleep, it helps to establish some basic sleeping routines. The bedroom should be reserved for sleep and intimacy, so it is best to keep items such as televisions, computers, and exercise equipment elsewhere. If the individual is not asleep within 15 minutes, they should get out of bed and go to another room to read, watch television, or listen to soft music. The client should return to bed when sleepy. If the person is not asleep in 15 minutes, the same process should be repeated.

Special consideration must be made for individuals who have been physically and sexually abused and who may be unable to put themselves in a vulnerable position (e.g., lying down in a room with other people or closing their eyes). These clients may need additional safeguards to help them sleep, such as a night light or repositioning of furniture to afford easy exit.

Nutritional Balance

The nutritional status of the person with BPD can quickly become a priority, particularly if the individual has coexisting eating disorders or substance abuse. Eating is often a response to stress, and clients can quickly become overweight. This is especially a problem when the individual has also been taking medications that can promote weight gain, such as antipsychotics, antidepressants, or mood stabilizers. Helping the client to learn the basics of nutrition, make reasonable choices, and develop other coping strategies is a useful intervention. If individuals are engaging in purging or severe dieting practices, teaching them about the dangers of both of these practices is important (see Chapter 25). Referral to an eating disorders specialist may be needed.

Prevention and Treatment of Self-Injury

Within inpatient settings, nurses may need to help clients with BPD (and other cluster B disorders) set limits on their behaviour. Limit setting should be accomplished in such a way that clients recognize that it is the behaviour that is unacceptable, and not them. This is key to the prevention of self-injury, which is frequently a major factor in the hospitalization of persons with BPD. Observing for antecedents of self-injurious behaviour and intervening before an episode is an important to the client's safety. Clients can learn to identify situations leading to self-destructive behaviour and develop preventive strategies. Because individuals with BPD are impulsive and may respond to stress by harming themselves, observation of the person's interactions and assessment of mood, level of distress, and agitation are important in determining the threat of self-injury.

Remembering that self-injury is an effort to self-soothe by activating endogenous endorphins, the nurse can assist the individual to find more productive and enduring ways to find comfort. Linehan (1993b) suggests using a self-soothing exercise and focusing on each of the five senses. For example, a client may try focusing in such ways as follows:

- Vision (e.g., look at photos of places one finds peaceful)
- Hearing (e.g., listen to music or the sounds of nature)
- Smell (e.g., use a drop of lavender oil on a pillow or handkerchief)
- Taste (e.g., drink a soothing, nonalcoholic, warm beverage)
- Touch (e.g., have a warm bath, pet a dog)

Pharmacologic Interventions

There is no specific drug available for the treatment of BPD, but medications for target symptoms may be used: selective serotonin reuptake inhibitors (SSRIs) for affective problems and aggressive impulses and low doses of an antipsychotic for symptoms related to cognitive–perceptive issues (Bateman et al., 2015). These should be on a short-term basis. Clients with BPD may be taking medications for a comorbid disorder, such as a mood disorder or a substance-related disorder.

TEACHING POINTS

Clients should be educated about any medications and their interactions with other drugs and substances. Interventions include teaching individuals about the medication and how and where it acts in the brain and body, helping establish a routine for taking prescribed medication, reporting side effects, and facilitating the development of positive coping strategies to deal with daily stresses, rather than relying on medications. Eliciting the client's partnership in care improves adherence and, thereby, outcomes.

Psychological Domain

Psychological Assessment

People with BPD have usually experienced significant losses in their lives that shape their view of the world. They experience inhibited grieving, "a pattern of repetitive, significant trauma and loss, together with an inability to fully experience and personally integrate or resolve these events" (Linehan, 1993a, p. 89). They may have unresolved grief that began years ago and avoid situations that evoke related feelings of separation and loss. During the assessment, the nurse can identify the losses (real or perceived) and explore the client's experience during these losses, paying particular attention to whether the individual has reached resolution. A history of physical or sexual abuse and an early separation from significant caregivers may provide important clues to the severity of the disturbances.

Mood fluctuations are common and can be assessed by any number of the depression and anxiety screening scales or by asking the following questions:

- What things or events bother you and make you feel happy, sad, and angry?
- Do these things or events trouble you more than they trouble other people?
- Do friends and family tell you that you are moody?
- Do you get angry easily?
- Do you have trouble with your temper?
- Do you think you were born with these feelings, or did something happen to make you feel this way?

Appearance and activity level generally reflect the person's mood and psychomotor activity. Many of those with BPD have been physically or sexually abused and thus should be assessed for depression. A dishevelled appearance can reflect depression or an agitated state. When feeling good, these individuals can be very engaging; they tend to be dramatic in their style of dress and attract attention, such as by wearing an unusual hairstyle or heavy makeup. Because physical appearance reflects identity, clients may experiment with their appearance and seek affirmation and acceptance from others. Body piercings, tattoos, and other adornments may provide a mechanism to define self.

Impulsivity

Impulsivity can be identified by asking clients if they do things impulsively or on the spur of the moment (e.g., "Have there been times when you were hurt by your actions or were sorry later that you acted in the way you did?"). Direct questions about gambling, choices in sexual partners, sexual activities, fights, arguments, arrests, and alcohol drinking habits can also help in identifying areas of impulsive behaviour. Teaching the client strategies to slow down automatic responses (e.g., deep breathing, counting to 10) allows time to think before acting.

Cognitive Disturbances

The mental status examination of those with BPD usually reveals normal thought processes that are not disorganized or confused, except during periods of stress. Those with BPD usually exhibit dichotomous thinking, or a tendency to view things as absolute—either black or white, good or bad—with no perception of compromise. Dichotomous thinking can be assessed by asking clients how they view other people. Evidence of dichotomous thinking is indicated with responses of "good" or "bad," "wonderful" or "terrible."

Dissociation and Transient Psychotic Episodes

Individuals with BPD may experience periods of dissociation and of transient psychotic episodes. Dissociation can be assessed by asking if there are times when they do not remember events or have the feeling of being separate from their body. Some individuals refer to this as "spacing out." By asking specific information about how often, how long, and when dissociation first was used, the nurse can get an idea of how important dissociation is as a coping skill. It is important to ask the person what is happening in the environment when dissociation occurs. Frequent dissociation indicates a highly habitual coping mechanism that will be difficult to change.

Because transient psychotic states occur, it is also important to elicit data regarding the presence of hallucinations or delusions along with their frequency and circumstances. Terms such as "pseudopsychotic" or "quasipsychotic" are misleading and should not be used (Schroeder et al., 2013).

Risk Assessment: Suicide or Self-Harm

It is critical that individuals with BPD be assessed for suicidal and self-damaging behaviours, including alcohol and drug abuse. Further information regarding suicide assessment is found in Chapter 20; substance use in Chapter 26. Suicide is a real risk; it is estimated that about 10% of clients with BPD will die of suicide, many before the age of 40 years (Hooley et al., 2012). An assessment should include direct questions, asking if the person thinks about or engages in self-injurious behaviours. If so, the nurse should continue to explore the behaviours: what is done, how it is done, its frequency, and the circumstances surrounding the self-injurious behaviour. It is helpful to explain briefly to the client that sometimes people cut, scratch, or pick at themselves as a way of bringing some relief and comfort. Although the behaviour brings temporary relief, it also places the person at risk for such things as infection and permanent disfigurement. Approaching the assessment in this way conveys a sense of understanding and is more likely to invite the individual to disclose honestly.

Monitoring changes in the stress levels of a client with BPD is important, as increased stress (or distress) can be a trigger for self-harming behaviours, including a suicide attempt. Common risk factors for suicide attempts remain true for clients with BPD: history of recent attempts and hospitalizations and a history of childhood sexual abuse (Links et al., 2013).

Nursing Care Foci Related to the Psychological Domain

It is important to determine whether observation for risk for self-mutilation is a necessary focus of nursing care because protecting the individual from self-injury is always a priority. If cognitive changes are present (dissociation and transient psychosis), two other nursing care foci may be appropriate: disturbances in thinking and difficulty coping. The disturbance in thinking needs to be a nursing focus of care when dissociative and psychotic episodes interfere with daily living. For example, an office assistant could not complete processing letters because they were unable to differentiate whether the voices on the dictating machine were being transmitted by the machine or by their hallucinations. The nurse helped them learn to differentiate the hallucinations from dictation. The client learned to take their headset off, take a deep breath, and listen to the external environment. When the client recognized "the voice" as their partner criticizing them, the client was able to use their cognitive reframing strategies to refocus on reality.

If the individual copes with stressful situations by dissociating or hallucinating, a care focus on the individual's difficulty in coping is necessary. The intended outcome would be the substitution of effective coping skills for the dissociations or hallucinations.

Assessment data informing the determination of nursing care foci in this domain include disturbance in identity, anxiety, grieving, low self-esteem, powerlessness, and spiritual distress. The related outcomes are dependent on the determined foci of care (see Fig. 27.1).

Interventions for the Psychological Domain

The greatest challenge of working with clients with BPD is engaging the individual in a therapeutic relationship that will survive its emotional ups and downs. Clients need to understand that the nurse is there to coach them to develop self-modulation skills. A relationship based on mutual respect and consistency is crucial for helping the person with those skills. Self-awareness skills, along with access to supervision and collaboration, are needed by the nurse. Research reveals, however, that nurses may struggle with negative attitudes towards clients with BPD and respond to them countertherapeutic ways (see Box 27.4, Therapeutic Dialogue).

Because individuals with BPD are frequently hospitalized, nurses in acute care settings have an opportunity to develop a long-term relationship (Fig. 27.2). A recovery-focused approach to change can be successful, including for persons with BPD who exhibit suicidal behaviours, if clients feel supported and that their experience of what it means to live with BPD is understood (Holm & Severinsson, 2011).

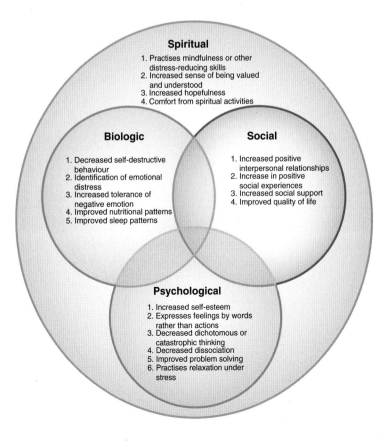

Figure 27.1 Bio/psycho/social/spiritual outcomes for individuals with BPD.

BOX 27.4 THERAPEUTIC DIALOGUE

Borderline Personality Disorder

Ineffective Approach

Client: Hey, you know what? You are my favourite nurse. That night nurse sure doesn't understand me the way you do.
Nurse: Oh, I'm glad you are comfortable with me. Which night nurse?
Client: You know, Sue.
Nurse: Did you have problems with her?
Client: She is terrible. She sleeps all night or she is on the telephone.
Nurse: Oh, that doesn't sound very professional to me. Anything else?
Client: Yeah, she said that you didn't know what you were doing. She said that you couldn't nurse your way out of a paper bag (smiling).
Nurse: She did, did she. (Getting angry.) She should talk.
Client: Well, I gotta go to group. Where will you be? I feel so much better if I know where you are. I don't know how I can possibly be discharged tomorrow.

Effective Approach

Client: Hey, you know what? You are my favourite nurse. That night nurse sure doesn't understand me the way you do.
Nurse: Tomorrow, you will be discharged, and I'm glad that you will be able to return home. (The nurse avoided responding to "favourite nurse" statement. Redirected the interaction to impending discharge.)

Client: That night nurse slept all night.
Nurse: What was your night like? (Redirecting the interaction to Sara's experience.)
Client: It was terrible. Couldn't sleep all night. I'm not sure that I'm ready to go home.
Nurse: Oh, so you are not quite sure about discharge? (Reflection.)
Client: I get so, so lonely. Then, I want to hurt myself.
Nurse: Lonely feelings are a bit of a trigger for you, aren't they? (Validation.)
Client: Yes, I'm very scared. I haven't cut myself for 1 week now.
Nurse: Do you have a plan for dealing with your lonely feelings when they occur?
Client: I'm supposed to start thinking about something that is pleasant—like spring flowers in the meadow.
Nurse: Does that work for you?
Client: Yes, sometimes.

CRITICAL THINKING QUESTIONS

- How did the nurse in the first scenario get sidetracked?
- How was the nurse in the second scenario able to keep the client focused on herself and her impending discharge?

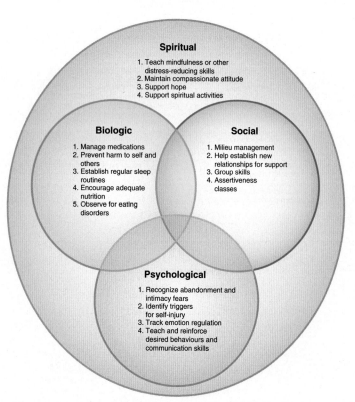

Figure 27.2 Bio/psycho/social/spiritual interventions for individuals with BPD.

A further challenge that may face nurses within this nurse–client relationship is maladaptive coping behaviour that persons with BPD may use that involves regarding a particular person as being all good or all bad, rather than seeing the person as a complex human being. This seeing others in terms of black and white, rather than in shades of grey, can create problems for individuals with BPD in maintaining their relationships. If this happens within the nurse–client relationship and/or affects the team approach to the client, it is important to respond professionally and appropriately, with understanding of the relationship dynamics.

Generalist nurses, including psychiatric and mental health nurses, do not function as the client's primary therapists, but they do need to establish a therapeutic relationship that strengthens the client's coping skills and self-esteem and supports individual psychotherapy. The therapeutic relationship helps the client to experience a model of healthy interaction with consistency, limit setting, caring, and respect for others (both self-respect and respect for the person). Clients who have low self-esteem need help in recognizing genuine respect from others and reciprocating with respect for others. In the therapeutic relationship, the nurse models self-respect by observing personal limits, being assertive, and clearly communicating expectations. Consistency is critical in building self-esteem (see Box 27.5 Challenging Dysfunctional Thinking).

Responding to Abandonment and Intimacy Fears

A key to helping individuals with BPD is recognizing their fears of both abandonment and intimacy. Informing the client of the length of the relationship as much as possible allows the individual to engage in and prepare for termination with the least pain of abandonment. If the client's hospitalization is time limited, the nurse overtly acknowledges the limit and reminds the person with each contact how many sessions remain.

In day treatment and outpatient settings, the duration of treatment may be indeterminate, but the nurse may not be available that entire time. The termination process cannot be casual; this would stimulate abandonment fears. However, some clients end prematurely when the nurse informs them of the impending end as a way to leave before being rejected. Anticipating premature closure, the nurse explores with the individual anticipated feelings, including the wish to run away. After careful planning, the nurse anticipates, in advance, the client's feelings, discusses how to cope with them, reviews the progress the individual has made, and summarizes what the person has learned from the relationship that can be generalized to future encounters.

Establishing Personal Boundaries and Limitations

Personal boundaries are highly context specific. Our personal physical space needs (boundaries) are distinct

BOX 27.5 Challenging Dysfunctional Thinking

Ms. S had worked for the same company for 20 years with a good job record. Following an accident, she made some minor mistakes in her work that she quickly corrected. She informed her company's nurse that her work was "really slipping" and that she was fearful of her coworkers' disapproval and getting fired from her job. The nurse asked her to keep a journal of coworkers' comments for the next week. At the next visit, the following dialogue occurred:

Nurse: I noticed that you received several compliments on your work. Even a close friend of your boss expressed appreciation for your work.

Ms. S: It was a light week at work. I really don't believe they meant what they said.

Nurse: I can see how you can believe that one or two comments are not genuine, but how do you account for four and five good reports on your work?

Ms. S: Well, I don't know.

Nurse: It looks like your beliefs are not supported by your journal entries. Now, what makes you think that your boss wants to fire you after 20 years of service?

from the behavioural and emotional limits which we have. These concepts apply to both the client and the nurse. Furthermore, limits may be temporary (e.g., "I can't talk with you right now, but after my meeting, I can be available for 30 minutes.") (see Chapter 7).

Testing limits is a natural way of identifying where the boundaries are and how strong they are. Therefore, it is necessary to state clearly the enduring limits (e.g., the written rules or contract) and the consequences of violating them. The limits must then be consistently maintained. Clarifying limits requires making explicit what is usually implicit. Despite the clinical setting (e.g., hospital, day treatment setting, outpatient clinic), the nurse must clearly state the day, time, and duration of each contact with the client and remain consistent in those expectations. This may mean having a standing appointment in day treatment or a mental health clinic or noting the time during each shift that the nurse will talk individually with the hospitalized client. The nurse should refrain from offering personal information, which is frequently confusing to the person with BPD. At times, the person may present in a somewhat arrogant and entitled way. It is important for the nurse to recognize such a presentation as reflective of internal confusion and dissonance. Responding in a very neutral manner avoids confrontation and a power struggle, which might also unwittingly reinforce the client's internal sense of inferiority.

Some additional strategies for establishing the boundaries of the relationship include the following:

• Documenting in the client chart the agreed-on appointment expectations
• Sharing the treatment plan with the client
• Confronting violations of the agreement in a nonpunitive way
• Discussing the purpose of limits in the therapeutic relationship and applicability to other relationships

When individuals violate boundaries, it is important to respond right away, but without taking the behaviour personally. For example, if a client is flirtatious, simply say something like, "It is important that we maintain a professional relationship so that I may help you."

Management of Dissociative States

The desired outcome for someone who dissociates is to reduce or eliminate the dissociative experiences. The natural tendency is to want to "fix it." Unfortunately, there are limited medications for dissociation, but because the SSRIs, dopamine antagonists, and serotonin–dopamine antagonists affect other target symptoms, the dissociative experiences decrease. Because dissociation occurs during periods of stress, the best approach is to help the individual develop other strategies to deal with stress.

The nurse can teach clients how to identify when they are dissociating and then to use some grounding strategies in the moment. Basic to grounding is planting both feet firmly on the floor or ground, then taking a deep abdominal breath to the count of four, holding it to the count of four, exhaling to the count of four, and then holding it to the count of four. This is called the four-square method of breathing. The benefit of this approach is to bring about a deep, slow breath that activates the calming mechanisms of the parasympathetic system. After the grounding exercise, the client uses one or more senses to make contact with the environment, such as touching the fabric of a nearby chair or listening to the traffic noise. As the client improves in self-esteem and the ability to relate to others, the frequency of dissociation should decrease.

A related evidence-based, trauma- and recovery-informed intervention is being used in mental health settings: sensory modulation. Sensory modulation is directed at enabling individuals to modify and self-regulate their response to the sensory stimuli of hearing, smell, sight, taste, and touch, as well as the senses of proprioception (body awareness) and vestibular sense (balance and spatial orientation). Achieving optimal arousal to sensory inputs means being able to pay attention to relevant stimuli without being distracted by that which is irrelevant—being "calmly alert" (Wright, 2016 as cited in Hitch et al., 2020). A spectrum of sensory thresholds exists, with individual responses ranging from hypersensitive (low arousal threshold) to hyposensitive (high

arousal threshold). Originating in occupational therapy, sensory modulation has specific strategies based on an individual's professionally assessed sensory profile and preferences. The individual learns to self-regulate through participating in behaviours and activities that engage the senses. Music, lighting and aromas are examples of intervention tools (Hitch et al., 2020).

The Use of Behavioural Interventions

The goal of behavioural interventions is to replace dysfunctional behaviours with positive ones. The nurse has an important role in helping individuals control emotions and behaviours by acknowledging and validating desired behaviours and by ignoring or confronting undesired behaviours. Clients often test the nurse for a response, and nurses must decide how to respond to particular behaviours. This can be challenging because even negative responses may act as positive reinforcement for the client. In some instances, if the behaviour is inappropriate but not harmful or demeaning, the best strategy is to ignore rather than focus on it. Seriously inappropriate and disrespectful behaviours must be addressed in a way that acknowledges the negative impact of such behaviours and incorporates a remedial response, such as an apology to those disrespected and/or changes in client privileges.

Such incidences are opportunities to help the client understand why the behaviour is inappropriate and how it can be changed. The nurse should explore with the client what happened, what events led up to the behaviour, what were the consequences, and what feelings were aroused. Advanced practice nurses or other therapists will explore the origins of the client's behaviours and responses, but the generalist nurse needs to help the person explore ways to change behaviours involved in the current situation.

Addressing Emotional Regulation

A major goal of cognitive therapeutic interventions is emotional regulation—recognizing and controlling the expression of feelings. Clients often have difficulty recognizing their feelings; instead, they respond quickly without regard for the consequences. Cognitive/behavioural strategies are useful in dealing with such immediacy of action to an emotional response (see Chapter 14). Viktor Frankl, psychiatrist and author of *Man's Search for Meaning* (see Chapter 9), shared a helpful image: "Between stimulus and response, there is a space. In this space is our power to choose a response. In our response lies our growth and our freedom." The nurse assists the client to use this "space" to choose.

The client needs help to identify feelings and gain control over expressions such as anger, disappointment, or frustration. The goal is for individuals to tolerate their feelings without being compelled to act upon them in ways that hurt another person or themselves.

A helpful technique for managing feelings is known as the **communication triad**. The triad provides a specific syntax and order for clients to identify and express their feelings and seek relief. The "sentence" consists of three parts:

- An "I" statement to identify the prevailing feeling
- A nonjudgmental statement of the emotional trigger
- What the individual would like differently or what would restore comfort to the situation

The nurse must emphasize with clients that they begin with the "I" statement. Beginning with "I" allows the client to identify and express the feeling first and take full ownership. For example, the individual who is angry with another client in the group might say, "Joe, I feel angry ('I' statement with ownership of feeling) when you interrupt me (the trigger), and I would like you to apologize and try not to do that with me (what the individual wants and the remedy)." This simple skill is easy to teach, is easy to reinforce and to encourage others to reinforce, and is a surprisingly effective way of moderating the emotional tone.

Another element of emotional regulation is learning to delay gratification. When clients want something that is not immediately available, the nurse can teach individuals to distract themselves, find alternate ways of meeting the need, and think about what would happen if they have to wait to meet the need.

The practice of thought stopping might also help the person to control the inappropriate expression of feelings. In thought stopping, the client identifies what feelings and thoughts exist together. For example, when the person is ruminating about a perceived hurt, the individual might say "Stop that" (referring to the ruminative thought) and engage in a distracting activity. Three activities associated with thought stopping are effective:

- Taking a quick deep breath when the behaviour is noted (this also stimulates relaxation)
- Visualizing a stop sign or saying "stop" when possible (this allows the person to hear externally and internally)
- Deliberately replacing the undesired behaviour with a positive alternative (e.g., instead of ruminating about an angry situation, thinking about a neutral or positive self-affirmation)

The sequencing and combining of the steps puts the person back in control.

Addressing Dysfunctional Thinking

The nurse can help the individual address their problematic, dysfunctional ways of thinking by encouraging the person to think about the event in a different way. This is termed reframing. The client learns to take a more positive, yet realistic, perspective on a situation or issue. When a client engages in catastrophic thinking, the nurse can address such thinking by asking, "What is the worst that could happen?" and "How likely would that be to occur?" For dichotomous thinking, as when the client fixates on one extreme perception or alternates between the extremes only, the nurse can ask the person to think about any examples of exceptions to the extreme. The point of the challenge is not to debate or argue with the individual but to provide different perspectives to consider. Encouraging clients to keep journals of real interactions to process with the nurse or therapist is another effective way of testing the reality of their thinking and anticipations, affording more choices and flexibility (Box 27.6).

BOX 27.6 Thought Distortions and Corrective Statements

Thought Distortion	Corrective Statement
Catastrophizing	
"This is the most awful thing that has ever happened to me."	"This is a sad thing, but not the most awful."
"If I fail this course, my life is over."	"If you fail the course, you can take the course again. You can change your major."
Dichotomizing	
"No one ever listens to me."	"Your husband listened to you last night when you told him…"
"I never get what I want."	"You didn't get the promotion this year, but you did get a merit raise."
"I can't understand why everyone is so kind at first and then always dumps me when I need them the most."	"It is hard to remember those kind things and times when your friends have stayed with you when you needed them."
Self-Attribution Errors	
"If I had just found the right thing to say, she wouldn't have left me."	"There is not a single right thing to say, and she left you because she chose to."
"If I had not made him mad, he wouldn't have hit me."	"He has a lot of choices in how to respond, and he chose hitting. You are responsible for your feelings and actions."

In problem-solving, the nurse might encourage the individual to debate both sides of the problem and then search for common ground. Practicing communication and negotiation skills through role-playing helps clients make mistakes and correct them without harm to their self-esteem. The nurse also encourages clients to use these skills in their everyday lives and report back on the results, asking individuals how they feel applying the skills and how doing so affects their self-perceptions. Success, even partial success, builds a sense of competence and self-esteem.

Management of Transient Psychotic Episodes

During psychotic episodes with auditory hallucinations, clients should be protected from harming themselves or others. In an inpatient setting, the client should be monitored closely and a determination made as to whether the voices are telling the person to engage in self-harm (command hallucinations). The client may be observed more closely and begin taking antipsychotic medications. In the community setting, the nurse should help the client develop a plan for managing the voices. For example, if the voices return, the individual contacts the clinic and returns for evaluation. There may be a friend or relative who should be contacted or a case manager who can help the person get the necessary protection if it is needed. In some instances, hearing the voices is a prelude to self-injury. Another person may be able to help the individual resist the voices. Once other aspects of the disorder are managed, the episodes of psychosis decrease or disappear.

Teaching and practicing distress tolerance skills help the individual have power over the voices and control intense emotions. When not experiencing hallucinations, the client can practice deep abdominal breathing, which calms the autonomic nervous system. Using brainstorming techniques, the individual identifies early internal cues of rising distress while the nurse writes them on an index card for the client to refer to later. Next, the nurse teaches some skills for tolerating painful feelings or events. To help the client, suggest the mnemonic "Wise Mind ACCEPTS" with the following actions:

- Activities to distract from stress
- Contributing to others, such as volunteering or visiting a sick neighbour
- Comparing yourself to people less fortunate than you
- Emotions that are opposite to what you are experiencing
- Pushing away from the situation for a while
- Thoughts other than those you are currently experiencing
- Sensations that are intense, such as holding ice in your hand (Linehan, 1993b, pp. 165–166)

BOX 27.7 Psychoeducation Checklist: Borderline Personality Disorder

When caring for the client with BPD, be sure to include the following topic areas in the teaching plan:

- ✓ Management of medication, if used, including drug action, dosage, frequency, and possible adverse effects
- ✓ Regular sleep routines
- ✓ Nutrition
- ✓ Safety measures
- ✓ Functional versus dysfunctional behaviours
- ✓ Cognitive strategies (distraction, communication skills, thought stopping)
- ✓ Structure and limit setting
- ✓ Social relationships
- ✓ Community resources

Client Education

Client education within the context of a therapeutic relationship is one of the most important, empowering interventions for the nurse to use. Teaching individuals skills to resist parasuicidal urges and self-harming behaviours, improve emotional regulation, enhance interpersonal relationships, tolerate stress, and enhance overall quality of life provides the foundation for long-term behavioural changes. These skills can be taught in any treatment setting as a part of the overall facility program (see Box 27.7). If nurses are practicing in a facility where DBT is the treatment model, they can be trained in DBT and can serve as group skills leaders.

Social Domain

Social Assessment

Some individuals with BPD can function very well except during periods when symptoms erupt. They hold jobs, are active in communities, and can perform well. During periods of stress, symptoms often appear. On the other hand, some individuals with severe BPD function poorly; they are always in a crisis, which they have often created.

Social Support Systems

The identification of social supports, such as family, friends, and religious organizations, is the purpose in assessing resources. Knowing how the person obtains social support is important in understanding the quality of interpersonal relationships. For example, some individuals consider their "best friends" to be their nurses, physicians, and other healthcare personnel. Because this is a false friendship (i.e., not reciprocal), it can lead to frustration and disappointment. Helping the individual find ways to meet other people and encouraging the client's efforts in developing meaningful relationships are more realistic.

Interpersonal Skills

An assessment of the person's ability to relate to others is important because interpersonal problems are linked to dissociation and self-injurious behaviour. Information about friendships, frequency of contact, and intimate relationships will provide data about the person's experience in relating to others. Some clients with BPD may be sexually active with several sexual partners. Their need for closeness clouds their judgment about sexual partners. They are at risk for entering into relationship with persons with antisocial personality disorder (discussed later in this chapter). During assessment, nurses should be self-aware regarding their personal response to the client. How the nurse responds to the individual may be a clue to how others perceive and respond to this person. For example, if the nurse feels impatient during the interview, it may be indicative that others respond to this person in this way; on the other hand, if the nurse feels empathy or closeness, the individual may evoke these feelings in others.

Self-Esteem and Coping Skills

Coping with stressful situations is one of the major problems for people with BPD. An assessment of their coping skills and their ability to deal with stressful situations is important. Because the individual's self-esteem is usually very low, an assessment of self-esteem can be done with a self-esteem assessment or by interviewing the client and analyzing the assessment data for evidence of personal self-worth and confidence. Clients with BPD perceive their families and friends as being weary of their numerous crises and their seeming unwillingness to break the cycle of self-destructiveness. Feeling rejected by their natural support system, these individuals may attempt to create one within the healthcare system. During periods of crisis or affective instability, especially during the late evening, early morning, or on weekends, they may call or visit the hospital, asking to speak to specific personnel who formerly cared for them. Sometimes, they bring gifts to nurses or call them at home. Because this attempt at a new social support system must fail as it cannot provide the desired support, the person continues to feel rejected. One of the goals of the treatment is to help the individual establish a natural support network.

Family Assessment

Family members may or may not be involved with the client. Individuals with BPD are often estranged from their families. In other instances, they are dependent on them, which is also a source of stress. If childhood abuse has occurred, the perpetrator may be a family member. Ideally, family members are interviewed for their perspectives on the client's problem. An assessment of any mental disorder in the client's family and of the current level of functioning is useful in understanding the client and identifying potential resources for support.

Nursing Care Foci for the Social Domain

Impaired coping, negative sense of self, problems in interpersonal interactions are potential foci of nursing care that address the social problems clients with BPD may face.

Interventions for the Social Domain: Modifying Coping Behaviours

Environmental management becomes critical in caring for a person with BPD. Because the unit can be structured to represent a microcosm of the individual's community, clients have an opportunity to identify relationship problems, boundary violations, and stressful situations. When these situations occur, the nurse can help the individual cope by finding alternative explanations for the situation and practicing new skills. Individual sessions help the client try out some skills, such as putting feelings into words without actions. Role-playing may help individuals experience different degrees of effectively relating feelings without the burden of hurting someone they care about. Day treatment and group settings are excellent places for clients to learn more effective feeling management and to practice these techniques with each other. The group helps members develop empathy and diffuses attachment to any one person or therapist.

Building Social Skills and Self-Esteem

Many women with a diagnosis of BPD are involved in abusive relationships and lack the ability to resolve these relationships because of their extreme anxiety regarding separating from those they love and their extreme need to feel connected. These women verbalize desires to leave, but they do not have the sense of safety self-confidence needed to leave. Exposing them to a different style of interaction as well as validation from other people increases their self-esteem and ability to separate from negative influences.

Exploring Social Supports

Dependency on family members is a problem for many people with BPD. In some families, a client's positive progress may be met with negative responses, and individuals in these situations need help in maintaining a separate identity while staying connected to family members for social support. Family support groups sometimes help. Usually, the nurse helps the person explore new relationships that can provide additional social contacts.

Teaching Effective Ways to Communicate

An important area of client education is teaching communication skills. Clients lack interpersonal skills in relating because they often had inadequate modelling and few opportunities to practice. The goals of relationship skill development are to identify problematic behaviours that interfere with relationships and to use appropriate behaviours in improving relationships. The starting point is with communication. The nurse teaches the individual basic communication approaches, such as making "I" statements, paraphrasing what the other party says before responding, checking the accuracy of perceptions with others, compromising and seeking common ground, listening actively, and offering and accepting reactions. Besides modelling the behaviours, the nurse guides clients in practicing a variety of communication approaches for common situations. When role-playing, the nurse needs to discuss not only what the skills are and how to perform them but also the feelings clients have before, during, and after the role-play.

In day treatment and outpatient settings, the nurse can give the client homework, such as keeping a journal, applying role-playing skills to actual situations, and observing behaviours in others. In the hospital, the individual can experience the same process, and the nurse is available to offer immediate feedback. Whatever the setting, or even the specific problems addressed, the nurse must keep in mind and remind the client that change occurs slowly. Thus, working on the problems occurs gradually, with severity of symptoms as the guide to deciding how fast and how much change to expect.

Spiritual Domain

In addressing the spiritual domain, the qualities of the nurse that have been identified as important include receptivity (e.g., being genuinely available to the client as a person), humanity (e.g., taking time for the "little things" when giving care), competency (e.g., demonstrating safe practice), and positivity (e.g., having a hopeful attitude and fostering a positive spirit) (Carr, 2008); (see Chapter 12). In nursing clients with BPD, enacting these qualities may be challenging, as characteristics of BPD involving self-dysregulation and interpersonal dysregulation can sometimes promote a negative response to the person in the nurse. If the nurse does not grasp that the client's personality patterns do comprise a mental disorder, they may become frustrated with the lack of client behaviour change and progress. As well, trying to understand the worldview of the client with BPD can be difficult. Spiritual care is particularly important for such clients as they struggle with issues of self and connection, purpose, and meaning. A review of the research on spirituality and persons with PDs, in fact, indicates that spiritual wellbeing may remain high for persons with borderline personality traits, even though general wellbeing is low (Bennett et al., 2013). Nurses can play an important role in helping clients sustain such wellbeing through respectful, knowledgeable, and supportive connection within a therapeutic relationship.

Evaluation and Outcomes

Evaluation and outcomes vary depending on the severity of the disorder, the presence of comorbid disorders, and the availability of resources. For a client with severe symptoms or continual self-injury, keeping the individual safe and alive may be a realistic outcome. Helping the person resist parasuicidal urges may take years. In contrast, individuals who rarely need hospitalization and have adequate resources can expect to recover from the self-destructive impulses and learn positive interaction skills that promote a fulfilling lifestyle. Most clients fall somewhere in between, with periods of symptom exacerbation and remission. In these individuals, increasing the symptom-free time may be the best indicator of outcomes.

Continuum of Care

Treatment of BPD is long term. Hospitalization is sometimes necessary during acute episodes involving parasuicidal or suicidal behaviour. Brief psychiatric hospitalization as an intervention has be found to be effective in preventing such behaviour and in facilitating quick return to the community. Such brief admission is goal directed (e.g., prevention of self-harm), with potential interventions and conditions for premature (i.e., forced) discharge identified on admission. As an intervention, it permits nurses to support the individual with BPD to actively cope with symptoms (Helleman et al., 2014). Ongoing treatment in the outpatient or day treatment setting is important as individuals with BPD may appear more competent and in control than they are. They need continued follow-up and therapy, including individual therapy, psychoeducation, and positive role models (see Box 27.8).

BOX 27.8   NURSING CARE PLAN

Client With BPD

EL is a 26-year-old woman, admitted to the hospital's psychiatric unit via the emergency department. The manager of EL's apartment building found her lying on floor of its entrance way, sobbing loudly and surrounded by her scattered mail. She had bleeding lacerations on both arms; the manager noticed faint scars on EL's arms, as well. When her attempts to assist EL to her apartment were met with physical resistance and cursing, the manager called the police. EL cooperated when the police wanted to transport her to the hospital. Assessment of EL by an emergency physician and a psychiatric resident determined that she had a history of self-harm, as well as one psychiatric admission for suicidal behaviour from which she was discharged with a diagnosis of BPD and a referral for psychotherapy. EL states that she went for psychotherapy but quit after a few months as it was not helpful. The therapist disliked her. Her current distress appears related to her new boyfriend's departure on a business trip. Despite her pleas, he refused to allow her to accompany him. EL works part-time as an office "temp." She has a married, younger brother living in another province. EL's mother died suddenly of an aneurysm when EL was 7 years old; she refuses to speak of her father, saying only that she has had nothing to do with him since she left home at 16 years of age. EL's lacerations were treated in the emergency department, and she was voluntarily admitted to the hospital's psychiatric unit.

Once on the psychiatric unit, EL is assigned a primary nurse, JK. During her unit admission and nursing assessment, EL begins to cry. Through tears, she laughs and tells JK, "I am just so relieved to be here and to have such a nice nurse like you. When I was here before, my primary nurse was so cold and critical of me." JK asks her to agree not to cut or harm herself in any way for the next 24 hours. EL shouts, "No! I can't promise that! If I could do that I wouldn't be here!" Observing EL's level of distress during her assessment and her inability to agree not to self-harm, JK decides that EL requires close observation. JK orients EL to the unit facilities. In the lounge area, EL smiles at other clients sitting there and readily joins in conversation with them.

Setting: Inpatient Psychiatric Unit in a General Hospital

Baseline Assessment: EL is a 26-year-old woman, admitted to the psychiatric unit through the emergency department where she was treated for self-inflicted lacerations on both forearms. She is distressed and angry that her new boyfriend refused to allow her to accompany him on a business trip. She appears to understand this as a lack of commitment to their relationship and is fearful that he may connect with other women on his trip and that he is intending to "dump" her. Her behaviour since being found by her apartment manager has fluctuated between being distressed, angry, and resistant to assistance to being cooperative and relieved at receiving help.

Psychiatric Diagnosis	Medications
Borderline personality disorder	Sertraline (Zoloft) 150 mg qd for anxiety.

Nursing Care Focus 1: Self-Harm

Defining Characteristics	Related Factors
Lacerations on forearms	Fears of abandonment secondary to boyfriend's departure on a business trip
Self-inflicted wounds	Inability to handle stress

Outcomes

Initial	Discharge
1. Remain safe and not harm herself.	4. Identify ways to respond to self-harming impulses if they return.
2. Identify feelings before and after cutting herself.	5. Verbalize alternate thinking with more realistic base.
3. Consider alternative response to self-harm to deal with feelings.	6. Identify community resources to provide structure and support.

Continued on following page

NURSING CARE PLAN (*Continued*)

Interventions

Interventions	Rationale	Ongoing Assessment
Monitor the client for changes in mood or behaviour that might lead to self-injurious behaviour.	Close observation establishes safety and protection of the client from self-harm and impulsive behaviours.	Document according to policy. Continue to observe for mood and behaviour changes.
Monitor for suicidal ideation.	Will indicate increased risk for suicide.	Document according to policy. Continue to observe for suicide risk.
Discuss with the client the need for close observation and rationale to keep her safe.	Explanation to the client for the purpose of nursing interventions helps her cooperate with the nursing activity.	Assess her response to the increasing level of observation.
Administer medications as prescribed and evaluate medication effectiveness in reducing anxiety and cognitive disorganization.	Allows for adjustment of medication dosage based on target behaviours and outcomes.	Observe for side effects.
Communicate information about the client's risk for self-harm and potential risk for suicide to other nursing staff.	The close observation should be continued throughout all shifts until the risk for self-harm has abated. Risk assessment includes distress level and presence of suicidal ideation.	Review the documentation of close observation for all shifts.
Teach relaxation techniques.	Provides an alternative way to deal with tension.	Support practice of techniques. Document.

Evaluation

Outcomes	Revised Outcomes	Interventions
Remained safe without further harming self. Identified fears of abandonment before cutting herself and relief of anxiety afterwards.	Will record her fears in a journal to gain further understanding of them.	Offer her a notebook to use as a journal.
Identified friends to call when fears return and hotlines to use if necessary.	Use hotlines or call friends if self-harm fears return.	Give the client hotline number. Advise her to record this number and her friends' contact numbers in an easily accessible place.
Notified staff when desire to self-harm occurred; discussed her feelings; used relaxation techniques to deal with tension.	Does not harm self for 3 days.	Remind her to call someone if urges return.
Enrolled in a day hospital program for 4 weeks.	Attend the day hospital program.	Follow-up on enrolment.

Nursing Care Focus 2: Motivation for Positive Change

Defining Characteristics	Related Factors
Wants to stop self-harming.	Desires a good relationship with boyfriend. Believes self-harming will negatively impact it.

NURSING CARE PLAN (*Continued*)

Outcomes

Initial	Discharge
Discuss her hopes for change.	Identify two strategies to enhance hope for change.
Identify desired positive changes.	Select one positive change as a goal. Record the goal in journal.

Interventions

Interventions	Rationale	Ongoing Assessment
Develop a therapeutic relationship.	Individuals with BPD are able to consider positive change within the structure of a therapeutic relationship.	Assess her ability to relate and the nurse's response to the relationship.
Discuss her past experience with making a positive change in behaviour.	By identifying barriers to change and elements of success, she can identify a realistic goal.	Assess her ability to accept challenges related to change.
Acknowledge that change takes time and that it is usual for setbacks to occur.	Acknowledging that making changes in one's life is possible even when setbacks occur and progress is slow will support hope for realistic change.	Assess whether she is accepting of the time and effort to make a behavioural change.
Teach her cognitive behavioural techniques.	Learning about ways of identifying and assessing negative thoughts will help the client recognize those which detract from sustaining hope for change.	Review understanding of the techniques. Encourage questions about it.

Evaluation

Outcomes	Revised Outcomes	Interventions
EL is able to express realistic hope for change of self-harming behaviour and wants to seek new opportunities for support, such as the day treatment program.	None	Continue to identify ways to enhance hope through resources such as those at Hope Studies Central at the University of Alberta (https://sites.google.com/a/ualberta.ca/hope-studies/). Use journal to record ideas and strategies.

Carpenito, L. J. (2017). *Handbook of nursing diagnoses* (15th ed.). Lippincott Williams & Wilkins.

Antisocial Personality Disorder

Clinical Course of Disorder

In the *DSM-5*, the essential feature of ASPD is "a pervasive pattern of disregard for, and violation of, the rights of others that begins in childhood or early adolescence and continues into adulthood" (APA, 2013, p. 659). Because of its association with conduct disorders, ASPD is listed there as well as with PDs in the *DSM-5*. A diagnosis of ASPD cannot be given until an individual is 18 years of age; however, there must be a history of symptoms of conduct disorder before the age of 15 years

(APA). Features of ASPD are discussed below, but for the official APA diagnostic criteria, see the DSM-5.

ASPD is related to, but not synonymous with, the older, broader term "psychopath." The work of Cleckley (1941), author of *The Mask of Sanity*, remains the greatest influence on contemporary understanding of psychopathy, but Cleckley's criteria have evolved by researchers such as Hare, who developed measures of psychopathy (e.g., Crego & Widiger, 2016; Hare, 1991). Although the DSM-5 criteria for ASPD include features essential to the psychopathy construct, these features are not required for an ASPD diagnosis to be given; most individuals with ASPD are not psychopathic, but most of those who are psychopathic meet ASPD diagnostic criteria (Hare & Neumann, 2009).

Individuals with ASPD fail to conform to the ethical and social standards of their community (e.g., deceitful, exploitive, callous). Although they can be superficially charming and facile communicators, in reality, they lack empathy and compassion. Easily irritated, they often act out aggressively without concerns for consequences and may end up in the correctional system. Although it has been suggested that, in forensic environments, an ASPD diagnosis indicates a higher risk for being a serious threat to others, research to date gives no credence to that claim (Edens et al., 2015). Most individuals with ASPD, however, do not come in conflict with the law; some find a niche in society, such as in business, the military, or politics, which rewards their competitive, tough behaviour (Millon et al., 2004). Given that ASPD is associated with low economic status in urban settings, the diagnosis may be misapplied when antisocial behaviour is an aspect of survival and protective strategies (APA, 2013, p. 662); criminal behaviour for gain without the personality features of ASPD does not meet ASPD diagnostic criteria.

Prevalence and Comorbidity

Sadock et al. (2019) in a review of ASPD reported that the prevalence in males as 3% (may be as high as 7%) and 1% in the female population. The prevalence among individuals with severe alcohol use disorder and/or in clinical and forensic settings is much higher, over 70% (APA, 2013).

Aetiology

There appears to be both genetic and environmental influences (shared and nonshared) involved in the aetiology of ASPD, but the weight of these influences and whether these influences act independently or together has yet to be concluded. Through behavioural genetics studies, particularly with twins, knowledge of the aetiology of ASPD is evolving. In an overview of the behavioural genetics of ASPD and psychopathy, Werner and colleagues (2015) noted that studies indicate both psychopathic personality traits and ASPD are influenced by additive genetic factors and nonshared environmental factors (i.e., factors not in common with siblings, such as friends, independent activities) without there being a significant contribution of shared environment (i.e., same home with its elements of culture, parenting). Rosenström and colleagues (2017) used structured interview data (i.e., DSM interview for PDs) and a population-based twin sample (n = 2,794) to investigate genetic and environmental factors associated with ASPD criteria. Both independent and common pathway biometric models were compared. These researchers concluded

that there is "a single, highly heritable common factor" liability for ASPD that may account for correlations among the ASPD criteria (Rosenström et al., 2017, p. 272). This finding challenges the results of other studies in this area.

Other research, which contributes to our understanding of the influences of nature (genetics) and nurture (environment) in ASPD, is a study of callous and unemotional behaviour in children (at 27 months of age) by Hyde and colleagues (2016). They used an adoption cohort of 561 families and assessed biologic mothers for a history of severe antisocial behaviour and observed the positive reinforcement behaviours of the adoptive mothers. Antisocial behaviour of biologic mothers predicted early callous–unemotional behaviours in their offspring, despite limited or no contact between them. High levels of adoptive mother positive reinforcement, however, appeared to buffer the effects of heritable risk. This finding has implications for prevention of ASPD, especially given that, for adults with severe antisocial behaviours, these behaviours begin in childhood (Hyde et al., 2016).

Individuals with antisocial and violent histories of offending behaviour have been found to have social cognition problems. Compared with members of a control group, offenders with ASPD had greater difficulty with mentalizing, such that mentalization scores predicted ASPD status. Specific impairments in "perspective taking, social cognition, and social sensitivity, as well as tendencies towards hypomentalizing and nonmentalizing" were greater in those with ASPD (Newbury-Helps et al., 2017, p. 232). Such findings point to mentalization-focused interventions as a potential means of helping persons with such histories in overcoming social cognitive impairment (see section Mentalization-Based Treatment earlier in this chapter).

Nursing Care

Persons with ASPD rarely seek mental health care for their disorder itself; instead, they may seek treatment for depression, substance misuse, or unmanaged and destructive anger, or be hospitalized in forensic psychiatric settings for evaluation. Key areas of assessment are determining the quality of relationships, impulsivity, and the extent of irritability and aggression. The characteristics of ASPD mean that individuals with a diagnosis of ASPD will be indifferent to rules and norms, as well as the rights and wellbeing of others. They may use manipulation, including lying, to get what they want. Counter to what is implied for the term "antisocial," these persons often make good first impressions and are socially adept. ASPD is often described as a disorder in which the distress is felt by others. Attention to the protection of other clients and staff from manipulative and sometimes abusive behaviours is necessary. Self-awareness is especially important for the nurse because of the charming quality of many of these individuals. A matter-of-fact approach to such clients is appropriate; vigilance regarding manipulation in terms of bending hospital rules (e.g., regarding smoking, visitors, use of street drugs) or providing unnecessary information about other clients, staff, or oneself is important. At the same time, nurses' self-protection against being manipulated should not translate into unfair treatment of clients with ASPD. Nursing care foci for clients with ASPD are related to their interpersonal detachment, lack of awareness of others, avoidance of feelings, impulsiveness, and discrepancy between their perception of themselves and others' perception of them. Outcomes should be short term and relevant to a specific problem. For example, if a person has been chronically unemployed, a reasonable short-term outcome would be to set up job interviews or work on interpersonal skills building, rather than obtain a job.

Therapeutic relationships are difficult to establish with an individual with ASPD; an alliance may be formed, however, that allows the objectives of care and treatment to move forward. The ability to make genuine commitments is not typical for the individual with ASPD and this should be expected. The goal of the therapeutic relationship is to assist the client in identifying dysfunctional thinking patterns and developing healthier problem-solving behaviours.

Self-responsibility facilitation (encouraging a person to assume more responsibility for personal behaviour) is useful with clients with ASPD. The nursing activities that are particularly helpful include holding clients responsible for their behaviours, monitoring the extent to which self-responsibility is assumed, and discussing the consequences of not dealing with responsibilities. The nurse needs to refrain from arguing or bargaining about the unit rules, such as time for meals, use of the television room, and smoking. Instead, positive feedback is given to the individual for accepting additional responsibility or changing behaviour.

Self-awareness enhancement (exploring and understanding personal thoughts, feelings, motivation, and behaviours) is another nursing intervention that is important in helping these individuals develop a sense of understanding about relating positively to the rest of the world (Bulechek et al., 2008). Encouraging clients to recognize and discuss thoughts and feelings helps the nurse understand how the person views the world. Bear in mind, however, that individuals with ASPD may be telling the nurse what they believe the nurse wants to hear. Communication techniques discussed in the section on BPD are also helpful with these clients. In teaching the client about positive healthcare practices, impulse control, and anger management, the best approach is to engage the individual in a discussion about the specific challenges faced and then to direct the topic to the major teaching points and avoid being sidetracked (Fisher et al., 2021). Refer further to Box 27.9.

> ## BOX 27.9 Psychoeducation Checklist: Antisocial Personality Disorder
>
> When caring for the client with ASPD, be sure to include the following topic areas in the teaching plan:
>
> ✓ Positive healthcare practices, including substance abuse control
> ✓ Effective communication and interaction skills
> ✓ Impulse control
> ✓ Anger management
> ✓ Group experience to help develop self-awareness and impact of behaviour on others
> ✓ Analyzing an issue from the other person's viewpoint
> ✓ Maintenance of employment
> ✓ Interpersonal relationships and social interactions

In an inpatient unit, interventions can be used to assist the individual in developing positive interaction skills and to experience a consistent environment. For example, the focus of nursing interventions may be the client's continual disregard of the rights of others. On one unit, a client continually placed orders for pizzas in the name of another person on the unit. This other person was genuinely afraid of the person with ASPD— and always paid for the pizza and gave it to the other client. When the nursing staff realized what was happening, they discussed the incident with the person with ASPD using facts (e.g., financial implications, respect for others, boundaries) and helped them to create a plan for future accountability for their actions. The nursing staff also discussed the incident with the other client and helped them identify strategies for future interactions with the person with ASPD.

Group interventions typically are more effective than individual modalities for persons with ASPD. Problem-solving groups that focus on identifying a problem and developing a variety of alternative solutions can be particularly helpful, as can groups with a focus on the development of empathy. Within group therapy, clients are able to confront each other with dysfunctional schemas or thinking patterns.

Milieu interventions, such as providing a structured environment with rules that are consistently applied to clients who are responsible for their own behaviour, are important. While living in close proximity to others, the individual with ASPD will demonstrate dysfunctional social patterns that can be identified and targeted for correction, such as the violation of unit rules.

Aggressive behaviour is often a problem for these individuals and their family members. Anger control assistance (helping to express anger in an adaptive, nonviolent manner) becomes a priority intervention; anger management techniques can be beneficial.

Social support for individuals with ASPD is often minimal as they have taken advantage of friends and relatives who no longer trust them. For new friendships to be developed and sustained and for re-engagement with family members to occur, new ways of interaction must be learned by the person with ASPD. As these ways of interaction need to include empathy and attachment, such goals may never become reality.

The outcomes of interventions for individuals with ASPD need to be evaluated in terms of management of specific problems, such as maintaining employment or developing a meaningful interpersonal relationship, as well as adherence to treatment recommendations and the development of healthcare practices for other healthcare issues (e.g., reduce smoking and alcohol consumption).

IN-A-LIFE 🏠

Ferdinand Waldo Demara (1921–1982)

THE GREAT IMPOSTOR

Public Persona

Ferdinand Waldo Demara spent much of his adult life using forged, stolen, or nonexistent credentials to gain employment in numerous and varied vocations. He became most famous for his masquerade as a commissioned Surgeon–Lieutenant in the Royal Canadian Navy in 1951, having stolen the identity of the Canadian physician Dr. Joseph Cyr. Demara was apparently competent in his role as a physician, relying on medical texts and a medical assistant. Demara had similar success in other branches of the military, as a psychologist in a college, as a prison warden, and as a well-respected schoolteacher.

Personal Realities

Demara's life was patterned by the establishment of personal connections with individuals (often in the context of a religious order), theft of this person's identity, and subsequent employment using these false credentials. Once caught, he would disappear, only to reappear claiming a new identity. It was a sense of emptiness and boredom that would kindle Demara's dreams and his need to act as an impostor to fulfill his seemingly well-intentioned passions. Source: Crichton, R. (1959). *The great impostor*. Random House.

Histrionic Personality Disorder

"Hysteria" (a term derived from the Greek for "uterus") is one of the oldest mental disorders. It was described by early Egyptian and Greek physicians as a female illness in which the womb "wandered," producing symptoms wherever it was in the body. The term's influence reached modern psychiatry: conversion hysteria, somatization disorder, and hysterical personality disorder. The latter became histrionic personality disorder (HPD) in the DSM-III. Currently, the argument is being made that HPD should be deleted from the Diagnostic and Statistical Manual system as it is infrequently seen in clinical practice (Novais et al., 2015) and research regarding its treatment is lacking (Paris, 2015).

Despite its roots in hysteria, HPD is not a female disorder: although more females may be diagnosed with HPD in clinical settings, its prevalence is similar across genders (APA, 2013). "Attention seeking" and "emotional" describe people with HPD, who are lively and dramatic and draw attention to themselves by their enthusiasm, dress, and apparent openness; they can be "the life of the party." Their speech, too, is dramatic; strong opinions without supporting facts are often expressed and readily changed. (A further historical note: "histrione" was used in ancient Rome to name actors in farces representing characters who were false and theatrical [Novais et al., 2015].) Persistent need for attention and approval is an aspect of this PD.

The person with HPD may be moody and experience a sense of helplessness when others are disinterested in them. Although they may be hypersensitive to the moods and thoughts of those they hope to please, individuals with HPD have difficulty achieving genuine intimacy in interpersonal relationships (Sadock et al., 2015). Their need for constant attention can quickly alienate others; without such attention they may become depressed.

As culture affects the norms for physical appearance, interpersonal behaviour, and emotional expressiveness, the traits expressed by an individual must be evaluated in context as to whether clinically significant impairment or distress exists before a diagnosis of HPD is made (APA, 2013). This disorder may co-occur with BPD, DPD (discussed later in this chapter), and ASPD, as well as anxiety disorders, substance abuse, and mood disorders (Millon et al., 2004).

Nursing Care

The ultimate treatment goal for individuals with HPD is to help them change the tendency to fulfill all their needs by focusing on others to the exclusion of themselves. In the nursing assessment, the nurse focuses on understanding the quality of the individual's interpersonal relationships. Those with HPD can be dissatisfied with spouses, partners, and friends as insufficiently supportive. During the assessment, the client may make statements that indicate low self-esteem. Because these individuals assume that they are incapable of handling life's demands and that they need a truly competent person to take care of them, they have not developed a positive self-concept or adequate problem-solving abilities.

The nursing care foci for clients diagnosed with HPD generally centred around chronic low self-esteem, coping impairment, and intimacy and sexuality. Outcomes focus on helping the individual develop autonomy, a positive self-concept, and mature problem-solving and coping skills.

A variety of interventions support the outcomes. A nurse–client relationship that allows the client to explore positive personality characteristics and develop independent decision-making skills forms the basis of the interventions. Reinforcing personal strengths, conveying confidence in the person's ability to handle situations, and examining negative perceptions of self can be done within the therapeutic relationship. Encouraging the client to act autonomously can also improve the individual's sense of self-worth. Assertiveness training may help increase the individual's self-confidence and improve self-esteem.

Narcissistic Personality Disorder

The use of the term "narcissism" for excessive self-love came from an ancient Greek myth. A young man, Narcissus, upon seeing his own reflection in a forest pool, fell in love and died pining for his own image: "Unwitting youth, himself/He wants;—at once beloving, and belov'd" (Ovid, 1807/2009, p. 949). Individuals with NPD possess a form of self-love that causes problems for themselves and affects their relationships with others. They present as having an inexhaustible need for admiration, a grandiose sense of their own importance, and a lack of empathy (Sadock et al., 2015). The latter symptom is being challenged, as analysis of clinical cases suggests that empathy is not absent in individuals but dysfunctional and can fluctuate in terms of motivational disengagement or affective experience (Baskin-Sommers et al., 2014). Persons with NPD have a sense of being very special, which leads them to be preoccupied with fantasies of unlimited success, power, beauty, or ideal love. Their benign arrogance is associated with a strong sense of entitlement. Behavioural features associated with NPD include "vulnerable self-esteem, feelings of shame, sensitivity, and intense reactions of humiliation, emptiness or disdain to criticism or defeat, and vocational irregularities due to difficulties tolerating criticism or competition" (Ronningstam, 2012, p. 536). Others' perceptions of a person with NPD may be very different from that individual's self-perception. Behind grandiose notions of self-importance, for example, there may be a sense of insecurity (Ronningstam, 2012).

The aetiology of NPD is believed to include inheritance, temperament, and psychological trauma (e.g., neglect, deeply humiliating or fearful experiences, sudden loss of relationships); reactivation of such trauma can be a factor in seeking treatment. In addition, change and unexpected life events can threaten the individual's self-esteem, stimulate emotional reactions, and severely impact their functioning (Ronningstam, 2017).

Treatment for NPD is usually some form of community-based psychotherapy.

Nursing Care

The nurse usually encounters persons with NPD in clinical settings due to another medical condition, or at times a coexisting psychiatric disorder. Within the nurse–client relationship, it is important to listen carefully and attempt to understand the person's own perceptions of experiences, bearing in mind that the person may not readily self-disclose. Understanding their sense of self-agency is helpful as it reflects self-awareness, self-esteem, and self-regulation; it allows for some differentiation regarding real competence and accomplishments from grandiose or self-devaluated ones (Ronningstam, 2012, 2017). Individuals with NPD tend to have a sense of entitlement and expect special consideration and "service"; a therapeutic response to such demands may be required. Nurses must pay close attention to their own reaction to the client: it will give clues as to the way others may respond to the client, as well as indicate any issues with therapeutic use of self that need to be addressed.

Cluster C Disorders

Avoidant Personality Disorder

AVPD is characterized by a desire for affiliation that is affected by a sense of personal inadequacy and intense fear of social rejection (Sanislow et al., 2012). The person with AVPD thus avoids social situations, including occupational activities, in which there is interpersonal contact with others. They engage in interpersonal relationships only when they are certain that they will receive approval and be liked. They appear timid, shy, and hesitant. They perceive themselves as socially inept and inadequate and avoid new activities as they may be a new source of embarrassment (Sadock et al., 2015). Fantasy may become a means to gratify needs and to feel confident; withdrawing into fantasies can be a means of dealing with frustration and anger. Persons with AVPD experience feelings of tension, sadness, and anger that vacillate between desire for affection, fear of rebuff, embarrassment, and numbness of feeling (APA, 2013; Millon et al., 2004). They may have a fulfilling family life with their relationships restricted primarily to family members (Sadock et al., 2015).

Nursing Care

An assessment of these individuals reveals a lack of social contacts, fear of being criticized, and evidence of chronic low self-esteem. The nursing care foci centres around chronic low self-esteem, social isolation, and coping impairment. The establishment of a therapeutic relationship is necessary to be able to help the client meet treatment outcomes. The nurse should expect the nurse–client relationship to take time to develop, as the individual is usually inexperienced in positive interpersonal relationships and will need time to trust that the nurse will not be critical and demeaning. Interventions should focus on assisting the client to identify positive responses from others, exploring previous achievements of success, and exploring reasons for self-criticism. The person's social dimension should be examined for activities that increase self-esteem and interventions focused on multiplying such activities. Social skills training may help reduce symptoms.

Dependent Personality Disorder

Individuals with dependent personality disorder (DPD) are desperate to keep others close and will be over willing to do anything to maintain closeness, including being submissive and without regard for self. Decision-making is difficult for persons with DPD, who adapt their behaviour to please those to whom they lean upon for guidance. Ingratiating to others but self-denigrating, the person with DPD's self-esteem is other determined. Behaviourally, they are fearful of adult responsibilities and seek nurturance and support from others. In interpersonal relationships, they need excessive advice and reassurance. They are compliant, conciliatory, and placating. They rarely disagree with others and are easily persuaded. Friends describe them as gullible. They are warm, tender, and noncompetitive. They timidly avoid social tension and interpersonal conflicts (APA, 2013; Sadock et al., 2015). DPD bears resemblance to HPD; individuals with DPD demonstrate high levels of self-attributed dependency needs, while those with HPD have a greater implicit dependency and will even argue against needing others (Sadock et al., 2019).

Nursing Care

Nurses can determine the extent of dependency by an assessment of self-worth, interpersonal relationships, and social behaviours. They should determine whether there is currently someone on whom the person relies (e.g., parent, spouse) or if there has been a separation from a significant relationship by death or divorce.

Nursing care foci that are usually generated from the assessment data include coping impairment, chronic low self-esteem, impaired interpersonal relationships, impaired activities of daily living, and fatigue. Activities of daily living, for example, may be a problem if the client does not have the necessary skills and has to make decisions related to finances, shopping, cooking, and cleaning. The challenge of caring for these individuals is to help them recognize their dependent patterns, motivate them to want to change, and teach them adult skills that have not been developed, such as managing online banking, planning a weekly menu, and paying bills.

Occasionally, if a client is extremely fatigued, lethargic, or anxious and the disorder interferes with efforts at developing more independence, antidepressants or anti-anxiety agents may be used.

These individuals readily engage in a nurse–client relationship and initially will look to the nurse to make all decisions. The nurse can support these individuals to make their own decisions by resisting the urge to tell them what to do. Ideally, these clients are in individual psychotherapy and working towards long-term personality changes. The nurse can encourage clients to stay in therapy and to practice the new skills that are being learned. Assertiveness training is helpful therapy. Persons with chronic illness may be more susceptible than others to developing this disorder (Sadock et al., 2015).

Obsessive–Compulsive Personality Disorder

Obsessive–compulsive personality disorder (OCPD) bears a close resemblance to obsessive–compulsive disorder (OCD). A distinguishing difference is that those with OCD tend to have obsessive thoughts and compulsions when anxious but less so when anxiety decreases. With OCPD, the person does not demonstrate obsessions and compulsions as much as an overall inflexibility, perfectionism, and need to be in mental and interpersonal control. In an attempt to maintain control, the individual is preoccupied with orderliness, details, rules, organization, schedules, and lists; they have difficulty delegating tasks and working with others who may not do things exactly as they do (APA, 2013; Sadock et al., 2015). Their perfectionism can interfere with completion of tasks. As they have difficulty adapting to change, they strive to maintain a highly structured, organized life. They may have difficulty accepting new ideas and customs and react to them with rigidity and stubbornness. Nevertheless, persons with OCPD can do well in occupations requiring routine and attention to detail (Sadock et al., 2015). Some individuals with OCPD have difficulty discarding useless objects, even those without sentimental value (APA, 2013).

Nursing Care

Clients with OCPD generally seek mental health care when they have attacks of anxiety, spells of immobilization, sexual dysfunction, and excessive fatigue. To change the compulsive pattern, psychotherapy is needed. For instance, a clinical case report of therapy for a client diagnosed with OCPD with perfectionism and self-criticism describes the client as symptom-free after 6 months of metacognitive interpersonal therapy and without OCPD at a 6-month follow-up (Cheli et al., 2020). Psychotherapy may be augmented with short-term adjunct pharmacologic intervention with an antidepressant or anxiolytic.

The nursing assessment focuses on the client's physical symptoms (sleep, eating, sexual), interpersonal relationships, and social problems. Typical nursing diagnoses include anxiety, risk for loneliness, decisional conflict, sexual dysfunction, disturbed sleep pattern, and impaired social interactions. People with OCPD realize that they can improve their quality of life, but they will find it extremely anxiety provoking to make the necessary changes. A supportive nurse–client relationship based on acceptance of the individual's need for order and rigidity will help the person have enough confidence to try new behaviours. Examining the person's belief that underlies the dysfunctional behaviours can set the stage for changing them through alterations in thinking patterns. The course of OCPD is typically fluctuating; when it begins in childhood, it tends to be more severe (Gorman & Abi-Jaoude, 2014).

Continuum of Care

Persons with cluster C PDs are typically treated with psychotherapy in the community, unless a coexisting disorder, such as depression, requires short-term hospitalization. Group and behaviour therapy can be helpful to augment positive changes.

Other Personality Disorders

Other PDs identified in the *DSM-5* but not addressed in this chapter are *General Personality Disorder, Personality Change Due to Another Medical Condition, Other Specified Personality Disorder* (does not meet full criteria for a PD), and *Unspecified Personality Disorder* (does not meet full criteria due to insufficient information or clinician's choice) (APA, 2013). See the DSM-5 for information about these PDs.

Disruptive, Impulse Control, and Conduct Disorders

Disruptive, impulse control, and conduct disorders are combined in the *DSM-5*. They are characterized by emotional and behavioural self-control problems that lead to violation of the rights of others or bring the person into conflict with societal norms or authority figures (APA, 2013). The underlying causes of these problems vary greatly, even among individuals with the same diagnosis (APA, 2013). The risk factors for them may be temperamental, genetic, epigenetic, physiologic, environmental, or an interaction among such factors.

These disorders, which often coexist with other disorders, are identified by the APA as follows:

- Oppositional defiant disorder
- Intermittent explosive disorder
- Conduct disorder
- Kleptomania
- Pyromania

Of these disorders, intermittent explosive disorder, **pyromania**, and **kleptomania** are considered in this chapter. Oppositional defiant disorder and conduct disorder are discussed in Chapter 30, "Psychiatric Disorders in Children and Adolescents." As previously noted, ASPD is listed in the *DSM-5* with the disruptive, impulse control, and conduct disorders as well as with the PDs. For official APA criteria of the disruptive, impulse control, and conduct disorders, please see the DSM-5.

Intermittent Explosive Disorder

Individuals with intermittent explosive disorder (IED) have outbursts of verbal and/or physical aggressiveness, out of proportion to provocation, that result in an assault of persons or animals or in the destruction of property. These episodes are over in minutes or hours with the individual usually experiencing remorse. Such behaviour not only affects interpersonal relationships but can have serious psychosocial consequences, such as job loss, school expulsion, automobile collisions, legal fines, or imprisonment. This diagnosis is given only after all other disorders with aggressive components (e.g., delirium, dementia, head injury, BPD, ASPD, substance abuse) have been excluded. Risk for suicide can be high. In a study of individuals with posttraumatic stress disorder (PTSD), IED, or comorbid PTSD and IED, it was found that those with both PTSD and IED had a high rate of suicide attempts, as well as aggressive behaviour (Fanning et al., 2016). There is some evidence that IED is associated with childhood exposure to interpersonal traumatic events (Nickerson et al., 2012).

CBT, addressing cognitive **reframing**, coping skills, and relaxation, has been used with some success, including via video conferencing (Osma et al., 2016). Psychopharmacologic agents, such as fluoxetine, have been used as an adjunct to psychotherapy, but such treatment requires further research (Grant & Leppink, 2015).

Kleptomania

In kleptomania, individuals cannot resist the urge to steal, and they independently steal items that they could easily afford and/or that are not particularly useful or wanted (APA, 2013). The underlying issue is the act of stealing. The term kleptomania was first used in 1838 to describe the behaviour of several kings who stole worthless objects (Goldman, 1992). Individuals with this disorder experience an increase in tension and then gain pleasure and relief with the theft; they usually experience much guilt and shame afterwards. It is a rare condition (0.3% to 0.6% of general population) and occurs in about 4% to 24% of arrested shoplifters (APA, 2013). In clinical settings, approximately two thirds of clients with kleptomania are female; it is concurrent with a range of other mental disorders, including a 24% concurrency rate with bulimia (Grant & Potenza, 2008).

The rate of suicide attempts found in a study of persons with kleptomania was high (24.3%), with the majority attributing their suicidality specifically to their kleptomania (Odlaug et al., 2012). Researchers (Kim et al., 2017) who examined the incidence of addictive disorders among individuals with kleptomania (*n* = 53) found that approximately 21% (*n* = 11) met the criteria for an addictive disorder (four for substance use disorder, four for behavioural addiction [e.g., sex addiction, Internet addiction], three for both). This suggests that assessment of kleptomania should include assessment for addictive disorder, as well as the need for further research in this area.

Kleptomania, which seems to have an early onset and a chronic trajectory, is poorly understood, difficult to detect (individuals with this disorder actively hide it from family and friends), and challenging to treat. There is inconsistent success with various individual, group, and behavioural therapies; CBT is recommended but this approach, too, awaits further research (Aboujaoude et al., 2004; Grant & Chamberlain, 2018).

Pyromania

Although pyromania has been recognized as a mental disorder for about 200 years, its inclusion in the DSM-5

did not occur without debate, as some believe that there is insufficient evidence that it is a distinct disorder; its incidence appears to be less than 1%. It was first defined as a distinct pathologic disorder in 1833 by Henri Marc and viewed as an uncontrollable impulse to set fires (Nanayakkara et al., 2015); this understanding is similar to that of today. To be regarded as a disorder, and thus noncriminal behaviour, this intentional fire setting must be motiveless, except to achieve the arousal or relief it brings to the individual who is fascinated with fire. The frequency of fire setting for persons with pyromania fluctuates over time; there may be comorbidity with other disorders in this category, as well as with substance use, gambling disorders, and depressive and bipolar disorders (APA, 2013). (See the DSM-5 for specific criteria for pyromania.) CBT is used to treat this disorder (Burton et al., 2012), as are social skills training and the prescribing of SSRIs, but evidence for treatment efficacy is lacking (Nanayakkara et al., 2015).

Continuum of Care

Hospitalization for disruptive, impulse control, and conduct disorders is rare, except when there are comorbid psychiatric or medical disorders.

🍁 Summary of Key Points

- Personality is a complex pattern of characteristics, largely outside of the person's awareness, that compose the individual's distinctive pattern of perceiving, feeling, thinking, coping, and behaving. The personality emerges from a complicated interaction of biologic dispositions, psychological experiences, and environmental situations.
- Personality disorder is an enduring pattern of inner experience and behaviour that deviates markedly from the expectations of the individual's culture, is pervasive and inflexible, has an onset in adolescence or early adulthood, is stable over time, and leads to distress or impairment.
- In the *DSM-5*, personality disorders are organized around three clusters: A, B, and C.
- In cluster A, paranoid personality disorder is characterized by a suspicious pattern, schizoid personality disorder by an asocial pattern, and schizotypal personality disorder by an eccentric pattern.
- People with cluster A personality disorders, whose odd, eccentric behaviours often alienate them from others, can benefit from interventions such as social skills training, environmental management, and cognitive skill building. Changing the patterns of thinking and behaving is difficult and takes time; client outcomes must, therefore, be evaluated in terms of small changes in thinking and behaviour. People with

- BPD (cluster B) have difficulties regulating emotion and have extreme fears of abandonment, leading to dysfunctional relationships; they often engage in self-injury.
- ASPD (cluster B) includes people who have no regard for and refuse to conform to social rules, including the law.
- Individuals with cluster B personality disorders often have difficulties with emotional regulation or being able to recognize and control the expression of feelings such as anger, disappointment, and frustration. The nurse can help these clients identify feelings and gain control over their feelings and actions by teaching communication skills and techniques, **thought-stopping** techniques, distraction, or problem-solving techniques.
- Cluster C personality disorders are characterized by anxieties and fears and include avoidant, dependent, and obsessive–compulsive disorders. The obsessive–compulsive personality disorder differs from the obsessive–compulsive anxiety disorder because the individual demonstrates an overall rigidity, perfectionism, and a need for control.
- For many persons with personality disorders, maintaining a therapeutic nurse–client relationship can be one of the most helpful interventions. Through this therapeutic relationship, the individual experiences a model of healthy interaction, establishing trust, consistency, caring, boundaries, and limitations that

help to build the client's self-esteem and respect for self and others. In some personality disorders, nurses will find it more difficult to engage the individual in a true therapeutic relationship because of the person's avoidance of interpersonal and emotional attachment (e.g., ASPD or PPD).

• Individuals with personality disorders rarely receive inpatient treatment, except during periods of destructive behaviour or self-injury. Treatment is delivered in

the community and over time. Continuity of care is important in helping the individual change lifelong personality patterns.

• Although not classified as personality disorders, the impulse control disorders share one of the primary characteristics of impulsivity, which leads to inappropriate social behaviours that are considered harmful to self or others and that give the individual excitement or gratification at the time the act is committed.

 ## Thinking Challenges

1. Your friend LR is applying for a summer job as a research intern in the psychology department of the university. As part of the job application, he is asked to describe his personality. LR knows that you have learned about personality in your mental health nursing classes and asks you for advice on how to approach describing himself. How would you suggest he frame his answer?

2. MA, a 36-year-old woman receiving inpatient care, was admitted for depression; she also has a diagnosis of BPD. After a telephone argument with her husband, she approaches the nurse's station with her wrist dripping with blood from cutting. What interventions

should the nurse use with the client once the self-injury is treated?

3. Name the five core components of maladaptive personality functioning that can be used to describe the severity of a personality disorder.

> Visit the**Point** to view suggested responses.
> Go to **thePoint.lww.com/activate** and use the activation code found in the front of this text to unlock answers to the "Thinking Challenges" and other online resources.

 ## Web Links

borderlinepersonalitydisorder.com/consumer-recovery-resources This site provides information about recovering from borderline personality disorder, reviewed by a committee of people who have had the diagnosis and who are family members of a loved one with the diagnosis and two dedicated professionals who work with individuals diagnosed with BPD.

bpdcentral.com The site of BPD Central provides consumer, family, and professional information and resources.

bpdworld.org This British website provides information, advice, and support for those affected by personality disorders and other related conditions. This includes carers and professionals, as well as persons with BPD.

camh.ca/en/hospital/health_information/a_z_mental_health_and_addiction_information/Personality-Disorder/Pages/default.aspx This is the site of the Centre for Mental Health and Addiction in Toronto that provides information about personality disorders and their treatment.

References

Aboujaoude, E., Gamel, N., & Koran, L. M. (2004). Overview of kleptomania and phenomenological description of 40 patients. *Primary Care Companion to the Journal of Clinical Psychiatry, 6*(6), 244–247.

American Psychiatric Association (APA). (2013). *Diagnostic and statistical manual of mental disorders* (5th ed.).

Bach, B., & First, M. B. (2018). Application of the ICD-11 classification of personality disorders. *BMC Psychiatry, 18*, 351. https://doi.org/10.1186/s12888-018-1908-3

Bartholomew, K., & Horowitz, L. (1991). Attachment styles among young adults: A test of a four-category model. *Journal of Personality and Social Psychology, 61*, 226–244.

Baskin-Sommers, A., Krusemark, E., & Ronningstam, E. (2014). Empathy in narcissistic personality disorder: From clinical and empirical perspectives. *Personality Disorders, Theory, Research, and Treatment, 5*(3), 323–333. https://doi.org/10.1037/per000006.1

Bateman, A., & Fonagy, P. (2016). *Mentalization-based treatment for personality disorders: A practical guide.* Oxford University Press.

Bateman, A. W., Gunderson, J., & Mulder, R. (2015). Treatment of personality disorder. *The Lancet, 385*, 735–743.

Bennett, K., Shepherd, J., & Janca, A. (2013). Personality disorders and spirituality. *Current Opinion in Psychiatry, 26*, 79–83.

Bohus, M., Haaf, B., Stiglmayr, C., Pohl, U., Böhme, R., & Linehan, M. (2000). Evaluation of inpatient dialectical-behavioral therapy for borderline personality disorder—A prospective study. *Behaviour Research and Therapy, 38*(9), 875–887.

Bulechek, G., Butcher, H., & McCloskey Dochterman, J. (Eds.). (2008). *Nursing interventions classification (NIC)* (5th ed.). Mosby.

Burton, P. R. S., McNiel, D. E., & Binder, R. L. (2012). Firesetting, arson, pyromania, and the forensic mental health expert. *The Journal of the American Academy of Psychiatry and the Law, 40*, 355–365.

Carr, T. (2008). Mapping the processes and qualities of spiritual nursing care. *Qualitative Health Research, 18*(5), 686–700.

Cheli, S., MacBeth, A., Popolo, R., & Dimaggio, G. (2020). Clinical case report: The intertwined path of perfectionism and self-criticism in a client with obsessive-compulsive personality disorder. *Journal of Clinical Psychology, 76*, 2055–2066. https://doi.org/10.1002/jclp.23051

Clarkin, J. F., Yeomans, F. E., & Kernberg, O. F. (2006). *Psychotherapy for borderline personality: Focusing on object relations.* American Psychiatric Press.

Cleckley, H. (1941). *The mask of sanity.* Mosby.

Cloninger, C., Bayon, C., & Svrakic, D. (1998). Measurement of temperament and character in mood disorders: A model of fundamental states as personality types. *Journal of Affective Disorders, 51*(1), 21–32.

Crego, C., & Widiger, T. A. (2016). Cleckley's psychopaths: Revisited. *Journal of Abnormal Psychology, 125*(1), 75–87.

Crichton, R. (1959). *The great impostor*. Random House.

David, D. O., & Freeman, A. (2015). Overview of cognitive-behavioral therapy of personality disorders. In A. T. Beck, D. D. Davis, & A. Freeman (Eds.). *Cognitive therapy of personality disorders* (3rd ed., pp. 16–26). Guilford.

Dickens, G. L., Lamont, E., & Gray, S. (2016). Mental health nurses' attitudes, behavior, experience and knowledge regarding adults with a diagnosis of borderline personality disorder: Systematic, integrative literature review. *Journal of Clinical Nursing, 25*, 1848–1875. https://doi.org/10.1111/jocn.13202

Dimaggio, G., & Brüne, M. (2016). Dysfunctional understanding of mental states in personality disorders: What is the evidence? *Comprehensive Psychiatry, 64*(1), 1–3. https://doi.org/10.1016/j.comppsych.2015.09.014

Dimaggio, G., Salvatore, G., MacBeth, A., Ottavi, P., Buonocore, L., & Popolo, R. (2017). Metacognition interpersonal therapy for personality disorders: A cases study series. *Journal of Contemporary Psychotherapy, 47*, 11–21. https://doi.org/10.1007/s10879-016-9342-7

Dokucu, M. E., & Cloninger, C. R. (2019). Personality disorders and physical comorbidities: A complex relationship. *Current Opinion in Psychiatry, 32*, 435–441. https://doi.org/10.1097/YCO.0000000000000536

Edens, J. F., Kelley, S. E., Lilienfeld, S. O., Skeem, J. L., & Douglas, K. S. (2015). Predictive validity in a prison. *Law and Human Behavior, 39*(2), 123–129.

Erikson, E. (1968). *Identity: Youth and crisis*. Norton.

Fanning, J. R., Lee, R., & Coccaro, E. F. (2016). Comorbid intermittent explosive disorder and posttraumatic stress disorder: Clinical correlates and relationship to suicidal behavior. *Comprehensive Psychiatry, 70*, 125–133. https://doi.org/10.1016/j.comppsych.2016.05.018

Feigenbaum, J. (2007). Dialectical behaviour therapy: An increasing evidence base. *Journal of Mental Health, 16*(1), 51–68.

Fisher, K. A., Hany, M., & Doerr, C. (2021). Antisocial Personality Disorder (Nursing). In *StatPearls*. StatPearls Publishing.

Fonagy, P. (1991). Thinking about thinking: Some clinical and theoretical considerations in the treatment of a borderline patient. *The International Journal of Psychoanalysis, 72*(4), 639–656.

Friedman, H. S., & Schustack, M. W. (2012). *Personality: Classic theories and modern research*. Allyn & Bacon.

Gamache, D., Savard, C., Leclerc, P., Payant, M., Berthelot, N., Côté, A., Faucher, J., Lampron, M., Lemieux, R., Mayrand, K., Nolin, M. -C., & Tremblay, M. (2021). A proposed classification of ICD-11 severity degrees of personality pathology using the self and interpersonal functioning scale. *Frontiers in Psychiatry, 12*, 628057. https://doi.org/10.3389/fpsyt.2021.628057

Gillard, S., Turner, K., & Heffgen, M. (2015). Understanding recovery in the context of lived experience of personality disorders: A collaborative, qualitative study. *BMC Psychiatry, 15*(183), 1–13. https://doi.org/10.1186/s12888-015-0572-0

Goldman, M. (1992). Kleptomania: An overview. *Psychiatric Annals, 22*(2), 68–71.

Gorman, D. A., & Abi-Jaoude, E. (2014). Obsessive-compulsive disorder. *Canadian Medical Association Journal, 186*(11), E435. Appendix 1. www.cmaj.ca/lookup/suppl/doi:10.1503/cmaj.131257/-/DC1

Grant, J. E., & Chamberlain, S. R. (2018). Symptom severity and its clinical correlates in kleptomania. *Annals of Clinical Psychiatry, 30*(2), 97–101.

Grant, J. E., & Leppink, E. W. (2015). Choosing a treatment for disruptive, impulse-control, and conduct disorders: Limited evidence, no approved drugs to guide treatment. *Current Psychiatry, 14*(1), 29–36.

Grant, J. E., & Potenza, M. N. (2008). Gender-related differences in individuals seeking treatment for kleptomania. *CNS Spectrums, 13*(3), 235–245.

Gutiérrez, F., Peri, J. M., Gárriz, M., Vall, G., Arqué, E., Ruiz, L., Condomines, J., Calvo, N., Ferrer, M., & Sureda, B. (2021). Integration of the ICD-11 and DSM-5 dimensional systems for personality disorders into a unified taxonomy with non-overlapping Traits. *Frontiers in Psychiatry, 12*, 591934. https://doi.org/10.3389/fpsyt.2021.591934

Hare, R. D. (1991). *The Hare Psychopathy Checklist-Revised*. Multi-Health Systems.

Hare, R. D., & Neumann, C. S. (2009). Psychopathy: Assessment and forensic implications. *Canadian Journal of Psychiatry, 54*(12), 791–802.

Hayward, B. A. (2007). Cluster A personality disorders: Considering the "odd-eccentric" in psychiatric nursing. *International Journal of Mental Health Nursing, 16*(1), 15–21.

Helleman, M., Goossens, P. J. J., Kaasenbrood, A., & van Achterberg, T. (2014). Evidence base and components of brief admission as an intervention for patients with borderline personality disorder: A review of the literature. *Perspectives in Psychiatric Care, 50*, 65–75.

Hess, N. (2016). On making emotional contact with a schizoid patient. *British Journal of Psychotherapy, 32*(1), 53–64. https://doi.org/10.111/bjp.12193.

Hitch, D., Wilson, C., & Hillman, A. (2020). Sensory modulation in mental health practice. *Mental Health Practice, 23*, 10–16. https://doi.org/10.7748/mhp.2020.e1422

Hoffman, P. D., Fruzzetti, A. E., & Buteau, E. (2007). Understanding and engaging families: An education, skills and support program for relatives impacted by borderline personality disorder. *Journal of Mental Health, 16*(1), 69–82.

Holm, A. L., & Severinsson, E. (2011). Struggling to recover by changing suicidal behaviour: Narratives from women with borderline personality disorder. *International Journal of Mental Health Nursing, 20*(3), 165–173.

Hong, V. (2016). Borderline personality disorder in the emergency department: Good psychiatric management. *Harvard Review of Psychiatry, 24*, 357–366.

Hooley, J. M., Cole, S. H., & Gironde, S. (2012). Borderline personality disorder. In T. A. Widiger (Ed.), *The Oxford handbook of personality disorders* (pp. 409–436). Oxford University Press.

Hopwood, C. J., & Thomas, K. M. (2012). Paranoid and schizoid personality disorders. In T. Widiger (Ed.), *The Oxford handbook of personality disorders* (pp. 582–602). Oxford University Press.

Hummelen, B., Pedersen, G., Wilberg, T., & Karterud, S. (2015). Poor validity of the DSM-IV Schizoid personality disorder construct as a diagnostic category. *Journal of Personality Disorders, 29*(3), 334–346.

Hyde, L. W., Waller, R., Trenacosta, C. J., Shaw, D. S., Neiderhiser, J. M., Ganiban, J. M., Reiss, D., & Leve, L. D. (2016). Heritable and nonheritable pathways to early callous-unemotional behaviors. *American Journal of Psychiatry, 173*(9), 903–909. https://doi.org/10.1176/appi.ajp.2016.15111381

Jacob, J. D., Gagnon, M., Perron, A., & Canales, M. K. (2021). Revisiting the concept of othering: A structural analysis. *Advances in Nursing Science, 44*(4), 280–290.

Jordan, J. V. (2004). Personality disorder or relational disconnection. In J. J. Magnavita (Ed.), *Handbook of personality disorders* (pp. 120–134). John Wiley.

Jovev, M., McKenzie, T., Whittle, S., Simmons, J. G., Allen, N. B., & Chanen, A. M. (2013). Temperament and maltreatment in the emergence of borderline and antisocial personality pathology during early adolescence. *Journal of the Canadian Academy of Child and Adolescent Psychiatry, 22*(3), 220–229.

Kim, H. S., Christianini, A. R., Bertoni, D., Medeiros de Oliveira, M. C., Hodgins, D. C., & Tavares, H. (2017). Kleptomania and co-morbid addictive disorders. *Psychiatry Research, 250*, 35–37. https://doi.org/10.1016/j.psychres.2017.01.048

Koenig, J., Thayer, J. F., & Kaess, M. (2016). Pain sensitivity in self-injury: A meta-analysis on pain. *Psychological Medicine, 46*, 1597–1612. https://doi.org/10.1017/50033291716000301

Krause, E. D., Mendelson, T., & Lynch, T. R. (2003). Childhood emotional invalidation and adult psychological distress: The mediating role of emotional inhibition. *Child Abuse and Neglect, 27*, 199–213.

Kulacaoglu, F., & Kose, S. (2018). Review: Borderline Personality Disorder (BPD): In the midst of vulnerability, chaos, and awe. *Brain Sciences, 8*, 201–211. https://doi.org/10.3390/brainsci8110201

Kwapil, T. R., & Barrantes-Vidal, N. (2012). Schizotypal personality disorder: An integrative review. In T. A. Widiger (Ed.), *The Oxford handbook of personality disorders* (pp. 437–477). Oxford University Press.

Langlois, K. A., Samokhvalov, A. V., Rehm, J., Spence, S. T., & Gorber, S. C. (2012, modified 2013). *Health state descriptions for Canadians*. Statistics Canada.

Leahy, R. L., & McGinn, L. K. (2012). Cognitive therapy for personality disorders. In T. A. Widiger (Ed.), *The Oxford handbook of personality disorders* (pp. 727–750). Oxford University Press.

Lee, J. L. (2017). Mistrustful and misunderstood: A review of paranoid personality disorder. *Current Behavioral Neuroscience Reports, 4*, 151–165. https://doi.org/10.1007/s40473-017-0116-7

Leichsenring, F., Leibing, E., Kruse, J., New, A. S., Leweke, F. (2011). Border line personality disorder. *The Lancet, 377*, 74–84.

Linehan, M. (1993a). *Cognitive-behavioral treatment of borderline personality disorder*. Guilford.

Linehan, M. (1993b). *Skills training manual for treating borderline personality disorder*. Guilford.

Links, P. S., Kolia, N. J., Guimond, T., & McMain, S. (2013). Prospective risk factors for suicide attempts in a treated sample of patients with borderline personality disorder. *Canadian Journal of Psychiatry, 58*(2), 99–106.

Lohman, M. C., Whiteman, K. L., Yeomans, F. E., Cherico, S. A., & Christ, W. R. (2017) Qualitative analysis of resources and barriers for borderline personality disorder in the U.S. *Psychiatric Services, 68*(2), 167–172. https://doi.org/10.1176/appi.ps.201600108

Lynch, T. R., & Cuper, P. F. (2012). Dialectical behavior therapy of borderline and other personality disorders. In T. A. Widiger (Ed.), *The Oxford handbook of personality disorders* (pp. 785–793). Oxford University Press.

Lyness, J. M. (2016). Psychiatric disorders in medical practice. In L. Goldman, & A. I. Schafer (Eds.), *Goldman-Cecil medicine* (25th ed., Vol. II, pp. 2346–2356, e2). Elsevier Saunders.

Mack, M., & Nesbitt, H. (2016). Staff attitudes towards people with border-line personality disorder. *Mental Health Practice, 19*, 28–32.

Magnavita, J. J. (Ed.). (2004). The relevance of theory in treating personality dysfunction. In *Handbook of personality disorders: Theory and practice* (pp. 56–77). John Wiley & Sons.

Mahler, M., Pine, F., & Bergman, A. (1975). *The psychological birth of human infant: Symbiosis and individuation.* Basic Books.

Martin-Blanco, A., Ferrer, M., Soler, J., Arranz, M. J., Vega, D., Calvo N., Elices, M., Sanchez-Mora, C., García-Martinez, I., Salazar, J., Carmona, C., Bauzà, J., Prat, M., Pérez, V., & Pascual, J. C. (2016). Role of the hypothalamus-pituitary-adrenal genes and childhood trauma in borderline personality disorder. *European Archives of Psychiatry and Clinical Neuroscience, 266*(4), 307–316.

McKenzie, K., Gregory, J., & Hogg, L. (2021). Mental health workers' attitudes toward individuals with a diagnosis of Borderline Personality Disorder: A systematic literature review. *Journal of Personality Disorders, 36*(1), 70–98. https://doi.org/10.1521/pedi_2021_35_528

McMain, S. F., Boritz, T. Z., & Leybman, M. J. (2015). Common strategies for cultivating a positive therapy relationship in the treatment of personality disorders. *Journal of Psychotherapy Integration, 25*(1), 20–29.

Meaney, R., Hasking, P., & Reupert, A. (2016). Prevalence of borderline personality disorder in university samples: Systematic review, meta-analysis and meta-regression. *PLoS One, 11*(5), e0155439. https://doi.org/10.1371/journal.pone.0155439

Meuldijk, D., McCarthy, A., Bourke, M. E., & Grenyer, B. F. S. (2017). The value of treatment for borderline personality disorder: Systematic review and cost-effectiveness analysis of economic evaluations. *PLoS One, 12*(3), e0171592. https://doi.org/10.1371/journal.pone.0171592

Millon, T. (2016). What is a personality disorder? *Journal of Personality Disorders, 30*(3), 289–306.

Millon, T., & Davis, R. (1999). *Personality disorders in modern life.* John Wiley.

Millon, T., Millon, C., Meagher, S., Grossman, S., & Ramnath, R. (2004). *Personality disorders in modern life* (2nd ed.). John Wiley.

Moran, P., Romaniuk, H., Coffey, C., Chanen, A., Degenhardt, L., Borschmann, R., & Patton, G. C. (2016). The influence of personality disorder on the future mental health and social adjustment of young adults: A population-based, longitudinal cohort study. *Lancet Psychiatry, 3*, 636–645. https://doi.org/10.1016/S2215-0366(16)30029-3

Moroni, F., Procacci, M., Pellecchia, G., Semerari, A., Nicolò, G., Carcione, A., Pedone, R., & Colle, L. (2016). Mindreading dysfunction in avoidant personality disorder compared with other personality disorders. *The Journal of Nervous and Mental Disease, 204*(10), 752–757.

Nanayakkara, V., Ogloff, J. R. P., & Thomas, S. D. M. (2015). From haystacks to hospitals: An evolving understanding of mental disorder and firesetting. *International Journal of Forensic Mental Health, 14*(1), 66–75. https://doi.org/10.1080/14999013.2014.974086

National Health and Medical Research Council. (2012). *Clinical practice guidelines for the management of borderline personality disorder.*

Nehls, N. (1999). Borderline personality disorder: The voice of patients. *Research in Nursing and Health, 22*(4), 285–293.

Newbury-Helps, J., Feigenbaum, J., & Fonagy, P. (2017). Offenders with antisocial personality disorder display more impairments in mentalizing. *Journal of Personality Disorders, 31*(2), 232–255.

Newton-Howes, G., Clark, L. A., & Chanen, A. (2015). Personality disorder across the lifespan. *The Lancet, 385*, 727–734.

Nickerson A., Aderka, I. M., Bryant, R. A., & Hofmann, S. G. (2012). The relationship between childhood exposure to trauma and intermittent explosive disorder. *Psychiatry Research, 197*, 128–134. https://doi.org/10.1016/j.psychres.2012.01.012

Novais, F., Araújo, A., & Godinho, P. (2015). Historical roots of histrionic personality disorder. *Frontiers in Psychology, 6*(1463), 1–5. https://doi.org/10.3389/fpsyg.2015.01463

Odlaug, B. L., Grant, J. E., & Kim, S. W. (2012). Suicide attempts in 107 adolescents and adults with kleptomania. *Archives of Suicide Research, 16*, 348–359.

Oltmanns, T. F., & Powers, A. D. (2012). Gender and personality disorders. In T. A. Widiger (Ed.). *The Oxford handbook of personality disorders* (pp. 206–218). Oxford University Press.

Osma, J., Crespo, E., & Castellano, C. (2016). Multicomponent cognitive-behavioral therapy for intermittent explosive disorder by videoconferencing: A case study. *Anales de psicologia, 32*(2), 424–432.

Ovid. (1807/2009). *The metamorphoses of Publius Ovidus Naso in English blank verse, Vols. I & II.* J. J. Howard (Trans.). Project Gutenberg EBook. http://www.gutenberg.org/files/28621/28621-h/28621-h.htm

Paris, J. (2005). Understanding self-mutilation in borderline personality disorder. *Harvard Review of Psychiatry, 13*(3), 179–185. https://doi.org/10.1080/10673220591003614

Paris, J. (2015). *A concise guide to personality disorders.* American Psychological Association. https://doi.org/10.1037/14642-009

Parmar, A., & Kaloiya, G. (2018). Comorbidity of personality disorder among substance use disorder patients: A narrative review. *Indian Jour-*

nal of Psychological Medicine, 40(6), 517–527. https://doi.org/10.4103/IJPSYM.IJPSYM_164_18

Pearce, J. M., Hulbert, C., McKechnie, B., McCutcheon, L., & Betts, J., & Chanen, A. M. (2017). Evaluation of a psychoeducational group intervention for family and friends of youth with borderline personality disorder. *Borderline Personality Disorder and Emotion Dysregulation, 4*(5), 1–7. https://doi.org/10.1186/s40479-017-0056-6

Pederson, L. D. (2015). *Dialectical behavior therapy: A contemporary guide for practitioners.* John Wiley & Sons.

Petersen, R., Brakoulias, V., & Langdon, R. (2016). An experimental investigation of mentalization ability in BPD. *Comprehensive Psychiatry, 64*, 12–21. https://dx.doi.org/10.1016/j.comppsych.2015.10.004

Putnam, S. P., & Gartstein, M. A. (2017). Aggregate temperament scores from multiple countries: Associations with aggregate personality traits, cultural dimensions, and allelic frequency. *Journal of Research in Personality, 67*, 157–170.

Reichl, C., & Kaess, M. (2021). Self-harm in the context of borderline personality disorder. *Current Opinion in Psychology, 37*, 139–144. https://doi.org/10.1016/j.copsyc.2020.12.007

Rogers, B., & Dunne, E. (2011). 'They told me I had this personality disorder … All of a sudden I was wasting their time': Personality disorder and the inpatient experience. *Journal of Mental Health, 20.* 226–233. https://doi.org/10.3109/09638237.2011.556165

Romeu-Labayen, M., Tort-Nasarre, G., Rigol Cuadra, M. A., Giralt Palou, R., & Galbany-Estragués, P. (2022). The attitudes of mental health nurses that support a positive therapeutic relationship: The perspective of people diagnosed with BPD. *Journal of Psychiatric and Mental Health Nursing, 29*(2), 317–326. https://doi.org/10.1111/jpm.12766

Ronningstam, E. (2012). Narcissistic personality disorder: The diagnostic process. In T. A. Widiger (Ed.), *The Oxford handbook of personality disorders* (pp. 527–549). Oxford University Press.

Ronningstam, E. (2017). Intersect between self-esteem and emotion regulation in narcissistic personality disorder—Implications for alliance building and treatment. *Borderline Personality Disorder and Emotion Dysregulation, 4*(3), 1–13. https://doi.org/10.1186/s40479-017-0054-8

Ronningstam, E., Simonsen, E., Oldham, J. M., Maffei, C., Gunderson, J., Chanen, A. M., & Millon, T. (2014). Studies of personality disorder: Past, present, and future in recognition of ISSPD's 25th anniversary. *Journal of Personality Disorders, 28*(5), 611–628.

Rosenström, T., Torvik, F. A., Ystrom, E., Czajkowski, N. O., Gillespie, N. A., Aggen, S. H., Krueger, R. F., Kendler, K. S., & Reichborn-Kjennerud, T. (2018). Prediction of alcohol use disorder using personality disorder traits: A twin study. *Addiction (Abingdon, England), 113*(1), 15–24. https://doi.org/10.1111/add.13951

Rosenström, T., Ystrom, E., Torvik, F. A., Czajkowski, N. O., Gillespie, G. A., Aggen, S. H., Krueger, R. F., Kendler, K. S., & Reichborn-Klennerud, T. (2017). Genetic and environmental structure of DSM-IV criteria for antisocial personality disorder: A twin study. *Behavior Genetics, 47*, 265–277. https://doi.org/10.1007/s10519-016-9833-z

Ruocco, A., & Carcone, D. (2016). A neurobiological model of BPD: Systematic and integrative review. *Harvard Review of Psychiatry, 24*(5), 311–329.

Saarinena, A., Rosenström, T., Hintsanen, M., Hakulinen, C., Pulkki-Råback, L., Lehtimäki, T., Raitakari, O. T., Cloninger, C. R., & Keltikangas-Järvinen, L. (2018). *Psychiatry Research, 261*, 137–142. https://doi.org/10.1016/j.psychres.2017.12.044

Sadock, B. J., Sadock, V. A., & Ruiz, P. (2015). *Kaplan & Sadock's synopsis of psychiatry: Behavioral sciences/clinical psychiatry* (11th ed.). Wolters Kluwer.

Sadock, B. J., Ahmad, S., & Sadock, V. A. (2019). Personality disorders. In B. J. Saddock, S. Ahmad, & V. A. Sadock (Eds.), *Kaplan & Sadock's Pocket Handbook of Clinical Psychiatry* (6th ed.). Lippincott Williams & Wilkins.

Sanislow, C. A., da Cruz, K. L., Gianol, M. O., & Reagan, E. M. (2012). Avoidant personality disorder, traits, and types. In T. A. Widiger (Ed.), *The Oxford handbook of personality disorders* (pp. 549–565). Oxford University Press.

Santangelo, P. S., Kockler, T. D., Zeitler, M. L., Knies, R., Kleindienst, N., Bohus, M., & Ebner-Priemer, U. W., et al. (2020). Self-esteem instability and affective instability in everyday life after remission from borderline personality disorder. *Borderline Personality Disorder and Emotion Regulation, 7*(1), 25. https://doi.org/10.1186/s40479-020-00140-8

Schroeder, K., Fisher, H. L., & Schäfer, I. (2013). Psychotic symptoms in patients with borderline personality disorder: Prevalence and clinical management. *Current Opinion in Psychiatry, 26*, 113–119.

Schore, A. N. (2017). Modern attachment theory. In S. N. Gold (Ed.), *APA Handbook of trauma psychology, Vol. 1 Foundations in Knowledge* (pp. 398–406). American Psychology Association.

Sheehan, L., Nieweglowski, K., & Corrigan, P. (2016). The stigma of personality disorders. *Current Psychiatry Reports, 18*(11), 1–7. https://doi.org/10.1007/s11920-015-0654-1

Silk, K. R. (2000). Borderline personality disorder. Overview of biologic factors. *The Psychiatric Clinics of North America, 23*(1), 61–75.

Silk, K. R., & Feurino III, L. (2012). Psychopharmacology of personality disorders. In T. Widiger (Ed.), *The Oxford handbook of personality disorders* (pp. 713–726). Oxford University Press.

Stepp, S. D., Scott, L. N., Morse, J. Q., Nolf, K. A., Hallquist, M. N., & Pilkonis, P. A. (2014). Emotion dysregulation as a maintenance factor of borderline personality disorder features. *Comprehensive Psychiatry, 55*(3):657–666. https://doi.org/10.1016/j.comppsych.2013.11.006

Stern, A. (1938). A psychoanalytic investigation and therapy in the borderline group of neuroses. *Psychoanalytic Quarterly, 7*, 467–489.

Stone, M. (2016). Borderline personality disorder: Therapeutic factors. *Psychodynamic Psychiatry, 44*(4), 505–540.

Swannell, S. V., Martin, G. E., Page, A., Hasking, P., & St John, N. J. (2014). Prevalence of nonsuicidal self-injury in nonclinical samples: Systematic review, meta-analysis and meta-regression. *Suicide & Life-Threatening Behavior, 44*(3), 273–303. https://doi.org/10.1111/sltb.12070

Turner B. J., Dixon-Gordon, K. L., Austin, S. B., Rodriguez, M. A., Zachary Rosenthal, M., & Chapman, A. L. (2015). Non-suicidal self-injury with and without borderline personality disorder: Differences in self-injury and diagnostic comorbidity. *Psychiatry Research, 230*(1), 28–35. https://doi.org/10.1016/j.psychres.2015.07.058

Tyrer, P., Reed, G. M., & Crawford, M. J. (2015). Classification, assessment, prevalence, and effect of personality disorder. *The Lancet, 385*, 717–725.

Van Wel, B., Kockmann, I., Blum, N., Pfohl, B., Black, D., & Heesterman, W. (2006). STEPPS group treatment for borderline personality disorder in the Netherlands. *Annals of Clinical Psychiatry, 18*(1), 63–67.

Vandyk, A., Bentz, A., Bissonette, S., & Cater, C. (2019). Why go to the emergency department? Perspectives from persons with borderline personality disorder. *International Journal of Mental Health Nursing, 28*(3), 757–765. https://doi.org/10.1111/inm.12580

Verheul, R., Andrea, H., Berghout, C. C., Dolan, C., Busschbach, J. J., van der Kroft, P. J., Bateman, A. W., & Fonagy, P. (2008). Severity indices of personality problems (SIPP-118): Development, factor structure, reliability, and validity. *Psychological Assessment, 20*(1), 23–34.

Via, E., Orfila, C., Pedreño, C., Rovira, A., Menchón, J. M., Cardoner, N., Palao, D. J., Soriano-Mas, C., & Obiols J. E. (2016). Structural alterations of the pyramidal pathway in schizoid and schizotypal cluster A personality disorders. *International Journal of Psychophysiology, 110*, 163–170. https://doi.org/10.1016/j.ijpsycho.2016.08.006

Waldeck, T. L., & Miller, L. S. (2000). Social skills deficits in schizotypal personality disorder. *Psychiatry Research, 93*(3), 237–246.

Watts, J. (2019). Problems with the ICD-11 classification of personality disorders. *Lancet Psychiatry, 6*, 461–463. https://doi.org/10.1016/S2215-0366(19)30127-0

Waugh, M. H., Hopwood, C. J., Krueger, R. F., Morey, L. C., Pincus, A. L., & Wright, A. G. C. (2017). Psychological assessment with the *DSM-5* alternative model for personality disorders: Tradition and innovation. *Professional Psychology: Research and Practice, 48*(2), 79–89.

Warrender, D. (2018). Borderline personality disorder and the ethics of risk management: The action/consequence model. *Nursing Ethics, 25*, 918–927. https://doi.org/10.1177/0969733016679467

Werner, K. B., Few, L. R., & Bucholz, K. K. (2015). Epidemiology, comorbidity, and behavioral genetics of antisocial personality disorder and psychopathy. *Psychiatric Annals, 45*(4), 195–199. https://doi.org/10.3928/00485713-20150401-08

Weston, D., Beton, E., & Defife, J. A. (2011). Identity disturbance in adolescence: Associations with borderline personality disorder. *Development and Psychopathology, 23*(1), 305–313.

Widiger, T. A. (Ed.). (2012). *The Oxford handbook of personality disorders.* Oxford University Press.

Widiger, T. A., & Costa Jr, P. T. (2013). Personality disorders and the five-factor model of personality: Rationale for the 3rd edition. In T. A. Widiger & P. T. Costa Jr (Eds.), *Personality disorders and the five-factor model of personality* (3rd ed., pp. 3–11). American Psychological Association.

Winsper, C., Bilgin, A., Thompson, A., Marwaha, S., Chanen, A. M., Singh, S. P., Wang, A., & Furtado, V. (2020). The prevalence of personality disorders in the community: A global systematic review and meta-analysis. *The British Journal of Psychiatry, 216*, 69–78. https://doi.org/10.1192/bjp.2019.166

Zanarini, M. C., Ruser, T., Frankenburg, F. R., & Hennen, J. (2000). The dissociative experiences of borderline patients. *Comprehensive Psychiatry, 41*(3), 223–227.

CHAPTER

28 Sleep–Wake Disorders

Anne Marie Creamer

LEARNING OBJECTIVES

After studying this chapter, you will be able to:

- Describe the phases of sleep and physiologic changes that occur during sleep.
- Discuss the bio/psycho/social/spiritual factors that impact sleep.
- Identify strategies used to assess sleep and sleep disturbances.
- Explain the impacts of commonly used psychiatric medications and other substances on the stages of sleep.
- Discuss the interaction between mental illness and sleep.
- Describe the role nurses play in the assessment and management of sleep problems and sleep disorders.

KEY TERMS

- circadian • electroencephalogram (EEG) • obstructive sleep apnea • polysomnography • sleep architecture • sleep efficiency • sleep hypnogram • sleep latency • slow-wave sleep • zeitgeber

KEY CONCEPTS

- insomnia • sleep • sleep hygiene

Nurses need to learn about sleep because understanding this fundamental human need is necessary across all areas of nursing practice. As well, as nurses often work during the night, they need to be cognizant of the effects sleep disturbances have on their own health. Insufficient sleep, including chronic insomnia symptoms, is associated with obesity, high cholesterol, diabetes, hypertension, and cardiovascular disease, including myocardial infarction (Yiallourou et al., 2018). This is because sleep duration and quality are closely linked with metabolic functions through a number of factors including insulin sensitivity and secretion, inflammatory processes, hormones such as ghrelin and leptin that impact satiety, and appetite and energy homeostasis. Obesity is linked with obstructive sleep apnea (OSA), and those who are obese without apnea experience more waking in the night and daytime sleepiness. In Canada alone, financial losses due to workers not getting enough sleep amount to about 12 billion dollars a year (Hafner et al., 2017). In this chapter, the question "What is sleep?" is answered, the phases of sleep are explained, and sleep patterns over the life span are described. Sleep–wake disorders and some of the strategies used to assess these common problems are identified. Because insomnia and OSA are so common, bio/psycho/social/spiritual approaches to nursing interventions for these disorders are delineated.

Historical Perspectives on Sleep and Dreams

Over time, beliefs about the roles and importance of sleep and dreams have changed. In ancient times, the Egyptians and Mesopotamians thought that dreams were how the gods communicated their wishes to mortals (Palagini & Rosenlicht, 2011). Joseph, one of the most famous dream interpreters in the Bible, influenced the decisions of the Pharaoh with his interpretations. In fact, the earliest known document of dream interpretation was written by the Egyptians around 1275 B.C.E., and this papyrus is found in the British Museum. In Greek mythology, Oneiros, the god of dreams, and Hypnos, the god of sleep, help reduce human suffering. Interestingly, the Greek philosopher Plato ascribed the site of dream prophecy to the liver and felt that humans express their bestial desires while dreaming. However, Aristotle rejected the idea that dreams were prophecies and posited that dreams were residual perceptions travelling through the bloodstream and activating the heart. In the second century, an "diviner" from Asia named Artemidorus Daldianus described more than 30,000 different types of dreams.

In more modern times, the 18th-century German philosopher Leibniz posited that dreams were a product of the mind. This concept was developed further in the late

729

19th century when Freud described dreams as expressions of human emotions and attempts by the unconscious to reconcile psychological conflicts. Freud also hypothesized a mind/brain model that included neurobiologic aspects of psychological activities (Palagini & Rosenlicht, 2011). When Hans Berger, a German psychiatrist, recorded electrical activity in the human brain in 1928, he demonstrated that different, identifiable wave forms occurred during sleep and waking times (Roehrs, 2011). These brain signal recordings were called **electroencephalograms** (EEG), and they allowed scientists to conduct more detailed studies of sleep without waking the person. By the late 1930s, the major elements of sleep brain wave patterns were described. However, it was not until the 1950s that the cyclical variation of EEG patterns during sleep was identified. With the discovery of the rapid eye movement (REM) stage and its characteristic features, it became clear that sleep consists of two very different states: REM and non-REM (NREM). These states are as different from each other as each is from the wake state. Since then, a tremendous amount of research has explained much of what happens during sleep; among the many important questions that remain though, is *why* we sleep.

What Is Sleep?

Until recently, it was thought that sleep was a resting period for the brain; with the decrease of sensory input, brain activities diminish and sleep occurred (Roehrs, 2011). However, several other theories have been suggested (Harrison, 2012). For example, sleep is thought to have an important relationship with visual processes. Compared with the other senses, vision requires a very large amount of processing capacity in the brain; with sleep, visual input to the brain is reduced. Another theory is that sleep is necessary for the maintenance and enhancement of memory, with REM and NREM sleep playing different roles. However, it is known that because humans can go for extended periods of time without REM sleep, as is seen when individuals take different medications like tricyclic antidepressants, NREM can play a role, albeit less efficiently, in memory processing. Animal studies have found that during critical periods in life, sleep is required for brain plasticity processes that support the maturation of certain brain circuits. It is dumbfounding that so much about sleep remains unclear considering that we spend about one third of our lives sleeping!

As mentioned, there are two distinct types of sleep: REM and NREM. The NREM stage is further subdivided into three stages according to depth:

- intermediate stage 1 (drowsiness and sleep onset)
- light stage 2
- deep stage 3 or **slow-wave sleep** (SWS)

Until recently, there were four stages of NREM sleep, but stages 3 and 4 have been consolidated.

There are several terms used in relation to describing sleep. The amount and distribution of the sleep type and stages is called **sleep architecture**. In healthy young people, sleep progresses fairly consistently each night through stages NREM 1 to 3 within 45 to 60 minutes. NREM sleep always precedes REM sleep unless there are certain pathologies (e.g., narcolepsy). **Sleep latency** is the length of time it takes to fall asleep once the person lies down to sleep. Although differences in individual sleepers exist, when asked how long it takes them to fall asleep, normal sleepers will report 15 to 30 minutes. This suggests that stage 2 is related to when the person believes their fell asleep. The first REM sleep episode occurs during the second hour of sleep, and a more rapid onset of REM sleep may suggest a health condition such as a depressive disorder. It normally takes 70 to 100 minutes for a young healthy person to move from stage 1 through REM sleep. The sleeper may complete up to five cycles in a regular 8-hour night. A **sleep hypnogram** is a graphic display of the individual's experience of moving through the stages of sleep during a sleep period (Fig. 28.1). Another measure, **sleep efficiency**, is the ratio of the time spent sleeping to the total amount of time spent in bed.

The duration of the NREM–REM cycle usually stays the same, but as the night progresses, the REM periods become longer and the NREM episodes become shorter. The SWS phase that occupied much of NREM during the first third of the night occupies less time as the night progresses. During the period of drowsiness, as the person transitions from wakefulness to sleep, events such as their response to someone who asks them a question are often forgotten. The first REM cycle of the night is usually very short, lasting 1 to 5 minutes. These differences are thought to be related to different processes at work. The circadian oscillator (see below) is thought to influence REM sleep while more SWS at the beginning of the night is related to the homeostatic sleep system (see below). A good sleeper may return to wakefulness several times a night, with many of these occurrences taking place when the brain is moving between REM and NREM sleep and with changes in body position. However, these awakenings are usually only 30 to 60 seconds long and are not remembered upon arising. When asked, the sleeper may report waking one to three times in the night.

A person's usual length of sleep is dependent on several factors, including personal choice, genetics, and the length of time one has been awake since the last sleep. Most young adults report sleeping about 7.5 hours on a weekday night and 8.5 hours on a weekend night. However, several changes in sleep patterns occur over the person's lifetime (see below, special populations). Some people are "short sleepers," meaning they may require less than the usual amount of sleep. In comparison with those with insomnia, they have no difficulty falling or staying asleep and are not troubled by daytime sleepiness. Similarly, some individuals require longer than usual sleep time.

HYPNOGRAMS

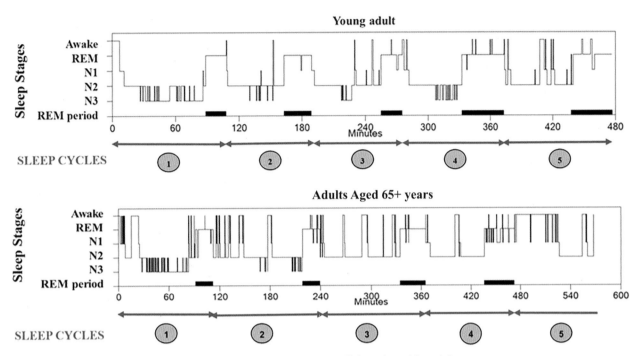

Figure 28.1 Comparing hypnograms of regular sleep seen in a young adult and an older adult. (Reprinted with permission from Sleeponitcanada. (2019). What is sleep? Sleep on it. https://sleeponitcanada.ca/all-about-sleep/what-is-sleep/)

Different events are occurring in the body during REM and NREM sleep (see Table 28.1). For example, during NREM sleep, the body can move and mental activity is usually associated with little or fragmented activity. In contrast, during REM sleep, the body is almost paralyzed except for episodes of eye movement and muscle twitches, and the brain is activated (Fig. 28.2). Therefore, someone walking about while dreaming is a sign of altered brain function.

KEY CONCEPT

Sleep is a behavioural and physiologic state of temporary disconnection from the environment, characterized by:

- Physical stillness characterized by no or few movements
- Stereotypical body postures (closed eyes, usually lying down)
- Reduced responsiveness to external stimulation
- Rapid reversibility between states, as compared with other states of altered vigilance like coma, hypothermia, or being anaesthetized (Landis, 2011; Peigneux et al., 2012).

▍ Dreaming

Initially, it was believed that dreaming occurred only during REM sleep, but now, it is believed that different types of dreaming occur throughout sleep from

"thought-like" brain activity that occurs in the early stages of NREM sleep to the vivid dreams typically reported in REM sleep (Mutz & Amir-Homayoun, 2017). The purpose of dreams is not yet known, but several theories have been suggested, some significantly different from others (Dubuc, n.d.). For example, Freud thought that our dreams are manifestations of our desires and motivation. In the 1970s, Hobson and McCarley (1977) proposed a model suggesting that dreams were the result of the brain's cortex being subjected to random stimulation by meaningless signals from the pons. However, we know that people who have injuries in different parts of the brain can still have REM sleep but not dream or not have REM sleep but report dreaming. Moreover, differences in REM and NREM dreams have been described. REM dreams tend to involve the senses and contain more emotional content whereas early night NREM dreams tend to be shorter, more fragmented, less vivid, more conceptual, and plausible. Interestingly, the dream experience has been compared to psychosis, especially the positive symptoms of schizophrenia, except that those with actual psychosis tend to judge their dreams as being less bizarre compared to those without psychosis. Figures 28.2 and 28.3 show which parts of the brain are activated during REM and NREM sleep. Research has found that people are better able to remember their dreams after taking a nap compared to remembering them after a normal night's sleep so it is hoped that studying dreams post naps will be more efficient. Dream therapy is practiced today as a

Table 28.1   Stages of Sleep

Stage	Percentage of Sleep Time During the Night	Physical Signs	Behavioural and Brain Activity
N1	2%–5%	Decrease in muscular activity; slow eye movement; pupils become smaller	Begin to fail to respond to auditory stimuli but easily awakened Awakened person reports not having been asleep
N2 Light NREM sleep	45%–55%	Eye movements stop; heart rate and respiration slow; body temperature, cerebral blood flow, and metabolism decrease.	Less likely to react to light or noise unless it is very bright or loud
N3 Slow-wave sleep (SWS); deepest stage of NREM sleep	13%–23%	Brain's temperature at its lowest; heart rate, respiration, and blood pressure decrease.	Harder to wake; possible confusion or disorientation after waking Will wake if the stimulus has strong personal meaning (e.g., mother hears her baby crying)
REM sleep	20%–25%	Rapid eye movements; general muscle tone is very low or absent; increased variability in pulse rate, blood pressure, and respiration Upper respiratory airway resistance increases; muscle tone in muscles associated with breathing is more flaccid. Body temperature is not regulated, no shivering or sweating. Partial or full penile erection	EEG waves look similar to waves seen in wakefulness. Waking is more likely to occur towards the end of REM sleep period. Cerebral blood flow and metabolism are restored to waking-state level. Dreaming occurs. High level of brain activity

form of psychotherapy that helps the dreamer increase self-awareness. However, "dream symbols," as found in popular books, do not have a scientific basis.

Biologic Processes

Process C and Process S

A two-process model provides a broad perspective on the sleep–wake cycle. These two processes oppose each other, enabling us to be awake during the daylight hours and sleep during the night. Process S, or homeostatic factor, represents sleep need. It drives how intensely we sleep, rising over the wake period and declining during sleep; the longer a person is awake, the stronger the drive to sleep. Additionally, loss of a specific phase of sleep results in a stronger drive to recover the lost phase. Adenosine, a brain compound, may be asleep-promoting substance that affects process S. Caffeine and theophylline, which is found in tea, act as antagonists at adenosine receptors and counter the effects of sleep deprivation.

Process C signifies circadian timing of the sleep–wake cycles in the day; the word "circadian" means "about the day." **Circadian** rhythms are biochemical, physiologic, and behavioural cycles (e.g., hormone function, body temperature changes) in the body, lasting between 24.2 and 25.5 hours. While the difference between a 24-hour day and 24.2- to 25.5-hour day does not seem significant, if the brain is unable to keep a consistent sched-

ule, over a 3-week period, this cycle would be reversed. Bodily processes normally occurring in the daytime would occur at night. Therefore, the body's ability to make adjustments to suit the individual's environment is essential.

Circadian rhythms are thought to be coordinated by molecular oscillations of neurons in the suprachiasmatic nuclei (SCN); two small areas in the left and right hypothalamus. Each SCN consists of a ventral SCN and a dorsal SCN. The neurons of the ventral SCN are believed to receive and respond to external inputs while the neurons of the dorsal SCN are believed to be the actual "clock." In order to maintain accuracy, these molecular oscillations are synchronized every day with external cues, also called **zeitgebers**. Examples of these cues include ambient temperature and noise, meal consumption, and the body's activity level. The strongest cue is the intensity of ambient light. These SCN neurons receive stimuli from specialized light-sensitive ganglion cells in the retina. Timing information from the SCN is then transmitted to the sleep–wake centres in the brain, including the pineal gland (Fig. 28.4). The neurons in the SCN also appear to release vasopressin in a cyclical pattern. This vasopressin acts only in the brain, impacting wakefulness, in contrast to pituitary vasopressin, which affects water metabolism throughout the body. There are also other oscillators located throughout the body, working at local levels.

The sleep–wake cycle is divided into two cycles, each about 12 hours long. The longest period of sleepiness

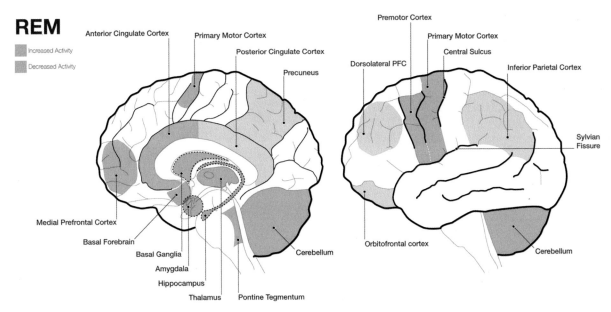

Figure 28.2 Brain areas activated in REM sleep. (From Muntz, J., & Amir-Homayoun, J. (2017). Exploring the neural correlates of dream phenomenology and altered states of consciousness during sleep. Neuroscience of Consciousness, 2017(1), 6. https://doi.org/10.1093/nc/nix009)

occurs when we normally go to bed in the evening and is deepest between 3:00 and 6:00 a.m. This is also when body temperature is at its lowest. A second period of sleepiness usually occurs between 2:00 and 4:00 p.m. It is interesting to note that if a person is exposed to bright light in the hours prior to the occurrence of minimum temperature, then the internal clock is reset to a later time. Alternatively, exposure to bright light after the body's lowest temperature is reached will move the clock earlier.

Several hormones fluctuate over the day, including melatonin, cortisol, and growth hormone. Melatonin is produced in the pineal gland under the control of signals from the SCN. Melatonin is released into the bloodstream, beginning in the midevening, 1 to 2 hours before the usual bedtime, and peaks between 2:00 and 4:00 a.m. The melatonin level begins to fall in the early morning because daylight inhibits the pineal gland's activity. As the level of melatonin rises, the need for sleep increases. Melatonin is thought to mediate dark signals and to stabilize and reinforce circadian rhythms.

The hormone *cortisol* is synthesized and released by the adrenal gland. Its levels are very low at bedtime but will rise as we sleep, reaching its peak at our usual wake time. Cortisol levels are minimally affected by whether we sleep during that time. Additionally, at the beginning of sleep and especially during SWS, the anterior pituitary releases a surge of *growth hormone*. The release of growth hormone will not occur if the person is not asleep, therefore of particular importance for children.

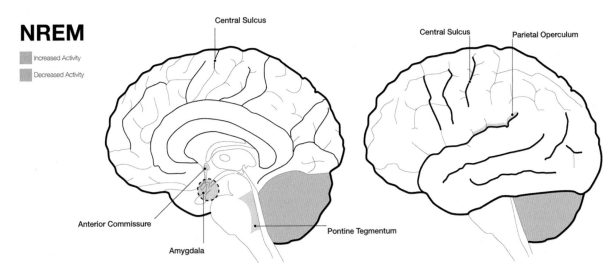

Figure 28.3 Brain areas activated in NREM sleep. (From Muntz, J., & Amir-Homayoun, J. (2017). Exploring the neural correlates of dream phenomenology and altered states of consciousness during sleep. Neuroscience of Consciousness, 2017(1), 7. https://doi.org/10.1093/nc/nix009)

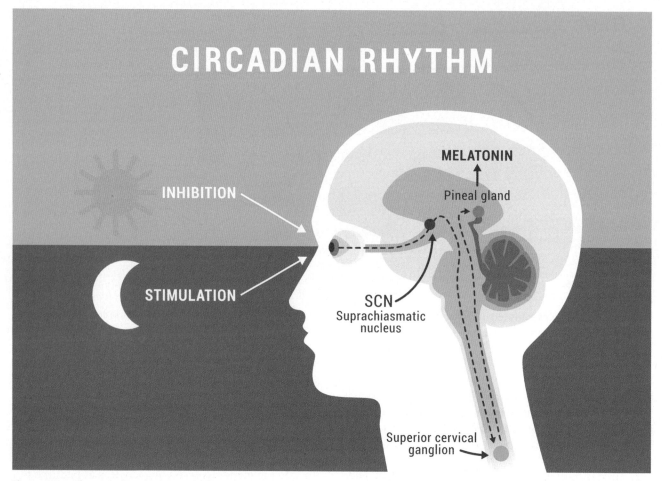

Figure 28.4 The circadian rhythm and affect of light on the sleep–wake cycle. (Shutterstock.com/elenabsl.)

Other hormones that are released during sleep or resting are prolactin, thyroid-stimulating hormone, and ghrelin and leptin, which are appetite-regulating hormones.

From a neurologic perspective, animal studies suggest that the medullary reticular formation, the thalamus, and the basal forebrain are involved in generating sleep, whereas the brain stem reticular formation, the midbrain, brain stem, thalamus, and the subthalamus are involved in generating wakefulness. Wakefulness is essential to survival and involves maintaining activation of the cortex. A complex network of neurons involving about 10 structures arising from the brain stem and progressing to the basal telencephalon supports the wake-promoting structures and the neurotransmitter acetylcholine plays a key role in the executive networks. Of note, Alzheimer disease is associated with a loss of cholinergic neurons and sleep disturbances.

The neurons associated with wakefulness and the phases of sleep are like switches: as neurons for one phase become active, another set ceases activity. When the wakefulness circuits are inhibited, the brain can transition through alternating periods of REM and NREM sleep. Additionally, different neurotransmitters involving the neural circuits are at work. The neurochemicals involved in sleep–wakefulness neural transmission include acetylcholine, histamine, norepinephrine, serotonin, hypocretin/orexin, dopamine, and glutamate (see Table 28.2). Other molecules that are involved in the sleep–wake process include adenosine, prostaglandin, cytokine, and GABAergic cells.

Recently, the glymphatic system has been described as a complex arrangement of molecular and fluid dynamics that plays a major role in waste removal in the brain (Shetty & Zantirati, 2020). This system is synchronized by the circadian rhythms and works primarily while we sleep. Research is showing that the accumulation of tau, one of the proteins implicated in Alzheimer disease, is regulated by the sleep–wake cycle. Sleep deprivation has been found to double the increase in tau and facilitates its spread to different parts of the brain including the hippocampus and locus coeruleus, areas involved in memory and maintaining wakefulness, respectively.

Normal sleep and several sleep disorders have been found to have genetic underpinnings, but a specific "sleep gene" has not been identified. Genome-wide association studies (see Epigenetics section in Chapter 10) have found many different areas on the human genome that are linked with sleep traits, such as timing of sleep, total daily sleep requirement, response to sleep deprivation, and several EEG measurements (Shi et al.,

Table 28.2 Neurobiology of Sleep

Neurochemical	Site of Synthesis	Wake (+) or Sleep (−)	Action
Acetylcholine (ACh)	Brain stem and anterior hypothalamus of the basal forebrain	+	ACh has high activity during wakefulness (especially the basal forebrain) and REM sleep and significantly lower activity during NREM sleep. Specific Ach-releasing neurons in the brain stem are selectively active during REM sleep to decrease muscle tone, thereby preventing motor activity during sleep. Basal forebrain Ach cells are involved in promoting wakefulness behaviours, especially attention, sensory processing, and learning.
Histamine (HA)	HA cells in the posterior hypothalamus project into wake-promoting areas in the brain stem and basal forebrain.	+	Neurons from this region are most active, and HA release is highest during periods of wakefulness; less so during NREM sleep and least so during REM sleep. HA improves attention and psychomotor performance. Lesions in this area of the brain produce a coma-like sleepiness.
Norepinephrine (NE)	Locus coeruleus of the pons. NE-producing neurons extend into the cerebral cortex, hippocampus, and amygdala.	+	NE neurons fire regularly during wakefulness, slow down during SWS, and are inactive during REM sleep. During REM sleep, their inactivity seems to be related to loss of muscle tone. NE may be in promoting arousal in stressful situations, while excess NE may contribute to insomnia.
Serotonin (5-HT)	The raphe nuclei in the brain stem	+ (?)	There are many sources of 5-HT in the body, with at least 15 different receptors to bind to, influencing various behaviours in the body. Its impact on brain arousal is unclear, but it is thought that 5-HT cells are very active during wakefulness and decreased in SWS. 5-HT is not active during, and may even suppress, REM sleep. 5-HT may play a role in regulating muscle tone during sleep.
Hypocretin/orexin	Lateral hypothalamus between sleep-initiating GABA cells in the anterior hypothalamus and the wake-initiating histamine cells in the posterior hypothalamus	+	Wakefulness is sustained by projections of these neurons into many of the primary wake-promoting systems in the brain. Loss of these cells is associated with narcolepsy. Orexin also increases arousal in motivating situations such as seeking food.
Dopamine	Substantia nigra compacta and ventral tegmental area in the midbrain	+	Extracellular concentrations of dopamine are increased during wake periods.
Glutamate	Mesencephalic reticular formation in the midbrain	+	Imaging techniques have shown that these cells are more active during wakefulness, supporting the proposal that they are important in maintaining wakefulness. Lesions in this region may cause a coma-like state of sleepiness.
Ghrelin and neuropeptide Y (NPY)	Hypothalamus	+	A hypothalamic NPY–orexin–ghrelin network is involved in integrating circadian, visual, and metabolic signals. The effects of ghrelin are less well understood. Sleep restriction to 4 hours a night is associated with increased plasma ghrelin levels and increased hunger.
GABA	Hypothalamus	−	GABA neurons are most active during NREM sleep, less so during REM sleep, and least so during wake periods. They are the most powerful sleep promoters in the brain. Bursts of GABA blocks transmission of signals into the cortex by inhibiting the histamine and cholinergic systems and serotonin and norepinephrine activity in the brain stem. Growth hormone–releasing hormone facilitates GABA.

Adapted from Peigneux, P., Urbain, C., & Schmitz, R. (2012). Sleep and the brain. In C. Morin & C. Espie (Eds.), *The Oxford handbook of sleep and sleep disorders* (pp. 11–37). Oxford University Press.

2017). Life processes such as aging and stressors such as sleep deprivation have been found to alter epigenome expression, or the way that the genes control how the body works (Gaine et al., 2018).

Sleep Pattern Changes Across the Life Span

Children

In the developing foetus, electrical patterns that can be associated with different sleep types are seen at about 28-week gestation (Graven & Browne, 2008). REM sleep, which takes up most of the sleep cycle at this early developmental phase, is thought to be associated with the development of the sensory systems. When the baby is full term, the REM and NREM phases comprise equal parts of sleep (50:50). The ratio of REM to NREM sleep time changes over the next year, with REM sleep making up 20% of total sleep time by 12 months of age. REM to NREM sleep time will remain at that ratio for the rest of the life span. The sleep cycle of a newborn lasts approximately 60 minutes, and it lengthens to 90 minutes with age. As the child ages, the need for sleep decreases from 16 to 20 hours a day in newborns to 10 to 11 hours a day in preschool and school-aged children. The 2016 ParticipACTION report card revealed that one third of 5- to 13-year-old children and 45% of 14- to 17-year-old youth in Canada have trouble falling or staying asleep (ParticipACTION, 2016). The role of sleep on brain development is still being studied, but there is evidence to suggest that sleep restriction seems to affect different parts of adult and child brains (Kurth et al., 2016). Additionally, children are more sensitive to light; melatonin suppression in children, by light at a typical indoor light level, is almost twice that of adults (LeBourgeois et al., 2017). Nurses can play an important role in educating families about the vital role sleep plays in children's development.

Another important role for nurses is to teach parents the importance of having infants sleep on their backs to minimize the risk of sudden infant death syndrome. Despite being the recommended practice, a survey of American mothers who were 2 to 6 months postpartum found that almost 22% of the mothers placed their babies in a sleep position other than on their backs (Bombard et al., 2018). A survey of Canadian women (*n* = 6,421) who had a baby between 5 and 9 months of age found that mothers with less than high school education were more than twice as likely to not put their babies on their backs to sleep (Smylie et al., 2014).

Adolescents

A change in the circadian rhythm system and a slower buildup of homeostatic sleep pressure are observed during puberty. Other environmental influences such as school and homework, social and extracurricular activities, employment, and increased electronic media exposure (screen time) impact the total sleep time adolescents are getting. Excessive screen time has been found to be associated with delayed bedtimes and less sleep among children and adolescents in more than 60 observational studies around the world (LeBourgeois et al., 2017).

In terms of sleep requirement per night, healthy children aged 11 to 13 years need 9 to 11 hours, those aged 14 to 17 years should have 8 to 10, and those 18 years and older require 7 to 9 hours. However, a survey of more than ten thousand Ontario middle and high school students found that 66.2% were not meeting those recommendations (Lien et al., 2020). Poor or insufficient sleep amongst adolescents has been found to be associated with an increased risk of depression (Fernandez, 2019).

Sleep disturbance (both broadly defined and that of specific sleep disorders such as insomnia, nightmares, and sleep apnea) is consistently found to be a risk factor for suicidal thoughts and behaviors. As it is a modifiable risk factor, screening for sleep disturbance is being recommended as a component of mental health assessment, such as using a general screening question, "Do you have trouble sleeping?" (Pigeon et al., 2020, April 30). Other increased risks associated with poor sleep include obesity, alcohol, cigarette and other substance use, and motor vehicle accidents caused by driving while drowsy. Nurses can help adolescents and their families by educating them about sleep hygiene and encouraging parents to be role models.

Women

Compared with men, women generally have more difficulty getting to sleep and staying asleep (Driver, 2012). Women tend to sleep 15 to 20 minutes longer than men (7 vs. 6 hours and 42 minutes); they may awaken more easily and have more difficulty falling back to sleep. Additionally, women tend to use hypnotics more frequently than men, especially among older adults. Hormonal changes seen with the menstrual cycle, pregnancy, and menopause can all negatively affect sleep. Some menopausal women find that hormone replacement therapy can help sleep problems. Insomnia symptoms are a known predictor for depression, especially among women.

Older Adults

It is recommended that older adults get 7 to 8 hours of sleep a night. However, sleep gradually changes as we age. Sleep becomes lighter: there is less slow-wave and REM sleep and more superficial sleep (See Fig. 28.1). The older person awakens more frequently in the night, especially in the latter part of the night, and awakenings last longer. The circadian rhythm may shift an hour earlier, resulting in earlier bedtimes and morning awakenings (Bishop et al., 2016). The decrease in SWS is thought to reflect age-related neuronal loss in the brain. However, compared with younger adults, tests of alertness and attention in older adults who have been sleep-deprived found that the older adults performed better.

Compared with matched controls, older people with sleep disorders have more problems with memory encoding and retrieval, and attention span. Some describe visuoperceptual and orientation difficulties. The prevalence of some sleep disorders, such as OSA, periodic leg movement, REM sleep behaviour disorder, and advanced sleep phase disorder, starts to increase from about the age of 40 years. As many as 50% of older adults report difficulty initiating or maintaining sleep (Bishop et al., 2016). Other contributing factors to poor sleep include medical or psychiatric illnesses, psychosocial factors, and medications. However, older adults are more vulnerable to sleeping medications because of slower drug absorption and elimination. In fact, many of the medications used for insomnia are on the BEERs list, a list published by the American Geriatric Society which identifies potentially inappropriate medications prescribed to older adults (Fixen, 2019).

Cultural and Racial Factors

Research into the impact cultural and racial factors have on sleep is in the early phases. Researchers have looked at several aspects of sleep, including sleep duration, sleep architecture, and specific sleep disorders among people of different races. However, for nurse researchers, areas that may be of particular interest include how sleep and sleep disorders are perceived, which sleep measurement tools are culturally and linguistically appropriate, and what sleep health promotion interventions are effective.

Consequences of Inadequate Sleep

Inadequate sleep can result in a number of cognitive and psychological deficits. These include impaired performance of tasks requiring intense or prolonged attention, as well as cognitive slowing. Inadequate sleep impairs information processing and learning, cognitive flexibility, and imagination. Further, it decreases insight and ability to assess risks. Mood may be impaired; the person may experience depression, irritability, and anxiety (see Fig. 28.5). Chronically disturbed sleep both increases the risk for developing a mental illness and hinders recovery. For example, alcohol is linked with poor sleep quality and insomnia is associated with an increased risk for alcohol dependence. Sleep loss is linked with increased risk of motor vehicle accidents and non–motor vehicle accidents; errors associated with sleep loss were linked with the *Exxon Valdez* oil tanker spill in 1989 (*Exxon Valdez* Oil Spill Trustee Council, 1990) and the Chernobyl nuclear reactor disaster in 1986 (Mitler et al., 1988).

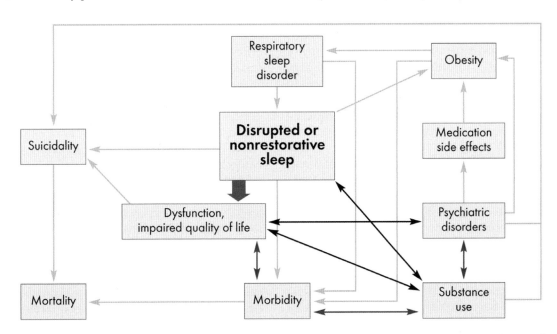

The primary effect of acute insomnia is daytime dysfunction, but when it is chronic, it is associated with psychiatric disorders that have a bidirectional relationship (coloured arrows) with sleep disturbance, substance use, dysfunction, and morbidity. Sleep deprivation, psychiatric disorders, and medication side effects can cause obesity that may cause or worsen a respiratory sleep disorder and directly or indirectly affect morbidity.

Figure 28.5 Interrelationship between disturbed sleep and dysfunction. (Source: Fleming, J. (2013). Psychiatric disorders and insomnia: Managing the vicious cycle. Insomnia Rounds, 2(1). https://css-scs.ca/wp-content/uploads/2020/09/150-007_Eng.pdf. Copyright © 2013 by the Canadian Sleep Society. Used with permission.)

Epidemiology: Canadian Sleep Habits

A survey of the sleep habits of Canadians aged 18 to 64 years between 2007 and 2013, found that men sleep on average 24 minutes less than women and individuals with a higher education and household income were more likely to sleep the recommended number of hours a night compared to those with less education and income (Chaput et al., 2017). However, among those 65 to 79 years of age, there was no difference in the length of time they slept. Women aged 18 to 79 experienced more trouble falling asleep when compared to men, "sometimes/most of the time or all the time."

Overview of Sleep–Wake Disorders

It is important to remember that occasionally having a disturbed sleep is a normal life experience, especially during times of stress. The sleep issue must cause clinically significant disturbances in a number of areas for a mental disorder diagnosis to be applied, and these disturbances must be attributed to dysfunctional processes that underlie mental functioning (American Psychiatric Association [APA], 2013). The *Diagnostic and Statistical Manual of Mental Disorders* (5th ed.) (*DSM-5*) (APA, 2013) lists 10 sleep–wake disorders. The category of sleep–wake disorders includes problems with staying awake when required. As with most mental disorder diagnoses, many of the sleep–wake disorders are further categorized by how long the symptoms have been present, the degree of severity, and whether another disorder or factor is playing a prominent role. The 10 disorders include insomnia disorder, hypersomnolence disorder, narcolepsy, breathing-related sleep disorders, circadian rhythm sleep–wake disorders, NREM sleep arousal disorders, REM sleep behaviour disorder, restless legs syndrome, and substance/medication-induced disorder. Additionally, the *DSM-5* has "Other Specified" and "Unspecified" categories that allow for diagnoses of conditions that have symptoms characteristic of a particular sleep–wake disorder but do not meet full criteria for the condition.

In contrast, the 3rd edition of the *International Classification of Sleep Disorders*, the most widely used system of sleep diagnoses, identifies 60 sleep disorders and provides an appendix that lists diagnoses of sleep disorders associated with medical and neurological disorders (Judd & Sateia, 2020). Detailed diagnostic criteria for each of these sleep disorders is beyond the scope of this chapter.

Sleep–wake disorders may accompany mental disorders such as anxiety and depression but, as previously noted, persistent sleep disturbances are also risk factors for the development of substance use and mental disorders. Furthermore, they may represent an early expression of an episode of mental illness. For example, a person with bipolar disorder may identify changes in sleep patterns as something that precedes an episode of mania. The nurse who is aware of this and intervenes early may prevent this person's hospitalization in addition to many other consequences of a manic episode. A study of 250 Canadians with a psychiatric diagnosis for at least one year determined that 27.6% of the participants had trouble going to, or staying asleep "all the time," compared with 6.8% of the general population (Schofield et al., 2016). Nurses should be aware of this relationship. Figure 28.5 demonstrates the links between impaired sleep substance use, morbidity, and impaired function (Fleming, 2013).

Other clinical disorders are also seen very commonly with sleep–wake disorders in particular, breathing-related sleep disorders, heart and lung disorders, neurodegenerative disorders (e.g., Alzheimer disease), and musculoskeletal disorders (e.g., osteoarthritis). How a person sleeps can affect how they are able to manage their other conditions. For example, people with chronic pain who sleep poorly have been found to have more difficulty coping with pain, decreased function, more emotional distress, lower positive affect, and more catastrophizing (Burgess et al., 2019). For this reason, it is essential to rule out and address contributors to sleep disturbances before assuming the issue can be addressed by a treatment for sleep complaints alone. Using the bio/psycho/social/spiritual framework, nurses can play an important role in identifying factors that affect sleep behaviours.

Sleep–Wake Assessments

Polysomnography is a sleep study that measures several variables associated with sleep (see Fig. 28.6). A sleep study can include an EEG, electrooculogram (EOG), electromyogram (EMG), and a video recording of the person sleeping. Other measures include oxygen saturation, electrocardiography, air flow, and respiratory effort. Based on the level of assessment required, different techniques are used. There are four levels of testing. A level 1 study includes many of the above measurements in a sleep lab, attended by a technician while a level 2 study records seven or more measures in a home sleep study. Level 3 sleep studies are frequently ordered by providers in primary care settings and records four to seven variables, including airflow and effort, pulse or ECG, and oxyhaemoglobin saturation, while a level 4 study involves recording one or two variables including oxyhaemoglobin saturation. Several factors can impact the results of these tests including fever, drugs, electrolyte imbalance, and hypoxemia.

EEGs measure electrical activity in the brain and record brain wave patterns. Electrodes are attached to the scalp using paste to pick up and record electrical signals produced by postsynaptic potentials in brain neurons. The signals are amplified, digitalized, and filtered then the result is examined for rhythms and transient

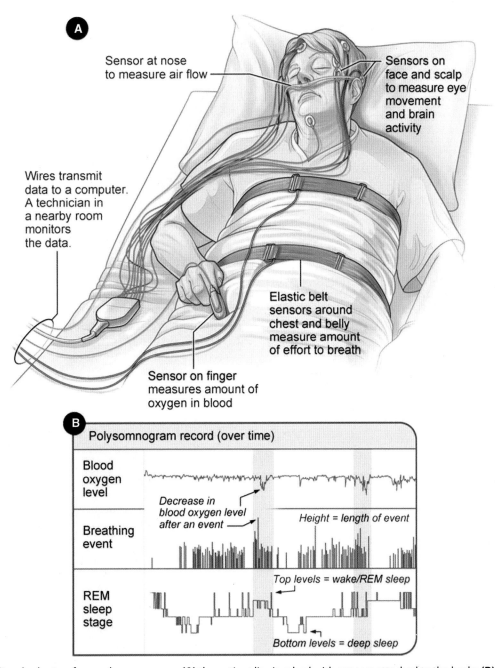

Figure 28.6 Standard setup for a polysomnogram: **(A)** the patient lies in a bed with sensors attached to the body; **(B)** the polysomnogram recording shows blood oxygen level, breathing event, and REM sleep stage over time. (Source: National Heart, Lung, and Blood Institute, U.S. Department of Health & Human Services. (2012). What to expect during a sleep study. www.nhlbi.nih.gov/)

events. The EEG plays a vital role in capturing the state of vigilance in the brain. In some settings, a cap with electrodes is worn. Other, newer technologies such as the ear—EEG sensors are being developed and tested in an effort to make EEG studies less cumbersome and costly, more user-friendly, and portable (Looney et al., 2016). Waveforms recorded by EEGs are specific to brain activity (Dubuc, n.d.). See Figure 28.7. For example, delta waves are seen in deep sleep and coma. Theta waves are seen when limbic system activity is noted; this would suggest that the emotions and memory are involved. Alpha waves occur when persons are alert, but the eyes

are closed and they are not actively processing information. Beta waves are seen when the person is alert and actively processing information; gamma waves may be related to communication between various parts of the brain when concepts are being formed. In NREM sleep, other waveforms called sleep spindles, K complexes, and high-voltage waves are seen. Paradoxically, the EEG waves of REM sleep are similar to those seen in someone who is awake.

Patients who are scheduled for an EEG should wash their hair with shampoo the night before the test but refrain from using other hair products like conditioners

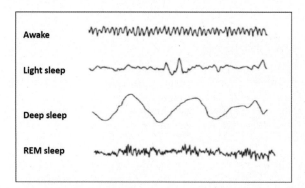

Figure 28.7 Recordings of waveforms recorded with the different stages of sleep. (Reprinted with permission from Sleeponitcanada. (2019). What is sleep? Sleep on it. https://sleeponitcanada.ca/all-about-sleep/what-is-sleep/)

and gels. They should not eat or drink anything containing caffeine for 8 hours prior to the test. Depending on the test's requirements, patients may or may not take their medications before the test. They may be asked to do certain things during the test, like look at a flashing light or breathe in and out deeply and quickly.

Eye movement in any direction generates electrical volt changes, and these changes are recorded with EOG testing. In essence, the moving eyeball acts like a small battery, and an electrode placed beside each eye records horizontal eye movements while an electrode placed above and below one of the eyes records vertical movements. Recorded eye movements will show when the person is in REM sleep.

An EMG records electrical activity generated with muscle activity. Electrodes are usually placed under the chin, where muscle tone changes associated with types of sleep are most apparent. The electrodes can also be placed on the limbs, most commonly the lower legs. As sleep approaches, muscles relax, and this change in activity is recorded. However, this test cannot show when sleep begins because, if the person is completely relaxed, there is no difference in the recording between sleep and being relaxed.

Respiratory and Cardiac Assessment

The person's efforts to breathe, and whether air is getting into the body, are assessed by different methods. Sensors pick up electrical or pressure changes and measure and record abdominal and/or chest movements. A sensor is placed in front of the person's nose and mouth to pick up changes in air temperature and pressure. Some sensors also pick up vibrations that occur with snoring. Measuring pulse oximetry using a sensor that fits over a finger or an earlobe provides information about respiratory functioning. Fingernail polish and acrylic nails can cause problems for recording for pulse oximetry. Sometimes, carbon dioxide levels in the exhaled air are also measured. Chest electrodes may be used to monitor the person's heart rate and cardiac rhythm.

Other Physiologic Measures

Orexin is a neural peptide that stimulates waking, is activated by emotional events, and inhibits sleep-promoting neurons. An orexin deficiency in cerebrospinal fluid levels is seen in narcolepsy. This peptide is inhibited during sleep by GABA. Melatonin level and minimum core body temperature measures are more likely to be used in research than in clinical practice.

Other Tests

Multiple Sleep Latency Test

The multiple sleep latency test (MSLT) measures the types (REM or NREM) of sleep a person has during the day. It is used to diagnose sleep disorders such as narcolepsy and idiopathic insomnia. In this test, the person is provided an opportunity to fall asleep in a dark, quiet room, four or five times over the course of a day. Brain activity and eye movements are recorded. In adults, average sleep latency (i.e., length of time it takes to fall asleep) is calculated. An average latency of less than 5 minutes indicates pathologic daytime sleepiness. An average latency of more than 10 minutes is normal. An average sleep latency of less than or equal to 8 minutes is one element in the diagnosis of narcolepsy.

Maintenance of Wakefulness Test

The maintenance of wakefulness test (MWT) is another daytime test that measures the person's ability to stay awake in a quiet setting for a period of time. It can be used to test for narcolepsy, response to medications, or the ability to stay awake for work or safety issues. In this test, the person sits quietly on a chair and is asked to stay awake for 40 minutes. These sessions are scheduled every 2 hours throughout the day.

Actigraphy

Actigraphy measures sleep–wake behaviour over several days and nights. The actigraph is a motion detector commonly worn on the wrist. It provides an indirect measure of several sleep–wake variables. The device is usually worn for about one week. This measurement tool can be helpful for populations that would be more difficult to assess using polysomnography, such as children and those with agitation or dementia. However, in some cases, it can overestimate sleep time, especially if the person is awake but not moving much. There are several commercially available trackers available on the market which claim to measure sleep and fitness.

Sleep Diary

A sleep diary to record information related to sleep over an identified period of time is a helpful tool in the assessment of sleep–wake patterns. Information collected may include waking time and time in bed, sleep latency, waking during sleep time, naps, lights-out time, medications, screen time, and caffeine, alcohol, and other substance intake.

Sleep Questionnaires

There are several questionnaires available for assessing sleep–wake disturbances for children and adults, including the Epworth Sleepiness Scale, Pediatric Sleep Questionnaire (PSQ), Children's Sleep Habits Questionnaire (CSHQ), Pittsburgh Sleep Quality Index, and Dysfunctional Beliefs and Attitudes about Sleep Scale (DBAS). As with all assessment tools, one needs to be aware of the tool's fit with the person's situation. For example, the Epworth Sleepiness Scale asks questions about driving a car, which are not always applicable.

Comorbid Mental Illnesses and Mental Health Problems

Sleep disturbances are commonly seen in the presentation of many psychiatric illnesses (Fleming, 2013). For example, one of the criteria of posttraumatic stress disorder is sleep disturbance, with 65% of people with this diagnosis experiencing significant problems such as insomnia and dreams and/or nightmares about the trauma. Those with generalized anxiety disorder (GAD) frequently experience difficulty falling or staying asleep, as well as a restless, unsatisfying sleep. Up to 70% of those with panic disorder can be awakened from sleep with a panic attack. Individuals with schizophrenia experience decreased latency to REM onset, more wake time in the night, less total and SWS sleep time, and taking longer to fall asleep. Disturbances noted in mood disorders include disruptions in sleep continuity, deficits in SWS, and REM sleep changes (Fleming, 2013). Approximately 80% of those with depression have insufficient sleep (see Fig. 28.8), while the other 20% sleep too much (Saleh et al., 2010). Many of the medications commonly used to treat psychiatric illnesses also affect sleep. See Table 28.3 for a list of medications used to treat other mental disorders and their impact on sleep.

Insomnia

Insomnia can be a symptom of mental disorders but when it is severe enough that it requires focused attention, it is classified as a comorbid illness. The fundamental characteristics of insomnia are being dissatisfied with sleep quantity or quality and having difficulty initiating and/or maintaining sleep. The *DSM-5* identifies several specific features of insomnia in addition to time and severity descriptors. Approximately 40% of people with insomnia also have a mental illness. Insomnia carries significant psychosocial, occupational, economic, and safety risks Numerous studies have demonstrated

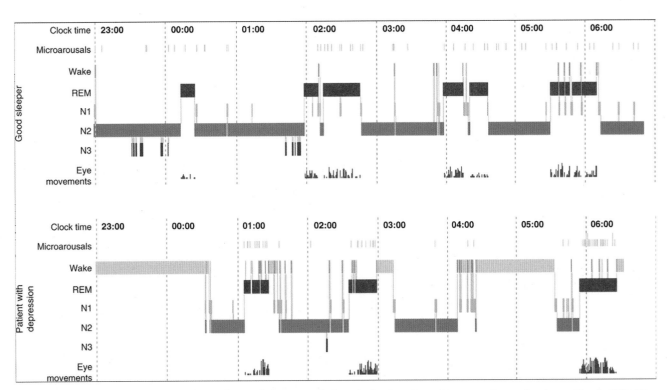

Figure 28.8 Comparing the hypnograms of a good sleeper and a hospitalized patient with severe depression (according to *DSM-IV*). Neither person had taken a psychotropic medication within the previous 14 days. (Adapted from Riemann, D., Krone, L. B., Wulff, K., & Nissen, C. (2020). Sleep, insomnia, and depression. Neuropsychopharmacology, 45(1), 75. https://doi.org/10.1038/s41386-019-0411-y)

Table 28.3   Effects of Commonly Used Psychiatric Drugs on Sleep and Waking

Drug Type	Examples	Pharmacologic Effect	Clinical Effects
Selective serotonin reuptake inhibitors (SSRIs)	Fluoxetine Fluvoxamine Citalopram	Increases extracellular levels of 5-HT, which inhibit REM sleep–producing cells	Decreased REM sleep Several SSRIs decrease sleep continuity and increase dreaming, nightmares, and sexual dreams.
Norepinephrine–dopamine reuptake inhibitors (NDRIs)	Bupropion	Inhibits reuptake of NE and DA into presynaptic neurons	Decreased REM latency and increased REM sleep; decreased slow-wave sleep
Serotonin–norepinephrine reuptake inhibitors (SNRIs)	Venlafaxine Duloxetine	Inhibits 5-HT and NE	Decreased sleep continuity and the percentage of REM sleep, vivid nightmares
Tricyclic antidepressants (TCAs)	Amitriptyline Nortriptyline Clomipramine Desipramine	Increases extracellular levels of 5-HT and NE, thereby inhibiting REM sleep–producing cells	Decreased REM sleep Some TCAs will increase slow-wave sleep.
Traditional amphetamine-like stimulants	Amphetamine Dextroamphetamine Methylphenidate	Increases extracellular levels of DA and NE	Increased wakefulness
Wake-promoting, nontraditional stimulants	Modafinil Armodafinil	Increases extracellular levels of DA	Increased wakefulness
Benzodiazepines	Diazepam Clonazepam Lorazepam Triazolam	Enhance GABA signalling via GABA$_A$ receptors	Shortened sleep latency, decreased nocturnal wake times, increased total sleep; decreased REM possible
Nonbenzodiazepine sedative–hypnotics	Zolpidem Zopiclone	Enhance GABA signalling via GABA$_A$ receptors, inhibiting the arousal systems	Improved sleep onset
Classic antihistamines	Diphenhydramine Triprolidine	Block HA H$_1$ receptors, reducing HA signalling	Increased NREM and REM sleep
Typical antipsychotics	Haloperidol Chlorpromazine	Block DA receptors, reducing DA signalling	Data inconclusive and inconsistent
Atypical antipsychotics	Clozapine Olanzapine Quetiapine Risperidone	See Chapter 13 for description of receptor-binding profile	Shortening of sleep onset latency (SOL), increases in sleep efficiency and total sleep time Olanzapine enhances slow-wave sleep and REM sleep
Mood stabilizers	Lithium	Exact mechanism unknown but may strengthen GABA inhibitory and reinforce serotonergic neurotransmission	Slowed circadian rhythms, increased slow-wave sleep and wake time after sleep onset, decreased REM sleep, increased sleep continuity
	Carbamazepine	Reinforces GABA and blocks excitatory glutamatergic neurotransmission	Increased sleep efficiency, decreased SOL, decreased wake time after sleep onset, increased slow-wave sleep
	Valproic acid	Similar to carbamazepine	Increased total sleep time and slow-wave sleep
	Lamotrigine	Similar to carbamazepine	Less well studied
Other mechanisms of action	Clonidine	Via α2-agonists, norepinephrine inactivates neurons in the locus caeruleus.	Increased NREM sleep
	Mirtazapine		Increased sleep continuity
	Trazodone		Increased slow-wave sleep and sleep continuity, suppressed REM sleep

Sources: España, R., & Scammell, T. (2011). Sleep neurobiology from a clinical perspective. *Sleep, 34,* 845–858; Mayers, A., & Baldwin, D. (2005). Antidepressants and their effect on sleep. *Human Psychopharmacology, 20,* 533–559; Riemann, D., & Nissen, C. (2012). Sleep and psychotropic drugs. In C. Morin & C. Espie (Eds.), *The Oxford handbook of sleep and sleep disorders* (pp. 190–220). Oxford University Press.

that nondepressed individuals with insomnia have double the risk of developing depression compared with those without insomnia. Nurses can perform an important role in assessing and supporting treatment. Additionally, they can serve critical roles as educators and participate in research and policy development.

Several factors and conditions are linked with insomnia. Medical conditions include psychiatric and substance use disorders, other sleep disorders, chronic pain, and cardiovascular, respiratory, neurologic, and urinary problems, to name a few. Treating insomnia in individuals with hypertension has been found to decrease the person's

BOX 28.1 Sleep Hygiene

Identify and break habits that disturb sleep:

- Set a bedtime and waking time. The brain will adapt to a fixed sleeping and waking time.
- Avoid daytime napping. Sleeping during the day will disrupt nighttime sleep. If a nap is necessary, limit it to 30 to 45 minutes.
- Avoid alcohol 4 to 6 hours prior to bedtime. While alcohol will induce sleep in the immediate term, sleep will be disrupted as the blood alcohol level decreases.
- Develop a bedtime routine. This may include a warm bath or shower, or consuming warm milk, which contains tryptophan, a protein thought to promote relaxation.
- Set aside time to relax prior to bedtime. This can consist of a formal activity, such as breathing or deep relaxation exercises, or more informal activities, such as listening to calming music or reading.
- Relaxation techniques can be helpful (see Box 28.4 for an example).
- Maintain a healthy diet. Eat moderately and at regular times throughout the day rather than eating a large meal in the evening. A light carbohydrate snack at bedtime might be helpful. Avoid greasy foods.
- Caffeine consumed later in the day or in the evening may disturb sleep.
- For those who wake hungry in the early morning, adding a snack at bedtime may promote a later sleep. Avoid sugary snacks and greasy foods at bedtime; consume food containing tryptophan or high in protein, which will take some time to digest and therefore maintain a more constant blood sugar level.
- Exercise regularly. Those who exercise vigorously in the morning sleep best.
- Go to bed and get up the same time every day, regardless of how much sleep is obtained. This will help set the biologic clock.
- Keep the bed only for sleep and intimacy time. Maintaining that space as an exclusive place strengthens the association between lying on the bed and sleeping. Using the bed for other daily activities, such as eating or surfing the internet, weakens the association between the bed and sleep.
- Keep a notepad and pen at the bedside to write down worries, thoughts, and plans that come to mind once in bed.
- Do not "try" to fall asleep or watch the clock if unable to sleep. This may make the problem worse. If unable to go to sleep, get up, leave the room, and do something boring.
- Ensure that the bedroom is comfortable (e.g., temperature, level of darkness, noise).
- Limit exposure to electronics before bedtime, and consider eliminating electronics from the bedroom.

blood pressure (Li et al., 2017). Frequently prescribed medications such as corticosteroids (e.g., prednisone), calcium channel blockers and beta-blockers (which are common antihypertensive medications), and decongestants are associated with insomnia. Examples of psychosocial stressors that are associated with insomnia include grief, job pressures, life changes, and the birth of a child.

Some behaviours perpetuate insomnia, such as drinking alcohol or consuming some other substances before bed, using the bed for tasks other than sleep and intimacy (e.g., eating, screen time), and ruminating about potential catastrophes (being fired, having an accident). Sleep hygiene is a term used to describe behaviours that promote healthy sleep habits. Box 28.1 reviews elements of sleep hygiene that nurses can include in educational programs.

KEY CONCEPT

Insomnia is "a subjective complaint of difficulty falling or staying asleep or poor sleep quality" (APA, 2013, p. 823).

KEY CONCEPT

Sleep hygiene is a term used to describe behaviours that promote healthy sleep habits (see Box 28.1).

Nursing Management: Insomnia

Nursing problems specific to sleep–wake disorders include insomnia and disturbed sleep pattern. When defining a nursing problem, several questions will help develop an understanding of what "normal" is for the patient and identify aspects of their sleep issues. The BEARS framework is a mnemonic that is helpful in guiding questions involved in assessing sleep (see Table 28.4). The person's medical and psychiatric history and collateral information from bed partners and family members need to be included in a comprehensive sleep assessment. See Figure 28.9 for the bio/psycho/social/spiritual outcomes of sleep loss.

Table 28.4 BEARS Sleep Screening Questionnaire	
Bedtime problems	Do you have any problems going to bed or falling asleep?
Excessive daytime sleepiness	Do you feel sleepy during the day? At work or school? Driving? Do you take naps during the day? When and for how long?
Awakenings during the night	Do you wake up during the night? What wakes you up? Do you have trouble getting back to sleep?
Regularity and duration of sleep	What time do you usually go to bed during the week? On weekends? How much sleep do you typically get?
Snoring and sleep-related breathing problems	Have you ever been told that you snore or seem to stop breathing in your sleep?

Adapted from *BEARS sleep screening questionnaire: Examples of developmentally appropriate trigger questions.* See Weiss, S., & Corkum, P. (2012). Pediatric behavioural insomnia—"Good night, sleep tight" for child and parent. *Insomnia Rounds, 1*(5). https://css-scs.ca/files/resources/insomnia-rounds/150-005_Eng.pdf

IN-A-LIFE

Charles Dickens (1812–1870)

PUBLIC PERSONA

Charles Dickens experienced significant episodes of insomnia during his lifetime (Horne, 2008). He walked the streets of London when he couldn't sleep, and drew inspiration from his encounters for many of his 15 major novels. He would return home to sleep exactly in the middle of his north-ward-pointed bed with his arms out and his hands equidistant from the bed's edges.

REALITIES

The term "insomniac" did not appear until 38 years after Dickens' time (Horne, 2008). In Victorian Britain, the usual remedies for sleeplessness were either alcohol (whiskey or brandy for those with higher incomes and gin for those with lower incomes) or opium. Laudanum, a solution of alcohol and morphine, was the most common form of opium consumed. It could be purchased easily and was so popular that Britain went to war with China to secure the free trade of opium. Another Victorian treatment for insomnia included embedding pillows with pieces of iron ore with magnetic polarity (called lodestones).

an eye mask, ear plugs, and a white noise machine to patients on a nonintensive care unit and then compared the effect of providing education on how to use the aids with those who were not educated about the aids found that patients who had the education used the aids more and had significantly less fatigue (Farrehi et al., 2016). See Box 28.2 for several nursing management strategies to promote a healthy sleep–wake cycle for hospitalized and institutionalized individuals.

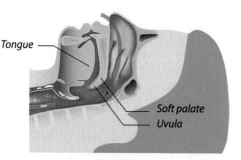

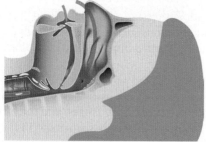

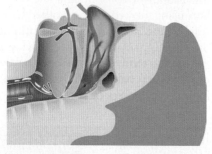

Figure 28.9 Normal airway, partial obstruction resulting in snoring and an obstructed airway seen in obstructive sleep apnea. (Shutterstock.com/Alila Medical Media.)

Hospital inpatient units are often guided by rigid routines that are directed by care providers' schedules. Someone who normally eats a snack, takes a shower, and then reads quietly in bed until they are tired enough to fall asleep will struggle settling to sleep when the routine is disrupted by being on a noisy, active unit with lights being turned on and off, doors opening and closing, and alarms and phones ringing. Quieter, more personalized settings are more conducive to promoting healthy sleep patterns. One study that provided sleep aids including

> **BOX 28.2 Nursing Management Strategies for Hospitalized and Institutionalized Patients**
>
> - Nursing and medical staff need to work together to minimize interruptions to patients' sleep at night.
> - Nursing stations are usually not soundproofed; nurses need to protect patient privacy and sleep. Noise reduction may be promoted with the use of a noise level monitor (e.g., Yacker Tracker) in the nursing station.
> - Promote specific quiet/sleep times for the nursing unit.
> - Identify the patient's normal sleep routines and facilitate maintaining them where possible.
> - Examine the medications the patient is taking to see if any might be affecting sleep; assess to see if any usual home medications have not been provided since admission.
> - Identify and manage barriers to sleep (e.g., pain, excessive fluid and caffeine intake) where possible.
> - Examine the environment for sources of possible disturbances: reduce alarm levels on equipment where possible; offer earplugs or headphones.
> - Offer light therapy, relaxation techniques, sleep education, back rubs, bedtime snacks, eye masks, and ear plugs.
>
> References: Gilsenan, I. (2012). Nursing interventions to alleviate insomnia. *Nursing Older People, 24*, 14–18.
> Graham, K., Ogbuji, G., Williams, Z., Crain, M., Rolin, B., Juala, J., Larbi, I., Bernard, N., Oster, C. A., Baird, M., & Gullatte, M. M. (2020). Challenges of implementing the choosing wisely guideline to promote sleep and rest at night for hospitalized patients. *Journal of Nursing Care Quality, 36*(1), 50–56. https://doi.org/10.1097/NCQ.0000000000000494

Biologic Domain

Insomnia is thought to be the result of an imbalance in the sleep–wake promoting systems of the brain, resulting in a state of hyperarousal. The consequence is an increase in body and brain metabolism, manifested by an increased heart rate and temperature and elevated cortisol, norepinephrine, and epinephrine levels. Factors that predispose an individual to chronic insomnia include genetic factors and biologic traits such as hyperactivity, hypervigilance, increased metabolic rate, and chronically elevated cortisol or reduced melatonin levels. Not only are sleep disorders linked to an increased risk of developing other physical illnesses, but physical illnesses such as congestive heart failure, neurologic diseases, breathing problems, and diabetes can precipitate or worsen insomnia. Many nonpharmacologic approaches may be helpful in the treatment of insomnia. These include acupuncture, exercise (including tai chi and yoga), massage, heat (sauna and hot tub), cooling (in hot environments), music and art therapy, and body and skin manipulations.

Pharmacologic Approaches to Insomnia

Historical Perspective

Over the ages, many different substances have been used to improve sleep (Riemann & Nissen, 2012). As mentioned, alcohol and opium products have long been used by some people to promote sleep. However, these substances are known to have high risk of abuse, dependence, overdose, and disruption to sleep architecture. Bromides were used in the early 20th century, but these

medications carried the risk of poisoning, nausea, rash, ataxia, and psychotic symptoms. Barbiturates were initially thought to be harmless, but they too were found to have a high risk of abuse, dependence, and overdose. Benzodiazepines (BZs) were introduced in the 1960s and initially they were thought to be effective and without risk of abuse, but evidence suggests that there is a risk of developing tolerance, rebound insomnia, and falls during the night. When zopiclone was introduced to Canada, it was claimed to carry less risk of falls, tolerance, and abuse. However, it has been found to have some risk of abuse and dependence. Lemborexant and suvorexant are dual orexin receptor antagonists (OX1R and OX2R), which is another new class of sleep medication. These medications promote sleep by decreasing the wake drive. (See Box 28.3 Research for Best Practice.)

Present-Day Pharmacotherapy

The benefit of sleep medication may be overestimated. A 2016 medical review of these medications found that evidence for important sleep outcomes was very limited (Wilt et al., 2016). Studies that compared effectiveness of the medications and how well they work in the long term are missing. Nurses need to keep in mind that not only can these medications cause cognitive and behavioural changes, but they have infrequently been associated with serious harm. A review of sleep preparations follows.

Herbal drugs sold OTC for sleep include humulus, passiflora, melissa, extractum cava, and valerian. Research on these products has not been comprehensive. Valerenic acid, thought to be the active ingredient

BOX 28.3 Research for Best Practice

Constantinescu, A., Warness, J., Virk, N., Perez, G., Shankel, M., & Holroyd-Leduc, J. (2019). Optimizing sleep for residents in long-term care without sedatives. *Annals of Long-Term Care, 27*(12), e7–e12. doi:10.25270/altc.2019.09.00086

Purpose: Sedatives for insomnia continue to be overprescribes despite several documented risks associated with their use in older adult populations. Warness, Virk, Shankel, and Holrody-Leduc sought to understand the effects of an evidenced-informed, educational intervention about older adult nighttime sedative use and sleep patterns for staff at a long-term care facility.

Method: A multifaceted educational intervention was implemented at a long-term care facility in Calgary, Alberta. Opinion leaders were developed among physician and nursing staff. Brief in-person nursing education and clinical decision support was offered, and physicians received letters explaining the project and sleep logs were maintained. Older adult residents living on five nursing units were involved in the study over 5 months.

Education addressed reasons for poor sleep and possible practical strategies to improve sleep. In addition to scheduled and as needed sedative–hypnotic use, nighttime sleep quality and quantity and daytime sleeping before and after educational intervention were measured.

Results: A nonsignificant reduction in the number of sedative–hypnotic bedtime tablets provided to the residents between the pre- and postintervention time periods was found. However, there was a significant decrease in the number of hours the residents slept in the daytime, while the number of hours slept in the nighttime increased.

Conclusions and Implications for Practice: Education for caregivers about nonpharmacological strategies to improve sleep for older adult residents in long-term care facilities has a positive effect on sleeping patterns. The entire healthcare team needs to be involved in addressing sleep concerns and nurses can play an important role in educating, advocating, and implementing sleep promotion strategies.

of valerian, may be related to benzodiazepine-like activity on the GABA receptors. The use of this product is not recommended near conception, during pregnancy, or during lactation, because of possible mutagenic effects. In randomized studies, valerian has been found to have more adverse effects, including liver toxicity (Neubauer, 2014). Overall, no clear evidence supports the use of herbal products for insomnia.

A list of commonly used medications, their dosages, onset of action, and half-life elimination is found in Table 28.5. Of note, first-generation antihistamines such as diphenhydramine and hydroxyzine are commonly used in OTC products for insomnia.

These medications have a 3- to 9-hour half-life, and CNS effects include sedation, decreased alertness, and slowed reaction times. Most drugs of this class also have some anticholinergic effects. The effects of these drugs on sleep have not been well studied and long-term use is not recommended. Other side effects include psychomotor impairment, dizziness, tinnitus, decreased appetite, nausea and vomiting, constipation, and weight gain.

Chloral hydrate has been used in the past for insomnia but is no longer recommended. It has been found to reduce sleep latency and improve sleep continuity without significant effect on REM or SWS. However, a serious

Table 28.5 Commonly Used Medications, Dosages, and Onset of Action and Half-Life Elimination

Medication	Dosage	Onset of Action	Half-Life Elimination[a]
Diphenhydramine (Benadryl)	12.5–50 mg	15–60 min 0–80 min	2.4–7 h
Doxepin (Silenor)	3–6 mg	30 min	15 h
Flurazepam (Dalmane)	15–30 mg	15 min or less	40–114 h
Hydroxyzine (Atarax)	50–100 mg	15–30 min	20–37 h
Ramelteon (Rozerem)	8 mg	45 min	1–2.6 h Metabolite MII: 2–5 h
Suvorexant (Belsomra)	10–20 mg	30 min	12 h
Temazepam (Restoril)	7.5–30 mg	30–60 min	9.5–12.5 h
Trazodone (Desyrel)	25–100 mg	1–3 h	7–10 h
Triazolam (Halcion)	0.125–0.25 mg	15–30 min	1.5–5.5 h
Zolpidem (Ambien)	5–10 mg	30 min	1.5–4.5 h
Zopiclone (Imovane)	5.0–7.5 mg (lower in older adults)	30 min	5–12 h

[a]Elimination can be affected by age and metabolic function.

potential side effect is the development of liver lesions and, because the range between therapeutic and toxic effect is narrow, overdosing can be fatal. Difficulties with tolerance, loss of effectiveness, and severe withdrawal syndromes on discontinuation have been reported.

Melatonin has been found to help with the symptoms of jet lag and have a mild reduction on sleep latency in those with delayed sleep-phase syndrome. In the short term (less than 4 weeks), the side effect profile is low, but caution is needed for those with liver impairment. There is minimal risk of abuse or tolerance. The recommended dose for OTC melatonin is 3 to 5 mg. L-Tryptophan, an essential amino acid in the human diet, is a precursor of serotonin and is thought to be metabolized to serotonin in the brain. It has been found to decrease sleep latency without affecting SWS or REM sleep. The recommended dose is 500 to 1,000 mg, and the half-life is 1 to 2 hours.

Benzodiazepines (BZs), such as lorazepam, and benzodiazepine receptor agonists (BZRAs) like zopiclone are probably the most commonly used medications for the treatment of insomnia. These medications work by binding to the GABA receptor site, thereby enhancing the flow of negatively charged chloride ions into the neuron and decreasing the postsynaptic neuron's capacity to generate an action potential. This effect is very powerful because $GABA_A$ receptors are the most widespread receptors in the inhibitory synapses, which constitute up to 30% of all synapses in the CNS. There are two types of $GABA_A$ receptors: type 1 is found in most parts of the brain, and type 2 is primarily located in the spinal cord motor nerves and hippocampus parental neurons. BZ medications bind to both type 1 and 2 receptors, while the BZRAs bind more specifically with type 1 receptors. This may explain why BZs have muscle relaxant, anxiolytic, and anticonvulsant effects and can cause nighttime falls that result from muscle relaxation. Other side effects of both the BZs and BZRAs include next-morning hangovers, next-day performance deficits, amnesia, sleepwalking, and nocturnal eating. Difficulty driving a car, attention problems, and hangover effects occur primarily with longer-acting BZs. Prescribers are encouraged to avoid using BZs and the BZRAs in the older population because there is an increased risk of cognitive impairment, falls, motor vehicle accidents, and delirium (Fixen, 2019).

The use of other psychotropic medications such as antidepressants and atypical antipsychotics as first-line treatment for insomnia has not been thoroughly studied and are not recommended primarily for sleep; the serious side effect profile for many of these medications will place patients at risk. However, other medications used to treat specific psychiatric conditions can impact sleep as a side effect; and indeed, this side effect should be considered when selecting a drug. For example, a side effect of mirtazapine, which is an antidepressant, is somnolence. This medication may be used for someone who has depression and insomnia.

Caffeine taken orally is absorbed rapidly; peak blood levels are reached after 30 to 75 minutes and the half-life of one dose of caffeine is 3 to 7 hours. With increasing amounts of caffeine intake, the duration of action is longer because the renal clearance of caffeine is delayed and paraxanthine, one of its metabolites, accumulates. Caffeine blocks adenosine receptors, which are found throughout the brain, blood vessels, kidneys, heart, and gastrointestinal tract. Adenosine is thought to promote sleep by inhibiting cholinergic neurons in the basal forebrain that normally mediate arousal. Anxiety, insomnia, and mood changes can occur with high doses of caffeine, in addition to high blood pressure, cardiac arrhythmias, and gastrointestinal effects. Taken 1 hour before sleep time, 77 to 322 mg of caffeine delays sleep onset, reduces total sleep time, and decreases SWS. No effect on REM sleep has been observed. Caffeine content in Tim Hortons' coffee in Canada can range from 140 to 330 mg per cup (Tim Hortons Research and Development, 2020). Caffeine has been found to improve vigilance, attention, reaction times, and several aspects of memory.

Many people use cannabis to help them to go to sleep, but this compound affects sleep in different ways (Kesner & Lovinger, 2020). Depending on whether the person is acutely intoxicated, chronically using it, or withdrawing from it, slow-wave and REM sleep are affected differently. See Table 28.6 for a description of the effects of cannabis on sleep.

Psychological Domain

Cognitive–behavioural models of insomnia posit that insomnia results from conditioning. Individuals with insomnia develop misperceptions and dysfunctional ideas about their sleep that affect their ability to initiate and maintain sleep. For example, a person can develop and retain an idea that they "will never sleep well," thereby perpetuating poor sleep. Some people with insomnia will complain of not sleeping at all, but polysomnography testing may show that in fact they do sleep. This is called a "sleep-state misperception"; it is thought to be caused by high-frequency EEG activity at sleep onset that may alter the person's perceptions of sleep and wake.

Table 28.6 Effects of Cannabinoid Type 1 on Slow-Wave and REM Sleep

	Acute Intoxication	Chronic Use	Withdrawal
Slow-Wave Sleep	Increased	Decreased	Decreased
REM	Decreased	Equivocal	Increased

Reference: Kesner, A. J. & Lovinger, D. M. (2020). Cannabinoids, endocannabinoids and sleep. *Frontiers in Molecular Neuroscience, 13*, 125. https://doi.org/10.3389/fnmol.2020.00125

Several psychological and behavioural approaches can be used to treat insomnia and other sleep–wake disorders. These include sleep hygiene education, relaxation training, and cognitive–behavior therapy (Garland et al., 2018), which includes stimulus control therapy, sleep restriction, and cognitive restructuring. Nurses have been involved in providing education about several of these therapies.

Stimulus Control Therapy

Stimulus control therapy involves implementing several behavioural strategies that promote conditioning the brain to associate the sleep environment with sleepiness. Strategies include using the bed for sleep and intimacy only (e.g., not screen time or eating), maintaining a regular wake-up time and bedtime, and avoiding napping. Other strategies include lying down only when sleepy, and getting out of bed if one cannot get to sleep within 15 to 20 minutes, and only returning to bed again when sleepy.

Sleep Restriction Therapy

Some people who are awake for long periods of time in the night will try to deal with poor sleep by sleeping later into the morning or going to bed earlier. This may lead to more difficulty falling asleep and subsequently, later sleep-ins. Sleep restriction helps to reset the sleep–wake cycle. It involves restricting the total time in bed at night to the average amount of time the person has been sleeping, as long as it is not less than 4 hours. Once the person maintains their sleep efficiency for that average number of hours for at least 85% of the time, the sleep window is expanded in 15 to 30-minute increments until no further time asleep is gained. The person is advised to maintain a consistent bedtime and waking schedule and avoid daytime naps. This will cause a partial sleep deprivation, making it easier to fall asleep the next night. Increasing daytime activity will help deal with any daytime sleepiness.

Cognitive Restructuring

One principle of cognitive therapy is that it is not the events themselves that are good or bad, but how we interpret the events. The goal of cognitive restructuring is to identify thoughts that contribute to the development or reinforcement of behaviors that disrupt sleep. These thoughts are then examined for accuracy and if needed, modified. Thought records are used to document the problematic thought and associated emotions (see Chapter 14).

Relaxation Training

Relaxation training involves learning and practicing several relaxation techniques that counteract muscle tension

---

BOX 28.4 The 5-4-3-2-1 Relaxation Technique

While lying in bed with eyes closed:

- Think of **5** things that you could see in your bedroom if your eyes were open. Then, listen for **5** things that you can hear. Once you have heard **5** things, identify **5** things that you can physically feel (e.g., your head on the pillow, one leg touching the other).
- Next, think of **4** things you can see, **4** you can hear, **4** you can feel.
- Then, think of **3** things…
- Then **2**…
- **1**…
- If you are still awake, begin again at **5**.

Adapted from O'Brien, D. (2017). *Self hypnosis: The Betty Erickson special.* http://ericksonian.info/therapeutic_scripts/self-hypnosis-the-betty-erickson-special/

---

and cognitive arousal. Examples of these include guided imagery, progressive muscle relaxation, and mindfulness. The 5-4-3-2-1 exercise is an example of a relaxation strategy that nurses can teach (see Box 28.4).

Social Domain

Social factors that predispose someone to chronic insomnia may include societal or bed partner demands that disrupt the person's sleep schedule. Low income, inadequate family support, and family and/or work stressors are all associated with insomnia. Daley et al. (2009) found insomnia cost the province of Quebec an estimated $6.5 billion, accounted for by healthcare visits ($191.2 million), prescription medications ($16.5 million), alcohol used as a sleep aid ($339.8 million), insomnia-related absenteeism ($970.6 million), and insomnia-related productivity losses ($5.0 billion). While dated, this suggests the many costs associated with insomnia.

Spiritual Domain

For some, spiritual distress can lead to insomnia. Conversely, insomnia can affect a person's capacity to address their personal spirituality. Some researchers have shown that engaging in spiritual activities is associated with improved sleep quality (Brewer-Smyth et al., 2020; Knowlden et al., 2018) while others believe that buffering factors confound this type of research. Bierman et al. (2018) examined sleep quality associated with levels of religious involvement among older people who chronically experienced discrimination, such as being treated as though they were less intelligent or as if others were afraid of them. They found that experiences of discrimination and sleep problems and level of religious involvement were not associated for men but there was a difference between groups of women. Regularly attendance at religious services acted as a protective factor for older women; they had fewer sleep problems compared to women who rarely attended services.

Obstructive Sleep Apnea

Obstructive sleep apnea (OSA) is the most common sleep-related breathing disorder. In 2016 and 2017, a Statistics Canada (2018) survey found that approximately 6.4% of Canadian adults have been told by a health professional that they have sleep apnea; with those between 60 and 79 years of age being three times more likely to be diagnosed with the disorder compared to younger adults. Men were twice as likely as women to have the disorder. However, the incidence of OSA is thought to be much higher; almost half of middle-aged men are thought to have OSA, with up to 82% of them being undiagnosed (Lang et al., 2017). Nurses can play an important role in helping identify people at risk for OSA, in addition to educating about and advocating for assessment and treatment. Also, nurses can help individuals identify factors that promote adherence to treatment and intercede.

Signs and symptoms of untreated OSA include snoring, witnessed apneas, morning headaches, poor concentration, irritability, erectile dysfunction, and restless sleep. A physical assessment may reveal an overweight person (although not always) and specific oronasopharyngeal characteristics such as a large tongue with or without a scalloping pattern on the lateral aspects and/or crowding in the posterior aspect of the pharynx, which may be erythematous and/or oedematous. Nurses can identify patients at risk for OSA by asking questions using the STOP and BANG mnemonics (see Table 28.7). Positive responses to at least three of the

Table 28.7	BANG and STOP Mnemonics for Assessment of Sleep Apnea
BANG	**STOP**
Body mass index greater than 35	Do you **S**nore?
Age greater than 50	Do you feel **T**ired, fatigued, or sleepy during the day?
Neck size greater than 40 cm	Has anyone **O**bserved your stopping breathing in your sleep?
Gender is male	Do you have high blood **P**ressure?

Adapted from Driver, H., Gottschalk, R., Hussain, M., Morin, C., Shapiro, C., & Van Zyl, L. (2012). *Insomnia in adults and children* (p. 35). https://css-scs.ca/files/resources/brochures/Insomnia_Adult_Child.pdf

eight questions suggest the need for a sleep assessment. Polysomnography is the best tool for assessing OSA but is not always available; portable home sleep studies are also used.

Nursing Management: Obstructive Sleep Apnea

Biologic Domain

In OSA, the person has partial and/or complete upper pharyngeal airway closure (see Fig. 28.10) accompanied by ongoing efforts to breathe, resulting in sporadic oxyhaemoglobin desaturation and broken sleep. Mixed apneas, which are apneas associated with and without respiratory efforts, are also common. Respiratory events are seen more frequently during stage 1 and 2 of NREM sleep and REM sleep as opposed to SWS. When the person has a respiratory event, they will arouse from sleep, thereby ending the respiratory event. A diagnosis is applied when there are more than five episodes in an hour of partial and/or complete airway obstruction, each resulting in at least 10 seconds of hypopnoea or apnea. Daytime symptoms include sleepiness and fatigue, impaired cognition and daily function.

Risk factors for developing OSA include increased body mass index (BMI), prevalence in men, craniofacial and upper airway abnormalities, and older age (Kline, 2020). Other possible risk factors include smoking cigarettes, consuming alcohol, and sedative and hypnotic medication use. Links have been found between OSA and pregnancy and specific medical conditions such as diabetes, polycystic ovary syndrome, hypertension, coronary artery disease, heart failure, and stroke. However, it is not known if the conditions are caused by OSA or contribute to their development.

There is not a lot of evidence to show a benefit in treating mild OSA, but untreated moderate and severe cases are linked with many negative consequences (Laratta et al., 2020). Treatments for OSA include continuous positive airway pressure therapy (CPAP) and other positive airway pressure strategies (e.g., Bi-PAP or APAP), surgical treatments, oral appliances, and weight loss. CPAP is most commonly used for treating OSA. It involves delivering a positive pressure into the person's airway through a nasal or full-face mask (see Fig. 28.11). This pressure will help maintain the patency of the airway. The use of CPAP therapy has been shown to reduce respiratory events and oxyhaemoglobin desaturation, but its impact on daytime outcomes is not consistent. There seems to be a different optimal CPAP use time for each particular outcome being assessed. Improvements have been found in subjective sleepiness (especially among those with severe OSA), quality of life measures, blood pressure, vigilance, OSA symptoms (e.g., snoring, dry mouth, morning headaches), and productivity after instituting CPAP treatment. However, adherence to CPAP is a

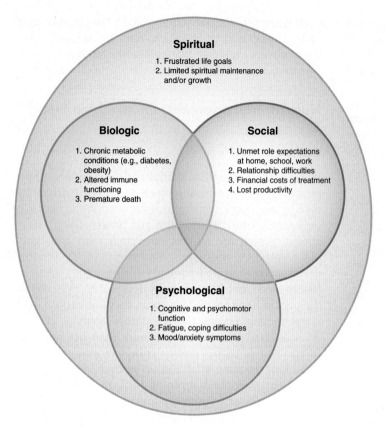

Figure 28.10 Bio/psycho/social/spiritual outcomes of sleep loss.

significant limitation to effective treatment; between 29% and 83% of CPAP users use this treatment fewer than 4 hours per night (Bakker et al., 2019). Behavioral therapies, motivational interviewing, cognitive–behavioral therapy group sessions, web-based interventions, and education sessions have been found to help adherence. Also, in Canada, it can be difficult for some individuals, including certain First Nations groups, to access CPAP therapy because of federal and provincial government policies (Marchildon et al., 2015). Nurses can serve a role in advocating for access to this treatment.

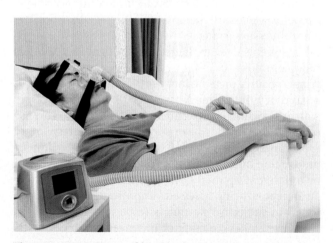

Figure 28.11 A variety of facial and nasal masks are used to treat obstructive sleep apnea. (Shutterstock.com/Chalermpon Poungpeth.)

Psychological Domain

Two of the main consequences of OSA are impaired cognitive performance and mood disturbance. Impaired executive function, including memory, mental flexibility, planning, organization, behavioural inhibition, and problem-solving can negatively impact work, school, and everyday life. The relationship between depression and OSA is complex; it varies depending on age, sex, and other health characteristics. Additionally, the risk of depression depends on the severity of the OSA and excessive daytime sleepiness; as these become more serious, the risk of depression rises. Being aware of these links, nurses may need to screen for depression when they see individuals who have OSA and excessive daytime sleepiness. Social cognitive theory has been used as a framework for understanding adherence to CPAP treatment (Sawyer et al., 2010). Commitment to long-term use of CPAP has been found to be determined by the person's experience with the treatment within the first week of starting treatment and a positive experience using CPAP correlated with commitment to using it. Helping the patient connect specific signs and symptoms with OSA is an important motivator for seeking assessment and treatment. Other beliefs and perceptions that affect commitment to CPAP included outcome expectations, treatment goals, self-efficacy, and treatment barriers/facilitators.

Social Domain

OSA has been associated with decreased work productivity, marital problems, and motor vehicle and work incidents. The risk of a motor vehicle incident for those with untreated OSA is twice as likely as for those without. Nurses need to ask individuals being assessed for OSA about their driving habits and occupational requirements. Questions should include the number of hours and days the person drives, history of vehicle incidents, and near misses caused by sleepiness. The criteria for when individual provincial and territorial transportation ministries need to be notified about the person's OSA varies across the country and the Canadian Medical Association has a driver's guide which delineates criteria for mandatory reporting in occupations which are safety-critical. Those suspected of having severe OSA should avoid driving or operating heavy equipment until their OSA is treated. Individuals who live alone and have had a recent traumatic life event have been shown to have decreased adherence to CPAP; attending support groups and having immediate social support promote adherence.

Spiritual Domain

While research that looks at the link between spirituality and OSA was not found in the literature, OSA has been found to be associated with a decreased quality of life (Laratta et al., 2020). Understandably, it would be difficult to develop and participate in spiritual experiences if the person is dealing with impaired executive functioning, mood disturbance, sleepiness, and other related physical complaints and social difficulties.

Common Circadian Rhythm Sleep–Wake Disorders

Shift Workers

Approximately 25% of workers in North America are engaged in shift work, and intolerance of being awake during the night hours is not uncommon (Government of Canada, 2020). For those trying to sleep during the day, typically sleep duration is shorter and the quality is less consolidated than nighttime sleep.

Among nurses, fatigue often related to altered sleep patterns, has been associated with a higher risk of making errors, burnout, and work-related injuries and accidents, including motor vehicle accidents (Halm, 2018). Moreover, the risk of making an error increases by three-fold if the shifts are longer than 12.5 hours.

Shift workers who drive a motor vehicle while sleepy have been found to have double the risk of having an accident (Bioulac et al., 2017). Caffeine, short breaks, and naps can provide temporary relief but there is no substitute for sleep. Several strategies can be used to help cope with sleepiness associated with shift work (see Box 28.5).

In 2010, the Canadian Nurses Association (CNA) released a position statement on nurse fatigue, which they defined as a "subjective feeling of tiredness (experienced by nurses) that is physically and mentally penetrative" (CNA, 2010, p. 1). This fatigue could not be "slept off" and so it is more than sleep deprivation, but circadian rhythm disturbances, sleepiness, and sleep habits were identified as contributing factors. The CNA has identified several systemic, organizational, and individual responsibilities to manage nurse fatigue. See the Web Links section at the end of the chapter for details regarding nurse fatigue and patient safety.

Jet Lag

Jet lag occurs when a person travels by air across several time zones in a short period of time, and the person's internal clock is out of phase with the light–dark cycle of the destination. It is not clear why this happens. Symptoms of jet lag include poor sleep at night and feeling

---

BOX 28.5 Behavioural Strategies to Manage Effects of Shift Work

- If working 8-hour rotating shifts, rotate the shifts clockwise, from days to evenings to nights.
- Avoid switching to different shifts rapidly within a short time period.
- Follow a regular sleep schedule regardless of the shift you are working.
- Keep your bedroom as dark as possible when you are sleeping.
- When awake, spend as much time as possible in brightly lit rooms.
- Wear sunglasses to block blue light on the way home from work in the morning.

- Avoid scheduling appointments during your daytime sleep hours.
- After the last night shift, sleep 4 hours and then get up.
- Avoid eating large meals within 4 hours of going to bed.
- Avoid caffeine and nicotine before sleep.

A short nap (15 to 20 minutes) during the night shift may reduce sleepiness and increase alertness.

Adapted from Rosenberg, R., & Doghramji, P. (2011). Is shift work making your patient sick? Emerging theories and therapies for treating shift work disorder. *Postgraduate Medicine, 123*(5), 106–115.

groggy during the day. Additionally, some travellers experience gastrointestinal upset and general malaise. Flying westbound is generally less challenging to adapt to than flying eastward. Because our internal clocks are a little longer than 24 hours, a person can move their internal clock *later* by approximately 2 hours a day but *earlier* by only 1 to 1½ hours a day. Other factors that can contribute to jet lag include sleep deprivation, the discomfort of airplane travel, and in-flight caffeine and/or alcohol intake.

Treating Circadian Rhythm Disorders

Treatments of circadian rhythm disorders include melatonin, strategic avoidance or exposure to light and napping, BZRA medications (e.g., zopiclone), strategically consumed stimulants such as caffeine and modafinil, and bright light therapy. The effectiveness of bright light therapy is dependent on when in the circadian cycle it is used. This therapy works through the action of the light on the eyes and retina; the person does not need to look directly at the light to benefit. The usual "dose" of light is 5,000 lux shortly after waking in the morning, typically obtained through exposure to a 10,000-lux light box for 30 minutes every day. A benefit can be felt within days. Eye damage due to this therapy has not been found, but nausea, headache, and nervousness can occur.

Narcolepsy

The best-known symptom of this disorder is the uncontrollable urge to fall asleep in any situation (Lord, 2019). While only about 0.05% of the population is diagnosed with narcolepsy, it is likely under diagnosed. Five of the most common symptoms include hallucinations

(usually visual) and sleep paralysis (i.e., being unable to speak or move for a few seconds or minutes) when transitioning to sleep or waking, severe daytime sleep attacks, interrupted nighttime sleep despite feeling rested when they awake and cataplexy. Cataplexy is often featured humorously in the media but can be a devastating symptom for the person when they experience a sudden loss of muscle control while awake. This loss of control can affect all or parts of muscles and be provoked by strong emotions, including positive feelings such as excitement and happiness. Ninety percent of those who have narcolepsy with cataplexy are found to have lower levels of orexin in their cerebral spinal fluid.

Sleep Terrors

Almost 40% of children are affected by night terrors by the time they reach adolescence. This is compared to less than 2% of adults (Lord, 2019). Night terrors and nightmares are sometimes confused, but night terrors occur less frequently and are diagnostically quite different. The person experiencing a night terror will, while still asleep, sit upright in bed, act upset, be inconsolable, scream or shout, breathe quickly, and have an elevated heart rate. The terror can last 1 to 5 minutes, sometimes longer in children, and occur usually early in the night during SWS. Once over, the person returns to sleep soundly and will not remember it the next day. Waking the person in the middle of a night terror can be frightening for the person, so it is better to avoid wakening and be available to monitor the person for safety risks. In contrast, nightmares often occur during the later part of the night during REM sleep and those experiencing nightmares can be woken to stop the dream and comforted.

🍁 Summary of Key Points

- The brain has three different naturally occurring states: wakefulness, REM sleep, and NREM sleep. Coma and anaesthesia are other physiologic brain states not discussed in this chapter.
- Physical, psychological, social, and/or spiritual disturbances can cause sleep problems and vice versa. Any assessment of sleep complaints needs to include a review of these possible influences.
- Sleep disorders are common comorbidities of many mental disorders. However, sleep disturbances can be

risk factors as well as early or prodromal symptoms for mental disorders.
- Nurses have an important role to play in assessing and helping people manage sleep difficulties.
- Many nurses are also at risk for sleep-related problems because of the nature of their work. It is important that nurses understand the risks and manifestations of these problems and develop strategies to prevent and manage the issues.

🧠 Thinking Challenge

A stocky 40-year-old patient, Drew, complains of disrupted sleep, daytime sleepiness, and feeling irritable for the past 2 months. This sleepiness is interfering with work to the point of threatening the loss of employment.

Drew reports that this threat is damaging their marital relationship. As a result, Drew is eating more and drinking more coffee. Additionally, Drew has been buying over-the-counter sleep products. Drew has been diagnosed with an anxiety disorder and been ordered testing for obstructive sleep apnea.

a. Explain how anxiety and obstructive sleep apnea (OSA) affect sleep.

b. How does the coffee and an antihistamine sleep aid affect sleep?

c. What role does education about sleep hygiene play in this case?

> Visit thePoint to view suggested responses. Go to **thePoint.lww.com/activate** and use the activation code found in the front of this text to unlock answers to the "Thinking Challenges" and other online resources.

 ## Web Links

css-scs.ca The Canadian Sleep Society (CSS)/Société Canadienne du Sommeil (SCS) has a website for clinicians, scientists, and technologists that promotes the advancement and understanding of sleep and its disorders.

sleepfoundation.org This is an American organization that provides information on a variety of sleep-related topics.

sleeponitcanada.ca/ Sleep on it! Dormez Là-Dessus! is a bilingual, Canadian site that promotes and educates about healthy and disordered sleep.

thebrain.mcgill.ca The Brain from Top to Bottom is a web site supported by McGill University. Refer to the module on sleep and dreams. It has several modules that provide information on the brain at beginner, intermediate, and advanced levels. The modules are organized for social, psychological, neurologic, cellular, and molecular content.

cna-aiic.ca Canadian Nurses Association web site. Their position statement, *Nursing Fatigue and Patient Safety*, can be found by conducting a search on the web site or at this exact URL: cna-aiic.ca/en/nursing-practice/evidence-based-practice/patient-safety/nurse-fatigue-and-patient-safety

Acknowledgements

Appreciation to Dr. Rachel Morehouse, past Medical Director of the Atlantic Sleep Centre, Saint John Regional Hospital, Saint John N.B., for sharing her knowledge about sleep and to Dr. Glen Sullivan, the present Director of the same centre. He generously read this work and offered suggestions for this latest version.

References

American Psychiatric Association. (2013). *Diagnostic and statistical manual of mental disorders* (5th ed.).

Bakker, J., Weaver, T., Parthasarathy, S., & Aloia, M. (2019). Adherence to CPAP. What should we be aiming for, and how can we get there? *Chest, 155*(6), 1272–1287.

Bierman, A., Lee, Y., & Schieman, S. (2018). Chronic discrimination and sleep problems in late life: Religious involvement as buffer. *Research on Aging, 40*(10), 933–955. https://doi.org/10.1177/0164027518766422

Bioulac, S., Micoulaud-Franchi, J. A., Arnaud, M., Sagaspe, P., Moore, N., Salvo, F., & Philip, P. (2017). Risk of motor vehicle accidents related to sleepiness at the wheel: A systematic review and meta-analysis. *Sleep, 40*(10). 10.1093/sleep/zsx134. https://doi.org/10.1093/sleep/zsx134

Bishop, T., Simons, K., King, D., & Pigeon, W. (2016). Sleep and suicide in older adults: An opportunity for intervention. *Clinical Therapeutics, 38,* 2332–2339.

Bombard, J. M., Kortsmit, K., Warner, L., Shapiro-Mendoza, C. K., Cox, S., Kroelinger, C. D., Parks, S. E., Dee, D. L., D'Angelo, D. V., Smith, R. A., Burley, K., Morrow, B., Olson, C. K., Shulman, H. B., Harrison, L., Cottengim, C., & Barfield, W. D. (2018). Vital signs: Trends and disparities in infant safe sleep practices—United States, 2009–2015. *Morbidity and Mortality Weekly Report, 67*(1), 39–46. https://doi.org/10.15585/mmwr.mm6701e1

Brewer-Smyth, K., Kafonek, K., & Koenig, H. G. (2020). A pilot study on sleep quality, forgiveness, religion, spirituality, and general health of women living in a homeless mission. *Holistic Nursing Practice, 34*(1), 49–56. https://doi.org/10.1097/HNP.0000000000000362

Burgess, H. J., Burns, J. W., Buvanendran, A., Gupta, R., Chont, M., Kennedy, M., & Bruehl, S. (2019). Associations between sleep disturbance and chronic pain intensity and function: A test of direct and indirect pathways. *Clinical Journal of Pain, 35*(7), 569–576. https://doi.org/10.1097/AJP.0000000000000711

Canadian Nurses Association. (2010). *Nurse fatigue and patient safety: Research report.* Executive summary. https://www.cna-aiic.ca/-/media/cna/page-content/pdf-en/20---fatigue_safety_2010_summary_e.pd

Chaput, J-P., Wong, S., & Michaud, I. (2017). *Duration and quality of sleep among Canadians aged 18 to 79.* Health Reports. https://www150.statcan.gc.ca/n1/pub/82-003-x/2017009/article/54857-eng.htm

Constantinescu, A., Warness, J., Virk, N., Perez, G., Shankel, M., & Holroyd-Leduc, J. (2019). Optimizing sleep for residents in long-term care without sedatives. *Annals of Long-Term Care, 27*(12), e7–e12. https://doi.org/10.25270/altc.2019.09.00086

Daley, M., Morin, C., LeBlanc, M., Grégoire, J. P., & Savard, J. (2009). The economic burden of insomnia: Direct and indirect costs for individuals with insomnia syndrome, insomnia symptoms, and good sleepers. *Sleep, 32,* 55–64.

Driver, H. (2012). Sleepless women: Insomnia from the female perspective. *Insomnia Rounds, 1*(6). https://css-scs.ca/files/resources/insomnia-rounds/150-006_Eng.pdf

Driver, H., Gottschalk, R., Hussain, M., Morin, C., Shapiro, C., & Van Zyl, L. (2012). *Insomnia in adults and children.* https://css-scs.ca/files/resources/insomnia-rounds/150-006_Eng.pdf

Dubuc, B. (n.d.). *The different types of sleep.* The Brain from Top to Bottom website. Retrieved January 15, 2020, from http://thebrain.mcgill.ca/flash/a/a_11/a_11_p/a_11_p_cyc/a_11_p_cyc.html

España, R., & Scammell, T. (2011). Sleep neurobiology from a clinical perspective. *Sleep, 34,* 845–858.

Exxon Valdez Oil Spill Trustee Council. (1990). *Details about the accident.* http://www.evostc.state.ak.us/index.cfm?FA=facts.details

Farrehi, P., Clore, K., Scott, J. R., Vanini, G., & Clauw, D. (2016). Efficacy of sleep tool education during hospitalization: A randomized controlled trial. *The American Journal of Medicine, 129,* 1329.e9–1329.e17.

Fernandez, S. (2019). Adolescent sleep: Challenges and solutions for pediatric primary care. *Pediatric Annals, 48*(8), e292–e295.

Fixen, D. (2019). 2019 AGS Beers Criteria for older adults. *Pharmacy Today, 25*(11), 42–54. https://www.pharmacytoday.org/action/showPdf?pii=S1042-0991%2819%2931235-6

Fleming, J. (2013). Psychiatric disorders and insomnia: Managing the vicious cycle. *Insomnia Rounds, 2*(1). https://css-scs.ca/files/resources/insomnia-rounds/150-007_Eng.pdf

Gaine, M. E., Chatterjee, S., & Abel, T. (2018). Sleep deprivation and the epigenome. *Frontiers in Neural Circuits, 12,* 14. https://doi.org/10.3389/fncir.2018.00014

Garland, S. N., Vargas, I., Grandner, M. A., & Perlis, M. L. (2018). Treating insomnia in patients with comorbid psychiatric disorders: A focused review. *Canadian Psychology/Psychologie canadienne, 59*(2), 176–186. https://doi.org/10.1037/cap0000141

Gilsenan, I. (2012). Nursing interventions to alleviate insomnia. *Nursing Older People, 24,* 14–18.

Government of Canada. (2020). *Shiftwork.* CCOHS: Canadian Centre for Occupation Health and Safety. https://www.ccohs.ca/topics/hazards/ergonomic/shiftwork/

Graham, K., Ogbuji, G., Williams, Z., Crain, M., Rolin, B., Juala, J., Larbi, I., Bernard, N., Oster, C. A., Baird, M., & Gullatte, M. M. (2020). Challenges of implementing the choosing wisely guideline to promote sleep and rest at night for hospitalized patients. *Journal of Nursing Care Quality, 36*(1), 50–56. https://doi.org/10.1097/NCQ.0000000000000494

Graven, S., & Browne, J. (2008). Sleep and brain development: The critical role of sleep in fetal and early neonatal brain development. *Newborn and Infant Nursing Reviews, 8*, 173–179.

Hafner, M., Stepanek, M., Taylor, J., Troxel, W., & van Stolk, C. (2017). *Why sleep matters: The economic costs of insufficient sleep.* RAND Europe. https://www.rand.org/content/dam/rand/pubs/research_briefs/RB9900/RB9962/RAND_RB9962.pdf

Halm, M. (2018). Night shift naps improve patient and workforce safety. *American Journal of Critical Care, 27*(2), 157–160. https://doi.org/10.4037/ajcc2018861

Harrison, Y. (2012). The functions of sleep. In C. Morin & C. Espie (Eds.), *The Oxford handbook of sleep and sleep disorders* (pp. 61–74). Oxford University Press.

Hobson, A., & McCarley, R. W. (1977). Brain as a dream state generator: An activation-synthesis hypothesis of the dream process. *American Journal of Psychiatry, 134*, 1335–1348.

Horne, J. (2008). Insomnia—Victorian style. *The Psychologist, 21*(10), 910–911.

Judd, B., & Sateia, M. (2020). Classification of sleep disorders. *UpToDate.* Retrieved December 6, 2020, from https://www.uptodate.com/contents/classification-of-sleep-disorders

Kesner, A., & Lovinger, D. (2020). Cannabinoids, endocannabinoids and sleep. *Frontiers in Molecular Neuroscience, 13*, 125. https://doi.org/10.3389/fnmol.2020.00125

Kline, L. (2020). Clinical presentation and diagnosis of obstructive sleep apnea in adults. *UpToDate.* Retrieved December 6, 2020, from https://www.uptodate.com/contents/clinical-presentation-and-diagnosis-of-obstructive-sleep-apnea-in-adults?search=risk%20factors%20obstructive%20sleep%20apnea&sectionRank=1&usage_type=default&anchor=H3055109064&source=machineLearning&selectedTitle=1~150&display_rank=1#H3055109064

Knowlden, A. P., Shewmake, M. E., Burns, M., & Harcrow, A. (2018). Sex-specific impact of spiritual beliefs and sleep quality on degree of psychological distress. *Journal of Religion and Health, 57*, 72–83. https://doi.org/10.1007/s10943-016-0342-4

Kurth, S., Dean, D., Achermann, P., O'Muircheartaigh, J., Huber, R., Deoni, S., & LeBourgeois, M. (2016). Increased sleep depth in developing neural networks: New insights from sleep restriction in children. *Frontiers in Human Neuroscience, 10*, 456. https://doi.org/10.3389/fnhum.2016.00456

Landis, C. (2011). Physiological and behavioral aspects of sleep. In N. Redeker & G. McEnany (Eds.), *Sleep disorders and sleep promotion in nursing practice* (pp. 1–18). Springer.

Lang, C., Appleton, S., Vakulin, A., McEnvoy, D., Vincent, A., Wittert, G., Martin, S. A., Grant, J. F., Taylor, A.W., Antic, N., Catcheside, P. G., & Adams, R. (2017). Associations of undiagnosed obstructive sleep apnea and excessive daytime sleepiness with depression: An Australian population study. *The Journal of Clinical Sleep Medicine, 13*, 575–582. https://doi.org/10.5664/jcsm.6546

Laratta, C, Ayas, N., Povitz, M., & Pendharkar, S. (2020). Diagnosis and treatment of obstructive sleep apnea. *Canadian Medical Association Journal, 189*(48), E1481–E1488. https://doi.org/10.1503/cmaj.170296

LeBourgeois, M. K., Hale, L., Chang, A-M., Akacem, L. D., Montgomery-Downs, H. E., & Buxton, O. M. (2017, November). Digital media and sleep in childhood and adolescence. *Pediatrics, 140*(Supplement 2), S92–S96. https://doi.org/10.1542/peds.2016-1758J

Li, Y., Yang, Y., Li, Q., Yand, X., Wang, Y., Ku, W., & Li, H. (2017). The impact of the improvement of insomnia on blood pressure in hypertensive patients. *Journal of Sleep Research, 26*, 105–114.

Lien, A., Sampasa-Kanyinga, H., Colman, I., Hamilton, H. A., & Chaput, J.-P. (2020). Adherence to 24-hour movement guidelines and academic performance in adolescents. *Public Health, 183*, 8–14. https://doi.org/10.1016/j.puhe.2020.03.011

Looney, D., Goverdovsky, V., Rosenzweig, I., Morrell, M., & Mandic, D. (2016). Wearable in-ear encephalography sensor for monitoring sleep: Preliminary observations from nap studies. *Annals of the American Thoracic Society, 13*, 2229–2233.

Lord, C. (2019). *Narcolepsy. Don't sleep on it!* Sleep On It-Dormez-Là Dessus! https://sleeponitcanada.ca/sleep-disorders/narcolepsy

Marchildon, G., Katapally, T., Beck, C., Abonyi, S., Episkenew, J., Pahwa, P., & Dosman, J. (2015). Exploring policy driven systemic inequities leading to differential access to care among indigenous populations with obstructive sleep apnea in Canada. *International Journal for Equity in Health, 14*, 148. https://doi.org/10.1186/s12939-015-0279-3

Mayers, A., & Baldwin, D. (2005). Antidepressants and their effect on sleep. *Human Psychopharmacology, 20*, 533–559.

Mitler, M. M., Carskadon, M. A., Czeisler, C. A., Dement, W. C., Dinges, D. F., & Graeber, R. C. (1988). Catastrophes, sleep, and public policy: Consensus report. *Sleep, 11*(1), 100–109.

Mutz, J., & Amir-Homayoun, J. (2017). Exploring the neural correlates of dream phenomenology and altered states of consciousness during sleep. *Neuroscience of Consciousness, 2017*(1), nix009. https://doi.org/10.1093/nc/nix009

Neubauer, D. N. (2014). New and emerging pharmacotherapeutic approaches for insomnia. *International Review of Psychiatry, 26*(2), 214–224. doi:10.3109/09540261.2014.888990. PMID: 24892896.

O'Brien, D. (2017). *Self hypnosis: The Betty Erickson special.* http://ericksonian.info/therapeutic_scripts/self-hypnosis-the-betty-erickson-special/

Palagini, L., & Rosenlicht, N. (2011). Sleep, dreaming, and mental health: A review of historical and neurobiological perspectives. *Sleep Medicine Reviews, 15*, 179–186.

ParticipACTION. (2016). *Are Canadian kids too tired to move? The 2016 ParticipACTION report card on physical activity for children and youth.* ParticipACTION. https://www.participaction.com/sites/default/files/downloads/2016%20ParticipACTION%20Report%20Card%20-%20Full%20Report.pdf

Peigneux, P., Urbain, C., & Schmitz, R. (2012). Sleep and the brain. In C. Morin & C. Espie (Eds.), *The Oxford handbook of sleep and sleep disorders* (pp. 11–37). Oxford University Press.

Pigeon, W. R. & Bishop, T. M. (2020, April 30). The strong relationship between sleep and suicide. *Psychiatric Times.* https://www.psychiatrictimes.com/view/strong-relationship-between-sleep-and-suicide

Riemann, D., & Nissen, C. (2012). Sleep and psychotropic drugs. In C. Morin & C. Espie (Eds.), *The Oxford handbook of sleep and sleep disorders* (pp. 190–220). Oxford University Press.

Roehrs, T. (2011). Normal sleep and its variations. In M. Kryger, T. Roth, & W. Dement (Eds.), *Principles and practice of sleep medicine* (5th ed., pp. 1–100). Elsevier Saunders.

Rosenberg, R., & Doghramji, P. (2011). Is shift work making your patient sick? Emerging theories and therapies for treating shift work disorder. *Postgraduate Medicine, 123*(5), 106–115.

Saleh, P., Ahmadi, N., & Shapiro, C. (2010). Sleep and psychiatric disease. In M. Kryger (Ed.), *Atlas of clinical sleep medicine* (pp. 254–260). Saunders Elsevier.

Sawyer, A., Deatrick, J., Kuna, S., & Weaver, T. (2010). Differences in perceptions of the diagnosis and treatment of obstructive sleep apnea and continuous positive airway pressure therapy among adherers and non-adherers. *Qualitative Health Research, 20*(7), 873–892.

Schofield, R., Forchuk, C., Montgomery, P., Rudnick, A., Edwards, B., Meier, A., & Speechley, M. (2016). Comparing health practices: Individuals with mental illness and the general Canadian population. *Canadian Nurse, 112*(5), 23–27.

Shetty, A., & Zantirati, G. (2020). The interstitial system of the brain in health and disease. *Aging and Disease, 11*(1), 200–211. https://doi.org/10.14336/AD.2020.0103

Shi, G., Wu, D., Ptáček, L. J., & Fu, Y. H. (2017). Human genetics and sleep behavior. *Current Opinion in Neurobiology, 44*, 43–49. https://doi.org/10.1016/j.conb.2017.02.015

Smylie, J., Fell, D., Chambers, B., Sauve, R., Royle, C., Allan, B., & O'Campo, P. (2014). Socioeconomic position and factors associated with use of a nonsupine infant sleep position: Findings from the Canadian Maternity Experiences Survey. *American Journal of Public Health, 104*, 539–547.

Statistics Canada. (2018). *Sleep apnea in Canada, 2016 and 2017.* https://www150.statcan.gc.ca/n1/pub/82-625-x/2018001/article/54979-eng.htm

Tim Hortons Research and Development. (2020). *Tim Hortons caffeine content.* https://company.timhortons.com/ca/en/menu/nutrition-and-wellness.php

Weiss, S., & Corkum, P. (2012). Pediatric behavioral insomnia—"Good night, sleep tight" for child and parent. *Insomnia Rounds, 1*(5), 1–6. https://css-scs.ca/files/resources/insomnia-rounds/150-005_Eng.pdf

Wilt, T., MacDonald, R., Brasure, M., Olson, C., Carlyle, M., Fuchs, E., Khawaja, I. S., Diem, S., Koffel, E., Ouellette, J., Butler, M., & Kane, R. (2016). Pharmacologic treatment of insomnia disorder: An evidence report for a clinical practice guideline by the American College of Physicians. *Annals of Internal Medicine, 165*, 103–112. https://doi.org/10.7326/M15-1781

Yiallourou, S. R., Maguire, G. P., Eades, S., Hamilton, G.S., Quach, J., & Carrington, M. J. (2018). Sleep influences on cardio-metabolic health in Indigenous populations. *Sleep Medicine, 59*, 78–87. https://doi.org/10.1016/j.sleep.2018.10.011

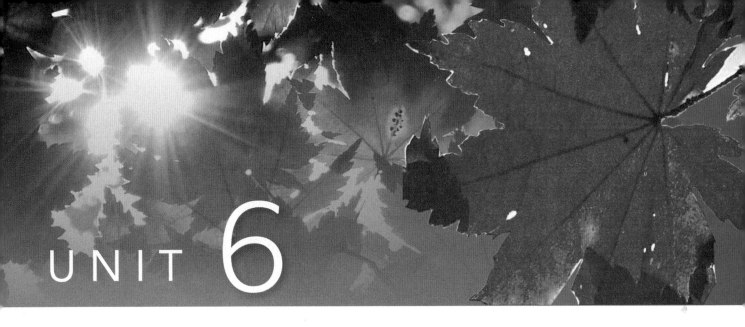

UNIT 6

Mental Health Across the Lifespan

Mental Health Promotion and Assessment: Children and Adolescents*

Patricia M. King and Cindy Peternelj-Taylor

LEARNING OBJECTIVES

After reading this chapter, you will be able to:

- Describe the protective factors in the mental health promotion of children and adolescents.
- Identify the risk factors for the development of child and youth psychopathology.
- Analyze the role of the nurse in mental health promotion with children and families.
- Define and apply the assessment process for children and adolescents.
- Discuss assessment data collection techniques used with children and adolescents.
- Discuss the synthesis of bio/psycho/social/spiritual assessment data for children and adolescents.
- Identify the responsibilities of nurses to recognize and assess the effects of maltreatment in children.

KEY TERMS

- bibliotherapy • childhood abuse/neglect
- developmental delays • disorganized attachment
- egocentrism • formal operations • maturation
- normalization • protective factors • psychoeducational programs • resilience • risk factors • self-concept • social skills training • support groups

KEY CONCEPTS

- attachment • grief • personal fable

Introduction

In this chapter, the importance of child and adolescent mental health is examined, the core prevention strategies and childhood stressors are identified, and guidelines for mental health promotion and risk reduction are provided. Assessment of the mental health of children and adolescents is outlined, including its components and the techniques required for an accurate, meaningful, and holistic result. The assessment of child abuse and neglect is addressed, as is Canadian nurses' legal responsibility to report maltreatment of this vulnerable population. Through their close contact with families in community and hospital-based healthcare settings, and their role as educators, nurses are in key positions to identify and intervene with children and adolescents at risk for psychopathology. Knowing the difference between normal child development and psychopathology helps parents view their children's behaviour realistically and respond appropriately.

Childhood and Adolescent Mental Health

The Child and Youth Advisory Committee of the Mental Health Commission of Canada (MHCC, 2016) have identified strategic directions for promotion, prevention, intervention and ongoing care, research, and evaluation to address the mental health needs of children and youth in their document, *The Mental Health Strategy for Canada: A Youth Perspective*. The committee's *Evergreen* framework (Kutcher & McLuckie, 2010) upholds the values of human rights; dignity, respect, and diversity; best available evidence; choice, opportunity, and responsibility; collaboration, continuity, and community; and access to information, programs, and services for all children, youth, and families. The framework is available to guide service providers, policy makers, and officials in creating mental health programs and services for children, youth, and families.

---

*Adapted from the chapter "Mental Health Promotion and Assessment: Children and Adolescents" by Lorelei Faulkner-Gibson, Kimberly Wong, Wendy Austin, and Cindy Peternelj-Taylor

In *The Health of Canada's Young People: A Mental Health Focus*, Freeman and associates (2010) reported on views of youth about health and wellbeing and the health behaviours of young people aged 11 to 15 years. The authors indicated that, while there are mental health issues specific to age and sex, positive relationships with adults in school and community and overall physical health are critical in the mental health of youth. Supportive social networks and positive childhood and adolescent experiences maximize the mental health of children and adolescents.

Children are more likely to be mentally healthy if they have normal physical and psychosocial development and a secure attachment at an early age. A secure, warm, responsive, and predictable attachment relationship between infants and their caregivers is critical to positive wellbeing and healthy development (Clinton et al., 2016). Parents play a critical role in preventing adverse outcomes in their children and, if needed, can be assisted to learn ways of being optimally responsive to their children.

KEY CONCEPT

Attachment is the bond between a child and a parent (or parental figure) that begins in infancy and, when secure, allows the child to explore the world without fear of rejection.

Families play a significant role in children and adolescents' lives as protectors, nurturers, mediators, and mentors for surviving and thriving in the world. Values are transmitted and interpreted within families. Children need to explore their world, play, and learn how to speak and listen to others: it is the family's role to provide the opportunities to do so. Communal conditions and efforts are also necessary. As the Nigerian proverb advises, "It takes a whole village to raise a child." When children enter the world, there will be protective and risk factors that shape their health and wellbeing over time. Nurses and other healthcare professionals are there to assist and guide them in growing up to be as healthy as possible.

Common Childhood Stressors

Stress is an inevitable part of life and may occur in one or many spheres of influence in a child's life. Stressors in each sphere of influence can include the following:

- Child: Temperament, birth difficulties (e.g., genetic anomalies, prematurity, developmental delay, failure to thrive), extreme sensitivity to sensory experiences, suspected abuse/neglect, loss of a significant caregiver, withdrawal, extreme activity level, aggressive behaviour and emotional dysregulation/reactivity, and substance use.
- Family: Primary caregivers may lack parenting knowledge, skills, and education. They may be experiencing unresolved loss/trauma, developmental delay, financial and marital stress, chronic health problems, mental health problems, and/or substance use resulting in negative attributions to the child. They may show insensitivity or rejection responses, angry or harsh discipline, frightening or threatening behaviour, and a failure to protect the child. Ultimately, the parent–child attachment may be negatively affected. Jones et al. (2018) noted that low income is linked with many other difficulties, such as inadequate nutrition and supportive parenting.
- Residential community: Neighbourhoods with lower socioeconomic status may be exposed to toxic or hazardous wastes, residential overcrowding, and low housing quality. They may also have limited access to services such as learning and recreation, child care, medical facilities, access to transportation, and employment opportunities. Additionally, exposure to negative social environments and smaller support networks also contribute to childhood adversities since it provides poor assistance for coping and buffering stresses (Jones et al., 2018).

Regardless of origin, stress can cause conflict and difficulty within family relationships. Stress responses can disrupt parenting behavior and the interactions between the parent and the child and can lead to short-term or long-term poor outcomes. The earlier these events begin in a child's life, and the longer that the disruption is sustained, the more risk a child experiences in terms of mental health and wellness. Psychological distress due to different childhood stressors, such as parental death, single parent household, poor child health, frequent change of residence or school, teenage parenthood, receiving household public assistant due to poverty, long-term parent unemployment, can put those individuals at risk for poor mental health in adulthood. When someone is exposed to a high number of these stress indicators, risk of psychological distress is also increased (Björkenstam et al., 2015). Epidemiological data from a World Health Organization (WHO) Survey demonstrate that some childhood adversities contribute to increased chances of developing post-traumatic stress disorder (McLauglin et al., 2017). Following a meta-analysis of the association between adverse child experiences (ACEs) and health outcomes, Petrucelli and associates (2019) categorized ACEs under three categories: (a) abuse (physical, emotional, sexual); (b) neglect (physical, emotional); and (c) household dysfunction (substance use, mental illness, domestic violence, incarceration, parental separation). Of note, each ACE score has the potential of equal contribution to poor mental health.

Nurses and other healthcare providers have an important role in providing routine education to parents and other care providers regarding adverse childhood experiences, ways to identify toxic stresses and their health impacts, and strategies to promote resilience (Koball et al., 2019).

Grief and Loss

Nurses need to recognize that grief and loss are universally experienced by children, and they are among the most common stresses they encounter. Children respond to loss and grief not as adults do but based on their developmental stage. The most common losses experienced are the death of a grandparent, parental divorce, family separation (parents who work away or who are ill for extended periods), death of a pet, and loss of friends through moving or changing schools. Learning to mourn losses can lead to a renewed appreciation of life's precious value and close relationships. Extensive research shows that both children and adults who experience significant losses are at risk for mental health problems, particularly if the natural grieving process is impeded. The grieving process differs somewhat between children and adults (see Table 29.1).

KEY CONCEPT

Grief is the subjective experience (i.e., the thoughts, feelings, body sensations, and behaviours) that accompanies the perception of a loss. Children grieve in stages, as do adults, but children's grief is shaped by developmental stages as well as by life experiences.

Children's responses to loss reflect their developmental level, as well as their previous experiences. As early as the age of 3 years, children can have some concept of death. For example, a pet goldfish's death provides an opportunity for the child to grasp the idea that the fish will never swim again. However, it is not until about age seven that most children understand the permanence of death. Before this age, they may verbalize that someone has "died," but in the next sentence, ask when the dead person will be "coming back." Even though death's finality is understood by early adolescence, adolescents sometimes flirt with death by engaging in risky behaviours, such as driving dangerously, as if they believe that they are immune to death. This phenomenon is a result of a *personal fable* (Elkind, 1967) wherein adolescents view themselves egocentrically as unique and invulnerable to other's consequences.

KEY CONCEPT

A personal fable is an aspect of egocentric thinking in adolescence, characterized by the belief that one is unique and invulnerable to harm. This belief may lead to risky social and health behaviours, such as unprotected sex, fast driving, and substance use.

Adults should be sensitive to the child's struggle to understand and cope with death. Research suggests that children want to be included in the rituals related to a death in the family (e.g., funerals, memorials) and thus recognized as mourners alongside adults. It allows them to participate in "saying good-bye" (Søfting et al., 2016). Most children closely watch their parents' response to grief and loss and use fantasy to fill the gaps in their understanding. In many cases, family members take turns grieving, and some children may sense that their parents are so overwhelmed by their own emotional

Table 29.1 Grieving in Childhood, Adolescence, and Adulthood		
Children	**Adolescents**	**Adults**
• View death as reversible: do not understand that death is permanent until about age 7 years • Experiment with ideas about death by killing bugs, staging funerals, acting out death in play • Mourn through activities (e.g., mock funerals, playing with things owned by the loved one); may not cry • May not discuss the loss openly but express grief through regression, somatic complaints, behaviour problems, or withdrawal • Need repeated explanations to fully understand the loss; it may be helpful to read children's books that explain death	• Understand that death is permanent but may flirt with death (e.g., reckless driving, unprotected sex) due to omnipotent feelings • May be fascinated by death, enjoy morbid books and movies, listen to rock music about death and suicide • Mourn by talking about the loss, crying, and reflecting on it, sometimes becoming dramatic (e.g., overidentifying with the lost person, developing poetic or romantic ideas about death) • Often withdraw when mourning or seek comfort through peer groups; may feel parents do not understand their feelings • Need permission to grieve openly because they may believe they should act strong or take care of the adults involved; need acceptance of their sometimes extreme reactions	• Understand that death is permanent: may struggle with spiritual beliefs about death • May try not to think about death, depending on cultural background • Mourn through talking about the loss, crying, reviewing memories, and thinking privately about it • Usually discuss loss openly, depending on the level of support available; may feel there is a "time limit" on how long it is socially acceptable to grieve • Need friends, family, and other supportive people to listen and allow them to mourn for, however, long it takes; need opportunities to review their feelings and memories

pain that they cannot bear the children's grief. Adults may attribute certain responses or reactions to the child that may not be accurate. It is important for the nurse to be aware of this when working with families who are experiencing grief and loss. Assessing and responding with sensitivity to differing familial and cultural norms is important.

Children and adolescents may experience complicated grief. *Complicated grief* is a form of bereavement-related distress that can include such symptoms as being preoccupied with thoughts of the deceased, including difficulty accepting the death, and numbness, bitterness, or a sense of futility. An indication that bereaved children may need mental health services is related to such things as level of functioning (e.g., extended period of depression), coping, self-esteem, and aspects of their family environment (e.g., stressors, parenting) (American Academy of Child & Adolescent Psychiatry, 2018).

Grief throughout childhood is shaped by developmental stages and life experiences. As with adults, children's grief is experienced in stages. Children's grief usually begins without understanding the full effects of the loss, and they experience some numbness or dulling of emotional pain. This stage progresses to a greater acceptance of the reality of the loss, which leads to more intense psychological pain. Finally, they undergo a reorganization of identity to incorporate the loved person, engaging in new activities and interests.

A parent's death in childhood or adolescence is a highly stressful event, and a risk factor for mental health problems, traumatic grief, lower self-esteem, and school performance difficulties. However, the remaining parent or caregiver may also struggle with their own grief, which may contribute to them being unavailable to provide the emotional support and attention that the child needs (Bergman et al., 2017). When the death is by suicide, the bereavement is particularly difficult with children fearing further abandonment. They may struggle with a sense of responsibility and guilt that they were somehow responsible. Such a death can "disenfranchise" a family from the community, causing isolation and a grief experience for a child significantly different from that experienced by a child whose parent died from natural causes (Schreiber et al., 2017). Adults have difficulty knowing how to respond to a bereaved child, especially when the death was by suicide. Good communication with the surviving parent and age-appropriate support, such as in a support group, can enhance the protective factors for children coping with suicide (Schreiber et al., 2017).

Loss and Preschool-Aged Children

The preschool-aged child may react more to a parent's distress about a death than to the death itself. Young children who depend totally on their parents may be frightened when they see their parents upset. Anything the parent can do to alleviate children's anxiety, such as reassuring them that the parent will be okay while maintaining their everyday routines (e.g., regular bedtimes, snacks, play times), will help the bereaved child to feel secure. Because preschool-aged children have limited ability to verbalize their feelings, they may need to express them through fantasy play and activities, such as mock funerals. Books that explain death, such as *Charlotte's Web* by E. B. White (1952), or The Ten Good Things about Barney by J. Viorst (1972), may also be helpful. Parents should take care not to use euphemisms that could fuel misconceptions of death, such as "He went to sleep" or "Jesus took him." Young children may interpret these messages literally and fear going to sleep (because they might die) or focus their natural, grief-related anger on the irrational idea that the person deliberately has not returned. The best approach is to honestly explain that the person has died and is not coming back, elicit the child's understanding and questions about what has happened, and to repeat the process continually as the child gradually begins to grasp the reality of the situation. Whether to take a small child to a funeral depends on the child's preference and the availability of adult support at the event; inclusiveness with the family can be a positive element in coping with death.

It is important to remember that children (especially those 3 to 6 years) think in very concrete terms. Any discussion about death should include concrete terms (e.g., cancer, died, death) and avoid euphemisms (e.g., "he passed away," "he is sleeping," "we lost him"), because they can confuse children and lead to misinterpretations. In response to death, children younger than five may regress and experience disturbances in eating, sleeping, and toileting.

Loss and School-Aged Children

School-aged children understand the permanence of death more clearly than do preschoolers, but they may be unable to express their feelings, not unlike many adults. Children in this age group may express their grief through somatic complaints. They may show signs of regression and find comfort in behaviours engaged in during earlier developmental stages. There may be behavioural reactions such as withdrawal or hostility toward parents. Children may think that others expect them to cry and react with immediate emotional intensity to the death; when they do not react this way, they may feel guilty.

Loss and Adolescents

Adolescents who are in Piaget's stage of formal operations can better understand death as an abstract concept. **Formal operations** are the period of cognitive development characterized by the ability to use abstract reasoning to conceptualize and solve problems. Because adolescents tend to be idealistic and to think in extremes, they may even have poetic or romantic notions about death. Some teenagers may become fascinated with morbid rock music, movies, and books. Although they may express their thoughts and feelings about death more clearly than younger children, they often are reluctant to do so for fear of being viewed as childish.

Adolescents, striving to gain independence, may be reluctant to share their feelings of grief and carefully choose with whom to share them. Their grief reactions may be more hidden but, most often, they want to be regarded as able to cope and not to be shielded from death of a friend or family member. Research indicates that bereavement can be a time of potential personal growth and maturation for adolescents (Andriessen et al., 2018). Sometimes, an adolescent will assume a parental role in the family after a death and deny their own needs. School settings may be conducive in providing group and individual support for grieving adolescents, particularly as a preventive intervention. Death education in high schools, when well-planned with formal and informal components, and thoughtfully presented, can be of significant benefit to students (Testoni et al., 2020).

Families

The diversity of Canadian families is a reflection of the people who comprise them. There are many diverse family forms; a nurse may work with families consisting of mother and father, those in same-sex marriages, others living in common-law relationships, and those embracing coparenting relationships. The nurse needs to clarify with the child/youth and care provider who *the family* of reference is and any unique, relevant contextual family circumstances. For example, a separated or divorced couple may continue to cohabitate, with one partner sleeping in a separate bedroom or living in a basement suite, to provide parental consistency and/or financial support. In contrast, others continue to coparent but live separately. Assessing each family's unique structure is key. Refer further to Chapter 16.

Separation and/or Divorce

Separation and/or divorce can be particularly stressful for families and children, and it is during these situational crises that children may present with mental health concerns.

Separation

Separation of families occurs for many reasons: marital/partner discord, parental mental or physical illness, work circumstances, ill extended family, or immigration. Many Canadian couples live in various complex situations to cope with financial, professional, and life circumstances. This can include "living apart together," that is, being in

an intimate relationship with someone living in another dwelling. In 2017, an estimated 1.5 million Canadians aged 25 to 64 were in a "living-apart-together" (LAT) relationship. Between 2006 and 2017, the share of LAT couples increased from 6% in 2006 to 9% in 2017, and more common in couples aged 25 to 34 years of age (Statistics Canada, 2019). The reasons couples gave for living apart were often dependent on contextual circumstances, including studying for school, financial circumstances, and work circumstances (25%), primarily for those under age 30. Individuals aged 40 to 49 identified "work circumstances" (32%). Regardless of circumstance, many couples are living separately yet together. As this becomes more common in our society, the impact on children and youth must be addressed for them to feel safe and secure.

One agency that is much attuned to this phenomenon is the Canadian Armed Forces. There are many support resources available for families in which parents are deployed away from home (see Web Links). The developmental age of children in military families will need to be taken into consideration regarding their understanding of where and what the parent may experience or how they may be upon return from a military mission. The child may also need support if there are critical events publicized in the media.

Divorce

Divorce can be one of the most stressful life events for both children and parents. Familial disruption and conflict before divorce may contribute to children and youths' overall functioning, so that when the actual divorce or separation occurs, it may or may not be perceived as an adverse event (Strohschein, 2012). During times of stress, the child's/youth's ability to cope is determined by their resilience and the overall family/parental coping and support behaviours.

Although many families adapt to separation and divorce without long-term adverse effects for the children, there are often temporary structural and functional difficulties dealing with this family change. Parental separation and divorce create changes in the family structure that can functionally result in a substantial reduction in the contact that children have with one of their parents. The child's response to divorce can be similar to the response to death. In some ways, divorce may be more challenging for the child to understand because the noncustodial parent is gone but still alive, and the parents have made a conscious choice to separate.

Analysis of data from Canada's Longitudinal Survey of Children and Youth shows that children who grow up in a married biologic-parent household do not have better short-term behavioural outcomes than those who do not (Wu et al., 2008). Instead, behavioural outcomes are linked to income, family dysfunction, and parental nurturance. The response to the loss that divorce imposes varies depending on the child's predivorce experience

(Kelly, 2012), the child's temperament; the parents' interventions; and the level of stress, change, and conflict surrounding the divorce (Hetherington & Kelly, 2002). Impactful changes in socioeconomic status, such as moving from a dual-earner status to single-parent family status, and changing residence may account for variation in levels of distress among divorcing families.

The first 2 or 3 years after the couple's breakup tend to be the most difficult. Typical childhood reactions include confusion, guilt, depression, regression, somatic symptoms, acting-out behaviours (e.g., stealing, disobedience), fantasies that the parents will reunite, fear of losing the custodial parent, and alignment with one parent against the other. After an initial adjustment period, children usually accept the reality of the situation and begin coping adaptively. If the divorced parents remarry new partners, this often imposes another period of coping difficulties for the children. Children

with stepparents and stepsiblings are at renewed risk for emotional and behavioural problems as they struggle to cope with the new relationships.

Protective factors against emotional and behavioural problems in children of divorce include parental nurturance, parents' mental health, joint custody, and low parental conflict (Kelly, 2012). For children of divorce and remarriage, protective factors also include a structured home and school environment with reasonable and consistent limit-setting and a warm and supportive relationship with stepparents (Hetherington & Kelly, 2002). Helpful interventions for children of divorce include education regarding children's reactions; promotion of regular and predictable visitation; reduction of conflict between the parents through counselling, mediation, and clear visitation policies; continuance of usual routines; and family counselling to facilitate adjustment after remarriage (Table 29.2). It may not be the divorce

Table 29.2 Play Therapy With a 4-Year-Old Child Whose Parents Are Divorcing

Child Statement	Nurse Response	Analysis and Rationale
(The child smashes two cars together and makes loud, crashing sound.)	That's a loud crash. They really hit hard.	The child may be expressing anger and frustration nonverbally through play. The nurse attempts to establish rapport with the child by relating at the child's level, using age-appropriate vocabulary.
Crrrash!	I know a boy who gets so mad sometimes that he feels like smashing something.	The child is engrossed in fantasy play, typical of preschoolers. Children often use toys as symbols of human figures. The nurse uses an indirect method of eliciting the child's feelings, because preschoolers often do not express feelings directly. Reference to another child's anger helps to normalize this child's feelings.
Yeah!	Sounds like you feel angry too sometimes … the same way the other boy feels.	The child is beginning to relate to the nurse and senses her empathy. The nurse reflects the child's feelings to facilitate further communication.
Yeah, when my mom and dad fight.	It's tough to listen to parents fighting. Sometimes, it's scary. You wonder what's going to happen.	The child is experiencing frustration and helplessness related to family conflict. The nurse expresses empathy and attempts to articulate the child's feelings, because preschool children have a limited ability to identify and label feelings.
My mom and dad are getting a divorce.	That's too bad. Children often feel mixed up when their parents get divorced. What's going to happen when they get the divorce?	The child has a basic awareness of the reality of the parents' divorce but may not understand this concept. The nurse expresses empathy and attempts to assess the child's level of understanding of the divorce.
Dad's not going to live in our house.	Oh, I guess you'll miss having him there all the time. It would be nice if you all could live together, but I guess that's not going to happen.	The preschool child focuses on the effects the divorce will have on him (egocentrism). The child seems to have a clear understanding of the consequences of the divorce. The nurse articulates the child's perspective and reinforces the reality of the divorce to avoid fuelling the child's possible denial and reconciliation fantasies.
(Silently moves cars across the floor.)	What do you think is the reason your parents decided to get a divorce?	The child expresses sadness nonverbally. The nurse further attempts to assess the child's understanding of the circumstances surrounding the divorce.
Because I did it.	What do you mean—you did it? How?	The child provides a clue that he may be feeling responsible. The nurse uses clarification to fully assess the child's understanding.
I made them mad because I left my bike in the driveway and Dad ran over it.	Do you think that's why they're getting the divorce?	The child uses egocentric thinking to draw a conclusion that his actions caused the divorce. The nurse continues to clarify the child's thinking. The goal is to elicit the child's perceptions so that misperceptions can be corrected.
Yeah, they had a big fight.	They may have been upset about the bike, but I don't think that's why they're getting a divorce.	The nurse goes on to explain why parents get divorced and to provide opportunities for the child to ask questions.
Why?	Because parents get divorced when they're upset with *each other*—when they can't get along—not when they're upset with their children.	

itself but rather the continuing conflict between the parents that is most damaging to the child. Conflict and discord affect parenting skills (Chang & Kier, 2016); parents need to remember that children identify with both parents and need to view both positively. Therefore, it is helpful for parents to reinforce each other's good qualities and focus on evidence of their former partner's love and respect for the child.

Sibling Relationships

The family often consists of various constellations of parents, children, and others. The family is whomever they define themselves to be. Within many families, siblings are an integral part of that constellation. Some parents prefer not to have the siblings present if they have brought one child in for a mental health assessment. It is helpful for the nurse to encourage the parents/care providers to include the siblings in the process, as they often add information that the parents may be unaware of. Nurses also need to be aware of siblings who may also be mentally unwell or experiencing distress due to an unwell sibling or parent. Shajani & Snell (2019) encourage nurses to consider the sibling "rank order— the position of children in the family in respect to age and gender" (p. 59). Depending on parental functioning (e.g., mental or physical illness), or cultural and ethnic background, sibling position may positively or negatively affect children's functioning. For example, older children may be put in a care provider role if both parents work outside the home. This role may create added stress on their ability to manage sibling care, domestic chores, and school work (or employment in the case of an adolescent).

The role of siblings in a child's development tends to be underemphasized, but there are several theoretical perspectives regarding relational development between siblings. Whiteman and colleagues (2011) present four perspectives within sibling research literature: psychoanalytic–evolutionary, social psychological, social learning, family–ecologic systems. No one theory is emphasized; however, because families function as a system and within the context of relationships, it would stand to reason that sibling relationships would be multidimensional and affected by numerous variables based on their development. Positive sibling relationships can be protective factors against the development of psychopathology, particularly in families in which the parents are emotionally unavailable. A Canadian longitudinal study revealed that sibling affection moderated the effects of stressful life events on "internalized symptomatology" (e.g., being anxious, depressive, over-controlled) (Gass et al., 2007).

Nurses working with families need to pay attention to the parent–child dynamic and also the sibling dynamic, assessing whether positive or negative behaviours are being modelled. Parents may need support in

modelling effective problem-solving to minimize sibling rivalry and maximize cooperative behaviour in the family system. Sibling rivalry can begin with the birth of the second child. It is a natural experience, and some sibling rivalry is inevitable. The birth of a sibling can be a surprise for the first child, who, up until then, was the sole focus of the parents' attention. The older sibling may react with anger and reveal not-so-subtle fantasies of getting rid of the new sibling. The child should be allowed to express both positive and negative feelings about the baby while being reassured of their special place in the family. Allowing the older child opportunities to care for the baby and reinforcing any nurturing or affectionate behaviour will promote positive bonding.

Physical Illness

Many children experience a major physical illness or injury. The experience of hospitalization and intrusive medical procedures can have a lasting and possibly acutely traumatic impact on many children. The likelihood of lasting psychological problems resulting from physical illness depends on the child's experiences during hospitalization, the child's developmental level, coping mechanisms, the family's level of functioning before, during, and after the illness, and the nature, trajectory, and severity of the illness. As with any significant stressor, the perception of the event (i.e., the meaning of the illness) will influence the family's ability to cope. The mental health effects of being physically compromised can begin at birth. For instance, early preterm children (born at 23 to 25 weeks' gestation), with or without neurodevelopmental disabilities, are at risk for anxiety and attention, social, and thought problems (Samuelsson et al., 2017). Common childhood reactions to physical illness include developmental regression (e.g., in toilet training, social maturity, autonomous behaviour), sleep and feeding difficulties, behavioural reactions (e.g., negativism, tantrums, withdrawal), somatic complaints that mask attempts at emotional expression (e.g., headaches, stomachaches), and depression. Infants and children younger than school age are particularly vulnerable to separation anxiety during illness and may regress to anxiety about strangers and become fearful of healthcare providers. Young children often have magical thinking about the illness, and their tendency to process information in concrete terms may lead to misperceptions about the illness and treatment procedures (e.g., dye = die; stretcher = stretch her) (Deering & Cody, 2002). Adolescents may be concerned about their body image and maintaining their sense of independence and control.

Nurses must remember that parents are the primary resource to the child and the experts who know their child's needs and reactions. Thus, nurses must maintain a collaborative approach in working with parents of both physically and mentally ill children. If the child is a sick infant, nurses should take care to allow the normal attachment process between parents and the infant to unfold, despite the healthcare professionals' efforts to assume some parenting functions. Parents who view their children as physically and emotionally fragile will feel disempowered in decision-making and boundary setting and may develop helpless or overprotective styles of dealing with their children.

Many parents react with fear and anxiety to an injury or illness and this can lead to feelings of parental guilt, especially if the illness is genetically based or partially due to their behaviour (e.g., drug or alcohol use during pregnancy). Parents may project their feelings onto each other or on healthcare professionals, lashing out in anger and blame. Nurses should view these responses as part of the grieving process and help parents move forward to confidently care for their children. Teaching parents about their children's health needs and reinforcing their caregiving skills will help parents adapt. For example, rather than reacting to what may appear to be an abdication of parenting responsibilities, nurses can instead use empathy to acknowledge the parent's feelings and discuss ways to help the parent regain a sense of control with comments such as the following:

> It is not always easy to know how to respond to your child's behaviour. Before receiving Sophie's diagnosis, you felt comfortable setting reasonable limits on her behaviour, but now that seems to have changed. Sometimes parents feel reluctant and are even afraid of setting limits because they know how sick their child is.… It may seem odd, but children actually feel safer and more secure when their parents let them know what the boundaries for their behaviour are.… Let's talk about some of the boundaries that you might feel most comfortable setting up for Sophie to help her feel safe and secure while she is so ill?

Chronic physical illness in childhood presents a unique set of challenges, with survival rates of previously fatal diseases at an all-time high. Although most children with chronic illnesses and their families are remarkably resilient and adjust to the stressors and regimens involved in their care, children with chronic health conditions are at higher risk for developing anxiety-related disorders, academic problems, and learning disabilities (Martinez & Ercikan, 2009). Conditions that affect the central nervous system (CNS) (e.g., infections, metabolic diseases, CNS malformations, brain and spinal cord trauma) are particularly likely to result in psychiatric difficulties. Nurses who understand these pathophysiologic processes are in a unique position to assess the interaction between biologic and psychological factors that contribute to mental health problems for chronically ill children (e.g., lethargy from high blood sugar levels or respiratory problems; mood swings from steroid use). Inactivity and a lack of sensory stimulation from hospitalization or bed rest may contribute to neurologic deficits and developmental delays.

The major challenge for a chronically ill child is to remain active despite the limitations of the illness and to become fully integrated into school and social activities. Children who view themselves as different or defective will experience low self-esteem and be more at risk for depression, anxiety, and behaviour problems. An earlier study by Anthony and colleagues (2003) found that parental perceptions of the child's vulnerability predicted greater adjustment problems, even after controlling for age and disease severity. Providing support for parents and helping them foster maximum independence within the limitations of their child's health problem is the key. For example, nurses might comment,

> Having kidney disease is no fun … and it must make you want to protect your son as much as possible. But too much protection will be a different sort of harm. Noah might feel he does not have possibilities in life like other children. We know he does. Even with all the limitations. What are the best things your son has going for him?

Physical and Developmental Challenges in Adolescence

Adolescence is a time of growing independence and, consequently, experimentation. Generally, emotional extremes prevail for teens. To adolescents, one day the world seems great and the next day, terrible; they perceive that people are either for them or against them. Adolescents are struggling to consolidate their abilities to control their impulses and react to the many "crises" that may seem trivial to adults but are very important to teens. Biologic changes (e.g., the onset of puberty, height and weight changes, hormonal changes), psychological changes (e.g., increased ability for abstract thinking), and social changes (e.g., dating, driving, increased autonomy) are all significant. The primary developmental task of identity formation leads teenagers to test different roles and struggle to define who they are. This process may include testing various peer groups to find one that fits their unfolding self-image.

Sexual Identity

In addition to the typical challenges associated with adolescence regarding sexuality and gender development, adolescents who identify as lesbian, gay, bisexual, two-spirited, transgender, intersex, or queer or questioning (LGBTQI2SA+) face additional challenges. Societal constructs and stigmatization of identities can put such youth at risk for adverse experiences (see Chapter 3). Beyond societal rejection, adolescents may experience a lack of acceptance of their gender identity and/or sexual orientation on the part of their family, peers, teachers, and others significant to their life.

Family response has an overwhelming effect on the mental health and wellbeing of LGBTQI2SA+ youth. Family acceptance is linked to improved health outcomes in this population and family rejection is often associated with suicidality, depression, and anxiety (Holt et al., 2016; McConnell et al., 2016; Olson et al., 2015). These youth are overrepresented in the homeless population, perhaps due to youth choosing to leave home to avoid family conflict, or being forced to leave. When families accept their child's sexual orientation and/or gender identity and respond through personal affirmation and advocacy, the risk of suicide attempts and depression are lower and risk-taking behaviour (e.g., substance use, risky sexual behaviour) is mitigated (McCormick & Baldridge, 2019).

Mental health risk for LGBTQI2SA+ youth occurs beyond the family. These youth also experience interpersonal violence at a higher rate and are at risk for problematic substance use and generalized anxiety (Schwartz et al., 2017). A state-wide American survey of a representative sample of high school students (ages 14 to 18) that included questions regarding sexual orientation, gender identity, and mental health found that all sexual and gender minority youth were at increased risk for depression, and that transgender youth and those questioning their sexuality or gender were at heightened risk for depression and suicidality. Researchers noted their findings point to ways that more inclusive cultures may be fostered in schools (Guz et al., 2021).

Nurses will need to reflect upon their own attitudes, values, and beliefs about sexual and gender identity if they are to support LGBTQI2SA+ youth and offer support to parents who are struggling to understand their child's sexual and/or gender identity. Psychoeducation and therapeutic dialogue regarding the importance of family efforts to their child's mental health can be helpful. It will be important for nurses to recognize that there may be ethnic, cultural, and religious influences shaping the family's response. Different religious and spiritual traditions hold various viewpoints on sexuality, and this affects how a youth perceives or predicts their family will react to their gender identity and sexual preferences. For example, a 13-year-old young woman might say "my family is ultra-religious and they would not be cool with me being attracted to girls so I am gonna keep it quiet; it's not worth the drama." It is not uncommon for youth to struggle with self-acceptance or with their family's religious context. Spiritual advisors, such as hospital chaplains, can offer support to LGBTQI2SA+ adolescents and their families to address religious-based stigma (Adelson & Walker-Cornetta, 2019).

Understanding pertinent family dynamics, expressive communication, and the family's response to their child's identity should be part of a family assessment.

Such information can inform a nurse's efforts to support a youth finding a voice within their family. Family response will evolve across the trajectory of the child's disclosures, coming out, or gender transition. There is some evidence in the literature indicating that early social transition for transgender children may result in positive improvements in mental health and psychosocial indicators (Durwood et al., 2017; Turban, 2017). Nevertheless, significant gaps remain regarding evidence-based models for promoting mental health and reducing mental health problems within this minority group (Russell & Fish, 2016). This is an area of research that needs further exploration.

Adolescence is a time of exploring social and personal boundaries. Youth may experiment with risk-taking behaviours and make choices which contribute to poor physical health, mental health problems, substance use or misuse, and/or high-risk behaviours (e.g., driving at excessive speeds, high-intensity sports). Exploration of sexual limits may lead to unsafe sexual behaviours and psychological distress. Knowledge about trends in teen pregnancy is important information for educators and policy makers, as these trends reflect the sexual and reproductive health and the overall wellbeing of Canadian teenagers. Nurses need to stay informed as they are often the first contact for teens with pregnancy concerns. Nurses can provide assessments, education, and, in some circumstances, intervention in relation to sexually transmitted and blood borne infections (STBBIs).

Substance Use

Among youth in later adolescence, approximately one in five, reports symptoms associated with a major mental disorder and nearly 1 in 10 report substance dependence (Centre for Addiction and Mental Health, 2012). Although most youths eventually become more conventional in their behaviour, some develop harmful behaviour patterns and addictions that endanger their mental and physical health. Adolescents whose psychiatric problems are developing are particularly vulnerable to engaging in risky behaviours because they may have limited coping skills, attempt to self-medicate their symptoms, or feel an increased pressure to fit in with other teens. Moreover, high-risk behaviours tend to be interrelated (Eggert et al., 2002).

Cannabis is a common substance for teen experimentation. Despite the Canadian Paediatric Association (Grant & Bélanger, 2017) expressing grave concerns, cannabis is legal for Canadians over the age of 19. According to the 2017 Canadian Cannabis Survey, 41% of respondents aged 16 to 19 and 45% of respondents aged 20 to 24 reported cannabis use in the past 12-months (Health Canada, 2017). Cannabis consumption is greater in this age demographic than others, in part because youth perceive minimal risks associated with its use (Porath-Walker et al., 2013). Research provides evidence of adverse consequences associated with cannabis use before the age of 25, including impaired cognitive functioning, mental health disorders, poor academic performance, risk of driving while intoxicated, and risk of dependency (George & Vaccarino, 2015; McInnis & Porath-Waller, 2016). With long-term, frequent use, the chemical compounds in cannabis can permanently alter the attention, memory, and learning centres of developing brains (Grant & Bélanger, 2017; McInnis & Porath-Waller, 2016). Mental health conditions, including psychotic symptoms, schizophrenia, depression, and risk of suicide, are more pronounced when cannabis use occurs before the age of 16 (George & Vaccarino, 2015; Melchior et al., 2017).

Comprehensive education is required if youths are to have the knowledge, skills, and attitudes to make confident, healthy, informed decisions about cannabis consumption that are grounded in evidence-based health information (Valleriani et al., 2018). **REACH** (Real Education About Cannabis and Health) is an innovative, comprehensive curriculum resource for youth, created by nurses and pharmacists for Saskatchewan schools (Fig. 29.1) (King et al., 2020). Resources are provided, incorporating health promotion, risk reduction, decision-making competence enhancement, and student engagement in learning. The program builds drug literacy and agency, key to its effectiveness (Reist & Asgari, 2018). Students are engaged in discussions and projects that facilitate critical thinking. This approach is crucial, as fear- and abstinence-based approaches do not resonate with youth (Valleriani et al., 2018).

Youth Health Promotion

Enhanced life skills and supportive school and family environments can mediate the effect of stressful life events. Programs that enhance the school environment are associated with improved behaviour and wellbeing. Interventions that teach cognitive skills help reduce one of the most prevalent mental health problems affecting adolescents—depression (Korczak, 2012). For an intervention to be sustainable, it must encompass multiple components across several levels, including the classroom, curriculum, whole school, and school–community boundaries. Several approaches to mental health promotion with adolescents are recommended. First, intervening at the peer group level through educational programs, alternative recreational activities, and peer counselling is most successful. Adolescents are skeptical of authority figures and tend to take cues from one another. Nurses working with teenagers find it helpful to use a conversational approach that encourages questioning and argument, as opposed to talking down to or at them (see Web Links).

Second, training in values clarification, decision-making, problem-solving, social skills, and assertiveness helps give adolescents the skills to cope with situations in which they are pressured by their peers. The impact of social norm messaging on youth behaviour is clear. Social psychological research shows that if just one person can find the strength to express an unpopular viewpoint in a group and decline to participate in a destructive activity, others will quickly follow. It takes enormous courage, as well as concrete knowledge and practice with assertiveness, to speak up in these situations.

A third type of intervention is a program that uses team efforts by teachers, parents, community leaders, and teen role models. These programs help at-risk youth by building self-esteem, setting positive examples, and involving and engaging youth in community activities. It is important to note that teaching interpersonal skills, including cognitive and problem-solving skills, should be coupled with promoting positive school and family environments to prevent mental health problems in young people, notably depression (Burns et al., 2002). Utilization of social media and other digital forms of communication to reach adolescents is essential in today's digital age. A recent online survey focused on virtual services for Ontario youth experiencing mental health and substance use challenges during the COVID-19 pandemic found that they preferred video calls, followed by phone/voice calls, and texting (Hawke et al., 2021). Overall, youth perceive these forms of communication as credible and impactful methods of communication in the context of public health programs. Public health interventions must continue to evolve and integrate new technologies to reach young people.

Development of Child Psychopathology

The factors that affect the development of child psychopathology are also factors that protect children. The issues presented are not independent components but are intertwined and interdependent, thus indicating that the care provided must be collaborative, holistic, and socially and culturally relevant to those involved. Creating a structure to describe the context in which child psychopathology develops is difficult, and one must remember that this is not a black and white process but that all aspects are systemically interwoven and affect the whole.

Protective Factors

Protective factors are attributes or conditions in individuals, families, communities, and society that diminish harm and mitigate risk by allowing for stressful occurrences to be addressed in healthy ways. Protective factors, identified as such for several decades, focus on

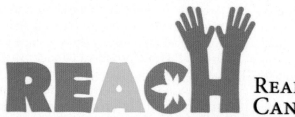

Health Education

Kids will learn reliable information about cannabis and its health impacts

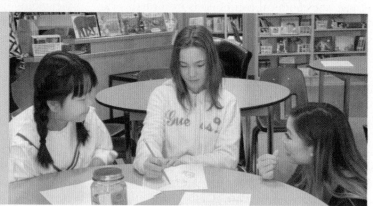

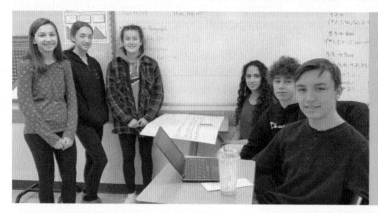

Meaningful Inclusion

Kids will have the opportunity to teach their peers

Engagement through Technology

Kids will collaborate to create an educational video

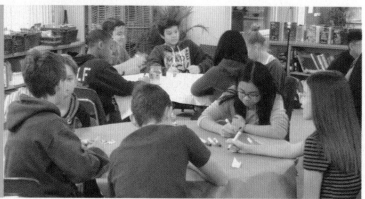

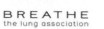

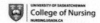

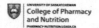

Figure 29.1 REACH—Real Education About Cannabis and Health. Printed with permission

children's and adolescents' ability to develop self-confidence, positive relationships, competencies (skills/strengths), self-regulation, and community involvement. In the family, low stress, stable employment, adequate child care resources, and higher socioeconomic status can serve as protective factors. In the community, protective factors include positive and cohesive families, schools, and neighbourhoods. All of the protective factors intertwine to create a context in which the child/youth thrives. Research on resilience provides insight and direction on where to focus attention and care when working with children/youth and their families.

Protective factors include the following:

- Individual attributes, such as problem-solving skills, sense of self-efficacy, accurate processing of interpersonal cues, positive social orientation, and self-regulation
- A supportive family environment, including an attachment with adults in the family, low family conflict, and supportive relationships
- Environmental supports, including those that reinforce and support coping efforts and recognize and reward competence

Resilience

Nurses will work with various children and youth and their families throughout their careers, but the majority will not have psychopathology. However, many will have experienced life circumstances that often lead to severe consequences, yet they function at or above what might be expected. These individuals have resilience. **Resilience** is the ability to overcome or rise above adversity, learn from the experience, and apply strategies and cope with other life events even when the situation dictates otherwise. Resilience refers to achieving positive outcomes despite challenging or threatening circumstances, coping successfully with traumatic experiences, and avoiding negative paths linked with risks (Zolkoski & Bullock, 2012). Resilience is commonly conceived as a state, depending on environmental and familial factors. "In the context of exposure to significant adversity, resilience is both the capacity of individuals to navigate their way to the psychological, social, cultural, and physical resources that sustain their wellbeing, and their capacity individually and collectively to negotiate for these resources to be provided in culturally meaningful ways" (Unger, 2013, p. 1). Therefore, resilience is not limited to the individual but can apply to a group or society's ability to move beyond adverse circumstances.

Risk Factors

A **risk factor** is a genetic, environmental, behavioural, or other influence that increases the probability of disease, disorder, or trauma. Risk factors inhibit resilience, while protective factors promote it. The number of stresses that children experience, the supports they have in place, and their developmental stage influence their ability to cope with stressors.

Biologic, social, and environmental risk factors include congenital disabilities, low birth weights, poverty, parental education level, negative life experiences such as abuse or neglect, minority status, and racial discrimination (Clinton et al., 2016; Zolkoski & Bullock, 2012).

Impact of Social Determinants of Health

The World Health Organization (see, e.g., Currie et al., 2011) has brought attention to the broad social factors that influence children's health and wellbeing. The health of young people and their families is generally determined less by lifestyle choices or application of medical knowledge than by the complex interaction of living conditions that often transcend the capacities of the individual. These include income and distribution of wealth, employment and working conditions, quality of food and housing, health care and other social services, and equitable access to education. Negative economic and social circumstances can pose significant risk to child wellbeing and may lead to short- and long-term implications for the individual and society (see Chapter 3).

Poverty

According to Statistics Canada (2020), approximately 3.2 million Canadians (8.7% of the population) lived below Canada's poverty line in 2018. The poverty rate for children under the age of 18 years during this same period was 8.2% (approximately 566,000 children). While this number is alarming, it does represent a downward trend, when compared to 1 million children living in poverty in 2012. The low-income rates for children vary significantly according to their family structure. For instance, children in lone-parent families continue to be more vulnerable to poverty. In 2018, 5.8% of children in two-parent families were in a low-income environment, while 26.2% for those in female lone-parent families faced this reality. First Nations children, however, "are far and away the most marginalized and economically disadvantaged" (Beedie et al., 2019, p. 3). In *Towards Justice: Tackling Indigenous Poverty in Canada*, the authors report that 47% of status First Nations children, 25% of Inuit children, 22% of Métis children, and 32% of nonstatus First Nations children live in poverty (Beedie et al., 2019).

Children, youth and families living in poverty are at increased risk of exposure to additional factors that contribute to childhood psychopathology. The effects of poverty on child development and family functioning are numerous and pervasive. The obstacles to overcoming the effects of poverty can seem insurmountable to young people. Lack of proper nutrition and lack of access to prenatal and mother–infant care can place children from impoverished families at risk for physical and mental health problems. Children from impoverished rural areas often lack access to educational and other community support resources. Children living in neighbourhoods with high rates of poverty experience vulnerabilities, including more exposure to violent crimes, crowded living conditions, and increased access to substances. Although crime, drug use, gang activity, and teenage pregnancy are seen in adolescents from all socioeconomic backgrounds, children living in poverty are more vulnerable to these problems because they may have limited opportunities, resources, and role models for change.

A primary focus of preventive nursing interventions for disadvantaged families involves forming a therapeutic relationship that conveys respect and willingness to advocate to assist clients' seeking out and accessing resources. In terms of Maslow's need hierarchy, due to their circumstances, families living in poverty may be more focused on survival needs (e.g., food, shelter) than on self-actualization needs (e.g., insight-oriented psychotherapy for themselves or their children). Unless the nurse can work as a partner with the family and address the issues most pressing for the family with an active problem-solving approach, other types of intervention may be fruitless. At the same time, it is inappropriate to assume that low-income families will be resistant to or unable to benefit from psychotherapies or other mental health interventions.

Homelessness

Homelessness is a complex phenomenon that reveals the failure of a society to ensure that systems and support are in place so that everyone has access to housing (Gaetz et al., 2016). Persons experiencing homelessness make up a heterogeneous population that includes adults of all genders, children, youth, families, new immigrants, people with mental illness, racial and ethnic minorities, and Indigenous Peoples. Youth homelessness refers to any youth without a home or who is at risk of experiencing homelessness. Youth may be found to be "couch-surfing" and so can be hidden from statistical data and reports. Many youths experiencing homelessness who don't live on the street and are among the hidden homeless live in temporary shelters or in unsafe or crowded conditions (Hulchanski et al., 2009). Parental conflict is an often reported factor contributing to homelessness in Canada; many youth have been "thrown out," experienced physical and sexual abuse, or were apprehended by a child protection agency. Youth also cite parental mental health or drug problems as reasons for leaving home (Gaetz et al., 2016). Parental drug and alcohol use is often associated with parental abandonment, family violence, and neglect. Youth in foster care and LGBTQI2SA+ youth are particularly susceptible to homelessness (Edidin et al., 2012).

For youth experiencing homelessness, there is an increased risk for physical health problems (e.g., nutritional deficiencies, infections, chronic illnesses, injuries as a result of violence, STIs), mental health problems (particularly **developmental delays** in language, fine or gross motor coordination, and social development; depression, anxiety, posttraumatic stress disorder, and psychotic symptoms; disruptive behaviour disorders; substance abuse), and educational underachievement (Gaetz et al., 2016). Many of these youth may have been physically or sexually abused, leading to elevated rates of externalizing disorders (e.g., antisocial behaviour) for males and internalizing disorders (e.g., anxiety, depression) for females. Their runaway experience compounds an already chronic history of trauma and disruption.

Unfortunately, responses to homelessness often result in greater social control measures (e.g., rendering panhandling illegal, excluding people experiencing homelessness from the community) rather than developing strategies to address the underlying causes of housing status. Street nurses are often one of the few resources available to marginalized populations who face various barriers accessing healthcare services. Not only do these youth experience mental health problems, they are at risk for involvement with the criminal justice system. Canadian research shows that youth who are unhoused are more likely to be victims of violent crime, including high rates of sexual assault when compared to the general public (Perri & Schwan, 2020).

Furthermore, they lack knowledge of specialized providers, transportation to service providers, and the ability to pay for prescriptions. They can also encounter provider discrimination and stigma (Self & Peters, 2005). However, street services for this population can be useful and effective because they are accessible and delivered wherever the person feels most comfortable: a school, youth centre, drop-in centre, mall, or simply on the street.

The living conditions of many shelters place children at risk for irregular patterns of sleep, feeding, play, and bathing, all of which are important for normal development. Nurses working with youth and families experiencing homelessness need to be aware of the effects of lack of housing on children. Nurturing one's children while living in homeless shelters is highly challenging for parents. Children's needs can be overlooked or underassessed in these settings. And while transition services for women and children who are victims of abuse are available across the country, they may remain inaccessible and ineffectual for some families.

While there is no evidence to date that Canada's efforts to reduce homelessness have had an overall positive effect, given the meaningful collaboration to address homelessness at the national, provincial, municipal, and community levels, there are reasons to be hopeful. (e.g., Homeless Partnering Strategy; Housing First) (see Chapter 2).

Table 29.3 Types of Abuse in Canada	
Type	**Description**
Neglect	Is often chronic and usually involves repeated incidents of failing to provide what a child needs for their physical, psychological, or emotional development and wellbeing
Physical abuse	May consist of just one incident or happen repeatedly. It involves deliberately using force against a child in such a way that the child either is injured or is at risk for being injured. Injuries may include bruises, lacerations, burns, and fractures caused by another person or object (e.g., belt, cords, cigarette)
Emotional abuse	Involves harming a child's sense of self. It includes acts (or omissions) that result in, or place a child at risk for, serious behavioural, cognitive, emotional, or mental health problems
Sexual abuse and exploitation	Involves using a child for sexual purposes, resulting in physical wounds such as bruises or bleeding of the genitals or rectum, STIs, sore throat, enuresis/encopresis, pregnancy, and foreign objects in the vagina or rectum. The child may also display sophisticated knowledge/behaviour/preoccupation with sexual activities, withdrawal, hypervigilance, or sleep difficulties

Child Abuse and Neglect

Family violence in Canada is a serious public health issue (Conroy, 2021). **Childhood abuse/neglect** and maltreatment affect an individual's overall growth and development, impacting their health and wellbeing, even when the individual is resilient (Blaustein & Kinniburgh, 2010). One in three Canadians state that they experienced abuse before the age of 15 years. Being male with Indigenous heritage and having been under the legal responsibility of the government at some time in childhood are associated with increased risk of abuse history (Hango, 2017). A biological parent is most often identified as the main perpetrator of physical abuse of children in Canada (Hango, 2017). Table 29.3 lists types of abuse of children in Canada. See also Chapter 34.

Childhood adversities, such as neglect and emotional, physical, and sexual abuse, have significant and long-term negative effects on child and adolescent health and wellbeing. Physical abuse is associated with lower social integration and competence levels and physical and mental health challenges among young adults. Such adverse experiences are a significant predictor of troubled sleep in adulthood (Baiden et al., 2015); a risk factor for diabetes (Shields et al., 2016); a risk factor for a higher probability, as an adult, of not being involved in education, training, or employment in the past year and for being victimized (Hango, 2017). Concerningly, as the number of adversities multiplies, the risk of becoming a serious, violent, and chronic juvenile offender (Fox et al., 2015) grows. Severe physical abuse can cause health conditions that continue in adulthood to limit, at least at times, daily living activities (Statistics Canada, 2017). See Research for Best Practice Box 29.1.

BOX **29.1** Research for Best Practice

CHILD ABUSE HOTLINE IN PANDEMIC TIMES

Ortiz, R., Kishton, R., Sinko, L., Fingerman, M., Moreland, D., Wood, J., & Venkataramani, A. (2021). Assessing child abuse hotline inquiries in the wake of COVID-19: Answering the call. *JAMA Pediatrics*, 175, 859–861. https://doi.org/10.1001/jamapediatrics.2021.0525

Question: How does the volume of calls and texts to a Child Abuse Hotline during the pandemic compare to the prior year?

Method: A cross-sectional study was conducted, using restricted-access data from Childhelp, a 24-h multilingual, national, American hotline focused on child abuse and neglect.

Study data included the number of inquiries, modality (call or text), and demographic characteristics (inquirer's age category, sex). [Users of Childhelp are connected to a crisis counsellor after having the optional opportunity to give anonymously demographic and relational information.]

Findings: Overall, inquiries increased by nearly 14% following school closures and quarantine orders associated with the COIVD-19 pandemic compared to overall inquiries in 2019 (2019 [$n = 16,599$]; 2020 [$n = 18,881$]). There were changes in the callers, as well, between these time periods: fewer calls came from teachers and school personnel while calls from neighbors or landlords, relatives, and friends increased. Text messaging, preferred by children and teenagers, expanded during the time of school closures, suggesting increased self-advocacy.

Implications: The higher rate of calls may reflect a higher rate of child-related distress and maltreatment during the restrictions and school closures required by the pandemic. Use of texts increased, suggesting children and teenagers may have needed to advocate for themselves when resources such as teachers and other school personnel were no longer available.

All types of child abuse exposure have been found to be associated with increased odds of suicidal ideation, plans, and attempts (Afifi et al., 2016). A Canadian study of child abuse exposure in the Canadian Armed Forces compared to the general population (Afifi et al., 2016) found that individuals with a history of child abuse were more likely to join the military; additive effects for past year suicide ideation and plans were noted between deployment-related trauma and child abuse exposure. The importance of recognizing the impact of trauma in children and families and the subsequent long-term effects is well established. Prevention, early detection, and intervention in the maltreatment of children are warranted. See Chapter 34.

Children in Care

The adjustment to an out-of-home placement can be viewed through the conceptual framework of Bowlby's stages of coping with parental separation. According to Bowlby (1960), the child initially responds to separation from parents with protest (crying, kicking, screaming, pleading, and attempting to elicit the parent's return). The child then moves to a state of despair (listlessness, apathy, and withdrawal, which lead to some acceptance of caregiving by others, but with reluctance to reattach fully). Finally, the child experiences detachment if the child and the foster parent cannot form an emotional bond. Because children often experience multiple placements, the potential for a disrupted attachment may be great when the child faces the prospect of a permanent family. After repeatedly undergoing separation and mourning, the child learns that rejection is inevitable and may automatically maintain distance from a new caregiver.

The trauma elicited, not only from the reason for children's placement but from their being exposed to multiple placements, can include detachment, diffuse rage, chronic depression, low self-esteem, and emotional dependency or insatiable need for nurturing and support (see Clinical Vignette). It takes knowledgeable, committed, and resilient care providers to work with a child challenged by these significant emotional and behavioural problems and struggles to reciprocate caring.

CLINICAL VIGNETTE

PREVENTIVE INTERVENTIONS WITH AN ADOLESCENT IN CRISIS

- Having been removed from their mother's care when she relapsed on cocaine and left them unattended, Aiden and Jenna have now been transferred to a second foster home. The plan is for the two children to return to their mother's home after she completes a 30-day drug treatment program. Aiden, who is in the 10th grade, is in the school nurse's office asking for aspirin for another headache.
- The nurse notices that Aiden's nose looks inflamed, he is sniffling, and seems more "hyper" than usual. In a concerned tone of voice, she asks Aiden if he has been using cocaine. "Just because my mother's a cokehead," he snaps, "doesn't give you the right to suspect me!" When the nurse gently says, "I'm sorry, I had no idea. Would you like to tell me about what's been happening with your mother?" Aiden responds less defensively and explains the situation about the foster home and their mother's drug problem. He says that if it were not for Jenna, his younger sister, he would have run away by now. Aiden notes that the foster parents are "making he and Jenna" go to school, but he plans on dropping out as soon as he returns to live with his mother. The only thing he likes about school is playing basketball; the basketball coach, who is his gym teacher, wants Aiden on the team.
- After a lengthy talk with Aiden, the nurse finishes the assessment interview and concludes that he is at risk for drug use, running away, and dropping out of school. Jaiden is also showing symptoms of depression, which he may be attempting to medicate with cocaine. Protective factors for Aiden include his strong attachment to his sister, his ability and willingness to express his thoughts and feelings, his interest in basketball, and a positive relationship with the basketball coach.
- The nurse discusses with Aiden what to do next. Using motivational interviewing strategies over several weeks, the nurse develops a plan with Aiden to attend the school's weekly drug and alcohol discussion group, so that he can talk with other teens from substance-abusing families and learn coping skills to prevent addiction. The nurse contacts the basketball coach, who agrees to find a student mentor who can shoot hoops with Aiden and help him to come up with a plan to stay in school, maybe find a part-time job, and join the basketball team. Aiden agrees to check in regularly with the nurse to report how the plan is working, and they can revise it if needed. The nurse feels optimistic that with support from their peers, coach, mentor, and herself, Aiden can reduce his risk for depression and addiction. Aiden shows signs of resilience, is motivated to "keep it together for Jenna," is capable of forming positive attachments, and willing to seek help, and knows where to find it.

Census data from 2011 and 2016 estimated that the numbers of children in foster care (0 to 14 years) were 29,500 and 28,300, respectively (Statistics Canada, 2017). The difficulty with identifying and tracking the numbers of children in care is that child welfare services fall under the provincial and territorial authorities and jurisdiction. The various provincial legislation directives can make it difficult to compare rates of children in out-of-home care across the country. In estimating the number of children in out-of-home care in Canada at year-end 2019, researchers from the Canadian Child Welfare Research Portal aggregated point-in-time data from each province and territory. Accordingly, the number of children in out-of-home care in Canada was 54,139, and 59,283 when informal kinship services were included. Provincial rates per 1,000 children varied significantly across the country, from 3.8 per 1,000 in Prince Edward Island to 33.2 per 1,000 in Manitoba (Saint-Girons et al., 2020). The overrepresentation of Indigenous children in care remains a significant concern, particularly in provinces and territories with an Indigenous child population over 25% (i.e., Manitoba, Nunavut, Northwest Territories, Saskatchewan, and Yukon) (Saint-Girons et al., 2020). Intergenerational trauma and the legacy of the residential school system continue to impact the lives of Indigenous Canadians (see Chapter 4). Nurses working with Indigenous children and families in community and hospital-based settings are in key positions to assist children and families at risk of child apprehension by adopting culturally safe practices. Eberl and Ogenchuk have concluded that, "Highlighting Indigenous values, and increasing the number of Indigenous policy-makers and consulting allies, would be huge first steps in creating a safer, more equitable child welfare system in Canada" (2019).

The Government of Canada, in collaboration with Indigenous Peoples, provinces and territories, recently codeveloped new legislation to reduce the overrepresentation of Indigenous children in care and to improve child and family services. The Act Respecting First Nations, Inuit and Métis children, Youth and Families came into force January 1, 2020 (Government of Canada, 2021) (see Web Links).

Parent With Mental Illness

A parent with mental illness can have profound effects on a child's growth and development. These effects can be experienced directly, through genetics, the intrauterine environment and antenatal stressors, and experience of the illness itself, or indirectly, due to socioeconomic issues such as poverty, and familial issues such as marital conflict, violence, substance use disorders, and lack or resources to buffer against negative outcomes (Majers, 2021; Reedtz et al., 2019).

IN-A-LIFE 🏠

Evelyn Lau (1971–)

Evelyn Lau is a noted poet, novelist, and short story writer. She was born in Vancouver, British Columbia, and wanted to pursue a career in the arts; however, this was not the desire of her traditional Chinese parents. Evelyn challenged her traditional family upbringing and left home when she was 14 years old. She spent much of the next 2 years living on the streets as a sex trade worker abusing addictive substances, resulting in suicide attempts. She has portrayed her experiences through her art, creating *Runaway: Diary of a Street Kid* (1989), which was later made into a CBC movie called *The Diary of Evelyn Lau* (1994) staring Sandra Oh. Subsequently, her first collection of poetry, *You Are Not Who You Claim* (1990), reflected much of that same time, and Evelyn was the recipient of the Milton Acorn People's Poetry Award. A second memoir, *Inside Out*, was published in 2001. To date, she has published thirteen books, and 8 volumes of poetry. Her eighth book of poetry *Pineapple Express* (2020) is a reflection on aging and anxiety, a synthesis of her public life and her professional life.

She was the youngest poet to receive a nomination for the Governor General's Award for *Oedipal Dreams*. She won the Air Canada Award in 1990 for Most Promising Writer under 30 and the Vantage Woman of Originality Award in 1999. Her book *Living Under Plastic* won the Pat Lowther Award for best book of poetry by a woman in Canada. From 2011 to 2014, Evelyn Lau was Vancouver's Poet Laureate. She has served as a writer-in-residence at the University of British Columbia, Kwantlen University, and Vancouver Community College.

Evelyn has spoken and written about her experiences and how this has created the work and person she has become. She does not make excuses for her choices and openly shares her feelings. Her story is one of how rigid traditional values can clash with youths' desires and dreams and of how she was fortunate that, for her, it resulted in a successful career. Unfortunately, this is not the case for many youths who find themselves living on the street in a life of drugs and prostitution.

A recent Canadian study that assessed symptoms of postpartum anxiety (PPA) and post partum depression (PPD) among women in Canada found that 14% of study participants ($n = 6,558$) had symptoms consistent with PPA, and 18% had symptoms consistent with PPD (Gheorghe et al., 2021). Postpartum depression can affect the parent–child bond and impact the attachment process for children. Therefore, nurses need to assess the parental history of stressors and physical and mental illness throughout the parent's pregnancy and assess the child during development.

Many children know that something is wrong when a parent has a mental illness, but they may not be able to identify the problem specifically (Gladstone et al., 2011). They feel alone, left out, distanced, and powerless to participate in decisions. They report feeling angry, sad, and that they are to blame for their parent's illness. They also worry that they may become ill, and they fear the stigma that surrounds mental illness. Fortunately, the likelihood or severity of these problems can be reduced or eliminated when families have the knowledge and support they need. Children need age-appropriate information, their questions answered, an opportunity to talk about how they feel, and routine childhood experiences. As with other family stressors, children need information as they are ready (Gladstone et al., 2011). Nurses can help parents get started by modelling. For example, "Mommy isn't feeling well. She feels sad. It's because of an illness and it's not her fault. It is a sad time for all of us, but I'm here to talk with you about it when you need to do so."

Given Canada's ethnic diversity, and the Canadian government's commitment in particular to the resettlement of refugees from the Middle East, nurses will inevitably come into contact with refugee families in their practice. Parental histories of pre- and postmigration trauma, anxiety, and depression, coupled with the stressors of learning a new language, seeking employment, and managing a household with limited resources and social networks, can weigh heavily on parents' ability to be responsive and nurturing. This may lead to inconsistencies in attachment with younger children and strained relationships with older children. Nurses need to be cautious that they do not prematurely judge parents' capabilities to parent, especially when older children have assumed many navigational roles (e.g., education system, healthcare system) as a result of their ease with communicating in a new language (Minhas et al., 2017).

Children with a mentally ill parent will usually need supportive relationships outside the home with someone (e.g., a teacher, coach, neighbour) who can provide a listening ear, extra support, and a measure of respite for the family. Children need to know that their routine in life will continue, including the fun times, and that their relationship with both parents is valued by the parents. Parents worry about how their mental illness will affect their child. Support and education need to be provided to all during these challenging times (Costea, 2011; Gladstone et al., 2011). Evidence shows that when children and their families are given information about the affected parent's mental illness, they show improved knowledge and long-standing positive effects in how they problem solve (a resilience-related quality) around parental illness (Gladstone et al., 2011). In a personal reflection, Majers (2021) explains how a parent's mental illness can have a profound impact on family members, and particularly on children, who are often too young to comprehend the losses they experience. Parental mental illness disrupts the communication between child and parent, as does the parent's potential unavailability due to hospitalization and/or custody issues, which ultimately may contribute to profound grief.

Parent With a Substance Use Problem

Exposure to parental addiction in childhood is common in Canada, with reported prevalence higher for women (20%) than for men (16%) (Langlois & Garner, 2013). Children whose parents are dependent on alcohol live in an unpredictable family environment and are more likely to experience abuse, and their efforts to cope with stress may disrupt their ability to perform in school and lead to other emotional problems (Maina et al., 2021). A study that examined the course of psychological distress among a nationally representative sample of Canadians (aged 18 to 74) revealed that those who experienced parental addictions had consistently higher distress scores than those who did not (Langlois & Garner, 2013). Such experience also appears associated with other childhood adversities, parental comorbidities, and a negative family environment; thus, understanding the effects of exposure to parental addiction on children requires further study (Langlois & Garner, 2013). In a recent Canadian study, Maina and colleagues (2021) found that for children growing up in homes where addiction use was profuse, participants adopted a variety of diverse coping strategies, including leaving home, using substances, and dropping out of school. Nurses working in schools and community settings are uniquely positioned to screen and intervene with children and youth at risk for substance use, homelessness, and dropping out of school.

Genetic factors are at least partly responsible for the well-documented increased risk for substance abuse. Studies are beginning to link a family history of mental disorders and alcoholism with genetically transmitted mental disorders, which may be a precursor to alcohol abuse. The precise mechanism of family transmission of alcoholism remains unknown. Children of those who abuse substances may inherit a predisposition to a nonspecific form of biologic dysregulation that may be expressed phenotypically, either as alcoholism or as some other psychiatric disorder (e.g., hyperactivity, conduct disorder, depression), depending on the individual's developmental history.

Children of persons who misuse substances are at high risk for both substance use and behaviour disorders (Maina et al., 2020, 2021; Mylant et al., 2002). Moreover, some evidence shows that in terms of alcohol use disorder, other factors related to addiction, such as family stress, violence, divorce, dysfunction, and other concurrent parental psychiatric disorders (e.g., depression, anxiety), are as important as the disorder itself in increasing this risk (Ritter et al., 2002). The experience of growing up in a family where the misuse of substances is prevalent is commonly marked by unpredictability, fear, and helplessness because of the cyclic nature of addictive patterns.

The literature on children of parents who have alcohol use disorder has described several typical roles that children assume, including the "hero" (overly responsible children who may ignore their own needs to take care of parents and other children), "scapegoat" (problem children who divert the attention away from the parent), "mascot" (family clowns who relieve tension and mask feelings through joking), and "lost child" (children who suffer in silence but may exhibit difficulties at school or in later life) (Veronie & Freuhstorfer, 2001). These roles, combined with the enabling behaviours of other family members who attempt to cover up and minimize the effects of the addiction, may become so rigid and effective in masking the problem that children of people who misuse substances may not come to the attention of mental health professionals until after the parent stops consuming the substance and family roles are disrupted.

The experience of growing up in this environment can lead to poor self-concept if children feel responsible for their parents' behaviour. The child becomes isolated and learns to mistrust their own perceptions as the family denies the reality of the addiction. There is, however, no uniform pattern of outcomes, and many children demonstrate resilience (Harter, 2000). As noted previously, resilience is the phenomenon by which some children at risk for psychopathology—because of genetic or experiential circumstances—attain good mental health, maintain hope, and achieve healthy outcomes (Masten, 2001). Again, individual protective factors and preventive interventions are paramount.

Addressing Risks and Challenges to Children's and Adolescents' Mental Health

Nurses and other healthcare professionals need to become aware of and use strategies to address negative impacts on a children's overall functioning. Professional nursing emphasizes a family-centred, interdisciplinary approach in which the nurse acts as the collaborator, coordinator, case manager, and advocate to establish linkages with physicians and nurse practitioners, teachers, speech and language specialists, social workers, and other professionals to develop and implement comprehensive preventative interventions. A view of parents as partners should be foremost. In the past, parents have been too often viewed as the culprits in creating children's mental health problems. Recent insights into the biological and genetic origins of psychiatric disorders have contributed to a shift from blaming parents to seeking their collaboration in treatment.

Trauma-and Violence-Informed Care for Children and Adolescents

Trauma- and violence-informed care is essential in the nursing care of children and adolescents, as it crosses all areas of practice (see Chapters 18 and 34). Universal trauma precautions ensure that care and treatment do not inadvertently retraumatize a patient nor trigger a trauma response (see Box 29.2). Attention is paid to reducing stigma and increasing safety and control.

The neurodevelopment of children exposed to traumatic events affects their cognitive and emotional development (De Bellis & Zisk, 2014). "These children may demonstrate hypervigilance, intrusive thoughts, nightmares, bed-wetting, excessive clinginess, inconsolable crying, and severe tantrums" (Arvidson et al., 2011, p. 41). Programs that emphasize establishing self-regulation strategies and attachment attunement and that work toward development or repair of cognitive skills have been shown to shift affected children toward better success and reduced psychopathology (Arvidson

---

BOX 29.2 Trauma and Violence-Informed Approaches

The implementation of trauma and violence-informed care involves the following:

a. Understanding that trauma and violence affect people's behavioral responses
b. Creating emotionally and physically safe environments to support engagement
c. Fostering opportunities for choices, collaboration and connection
d. Providing a strength based, asset approach to support capacity building, coping, and resilience

Government of Canada. (2018). *Trauma and violence-informed approaches to policy and practice.* https://www.canada.ca/en/public-health/services/publications/health-risks-safety/trauma-violence-informed-approaches-policy-practice.html et al., 2011). An example is the Attachment, Self-Regulation, and Competency program that teaches both the healthcare provider and parent how to modulate their emotional responses, attune to the child, and assist with their self-regulation. "Caregivers and clinicians play an essential role in restoring a sense of safety and security to traumatized children by developing predictable routines and rituals in their lives" (Arvidson et al., 2011, p. 42). Once the child is better able to self-regulate, they are more open to learning and experiencing the world from a safer perspective (Blaustein & Kinniburgh, 2010). A trauma-informed approach has been shown to benefit children attending inpatient settings and outpatient settings, as well as schools and residential care homes (Arvidson et al., 2011). Resources for such an approach are increasingly available. For instance, in British Columbia, the Child and Youth Mental Health and Substance Use Collaborative offers a "Trauma Informed Practice and Trauma Informed Services Resources List" (2017) for accessing provincial, national, and international resources (see Chapter 18).

At the individual level, such factors as secure attachment, good parenting, friendship and social support, meaningful employment and social roles, adequate income, and physical activity will strengthen mental health and, indirectly, reduce the impact or incidence of some mental health problems. At a system level, strategies that create supportive environments, strengthen community actions, develop personal skills, and orient health services can ensure that the population has some control over the psychological and social determinants of mental health. A Canadian qualitative study of a community based drop-in psychosocial mental health centre designed specifically for youth struggling with mental health issues was conducted to identify program features that promoted or discouraged engagement. Overall, the researchers found that approaching youth with a trauma-informed and healing-centred lens can increase the engagement in and impact of programming in such centres. Creating a safe space, building trust, encouraging growth, and facilitating connections and transitions promoted engagement in programming efforts (Creamer et al., 2020).

Promotion and Prevention Programs

Promotion and prevention programs incorporate a range of techniques to provide reassurance and education, skills training, or direct intervention. The programs may use face-to-face techniques (e.g., home visits, educational groups), literature (e.g., pamphlets, books), phone (e.g., crisis lines), or electronic mechanisms (e.g., internet, telehealth).

Psychoeducational Programs

Psychoeducational programs are a particularly effective form of mental health promotion and intervention. These programs are designed to teach parents and children necessary coping skills for dealing with various stressors. Among other techniques, they use the process of **normalization** (i.e., teaching families what are typical behaviours and expected responses) and provide families with information about normal child development and expected reactions to various stressors so that the families will feel less isolated, know what to expect, and put their reactions into perspective. For example, if families learn that anger is a natural part of grieving, they will be less likely to view it as abnormal and more likely to accept and cope with it constructively.

An excellent example is *Transitions*, a downloadable resource for teenagers and their families developed by a Canadian expert in adolescent mental health, Stanley Kutcher, Dalhousie University, and his colleagues. *Transitions* is focused on helping youth transition from high school to university and covers topics ranging from study tips, time management, and exams to sexuality and dating to mental illness, unhealthy behaviours (e.g., violence), substance use, and suicide (Kutcher, 2019). See Web Links—Mental Health Literacy.

Psychoeducational approaches that utilize parallel curricula, established with concurrent psychoeducational groups for adults and children, are helpful. Most foster care agencies now provide a program of education and training for prospective foster parents to help them know what to expect and how to help the child adjust to placement.

Social Skills Training

Social skills training is one psychoeducational approach that has been useful with youth who have low self-esteem, aggressive behaviour, or high risk for substance abuse. **Social skills training** involves instruction, feedback, support, and practice with learning behaviours that help children interact more competently with peers and adults. When combined with assertiveness training, social skills training can help provide children with coping skills to resist engaging in addictive or antisocial behaviours and prevent social withdrawal under stress. Social skills training may be particularly beneficial for children dealing with peer rejection, marginalization, or lagging social integration.

Bibliotherapy

Bibliotherapy is the therapeutic use of books, stories, and other reading material to facilitate emotional growth and healing. It can help children, adolescents, and families gain information and understanding about life stressors, illness, and recovery. Stories provide a catalyst for change and are a particularly potent form of intervention as they have the potential to provide other perspectives, gain insight into issues, and facilitate ways to learn and develop coping mechanisms (Gregory & Vessey, 2004; Heath et al., 2005). A wide variety of books are available to help children understand issues such as death, divorce, chronic illness, stepfamilies, adoption, and a sibling's birth.

Children and adolescents can find comfort and increased understanding through stories that reflect their own experiences. Parents can use stories as a way to learn about their children's concerns: the adventures and/or tribulations of a story's characters can be a means to discover their child's thoughts and feelings about an experience. Some health centres and hospitals have patient library services available. Many mental health organizations such as the Canadian Mental Health Association, public health agencies, and Health Canada have pamphlets or website information designed for parents or children and youth about various physical and psychological problems. In addition to providing factual information and advice, these reading materials help to reduce anxiety by pointing out common reactions to the various stressors so that families do not feel alone.

Support Groups

Support groups, groups composed of people with a similar experience or problem who meet regularly to sustain and support one another, are available for just about every kind of stressor that a family can experience, including substance abuse, death, divorce, and coping with a chronic illness. Both parents and children in groups can experience Yalom's (1985) healing effects of group therapy, including group cohesiveness, universality (awareness of the normalcy and commonality of one's reactions), catharsis, hope, and altruism (being able to help others; see Chapter 15).

Early Intervention Programs

Early intervention programs, possibly the most important form of primary prevention available to children and families, offer regular home visits, support, education, and concrete services to those in need. The assumption underlying these programs is that parents are the most consistent and influential figures in children's lives, and they should be allowed the opportunity to define their own needs and priorities. With support and education, parents will be empowered to respond more effectively to their children.

Canada invests in early intervention to promote healthy child development by enhancing such programs as paid parental leave, child care, family resource centres, and early learning. A number of jurisdictions have introduced promotion and prevention programs around the birth of a newborn, for example, Healthy Beginnings Postpartum Program in Alberta in which mothers and babies are visited by a nurse following discharge from a hospital birth and Healthy Beginnings: Enhanced Home Visiting in Nova Scotia where a home visitor shares information about child development to support families in making healthy choices. Intensive postpartum support (more than antenatal support) provided by a healthcare professional can help prevent postpartum depression (Werner et al., 2015). Early intervention, especially when initiated prenatally, can be effective in preventing child abuse. Early intervention can contribute to developmental benefits in terms of cognition and reduce behavioural problems in older children (Peacock et al., 2013). Population-based early intervention initiatives aimed at socioeconomically disadvantaged communities are directed toward the child (e.g., classroom enrichment, quality childcare), parent (e.g., home visiting, parent help/information/crisis phone lines, parent–child play groups), and neighbourhood (information that engages families and connects them to community supports), with an emphasis on providing intensive services that benefit children directly. They have demonstrated improvements in children's emotional problems, behavioural problems, social skills, and a decreased need for special education during the early years (ages 4 to 8) (Peters et al., 2003).

Programs designed for adolescent mental health should support and educate youth (e.g., through peer mentoring in community organizations and schools); enhance self-help and self-responsibility, coping skills, self-esteem, and skill development in ways that foster mental health; and teach youth when and how to seek assistance for problems. Since youth are often influenced by peers, particular emphasis has been placed on the creation of healthy youth images related to gender, body image, empowerment, and youth engagement.

Historically, nurses have been underused in school-based mental health efforts, although schools are good locations for other early intervention programs because they are physically near the families they serve and are less intimidating than mental health centres. Programs can be targeted for very young children before symptoms have time to develop. Recognizing the importance of early intervention and interprofessional collaboration, nursing programs across Canada are placing senior nursing students in schools (elementary and high schools), and together with school officials, they work to promote mental health from a holistic perspective. Refer further to Eberl and Ogenchuk (2019) and King et al. (2020).

Electronic Media Services

The number of promotion and early intervention mental health services provided through electronic media (e.g., internet, telehealth) is growing. Targeted support groups are increasingly available through the internet. Dedicated websites providing both universal mental health information and confidential intervention services by e-mail are also available through some school systems. Similar services around specific mental health issues are also being tested with high-risk populations. Telehealth involves telephone and video support to rural and remote Canada (see Chapter 6).

Comprehensive Approaches

Undertaking interventions to promote the mental health of children and adolescents is time and effort well spent. Many adult mental health problems can be prevented, coped with more effectively, or at least reduced in their scope and severity through focused intervention with children, youth, and families. Children and youth lack the power and voice to fight for their own needs, making them one of the most vulnerable groups in society. By virtue of their close interaction with families, nurses are in a key position to identify children's and youth's mental health needs and intervene, particularly in times of crisis.

Community-Based Mental Health Promotion

Mental health promotion with children and youth can occur at individual, familial, community, and global levels. Multiple factors affect mental wellbeing; mental health does not equate to a lack of mental illness and is affected by the social determinants of health (See Chapters 2 and 3). Mental health promotion initiatives need to be tailored to the individual children and youth with whom nurses work (including their familial and social resources). Nurses must be sensitive to context and must incorporate the latest empirical and theoretical developments. Among children and youth, in addition to the health and social services systems, the education system can be among the sites where mental health promotion initiatives take place.

Mental Health Assessment of Children and Adolescents

The assessment of children and adolescents generally follows the same format as that for adults (see Chapter 11), but there are significant differences. In working with children, adolescents, and families, nurses must recognize that the perspective of each person involved. Children think in more concrete terms; the nurse needs to ask specific questions and use fewer open-ended questions than would typically be asked of adults. Simple phrasing should be used because children have a narrower vocabulary than do adults. Examples include saying "sad" instead of "depressed" or "nervous" or "worried" instead of "anxious." Corroborate information that children offer with more sources (e.g., parents, teachers) than might be needed with adults. Artistic and play media (e.g., puppets, family drawings) can be used to engage children and evaluate their perceptions, inner worlds, fine motor skills, and intellectual functions. Children have a less specific sense of time and a less developed memory than do adults. When children are asked about a sequence of events or specific times when events occurred, they may not provide accurate information.

Adolescents must be assessed within their range of cognitive and developmental functioning. Adolescents may or may not be willing participants in the assessment process, depending on why they have been referred and who has referred them. It is essential to meet with adolescents separate from their care providers. It is critical to ensure what level of confidentiality can be provided to the youth in the context of an individual interview. For example, issues of safety, such as suicidality, would need to be revealed to care providers, whereas issues of sexual identity are less immediately urgent. There is usually time to determine when or if this issue should be shared collaboratively with the child's/youth's care providers. Mental health assessment involves much more than completing assessment tools and considers far more than the individual. A conceptual framework used as a guide can assist in planning the goals of the assessment, as well as identifying the factors, types of information and sources, and the elements within the environment to be considered. Frameworks that shape the mental health assessment of children and youth in Canada are identified and described below.

The Canadian Mental Health Association's (CMHA) Framework for Support

The CMHA's Framework for Support identifies three resource bases important to mental health assessment: the *Community Resource Base, the Knowledge Resource Base, and the Personal Resource Base.* This framework helps focus assessment on outcomes that play a critical role in recovery from mental illness. Specifically, it supports an assessment of whether a child has access to the social determinants of good mental health (housing, school, family, friends, a sense of purpose), feels well and has a sense of personal control, and has various personal resources in place and ways to connect with the formal service system if needed. Finally, the framework assesses how the individual's age (child or youth) and life circumstances (e.g., breakup or death in the family, being cut from a sports team) have challenged the child. By focusing on the *Community Resource Base,* an understanding is gained of the many factors and social determinants that affect the everyday life of children and youth

The *Community Resource Base* acknowledges the importance of both formal services (mental health services, generic community services) and the network of natural supports (family and friends, self-help, and consumer organizations) available to promote mental health and recovery. Equally important, this framework recognizes the person (child or youth) as having the power (age appropriate) to make choices about which resources to use, if any, and to participate fully in decision-making related to their care. By focusing on the *Knowledge Resource Base*, consideration is given not only to medical–clinical and social science knowledge but also to experiential knowledge (firsthand experience) and traditional knowledge (cultural ways). How children experience mental illness and how the family and community accept through its public attitudes and conventional wisdom are noted in the assessment. A critical analysis of such information helps build a rich understanding of children and guards the nurse against drawing inaccurate assumptions. It can also identify inaccuracies and misconceptions that may be held within the family or community about mental illness. Focusing on the *Personal Resource Base* acknowledges that the child/youth is far more than a repository of illness and symptoms and that positive change builds on existing strengths. Hence, when approaching assessment, their understanding of their mental health problem/illness and their self-esteem, their sense of belonging (within their family and community), and a sense of purpose and meaning in the world are considered. The child/youth's skills and capacities (sense of personal control, confidence, resilience, hope) to confront illness are assessed (Trainor et al., 2004).

Evergreen: A Child and Youth Mental Health Framework for Canada

The Mental Health Commission of Canada's (MHCC) Evergreen Framework provides values and strategic directions for child and youth mental health care in Canada (Kutcher & McLuckie, 2010). The values identified are as follows:

- Human rights
- Dignity, respect, and diversity
- Best available evidence
- Choice, opportunity, and responsibility
- Collaboration, continuity, and community
- Access to information, programs, and services

Health professionals should be cognizant of human rights documents in a way that informs their practice. These documents include the United Nation's (UN) *Convention on the Rights of the Child* and the *Convention on the Rights of Persons with Disabilities*, as well as *A Canada Fit for Children* that is Canada's response to the UN's *A World Fit for Child*ren. Valuing dignity, respect, and diversity involves striving for equal access to services and programs for all children and their families in Canada. Ongoing commitment is necessary for best evidence-based programs to evolve; children and families

need to make informed choices about what best fits their needs. Collaboration among all those who have a significant role in a child's life allows for meaningful networks of support. Publicly accessible mental health information and the promotion of access to programs and services are crucial to an equitable healthcare system. These explicitly stated values contribute to a shared vision for the evolution of child and adolescent mental health in Canada.

Four categories of strategic directions are identified in the Evergreen Framework, envisioned as separate but overlapping categories: *promotion, prevention, intervention and ongoing care*, and *research and evaluation*. Within the Evergreen Framework, specific strategies for each category are identified.

The Bio/Psycho/Social/Spiritual Model

The holistic, integrated approach of the bio/psycho/social/spiritual model of health used throughout this textbook is applicable to child and adolescent care. Comprehensive assessment should include a bio/psycho/social/spiritual history, mental status examination, additional testing (e.g., cognitive or neuropsychological), and, if necessary, records of the child's school performance and medical–physical history and information from other agencies that may be providing services (e.g., department of child and family services, juvenile court). Various assessment and screening tools can be used to facilitate evaluation and intervention strategies (see Web Links—Canadian Paediatric Society: Mental Health: Screening tools and rating scales).

Collection of Assessment Data

Comprehensive collection of meaningful data is crucial to an accurate, holistic assessment of the mental health of a child or youth. Components of assessment data and the necessary nursing skills necessary are addressed here. (Note: where appropriate, "child" will be the term used to refer to both children and adolescents).

The Clinical Interview

The clinical interview is the primary assessment tool used in child and adolescent mental health nursing. A unique set of skills is necessary for interviewing children and adolescents. How the nurse obtains mental health information depends on each child's developmental level explicitly considering the child's language and cognitive, social, and emotional skills. For example, the nurse should simplify questions for young children or children with developmental delays or communication issues (e.g., autism spectrum disorder, hearing impairment, English as an additional language) so these children can understand and respond accordingly.

The assessment interview may be the initial contact between the child and parent/guardian and the nurse. The first step is to establish a connection and rapport to build a relationship, and the second is to assess the interactions between the child and their caregivers. It is important to understand that children cannot be considered apart from their caregivers and the context in which they live. However, defining the caregiving context is sometimes a challenge. The nurse needs to identify the child's primary caregivers, the patterns of current caregiving relationships (e.g., how often the child goes to other caregivers), and the history of these relationships (e.g., multiple transitions, abrupt losses). The nurse should also explore the family's definition of *family* and identify those included in the family constellation This would include the biological, psychosocial, and spiritual relationships the child experiences (e.g., uncle, Big Brother/Big Sister volunteer, friends, neighbours, godmother) (Shajani & Snell, 2019) (see Chapter 16).

Building Rapport

Building rapport is fundamental to any mental health assessment. To reduce anxiety and establish trust during the assessment, the nurse strives to develop rapport with the family members. The nurse can establish a relationship with the child/youth and family by recognizing the child's individuality and showing respect and concern consistently. The nurse should demonstrate sensitivity, objectivity, and confidentiality. Children will be more forthcoming if they believe that the nurse is listening carefully and is interested in what they have to say. Establishing rapport can be facilitated by making and maintaining eye contact (as culturally relevant); speaking slowly, clearly, and calmly, with friendliness and acceptance; using a warm and expressive tone; reacting to communications objectively; showing interest in what families are saying; and making the interview a joint undertaking (see Chapter 7).

The information in Box 29.3 can serve as a guide to asking specific questions during a child's comprehensive assessment. The Community Resource Base of the Framework for Support (Trainor et al., 2004) provides a useful guide for identifying a range of stakeholders from the child's daily living activities (e.g., parent, school, daycare, recreation, arts) as well as services (formal or informal) that might be consulted (with family permission) for related information about the various contexts in which the child interacts. These stakeholders can provide complementary information (formal or informal) about how the child functions in critical developmental

---

BOX 29.3 Semistructured Interview With School-Aged Children

This guide identifies a range of areas and sample questions that can be addressed during an interview with a school-aged or adolescent child. The nurse should note that children generally prefer to be engaged in a conversation rather than peppered with questions. The interview should be tailored in a way that is comfortable and relevant for the child. Although some direct questions are inevitable, open-ended questions are preferable. Similarly, phrasing questions to get at what a child is thinking (e.g., "I can see you are trying to tell me something" or "Tell me more") is preferable to asking "why" questions that tend to put people on the defensive. Note that in the guide, "Explain" means to explore an explanation; it does not indicate giving the command "explain" to the child or adolescent. Finally, trying to match the child's emotional state (unless hostile) helps people feel understood. The interview can begin with a simple greeting, such as the following: "Hi, I am (your name and title). You must be Tom Brown. Come in."

FOR ALL SCHOOL-AGED CHILDREN

Presenting Concern

Thank you for coming to talk with me today. To begin, it would help me if I knew what, if anything, you have been told about why you are here or what will go on today.... Can you tell me *your* story of how you came to be here today? (If necessary, probe with specific questions below. Let the child take the lead and explore issues as they raise them. If the child raises a problem, explore it in detail.)

Demographic Information

I'd like to know you better. Could you tell me about yourself?

Probes

1. How old are you?
2. When is your birthday?
3. Where do you live? (address)
4. And your telephone number is...?

School

Tell me about your school.

Probes

5. Which school do you go to? Is it close to your home? How do you get there each day?
6. Where do you go after school (home, sitter, etc.)... and who is there (parent/relative, sitter, no one)?

BOX 29.3 Semistructured Interview With School-Aged Children (Continued)

7. What do most kids think about your school? … What is it like for you?

8. What grade are you in? What do most kids think about it? … What is it like for you?

9. What subjects do you like the best? … Like least?

10. What subjects give you the least trouble? … Most trouble?

11. How well do you do in school—about the same as, better than, or not as well as other kids in your class?

12. On the whole, would you say that you are doing better or worse than last year?

13. What activities do you participate in at school?

14. How well do you get along with your classmates?

15. How well do you get along with your teachers?

16. Tell me how you spend a usual day at school.

HOME AND FAMILY

To help me understand your family, can you name each of the people who live with you … and then other important family members who live somewhere else … and I'll put them into a picture…. Now, using the picture, tell me a little about your family.

A genogram provides a useful diagram of family relationships. It resembles a family tree but includes additional relationships among individuals. It permits the nurse and the child to quickly see patterns in family history. It maps relationships and traits that may otherwise be missed and includes basic information about number of families, number of children in each family, birth order, and deaths. Some genograms include information on disorders running in the family such as alcoholism, depression, diseases, alliances, and living situations. Older children can provide additional information (e.g., about separation/divorce, death) for understanding family dynamics. (See Chapter 16 for detailed information regarding creating a genogram.)

Probes

17. Tell me a little about each of them.
   - Who makes you happy and who makes you sad/angry/worried? Explain.
   - Do you have a favourite photo of you and your family? Tell me about it … and why you like it.

18. What does your father do during the day—does he work? (Other activities at home/with friends?)

19. What does your mother do during the day—does she work? (Other activities at home/with friends?)

20. Tell me what your home is like.

21. Tell me about your room at home.

22. What chores do you do at home?

23. How do you get along with your father?

24. What does he do that you like? … Don't like?

25. How do you get along with your mother?

26. What does she do that you like? … Don't like?

27. (Where relevant) Some brothers and sisters get along well, whereas others don't get along at all … How do you get along with your brothers and sisters?

28. What do (does) they (he/she) do that you like? … That you don't like?

29. Who handles the discipline at home?

30. Tell me about how they (he/she) handle (handles) it.
   - When you do something good, what happens and who is involved?
   - When you get in trouble, what happens and who is involved?
   - If you want to do something different from the rest of your family, would that be okay? Explain … Who would support you?
   - If you need help, what would you do? Would someone support you? Explain.
   - Are there other relatives who are important to you? Tell me about who they are and how they connect with you (if not already discussed with the genogram).
   - Would you say that your family is like most other families in your school/neighbourhood or different? Explain. Does that make it easy or difficult for you/your family … and in what ways and in what types of situations? This question gets at culture (ethnicity, socioeconomic status, language, beliefs/values, etc.) in a broad way.

INTERESTS

Now let's talk about the things you like to do.

Probes

31. What hobbies and interests do you have?

32. What do you do in the afternoons/evenings after school?

33. Tell me what you usually do on Saturdays and Sundays.
   - What do you do on special holidays? Tell me about the best holiday you ever had.
   - When you are having fun, what are you doing, who are you with? Tell me about a time when you were really having a good time.

(Continued)

BOX 29.3 Semistructured Interview With School-Aged Children *(Continued)*

Friends

Tell me about your friends.

Probes

34. What do you like to do with your friends?
    • Any best friends?
    • If you needed help, could you count on them to support you? Give an example.
    • If you wanted to do something different from them, would that be okay?

MOODS AND FEELINGS

Probes

35. Everybody feels happy at times. What things make you feel happiest?
36. What are you most likely to get sad about?
37. What do you do when you are sad?
38. Everybody gets angry at times. What things make you angriest?
39. What do you do when you are angry?

FEARS AND WORRIES

Probes

40. All children get scared sometimes about some things. What things make you feel scared?
41. What do you do when you are scared? … What takes away the fear?
    • How well does that work?
42. Tell me what you worry about … What takes away the worry?
    • How well does that work?
43. Any other things?

SELF-CONCERNS

Probes

44. What do you like best about yourself? … Anything else?
45. What do you like least about yourself? … Anything else?
46. Tell me about the best thing that ever happened to you.
47. Tell me about the worst thing that ever happened to you.
    • What did you do about this situation?
    • How well does that work?
    • Overall, how much would you say you believe in yourself?

SOMATIC CONCERNS

Probes

48. Do you ever get headaches?
49. (If yes) Tell me about them. (How often? What do you usually do?)
50. Do you get stomachaches?
51. (If yes) Tell me about them. (How often? What do you usually do?)
52. Do you get any other kinds of body pains?
53. (If yes) Tell me about them.
    • What do you do to ease these problems?
      • How well does that work?

THOUGHT DISORDER

Probes

54. Do you ever hear things that seem funny or unusual?
55. (If yes) Tell me about them. (How often? How do you feel about them? What do you usually do?)
56. Do you ever see things that seem funny or unreal?
57. (If yes) Tell me about them. (How often? How do you feel about them? What do you usually do?)

HELP-SEEKING

Probes

58. Tell me about a time when you have needed help. What did you do? Whom did you ask for help? What kind of help did you get? How did things work out?
59. Have you ever gone to see a counsellor before? Explain. Did it help?

MEMORIES AND FANTASY

Probes

60. What is the first thing you can remember from the time when you were a very little baby?
61. Tell me about your dreams.
62. Which dreams come back again?
63. Who are your favourite television characters?
64. Tell me about them.
65. What animals do you like best?
66. Tell me about these animals.
67. What animals do you like least?
68. Tell me about these animals.
69. What is your happiest memory?
70. What is your saddest memory?
71. If you could change places with anyone in the whole world, who would it be?

BOX 29.3 Semistructured Interview With School-Aged Children *(Continued)*

72. Tell me about that.
73. If you could go anywhere you wanted to right now, where would you go?
74. Tell me about that.
75. If you could have three wishes, what would they be?
76. What things do you think you might need to take with you if you were to go to the moon and stay there for 6 months?

ASPIRATIONS

77. What do you plan on doing when you become an adult?
78. What things will help you be successful? Is there anything standing in the way of you being successful?
    - How hopeful are you that you might be successful? (Suggestion—using a visual analogue with a series of faces on a line [sad face to very happy face], ask child to choose the face that best describes their hopefulness.)
79. If you could do anything you wanted when you become an adult, what would it be?

CONCLUDING QUESTIONS

80. Do you have anything else that you would like to tell me about yourself?
81. Do you have any questions that you would like to ask me?
    - What are you hoping will happen as a result of our talking today?

FOR ADOLESCENTS
SEXUAL RELATIONS

Adolescence is a very confusing time emotionally. Our bodies change as we begin to look more like adults. Our relationships also change. While our sexual relationships are new and exciting, they can also be puzzling, frustrating, or even frightening.

1. Do you have any romantic feelings or relationship(s) with guys or girls? Do you feel comfortable talking about them? With girls/guys/or both?
2. What makes you feel good about it/them?
3. What makes you feel not so good about them?
4. Do you have any special girlfriend or boyfriend?
5. (If yes) Tell me about her (him). Most people have lots of questions about their sexual relationships and yet are not sure whom to trust to talk openly.
6. What kind of sexual concerns do you have?
7. (If present) Tell me about them.
8. (If applicable) What do you think might be helpful to do about your concerns? (getting information, talking to someone, getting a checkup/some medication)
9. Are you interested in getting help? Would you like me to help you make the right connections?

DRUG AND ALCOHOL USE

10. Do your parents/sister/brothers drink?
11. (If yes) Tell me about their drinking. (How much, how frequently, and where?)
12. Do your friends drink alcohol?
13. (If yes) Tell me about their drinking.
14. Do you drink alcohol?
15. (If yes) Tell me about your drinking.
16. Do your parents use drugs?
17. (If yes) Tell me about the drugs they use. (How much, how frequently, and for what reasons?)
18. Do your friends use drugs?
19. (If yes) Tell me about the drugs they use.
20. Do you use drugs?
21. (If yes) Tell me about the drugs you use
22. Are you worried about the way your parents/siblings/friends use alcohol or drugs?
23. Are you worried about the way you use alcohol/drugs?
24. (If yes) Are you interested in getting help?
25. (If applicable) What do you think might be helpful to do regarding your concerns?

domains (language and literacy, physical, cognitive, social, and emotional). They also provide an understanding of how the child is treated within, and copes with, various peer environments involving diverse cultures (e.g., ethnic, socioeconomic, language) and activities (e.g., scholastic, recreational, artistic). This information can help the nurse formulate a well-balanced and integrated mental health assessment (strengths and limitations from multiple contexts) of the child.

Child and Parent Observation

Because the child's immediate environment is often with the parent, child–parent interactions provide important data about the child–parent attachment and parenting practices. As discussed earlier, attachment is the term used to name the emotional bonds between a child and parent (or parental figure) that begin in infancy. The nurse's observations focus on both the child alone and the child within the family. The nurse can make some of these observations while the family is in the waiting area, noting behaviours. Barnard's (1994) observations remain relevant to contemporary nursing practice.

• Sensitivity/clarity/responsiveness to cues
• How the child and parent get each other's attention
• How parent and child interact with and talk to each other (clarity of cues)
• How frequently each initiates conversation and how promptly each responds
• How the child and parent separate
• Whether the parent and child play together
• How responsive the parent is to the child's attention-seeking initiatives
• How the parent and child show affection to each other
• How attached the parent and the child appear
• Response to distress
• Whether the parent starts/stops/notes the distress/changes in activity
• How the parent consoles the child
• How the parent disciplines the child (clear directive voice, yells, hits)
• Use of talking, smiling, laughing, singing, touching (praising or criticizing)
• Parent talks about/describes objects/ideas using developmentally appropriate and stimulating language
• Parent provides their child with/points out objects of interest
• Parent encourages and/or allows the child to explore

Interview Techniques

To get an accurate picture of the child, the nurse should interview the child and parent individually for some part of the session because each can provide unique, meaningful information. Often, disagreement between child and parent regarding signs and symptoms relevant to diagnostic criteria emerges in separate interviews. Generally, children provide better information about internalizing symptoms (e.g., mood, sleep, suicide ideation), and parents provide better information about externalizing symptoms (e.g., behaviour disturbances, oppositionality, relationship with parents).

Discussion With the Child

After talking with the parent and child together, the nurse should ask to speak with the child alone for a while. Young children may fear separating from their parents. The nurse can reassure children by showing them where the waiting area is and telling them, "Mommy and

Daddy will be waiting right here for you. You and I are going to be in a room close by. But if you get worried, we can come back out here to check on them." Introducing a toy or game or giving the child a transitional object to hold may help. For example, young children often like holding the family house or car keys, knowing that their parents cannot go anywhere without them. Remember that observing how the child separates from the parent is part of the data needed to complete the assessment.

Adolescents may act indifferent or even hostile when the nurse asks to speak with them alone. Remember that this may cover anxiety and fear. Teens tend to be skeptical that adults can really understand their experience, suspicious that they will be blamed for their problems, and fearful that their thoughts and feelings are abnormal. The nurse should be patient with adolescents and show empathy for their concerns through comments such as, "I can see that you're pretty angry about being here. There might be a way that I can help.... But to help, I need to know from *you* what is going on that is making you so angry. I want to assure you that I am not here to judge or blame. I can also promise you that if you tell me anything that I think needs to be shared with your parents, then I will tell you first." If the youth is particularly silent, the nurse might comment, "You've been pretty quiet during the last few minutes.... I'm not sure if that means you're having trouble expressing yourself...." The nurse should allow the adolescent ample time to respond and then offer other prompts. "That can be really frustrating. If that is the case, then, maybe if you just start talking, we can try to find some words together to express your ideas...." "You may be wondering if it is safe to tell me what you're thinking. It can be frightening to trust a stranger with your most private thoughts...." "You may be wondering whether I really meant what I said about confidentiality/keeping things private.... or about not judging you.... I guess the dilemma/problem is whether it is safer to keep troubling thoughts and feelings to oneself or to take a chance that someone might be able to help."

The child's initial assessment begins with an introduction by the nurse, including a brief explanation of what the nurse and the child will be doing together. For children younger than 11 years of age, an additional explanation that the nurse helps worried or upset children by talking, playing, and getting together with their parents to think of ways to make things better is helpful. It is important to determine the child's understanding of the reason why the child is there. This helps to identify children's misconceptions (e.g., believing the nurse is going to give them an injection, thinking that they have done something bad) that could create barriers to working with them.

The nurse will require several releases of information from the child's guardian to obtain corroborating reports, such as the child's physical assessment from the paediatrician or paediatric nurse practitioner; the school's report about the child's academic (report card) and behavioural performance (interactions with peers and adults); and records of diagnosis and treatment from any previous psychiatric provider. Adolescents are often very sensitive when reports are requested from their school. They worry about repercussions if they have had prior difficulties (e.g., disciplinary problems). The nurse must explain how these reports will be used, whether the school will be involved in the development of treatment plans, and how the youth and family will participate.

Communication needs to be adapted to the child's age level (Box 29.4). The challenge is to avoid using overly complex vocabulary or talking down to children. Young children often express themselves more quickly in the context of play than through adult-like conversation. For example, a child may use puppets to re-enact a conversation that they had with a sibling or parent. Children respond well to third-person conversation prompts, such as "Some kids don't like being compared to their brothers and sisters" or "I know a kid who was so sad when he lost his dog that he thought he would never be happy again."

Early in the interview, the goal is to explain the nurse's purpose, elicit any concerns the child may have about what is happening, and establish rapport with the child by engaging in nonthreatening conversation. Many adults rarely ask children about things that genuinely interest them but expect children to respond readily to adult conversation. The nurse can establish a high degree of credibility simply by taking note of and asking about things that are obviously important to children

(e.g., a sport that they participate in, a rock group displayed on a shirt, a toy they have brought with them). However, children have an uncanny natural "radar" for dishonest adult behaviour. Attempts to establish rapport work only when the nurse is genuinely interested in the child's life.

Discussion With the Parents

After meeting with the child alone, the nurse lets the child know that it is the parents' turn to meet with the nurse. It needs to be emphasized that no one is being judged and that these meetings are about helping. The child should have a safe place to wait and be given age-appropriate activities. With the parents, the expectations should be reviewed. Reassurances around confidentiality, building trust, and being nonjudgmental must be provided.

Parents should be given opportunity to describe their view of the child's problem. When alone, parents often feel more comfortable discussing their children in depth and sharing their frustrations and fears. Parents need this opportunity to speak freely, without being constrained by concern for the child's feelings. Although children often have a pretty good sense of their parents' reactions, it may not be constructive for them to hear the full force of the parents' complaints and feelings, such as their sense of helplessness, anger, or disappointment. Parents sometimes feel guilty and need permission to express their negative feelings without feeling judged. This session is an opportunity to enlist parent's help as partners in understanding and addressing the child's problem. This is also a suitable time to fill in gaps

---

BOX 29.4 Strategies for Interviewing Children

- Use a simple vocabulary and short sentences tailored to the child's developmental and cognitive levels.
- Be sure that the child understands the questions and that you do not lead the child to give a particular response. Presenting polar opposite choices (never … or all the time) or scaled questions (1 to 10) is helpful. For example, "Some people feel angry all the time, some only feel angry at certain times, and others don't seem to feel angry at all. On a scale of 1 to 10, where 1 means never and 10 means all the time, how often do you feel angry?" If the child chooses a number greater than 1, she can be asked to describe times when she is angry.
- Select the questions for your interview on an individual basis, using judgment and discretion and

considering the child's age and developmental level.
- Be sure that the manner and tone of your voice do not reveal any personal biases.
- Speak slowly and quietly, and try to allow the interview to unfold, using the child's verbalizations and behaviour as guides.
- Use simple terms (e.g., "sad" for "depressed") in exploring affective reactions, and ask the child to give examples of how they behave or how other people behave when emotionally aroused.
- Assume an accepting and neutral attitude toward the child's communications.
- Learn about children's current interests (e.g., by looking at Saturday morning television programs, talking with parents, visiting toy stores).

in the history and clarifying the data obtained from the interview with the child.

Parents need the chance to describe the presenting problem in their own words. They can be encouraged to verbalize through comments such as "It is not easy for parents to recognize that childhood is sometimes unhappy and that their child needs help. A child's emotions and behaviour can be pretty confusing, even frightening, and many parents hope that, with time, the problems will disappear on their own. Unfortunately, that is sometimes not the case; and if left unattended over time, the problems can worsen. It takes great courage to seek help, and you took a big step in coming here today. I hope that by working together with your child, we will find some ways of assisting. I am interested in *your* story. Tell me what brings *you* here *today*." The nurse should then listen carefully and reflect upon the parent's understanding of the problem, showing empathy and respect for both parent and child.

If the parents have very different perspectives about the problem, it is helpful to ask each of them to provide a viewpoint. Asking other family members about their view of the problem is a way to clarify discrepancies, obtain additional data, and communicate awareness that different family members experience the same problem in different ways (Shajani & Snell, 2019).

Child and Adolescent Screening and Rating Scales

There are a number of instruments available for conducting bio/psycho/social/spiritual assessments. They vary according to age and target areas of interest as well as purpose and often require trained or credentialed clinicians who are able to administer and interpret the evaluations. Observational assessment and parent-report questionnaires are generally used for screening, whereas in-depth surveys and interviews help formulate diagnoses of psychopathology. Screening for early problems is both feasible and effective in improving rates of referral for mental health services. Screening can be administered in stages starting with short screens of groups of children (e.g., in clinics, daycare, school) followed by more in-depth screens involving parents and observations of those identified as elevated risk.

It is important to remember that screening measures are most effective in evaluating the level of risk for children with socioemotional problems within a population (e.g., a community, school) and are less effective in identifying with certainty an individual at risk (Costello et al., 2005). This means that the nurse should not rely on one source of evidence but, instead, use multiple sources of data to understand a child's mental health and wellbeing. The Canadian Paediatric Society's Mental Health Task Force has compiled a list of screening tools and rating scales for use by pediatricians and other child health providers. Each instrument was evaluated on a number of criteria, including age range to which it applies, time required to complete, and who completes the questionnaire. Clinicians can look through the tools and scales by a number of filters such as general assessment tools, general developmental screening measures, condition (e.g., anxiety, depression, substance use, suicide risk), and age (Canadian Paediatric Society, 2021). Refer to the Canadian Paediatric Society's Mental Health: Screening Tools and Rating Scales for children and youth in the Web Links.

Assessment Within Age Groups

Assessment techniques vary with the age and developmental stage of the child.

Preschool-Aged Children

Preschool-aged children may have difficulty putting feelings into words and provide assistance (e.g., "When I see your face all wrinkled up, it tells me that you are mixed up—confused"). Language should be kept simple and tailored to the child's developmental level. Rapport with preschool-aged children can be achieved by joining their world of play. Play is an activity by which the child transforms an experience from real life into a symbolic, nonliteral representation. Play encourages verbalizations, promotes manual strength, teaches rules and problem-solving, and helps children master control over their environment. Useful materials are paper, pencils, crayons, paints, paintbrushes, easels, clay, blocks, balls, dolls, dollhouses, puppets, animals, dress-up clothes, and a water supply.

When observing the child in a free play setting, attention needs to be paid to initiation of play, energy level, manipulative actions, tempo, body movements, tone, integration, creativity, products, age appropriateness, and attitudes toward adults. In addition, themes of play, expression of emotions, and temperament are important to observe. The nurse must allow children to direct and initiate these themes. When evaluating the young child's peer relationships through play therapy in a play group or school setting, observe play settings and themes, initiation of play, response to peer initiations of play, integration of affect and action during play, resolution of conflicts, responses to suggestions of others during play, and the ability to engage in role taking and role reversals (Pietrangelo, 2019).

The nurse should be a good listener, use appropriate vocabulary, tolerate a child's anxious, angry, or sad behaviour, and use thoughtful comments about the child's play. Through play, the nurse can assess the child's sensorimotor skills, cognitive style, adaptability, language functioning, emotional and behavioural

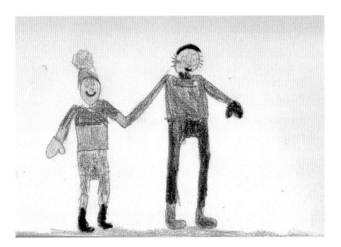

Figure 29.2 Me and my Papa walking to school in the snow. Drawing by a 6-year-old girl.

responsiveness, social level, moral development, coping styles, problem-solving techniques, and approaches to perceiving and interpreting the surrounding world. In any assessment, both strengths and limitations need to be addressed, with strengths then built upon to address the child's problem areas. For example, the nurse might engage a preschooler with the comment, "Sara, you are a great storyteller; I wonder if you could tell me a story about this doll, Jane, who is afraid at day care just like you." Drawings are also used in child assessment to illuminate the child's intellect, creative talents, neuropsychological deficits, body image difficulties, and perceptions of family life (Fig. 29.2).

School-Aged Children

Unlike preschool-aged children, school-aged children (5 to 11 years) can use more constructs, provide longer descriptions, make better inferences of others, and acquire more complete conceptions of various social roles. Children in middle school are more capable of verbal exchange and can tolerate limited periods of direct questioning. The nurse can establish rapport with school-aged children by using competitive board games, such as checkers and playing cards, or by colouring a picture or poster together with felt pens. A therapeutic thinking-feeling-doing game is a useful technique that can solidify rapport between the nurse and child while revealing the child's perceptions, cognition, and emotions. In this game, the clinician and the child take turns drawing cards that pose hypothetical situations and ask what a person might think, feel, or do in such scenarios. For example, one card might say, "Ethan has something on his mind that he is afraid to tell his father. What is he scared to talk about?" Another might read, "Kim heard her parents fighting. What were they fighting about? What was Kim thinking while she listened to her parents?"

Adolescents

Adolescents have an increased command of language concepts and have developed abstract and formal operations thinking capacity. Their social world is complex. "Identity" is a core psychosocial developmental task of this phase of life (Erikson, 1968). Some early adolescents may assume that their subjective experiences are real and congruent with objective reality, leading to egocentrism. **Egocentrism** is a preoccupation with one's own appearance, behaviour, thoughts, and feelings. For example, a preteen may think that he caused his parents to divorce because he fought with his father the day before the parents announced their decision to separate. Because teenagers have a new, heightened sense of self-consciousness, they may be preoccupied during the interview with applying makeup or other self-grooming tasks.

During early adolescence, cognitive changes include increased self-consciousness, fear of being shamed, and demands for privacy and secrecy. An adolescent's willingness to talk to a nurse will depend partly on their perception of the degree of rapport between them. The nurse's ability to communicate respect, cooperation, honesty, and genuineness is important. Rejection by the adolescent, even outright hostility, during the first few interactions is not uncommon, especially if the teen is having behaviour problems at home, at school, or in the community. The nurse should be patient and avoid jumping to conclusions. Hostility or defiance may help the teen gauge how much they can trust the nurse, a defense against anxiety, or a transference phenomenon (see Chapter 9).

Adolescents are likely to be defensive in front of their parents and concerned with confidentiality. At the start of the interview, the nurse should clearly convey to the adolescent what information will and will not be shared with parents. Adolescents generally prefer a straightforward, candid approach to the interview because they often distrust those in authority. Making a commitment to adolescents that they do not have to discuss anything they are not ready to reveal is important so that they will feel in control while they gradually build trust.

Bio/Psycho/Social/Spiritual Psychiatric Nursing Assessment of Children and Adolescents

The comprehensive assessment of the child or adolescent includes interviews with the child and parents, child alone, and parents alone. After completing these assessment interviews, the child and parents are brought back together to receive a summary of the assessment and an opportunity to respond as to whether it fits with their perceptions. The family must have a chance to share additional information and ask questions. They should be then thanked for their willingness to talk; an indication of the next steps should be given. The use of an assessment tool is helpful in organizing data for mental health planning and intervention (see Box 29.5). Feedback on

BOX 29.5 Bio/Psycho/Social/Spiritual Psychiatric Nursing Assessment of Children and Adolescents

1. **Identifying information**
   Name
   Sex
   Date of birth
   Age
   Birth order
   Grade
   Ethnic background
   Religious preference
   List of others living in household

2. **Major reason for seeking help**
   Description of presenting problems or symptoms
   When did the problems (symptoms) start?
   Describe both the child's and the parent's perspectives.

3. **Psychiatric history**
   Previous mental health contacts (inpatient and outpatient)
   Other mental health problems or psychiatric diagnosis (besides those described currently)
   Previous medications and compliance
   Family history of depression, substance abuse, psychosis, etc., and treatment

4. **Current and past health status**
   Medical problems
   Current medications
   Surgery and hospitalizations
   Allergies
   Diet and eating habits
   Sleeping habits
   Height and weight
   Hearing and vision
   Menstrual history
   Immunizations
   If sexually active, birth control method used
   Date of last physical examination
   Paediatrician or nurse practitioner's name and telephone number

5. **Medications**
   Prescription (dosage, side effects)
   OTC drugs

6. **Neurologic history**
   Right handed, left handed, or ambidextrous
   Headaches, dizziness, fainting
   Seizures
   Unusual movement (tics, tremors)

   Hyperactivity
   Episodes of weakness or paralysis
   Slurred speech, pronunciation problems
   Fine motor skills (eating with utensils, using crayon or pencil, fastening buttons and zippers, tying shoes)
   Gross motor skills and coordination (walking, running, hopping)

7. **Responses to mental health problems**
   What makes problems (symptoms) worse or better?
   Feelings about those experiences (what helped and did not help)
   What interventions have been tried so far?
   Major losses or changes in the past year
   Fears, including punishment

8. **Mental status examination**
   Appearance, gait, posture, dress, nutrition, gestures
   Motor/motility
   Interaction with nurse, eye contact
   Psychosis, hallucinations, delusions
   Mood, affect, anxiety
   Speech (clarity, speed, volume), language (articulation, tone, modulation, coherence)
   Writing/reading (comprehension), content
   Thought patterns (organization, thought content)
   Intellectual ability, judgment, insight, general knowledge, orientation to date, time, person
   Activity level, stereotypes, mannerisms, obsessions or compulsions, attention, phobia

9. **Developmental assessment**
   Mother's pregnancy, delivery
   Child's Apgar score, whether preterm or full-term, weight at birth
   Physical maturation
   Psychosocial
   Language
   Developmental milestones: walking, talking, toileting

10. **Attachment, temperament/significant behaviour patterns**
    Attachment
    Concentration, distractibility
    Eating and sleeping patterns
    Ability to adjust to new situations and changes in routine
    Usual mood and fluctuations

BOX 29.5 Bio/Psycho/Social/Spiritual Psychiatric Nursing Assessment of Children and Adolescents *(Continued)*

Excitability

Ability to wait, tendency to interrupt

Responses to discipline

Lying, stealing, fighting, cruelty to animals, fire setting

11. Self-concept

Beliefs about self

Body image

Self-esteem

Personal identity

12. Risk assessment

History of suicidal thoughts, previous attempts

Suicide ideation, plan, lethality of plan, accessibility of plan

History of violent, aggressive behaviour

Homicidal ideation

13. Family relationships

Relationship with parents

Deaths/losses

Family strengths and conflicts (nature and content)

Nurturing and disciplinary methods

Quality of sibling relationship

Sleeping arrangements

Who does the child relate to or trust in the family?

Relationships with extended family

14. School and peer adjustment

Learning difficulties and strengths

Behaviour problems and strengths at school

School attendance

Relationship with teachers

Special classes

Best friend

Relationships with peers

Dating

Drug and alcohol use

Participation in sports, clubs, other activities

After-school routine

15. Community resources

Professionals or agencies working with child or family

Day care resources

16. Functional status

See Functional Status section of this chapter.

17. Stresses and coping behaviours

Psychosocial stresses

Coping behaviours (strengths)

18. Summary of significant data

---

the suggested next steps should be requested of both child and parents and any areas of disagreement discussed. A plan with which all can live is the goal.

When interviewing both child and parents, directly asking the child as many questions as possible is generally the best way for the nurse to get accurate, firsthand information and to reinforce interest in the child's viewpoint. Asking the child questions about the history of the current problem, previous psychiatric experiences (both good and bad), family psychiatric history, medical problems, developmental history (to get an idea of what the child has been told), school adjustment, peer relationships, and family functioning is particularly important. Adolescents, particularly in Western societies, are often preoccupied with love and romance. Although it tends to be considered "puppy love" by adults, unrequited love or a romantic relationship with a peer may be an important aspect of the adolescent's life and needs to be gently explored along with other peer relationships (Austin, 2003).

If necessary, the nurse can ask some or all of these same questions of the parents to get consensus or another opinion about the matter, attain supplemental information, or both. Keep in mind that developmental research shows moderate to low correlation between parent and child reports of family behaviour. It is helpful to discuss openly with the family the fact that different perspectives exist and to note that the nurse's role is not to judge or side with one view but rather to understand the different perspectives and how they might be affecting the family.

Biologic Domain

Nurses should include a thorough history of psychiatric and medical problems in any comprehensive assessment. A physical assessment is necessary to rule out any medical problems that could be mistaken for psychiatric symptoms (e.g., weight loss resulting from diabetes, not depression; drug-induced psychosis). Pharmacologic assessment should include prescription and over-the-counter (OTC) medications. Nurses should ask about any allergies to food, medications, or environmental triggers.

Genetic Vulnerability

Research increasingly shows that major psychiatric disorders (e.g., depression, anxiety disorder, schizophrenia, bipolar disorder, substance abuse) can run in families (see Chapter 30). Thus, having a parent or sibling with a psychiatric disorder may indicate an increased risk for the same or another closely related disorder in a child or adolescent. In addition, many psychiatric disorders appearing in childhood, such as autism spectrum disorder, intellectual developmental disorder, some language disorders, attention deficit hyperactivity disorder (ADHD), Tourette syndrome, enuresis, and trisomy disorders (e.g., Down syndrome), have genetic factors associated with their aetiology (American Psychiatric Association, 2013).

Neurologic Examination

A full neurologic evaluation is beyond the scope of practice for a baccalaureate-level or master's-level nurse without specific neuropsychiatric training. However, a screening of neurologic soft signs can help establish a database that will clarify the need for further neurologic consultation. The nurse should ask the child directly the brief neurologic screening questions suggested in Box 29.5 and note any soft signs of neurologic dysfunction, such as slurred speech, unusual movements (e.g., tics, tremors), hyperactivity, and coordination problems. The nurse can ask young children to hop on one foot, skip, or walk from toe to heel to assess their gross motor coordination and to draw with a crayon or pencil or to play pickup sticks or jacks to assess their fine motor coordination.

Psychological Domain

Children can usually identify and discuss what improves or worsens their problems. Their perspectives are important to genuine understanding of their issues. The assessment may be the first time that someone has asked the child to explain their view of the problem. It is also a perfect opportunity to discuss any life changes or losses (e.g., death of grandparents or pets, parental divorce) and fears.

Mental Status Examination

The mental status examination combines observation and a clinical interview (Chapter 11). The exam is conducted taking into account the child or youth's age and developmental level and presenting problems. The establishment of therapeutic rapport and the nurse's observational skills are the foundations of the assessment. The nurse should note the child's general appearance, including age (actual and apparent), self-care/hygiene, and dress. The nurse also should note the child's nonverbal behaviour, including posture, tone of voice, eye contact, and affect. What is the child or youth's attitude toward the interviewer, others involved, and the interview process itself? How active is the child? Does the child seem to have difficulty focusing on the interview, sitting still, refraining from impulsive behaviour, and listening without interrupting? Does the child seem underactive, lethargic, distant, or hopeless?

The child's sentence structure and vocabulary needs to be observed for a general sense of their intellectual functioning. Speech patterns, such as rate (overly fast or slow), clarity, and volume, and any speech disfluencies (e.g., stuttering, halting) are important in screening for mood disorders (e.g., depression, mania), language disorders, psychotic processes, and anxiety disorders.

Asking children general questions about their everyday lives and observing the content and process of their play (e.g., ability to focus on an activity, play themes, boundaries between themselves and others) help reveal the level of organization and content of their thinking. The level of speech organization should be noted. Young children normally shift subjects rather abruptly, but adolescents should continue with one train of thought before moving to another. Any morbid or eccentric thoughts, violent fantasies, and self-deprecating statements that could reflect a poor self-concept should also be noted. Assessment of preteens and adolescents should address substance use and sexual activity, because responses may provide useful information about high-risk behaviour or harmful substance use. The nurse should also inquire about any obsessions or compulsions (e.g., worries about germs, severe hand washing, obtrusive thoughts).

Developmental Assessment

A developmental assessment is one of the core components of any psychiatric evaluation. Determining psychopathology involves evaluating the extent to which behaviours and experiences are appropriate for a child's age and stage of development. Developmental disorders are commonly associated with psychiatric and behavioural disorders.

Disorders characterized by intellectual disabilities (mild, moderate, severe, and profound forms) are distinguished from disorders that affect specific functional domains (communication disorders, specific learning disorders, ADHD, or motor disorders), as well as from an autism spectrum disorder that exhibits a distinctive pattern of deviation from the normal developmental trajectory. The conditions are not mutually exclusive, and comorbidity is common. Therefore, it is necessary to evaluate both the extent to which development is progressing at the right rate and the extent to which it is following the correct path.

It is best to obtain information from various sources (parents, teachers, other professionals) and use a number of different methods of gauging progress (developmental history, current functioning by report and on specific tests) to ensure an accurate developmental picture. A comprehensive assessment may require input from a range of professionals (psychiatrists, psychologists, speech/language and occupational therapists, physiotherapists) and entail some form of multidisciplinary evaluation The key areas for assessment include maturation, psychosocial development, and language.

Maturation

Healthy development of the brain and nervous system during childhood and adolescence provides the foundation for successful functioning throughout life. Such development, called **maturation**, unfolds through sequential and orderly growth processes. These processes are biologically and genetically based but depend on constant interactions with a stimulating and nurturing environment.

If trauma impairs the process of normal biologic maturation, developmental delays and disorders that may not be fully reversible can result. Trauma is defined as experiences that overwhelm an individual's capacity to cope. Trauma early in life, including child abuse, neglect, witnessing violence, and disrupted attachment, as well as later traumatic experiences such as violence, accidents, natural disaster, war, sudden unexpected loss, and other life events that are out of one's control can be devastating. There are a number of dimensions of trauma, including magnitude, complexity, frequency, duration, and whether it occurs from an interpersonal or external source (BC Provincial Mental Health and Substance Use Planning Council, 2013). Refer further to Chapters 18 and 34.

The nurse can assess for developmental delays by asking questions from specific sections of the mental status examination:

- *Intellectual functioning*: Evaluate the child's creativity, spontaneity, ability to count money and tell time, academic performance, memory, attention, frustration tolerance, and organization.
- *Gross motor functioning*: Ask the child to hop on one foot, throw a ball, walk up and down the hall, and run.
- *Fine motor functioning*: Ask the child to draw a picture or play pick-up sticks.
- *Cognition*: Evaluate the child's general level of cognition by assessing the child's vocabulary, level of comprehension, drawing ability, and responsiveness to questions. Testing, such as the Wechsler Intelligence Scale for Children (WISC-III), provides measures of intelligence quotient. A psychologist usually performs

such tests. Request cognitive testing if there are concerns about developmental delays or learning disabilities.
- *Thinking and perception*: Evaluate level of consciousness; orientation to date, time, and person; thought content; thought process; and judgment.
- *Social interactions and play*: Assess the child's organization, creativity, drawing capacity, and ability to follow rules. Children experiencing developmental delays may remain engaged solely in parallel play instead of moving to reciprocal play. They may consistently play with toys designed for younger children, draw crude body pictures, or display receptive (understanding) or expressive (communicative) language problems.

Psychosocial Development

Assessment of psychosocial development is very important for children with mental health problems. Various theoretical models are available from which to choose; the most commonly used model is Erikson's stages of development (see Chapter 9). When considering this model, the child's gender identity and cultural background may be variables.

Language

At birth, infants can emit sounds of all languages. Maturation of language skills begins with babbling, or the utterance of simple, spontaneous sounds. By the end of the first year, children can make one-word statements, usually naming objects or people in the environment. By age 2 years, they should speak in short, telegraphic sentences consisting of a verb and noun (e.g., "want cookie"). Between ages 2 and 4, vocabulary and sentence structure develop rapidly. In fact, the preschooler's ability to produce language often surpasses motor development, sometimes causing temporary stuttering when the child's mind literally works faster than the mouth.

Language development depends on the complex interaction of physical maturation of the nerves, development of head and neck musculature, hearing abilities, cognitive abilities, exposure to language, educational stimulation, and emotional wellbeing. Social needs create a natural inclination toward communication, but the child needs reinforcement to develop correct pronunciation, vocabulary, and grammar.

Before a diagnosis of a communication disorder (i.e., impairment in language expression, comprehension, or both) can be made, the child must be tested to rule out hearing, visual, or other neurologic problems. Brain damage, especially to the left hemisphere (dominant for language in most individuals), can seriously impair the development of communication abilities in children. Any child who has experienced brain damage from anoxia at birth, congenital trauma, head injury, infection, tumour, or drug exposure should be closely monitored for signs of a communication disorder.

Before the age of 5 years, the brain has amazing plasticity; sometimes, other intact areas of the brain can take over functions of damaged areas, especially with immediate speech therapy. Genetically based disorders such as autism can cause language delays that are sometimes permanent and severe. Children with language delays need particular encouragement to communicate in a way that others can understand, because they tend to compensate by using nonverbal signals (Tanguay, 2000).

The nurse must recognize normal variations in child development and assess lags in the development of vocabulary and sentence structure during the critical preschool years (Table 29.4). Delays in this area

Table 29.4	Milestones for Normal Language Development in the Preschool Years
Age	Milestones
Birth to 3 months	Makes cooing sounds
	Has different cries for different needs
	Startles to loud sounds
	Soothed by calm, gentle voices
4–6 months	Babbles and makes different sounds
	Makes sounds back when you talk
	Turns his/her eyes toward a sound source
	Responds to music or toys that make noise
7–12 months	Waves hi/bye
	Responds to his/her name
	Lets you know what he/she wants using sounds and/or actions like pointing
	Begins to follow simple directions (e.g., Where is your nose?)
	Localizes correctly to sound by turning his/her head toward it
	Pays attention when spoken to
By 12–18 months	Uses common words and starts to put words together
	Enjoys listening to storybooks
	Points to body parts or pictures in a book when asked
	Looks at your face when talking to you
By 18–24 months	Understands more words than he/she can say
	Says two words together (e.g., More juice)
	Asks simple questions (e.g., What's that?)
	Takes turns in a conversation
2–3 years	Uses sentences of three or more words most of the time
	Understands different concepts (e.g., in/on, up/down)
	Follows two-part directions (e.g., Take the book and put it on the table)
	Answers simple questions (e.g., Where is the car?)
	Participates in short conversations
3–4 years	Tells a short story or talks about daily activities
	Talks in sentences with adult-like grammar
	Generally speaks clearly so people understand
	Hears you when you call from another room
	Listens to TV at the same volume as others
	Answers a variety of questions

Source: Speech-Language & Audiology Canada. (2014). *Speech, language and hearing milestones.* www.sac-oac.ca

can seriously affect other areas, such as cognitive, educational, and social development. Many children who receive psychiatric treatment have speech and language disorders that are sometimes undetected, either leading to or compounding their emotional problems.

By the time children reach the age of 4 to 5 years, they will have a vocabulary of approximately 2,000 words, will be able to listen well, and 90% to 100% of their speech will be understandable. By school age, a child should be able to speak in complete sentences with minor grammatical errors. A child's language skills continue to develop through the school years. From about age 9 to 19, most growth occurs in the area of written language (Canadian Association of Speech-Language Pathologists and Audiologists, 2000).

Attachment: The Caregiving Context

Researchers and clinicians who assess early emerging social–emotional and behavioural problems tend to believe that children must be evaluated in relation to their primary caregivers (Shajani & Snell, 2019). Although parents usually serve as the primary caregivers, in today's world, other family members (biologically or psychologically related), babysitters, day care, and club activity staff, to name a few, often play a significant role in the development of child attachment and should be assessed. In addition, recognizing that children respond differently in different situations, the routine environments in which the child interacts need to be evaluated. Finally, the nurse considers the contexts of culture, class, ethnicity, language, stigma, and social exclusion on the therapeutic process and negotiates care that is sensitive to these influences as suggested by the Canadian Federation of Mental Health Nurses (2014), in the *Standards of Psychiatric-Mental Health Nursing*.

Secure Attachment

Secure attachments in early childhood produce cooperative, harmonious parent–child relationships in which the child is responsive to the parents' socialization efforts and likely to adopt the parents' viewpoints, values, and goals. Securely attached young children tend to socialize competently, be popular with well-acquainted peers during the preschool years, and have warm relationships with important adults in their lives. They see themselves and others constructively and have relatively sophisticated emotional and moral understanding (Thompson, 2002).

Mothers and fathers foster security of attachment and exploration and thus provide psychological security for the child. Security of attachment involves tender loving care, comfort and consolation, and external help with emotion regulation. Security of exploration, based on sensitive support from both mother and father, allows a child to explore to gain knowledge and skills. The quality of the emotional bond between the infant and parental or caregiver figures provides the groundwork for future relationships.

The need to touch and be close to a parental figure appears biologically driven and has been demonstrated in classic studies of monkeys who bonded with a terry-cloth surrogate mother (Harlow et al., 1971). A secure attachment is based on the caretaker's consistent, appropriate response to the infant's attachment behaviours (e.g., crying, clinging, calling, following, protesting). Children who have developed a secure attachment protest when their parents leave them (beginning at about age 6 to 8 months) seek comfort from their parents in unfamiliar situations and playfully explore the environment in the parent's presence. If the child develops an insecure attachment, perhaps due to unresponsiveness or mixed responses to a child's attachment behaviours on the part of parents, it is evidenced by clinging and lack of exploratory play when the parent is present and intense protest when the parent leaves (Thompson, 2002).

Disrupted Attachments

Disrupted attachments resulting from deficits in infant attachment behaviours, lack of responsiveness by caregivers to the child's cues, or both may lead to a diagnosis of reactive attachment disorder, feeding disorder, failure to thrive, or anxiety disorder. A reactive attachment disorder may exist when a child, before the age of 5 years, demonstrates a pattern of markedly disturbed and developmentally inappropriate attachment behaviours in which they rarely or minimally turns preferentially to an attachment figure for comfort, support, protection, and nurturance (APA, 2013). Infants with **disorganized attachment** appear to be unable to maintain the strategic adjustments in attachment behaviour, represented by organized avoidant or ambivalent attachment strategies, with the result that an alteration in both behavioural and physiologic behaviour occurs. Preschoolers with disorganized attachment manifest behaviours of fear, contradictory behaviour, or disorientation or disassociation in the caregivers' presence.

Attachment Theory

Attachment theory describes a disorganized attachment as a consequence of extreme insecurity that results from a disrupted attachment from the primary caregiver (Solomon & George, 1999). Emotional or physical separation can result from parental mental health problems, such as substance use or depression, or from frequently changing caregivers such as may be experienced by a child in foster care.

Bowlby's early studies (Bowlby, 1969) of maternal deprivation formed the initial framework for attachment theory, based on the notion that the infant tends to bond to one primary parental figure, usually the mother. Nursing theories, such as Barnard's (1994) parent–child

interaction model, have stressed the importance of the interaction between the child's spontaneous behaviour and biologic rhythms and the mother's ability to respond to cues that signal distress (Pokorny 2022.). The model provides the foundation for the development of several scales measuring dimensions of attachment. These standardized, observational assessment scales use routine parent–child interaction activities involving feeding (the Nursing Child Assessment of Feeding Scale, or NCAFS—76 items, birth to 1 year) and teaching (NCATS scale—73 items, birth to 3 years) to assess a dyad's strengths and limitations during the early years. Areas assessed include contingency (reciprocal communication patterns between caregiver and child), positioning (caregiver's sensitivity to child developmental stage and needs), verbalness (ability to stimulate language development), sensitivity (psychological availability and responsivity to the child), affect (positive or negative quality of communication patterns), and attention regulation (engaging and disengaging behaviours). Such measures can provide informed assessments to nurses in a variety of settings, such as postpartum hospital care, the home (e.g., public health newborn visits), or primary care settings (e.g., mental health nurse in community health centre) (Hodges et al., 2007, 2009). A more recent study has confirmed that the Nursing Child Assessment Satellite Training (NCAST) Parent-Child Interaction (PCI) Teaching and Feeding Scales satisfactorily identify at-risk families and can help direct interventions to promote optimal parent–child relationships and ultimately child development (Letourneau et al., 2018).

Nicole Letourneau, Professor of Nursing, and former Canada Research Chair in Healthy Child Development, University of Calgary has dedicated her research and scholarship to the intersections among parental mental health, adversity, and child behavioural development. In a systematic review addressing the associations between neurodevelopmental disorders (NDDs) (i.e., autism spectrum disorder, intellectual disability, or developmental language disorder) and attachment patterns in preschool children, Letourneau and fellow researchers found that secure attachments could be found in 42% to 50% of children with NDDs compared to 62% in neurotypical children. Factors influencing attachment patterns were autistic symptoms, developmental level, maternal sensitivity, and maternal insightfulness. And while the study demonstrated that children with NDDs are able to develop a secure attachment with their caregivers, given the importance of secure attachment for brain health and organ development, the researchers concluded that additional research is required to investigate attachment patterns with children with various other NDDs as well as other co-occurring disorders (Potter-Dickey et al., 2020).

Self-Concept

Self-concept is a child's knowledge about self. For young children, eliciting their view of themselves and the world through projective techniques is helpful. For example, the answers to "What would you wish for if you had three wishes?" can be revealing. An inability to wish for anything beyond a nice meal or place to live may reflect hopelessness, whereas wishes to conquer the world or put one's teacher in jail may indicate feelings of grandiosity. Another technique is to tell a story and ask the child to make up an ending for it. For example, a baby bird fell out of a nest—"What happened to it?" Or a little girl went to the mall with her mother but got lost—"What happened to her?" The nurse may design stories to elicit particular fears or concerns that based on what may be relevant for the individual child.

Drawings also provide an excellent window into the child's internal world (Fig. 29.3). Asking the child to draw a self-portrait, or picture of a person, can provide data about the child's self-concept, sexual identity, body image, and developmental level. By age 3 years, children should be able to draw some facial features and limbs, but their drawings may have an "x-ray" quality, in which clothing is transparent and the body can be seen underneath. Older children should produce more sophisticated drawings, unless they are resistant to the task. After the child has finished the drawing, the nurse can ask what the person in the drawing is thinking and feeling, using this device to assess the child's mental processes. For example, one adolescent with school phobia drew a person fully dressed, in great detail, but with no feet. When asked about the drawing, he said that the boy could not go anywhere because his mother was afraid to let him leave home.

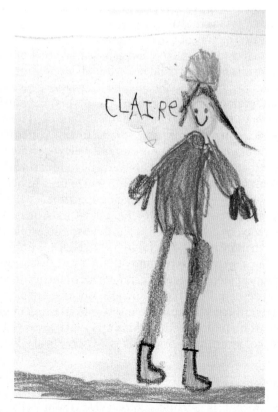

Figure 29.3 Winter self-portrait of girl, age 5.

Other ways to assess children's self-concepts include asking them what they want to do when they grow up, what their best subjects are in school, what things they are really good at, and how well liked they are at school. Before concluding an individual interview with a child, it is important to ask whether the child has any other information to share and whether they have any questions.

Nurses need to recognize the difference between self-concept and self-esteem. Self-esteem is a child's general attitude about themselves. Self-concept and self-esteem have a lot in common and can be similarly assessed. Both are reflective processes that are also influenced by comparison with others around you and how others respond to you. The main difference in self-esteem is the addition of feelings.

Although relatively rare, some children's sense of self is affected by gender dysphoria; that is, they strongly feel that there is a discrepancy between the sex they were assigned at birth and their own sense of gender. For instance, a child assigned female at birth may feel she is a boy, even though her body appears female. This gender confusion can occur at a young age and may or may not be temporary. If it causes significant distress for the child or youth, parents may wish for an assessment from a paediatric endocrinologist or from a nurse clinician, psychiatrist, or psychologist with expertise in this area.

Risk Assessment

The child should be asked about any suicidal or violent thoughts. The best way to assess these areas is to ask straightforward questions, such as, "Have you ever thought about hurting yourself? Have you ever thought about hurting someone else? Have you ever acted on these thoughts? Have you thought about how you would do it? What did you think would happen if you hurt yourself? Have you ever done anything to hurt yourself before?" Contrary to popular belief, talking about suicide with someone who can help can provide great relief to a child or youth. Further, no age should be exempt from assessment because even young children attempt suicide, and they are capable of violent acts toward other children, adults, and animals. An assessment of lethality and access to means must also be assessed to determine risk. Questions such as "Do you have a plan to hurt yourself (or others)? How would you go about hurting yourself (or others)?" and "Do you have access to guns, knives, pills … (or whatever means the child has identified)?"

The Tool for Assessment of Suicide Risk for Adolescents (TASR-A) is a clinical tool that assists in the evaluation of adolescents at imminent risk for suicide. A semistructured measure, it helps clinicians ensure that in their evaluation of an adolescent, the most common risks factors are assessed. It was derived from the adult TASR that was developed for use in emergency room, hospitals, and outpatient settings (Chehil & Kutcher, 2012).

When a child shares the intent to commit a suicidal or violent act, the nurse must inform the child that the nurse will have to discuss this concern with the parent to keep the child and others safe. It is helpful to ask the child if there is anything in particular to be said to the parent and the child wants to be present when the nurse talks with the parents. Although painful, such conversations can serve as an abrupt halt to the charade of happiness that the child may feel forced to portray to the outside world and often open honest dialogue within a family in which none has occurred for some time. Alternatively, the conversation can sometimes give words to what the family feared but were without the skills or courage to break the silence. The nurse provides a safe environment for the family to begin to face the issues.

Substance Use

Substance use disorders across the lifespan account for more deaths, illness, and disabilities than any other preventable health condition. Screening for potential use and misuse of substances is becoming a priority in mental health assessment of adolescents. An interview guide has been adapted from questions on substance use developed by Adlaf (Adlaf & Zdanowicz, 1999) to serve as a useful screen for identifying substance use problems in youth. Other screening tools for clinicians include the SACS: Substances and Choices Scale (Christie et al., 2007) and the CAGE questionnaire for alcohol use (Ewing, 1984). Given that many younger children engage in substance use (see Chapter 26), assessing younger children should be considered, as well (Box 29.6). Inhalant misuse, also known as sniffing, huffing, or bagging, is the deliberate inhalation of a volatile substance to achieve an altered mental state. Although a worldwide phenomenon, in Canada, it often affects younger children when compared to other forms of substance misuse, likely due to the ease of availability. Common products used as inhalants include solvents (e.g., paint thinners), aerosols (e.g., spray paint, hairspray), gases (e.g., butane lighters), and nitrates (e.g., room deodorizer) (Maina et al., 2020; National Institute on Drug Abuse, 2020). Alberta Health Services (2018) estimates that between 1% and 3% of children and youth seeking substance use treatment is due to inhalant abuse. Prevention efforts are critically important, as long-term chronic use has been shown to cause irreversible neurologic and neuropsychological effects (Baydala, 2010). It is estimated that Indigenous youth in Canada are more likely to engage in early-onset substance use when compared to their non-Indigenous counterparts, due largely to the legacies of colonization and intergenerational trauma (Maina et al., 2020). Nurses in collaboration with other professionals, families, and community members need to advocate for appropriate culturally responsive education to prevent substance misuse among children and adolescents, consider appropriate treatment strategies, and contribute to increased understanding of this issue through research (Baydala, 2010; Maina et al., 2020).

Social Domain

Nurses addressing the social domain when working with children and youth are particularly concerned with family relationships, school functioning, and community involvement.

Family Relationship

Children depend on adults to create a safe, nurturing, and appropriate environment to support their development. The quality of the home in terms of its ability to provide appropriate physical space (living space, sleeping arrangements, safety, cleanliness), childcare arrangements (age-appropriate supervision), and stimulation (activities or resources) should be assessed, either through a home visit or by discussing these issues with the family. When gathering a family history, a genogram and timeline are also useful tools to map family members according to birth order and medical and psychiatric histories; family roles, norms, boundaries, strengths, and subgroups; birth dates, deaths, and relationships; stage in the family cycle; and critical events. To understand fully the family's values, goals, and beliefs, the nurse must consider the family's ethnic, cultural, and economic background throughout the assessment (Shajani & Snell, 2019). A comprehensive family assessment should be considered (see Chapter 16 for assessment guidelines and how to create a genogram).

School Functioning

The child's adjustment to school is also significant. Often, children are referred for a mental health assessment as a result of changes in behaviour at school or lagging social competence. Failing grades, loss of interest in normal activities, decreased concentration, or withdrawal from or aggression toward peers may indicate that the child is experiencing emotional problems. It is very important to obtain signed permission from the parents to talk to the child's teacher about observations of the child. The nurse may want to observe the child in school, if feasible, to see how the child socially and interpersonally functions. The parent can request a treatment planning conference in which the teacher, parent, and nurse discuss the child's school performance and plan ways to promote the child's emotional, cognitive, and social functioning in school.

In such interprofessional endeavors, the nurse can use group leadership skills to facilitate accurate assessments, dialogue, goal setting, and program planning to meet the needs of a child and build social competence

---

BOX 29.6 An Interview Protocol for Reviewing Substance Use in Youth

As with other topics, questions about substance use are interactive—the answers given determine, to some extent, the subsequent questions. The questions can be used for investigating the use of tobacco, alcohol, and drugs.

TOBACCO

- Many youth smoke, do you?
- Do you ever feel you should smoke less?
- Do you wish you could smoke less than you do now?
- Have others bothered you by complaining about your smoking?
- Have you felt bad or guilty because of your smoking?
- Have you thought you had a problem because of your smoking?
- Have you ever had a medical problem as a result of your smoking?
- Have you been in hospital because of your smoking?
- Have you gone to anyone for help for a smoking problem?
- How many of your friends smoke occasionally/regularly?
- How many of your family smoke occasionally/regularly?

ALCOHOL

- Many youth drink, do you?
- Are you always able to stop drinking when you want?
- Have you felt you should drink less?
- Have others bothered you by complaining about your drinking?
- Have you felt bad or guilty because of your drinking?
- Have you been arrested or warned by police because of your drinking?

- Have you ever had "blackouts" or "flashbacks" due to your drinking?
- Have you drunk in the early morning or drunk to get rid of a hangover?
- Have you ever had any medical problem as a result of your drinking?
- Have you been in hospital because of your drinking?
- Have you gone to anyone for help for a drinking problem?
- How many of your friends drink occasionally/regularly?
- How many of your family drink occasionally/regularly?

DRUGS

- Many youth use drugs, do you?
- Do you ever feel concerned about your drug use?
- Are you always able to stop using drugs when you want?
- Have you been arrested or warned by police because of your drug use?
- Have you ever had "blackouts" or "flashbacks" due to your drug use?
- Do you wish you could use fewer drugs than you do now?
- Have you ever had any medical problems as a result of your drug use?
- Have you gone to anyone for help for a drug problem?
- Have you ever seen a doctor or been in the hospital because of your drug use?
- How many of your friends use drugs occasionally/regularly?
- How many of your family use drugs occasionally/regularly?

Adapted from Adlaf, E. M., & Zdanowicz, Y. M. (1999). A cluster-analytic study of substance problems and mental health among street youths. *American Journal of Drug and Alcohol Abuse, 25*(4), 639–660.

---

capacities. Families and students should be provided with pertinent mental health education and information as referrals are initiated (DeFehr, 2020). Referrals are a valuable component of the process and may include referral and/or consultation with occupational therapy, learning assistance, social workers, school chaplains, restorative action workers, school psychologists, and speech and language professionals. A comprehensive program plan for a child will include the support of a multilayered and diverse interprofessional intervention team.

It is critical that children feel consulted and have an opportunity to participate in the planning processes when it is age appropriate. Although such involvement is not always comfortable or even desired by all parties, it provides formal recognition of each participant involved in the change process. Suggestions emanating from planning sessions may range from having the child tested (e.g., for learning disabilities) to designing strategies for addressing predictable situations that routinely dissolve into chaos, in which rewards result for each party (e.g., extra computer time for the child, quiet time for the parent) for improved functioning. Setting realistic timelines and evaluation indicators is crucial to evaluate progress and celebrate successes.

Community

Assessing the child's economic status, access (psychologically, geographically, economically) to health and other services, housing and home environment, exposure to environmental toxins (e.g., lead), neighbourhood safety, and exposure to violence is important in understanding the social context of children and families. Children and adolescents function better if they are linked to community supports, such as churches, recreational programs, park district programming, and after-school programming. A number of voluntary organizations such as the YMCA/YWCA or Big Brothers and Big Sisters offer mentoring relationship programs for children in communities. Before making a commitment, a family should visit the organization and talk with staff to ensure that the programs are well organized and monitored by trained staff. The mentor may perform a wide range of services, from taking a child to community events, helping with homework, or talking about how the child can achieve their dreams and goals. Some towns offer community-based juvenile justice programs to rehabilitate children who have had an altercation with the legal system. Juvenile justice programs provide support, such as individual and family counselling and prosocial recreational activities; teach children how to make positive choices about spending free time; and closely monitor their behaviours.

Stresses and Coping Behaviours

Biologic, behavioural, and personality predispositions, family, and community environment may affect a child's ability to cope with stressful life events. As discussed throughout this chapter, stressful experiences for children include the death of a loved person or pet, parental divorce, violence, physical illness (especially chronic illness), mental illness, social isolation, racial discrimination, neglect, and physical and sexual abuse.

Spiritual Domain

Spiritual beliefs (the way spirituality is understood by an individual) are shaped by experience, family, friends, community, culture, and religious affiliation. With children and adolescents in particular, developmental level is a significant factor. This can be seen in children's response to loss, for instance. In addressing the spiritual domain with children and adolescents, openness and receptivity to their questions and concerns, as well as

sensitivity to their level of understanding, are important. Nurses can use stories to open discussion about the way a child or an adolescent understands and gives meaning to their experiences. There is a wide range of classic and contemporary literatures (across levels of development) that address spiritual concerns such as loneliness, illness, injury, disability, and death. Adolescents may be particularly hesitant to raise their spiritual concerns unless they feel safe and comfortable. Importantly, paediatric nurses describe approaching the spiritual domain primarily at the family level (Whitehead, 2008). There is recognition that establishing a relationship with the family as well as the child is foundational to understanding spiritual beliefs, values, and needs (see Chapter 16).

Spiritual assessment is another important, but sometimes overlooked, aspect of the assessment of children and adolescents. Measuring spirituality, even with adults, continues to have its challenges and limits. Rubin and colleagues (2009) assessed the applicability of two adult scales (the Spiritual Involvement and Beliefs Scale, the Spirituality Well-Being Scale) with chronically ill and healthy adolescents and their parents. The conclusion made was that there is a need to develop a specific spirituality scale for adolescents, as less than half of the adolescents in the study considered either scale as an effective measure of their spiritual wellbeing. Parents, too, did not feel the scales to be adequate measures of their own spirituality. More recently, Michaelson and colleagues (2019) reported on a study conducted in Canada, England, and Scotland. The researchers found strong associations between mental health and higher scores on the four domains of spirituality (i.e., connections to self, others, nature, and the transcendent), but connections to others, nature, and transcendent are sometimes influenced by connection to the self. The researchers concluded that their findings provided insight into protective factors and identified implications for future interventions to address mental health and emotional wellbeing.

Spiritual assessment, including the expressed values and beliefs of children, youth, and families, should be appropriately documented so that other health professionals can be involved in spiritual care. Pastoral care services are a resource in many health services, and representatives of the family's religious or cultural community may be utilized as a resource under the family's direction. For example, Indigenous elders and/or cultural workers have been described by paediatric nurses as being very helpful in the provision of spiritual care to Indigenous families (Whitehead, 2008).

Evaluation of Child Abuse

The CFMHN's (2014) *Standards of Psychiatric-Mental Health Nursing* identifies nurses' roles in the assessment of clients at risk for violence and abuse. There are Canadian children who suffer maltreatment (intentional physical or emotional abuse, neglect, or sexual exploitation) each year as the result of their parents' action or inaction. The harmful psychiatric and behavioural effects of children's maltreatment are broad and similar across types of abuse, with treatment having the potential for comprehensive psychological benefit (Vachon et al., 2015).

The 2008 Canadian Incidence Study of Reported Child Abuse and Neglect (Trocmé et al., 2010), the first national report on this issue, revealed an incidence rate of 16.19 substantiated investigations per 1,000 children. The three most common categories of substantiated maltreatment were exposure to domestic violence (31%), neglect (28%), and physical abuse (15%). Emotional maltreatment accounted for another 6% of cases, whereas sexual abuse cases represented only 2% of all substantiated investigations. Most referrals (68%) came from professionals (e.g., police and school). The Ontario Incidence Study of Reported Child Abuse and Neglect 2013 notes that 78% (97,951) of the investigations were for abuse or neglect concerns with 22% (27,330) related to concerns for future maltreatment. Thirty-four percent of all maltreatment investigations were substantiated. There were differences in substantiation based on subtype of sexual abuse: those involving noncontact (e.g., sex talk, voyeurism, exploitation) had the highest rate; the least involved children referred to a child protection agency due to their behaviour or contact with a known perpetrator (Fallon et al., 2017).

Despite the need for vigilance regarding child maltreatment on the part of frontline healthcare practitioner, barriers to the identification of maltreated children exist: lack of confidence and certainty, inadequate training, concerns regarding communicating with parents, and complicated disclosure processes (Eniola & Evarts, 2017; Kraft et al., 2017). There is less confidence in identifying and reporting abuse that is less overt in nature, such as emotional abuse or neglect; apprehension regarding institutional support (or its lack) is also a barrier (McTavish & MacMillan, 2019). All health practitioners require adequate preparation to recognize potential signs of child maltreatment and knowledge of how to follow up appropriately. Those in emergency departments need to follow an established clinical pathway for the evaluation of nonaccidental injuries in children: early recognition can prevent further injury and even death (Tiyyagura et al., 2017).

Assessment of child abuse needs to take into consideration the child's current developmental level and understands that compromises to early development may continue in various ways through all the developmental stages that follow. It is child centred (child welfare is critical) and family focused (most child abuse occurs within the family), has a community context (forms a key part of the child's environment), and is culturally sensitive (the nurse must be culturally competent). It also involves gathering information from a number of stakeholders and ensures that information is gathered in a coordinated way to maximize the integrity of the data collection.

In a review of the literature focused on physical, sexual, and psychological abuse and neglect of children, Hoft and Haddad (2017) concluded that a comprehensive screening tool or protocol for capturing all forms of child abuse and neglect has yet to be developed. No screening tool for psychological abuse was found; the one tool to identify neglect was without empirical support. Scales to assess physical abuse were noted, but for use in specific environments: the "Escape Form" (for all ages in the emergency room) and the "TEN-4 Bruising Clinical Decision Rule" (children under 48 months in paediatric intensive care) (Hoft & Haddad, 2017).

Nurses must understand the forensic implications of an assessment of a child for abuse. The information gathered needs to be such that it will have validity in court, if necessary. Language and vocabulary that are age-appropriate (e.g., anatomical terms) and nonleading questions must be used. Immediate referral to or consultation with a nurse or physician trained in this area, including the use of anatomically correct dolls in obtaining information, is recommended.

Nurses are ethically and legally responsible for reporting abuse to the appropriate provincial/territorial child protection systems. Mandated reporting laws are designed to allow the provinces and territories and child protection systems to investigate the possibility of abuse, provide protection to children, and link families with the support and services that they need to reduce the risk for further abuse.

Once agencies intervene to establish the child's safety, a family system approach that is supportive of the whole family unit is most effective.

Experts recommend that, when possible, nurses report abuse in the presence of the parents, preferably with the parent initiating the telephone call, and that the professional should explain the reporting as necessary to provide safety for the child and to obtain services for the family. If the parents cannot be present when the report is made, the nurse should, at minimum, notify the family that the report was made and explain the reasons. A major protective factor against psychopathology stemming from abuse and neglect is the establishment of a supportive relationship with at least one adult who can provide empathy, consistency, and caring for the child.

The decision to report abuse sometimes poses an ethical dilemma for nurses as they try to balance the need to maintain the family's trust against the need to protect the child. This decision is further complicated because, if temporary out-of-home placement is necessary, the placement's effect may also contribute to the child's and family's suffering. However, with interventions that support and attend to the parents with physical, financial, mental health (with respect to parents' own trauma history), and medical resources that will reduce stress within the family system, further distress, harm, and abuse can be prevented. See Chapter 34 for additional understanding of caring for abused persons.

🍁 Summary of Key Points

- Nurses working with children and adolescents are in a key position to identify risk and protective factors for psychopathology and to intervene to reduce risk.
- Nurses who are aware of normal developmental processes can educate parents about their children's behaviours, help them better understand their children's reactions to stress, and decide when intervention may be warranted.
- If the process of normal biologic maturation in childhood is disrupted through trauma or neglect, developmental delays and disorders can occur, some of which may have irreversible effects.
- From early infancy, children exhibit different kinds of temperaments that are at least partially biologically determined.
- Studies of attachment show that the quality of the emotional bond between the child and the parental figure is an important determinant of the success of later relationships.
- Research shows that children who experience major losses, such as death or divorce, are at risk for developing mental health problems.
- Sibling relationships have significant effects on personality development. Positive sibling relationships can be protective factors against the development of mental health problems.
- Medical problems in childhood and adolescence may cause psychological problems when illness leads to behaviours common to an earlier developmental stage (regression) or lack of full participation in family, school, and social activities.
- Striving for identity and independence may lead adolescents to participate in high-risk activities (e.g., substance use, including tobacco; unprotected sex; delinquent behaviours) that may lead to mental health problems.
- Poverty, homelessness, abuse, neglect, and parental alcoholism all create conditions that undermine a child's ability to make normal developmental gains and contribute to the child's vulnerability for various emotional and behavioural problems.
- Children who experience disrupted attachments because of out-of-home placements may have difficulty forming close relationships with their new parents and trusting others.
- Family support services and early intervention programs are designed to prevent the removal of the child from the family as a result of abuse or neglect and to maintain a strong, nurturing family system.
- Mental health assessment of children and adolescents includes evaluating the child's biologic, psychological, social, and spiritual factors.
- Assessment of children and adolescents differs from assessment of adults in that the nurse must consider the child's developmental level, specifically addressing the child's language, cognitive, social, and emotional skills. Establishing a treatment alliance and building rapport are essential to obtaining a good mental health history.
- The mental status examination includes observations and questions about the child's appearance, speech, language, vocabulary, orientation, knowledge base (including reading, writing, and math skills), attention level, activity level, memory, social skills, peer relationships, relationship to interviewer, mood, affect, suicidal or homicidal tendencies, thinking (presence or absence of hallucinations or delusions), substance use, and behaviours.
- Assessment of the child and caregiver together provides important information regarding child–parent attachment and parenting practices.
- A child's self-concept can be evaluated using tools such as play, stories, asking three wishes, and asking the child to draw a picture of himself or herself.
- If a child reveals suicidal ideation in the interview, the nurse must determine whether the child has a plan, let the parent know the child is suicidal, and make a plan to keep the child safe, including consideration of inpatient hospitalization.
- If a child reports to the nurse neglect or physical or sexual abuse, the nurse must by law report the child's disclosure to Child Protection Services.
- Protective factors that promote resiliency in children are active coping and the ability to solve problems, a sense of self-efficacy, self-esteem, accurate processing of social cues, supportive family environment, peer acceptance, and environmental supports that promote coping efforts and recognize and reward competence.

 ## Thinking Challenges

You are starting your first clinical rotation in community mental health nursing. You have been placed at a high school with approximately 600 students.

In this school, nursing students offer student supports during lunch hour. This is done in collaboration with the school psychologist, guidance counsellors, social worker, and the RAP (restorative action planning) worker. On your third day in the noon hour service, a student approaches you and says, "Hey, I'm Taylor; I need to talk to a nurse who isn't judgmental!" You welcome Taylor into a private office where you close the door. Taylor slumps into one of the recliners and you sit in an office chair, facing them to begin the visit. As soon as you sit down Taylor says angrily, "I hate this school. No one gets me or accepts me;

not even my family! They kicked me out last night. I feel so alone and sometimes I want to just go get wasted or even die. And, on top of all this my partner wants me to get on PrEP (preexposure prophylaxis)." Taylor's speech is direct and matter of fact. You immediately feel like the teen is testing you to see how or if you would react. Taylor's arms were crossed. There is hesitancy to make much eye contact, and you notice there are tears in Taylor's eyes.

a. How would you respectfully and professionally navigate this conversation with Taylor?

b. Which vulnerabilities does Taylor present with during this first encounter?
c. What assessments would you complete?

Visit the**Point** to view suggested responses. Go to **thePoint.lww.com/activate** and use the activation code found in the front of this text to unlock answers to the "Thinking Challenges" and other online resources.

Web Links

https://kidshelpphone.ca/ This website is an excellent resource for children and adolescents, family members, and teachers on topics such as bullying and abuse, eating disorders, LGBTQ2S+, self-injury and suicide, etc. The site features articles, videos, and first person accounts.

Cwrp.ca/infosheets Information sheets about provincial reporting legislation on reporting child abuse and neglect are available at this site.

forces.gc.ca/en/caf-community-health-services-r2mr-deployment/deployment-resources-family-members.page Deployment resources for family members of the Canadian military.

https://www.cps.ca/en/mental-health-screening-tools Canadian Paediatric Society: Mental Health: Screening tools and rating scales. The Canadian Paediatric Society's Mental Health Task Force has compiled a list of screening tools and rating scales for use by paediatricians and other child health providers.

medicine.usask.ca/documents/psychiatry/WHO-DAS2_20150123-1.pdf The WHODAS2 assessment form can be found at this site.

https://www.rainbowhealthontario.ca/ Rainbow Health Ontario (RHO) is a province-wide program working to improve access to services and promote the health of lesbian, gay, bisexual, trans, two-spirited, and queer (LGBT2SQ) communities. [Intersex individuals are not specifically identified as users of RHO services.] RHO is a valuable resource for a number of stakeholders, including community groups, service providers, researchers, policy makers, and educators.

https://www.cdc.gov/lgbthealth/youth-resources.htm The Centers for Disease Control and Prevention (CDC) hosts LGBT Youth Resources. Here, readers will find particularly relevant resources from the CDC, other government agencies, and community organizations that support positive environments for LGBT youth, their friends, educators, parents, and family members.

http://iacapap.org/iacapap-textbook-of-child-and-adolescent-mental-health "Promoting the mental health and development of children and adolescents through policy, practice, and research" is the mandate of the International Association for Child and Adolescent Psychiatry and Allied Professionals (IACAPAP). Here, readers will find *The IACAPAP Textbook of Child and Adolescent Mental Health,* a comprehensive and innovative open access publication, complete with relevant pictures, graphics, video links, and PowerPoints for teaching purposes.

https://www.youthmentalhealth.ca/ Youth Mental Health Canada is a grassroot youth-driven and youth-led nonprofit organization that advocates for "greater funding of publicly funded, culturally sensitive, needs-based, innovative supports and services in health care and education."

http://www.caringforkids.cps.ca/ This easily accessible reliable parenting resource, developed by the Canadian Paediatric Society, is an excellent resource for parents and healthcare professionals alike. The site features resources related to growth and development, news to use (timely current events), helpful tips (e.g., communicating with teens), and an informative video library with many relevant titles specific to child and adolescent mental health.

http://www.kidsnewtocanada.ca/ Caring for Kids New to Canada is an excellent resource for health professionals working with immigrant and refugee families including resources dedicated to assessment and screening, mental health and development, and culture and health.

https://imhpromotion.ca/ "Supporting Healthy Minds from the Beginning" is the mandate for Infant and Early Mental Health Promotion, a program of SickKids. This site is an excellent source for information included in their learning centre, resource library, and research and innovation portal.

https://www.sac-isc.gc.ca/eng/1541187352297/1541187392851 Here readers will find the Government of Canada's—Reducing the number of Indigenous children in care—illustrates the codevelopment of new legislation to reduce the number of children and youth in care and to improve family services.

https://mentalhealthliteracy.org/ This Canadian based organization is committed to mental health literacy information, research, education, and resources—including videos, animations, brochures, e-books, face-to-face training programs, and online training.

References

Adelson, S. L., Walker-Cornetta, E., & Kalish, N. (2019). LGBTQ Youth, mental health and spiritual care: Psychiatric Collaboration with health care chaplains. *Journal of the American Academy of Child and Adolescent Psychiatry, 58*(7), 651–655. https://doi.org/10.1016/j.jaac.2019.02.009

Adlaf, E. M., & Zdanowicz, Y. M. (1999). A cluster-analytic study of substance problems and mental health among street youths. *American Journal of Drug and Alcohol Abuse, 25*(4), 639–660. https://doi.org/10.1081/ada-100101884

Afifi, T. O., Taillieu, T., Zamorski, M. A., Turner, S., Cheung, K., & Sareen, J. (2016). Association of child abuse exposure with suicidal ideation, suicide plans, and suicide attempts in military personnel and the general population in Canada. *JAMA Psychiatry, 73*(3), 229–238. https://doi.org/10.10.1001/jamapsychiatry.2015.2732

Alberta Health Services. (2018). *Solvents/inhalants information for health professionals.* Alberta Addiction and Mental Health Research Partnership Program. https://crismprairies.ca/wp-content/uploads/2018/12/SolventsInhalants_V02-2018-11-13.pdf

American Academy of Child & Adolescent Psychiatry. (2018). *Grief and children.* https://www.aacap.org/AACAP/Families_and_Youth/Facts_for_Families/FFF-Guide/Children-And-Grief-008.aspx

American Psychiatric Association. (2013). *Diagnostic and statistical manual of mental disorders* (5th ed.).

Andriessen, K., Mowll, J., Lobb, E., Draper, B., Dudley, M., & Mitchell, P. B. (2018). "Don't bother about me". The grief and mental health of bereaved adolescents. *Death Studies, 42,* 607–615. https://doi.org/10.1080/07481187.2017.1415393

Anthony, K. K., Gil, K. M., & Schanberg, L. E. (2003). Parental perceptions of child vulnerability in children with chronic illness. *Journal of Pediatric Psychology, 28*(3), 185–190. https://doi.org/10.1093/jpepsy/jsg005

Arvidson, J., Kinniburgh, K., Howard, K., Spinazzola, J., Strothers, H., Evans, M., Andres, B., Cohen, C., & Blaustein, M. (2011). Treatment of complex trauma in young children: Developmental and cultural considerations in application of the ARC intervention model. *Journal of Child and Adolescent Trauma, 4,* 34–51. https://doi.org/10.1080/19361521.2011.545046

Austin, W. (2003). *First love: The adolescent experience of amour.* Peter Lang Publishing Inc.

Baiden, P., Fallon, B., den Dunnen, W., & Boateng, G. O. (2015). The enduring effects of early childhood adversities and troubled sleep among Canadian adults: A population-based study. *Sleep Medicine, 16,* 760–767. http://doi.org.10.1016/j.sleep.2015.02.527

Barnard, K. E. (1994). The Barnard model. In G. Sumner & A. Spitz (Eds.), *NCAST caregiver/parent–child interaction feeding manual* (pp. 6–14). NCAST Publications, University of Washington, School of Nursing.

Baydala, L. (2010). Inhalant abuse. *Paediatrics & Child Health, 15*(7), 443–448. https://doi.org/10.1093/pch/15.7.443

BC Provincial Mental Health and Substance Use Planning Council. (2013). *Trauma-informed practice guide.* http://bccewh.bc.ca/publications-resources/documents/TIP-Guide-May2013.pdfdivorce

Beedie, N., Macdonal, D., & Wilson, D. (2019). *Towards justice: Tackling indigenous child poverty in Canada.* https://www.afn.ca/wp-content/uploads/2019/07/Upstream_report_final_English_June-24-2019.pdf

Bergman, A. S., Axberg, U., & Hanson, E. (2017). When a parent dies—a systematic review of the effects of support programs for parentally bereaved children and their caregivers. *BMC Palliative Care, 16*(1), 39. https://doi.org/10.1186/s12904-017-0223-y

Björkenstam, E., Burström, B., Brännström, L., Vinnerljung, B., Björkenstam, C., & Pebley, A. R. (2015). Cumulative exposure to childhood stressors and subsequent psychological distress. An analysis of US panel data. *Social Science & Medicine (1982), 142,* 109–117. https://doi.org/10.1016/j.socscimed.2015.08.006

Blaustein, M. E., & Kinniburgh, K. M. (2010). *Treating traumatic stress in children and adolescents: How to foster resilience through attachment, self-regulation, and competency.* Guilford Press.

Bowlby, J. (1960). Grief and mourning in infancy and early childhood. *Psychoanalytic Study of the Child, 15,* 9–52.

Bowlby, J. (1969). *Attachment* (Vol. 1 of Attachment and loss). Basic Books.

Burns, J. M., Andrews, G., & Szabo, M. (2002). Depression in young people: What causes it and can we prevent it? *Medical Journal of Australia, 177*(Suppl.), S93–S96. https://doi.org/10.5694/j.1326-5377.2002.tb04864.x

Canadian Association of Speech-Language Pathologists and Audiologists. (2000). *School age speech & language development fact sheet.* http://www.saslpa.ca/school_age_speech_and_language.pdf

Canadian Federation of Mental Health Nurses. (2014). *The Canadian standards for psychiatric-mental health nursing* (4th ed.).

Canadian Paediatric Society. (2021). *Mental health: Screening tools and rating scales.* https://www.cps.ca/en/mental-health-screening-tools

Centre for Addiction and Mental Health. (2012). *Mental health and addiction statistics.* http://www.camh.ca/en/hospital/about_camh/newsroom/for_reporters/Pages/addictionmentalhealthstatistics.aspx

Chang, J., & Kier, C. A. (2016). Introduction to the special issue: Divorce in the Canadian context—Interventions and family processes. *Canadian Journal of Counselling and Psychotherapy, 50*(3S), S1–S4. https://cjc-rcc.ucalgary.ca/article/view/61148

Chehil, S., & Kutcher, S. P. (2012). *Suicide risk management: A Manual for health professionals.* Wiley.

Christie, G., Marsh, R., Sheridan, J., Wheeler, A., Suaalii-Sauni, T., Black, S., & Butler, R. (2007). The substances and choices scale (SACS)—the development and testing of a new alcohol and other drug screening and outcome measurement instrument for young people. *Addiction, 102*(9), 1390–1398. https://doi.org/10.1111/j.1360-0443.2007.01916.x

Clinton, J., Feller, A. F., & Williams, R. C. (2016). The importance of infant mental health. *Paediatrics & Child Health, 21*(5), 239–241.

Conroy, S. (2021). *Family violence in Canada: A statistical profile, 2019.* Statistics Canada. https://www150.statcan.gc.ca/n1/en/pub/85-002-x/2021001/article/00001-eng.pdf?st=PQ238In-

Costea, G. O. (2011). Considering the children of parents with mental illness: Impact on behavioral and social functioning. *Brown University Child and Adolescent Behavior Letter, 27*(4), 1–6.

Costello, E. J., Egger, H., & Angold, A. (2005). Ten-year research update review: The epidemiology of child and adolescent psychiatric disorders. I. Methods and public health burden. *Journal of American Academy of Child and Adolescent Psychiatry, 44*(10), 972–986. https://doi.org/10.1097/01.chi.0000172552.41596.6f

Creamer, A. M., Hughes, J., & Snow, N. (2020). An exploration of facilitators and challenges to young adult engagement in community-based program for mental health promotion. *Global Qualitative Nursing Research,* (7), 1–14. https://doi.org/10.1177/2333393620922828

Currie, C., Zanotti, C., Morgan, A., Currie, D., de Looze, M., Roberts, C., … Barkenow, V. (Eds.) (2011). *Social determinants of health and well-being among young people. Health Behaviour in School-aged Children (HBSC) study: International report from the 2009/2010 survey.* World Health Organization Regional Office for Europe.

De Bellis, M. D., & Zisk, A. (2014). The biological effects of childhood trauma. *Child and Adolescent Psychiatric Clinics of North America, 23*(2), 185–222. https://doi.org/10.1016/j.chc.2014.01.002

Deering, C. G., & Cody, D. J. (2002). Communicating effectively with children and adults. *American Journal of Nursing, 102*(3), 34–42.

DeFehr, J. N. (2020) "Voluntarily, knowingly, and intelligently": Protecting informed consent in school-based mental health referrals. *Brock Educational Journal, 29*(1), 6–23.

Durwood, L., McLaughlin, K. A., & Olson, K. R. (2017). Mental health and self-worth in socially transitioned transgender youth. *Journal of the American Academy of Child and Adolescent Psychiatry, 56*(2), 116–123. https://doi.org/10.1016/j.jaac.2016.10.016

Eberl, C., & Ogenchuk, M. (2019, September 30). Foster care—a social determinant of health. *Canadian Nurse.* https://www.canadian-nurse.com/en/articles/issues/2019/september-2019/foster-care-a-social-determinant-of-health

Edidin, J. P., Ganim, Z., Hunter, S. J., & Karnik, N. S. (2012). The mental and physical health of homeless youth: A literature review. *Child Psychiatry and Human Development, 43*(3), 354–375. https://doi.org/10.1007/s10578-011-0270-1

Eggert, L. L., Thompson, E. A., Randell, B. P., & Pike, K. (2002). Preliminary effects of brief school-based prevention approaches for reducing youth suicide: Risk behaviors, depression, and drug involvement. *Journal of Child and Adolescent Psychiatric Nursing, 15*(2), 48–64. https://doi.org/10.1111/j.1744-6171.2002.tb00326.x

Elkind, D. (1967). Egocentrism in adolescence. *Child Development, 38,* 1025–1034.

Eniola, K., & Evarts, L. (2017). Diagnosis of child maltreatment: A family medicine physician's dilemma. *Southern Medical Journal, 110*(5), 330–336. https://doi.org/10.14423/SMJ.0000000000000644

Erikson, E. (1968). *Identity, youth and crisis.* Norton.

Ewing, J. A. (1984). Detecting alcoholism: The CAGE questionnaire. *Journal of the American Medical Association, 252*(14), 1905–1907.

Fallon, B., Collin-Vézina, D., King, B., Houston, E., Joh-Carnella, N., & Black, T. (2017). *Sexual abuse substantiation by sub-types and outcomes of sexual abuse investigations by gender.* CWRP Information Sheet # 188E. Canadian Child Welfare Research Portal.

Foster, K., O'Brien, L., & Korhonen, T. (2012). Developing resilient children and families when parents have mental illness: A family-focused approach. *International Journal of Mental Health Nursing, 21*(1), 3–11.

Fox, B. H., Perez, N., Cass, E., Baglivio, M. T., & Epps, N. (2015). Trauma changes everything: Examining the relationship between adverse childhood experiences and serious, violent and chronic juvenile offenders. *Child Abuse & Neglect, 46,* 163–173. http://doi.org/10.1016/j.chiabu.2015.01.011

Freeman, J. G., King, M., Pickett, W., Craig, W., Elgar, F., Janssen, I., & Klinger, D. (2010). *The health of Canada's young people: A Mental health focus.* http://www.phac-aspc.gc.ca/hp-ps/dca-dea/publications/hbsc-mental-mentale/assets/pdf/hbsc-mental-mentale-eng.pdf

Gaetz, S., O'Grady, B., Kidd, S., & Schwan, K. (2016). *Without a home: The National youth homelessness survey.* Canadian Observatory on Homelessness Press.

Gass, K., Jenkins, J., & Dunn, J. (2007). Are sibling relationships protective? A longitudinal study. *Journal of Child Psychology and Psychiatry, 48*(2), 167–175.

George, T., & Vaccarino, F. (Eds.). (2015). *Substance abuse in Canada: The effects of cannabis use during adolescence.* Canadian Centre on Substance

Abuse. http://www.ccsa.ca/Resource%20Library/CCSA-Effects-of-Cannabis-Use-during-Adolescence-Report-2015-en.pdf

Gheorghe, M., Varin, M., Wong, S. L., Baker, M., Grywacheski, V., & Orpana, H. (2021). Symptoms of postpartum anxiety and depression among women in Canada: Findings from a national cross-sectional survey. *Canadian Journal of Public Health, 112*, 244–252. https://doi.org/10.17269/s41997-020-00420-4

Gladstone, B. M., Boydell, K. M., Seeman, M. V., & McKeever, P. D. (2011). Children's experiences of parental mental illness: A literature review. *Early Intervention in Psychiatry, 5*(4), 271–289. https://doi.org/10.1111/j.1751-7893.2011.00287.x

Government of Canada. (2018). *Trauma and violence-informed approaches to policy and practice.* https://www.canada.ca/en/public-health/services/publications/health-risks-safety/trauma-violence-informed-approaches-policy-practice.html

Government of Canada. (2021). *Reducing the number of Indigenous children in care.* https://www.sac-isc.gc.ca/eng/1541187352297/1541187392851

Grant, C. N., & Bélanger, R. E. (2017). Position Statement: Cannabis and Canada's children and youth. *Paediatrics & Child Health, 22*(2), 98–102. https://doi.org/10.1093/pch/pxx017

Gregory, K. E., & Vessey, J. A. (2004). Bibliotherapy: A strategy to help students with bullying. *The Journal of School Nursing, 20*, 127–133. https://doi.org/10.1177/10598405040200030201

Guz, S., Kattari, S. K., Atteberry-Ash, B., Klemmer, C., Call, J., & Kattari, L. (2021). Depression and suicide risk at the cross-section of sexual orientation and gender identity for youth. *Journal of Adolescent Health, 68*, 317–323. https://doi.org/10.1016/j.jadohealth.2020.06.008

Hango, D. (2017, September). *Childhood physical abuse: Difference by birth cohort.* Insights on Canadian society. Statistics Canada Catalogue no. 75-006-X.

Harlow, H. F., Harlow, M. K., & Suomi, S. J. (1971). From thought to therapy: Lessons from a private laboratory. *American Scientist, 59*(5), 538–549.

Harter, S. (2000). Psychosocial adjustment of adult children of alcoholics: A review of recent empirical literature. *Clinical Psychology Review, 20*(3), 311–337.

Hawke, L. D., Sheikhan, N. Y., MacCon, K., & Henderson, J. (2021). Going virtual: youth attitudes toward and experiences of virtual mental health and substance use services during the COVID-19 pandemic. *BMC Health Services Research, 21*, 340. https://doi.org/10.1186/s12913-021-06321-7

Health Canada. (2017). *Canadian cannabis survey 2017—summary.* Government of Canada. https://www.canada.ca/en/health-canada/services/publications/drugs-health-products/canadian-Cannabis-survey-2017-summary.html

Heath, M. A., Sheen, D., Leavy, D., Young, E., & Money, K. (2005). Bibliotherapy: A resource to facilitate emotional healing and growth. *School Psychology International, 26*(5), 563–580. https://doi.org/10.1177/0143034305060792

Hetherington, E. M., & Kelly, J. (2002). *For better or for worse: Divorce reconsidered.* WW Norton.

Hodges, E. A., Houck, G. M., & Kindermann, T. (2007). Reliability of the nursing child assessment feeding scale during toddlerhood. *Issues in Comprehensive Pediatric Nursing, 30*(3), 109–130. https://doi.org/10.1080/01460860701525204

Hodges, E. A., Houck, G. M., & Kindermann, T. (2009). Validity of the nursing child assessment feeding scale during toddlerhood. *Western Journal of Nursing Research, 31*(5), 662–678. https://doi.org/10.1177/0193945909332265

Hodgson, K. J., Shelton, K. H., van den Bree, M. B., & Los, F. J. (2013). Psychopathology in young people experiencing homelessness: A systematic review. *American Journal of Public Health, 103*(6), e24–e37. https://doi.org/10.2105/AJPH.2013.301318

Hoft, M., & Haddad, L. (2017). Screening children for abuse and neglect: A review of the literature. *Journal of Forensic Nursing, 13*(1), 26–32. http://doi:10.1097/JFN.0000000000000136

Holt, V., Skagerberg, E., & Dunsford, M. (2016). Young people with features of gender dysphoria: Demographics and associated difficulties. *Clinical Child Psychology and Psychiatry, 21*, 108–118.

Hulchanski, J. D., Campsie, P., Chau, S. B. Y., Hwang, S. H., & Paradis, E. (Eds.) (2009). *Finding home: Policy options for addressing homelessness in Canada.* http://www.homelesshub.ca/library/finding-home-policy-options-for-addressing-homelessness-in-canada-45761.aspx

Jones, T. M., Nurius, P., Song, C., & Fleming, C. M. (2018). Modeling life course pathways from adverse childhood experiences to adult mental health. *Child Abuse & Neglect, 80*, 32–40. https://doi.org/10.1016/j.chiabu.2018.03.005

Kelly, J. B. (2012). Risk and protective factors associated with child and adolescent adjustment following separation and divorce: Social science applications. In K. Kuehnle & L. Drozd (Eds.), *Parenting plan evalua-*

tions: *Applied research for the family court* (pp. 49–84). Oxford University Press. https://doi.org/10.1093/med:psych/9780199754021.003.0003

King, P. M., Klemmer, J., Mansell, K., Alcorn, J., & Mansell, H. (2020). Development of the REACH (real education about cannabis and health) program for Canadian youth. *Journal of Nursing Education, 59*(8), 465–469. http://dx.doi.org/10.3928/01484834-20200723-09

Koball, A. M., Rasmussen, C., Olson-Dorff, D., Klevan, J., Ramirez, L., & Domoff, S. E. (2019). The relationship between adverse childhood experiences, healthcare utilization, cost of care and medical comorbidities. *Child Abuse & Neglect, 90*, 120–126. https://doi.org/10.1016/j.chiabu.2019.01.021

Korczak, D. (2012). Identifying depression in childhood: Symptoms, signs and significance. *Pediatrics & Child Health, 17*(1), 572. https://doi.org/10.1093/pch/17.10.572

Kraft, L. E., Rahm, G., & Erikkson, U. (2017). The school nurse's ability to detect and support abused children: A trust-creating process. *The Journal of School Nursing, 33*(2), 133–142.

Kutcher, S. (2019). *Transitions: Making the most of your campus experience.* https://mentalhealthliteracy.org/wp-content/uploads/2019/05/FINAL-Transitions-MAY-2019-Full-Online.pdf

Kutcher, S., & McLuckie, A. (2010). *Evergreen: A child and youth mental health framework for Canada.* Mental Health Commission of Canada.

Langlois, K. A., & Garner, R. (2013). Trajectories of psychological distress among Canadian adults who experienced parental addiction in childhood. *Health Reports, 24*(3), 14–21.

Letourneau, N. L., Tryphonopoulos, P. D., Novick, J., Hart, J. M., Giesbrecht, G., & Oxford, M. L. (2018). Nursing child assessment satellite training parent-child interaction scales: Comparing American and Canadian normative and high-risk samples. *Journal of Pediatric Nursing, 40*, 47–57. https://doi.org/10.1016/j.pedn.2018.02.016

Maina, G., Mclean, M., Mcharo, S., Kennedy, M., Djiometio, J., & King, A. (2020). A scoping review of school based indigenous substance use prevention in preteens (7-13 years). *Substance Use Treatment, Prevention, and Policy, 15*, 74. https://doi.org/10.1186/s13011-020-00314-1

Maina, G., Ogenchuk, M., & Gaudet, S. (2021). Living with parents with problematic substance use: Impacts and turning points. *Public Health Nursing (Boston, Mass.), 38*, 730–737. https://doi.org/10.1111/phn.12888

Majers, S. J. (2021). When I complicated understood loss and grief. *The Journal of Psychiatric and Mental Health Nursing, 28*(2), 268–270. https://doi.org/10.1111/jpm.12641

Martinez, Y., & Ercikan, K. (2009). Chronic illnesses in Canadian children: What is the effect of illness on academic achievement, and anxiety and emotional disorders? *Child: Care, Health and Development, 35*(3), 391–401. https://doi.org/10.1111/j.1365-2214.2008.00916.x

Masten, A. S. (2001). Ordinary magic: Resilience processes in development. *American Psychologist, 56*(3), 227–238. https://doi.org/10.1037//0003-066x.56.3.227

McConnell, E. A., Birkett, M., & Mustanski, B. (2016). Families matter: Social support and mental health trajectories among lesbian, gay, bisexual, and transgendered youth. *Journal of Adolescent Health, 59*, 674–680. https://doi.org/10.1016/j.jadohealth.2016.07.026

McCormick, A., & Baldridge, S. (2019). Family acceptance and faith: understanding the acceptance processes of parents of LGBTQ youth. *Social Work & Christianity, 46*(1), 32–40. https://doi.org/10.1016/j.pcl.2016.07.005

McInnis, O. A., & Porath-Waller, A. (2016). *Clearing the smoke on cannabis: Chronic use and cognitive functioning and mental health—An update.* Canadian Centre on Substance Abuse. https://aventa.org/wp-content/uploads/2016/10/CCSA-Chronic-Cannabis-Use-Effects-Report-2016-en.pdf

McLaughlin, K. A., Koenen, K. C., Bromet, E. J., Karam, E. G., Liu, H., Petukhova, M., Ruscio, A. M., Sampson, N. A., Stein, D. J., Aguilar-Gaxiola, S., Alonso, J., Borges, G., Demyttenaere, K., Dinolova, R. V., Ferry, F., Florescu, S., de Girolamo, G., Gureje, O., Kawakami, N., … Kessler, R. C. (2017). Childhood adversities and post-traumatic stress disorder: Evidence for stress sensitisation in the World Mental Health Surveys. *The British Journal of Psychiatry: The Journal of Mental Science, 211*(5), 280–288. https://doi.org/10.1192/bjp.bp.116.197640

McTavish, J. R., & MacMillan, H. L. (2019). *Briefing Note: Mandatory reporting of child maltreatment.* VEGA Project. McMaster University. https://vegaproject.mcmaster.ca/docs/default-source/pdf/vega-cm-briefing-note-mandatory-reporting.pdf?sfvrsn=d38adae4_4

Melchior, M., Bolze, C., Fombonne, E., Surkan, P. J., Pryor, L., & Jauffret-Roustide, M. (2017). Early cannabis initiation and educational attainment: Is the association casual? *International Journal of Epidemiology, 46*, 1641–1650. https://doi.org/10.1093/ije/dyx065

Mental Health Commission of Canada. (2016). *The mental health strategy for Canada: A youth perspective.* https://www.mentalhealthcommission.ca/sites/default/files/2016-07/Youth_Strategy_Eng_2016.pdf

Michaelson, V., King, N., Inchley, J., Currie, D., Brooks, F., & Pickett, W. (2019). Domains of spirituality and their associations with positive mental health: A study of adolescents in Canada, England and Scotland. *Preventive Medicine, 125*, 12–18. https://doi.org/10.1016/j.ypmed.2019.04.018

Minhas, R. S., Graham, H., Jegathesan, T., Huber, J., Young, E., & Barozzino, T. (2017). Supporting the development health of refugee children and youth. *Paediatrics & Child Health, 22*(2), 68–71.

Mylant, M. L., Ide, B., Cuevas, E., & Meehan, M. (2002). Adolescent children of alcoholics: Vulnerable or resilient? *Journal of the American Psychiatric Nurses Association, 8*(2), 57–64.

National Institute on Drug Abuse. (2020). *Inhalants drug facts.* https://www.drugabuse.gov/publications/drugfacts/inhalants

Olson, J., Schrager, S. M., Belzer, M., Simons, L. K., & Clark, L. F. (2015). Baseline physiologic and psychosocial characteristics of transgender youth seeking care for gender dysphoria. *Journal of Adolescent Health, 57*, 374–380.

Peacock, S., Konrad, S., Watson, E., Nickel, D., & Muhajarine, N. (2013). Effectiveness of home visiting programs on child outcomes: A systematic review. *BMC Public Health, 13*, 17. http://doi.org/10.1186/1471-2458-13-17

Perri, M., & Schwan, K. (2020). *Criminal justice involvement amongst youth experiencing homelessness in Canada: Reflections during a pandemic.* Homeless Hub. https://www.homelesshub.ca/blog/criminal-justice-involvement-amongst-youth-experiencing-homelessness-canada-reflections-during#:~:text=Further%2C%20research%20shows%20that%20young,7.6%25%20of%20the%20general%20public

Peters, R., Petrunka, K., & Arnold, R. (2003). The better beginnings, brighter futures project: A universal, comprehensive, community-based prevention approach for primary school children and their families. *Journal of Clinical Child and Adolescent Psychology, 32*, 215–227. https://doi.org/10.1207/S15374424JCCP3202_6

Petruccelli, K., Davis, J., & Berman, T. (2019). Adverse childhood experiences and associated health outcomes: A systematic review and meta-analysis. *Child Abuse & Neglect, 97*, 104127. https://doi.org/10.1016/j.chiabu.2019.104127

Pokorny, M. E. (2022). Nursing theorists of historical significance. In M. R. Alligood (Ed.), *Nursing theorists and their work* (10th ed.) Elsevier.

Pietrangelo, A. (2019, October 2019). How play therapy treats and benefits children and some adults. *Healthline.* https://www.healthline.com/health/play-therapy

Porath-Walker, A., Brown, A., Frigon, A., & Clark, H. (2013). *What Canadian youth think about cannabis.* Canadian Centre on Substance Abuse. http://www.ccsa.ca/Resource%20Library/CCSA-What-Canadian-Youth-Think-about-Cannabis-2013-en.pdf

Potter-Dickey, A., Letourneau, N., & de Koning, A. P. J. (2020). Associations between neurodevelopmental disorders and attachment patterns in preschool-aged children: Systematic review. *Current Developmental Disorders Reports, 7*, 277–289. https://doi.org/10.1007/s40474-020-00219-5

Public Health Agency of Canada. (2016). *A focus on family violence in Canada.* https://www.canada.ca/content/dam/canada/public-health/migration/publications/department-ministere/state-public-health-family-violence-2016-etat-sante-publique-violence-familiale/alt/pdf-eng.pdf

Reedtz, C., Lauritzen, C., Stover, Y. V., Freili, J. L., & Rognmo, K. (2019). Identification of children of parents with mental illness: A necessity to provide relevant support. *Frontiers in Psychiatry, 9*, 728. https://doi.org/10.3389/fpsyt.2018.00728

Reist, D., & Asgari, M. (2018). *Drug education as health promotion.* Canadian Institute for Substance Use Research. https://www.uvic.ca/research/centres/cisur/assets/docs/hs-drug-education-as-health-promotion.pdf

Ritter, J., Stewart, M., Bernet, C., Coe, M., & Brown, S. A. (2002). Effects of childhood exposure to familial alcoholism and family violence on adolescent substance use, conduct problems, and self-esteem. *Journal of Traumatic Stress, 15*(2), 113–122.

Rubin, D., Dodd, M., Desai, N., Pollock, B., & Graham-Pole, J. (2009). Spirituality in well and ill adolescents and their parents: The use of two assessment scales. *Pediatric Nursing, 35*(1), 37–42.

Russell, S. T., & Fish, J. N. (2016). Mental health in lesbian, gay, bisexual, and transgender (LGBT) youth. *Annual Review of Clinical Psychology, 12*, 465–487. http://doi.org/10.1146/annurev-clinpsy-021815-093153

Saint-Girons, M., Trocmé, N., Esposito, T., & Fallon, B. (2020). *Children in out-of-home care in Canada in 2019.* CWRP Information Sheet #211E. Canadian Child Welfare Research Portal.

Samuelsson, M., Holsti, A., Adamsson, M., Serenius, F., Häggöi, B., & Farooqi, A. (2017). Behavioral patterns in adolescents born at 23 to 25 weeks of gestation. *Pediatrics, 140*(1), e20170199. http://doi.org/10.1542/peds.2017-0199f

Schreiber, J. K., Sands, D. C., & Jordan, J. R. (2017). The perceived experience of children bereaved by parental suicide. *Omega: Journal of Death & Dying (OMEGA), 75*(2), 184–206. https://doi.org/10.1177/0030222815612297

Schwartz, C., Waddell, C., Andres, C., Yung, D., & Gray-Grant, D. (2017). Supporting LGBTQ+ youth. *Children's Mental Health Research Quarterly, 11*(2), 1–16. Children's Health Policy Centre, Faculty of Health Sciences, Simon Fraser University.

Self, B., & Peters, H. (2005). Street outreach with no streets. *Canadian Nurse, 101*(1), 20–24.

Shields, M. E., Hovdestad, W. E., Pelletier, C., Dykxhoorn, J. L., O'Donnell, S. C., & Tonmyr, L. (2016). Childhood maltreatment as a risk factor for diabetes: Findings from a population-based survey of Canadian adults. *BMC Public Health, 16*(879), 1–12. https://doi.org/10.1186/s12889-016-3491-1

Shajani, Z., & Snell, D. (2019). *Wright & Leahey's nurses and families: A guide to family assessment and intervention* (7th ed.). F. A. Davis.

Søfting, G. H., Dyregro, A., & Dyregrov, K. (2016). Because I'm also part of the family, children's participation in rituals after the loss of a parent or sibling: A qualitative study from the children's perspective. *OMEGA—Journal of Death and Dying, 73*(2), 141–158. https://doi.org/10.1177/0030222815575898

Statistics Canada. (2017). *Portrait of children's family life in Canada, 2016.* No. 88-200-X2016006. https://www12.statcan.gc.ca/census-recensement/2016/as-sa/98-200-x/2016006/98-200-x2016006-eng.pdf

Statistics Canada. (2019, February 20). Family matters: Couples who live apart. *The Daily.* https://bit.ly/2GAscHs.

Statistics Canada. (2020). *Canadian income survey, 2018.* https://www150.statcan.gc.ca/n1/daily-quotidien/200224/dq200224a-eng.htm?HPA=1

Strohschein, L. (2012). Parental divorce and child mental health: Accounting for predisruption effects. *Journal of Divorce and Remarriage, 53*(6), 489–502. https://doi.org/10.1080/10502556.2012.682903

Solomon, J., & George, C. (1999). *Attachment disorganization.* Guilford Press.

Speech-Language & Audiology Canada. (2014). *Speech, language and hearing milestones.* https://sac-oac.ca/sites/default/files/resources/SAC-Milestones-TriFold_EN.pdf

Tanguay, P. (2000). Pervasive developmental disorders: A 10-year review. *Journal of the American Academy of Child and Adolescent Psychiatry, 39*, 1079–1095. https://doi.org/10.1097/00004583-200009000-00007

Testoni, I., Palazzo, L., De Vincenzo, C., & Wieser, M. A. (2020). Enhancing existential thinking through death education: A qualitative study among high school students. *Behavioral Sciences, 10*, 113. https://doi.org/10.3390/bs10070113

Thompson, R. (2002). Attachment theory and research. In M. Lewis (Ed.), *Child and adolescent psychiatry: A comprehensive textbook* (3rd ed.). Lippincott Williams & Wilkins.

Tiyyagura, G., Beucher, M., & Bechtel, K. (2017). Nonaccidental injury in pediatric patients: Detection, evaluation, and treatment. *Pediatric Emergency Medicine Practice, 14*(7), 1–20.

Trainor, J., Pomeroy, E., & Pape, B. (2004). *A framework for support* (3rd ed.). Canadian Mental Health Association.

Trocmé, N., Fallon, B., MacLaurin, B., Sinha, V., Black, T., Fast, E., Felstiner, C., Hélie, S., Turcotte, D., WEghtman, P., Douglas, J., & Holroyd, J. (2010). *Canadian Incidence Study of reported child abuse and neglect—2008: Major findings.* Public Health Agency of Canada.

Turban, J. L. (2017). Transgender youth: The building evidence base for early social transition. *Journal of the American Academy of Child & Adolescent Psychiatry, 56*(2), 101–102. https://doi.org/10.1016/j.jaac.2016.11.008

Unger, A. (2013). Children's health in slum settings. *Archives of Disease in Childhood, 98*(10), 799–805. https://doi.org/10.1136/archdischild-2011-301621

Vachon, D. D., Krueger, R. F., Rogosch, F. A., & Cicchetti, D. (2015). Assessment of the harmful psychiatric and behavioral effects of different forms of child maltreatment. *JAMA Psychiatry, 72*(11), 1135–1142. http://doi:10.1001/jamapsychiatry.2015.1792

Vallerioni, J., Maghsoudi, M., Nguyen-Dang, M., Lake, S., Thiessen, M., Robinson, J., & Pavlova, D. (2018). *Sensible cannabis education: A toolkit for educating youth.* Canadian Students for Sensible Drug Policy (CSSDP). https://cssdp.org/uploads/2018/04/Sensible-Cannabis-Education-A-Toolkit-for-Educating-Youth.pdf

Veronie, L., & Freuhstorfer, D. B. (2001). Gender, birth order and family role identification among children of alcoholics. *Current Psychology: Developmental, Learning, Personality, Social, 20*(1), 53–67. https://doi.org/10.1007/s12144-001-1003-6

Viorst, J. (1972). *The ten good things about Barney.* Simon & Schuster.

Werner, E., Miller, M., Osborne, L. M., Kuzava, S., & Monk, C. (2015). Preventing postpartum depression: Review and recommendations. *Archives of Women's Mental Health, 18*(1), 41–60. https://doi.org/10.1007/s00737-014-0475-y

White, E. B. (1952). *Charlotte's web.* HarperCollins.

Whitehead, M. (2008). *Pediatric nurses' perspectives of spirituality and spiritual care within nurse-patient relationships: An interpretive description.* Unpublished Master Thesis. University of Alberta, Canada.

Whiteman, S. D., McHale, S. M., & Soli, A. (2011). Theoretical perspectives on sibling relationships. *Journal of Family Theory and Review, 3,* 124–139. https://doi.org/10.1111/j.1756-2589.2011.00087.x

Wu, Z., Hou, F., & Schimmele, C. (2008). Family structure and children's psychosocial outcomes. *Journal of Family Issues, 29*(12), 1600–1624.

Yalom, I. D. (1985). *The theory and practice of group psychotherapy* (2nd ed.). Basic Books.

Zolkoski, S. M., & Bullock, L. M. (2012). Resilience in children and youth: A review. *Children and Youth Services Review, 34*(12), 2295–2303.

CHAPTER 30

Psychiatric Disorders in Children and Adolescents*

Hua Li

LEARNING OBJECTIVES

After studying this chapter, you will be able to:

- Identify the common psychiatric disorders usually first diagnosed in infancy, childhood, or adolescence.
- Describe aspects of the nursing care of psychotic, bipolar, depressive, anxiety, and obsessive–compulsive disorders.
- Discuss the prevalence, possible causes, and nursing interventions for trauma- and stressor-related disorders.
- Identify the bio/psycho/social/spiritual nursing domains in the care of children with neurodevelopmental disorders, particularly autism spectrum disorder.
- Relate the assessment data of children with attention deficit hyperactivity disorder (ADHD) to the development of nursing diagnoses, interventions, and evaluation of outcomes.
- Compare the disruptive, impulse control, and conduct disorders.
- Using Tourette syndrome as an example, explain the challenges facing children and adolescents with motor disorders.
- Discuss the behavioural intervention strategies for the treatment of enuresis and encopresis.

KEY TERMS

- communication disorders • compulsions • concordant • encopresis • enuresis • externalizing disorders • habit reversal training • internalizing disorders • learning disorders • obsessions • school phobia • stereotypic behaviour • tic disorders

KEY CONCEPTS

- attention • autism spectrum disorder • developmental delay • hyperactivity • impulsiveness

Child and adolescent mental health is a relatively new phenomenon in the field of psychiatry. As research into the neurobiology and genetics of human development advances, the various categories and diagnoses identified will evolve. The understanding of child psychiatric disorders has benefited from advances in several fields, including developmental biology, neuroanatomy, psychopharmacology, genetics, and epidemiology.

The *Diagnostic and Statistical Manual of Mental Disorders-5* (5th ed.; *DSM-5*; American Psychiatric Association [APA], 2013) integrates current evidence relevant to nurses' practice with children and families, in a way that

will not only guide their practice but also impact future research. The classifications of child and adolescent psychiatric disorders discussed in this chapter include schizophrenia spectrum and other psychotic disorders; bipolar and related disorders; depressive disorders; anxiety disorders; obsessive–compulsive disorder (OCD); trauma- and stressor-related disorders; neurodevelopment disorders of childhood; disruptive, impulse control, and conduct disorders; motor disorders; and elimination disorders.

Approximately one in five Canadians lives with a mental illness (Mental Health Commission of Canada

---

*Adapted from the chapter, "Psychiatric Disorders in Children and Adolescents," by Lorelei Faulkner-Gibson and Kimberly Wong

803

[MHCC], 2012), and for most, the onset will occur during childhood, adolescence, or young adulthood (Kim-Cohen et al., 2003). The prevalence of child and adolescent psychiatric disorders varies. According to the British Columbia Provincial School Survey of 2013, at least 15% of students who are young men and 22% of students who are young women from grade 7 to grade 12 reported at least one mental health condition (Smith et al., 2014). In Ontario, 25% of grade 7 to grade 12 students visited a mental healthcare professional at least once in 2017 (Center for Addiction and Mental Health [CAMH], 2018). According to the Saskatchewan Youth Health Survey in 2015, 22% of grade 7 to grade 12 students had harmed themselves (12% of young men and 32% of young women), while almost 1 in 5 (19%) students had considered suicide in the previous 12 months (Saskatchewan Alliance for Youth & Community Wellbeing, 2016). While these prevalence rates vary across the country, they highlight the importance of prompt identification, referral, and treatment for children experiencing illness.

Mental health illness in children and adolescents represents a critical window for early detection and intervention that can improve long-term outcomes. However, only 1 in 11 Canadian youth received medical treatment for their mood and anxiety disorders or antipsychotic symptoms in 2018–2019 (Canadian Institute for Health Information, 2020). This discrepancy appears to be the result of limited access to treatment and appropriate mental health services, as well as the reality that psychiatric problems are less easily diagnosed in children than they are in adults. One factor contributing to this difference is that sometimes the symptoms of disorders are difficult to distinguish from the turbulence of normal growth and development.

An overview of the psychiatric disorders diagnosed in children and adolescents that a nurse may encounter in practice, and the bio/psycho/social/spiritual domains of nursing care for this population experiencing these mental health challenges, is presented. The spiritual domain of nursing care for child and adolescent psychiatric disorders is presented separately. All of the psychiatric disorders of childhood and adolescence should be viewed within the context of growth and development models (Box 30.1). Safety and self-esteem are priority considerations. A more in-depth look at ADHD with respect to assessment, management, and follow-up is provided. The various aspects of family dynamics are incorporated within this overview.

Schizophrenia Spectrum and Other Psychotic Disorders

The symptoms of psychotic disorders cluster into five common domains, often referred to as positive symptoms: delusions, hallucinations, disorganized thinking

---

> **BOX 30.1 History and Hallmarks of Childhood and Adolescent Disorders**
>
> - Maternal age and health status during pregnancy
> - Exposure to medication, alcohol, or other substances during pregnancy
> - Course of pregnancy, labour, and delivery
> - Infant's health at birth
> - Eating, sleeping, and growth in first year
> - Health status in first year
> - Interest in others in first 2 years
> - Motor development
> - Mastery of bowel and bladder control
> - Speech and language development
> - Activity level
> - Response to separation (e.g., school entry)
> - Regulation of mood and anxiety
> - Medical history in early childhood
> - Social development
> - Interests

(speech), grossly disorganized or abnormal motor behaviour (including catatonia), and negative symptoms. Negative symptoms typically are deficits of normal emotional responses or other thought processes and commonly include flat or blunted affect and emotion, poverty of speech (alogia), inability to experience pleasure (anhedonia), lack of desire to form relationships (asociality), and lack of motivation (avolition). Research suggests that negative symptoms may contribute to a poorer quality of life, functional disability, and burden on others when compared to positive symptoms, and unfortunately, they respond less well to antipsychotic medication (refer further to Chapter 21).

Brief Psychotic Disorder

In children and youth, what is commonly observed and diagnosed is either "brief psychotic disorder" or "substance/medication-induced psychotic disorder," prior to a confirmed diagnosis of schizophrenia or other related psychotic disorder. Although psychosis can occur in children under 13 years, it is rare (APA, 2013).

Treatment Interventions

Most psychoses, including schizophrenia, are treated with antipsychotic medications. These medications often cause unpleasant side effects, which is a contributing factor to clients either stopping their medication altogether or being inconsistent in their adherence to their medication regimen. This affects the duration and prognosis of the illness. For example, with the advent of second-generation antipsychotic medications, the increase in metabolic illnesses has increased. Many adolescents experience substantial weight gain, which can further contribute to stigma and illness (Emmer et al., 2020). Nurses working with clients need to provide support and work to mitigate these side effects while supporting medication adherence. Reducing the duration of untreated psychosis is critical to remission and recovery.

Nursing Care

The nursing care priority for a child or adolescent with a diagnosis of psychosis is to ensure safety. Altered perceptions affect the individual's organization and thus affect adequate intake, output, and general hygiene and health. Providing education of the child or adolescent experiencing psychosis and their family regarding signs and symptoms of relapse is important. Encouragement of daily exercise, healthy nutrition, and the maintenance of social connections will assist in the promotion of recovery and the prevention of an illness relapse. Monitoring of medication adherence and follow-up is critical. Engaging families in support programs also alleviates the stigma associated with psychotic illnesses.

Biologic Domain

It is well established that schizophrenia spectrum disorders typically have a neurologic basis with some linkages to genetics. No definitive cause has been identified to date. There is strong evidence that first-degree relatives of individuals with schizophrenia are at higher risk of developing the disorder. In relation to brief psychotic disorder, there may be evidence of a marked stressor, or postpartum onset, or it may be related to catatonia (APA, 2013). The incidence is approximately 9% of first-onset psychosis. The symptoms typically dissipate within 1 month; however, if the duration is longer, the diagnosis may be altered. See Box 30.2 for early warning signs of psychosis.

Psychosocial Domain

A lack of insight is often experienced by those with a psychotic disorder, and children and adolescents often do not recognize that they are ill, or if they do, then they often do not tell their families or friends out of fear of stigma. Many families may not be aware of symptoms until they become overtly severe. The earlier the symptoms are identified and treated, the more likely the illness will move into remission. The better the medical and psychosocial management is, the better chance of remission and recovery. Family education and support are critical to prognosis and remission. Early psychosis intervention (EPI) programs are available in most

> ## BOX 30.2 Early Warning Signs of Psychosis
>
> - Withdrawal from activities and social contacts
> - Irrational, angry, or fearful responses to friends and family
> - Sleep disturbances
> - Deterioration in studies or work
> - Inappropriate use of language—words that do not make sense
> - Sudden excesses, such as extreme religiosity and extreme activity
> - Deterioration in personal hygiene
> - Difficulty controlling thoughts and difficulty concentrating
> - Hearing voices or sounds others don't hear
> - Seeing people or things others don't see
> - A constant feeling of being watched
> - Inability to turn off the imagination, delusions, and off-the-wall ideas
> - Mood swings and increased anxiety
> - Somatic symptoms: weakness, pains, and bizarre body sensations

provinces to provide support, education, and group or individual support (Nolin et al., 2016) (see Web Links).

Bipolar and Related Disorders

Bipolar disorder often first presents during adolescence. Symptoms include periods of mania (extreme optimism, euphoria, and feelings of grandeur; rapid, racing thoughts and hyperactivity; a decreased need for sleep; increased irritability; impulsiveness and possibly reckless behaviour; and alternate periods of depression) (Canadian Mental Health Association, 2014a, 2014b). This can be a very difficult experience for both adolescents and their families, as the youth may engage in behaviours that contribute to ongoing stigma about mental illness (Leibenluft, 2011). Bipolar disorder is rare in children, and the observed symptoms may fall into a diagnosis of ADHD, oppositional defiant disorder (ODD), or disruptive mood regulation disorder (see section "Disruptive Mood Regulation Disorder").

Treatment Intervention

Working with healthcare providers, a treatment plan can be developed for children and adolescents with bipolar disorder that aims to manage symptoms and improve the quality of life. Several types of medications are used to treat the symptoms and, depending on the responses to the medication, children and adolescents may have to try different medications to find out which medication works best for them. The goal is the client is taking the fewest number of medications with the lowest dosage as possible. Psychosocial therapies can help families and their child manage symptoms by providing information, support, education, and guidance (Black & Andreasen, 2014).

Nursing Care

Biologic Domain

A family history of bipolar disorder is correlated with a "10-fold increased risk among adult relatives" (APA, 2013, p. 130). Various mood stabilizer medications are used, with most clients requiring daily or weekly blood tests to assess for therapeutic levels until stable.

Psychosocial Domain

The risk of suicide among the population of individuals with bipolar disorder is 15 times the general population. With suicide being the leading cause of nonaccidental death in individuals 15 to 24 years of age (Government of Canada, 2020), it is critical to assess for risk and intent with this group. Bipolar illness can affect various relationships in an individual's life. Education for friends and school assists the youth. (See Web Links for an online educational resource.)

Depressive Disorders

As noted in Chapter 29, many children and adolescents have lived experience of mental illness. Children and youth are often challenged by disturbances in mood. According to the 2012 Canadian Community Health Survey—Mental Health, approximately 7% of 15- to 24-year-olds reported having depression in the past 12 months, compared with 5% those of aged 25 to 64 years, and 2% of people aged 65 years or older (Findlay, 2017). Treatment for depressive disorders is multimodal, depending on the child's age and symptom presentation (Public Health Agency of Canada, 2016).

Assessing children and adolescents for depression can be especially challenging for nurses and other mental health clinicians. Children may not be able to tell the clinician how they feel, and some adolescents may simply be reluctant to talk about how they are feeling.

As a result, some clinicians purport that depressive disorders in children and adolescents are among the most underdiagnosed mental health disorders. Children and adolescents with a depressive disorder may demonstrate physical symptoms of headaches and stomachaches or avoid situations in which they are feeling overwhelmed or begin to slowly withdraw from social activities (CMHA, 2016). The onset of depression in childhood often persists, recurs, and continues into adulthood, most likely in a more severe form. Depression in young people is frequently accompanied by somatic or psychological symptoms, behavioural issues, or other mental illnesses such as anxiety disorders and substance abuse. Before puberty, there is no gender difference in prevalence; however, after puberty, a gender ratio of 2:1 girls to boys has been documented (Kelvin, 2016).

Major Depressive Disorder

Depressive disorders have prevalence rates of up to 3% in children, and a lifetime prevalence of 11% in adolescence (Avenevoli et al., 2015; Zinck et al., 2009). Suicidal ideation and suicidal behaviour have been associated with severe depression. According to the 2012 Canadian Community Health Survey—Mental Health, one in five adolescents reported suicidal ideation in the past 12 months; suicide is the second leading cause of death among young Canadians, accounting for nearly one quarter of all deaths for those aged 15 to 24 years (Findlay, 2017; Government of Canada, 2020).

Disruptive Mood Dysregulation Disorder

This diagnostic category is new for the *DSM-5* and especially for the assessment of children. The category was developed to better distinguish bipolar disorder in children from other related disorders. The incidence of this disorder is estimated to be 2% to 5% of children, who demonstrate a chronically irritable temperament, and the majority of whom are boys (Black & Andreasen, 2014). "In severe mood dysregulation, irritability is defined as having two components: (a) temper outbursts that are developmentally inappropriate, frequent, and extreme; and (b) negatively balanced mood (anger or sadness) between outbursts" (Leibenluft, 2011, p. 4). According to a study review by Shanahan and colleagues (2014), there appears to be an overlap with childhood diagnoses of depression and/or ODD. As this new category for children unfolds, it will be important that nurses work closely with children and families to ensure that they access the best and most appropriate interventions.

Treatment Interventions

Cognitive–behavioural therapy (CBT) is the treatment of choice for most children and youth experiencing depression, which requires training for most individuals to implement. The use of mindfulness, for a variety of circumstances, is also an easily accessible treatment for most children, adolescents, and their families. See Chapter 14 for cognitive–behavioural interventions and mindfulness, as well as Web Links for a link to the Beck Institute for Cognitive Behavior Therapy. Pharmaceutical intervention is not typically used unless the symptoms observed are interfering with social functioning and are unresponsive or limited in response to other therapeutic interventions.

BOX 30.3 Research for Best Practice

MOTHERS AND ADOLESCENTS WITH DEPRESSION

Armitage, S., Parkinson, M., Halligan, S., & Reynolds, S. (2020). Mothers' experiences of having an adolescent child with depression: An interpretative phenomenological analysis. *Journal of Child and Family Studies, 29*(6), 1617–1629.

Questions: What are mothers' experiences of raising an adolescent child with depression?

Methods: Semi-structured individual interviews were conducted with eight mothers. Data analysis was guided by Interpretative Phenomenological Analysis (IPA), which offers insights into how individuals make sense of their personal and social world. The thoughts, feelings, and experiences related to having an adolescent child with depression were explored.

Findings: Five themes emerged: (a) finding a reason, something to blame (i.e., blaming oneself, feeling blamed, and/or judged by others), and blaming external factors (i.e., chemical imbalance, education system); (b) living with uncertainty including living with fear (i.e., child's self-harm and suicidal ideation), the long-term

impact of depression (i.e., child's education and future employment), the unpredictability of child's challenging behaviour described as "living in a minefield," and adapting parenting described as "walking on eggshells"; (c) feeling of helplessness and frustration (i.e., not knowing how to help and who could help); (d) depression causes change including loss of connection with child, witness a change of personality in their child described as "loss of spirit," and change in family interactions (i.e., no longer wanting to participate in family things); and (e) hiding own emotions and needs described as mothers had to remain positive and to keep their emotions hidden and under control in order to help the situation.

Implications for Nursing Practice: Growing evidence shows that the mental health of adolescents is significantly affected by their caregivers' wellbeing, so the caregivers' wellbeing should be placed as a priority in improving the quality of care for children and adolescents with mental health disorders through professional and peer support including information, education, learning coping skills, and engaging formal or informal social networks.

Nursing Care

Nurses will need to ensure that they are assessing levels of mood in a developmentally conducive manner and that risk assessments have been conducted to rule out concerns of suicidality. The child's functioning will be impacted by numerous factors, including knowledge and support of the education system, family capacity for coping and seeking treatment, and the child's or adolescent's understanding and motivation to participate in treatment.

Nurses need to develop comfort and confidence in assessing children and youth regarding suicidal thoughts and intention. Various age-appropriate tools are available to assist the nurse with those assessments. Education and support are needed for parents and caregivers to understand that asking about suicide does not increase the risk of suicide. Mothers' experiences of living with a child with a diagnosis of depression can be particularly challenging. Refer to Research for Best Practice Box 30.3.

Biologic Domain

Depression has been demonstrated to have a familial or genetic link. Depression can also be caused by stressful events or experiences, medical illness, or medications. Regardless of the cause, depression can look very

different in children and youth than it does in adults. Young children may become withdrawn, have trouble sleeping, regress in certain behaviours (e.g., bed wetting), or become irritable. Older children may start to report headaches and stomachaches or withdraw from activities and friends. Adolescents may be better able to articulate what is happening for them, but they may not necessarily report directly to parents. They may experience sadness and become withdrawn and may exhibit increases or decreases in sleep and appetite (Health-LinkBC, 2017).

Psychosocial Domain

Depression has been linked with life stressors (Box 30.4). Stressors for children can include the death or loss of a pet, parental separation or divorce, or household relocation. There is also evidence that depression (and anxiety) is higher in children who have suffered maltreatment and demonstrated poor coping skills or other life stressors such as "substance abuse, emotional maltreatment, primary caregivers' mental illness, sexual abuse, and numerous moves in a year" (Tonmyr et al., 2011, p. 497). The most serious concern regarding children and youth with depression is their risk of suicide. Suicide screening and assessment needs to start with children as young as 10 years and increase over

BOX 30.4 Questions, Choices, and Outcomes

Mrs. S has just returned with her son, Jared, to the child psychiatric inpatient services following an overnight pass. She reports that the visit did not go well due to Jared's anger and defiance. She remarked that this behaviour was distressingly similar to his behaviour before the hospitalization. She expressed additional concern because of the upcoming discharge from the hospital. After saying goodbye to Jared,

she pulled the nurse aside and stated that she had decided to file for divorce.

Mrs. S indicated that she had not told her husband or the family therapist. When asked whether Jared knew about her decision, Mrs. S suddenly realized that he may have overheard her discussing the matter with her sister on the telephone during this home visit.

How should the nurse approach this situation?

Choice	Possible Outcomes
Discuss her hypothesis about Jared's behaviour and his uncertainty.	Mother can see the relationship between Jared's behaviour and her plan for divorce.
	Mother ignores the nurse.
	Mother is interested but does not see the connection.
Ignore the statement.	Child and family did not learn about the connection between Jared's behaviour and the events at home.
Encourage mother to sort out her problems.	The focus is then on mother's problems.

Analysis

The best response is focusing on the possible relationship between Jared's recent behavioural deterioration and his uncertainty of his family's future. If the nurse ignores the statement or focuses on the mother's interpretation of Jared's behaviour, then the mother is less likely to

appreciate the connection between pending divorce and Jared's behaviour. The nurse should also emphasize the importance of discussing the matter in family therapy. An additional factor may be that individuals can briefly and unintentionally react to an upcoming discharge by reverting to their original problematic behaviour.

---

adolescence (see Chapter 29). Children often report feeling relieved when finally asked about their feelings.

Anxiety Disorders

Anxiety disorders are the most prevalent mental illness in Canadian children between 4 and 17 years of age. Approximately 4 in 100 children have severe problems with worries and fears warranting a clinical diagnosis (Waddell et al., 2014). Many childhood fears are developmentally normal: it is common for toddlers to fear the dark, for school-aged children to fear animals, and for adolescents to worry about relationships with peers. These typical anxiety experiences do not usually interfere with the child's development and functioning (Black & Andreasen, 2014). Children with anxiety disorders experience excessive, prolonged, or recurrent fears or symptoms of anxiety, with accompanying impairment in age-appropriate functioning at home, at school, and with peers (Essau et al., 2018). Mood and anxiety disorders often coexist; therefore, it is important to assess for both especially in children.

To screen quickly for one or more anxiety disorders in children, the following questions may be useful:

• Does the child worry or ask for parental reassurance every day?

• Does the child consistently avoid age-appropriate situations or activities or avoid doing them without a parent?
• Does the child have frequent episodes of stomachaches, headaches, or hyperventilation?
• Does the child have daily repetitive rituals?

These four questions address the main thoughts, behaviours, and feelings related to anxiety seen in children (Manassis, 2004).

The following are the main types of anxiety disorders: generalized anxiety disorder (GAD), specific phobias, posttraumatic stress disorders (PTSDs), panic disorder, and agoraphobia, which are more common in females and usually develop in childhood through early adulthood (Public Health Agency of Canada, 2016). The focus in this chapter will be on the more common childhood diagnoses. Separation anxiety, a disorder diagnosed in childhood, as well as GAD, which occurs in both adults and children (see Chapter 23), will be discussed.

Generalized Anxiety Disorder

GAD is characterized by excessive anxiety and worry about many events or activities. The intensity, duration, or frequency of the anxiety and worry is out of proportion to the actual likelihood or impact of the anticipated event. Children tend to worry excessively about their competence or the quality of their performance, such as academic performance or athletic prowess on sports teams. However, the focus of the worry can change over time. In addition to the excessive and debilitating anxiety and worry, the child may experience feeling on edge and being easily fatigued, have difficulty concentrating, and experience irritability, muscle tension, and disturbed. For the full diagnostic criteria for GAD, see the *DSM-5* (APA, 2013).

GAD affects an estimated 1 out of 150 school-aged children in Canada (Waddell et al., 2014). Risk for developing GAD includes a genetic predisposition as evidenced by a family history of anxiety and environmental factors including experiencing stressful or traumatic events. Many individuals with GAD report that they have felt anxious and nervous all of their lives (APA, 2013).

Treatment Interventions

Cognitive therapy and pharmacotherapy (monotherapy or combination) have been reported to be most effective in treating anxiety disorders. In a systematic review and meta-analysis of 27 randomized control trials, participants (aged from 6 to 16 years old) were randomly assigned to experimental groups and control groups in CBT (20 studies with 3,790 participants) and pharmacotherapy (7 studies with 1,628 participants) (Schwartz et al., 2019). The study findings indicate a positive correlation between participating in a variety of CBT interventions in homes, communities/schools, and clinics, and a significant reduction of anxiety symptoms in students from preschool to high school. For pharmacological treatment, selective serotonin reuptake inhibitors (SSRIs) were significantly linked to improvement in symptoms. Another study found that the combination of CBT and pharmacotherapy (i.e., SSRIs) was significantly more effective than either CBT or medication alone in treating anxiety among children and adolescents (Piacentini et al., 2014).

Separation Anxiety Disorder

Separation anxiety disorder (SAD) is excessive anxiety on separation from home or a major attachment figure before adulthood (taken as the age of 18 years). It is manifested by acute distress, frequent nightmares about separation, and reluctance or refusal to separate. It causes clinically significant impairment in social or academic functioning (APA, 2013). SAD may be the childhood equivalent of panic disorder in adults. Although many children experience some discomfort on separation from their mothers or major attachment figures, children with SAD suffer great distress when faced with ordinary separations, such as going to school. In most cases, the mother is the focus of the child's concern, but

this may not be so, especially if the mother is not the primary caregiver. The child may exhibit extraordinary reluctance or even refusal to separate from the primary caregiver. When asked, most children with SAD will express worry about harm or permanent loss of their major attachment figure. Other children may express worry about their own safety (Phillips et al., 2020).

Epidemiology and Aetiology

The prevalence of SAD is estimated at 4% of school-aged children; thus, it is relatively common. Anxiety disorders run in families, and it appears that both environmental and genetic factors affect the risk for SAD. For example, it may emerge after a move, change to a new school, or death of a family member or pet. Traits such as shyness and behavioural inhibition (reluctance in new situations) are believed to be inherited (Poole & Schmidt, 2020). Furthermore, not only are children with an enduring "inhibited" temperament at greater risk for anxiety disorders but also their immediate family members are at greater risk for anxiety disorders, when compared with a psychiatric control group. Others have argued in favour of environmental determinants of separation anxiety, contending that anxious parents communicate to the child that the world is inhospitable and menacing in order to keep the child near. Available data suggest that childhood SAD is significantly associated with other psychiatric disorders in the same population (Mohammadi et al., 2020) and is a strong predictor for panic disorder and any anxiety disorders later in life (Silove et al., 2016).

Treatment Interventions

For treatment choices, CBT as an effective evidence-based treatment for childhood anxiety disorders and has been used in the treatment of SAD, while SSRIs have been indicated as first line of pharmacological treatment (Wehry et al., 2015). CBT includes psychoeducation of the disorder, relaxation technique training, cognitive restructuring, and problem-solving skill practice. Fluvoxamine and sertraline have been shown to be effective in treating SAD (Wehry et al., 2015). In addition to the combination of CBT and medication intervention, a close collaboration with the family and the school is critical in treating SAD.

Nursing Care

The child's developmental history and response to new situations and prior separations provide essential background information for understanding the child's current separation anxiety. The assessment should also include a review of recent life events and the methods the family has used to promote the child's return to school. Finally, family history with respect to anxiety, panic attacks, or phobias is also informative.

A common manifestation of anxiety is **school phobia,** in which the child refuses to attend school, preferring to stay at home with the primary attachment figure. However, it should be noted that school phobia is a common presenting complaint in child psychiatric clinics and may be part of SAD, general anxiety disorder, social phobia, OCD, depression, or conduct disorder (Shanahan et al., 2014).

School phobia or avoidance is often what prompts the family to seek consultation for the child. The onset of school refusal may be gradual or acute. School phobia can be a behavioural manifestation of several different child psychiatric disorders, so it requires careful assessment. Issues to consider include whether the parents have been aware that the child is avoiding school (separation vs. truancy), what efforts the family has made to return the child to school, the presence of significant subjective distress in the child with anticipation of going to school, sleep problems, and whether school refusal occurs in the context of other behavioural, social, or emotional problems (Fox-Lopp & McLaughlin, 2015; Shanahan et al., 2014) (see Clinical Vignette Box).

▌ Obsessive–Compulsive Disorder

As with anxiety disorders, OCD occurs in both adults and children. OCD is characterized by intrusive thoughts that are difficult to dislodge (**obsessions,** i.e., unwanted persistent, intrusive thoughts, impulses, or images related to anxiety) or by ritualized behaviours that the child feels driven to perform (**compulsions,** i.e., unwanted behavioural acts or patterns) to prevent or reduce anxiety. The most common obsessions in children are fears of contamination. Worries about personal and family safety are also frequent. The most common compulsions are excessive washing, cleaning, and checking actions. In earlier editions of the *DSM*, OCD was classified as an anxiety disorder; however, in 2013, OCD was classified as a distinct disorder within the classification of OCD and Related Disorders (see Chapter 23).

Epidemiology and Aetiology

OCD is common not just in adults but also in children and adolescents. One study estimated that the prevalence of OCD in ages 4 to 17 years is approximately 0.4%

CLINICAL VIGNETTE ✚

EMILY AND SEPARATION ANXIETY DISORDER

Emily, a 13-year-old eighth-grader, comes for an evaluation because her parents and teacher have become increasingly concerned about her missed 97 days of school during her eighth-grade due to various somatic complaints including nausea, vomiting, headache, stomach discomfort, and shortness of breath. During the interview, her mother commented that Emily was an excellent student before the family's relocation; her school avoidance behaviour started when she was transferred to a different school in seventh grade, with her school performance since declining. She is the only child in the family and has a close relationship with her father; however, her father works away from home. Emily sees him once a week. Her mother described Emily's anxiety-related symptoms as nervousness, worrying, and self-consciousness. She also displays other symptoms including sadness, fatigue, being argumentative and demanding attention, and an inability to concentrate.

At the evaluation, Emily describes getting nervous, anxious, and overwhelmed when she goes to school, where she feels that she doesn't belong. She is afraid of failing in school. When she is in school, she often stays in the bathroom until being found by school staff; does not want to make new friends, and barely eats. She expresses that she loved her former school where she got along with almost everyone. She had a lot of friends and misses them terribly. When her father left for work, she became depressed and felt emotionally numb for a long time, and remarked that "a part of me is dead." She fights with her mother a lot. Emily reveals that she has trouble getting to sleep and frequently awakens with nightmares, at least three times a week. She feels her worries about something bad happening to her father may cause her bad dreams.

Emily's medical history is negative for serious mental and physical illness or injury. She was born after an uncomplicated pregnancy, labour, and delivery, with her developmental milestones met within the appropriate time frame. Indeed, her mother describes Emily as conscientious and "a bit of a worrier." Her mother revealed a history of anxiety and experienced several panic attacks in the past, but the family history is otherwise negative for other mental health disorders, including separation anxiety.

(Waddell et al., 2014) while other studies reported approximately 1.39% (Politis et al., 2017) and 3.3% (Vivan et al., 2014) in adolescents, respectively. It is estimated that, for 8 in 10 adults with an OCD diagnosis, symptoms initiate by 18 years of age (Veale & Roberts, 2014).

Family studies and twin studies indicate that genetic determinants play a significant role in the aetiology of OCD, as well as anxiety disorders, and recur with a greater than expected frequency in the families of clients with OCD or Tourette disorder (Nazeer et al., 2020). Many biologic theories of OCD hypothesize dysfunctions in the brain including frontoparietal-limbic and orbitofrontal areas (Nazeer et al., 2020). The alternations of serotonergic–dopaminergic pathway have been indicated in OCD (Goodman et al., 2014). The quality of life for children and adolescents with OCD can be compromised depending on different factors, including the age of onset, severity of the OCD symptoms, family environment, undiagnosed or underdiagnosed, and comorbidities.

Treatment Interventions

Research findings support the treatment of OCD using SSRIs and CBT in children and adolescents, often used in combination. The goals focus on reducing the obsessions and compulsions and their effects on the development of children and adolescents. CBT, particularly exposure and response prevention, was found to be an effective intervention in children with OCD (Torp et al., 2015). Exposure consists of gradual confrontation with events or situations that trigger obsessions and cause the urge to ritualize. According to the theory behind exposure and response prevention therapy, repeated exposure works because clients learn that the immediate anxiety will subside even if they do not complete the ritual. To have successful outcomes with CBT, parents should be involved in their child's treatment plan and should reduce their involvement in ritualized behaviour. Pharmacotherapy of SSRIs including fluvoxamine, sertraline, and paroxetine has been shown to be effective in treating OCD (Nazeer et al., 2020).

Nursing Care

Recurrent worries and ritualistic behaviour can occur normally in children at stages of development. The first step in the assessment of OCD in children is to distinguish between normal childhood rituals and worries and pathologic rituals and obsessional thoughts (Cameron, 2007). Obsessional thoughts are recurrent, nagging, and bothersome. Although children may describe obsessions as occurring "out of the blue," external events may trigger obsessions. For example, a child may fear contamination whenever they are in contact with a certain person or object. Likewise, compulsions waste time, cause distress, and interfere with daily living.

The severity of the child's and family's response to OCD will determine the appropriate nursing diagnoses. The amount of distress within the family context can be quite detrimental to overall family and individual functions (Stewart et al., 2017). When the obsessions and compulsions emerge, children or adolescents are in distress because of the disturbing and relentless nature of the symptoms. What distinguishes families experiencing OCD from families of children with other mental disorders is the inextricable way that they are brought into the illness. Parents may be pulled into the child's rituals. The term *family accommodation* is often used to refer to family responses that are direct (e.g., participation in or assistance with the ritual) or indirect (e.g., modification in the family's lifestyle around the OCD symptomatology) (Caporino et al., 2012). Ineffective coping, compromised family coping, and ineffective role performance are likely nursing diagnoses for these families.

Trauma- and Stressor-Related Disorders

It is well documented that early chronic stress or trauma affects how the developing brain grows and evolves (Bellis & Zisk, 2014). Childhood trauma can be the result of a number of factors that can include physically or emotionally absent parent(s), erratic or inconsistent caregiving, abuse (verbal, sexual, or emotional), neglect, violence in the home or community, and war or disasters (Goldbeck & Jensen, 2017). Traumatic reactions may occur with unexpected events that may be a one-time incident, or ongoing, such as frequent hospitalizations for chronic illness contributing to a child experiencing traumatic effects (Afifi et al., 2015).

There is increasing awareness of the intergenerational transfer of stressor and traumatic effects onto children. A child may be affected by traumatic events that happened to a parent or to a community. Collective trauma occurs when a significant number of members of a social group are exposed to a traumatic event (e.g., a natural disaster, or a political event, or residential school). Historical trauma occurs when cumulative psychosocial wounding occurs across generations due to mass group trauma experiences (e.g., the colonization of Indigenous Peoples), and can have long-term effects on children born into such communities (Bombay et al., 2014). Trauma- and violence-informed care in child and adolescent mental health settings is increasingly being recommended (see Chapter 18).

The brains of children and adolescents with trauma histories prepare them to live in a state of neurologic hyperarousal in order to be alert and safe in their environment, even when they are in a situation that is perceived to be "safe" (Mulvihill, 2005). While trauma or maltreatment during childhood is known to be a risk factor for the development of mental health disorders in adulthood, researchers in a recent study concluded that adverse childhood experiences had negative effects on the basolateral amygdala and the CA1-3 hippocampal sub-field in adults with major depressive disorder (Agham-ohammadi-Sereshki et al., 2021). Traumatized children often have difficulty regulating emotions such as anger, sadness, and anxiety, while traumatic stress is likely to evoke emotional experiences in two extremes: feeling overwhelmed or feeling indifferent (Center for Substance Abuse Treatment, 2014). There are many triggers—loud noises, tone of voice, nonverbal behaviours, gender, the environment, the gender stance, intonation, or touch of others—that can initiate a hyperarousal response. The reactivity is in the form of automatic fight-or-flight system and can take the form of overt aggression or internal withdrawal and may impact the child's/youth's ability to reach their developmental milestones (Thakur et al., 2016). Adolescents may rely on negative coping strategies and engage in substance use, cutting, sensory-seeking behaviours, or sexual behaviours. Self-esteem and self-awareness are affected, leaving the individual without a positive sense of self-identity (Blaustein & Kinniburgh, 2010). When nurses work with children/youth or families in these circumstances, they need to be aware of what the triggers may be, how to mitigate them, and how to access the families' coping strategies when possible.

Reactive Attachment Disorder

Attachment disorders are typically identified prior to the age of 5 years. Previously, Mary Ainsworth's (1979) work on attachment described four types: secure, insecure avoidant, insecure ambivalent/resistant, and disorganized. It is recognized that children without secure attachment will struggle with relationships throughout their lives if difficulties with attachment are not addressed early in development (Lehmann et al., 2020). The *DSM-5* diagnosis of disinhibited social engagement disorder is similar to Ainsworth's insecure–ambivalent–resistive attachment style; it occurs in about 20% of severely neglected children. The behaviours seen with this disorder include a lack of social or cultural boundaries and overfamiliarity with strangers (APA, 2013). The *DSM-5* diagnosis of reactive attachment disorder (RAD) is most similar to Ainsworth's disorganized attachment style, the style most likely to develop into later psychopathology without early intervention (Glowinski, 2011). The focus here will be on RAD.

Epidemiology and Aetiology

The prevalence of RAD is unknown. Research suggests that children who have experienced severe neglect and adverse caregiving environments are at a higher risk of developing RAD in comparison with children who are raised in lower-risk environments (Gleason et al., 2011).

Treatment Intervention

Some of the interventions used for treating RAD are relevant for PTSD and acute traumatic stress response, depending on the context and situation. Currently, there is no medication treatment for RAD. Medications often are used to treat comorbidity issues of RAD, such as anxiety and sleeping disturbances.

The first component of intervention is to explore the rationale for the various behaviours being expressed by the child/youth and that the caregivers are experiencing. The nurse works with the caregivers to learn the child's language of emotional expression (verbal and nonverbal). The caregiver begins to attune to the child's expressions of need and reciprocate to meet that need; the pattern of coregulation begins. The caregiver then develops a consistent response to the child that is predictable. From this point, the caregiver and child learn self-regulation strategies to calm or arouse the child as reflective of the circumstance at hand. As the child and caregiver develop competence in these areas, the child will be increasingly free to develop and to learn new skills. This is not a "quick-fix" process and may take several months to years for some families. The nurse may determine that the parents may be struggling with their own issues of attachment and trauma histories. In order to work with the child, the care provider will need support and educate the parents regarding regulation and attunement of their own emotions as they attend to the child's. There are several programs that work with families on these issues, for example, Attachment, Self-Regulation and Competencies (Blaustein & Kinniburgh, 2010) and the CASA Trauma program (Ashton et al., 2015).

Nursing Care

Care for a family with a child or adolescent with RAD is complex. The first component of intervention is the provision of psychoeducation about the disorder, context, and strategies of therapy. Interventions will depend on the age of the child/youth, symptoms being expressed, and severity of the attachment dysfunction at the time. Relational therapy between the therapist and child is paramount to establish trust and rapport, as well as with the family. Some interventions will include specific behavioural management components such as the Incredible Years by Webster-Stratton and Reid (Webster-Stratton, 2011) or Parent–Child Interaction Therapy by Eyberg and Boggs (Buckner et al., 2008). The use of these programs will depend greatly on the caregivers' ability to participate and the overall issues facing the child. Family or individual therapy is recommended; pharmacotherapy is used only if required for a coexisting diagnosis (Mayo Clinic, 2017a).

Biologic Domain

There do not appear to be specific biologic factors attributed to the development of RAD; however, parents who may be compromised neurologically or psychologically may create an environment in which RAD could develop.

Psychosocial Domain

RAD can also develop from unpredictable care providers who create a sense of fear in the child to the extent that they are unsure of where their safety net may be (Zeanah et al., 2016). Children with RAD do not typically turn to their primary attachment figure for "comfort, support, protection, or nurturance" (APA, 2013, p. 266). The nurse may suspect potential for attachment concerns if the primary caregiver is being seen because the child has non-organic failure to thrive or if the primary caregiver has an active psychiatric illness such as postpartum depression (Zeanah et al., 2016). Children placed in institutional care for extended periods of time are more likely to develop RAD than those in a consistent, reliable, and predictable care environment (Humphreys et al., 2017).

Disinhibited Social Engagement Disorder

The child will demonstrate behaviours towards strangers or adults unfamiliar to the child that puts the child at increased risk of further exposure to abusive situations or abduction. The child appears to have a blatant disregard of social inhibition when approaching strangers both verbally and physically, may go with the stranger, and does not check back with primary caregiver before heading off. Understanding of this behaviour needs to be taken in the context of other diagnoses such as developmental delay or impulsivity.

The prevalence of this disorder remains unknown; however, in high-risk populations, the incidence is about 20% of children. Causes are similar to RAD, and this may cause challenges with diagnosis. Contributing factors include repeated changes of primary care providers such as children in foster or institutional care or situations of severe neglect (Smyke et al., 2012). As with RAD, pharmacologic intervention is not used except for symptom management. See Nursing Care section of RAD for guidance regarding care of disinhibited social engagement disorder.

Posttraumatic Stress Disorder and Acute Stress Disorder

Children's exposure to one or more traumatic events in their lives can lead to a trauma response or PTSD. In the United States, the National Child Traumatic Stress Network (NCTSN, n.d.) identifies that one in four children will be exposed to trauma prior to the age of 16 years. A child may have been exposed to domestic violence, community violence, war, natural disasters, or various forms of abuse and neglect. All of these events put a child/youth and family at risk of developing PTSD. Children experience and express their symptoms of PTSD differently from adults. For example, expression of recurrent involuntary distressing memories may manifest in repetitive play themes, as nightmares, or as reenactment of the event in a dissociative space or in play or in regression of otherwise acquired skills (e.g., bed wetting) (APA, 2013; NCTSN, 2013). The *DSM-5*

criteria for PTSD apply to adults, adolescents, and children over 6 years, with notations regarding children's symptom expression (APA, 2013). There are separate PTSD criteria for children 6 years and younger. *DSM-5* criteria for acute stress disorder apply to adults, adolescents, and children, with notations regarding children's symptom expression (APA). See Chapters 18 and 34.

Treatment Intervention

Trauma-focused CBT is most effective in treating PTSD. Approaches of trauma-focused CBT include psychoeducation regarding the disorder, parental skills, relaxation strategies, feeling identification, and cognitive processing (see also Chapter 18). Although SSRIs have been shown to be effective in treating symptoms of PTSD in adults, their efficacy for children and adolescents is not evidenced. Pharmaceutical intervention is used to treat comorbid symptoms including anxiety, mood symptoms, and sleeping issues (Thakur et al., 2016).

Nursing Care

Creating safety, support, guidance, and education for the child/youth and family, regardless of the cause of the trauma, will be the primary focus for the nurse.

Biologic Domain

Over the past 20 years, research regarding the neurodevelopmental effects of trauma and neglect on the developing brain has been evolving (Aghamohammadi-Sereshki et al., 2021; Bellis & Zisk, 2014; Blaustein & Kinniburgh, 2010). Although there may not be an overt genetic pathway, the environmental exposures that create a brain sensitive and receptive to developing PTSD are clear. Other risk factors include gender and age. Women are at an increased risk for PTSD while the younger the age of trauma exposure, the greater the risk of developing PTSD (APA, 2013). Temperament and preexisting psychopathology may also increase the risk for anxiety or panic disorders and depression (Thakur et al., 2016).

Psychosocial Domain

Children exposed to various life stressors, who live in communities where violence and/or war exists, and those who are deprived of the basic determinants of health (nutrition, housing, safety) are at risk. Resilience may be a protective factor; however, depending on the circumstance/event, it is not absolute.

In the event of a natural disaster where the family home may no longer exist, it will be important for the parent/primary caregivers to create an atmosphere of as much normalcy as possible. Supporting the child's/youth's and family's return to regular routines as much as possible will help with recovery and general wellness. Activities such as regular exercise, relaxation, a balanced diet, positive relationships, stress management, adequate

---

BOX 30.5 Tips for Caregivers Managing a Child's Symptoms of PTSD

- Maintain a calm, structured home environment (e.g., practice relaxation, develop routines).
- Keep your routines the same (morning, school, homework, bedtime).
- Provide clear expectations, limits, and consequences.
- Help your child learn about and identify feelings.
- Pay attention to your child's feelings.
- Remain calm when your child is anxious.
- Hold realistic expectations for your child's age—change them if you need to.
- Plan for transitions (e.g., getting to school).
- Focus on the here and now—use the sense to notice what is going on in the moment (e.g., your child describes what they hear, see). PTSD anxiety forces children to be focused on the future.

- Show your child the way you identify and accept your feelings.
- Show your child how to solve problems.
- Take care of your own needs—parenting an anxious child can be challenging.
- Talk to others for support, and ask for help when you need it.
- Be aware of and manage your own reactions. Seek help if you are struggling with this.
- Praise effort and provide rewards for effort.

BC Children's Hospital's Kelty Mental Health Resource Centre (Adapted with permission). (2018). *Post-traumatic stress disorder*. Retrieved from http://keltymentalhealth.ca/mental-health/disorders/post-traumatic-stress-disorder

---

sleep, community involvement, and social support are very important in managing anxiety in relation to PTSD or acute stress response and for general wellness (see Box 30.5). Children or youth may need the assistance of medication during this time; however, that is a collaborative conversation between the family, child/youth, and therapist and physician involved.

Neurodevelopmental Disorders of Childhood

Under the primary influences of genes and environment, development may be said to proceed along several pathways, such as attention, cognition, language, affect, and social and moral behaviours. The common feature of **neurodevelopmental disorders** is significant developmental delays or deficits in one or more areas. These deficits can be closely interwoven. For example, a language delay can interfere with a child's social development and contribute to behaviour problems (Marrus et al., 2018). There are several categories of these childhood disorders in the *DSM-5* (APA, 2013): intellectual disability, communication disorders (e.g., childhood-onset fluency disorder [stuttering]), autism spectrum disorder (ASD), ADHD, specific learning disorder, and motor disorders (e.g., tic disorders; APA).

KEY CONCEPT

Developmental delay is the development of a child that is outside the norm, including delayed socialization, communication, peculiar mannerisms, and idiosyncratic interests.

Autism Spectrum Disorder

Autism has been a subject of considerable interest and research effort since its original description more than 70 years ago, when Kanner (1943) described the profound isolation of these children and their extreme desire for sameness. The impairment in communication can be severe and affect both verbal and nonverbal communication (APA, 2013). Children with autism manifest delayed and deviant language development, as evidenced by *echolalia* (repetition of words or phrases spoken by others), and a tendency to be extremely concrete in the interpretation of language. Pronoun reversals and abnormal intonation are also common. Other common features of severe autism categorized as **stereotypic behaviour** (i.e., behaviour patterns that are repetitive and unchanging) include repetitive rocking, hand flapping, and an extraordinary insistence on sameness. The child may also engage in self-injurious behaviour, such as hitting, head banging, or biting. For some children, their unusual interests may evolve into fascination with specific objects, such as fans or air conditioners, or a particular topic, such as Prime Ministers of Canada.

Children with autism spectrum disorder (ASD) commonly show an uneven pattern of intellectual strengths and weaknesses. They can show a lifelong pattern of being rigid in style, being intolerant of change, and be prone to behavioural outbursts in response to environmental demands or changes in routine. ASD is diagnosed with a severity level requiring support (level 1), substantial support (level 2), or very substantial support (level 3) in the areas of social communication and restricted, repetitive behaviours. Children may or may not have accompanying intellectual impairment;

language impairment; association with a known medical or genetic condition or environmental factor; association with another neurodevelopmental, mental, or behavioural disorder; and catatonia.

KEY CONCEPT

An **autism spectrum disorder** is a neurodevelopmental disorder that is distinguished by a marked impairment of development in social interaction and communication with a restrictive repertoire of repetitive activity and interest.

The literature quite clearly supports the need for early screening and referral programs to promote early diagnosis and treatment (Magán-Maganto et al., 2017). Some early developmental indicators that suggest that a child should be referred for a full assessment include lack of babbling or gestures at 12 months, lack of single words by 16 months, lack of two-word combinations by 18 months, and any regression or loss of words or skills. Other developmental indicators include lack of joint attention (pointing to show), lack of response to name, unusual or absent eye contact, uses few or no gestures, and does not show facial expression (Centers for Disease Control and Prevention, 2021). Parents who report concerns about their child's development should be taken seriously. Early identification through screening followed by psychosocial support and education about the disorder and treatment options can help families to adjust and cope (Magán-Maganto et al., 2017). Nursing has a pivotal role to play in all these areas.

Epidemiology and Aetiology

There has been a dramatic rise in the incidence of ASD, from 6.7 per 1,000 children aged 8 years in 2000 to 16.8 per 1,000 in 2014, according to the Centers for Disease Control and Prevention's (CDC) Autism and Developmental Disabilities Monitoring Network, for 11 sites in the United States (Baio et al., 2018). The contributing factors to the increased estimated prevalence include diagnostic criteria changes, enhanced ASD services access, and children with few or mild ASD symptoms and high intellectual functioning being included (Baio et al., 2018). ASD occurs more often in boys than in girls, with the ratio ranging from 2:1 to 5:1. However, when girls are affected, they are often diagnosed later than boys. Researchers have attributed this to differences between the sexes in autism symptoms. They found that girls have less severe autistic mannerisms (Hiller et al., 2014). About half of children with ASD are intellectually disabled, and about 25% have seizure disorders.

The specific cause of ASD remains elusive, though research continues in the areas of genetics, neurology, and metabolic disorders. Numerous theories suggest various causes for autism, including genetics, perinatal insult,

neonatal complications, and preterm birth (Baio et al., 2018). It is estimated that 15% to 20% of younger siblings of children with autism, and monozygotic twins are more likely to be **concordant** (mutually affected) than are dizygotic twins. Other proposed causes include perinatal complications, such as exposure to infectious agents or medications during gestation, prematurity, and gestational bleeding. The role of environment in autistic disorders has been conclusively demonstrated only for prenatal or perinatal exposure to viral agents, such as rubella and cytomegalovirus, and prenatal exposure to thalidomide and valproic acid. Vaccinations, especially the MMR vaccine, have also drawn attention as a possible causative factor. However, recent epidemiologic studies and meta-analyses have excluded a widespread causal role for vaccines in autism (Taylor et al., 2014). The specific cause remains unknown and may result from multiple factors. Studies of genetic, epigenetic, and environmental factors are finally beginning to provide some insights into solving the complexities of autistic disorder (Anagnostou et al., 2014; Volkar et al., 2014). Structural and functional imaging studies also provide intriguing leads for future inquiry (Fig. 30.1).

Nursing Care

The nursing assessment is an ongoing process in which attention is given to establishing a positive relationship with the child and the family. The assessment should include a review of the child's capacity for self-care and maladaptive behaviours (Anagnostou et al., 2014). Self-injury and aggression are sometimes present, and children may need to be protected from hurting themselves and others. Inquiry should also include the presence of perseverative behaviours and preoccupation with restricted interests. These odd behaviours may not necessarily cause a problem, but they often interfere with the child's relationships.

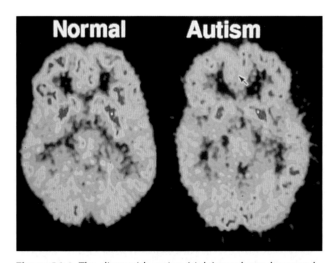

Figure 30.1 The client with autism (*right*) may have decreased metabolic rates in the cingulate gyrus and other associated areas; however, wide heterogeneity in brain metabolic patterns is seen in clients with autism. (Courtesy of Monte S. Buchsbaum, MD, Mount Sinai Medical Centre and School of Medicine, New York, NY.)

Assessment data generate a variety of potential nursing care foci, including social isolation. Because of the long-term nature of these disorders, the aims of treatment may change with time. However, throughout childhood, the focus should be on the development of age-appropriate adaptive and social skills. The family may be grieving the loss of a "normal" child it had expected and is trying to cope with the multitude of problems inherent in raising a child with a disability. Therefore, an important domain to consider in the nursing assessment is the effect of the child's developmental delays on the family. Having a child with ASD is bound to influence family interaction and responding to the child's needs may adversely affect family functioning. For example, sleep disruption in family members who care for children with ASD may increase family stress.

Biopsychosocial Domain

Planning interventions for children and youth with severe developmental problems need to consider the child, family, and community supports, such as schools, rehabilitation centres, mental health centres, or group homes, and availability of respite services. First and foremost, the various clinicians involved in the child's treatment should collaborate with the family to promote reaching the same general goals. As the number of clinicians and educators involved increases, the chance of fragmentation in treatment planning also increases. The nurse can serve as a case coordinator to ensure that the plan of care is both comprehensive and appropriate in meeting the needs of both the child and the family.

Continuum of Care

ASD is chronic and usually requires long-term care at various levels of intensity. Children and adolescents with autism are a heterogeneous group, and as such, they have diverse needs. It is essential that intervention treatment plans be based on individual patterns of strengths and limitations (Anagnostou et al., 2014). Intervention treatment consists of designing academic, interpersonal, and social experiences that support the child's development. Children with autism, even those who are severely affected, are increasingly able to attend public schools with accommodations, often with the support of an educational assistant. Other outpatient services may include family counselling, home care, and medication. As the child moves towards adulthood, living at home may become more difficult, given the appropriate need for greater independence. The level of structure required depends primarily on IQ and adaptive functioning. Ongoing support and respite for the family are critical and an essential part of the intervention treatment plan in which nursing plays an integral role. Autism services in some communities facilitate residential and supported living care.

Promoting Interaction

Many of the core deficits in ASD fall within the domain of social development, regardless of the level of cognitive functioning of the particular child or youth. The goal of intervention in the social domain is to increase meaningful relationships by teaching skills that support the development of social interest, social initiation, social responsiveness, empathy, and understanding of the other's perspective. It is critical that intervention treatment plans include strategies to enhance social understanding, social relating, and play skills and that these strategies take into account the individual's cognitive, learning, linguistic, and developmental abilities (Anagnostou et al., 2014; Baio et al., 2018). Interventions fostering nonverbal social interactions may sometimes be more useful than those based on speech. For higher-functioning children, activities such as getting the mail, passing out snacks, or taking turns in the context of simple games can engage them in social activities without requiring the use of their limited language skills. Structuring social interactions so that the child has to share a task with another (e.g., carrying a load of books) may help to boost confidence in relating to others.

Ensuring Predictability and Safety

When children with ASD are hospitalized, milieu management—a consistent, structured environment with predictable routines for activities, mealtimes, and bedtimes—is necessary for successful treatment. Changes in routine may provoke disorganization in the child with ASD, leading to emotional disequilibrium and explosive behaviour. The safety of the inpatient unit offers an opportunity to try behavioural strategies, such as rewards for managing transitions. Healthcare professionals can explore with family the strategies that have been successful for managing behaviours in the past and can also share new successful strategies with parents or primary caregivers.

Self-Care

In teaching self-care skills, the nurse needs to consider the child's current adaptive skills and language limitations. Developing a list of activities for children to post in their bedroom may be effective. Drawings or symbols may be useful for nonverbal children. Physical safety is an important concern for children who are cognitively delayed and may have impaired judgment.

Supporting Family

Autism and related disorders are chronic conditions that call for extraordinary patience and determination. Unfortunately, lack of integration of medical, psychiatric, social, and educational services can add to the family's burden. Family stress research has repeatedly demonstrated that parents (especially mothers) of children with ASDs experience greater stress, depression, and mental health difficulties than parents of children with other types of disability (Pastor-Cerezuela et al., 2016). Parents may manifest feelings of denial, grief, guilt, anger, and sorrow at various points as they adjust to their child's disability. The nurse can offer parents the opportunity to express their frustrations and disappointments and can be alert for indications that parents are in need of additional assistance, such as parent support groups or respite care. Residential and respite care may be necessary in some cases. After making the decision to place a child into someone else's care, family members may experience guilt, loss, and a sense of failure concerning their inability to care for the child at home.

Family interventions include support, education, counselling, and referral to self-help groups. Whenever possible, the nurse provides education to help parents determine appropriate expectations for their child with ASD and to meet the child's special needs. The following are examples of potentially useful nursing interventions focusing on the family:

- interpreting the treatment plan for parents and the child
- modelling appropriate behaviour modification techniques

- including the parents as co-therapists for the implementation of the care plan
- assisting the family members in identifying and resolving their sense of loss related to the diagnosis
- coordinating support systems for parents, siblings, and family members
- maintaining interdisciplinary collaboration
- facilitating access to and encouraging families to use formal support services such as respite care
- assisting parents to advocate/lobby on behalf of their child and children with disabilities

There are a number of support services in Canada and throughout the provinces; however, it is best that parents access services through legitimate agencies and organizations. For examples of these, see Web Links.

Evaluation of client and family outcomes is an ongoing process. Short-term outcomes might consist of discrete behavioural improvements, such as reducing self-injurious behaviour by 50%. The long-term goal is for the client to achieve the highest level of functioning. The prognosis depends on the severity of the impairments, the interventions available, and the cognitive ability of the child.

IN-A-LIFE

Greta Thunberg (2003-)

CLIMATE ACTIVIST AND A PERSON WITH AUTISM SPECTRUM DISORDER

Public Persona

Greta Thunberg is a climate activist and was named person of the year in 2019 by *Time* magazine with the notation, "The Power of Youth" (Alter et al., 2019). She is a Swedish young adult who has inspired an international movement to fight climate change, which is building real momentum. The "Greta Thunberg effect" has been translated into a growing number of children engaging in online activism; young people pushing communities, governments, and corporations to take action on the climate change crisis (Wood, 2020).

Personal Realities

At the age of 11, Greta Thunberg was diagnosed with Asperger syndrome, now a part of autism spectrum disorder. At the onset of her symptoms, she cried at school and during the night and also experienced disordered eating. Her mother described Greta at that time as slipping into darkness gradually; she appeared to stop functioning. Greta has shared that Asperger syndrome held her back previously; however, now she believes her Asperger syndrome as a

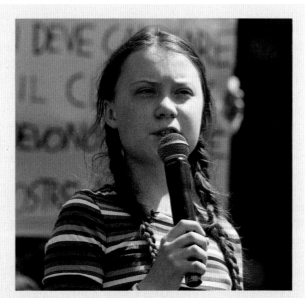

Source: shutterstock.com/Daniele COSSU

"gift" since "thinking outside of the box" is a common feature among individuals with Asperger syndrome. Greta has a powerful message: "We can't just continue living as if there was no tomorrow because there is a tomorrow" (Alter et al., 2019; Gallagher, 2020).

Attention Deficit Hyperactivity Disorder

All children have occasional experiences with inattention and high energy levels. For most children, these occurrences do not interfere with daily life. However, children with ADHD demonstrate physically overactive, inattentive, impulsive, distractible, and difficult to manage behaviours. ADHD is a neurodevelopmental disorder defined by two broader categories based on symptoms: inattention, hyperactivity, and impulsivity (Black & Andreasen, 2014). It affects 5% to 12% of school-aged children, 8% to 10% of boys under the age of 18, and 3% to 4% of girls under 18 (Canadian ADHD Resource Alliance [CADDRA], 2013a). It is associated with functional impairments such as school challenges, peer problems, and family conflict. Parents and teachers describe children with ADHD as restless, always on the go, highly distractible, unable to wait for their turn, heedless, and frequently disruptive. Often, it is their disruptive behaviour that brings these children into treatment. Children with inattentive symptoms often are missed and do not receive a diagnosis until later in life. Children and youth with ADHD can struggle in a multitude of domains at different times throughout their development. It is likely that, at some point in their career, nurses will work with children, adolescents, and adults with ADHD. See the *DSM-5* for APA diagnostic criteria for ADHD (APA, 2013).

Both clinical observations and laboratory studies support the conclusion that children with ADHD can be prone to impulsiveness and risk-taking behaviours (Sørensen et al., 2017). In behavioural terms, children with ADHD often fail to consider the consequences of their actions, exercise poor judgment, and tend to have more than the usual lumps, bumps, and bruises because of their risk-taking behaviour. They often require a high degree of structure and supervision. In many cases, it is the hyperactivity that prompts the search for treatment. Parents typically report that the child's hyperactivity started early in life and is evident in most situations. These behaviours, although challenging, often are not deemed problematic until the child enters a more structured environment, such as day care, kindergarten, or school.

The diagnosis of ADHD is based upon the ability to observe symptoms that seem to occur consistently in at least two different environments, such as home and school. For the diagnosis to be given, there must be at least some symptoms present before the age of 12 years and they must be present for at least 6 months (APA, 2013). A physical examination should be performed, as well as a hearing and eyesight test, to rule out any physical reasons for the symptoms. A psychoeducational assessment is recommended to determine whether other learning disabilities coexist with the ADHD or cause the symptoms (CADDRA, 2013b).

Longitudinal studies that followed groups of children with ADHD into adulthood have shown the persistence of symptoms (Uchida et al., 2018). There is change in symptom presentation as an individual grows and

develops and perhaps acquires compensatory strategies; however, even when symptoms are not prominent, they remain associated with clinically significant impairments (Centre for ADHD Awareness, Canada, 2013). Older adolescents and young adults with a history of ADHD may struggle with staying in school and keeping a job and maintaining relationships and have more traffic violations and accidents than individuals without the diagnosis of ADHD (CADDAC, 2013).

 KEY CONCEPT

Attention is a complex process that involves the ability to concentrate on one activity to the exclusion of others and the ability to sustain that focus.

 KEY CONCEPT

Impulsiveness refers to acting in the moment without considering the consequences of the act, which may be potentially highly harmful, and without considering alternative actions.

 KEY CONCEPT

Hyperactivity refers to excessive motor activity, movement, and/or utterances when it is not appropriate and may be purposeless (e.g., fidgeting, tapping, or talkativeness) (APA, 2013).

Epidemiology and Aetiology Factors

From the 20th century, scientific investigation of its validity and clarification of clinical controversies has been ongoing. Nevertheless, the aetiology of ADHD remains unclear. No single factor is sufficient to cause the disorder, and multifactorial risks have been suggested including genetic, prenatal, and environmental factors. Strong evidence from family, twin, and adoption studies indicates that aetiology of ADHD is highly influenced by genetic factors. Although heritability is estimated between 70% and 90% (Larsson et al., 2014), identification of genes responsible for ADHD has been challenging due to multiple genetic variants contributing to the aetiology (Klein et al., 2017).

Neuroimaging studies have hypothesized brain differences observed in ADHD to be partly contributable to a delay in maturational processes (Klein et al., 2017). Based on volumetric and functional MRI studies, differences are found in the structural development and functional activation in the prefrontal cortex, basal ganglia, anterior cingulate cortex, and cerebellum between children with ADHD and control groups (Klein et al., 2017).

Risk factors of pregnancy and birth complications for ADHD are mixed; however, study findings support that there is an increased risk for developing ADHD following in utero exposure to alcohol (Eilertsen et al., 2017), tobacco (He et al., 2020), low birth weight (<2,500 g) (Franz et al., 2018), or prenatal stress (i.e., financial difficulties, divorce, or loss of a loved one) (VinayaKumar, 2019). Numerous environmental exposures to toxins (specifically lead, organophosphate pesticides, and polychlorinated biphenyls) have been linked to ADHD symptoms (Hong et al., 2015; Peterson et al., 2015).

Treatment Interventions

A multimodal approach combining behaviour management and pharmacotherapy intervention has proven to be effective in treating children and adolescents affected by ADHD. For children under 6 years of age, nonpharmacotherapy intervention has been recommended as first line of treatment (CADDRA, 2020). Nonpharmacological interventions for children and adolescents with ADHD include psychoeducation, shared decision-making, parent behaviour training, social skills training, cognitive training, and behavioural peer interventions (Feldman et al., 2018). When initiating pharmacological intervention of stimulant medications, the Canadian Paediatric Society recommends:

1. symptom reduction and function improvement are the outcome goals;
2. treatment response should be monitored by obtaining information from multiple sources including school and parents;
3. stimulant medication of either from the methylphenidate (MPH) or amphetamine/dextroamphetamine (DEX) subclass is recommended; and
4. in combination with nonpharmacological interventions, immediate-release stimulants are recommended

as first-line treatment for the majority of children and adolescents with ADHD (Feldman et al., 2018).

A combined behavioural–psychosocial and pharmaceutical approach allows for significantly lower doses of medication than a medication-only approach in achieving treatment outcomes and decreasing the risk of side effects (Feldman et al., 2018). Medication can mitigate the symptoms of hyperactivity, impulsiveness, and inattention; therefore, teaching the parent, child, and school personnel about the importance of the medication in ADHD and the potential side effects is a place to begin. Explaining to the child that the medication improves concentration and the ability to sit still can help strengthen motivation and adherence to treatment; however, nonadherence is typically more a matter of forgetting than one of deliberate avoidance.

Nursing Care

The primary focus of the assessment is the impact of ADHD symptoms on academic and social functioning. The nurse tries to determine the contribution of symptoms of ADHD with the acute psychiatric problem. Assessment data are collected through direct interview, observation of the child and parent, and teacher ratings. Because children with ADHD may have difficulty sitting through long sessions, interviews are typically brief or involve an activity to engage the child. Parents and teachers are extremely important sources for assessment data. To this end, the nurse can make use of several standardized instruments. Refer further to Box 30.6.

The association of ADHD with other psychiatric disorders warrants a careful and fulsome assessment.

BOX 30.6 Standardized Tools for ADHD Diagnosis

The Conners Parent Questionnaire is a 48-item scale that a parent completes about their child. Each item is a statement that the parent rates on a four-point scale from 0 (not at all) to 3 (very much). The Conners Teacher Questionnaire is a 28-item questionnaire that the child's teacher completes according to the same four-point scale as the parent questionnaire. Both questionnaires have been standardized by age and gender for a mean of 50 and a standard deviation of 10 (Conners, 1989; Goyette, Conners, & Ulrich, 1978).

The ADHD Rating Scale asks parents or teachers to respond directly to 18 items (see Barkley, 1998, for a description of this scale). A similar scale called the SNAP-IV is available online for free at www.adhd.net. The SNAP-IV was used as the primary outcome measure in the MTA Cooperative Group Study (1999).

The Child Behaviour Checklist (CBCL) is a 118-item questionnaire that a parent completes. In addition to the 118 questions about specific behaviours and psychiatric symptoms, the CBCL also includes questions concerning the child's competence in social and academic spheres as well as age-appropriate activities. Normative data are available allowing the conversion of raw scores to standard scores for age and gender. There is also a teacher version of this scale.

Note that the diagnosis of ADHD is not made on the basis of questionnaires alone. Data from these rating scales augment the information gathered through interview and observation. These questionnaires can be especially useful before and after initiating a treatment plan to measure the change.

Medical history is essential, consisting of perinatal course, childhood illnesses, hospital admissions, injuries, seizures, tics, physical growth, overall health status, and timing of the child's last physical examination. Family history is also an important part of assessment data.

Children with ADHD can be very active; they struggle to sit still and often fidget or bounce their legs to keep moving. They may be more active during sleep than children without the disorder. A functional assessment of eating, sleeping, and activity patterns is therefore essential. Assessing daily food intake, typical diet, and frequency of eating will help identify any nutrition problems. Caffeinated products can contribute to hyperactivity. Sleep is often disturbed for children with ADHD and, consequently, the family. A detailed sleep assessment can provide points for interventions and help the interpretation of drug effects.

With the severity of the responses, regarding family functioning and school environment, several nursing diagnoses could be generated from the assessment data, including self-care deficit, risk for imbalanced nutrition, risk for injury, and disturbed sleep pattern. The outcomes should be individualized to the child (see Fig. 30.2).

Psychosocial

ADHD often occurs in the context of psychosocial adversity. It is important to review the family situation, including parenting style, stability of household membership, consistency of rules and routines, and life events, such as divorce, moves, deaths, and job loss. Identification of these factors can be useful in shaping a care plan that builds on potential strengths and mitigates the effects of environmental factors that may perpetuate the child's disruptive behaviour. Data regarding school performance, behaviour at home, and comorbid psychiatric disorders are essential for developing school interventions and behaviour plans and establishing the baseline severity for medication.

Parents of children with ADHD report more frequent and severe interparental discord and child-rearing disagreements, more negative parenting practices, greater

caregiver strain, and more psychopathology themselves. With the added burden that ADHD is highly heritable, one or both parents may also suffer from symptoms that can contribute to family dysfunction (Schachar, 2014). Children with ADHD (impulsive/hyperactive) can be bossy, intrusive, immature, boisterous, aggressive, and less aware of social cues. Such behaviours affect social function, making and keeping friends, and can contribute to parental unwillingness to take their ADHD child on social outings or vacations.

Behavioural programs should focus on creating success and achievement for the child or adolescent. The system should be based on acknowledgment for positive behaviour, such as waiting or completing chores. Interventions may also include specific cognitive–behavioural techniques in which the child learns to "stop, look, and listen" before acting. Depending on the severity of the child's symptoms, family situation, and school environment, several nursing diagnoses could be generated from the assessment data, including impaired social interaction, ineffective role performance, and compromised family coping. Short-term outcomes, such as decreasing the number of times a student is asked to leave the classroom within a 2-week period, may be useful for one child, whereas reducing the frequency and amplitude of angry outbursts at home may be relevant to another child. Building on the child's strengths and capacity, children with ADHD may function better in individualized sports or activities. Removal of these activities as consequences for unacceptable behaviour is not necessarily productive for changing behaviour.

Family treatment is nearly always a component of cognitive–behavioural treatment approaches with the child. This may involve parent education training that focuses on the principles of creating a home environment that has increased predictability and structure. This may prove to be a challenge for parents who have ADHD themselves. At times, the institution of a more formal behaviour management strategy may be required, such as boundary setting and the use of reward systems, as well as revised expectations about the child's behaviour. School programming often involves increasing structure in the child's school day to offset the child's tendency to act without forethought and to be easily distracted by extraneous stimuli. Specific remediation is required for the child with comorbid deficits in learning or language. Some children may require specialized self-contained classrooms; however, they typically have coexisting challenges such as learning disabilities and oppositional defiant or conduct disorder (Centers for Disease Control and Prevention, 2020).

The planning of nursing interventions must be done within the context of the family, treatment setting, and school environment. With the parents, clinical team members, and school personnel, the nurse participates in designing a plan of care that fits the child's and family's needs. Resiliency support and focus on strength, for all members of the family, is important and the child moves through life stages (see Box 30.7).

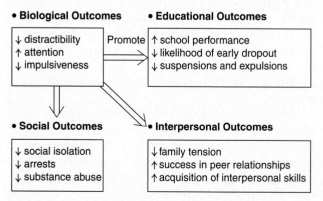

Figure 30.2 Long-term outcomes of optimal treatment for clients with attention deficit hyperactivity disorder.

BOX 30.7 NURSING CARE PLAN

Attention Deficit Hyperactivity Disorder

James is a 6-year-old student in grade 1 and comes to the mental health clinic with his mother, Linda, because of concerns raised by his teacher. James has difficulties with concentration and is distracted and disruptive in class, displays restlessness, and often requires reminders to help him stay on task. Linda explains that James was able to adjust to kindergarten, but since his entry into first grade this year, his teacher has reported that he has behaviour issues, such as not waiting his turn and interrupting other students in the classroom. James recognizes that he is able to "hyper-focus" on some activities of interest; however, he often has difficulty sustaining his attention at school.

James' medical history is unremarkable. Linda's pregnancy with James was her first and without complications, although the labour was long and resulted in a caesarean section. Linda notes that a marital problem with James' father started during the pregnancy, culminating in divorce before James' first birthday. James was healthy at birth and grew normally, without developmental delays. He is a nice and caring young boy who genuinely wants to play with other children, but his intrusive style and inability to wait

his turn can create frequent conflicts with them. There is an extended family history of ADHD and mental health and addiction issues including his father's. James' father is inconsistent in his visits with his son.

During the two evaluation sessions, James is active but cooperative. His speech is fluent and normal in tone and tempo, if somewhat loud. His discourse is coherent, but at times, he makes rather abrupt changes in conversation without warning his listeners. Psychological testing at the school revealed average to above average intelligence. Parent and teacher questionnaires concurred that James was overactive, impulsive, inattentive, and quarrelsome but not defiant.

Setting: Mental Health Centre, Child and Adolescent Services

Baseline Assessment: James is a 6-year-old boy with prominent hyperactivity and disruptive behaviour. These problems interfere with his interpersonal relationships and academic progress. He lives with his mother, Linda, in a household with one parent. Linda has difficulties in managing James' behaviour.

Associated Psychiatric Diagnosis	Treatments
ADHD Other issues of note: • Educational problems (peer conflict) • Low income (mother in an entry-level job) • Disruption of the family by divorce (father inconsistent in visitation routine)	Methylphenidate 5 mg at breakfast and lunch (i.e., at 8 a.m. and 12 noon) and then adding 5 mg at 4 p.m.

Nursing Care Focus 1: Impaired Social Interaction

Defining Characteristics	Related Factors
• Cannot establish and maintain developmentally appropriate social relationships • Has interpersonal difficulties at school • Is not well accepted by peers • Interrupts others	• Impulsive behaviour • Overactive • Failure to recognize the effects of his behaviour on others

Goals of Care

Initial	Long Term
• James will participate in social skill training. • Decrease the frequency of conflicts with peers.	• Improve capacity to identify alternative responses in conflicts with peers. • James will be able to interact with peers appropriately without discomfort.

Continued on following page

BOX 30.7 NURSING CARE PLAN (*Continued*)

Interventions

Interventions	Rationale	Ongoing Assessment
Social skill group training session twice-a-week.	Social skills are often impaired in children with ADHD. Social skill training with a small group will provide a safe environment for children to learn how to interact with peers appropriately including providing immediate and frequent feedback about inappropriate behaviour or social miscues, and role-playing to teach, model, and practice positive social skills, and the ways to respond to challenging situations like teasing.	Assess James' progress in social skill group training.
Create opportunities for friendship development by identifying one or two classmates James enjoys playing with to have supervised play dates.	Parents supervised play and structuring activities ensure the child with ADHD receives clearly defined expectations and early interventions when problems arise.	Determine any improvement or issues in interacting with peers.
Encourage participation in school and community activities.	Social skills will be improved and confidence will be built by participating in peer-group activities such as community hockey team through improving the interpretation of motives and behaviours of others and excising appropriate behaviours, and ultimately, improve the acceptance of peers.	Assess James' perspective of the activities including positive and negative experiences, and how to improve the experience next time.
Provide support and advocate for James and his mother as needed.	To identify and utilize resources at home, in school, and community can provide support and assistant.	Continue to assess: whether James and his mother are able to access services and identify any service gaps and unmet needs.

Evaluation

Outcomes	Revised Goals of Care	Interventions
James will complete the social skill training sessions.	Improved the ability to identify inappropriate behaviours or social miscues and also appropriate behaviours.	Encourage James to attend the training sessions. Help James to practice appropriate behaviours at home and school. Communicate with James and the training program about James' progress.
James will demonstrate appropriate social interactions with peers at school and in the community.	Improved social skills.	Help James learn a set of responses for the given situation in an appropriate way.

Nursing Care Focus 2: Alteration in Attention and Hyperactivity

Defining Characteristics	Related Factors
• Easily distracted by external stimuli • Fail to give close attention • Difficulty in sustaining attention • Has difficulty waiting for their turn • Often interrupts or intrudes on others • Is often "on the go"	Alternations in brain activities

BOX 30.7 NURSING CARE PLAN (*Continued*)

Goals of Care

Initial	Long Term
Decrease hyperactivity and disruptive behaviour and improve attention.	Improved ability to concentrate and sustain attention, strengthen good behaviours, and decreased disruptive or intrusive behaviours.

Interventions

Interventions	Rationale	Ongoing Assessment
Set expectations and implement classroom interventions to manage James' behaviour by developing behaviour modification plans with a reward system to recognize positive behaviours.	Children respond positively to structure and rules. The behaviour modification plans involved in teacher, James, and his mother clearly indicate the responsibilities and consequences of James' behaviours.	Assess whether James identifies options of appropriate behaviour.
Educate the mother about ADHD and the use of stimulant medication. Provide written information about ADHD, which Linda may share with the teacher and school.	Better understanding helps to ensure adherence; parents and teachers are often miscast children with ADHD as "troublemakers."	Determine the extent to which parent or teacher "blames" James for his problems.
Monitor and assess response to medication.	Each child responds to medication treatment differently. Especially during the early phase of treatment, monitoring response and adjustment of the treatment regime are often required to achieve optimal results.	Monitor and assess any side effects (appetite, sleep, and irritability) and symptoms reduction.
Monitor adherence to the treatment regime.	Medication nonadherence may contribute to a relapse of symptoms.	Assess behaviours through the day, and maintain communication between teacher and parents.

Outcomes

Outcomes	Revised Goals of Care	Interventions
James will show decreased hyperactivity and less disruption in the classroom	Improved the ability to identify disruptive behaviours, and demonstrate appropriate behaviours	Initiate a point system to reward appropriate behaviour.
James will complete assignments in class in an allotted time frame.	Improved academic performance overall.	Preferential seating with less external stimuli that helps James focus. Provide alternative ways to complete assignments.

Specific Learning Disorders

Specific **learning disorders** (also called learning disabilities) are among the most common neurodevelopmental disorders in children and are defined as difficulties in learning and using academic skills. They are important causes of poor school performance. For this diagnosis to be given, a child must have specific difficulties for over 6 months. These need to be significantly different from what is expected for their age and interfere with their performance in school or work. See the *DSM-5* for the APA (2013) diagnostic criteria.

Communication Disorders

Communication disorders involve deficits in speech, language, and communication. *Speech* refers to the motor aspects of making sounds and includes "articulation, fluency, voice, and resonance quality" (APA, 2013, p. 41). *Language* consists of higher-order aspects of formulating and comprehending a conventional system of symbols (e.g., spoken words, sign language, pictures) (APA). *Communication* involves verbal and/or nonverbal behaviour (whether or not intentional) that influences another person (APA). Communication disorder in the *DSM-5* includes "language disorder, speech sound disorder, childhood-onset fluency disorder (stuttering), social (pragmatic) communication disorder, and other specified and nonspecified communication disorders" (APA, 2013, p. 41).

Nursing Care Related to Learning Disabilities and Communication Disorders

For children with learning disabilities, the negative effects of low achievement or failure may be manifested in low self-esteem and reduced academic effort. Some children and adolescents may also exhibit difficulties in age-appropriate social interactions. Postsecondary students with learning disabilities have been observed to exhibit poor self-concept, have difficulties with interpersonal skills, and have deficits in processing and study skills (Lightfoot et al., 2018). Research also suggests that children and adolescents with learning disorders experience more feelings of loneliness, depression, stress, and suicidal ideations than their peers without learning disabilities (Fletcher et al., 2018). For the child/adolescent with learning disabilities, nurses can focus on building self-confidence and helping the family connect with guidance and educational resources that support their ongoing development.

Communication disorders are an area in which assessments must be absolutely relevant to the cultural and linguistic background of the individual, if they are to be valid. Speech pathologists conduct the diagnostic assessment. Services such as speech therapy (directed at the motor aspects of speaking) or social skills groups (directed at the social and interpersonal aspects of language) may be available in some school districts and can be obtained if a speech or language disorder has been identified. For some children with communication disorders, the services offered by the school may be insufficient. In such cases, the nurse can help the family locate resources that can provide these needed services.

For the child with a communication disorder, interventions focus on fostering social and communication skills, identifying and addressing low self-esteem, and making referrals for specific speech or language therapy. Modelling appropriate communication in spontaneous situations with the child can be a useful intervention for some children. As with other neurodevelopmental disorders, education and support of the parents are a key intervention.

Neurobehavioural Disorder Associated With Prenatal Alcohol Exposure and Foetal Alcohol Spectrum Disorder

Neurobehavioural disorder associated with prenatal alcohol exposure (ND-PAE) is identified by the APA as a condition needing further study (APA, 2013). It is intended as a classification that can include the range of developmental disabilities arising due to exposure to alcohol in utero (APA). Its broader criteria could increase treatment options for those affected by its symptoms (Cook et al., 2016). See the *DSM-5* for the symptoms of ND-PAE. Foetal alcohol spectrum disorder (FASD) is a set of effects due to prenatal alcohol exposure. Its diagnosis requires physical and neurodevelopment assessments by an interprofessional team. For a diagnosis of FASD to be made, pervasive brain dysfunction needs to be indicated in at least three of these neurodevelopmental areas: "motor skills; neuroanatomy/neurophysiology; cognition; language; academic achievement; memory; attention; executive function, including impulse control and hyperactivity; affect regulation; and adaptive behaviour, social skills or social communication" (Cook et al., 2016, p. 193). There are sentinel facial features that can warrant the diagnosis without confirmation of the mother's intake of alcohol during pregnancy due to their specific association with FASD. Good evidence of the mother's prenatal alcohol use is sufficient for an "at-risk" diagnosis for FASD (Cook et al., 2016).

Epidemiology and Aetiology

The prevalence of ND-PAE is estimated to be between 2% and 5% in the United States (APA, 2013). The prevalence of FASD is approximately 1% in Canada. The amount of alcohol needed to have negative effects on the developing foetus is unknown. There is no safe amount or safe time in the gestational period for alcohol consumption.

Treatment Interventions

There are no medications approved specifically to treat ND-PAE or FASD. However, several medications can help improve some of the symptoms; medication might help manage high energy levels, inability to focus, aggression, anxiety, or depression. Medications can affect each child differently. For example, one medication might work well for one child but not for another. To find the right treatment, a trial of different medications and doses may be explored. It is important for the nurse to work closely with the child and family to monitor both negative and positive effects of medication prescribed.

Nursing Care

The bio/psycho/social/spiritual care of the child with ND-PAE or FASD can be complex; therefore, each child or adolescent must be reviewed individually to determine what symptoms are causing dysfunction. Most interventions focus on providing support with executive functioning, social skills teaching and practice, self-regulation skills, and positive behavioural supports. The coexisting or predominant symptoms of the disorder will determine the intervention strategies employed. For example, if the child or adolescent has challenges of impulsiveness and hyperactivity, interventions similar to those used with a child with ADHD may be beneficial. Factors of cognitive processing may impact the effectiveness of interventions used. Each child will need to be assessed and worked with individually to truly identify the best approach.

Disruptive, Impulse Control, and Conduct Disorders

The disruptive behaviour disorders within the *DSM-5* include ODD, conduct disorder, intermittent explosive disorder, kleptomania, and pyromania (APA, 2013). For purposes of this text, we will focus on ODD and conduct disorder, syndromes marked by significant problems of conduct. These **externalizing disorders** contrast with disorders of depressive and anxiety disorders, which are referred to as **internalizing disorders** because the symptoms tend to be within the child.

Oppositional Defiant Disorder

Unfortunately, some children are labeled oppositional if they challenge authority or have temper tantrums. To be diagnosed as a disorder, however, the argumentative, defiant, and angry behaviour needs to be continual over a period of months and be present with more than family members. There cannot be another mental health disorder that accounts for it, such as substance use disorder or psychosis. There is some discourse that ODD may be a disorder of emotional dysregulation. Further research will need to be conducted to affirm this aspect of the diagnosis (Cavanagh et al., 2017).

Treatment Interventions

The nurse will need to work with the child and family to attend to coexisting conditions such as ADHD, anxiety disorder, or depression. Specific interventions to support the child coping with anxiety may alleviate some of the oppositional traits. Similarly, if the ADHD is treated medically or structurally, the symptoms of ODD may be alleviated. The nurse will need to provide additional teaching and direction regarding ODD to support groups and agencies primarily focused on working with children with ADHD and depressive and anxiety disorders (Ollendick et al., 2016).

Nursing Care

Families of children who have ODD may be frustrated and focused on the negative behaviour challenges of the child. The nurse's task is to assist the family to refocus and find the child's strengths and skills, as well as learn to respond to negative behaviours in ways that promote positive change. Similar to working with a child with a trauma history, the caregivers work to develop strategies to attune to their child and understand the child's emotional triggers. The family is taught to work with the child to recognize those feelings and develop new coping skills that allow the child to socialize with others in a more positive manner (eMentalHealth, 2017). Depending on the child's age and family circumstances, some programs take a behavioural modification approach. The evidence for successful outcomes with this approach is inconsistent. Mindfulness is being used in some programs as a strategy; others are incorporating technology, such as computer games, to teach children emotional regulation (Boston Children's Hospital, n. d.).

Biologic Domain

The aetiology of ODD is complex; however, there is growing evidence that indicates both genetic and environmental components (Bonham et al., 2020). Complicating a diagnosis of ODD is often a coexisting condition such as ADHD, a learning disability, internalizing disorder, and/or trauma disorder (Shanahan et al., 2014). If ODD persists into adulthood, then the challenges the youth and adult face may be significant (Burke et al., 2014).

Psychosocial Domain

Children with ODD that persists across their development struggle socially: they experience frequent conflicts with peers, teachers, siblings, and caregivers. The child may have experienced negative parenting (e.g., neglectful, punitive, erratic), perhaps due to parental frustration or a parent's own oppositional traits. The child may have experienced bullying or may be the bully. If the challenges are significant, then the family will need to consider if the child's recovery will be better supported in a new school environment. The nurse will need to work closely with those involved with the child to create an environment where the child learns new communication strategies and others learn ways to respond to the child that are helpful and supportive of change. Evaluation for secondary contributing disorders such as ADHD, anxiety, or depression will need to occur (Burke & Romano-Verthelyi, 2018).

Conduct Disorder

Conduct disorder is a repetitive and persistent pattern of behaviour in children or adolescents and is characterized by disregard for the rights of others or basic social rules violation (APA, 2013). Conduct disorder is considered antecedent to antisocial personality disorder in adults. It is estimated that 8% of boys and 3% of girls meet the criteria for conduct disorder, in which, about 40% of boys and 25% of girls will eventually be diagnosed with antisocial disorder (Black & Andreasen, 2014). Childhood-onset conduct disorder may have a poorer prognosis than adolescent onset. The disorder typically occurs in boys and may or may not have precursor conditions such as ODD, ADHD, or internalizing disorders. There is some indication that a traumatic childhood or poor attachment may also lead to the development of conduct disorder symptoms.

Nursing Care

Determining what the child/youth and family are ready to address is critical with this population. There are several family-based treatments that have demonstrated success over time. The challenge for the nurse is engaging the child/youth and family in the process (Clinical Vignette box). For example, multisystem therapy is an intensive family- and community-based treatment program that focuses on addressing all environmental systems—home, school, neighbourhood—and works towards affecting change in all domains. The primary focus is developing the child's/youth's relationships, identifying and building on strengths, developing responsibility and accountability, and promoting success (Henggeler & Sheidow, 2012).

Biologic Domain

The aetiology of conduct disorder is multifactorial. For instance, the risk for conduct disorder is increased in the offspring of individuals with antisocial personality disorder, mood disorders, substance use disorders, and learning disorders. The effects of a traumatic home environment that includes family disruption, parental mental illness, poverty, community violence, and abuse

CLINICAL VIGNETTE

LEON (CONDUCT DISORDER)

Leon, a 14-year-old boy, was admitted to the child psychiatric inpatient service from the emergency department after a fight with his mother. His mother reported that she and Leon had argued earlier in the evening and that he stormed out of the house screaming and vowing that he would never return. Several hours later, Leon came back, yelling and demanding entry into the apartment. Leon's father was working and not at home. While his mother was getting up to open the door, Leon continued to yell and scream, waking the neighbours. This led to further arguing between Leon and his mother. Before long, the police were called, and Leon was taken to the emergency department.

The admission interview revealed that Leon had run away on several occasions and had even stayed away overnight. Although he strongly denied drug use, he had gotten drunk on several occasions. He had also been in several fights, the latest of which resulted in an expulsion from school. Three months before admission, he was caught trying to steal a CD from a music store. More recently, he boasted that he and his friends had snatched a purse at an outdoor concert and had broken into a car to steal its contents. Leon's school performance has been declining; he was truant on several occasions and will probably have to repeat ninth grade.

Leon was born in Cape Breton, N.S., and is the oldest of three children. His family moved to Toronto shortly after his birth. His father is employed as a janitor and is illiterate. His mother works as a secretary and has recently completed a BA in English. There is much marital discord at home. Leon has received no treatment except for consultation with the school social worker.

WHAT DO YOU THINK?

- When conducting a nursing assessment, what would you want to learn about Leon's school performance?
- What information could you provide Leon's parents about pharmacotherapy? About behaviour management?
- How would you present the material so it meets the learning needs of both parents?

also increase the risk for conduct disorder in biological and adopted children (Bornovalova et al., 2010). Conduct disorder in children and adolescents is highly comorbid with ADHD and mood and anxiety disorders (Black & Andreasen, 2014). Research has been examining the neurodevelopment of children with conduct disorder and found that impairments in neural structure and function (i.e., decreased size and functioning of the amygdala and prefrontal cortex, and reduced connectivity of the default mode network), which are related to emotional regulation and intellectual or executive functions (Junewicz & Billick, 2020). Lower than average intelligence, verbal IQ in particular, may be contributory to the diagnosis. Boys with conduct disorder often exhibit more overt aggression, whereas girls tend to be more subversive in their aggression (APA, 2013).

Psychosocial Domain

Children/youth with conduct disorder are often in trouble with the law, school authorities, and family. They often experience rejection from caregivers, school, and their community. They may also be exposed to abusive home environments if parents also have conduct traits or there are environmental contributors such as poverty or violence. The context in which a diagnosis is applied needs to be taken into account if it is considered normative for the community and general survival. Coexisting disorders that are often associated with conduct disorder are ODD, ADHD, learning and/or communication disorders, as well as internalizing disorders such as anxiety, depression, and likely PTSD.

Motor Disorders: Tourette Disorder

Motor disorders include developmental coordination disorder, stereotypic movement disorder, and **tic disorders**. Tic disorders consist of Tourette disorder, persistent motor or vocal tic disorder, provisional tic disorder, other specified tic disorder, and unspecified tic disorder (APA, 2013). Tourette disorder involves both motor (shrugs, blinks, grimaces to smelling, touching objects or people) and vocal (humming, yelling a word) tics and exhibits a waxing and waning course. Regarding prognosis: by late adolescence/early adulthood, the disorder will have disappeared for one third of those diagnosed with it, improved for another one third, and continue to fluctuate for the remaining third (Singer, 2013).

Tourette disorder is undetectable in CAT, PET, and MRI scans (Murray, 2008), and there are no diagnostic laboratory tests for it. The Yale Global Tic Severity Scale has been found to be a reliable and valid instrument for the assessment of paediatric Tourette syndrome (Stern, 2018).

Epidemiology and Aetiology

The prevalence of Tourette disorder is estimated to be from 3 to 8 per 1,000 in school-aged children, with boys being affected more than girls at a 2:1 to 4:1 ratio (APA, 2013). Named after George Gilles de la Tourette, a French neurologist who described "maladie des tics" in the late 1880s, Tourette syndrome was originally deemed psychological in origin—Freud considered it a form of hysteria—with treatment thus being psychoanalytic therapy and/or hypnosis (Bennett et al., 2013). In the 1960s, a biologic aetiology became the preferred causal explanation, supported by the efficacy (although limited) of treatment with antipsychotics (e.g., chlorpromazine and haloperidol). Today, innovations in neuroscience and genetics have moved the understanding of this disorder further: it is viewed as the result of an interplay of the brain, behaviour, and environment. The individual with tic disorder is seen as having a biologic (genetic) vulnerability that is affected by physiologic arousal related to stress (personal, environmental) (Bennett et al., 2013).

Treatment Interventions

A Canadian review of evidence-based treatment of tic disorders that made recommendations regarding pharmacotherapy concluded that behaviour therapy and the alpha-2-adrenergic antagonists are the first line of therapy for children with tic disorders (Pringsheim et al., 2012; 2019). A similar review but focused on behavioural and other therapies (e.g., brain stimulation) strongly recommended habit reversal therapy with accompanying psychoeducation and with or without pharmacotherapy (Steeves et al., 2012).

Nursing Care

A major focus of the nursing care of a child or adolescent with Tourette disorder is the careful exploration of the way that tics are affecting the individual's physical, psychological, social, and academic wellbeing. The way the family members are dealing with the symptoms is important information, as well. Completion of a family history of tic disorder may also provide critical assessment data.

To get a clear understanding of an individual child's manifestation of the disorder, a functional assessment is required. Specific information is needed regarding when tics occur and when their severity decreases (usually when the child is calm, asleep, concentrating, or focused on an activity) and when severity increases (usually when the child is excited, emotionally upset, fatigued) (Bennett et al., 2013). As the child can suppress the tics for brief periods, it is not uncommon to learn that the child has more frequent tics at home than at school. It is helpful to explore, however, the times in class that are associated with increased severity of the tics. For instance, is it when new material is being taught or when the child is called upon to speak? Older children and adults may describe a "premonitory urge" or a physical sensation before having a tic and a sense of tension reduction afterward (APA, 2013). This cycle of tension–tic–tension reduction makes it possible to envision tics as goal-directed behaviours (Singer, 2013). This is an important perspective for treatment of the disorder.

Biologic Domain

Although twin and family studies suggest that Tourette disorder is inherited, the pattern of inheritance is complex (Black & Andreasen, 2014). Aetiologic underpinnings for Tourette disorder indicate abnormality of CNS, including dopamine metabolism, frontal lobe, striatum, globus pallidus, thalamus, the connections of the basal ganglia and cortical areas (Greydanus & Tullio, 2020). It is recognized that "Obstetrical complications, older parental age, lower birth weight, and maternal smoking during pregnancy are associated with worse tic severity" (APA, 2013, p. 83).

Psychosocial Domain

The *psychoeducation* component of addressing Tourette syndrome is crucial. It involves providing the child and family general information about Tourette disorder that includes its prevalence, course, and aetiology. The behavioural model of treatment should be explained. They will need to learn about the role of context and consequences in the expression and maintenance of the child's tics. It is in the modification of these, targeting internal and external reinforcements of the tics, that forms the basis of the functional intervention. The *functional assessment*, described earlier, allows for the identification of tic triggers and consequences specific to the child and for *functional interventions* to reduce or eliminate them to be developed (Bennett et al., 2013). There is good-to-moderate efficacy for reduction of the expression and severity of tics with the use of behavioural interventions.

Teachers, guidance counsellors, and school nurses will need current information about Tourette disorder and related problems. Discussions with school personnel often include issues such as how to deal with tic behaviours if they are disruptive in the classroom (Box 30.8), how to manage teasing from other children, and how to deal with medication side effects. In some situations, a brief presentation about Tourette disorder to the class/school can reduce teasing and help both teachers and classmates tolerate the tic symptoms (Ramsey et al., 2020). Psychoeducation about Tourette syndrome may be necessary for some health professionals, as well. A qualitative study of parents' and caregivers' daily

---

BOX 30.8 Tics and Disruptive Behaviours

INEFFECTIVE APPROACH

Teacher: I see the tics. He jerks his head, makes faces, and flicks his hands.

Nurse: What do you do about them?

Teacher: What can I do? If he isn't disrupting the class, I leave him alone, even when he is throwing spitballs.

Nurse: Spitballs! He shouldn't be allowed to throw spitballs.

Teacher: Oh, I thought that was a part of his problem.

Nurse: Well, throwing spitballs has nothing to do with tics.

EFFECTIVE APPROACH

Teacher: I see the tics. He jerks his head, makes faces, and flicks his hands.

Nurse: He cannot help the tics that you are seeing. Tic disorders can exhibit a wide range of severity, from mild to severe and from simple to complex. Some complex tics may be difficult to distinguish from habits or rituals.

Teacher: What about things like throwing spitballs? When he does things like that, I try to ignore that behaviour.

Nurse: Sounds like you give him the benefit of the doubt. (Validation) However, throwing a spitball is not a tic behaviour.

Teacher: What should I do?

Nurse: How do you usually handle that type of behaviour? (A modification of reflection)

Teacher: I'd ask him to stop and sometimes to go into the hall.

Nurse: Disruptive behaviour that is voluntary in a student with a tic disorder should be handled as you would handle any other child.

Compare the responses of the nurse in these scenarios. What made the difference in the teacher's responsiveness to the nurse?

experiences and challenges revealed that they found little understanding or support from some health professionals and suggested that more training was required (Ludlow et al., 2018).

There are videos and information pamphlets available to use as resources; see Tourette Syndrome Foundation, in Web Links. Informative presentations foster openness and understanding and help students with this disorder feel included. Before initiating these interventions, it is essential to identify the child's needs and to pursue these strategies in collaboration with the family and other clinical team members. If evidence shows that Tourette disorder is hindering academic progress, the nurse can help families negotiate with the school to obtain appropriate services.

Comprehensive Behavioural Intervention for Tics (CBIT) is a treatment whose efficacy has been measured in randomized control trials. This behavioural approach is based on the assumption that, while tics are neurologic in origin, their expression is determined by the interplay of biological and environmental factors (Yang et al., 2016). The components of CBIT include psychoeducation, habit reversal training (HRT), and functional intervention (Pringsheim et al., 2019). In CBIT, the child with Tourette disorder is coached in HRT. This is based on the fact that a premonitory urge occurs prior to tic expression and then the expression of the tic relieves the tension. This positively reinforces the tic behaviour. HRT involves using a competing response (i.e., one that is incompatible with tic expression) to diminish the habitual undesired behaviour (tic). Deep breathing is one such competing behaviour (Bennett et al., 2013). Children and adolescents can be taught how to deep breathe when they feel tic expression is imminent. Using HRT to manage symptoms and to maintain their everyday routine despite tic expression can bring rewards for the child (positive reinforcement) in the form of a sense of achievement and self-efficacy, as well as increased opportunities to stay active and engaged with others (Bennett et al., 2013).

CBIT also involves recognizing the positive consequences or secondary gains of tics for the child, such as no chores when tics occur, mom giving massages and sympathy, or teacher excusing homework. Such positive consequences reinforce the tic "behaviour," and thus, the severity and frequency of tics can increase (Bennett et al., 2013). It is important to ensure that parents do not misinterpret behavioural interventions as indicating that tics are voluntary; this could create inappropriate expectations of the child. Nurses need to be knowledgeable about CBIT in order to assist and support the child and family in enacting this treatment and to appropriately monitor changes in the frequency, intensity, complexity, and interference of the tics as they occur. They may serve as consultants with the child's school.

Elimination Disorders

Enuresis

Enuresis means involuntary or intentional voiding of urine in inappropriate places. It may occur at night (nocturnal) or during the day (diurnal) or both. See the *DSM-5* (APA, 2013) for diagnostic criteria for enuresis. The behaviour cannot be attributed to a medication side effect or to another medical condition. Even without treatment, 50% of these children can achieve dryness by the age of 10 years.

Epidemiology and Aetiology

The prevalence of nocturnal enuresis is estimated more than 15% to 20% of children by the age of 5, and with a spontaneous recovery rate of 14% per year, 1% to 2% by the age of 17 (Arda et al., 2016). Most children with nocturnal enuresis are urologically normal. Although the aetiology of enuresis is unknown, multifactorial risk factors are suggested. Research found that boys are at an elevated risk to have enuresis while children with constipation or whose parents previously had enuresis are more likely to experience enuresis (Arda et al., 2016).

Treatment Interventions

Standard first-line treatments for enuresis are recommended to be alarm therapy or desmopressin (Caldwell et al., 2018). A moisture alarm can be connected to a moisture sensitive pad on a child's pajamas or bedding, and it will go off when the pad senses wetness. However, it takes time to achieve dry night (up to 16 weeks) (Mayo Clinic, 2017a). Desmopressin (a synthetic analogue of vasopressin) decreases the nighttime urine production, thus reducing the need to wake to void. Anticholinergic medications such as oxybutynin (Ditropan XL) are also used to treat enuresis. They help reduce bladder contractions and increase bladder capacity when other treatments have failed (Mayo Clinic, 2017a). Tricyclic antidepressants (TCAs) are also sometimes used to treating enuresis. The mechanisms of action of TCAs are not well understood, but they are suggested to be related to the anticholinergic effect on the bladder (Caldwell et al., 2018).

Simple behavioural interventions are undemanding strategies that the child may achieve with help from parents. They include reward for "staying dry," such as receiving a sticker on a chart, although this belies the nature of unintentional enuresis and suggests the child has some control. Other interventions include being wakened to urinate at night, retention control training to enlarge the bladder, and fluid restriction. Families can be educated to intervene in the following ways: limiting fluid intake in the evening, avoiding beverage and foods containing caffeine, encouraging voiding before preparing for going to bed and before falling asleep (Mayo Clinic, 2017a).

Family coping and support are very important for their child with enuresis. While working together with their child to manage the disorder, parents need to be patient and sensitive to their child's feelings by encouraging them to express themselves, offering support by planning for easy cleanup, and praising their child's efforts (Mayo Clinic, 2017a).

Nursing Care

The nursing assessment should include the child's developmental history, the onset and course of enuresis, prior treatment, presence of emotional problems, medical history, and family history of enuresis, diabetes, or kidney disease. Psychosocial issues such as a change in living arrangements, a new child in the family, or a death should also be documented because stress can be a contributing factor to the problem (Caldwell et al., 2018). Nurses should also explore the family's home environment and family attitudes about the child/s enuresis. Routine laboratory tests such as urinalysis and a urine culture are used to determine the presence of infection; nurses should obtain baseline data regarding toileting habits, including daytime incontinence, urinary frequency, and constipation, and they should refer children with persistent daytime enuresis for consultation with a urologist (Caldwell et al., 2018).

The nurse can explore and dispel myths and a misconception that parents may have about bed wetting, such as that the child is lazy, defiant, attention seeking, or misbehaving (Schlomer et al., 2013). In addition, education about bed wetting and its causes may help to alleviate parents' feelings of frustration and the child's feelings of humiliation and shame.

Encopresis

Encopresis involves soiling clothing with feces or depositing feces in inappropriate places, whether involuntarily or intentionally. See the *DSM-5* (APA, 2013) for the diagnostic criteria for encopresis. The diagnosis is made only if soiling is not the result of a medical disorder, such as aganglionic megacolon (Hirschsprung disease). The most common form of encopresis is fecal impaction accompanied by leakage around the hardened mass of stool. Because of the loss of muscle tone in the lower bowel, the child loses the usual urge to defecate and may not feel the leakage. Surprisingly, the child may not detect the smell of the stool because the olfactory apparatus becomes accustomed to the odour. If left untreated, then this problem generally resolves independently by middle adolescence (Jackson et al., 2020).

Encopresis can affect the lives of children in the following areas: physical, psychological, educational, social, emotional, and in the area of self-esteem.

Epidemiology and Aetiology

The problem of encopresis has received less attention in paediatric literature compared with enuresis. The prevalence of encopresis is estimated to be 1% to 4% in children greater than 4 years old, 1% to 2% in children aged 7 years, and 1.6% in 10- and 11-year-old children, with boys three to six times more likely to have encopresis than girls (Vuletic, 2017). The diagnosis of encopresis includes both retentive fecal incontinence

---

TEACHING POINTS

Effective intervention begins with educating the parents and the child about normal bowel function and the self-perpetuating cycle of fecal impaction and leakage of stool around the hardened mass of feces. The short-term goal of this educational effort is to decrease the anger and recrimination that often complicate the picture in these families. It is important for parents to understand that soiling from overflow incontinence is not a willful and defiant manoeuvre. Parents are encouraged to maintain a consistent, positive, and supportive attitude in all aspects of treatment (Vuletic, 2017). Because encopresis often results in a loss of bowel tone, it may help to motivate children by emphasizing the need to strengthen their muscles. In many cases, cleaning out the bowel is necessary before initiating behavioural treatment. Disimpaction may be accomplished with the use of oral cathartics such as polyethylene glycol. Once the colon has been evacuated, long-term laxative use is often continued during the bowel retraining program. A high-fibre diet is also recommended.

The behavioural treatment program involves daily sitting on the toilet after each meal for a predetermined period (e.g., 5 to 10 minutes). The child and parents can measure the time with an ordinary kitchen timer, and the parents can encourage the child to read or look at picture books while sitting. They can give the child rewards in the form of stars, stickers, or points for complying with the retraining program. Children with nonretentive fecal incontinence should not be treated with laxatives. After the exclusion of underlying organic diseases, the recommended treatments for encopresis in children focus on education, toilet training, and positive motivation (Vuletic, 2017).

and nonretentive fecal incontinence, which present as a single symptom without any organic cause or signs of constipation (Bongers et al., 2007). The reasons for withholding stool and starting the cycle of fecal impaction are unclear but are usually not the result of physical causes. However, as noted, once the fecal impaction occurs, there is a loss of tone in the bowel and leakage.

Nursing Care

The assessment includes a detailed interview with the child and parent regarding the pattern of the encopresis. A calm, matter-of-fact approach can help to reduce the child's embarrassment. A physical examination is also necessary; collaboration with the child's family physician or consulting paediatrician is therefore essential. The presence of encopresis does not necessarily signal severe emotional or behavioural disturbances, but the nurse should inquire about other psychiatric disorders. The diagnosis of encopresis is presumed given a history of intermittent constipation and soiling. Collaboration with the family physician and paediatrician often is helpful to rule out rare medical conditions, such as Hirschsprung disease.

■ Spiritual Domain of Nursing Care

Spirituality is a universal human phenomenon with an assumption of the wholeness of individuals and their connectedness to a higher being that integrates the quest for meaning and purpose in life. Religion is both the organized expressions of one's spirituality and the practice of worship. Spirituality supports a sense of hope, comfort, and strength and serves as a coping mechanism especially in times of illness (Dilmaghani, 2018). Nurses recognize that those in their care, from the youngest child to the oldest adult, are integral beings with spiritual needs requiring the support of their families (Veloza-Gomez et al., 2017).

Regardless of the child's or adolescent's psychiatric diagnosis, the nurse includes in the plan of care an assessment of the client and family's spirituality. The nurse must feel comfortable asking spiritual assessment questions and be nonjudgmental, open, and honest. The family's beliefs, practices, and spiritual needs are identified by asking open-ended questions that are not specific to the client's and family's religious background. The child's or youth's developmental stage, cognitive abilities, and social interactions are important components of an accurate assessment. It is important to understand whether and how the family's and/or caregivers' spirituality is helping them make sense of the child's illness and its effect on their coping. Spirituality

may influence the response of both the child and adolescent and the family to treatment, including acting as a barrier to it. This can occur, for instance, if psychiatric illness is not accepted as real, caused by sin, or a sign of bad faith. Children and adolescents may be fearful of repercussions of sharing information with family if they have experienced conflict between traditional belief systems and their own beliefs. If the child or adolescent has a history of trauma that involves a religious institution or an individual within such an institution, the spirituality assessment will be particularly important.

Based on the nurse's assessment of a child's or adolescent's spiritual needs, spiritual care is provided within the context of a therapeutic relationship. The nurse uses active listening to build rapport in addition to gathering information (Nash et al., 2015), with the aim to build trust and to provide consistency in meeting the young client's need for safety and security. This need for safety and security is one of the first spiritual needs of children. Specifically, the nurse can help to minimize the separation of the child from family and try to ensure the same nurse cares for the child daily whenever possible. Developing and adhering to a routine with a child and family also help to provide predictability. Religious practices that are carried out at the same time every day can be scheduled into the plan of care. A referral to clergy or other spiritual support can be offered to the family, as well as to an adolescent. Incorporating spiritual care into the plan of care is essential for optimal health and for positive outcomes when resolving crises.

The spiritual issues of a child or adolescent may be shaped by their psychiatric illness and/or the family's and community's response to it. For instance, children or adolescents experiencing suicidal ideation may be influenced by what they or their family believe will happen after death to those who commit suicide. Would they go to a better place, or find enlightenment, or be punished (Preet, 2007)? For those with a psychotic disorder, the beliefs about hallucinations and delusions of the family and community matter. Psychosis has been viewed as a sign of a spiritual inhabitation (positive or negative) or as a curse, a perspective that should be explored in the spiritual assessment. The therapeutic relationship with the family will be an asset in understanding the situation, protecting the child from any potential harm, and supporting the family. The ADHD symptoms of a child or adolescent may not be tolerated within the setting of the family's religious worship. This rejection has the potential to cut the child or adolescent and the family from important emotional and social support. Education for all those involved by a representative of the healthcare team, such as the nurse, can be a helpful intervention.

Summary of Key Points

- Improved methods of assessing and defining psychiatric disorders have enhanced appreciation for the frequency of psychiatric disorders in children and adolescents.
- An estimated 14% of children 4 to 17 years of age (more than 800,000) in Canada experience mental disorders that cause significant distress and impairment at home, at school, and in the community.
- The developmental disorders include intellectual disability, ASDs, and specific developmental disorders. Assessment findings should guide nursing management. Specific developmental disorders include communication disorders and learning disorders. These disorders are fairly common in the general population, but they are more common in children with other primary psychiatric disorders.
- Child psychiatric disorders can be divided into externalizing and internalizing disorders. Externalizing disorders include the disruptive behaviour disorders: ODD and conduct disorder. Internalizing disorders include depression and anxiety disorders.
- ADHD is defined by the presence of inattention, impulsiveness, and, in most cases, hyperactivity. This heterogeneous disorder affects boys more often than girls.

- Effective treatment of ADHD often involves multiple approaches, including medication and parent teaching.
- Assessment of children involves securing data from multiple sources, including the child, parents, and school personnel.
- Standardized rating instruments can assist data collection from multiple informants.
- Separation anxiety is a relatively common anxiety disorder in school-aged children. OCD is more common in adolescents.
- Treatment of separation anxiety and OCD may include medication, behavioural therapy, or a combination of these treatments.
- Major depression in children/youth is believed to be similar to major depression in adults; however, it may be expressed differently.
- The efficacy of antidepressant medications is less well established in children and adolescents than in adults.
- Childhood schizophrenia is a rare disorder.
- Elimination disorders include encopresis and enuresis. Behavioural therapy approaches are the most effective treatment for these disorders. Medication may also be used.
- Attention to the spiritual needs of children and adolescents is a basic element of their nursing care plan.

Thinking Challenges

During lunch, a 6-year-old girl presents to the principal's office indicating she has a stomachache and wants to go home because she misses her mother and her new puppy. For the past 2 weeks now, she has shared with her teacher that she is experiencing a number of somatic concerns. She starts crying when her mother picks her up from school. The principal asks the nursing student for assistance in working with this child.

a. How does anxiety manifest in the child diagnosed with separation anxiety disorder?

b. What is the prevalence of separation anxiety disorder in children?
c. How can this disorder be treated effectively?

> Visit thePoint to view suggested responses.
> Go to thePoint.lww.com/activate and use the activation code found in the front of this text to unlock answers to the "Thinking Challenges" and other online resources.

Web Links

autismcanada.org This site of Autism Canada has screening tools, educational videos, and ways to connect with interested others regarding autism.

autismspeaks.ca *Autism Speaks Canada*, along with the international *Autism Speaks*, supports research and services on autism spectrum disorder, including Asperger syndrome. Information about this developmental brain disorder can be found at this site.

www.caddra.ca The *Canadian ADHD Resource Alliance* offers healthcare professionals of all disciplines resources such as practice guidelines, assessment toolkits, and training courses.

caddra.ca/pdfs/Medication_Chart_English_CANADA.pdf The CADDRA Guide to ADHD Pharmacological Treatments

is available at this site in chart format, including coloured images of the medication.

camh.ca/en/health-info/mental-illness-and-addiction-index/cognitive-behavioural-therapy#:~:text=CBT%20is%20a%20structured%2C%20time,reactions%20that%20cause%20them%20difficulty This is where the Centre for Addiction and Mental Health's overview of cognitive–behaviour therapy is to be found.

cmha.ca/documents/children-youth-and-depression The Canadian Mental Health Association's site with information about children and depression.

canfasd.ca/2015/12/14/new-canadian-guideline The Canadian guidelines for diagnosing fetal alcohol spectrum disorder (FASD) are available at this website of the Canada FASD Research Network.

chadd.org Children and Adults with Attention-Deficit/ Hyperactivity Disorder is an American support and advocacy organization whose website features blogs and chat rooms as well as training and continuing education opportunities for parents, teachers, and health professionals.

www.earlypsychosis.ca Early Psychosis Intervention was created with the intent of providing a collective resource about Early Psychosis Intervention (EPI) for the province of British Columbia (BC).

keltymentalhealth.ca/mental-health/disorders/bipolar-disorder Information about bipolar disorder, including that of children, can be found at this site. Information regarding suicide is also available here.

nctsnet.org The National Child Traumatic Stress Network provides information and resources for children and their families who have been exposed to traumatic events.

teenmentalhealth.org Based at Dalhousie University, this site offers free downloadable learning modules on child and adolescent health designed for first contact health providers, such as family physicians. Although beyond the practice scope of preregistration nursing students, the modules on child anxiety disorders, adolescent anxiety disorders, child and adolescent depression (MDD), and ADHD are informative, overviewing identification, diagnosis, and treatment of the disorders.

tourette.ca The Tourette Syndrome Foundation is a Canadian advocacy and support network currently developing a "virtual community" for individuals and families living with Tourette disorder. The site offers resources such as videos and a book for the newly diagnosed.

References

Afifi, T. O., MacMillan, H. L., Taillieu, T., Cheung, K., Turner, S., Tonmyr, L., & Hovdestad, W. (2015). Relationship between child abuse exposure and reported contact with child protection organizations: Results from the Canadian Community Health Survey. *Child Abuse and Neglect, 46*, 198–206. https://doi.org/10.1016/j.chiabu.2015.05.001

Aghamohammadi-Sereshki, A., Coupland, N. J., Silverstone, P. H., Huang, Y., Hegadoren, K. M., Carter, R., Seres, P., & Malykhin, N. V. (2021). Effects of childhood adversity on the volumes of the amygdala subnuclei and hippocampal subfields in individuals with major depressive disorder. *Journal of Psychiatry & Neuroscience, 46*(1), E186–E195. https://doi.org/10.1503/jpn.200034

Ainsworth, M. D. S. (1979). Infant–mother attachment. *American Psychologist, 34*, 932–937. https://doi.org/10.1037/0003-066X.34.10.932

Alter, C., Haynes, S., & Worland, J. (2019, December 04). 2019 Person of the Year: Greta Thunberg. In *Time*. https://time.com/person-of-the-year-2019-greta-thunberg/

American Psychiatric Association. (2013). *Diagnostic and statistical manual of mental disorders (DSM-5®)*.

Anagnostou, E., Zwaigenbaum, L., Szatmari, P., Fombonne, E., Fernandez, B. A., Woodbury-Smith, M., Brian, J., Bryson, S., Smith, I. M., Drmic, I., Buchanan, J. A., Roberts, W., & Scherer, S. W. (2014). Autism spectrum disorder: Advances in evidence-based practice. *Canadian Medical Association Journal, 186*(7), 509–519. https://doi.org/10.1503/cmaj.121756

Arda, E., Cakiroglu, B., & Thomas, D. T. (2016). Primary nocturnal enuresis: A review. *Nephro-urology Monthly, 8*(4), e35809. https://doi.org/10.5812/numonthly.35809

Armitage, S., Parkinson, M., Halligan, S., & Reynolds, S. (2020). Mothers' experiences of having an adolescent child with depression: An interpretative phenomenological analysis. *Journal of Child and Family Studies, 29*(6), 1617–1629. https://doi.org/10.1007/s10826-020-01705-5

Ashton, C. K., O'Brien-Langer, A., & Silverstone, P. H. (2015). The CASA trauma and attachment group (TAG) program for children with have attachment issues following early developmental trauma. *Journal of the Canadian Academy of Child and Adolescent Psychiatry, 25*(1), 35–42.

Avenevoli, S., Swendsen, J., He, J.-P., Burstein, M., & Merikangas, K. R. (2015). Major depression in the National Comorbidity Survey–Adolescent Supplement: Prevalence, correlates, and treatment. *Journal of the American Academy of Child & Adolescent Psychiatry, 54*(1), 37–44. e32. https://doi.org/10.1016/j.jaac.2014.10.010

Baio, J., Wiggins, L., Christensen, D. L., Maenner, M. J., Daniels, J., Warren, Z., Kurzius-Spencer, M., Zahorodny, W., Rosenberg, C. R., & White, T. (2018). Prevalence of autism spectrum disorder among children aged 8 years—autism and developmental disabilities monitoring network, 11 sites, United States, 2014. *MMWR Surveillance Summaries, 67*(6), 1. https://doi.org/10.15585/mmwr.ss6706a1

Barkley, R. A. (1998). *Attention deficit hyperactivity disorder: A handbook for diagnosis and treatment* (2nd ed.). Guilford.

Bellis, M. D., & Zisk, A. (2014). The biological effects of childhood trauma. *Child and Adolescent Psychiatric Clinics of North America, 23*, 185–222. https://doi.org/10.1016/j.chc.2014.01.002

Bennett, S. M., Keller, A. E., & Walkup, J. T. (2013). The future of tic disorder treatment. *Annals of the New York Academy of Sciences, 1304*(1), 32–39. https://doi.org/10.1111/nyas.12296

Black, D. W., & Andreasen, N. C. (2014). *Introductory textbook of psychiatry*. American Psychiatric Pub.

Blaustein, M., & Kinniburgh, K. (2010). *Treating traumatic stress in children and adolescents: How to foster resilience through attachment, self-regulation, and competency*. Guilford Press.

Bombay, A., Matheson, K., & Anisman, H. (2014). The intergenerational effects of Indian Residential Schools: Implications for the concept of historical trauma. *Transcultural Psychiatry, 51*(3), 320–338. https://doi.org/10.1177/1363461513503380

Bongers, M., Tabbers, M., & Benninga, M. (2007). Functional nonretentive fecal incontinence in children. *Journal of Pediatric Gastroenterology and Nutrition, 44*(1), 5–13. https://doi.org/10.1097/01.mpg.0000252187.12793.0a

Bonham, M. D., Shanley, D. C., Waters, A. M., & Elvin, O. M. (2020). Inhibitory control deficits in children with oppositional defiant disorder and conduct disorder compared to attention deficit/hyperactivity disorder: A systematic review and meta-analysis. *Research on Child and Adolescent Psychopathology, 49*(1), 39–62. https://doi.org/10.1007/s10802-020-00713-9

Bornovalova, M., Hicks, B., Iacono, W., & McGue, M. (2010). Familial transmission and heritability of childhood disruptive disorders. *American Journal of Psychiatry, 167*, 1066–1074. https://doi.org/10.1176/appi.ajp.2010.09091272

Boston Children's Hospital. (n.d.). Oppositional Defiant Disorder. https://www.childrenshospital.org/conditions/oppositional-defiant-disorder#

Burke, J. D., Rowe, R., & Boylan, K. (2014). Functional outcomes of child and adolescent oppositional defiant disorder symptoms in young adult men. *Journal of Child Psychology and Psychiatry, 55*(3), 263–272. https://doi.org/10.1111/jcpp.12150

Burke, J. D., & Romano-Verthelyi, A. M. (2018). Oppositional defiant disorder. In M. Martel (Ed.) *Developmental Pathways to Disruptive, Impulse-Control and Conduct Disorders* (pp. 21–52). Elsevier.

Buckner, J., Lopez, C., Dunkel, S., & Joiner, T. (2008). Behaviour management training for the treatment of reactive attachment disorder. *Child Maltreatment, 13*(3), 289–297. https://doi.org/10.1177/1077559508318396

Caldwell, P. H., Lim, M., & Nankivell, G. (2018). An interprofessional approach to managing children with treatment-resistant enuresis: An educational review. *Pediatric Nephrology, 33*(10), 1663–1670. https://doi.org/10.1007/s00467-017-3830-1

Canada Fetal Alcohol Spectrum Disorder Research Network. (2016). Fetal alcohol spectrum disorder: A guideline for diagnosis. *Canadian Medical Association Journal, 188*(3), 191–197.

Cameron, C. L. (2007). Obsessive-compulsive disorder in children and adolescents. *Journal of Psychiatric and Mental Health Nursing, 14*(7), 696–704. https://doi.org/10.1111/j.1365-2850.2007.01162.x

Canadian ADHD Resource Alliance. (2013a). *Adult ADHD*. http://www.caddra.ca/public-information/adults

Canadian ADHD Resource Alliance. (2013b). *Information for educators*. https://www.caddra.ca/public-information/educators/

Canadian ADHD Resource Alliance (ADDRA). (2020). *Canadian ADHA Practice Guidelines* (4.1 ed.). Canadian ADHD Resource Alliance.

Canadian Institute for Health Information. (2020). *Child and youth mental health in Canada -Infographic*. https://www.cihi.ca/en/child-and-youth-mental-health-in-canada-infographic

Canadian Mental Health Association. (2014a). *Bipolar disorder*. http://www.cmha.ca/mental-health/understanding-mental-illness/bipolar-disorder/

Canadian Mental Health Association. (2014b). *Mental illness in children and youth.* https://cmha.bc.ca/documents/mental-illnesses-in-children-and-youth-2/

Canadian Mental Health Association (CMHA). (2016). *Children, youth, and depression.* https://cmha.ca/documents/children-youth-and-depression

Caporino, N. E., Morgan, J., Beckstead, J., Phares, V., Murphy, T. K., & Storch, E. A. (2012). A structural equation analysis of family accommodation in pediatric obsessive-compulsive disorder. *Journal of Abnormal Child Psychology, 40*(1), 133–143. https://doi.org/10.1007/s10802-011-9549-8

Cavanagh, M. Quinn, D., Duncan, D., Graham, T., & Balbuena, L. (2017). Oppositional defiant disorders is better conceptualized as a disorder of emotional dysregulation. *Journal of Attention Disorders, 21*(5), 381–389. https://doi.org/10.1177/1087054713520221

Centre for ADHD Awareness, Canada. (2013). *Adult attention deficit hyperactivity disorder.* http://www.caddac.ca/cms/page.php?82%29.

Centre for Addiction and Mental Health. (2018). *The Mental Health and Well-Being of Ontario Students.* https://www.camh.ca/-/media/files/pdf---osduhs/mental-health-and-well-being-of-ontario-students-1991-2017---summary-osduhs-report-pdf.pdf

Center for Substance Abuse Treatment (US). (2014). Understanding the impact of trauma. In *Trauma-informed care in behavioral health services* (pp. 59–90). Substance Abuse and Mental HealthServices Administration.

Centers for Disease Control and Prevention. (2020). *Treatment of ADHD.* https://www.cdc.gov/ncbddd/adhd/treatment.html

Centers for Disease Control and Prevention. (2021). *Signs and symptoms of autism spectrum disorders.* https://www.cdc.gov/ncbddd/autism/signs.html

Conners, C. K. (1989). *Conners' Rating Scales Manual.* Multi-Health Systems.

Cook, J. Green, C., Lilley, C., Anderson, S., Baldwin, M., Chudley, A., Conry, J. L., LeBlanc, N., Loock, C. A., Lutke, J., Mallon, B. F., McFarlane, A. A., Temple, V. K., & Rosales, T.; Canada Fetal Alcohol Spectrum Disorder Research Network. (2016). Fetal alcohol spectrum disorder: A guideline for diagnosis across the lifespan. *Canadian Medical Association Journal, 188*(3), 191–197. https://doi.org/10.1503/cmaj.141593

Dilmaghani, M. (2018). Importance of religion or spirituality and mental health in Canada. *Journal of Religion and Health, 57*(1), 120–135. https://doi.org/10.1007/s10943-017-0385-1

Eilertsen, E. M., Gjerde, L. C., Reichborn-Kjennerud, T., Ørstavik, R. E., Knudsen, G. P., Stoltenberg, C., Czajkowski, N., Røysamb, E., Kendler, K. S., & Ystrom, E. (2017). Maternal alcohol use during pregnancy and offspring attention-deficit hyperactivity disorder (ADHD): A prospective sibling control study. *International Journal of Epidemiology, 46*(5), 1633–1640. https://doi.org/10.1093/ije/dyx067

eMentalHealth.ca/PrimaryCare. (2017). *Oppositional defiant disorder (ODD): Information for primary care.* https://primarycare.ementalhealth.ca/index.php?m=fpArticle&ID=48957

Emmer, C., Bosnjak, M., & Mata, J. (2020). The association between weight stigma and mental health: A meta-analysis. *Obesity Reviews, 21*(1), e12935. https://doi.org/10.1111/obr.12935

Essau, C. A., Lewinsohn, P. M., Lim, J. X., Moon-ho, R. H., & Rohde, P. (2018). Incidence, recurrence and comorbidity of anxiety disorders in four major developmental stages. *Journal of Affective Disorders, 228,* 248–253. https://doi.org/10.1016/j.jad.2017.12.014

Feldman, M. E., Charach, A., & Bélanger, S. A. (2018). ADHD in children and youth: Part 2—Treatment. *Paediatrics & Child Health, 23*(7), 462–472. https://doi.org/10.1093/pch/pxy113

Findlay, L. (2017, January 18). *Health Reports: Depression and Suicidal ideation among Canadians aged 15 to 24.* https://www150.statcan.gc.ca/n1/pub/82-003-x/2017001/article/14697-eng.htm

Fletcher, J. M., Lyon, G. R., Fuchs, L. S., & Barnes, M. A. (2018). *Learning disabilities: From identification to intervention.* Guilford Publications.

Fox-Lopp, J., & McLaughlin, T. (2015). The effects of classroom interventions on anxiety disorders in elementary school children: A brief review. *International Journal of Multidisciplinary Research and Development, 2*(1), 10–15.

Franz, A. P., Bolat, G. U., Bolat, H., Matijasevich, A., Santos, I. S., Silveira, R. C., Procianoy, R. S., Rohde, L. A., & Moreira-Maia, C. R. (2018). Attention-deficit/hyperactivity disorder and very preterm/very low birth weight: A meta-analysis. *Pediatrics, 141*(1), e20171645. https://doi.org/10.1542/peds.2017-1645

Gallagher, S. (2020, February 24). Greta Thunberg was nearly hospitalized due to disordered eating, says mother. In *Independent.* https://www.independent.co.uk/life-style/health-and-families/greta-thunberg-aspergers-eating-disorder-malena-ernman-interview-a9355201.html

Gleason, M. M., Fox, N. A., Drury, S., Smyke, A., Egger, H. L., Nelson III, C. A., Gregas, M. C., & Zeanah, C. H. (2011). Validity of evidence-derived criteria for reactive attachment disorder: Indiscriminately social/dis-inhibited and emotionally withdrawn/inhibited types. *Journal of the American Academy of Child & Adolescent Psychiatry, 50*(3), 216–231. e213. https://doi.org/10.1016/j.jaac.2010.12.012

Glowinski, A. L. (2011). Reactive attachment disorder: An evolving entity. *Journal of the American Academy of Child and Adolescent Psychiatry, 50*(3), 210–212. https://doi.org/10.1016/j.jaac.2010.12.013

Goldbeck, L., & Jensen, T. K. (2017). The diagnostic spectrum of trauma-related disorders in children and adolescents. In M. A. Landolt, M. Cloitre, & U. Schnyder (Eds.), *Evidence-based treatments for trauma related disorders in children and adolescents* (pp. 3–28). Springer.

Goodman, W. K., Grice, D. E., Lapidus, K. A., & Coffey, B. J. (2014). Obsessive-compulsive disorder. *Psychiatric Clinics of North America, 37*(3), 257–267. https://doi.org/10.1016/j.psc.2014.06.004

Government of Canada. (2020). *Suicide in Canada: Key statistics (infographic).* https://www.canada.ca/en/public-health/services/publications/healthy-living/suicide-canada-key-statistics-infographic.html

Goyette, G. H., Conners, C. K., & Ulrich, R. F. (1978). Normative data on the revised Connors parent and teacher rating scales. *Journal of Abnormal Child Psychology, 6*(2), 221–236. https://doi.org/10.1007/BF00919127

Greydanus, D. E., & Tullio, J. (2020). Tourette's disorder in children and adolescents. *Translational Pediatrics, 9*(Suppl 1), S94. https://doi.org/10.21037/tp.2019.09.11

He, Y., Chen, J., Zhu, L.-H., Hua, L.-L., & Ke, F.-F. (2020). Maternal smoking during pregnancy and ADHD: Results from a systematic review and meta-analysis of prospective cohort studies. *Journal of Attention Disorders, 24*(12), 1637–1647. https://doi.org/10.1177/1087054717696766

HealthLinkBC. (2017). *Depression in children and teens.* http://www.healthlinkbc.ca/kb/content/major/ty4640.html

Henggeler, S. W., & Sheidow, A. J. (2012). Empirically supported family-based treatments for conduct disorder and delinquency in adolescents. *Journal of Marital and Family Therapy, 38*(1), 30–58. https://doi.org/10.1111/j.1752-0606.2011.00244.x

Hiller, R. M., Young, R. L., & Weber, N. (2014). Sex differences in autism spectrum disorder based on DSM-5 criteria: Evidence from clinician and teacher reporting. *Journal of Abnormal Child Psychology, 42*(8), 1381–1393. https://doi.org/10.1007/s10802-014-9881-x

Hong, S.-B., Im, M.-H., Kim, J.-W., Park, E.-J., Shin, M.-S., Kim, B.-N., Yoo, H.-J., Cho, I.-H., Bhang, S.-Y., & Hong, Y.-C. (2015). Environmental lead exposure and attention deficit/hyperactivity disorder symptom domains in a community sample of South Korean school-age children. *Environmental Health Perspectives, 123*(3), 271–276. https://doi.org/10.1289/ehp.1307420

Humphreys, K. L., Nelson, C. A., Fox, N. A., & Zeanah, C. H. (2017). Signs of reactive attachment disorder and diminished social engagement disorder at age 12 years: Effects of institutional care history and high quality foster-care. *Development and Psychopathology, 29*(2), 675–684. https://doi.org/10.1017/S0954579417000256

Jackson, M. L., Williams, W. L., Rafacz, S. D., & Friman, P. C. (2020). Encopresis and enuresis. In P. Turmey (Ed.), *Functional Analysis in Clinical Treatment* (pp. 199–225). Elsevier.

Junewicz, A., & Billick, S. B. (2020). Conduct disorder: Biology and developmental trajectories. *Psychiatric Quarterly, 91*(1), 77–90. https://doi.org/10.1007/s11126-019-09678-5

Kanner, L. (1943). Autistic disturbances of affective contact. *Nervous Child, 2,* 217–250.

Kelvin, R. (2016). Depression in children and young people. *Paediatrics and Child Health, 26*(12), 540–547. https://doi.org/10.1016/j.paed.2016.08.008

Kim-Cohen, J., Caspi, A., Moffitt, T. E., Harrington, H., Milne, B. J., & Poulton, R. (2003). Prior juvenile diagnoses in adults with mental disorder: Developmental follow-back of a prospective-longitudinal cohort. *Archives of General Psychiatry, 60*(7), 709–717. https://doi.org/10.1001/archpsyc.60.7.709

Klein, M., Onnink, M., van Donkelaar, M., Wolfers, T., Harich, B., Shi, Y., Dammers, J., Arias-Vásquez, A., Hoogman, M., & Franke, B. (2017). Brain imaging genetics in ADHD and beyond–mapping pathways from gene to disorder at different levels of complexity. *Neuroscience & Biobehavioral Reviews, 80,* 115–155. https://doi.org/10.1016/j.neubiorev.2017.01.013

Larsson, H., Chang, Z., D'Onofrio, B. M., & Lichtenstein, P. (2014). The heritability of clinically diagnosed attention-deficit/hyperactivity disorder across the life span. *Psychological Medicine, 44*(10), 2223. https://doi.org/10.1017/S0033291713002493

Lehmann, S., Monette, S., Egger, H., Breivik, K., Young, D., Davidson, C., & Minnis, H. (2020). Development and examination of the reactive attachment disorder and disinhibited social engagement disorder assessment interview. *Assessment, 27*(4), 749–765. https://doi.org/10.1177/1073191118797422

Leibenluft, E. (2011). Severe mood dysregulation, irritability, and the diagnostic boundaries of bipolar disorder in youths. *American Journal of Psychiatry*, 162(2), 129–142. https://doi.org/10.1176/appi.ajp.2010.10050766

Lightfoot, A., Janemi, R., & Rudman, D. L. (2018). Perspectives of North American postsecondary students with learning disabilities: A scoping review. *Journal of Postsecondary Education and Disability*, 31(1), 57–74.

Ludlow, A., Brown, R., & Schulz, J. (2018). A qualitative exploration of the daily experiences and challenges faced by parents and caregivers of children with Tourette's syndrome. *Journal of Health Psychology*, 23(14), 1790–1799. https://doi.org/10.1177/1359105316669878

Magán-Maganto, M., Bejarano-Martín, Á., Fernández-Alvarez, C., Narzisi, A., García-Primo, P., Kawa, R., Posada, M., & Canal-Bedia, R. (2017). Early detection and intervention of ASD: A European overview. *Brain Sciences*, 7(12), 159. https://doi.org/10.3390/brainsci7120159

Manassis, K. (2004). Childhood anxiety disorders: Approach to interventions. *Canadian Family Physician*, 50, 379–384.

Marrus, N., Hall, L., Paterson, S., Elison, J. T., Wolff, J. J., Swanson, M., Parish-Morris, J., Eggebrecht, A., Pruett, J., & Hazlett, H. (2018). Language delay aggregates in toddler siblings of children with autism spectrum disorder. *Journal of Neurodevelopmental Disorders*, 10(1), 29. https://doi.org/10.1186/s11689-018-9247-8

Mayo Clinic. (2017a). *Reactive attachment disorder*. https://www.mayoclinic.org/diseases-conditions/reactive-attachment-disorder/symptoms-causes/syc-20352939

Mayo Clinic. (2017b). *Bed wetting*. https://www.mayoclinic.org/diseases-conditions/bed-wetting/diagnosis-treatment/drc-20366711

Mental Health Commission of Canada. (2012). *The Mental Health Strategy for Canada*. https://www.mentalhealthcommission.ca/English/resources/mhcc-reports/mental-health-strategy-canada

Mohammadi, M. R., Badrfam, R., Khaleghi, A., Hooshyari, Z., Ahmadi, N., & Zandifar, A. (2020). Prevalence, comorbidity and predictor of separation anxiety disorder in children and adolescents. *The Psychiatric Quarterly*, 91(4), 1415–1429. https://doi.org/10.1007/s11126-020-09778-7.

MTA Cooperative Group. (1999). A 14-month randomized clinical trial of treatment strategies for attention-deficit/hyperactivity disorder. Multimodal treatment study of children with ADHA. *Archives of General Psychiatry*, 56(12), 1073–1086. https://doi.org/10.1001/archpsyc.56.12.1073

Mulvihill, D. (2005). The health impact of childhood trauma: An interdisciplinary review, 1997– 2003. *Issues in Comprehensive Pediatric Nursing*, 28(2), 115–136. https://doi.org/10.1080/01460860590950890

Murray, B. (2008). Disorders diagnosed in infancy, childhood or adolescence. In P. O'Brien, W. Kennedy, & K. Ballard (Eds.), *Psychiatric mental health nursing: An introduction to theory and practice* (pp. 207–234). Jones and Bartlett Publishers.

Nash, P., Darby, K., & Nash, S. (2015). *Spiritual care with sick children and young People: A handbook for chaplains, paediatric health professionals, arts therapists, and youth workers*. Jessica Kingsley Publishers.

National Child Traumatic Stress Network. (n. d.). *About child trauma*. https://www.nctsn.org/what-is-child-trauma/about-child-trauma

National Child Traumatic Stress Network. (2013). *Effective treatments for youth trauma*. http://www.nctsn.org/resources/audiences/parents-caregivers/treatments-that-work

Nazeer, A., Latif, F., Mondal, A., Azeem, M. W., & Greydanus, D. E. (2020). Obsessive-compulsive disorder in children and adolescents: Epidemiology, diagnosis and management. *Translational Pediatrics*, 9(Suppl 1), S76. https://doi.org/10.21037/tp.2019.10.02

Nolin, M., Malla, A., Tibbo, P., Norman, R., & Abdel-Baki, A. (2016). Early intervention for psychosis in Canada: What is the state of affairs? *Canadian Journal of Psychiatry*, 61(3), 188–194. https://doi.org/10.1177/0706743716632516

Ollendick, T. H., Greene, R. W., Austin, K. E., Fraire, M. G., Halldorsdottir, T., Allen, K. B., Jarrett, M. A., Lewis, K. M., Whitmore Smith, M., Cunningham, N. R., Noguchi, R. J., Canavera, K., & Wolff, J. C. (2016). Parent management training and collaborative & proactive solutions: A randomized control trial for oppositional youth. *Journal of Clinical Child & Adolescent Psychology*, 45(5), 591–604. https://doi.org/10.1080/15374416.2015.1004681

Pastor-Cerezuela, G., Fernández-Andrés, M. I., Tárraga-Mínguez, R., & Navarro-Peña, J. M. (2016). Parental stress and ASD: Relationship with autism symptom severity, IQ, and resilience. *Focus on Autism and Other Developmental Disabilities*, 31(4), 300–311. https://doi.org/10.1177/1088357615558347

Peterson, B., Rauh, V. A., Bansal, R., Hao, X., Toth, Z., Nati, G., Walsh, K., Miller, R. L., Arias, F., & Semanek, D. (2015). Effects of prenatal exposure to air pollutants (polycyclic aromatic hydrocarbons) on the development of brain white matter, cognition, and behavior in later childhood. *JAMA Psychiatry*, 72(6), 531–540. https://doi.org/10.1001/jamapsychiatry.2015.57

Phillips, K. E., Norris, L. A., & Kendall, P. C. (2020). Separation anxiety symptom profiles and parental accommodation across pediatric anxiety disorders. *Child Psychiatry & Human Development*, 51, 377–389. https://doi.org/10.1007/s10578-019-00949-7

Piacentini, J., Bennett, S., Compton, S. N., Kendall, P. C., Birmaher, B., Albano, A. M., March, J., Sherrill, J., Sakolsky, D., & Ginsburg, G. (2014). 24-and 36-week outcomes for the Child/Adolescent Anxiety Multimodal Study (CAMS). *Journal of the American Academy of Child & Adolescent Psychiatry*, 53(3), 297–310. https://doi.org/10.1016/j.jaac.2013.11.010

Politis, S., Magklara, K., Petrikis, P., Michalis, G., Simos, G., & Skapinakis, P. (2017). Epidemiology and comorbidity of obsessive–compulsive disorder in late adolescence: A cross-sectional study in senior high schools in Greece. *International Journal of Psychiatry in Clinical Practice*, 21(3), 188–194. https://doi.org/10.1080/13651501.2017.1324038

Poole, K. L., & Schmidt, L. A. (2020). Adaptive shyness: A developmental perspective. In L. A. Schmidt, & K. L. Poole *Adaptive Shyness* (pp. 25–40). Springer.

Preet, J. (2007). Suicide and spirituality: A clinical perspective. *Southern Medical Journal*, 100(7), 752–755. https://doi.org/10.1097/SMJ.0b013e318073c757

Pringsheim, T., Okun, M. S., Müller-Vahl, K., Martino, D., Jankovic, J., Cavanna, A. E., Woods, D. W., Robinson, M., Jarvie, E., & Roessner, V. (2019). Practice guideline recommendations summary: Treatment of tics in people with Tourette syndrome and chronic tic disorders. *Neurology*, 92(19), 896–906. https://doi.org/10.1212/WNL.0000000000007466

Pringsheim, T., Doja, A., Gorman, D., McKinlay, D., Day, L., Billinghurst, L., Carroll, A., Dion, Y., Luscombe, S., Steeves, T., & Sandor, P. (2012). Canadian Guidelines for evidence-based treatment of tic disorders: Pharmacotherapy. *Canadian Journal of Psychiatry*, 57(3), 133–143. https://doi.org/10.1177/070674371205700302

Public Health Agency of Canada. (2016). *Report from the Canadian chronic disease surveillance system: Mood and anxiety disorders in Canada 2016*. https://www.canada.ca/content/dam/canada/health-canada/migration/healthy-canadians/publications/diseases-conditions-maladies-affections/mood-anxiety-disorders-2016-troubles-anxieux-humeur/alt/mood-anxiety-disorders-2016-troubles-anxieux-humeur-eng.pdf

Ramsey, K. A., Essoe, J. K.-Y., Storch, E. A., Lewin, A. B., Murphy, T. K., & McGuire, J. F. (2020). The role of affect lability on tic severity and impairment in youth with Tourette's disorder. *Journal of Obsessive-Compulsive and Related Disorders*, 27, 100578. https://doi.org/10.1016/j.jocrd.2020.100578

Saskatchewan Alliance for Youth & Community Well-being. (2016). *SAYCW Youth Health Survey*. https://selu.usask.ca/documents/research-and-publications/SAYCW-Youth-Health-Survey_2016.pdf

Schachar, R. (2014). Genetics of attention deficit hyperactivity disorder (ADHD): Recent updates and future prospects. *Current Developmental Disorders Report*, 1, 41–49. https://doi.org/10.1007/s40474-013-0004-0

Schlomer, B., Rodriguez, E., Weiss, D., & Copp, H. (2013). Parents' beliefs about nocturnal enuresis causes, treatments, and the need to seek professional medical care. *Journal of Pediatric Urology*, 9, 1043–1048. https://doi.org/10.1016/j.jpurol.2013.02.013

Schwartz, C., Barican, J. L., Yung, D., Zheng, Y., & Waddell, C. (2019). Six decades of preventing and treating childhood anxiety disorders: A systematic review and meta-analysis to inform policy and practice. *Evidence-Based Mental Health*, 22(3), 103–110. http://dx.doi.org/10.1136/ebmental-2019-300096

Shanahan, L., Copeland, W. E., Angold, A., Bondy C. L., & Cosello, J. (2014). Sleep problems predict and are predicted by generalized anxiety/depression and oppositional defiant disorder. *Journal of the American Academy of Child and Adolescent Psychiatry*, 53(5), 550–558. https://doi.org/10.1016/j.jaac.2013.12.029

Silove, D., Manicavasagar, V., & Pini, S. (2016). Can separation anxiety disorder escape its attachment to childhood? *World Psychiatry*, 15(2), 113–115. https://doi.org/10.1002/wps.20336

Smith, A., Stewart, D., Poon, C., Peled, M., & Saewyc, E. (2014). *From Hastings Street to Haida Gwaii: Provincial results of the 2013 BC Adolescent Health Survey*. M. C. Society. https://apsc- saravyc.sites.olt.ubc.ca/files/2018/04/From_Hastings_Street_To_Haida_Gwaii.pdf

Singer, H. S. (2013). Motor control, habits, complex motor stereotypies, and Tourette syndrome. *Annals of the New York Academy of Sciences*, 1304(1), 22–31. https://doi.org/10.1111/nyas.12281

Smyke, A. T., Seanah, C. H., Gleason, M. M., Drury, S. S., Fox, N. A., Nelson, C. A., & Guthrie, D. (2012). A randomized controlled trail comparing foster care and institutional care for children with signs of reactive attachment disorder. *American Journal of Psychiatry*, 169, 508–514. https://doi.org/10.1176/appi.ajp.2011.11050748

Sørensen, L., Sonuga-Barke, E., Eichele, H., van Wageningen, H., Wollschlaeger, D., & Plessen, K. J. (2017). Suboptimal decision making by children with ADHD in the face of risk: Poor risk adjustment and delay aversion rather than general proneness to taking risks. *Neuropsychology*, 31(2), 119–128. https://doi.org/10.1037/neu0000297.

Steeves, T., McKinlay, B. D., Gorman, D., Billinghurst, L., Day, L., Carroll, A., Dion, Y., Doja, A., Luscombe, S., Sandor, P., & Pringsheim, T. (2012). Canadian guidelines for evidence-based treatment of tic disorders: Behavioural therapy, deep brain stimulation, and transcranial magnetic stimulation. *Canadian Journal of Psychiatry, 57*(3), 144–151. https://doi.org/10.1177/070674371205700303

Stern, J. S. (2018). Tourette's syndrome and its borderland. *Practical Neurology, 18*(4), 262–270. https://doi.org/10.1136/practneurol-2017-001755

Stewart, S. E., Hu, Y., Leung, A., Chan, E., Hezel, D. M., Lin, S. Y., Belschner, L., Walsh, C., Geller, D. A., & Pauls, D. L. (2017). A multisite study of family functioning impairment in pediatric obsessive-compulsive disorder. *Journal of the American Academy of Child and Adolescent Psychiatry, 56*(3), 241–249.e3. https://doi.org/10.1016/j.jaac.2016.12.012

Taylor, L. E., Swerdfeger, A. L., & Eslick, G. D. (2014). Vaccines are not associated with autism: An evidence-based meta-analysis of case-control and cohort studies. *Vaccine, 32*(29), 3623–3629. https://doi.org/10.1016/j.vaccine.2014.04.085

Thakur, A., Creedon, J., & Zeanah, C. H. (2016). Trauma-and stressor-related disorders among children and adolescents. *FOCUS (American Psychiatric Publishing), 14*(1), 34–45. https://doi.org/10.1176/appi.focus.20150026

Tonmyr, L., Williams, G., Hovdestad, W. E., & Draca, J. (2011). Anxiety and/or depression in 10–15 year-olds investigated by child welfare in Canada. *Journal of Adolescent Health, 48*(5), 493–498. https://doi.org/10.1016/j.jadohealth.2010.08.009

Torp, N. C., Dahl, K., Skarphedinsson, G., Thomsen, P. H., Valderhaug, R., Weidle, B., Melin, K. H., Hybel, K., Nissen, J. B., & Lenhard, F. (2015). Effectiveness of cognitive behavior treatment for pediatric obsessive-compulsive disorder: Acute outcomes from the Nordic Long-term OCD Treatment Study (NordLOTS). *Behaviour Research and Therapy, 64*, 15–23. https://doi.org/10.1016/j.brat.2014.11.005

Uchida, M., Spencer, T., Faraone, S., & Biederman, J. (2018). Adult outcome of ADHD: An overview of results from the MGH longitudinal family studies of pediatrically and psychiatrically referred youth with and without ADHD of both sexes. *Journal of Attention Disorders, 22*(6), 523–534. https://doi.org/10.1177/1087054715604360

Veale, D., & Roberts, A. (2014). Obsessive-compulsive disorder. *BMJ, 348*, g2183. https://doi.org/10.1136/bmj.g2183

Veloza-Gomez, M., Munoz de Rodriguez, L., Guevara-Armenta, C., & Mesa-Rodriguez, S. (2017). The importance of spiritual care in nursing practice. *Journal of Holistic Nursing, 35*(2), 118–131. https://doi.org/10.1177/0898010115626777

VinayaKumar, N. (2019). Impact of prenatal maternal stress on incidence of ADHD in children of Thiruvananthapuram district. *EPRA International Journal of Research and Development, 4*(11). https://doi.org/10.36713/epra2016

Vivan, A. d. S., Rodrigues, L., Wendt, G., Bicca, M. G., Braga, D. T., & Cordioli, A. V. (2014). Obsessive-compulsive symptoms and obsessive-compulsive disorder in adolescents: A population-based study. *Brazilian Journal of Psychiatry, 36*(2), 111–118. https://doi.org/10.1590/1516-4446-2013-1113

Volkar, F. R., Siegel, M., Woodbury-Smith, M., King, B., McCracken, J., & State, M. (2014). Practice parameter for the assessment and treatment of children and adolescents with autism spectrum disorder. *Journal of the American Academy of Child and Adolescent Psychiatry, 53*(2), 237–257. https://doi.org/10.1016/j.jaac.2013.10.013

Vuletic, B. (2017). Encopresis in children: An overview of recent findings. *Serbian Journal of Experimental and Clinical Research, 18*(2), 157–161. https://doi.org/10.1515/sjecr-2016-0027

Waddell, C., Shepherd, C. A., Schwartz, C., & Barican J. (2014). *Child and youth mental disorders: Prevalence and evidence-based interventions.* Children's Health Policy Centre, Simon Fraser University. http://childhealthpolicy.ca/wp-content/uploads/2014/06/14-06-17-Waddell-Report-2014.06.16.pdf

Webster-Stratton, C. (2011). *The incredible years: Parents, teachers and children's training series. Program content, methods, research and dissemination 1980–2011.* Incredible Years, Inc.

Wehry, A. M., Beesdo-Baum, K., Hennelly, M. M., Connolly, S. D., & Strawn, J. R. (2015). Assessment and treatment of anxiety disorders in children and adolescents. *Current Psychiatry Reports, 17*(7), 52. https://doi.org/10.1007/s11920-015-0591-z

Wood, C. (2020, February 04). *The UK media regulator says a 'Greta Thunberg effect' means more children are engaging in online activism.* Business Insider. https://www.businessinsider.com/greta-thunberg-effect-uk-children-online-activism-spikes-2020-2

Yang, C., Hao, Z., Zhu, C., Guo, Q., Mu, D., & Zhang, L. (2016). Interventions for tic disorders: An overview of systematic reviews and meta-analyses. *Neuroscience and Biobehavioral Reviews, 63*, 239–255. https://doi.org/10.1016/j.neurobiorev.2015.12.0.013

Zeanah, C. H., Chesher, T., Boris, N. W., Walter, H. J., Bukstein, O. G., Bellonci, C., Benson, R. S., Bussing, R., Chrisman, A., & Hamilton, J. (2016). Practice parameter for the assessment and treatment of children and adolescents with reactive attachment disorder and disinhibited social engagement disorder. *Journal of the American Academy of Child & Adolescent Psychiatry, 55*(11), 990–1003. https://doi.org/10.1016/j.jaac.2016.08.004

Zinck, S., Bagnell, A., Bond, K., & Newton, A. S. (2009). The Cochrane library and the treatment of major depression in children and youth: An overview of reviews. *Evidence-Based Child Health: A Cochrane Review Journal, 4*(4), 1336–1350. https://doi.org/10.1002/ebch.439

Mental Health of Older Adults: Promotion and Assessment*

Barbara Tallman and Wendy Austin

LEARNING OBJECTIVES

After studying this chapter, you will be able to:

- Explain how a health promotion focus relates to the assessment of the older adult.
- Discuss the relationship between mental health and healthy aging.
- Discuss the bio/psycho/social/spiritual domains in relation to late adulthood.
- Describe how health promotion can reduce the risks associated with chronic illness.
- Identify the importance of a functional ability assessment of the older adult.
- Describe the uniqueness of the older adult's presentation of health-related problems, such as frailty, depression, and risk for suicide.
- Analyze the nurse's role in mental health promotion with older adults and their families.
- Discuss mental health promotion and illness prevention interventions appropriate to the health challenges of older adults.
- Identify various techniques in the assessment of older adults presenting with functional changes.

KEY TERMS

- apraxia • cognitive reserve • deprescribing
- frailty • functional status • geriatric syndromes
- gerotranscendence • life expectancy • middle-old
- neuroplasticity • old-old • polypharmacy • young-old

KEY CONCEPTS

- age friendly • bio/psycho/social/spiritual nursing assessment: older adult • healthy aging • late adulthood

Introduction

"As holistic healthcare practitioners, nurses utilize their skills to care for the mental health and wellbeing of Canadians across the nation. Nurses are well positioned to drive improvements in mental health services delivery across all aspects of Canadian health care" (Canadian Nursing Association, 2021).

An area of health services that requires nurses' attention is that of healthy aging. The World Health Organization (WHO) has declared the years between 2021 and 2030 as *The Decade of Healthy Ageing* (WHO, 2021a). There are slightly more than 1 billion older adults globally, about 13.5% of the global population and, by 2030, 1 in 6 humans will be 60 years of age or older (WHO, 2021b). In their global strategy on aging, the WHO highlights the need to promote and maximize the health of the older population, identifying four action areas: age-friendly environments, combating ageism, integrated care, and long-term care. In a global systematic review on the impacts of ageism on health (422 studies from 45 countries), part of the WHO's *Global Report on Ageism* (2021b), it was found that ageism was associated with the worst outcomes in all health domains in 96% of the studies.

In Canada, seniors are defined as those individuals aged 65 years and older. Those over the age of 85 years are increasing in number, as older adults live longer and healthier with the average **life expectancy** being 82 years (Statistics Canada, 2021). It is predicted that older adults will make up more than 30% of the population by the year 2050 (Public Health Agency of Canada [PHAC], 2020a).

---

*Adapted, in part, from the chapter "Mental Health Assessment of the Older Adult: Promotion and Assessment" by Sharon L. Moore

Age friendly is a term used to describe practices and environments (including institutions, communities, and cities) that foster healthy, active aging through optimizing opportunities for a meaningful life and for safe, respectful engagement with others, participation in one's community, and opportunities to contribute to society.

In this chapter, the focus is on the mental health promotion and assessment of older adults and the related nursing strategies. It is based in *upstream thinking*, addressing the determinants of health of older adults before disease or injury occur. (*Downstream thinking* addresses care and treatment disease or injury do occur. See Chapter 32.) The bio/psycho/social/spiritual domains frame the factors that influence the mental health of older adults and shape their circumstances. This model structures holistic assessments and wellness strategies appropriate to the older adult. Nurses bring considerable skills to the promotion of the mental health of the older adult. The ability to develop and sustain sensitive, nonjudgmental interactions with these clients and those who are close to them is an important aspect of this skill set. The therapeutic nurse–client interaction is a key strategy that can foster hope and support older adults in sustaining meaning in life (Wiechula et al., 2016).

Goals for nurses working with this population include the promotion of wellness, optimization of functioning, and facilitation of quality of life to life's end (Melillo, 2017). Nurses, as members of interdisciplinary teams, work to optimize the strengths and functioning of older adults and to reduce or modify risk factors associated with mental illness (Clements-Cortés & Yip, 2020). They do so in a range of sectors in society: on the front lines, developing programs, educating clients about resources and their acquisition, and monitoring clients' physical and mental status to promote health and wellness.

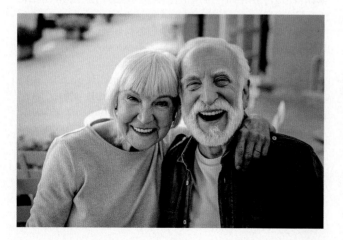

Mental Health Promotion of the Older Adult

First Nations Peoples in Canada have articulated a description of mental wellness that is meaningful across the life span and that focuses on strengths and resilience rather than deficits. As per the *First Nations Mental Wellness Continuum Framework*, mental wellness is described as a balance of the mental, physical, spiritual, and emotional. This balance is enriched as individuals have *purpose* in their daily lives, whether it is through education, employment, care giving activities, or cultural ways of being and doing; *hope* for their future and those of their families that is grounded in a sense of identity, unique indigenous values, and having a belief in spirit; a sense of *belonging* and connectedness within their families, to community, and to culture; and finally, a sense of *meaning* and an understanding of how their lives and those of their families and communities are part of creation and a rich history (Health Canada and Assembly of First Nations, 2015, p. 1). The Framework represents a call for nurses and all healthcare professionals to recognize that "cultural values, sacred knowledge, language, and practices of First Nations are essential determinants of individual, family, and community health and wellness" (Health Canada and Assembly of First Nations, 2015, p. 22). This framework captures well the concepts of mental wellness (as balance) and health promotion (as a focus on strength and resilience) and reflects the ideas and information shared in this chapter.

Mental health does involve the capacity to feel, think, and act in ways that enhance enjoyment of life and coping with challenges (PHAC, 2020a, 2021). Health is a state of physical, mental, and social wellbeing, not merely the absence of disease or infirmity. The WHO describes the outcome of a healthy aging process as the maintenance of functional ability that enables wellness in older age (WHO, 2017a). A challenge to this, however, is the projection that by 2041, adults between 70 and 89 years of age will have higher rates of mental illness and disorders (including dementia) than any other age group (MHCC, 2012). Urgent action in the promotion of mental health and the prevention of mental health issues is required for healthy aging to occur.

Healthy aging is a process that recognizes the life course as shaping health as we age. While there are changes, including some physical decline, such as decrease in sensory abilities and in pulmonary and immune functions, much does not change. The aim of healthy aging is for the adult to maintain functional ability that enables wellness in late adulthood.

Health promotion focuses on improving opportunities for people to embrace behaviours that promote optimal health and change those behaviours that increase risk for illness (WHO, 2021c). Promotion of mental health for those in late adulthood involves not only prevention of illness but support of maximum functioning and quality of life, including for those with preexisting mental illness. Characteristics of older adults are more varied than for other age groups, as they not only have varied genetic make-up and personalities, but differing experiences and challenges over the course of their lives. Although many Canadian older adults are living with a chronic health condition (Wengel et al., 2018), seventy percent report that they are in very good or excellent health, even when living with chronic disease (Statistics Canada, 2021).

Promotion of mental health in late adulthood involves consideration of the age category of the older adult, as well as the level of **functional status**, the ability to live independently. Distinctions exist between the **young-old** (65 to 74 years), **middle-old** (75 to 84 years), and **old-old** (85 years and older). The young-old and the middle-old benefit from programs that prevent chronic illness or that aim to reduce the symptoms of specific conditions, while the old-old, 50% of whom are categorized as frail, require support for increased vulnerability related to decline (Diehl et al., 2020). Chronological age can be an inaccurate description of the older adult because of their varied presentation. Functional status is a better descriptor.

When functional status declines, vulnerability to health risks increases. Such vulnerability was made very evident by the COVID-19 virus as seniors were inherently at risk for serious outcomes due to age-related decline in immunity and underlying chronic diseases and conditions (PHAC, 2021). The life situation of the older adult may need to change when functional status lessens to ensure that their environment can sustain their healthiest living. Options for older adults include home care, possibly with changes to the home (e.g., stair lifts); living with a family member; a suite in a retirement residence community with access to meals and other services; or long-term care, if supervised care is required (Feder, 2020). Financial costs will be a factor in any choice. According to the most recent data, the majority of Canadian seniors (92.1%) live in private dwelling in their community with almost one third of these living alone, while about 7.9% live in residential care facilities (i.e., residences for seniors; healthcare facility) (PHAC).

KEY CONCEPT

Late adulthood can be divided into three chronologic groups: *young-old* (ages 65 to 74 years), *middle-old* (ages 75 to 84 years), and *old-old* (age 85 years and older).

Ageism, unfortunately, is prevalent in Canadian society and worldwide (WHO, 2017a). It is represented in the negative stereotypes and myths associated with aging and in policies that do not consider the unique physical, social, and psychological needs of the older adult. Ageism is tolerated in Canadian society more than is prejudice related to gender or race. Most often—according to older adults—it takes the form of ignoring older adults or assuming that they are incompetent with nothing to contribute to society (Sheridan Centre for Elder Research, 2016). Such perspectives increase vulnerability and negatively impact the self-image of those in late adulthood, as does disparaging language used in descriptions of older adults, such as "being senile" (Ravary et al., 2020). A survey of over 1,500 Canadians found that 78% of older adults surveyed had experienced their complaints dismissed by healthcare professionals as simply part of aging (Sheridan Centre for Elder Research). This may be a factor in ageism's association with increased risk for chronic illness, including mental illness. For guidance in communicating effectively with older adults, see Box 31.1.

The capacity to feel, think, and act in ways that enhance enjoyment of life and coping with challenges is determined by the older adults' attributes and by their life circumstances. A life course perspective involves recognition that an individual's past experiences shape their understanding of their physical and mental status and of their social situation, as well as their perceptions of mental health and illness (WHO, 2017b). Older adults benefit from health promotion strategies at the social level as well as the personal level, including activities that promote age-friendly communities. The WHO's initiative for age-friendly cities involves policies, services, settings, and structures that support and enable active aging (Menec, 2017).

Health Promotion Strategies With the Older Adult

Health promotion strategies for the older adult can significantly impact their life trajectory. If the onset of chronic illness can be delayed, reducing its lifetime burden, it will extend the individual's years of healthy life. In other words, there will be a "compression of morbidity" (Fries et al., 2011). Addressing smoking and obesity, increasing exercise, promoting healthy eating, and moderating risks related to diabetes, heart disease, and hypertension, responsible use of substances, such as alcohol and cannabis, and attention to oral hygiene are ways to sustain health. The importance of physical activity (particularly aerobic activity) in middle-aged and older adults in reducing functional limitations and disability in later years has been known for some time (Paterson & Warburton, 2010). In Canada, there are resources to facilitate engagement in physical

BOX 31.1 Communicating With Older Adults

- Greet the older person by name.
- Invest time in a caring and respectful interaction.
- Focus the person's attention on the exchange of communication; the older adult may need extra time to begin to process information.
- Face the person when speaking to them.
- Minimize distractions in the room, including other people, objects in your hands, noise, and other activities.
- Reduce glare from room lighting by dimming too-bright lights. Conversely, avoid sitting in shadows.
- Speak slowly and clearly. Older adults may depend on lip reading, so ensure that the individual can see you. Speak loudly, but do not shout. It is not necessary to over enunciate with exaggerated lip movements.
- Use short, simple sentences and be prepared to repeat or revise what you have said.
- Limit the number of topics discussed at one time to prevent information overload.
- Ask one question at a time to minimize confusion. Allow plenty of time for the person to answer and express ideas.
- Frequently summarize the important points of the conversation to improve understanding and comprehension.
- Avoid the urge to finish sentences.
- If the communication exchange is going poorly, postpone it for another time.
- Encourage connectedness with like-minded persons.

activity, such as CSEP's Canadian guidelines of 24-hour movement for the adult 65 and over (see Web Links). Other ways to assist the older adult remain or become healthy are being explored. For instance, a home-based progressive resistance training program explored building muscle strength, muscle mass, and physical function in dynapenic older adults with low protein intake and included nutritional supplementation (de Carvalho Bastone et al., 2020).

While these strategies impact the older adult's mental health in positive ways, there are more focused strategies. A number of studies demonstrate that there is a relationship between health behaviours and improved cognitive functioning, as well as mood and wellbeing. As physical mobility, life satisfaction, and wisdom are attributes of the older adult associated with good cognitive function (Jeste, 2019), positive changes to cognition are highly desirable. Meditation-based training promotes healthy aging, particularly in the domains of emotions, cognition (e.g., attentional processes), and the preservation of related brain structures (e.g., grey matter brain structure) (Klimecki et al., 2019). Meditation with prayer and other spiritual practices have been found to help sustain or improve cognitive function, such as memory (Laird et al., 2018).

Other ways of sustaining cognitive functioning include "reminiscence" or "life story" opportunities for older adults to share aspects of their past and perhaps consider its effect on the present. Technologies such as conversational bots, or "chatbots," are being investigated for effectiveness in improving memory function. A chatbot is a computer program that supports interaction between people and technology. Originally, the communication was only text based. Now interaction by touch and voice is possible, such that chatbots, which are able to recognize voices, can simulate conversation. When chatbots were programmed to be humorous, memory recognition improved for the older adults interacting with them (Mundhra et al., 2021).

Life-long learning contributes to **neuroplasticity** and **cognitive reserve**. There are various approaches to fostering the different learning abilities and styles of the older adult to enable them to flourish in learning environments. The intergenerational classroom, for instance, provides an environment to expand the older adult's use of social media (Harvey et al., 2019). Older adults have shown a preference for human teachers; a study comparing older adults' recall and accuracy following learning from a computer versus learning from a human found that those taught by a human performed better (Crompton & Macpherson, 2019). Although there are not age-related differences in processing knowledge to learn a skill, older adults appear to engage differently with the material they are learning. They are more selective, requiring motivation ("How important is this information?"); desire meaningful content ("Why do I need to know this?"), and want familiarity with the idea or content.

In the Greek myth wherein Pandora gives in to her curiosity and opens the box that was a gift from the gods, releasing disease and pestilence upon the world, hope still remained. That was fortunate for us: hope is good for our health. In their meta-synthesis of hope, older adults, and chronic illness, Duggleby et al. (2012) found transcendence beyond current difficulties to be a major theme in how older persons coped and hoped.

Psychological interventions of hope/hopelessness in older adults have been systematically reviewed (*n* = 36 studies) with the conclusion that interventions based on cognitive–behavioural therapy (with or without antidepressants) and life review (including for those depressed, bereaving, or medically ill) significantly decreased hopelessness. Little to no support was evidenced for exercise, educational interventions (with medically ill individuals), or dignity therapy (with palliative care patients). Reviewers note that treating hope and hopelessness as separate but related constructs could further our knowledge of their trajectories and responses to intervention (Hernandez & Overholser, 2021). Nurses, when working with older adults on maintaining or improving their functional status and enjoying their lives, must remember the power of hope: it provides a reason to live, allowing the smallest ray of light to shine when the world looks its darkest.

Bio/Psycho/Social/Spiritual Mental Health Nursing Assessment: The Older Adult

A bio/psycho/social/spiritual assessment for older adults is similar to the assessment process presented in Chapter 11 but informed by a geriatric focus. A comprehensive assessment includes a health history and physical examination. Functional and cognitive abilities, as well as environmental and social supports, including housing, are noted. The identification of risk factors amenable to diet and behavioural change is an important strategy for optimizing the older adult's wellbeing.

KEY CONCEPT

A **bio/psycho/social/spiritual mental health nursing assessment for the older adult** is the comprehensive, deliberate, and systematic collection and interpretation of bio/psycho/social/spiritual data that are based on the special needs and problems of those in later adulthood to determine current and past health, functional status, and responses to mental health problems, both actual and potential.

Nurses need to be aware that in later adulthood, there is a potential for **geriatric syndromes**: "multifactorial health conditions that occur when the accumulated effect of impairments in multiple systems renders an older person vulnerable to situational challenges" (Stevenson et al., 2019, p. 8). These can complicate a comprehensive assessment as such conditions can go unrecognized, including frailty, sarcopenia (muscle wasting), anorexia and weight loss, depression, delirium, falls, cognitive dysfunction, and caregiver stress (Morley, 2017). Medication-related harm has been

added to the list of geriatric syndromes (Stevenson et al., 2019).

The geriatric syndrome of **frailty** is complex and describes the increased vulnerable state of the older adult. It is a result of the increasing impact of chronic illness (including chronic mental illness) and various other social and psychological factors (Jeste et al., 2021). Frailty increases the risk of injury related to falls, disability, depression, cognitive impairment, increased risk of hospitalization, and morbidity (CIHR, 2020). The frail older adult is often identified as having "nonintentional weight loss, exhaustion, low levels of physical activity, and slow gait" (Pinheiro et al., 2019, p. 597). Sarcopenia (the decrease in muscle mass) and dynapenia (loss of muscle strength) are changes in muscle not associated with neurological or muscle-related illness that contribute to frailty (O'Hoski et al., 2020; Sampaio et al., 2020). Older adults need to be assessed for frailty so it can be identified at prefrail and early frail levels, when the condition may be reversible. Addressing factors such as nutritional status can reduce the risks associated with frailty (Gonzalez-Colaço Harmand et al., 2017), as can identifying appropriate activities that have the potential to improve health status (Pilotto et al., 2020).

With life expectancy increasing, the prevalence of most chronic diseases in older adults will increase too, as will acute illness and functional decline (PHAC, 2021). These increases will be associated with increased risk for mental illness. Health promotion aims to decrease this risk and to extend optimal wellness and life. It intends to do so by preventing disease, disability, and frailty; managing comorbidities; and providing quality of life and dignity to those older adults requiring institutionalization (WHO, 2017b).

The Assessment Process

The first assessment step is to appraise whether or not the older client understands the nature and purpose of the assessment. An assessment report form is a useful aid. See Box 31.2 for an example of a bio/psycho/social/spiritual mental health nursing assessment form. The mental status assessment (MSA), as a "snapshot" of an individual's appearance, affect, behaviour, and cognitive function, remains an important tool. (Refer to Chapter 11 for an outline of the components of the MSA.) Box 31.2 contains a representative listing of common physiologic causes of changes in mental status. Self-report standardized tests, such as depression and cognitive functioning tools, may be part of the assessment process, as may laboratory tests (e.g., urinalysis may detect a urinary tract infection that is affecting a client's cognitive status).

Note that when diagnostic tests are used that a high *sensitivity* rating for the test indicates how confident we can be that those who test negative do not have the

BOX 31.2 Bio/Psycho/Social/Spiritual Geriatric Mental Health Nursing Assessment

I. Major reason for seeking help _____

II. Initial information

Name _____

Age _____ Current marital status _____

Gender identity _____ Caregiver (or N/A) _____

Living arrangements

III. Level of independence:

High (needs no help) _____

Moderate (lives independently but needs some help with instrumental activities) _____

Low (relies on others for help in meeting functional and instrumental activities) _____

Physical limitations _____

Level of education completed _____

	Normal	Treated	Untreated
Physical functions: system review	☐	☐	☐
Activity/exercise	☐	☐	☐
Sleep patterns	☐	☐	☐
Appetite and nutrition	☐	☐	☐
Hydration	☐	☐	☐
Elimination	☐	☐	☐
Existing physical illnesses	☐	☐	☐

List any chronic illnesses

Presence of pain (Use standardized instrument if pain is present.) No _____ Yes _____

Score _____ Treatment of pain _____

Medication (Prescription and Over the Counter)	Dosage	Side Effects	Frequency of Side Effects

Significant Laboratory Tests	Values	Normal Range

IV. Responses to mental health problems

Major concerns regarding mental health problem _____

Major loss/change in past year: No _____ Yes _____

Fear of violence: No _____ Yes _____

If yes, type of violence Source of violence _____

Strategies for managing problems/disorder _____

V. Mental status examination _____

General observation (appearance, psychomotor activity, attitude) _____

Orientation (time, place, person)

Mood, affect, emotions (Geriatric Depression Scale should be used if evidence of depression) _____

Speech (verbal ability, speed, use of words correctly) _____

Thought processes (hallucinations, delusions, tangential, logic, repetition, rhyming of words, loose connections, disorganized) (*Describe the content of hallucinations, delusions.*)

Cognition and intellectual performance (*Use standardized test scores as well as observations.*)

Attention and concentration _____

Abstract reasoning and concentration _____

Memory (recall, short term, long term) _____

Judgment and insight _____

(MMSE, CASI scores) _____

VI. Significant behaviours (psychomotor, agitation, aggression, withdrawn) (*Use standardized test if behaviours are problematic.*) _____

When did problem behaviour begin? Has it gotten worse?

VII. Self-concept (beliefs about self: body image, self-esteem, personal identity)

VIII. Risk assessment

Suicide: High _____ Moderate _____ Low _____

Assault/homicide: High _____ Low _____

Suicide thoughts or ideation: No _____ Yes _____

Current thoughts of harming self _____ Plan _____

Means _____

Means available

Assault/homicide thoughts: No _____ Yes _____

What do you do when angry with a stranger? _____

What do you do when angry with family or partner? _____

Have you ever hit or pushed anyone as an adult? No _____ Yes _____

Have you ever been arrested for assault? No _____ Yes _____

Current thoughts of harming others

IX. Functional status (*Use standardized test such as Functional Assessment Questionnaire.*) _____

X. Cultural assessment

Cultural group _____

Cultural group's view of health and mental illness _____

By what cultural rules do you try to live? _____

Special, cultural foods that are important to you _____

XI. Stresses and coping behaviours

Social support _____

Family members _____

Which members are important to you? _____

On whom can you rely? _____

Community resources _____

XII. Spiritual assessment _____

What brings happiness to your life? _____

Do you feel connected with the world? _____

Do you participate in religious activities or belong to a religious group or community? If so, would you like to include that information in this assessment? _____

Is there anything you would like to add about your spiritual needs or interests? _____

XIII. Economic status _____

XIV. Legal status _____

XV. Quality of life _____

Summary of significant data that can be used in formulating a nursing diagnosis:

SIGNATURE/TITLE _____ Date _____

disease; a high *specificity* rating indicates the degree of confidence we can have that those who test positive do have the disease. In addition, medical records from other healthcare providers are useful in developing a complete picture of the client's health status. Family members' descriptions of the older adult's health and lifestyle can be valuable: it adds relevant information and provides some insight into their concerns or lack of them. It is not uncommon, however, for the older adult and their family to offer contradictory information on the older adult's health status.

At the beginning of the assessment, the client's ability to participate needs to be assessed. For example, determine whether there are physical limitations, such as the client requiring the use of a wheelchair, that require adaptation of the assessment process. A client with compromised hearing will require the nurse to attend to voice projection and volume, lowering the pitch of their voice (higher-pitched sounds can be lost due to age-related hearing loss in both ears [presbycusis]), and to use clear enunciation while facing the client. Any aid to hearing should be in place and turned on. The pace of the interview is set by the client's ability to participate.

Techniques of Data Collection

It is essential in an assessment that the nurse sees the client alone for a period of time. This provides the client an opportunity to reveal concerns and issues, which they may not want to share with their family or caregiver. Aspects of the assessment (e.g., sexual health, intimate relationships, suicidal thoughts, paranoid ideas) are more readily completed one-to-one with the client. Exploring suspicions of neglect or abuse can take place at this time.

The mental health assessment of the older adult is addressed for each bio/psycho/social/spiritual domain within the following overview of the domains. It is important to recognize that a mental health assessment involves all domains. For instance, falls related to changes in the musculoskeletal system of an older adult may significantly affect mental health if they cause chronic pain, need for surgery, social isolation, or changes in living situation. A holistic approach to health assessment promotes a more genuine understanding of a client, allowing for appropriate treatment and care.

See Box 31.3 for an example of a therapeutic dialogue during an assessment interview.

The Bio/Psycho/Social/Spiritual Domains and the Older Adult

Overview of the Biologic Domain

Aging is a natural process and each stage of the process involves adapting to differing biological circumstances. The physiological and physical changes associated with

aging are interdependent with the familial, cultural, and societal messages transmitted through everyday life (see the Positive Mental Health Surveillance Framework in Chapter 2). Recognition of the adaptability and resilience of the older adult within their circumstances can foster their optimal functioning and mental health (Stephens et al., 2015). The biologic domain in late adulthood encompasses age-related changes, chronic health conditions and their atypical presentation, and the geriatric syndromes discussed above.

It has been found that 50% of older adults between 50 and 61 years of age are living with up to 3 chronic illnesses; 68% between 61 and 70 years are living with chronic conditions; and 81% over 71 years are doing so (Statistics Canada, 2021). Assessment of the older adult allows identification of changes in functional ability that can be key to recognizing and treating physical and/or environmental factors impacting their health. Of particular interest here is the impact on mental health. For instance, the anxiety disorders are associated with multi-morbidities, chronic pain, as well as lifetime smoking and other unhealthy behaviours (Davison et al., 2020). Following are selected examples of age-related changes and how they may affect the quality of life and mental health in older adulthood.

Coronary Artery Changes

Hypertension is diagnosed in 44% of Canadians over the age of 65 years (Statistics Canada, 2021). Hypertension increases the older adult's risk for depression; reducing hypertension can reduce such risk (Boima et al., 2020). Plaque buildup in the arteries, an age-related change, starts when people are about 30 years of age, causing pathological conditions such as atherosclerosis and coronary artery disease (CAD). Research indicates that strategies to reduce the symptoms of hypertension and improve self-management can be successful. For instance, a nurse-led study demonstrated that a 20-week program of educational and motivational sessions for older adults led to significant reduction of blood pressure, improved medication adherence, improved quality of life, and reduced weight of intervention group participants when compared to the control group (Kolcu & Ergun, 2020).

Hearing and Vision Changes

There are age-related deficits in hearing and vision that can have a significant impact on the older adult's function and quality of life, as well as increase risk for dementia and delirium (Livingston et al., 2020). Age-related changes in the auditory system (e.g., increased keratin production leads to impacted wax in the ear canal; stiffer, less responsive tympanic membranes leads to decreased capacity for full range of sounds) create communication problems, which ultimately affect social interaction.

BOX 31.3 THERAPEUTIC DIALOGUE

Assessment Interview

Tom, 79 years old, is being seen for the first time in a geriatric mental health clinic because of recent changes in his behaviour and his accusations that family members are trying to steal his house and car. He locked his wife out of the house, accusing her of being unfaithful. When Susan, the nurse assigned to his case, is conducting the assessment interview, Tom cooperates and is very pleasant until the nurse begins to assess the psychological domain.

Ineffective Approach

Nurse: Have there been times when you have had problems with any members of your family?

Client: No. (Silence)

Nurse: Have you noticed that lately you have been getting more upset than usual?

Client: No. Who has been talking to you?

Nurse: Your wife seems to think that you may be getting a little more upset than usual.

Client: You are just like her. She keeps telling me something is wrong with me. (Getting very agitated.)

Nurse: Please, I'm trying to help you. I understand that you locked your wife out of the house last week.

Client: Leave me alone. (Gets up and leaves.)

Effective Approach

Nurse: How have things been going at home?

Client: All right.

Nurse: (Silence)

Client: Well, my wife and I sometimes argue.

Nurse: Oh. Most husbands and wives argue. Any special arguments?

Client: No. Just the usual. I don't pick up after myself enough. I don't dress right to suit her. But, lately, she's gone a lot.

Nurse: She is gone a lot?

Client: Yeah! A lot.

Nurse: The way you say that, it sounds like you have some feelings about her being gone.

Client: You're damned right I do—and you would, too.

Nurse: I'm missing something.

Client: Well, if you must know, I think she's having an affair with the man next door.

Nurse: Really? That must upset you to think your wife is having an affair.

Client: I am devastated. I feel so bad.

Nurse: Would you say that you are depressed?

Client: Well, wouldn't you be? Yes, I'm feeling pretty low.

CRITICAL THINKING CHALLENGE

- How do the very first questions differ in the two interviews?
- What therapeutic techniques did the nurse use in the second interview to avoid the pitfalls the nurse encountered in the first scenario?
- How did the nurse in the second scenario elicit the client's delusion about his wife's affair?
- From the data that the second nurse gathered, how many of the client's problems can be identified?

Among individuals being treated at a memory clinic, researchers found that severity of hearing loss was associated with greater and more severe neuropsychiatric symptoms (NPS), as well as more severe depressive symptoms. Hearing aid use was correlated with fewer NPS, lower severity, and less severe depressive symptoms. Addressing hearing loss appears to be a low-risk, nonpharmacological way to prevent and treat NPS (Kim et al., 2021).

Age-related vision changes promote cataract formation, reported in 18.2% of older adults, with cataract surgery being the most common surgery in Canada (Statistics Canada, 2021). Assessing for retinopathy (particularly in those with diabetes), macular degeneration, glaucoma, and retinal detachment promotes early identification, which can decrease their impact on daily life.

Musculoskeletal System

Degenerative changes in the bones, muscles, joints, and connective tissue come with age and affect the mobility,

and thus lifestyle, of many older adults. Osteoarthritis—which 47% of Canadians over 65 report having—is associated with increased risk for falls (Quach & Burr, 2018). An evidence-based, preventive strategy for age-related falls is exercise (Grossman et al., 2018; Teng et al., 1994; see Web Links for further information at The Arthritis Society of Canada's website). Loss of bone mass (osteoporosis) increases the risk of fragility fractures and is the cause of 80% of fractures in adults over 50 (Osteoporosis Canada, 2019).

Age-Related Increase in Other Health Risks

Changes to the production of insulin increases the older adult's risk for diabetes, which in turn increases their risk for a number of other chronic illnesses, negatively affecting quality of life. **Polypharmacy** and alcohol consumption affect liver and kidney functioning, which, in turn, increases risk for adverse medication events. Polypharmacy is the term used when a person is taking five or more medications, taking unnecessary medications, or taking medications that cause more harm than benefits (Canadian Deprescribing Network, 2019). Polypharmacy can cause significant side effects, such as confusion, hypertension, falls, blurred vision, constipation, urinary retention, cognitive impairment, and other adverse reactions. Adverse drug interactions may cause delirium in older adults and constitute a medical emergency that may result in death (see Chapter 32).

The internationally recognized Beers Criteria identifies, in relation to older adults, potentially inappropriate medication, which needs to be used with much caution, harmful medication interactions, and medication, which may be adverse for those with poor renal function (American Geriatrics Society, 2015). An alternative to a medication on the Beers list may not be an alternative medication, but rather a nonpharmacologic strategy, such as a lifestyle change (Steinman et al., 2015).

Deprescribing involves the systematic assessment of the older adults' need for medication. This optimally results in a decrease in medications and medication-related adverse effects with improvement in quality of life (Canadian Deprescribing Network, 2019).

Alcohol consumption by older adults may be a means of managing pain (Brennan & Soohoo, 2013) or dealing with life stresses (e.g., health issues, retirement, loss of independence). Alcohol's effects on older adults vary related to age, health problems, and use of other medications. The Canadian Community Health Survey of 2019 revealed that, among Canadian 65 years and older, 10% of males and 4% of females met the definition of "heavy drinker"—5 or more drinks on one occasion if male; 4 or more if female—at least once a month over the past year (Statistics Canada, 2021). Physiological vulnerability and the incompatibility of alcohol with many medications taken by older adults increase the health risks of excessive drinking (National Institute on Aging, 2017b). Even low consumption of alcohol can be dangerous when taken with certain medications, and older adults may be taking multiple.

Sleep

Healthy older adults need 7 to 8 hours of sleep (National Sleep Foundation, 2021). Change in sleep patterns is part of aging, but recent changes in the sleep patterns of the older adult should be evaluated as to whether they are symptomatic of an underlying disorder. Sleep problems may be linked to the use of alcohol or other drugs and to psychiatric diagnosis. Insomnia, the inability to fall or remain asleep throughout the night, can be related to depression. Individuals with insomnia do not feel rested upon wakening and tired throughout the day, often leading to regular use of sleep medications. Clients with insomnia report that they cannot sleep at night and do not feel rested in the morning. (See Chapter 28.)

Sexual Health

Many older adults continue to have active and fulfilling sex lives (Mayo Clinic, 2020). There are physical changes that can affect one's ability to have and enjoy sex (e.g., vaginal dryness in women, often relieved by using a lubricant, and impotence or erectile dysfunction in men, often relieved by medication) (National Institute on Aging [NIA], 2017a). Consultation with a family physician or nurse can be useful as those in later adulthood may be reassured that sexual health issues are common at this stage of life, but most often are remediable. There are physical illnesses, disabilities, and medications that can cause sexual problems (NIA, 2017a, 2017b), such as arthritis, chronic pain, dementia, diabetes, heart disease, incontinence, surgery, mastectomy, and prostatectomy. There are strategies for each of these conditions that may alleviate worrisome symptoms and increase pleasure, performance, and desire. Research shows that sexually transmitted infections among the older population are rising, emphasizing that practicing safe sex is as important for older persons as for younger persons (Brandon, 2016).

As is true across the life span, the biologic domain of the older adult is shaped and influenced by each of the other domains, from having a positive attitude towards aging to possessing sufficient social support to sustaining a sense that one's life is meaningful. See Research for Best Practice Box 31.4.

Assessment of the Biologic Domain

A mental health assessment of an older adult in terms of the biologic domain involves conducting a physical and neurological assessment to rule out causes for changes in mental status. Results of laboratory tests are informative (e.g., urinalysis can detect a urinary tract infection that can affect cognitive status) and the client's medical records, including from other healthcare practitioners, are useful in developing a more complete picture of health status. A wide variety of physiologic disorders can cause changes in mental status for older adults (see Box 31.5). Coexisting medical problems and treatments add complexity to an assessment, as many symptoms of somatic disorders mimic or mask psychiatric disorders. (For example, fatigue may be related to anemia, but it also may be symptomatic of depression.) As older individuals are more likely to report somatic symptoms than psychological ones, the identification of a mental disorder becomes even more difficult (Wengel et al., 2018).

A thorough review of medications is essential in a geriatric assessment. A review of the medications of the older adult client, including over-the-counter medications, herbal supplements, and vitamins, is an important aspect of a biologic assessment. This is facilitated by asking the older adult for a complete list, including

BOX 31.4 Research for Best Practice

HOW DO VISUAL ART ACTIVITIES AND PHYSICAL EXERCISE AFFECT THE WELLBEING AND MOOD OF OLDER ADULTS?

Roswiyani, K., Kwakkenbos, L., Spijker, J., & Witterman, C. L. (2019). The effectiveness of combining visual art activities and physical exercise for older adults on wellbeing or quality of life and mood: A scoping review. *Journal of Applied Gerontology, 38*(12), 1784–1804. doi. org/10.1177/0733464817743332

The Question: What is understood about the effectiveness of the combination of visual art activities and physical exercise on older adults' wellbeing or quality of life and mood?

Methods: A scoping review of studies that focused on a combination of visual art activities and physical exercise for older adults was conducted within the following data bases: Embase, CINAHL, Ovid Medline, PsycINFO, and Web of Science. Examples of key words searched were *quilting, art therapy, painting, sculpting, crafts* and *Tai Chi, Qigong, exercise, yoga.* The research studies were critiqued. Of the 157 full-text articles assessed for eligibility, 10 articles met inclusion criteria. The primary outcomes of interest in the studies were physiological functioning,

cognitive performance, and pain reduction; secondary outcomes were wellbeing or quality of life or mood.

Findings: The health professionals delivering the interventions in the studies included physiotherapists, certified art psychotherapists, art therapists, nurses, physical trainers, or fitness instructors. This scoping review provided some empirical evidence for the usefulness of a combination of art activities and physical activities to improve the wellbeing or quality of life of the older adult. Evidence was found that depressive symptoms may be reduced with these strategies. The researchers note that the short duration of the interventions (1 to 2 hours, once or twice/week for 6 to 18 weeks) were suitable for the physical limitations of older adults.

Implications for Nursing: Older adults benefit from activities that foster their social engagement, their positive sense of self, and their agency. The value of appropriate physical and psychosocial interventions to support the mental health of the older adult needs to be recognized and adapted.

times taken. Information regarding any medication which clients have been taking until recently is also important; for example, they may have been using a monoamine oxidase inhibitor or suddenly stopped taking a prescribed medication such as a benzodiazepine or a selective serotonin reuptake inhibitor (see Chapter 13). Psychiatric medications have potentially serious side effects, such as lowering the seizure threshold, orthostatic hypotension, weight gain, sexual problems, and movement disorders (e.g., tremors, abnormal movements, shuffling). Conventional antipsychotics can cause tardive dyskinesia (TD) over time; early iden-

tification of this side effect is crucial to limiting it (refer further to Chapter 13). The Simplified Diagnoses for TD is to be found in Appendix D.

A further query is necessary regarding grapefruit juice. It contains naringin, a compound that inhibits the CYP3A4 enzyme involved in the metabolism of many medications (e.g., antidepressants, antiarrhythmics, erythromycin, several statins).

Box 31.6 provides a guide for nurses in the provision of drug therapy interventions with older adults.

Functional Status

Standardized assessments of activities of daily living (ADLs; e.g., dressing, grooming, walking) and instrumental activities of daily living (IADLs; e.g., managing finances, shopping, transportation) provide a description of the dependencies of the older adult being assessed, as well as baseline information to determine if treatment plans are improving their health. There are various approaches to determining the ADLs and IADLs of an individual. When possible, observation is best, rather than self-report or report of the family.

Common functional status assessment tools include the *Index of Independence in ADLs and the IADLs* (Katz & Akpom, 1976). *The Functional Activities Questionnaire (FAQ)* is based on the family's and caregiver's information and rates 10 complex, higher-order activities, such

BOX 31.5 Changes That Affect Mental Status

- Acid–base imbalance
- Dehydration
- Drugs (prescribed and over the counter)
- Delirium
- Electrolyte changes
- Hypothyroidism
- Hypothermia and hyperthermia
- Hypoxia
- Infection and sepsis

BOX 31.6 A Guide to Drug Therapy Interventions

- Administer priority/life essential medications first.
- Minimize the number of drugs that the person uses, keeping only those drugs that are essential.
- Always consider alternatives among different drug classifications or dosage forms that are more suitable for older adults. Monitor the claim trends for Beers drugs.
- Implement preventive measures to reduce the need for certain medications. Such prevention includes health promotion through proper nutrition, exercise, and stress reduction.
- Most age-dependent pharmacokinetic changes lead to potential accumulation of the drug; therefore, medication dosage should start low and go slow.
- Exercise caution when administering medication with a long half-life or in an older adult with impaired renal or liver function. Under these conditions, the time may be extended between doses.
- Be knowledgeable of each drug's properties, including such factors as half-life, excretion, and adverse effects. For example, venlafaxine HCl

(Effexor), a structurally novel antidepressant that inhibits the reuptake of serotonin and norepinephrine, requires regular monitoring of the older person's blood pressure.
- Assess the individual's clinical history for physical problems that may affect excretion of medications to assess for orthostatic hypotension and the potential for falls.
- Monitor laboratory values (e.g., creatinine clearance) and urinary output in clients receiving medications eliminated by the kidneys.
- Monitor plasma albumin levels in clients receiving drugs that have high binding affinity to protein.
- Regularly monitor the older person's reaction to all medications to ensure a therapeutic response.
- Look for potential drug interactions that may complicate therapy. Antacids lower gastric acidity and may decrease the rate at which other medications are dissolved and absorbed.
- Remind older adults to consult with their healthcare provider before taking any over-the-counter medications.

as writing cheques, assembling tax records, and driving (Pfeffer et al., 1982). *The Functional Autonomy Measuring System* (Hebert et al., 2002; McKye et al., 2009) is designed for use in a community setting and measures a person's actual performance on a task (e.g., performs task alone; with cueing or help; total help needed). Client and family reports can be used in completing it.

Overview of the Psychological Domain

In his psychosocial development model, the psychologist Erik Erikson identified "integrity versus despair" as a developmental task specific to late adulthood. An extension of his theory by his wife Joan Serson Erikson included old age as a ninth stage, **gerotranscendence** (Erikson & Erikson, 1997). Gerotranscendence (i.e., transcending being old), developed further by Tornstam (1989), is a psychosocial theory that regards aging as the final stage in a "possible natural progression towards maturation and wisdom" that can bring satisfaction and meaning in life (Tornstam, 2005, p. 1). Opportunities for continued development in dimensions such as inner strength and spirit are its focus, while losses in physical capacity and function and the possibility of despair are not addressed. The promotion of gerotranscendence for older adults suffering from depression needs to be explored (Rajani, 2015).

Cognitive Function

Cognition is "the mental action or process of acquiring knowledge and understanding through thought, experience, and the senses," with six key areas: perceptual motor function, language, learning and memory, social cognition, complex attention, and executive function (Giddens, 2021, p. 320). Changes in cognition are viewed primarily as the result of structural and functional changes in the brain, but external factors, including activity levels, socioeconomic status, education, personality, as well as adverse life events (e.g., death of a parent), may modify the development or the expression of age-related changes in cognition (Gold et al., 2021). While neuroimaging research has greatly advanced our knowledge of cognition, understanding age-related changes and differences in brain structure, activation, and functional connectivity remains highly challenging (Cabeza et al., 2018) and the relationship between these changes and brain functioning is not clear (Radanovic, 2020).

Memory declines occur in older adulthood. Working memory, the available information that can be used to solve problems, reason, and learn (Mattys & Baddeley, 2019), appears to decline in older adulthood. Episodic memory, which links conscious memories of an event to past, present, and future events, appears to decline as well (Shing & Lindenberger, 2011). However, semantic memory, memory related to knowledge gained through life's experience, remains stable or can improve (Rizzo et al., 2018). Most older adults are able to adjust to age-related changes, sustaining their functional status and carrying out day-to-day activities. This is possible through neuroplasticity, the brain's capacity to modify its connections and to regenerate and repair—essentially, to rewire itself. Neuroplasticity enables us to adapt and function in complex, changing environments as we learn from experience. It also aids brain recovery from damages due to stroke or traumatic injury (Mateos-Aparicio & Rodriguez-Moreno, 2019).

There is significant variability across individuals' cognitive aging trajectories, evidenced in longitudinal studies and most likely related to genetic and environmental differences (Cabeza et al., 2018). A reserve against brain impairment, **cognitive reserve**, is associated with increased strength in neural nets improving the brain's functional connectivity (Radanovic, 2020). Continuous lifelong learning and improved vascular health are associated with maintaining cognitive function (Cabeza et al.). Studies of cognitive function in the older adult are exploring how changes in motor performance speed (e.g., hand skill in a paper and pencil tasks) and impaired vision and hearing can influence measures of cognition (Ebaid et al., 2017).

Evidence that meditation-based training promotes healthy aging, particularly in the domains of emotions, cognition (e.g., attentional processes), and the preservation of related brain structures (e.g., grey matter structure) is building. However, more longitudinal research is required (Klimecki et al., 2019).

Memory

Age-related memory alterations are a widely studied aspect of cognition. Contrary to popular belief, memory loss is not a normal part of aging. To remember events, individuals must first attend to information and process it. Older adults may well dismiss information that is not important to them ("Why do I need to know this?"). Memory problems in later life are believed to result from encoding problems or "getting" the information in the first place. This problem may be related to sensory problems, not paying attention, or a general failure to link the "to-be-remembered" information to existing knowledge through association or to strengthen the memory through repetition. It is important not to confuse decline with deficit. Although a decline in memory ability may be frustrating for the older individual, it does not necessarily hamper their ability to function daily. Threats to memory include medications, depression (impairs concentration and attention), poor nutrition, infection, heart and lung disease (results in lack of oxygen), thyroid problems (can cause depressive symptoms or confusion mimicking memory loss), alcohol use, and sensory loss (interferes with perception).

Resiliency

Resiliency is a trait characterized by the ability to adjust to the challenging circumstances of life (Constantino, 2020). It is associated with self-efficacy, a belief that one's actions can lead to goal achievement. Older adults, perhaps because of life experience, tend to show as much or more resilience than younger adults. A systematic review of the research found that previous experience, social support, and spirituality were the common factors related to resilience in older adults following a disaster (Timalsina & Songwathana, 2020). Research has noted that after a disaster, spirituality was a predictor among older adults of resilience, decreasing vulnerability and trauma levels, and enhancing a sense of self-worth (Almazan et al., 2018). Higher levels of neuropsychological functioning in older adults are associated with more frequent use of compensation strategies. Behaviours aimed at mitigating or adapting to loss such as writing lists, proactively seeking assistance, or performing tasks in an alternate manner support memory and executive function. Significantly, higher frequency of compensation strategies in daily life (observed by a knowledgeable informant) correlate with higher levels of independent functioning, even when level of cognition is controlled as a factor (Farias et al., 2018).

Depression

Depression is not a normal part of aging, yet it is the most common mental disorder in older adults (Centers for Disease Control and Prevention [CDC], 2021) and is associated with the following risk factors: loss of spouse, physical illness, education below high school, impaired functional status, and heavy alcohol consumption. In older people, other disorders may mask depression. When symptoms are present, they may be attributed to aging or atherosclerosis or other age-related problems. Older clients are less likely to report feeling sad or worthless than are younger clients. As a result, family members and primary care providers may overlook depression in older adults. Depressive symptoms are much more common than a full-fledged depressive disorder, as characterized by the *Diagnostic and Statistical Manual of Mental Disorders-5* (American Psychiatric Association, 2013). Untreated depression in older adults may result in the overuse of healthcare services, longer hospital stays, decreased treatment compliance, and increased morbidity and mortality (Gilmour & Ramage-Morin, 2020).

Assessment of the Psychological Domain

Cognitive Functioning

An assessment of the cognition of the older adult is recommended as part of the regular clinical care of the older adult (Nguyen & Lee, 2020). Older adults are often aware of changes in working memory and episodic memory. Subjective recognition of memory changes should be assessed as a condition called mild cognitive impairment (MCI), which may be a prodromal sign of dementia. There is increasing evidence that early identification of MCI can lead to risk reduction strategies that inhibit further decline (Chehrehnegar et al., 2020). While there is no standard measure to detect MCI, the Montreal Cognitive Assessment is used to screen for cognitive decline and sensitive to early changes (Rosenweig, 2022). A commonly used screening tool is the Mini Mental State Exam (MMSE) for which a score below 24 of 30 has sensitivity (80% to 90%) and specificity (80%) for discriminating between those with and without dementia. Research indicates that education may have a protective effect against cognitive decline in early-stage MCI, but that this effect disappears in late-stage MCI (Ye et al., 2013).

When interpreting the score, a cognitive assessment must take into account the older adult's educational and cultural background and first language when interpreting the score. Older adults with depression or depressed symptoms can score lower on a test score than is their actual ability. A screening test is one step in the assessment process. Further assessment of cognitive function using more detailed testing by a psychologist may be important. (For assessment of the critical cognitive disorder of delirium and the debilitating disorder of dementia, see Chapter 32.)

Behaviour Changes

Behaviour changes in older adults can indicate neuropathologic processes. Such changes will be likely noticed by family members, before the older adult does. **Apraxia** (the inability to execute a voluntary movement despite normal muscle function) is not attributed to age but indicates an underlying disease process, such as Alzheimer disease, Parkinson disease, or other disorders. Behaviour problems associated with psychiatric disorders in older individuals include irritability, agitation, apathy, and euphoria. Wandering and aggressive behaviours are sometimes noted in older adults experiencing psychiatric problems.

Depression

With older adults, it may be challenging to distinguish symptoms of depression from other common medical conditions. While low energy is associated with depression in the older adult, it is associated with a myriad of other conditions common to older adults. There can be unique presentation of somatic symptoms (e.g., abdominal pain, musculoskeletal pains, headaches). Diagnosing depression does not, therefore, focus only on mood and cognition. A complete medical examination and evaluation is required. A first diagnosis of depression for an individual in late adulthood has some serious implications. It is associated with a twofold increased risk for Alzheimer disease (Wengel et al., 2018), as well as increased odds for adverse outcomes such as admission to long-term care and death of the depressed individual (Strauss et al., 2020).

The CDC (2017) reports that "Someone who is depressed has feelings of sadness or anxiety that last for weeks at a time. They may also experience

- Feelings of hopelessness and/or pessimism
- Feelings of guilt, worthlessness and/or helplessness
- Irritability, restlessness
- Loss of interest in activities or hobbies once pleasurable
- Fatigue and decreased energy
- Difficulty concentrating, remembering details and making decisions
- Insomnia, early morning wakefulness, or excessive sleeping
- Overeating or appetite loss
- Thoughts of suicide, suicide attempts
- Persistent aches or pains, headaches, cramps, or digestive problems that do not get better, even with treatment" (p. 3)

The Geriatric Depression Scale (GDS) is a useful screening tool with demonstrated validity and reliability (Hyer & Blount, 1984). The GDS was designed as a self-administered test, although it has been used in observer-administered formats. One advantage of the test is its "yes/no" format, which may be easier for older adults than the Hamilton Rating Scale for Depression (see Appendix E), which uses a scale from 0 to 4. This tool is easy to administer and provides valuable information about the possibility of depression (Box 31.7). If results are positive, the nurse should refer the client to a psychiatrist or advanced practice nurse for further evaluation.

Among residents in long-term care facilities, the usefulness of the GDS depends on the degree of cognitive impairment. Residents who are mildly impaired may be able to answer yes/no questions; however, moderately to severely impaired older adults will be unable to do the same. A well-validated scale for individuals with dementia is the Cornell Scale for Depression in Dementia (CSDD) (Alexopoulos et al., 1988). The CSDD is an interview-administered scale that uses information from both the client and an outside informant (Refer also to Chapter 22).

Thought Processes

Thought processes and content are critical in the cognitive assessment of older adults. Can the client express

1. Are you basically satisfied with your life?	Yes	No
2. Have you dropped many of your activities and interests?	Yes	No
3. Do you feel that your life is empty?	Yes	No
4. Do you often get bored?	Yes	No
5. Are you in good spirits most of the time?	Yes	No
6. Are you afraid that something bad is going to happen to you?	Yes	No
7. Do you feel happy most of the time?	Yes	No
8. Do you often feel helpless?	Yes	No
9. Do you prefer to stay at home rather than go out and do new things?	Yes	No
10. Do you feel you have more problems with memory than most?	Yes	No
11. Do you think it is wonderful to be alive now?	Yes	No
12. Do you feel pretty worthless the way you are now?	Yes	No
13. Do you feel full of energy?	Yes	No
14. Do you feel that your situation is hopeless?	Yes	No
15. Do you think that most people are better off than you are?	Yes	No

*Score:*____/15 One point for "No" to questions 1, 5, 7, 11, 13

One point for "Yes" to other questions

Normal	3 ± 2
Mildly depressed	7 ± 3
Very depressed	12 ± 2

Adapted from Sheikh, J. I., & Yesavage, J. A. (1986). Geriatric Depression Scale (GDS): Recent evidence and development of a shorter version. In T. L. Brink (Ed.), *Clinical gerontology: A guide to assessment and intervention* (pp. 165–173). Haworth Press. © By the Haworth Press, Inc. All rights reserved. Reprinted with permission.

ideas and thoughts logically, as well as understand questions and follow the conversation of others? If there is any indication of hallucinations or delusions, the content of these should be explored. If the client has a history of mental illness, such as schizophrenia, these symptoms may not be new and further information from health records, family, or caregivers will be required. Suspicious and delusional thoughts may characterize dementia.

Stress and Coping Patterns

Identifying stresses and coping patterns is important across all age groups. Unique stresses for older clients include living on a fixed income, handling declining health and abilities, losing partners and friends, and ultimately confronting death. Coping ability varies depending on the clients' unique circumstances, as is true for everyone. The range of response to severe stress by older adults is from amazing adaptability to becoming depressed and suicidal (MHCC, n.d.).

Suicide Risk Assessment

Older adults at risk for suicide often seek medical help prior to their decision to suicide. Most older individuals who die by suicide have visited their family physician within the month of their death (Gregg et al., 2013). When caring for the older client with mental health problems, the individual's potential to die by suicide must always be considered. Depression is the greatest risk factor for suicide (see Chapters 20 and 22). The following characteristics are indications of high risk for committing suicide:

- Depression
- Previous suicide attempts
- Family history of suicide
- Firearms in the home
- Abuse of alcohol or other substances
- Unusual stress
- Chronic medical condition (e.g., cancer, neuromuscular disorders)
- Feelings of helplessness and hopelessness
- Feelings of being a burden to others
- Social isolation

Overview of the Social Domain

The social domain are those aspects of the older adult's circumstances that are structured by society. Retirement is an example. Work significantly structures an individual's life and in some ways may define them. In Canada, it is not unusual, when getting acquainted with someone new, to ask early in the conversation: "So, what do you do?" This is essentially asking, "Who are you?" Work allows one to make a contribution to society and becomes a component of one's self-esteem. It can become significant to one's social life, particularly if most friends are workmates. Although support for delaying retirement is increasing (e.g., pension incentives), ageism and the social expectation that one retires when they reach late adulthood still exists. In some workplaces ageist attitudes may survive, particularly if there are not policies that support intergenerational dialogue and integration. Employers need to be sensitive to the presence of aging stereotypes that can be detrimental to all workers (Lagacé et al., 2019). Research has found that ageism created lower job satisfaction, lower self-rated health, and a higher level of symptoms of depression for older adult employees; policies that can help prevent ageism from occurring will contribute to workplace efficiency, as well (Marchiondo et al., 2019).

Social Connection

Social connectedness is "a subjective evaluation of the extent to which one has meaningful, close, and constructive relationships with others (i.e., individuals, groups, and/or society)" (O'Rourke & Sidani, 2017, p. 43). It is the opposite of social isolation and loneliness. Aging, however, brings many identity and social changes. An ability to express oneself in a way that fosters new and continuing social connections is an asset for older adults in sustaining an ongoing sense of identity. When cognitive and/or physical decline begins to occur, some older adults experience lower self-worth, which can negatively affect wellbeing and create stress. Those with the ability to selectively attend to positive aspects of their social environment will be able to adjust more readily to changes than those who do not (Ravary et al., 2020).

The Government of Canada's Working Group on Social Isolation and Social Innovation acknowledges that "the social and economic contributions of older adults will likely be increasingly connected to the success of the entire country" (Government of Canada, 2017, p. 4). Strategies to prevent and mitigate social isolation of older adults will benefit everyone.

Does one's social community impact daily living? Research from 2011 to 2018 with over 7,400 participants in the National Health and Aging Trend Study, USA, explored whether neighbourhoods' social cohesion or physical disorder (litter on sidewalks; graffiti on walls; vacant homes or stores) affected ADL and IADL. The answer is that neighbourhood social cohesion is associated with fewer limitations in ADL and IADL, while physically disordered neighbourhoods are associated with more IADL limitations. The conclusion drawn from these results was that the social and physical aspects of neighborhood environment impact the daily lives and activities of older adults (Qin et al., 2021).

Relationships

Belonging to a family is a significant aspect of an individual's life. For older adults, families can be a valuable resource as a significant sense of connection, relatedness, and belonging, as well as a source of support and caregiving as one approaches closer to life's end. A sense of being valued and needed can be found among families, such as when caring for grandchildren or providing a place of respite for troubled relatives. This is true, as well, for those who, due to loss or by choice, create a family from close friends. As family relationships change due to physical and social distance, death, divorce, or other factors, new relationships may evolve. The composition of the family transitions over time and is context specific. Those who have been socially excluded across their lifetime, due to being viewed "different" in some way (such as due to race, culture, sexuality, gender identity, or other social factors; see Chapter 3), may have found or created a supportive community outside of the mainstream population that will be significant to them, including as older adults.

Dating is a strategy many older adults are exploring. Online dating sites are potential facilitators of this strategy, increasing the number of contacts who are identified as compatible prior to meeting in-person. Dating sites used by Canadian older adults include Zoosk, Elite Single, Match, eHarmony, and OurTime, with many of these sites with filters to enable searching for faith-based or gay and lesbian matches. Online connections, however, are not without risk. Personal information can be compromised, opening the individual up to various scams, including financial scams (e.g., initiating an online relationship for a few months and then asking for money for an emergency or for trip expenses to meet the person; Wion & Loeb, 2015). Nurses can offer an older adult ways to be safer online, if during an assessment the question, "Are you dating or interested in dating?" receives a positive reply. For example, they can recommend the use of an easily discarded email address that does not reveal personal information and/or the use of a public place for a first meeting. Nurses need to reflect on their own biases regarding dating and romance for seniors to ensure that they are not acting in a judgmental way.

Loneliness

Loneliness is defined as distress resulting from differences between actual and desired social relationships (Hawkley & Cacioppo, 2010). Social isolation and loneliness are related, but individuals may be socially isolated and not lonely (Yu et al., 2020). Loneliness is associated with increased risk for mental illness—and mental illness can put one at risk for loneliness. Loneliness can shorten one's life. There are several risk factors for loneliness and social isolation: living alone, being age 80+, having compromised health status or multiple chronic health problems, having no children or contact with family, lacking access to transportation, and living on a low income. Females are more likely to be lonely than males (PHAC, 2020a, 2021). If one's spouse, partner, siblings, and friends are members of the older adult's generation and have reached older adulthood, too, the likelihood of loss and bereavement is more likely for the individual.

The health problem of loneliness impacts health services: lonely people have increased use of inpatient care, more healthcare provider visits, increased rehospitalizations, and longer lengths of stay. There is a role for healthcare practitioners to play in the identification of those at risk for or already experiencing isolation and/or loneliness (National Academies of Sciences, Engineering, and Medicine, 2020; WHO, 2021d). There are healthcare interventions to address such risk: cognitive–behavioural interventions, social training, and befriending, in person or by digital means, can be helpful. There are system-level interventions as well, including improving infrastructure to make connection via transport or digital means readily available for all; the promotion of age-friendly communities; and policies and laws to support such changes (WHO, 2021c).

Diversity

The Canadian population is becoming more culturally diverse and heterogeneous. First Nations, immigrants, refugees, ethnocultural and racialized groups, as well as historically marginalized identities such as Black, Indigenous, People of Colour (BIPoC), and lesbian, gay, bisexual, trans, queer (or questioning), intersex, two-spirit, and asexual (LGBTQI2SA+) are becoming more visible in Canadian society. This is, of course, increasingly true for the senior community and for healthcare personnel. Canadian healthcare professionals and workers have the obligation to perform their responsibilities in safe and appropriate ways, adapting care as much as possible to the personal, familial, social, and cultural needs of the client.

Poverty

The average income (after tax) of senior families (highest earner: 65 years plus) was $63,500 in 2018 (Statistics Canada, 2020). Canada's aim to reduce poverty resulted in the development of *Opportunity for All—Canada's First Poverty Reduction Strategy 2018*, with targets aligned with the United Nations Development goals to end poverty (Employment and Social Development Canada [ESDC], 2018). According to ESDC, based on the 2018 Canadian Income Survey, over 1 million Canadians, including 73,000 seniors, have risen out of poverty since 2015, with the poverty rate continuing its downward trend. Actions taken since 2018 include an increase to the Guaranteed Income Supplement top-up benefit, to improve the financial security of vulnerable

IN-A-LIFE 🏠

Lynne Mitchell-Pedersen, Outstanding Canadian Nurse

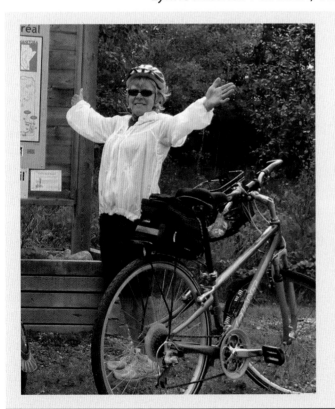

LYNNE MITCHELL-PEDERSEN

Lynne is a trail blazer in Canadian Gerontological Nursing. As the founding president of the Canadian Gerontological Nursing Association (CGNA) in 1983, Lynne has profoundly influenced and shaped the history of Gerontological nursing in Canada, an achievement noted when she was selected as a keynote speaker for the 2017 CGNA biennial conference. She along with Dr. Colin Powell and her nursing colleagues were instrumental in orchestrating the diminution of the use of physical restraints in the care of older people. Lynne brought a world of compassion and caring to understanding and problem-solving around "vocalizing" behaviour of residents in personal care, facilitating more responsive staff caring to the so-called difficult behaviour. Lynne did the Ascent for Alzheimer's, a climb of Mount Kilimanjaro in Africa, the highest free-standing mountain in the world. Lynne loves the great outdoors and, at the age of 75 years, completed a 1,400 km bike trip on the Trans Canada Trail across Manitoba. Lynne continues to inspire nurses, colleagues, family, and friends as she continues to make a difference in the world.

seniors (close to 900,000). Nevertheless, the organization, Canada Without Poverty, reports on their website that nearly 15% of single older adults in Canada live in poverty. Poverty has significant effects on those in late adulthood, including increased health problems and mortality rates and lower health-related quality of life.

Assessment of the Social Domain

An assessment of the social domain includes understanding the client's social resources, including relationships with family, friends, and neighbours—or the lack of them. Does the client live alone or with others, reside in a single dwelling, in a retirement community, in an assisted living facility, or in long term care? The characteristics of the community in which the client resides (e.g., safe; cohesive; disordered) and the way it impacts the client's daily life are important to understand as it informs the nurse regarding their day-to-day challenges. How does the client feel about their way of life?

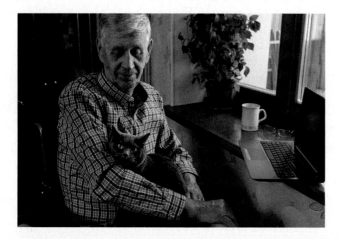

Social Support

The role of social support is critical to assess in this age group. Connections with others can be affected by such factors as location (ease of access, safety, availability of transport and means of communication); health (mobility, self-esteem, shyness); and socioeconomics (potential for poverty, shame, fear). During the isolation of COVID-19, Canadian communities were reminded to be aware of the wellbeing of their older adult neighbours and their potential need for support and assistance (e.g., access to groceries and health care) (Miller, 2020). Communication can be supported by telephone, online connections, and postal services; the internet, radio, and television offer connection to news, weather, and entertainment. The ability to afford the necessary technology and service charges, however, can be a significant factor for some older adults.

For specific information regarding the social support available to the client, the following questions can be helpful, if asked with genuine interest and not in an intrusive way.

- Who are the people that you see or speak with most often? Do you get to connect with family members regularly? With friends? Do you reach out to others?
- Do you have a special person you can call or contact if you need help? Who would that be? Do you have a neighbour with whom you are comfortable in asking for assistance? (For instance, for a ride to your physician's office for an appointment, or to help you carry something?)

Opening dialogue about the quality of relationships with family and others will allow a deep understanding of the client's social support. Tallman (2019), in a study focused on the relationships of couples where one spouse experienced dementia, found that couples make efforts toward mutuality in their relationships with one another. Relational practice is suggested as a strategy to promote the wellbeing of couples living with dementia. Furthermore, it is important to understand the individual's assessment will be influenced by their expectations of others. For instance, a person whose attentive daughter visits her daily may feel neglected, while another person whose son lives out-of-province feels well connected and "only a phone call away!" For older clients who are isolated with few social contacts, there will be resources and community services which nurses can use to improve the individual's access to social support.

Older adults who believe that they can and do contribute to the welfare of others are most likely to remain mentally healthy. For this reason, pets are often "life-savers" for older adults who live alone. Robotic animals (e.g., dogs, cats, rabbits, and seals) have been designed to respond with gestures and sounds to interact with older adults, including those with cognitive impairment. Pet robots can have a positive effect (e.g., reduce feelings of loneliness and stress and improve quality of life) on older adults living in nursing homes when compared with control groups without actual animal pets. Sensors can be included in the robotic pet that permit the assessment of the older adult, including an alarm system when deterioration is noted (Preuß & Legal, 2017).

Social Systems

Community resources are essential to an older adult's ability to maintain mental health and wellness, as well as to their ability to remain in place throughout the later years. Senior centres are community resources that provide an array of services to Canada's older population. Healthy, balanced daily meals at a nominal cost may be available, as well as opportunities for socialization, vaccine clinics, and educational events on health topics (e.g., health promotion strategies) and other selected topics of interest (e.g., travel, books, local political issues). Some centres will have programs such as geriatric assessment clinics and adult day programs.

The financial sources and situation of an older adult client may be directly affecting their health. The amount available to the older adult may be inadequate to support healthy living; finances may be a source of worry and stress. This is the reason for its assessment and should be explained to the client so the request for this information does not come as an invasion of privacy. A number of older adults rely on Canada Pension Plan (or for older adults living in Quebec, the Quebec Pension Plan), Old Age Security, and Guaranteed Income Supplement as their only source of income. If financial assistance is required, an appropriate referral for guidance (e.g., social work; public trustee) should be made.

The nurse should ask the client about accessible healthcare facilities; available transportation to and from healthcare facilities; formal supports such as physicians, nurses, and other healthcare professionals; and the client's ability to pay for medications and health aids. Information about available healthcare resources beyond standard provincial healthcare (e.g., plans to pay for additional services such as medications or foot care) will alert the nurse to what services the client currently can and cannot access. In urban areas that are likely to have adequate healthcare resources, cultural and language barriers may prohibit access. People who live in rural areas where healthcare resources are limited are less likely to enjoy the full range of healthcare resources than are those in urban areas. Initiatives of the Mental Health Commission of Canada (MHCC) and its Seniors Advisory Committee involve strategies aimed at reducing the stigma of mental illness and aging.

Legal Status

A growing trend in Canada and the United States is to view older adults as a special population whose rights deserve increased attention and protection. Elder abuse (psychological and/or physical) and neglect is a serious issue and nurses must be vigilant in recognizing their signs, such as unexplained injuries (see Chapter 34). At times there are attempts, usually on the part of a family member, to usurp the rights of the older adult. Note that unless the senior is medically and legally determined to be incompetent, they have all the rights to personal decision-making as any other adult, including the right to refuse treatment. See Web Links for access to the Canadian government's Department of Justice's explanation of the legal definitions of abuse and neglect across Canada.

Overview of the Spiritual Domain

Victor Frankl (1963) proposed in his landmark work, *Man's Search for Meaning*, that this search was the main purpose of human life, achieved through experiences and accomplishments in the world and by our attitude towards suffering. Spirituality can be understood as an intimate relation with a transcendent force that brings respect and value to oneself and to relations with others (Tomás et al., 2016). For many, it is expressed through commitment to organized religion, but others find different means of expression. Aging is a process that can bring individuals closer to understanding the finite nature of existence, evoking an awareness of their spiritual needs. With advanced age, many people begin to reflect on their successes and failures. During such reflection, many seek out God or a higher being to make sense of the past and establish hope for the future. Nurses can support the client in exploring the meanings that a particular life change has for them. In later life, existential issues, such as experiencing losses, redefining meanings in existence, and finding and nurturing hope, replace, on the whole, the performance and future orientation that characterize earlier adulthood. There is growing evidence of the significance that spirituality plays in successful aging (Harrington, 2016).

Spiritual care in nursing is situated within the nurse–client relationship and involves a sense of being-with and being-for the client as a means of promoting spiritual comfort, hope, and wellbeing (see Chapter 12). Recognition of the significance of older adults' spiritual practices is an important component of their care and fosters wellness.

Assessment of the Spiritual Domain

While some nurses may hesitate to engage with older adults regarding their spiritual needs, the process of spiritual assessment primarily involves active listening, thoughtful observing, and sensitive questioning. When clients raise existential questions (e.g., about the meaning of suffering, forgiveness, or life's worth), they are not expecting a "right" answer. Primarily such questions are asking for a conversation, a sharing of thoughts about life and death that do not come up in everyday conversation. While a referral to pastoral care may be offered, nurses should not avoid engaging with the client at such times. Responses such as, "You seem to have thought about this for a while; will *you* share with me what *you* think?" may deepen understanding of the client's spiritual needs.

There are helpful spiritual resources. *The FICA History Tool*—developed to be used by hospital-based nurses and recommended by the Hartford Institute for Geriatric Nursing in their "Try This: Series"—is freely available (see Web Links). A spiritual assessment allows exploration of the individual's need for spiritual resources (e.g., a prayer rug; an icon) or support (e.g., a clerical visit; a ritual).

🍁 Summary of Key Points

- The aging of the Canadian population is a significant force shaping our society.
- Late adulthood is conceived as having three chronologic groups: young-old (65 to 74 years), middle-old (75 to 84 years), and old-old (85 years and older).
- Aging is associated with some physical decline, but most functions do not change. Intellectual functioning, capacity for change, and productive engagement with life remain.
- Cognitive changes with aging are, for the most part, accounted for by structural and functional changes in the brain, with external factors (e.g., activity levels, socioeconomic status) also having an effect.
- Threats to memory in older persons include medications, depression, poor nutrition, infection, heart and lung disease, thyroid problems, alcohol use, and sensory loss.
- Nurses need to recognize that older persons may need more time to process information and that they tend to focus on accuracy in their answers rather than on giving a prompt reply.
- Aging affects pharmacokinetics, including drug absorption, distribution, metabolism, and excretion, and nurses need to know the drug therapy implications of such changes.
- Gerotranscendence is a concept related to aging in which spiritual growth and the development of inner strength is emphasized over decrements in functioning.
- The majority of Canadian seniors wish to "age in place" and need adequate support to do so.
- Risks to health during this phase of the life span include chronic illness, polypharmacy, loss and bereavement, poverty, and social isolation. The latter has been associated with suicide.
- Older persons experience many physical changes, but they can remain sexually active.

- Mental health assessments are necessary when older clients face psychiatric or mental health issues. The bio/psycho/social/spiritual geriatric mental health nursing assessment examines many sources of data, including self-reports, laboratory test results, and reports from family members.
- The bio/psycho/social/spiritual geriatric mental health nursing assessment is based on the special needs and problems of older individuals. This assessment examines current and past health, functional status, and human responses to mental health problems taking into account social support, spiritual needs, legal issues, and quality of life.
- The assessment of the biologic domain involves collecting data about the past and present health status, physical examination findings, physical functions (i.e., nutrition and eating, elimination patterns, sleep), pain, exercise, and pharmacologic information.
- The assessment of the psychological domain includes the client's responses to mental health problems, mental status examination, behavioural changes, stress and coping patterns, and risk assessment.
- There are a number of screening tools that nurses can use to complement a comprehensive assessment (for activities of daily living and cognitive and mental health issues).
- Coping with stresses and transitions vary among older adults. Determining stresses and coping skills along with the meaning of these stresses is important.
- Assessing and intervening with older adults should always occur within a climate of respect and recognition for his/her life history and experience and ability to be part of the process.
- Nurses can play a significant role in the mental health promotion of older persons and in supporting them and their families in living meaningful, hopeful lives.

🧠 Thinking Challenges

1. Gerald is 72 years old, living alone since his wife, Maureen, died 2 years ago. The community nurse wants to promote Gerald to become more active, not only physically, but socially as well. Gerald has continued to attend church services on Sunday but no longer goes to other activities for the congregation. If you were the community nurse, what would your initial plan be to help Gerald get physically moving and socially connecting with others?
2. As a nurse you have made a home visit to Gerta, who is 79 years old and lives with her daughter, Heidi, and her family. You find Gerta to be thriving, keeping active through walking and yoga, eating well, and socializing with neighbours and friends. As you leave, Heidi asks to speak with you and takes you aside. She is very worried about her mother and appears upset as she discovered that she was searching dating sites on the computer. How would you approach this situation with Heidi? What would you tell her?
3. Describe what you would take into consideration when completing a mental status examination with an older adult.

Visit thePoint to view suggested responses. Go to thePoint.lww.com/activate and use the activation code found in the front of this text to unlock answers to the "Thinking Challenges" and other online resources.

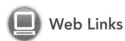 Web Links

alzheimer.ca/en Alzheimer Society of Canada website includes information about the society, Alzheimer disease (AD), how to care for someone with AD, and research updates.

AgeIsMore.com The Revera reports on ageism and other resources are found at this site.

hign.org/consultgeri/try-this-series/2019-american-geriatrics-society-updated-beers-criteria-r-potentially The American Geriatrics Society's updated Beers Criteria can be found at this site.

cwp-csp.ca/poverty/just-the-facts/ Canada Without Poverty.

www.cagp.ca/ Canadian Academy of Geriatric Psychiatry Dedicated to promoting mental health in the Canadian older adults population through the clinical, educational, and research activities of its members.

cgna.net/ Canadian Gerontological Nursing Association represents nurses who work with and for older adults in a wide variety of settings. Its interests include education, research, and clinical practice. It encourages and supports members through research grants, scholarships, conference funding, and certification study sessions.

www.cmhc-schi.gc.ca Canada Mortgage and Housing Corporation (CMHC) website provides information about how older adults can adapt their homes for increasing disabilities and financial assistance programs for housing for older adults.

ccsmh.ca/projects/suicide/ Canadian Coalition for Seniors' Mental Health was established in 2002 and has its goal supporting collaborative initiatives that will facilitate positive mental health for seniors through innovation and dissemination of best practices. See resources for suicide prevention and intervention. National evidence-informed guidelines can be downloaded (Depression, Suicide, Delirium, and Mental Health Issues in Long-term Care).

csepguidelines.ca/adults-65/ CSEP's Canadian 24-hour movement guidelines for adults ages 65 years and older: an integration of physical activity, sedentary behaviour, and sleep can be found at this site.

www.hope-lit.ualberta.ca/ Site of the Hope-Lit Database, a comprehensive index of hope research and literature (English), is supported by the Hope Foundation of Alberta and the University of Alberta.

www.mentalhealthcommission.ca/English Mental Health Commission of Canada's excellent website contains a multitude of current information, publications, and what's new in Canada. The Mental Health Strategy for Canada and the Guidelines for Seniors Mental Health can be downloaded.

https://www.canada.ca/en/national-seniors-council.html National Seniors Council: This is the website of the National Seniors Council in Canada (formerly the National Advisory Council on Aging). It advises the Canadian Government on all matters related to wellbeing and quality of life for seniors.

https://www.nia-ryerson.ca/ National Institute on Aging has a website dedicated to the scientific effort to understand the nature of aging and to extend healthy, active years of life.

www.nicenet.ca/ National Initiative for the Care of the Elderly (NICE), an international network of researchers, practitioners, and students dedicated to improving the care of older adults in Canada and abroad.

www.justice.gc.ca/eng/rp-pr/cj-jp/fv-vf/elder-aines/def/p23.html At this site is a discussion of the legal definitions of Elder Abuse and Neglect used across Canada by the Government of Canada's Department of Justice.

https://www.canada.ca/en/public-health.html Public Health Agency of Canada: Mental health promotion website for the Public Health Agency of Canada.

www.mentalhealthcommission.ca/English/document/269/seniors-mental-health-policy-lens-toolkit The Seniors Mental Health Policy Lens (SMHPL) was developed as part of a national project, "Psychosocial Approaches to the Mental Health Challenges of Late Life," awarded to the BC Psychogeriatric Association by Health Canada, Population Health Fund. This site contains the SMHPL toolkit.

Wongbakerfaces.org : Information regarding the Wong-Baker FACES Pain Rating Scale and its use can be found at this site.

References

Alexopoulos, G. S., Abrams, R. C., Young, R. C., & Shamoian, C. (1988). Cornell scale for depression in dementia. *Biological Psychiatry, 23*, 271–284. https://doi.org/10.1016/0006-3223(88)90038-8

Almazan, J. U., Cruz, J. P., Alamri, M. S., Alotaibi, J. S. M., Albougami, A. S. B., Gravoso, R., Abocejo, F., Allen, K., & Bishwajit, G. (2018). Predicting patterns of disaster-related resiliency among older adult Haiyan Typhoon survivors. *Geriatric Nursing, 39*, 629–634.

American Geriatrics Society. (2015). Updated Beers Criteria for potentially inappropriate medication use in older adults. *Journal of the American Geriatrics Society, 63*(11), 2227–2246. https://doi.org/10.1111/jgs.13702

American Psychiatric Association. (2013). *Diagnostic and statistical manual of mental disorders* (5th ed.).

Boima, V., Tetteh, J., Yorke, E., Archampong, T., Mensah G., Biritwum R., & Yawson, A. E. (2020). Older adults with hypertension have increased risk of depression compared to their younger counterparts: Evidence from the World Health Organization study of Global Ageing and Adult Health Wave 2 in Ghana. *Journal of Affective Disorders, 277*, 329–336. https://doi.org/10.1016/j.jad.2020.08.033

Brandon, M. (2016). Psychosocial aspects of sexuality with aging. *Geriatric Rehabilitation, 32*(3), 151–155. https://doi.org/doi: 10.1097/TGR.0000000000000116

Brennan, P. L., & Soohoo, S. (2013). Pain and use of alcohol in later life: Prospective evidence from the health and retirement study. *Journal of Aging and Health, 25*(4), 656–677.

Cabeza, R., Albert, M., Belleville, S., Craik, F., Duarte, A., Grady, C., Lindenberger, U., Nyberg, L., Park, D., Reuter-Lorenz, P., Rugg, M., Steffener, J., & Rajah, M. (2018). Maintenance, reserve and compensation: The cognitive neuroscience of healthy ageing. *Nature Reviews Neuroscience, 19*(11), 701–710. https://doi.org/10.1038/s41583-018-0068-2

Canadian Deprescribing Network. (2019). *A focus on appropriate medication use in Canada: Annual report.* https://static1.squarespace.com/static/5836f01fe6f2e1fa62c11f08/t/5e1612f4fbdebd1ecdb8460c/1578504951798/CaDeN+Annual+Report+2019_Eng.pdf

Canadian Institutes of Health Research (CIHR). (2019). *Living longer, living better: Canadian Institutes of Health Research Institute of Aging 2019–2021 strategic plan.* https://cihr-irsc.gc.ca/e/51447.html

Canadian Nursing Association. (2021). *Mental health.* https://www.cna-aiic.ca/en/nursing-practice/the-practice-of-nursing/health-human-resources/mental-health

Centers for Disease Control and Prevention. (2021). *How is depression different for older adults.* https://www.cdc.gov/aging/depression/

Chehrehnegar, N., Nejati, V., Shati, M., Rashedi, V., Lotfi, M., Adelirad, F., & Foroughan, M. (2020). Early detection of cognitive disturbances in mild cognitive impairment: A systematic review of observational studies. *Psychogeriatrics, 20*(2), 212–228. https://doi.org/10.1111/psyg.12484

Clements-Cortés, A., & Yip, J. (2020). Social prescribing for an aging population. *Activities, Adaptation & Aging, 44*(4), 327–340. https://doi.org/10.1080/01924788.2019.1692467

Constantino, R. (2020). Matters of HEARTS: Health, experience of abuse, resilience, technology use, and safety of older adults. *Educational Ger-*

ontology, 46(7), 367–381. https://doi.org/10.1080/03601277.2020.175 7588

Crompton, C. J., & MacPherson, S. (2019). Human agency beliefs affect older adults' interaction behaviours and task performance when learning with computerised partners. *Psychology, 101,* 60–67. https://doi.org/10.1016/j.chb.2019.07.006

Davison, L., Lin, S., Tong, H., Kobayashi, K., Mora-Almanza J. G., & Fuller-Tomson, E. (2020). Nutritional factors, physical health and immigrant status are associated with anxiety disorders among middle-aged and older adults: Findings from baseline data of the Canadian Longitudinal Study on Aging (CLSA). *International Journal of Environmental Research and Public Health, 17*(5), 1493. https://doi.org/10.3390/ijerph17051493

de Carvalho Bastone, A., Nobre, L. N., de Souza Moreira, B., Rosa, I. F., Ferreira, G. B., Santos, D. D. L., Monteiro, N. K. S. S., Alves, M. D., Gandra, R. A., & de Lira, E. M. (2020). Independent and combined effect of home-based progressive resistance training and nutritional supplementation on muscle strength, muscle mass and physical function in dynapenic older adults with low protein intake: A randomized controlled trial. *Archives of Gerontology and Geriatrics, 89,* 104098. https://doi.org/10.1016/j.archger.2020.104098

Diehl, M., Smyer, M. A., & Mehrotra, C. M. (2020). Optimizing aging: A call for a new narrative. *The American psychologist, 75*(4), 577–589. https://doi.org/10.1037/amp0000598

Duggleby, W., Hicks, D., Nekolaichuk, C., Holtslander, L., Williams, A., Chambers, T., & Eby, J. (2012). Hope, older adults, and chronic illness: A metasynthesis of qualitative research. *Journal of Advanced Nursing, 68*(6), 1211–1223. https://doi:10.1111/j.1365-2648.2011.05919.x

Ebaid, D., Crewther, S. G., MacCalman, K., Brown, A., & Crewther, D. P. (2017). Cognitive processing speed across the lifespan: Beyond the influence of motor speed. *Frontiers in Aging Neuroscience, 9,* 62. https://doi.org/10.3389/fnagi.2017.00062

Employment and Social Development Canada. (2018). *Opportunity for all—Canada's first poverty reduction strategy 2018.* Government of Canada. www.canada.ca/content/dam/canada/employment-social-development/programs/poverty-reduction/reports/poverty-reduction-strategy-report-EN

Erikson, E. H., & Erikson, J. M. (1997). *The lifecycle completed, extended version.* WW Norton.

Farias, S. T., Schmitter-Edgecombe, M., Weakley, A., Harvey, D., Denny, K. D., Barba, C., Gravano, J. T., Giovannetti, T., & Willis, S. (2018). Compensation strategies in older adults: Association with cognition and everyday function. *American Journal of Alzheimer's Disease & Other Dementias, 33,* 184–191. https://doi.org/10.1177/1533317517753361

Feder, J. (2020). COVID-19 and the future of long-term care: The urgency of enhanced federal financing. *Journal of Aging & Social Policy, 32*(4–5), 350–357. doi.org/10.1080/08959420.2020.1771238

Frankl, V. (1963). *Man's search for meaning: An introduction to logotherapy.* Pocket Books.

Fries, J. F., Bruce, B., & Chakravarty, E. (2011). Compression of morbidity 1980–2011: A focused review of paradigms and progress. *Journal of Aging Research, 11,* 1–10. https://doi.org/10.4061/2011/261702

Giddens, J. F. (2021). *Concepts for nursing practice* (3rd ed.). Elsevier.

Gilmour, H., & Ramage-Morin, P. L. (2020, June). Social isolation and mortality among Canadian seniors. *Health Reports, 31,* 27–38. Statistics Canada. Catalogue no. 82-003-X

Gold, A. L., Meza, E., Ackley, S. F., Mungas, D. M., Whitmer, R. A., Mayeda, E. R., Miles, S., Eng, C. W., Gilsanz, P., & Glymour, M. (2021). Are adverse childhood experiences associated with late-life cognitive performance across racial/ethnic groups: Results from the Kaiser Healthy Aging and Diverse Life Experiences study baseline. *BMJ Open, 11*(2), e042125. https://doi.org/10.1136/bmjopen-2020-042125

Gonzalez-Colaço Harmand, M., Meillon, C., Bergua, V., Tabue Teguo, M., Dartigues, J.-F., Avila-Funes, J. A., & Amieva, H. (2017). Comparing the predictive value of three definitions of frailty: Results from the three-city study. *Archives of Gerontology and Geriatrics, 72,* 153–163. https://doi.org/10.1016/j.archger.2017.06.005

Government of Canada. (2017). *Social isolation of seniors—Volume 1: Understanding the issue and finding solutions.* https://www.canada.ca/en/employment-social-development/corporate/partners/seniors-forum/social-isolation-toolkit-vol1.html

Gregg, J. J., Fiske, A., & Gatz, M. (2013). Physician's detection of late-life depression: The roles of dysphoria and cognitive impairment. *Aging and Mental Health, 13*(45), 1–11. https://doi.org/10.1080/13607863.2013.805403

Grossman, D. C., Curry, S. J., Owens, D. K., Barry, M. J., Caughey, A. B., Davidson, K. W., Doubeni, C. A., Epling Jr, J. W., Kemper, A. R., Krist, A. H., Kubik, M., Landefeld, S., Mangione, C. M., Pignone, M., Silverstein, M., Simon, M. A., & Tseng, C.-W. (2018). Interventions to prevent falls in community-dwelling older adults: US Preventive Services Task Force

recommendation statement. *JAMA, 319*(16), 1696–1704. https://doi.org/10.1016/j.archger.2017.06.005

Harrington, A. (2016). The importance of spiritual assessment when caring for older adults. *Ageing and Society, 36*(1), 1–16. https://doi.org/10.1017/S0144686X14001007

Harvey, J., Beck, A., & Carr, C. T. (2019). A cognitive social media training program and intergenerational learning: A pilot study with older adults and speech-language pathology graduate students. *Perspectives of the ASHA Special Interest Groups, 4*(4), 683–695. https://doi.org/10.1044/2019_PERS-SIG15-2018-0004

Hawkley, L. C., & Cacioppo, J. T. (2010). Loneliness matters: A theoretical and empirical review of consequences and mechanisms. *Annals of Behavioral Medicine, 40*(2), 218–227. https://doi.org/10.1007/s12160-010-9210-8

Health Canada and Assembly of First Nations. (2015). *First Nations mental wellness continuum framework.* http://publications.gc.ca/collections/collection_2015/sc-hc/H34-278-1-2014-eng.pdf

Hebert, R., Guilbeault, J., & Pinsonnault, E. (2002). *Functional autonomy measuring system user guide.* Centre d'expertise de l'Institut universitaire de geriatrie de Sherbrooke.

Hernandez, S. C., & Overholser, J. C. (2021). A systematic review of interventions for hope/hopelessness in older adults. *Clinical Gerontologist, 44,* 97–111. doi:10.1080/07317115.2019.1711281

Hyer, L., & Blount, J. (1984). Concurrent and discriminant validities of the geriatric depression scale with older psychiatric inpatients. *Psychological Reports, 54,* 611–616. https://doi.org/10.2466/pr0.1984.54.2.611

Jeste, D. (2019). Frailty and mental health: Association with cognition, sleep, and well-being in older adults. *International Psychogeriatrics, 31*(6), 755–757. https://doi.org/10.1017/S1041610219000863

Jeste, D. V., Thomas, M. L., Liu, J., Daly, R. E., Tu, X. M., Treichler, E. B., Palmer, B. W., & Lee, E. E. (2021). Is spirituality a component of wisdom? *Journal of Psychiatric Research, 132,* 174–181. https://doi.org/10.1016/j.jpsychires.2020.09.033

Katz, S. & Akpom, C. A. (1976). A measure of primary sociobiological functions. *International Journal of Health Service, 6*(3), 493–508.

Kim, A. S., Garcia Morales, E. E., Amjad, H., Cotter, V. T., Lin, F. R., Lyketsos, C. G., Nowrangi, M. A., Mamo, S. K., Reed, N. S., Yasar, S., Oh, E. S., & Nieman, C. L. (2021). Association of hearing loss with neuropsychiatric symptoms in older adults with cognitive impairment. *American Journal of Geriatric Psychiatry, 29*(6), 544–553. https://doi.org/10.1016/j.jagp.2020.10.002

Klimecki, O., Marchant, N. L., Lutz, A., Poisnel, G., Chételat, G., & Collette, F. (2019). The impact of meditation on healthy ageing—The current state of knowledge and a roadmap to future directions. *Current Opinion in Psychology, 28,* 223–228. https://doi.org/10.1016/j.copsyc.2019.01.006

Kolcu, M., & Ergun, A. (2020). Effect of a nurse-led hypertension management program on quality of life, medication adherence and hypertension management in older adults: A randomized controlled trial. *Geriatrics & Gerontology International, 20*(12), 1182–1189. https://doi.org/10.1111/ggi.14068

Lagacé, M., Van de Beeck, L., & Firzly, N. (2019). Building on intergenerational climate to counter ageism in the workplace? A cross-organizational study. *Journal of Intergenerational Relationships, 17,* 201–219. doi.org/10.1080/15350770.2018.1535346

Laird, K. T., Paholpak, P., Roman, M., Rahi, B., & Lavretsky, H. (2018). Mind-body therapies for late-life mental and cognitive health. *Current Psychiatry Reports, 20*(1), 1–12. https://doi.org/10.1007/s11920-018-0864-4

Livingston, G., Huntley, J., Sommerlad, A., Ames, D., Ballard, C., Banerjee, S., Brayne, C., Burns, A., Cohen-Mansfield, J., Cooper, C., Costafreda, S., Dias, A., Fox, N., Gitlin, L., Howard, R., Kales, H., Kivimäki, M., Larson, E., Ogunniyi, A., … Mukadam, N. (2020). Dementia prevention, intervention, and care: 2020 report of the Lancet Commission. *The Lancet (British Edition), 396*(10248), 413–446. https://doi.org/10.1016/S0140-6736(20)30367-6

Marchiondo, L. A., Gonzales, E., & Williams, L. J. (2019). Trajectories of perceived workplace age discrimination and long-term associations with mental, self-rated, and occupational health. *The Journals of Gerontology, 74,* 655–663. https://doi.org/10.1093/geronb/gbx095

Mateos-Aparicio, P., & Rodríguez-Moreno, A. (2019). The impact of studying brain plasticity. *Frontiers in Cellular Neuroscience, 13,* 66. https://doi.org/10.3389/fncel.2019.00066

Mattys, S. L., & Baddeley, A. (2019). Working memory and second language accent acquisition. *Applied Cognitive Psychology, 33*(6), 1113–1123. https://doi.org/10.1002/acp.3554

Mayo Clinic. (2020, October 1). *Sexual health and aging: Keep the passion alive.* https://www.mayoclinic.org/healthy-lifestyle/sexual-health/in-depth/sexual-health/art-20046698

McKye, K. A., Naglie, G., Tierney, M., & Jaglal, S. (2009). Comparison of older adults' and occupational therapists' awareness of functional abilities at discharge from rehabilitation with actual performance in the home. *Physical and Occupational Therapy in Geriatrics*, *27*(3), 229–244. https://doi.org/10.1080/02703180802547394

Melillo, K. (2017). Geropsychiatric nursing: What's in your toolkit? *Journal of Gerontological Nursing*, *43*(1), 3–6. https://doi.org/10.3928/00989134-20161215-01

Menec, V. H. (2017). Conceptualizing social connectivity in the context of age-friendly communities. *Journal of Housing for the Elderly*, *31*(2), 99–116. https://doi.org/10.1080/02763893.2017.1309926

Mental Health Commission of Canada. (n.d.). *Fact sheet: Older adults and suicide*. https://www.mentalhealthcommission.ca/wp-content/uploads/drupal/2019-05/Older%20adults%20and%20suicide%20fact%20sheet.pdf

Mental Health Commission of Canada. (2012). *Changing directions: Changing lives: The mental health strategy for Canada*. http://www.mentalhealthcommission.ca/English/node/721

Miller, E. A. (2020). Protecting and improving the lives of older adults in the COVID-19 era. *Journal of Aging & Social Policy*, *32*(4–5), 297–309. https://doi.org/10.1080/08959420.2020.1780104

Morley, J. (2017). The importance of geriatric syndromes. *Missouri Medicine*, *114*(2), 99–100. https://www.ncbi.nlm.nih.gov/pmc/articles/PMC6140017/

Mundhra, R., Lim, T. J., Duong, H. N., Yeo, K. H., Niculescu, A. I. (2021). Towards a humorous chat-bot companion for senior citizens. In L. F. D'Haro, Z. Callejas, & S. Nakamura (Eds.), *Conversational dialogue systems for the next decade. Lecture notes in electrical engineering*, Vol. 704. Springer. https://doi.org/10.1007/978-981-15-8395-

National Academies of Sciences, Engineering, and Medicine. (2020). *Social isolation and loneliness in older adults: Opportunities for the health care system*. The National Academies Press.

National Institute on Aging. (2017a). *Sexuality in later life*. U.S. Department of Health and Human Services. https://www.nia.nih.gov/health/sexuality-later-life

National Institute on Aging. (2017b). *Facts about aging and alcohol*. https://www.nia.nih.gov/health/facts-about-aging-and-alcohol

National Sleep Foundation. (2021). *Sleep health topics*. https://www.thensf.org/sleep-health-topics/

Nguyen, A., & Lee, G. (2020). Cognitive screening for early detection of mild cognitive impairment. *International Psychogeriatrics*, *32*(9), 1015–1017. https://doi.org/10.1017/S1041610219000991

O'Hoski, S., Bean, J. F., Ma, J., So, H. Y., Kuspinar, A., Richardson, J., Wald, J., & Beauchamp, M. K. (2020). Physical function and frailty for predicting adverse outcomes in older primary care patients. *Archives of Physical Medicine and Rehabilitation*, *101*(4), 592–598. https://doi.org/10.1016/j.apmr.2019.11.013

O'Rourke, H., & Sidani, S. (2017). Definition, determinants, and outcomes of social connectedness for older adults: A scoping review. *Journal of Gerontological Nursing*, *43*(7), 43–52. https://doi.org/10.3928/00989134-20170223-03

Osteoporosis Canada. (2019). https://osteoporosis.ca/about-the-disease/

Paterson, D. H., & Warburton, E. R. (2010). Physical activity and functional limitations in older adults: A systematic review related to Canada's physical activity guidelines. *International Journal of Behavioral and Nutrition and Physical Activity*, *7*, 38. https://doi.org/10.1186/1479-5868-7-38

Pfeffer, R., Kurosaki, T., Harrah, C., Chance, J., & Filos, S. (1982). Measurement of functional activities in older adults in the community. *Journal of Gerontology*, *37*(3), 323–329. https://doi.org/10.1093/geronj/37.3.323

Pilotto, A., Custodero, C., Maggi, S., Polidori, M. C., Veronese, N., & Ferrucci, L. (2020). A multidimensional approach to frailty in older people. *Ageing Research Reviews*, *60*, 101047. https://doi.org/10.1016/j.arr.2020.101047

Pinheiro, I. M., de Aguiar, D. S., Dos Santos, D. M., de Jesus, M., da Silva, F. M., Costa, D. F., da Silva Ribeiro, N. M., & Nóbrega, A. C. (2019). Biopsychosocial factors associated with the frailty and pre-frailty among older adults. *Geriatric Nursing*, *40*(6), 597–602. https://doi.org/10.1016/j.gerinurse.2019.06.002

Preuß, D., & Legal, F. (2017). Living with the animals: Animal or robotic companions for the elderly in smart homes. *Medical Ethics*, *43*, 407–410. https://doi.org/10.1136/medethics-2016-103603

Public Health Agency of Canada (PHAC). (2020a). *Aging and chronic disease. A profile of Canadian seniors*. Cat.: HP35-137/1-2020E-PDF ISBN: 978-0-660-35370-8 Pub.: 200117

Public Health Agency of Canada (PHAC). (2021). *The Chief Public Health Officer's report on the state of public health in Canada 2021: A vision to transform Canada's Public Health System*. Cat.: HP2-10E-PDF ISBN: 1924-7087 Pub: 210338.

Qin, W., Wang, Y., & Cho, S. (2021). Neighborhood social cohesion, physical disorder, and daily activity limitations among community-dwelling older adults. *Archives of Gerontology and Geriatrics*, *93*, 1–8. https://doi.org/10.1016/j.archger.2020.104295

Quach, L. T., & Burr, J. A. (2018). Arthritis, depression, and falls among community-dwelling older adults: Evidence from the health and retirement study. *Journal of Applied Gerontology*, *37*(9), 1133–1149. https://doi.org/10.1177/0733464816646683

Radanovic, M. (2020). Cognitive reserve: An evolving concept. *International Psychogeriatrics*, *32*(1), 7–9. https://doi.org/10.1017/S1041610219001947

Rajani, F. (2015). Theory of gerotranscendence: An analysis. *European Psychiatry*, *30*(Suppl), 28–31. doi.org/10.1016/S0924-9338(15)31138-X

Ravary, A., Stewart, E. K., & Baldwin, M. W. (2020). Insecurity about getting old: Age-contingent self-worth, attentional bias, and well-being. *Aging & Mental Health*, *24*(10), 1636–1644. https://doi.org/10.1080/13607863.2019.1636202

Rizzo, M., Anderson, S., & Fritzsch, B. (2018). *The Wiley handbook on the aging mind and brain*. Wiley Blackwell.

Rosenweig, A. (2022, January 29). *Montreal Cognitive Assessment (MoCA) Test for Dementia*. Very Well website. www.verywellhealth.com/alzheimers-and-montreal-cognitive-assessment-moca-98617

Roswiyani, K., Kwakkenbos, L., Spijker, J., & Witterman, C. L. (2019). The effectiveness of combining visual art activities and physical exercise for older adults on well-being or quality of life and mood: A scoping review. *Journal of Applied Gerontology*, *38*(12), 1784–1804. https://doi.org/10.1177/0733464817743332

Sampaio, R. A. C., Sewo Sampaio, P. Y., Uchida, M. C., & Arai, H. (2020). Management of dynapenia, sarcopenia, and frailty: The role of physical exercise. *Journal of Aging Research*, *2020*, 8186769. https://doi.org/10.1155/2020/8186769

Sheikh, J. I., & Yesavage, J. A. (1986). Geriatric Depression Scale (GDS): Recent evidence and development of a shorter version. In T. L. Brink (Ed.), *Clinical gerontology: A guide to assessment and intervention* (pp. 165–173). Haworth Press.

Sheridan Centre for Elder Research. (2016). *Revera report on ageism: Independence and choice as we age*. Revera. www.ageismore.com

Shing, Y. L., & Lindenberger, U. (2011). The development of episodic memory: Lifespan lessons. *Child Development Perspectives*, *5*(2), 148–155. https://doi.org/10.1111/j.1750-8606.2011.00170.x

Statistics Canada. (2020, February 24). *Canadian Income Survey*. https://www150.statcan.gc.ca/n1/daily-quotidien/200224/dq200224a-eng.htm

Statistics Canada. (2021). *Chronic conditions among seniors 65 and older*. https://www150.statcan.gc.ca/t1/tbl1/en/tv.action?pid=1310078801

Steinman, M. A., Beizer, J. L., DuBeau, C. E., Laird, R. D., Lundebjerg, M. E., & Mulhausen, P. (2015). Geriatrics Society 2015 Beers Criteria—A guide for patients, clinicians, health systems, and payors. *Journal of the American Geriatrics Society*, *65*(11), e1–e7. https://doi.org/10.1111/jgs.13701

Stephens, C., Breheny, M., & Mansvelt, J. (2015). Healthy ageing from the perspective of older people: A capability approach to resilience. *Psychology and Health*, *30*(6), 715–731. doi.org/10.1080/08870446.2014.904862

Stevenson, J. M., Davies, G., & Martin, F. C. (2019). COMMENTARY Medication-related harm: A geriatric syndrome. *Age and Ageing*, *49*, 7–11. https://doi.org/10.1093/ageing/afz121

Strauss, R., Kurdyak, P., & Glazier, R. H. (2020). Mood disorders in late life: A population-based analysis of prevalence, risk factors, and consequences in community-dwelling older adults in Ontario. *The Canadian Journal of Psychiatry*, *65*, 630–640. https://doi.org/10.1177/0706743720927812

Tallman, B. (2019). *The couple living with dementia in the Community: Accomplishing life together through their efforts toward mutuality*. University of Manitoba.m-space. https://mspace.lib.umanitoba.ca/bitstream/handle/1993/34289/tallman_barbara.pdf?sequence=1

Teng, E., Kazuo Hasegawa, K., Homma, A., Imai, Y., Larson, E., Graves, A., Sugimoto, K., Yamaguchi, T., Hideo, S., Chiu, D., & White, L. R. (1994). The Cognitive Abilities Screen Instrument (CASI): A practical test for cross-cultural epidemiological studies of dementia. *International Psychogeriatrics*, *6*(1), 45–58. https://doi.org/10.1017/s1041610294001602

Timalsina, R., & Songwathana, P. (2020). Factors enhancing resilience among older adults experiencing disaster: A systematic review. *Australasian Emergency Care*, *23*, 11–22. https://doi.org/10.1016/j.auec.2019.12.007

Tornstam, L. (1989). Gero-transcendence: A theoretical and empirical reformulation of the disengagement theory. *Aging Clinical and Experimental Research*, *1*, 55–63. https://doi.org/10.1007/BF03323876

Tornstam, L. (2005). *Gerotranscendence: A developmental theory of positive aging*. Springer.

Tomás, J. M., Sancho, P., Galiana, L., & Oliver, A. (2016). A double test on the importance of spirituality, the "forgotten factor", in successful aging. *Social Indicators Research*, *127*, 1377–1389. https://doi.org/10.1007/s11205-015-1014-6

Wengel, S. P., Burke, W. J., & Cervantes, R. F. (2018). Psychiatric disorders. In Rizzo, M., Anderson, S., & Fritzsch, B. (Eds.), *The Wiley handbook on the aging mind and brain* (pp. 541–552). Wiley Blackwell.

Wiechula, R., Conroy, T., Kitson, A., Marshall, R. J., Whitaker, N., & Rasmussen, P. (2016). Umbrella review of the evidence. What factors influence the caring relationship between a nurse and patient? *Journal of Advanced Nursing*, *72*(4), 723–724. https://doi.org/10.1111/jan.12862

Wion, R. K., & Loeb, S. J. (2015). Older adults engaging in online dating: What gerontological nurses should know. *Journal of Gerontological Nursing, 41*, 25–35. https://doi.org/10.3928/00989134-20150826-67

World Health Organization. (2017a). *Global strategy and action plan on ageing and health.* Licence: CC BY-NC-SA 3.0 IGO.

World Health Organization. (2017b). *Integrated care for older people: Guidelines on community-level interventions to manage declines in intrinsic capacity.* Licence: CC BY-NC-SA 3.0 IGO.

World Health Organization. (2021a). Decade of healthy ageing: Baseline report. Summary. Licence CC BY-NC-SA 3.0 IGO

World Health Organization. (2021b). *Global report on ageism.* CC BY-NC-SA 3.0 IGO.

World Health Organization. (2021c). *Health topics: Health promotion.* https://www.who.int/health-topics/health-promotion#tab=tab_1

Ye, B. S., Seo, S. W., Cho, H., Kim, S. Y., Lee, J. S., Kim, E. J., Lee, Y., Back, J. H., Hong, C. H., Choi, S. H., Park, K. W., Ku, B. D., Moon, S. Y., Kim, S., Han, S.-H., Lee, J.-H., Cheong, H.-K., & Na, D. L. (2013). Effects of education on the progression of early versus late-stage mild cognitive impairment. *International Psychogeriatrics, 25*(4), 597–606. https://doi.org/10.1017/S1041610212002001

Yu, B., Steptoe, A., Chen, Y., & Jia, X. (2020). Social isolation, rather than loneliness, is associated with cognitive decline in older adults: The China Health and Retirement Longitudinal Study. *Psychological Medicine, 51*(14), 2414–2421. https://doi.org/10.1017/S0033291720001014

CHAPTER

32

Neurocognitive Disorders: Delirium and Dementia*

Kathleen F. Hunter

LEARNING OBJECTIVES

After studying this chapter, you will be able to:

- Distinguish the clinical characteristics, onset, and course of the neurocognitive disorders (NCDs) of delirium and dementia.
- Describe the biologic, psychological, social, and spiritual factors that relate to NCDs in older adults.
- Discuss the emotional impact of dementia for the individual, family, and caregiver.
- Formulate nursing care focuses based on a bio/psycho/social/spiritual assessment of individuals with impaired cognitive function.
- Identify the expected outcomes and nursing interventions and provide an evaluation for individuals with impaired cognition.

KEY TERMS

- agnosia • Alzheimer disease • aphasia • apraxia • bradykinesia • catastrophic reactions • cortical dementias • delirium superimposed on dementia • disinhibition • hyperactive delirium • hypoactive delirium • mild cognitive impairment • mixed delirium • neurofibrillary tangles • neuropsychiatric symptoms • oxidative stress • postoperative delirium • responsive behaviours • subcortical dementia

KEY CONCEPTS

- cognition • delirium • dementia • memory

Cognition and memory as a part of cognition are important in many psychiatric disorders, but in this chapter on neurocognitive disorders (NCDs), they are the key concepts (American Psychiatric Association [APA], 2013). Cognition is the ability to think, know, and act. The definition is further refined to be understood as a relatively high level of intellectual processing in which perceptions and information are acquired, used, or manipulated. Specific functions include the acquisition and use of language, the ability to be oriented in time and space, judgment, reasoning, attention, comprehension, concept formation, planning, and the use of symbols, such as numbers and letters used in mathematics and writing. Cognition and behaviour are so closely linked that even mild cognitive impairment (MCI) can affect a person's daily functioning (Anderson, 2019). MCI is the name given to subjective cognitive decline (SCD) paired with objective cognitive impairment, but without substantial functional impairment being present. It is viewed as a transitional stage between usual aging and dementia (Anderson, 2019).

People who have memory impairment as part of the MCI presentation (amnestic MCI) are twice as likely to progress to dementia as those who do not have early memory impairment (nonamnestic MCI) (Glynn et al., 2020). Memory, one facet of cognition, refers to the ability to recall or reproduce what has been learned or experienced. It is more than simple storage and retrieval; it is a complex cognitive mental function that includes most areas of the brain, especially the hippocampus, which is believed to be essential to the transfer of some memories from short-term to long-term storage. Defects of memory are an essential feature of many cognitive disorders, particularly dementia.

The NCDs discussed in this chapter, delirium and dementia, are characterized by deficits in cognition or memory that represent a clear-cut deterioration from a previous level of functioning. Delirium is a disorder of acute cognitive impairment and can be caused by a medical condition (e.g., infection) or substance abuse, or it may have multiple aetiologies. Dementia is characterized by chronic cognitive impairments and

*Adapted from the chapter "Neurocognitive Disorders: Delirium and Dementia" by Dorothy Forbes and Wendy Austin

861

is differentiated by the underlying cause, not by symptom patterns, which are often similar. Although most dementias are irreversible and progressive, some conditions that present with symptoms of cognitive decline can be reversed with timely recognition and treatment. Examples are vitamin B12 deficiency and normal pressure hydrocephalus (Little, 2018).

Delirium is an acute disorder of attention with a fluctuating course, impaired level of consciousness, and disorganization of thought (APA, 2013; Oh et al., 2017). Predisposing factors include advanced age, previous delirium, dementia, and sensory impairments; precipitating factors can be alcohol or drug withdrawal, surgery and anaesthesia, infection, intracranial insults, or fluid–electrolyte imbalances (Oh et al., 2017). (For delirium tremens, the delirium that occurs after untreated withdrawal from a substance such as alcohol, see Chapter 26.)

Cortical dementias, such as Alzheimer disease (AD) and prion disease, result from a disease process that globally afflicts the cortex. **Subcortical dementia** is caused by dysfunction or deterioration of deep grey- or white-matter structures inside the brain and brain stem. Symptoms of subcortical dementia may be more localized and tend to disrupt arousal, attention, and motivation, but they can produce a variety of clinical behavioural manifestations. Examples of subcortical dementias include those due to Huntington disease, Parkinson disease, and HIV infection. In this chapter, AD is highlighted because it is the most prevalent form of dementia in Canada.

KEY CONCEPT

Cognition involves multiple brain processes that enable an individual to perceive, learn, and recall specific information for the purpose of reasoning or problem-solving. It is based on a system of complex interrelated abilities, such as perception, reasoning, judgment, intuition, and memory, which allow one to be aware of oneself and one's surroundings. Impairments in these abilities can result in a failure of the afflicted person to recognize that he or she is not well and is in need of treatment.

KEY CONCEPT

Memory is a facet of cognition concerned with retaining and recalling past experiences, whether they occurred in the physical environment or internally as cognitive events.

KEY CONCEPT

Delirium is a temporary disorder of physical origin with an abrupt onset characterized by fluctuating consciousness and attention.

KEY CONCEPT

Dementia is a condition characterized by chronic, progressive neurocognitive impairment and is differentiated by affected areas in the brain, by underlying cause, and by symptom patterns.

Delirium

Clinical Course of the Disorder

Delirium is an acute disorder of physical origin that develops over a short period of time and it is characterized by fluctuating consciousness and attention. The individual with delirium has reduced ability to focus, sustain, or shift attention, which is marked by a decline in cognitive function (memory, orientation, speech, thinking), perceptual abnormalities, circadian disruption, and psychomotor disturbances. Delirium is usually reversible if treated promptly, but it is a serious disorder associated with high morbidity and mortality. Delirium occurs across all care settings, community to hospital (DeWitt & Tune, 2018). It often follows acute illness, surgery, or a hospitalization episode (Oh et al., 2017). Delirium is associated with longer duration of hospitalization and increased mortality in children (Bettencourt & Mullen, 2017) and older persons (Geriatric Medicine Research Collaborative, 2019). The pathophysiologic mechanisms leading to delirium remain largely unknown despite its immense impact and life-threatening nature.

EMERGENCY

Delirium is an acute neuropsychiatric disorder that develops rapidly and has potentially severe consequences, including brain damage and death, if it goes unrecognized and without appropriate intervention. It is considered a medical emergency (Paulo et al., 2017).

Diagnostic Criteria

Impaired consciousness, in the form of inattention, is the key feature of delirium (DeWitt & Tune, 2018). Impacted individuals become less aware of their environment and lose the ability to focus, sustain, and shift attention. Associated cognitive changes typically include problems in memory, orientation, and language. They may not know where they are, may not recognize familiar objects, or may be unable to carry on a conversation. Delirium presents in hyperactive, hypoactive, and mixed forms. Hypoactive delirium in which the person's cognitive and motor responses are slowed and reduced is not uncommon but may be overlooked (Guthrie et al., 2018;

RNAO, 2016). Delirium may be confused with dementia, depression, or psychosis (Oh et al., 2017). It is possible to have a **delirium superimposed on dementia (DSD)**.

An important diagnostic indicator is that delirium develops rapidly, usually over hours or days. There can be rapid improvement when its underlying cause is identified and removed (DeWitt & Tune, 2018). Nurses are in a unique position to plan, implement, and evaluate care for these patients. Despite this key role, nurses too often do not recognize delirium in their patients. Factors that contribute to such under recognition include the fluctuating nature of delirium, lack of knowledge regarding delirium, inadequate use of delirium assessment tools, and the challenge of distinguishing among delirium, dementia, and DSD (El Hussein et al., 2019). (For the American Psychological Association criteria for delirium, please see the *Diagnostic and Statistical Manual of Mental Disorders*, 5th Revision [DSM-5].)

Delirium in Special Populations

Children

Delirium can occur in infants, children, and adolescents and is most often associated with critical illness (Bettencourt & Mullen, 2017). In addition to physiological contributors such as sepsis, metabolic disturbances, and complex illness, an environment unfamiliar to children can be a contributor. Delirium in the young can be challenging to diagnose, especially if the child is at a preverbal developmental stage, and symptoms may be mistaken for uncooperative behaviour. A child in a **hypoactive delirium** may be lethargic whereas one in a **hyperactive delirium** can be irritable and restless (Bettencourt & Mullen, 2017). Care of paediatric patients needs to include delirium hygiene (e.g., limiting changes and noise, monitoring medication response), alertness to indicators of delirium, and timely intervention if it occurs.

Older Adults

Although delirium may occur in any age group, it is most common among older adults,[†] although it may go unrecognized (DeWitt & Tune, 2018). Increasing age, dementia, and frailty are strongly associated with delirium in older persons (Geriatric Medicine Research Collaborative, 2019). Delirium in older adults is associated with poor outcomes, including increased length of stay, greater use of physical restraints, overuse of sedation, and higher mortality rates (Oh et al., 2017). Delirium increases the cost of care through persistent functional

and cognitive decline, increased nursing care and length of hospital stay, and need for nursing home placement (Kinchin et al., 2021). Early diagnosis and resolution are critical to achieving favourable outcomes. Older adults often present with multiple medical comorbidities and higher risk for postoperative complications. **Postoperative delirium** in the older adult is associated with increased length of hospital stay, rise in morbidity rates, decline in function, and greater risk of death. Screening for delirium, and potential functional loss, should be considered as part of the clinical routine for older adults on medical units and on surgical units. Nurses must be vigilant in assessment for delirium, recognizing that delirium, dementia, and depression present with overlapping clinical features and may coexist in the older adult (Guthrie et al., 2018; RNAO, 2016).

CLINICAL VIGNETTE

DELIRIUM

Mrs. Campbell, a widowed 72-year-old woman living in her own home, has been having trouble sleeping. Her daughter visits and suggests that she try an over-the-counter sleeping medication. Mrs. Campbell has also been taking antihistamines for allergies and the antidepressant amitriptyline. Three nights later, a neighbour calls the daughter, concerned because she encountered Mrs. Campbell wandering the streets, unable to find her home. When the neighbour approached Mrs. Campbell to help her home, she began to scream and strike out at the neighbour.

The daughter visits immediately and discovers that her mother does not recognize her, does not know what time it is, appears dishevelled, and is suspicious that people have been in her home stealing the things she cannot find. Mrs. Campbell does not recall taking any medication, but when her daughter investigates, she finds that 10 pills of the new sleeping aid have already been used. Mrs. Campbell is irritable and refuses to go to the hospital, but over the course of a few hours, she appears to calm down, and the following morning her daughter is able to take her to see her physician. After hearing the history, the physician hospitalizes Mrs. Campbell, withholds all medication, and provides intravenous hydration. Within 3 days, she is again able to recognize her daughter, and her mental status appears to be greatly improved.

WHAT DO YOU THINK?

- Identify risk factors that may have contributed to Mrs. Campbell's experiencing delirium.
- How could the addition of an OTC sleeping medication interact with the antihistamine and antidepressant to be responsible for her delirium?

[†]An older person is defined by the United Nations as a person who is over 60 years of age. However, families and communities often use other socio-cultural referents to define age, including family status (grandparents), physical appearance, or age-related health conditions.

Epidemiology and Risk Factors

Statistics concerning the prevalence of delirium are based primarily on older individuals in acute care settings. Estimated prevalence rates range greatly from 3.2% to 27.5% among older patients across surgical specialties at different hospitals (Berian et al., 2018) and 25% on acute stroke units (Shaw et al., 2019). In one study of nursing home residents, the point prevalence of delirium was reported as 36.8% (Morichi et al., 2018a). Delirium is also common in terminally ill patients nearing death. Variation in rates may be due in part to the assessment method (Shaw et al., 2019) as well as risk factors present in different patient populations.

The most powerful risks for developing delirium in adults, however, are present before admission: for example, older age, severe illness, preexisting dementia, visual/hearing impairments, polypharmacy, alcohol abuse, fracture, infection, pain, and renal impairment. Among children, the youngest patients are at greater risk (Barnes et al., 2020). Mechanical ventilation has been identified as the strongest risk factor for delirium in adult (Von Rueden et al., 2017) and pediatric (Barnes et al., 2020) critically ill patients. Some drugs taken by patients can also increase risk (DeWitt & Tune, 2018). Table 32.1 identifies delirium risk factors and related interventions. Box "Clinical Vignette: Delirium" presents a vignette of an individual who experienced delirium after using an over-the-counter (OTC) sleeping medication.

Aetiology

The aetiology of delirium is complex and usually multifaceted. A lack of generally accepted theories of causation has resulted in considerable variability in the research. Integrating the research and applying it to practice have been difficult. To date, studies focus almost exclusively on biologic causes of delirium, with psychosocial factors viewed as contributing or facilitating. Because environmental and psychosocial factors have been explored only in small, uncontrolled studies, conclusions cannot yet be drawn about these factors. For this reason, the following discussion of aetiology focuses on biologic theories of cause.

The most commonly identified causes of delirium, in order of frequency, are the following:

- Medications
- Infections (particularly urinary tract and upper respiratory)
- Fluid and electrolyte imbalance; metabolic disturbances

The probability of the syndrome's developing increases with the presence of predisposing factors such as very young or advanced age, brain damage, or dementia. Sensory overload or underload, immobilization, sleep deprivation, and psychosocial stress also contribute to delirium.

Because delirium has multiple causes, a wide variety of brain alterations may also be responsible for its development. Delirium may be the only manifestation of an underlying medical problem needing immediate attention, especially in frail older persons who may have an altered presentation of illness (Geriatric Medicine Research Collaborative, 2019). Several theories of delirium causation have been proposed including aging of neurons, inflammation, and changes to neurotransmitter function. Maldonado (2017) proposed that in older persons who are at increased risk of delirium, many of these hypotheses overlap in a complex web identified as the Systems Integration Failure hypothesis of acute brain failure. Some of the interacting pathophysiological factors in this hypothesis include the following:

- Neuronal aging (increased brain inflammation and susceptibility to oxidative damage)
- Neuroinflammation (increased circulating inflammatory mediator, e.g., cytokines)
- Oxidative stress (damage from free radicals)
- Neuroendocrine hypothesis (increased circulating stress hormones, e.g., glucocorticoids)
- Circadian rhythm dysregulation (disruptions to sleep–wake cycles)
- Neurotransmitters (changes in neurotransmitter activity in the central nervous system)

Similar complexity of delirium causation in children has been identified (Traube, 2019). In addition to increased understanding how pathophysiological factors interact, genetic studies and methods for brain research in humans offer new possibilities for studies related to delirium. For example, older surgical patients who are apolipoprotein ε4 (APOE ε 4) allele carriers are more likely to have severe, prolonged delirium in the presence of an elevation of the inflammatory marker C-reactive protein as compared with those individuals who were not APOE ε4 carriers (Vansunilashorn et al., 2020). APOE ε4 is also a genetic risk factor for late-onset Alzheimer disease and delayed recovery from head injury. Although research is ongoing, diagnostic and monitoring biomarkers for delirium are yet to be identified (Oh et al., 2017).

Prevention

Due to the profound negative consequences that an episode of delirium has on an individual, there is a growing emphasis on its prevention. Delirium prevention through nonpharmacological strategies includes orientation and cognitive stimulation, adequate fluid and nutritional intake, mobilization, ensuring sensory aids

Table 32.1 Delirium Risk Factors and Interventions

Risk Factor	Sample Intervention
Cognitive impairment, dementia, disorientation	Cognitive orientation/reorientation Environmental aids: • Adequate lighting • Clear signage • Clock • Calendar Avoid unnecessary room changes Use clear communication
Sensory deprivation, isolation	Therapeutic or cognitively stimulating activities: • Personally valued activities and familiar background stimulation • Reminiscence • Family/friend visits Note: Avoid unnecessary isolation, sensory deprivation, and sensory overload.
Sensory impairment (e.g., hearing or vision impairment)	Optimize sensory function by: • Ensuring hearing and visual aids are available and working • Ensuring adequate lighting • Resolving reversible causes of impairment (e.g., impacted ear wax)
Infection, fever	Look for and treat infection
Presence of urinary catheter	Avoid unnecessary catheterization Screen for and treat urinary tract infection Remove indwelling catheters ASAP Consider in-and-out catheterization over indwelling catheterization
Dehydration and/or constipation Electrolyte abnormalities (hyper- or hyponatremia) Sodium and/or potassium and/or calcium abnormalities	Monitor nutrition, hydration, and bladder/bowel function Prevent electrolyte disturbance/dehydration by: • Ensuring adequate fluid intake • Considering offering subcutaneous or intravenous fluids if necessary • Restoring serum sodium, potassium, and glucose levels to normal limits Pay attention to those who are at increased risk for dehydration (i.e., taking diuretics, diarrhoea, pneumonia, UTI, etc.)
Poor nutrition	Follow nutrition support advice Maintain adequate intake of nutrients and glucose Ensure proper fit of dentures Take time to open food packaging/set up tray Encourage families to be present at mealtimes to assist with feeding
Anaemia	Identify and manage treatable causes of anaemia
Hypoxia	Optimize oxygenation and monitor oxygen saturation levels
Inadequately controlled pain	Assess, monitor, and control pain
Sleep deprivation or disturbance	Promote high-quality sleep Use nonpharmaceutical sleep enhancement methods. Avoid nursing or medical procedures during sleeping hours, and schedule medication rounds to avoid disturbing sleep if possible. Reduce noise and light to a minimum during sleeping hours
Immobilization or limited mobility • Use of restraints • Prolonged bed rest or sedation, immobility after surgery Poor functional status/functional impairment	Avoid use of restraints Minimize use of medical devices (e.g., IV lines, catheters) that may restrict mobility or function Encourage mobilization, including: • Walking, if possible • Getting out of bed • Range-of-motion exercises • Self-care activities Provide appropriate walking aids if needed Encourage mobilization soon after surgery Physical and occupational therapy as needed (after surgery)
Polypharmacy and use of high-risk medications (e.g., psychoactive medications, sedative–hypnotics, benzodiazepines, anticholinergics, antihistamines, meperidine)	Carry out medication reviews for people taking multiple drugs, and modify dosage or discontinue drugs that increase the risk of delirium when possible

Adapted with permission from Registered Nurses' Association of Ontario. (2016). *Delirium, dementia, and depression in older adults: Assessment and care* (2nd ed.) Toronto, ON: Registered Nurses' Association of Ontario.

(glasses, hearing aids) are used, enhancing sleep (adjusting lighting, minimizing noise), preventing infection (avoiding unnecessary catheterization), pain management, adequate oxygenation, and review of potentially psychoactive medications (Oh et al., 2017). Nurses have a significant role to play in all of these interventions.

Single interventions have not yet been established as effective in preventing delirium, but multicomponent interventions including early mobilization, hydration and nutrition, adequate oxygenation, delivery, pain control, attention to bladder and bowel function and prevention, and early detection/treatment of postoperative complications have established efficacy in older surgical patients (Salvi et al., 2020). Among older medical patients, multicomponent interventions including reorientation (supported by trained family members) and strategies to address sleep deprivation, immobility, sensory impairment, and dehydration along with staff education are effective. Interventions to prevent delirium can reduce the length of stay in health facilities.

Interprofessional Recognition, Treatment, and Priority Care

The interprofessional team needs to act promptly to identify and intervene in delirium. Early recognition of delirium is key, and protocols to ensure regular screening for delirium have been recommended as a care standard in high-risk populations such as older hospital patients (Geriatric Medicine Research Collaborative, 2019) and across many settings from critical care (Devlin et al., 2018) to nursing homes (Morichi et al., 2018b). Although a number of screening tools have been developed, one of the common instruments used to screen for delirium is the Confusion Assessment Method (CAM) (Inouye et al., 1990). Nurses and other members of the interprofessional team need to be knowledgeable about the patient's baseline function and cognitive status to identify an acute change.

When developing a treatment plan for a patient in whom delirium is suspected, close attention must be paid to correcting any organic or disease-related factors. Initially, life-threatening illnesses must be ruled out or corrected, such as cerebral hypoxia, hypertensive encephalopathy, intracranial haemorrhage, meningitis, severe electrolyte and metabolic imbalances, hypoglycaemia, and intoxication. If possible, the use of all suspected medications should be stopped and vital signs monitored at least every 2 h. Many patients with delirium are seriously ill, thus necessitating close or constant nursing care. The plan of care requires close observation for changes in vital signs, behaviour, and mental status. Patients are monitored until the delirium subsides. If the delirium still exists at discharge, it is critical that referrals be implemented for postdischarge follow-up assessment and care.

Nursing Management: Human Response to Delirium

By definition, a biologic insult must be present for delirium to occur, but psychological and environmental factors are often involved. Because delirium develops in a matter of hours or days and has been associated with increased mortality, nurses should be particularly vigilant in assessing patients who are at increased risk for this syndrome. (If the patient is a child, the assessment process presented in Chapter 29 should be used.) If the patient is an older person, the assessment that follows will serve as a guide. Special efforts should be made to include family members in the nursing process.

Biologic Domain

Biologic Assessment

The onset of symptoms is typically signalled by a rapid or acute change in behaviour. To assess the symptoms, the nurse needs to know what is normal for the individual. Caregivers, family members, or significant others may be the only resource for accurate information on previous cognitive and physical function and should be interviewed.

Current and Past Health Status

History should include a description of the onset, duration, range, and intensity of associated symptoms. Chronic physical illness, dementia, depression, other psychiatric illnesses, referrals, and any past hospitalizations should be identified. Sorting out historical information may be particularly problematic when delirium accompanies acute illness, recent surgery, or infection.

Physical Examination and Review of Systems

In an attempt to discover the underlying cause of suspected delirium, monitoring of vital signs is crucial. An examination of body systems needs to be conducted. Laboratory data are gathered, including complete blood count, blood/urine glucose, blood urea nitrogen, creatinine, serum electrolyte analyses, liver function, and oxygen saturation levels. Fluid balance and bowel action disturbances relating to constipation or a recent history of diarrhoea should be assessed.

Physical Functions

A functional assessment includes physical functional status (activities of daily living [ADL]), the use of sensory aids (eyeglasses, contact lenses, and hearing aids), mobility aids, dentures/braces, sleep pattern, usual activity level and any recent changes, and pain assessment. Sleep disturbances are a symptom of delirium and may precipitate confusion. Often, the sleep–wake cycle of the patient becomes reversed, with the individual attempting to sleep during the day and be awake at night. Restoration of a normal sleep cycle is extremely important.

Pharmacologic Assessment

A substance use history (including alcohol intake and tobacco use) should be obtained (see Chapters 26 and 33). Information regarding medication use must be obtained, with particular attention given to new medications or changes in the dose or strength of current medications. Table 32.2 lists some of the drugs that can cause delirium, many of which are anticholinergics or have anticholinergic properties. Special attention should be given to combinations of medications because drug interactions can cause delirium.

Information regarding OTC medications should be included in this assessment. OTC medications are often thought of as harmless, but several medications, such as cold medications, taken in sufficient quantities may produce restlessness and confusion, especially in children and older individuals.

Findings from the medication and physical assessments are integrated and analyzed with a focus on improving health outcomes. Chronic pain may lead an individual to use more medication than has been intended and this increase in medication may then result in delirium. Careful monitoring of the effectiveness of pain medications may be supportive in the order of a more effective medication that results in less potential misuse. Because many classes of medications have been associated with delirium, the focus is on changes in the type and number of medications and how medications relate to other findings in the history and physical assessment.

Nursing Care Focus for the Biologic Domain

The nursing care focus typically generated from assessment data includes the risk or presence of acute delirium. However, astute nurses will also use their observations to focus on related indicators such as hyperthermia, fluid and electrolyte disturbances (including dehydration), cyanosis, acute pain, risk for infection, and disturbed sleep pattern. Observation skills are most needful in critically ill/lethargic patients who are voiceless due to the effects of intubation and mechanical ventilation.

Interventions for the Biologic Domain

Important interventions for a patient experiencing acute confusion include providing a safe, calm, and therapeutic environment; removing the stressor (if possible); and maintaining fluid and electrolyte balance. Nurses are often involved in the assessment of vital signs, blood glucose levels, pulse oximetry monitoring, and interpretation of laboratory or diagnostic profiles related to chemistry studies, drug levels, urinalysis, and arterial blood gas analysis. Other interventions include ensuring adequate nutrition, preventing aspiration and decubitus ulcers, and those that focus on individual symptoms and underlying causes—for example, for patients requiring protocols to enhance sleep patterns (see Chapter 28).

Table 32.2 Drugs That May Contribute to Delirium

Drug Class	Examples
Anticholinergics and drugs with anticholinergic side effects	**Antiarrhythmic agents**—disopyramide **Antipsychotics**—loxapine, risperidone, olanzapine **Antidepressants (SSRI)**—paroxetine **Antidepressants (tricyclic)**—amitriptyline, nortriptyline desipramine, imipramine, chlorpromazine, clozapine, desipramine, imipramine **Antiparkinson agents**—benztropine, trihexyphenidyl **Antispasmodics**—scopolamine (nonophthalmic), atropine (nonophthalmic) **Bladder antimuscarinics**—oxybutynin, tolterodine, fesoterodine, solifenacin **Skeletal muscle relaxants**—cyclobenzaprine, orphenadrine **Over-the-counter cold preparations**—antihistamines (e.g., diphenhydramine), decongestants
Benzodiazepines/ sedative hypnotics	Lorazepam, nitrazepam, flurazepam, diazepam, temazepam
Opioids	Meperidine, high doses of morphine, hydromorphone

Sources: American Geriatrics Society Beers Criteria Update Expert Panel. (2019). American Geriatrics Society 2019 Updated AGS Beers criteria for potentially inappropriate medication use in older adults. *Journal of the American Geriatrics Society, 67,* 674–694. https://doi.org/10.1111/jgs.15767. https://doi.org/10.1111/jgs.15767; Egberts, A., Moreno-Gonzalez, R., Alan, H., Ziere, G., & Mattace-Raso, F. (2021). Anticholinergic drug burden and delirium: A systematic review. *JAMDA: Journal of the American Medical Directors Association, 22,* 65–73. https://doi.org/10.1016/j.jamda.2020.04.019; Oh, E.S., Fong, T.G., Hshieh, T.T. & Inouye, S.K. (2017). Delirium in older persons: Advances in diagnosis and treatment. *Journal of the American Medical Association, 318*(12), 116–1173. Doi:10.1001/jama.2017.12067

Safety Interventions

Behaviours exhibited by the delirious patient, such as hallucinations, delusions, illusions, aggression, or agitation (restlessness or excitability), may pose safety problems. The patient must be protected from physical harm through the use of low beds, padded guardrails (use with caution when putting up both bedrails, as a confused person may try to climb over the rail), bed alarms, and careful supervision. Risk for injury is of high priority because individuals with delirium are more likely to fall or injure themselves during a confused state. "Prevention of Falls and Fall Injuries in the Older Adult" (RNAO, 2017) is a good resource to use for assessment and response to risk for falls.

Pharmacologic Interventions

Pharmacologic treatment of delirium, commonly directed at managing agitation and related psychosis, is the use of antipsychotic medication although the benefits of using these agents in older persons experiencing delirium are not clear and use may increase the risk of poor outcomes (Oh et al., 2017). The decision to use medications should be based on the specific symptoms such as severe agitation or hallucinations. Dosages must be kept low and usage of short duration. Medications should be chosen with reference to potential side effects (particularly anticholinergic effects, extrapyramidal side effects, oversedation, hypotension, and respiratory suppression) (see Box 32.1 for research on nurses' use of PRN psychotrophic medications for hospitalized older patients).

Nurses who are making a decision to administer an antipsychotic agent ordered PRN (as needed) must clearly identify the symptom it is prescribed for and its potential side effects. In some patients, the sedation effect may further impair cognition or paradoxic agitation. Antipsychotics such as haloperidol are no longer recommended for delirium prevention (Devlin et al., 2018; Oh et al., 2017). For treatment of a patient with severe agitation associated with delirium, the atypical antipsychotics such as risperidone, olanzapine, or quetiapine at low doses may be ordered short term in select cases, although more research is needed to establish their efficacy and safety. Haloperidol at low dose has been used for delirium, but it is an older agent with a riskier side effect profile (Riviere et al., 2019). Because of high extrapyramidal side effects, haloperidol should not be used in patients with underlying Lewy body dementia or Parkinson disease. Melatonin given to improve the sleep–wake cycle in delirious patients does not appear to have robust effect in studies to date (Oh et al., 2017). In critical care, lighter sedation for mechanically ventilated patients using a nonbenzodiazepine sedative such as propofol or dexmedetomidine is now recommended for agitation, rather than deep sedation (Devlin et al., 2018). To avoid worsening the patient's condition, benzodiazepines should be used only when the delirium is related to alcohol or benzodiazepine withdrawal. The use of antipsychotic agents in older individuals is discussed in greater detail later in the chapter.

BOX 32.1 Research for Best Practice

NURSE DECISION-MAKING IN PRN PSYCHOTROPHIC DRUG ADMINISTRATION

From Walsh, B., Dahlke, S., O'Rourke, H., & Hunter, K. F. (2020). Exploring acute care nurses' decision making in psychotrophic PRN use in hospitalized people with dementia. *Journal of Clinical Nursing*. Online ahead of print Aug 28. https://doi.org/10.1111/jocn.15477

The Objective: To understand how acute care nurses decided when to administer PRN psychotrophic medications to persons living with dementia.

Methods: A qualitative descriptive design was used to explore nurse decision-making. Eight nurses from medical units in a large hospital in Canada participated in semistructured interviews. Content analysis was used to guide the data analysis.

Findings: The authors identified three themes. The first was *Legitimizing control*, in which nurses medicated "undesirable" behaviours in an attempt to meet organizational expectations for safety, such as preventing falls.

The second theme, *Making the patient fit*, addressed the nurses attempts to maintain their work routines and the preferred order. Lastly, the theme *Future telling* concerned the use of medication to pre-empt undesirable behaviours. The participants did not describe any approach to assessment of the potential causes of behaviours such as delirium in hospitalized older people with dementia. Rather, they tended to use psychotrophic medications as a chemical restraint alternative to physical restraints.

Implications for Nursing: This study highlights the gaps in nurses' knowledge regarding appropriate psychotrophic medication use in hospitalized older people who are at risk of delirium. Given the serious potential side effects of psychotrophic medications, nurses need to be educated on their use. Further research is needed on the complex nature of decision-making for PRN use by nurses, and how best to promote evidence-based practice in the context of acute care units.

Administering and Monitoring Medications

Patients experiencing delirium may resist taking medications because of their confusion. If a medication is given, ideally, it should be oral. Medications should *not* be hidden in food.

Monitoring and Managing Side Effects

Monitoring drug action and side effects is especially important because the cause of the delirium may not be known, and the patient may inadvertently be affected by the medication. All antipsychotic medications have some degree of anticholinergic and extrapyramidal side effects (Riviere et al., 2019). Patients should be monitored for sedation, hypotension, anticholinergic, or extrapyramidal symptoms. Anticholinergic side effects include dry mouth, urinary retention, constipation, worsening confusion, mydriasis, and sinus tachycardia. Extrapyramidal symptoms include dystonia; repetitive, involuntary muscle movements (e.g., lip smacking); and/or an extreme urge to be moving constantly (akathisia). Although mental status often fluctuates during delirium, it may also be influenced by these medications, particularly those with anticholinergic side effects. Any changes or worsening of mental status after the administration of the medication should be reported immediately to the prescriber. For example, akathisia (see Chapter 13) may appear to be agitation or restlessness. The patient's physical condition and concurrent medication regimen may also influence the bioavailability, metabolism, distribution, and elimination of these medications. Adequate hydration and nutrition must be maintained. When using antipsychotic medications, closely monitor the patient for symptoms of neuroleptic malignant syndrome (see Chapter 13). The appearance of these symptoms may be confused with those related to delirium and therefore missed.

The use of medications to treat symptoms related to delirium should be discontinued as soon as possible. Benzodiazepines should be withdrawn gradually over a period of several days or weeks.

Identifying Drug Interactions

The aetiology of delirium is often a drug–drug interaction. OTC sleeping, cold, or allergy medication may be the cause. It is the nurse's responsibility to critically review each patient's medication record and discuss findings with the attending physician/nurse practitioner to avoid drug overdosage and intoxication, which can worsen symptoms. If medication is the underlying cause, it is important to identify accurately which medications are involved before administering any other drugs. Consultation with a clinical pharmacist may also be helpful. Exploring a patient's medication history in a physical assessment allows access to relevant data for guiding the care plan. Many of the medications used to treat symptoms of delirium (e.g., restlessness, altered sleep cycle) may in fact have potential side effects that worsen symptoms (Riviere et al., 2019).

Teaching Points

To prevent future occurrences, the nurse needs to educate the patient, family, and caregivers about the underlying causes and predisposing factors related to delirium. If the delirium is not resolved before discharge, caregivers need to know how to care for the patient at home and offer information on where to receive additional health, community, or social support.

Psychological Domain

Assessment

The psychological assessment of the individual with delirium focuses on cognitive changes revealed through the mental status examination as well as the resulting behavioural manifestations. Nurses are with patients around the clock and are the key interprofessional team members who first notice when the patient is experiencing a change in mental status or other indications of distress such as pain, anxiety, and behavioural changes. Effective communication from shift to shift between nurses and to other members of the interprofessional team is essential. A needs-based care plan can then be implemented to promote the patient's comfort and safety. Changes in mental status must be monitored frequently for an early detection of delirium, especially in vulnerable individuals.

Mental Status

Rapid onset of global cognitive impairment that affects multiple aspects of intellectual functioning is the hallmark of delirium. An essential nonpharmacologic nursing intervention for a patient experiencing delirium is to identify and help correct any unstable physiologic and haemodynamic conditions that evoke an acute change in mental status, such as sepsis, poisoning, or drug intoxication. Mental status evaluation usually reveals several changes such as the following:

- Fluctuations in the level of consciousness with a reduced awareness of the environment
- Difficulty focusing and sustaining or shifting attention
- Severely impaired memory, especially immediate and recent memory

Patients may be disoriented to time and place but rarely to person. Environmental perceptions are often disturbed. The patient may believe that shadows in the room are really people. Thought content is often illogical, and speech may be incoherent or inappropriate to context. Each variation in mental status tends to fluctuate over the course of the day. On any given day, an individual with delirium may appear confused and uncooperative but later may be lucid and able to follow instructions. Calculations, orientation (especially to time), and recall are most affected in delirium, whereas naming and registration are relatively preserved. Several rating scales are available for use in assessing the cognitive and behavioural fluctuations of delirium (Box 32.2). Nurses must assess and document the cognitive status of the individual throughout the day so that interventions can be modified accordingly.

Behaviour

Delirious patients exhibit a wide range of behaviours, complicating the process of determining a nursing care focus and planning interventions. At times, the individual may be restless or agitated and at other times lethargic and slow to respond. Precautions to prevent falls, aspiration, and accidental self-inflicted injuries should be established to ensure patient safety. Delirium can be categorized into three types:

- Hyperactive delirium involves behaviours such as being overly alert, exhibiting disturbing episodes of psychomotor hyperactivity, and marked excitability (may hallucinate). The patient may scream out in fear, describe hallucinations, pull at tubes, attempt to climb out of bed, and may attempt to hit staff (Oh et al., 2017).
- Hypoactive delirium is marked by lethargy, sleepiness, apathy, and psychomotor slowing; this is the "quiet" patient for whom the diagnosis of delirium often is missed (especially in seriously ill patients), as such patients often remain withdrawn or lie quietly in bed.
- **Mixed delirium** involves behaviour that fluctuates between the hyperactive and the hypoactive states over brief or long periods.

Nursing Care Focus for the Psychological Domain

Although the underlying cause of acute confusion is physiologic, which can be associated with impaired cognitive functioning, nursing care should focus on the psychological domain as well as the physical. Also related to the psychological domain, the nurse should be attentive to include the risk for acute confusion, disturbed thought process, ineffective coping, disturbed personal identity, and deficient knowledge.

Interventions for the Psychological Domain

Nurses should have frequent interactions with patients and support them with institutional and community resources if they are confused, experiencing illusions, or hallucinating. Patients should be encouraged to express their fears and discomforts that result from frightening or disconcerting psychotic experiences. Adequate lighting, easy-to-read calendars and clocks, a quiet noise level, and frequent verbal orientation may reduce this frightening experience. If the patient wears eyeglasses or uses a hearing aid, these devices should be used. Including familiar personal possessions such as favourite clothing and footwear, or wall paintings in the environment, may also help. Interventions that may be useful for these individuals are discussed in detail later in the chapter (see the section on dementia).

Social Domain

Assessment

Discussions should be initiated with the family to determine whether the patient's behaviours are new. An assessment of living arrangements may provide information about sensory stimulation or social isolation. Cultural and educational background must be considered when the patient's mental capacity is evaluated. New immigrants and individuals from certain ethnic backgrounds may not be familiar with the information used in tests of general knowledge (e.g., names of prime ministers, geographic knowledge), or in testing memory (e.g., date of birth in cultures that do not routinely celebrate birthdays), or orientation (e.g., sense of placement and location may be conceptualized differently in some cultures). Some cultural practices may involve using substances such as elixirs that contain chemicals that may

---

BOX 32.2 Rating Scales for Use With Delirium

THE CONFUSION ASSESSMENT METHOD (CAM)

Inouye, S. K., van Dyck, C. H., Alessi, C. A., Balkin, S., Siegal, A. P., & Horwitz, R. I. (1990). Clarifying confusion: The confusion assessment method. *Annals of Internal Medicine, 113*, 941–948.

DELIRIUM RATING SCALE (DRS)-R-98

Trzepacz, P. T., Mittal, D., Torres, R., Kanary, K., Norton, J., & Jimerson, N. (2001). Validation of the Delirium Rating Scale-revised-98: Comparison with the delirium rating scale and the cognitive test for delirium. *Journal of Neuropsychiatry and Clinical Neurosciences, 13*, 229–242.

NEECHAM CONFUSION SCALE

Miller, J., Neelon, V., Champagne, M., Bailey, D., Ng'andu, N., Belyea, M., Jarrell, E., Montoya, L., & Williams, A. (1997). The assessment of acute confusion as part of nursing care. *Applied Nursing Research, 10*(3), 143–151.

exacerbate delirium. The assessment should be language-specific and address such practices, as well as include exploring other relevant culture-specific practices.

Family Roles

Delirium is a burden not only for the patient but also for the patient's family caregivers (Shrestha & Fick, 2020). Family support for the individual and understanding of the disorder must, therefore, be assessed. The behaviours exhibited by the person experiencing delirium may be frightening or at least confusing for family members and significant others. Some family members may actually contribute to the patient's increased agitation. Observing and assessing family interactions and family members' ability to understand delirium is important. Family members often want to be involved in prevention and management of delirium.

Nursing Care Focus for the Social Domain

Among the several areas where nursing may become focused in the social domain, the most dominant involve risks for injury and supports for families.

Interventions for the Social Domain

The environment needs to be safe to protect the patient from injuries. A predictable, orienting environment will help to reestablish order to the patient's life. That is, a calendar, clock, music, and other items may be provided to help orient the patient to time, place, and person. If the patient is agitated, de-escalation techniques should be used (see Chapter 12). Physical restraint should be avoided as much as possible.

Support for Families

Families can be encouraged to work with staff members to reorient the patient and provide a supportive environment. Families need to understand that important decisions requiring the patient's input should be delayed if possible until the patient has fully recovered. Although patients may be able to participate in decision-making, they may not remember the decision later; it is, therefore, important to have several witnesses present and to document and keep record of any images and information in an ethical manner.

Spiritual Domain

Because delirium involves global cognitive impairment, including fluctuations in the level of consciousness and severely impaired memory, and may include agitation or lethargy, persons with delirium are very dependent on others for their comfort, dignity, and spiritual well-being. Communication and connection with others

is often seriously affected, and the nurse will need to enact well the critical qualities of spiritual care: receptivity, humanity, competency, and positivity (see Chapter 12). Patients experiencing hallucinations, delusions, and/or illusions in delirium may understand them as having a spiritual cause or ancestral connection or purpose. This can make them more or less frightening at the time, depending on the meaning attributed to them, particularly if a family member had undergone a similar experience ending in a poor outcome. The patient may benefit from a visit offered by their spiritual leader. Once the delirium passes, the patient may want to discuss such experiences (if remembered). The confusion of delirium necessitates, for the most part, that spiritual care of the patient is intensively "in the moment," as the nurse strives to sustain the person through the episode with family and religious support.

Evaluation and Treatment Outcomes

The primary treatment goal is the prevention or resolution of the delirious episode with return to previous cognitive status. Outcome measures include

- Correction of the underlying physiologic alteration
- Resolution of confusion
- Family member verbalization of understanding of confusion
- Prevention of injury

Resolution of confusion is the primary goal; however, the nurse makes important contributions to all four of these outcomes. The end result of delirium can be full recovery, incomplete recovery, incomplete recovery with some residual cognitive impairment, or a downward course leading to death.

Continuum of Care

The nurse may encounter patients with delirium in a number of management settings (e.g., home, nursing home, ambulatory care, day treatment, outpatient setting, hospital). Patients usually are admitted to an acute care setting for rapid evaluation and treatment of the underlying aetiology. An abrupt change in cognitive status can also occur while the patient is hospitalized for another reason. Delirium often persists beyond discharge from the hospital. Discharge planning should routinely include family education and referrals to community healthcare providers and social supports. If the patient will return to a residential long-term care setting, communication with facility staff about the patient's hospital stay, family support, and treatment regimen is crucial. Education of family members of persons with delirium (reversible or irreversible) is important across settings (Shrestha & Fick, 2020). For a checklist of psychoeducational topics to guide teaching of caregivers of individuals with delirium, see Box 32.3.

BOX 32.3 Psychoeducation Checklist: Delirium

When caring for the patient with delirium, be sure to include the caregivers, as appropriate, and address the following topic areas in the teaching plan:

✓ Psychopharmacologic agents, if used, including drug action, dosage, frequency, and possible adverse effects
✓ Underlying cause of delirium
✓ Mental status changes
✓ Safety measures
✓ Hydration and nutrition
✓ Avoidance of restraints
✓ Decision-making guidelines

DSD occurs when a patient with dementia develops a delirium (Caplan, 2019). DSD is often poorly identified or misdiagnosed because symptoms may appear to overlap. The co-occurrence of delirium and dementia (overlap syndrome) substantially impairs functional recovery from acute illness and hospitalization, as compared with those affected by depression or delirium alone. This suggests that depression and delirium act in an additive and independent fashion to produce higher rates of adverse outcomes. The overlap syndrome can be prolonged and carries significant risk for functional decline (Morandi et al., 2017). Nurses need to be alert for changes in persons living with dementia that might suggest delirium and work with the interprofessional team to assess and manage DSD effectively.

Mild Cognitive Impairment

MCI is a transitional stage between normal cognition and dementia (Tang-Wai et al., 2020). According to the Alzheimer's Association (2021b), long-term studies suggest that 15% to 20% of those aged 65 years and older may have MCI. The diagnostic criteria for MCI include a change in cognition over time in comparison with the person's previous level of performance. In addition, the cognitive performance is lower than expected for the person's age and education level. This change can occur in a variety of cognitive domains, including memory, executive function, attention, language, and visuospatial skills.

There are two types of MCI: amnestic (primarily affecting memory) and nonamnestic (affecting cognitive skills other than memory) (Glynn et al., 2020). Those with the amnestic type are twice as likely to progress to dementia. Persons with MCI commonly have mild problems performing complex functional tasks such as paying bills, preparing a meal, or shopping. They may take more time, be less efficient, and make more errors at performing such activities than in the past. Nevertheless, they generally maintain their independence of function in daily life, with minimal aids or assistance.

It is not yet possible to tell for certain what the outcome of MCI will be for a specific person or to determine the underlying cause of MCI from a person's symptoms (Alzheimer's Association, 2021b). Recently, an earlier potential manifestation on the MCI and dementia spectrum, SCD, has been proposed (Tang-Wai et al., 2020). This involves individuals identifying cognitive changes in themselves while objective cognitive testing remains normal. Persons identifying such concerns should be evaluated, and the possibility of presence of other psychiatric symptoms and conditions (e.g., anxiety, depression) should be taken into account because these too can contribute to a subjective sense of cognitive change.

Dementia

Dementia is an irreversible syndrome characterized by ongoing decline in intellectual functioning sufficient to disrupt physical, social, and/or occupational functioning. Dementia falls within three categories: early-onset familial AD (FAD); rapidly progressive dementia such as Creutzfeldt-Jakob disease (CJD), which is a mandatory reportable condition in Canada; and later-onset dementia, which includes four primary types of dementia: AD, vascular dementia, dementia with Lewy bodies (DLB), and frontotemporal dementia (FTD). Dementia may be preceded by **mild cognitive impairment** (MCI).

Dementia and Alzheimer Disease

The terms dementia and **Alzheimer disease (AD)** are often used interchangeably but there are distinct differences. The Alzheimer's Association clarifies that "dementia is a general term for a decline in mental ability severe enough to interfere with daily life. Alzheimer's is the most common cause of dementia. Alzheimer's is a specific disease. Dementia is not" (Dementia vs. Alzheimer Disease: What is the Difference? n.d.).

In 1901, Alois Alzheimer observed Auguste Deter, a 51-year-old patient at the Frankfurt Asylum, who exhibited strange behavioural symptoms and memory disturbance. When the patient died 5 years later, Alzheimer studied her brain and identified unusual pathological changes. Such changes came to be known as the plaques and tangles associated with Alzheimer disease (Petretto et al., 2021). However, the exact complex mechanism of the disease expression is still being studied as plaques and tangles have been found in people with normal cognitive function as well as those with AD.

Clinical Course of Alzheimer Disease

AD is a progressive neurodegenerative disorder characterized by irreversible memory loss and decline in other areas of cognition including language, praxis, visual/spatial ability, and executive functioning (Love & Geldmacher, 2018). The person's ability to function gradually declines, although their physical status often remains intact until late in the disease. Behavioural symptoms often develop. AD is a terminal illness.

Two subtypes of AD have been identified: the less common early-onset AD (a familial form starting before age 65) and late-onset AD (older than 65 years). AD is also routinely conceptualized in terms of three stages: early, middle, and late. Signs and symptoms of AD change as the person passes from one stage of the illness to another (Table 32.3). Persons living with AD tend to pass through a progressive sequence of deterioration and symptoms (Atri, 2019). Staging (i.e., identifying the stage the person is experiencing) is a useful technique for determining the person's current cognitive status and provides a sound basis for decisions in clinical management. People with AD live an average of 8 years with the disease, but some people may survive up to 20 years. The course of the disease depends, in part, on age at diagnosis and whether a person has other health conditions (Alzheimer's Association, 2021a).

Diagnostic Criteria of Dementia and Alzheimer Disease

The Canadian diagnostic criteria for dementia were reevaluated in 2019 by the fifth Canadian Consensus Conference on the Diagnosis and Treatment of Dementia (CCCDTD5) (Ismail et al., 2020). New criteria are based on recommendations made at this conference, those of the National Institute on Aging (NIA), and the Alzheimer's Association. Although a biological definition and biomarkers have emerged for research, the clinical criteria for AD include cognitive and/or behavioural symptoms that (a) interfere with the ability to function at work or at usual activities; (b) represent a decline from previous levels of functioning and performing; and (c) are not related to delirium or a major psychiatric disorder.

Screening for MCI and dementia in nonsymptomatic adults is not recommended. However, primary care healthcare professionals should watch for possible cognitive changes and if these occur, initiate assessment of cognition, function (activities of daily living), and behaviours with appropriate tools. This is especially important for those in categories such as advanced age, preexisting NCDs (e.g., Parkinson's) or other disorders that increase risk (e.g., diabetes, hypertension, stroke) (Ismail et al., 2020). Cognitive impairment is detected

Table 32.3 Stages of Dementia

Early Stage
Forgetfulness
Problems with orientation (e.g., cannot follow directions)
Communication difficulties
Limited attention span
Difficulty learning new things
Changes in mood and behaviour
May understand how they are changing and may wish to help plan and direct future care

Middle Stage
Memory problems are obvious (e.g., does not know address, own history)
Restlessness (e.g., wandering, pacing)
Spatial problems that may affect mobility
Confused, difficulty following a topic of conversation
Problems understanding verbal and written language
Changes in wake–sleep patterns; lack of appetite
Apprehensive and/or withdrawn
Uninhibited behaviour
Delusions and hallucinations

Late Stage
Severe cognitive impairment (memory, information processing, orientation)
Loses capacity for recognizable speech
Needs help with eating, toileting; may be incontinent
Loses ability to walk without assistance, to sit without support, to smile, hold head up
May have impaired swallowing and loss of weight

End of Life
Changes in blood circulation; skin breakdown
No longer accepting food and drink
Increased sleepiness; changes in breathing
Agitation
May have buildup of secretions; fever
Still experiences and senses emotion
Spiritual experience may be important

Adapted from Alzheimer Society of Canada. (2021a). *Stages of Alzheimer's disease.* http://www.alzheimer.ca/en/About-dementia/Alzheimer-s-disease/Stages-of-Alzheimer-s-disease. Refer to this site to see strategies for responding to the symptoms of each stage

and diagnosed through a combination of history taking from the person, a knowledgeable informant, and an objective cognitive assessment, such as the Mini-Mental State Exam (Folstein et al., 1975), Montreal Cognitive Assessment (MOCA) (Nasreddine et al., 2005), or other standardized tools recognized in the guideline. Those with positive corroborative history of cognitive decline from a reliable informant or care partner should be referred to a specialist memory clinic for further investigation using laboratory tests, neuroimaging, and more extensive neuropsychiatric testing (Ismail et al., 2020).

The cognitive and/or behavioural impairment can be apparent in any of the following domains: (a) impaired

Diagnostic Criteria	Symptoms
Impaired ability to acquire and remember information	Repetitive questions or conversations, misplacing personal belongings, forgetting events or appointments, getting lost on a familiar route
Impaired reasoning and handling of complex tasks, poor judgment	Poor understanding of safety risks, inability to manage finances, poor decision-making ability, inability to plan complex or sequential activities
Impaired visuospatial abilities	Inability to recognize faces or common objects or to find objects in direct view despite good visual acuity, inability to operate simple implements, or orient clothing to the body
Impaired language functions (speaking, reading, writing)	Difficulty thinking of common words while speaking, hesitations; speech, spelling, and writing errors
Changes in personality, behaviour, or comportment	Uncharacteristic mood fluctuations such as agitation; impaired motivation, initiative, apathy; loss of drive; social withdrawal; decreased interest in previous activities; loss of empathy; compulsive or obsessive behaviours; socially unacceptable behaviours

Table 32.4   Key Diagnostic Characteristics of Alzheimer Disease

Sources: Ismail, Z., Black, S. E., Camicioli, R, Chertkow, H., Herrmann, N., Laforce, R., Montero-Odasso, M., Rockwood, K., Rosa-Neto, P. Seitz, D., Sivananthan, S., Smith, E. E., Soucy, J.-P., Vedel, I., & Gauthier, S. (2020). Recommendations of the 5th Canadian Consensus Conference on the diagnosis, treatment of dementia. *Alzheimer's & Dementia, 16*(8), 1182–1195; Tang-Wai, D. F., Smith, E. E., Bruneau, M. A., Burhan, A. M., Chatterjee, A., Chertkow, H., Choudhury, S., Dorri, E., Ducharme, S., Fischer, C. E., Ghodasara, S., Herrmann, N., Hsiung, G.-Y. R., Kumar, S., Laforce, R., Lee, L., Massoud, F., Shulman, K.I., Stiffel, M., Gauthier S. & Ismail, Z. (2020). CCCDTD5 recommendations on early and timely assessment of neurocognitive disorders using cognitive, behavioral, and functional scales. *Alzheimer's & Dementia, 6*(1), e12057.

ability to acquire and remember new and retained information; (b) impaired reasoning and handling of complex tasks and poor judgment; (c) impaired visuospatial abilities; (d) impaired language functions (speaking, reading, writing); and (e) changes in personality, behaviour, or comportment. Table 32.4 lists examples presenting symptoms related to each of these criteria. If changes are identified, they should be further assessed using validated assessment tools for cognition, behaviours, and function (Ismail et al., 2020). Box 32.4 lists 10 warning signs of AD.

Clinical diagnosis is based on the person's detailed history, a comprehensive physical and neurologic examination, scores on validated tools, and the application of established diagnostic criteria that are reliable and valid. Diagnosis may be supported through neuropsychological testing and diagnostic investigations, such as neuroimaging of the brain to detect and monitor progressive atrophy. Magnetic resonance imaging (MRI) is recommended over computed tomography (CT) because of its greater sensitivity in detecting vascular lesions and some subtypes of dementia (Ismail et al., 2020). Specialist investigation to differentiate the type of dementia may involve more advanced diagnostic imaging such as FDG-PET scan or amyloid imaging. Noncognitive markers of dementia, such as slowed gait speed, are under investigation. There are currently no validated biomarkers for AD but researchers are investigating several promising candidates, including proteins in cerebrospinal fluid, proteins in blood, and genetic risk profiling.

Epidemiology and Risk Factors

Currently, 432,000 Canadians aged 65 and older are living with dementia. This does not include the number of people under 65 who are affected. In 15 years, this figure will increase to close to 1 million. The annual cost to Canadians to care for those living with dementia is over $8 billion dollars, projected to rise to 16.6 billion by 2031 (Public Health Agency of Canada, 2020). In 2019, the Government of Canada released a national dementia strategy to direct policy and research in prevention of dementia, advancing therapies and finding a cure and improving quality of life for people living with dementia and their care partners (Public Health Agency

---

BOX 32.4 Ten Warning Signs of Alzheimer Disease

To help the public know the warning signs of AD, the Alzheimer Society of Canada lists the following:

1. Memory loss that affects day-to-day function
2. Difficulty performing familiar tasks
3. Problems with language
4. Disorientation in time and place
5. Impaired judgment
6. Problems with abstract thinking
7. Misplacing things
8. Changes in mood and behaviour
9. Changes in personality
10. Loss of initiative

For more information, see https://alzheimer.ca/sites/default/files/documents/10-warning-signs.pdf (Alzheimer Society of Canada, 2018).

of Canada, 2019). Several provinces have also developed their own dementia strategies.

Age is the most acknowledged risk factor for developing dementia. It is estimated that dementia affects 1 in 14 people over the age of 65 and 1 in 6 over the age of 80. Women are at higher risk, even discounting the fact that they tend to live longer. People who experience severe or repeated head injuries are also at increased risk. It is also possible to inherit genes that cause dementia such as familial early-onset AD and Huntington disease. Conditions that affect the heart, arteries, or blood circulation all significantly affect a person's chances of developing dementia, particularly vascular dementia. These conditions include diabetes, midlife high blood pressure, high blood cholesterol levels, midlife obesity, heart problems, and stroke. Indeed, a history of stroke doubles the risk in older adults. On the other hand, there is evidence that lifestyle factors such as a Mediterranean diet, regular physical activity, zero to moderate (250 to 500 mL per day) amounts of alcohol, and social and mental activities may reduce the risk of dementia (Ismail et al., 2020).

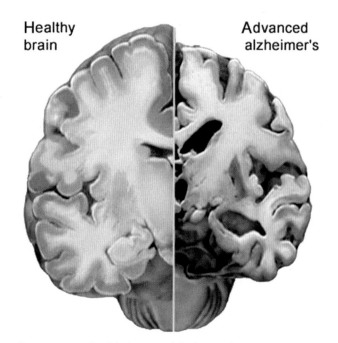

Healthy brain   **Advanced alzheimer's**

Figure 32.1 A healthy brain and the brain of a person in advanced Alzheimer disease. (Courtesy of National Institute on Aging.)

Aetiology

Researchers have yet to identify a definitive cause of AD; the causal pathway is likely complex. In the brain of a person with AD, the cortex shrivels up, thereby damaging areas involved in thinking, planning, and remembering. Shrinkage is especially severe in the hippocampus, which plays a key role in forming new memories. Ventricles (fluid-filled spaces within the brain) grow larger (Fig. 32.1). See Chapter 10 for the biological basis of dementia.

Magnetic resonance imaging and cerebrospinal fluid and/or amyloid positron emission tomography have been found supportive in identifying or ruling out the presence of AD pathology or differentiating it from other types of dementia. These differentiating results provide opportunities for improving diagnostic sensitivity and specificity (Ismail et al., 2020).

Beta-Amyloid Plaques

Following Alois Alzheimer's discovery of neuritic plaques and **neurofibrillary tangles**, accumulations of two separate proteins in the brain—beta-amyloid peptide and tau proteins—have been associated with AD (Love & Geldmacher, 2018). The pathophysiological changes start many years before the onset of symptoms (Atri, 2019). Microscopic plaques are made largely of a protein called beta amyloid (A-beta) (Love & Geldmacher, 2018). In low concentrations, A-beta may be part of the body's defences against invading bacteria and

other microbes. However, in AD, A-beta accumulates in the brain to a level that overwhelms the enzymes and other molecules that clear away A-beta and the plaques. Both the production of A-beta and, especially, the processes that clear it away appear to be defective, at least in part because the impaired blood vessels in the brain cannot adequately pick up and remove the A-beta. There is evidence that these fine blood vessels proliferate and become leaky, possibly allowing hazardous substances to get into the brain. The accumulating individual A-beta molecules begin to clump together to form small aggregates called oligomers, which are now linked to widespread loss of cortical synapses. Their continuing aggregation eventually leads to the formation of the amyloid plaques. However, it is the oligomers, not the plaques, that are the real problem: they are toxic to the brain's nerve cells. By the time enough A-beta molecules have stuck together to form the plaques, the damage has already been done (Fig. 32.2). What triggers the amyloid cascade and why is still under debate.

Neurofibrillary Tangles

Neurofibrillary tangles are made of a protein called tau (Love & Geldmacher, 2018). Tau is present in normal nerve cells, but in AD, it becomes chemically altered (phosphorylated) and tends to pile up as threadlike tangles, preventing its normal functions. A critical function is to provide a kind of railroad track system inside the nerve cells and along the nerve fibres that are spun off from the cell body. The tau pathways are inside the

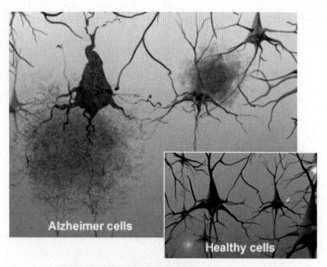

Figure 32.2 The beta-amyloid plaques and neurofibrillary tangles of Alzheimer disease compared with healthy neurons. (Courtesy of National Institute on Aging.)

nerve cells and fibres. Their main role in fibres is to convey essential nutrient and instructional chemicals and tiny organelles (structures) up and down the fibres in both directions. In AD, neurofibrillary tangles are made up of abnormal filaments with a unique paired helical structure (Love & Geldmacher, 2018). They are found

---

IN-A-LIFE 🏠

Dame Iris Murdoch (1919–1999)

PUBLIC PERSONA

Born in Dublin, Ireland, Dame Iris Murdoch became a much-loved philosopher and writer, the author of 36 novels, several plays, essays, and philosophical works, and engaged in a critical study of Jean-Paul Sartre. Over her life, she filled 95 diaries with her aspirations and analysis of her own shortcomings. Her book, *The Sea, The Sea*, won the Booker Prize in 1978. Iris Murdoch was elected as a fellow to St. Anne's College, Oxford, in 1948 and remained a tutor there until 1963.

PERSONAL REALITIES

Iris Murdoch married John Bayley in 1956. In the mid-1990s, she began to show signs of AD. Her extensive vocabulary became diminished; she had difficulty answering questions, and there was a noticeable decline in the quality of her last book, *Jackson's Dilemma*. She died of AD in 1999. Her husband's book about her life, an *Elegy for Iris* (1999), was made into a movie, *Iris*, in 2001.

---

in a number of brain structures including the forebrain and substantia nigra. When tangles develop, there is interference with normal function of the neuron due to loss of axonal transport. The density of the tangles correlates with neuronal loss. These pathophysiological changes and neuronal cell death result in deficiencies in neurotransmitters, including acetylcholine, norepinephrine, and GABA.

With the advent of advanced imaging techniques, we now understand that in those diagnosed clinically with AD, the spread of plaques and tangles through the brain occurs in what is now recognized as a predictable pattern, from areas involving memory and planning to areas affecting speech and position sense to the point of where most of the cortex is affected (Alzheimer's Association, 2021a).

Inflammation

An inflammatory response is normal whenever and wherever the body suffers trauma or is attacked by some kind of potentially threatening influence, such as an infection or a toxin. Normally, acute inflammation resolves. Neuroinflammation is the inflammatory response that occurs in the brain of the person with AD. It is hypothesized that in AD, this inflammatory immune response can become excessive and does not resolve (Whittington et al., 2017). The result is an exacerbation of the A-beta and neurofibrillary pathology.

Oxidative Stress and the Role of Antioxidants

Oxidative stress refers to the threatening situation created when reactive oxygen species (ROS) begin to accumulate faster than the body can get rid of them. ROS are normal products of metabolism. However, if ROS are allowed to build up, they become damaging, poisoning the cells of the body, including those of the brain. Normally, this is prevented by the body's antioxidants. Natural antioxidants also occur in food, such as vitamins C and E.

Oxidative stress has been identified as a contributor to aging, AD, and other neurodegenerative diseases. Synaptic activity is affected by increased production of ROS, altered metal homeostasis, and reduced antioxidant defence (Tönnies & Trushina, 2017). Risk factors for AD and the accumulation of A-beta protein likely contribute to the increased production of ROS. Although antioxidant treatment has been investigated, the results have not yet been robust.

Genetic Factors

The gene called apolipoprotein E (ApoE) has been shown to play a small part in the development of vascular dementia and late onset AD. Specifically, the ApoE4 variant is believed to preferentially promote production of the A-beta protein, constituting a significant risk for development of AD and other dementias (Atri, 2019). Other causative genes have been identified that affect inflammation, the amyloid pathway, lipid metabolism, and synaptic function (Ghani et al., 2018), demonstrating the complexity of dementia etiology.

The rare early onset familial form of AD (FAD) is almost totally attributable to genes that have mutated to an extent that makes them function abnormally, and the abnormal functions are responsible for the disease. This form of AD can result from mutations in one of three genes, *APP, PSEN1, or PSEN2* (Ghani et al., 2018). The abnormal genes are passed from generation to generation in an autosomal dominant mode.

Interprofessional Treatment of Dementia and Alzheimer Disease

The nature and range of information and services needed by persons living with dementia and AD, and their families throughout their journey can vary dramatically at different stages. In designing services and interventions, the interprofessional team must keep in mind that AD has a progressively deteriorating clinical course and that the anatomic and neurochemical changes that occur in the brain are accompanied by impairments in cognition, affect, behaviour, and psychosocial functioning. Pharmacologic intervention modestly improves cognitive symptoms and may subsequently decrease the rate of disease progression, typically at the early stage of AD (Ismail et al., 2020).

For a variety of reasons (e.g., stigma, reluctance of family physicians to make a diagnosis as they believe little can be done), many persons living with dementia are never formally diagnosed, thus limiting their ability to receive appropriate treatment and services. Heightening awareness of the importance of receiving an informed diagnosis, possibly from a neurologist or geriatrician, is strongly recommended. Initial assessment of the person suspected of having dementia has three main objectives: (a) confirmation of the diagnosis through neuropsychological testing and diagnostic investigations, such as neuroimaging of the brain type and severity of dementia; (b) establishment of baseline levels in a number of functional spheres; and (c) establishment of a therapeutic relationship with the patient and family that will continue through subsequent phases of the disease. Treatment efforts currently focus on managing the cognitive symptoms, delaying the cognitive decline (e.g., memory loss, confusion, and problems with learning, speech, and reasoning), treating the noncognitive symptoms (e.g., psychosis, mood symptoms, agitation), and supporting the caregivers as a means of improving the quality of life for both persons living with dementia and their family and friend caregivers.

Priority Care Issues

The priority of care for dementia will change throughout the course of the disease. Prorock and colleagues (2013) identified four phases of healthcare experience for persons living with dementia and their caregivers, each with health service implications, which remains a relevant framework. In the first phase, *seeking information and understanding*, there is distress regarding the changes in the individual and uncertainty about what is happening, a situation that public awareness and education could, at least in part, relieve. *Identifying the problem* comes with the formal diagnosis of dementia, bringing anxiety but also relief as understanding of the changes is achieved. The *role transition* phase includes both the person living with dementia and their caregivers beginning to prepare for coping with the illness. It is important that informed support is available to them and goals and potential treatments are discussed. The final phase, *living with change*, evolves as current and future care needs are focused upon.

What might living with such changes be like? Persons with dementia usually experience difficulties remembering the last meal taken or how to use a knife and fork and confuse names of even close relations, house addresses, or significant dates. Impaired self-care (loss of ability to perform routine household chores, bathing, dressing, and eating) becomes prominent as the disease progresses. Often, they may ask the same questions repetitively, despite answers being previously given. The disease places the person at an increased risk of getting lost, even inside the home. Close observation is necessary outside the home. As the disease progresses, the person becomes highly dependent due to deterioration in physiologic functions (e.g., incontinence, ADL dependence) added to the existing cognitive challenges. Initially, the priority is delaying cognitive decline and supporting family members. Later, the priority changes to protecting the person from injury. Near the end, the physical and emotional needs of the person living with dementia are the focus of care.

Family Response

Families are often the first to be aware of the cognitive problems of a loved one. The person living with dementia may be unaware of the extent of memory impairment. A diagnosis of dementia means long-term care responsibilities, while the essence of the person living with dementia diminishes day by day. Most families wish to keep their relative at home as long as possible to maintain contact and to avoid costly nursing home placement. The symptoms that often result in placement are incontinence that cannot be managed and behavioural problems, such as wandering, especially at night, and aggression. Across care settings, nurses need to support the individual and their families with education about treatment and choices as well as healthy coping strategies. To do this, nurses require better preparation in dementia and gerontological competencies (Boscart et al., 2019).

The needs of family members should also be considered. Caring for a family member with dementia takes its toll. Caregivers' health is often compromised, and normal family functioning is threatened. Caregiver distress is a major health risk for the family, and "caregiver burnout" is a common cause of the institutionalization of persons living with dementia.

Nursing Management: Human Response to Dementia

The development and implementation of appropriate, effective, and safe nursing care and services that support persons living with dementia and their families are a particular challenge because of the complex nature of the illness. Although the condition is caused by biologic changes, the psychological and social domains are seriously affected by this disorder (see Box 32.4). The assessment of the person with dementia needs to follow the geriatric mental health nursing assessment found in Chapter 31.

Biologic Domain

Assessment

Nursing assessment provides a foundation for the creation of a needs-specific patient care plan since the gathered data serve as evidence for appropriate interventions. The nursing assessment should include a review of the medical history, current medication profile (prescription and OTC medications), home and traditional remedies, substance use history (including alcohol intake and smoking history), chronic physical or psychiatric illness, and a description of the onset, duration, range, and intensity of symptoms associated with dementia. A history of hospitalization and the respective reasons must be noted. The onset of symptoms is typically gradual, with insidious changes in behaviour. To conduct a thorough assessment of the patient, the nurse needs to know what is typical for the individual; therefore, caregivers, family members, and significant others can be sources of valuable information.

Physical Examination and a Review of Body Systems

A review of body systems must be conducted on each person suspected of experiencing dementia. Specific biologic assessment parameters include vital signs, neuromuscular status, nutritional and weight status, bladder and bowel function, hygiene, skin integrity, rest and activity level, sleep patterns, and fluid and electrolyte balance. The neurologic function is usually preserved through the early and middle stages of dementia, although seizures, gait disturbances, and tremors may occur at any time. In the later stages of the disease, neurologic signs such as flexion contractures and primitive reflexes are prominent features.

Physical Functions

At first, limitations may primarily involve instrumental activities, such as shopping, preparing meals, and performing other household chores. Later in the disease process, basic physical dysfunctions occur, such as incontinence, ataxia, dysphagia, and contractures. Incontinence can be a major source of stress and a considerable burden to family caregivers. Assessment of physical functions includes ADL, recent changes in functional abilities (dressing, toileting, and feeding), use of sensory aids (eyeglasses and hearing aids), activity level, and assessment of pain.

Self-Care

Associated alterations in the central nervous system (CNS) impair the person living with dementia's ability to retrieve information from the environment and from memories, retain new information, and give meaning to current situations. Therefore, persons living with dementia often neglect self-care activities such as bathing, eating, and oral and skin care.

Sleep–Wake Disturbances

Sleep disruption among older adults with dementia and AD is common. The sleep–wake disturbances that commonly occur in persons with dementia are hypersomnia, insomnia, and reversal of the sleep–wake cycle. The disruptions in sleep at night are particularly difficult for family caregivers. In AD, degeneration of nerve cells in the suprachiasmatic nucleus as well as decreased melatonin levels have been identified. Sleep disruption has been identified as a potential factor in accelerating AD progression due to impaired clearing of A-beta proteins (Malhotra, 2018).

Persons with dementia may nap frequently in the daytime. Their nighttime periods of wakefulness mean that they have reduced rapid eye movement sleep. Sleep disturbances often increase as dementia advances. Where the person is unable to provide a reliable sleep history, the nurse must obtain the information from the person's caregiver. Such history usually encompasses sleep hygiene measures, use of sleep-promoting medications, and history of any sleep difficulties or underlying medical conditions. Increasing daylight exposure, engaging in daytime activities and exercises, and adhering to basic sleep hygiene measures can enhance nighttime sleep.

Activity and Exercise

Despite being physically capable, people in the early phase of AD often withdraw from normal activities due to the developing symptoms of memory loss, decrease in self-motivation, and, possibly, depression.

Nutrition

Eating can become a problem for persons with dementia because they may develop difficulty chewing and swallowing. As the disease progresses, they may lose the ability to feed themselves or recognize what is offered as food. The hyperactive patient requires frequent feedings of a high-protein, high-carbohydrate diet in the form of finger foods (which they can carry while on the go). Most persons with dementia prefer to feed themselves with their fingers when appropriate rather than have someone feed them. Weight loss is a common consequence. It is important to monitor persons with altered appetites for hydration and electrolyte imbalances.

Pain

Assessment and documentation of any physical discomfort or pain the person living with dementia may be experiencing should be included in the psychogeriatric nursing assessment (see Chapter 31). Although not usually thought of as a physically painful disorder, individuals with dementia often have other comorbid physical diseases. In the early stages of their disease, the individual can usually respond to verbal questions regarding pain. Later, it may be difficult to assess the comfort level objectively, especially if the person cannot communicate. However, pain should be assessed through physical examination and use of a pain assessment scale (see Web Link on managing pain).

Nursing Care Focus for the Biologic Domain

The unique and changing needs of persons with dementia present a challenge for nurses in all settings. A sample of common nursing care foci include imbalanced nutrition: feeding concerns, impaired swallowing, bathing/hygiene self-care deficit, dressing/grooming self-care deficit, toileting issues such as constipation (or perceived constipation), bowel incontinence, impaired urinary elimination, functional incontinence, total incontinence, deficient fluid volume, risk for impaired skin integrity, impaired physical mobility, activity intolerance, fatigue, disturbed sleep, and pain.

Interventions for the Biologic Domain

The numerous interventions for the biologic domain vary throughout the course of the disease. Initially, the person with dementia requires simple directions for self-care activities and initiation of psychopharmacologic treatment. At the end of the disorder, total care is required.

Self-Care Interventions

Promotion of self-care supports cognitive functioning and a sense of independence. In the early stages, the nurse (and family members) should maximize normal perceptual experiences by ensuring that the person with dementia has appropriate eyeglasses and working hearing aids. If eyeglasses and hearing aids are needed, but not used, persons with dementia are more likely to have false perceptual experiences. Ongoing monitoring of self-care is necessary throughout its course. Oral hygiene can be a problem and, although this may be difficult, requires excellent basic nursing care. Aging and many medications reduce salivary flow, leading to a painfully dry and cracking oral mucosa. Drugs that have xerostomia (dry mouth) as a side effect and are commonly prescribed for persons with progressive dementia include antidepressant, antispasmodic, antihypertensive, bronchodilator, and some antipsychotic agents. For persons experiencing xerostomia, hard candy or chewing gum may stimulate salivary flow, or modification of the drug regimen may be necessary. Glycerol mouthwash may also provide some relief from xerostomia.

Nutritional Interventions

Maintenance of nutrition and hydration are essential nursing interventions. The person's weight, oral intake, and hydration status should be monitored carefully. They need to eat well-balanced meals that are appropriate to their activity level and eating abilities, with special attention given to electrolyte balance and fluid intake.

The dining environment should be calm and food presentation appealing. If the person eats only a small portion of food at one meal, reduce the presentation of food in terms of the amount and number of choices. One-dish meals (e.g., a casserole) are ideal. If the person is distressed, delay feeding because eating, chewing, and swallowing difficulties are accentuated and choking becomes a risk.

Persons living with dementia should be presented food that is appropriate for their individual needs. When swallowing is a problem, thick liquids or semisoft foods are more effective than are traditionally prepared foods. If the individual is likely to choke or aspirate food, semisolid foods should be offered, because liquids flow into the pharyngeal cavity more quickly and may cause choking. In the later stages, some individuals hoard food in their mouths; others swallow too rapidly or fail to chew their food sufficiently before attempting to swallow. The nurse needs to watch for swallowing difficulties that place the person at risk for aspiration and asphyxiation. Swallowing difficulties may result from changes in oesophageal motility and decreased secretion of saliva.

As dementia progresses, and food intake is low, oral-assisted feedings are encouraged and vitamin and mineral supplements may be indicated. Percutaneous feeding tubes in persons with advanced dementia are not recommended. Careful hand-feeding is at least as good as tube feeding for the outcomes of death, aspiration pneumonia, functional status, and comfort. Tube feeding is associated with agitation, increased use of physical and chemical restraints, and worsening pressure ulcers (see Web Link on *Meal Times* for additional information).

Supporting Bowel and Bladder Function

Urinary or bowel incontinence affects many persons with dementia. Urinary urgency may be an early indicator of cognitive decline as central control of continence is governed by some of the same brain structures as executive function. Older persons with urgency have impaired executive function when compared with those without urgency (Gibson et al., 2020). During the middle stage of the disease, incontinence may be caused by the person's apathy or inability to communicate the need to use the toilet or locate a toilet quickly, undress appropriately to use the toilet, or recognize the sensation of fullness signalling the need to urinate or defecate. For the person who is incontinent because of an inability to locate the toilet, reorientation may be helpful. Displaying pictures or signs on bathroom doors provides visual cues, and verbal prompts promote reorientation to the environment.

Getting to know the person's habits and moods can help the nurse identify signals that indicate a need to void. The person can then be assisted to reach the bathroom in time. Positioning the person near the toilet or placing a portable commode nearby may help if the person cannot reach a toilet quickly. If the person demonstrates dressing **apraxia** (cannot undress appropriately), clothing can be modified with easy-to-open fasteners in place of zippers or buttons. For nocturnal incontinence, limiting the amount of fluid consumed after the evening meal, keeping lower leg edema under control, and taking the person to the toilet just before going to bed or upon awakening during the night may reduce or eliminate nocturia.

Indwelling urinary catheters are contraindicated in persons with dementia, because they are generally not well tolerated and because hand restraints are often needed to prevent them from removing the catheter. Indwelling urinary catheters foster the development of urinary tract infections and may compromise the person's dignity and comfort. Urinary incontinence can be managed with the use of disposable absorbent incontinent products.

Persons with dementia often experience constipation, although they may not be able to report this change. Therefore, subtle signs such as lethargy, reduced appetite, and abdominal distension need to be assessed frequently. Medications, decreased food and liquid intake, lack of motor activity, and decreased intestinal motility contribute to developing constipation. The person's diet should be rich in fibre, including bran or whole grains, vegetables, and fruit. Adequate oral intake (minimum of 1,500 to 2,000 mL per day) helps to prevent constipation. A gentle laxative such as milk of magnesia is commonly used to promote bowel elimination. Enemas and harsher chemical cathartics should be avoided because they may increase pain or discomfort.

Sleep Interventions

Disturbed sleep cycles are particularly stressful to the person with dementia, family, caregivers, and nursing staff. Disturbed sleep is difficult to manage from a behavioural perspective, and the person's overall level of health may suffer because sleep serves a restorative function. Bright light therapy using table-mounted "light boxes" have shown promise in improving sleep in persons with dementia by regulating the sleep–wake cycle (Hjetland et al., 2020). However, the best source of bright light is natural daylight. Physical activity such as walking and socializing outdoors has been shown to improve nighttime sleep.

Other sleep hygiene interventions that are helpful include having a fixed bedtime and awakening time that are the same every day; having certain activities that are always associated with going to bed (e.g., a particular piece of music or putting on a specific body lotion); avoiding napping during the day; avoiding alcohol 4 to 6 h before bedtime; and having lots of fluids during the day but not a few hours before going to bed. In addition, rest periods (in reclining chairs) in the morning and afternoon may help to eliminate late-day confusion (sundowning) and nighttime awakenings. Multicomponent interventions to enhance sleep seem to be the most effective (Kinnunen et al., 2017).

Benzodiazepines or other sedative–hypnotics should be the last choice for insomnia (American Geriatrics Society, 2019). These drugs may be prescribed for a short time for restlessness or insomnia, but they may also cause a paradoxic reaction of agitation and insomnia. They also increase the risk of falls.

Activity and Exercise Interventions

Activity and exercise programs appear to have a significant impact on improving balance, strength, and mobility in people with dementia (Lam et al., 2018). To promote a feeling of success, any activity or exercise plan must be culturally sensitive and adapted to the person's functional ability and interests. The activity or exercise must be designed to prevent excess stress (both physical and psychological). If the program of rest, activity, and exercise is truly individualized, the resultant feelings of value and competency may enhance the person's functional ability, cognition, and sleep pattern.

Pain and Comfort Management

Nursing care of noncommunicative persons with dementia and pain can be challenging. Common behaviours associated with pain may be difficult to interpret or absent. Signs to watch for that may indicate pain include body language and nonverbal signs that may indicate the person is uncomfortable; changes in behaviour (especially anxiety, agitation, shouting, and sleep disturbances); pale or flushed skin tone; dry, pale gums; mouth sores; vomiting; feverish skin; and swelling of any part of the body. Because of the difficulty in identifying and monitoring pain, persons with dementia are often undertreated. Undertreatment of pain may result in further cognitive and behavioural problems.

Relaxation

Approaching the person living with dementia in a calm, confident, unhurried manner; maintaining a soothing, quiet environment; avoiding unnecessary noise or chatter around them and lowering vocal tone and rate when addressing them; maintaining eye contact; and using touch judiciously are likely to promote a sense of security conducive to relaxation and comfort. Simple relaxation exercises can be used by the person to reduce stress.

Administering and Monitoring Medications

In the last two decades, the discovery of successful dementia medications has been challenged by lack of research funding and the high degree of brain deterioration at the time of diagnosis that is likely not reversible. Given this, more recent trials focus on people who have presymptomatic or mild disease (Wolters & Ikram, 2018). Thus, because no medication can cure those with established AD, psychopharmacologic interventions have two goals: maintain cognitive function and treat related psychiatric and behavioural disturbances that cause discomfort for the individual, interfere with treatment, or worsen the individual's functional and/or cognitive status. Medications for AD must be used with caution. Doses must be kept extremely low, and individuals should be monitored closely for any side effects or worsening of cognitive status. "Start low and go slow" is the principle guiding the administration of psychopharmacologic agents to older adults.

Often, convincing the person living with dementia to take the medication is one of the biggest nursing challenges. They may be unwilling, even though they previously agreed to take the drugs. The nurse will need to investigate and hypothesize the reason(s) for their reluctance to take medication. It may be because of difficulty swallowing pills, paranoid ideas, or lack of

understanding. The underlying reason(s) for medication refusal will determine the strategy. If the person has difficulty swallowing, most medications come in concentrate liquid form and can be easily swallowed. Medications should never be mixed in food without the person being made aware. If suspicion or paranoia is the reason, the nurse will need to try to identify the conditions under which the person feels safe to take the medication, such as in the presence of a favourite nurse or relative.

Cholinesterase Inhibitors

In Canada, three cholinesterase inhibitors (CIs) are approved: donepezil (Aricept), rivastigmine (Exelon), and galantamine (Reminyl). These medications are believed to work by preventing the breakdown of acetylcholine, which is important for learning and memory. The medications may temporarily ease of stabilize some of the symptoms of AD and can also be considered for treatment in vascular dementia (Ismail et al., 2020). Some people are affected by the side effects from CIs, which include diarrhoea, insomnia, nausea, infection, and bladder problems. To avoid side effects, CIs are contained in a skin patch, allowing the drug to be absorbed directly into the body.

N-Methyl-D-Aspartate Antagonists

Overstimulation of the N-methyl-D-aspartate receptor by glutamate (excitatory neurotransmitter) is considered to have a role in AD. The drug Ebixa (memantine hydrochloride) acts by blocking the glutamate receptors and preventing the reuptake of toxic amounts of the glutamate into the nerve endings. The combination of memantine with the CI galantamine has shown benefits for cognition as well as some behavioural and **neuropsychiatric symptoms** such as psychosis (Koola, 2020).

Antipsychotic Agents

Antipsychotic drugs have historically been used to treat the severe distortions in thought, perception, and emotion that characterize psychosis and have increasingly been used to treat the behavioural and psychological symptoms (e.g., delusion, aggression, and agitation) in persons with dementia. The adverse effects include sedation, higher risks of falls and hip fractures, Parkinson disease–type symptoms, cardiovascular events (stroke and heart attack), and the greater risk of death. Judicious short-term use of antipsychotics such as risperidone, olanzapine, and aripiprazole may be carefully considered for specific neuropsychiatric symptoms such as agitation or psychosis, but risk, especially for stroke, may outweigh benefit (Mueller et al., 2021). Nurses should focus on identifying and addressing the causes of behaviours and nonpharmacological management, which can make drug treatment unnecessary (Ismail et al., 2020).

Antidepressant Agents and Mood Stabilizers

A depressed mood is common in persons living with dementia. However, they often respond with improved mood to physical activity such as a walk outdoors, engagement in a group activity, and psychotherapeutic intervention (individual or group therapy), and if necessary, in combination with pharmacotherapy. Low doses of selective serotonin reuptake inhibitors (SSRIs) are often used for people with Alzheimer disease and depression because they have less anticholinergic and antiadrenergic effects than tricyclic antidepressants, which may reduce risk of causing confusion or falls. However, a research Cochrane review showed little evidence that any antidepressants were efficacious in treating depression in dementia (Dudas et al., 2018).

Antianxiety Medications (Sedative–Hypnotics)

Antianxiety medications, also known as benzodiazepines, should only be used as a last resort for insomnia, agitation, or delirium (American Geriatrics Society, 2019). Large-scale studies consistently show that the risk of motor vehicle accidents, falls, and hip fractures leading to hospitalization and death can more than double in older adults taking benzodiazepines and other sedative–hypnotics. Sedative–hypnotic agents may be prescribed for a short time for restlessness or insomnia, but they may also cause a paradoxical reaction of agitation and insomnia (especially in older adults).

Other Medications

Clinical observations indicate that persons with dementia are more vulnerable to the effects of anticholinergic drugs that can cause confusion and amnesia. Anticholinergic medications should be avoided for them if at all possible due to the CNS effects. There is emerging evidence that exposure to some drug classes that are strongly anticholinergic may increase risk of dementia (Coupland et al., 2019). See Box 32.5 for examples of medications that should not be taken by persons living with dementia if at all possible.

Psychological Domain

Psychological Assessment

As the disease progresses, personality changes can take the form of either an accentuation or a marked alteration from a person's previous lifelong character traits. The neural substrates underlying personality change in AD are not understood, but researchers have identified two contrasting patterns. One is marked by apathy, lack of spontaneity, and passivity. The other involves growing irritability, sarcasm, self-preoccupation, and intolerance of and lack of concern for others.

Cognitive Status

Cognitive disturbance is the clinical hallmark of dementia. A commonly used cognitive assessment instrument is the Mini-Mental State Examination, although it is not specific to dementia. Other instruments more specific to MCI, dementia, and assessment of behaviours are increasingly used (Box 32.6). If cognitive deterioration occurs rapidly, delirium should be suspected. The patient should be quickly evaluated by a nurse practitioner or physician because delirium calls for immediate attention to diagnose and treat the underlying cause.

Memory

The most dramatic and consistent cognitive impairment is in memory. Persons with early-stage dementia appear mildly forgetful and repetitive in conversation. They misplace objects, miss appointments, and forget what they were just doing. They may lose track of a conversation or television story. Initially, they may complain of memory problems, but in the course of the illness, insight is lost and they become unaware of what is lost. Sometimes, they may confabulate, making what appears to be an appropriate explanation of why the information or object is missing. Eventually, all aspects of memory are impaired. Short-term memory loss is usually readily evident by the person's inability to recall three or four words given to him or her at the beginning of an assessment. Often, the earliest symptom of AD is the inability to retain new information.

Language

Language is progressively impaired. Individuals with dementia or AD may initially have **agnosia**, difficulty finding a word in a sentence or in naming an object. They may be able to talk around it, but the loss is noticeable. Later, fluent **aphasia** develops, comprehension diminishes, and, finally, they become mute and unresponsive to directions or information.

Visuospatial Impairment

Deficits in visuospatial tasks that require sensory and motor coordination develop early; drawing is abnormal, and the ability to write may change. Inaccurate drawing, such as clock drawing, is seen. Sequencing tasks, such as cooking or other self-care skills, become impaired. The individual becomes unable to complete complex tasks that require calculations, such as balancing a chequebook.

Executive Functioning

Judgment, reasoning, and the ability to problem solve or make decisions are also impaired in the later stages of AD. It is hypothesized that as the disease progresses, the degeneration of neurons is spread diffusely throughout the neocortex.

BOX 32.5 Medications to Avoid for Persons Living With Dementia

Antispasmodic medications	• Atropine • Belladonna alkaloids • dicyclomine (Bentyl) • hyoscyamine (Levsinex) • oxybutynin (Ditropan) • scopolamine • tolterodine (Detrol)
Antihistamines	• brompheniramine (Dimetane) • carbinoxamine, chlorpheniramine (Chlor-Trimeton) • clemastine (Tavist) • cyproheptadine (Periactin) • dexchlorpheniramine (Polaramine) • diphenhydramine (Benadryl or Sominex) • hydroxyzine (Atarax) • phenindamine (Nolahist) • meclizine • triprolidine (Actifed/Myidyl)
Antiparkinson agents	• benztropine mesylate (Cogentin) • trihexyphenidyl HCl (Artane)
Barbiturates	• phenobarbital (Luminal Sodium)
Benzodiazepines	• Short-acting benzodiazepines: triazolam (Halcion) and midazolam (Versed) • Intermediate-acting benzodiazepines: lorazepam (Ativan), temazepam (Restoril), alprazolam (Xanax), oxazepam (Serax), estazolam (ProSom) • Longer-acting benzodiazepines: diazepam (Valium), chlordiazepoxide (Librium), clorazepate (Tranxene), halazepam (Paxipam), prazepam (Centrax), quazepam (Doral) and clonazepam (Klonopin), flurazepam (Dalmane)
CNS stimulants	• amitriptyline (Limbitrol or Limbitrol DS): used to treat symptoms of depression • fluoxetine (Prozac, Prozac Weekly): used to treat depression, obsessive–compulsive disorder, some eating disorders, and panic attacks
Antimuscarinics	• oxybutynin • tolterodine • trospium
Tricyclic antidepressants	• amitriptyline (Elavil) • clomipramine (Anafranil) • desipramine (Norpramin or Pertofrane) • doxepin (Sinequan) • imipramine (Tofranil) • protriptyline (Vivactil) • trimipramine (Surmontil)

Sources: Adapted from American Geriatrics Society Beers Criteria Update Expert Panel. (2019). American Geriatrics Society 2019 Updated AGS Beers criteria for potentially inappropriate medication use in older adults. *Journal of the American Geriatrics Society, 67,* 674–694. DOI: 10.1111/jgs.15767; Green, A. R., Segal, J., Tian, J., Oh, E., Roth, D. L., Hilson, L. … Boyd, C.M. (2017). Use of bladder antimuscarinics in older adults with impaired cognition. *Journal of the American Geriatrics Society, 65*(2), 390–394. doi:10.1111/jags.14498

Behaviours and Emotions in Dementia

There are many behavioural and emotional changes associated with AD and other dementias (Love & Geldmacher, 2018). These have been variously grouped and termed as behavioural symptoms or disturbances, neuropsychiatric symptoms, behavioural and psychological symptoms of dementia (BPSD), and responsive behaviours (Gilmore-Bykovski et al., 2020). In the following

BOX 32.6 Cognitive Assessment Tools for Use With Persons Living With Dementia

MENTAL STATUS QUESTIONNAIRES

Mini-Mental State Examination

Folstein, M. F., Folstein, S. E., & McHugh, P. R. (1975). Mini-Mental state: A practical method for grading the cognitive state of patients for the clinician. *Journal of Psychiatric Research, 12*, 189–198. See Chapter 10 for components of the mental status examination.

Cognitive Abilities Screening Instrument

Teng, E. L., Hasegawa, K., Homma, A., Imai, Y., Larson, E., Graves, A., Sugimoto, K., Yamaguchi, T., Sasaki, H., & Chiu, D. (1994). The Cognitive Abilities Screening Instrument (CASI): A practical test for cross-cultural epidemiological studies of dementia. *International Psychogeriatrics, 6*, 45–58.

Montreal Cognitive Assessment

Nasreddine, Z. S., Phillips, N. A., Bedirian, V., Charbonneau, S., Whitehead, V., Collin, I., Cummings, J. L., & Chertkow, H. (2005). The Montreal Cognitive Assessment, MoCA: A brief screening tool for mild cognitive impairment. *Journal of the American Geriatrics Society, 53*(4), 695–699. See www.mocatest.org for more details.

COMBINATION OF COGNITIVE AND FUNCTIONAL ASSESSMENT

Brief Cognitive Rating Scale

Reisberg, B., Schneck, M. K., & Ferris, S. H. (1983). The Brief Cognitive Rating Scale (BCRS): Findings in primary degenerative dementia. *Psychopharmacology Bulletin, 19*, 47–50.

Includes five scales: concentration, recent memory, remote memory, orientation, and functioning and self-care.

Agitation Scale

Rosen, J., Burgio, L., Kollar, M., Cain, M., Allison, M., Fogleman, M., Michael, M., & Zubenko, G. S. (1994). The Pittsburgh agitation scale: User-friendly instrument for rating agitation in dementia patients. *The American Journal of Geriatric Psychiatry, 2*(1), 52–59.

RATING SCALES OF ACTIVITIES OF DAILY LIVING

Progressive Deterioration Scale

DeJong, R., Osterlund, O. W., & Roy, G. W. (1989). Measurement of quality-of-life changes in patients with Alzheimer's disease. *Clinical Therapeutics, 11*, 545–554.

Dependence Scale

Stern, Y., Albert, S. M., Sano, M., Richards, M., Miller, L., Folstein, M., Albert, M., Bylsma, F. W., & Lafleche, G. (1994). Assessing patient dependence in Alzheimer's disease. *Journal of Gerontology, 49*, M216–M222.

RATING SCALE OF QUALITY OF LIFE

Quality of Life–Alzheimer Disease

Thorgrimsen, L., Selwood, A., Spector, A., Royan, L., de Madariaga Lopez, M., Woods, R. T., & Orrell, M. (2003). Whose quality of life is it anyway?: The validity and reliability of the Quality of Life-Alzheimer's Disease (QoL-AD) scale. *Alzheimer Disease and Associated Disorders, 17*(4), 201–208.

RATINGS SCALES FOR RELATIVES

Geriatric Evaluation by Relatives Rating Scale Instrument

Schwartz, G. E. (1983). Development and validation of the Geriatric Evaluation by Relatives Rating Instrument (GERRI). *Psychological Reports, 53*, 478–488.

---

sections, these symptoms and behaviours are discussed in three groups: psychotic symptoms, mood changes, and responsive behaviours. Some of these symptoms (paranoia/delusions, hallucinations, aggression, anxiety, depression) may respond in part to pharmacological interventions, whereas others (e.g., sleep disorders, repetitive questions, calling out or vocalizing, wandering) are not usually amenable to medications (Nash, 2019). In this case, the nurse must try to understand the meaning of the behaviour to the person and meet the need being expressed.

Neuropsychiatric Symptoms

Suspiciousness, Delusion, and Illusions

During the early and middle stages of dementia, many persons are aware of their cognitive losses and compensate with hyperalertness. In a hyperalert state, one becomes aware of many environmental stimuli one does not readily understand. Illusions (mistaken perceptions) are common with dementia. These experiences can be very frightening for the person living with dementia and their family. A kind, caring approach is needed.

As the disease progresses, delusions frequently develop. These characteristic delusions are different from those discussed in the psychotic disorders. Common delusional beliefs include the following:

- Belief that their partner is engaging in marital infidelity
- Belief that other patients or staff are trying to hurt them
- Belief that staff or family members are impersonators
- Belief that people are stealing their belongings
- Belief that strangers are living in their home
- Belief that people on television are real

Hallucinations

Hallucinations occur frequently in dementia and are usually visual or tactile (they can also be auditory, gustatory, or olfactory). A frequent concern is that children, adults, or strange creatures are entering the house or the person's room. These hallucinations may not seem unusual to the person. If possible, the content and form of hallucination should be ascertained because this information may suggest a treatable disorder. For example, an auditory hallucination commanding the person to commit suicide may be caused by a treatable disorder and not dementia.

Mood Changes

Recognition of coexisting (and often treatable) psychiatric disorders in persons with dementia is often missed. One of the challenges of caring for them is when there is the coexistence of depression. There is a correlation between late life depression and AD, and research has suggested that severe depression may be a factor in the conversion of MCI to AD (Kim & Kim, 2021). Depression is characterized by alterations in sleep, lack of eye contact, feelings of sadness, expression of somatic concerns, and decrease in self-care. A person with dementia may experience one or more depressive episodes with symptoms such as psychomotor retardation, anxiety, feelings of guilt and worthlessness, sadness, frequent crying, insomnia, loss of appetite, weight loss, and suicidal rumination. Depressive symptoms are most prevalent in the early stages of dementia, which may be attributed to the person's awareness of cognitive changes, memory loss, and functional decline. However, dysphoric symptoms can occur at any stage, even in the most disoriented older person. In more advanced stages of dementia, an assessment of depression depends more on changes in behaviour than on the verbal expression of concerns.

Anxiety

It is common to observe symptoms of anxiety with depression; therefore, it is important to assess for depression when signs of anxiety appear. Moderate anxiety is a natural reaction to the fear engendered by gradual deterioration of intellectual function and the realization of impending loss of control over one's life. Becoming unsure of one's surroundings and the expectations of others and failing to complete a task once regarded as simple creates a source of anxiety in a person. It is believed that anxious behaviour occurs when the person is pressed to perform beyond their ability.

Catastrophic Reactions

Catastrophic reactions are overreactions or extreme anxiety reactions to everyday situations. Catastrophic responses occur when environmental stressors are allowed to continue or increase beyond the person's threshold of stress tolerance. Behaviours indicative of catastrophic reactions typically include verbal or physical aggression, violence, agitated or anxious behaviour, emotional outbursts, noisy behaviour, compulsive or repetitive behaviour, agitated night awakening, and other behaviours in which the person is cognitively or socially inaccessible. Factors that contribute to catastrophic responses in persons with progressive cognitive decline include fatigue, change in routine (pace or caregiver), demands beyond the person's ability, overwhelming sensory stimuli, and physical stressors, such as pain or hunger.

Responsive Behaviours

Responsive behaviours reflect the ways in which a person living with dementia responds to circumstances or events that are negative, frustrating, or confusing to them (Alzheimer Society of Canada, 2021b).

Apathy and Withdrawal

Apathy, the inability or unwillingness to become involved with one's environment, is common in dementia, especially in moderate to late stages. Apathy leads to withdrawal from the environment and a gradual loss of empathy for others. The lack of empathy is very difficult for families and friends to understand.

Restlessness, Agitation, and Aggression

Restlessness, agitation, and aggression become more prominent in the middle to late stages of dementia. Restlessness should be further evaluated to determine its underlying cause. If the restlessness occurs during medication change or adjustment, side effects should be suspected.

Agitation and aggressive physical contacts are among the most dangerous behaviour management problems encountered in any setting. They often result in the placement of the person with dementia in a nursing home. Careful evaluation of the antecedents of the behaviour enables the nurse to plan nursing care that prevents future occurrences.

Repetitive Vocal and Motor Behaviour

Symptoms such as fidgeting, picking at clothing, wringing hands, loud vocalizations, and wandering may all be signs of underlying conditions such as dehydration, medication reaction, pain, or infection (suggesting delirium). One of the most difficult behaviours for which to determine an underlying cause is hypervocalization: the screams, curses, moans, groans, and verbal repetitiveness that are common in the later stages of dementia. In the assessment of these hypervocalizations, it is important to identify when the behaviour is occurring and any antecedents to the behaviour.

Disinhibition

One of the most frustrating symptoms of dementia and AD is **disinhibition**, which can include impulsiveness, impetuous comments, and irritability (Torrisi et al., 2017). Disinhibition can take many forms, from undressing in a public setting to touching someone inappropriately to making cruel statements. This behaviour is extremely disconcerting to family.

Hypersexuality

A closely related symptom to disinhibition is hypersexuality sexual behaviour that is perceived as inappropriate and socially unacceptable. The person may begin talking and behaving in ways that are uncharacteristic of premorbid behaviour. This behaviour is complicated by a preconception that older people are asexual (Torrisi et al., 2017). In congregate living settings, a balance between normal sexual expression and the prevention of inappropriate behaviours needs to be sought.

Stress and Coping Skills

Persons living with dementia seem extremely sensitive to stressful situations and often do not have the coping abilities to deal with the situation. A careful assessment of the triggers that precede stressful situations will help in understanding and preventing a future event.

Nursing Care Focus for the Psychological Domain

A multitude of potential nursing care foci can be identified for the psychological domain of this population. A sample of common concerns are chronic confusion, impaired environmental interpretation syndrome, risk for violence (self-directed or directed at others), risk for loneliness, risk for caregiver role strain, and concerns regarding coping, hopelessness, and powerlessness.

Interventions for the Psychological Domain

The therapeutic relationship is the basis for assessing and recommending interventions for the person living with dementia and their family members. Care entails a long-term relationship, much support, and expert nursing care.

Cognitive Impairment

Validation Therapy

Validation therapy emerged in the 1970s as a method for communicating with persons with AD. It was developed as a contrast to reality therapy, which attempted to provide a here-and-now, factual focus to the interaction. Validation therapy focuses on the emotions and subjective reality of the persons using an empathic approach. In validation therapy, individuals with cognitive impairment are viewed on one of four stages of a continuum: malorientation, time confusion, repetitive motion, and vegetation. The benefits of validation therapy are reported as restoration of self-worth, less withdrawal from the outside world, communication and interaction with other people, reduction of stress and anxiety, help in resolving unfinished life tasks, and facilitation of independent living for as long as possible. These outcomes are highly desirable; however, the research is inconclusive regarding the effectiveness of validation therapy (Heerema, 2017). Validation therapy is a useful model for nursing care of persons with dementia. The nurse does not try to reorient the person but rather respects the individual's sense of reality.

Memory Enhancement

Interventions for progressive memory impairment should always be a part of the treatment plan. The sooner the persons living with dementia begin taking a CI, the slower the cognitive decline. However, pharmacologic agents are only a small part of the intervention picture. The nursing goal is to maintain memory functioning as long as possible. The nurse should make a concerted effort to reinforce short- and long-term memory. For example, reminding persons with dementia what they had for breakfast, which activity was just completed, or who their visitors were a few hours ago will reinforce short-term memory. Encouraging individuals to tell the stories of their earlier years will help bring long-term memories into focus. In the earlier stages of AD, there is considerable frustration when the person realizes that they have short-term memory loss. In a matter-of-fact manner, the nurse should "fill in the blanks" and then redirect to another activity. Pictures of familiar people, places, and activities are also important tools in memory retrieval. Using scents (perfume, shaving lotions, spices, different foods) to stimulate memory retrieval and asking persons with dementia to relate memories are also useful strategies. Formalized reminiscence groups also help them relive their earlier experiences and support long-term memories.

Orientation Interventions

To enhance cognitive functioning, attempts should be made to remind persons with dementia of the day, time, and location. However, if the person begins to argue that they are really at home or that it is really 1992, the person need not be confronted by facts. Any confrontation could easily escalate into an argument. Instead, the nurse should either redirect the person or focus on the topic at hand (see Box 32.7).

Maintaining Language

Losing the ability to name an object (agnosia) is frustrating. For example, the person living with dementia may describe a flower in terms of colour, size, and fragrance but never be able to name it a flower. When this happens, the nurse should immediately say the name of the item. This reinforces cognitive functioning and prevents disruption in the interaction. Referral to speech therapists may also be useful if the language impairment impedes communication.

Supporting Visuospatial Functioning

The person living with dementia with visuospatial impairments loses the ability to sequence automatic

BOX 32.7 THERAPEUTIC DIALOGUE

The Person With Alzheimer Disease

Lois's daughter has told the home care nurse that on several occasions Lois has been found cowering and fearful under the kitchen table, saying she was hiding from voices. The nurse knows that Lois denies having any difficulty with her memory or her ability to care for herself.

Ineffective Approach

Nurse: I'm here to see you about your health problems.
Patient: I have no problems. Why are you here?
Nurse: I'm here to help you.
Patient: I do not need any help. I think there is a mistake.
Nurse: Oh, there is no mistake. Your name is Lois isn't it?
Patient: Yes, but I don't know who you are or why you are here. I'm very tired, please excuse me.
Nurse: OK. I will return another day.

Effective Approach

Nurse: Hello, my name is Susan Miller. I'm the home health nurse and I will be spending some time with you.
Person with dementia (PWD): Oh, alright. Come in. Sit here.
Nurse: Thank you.
PWD: There is nothing wrong with me, you know.
Nurse: Are you wondering why I am here? Tell me what is on your mind (open-ended statement).
PWD: I know why you are here. My children think that I cannot take care of myself.
Nurse: You're feeling concerned and perhaps a little worried your family seems to think you need more help at home?
PWD: Of course I can care for myself. When people get older, they slow down. I'm just a little slower now and that upsets my children.
Nurse: You are a little slower, and that's what you think is concerning your children.

PWD: I sometimes forget things.
Nurse: Such as… (open-ended statement)
PWD: Sometimes, I cannot remember a telephone number or a name of a food.
Nurse: … and that causes problems.
PWD: According to my children, it does!
Nurse: What about you? What causes problems for you?
PWD: Sometimes the radio says terrible things to me.
Nurse: That must be frightening to experience while listening to the radio.
PWD: It's terrifying. Then, my daughter looks at me as if I am crazy. Am I?
Nurse: Some people, when they become older, experience challenges with their memory. Also, for some people, the daily living tasks that used to be carried out easily become more challenging. For you, it seems doubly scary because you doubt yourself and you're afraid your daughter doesn't understand.
PWD: Oh, OK. Will you tell my daughter that I am not crazy?
Nurse: Sure, I would be happy to meet with both you and your daughter if you would like (acceptance).

THINKING CHALLENGE

- How did the nurse's underlying assumption that the person living with dementia would welcome the nurse in the first scenario lead to the nurse's rejection by the person?
- What communication techniques did the nurse use in the second scenario to open communication and set the stage for the development of a sense of trust?

behaviours, such as getting dressed or eating with silverware. For example, persons living with dementia often put their clothes on backward, inside out, or with undergarments over outer garments. Once dressed, they become confused as to how they arrived at their current state. If this happens, the nurse should begin to place clothes for dressing in a sequence so that the person can move from one article to the next in the correct sequence. This same technique can be used in other situations, such as eating, bathing, and toileting.

Managing Suspicions, Illusions, and Delusions

Persons' suspiciousness and delusional thinking must be addressed to be certain that they do not endanger themselves or others. Often, delusions are verbalized when persons living with dementia are placed in a situation they cannot master cognitively. The principle of nonconfrontation is most important in dealing with suspiciousness and delusion formation. No efforts should be made to ease the person's suspicions directly or to correct delusions. Efforts should be directed at determining the circumstances that trigger suspicion or delusion formation and creating a means of avoiding these situations.

Frequent causes of suspicion are changes in daily routine and strangers. The common accusations that "Someone has entered my room" or "Someone has changed my room" can be managed by asking, "Do you want to see if anything is missing?" Such accusations usually arise when the person cannot remember what the room looked like or when the room was rearranged or cleaned.

Persons with dementia often hide or misplace their belongings and later complain that the item is missing. It is helpful if the nurse and other caregivers pay attention to the person's favourite hiding places and communicate this so that objects can be more easily retrieved. An outburst of delusional accusations after a social outing or other activity may indicate that the activity was too long, the setting was too stimulating, there was too much activity, or the pace was too fast for the person. All these elements can be modified, or it may be necessary to engage the person in quieter activities.

Persons with dementia may have delusions that a spouse, child, or other significant person is an impostor. If this situation occurs, it is important to assert in a matter-of-fact manner, "This is your wife Barbara" or "I am your daughter Jenny." More vigorous assertions, such as offering various types of proof, tend to increase puzzlement as to why a person would go so far to impersonate the spouse or child.

When persons experience illusions, the nurse needs to find the source of the illusion and remove it from the environment if possible. For example, if the person is watching a program featuring animals and then verbalizes that the animal is in the room, switch the program and redirect the conversation. Some persons living with dementia may no longer recognize the reflection in the mirror as self and become agitated, thinking that a stranger is staring at them. Potentially misleading or disturbing stimuli, such as mirrors or artwork, can be easily covered or removed from the environment.

Managing Hallucinations

Reassurance and distraction may be helpful for the person living with dementia who is hallucinating. For example, an 89-year-old person with AD in a residential care facility might get up each night, walk to the nursing station, and whisper to the nurses, "There's a man in my bed who won't let me sleep. You should patrol this place better!" If the hallucination is not too disturbing for the person, it can often be dismissed calmly with diversion or distraction. Because this person did not seem too concerned by the man in her bed, the nurse may gently respond by saying, "I'm sorry you have to put up with so much. Just wait here (or come with me) and I'll make sure your room is ready for you." The nurse should then take the person back to her room and help her into bed.

Frightening hallucinations and delusions should be first dealt with by decreasing the perceptual cues (cover mirrors or turn off the television) and by encouraging the person living with dementia to stay physically close to their caregivers. For example, one person complained to her nurse that she was being poisoned by deadly bugs that crawled up and down her arms and legs while she tried to sleep at night. Reassurance and protection should be provided. Persons often benefit if nurses give them a specific distracting intervention to alleviate anxiety and to help diminish the hallucination, such as applying moisturizing lotion to their legs and arms to repel the bugs at night. The nurse does not agree with the person's hallucination or delusion but lets the person know that the feelings are justified based on their perception of the threat. If these strategies are not effective, as a last resort, antipsychotic medication may help this person sleep at night.

Interventions for Mood Changes

Managing Depression

Psychotherapeutic nursing interventions for depression that accompanies dementia are similar to interventions for any depression. It is important to spend time alone with the person living with dementia and to personalize their care as a way of communicating the person's value. Encouraging the expression of negative emotions is helpful because they can talk honestly to a nonjudgmental person about their feelings. Depressed persons, especially in the early stage of dementia, may attempt and commit suicide. It is wise to remove potentially harmful objects from the environment.

Do not force the person to interact with others or participate in activities, but encourage activity and exercise.

One of the psychogenic aspects of depression is a sense of lowered worth related to the person's actual decreased competence to work and to deal with the problems of daily living. Therefore, it may be helpful to involve the person in a simple repetitive task or project (such as folding linens or setting the table), especially one that involves helping someone else. Assist the person to meet self-care needs while encouraging independence when possible.

Managing Anxiety

Cognitively impaired persons are particularly vulnerable to anxiety. As persons with dementia become increasingly unsure of their surroundings or what is expected of them, they tend to react with fear and distress. They may feel lost, insecure, and left out. Failure to complete a task once regarded as simple creates anxiety and agitation. Often, they cannot explain the source of their anxiety. The difficulty in developing interventions for the anxious person living with dementia is that the symptoms may also be a sign of underlying illnesses, such as depression, pain, infection, or other physical illnesses.

In many cases, lowering the demands, or perceived demands, on the person will be conducive to promoting comfort. Although maintaining autonomy in any remaining function is a high priority in nursing care, it may decrease persons' anxieties or stress levels to have things done for them at certain points along the illness continuum. Frequently, as the day progresses and they become more fatigued, their ability to cope with stressors is increasingly challenged. Many persons living with dementia experience "sundowning" where they have an increased restlessness and agitation as the day draws to a close. In addition, being sensitive to the pronounced startle reflexes and potential hypersensitivity to touch also helps reduce stress.

The threshold for stress is progressively lowered in AD and other progressive dementias. A healthy person frequently uses cognitive coping strategies when under stress, whereas the person with dementia can no longer use many of these strategies. Effective nursing interventions include simplifying routines, making routines as consistent and predictable as possible, reducing the number of choices the person must make, identifying areas in which control can be maintained, and creating an environment in which the person feels safe. With any of the therapeutic interventions discussed, the nurse is reminded that each person has relative strengths and weaknesses and that sound nursing judgment must be used in each situation.

Commonly used therapeutic approaches may exacerbate anxiety in a person living with dementia. For example, reality orientation is contraindicated in the later stages of dementia because it is possible that the person's disoriented behaviour or language has inherent meaning. If the disoriented behaviour or language is continuously neglected or corrected by the nurse, the person's sense of isolation and anxiety may increase.

Another therapeutic intervention that may (or may not) be contraindicated in persons with dementia is providing the person with information before a difficult or painful procedure. Anticipatory preparation for nonroutine events may produce anxiety because the person is unable to retain information, use reasoning skills, or make sound judgments. Telling persons with dementia that they are scheduled for an upcoming diagnostic test only communicates, on an emotional level, that something distressing is about to happen. A simple explanation immediately before the event may be more helpful.

Managing Catastrophic Reactions

If persons living with dementia react catastrophically, the nurse needs to remain calm, minimize environmental distractions (quiet the environment), get their attention, and softly assure them that they are safe. Give information slowly, clearly, and simply, one step at a time. Let the person know that you understand the fear or other emotional response, such as anger or anxiety.

As the nurse becomes skilled at identifying antecedents to the person's catastrophic reactions, it becomes possible to avoid situations that provoke such reactions. Persons living with AD often respond poorly to change and respond well to structure. Attempts to argue or reason with them only escalate their dysfunctional responses.

Interventions for Responsive Behaviours

Managing Apathy and Withdrawal

As the person living with dementia withdraws and becomes more apathetic, the nurse is challenged to engage the person in meaningful activities and interactions. To provide this level of care, the nurse must know the premorbid functioning of the person. Close contact with family helps give the nurse ideas about meaningful activities. For example, using a multisensory room or getting the person involved with music, art therapy, or some psychomotor activity (Ismail et al., 2020) are recommended approaches.

Managing Restlessness and Wandering

Restlessness and wandering are major concerns for family caregivers in the home setting and for staff in long-term care settings. The principal means of dealing with restless persons with dementia who wander into other patients' rooms or out the door in a long-term care setting is to have an adequate number of staff to provide supervision. Electronic security systems and bed occupancy sensors are other strategies that can be used in homes and long-term care settings. An easy strategy is hanging bells on an exit door handle.

Wandering behaviour may be interrupted in more cognitively intact persons by distracting them verbally or visually. Persons who are beyond verbal distraction may be distracted by physically joining them on their walk and then interrupting their course of action and gently redirecting them back to the house or facility. In a long-term care setting, colour and structure of the setting can serve as cues and window boxes that contain photographs of family, personal mementoes, or pieces of art may cue a person living with dementia to identify their room.

Managing Repetitive Behaviour

When persons living with dementia are picking in the air or wringing their hands, simple distraction may work. Hypervocalizations have meaning to the person. The nurse should develop strategies to try to reduce the frequency of vocalizations such as offering comfort measures (change of position, a snack or drink, a warm facecloth to refresh the person's hands and face, toileting assistance). Research is needed to identify and test person-centred interventions for persistent vocalization to meet the comfort needs of the person living with dementia and reduce the stress of caregivers (Sefcik et al., 2019).

Managing Agitated Behaviour

The Alzheimer's Association (2021c) provides suggestions on working with persons who have dementia or AD and are experiencing agitation. These are paraphrased below:

- Listen to what may be causing the agitation, and try to understand.
- Provide reassurance by using phrases that are calming, reassuring the person that they are safe and that you will stay with them.
- Engage the person in activities such as art and music, which help with diverting attention.
- Modify the environment by reducing noise and distractions or by relocating the person to another space.
- Identify ways for the person to use their energy by assisting them to find something to do. Physical activity such as walking or other activity can be helpful.
- Be aware of your reaction and stay calm. Avoid raising your voice, showing alarm or offence. Do not corner, crowd, restrain, or argue with the person.

See box "Clinical Vignette: A Nurse's Dilemma."

CLINICAL VIGNETTE ✚

A NURSE'S DILEMMA

It is 8 a.m. and you are working as a nurse on an inpatient general medical unit of a large urban hospital. A 72-year-old man is admitted to your unit with symptoms of disorientation to time and place, and he is intermittently exhibiting signs of agitation. He thinks you are his child, and he falls asleep while you ask him questions about his symptoms. When you ask him to sign a consent form and hand him a pen, he looks at you as if he didn't understand your request.

The patient's wife tells you that he has had trouble with his memory for the past 3 or 4 years but that her husband has been "acting strange for the past 4 days." The patient's wife denies any history of substance abuse or head injury but states that her husband has been recently diagnosed as having dementia of the Alzheimer's type.

The patient's physician gives a verbal order to restrain the patient "as needed" while writing orders for laboratory tests.

WHAT DO YOU THINK?

- What assessment techniques would you use to determine whether this patient has dementia, delirium, or both?
- What nursing care focus should be included in the patient's plan of care?
- What nursing interventions would promote comfort and safety for this patient?
- Is this patient able to give consent?
- What would be the possible outcomes of physically restraining this patient (e.g., would restraints be helpful or harmful for the patient)?

Reducing Disinhibition

Anticipation of disinhibiting behaviour is the key to nursing interventions for this problem, as is remaining calm. With keen behavioural assessment of the person with dementia, the nurse should be able to anticipate the likely socially inappropriate behaviour and redirect the person or change the context of the situation. If the person starts undressing in the dining room, offering a robe and gently escorting him or her to another part of the room might be all that is needed. If the person is trying to fondle a staff member or another patient, having the person leave the immediate area or redirecting the patient may alleviate the situation.

Social Domain

Social Assessment

Dementia interferes with a person's ability to interact socially as much as it disrupts intellectual functioning. The social domain assessment should include those areas explained in Chapter 31, including functional status, social systems, legal status, and quality of life.

The person's whole social network is affected by dementia, and the needs of the primary caregiver also need to be considered. It is important to assess family caregiver's health status and willingness to use supportive resources to maintain their own health throughout the dementia journey.

The extent of primary caregiver's personal, informal, and formal support systems must also be assessed, as well as personal resources, skills, and stressors. The assessment of the social domain provides objective data on the person's social circumstances and impressions of their family structure, sociocultural beliefs, attitudes toward health and disease, myths about dementia, patterns of communication, and degree of psychopathology (such as potential for abuse). When persons with dementia reside in the community, home visits will prove useful because it gives the nurse information about the person in their own environment. From this assessment, the nurse can identify the situational and psychosocial stressors that affect the family and patient and can begin to develop relationships and interventions to strengthen coping strategies.

Nursing Care Focus for the Social Domain

Typical nursing care foci for the social domain include concerns regarding the type and quality of activities, social interactions, risks for isolation or loneliness, and the need for caregiver respite.

Interventions for the Social Domain

Safety Interventions

One of the primary concerns of the nurse should be safety for the person with dementia. In the early stages of the illness, safety may not seem to be a prime concern. However, early behaviours suggesting dementia are often related to safety, such as the person getting lost while driving or going the wrong way on a highway. Determining the ability of persons with dementia to drive and taking away their drivers' licences are recognized as challenges for family caregivers and healthcare providers. Safety may be an issue in the home when the person engages in unsupervised cooking, cleaning, or household tasks. (For resources and suggestions, see Web Links). Day care centres provide a safe and structured environment for these individuals. Family members should be encouraged to continually assess the abilities of the person to live at home safely and to implement appropriate responses and safety strategies.

In hospital and long-term care settings, the safety issues are different. By the time persons with dementia are admitted to a facility, they are in the middle to late stage of their illness. Cognitive impairments are more pronounced, and safety is of greater concern. Most psychogeriatric units are locked, and in a dementia unit, there often is an electronic alarm system to alert the staff of persons attempting to leave the secured floor. Staff and visitors need to be vigilant of unsafe situations.

Environmental Interventions

The need for stimulation varies from individual to individual and can change, depending on many factors, including cognitive intactness, alertness, emotional state, and physical state. The amount of stimulation received also influences each person's behaviour. Lack of stimulation or intense stimulation may cause emotional distress and aggression. Generally speaking, the more severe the dementia, the less stimulation can be integrated. The nurse should attempt to determine each person's optimal level of stimulation at various times of the day. Cognitive stimulation therapy—interventions that include enjoyable activities that stimulate memory, concentration, and thinking—recommended by the 5th Canadian Consensus Conference on the Diagnosis and Treatment of Dementia CCCDTD5 (Vedel et al., 2020).

Socialization Activities

Overlearned social skills are rarely lost with having dementia. It is not unusual for the person to respond appropriately to a handshake or smile well into the disease process. Even persons who are no longer able to communicate coherently will carry on long discussions with people who are willing to listen and respond. There is a strong risk for social isolation because of communication difficulties. Reinforcing social remarks and gestures, such as eye contact, smiling, greetings, and farewells, can promote a sense of competency and self-esteem (Box 32.8). Pet therapy may enhance social interaction in cognitively impaired individuals. It is

BOX 32.8 Psychoeducation Checklist: Tips for Caregivers of Persons With Dementia

When caring for the person living with dementia, be sure to include the caregivers, as appropriate, and address the following topic areas in the teaching plan:

✓ Psychopharmacologic agents, if used, including drug action, dosage, frequency, and possible adverse effects
✓ Rest and activity
✓ Consistency in routines
✓ Nutrition and hydration
✓ Sleep and comfort measures
✓ Protective environment
✓ Communication and social interaction
✓ Diversional measures
✓ Community resources

important to remember that the ability to laugh and play is not lost, and the psychosocial benefits of humour are well known.

The nurse who engages a person with dementia in an activity is encouraged to (a) avoid confrontation, (b) allow the level of autonomy best tolerated by the person, (c) simplify activities and directions to the point that they can be mastered, (d) provide adequate structure, and (e) recognize that instructions may not be carried out correctly. It is important to monitor the length of time, crowding, and noise level when the person participates in a group activity because all these factors may increase their stress level.

Activities that elicit pleasant memories from an earlier time in the person's life (reminiscence) may produce a soothing effect. Eliciting pleasant memories may be enhanced by gentle stimulation of the person's senses, for example, viewing and discussing photo albums, looking at personal memorabilia, providing a favourite food item, playing a musical instrument, or listening to music the person preferred in younger years.

It may be useful to incorporate movement or dance along with a singing exercise. If the person with dementia resists structured exercise, it may be because of a fear of falling or injury or of demonstrating to others that their health is failing. Persons often forget how to move or how to coordinate their movements in relation to objects. Therefore, exercise should be light and enjoyable. Encourage the person to participate and to take rest periods at intervals throughout the activity in an effort to minimize stress (see Web Link on Power of Music).

Home Visits

Recognizing the importance of supporting persons with dementia to remain at home for as long as possible and support their family caregivers in sustaining their role, cost-effective in-home and community-based long-term care services are expanding. Their goals are to maintain such persons in a self-determining environment that provides the most homelike atmosphere possible, to allow maximum personal choice for care recipients and caregivers, and to encourage optimal family caregiving involvement without overwhelming the resources of the family network. All services for these persons and their families are provided within a context of continuity of care, a concept that mandates access to a variety of health and supportive services over an unpredictable and changing clinical course.

Community Actions

Home care nurses and community public health nurses working with persons with dementia are especially knowledgeable about all aspect of the illness and care. These nurses often consult with local organizations, such as the Alzheimer Society of Canada, and participate on interprofessional teams. Issues of care, safety, and access to services often require professional expertise and influence.

Family Interventions

Family caregivers are faced with extreme challenges. Caregivers are either spouses of the person or children, usually a daughter, who may also have other responsibilities, such as children and a job. The caregiver often feels isolated, frustrated, and trapped. The potential for abuse of the person with dementia is significant, especially if agitated and aggressive behaviours are present. The use of home care services may assist in decreasing the burden and depression in family caregivers.

In Canada, about one in four people aged 15 years and older provided help or care to a relative or friend with a chronic health problem in 2018 (Statistics Canada, 2018). Almost half of these reported providing care for parents or parents-in-law, with 13% reporting providing care to a spouse or caregiver. It is important that the nurse recognize and assess the needs of the caregivers for support and relief from the 24-h responsibility. Determining the availability of family members or friends to assist with personal care of the person with dementia should be included in the assessment (see Box 32.9). Home care may assist with personal care needs of the person and provide respite for the caregiver. Caregivers should be encouraged to attend support groups and carve out personal time. Educational and training programs may help in understanding the complex nature of dementia. Community resources, such as day care centres, home care agencies, and other community services, can be an important aspect of nursing care for the person and their family caregivers (see Box 32.9).

BOX 32.9 Research for Best Practice

IMPROVING DEMENTIA CARE FOR GITXSAN FIRST NATIONS PEOPLE

From McAtackeny, D., Gaspard, G., Sullivan, D., Bourque-Bearskin, L., & Sebastian, M; for the Gitxsan Health Society and First Nations Health Authority. (2021). Improving dementia care for Gitxsan First Nations people. *International Journal of Indigenous Health, 16*(1), 118–145. https://doi.org/10.32799/ijih.v16i1.33225

Background and aim: Concerns regarding a lack of geriatric nursing knowledge need to meet the needs of Gitxsan people living with dementia were raised by the local health society. The study sought to understand how culturally relevant place-based learning for nurses, families, and the community could enrich the care provided to community elders living with dementia.

Methods: Guided by community partners, Elder from the Advisory Council and an Indigenous nurse researcher, a participatory action research-based inquiry was initiated with four parts: perspective gathering, cultural learning experiences for non-Indigenous nurses, dementia co-learning experience guided by cultural advisers, and a sharing circle with the community. Data collection included a variety of sources including interviews, a learning circle, and nurse education workshop/mentorship/mentorship meeting.

Findings: Three major themes from the interviews and learning circle were identified: *Loss* (including complex grief), *Relationality* (personal relationships), and *Access and Connections* (formal information and supports). Participants at the nurse education workshop had increased knowledge of dementia post workshop. The themes from the final sharing circle were *Reflections on the past, Learning and Action.*

Implications for Nursing: Non-Indigenous nurses working in Indigenous communities can benefit from better understanding of dementia, learning about the types of supports and information people in the community need, and being open to receiving information about requirements to consider when providing care for the Gitxsan person who is living with dementia, and their family. Understanding community ways of knowing can facilitate nurses' incorporating culturally safe practices.

Spiritual Domain

The changes in cognition and ability to communicate that occur in dementia may discourage some nurses from attempting to provide individualized spiritual care. Yet despite communication impairment, the need to be respected, to have hope, and to connect with others and, perhaps, a higher power does not diminish. If the spiritual domain is neglected in care, the person with dementia may be denied important comforting and supportive measures. It is important to understand the person's spiritual beliefs as early as possible in the progression of dementia when they may be better able to explain what has spiritual importance for them. Their religious beliefs, rituals, and their participation in a religious community can be explored at this time. The diagnosis of dementia may have brought despair that challenged the person's existing spiritual beliefs. This needs to be recognized, and opportunities for the person to express spiritual distress should be created.

For nurses, understanding the spiritual needs of the person with dementia can be challenging (Toivonen et al., 2018). Gaining information about the spiritual needs of the person living with dementia helps the nurse to provide person-centred, individualized care. Such information can come from direct and indirect verbal expressions of spiritual need. Direct expression may be asking to sing a favourite hymn or read from a religious text. Indirect expressions might include hearing the person praying or experiencing the calm brought on by attending a religious service. This is an area of care that needs further research.

Evaluation and Treatment Outcomes

The objectives of nursing interventions are to help the person living with dementia remain as independent as possible and to function at the highest cognitive, physical, emotional, spiritual, and social levels. The maximum level of functional ability can be promoted when nursing care is related to and based on the remaining abilities of the person. Those who receive diagnoses of AD or other types of dementia still have a wide and varying range of functional abilities. As cognitive decline progresses, there is a tendency for caregivers to perform more and more tasks for the person. It is essential to assess for strengths and to assist in the maintenance of existing skills. Adaptive and appropriate behaviours continue to some degree, even in the presence of increasing cognitive decline. It is important for nursing interventions to focus on more than the maintenance of optimal physical functional ability; interventions also must focus on meeting psychological, social, and spiritual needs of the person.

Nurses can maintain quality of life if they protect a person's overall wellbeing by balancing physical, mental, social, and spiritual health. Figure 32.3 illustrates the truly bio/psycho/social/spiritual aspects of the treatment of individuals with dementia by summarizing potential outcomes of nursing care.

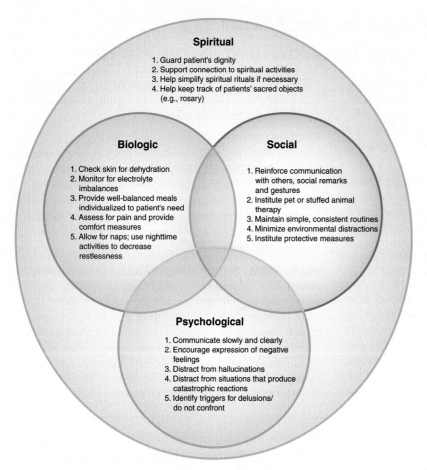

Spiritual
1. Guard patient's dignity
2. Support connection to spiritual activities
3. Help simplify spiritual rituals if necessary
4. Help keep track of patients' sacred objects (e.g., rosary)

Biologic
1. Check skin for dehydration
2. Monitor for electrolyte imbalances
3. Provide well-balanced meals individualized to patient's need
4. Assess for pain and provide comfort measures
5. Allow for naps; use nighttime activities to decrease restlessness

Social
1. Reinforce communication with others, social remarks and gestures
2. Institute pet or stuffed animal therapy
3. Maintain simple, consistent routines
4. Minimize environmental distractions
5. Institute protective measures

Psychological
1. Communicate slowly and clearly
2. Encourage expression of negative feelings
3. Distract from hallucinations
4. Distract from situations that produce catastrophic reactions
5. Identify triggers for delusions/ do not confront

Figure 32.3 Bio/psycho/social/spiritual interventions for persons with dementia.

Harding and colleagues (2019) developed a list of core outcomes to evaluate community-based, nonpharmacological health and social outcomes for people with dementia. They interviewed a variety of people including persons living with dementia, their caregivers, health and social care professionals, policymakers, and researchers. They also reviewed studies of nonpharmacological interventions. They identified 54 unique outcomes under four themes: (a) self-managing dementia symptoms, (b) independence, (c) friendly neighbourhood and home, and (d) quality of life. Further work on distilling this list and identifying measurement instruments is planned.

Continuum of Care

Community Care

Using the 2015/16 Canadian Community Health Survey data, Gilmore (2018) reported that 3.3% 18 years of age and older received home care services in the previous year. Women, older persons, and those living alone were more likely to receive home care or identify an unmet home care need. More often the identified need was for support services (e.g., bathing, housekeeping, or meal preparation), rather than home health care (e.g., nursing and other health services or equipment). This analysis

illustrates the need for greater investment in Canadian home care services, including support services.

Service delivery models vary across the country, with services provided through the public sector and/or contracted with private sector providers. Most home care programs provide case management, nursing, and personal care. There is a wide variation in the provision of therapies such as physiotherapy, occupational therapy, speech and language pathology, respiratory therapy, dietetic care, and social work. Similarly, home care programs vary in the range of and access to homemaking services such as cleaning, laundry, meal preparation, and, very rarely, assistance with transportation, shopping, and banking. The Canadian Home Care Association (2018) has identified home care principles of home care standards as part of a call for national standards. These include care that is person- and family-centred care, accessible, accountable, evidence-informed care that is integrated across care settings and sustainable. For more information on caring for the person with dementia in the home, see Box 32.10.

Acute Care Setting

Although admission to an acute care setting is not likely related to dementia, older adults with other conditions

Box 32.10 NURSING CARE PLAN

Person Living With Dementia

LW is a 76-year-old widow who lives with her oldest son. He is with her during the evening and night. Recently her children have noticed that she is becoming more forgetful and seems to have periods of confusion. LW refuses to see a healthcare provider but did agree to go in for a routine checkup. Her daughter helped her get dressed and took her to the primary healthcare clinic.

Setting: Primary Healthcare Clinic

Baseline Assessment: A well-groomed woman is accompanied by her daughter. LW says there is nothing wrong, but her daughter disagrees. A review of body systems reveals poor hearing and vision but is otherwise unremarkable. MMSE score is 19. Daughter reports that LW has become very suspicious of neighbours and has changed her locks several times.

Associated Diagnoses	Medications
Probable dementia of the Alzheimer's type (some memory problems) History of breast cancer, unilateral mastectomy, arthritis Other relevant factors: Social problems (suspiciousness)	galantamine (Reminyl) 4 mg bid, titrate to 8 mg bid over 4 wk

Nursing Care Focus 1: Impaired Memory

Defining Characteristics	Related Factors
Inability to recall information Inability to recall past events Observed instances of forgetfulness Forgets to perform daily activities	Neurocognitive changes associated with dementia

Outcomes

Initial	Long Term
Maintain or improve current memory.	Delay cognitive decline associated with dementia.

Interventions	Rationale	Ongoing Assessment
Develop memory cues in home. Have clocks and calendars well displayed. Make lists for person living with dementia.	Maintaining current level of memory involves providing cues that will help person recall information.	Contact family members for the person's ability to use memory cues.
Teach the person and family about taking an acetylcholinesterase inhibitor. Review expected effects, side effects, and adverse effects. Develop a titration schedule with family to decrease the appearance of side effects.	Confidence and self-esteem improve when a person feels better.	Monitor response to medications and suggestions.
Observe the person for visuospatial impairment. If present, sequence habitual activities, such as eating, dressing, bathing, etc.	Visuospatial impairment is one of the symptoms of dementia.	Observe for appropriate dress, bathing, eating, etc.

Evaluation

Outcomes	Revised Outcomes	Interventions
LW did have some improvement in memory. Suspiciousness and grooming improved.	Continue maintaining memory.	Continue with memory cues and galantamine.

may have symptoms of dementia. Unfortunately, care for persons with dementia in hospital is often less than optimal because of such factors as inadequate knowledge of dementia on the part of healthcare professionals, stigma towards those with dementia, and environments that are confusing and unsafe for the person with dementia (Handley et al., 2017). A call for more dementia-friendly acute care environments has been made. This includes a comprehensive admission assessment that encompasses dementia, followed by the development of an individualized (and constantly updated) care plan that involves the person with dementia, their family, and the interprofessional team and serves as the foundation of an effective and efficient care in hospital and transition home. Attention to all aspects of this process is necessary for continuity of care. The hospital-based nurse needs to engage the family in hospital care and discharge planning for persons with dementia.

Long-Term Care

As dementia progresses, most family members can no longer manage the symptoms, such as wandering at night and incontinence. A long-term care setting (nursing home) may be necessary where care is usually provided by personal care aides, who need support and direction from other healthcare professionals. Persons with dementia require complex nursing care, yet the skill level of people providing the direct care is often minimal, making education and support of the care providers a significant focus for nursing homes. Nurses in long-term care settings need to be knowledgeable in dementia care and leadership.

Other Major NCDs (Dementias)

Dementia symptoms may occur as a result of a number of NCDs and underlying aetiologies. The subsequent sections provide a brief description of some of the aetiologic subtypes identified in the *Diagnostic and Statistical Manual of Mental Disorders* (5th edition) (APA, 2013). In each case, significant cognitive decline must be evident in one or more cognitive domains (e.g., language, learning and memory, social cognition); the cognitive deficits affect independence in everyday life, and they do not occur exclusively with delirium (APA, 2013, p. 602). Nursing interventions for the subtypes of major NCDs are similar to those described for individuals with AD.

Vascular Neurocognitive Disorder

Vascular dementia is the second most common form of dementia after AD. More than 20% of all those who have dementia have vascular dementia. When AD and vascular dementia occur at the same time, the condition is called mixed dementia. Vascular dementia occurs from multiple cerebral infarctions (transient ischemic

attacks [TIAs]) or a stroke. These occur when blood flow in the brain is blocked or a blood vessel bleeds, preventing the blood from flowing properly through the vessel. Certain medical conditions such as type II diabetes, high blood pressure, and an unhealthy lifestyle are all contributory factors to developing vascular dementia. It is essential that anyone who demonstrates symptoms of dementia or who has a history of stroke have a complete physical examination that includes diet, smoking, medication history, review of recent stressors, and an array of laboratory tests.

The behaviour changes that result from vascular dementia are similar to those found in AD, such as loss of memory, judgment and reasoning, depression, emotional lability, wandering or getting lost in familiar places, bladder or bowel incontinence, difficulty in following instructions, gait changes, and problems handling daily activities. However, these symptoms usually begin more suddenly, rather than developing slowly, as is the case in AD. Often, the neurologic symptoms associated with a TIA are minimal (slight weakness in an extremity, dizziness, or slurred speech) and may last only a few minutes or hours but leave underlying damage. The clinical progression may be more steplike, with the person's cognitive and functional status plateauing for a period of time, followed by a rapid decline in function after further strokes. Treatment aims to reduce the primary risk factors for vascular dementia, including hypertension, diabetes, and additional strokes. Interventions that reduce the tendency of the blood to clot and of platelets to aggregate include lifestyle changes (diet, exercise, and smoking cessation) and using appropriate medications. Control of hypertension and stroke risk with antihypertensive and anticoagulant medications as guided by hypertension guidelines is imperative (Ismail et al., 2020). Cholinesterase inhibitor (CI) medications used in AD can be considered for some patients with vascular cognitive impairment.

Dementia With Lewy Bodies

The clinical features of DLB and Parkinson disease dementia (PDD; see later in this chapter) often overlap because of the related pathophysiology of cortical and subcortical α-synuclein (Lewy bodies) plus β-amyloid and tau pathologies (Jellinger & Korczyn, 2018). DLB is often diagnosed when the pattern of cognitive decline occurs before or concurrently with motor symptoms of PDD. In addition, AD and DLB frequently coexist. Persons with DLB may have symptoms much like those of both Parkinson disease and AD, making diagnosis challenging.

DLB usually progresses quickly. Symptoms include a progressive loss of memory, language, reasoning, and other higher mental functions, and occasionally, depression, anxiety, and apathy. Obvious changes in alertness may also happen. The person may be sleepy during the day but wide awake at night, unable to sleep. Visual hallucinations are common and can be worse during times of increased confusion. The visual hallucinations often come back repeatedly and typically are of people, children, or animals. People with the disease may also make errors in perception, for example, seeing faces in a carpet pattern. Parkinsonian features of DLB, rigidity and slow movement (**bradykinesia**), may develop. These can also develop as a result of use of medications with extrapyramidal side effects (neuroleptic sensitivity). For this reason, use of antipsychotic medications should be avoided, with the atypical antipsychotic agent quetiapine being one with less likelihood of adverse effects.

Parkinson Disease Dementia

Parkinson disease dementia (PDD) can be diagnosed when there is well-established Parkinson disease followed by gradual onset of cognitive decline. Parkinson disease is a neurodegenerative disease with the hallmark abnormality of Lewy bodies, deposits of a protein called alpha-synuclein, in a specific brain region critical for control of movement. The most common symptoms affect movement such as bradykinesia (the slowing of body movements), rigidity, resting tremor, and postural changes. The person's gait is unstable, resulting in frequent falls. Annually, approximately 10% of people with Parkinson disease will develop PDD, usually 10 to 20 years following a diagnosis of Parkinson disease. People can live with Parkinson's for years, although currently there is no cure. Medical treatment of Parkinson disease typically is with dopamine agonists. Anticholinergic medications may cause adverse mental effects (e.g., confusion, memory problems, restlessness, and hallucinations) and, as in DLB, antipsychotic agents should be avoided (Jellinger & Korczyn, 2018).

Frontotemporal Dementia

FTD tends to occur at a younger age than AD and is an umbrella term for a group of rare disorders that primarily affect the frontal and temporal lobes of the brain, the areas generally associated with personality and behaviour. With this form of dementia, a person may have symptoms such as behaviour changes, impaired executive function, or difficulties with speech and movement. There is often sparing of the memory and visuospatial function, but motor (movement) symptoms may develop over time (Kercher & Rosenbloom, 2018). Pathophysiology is diverse and can be characterized by aggregation of abnormal proteins such as "Pick bodies" in the frontal and temporal regions of the brain. Pick disease is an example of a subtype of FTD that has these specific abnormalities.

Because the frontal and temporal areas of the brain are affected, early symptoms of FTD often involve behaviour and/or speech. Changes in behaviour may include becoming either withdrawn and apathetic or disinhibited and impulsive. The person may lose interest in personal hygiene, become easily distracted, or repeat the same action over and over again. Overeating or compulsively putting objects in the mouth may occur. Sometimes incontinence is an early symptom of FTD. There may be significant decline in language ability (e.g., speech production, word finding, object naming, grammar, or word comprehension) (APA, 2013).

A person with FTD may have changes in personality but continue to manage the running of a home and manage the psychomotor and spatial skills needed to maintain employment. However, the person often loses their position due to changes in personality. The individual may become easily irritated, loud, and argumentative. This is particularly distressing to a family if they do not understand that these are symptoms of FTD.

Dementia Caused by Other General Medical Conditions

People of any age, race, or gender are at risk for dementia caused by a medical condition known to cause cerebral pathology. Older adults are particularly vulnerable to the development of dementia caused by general medical conditions because so many are affected by one or more of these illnesses. Strong relationships have been reported between the following chronic medical illness and the development of dementia.

Dementia Caused by HIV Infection

The NCD of dementia associated with HIV infection is known as AIDS dementia complex (ADC). ADC has been observed in 15% to 55% of persons with AIDS in the era of antiretroviral therapy (Sacktor, 2018). HIV-1 directly invades the CNS and allows opportunistic infections of the CNS and other organ systems. Although there has been a proportional increase in ADC at AIDS diagnosis, survival has improved markedly in the era of highly active antiretroviral therapy (HAART). The essential features of ADC are disabling cognitive impairment accompanied by motor dysfunction, speech problems, and behavioural change. Dementia only exists when neurocognitive impairment in the person is severe enough to interfere markedly with day-to-day function.

Dementia Due to Traumatic Brain Injury

Traumatic brain injury can occur from a variety of causes including a single injury from a fall or motor vehicle accident or repeated injury with or without loss of consciousness from some sports activities. The degree and type of cognitive impairment or behavioural disturbances demonstrated by a person with head trauma depend on the location and extent of the brain injury.

When head trauma occurs in the context of a single traumatic injury, the resulting dementia is usually not progressive, but repeated head injury (e.g., from the sports of boxing or football) may lead to a progressive dementia called chronic traumatic encephalopathy. Features such as memory impairment, speech hesitancy, and slowing of movement appear and worsen over time (Perry et al., 2020).

When the nurse observes progressive decline in intellectual functioning after a single incident of head trauma, the possibility of another superimposed process must be considered. Head injury associated with a prolonged loss of consciousness (days to months) may be followed by delirium, dementia, or a profound alteration in personality. Falls are a common cause of head injury in the older adult. Subarachnoid haemorrhage is often a result of an unwitnessed fall and often gets missed, leading to the potential for permanent brain damage and/or death. Subarachnoid haemorrhage is treatable if caught early.

Dementia Due to Huntington Disease

Huntington disease is a progressive, genetically transmitted autosomal-dominant disorder. Anyone with a parent with Huntington's has a 50% chance of inheriting the gene. People are born with the defective gene, but symptoms usually do not appear until middle age. Symptoms include the following: involuntary movements such as twitches and muscle spasms (dystonia); balance problems; personality changes such as irritability, depression, and mood swings; difficulties with memory, concentration, learning new things, or making decisions; and, in late stage, difficulty concentrating, gait abnormalities, eating independently, or swallowing. Medications such as antipsychotics for psychosis or serotonin reuptake inhibitors (SSRIs) for obsessive–compulsive/repetitive behaviours can help manage symptoms, but cannot slow down or stop the disease, and there is currently no cure for Huntington disease (Anderson, 2018).

Dementia Due to Prion Disease

Prion disease is a rare form of deadly dementia that is caused by misfolded proteins known as *prions (PrP)*. Prion diseases affect both humans and other mammals. There are many types of prion disease, including CJD, fatal familial insomnia, and Gerstmann-Straussler-Scheinker disease (GSS). Some, like the variant form CJD, can occur from ingesting affected meat. The other forms CJD and GSS are genetic. In all of these, the misfolding protein (the prion) spreads in a cascade of damage resulting in a rapid clinical course and death.

Although no disease-modifying treatment currently exists, research on agents to reduce PrP is ongoing (Vallabh et al., 2020).

Because of the rapid clinical course of this disease, an important nursing role is assisting family members to understand and come to terms with the illness and to make decisions related to treatment setting and life-sustaining treatments.

Substance-/Medication-Induced Dementia

If dementia results from the persisting effects of a substance (e.g., abuse of drugs, a medication, or exposure to toxins), the person is diagnosed with substance-/medication-induced dementia. Other causes of dementia (e.g., dementia caused by a general medical condition) must always be considered, even in a person with exposure to or dependence on a substance. For example, head injuries often result from substance use and may be the underlying cause of the NCD.

There are many psychoactive substances, including alcohol, cannabis, opioids, benzodiazepines, and hallucinogens, that are used repeatedly by individuals, and a number of theories exist that attempt to explain recurrent hazardous use of such substances that can result in NCDs (Saunders & Latt, 2021). One example is the dementia resulting from chronic alcohol abuse. Understanding the cognitive deficits associated with chronic alcohol consumption is complicated. Alcoholic dementia is directly related to the toxic effects of alcohol, although the vitamin deficiencies associated with alcoholism (thiamine and niacin) are also known to be aetiologically related to dementia. Individuals with alcoholism also have a high incidence of systemic illnesses that can affect cognition (e.g., cirrhosis, cardiomyopathy), and they are susceptible to repeated head injuries, which carry cognitive consequences of their own.

Drugs of abuse are the most common toxins in young adults, and prescription drugs are the most common toxins in older people. In older persons, dementia results from the use of long-acting benzodiazepines, barbiturates, meprobamate, and a host of other drugs depending on their dose and the length of time they have been used. Drugs such as flurazepam (Dalmane), with a half-life of more than 120 h, accumulate rapidly in a person's body. Other drugs accumulate more slowly or require relatively high doses for toxicity to develop. A toxic aetiology should be suspected in every person with a probable diagnosis of dementia. The nurse should inquire about exposure to drugs and toxins (exposure to toxins at work sites, medication use, and recreational drug use), and any substances known to be potentially injurious to the nervous system should be withdrawn if possible.

Chemicals and organic compounds that impair functioning of the CNS usually have their primary effects on other body systems: the gastrointestinal, renal, hepatic, blood-forming, and peripheral nervous systems. For example, metal poisonings generally produce gastrointestinal symptoms and peripheral neuropathy. Cognitive changes with poisoning tend to be more characteristic of delirium than dementia, with altered levels of consciousness a prominent feature. Many adolescents and indigent adults engage in the act of "huffing" because the cost of purchasing spray paint, hair spray, glue, and other aerosol products is relatively inexpensive (com-

pared with illicit street drugs). The nurse is reminded to evaluate people who abuse drugs for signs of cognitive impairment because neural and cognitive symptoms tend to appear before permanent brain damage occurs. It is also important to realize that the person's cognitive status may not immediately improve after discontinuation of use of the offending agent. The effects of drugs taken for a long period may be long lasting, and improvement may be slow after discontinuation of drug use.

Summary of Key Points

- NCDs, such as delirium and dementia, are characterized clinically by significant deficits in cognition or memory that represent a clear-cut change from a previous level of functioning. In some disorders, the loss of cognitive function is progressive, such as in AD.
- Two major syndromes of cognitive impairment in older adults are delirium and chronic cognitive impairments, such as dementia. It is crucial to recognize the differences because the interventions and expected outcomes of the two syndromes differ vastly.
- The symptoms of depression can overlap with the symptoms of both delirium and dementia. One individual may have one, two, or three of the conditions in the triad of delirium, dementia, and depression simultaneously.
- Delirium is characterized by a disturbance in attention (e.g., ability to focus) and awareness (reduced orientation to environment) that develops over a short period of time. It requires rapid detection and treatment because in 25% of cases, it is a sign of impending death.
- Usually, delirium is caused by a combination of precipitating factors. The most commonly identified causes are medications, infections (particularly urinary tract and upper respiratory tract infections), fluid and electrolyte imbalance, and metabolic disturbances such as electrolyte imbalance or poor nutrition. Other important predisposing factors include very young or advanced age, brain damage, preexisting dementia, and bio/psycho/social/spiritual stressors.

- The primary goal of treatment of delirium is prevention or resolution of the acute confusional episode with return to previous cognitive status and interventions focusing on (a) elimination or correction of the underlying cause and (b) symptomatic, safety, and supportive measures.
- Dementia is characterized by the gradual onset of decline in cognitive function, especially memory, usually accompanied by changes in behaviour and personality. Neurologic changes and damage in the brain may be present for many years before symptoms present. Although there are many proposed reasons for these changes, they are not entirely understood. Thus, cures for specific types of dementia have not been discovered.
- AD is an example of a progressive, degenerative dementia. Treatment efforts currently focus on the reduction of cognitive symptoms (e.g., memory loss, confusion, and problems with learning, speech, and reasoning) in attempts to improve the quality of life for both the person living with dementia and their family caregivers.
- Symptoms of dementia may occur as a result of a number of other types of NCDs including vascular dementia, DLB, PDD, and FTD. Symptoms of dementia may also be related to other conditions such as HIV infection, traumatic brain injury, Huntington disease, and prion disease.
- Educating families and caregivers about what to expect related to the progressive cognitive decline and behaviour changes, safety issues, and available community resources is essential to ensuring appropriate and adequate care.

Thinking Challenges

1. A long-term care nurse is caring for a client diagnosed with early-onset familial Alzheimer disease.
   a. Differentiate delirium from dementia.
   b. What is the clinical course of Alzheimer disease?
   c. How is neurobiology implicated in the diagnosis of Alzheimer disease?

Visit thePoint to view suggested responses Go to thePoint.lww.com/activate and use the activation code found in the front of this text to unlock answers to the "Thinking Challenges" and other online resources.

Web Links

https://www.the4at.com A brief clinical instrument for delirium detection, developed in the United Kingdom, can be found at this site. It is free to download and use. A link to references regarding its validation is provided.

https://alzheimer.ca/en The Alzheimer Society of Canada website provides information and resources related to AD.

https://alzheimer.ca/en/help-support/im-caring-person-living-dementia/end-life-care/what-do-i-need-know-about-caring-person This site provides detail and a rating scale for managing pain in persons with AD.

https://alzheimer.ca/en/help-support/im-caring-person-living-dementia/providing-day-day-care/meal-time A person-centred approach including strategies for dealing with mealtimes for persons with AD is addressed at this site.

https://alzheimer.ca/en/help-support/dementia-resources/video-resources This is the link to the Power of Music video discussed in this chapter.

https://www.alz.org The Alzheimer's Association website provides information, resources, and consumer and caregiver support. This is a U.S.-based organization.

https://www.alzheimers.org.uk/get-support/help-dementia-care The Alzheimer's Society, UK, website provides information about dementia, symptoms and diagnosis of dementia, living with dementia, caring for a person with dementia, and the latest research on dementia.

https://brainxchange.ca/public/home This website describes the latest resources and upcoming knowledge exchange opportunities. Topics of interest can be discussed by connecting with others in the network or through support from brainXchange staff.

https://uwaterloo.ca/living-well-with-dementia/care-and-support This site addresses strategies and support for persons living with dementia.

https://radar.fsi.ulaval.ca/documents/Formulaire_RADAR_en_2014-Autv4.pdf RADAR stands for *Recognize Active Delirium As* part of *Routine* and is a 3-step process to identify delirium in older adults developed at Laval University.

https://rnao.ca/bpg/guidelines/assessment-and-care-older-adults-delirium-dementia-and-depression A best practice guideline on the assessment of care of delirium, dementia, and depression in older adults can be found at this site.

References

Alzheimer's Association. (2021a). *Inside the brain: Alzheimer's brain tour.* http://www.alz.org/research/science/alzheimers_brain_tour.asp

Alzheimer's Association. (2021b). *Mild cognitive impairment.* http://www.alz.org/dementia/mild-cognitive-impairment-mci.asp

Alzheimer's Association. (2021c). *Anxiety and agitation.* https://www.alz.org/care/alzheimers-dementia-agitation-anxiety.asp

Alzheimer Society of Canada. (2018). *Ten warning signs of AD.* https://alzheimer.ca/sites/default/files/documents/10-warning-signs.pdf

Alzheimer Society of Canada. (2021a). *Stages of Alzheimer's disease (what happens).* http://www.alzheimer.ca/en/About-dementia/Alzheimer-s-disease/Stages-of-Alzheimer-s-disease

Alzheimer Society of Canada. (2021b). *Understanding symptoms: Responsive and reactive behaviours.* https://alzheimer.ca/en/help-support/im-caring-person-living-dementia/understanding-symptoms/responsive-reactive-behaviours#Tips_and_strategies

American Geriatrics Society Beers Criteria Update Expert Panel. (2019). American Geriatrics Society 2019 Updated AGS Beers criteria for potentially inappropriate medication use in older adults. *Journal of the American Geriatrics Society, 67,* 674–694. https://doi.org/10.1111/jgs.15767

American Psychiatric Association. (2013). *Diagnostic and statistical manual of mental disorders* (5th ed.).

Anderson, K. E. (2018). Huntington's disease. In D. B. Arciniegas, S. C. Yudofksy, & R. E. Hales (Eds.), *The American Psychiatric Association publishing textbook of neuropsychiatry and clinical neurosciences* (6th ed.). American Psychiatric Association. https://doi.org/10.1176/appi.books.9781615372423

Anderson, N. D. (2019). State of the science on mild cognitive impairment (MCI). *CNS Spectrum, 23,* 78–87. https://doi.org/10.1017/S1092852918001347

Atri, A. (2019). The Alzheimer's disease clinical spectrum. *Medical Clinics of North America, 103,* 263–293. https://doi.org/10.1016/j.mcna.2018.10.009

Barnes, S. S., Gabor, C., & Kudchadkar, S. R. (2020). Epidemiology of delirium in children: Prevalence, risk factors and outcomes. In C. Hughes, P. Pandharipande, & E. Ely (Eds.), *Delirium: Acute brain dysfunction in the critically ill* (pp. 93–102). Springer. https://doi.org/10.1007/978-3-030-25751-4_7

Berian, J., Zhou, L., Russell, M. M., Hornor, M., Cohen, M. E., Finlayson, E., Ko, C. Y., Rosenthal, R. A., & Robinson, T. N. (2018). Postoperative delirium as a target for surgical quality improvement. *Annals of Surgery, 268*(1), 93–99. https://doi.org/10.1097/SLA.0000000000002436

Bettencourt, A., & Mullen, J. E. (2017). Delirium in children: Identification, prevention and management. *Critical Care Nursing, 37*(3), e9–e18. https://doi.org/10.4037/ccn2017692

Boscart, V., McNeill, S., & Grinspun, D. (2019). Dementia care in Canada: Nursing recommendations. *Canadian Journal on Aging / La Revue Canadienne du Vieillissement, 38*(3), 407–418. https://doi.org/10.1017/S071498081800065X

Canadian Home Care Association (CHCA). (2018). *A framework for national principle-based home care standards.* https://www150.statcan.gc.ca/n1/pub/82-003-x/2018011/article/00002-eng.htm

Caplan, G. A. (2019). Delirium superimposed upon dementia. *Journal of the American Medical Directors Association, 20*(11), 1382–1383. https://doi.org/10.1016/j.jamda.2019.09.019

Coupland, A. C., Hill, T., Dening, T., Morriss, R., Moore, M., & Hippisley-Cox, M., (2019). Anticholinergic drug exposure and the risk of dementia: A nested case-control study. *Journal of the American Medical Association JAMA Internal Medicine, 179*(8), 1084–1093. https://doi.org/10.1001/jamainternmed.2019.0677

DeJong, R., Osterlund, O. W., & Roy, G. W. (1989). Measurement of quality-of-life changes in patients with Alzheimer's disease. *Clinical Therapeutics, 11,* 545–554.

Dementia vs. Alzheimer's Disease: What is the Difference? (n.d.). *Alzheimer's Association.* https://www.alz.org/alzheimers-dementia/difference-between-dementia-and-alzheimer-s

Devlin, J. W., Skrobik, Y., Gélinas, C., Needham, D. M., Slooter, A. J. C., Pandharipande, P. P., Watson, P. L., Weinhouse, G. L., Nunnally, M. E., Rochwerg, B., Balas, M. C., van den Boogaard, M., Bosma, K. J., Brummel, N. E., Chanques, G., Denehy, L., Drouot, X., Fraser, G. L., Harris, J. E., ... Alhazzani, W. (2018). Clinical practice guideline for the prevention and management of pain, agitation/sedation, delirium, immobility and sleep disruption in adults patients in the ICU. *Critical Care Medicine, 46*(9), e825–e873. https://doi.org/10.1097/CCM.0000000000003299

DeWitt, M. A., & Tune, L. E. (2018). Delirium. In D. B. Arciniegas, S. C. Yudofksy, & R. E. Hales (Eds), *The American Psychiatric Association publishing textbook of neuropsychiatry and clinical neurosciences* (6th ed.) https://doi.org/10.1176/appi.books.9781615372423

Dudas, R., Malouf, R., McCleery, J., & Dening, T. (2018). Antidepressants for treating depression in dementia. *Cochrane Database of Systematic Reviews, 8,* CD003944. https://doi.org/10.1002/14651858.CD003944.pub2

Egberts, A., Moreno-Gonzalez, R., Alan, H., Ziere, G., & Mattace-Raso, F. (2021). Anticholinergic drug burden and delirium: A systematic review. *Journal of the American Medical Directors Association, 22,* 65–73. https://doi.org/10.1016/j.jamda.2020.04.019

El Hussein, H., Hirst, S., & Osuji, J. (2019). Professional socialization: A grounded theory of clinical reasoning processes that RNs and LPNs use to recognize delirium. *Clinical Nursing Research, 28*(3), 321–339. https://doi.org/10.1177/1054773817724961

Folstein, M. F., Folstein, S. E., & McHugh, P. R. (1975). Mini-mental state: A practical method for grading the cognitive state of patients for the clinician. *Journal of Psychiatric Research, 12,* 189–198.

Gilmore-Bykovski, A., Mullen, S., Block, L., Jacobs, A., & Werner, N. E. (2020). Nomenclature used by family caregivers to describe and characterize neuropsychiatric symptoms. *The Gerontologist, 60*(5), 896–904.

Geriatric Medicine Research Collaborative. (2019). Delirium is prevalent in older hospital inpatients and associated with adverse outcomes: Results of a prospective multi-centre study on World Delirium Awareness Day. *BMC Medicine, 17,* 229. https://doi.org/10.1186/s12916-019-1458-7

Ghani, M., Reitz, C., St George-Hyslop, P., & Rogaeva, E. (2018). Genetic complexity of early-onset Alzheimer's disease. In D. Galimberti & E. Scarpini (Eds.), *Neurodegenerative diseases* (pp. 29–50). Springer. https://doi.org/10.1007/978-3-319-72938-1_3

Gibson, W., Makhani, A., Hunter, K. F., & Wagg, A. (2020). Do older adults with overactive bladder demonstrate impaired executive function compared to their peers without OAB? *Canadian Geriatrics Society Journal, 23*(4), 330–334. https://doi.org/10.5770/cgj.23.423

Gilmore, H. (2018). *Unmet home care need in Canada.* Statistics Canada Publication 82-003-X. https://www150.statcan.gc.ca/n1/pub/82-003-x/2018011/article/00002-eng.htm

Glynn, K., O'Callaghan, M., Hannigan, O., Bruce, I., Gibb, M., Cohen, R., Lawlor, B. A., & Robinson, D. (2020). Clinical utility of mild cognitive impairment subtypes and number of impaired cognitive domains at predicting progression to dementia: A 20-year retrospective study. *International Journal of Geriatric Psychiatry, 36*(1), 31–37. https://doi.org/10.1002/gps.5385

Green, A. R., Segal, J., Tian, J., Oh, E., Roth, D. L., Hilson, L., Dodson, J. L., & Boyd, C. M. (2017). Use of bladder antimuscarinics in older adults with impaired cognition. *Journal of the American Geriatrics Society, 65*(2), 390–394. https://doi.org/10.1111/jags.14498

Guthrie, P. F., Rayborn, S., & Butcher, H. K. (2018). Evidence-based practice guideline: Delirium. *Journal of Gerontological Nursing, 44*(2), 14–24. https://doi.org/10.3928/00989134-20180110-04

Handley, M., Bunn, F., & Goodman, C. (2017). Dementia-friendly interventions to improve the care of people living with dementia admitted to hospitals: A realist review. *BMJ Open, 7,* e015257. https://doi.org/10.1136/bmjopen-2016-015257

Harding, A. J. E., Morbey, H., Ahmed, F., Opdebeeck, C., Lasrado, R., Williamson, P. R., Swarbrick, C., Leroi, I., Challis, D., Hellstrom, I., Burns, A., Keady, J., & Reilly, S. (2019). What is important to people living with dementia?: The 'long-list' of outcome items in the development of a core outcome set for use in the evaluation of nonpharmacological community-based health and social care interventions. *BMC Geriatrics, 19,* 94. https://doi.org/10.1186/s12877-019-1103-5

Heerema, E. (2017). *Using validation therapy for people with dementia.* https://www.verywell.com/using-validation-therapy-for-people-with-dementia-98683

Hjetland, G. J., Pallesen, S., Thun, E., Kolberg, E., Nordhus, I. H., & Flo, E. (2020). Light interventions and sleep, circadian, behavioral, and psychological disturbances in dementia: A systematic review of methods and outcomes. *Sleep Medicine Reviews, 52,* 101310. https://doi.org/10.1016/j.smrv.2020.101310

Inouye, S. K., van Dyck, C. H., Alessi, C. A., Balkin, S., Siegal, A. P., & Horwitz, R. I. (1990). Clarifying confusion: The confusion assessment method. *Annals of Internal Medicine, 113,* 941–948.

Ismail, Z., Black, S. E., Camicioli, R., Chertkow, H., Herrmann, N., Laforce, R., Montero-Odasso, M., Rockwood, K., Rosa-Neto, P., Seitz, D., Sivananthan, S., Smith, E. E., Soucy, J.-P., Vedel, I., & Gauthier, S. (2020). Recommendations of the 5th Canadian Consensus Conference on the diagnosis, treatment of dementia. *Alzheimer's & Dementia, 16*(8), 1182–1195.

Jellinger, K. A., & Korczyn, A. D. (2018). Are dementia with Lewy bodies and Parkinson's disease the same disease? *BMC Medicine, 16,* 34. https://doi.org/10.1186/s12916-018-1016-8

Kercher, G. A., & Rosenbloom, M. H. (2018). Frontotemporal dementia. In D. B. Arciniegas, S. C. Yudofsky, & R. E. Hales (Eds.), *The American Psychiatric Association publishing textbook of neuropsychiatry and clinical neurosciences* (6th ed.). https://doi.org/10.1176/appi.books.9781615372423

Kim, J., & Kim, Y.-K. (2021). Crosstalk between depression and dementia with resting-state fMRI studies and its relationship to cognitive functioning. *Biomedicines, 9,* 82. https://doi.org/10.3390/biomedicines9010082

Kinchin, I., Mitchell, E., Agar, M., & Trepel, D. (2021). The economic cost of delirium: A systematic review and quality assessment. *Alzheimer's & Dementia: The Journal of the Alzheimer's Association, 17,* 1026–1041. https://doi.org/10.1002/alz.12262

Kinnunen, K. M., Vikhanova, A., & Livingston, G. (2017). The management of sleep disorders in dementia: An update. *Current Opinion in Psychiatry, 30*(6), 491–497. https://doi.org/10.1097/YCO.0000000000000370

Koola, M. M. (2020). Galatamine-memantine combination in the treatment of Alzheimer's disease and beyond. *Psychiatry Research, 293,* 113409. https://doi.org/10.1016/j.psychres.2020.113409

Lam, F. M. H., Huang, M. Z., Liao, L. R., Chung, R. K., Kwok T. C. Y., & Pang, M. Y. C. (2018). Physical exercise improves strength, balance, mobility and endurance in people with cognitive impairment and dementia: A systematic review. *Journal of Physiotherapy, 64*(1), 4–15. https://doi.org/10.1016/j.jphys.2017.12.001

Little, M. O. (2018). Reversible dementias. *Clinics in Geriatric Medicine, 34,* 537–562. https://doi.org/10.1016/j.cger.2018.07.001

Love, M. C. N., & Geldmacher, D. S. (2018). Alzheimer's disease. In D. B. Arciniegas, S. C. Yudofksy, & R. E. Hales (Eds.), *The American Psychiatric Association publishing textbook of neuropsychiatry and clinical neurosciences* (6th ed.). https://doi.org/10.1176/appi.books.9781615372423

Maldonado, J. R. (2017). Delirium pathophysiology: An updated hypothesis of the etiology of acute brain failure. *International Journal of Geriatric Psychiatry, 33,* 1428–1457. https://doi.org/10.1002/gps.4823

Malhotra, R. K. (2018). Neurodegenerative disorders and sleep. *Sleep Medicine Clinics, 13,* 63–70. https://doi.org/10.1016/j.jsmc.2017.09.006

McAtackeny, D., Gaspard, G., Sullivan, D., Bourque-Bearskin, L., Sebastian, M.; for the Gitxsan Health Society and First Nations Health Authority. (2021). Improving dementia care for Gitxsan First Nations people. *International Journal of Indigenous Health, 16*(1), 118–145. https://doi.org/10.32799/ijih.v16i1.33225

Morandi, A., Davis, D., Belleli, G., Arora, R., Caplan, G. A., Kamholz, B., Kolanowski, A., Fick, D. M., Kreisel, S., MacLullich, A., Meagher, D., Neufeld, K., Pandharipande, P. P., Richardson, S., Slooter, A. J. C., Taylor, J. P., Thomas, C., Tieges, Z., Teodorczuk, A., … Rudolph, J. L. (2017). The diagnosis of delirium superimposed on dementia: An emerging challenge. *Journal of the American Medical Directors Association, 18,* 12–18. http://dx.doi.org/10.1016/j.jamda.2016.07.014

Morichi, B., Fedecostante, M., Morandi, A., Di Santo, S. G., Mazzone, A., Mosello, E., Bo, N., Bianchetti, A., Rozzini, R., Zanetti, E., Musicco, M., Ferrari, A., Ferrara, N., Trabucchi, M., Cherubini, A., & Bellelli, G. (2018a). A point prevalence study of delirium in Italian nursing homes. *Dementia and Geriatric Cognitive Disorders, 46,* 27–41. https://doi.org/10.1159/000490722

Morichi, V., Fedecostante, M., Morandi, A., & Malhotra, R. K. (2018b). Neurodegenerative disorders and sleep. *Sleep Medicine Clinics, 13,* 63–70. https://doi.org/10.1016/j.jsmc.2017.09.006

Mueller, C., John, C., Perera, G., Aarsland, D., Ballard, C. & Stewart, R. (2021). Antipsychotic use in dementia: The relationship between neuropsychiatric symptoms and adverse outcomes. *European Journal of Epidemiology, 36,* 89–101. https://doi.org/10.1007/s10654-020-00643-2

Nash, M. C. (2019). Neuropsychiatric symptoms are a core feature of neurocognitive disorders. In M. Nash & S. Foidel (Eds.), *Neurocognitive behavioral disorders* (pp. 1–12). Springer. https://doi.org/10.1007/978-3-030-11268-4_1

Nasreddine, Z. S., Phillips, N. A., Bedirian, V., Charbonneau, S., Whitehead, V., Collin, I., Cummings, J. L., & Chertkow, H. (2005). The Montreal Cognitive Assessment, MoCA: A brief screening tool for mild cognitive impairment. *Journal of the American Geriatrics Society, 53*(4), 695–699.

Oh, E. S., Fong, T. G., Hshieh, T. T., & Inouye, S. K. (2017). Delirium in older persons: Advances in diagnosis and treatment. *Journal of the American Medical Association, 318*(12), 116–1173. https://doi.org/10.1001/jama.2017.12067

Paulo, M., Scruth, E. A., & Jacoby, S. (2017). Dementia and delirium in the elderly hospitalized patient. *Clinical Nurse Specialist, 31*(2), 66–69. https://doi.org/10.1097/NUR.0000000000000271

Perry, B. N., Collins, K., O'Conor, E., Weeks, S. R., & Tsao, J. W. (2020). Sports concussion. In J. Tsao (Ed.), *Traumatic brain injury.* Springer, Cham. https://doi.org/10.1007/978-3-030-22436-3_5

Petretto, D. R., Carrogu, G. P., Gaviano, L., Pili, L., & Pili, R. (2021). Dementia and major neurocognitive disorders: Some lessons learned one century after the first Alois Alzheimer's clinical notes. *Geriatrics, 6*(1), 5. https://doi.org/10.3390/geriatrics6010005

Prorok, J. C., Horgan, S., & Seitz, D. P. (2013). Health care experiences of people with dementia and their caregivers: A meta-ethnographic analysis of qualitative studies. *Canadian Medical Association Journal, 185*(14), E669–E680.

Public Health Agency of Canada. (2019). *A dementia strategy for Canada: Together we aspire.* Government of Canada. https://www.canada.ca/en/public-health/services/publications/diseases-conditions/dementia-strategy.html

Public Health Agency of Canada. (2020). *A dementia strategy for Canada: Together we achieve. 2020 annual report.* Government of Canada. https://www.canada.ca/en/public-health/services/publications/diseases-conditions/dementia-strategy-annual-report-parliament-june-2020.html

Registered Nurses Association of Ontario. (2016). *Delirium, dementia and depression in older adults: Assessment and care.*

Registered Nurses Association of Ontario. (2017). *Preventing falls and reducing injury from falls* (4th ed.). https://rnao.ca/bpg/guidelines/prevention-falls-and-fall-injuries

Reisberg, B., Schneck, M. K., & Ferris, S. H. (1983). The Brief Cognitive Rating Scale (BCRS): Findings in primary degenerative dementia. *Psychopharmacology Bulletin, 19,* 47.

Riviere, J., van der Mast, R. C., Vandenberghe, J., & Van Den Eede, F. (2019). Efficacy and tolerability of atypical antipsychotics in the treatment of delirium: A systematic review of the literature. *Psychosomatics, 60*(1), 18–26.

Rosen, J., Burgio, L., Kollar, M., Cain, M., Allison, M., Fogleman, M., Michael, M., & Zubenko, G. S. (1994). The Pittsburgh agitation scale: User-friendly instrument for rating agitation in dementia patients. *The American Journal of Geriatric Psychiatry, 2*(1), 52–59.

Sacktor, N. (2018). Changing clinical phenotypes of HIV-associated neurocognitive disorders. *Journal of Neurovirology, 24,* 141–145. https://doi.org/10.1007/s13365-017-0556-6

Salvi, F., Young, J., Lucarelli, M., Aquilano, A., Luzi, R., Dell'Aquila, G., & Cherubini, A. (2020). Non-pharmacological approaches in the prevention of delirium. *European Geriatric Medicine, 11,* 71–81. https://doi.org/10.1007/s41999-019-00260-7

Saunders, J. B., & Latt, N. C. (2021). Diagnostic definitions and classification of substance use disorders. In: N. el-Guebaly, G. Carrà, M. Galanter, & A. M. Baldacchino (Eds.), *Textbook of addiction treatment.* Springer. https://doi.org/10.1007/978-3-030-36391-8_8

Schwartz, G. E. (1983). Development and validation of the Geriatric Evaluation by Relatives Rating Instrument (GERRI). *Psychological Reports, 53,* 478–488.

Sefcik, J. S., Ersek, M., Harnett, S. C., & Cacchione, P. Z. (2019). Integrative review: Persistent vocalizations among nursing home residents with dementia. *International Psychogeriatrics, 31*(5), 667–683. https://doi.org/10.1017/S1041610218001205

Shaw, R., Walker, G., Elliott, E., & Quinn, T. J. (2019). Occurrence rate of delirium in acute stroke settings: Systematic review and meta-analysis. *Stroke, 50,* 3028–3036. https://doi.org/10.1161/STROKEAHA.119.025015

Shrestha, P., & Fick, D. M. (2020). Family caregiver's experience of caring for an older adult with delirium: A systematic review. *International Journal of Older People Nursing, 15*(4), e12321. https://doi.org/10.1111/opn.12321

Statistics Canada. (2018). *Caregivers in Canada 2018.* https://www150.statcan.gc.ca/n1/en/daily-quotidien/200108/dq200108a-eng.pdf?st=BJvzNvEB

Stern, Y., Albert, S. M., Sano, M., Richards, M., Miller, L., Folstein, M., Albert, M., Bylsma, F. W., & Lafleche, G. (1994). Assessing patient dependence in Alzheimer's disease. *Journal of Gerontology, 49,* M216–M222.

Tang-Wai, D. F., Smith, E. E., Bruneau, M. A., Burhan, A. M., Chatterjee, A., Chertkow, H., Choudhury, S., Dorri, E., Ducharme, S., Fischer, C. E., Ghodasara, S., Herrmann, N., Hsiung, G.-Y. R., Kumar, S., Laforce, R., Lee, L., Massoud, F., Shulman, K. I., Stiffel, M., … Ismail, Z. (2020). CCCDTD5 recommendations on early and timely assessment of neurocognitive disorders using cognitive, behavioral, and functional scales. *Alzheimer's & Dementia, 6*(1), e12057.

Teng, E. L., Hasegawa, K., Homma, A., Imai, Y., Larson, E., Graves, A., Sugimoto, K., Yamaguchi, T., Sasaki, H., & Chiu, D. (1994). The Cognitive Abilities Screening Instrument (CASI): A practical test for cross-cultural epidemiological studies of dementia. *International Psychogeriatrics, 6,* 45–58.

Thorgrimsen, L., Selwood, A., Spector, A., Royan, L., de Madariaga Lopez, M., Woods, R. T., & Orrell, M. (2003). Whose quality of life is it anyway?: The validity and reliability of the Quality of Life-Alzheimer's Disease (QoL-AD) scale. *Alzheimer Disease and Associated Disorders, 17*(4), 201–208.

Toivonen, K., Charalambous, A., & Suhonen, R. (2018). Supporting spirituality in the care of older people living with dementia: a hermeneutic phenomenological inquiry into nurses' experiences. *Scandinavian Journal of Caring Sciences, 32*(2), 880–888. https://doi.org/10.1111/scs.12519

Tönnies, E., & Trushina, E. (2017). Oxidative stress, synaptic dysfunction, and Alzheimer's disease. *Journal of Alzheimer's Disease, 57*(4), 1105–1121. https://doi.org/10.3233/JAD-161088

Torrisi, M., Cacciola, A., Marra, A., De Luca, R., Bramanti, P., & Calabro, R. S. (2017). Inappropriate behaviours and hypersexuality in individuals with dementia: An overview of a neglected issue. *Geriatrics and Gerontology International, 17,* 865–874. https://doi.org/10.1111/ggi.12854

Traube, C. (2019). Delirium. In C. Duncan, J. A. Talano, & J. McArthur (Eds.), *Critical care of the pediatric immunocompromised hematology/oncology patient.* Springer. https://doi.org/10.1007/978-3-030-01322-6_18

Trzepacz, P. T., Mittal, D., Torres, R., Kanary, K., Norton, J., & Jimerson, N. (2001). Validation of the Delirium Rating Scale-revised-98: Comparison with the delirium rating scale and the cognitive test for delirium. *Journal of Neuropsychiatry and Clinical Neurosciences, 13,* 229–242.

Vallabh, S. M., Minikel, E. V., Schreiber, S. L., & Lander, E. S. (2020). Towards a treatment for genetic prion disease: Trials and biomarkers. *The Lancet Neurology, 19*(4), 361–368. https://doi.org/10.1016/S1474-4422(19)30403-X

Vasunilashorn, S. M., Ngo, L. H., Inouye, S. K., Fong, T. G, Jonees, R. N., Dillon, S. T., Libermann, T. A., O'Connor, M., Arnold, S. E., Xie, Z., & Marcantonio, E. R. (2020). Apolipoprotein E genotype and the association between C-reactive protein and postoperative delirium: Importance of gene-protein interactions. *Alzheimer's & Dementia, 16*(3), 572–580. https://doi.org/10.1016/j.jalz.20

Vedel, I., Sheets, D., McAiney, C., Clare, L., Brodaty, H., Mann, J., Anderson, N., Liu-Ambrose, T., Rohas-Rozo, L., Loftus, L., Gauthier, S., & Sivananthan, S. (2020). CCCDTD5: Individual and community-based psychosocial and other non-pharmacological interventions to support persons living with dementia and their caregivers. *Alzheimer's and Dementia: Translational Research & Clinical Interventions, 6,* e12086. https://doi.org/10.1002/trc2.12086

Von Rueden, K. T., Wallizer, B., Thurman, P., McQuillan, K., Andrews, T., Merenda, J., & Son, H. (2017). Delirium in trauma patients: Prevalence and predictors. *Critical Care Nurse, 37*(1), 40–47.

Walsh, K., Dahlke, S., O'Rourke, H., & Hunter, K. F. (2020). Exploring acute care nurses' decision making in psychotropic PRN use in hospitalized people with dementia. *Journal of Clinical Nursing.* 1–12. https://doi.org/10.1111/jocn.15477

Whittington, R. A., Planel, E., & Terrando, N. (2017). Impaired resolution of inflammation in Alzheimer's disease: A review. *Frontiers of Immunology, 8,* 1464. https://doi.org/10.3389/fimmu.2017.01464

Wolters, F. J., & Ikram, M. (2018). Epidemiology of dementia: The burden on society, the challenges for research. In R. Perneczky (Ed.), *Biomarkers for Alzheimer's Disease drug development. Methods in molecular biology* (Vol. 1750). Humana Press. https://doi.org/10.1007/978-1-4939-7704-8_1

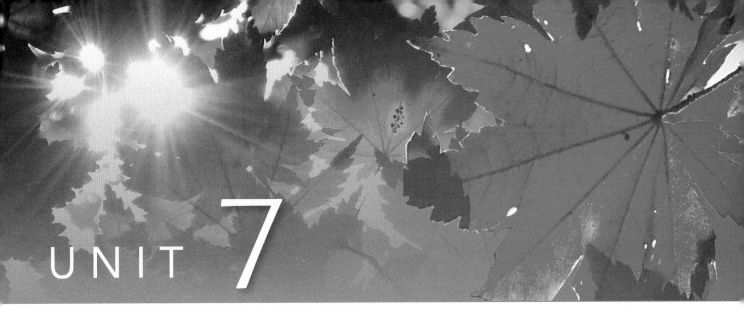

UNIT 7

Care of Persons With Additional Vulnerabilities

Care of Persons With Concurrent Substance-Related, Addictive, and Other Mental Disorders*

Diane Kunyk

LEARNING OBJECTIVES

After studying this chapter, you will be able to:

- Explain the common phenomenon described by the term concurrent disorders.
- Discuss the epidemiology of concurrent disorders.
- Appreciate the aetiologic theories on the development of concurrent disorders.
- Describe the effects of substances on mental status.
- Describe the most common concurrent disorders.
- Outline assessment approaches to concurrent disorders.
- Outline care and treatment approaches specific to concurrent disorders.
- Appreciate the opportunities and challenges in the care and treatment of concurrent disorders.
- Identify some future directions for research and care in the field of concurrent disorders.

KEY TERMS

- integrated care • integrated care pathways • parallel care • stress • substance-related/addictive disorder • trauma

KEY CONCEPT

- concurrent disorders

Numerous epidemiologic and clinical studies report the co-occurrence of **substance-related/addictive disorders** with psychiatric (mental) disorders—a common phenomenon referred to as concurrent disorders. The 5th edition of the *Diagnostic and Statistical Manual of Mental Disorders (DSM-5)* (American Psychiatric Association [APA], 2013) lists the symptoms of more than 300 psychiatric conditions, and it divides substances into 10 categories. The number of possible combinations of concurrent disorders is enormous and tends to be heterogeneous. The most salient examples of combinations of substance-related/addictive disorders with other mental disorders in the literature, which are discussed in detail in this chapter, include the following:

- Co-occurring addictive and mood disorders
- Co-occurring addictive and anxiety disorders
- Co-occurring addictive and posttraumatic stress disorder (PTSD)
- Co-occurring addictive and attention deficit hyperactivity disorders (ADHDs)

- Co-occurring addictive and psychotic disorders
- Co-occurring addictive and personality disorders

Aside from intoxication with or withdrawal from substances, substances themselves may mimic a range of bona fide psychiatric conditions. These are the substance-induced mental disorders, which *are not synonymous* with the co-occurrence of psychiatric and substance-related/addictive disorders. Examples include the following conditions (the first three of which were previously referred to as "organic brain syndrome") (Yuodelis-Flores et al., 2019):

- Substance-induced delirium
- Substance-induced major or mild neurocognitive disorder
- Substance-induced amnestic disorder
- Substance-induced psychotic disorder
- Substance-induced depressive disorder
- Substance-induced bipolar and related disorder
- Substance-induced obsessive–compulsive and related disorder

---

*Adapted from the chapter "Care of Persons with Concurrent Substance-Related, Addictive, and Other Mental Disorders by Charl Els and Diane Kunyk

- Substance-induced anxiety disorder
- Hallucinogen persisting perceptual disorder
- Substance-induced sexual dysfunction
- Substance-induced sleep disorder

Substance-associated suicidal behaviour may also occur and incur serious risk. Although these conditions frequently dissipate in the absence of ongoing substance use, suicidal behaviour may persist beyond the substance intoxication or withdrawal period. Distinguishing symptoms of substance-induced disorders from mental disorders is often difficult.

Concurrent disorders have also been called *dual disorders, comorbidity, co-occurring substance use and mental health problems, mentally ill chemical abuser,* and *dual diagnosis.* In many jurisdictions, however, the term dual diagnosis is reserved for persons with an intellectual disability and a mental health problem. The term *trimorbidity* has been utilized in the context of the co-occurrence of PTSD, traumatic brain injury, and a substance-related/addictive disorder.

The co-occurrence of mental and substance-related/addictive disorders represents a prevalent, pervasive, and urgent health issue. Given that concurrent disorders are associated with more severe adverse outcomes than either condition alone, identifying and treating individuals with concurrent disorders are high priorities. These negative outcomes include, among others, increased rates of rehospitalization and incarceration, disruption of family and social relationships, homelessness, depression, suicide, comorbid medical problems, relapse, and treatment dropout (McKee, 2017). These individuals are among the most complex and challenging clinical scenarios in health care. One ubiquitous problem concerning this heterogeneous and complex population is that "these patients typically have many disorders and severe life problems in addition to mental illness and substance use disorders" (Drake & Green, 2013, p. 105).

A pervasive problem in Canada is that the disease burden associated with concurrent mental health and substance-related/addictive disorders is insufficiently matched by the allocation of healthcare resources. Further, one of the most salient challenges has been that healthcare systems tend to be organized for the care and treatment delivery of single disorders, for example, either for mental disorders or for substance-related/addictive disorders, but not for both simultaneously. Despite the integration of mental health and addiction services in many of Canada's care systems, service provision may remain compartmentalized. This can result in persons with concurrent disorders not fitting well into either mental health or addiction services, and hence "falling through the cracks," unable to access holistic care and effective treatment. In the report by the Mental Health Commission of Canada (MHCC, 2016), *Advancing the Mental Health Strategy for Canada: A Framework for Action (2017–2022),* it is acknowledged that integration

of addiction and mental health services presents challenges to Canadians. One key recommendation from this document is to improve collaboration in the delivery of services to people with concurrent disorders (MHCC, 2016). It is postulated that nursing is the best discipline to reconcile the differences between mental health and substance use care in Canada because of the holistic approach nurses take (Danda, 2020).

The knowledge and practice related to the care and treatment of concurrent disorders is a dynamic, complex, challenging, and evolving area in health care. Increasing nursing knowledge and enhancing skills in caring for persons with concurrent disorders has the potential to improve outcomes for this vulnerable population. It is important for nurses to recognize that treatment is effective, harm can be reduced, and many individuals have the potential for recovery. Excess healthcare costs to society can also be curbed.

This chapter outlines the concept of concurrent disorders and the aetiologic models for concurrent substance-related, addictive, and other mental disorders. The general principles of care and treatment are outlined and nursing strategies and interventions specific to this population are recommended. Given the vast number of possible combinations of mental illness and addiction, only the most prevalent and clinically meaningful examples of concurrent disorders are discussed. This chapter focuses on an integrated approach to care and treatment, in contrast to sequential or parallel models, aimed at the prevention of these disorders and reduction of the severity and progression of existing concurrent conditions. See Chapter 26 for a comprehensive presentation of substance-related and addictive disorders.

■ Epidemiology of Concurrent Disorders

People with mental disorders are more likely to experience substance-related/addictive disorders than those not affected by mental illness (Substance Abuse and Mental Health Services Administration, 2020). It is estimated that approximately 50% of persons seeking help for substance-related/addictive disorders also suffer from a mental disorder, while 15% to 20% of persons with mental disorders also suffer from a substance-related/addictive disorder (United States Department of Health and Human Services, Substance Abuse and Mental Health Services Administration, 2015).

In persons with severe and persistent mental illness, the rates of addiction tend to be much higher. Lifetime substance use is particularly high in persons suffering from psychotic disorders (Margolese et al., 2004). For instance, one study determined that one half (51.7%) of individuals presenting with first episode psychosis met criteria for any lifetime alcohol or drug use disorder (Brunette et al., 2018). This finding echoes international estimates that substance use disorders, extending across a number of drug classes such as nicotine, cannabinoids, and alcohol, affect nearly 50% of individuals with schizophrenia (Menne & Chesworth, 2020).

Individuals with concurrent disorders are known to have poorer outcomes when compared with those presenting with a single diagnosis. For instance, an analysis of the Canadian Community Health Survey—Mental Health (2012) was conducted to compare the outcomes for individuals who presented with at least one mood/anxiety disorder, substance use disorder, or concurrent disorder (having both a mood/anxiety disorder and a substance use disorder). The individuals with concurrent disorders in this study had consistently poorer psychological health outcomes and higher use of health services when compared with those who either had only a mood/anxiety disorder or a substance use disorder (Kahn, 2017).

The high prevalence rates of mental disorders among incarcerated individuals, when compared with the general population, have been well established. Newly admitted male offenders entering the federal correctional system in Canada were examined for prevalence rates of major mental disorders. The study findings revealed that most (73%) met the criteria for any current mental disorder, and 38% of all admissions met the criteria for both a current mental disorder and one of the substance use disorders (Beaudette & Stewart, 2016). This finding draws attention to the vulnerability of incarcerated individuals and supports the movement towards increasing the access of healthcare services in forensic settings. (See Chapter 35 on the care of persons under forensic purview for a deeper discussion.)

KEY CONCEPT

The term concurrent disorder is used when an individual has at least one substance-related/addictive disorder co-occurring with at least one other mental disorder. It is established that about half the number of persons presenting with a substance-related/addictive disorder also experience a mental disorder; one in five persons presenting with a mental disorder also suffers from a substance-related/addictive disorder. Nurses must be attentive to the possibility that individuals presenting with either a substance-related/addictive disorder or another mental disorder may have more than one condition, that is, a concurrent disorder. Screening for a concurrent mental disorder or substance-related/addictive disorder is recommended with the presentation of either condition.

▌ Development of Concurrent Disorders

Four general models to explain the aetiology of co-occurrence of substance-related/addictive disorders with other mental disorders have emerged with varying degrees of empirical support for each model's validity: (a) common aetiology model, (b) secondary substance use disorder models (including supersensitivity and self-medication models), (c) secondary mental disorder model, and (d) bidirectional feedback models (Mueser et al., 1998).

The *common aetiology model* suggests that the same set of variables may contribute to an increased risk for the development of substance-related/addictive and other mental disorders. The cited risk factors may be biologic, psychological, social, or environmental. There is some degree of support for this theory in that the current evidence suggests that individuals with co-occurring disorders are likely to differ from those with either substance-related/addictive disorders or psychiatric disorders alone on various neurobiologic aspects (Balhara et al., 2017).

The *secondary substance use disorder model* proposes that mental health conditions increase the relative risks of developing a substance use disorder. This model includes the *supersensitivity model*, which proposes that there is an existing vulnerability in persons suffering from psychiatric disorders that result in their sensitivity to even small amounts of substances. The *self-medication* model suggests that people use substances to relieve subjective distress related to their mental illness. It has also been suggested that the accumulation of multiple risk factors related to mental illness, including subjective distress, may indeed increase the relative risk of a substance-related/addictive disorder.

The *secondary mental disorder model* suggests that the use of substances may precipitate mental health conditions in persons who would not otherwise have developed them. It should be noted that substance use is *associated* with the development of certain psychiatric symptoms. For example, amphetamines can cause psychotic symptoms, and alcohol may cause depressive symptoms. The evidence to suggest that substance use is *causally* linked to the development of a mental disorder is not as robust. However, there is an emerging body of evidence examining the link between cannabis and the development of a mental disorder. An overview of five systematic reviews concluded that cannabis use is likely to increase the risk of developing schizophrenia and other psychoses; the higher the use, the greater the risk (National Academies of Sciences, Engineering, and Medicine, 2017). There is also evidence suggesting that regular cannabis use is associated with increased risk for developing anxiety in the long term; however, given the variability of the studies reviewed, a causal relationship cannot be determined (Xue et al., 2021).

The *bidirectional feedback model* posits a two-way aetiologic process whereby substance-related/addictive disorders and other mental illnesses increase the risk for the development of other conditions. For instance, an increased use of substances in adolescence may, because of neurocircuitry vulnerability, increase risk for developing a substance-related/addictive disorder and is also a risk factor for psychotic symptoms (Otasowie, 2020).

The U. S. National Institute on Drug Abuse (2020) has identified that common risk factors for developing concurrent disorders include genetic vulnerability, epigenetics, environmental influences, **stress**, and **trauma** and adverse childhood experiences in one pathway. For instance, individuals who have been exposed to traumatic events may increase substance use, which can in turn lead to new traumatic exposures, which may perpetuate the stress–substance use cycle. Both acute stress and chronic stress lead to changes in the natural neurochemical homeostasis, modulated by numerous factors, which may increase the risk of the development of substance-related/addictive disorders. There is some evidence to suggest that the stress associated with the global pandemic has increased the potential in some individuals for developing concurrent disorders. (See Box 33.1.)

Assessment Approaches Specific to Concurrent Disorders

Assessment of persons with concurrent disorders follows the principles of assessment for each category of the mental disorder encountered, as well as for substance use patterns and complications. The protocols

for screening for tobacco use, illicit substance use, substance use disorders, at-risk drinking, and alcohol use disorders are discussed in Chapter 26.

Treatment planning for persons with concurrent disorders is based on the principle of treatment matching, that is, utilizing the least restrictive level of care that is proven to be safe and likely to be effective. The criteria for placement of a person on a certain level of care are predominantly based on consensus best practices of care and treatment. To allow for adequate treatment planning and appropriate utilization of resources in persons with concurrent disorders, assessment of the following six domains is recommended: (a) acute intoxication and/or withdrawal potential, (b) biomedical conditions and complications, (c) emotional/behavioural/cognitive conditions and complications, (d) readiness to change, (e) relapse/continued use/continued problem potential, and (f) recovery environment.

Care and Treatment Approaches Specific to Concurrent Disorders

Care and treatment for concurrent disorders should include screening and comprehensive assessment for both substance-related/addictive disorders and other mental health disorders, psychosocial and pharmacologic interventions, and a plan for coordinated care. Because this population is highly heterogeneous, there does not appear to be a single approach or set of interventions that is proven to be effective for all persons with

BOX 33.1 Research for Best Practice

ANXIETY AND DEPRESSION IN CANADA DURING THE COVID-19 PANDEMIC: A NATIONAL SURVEY

Dozois, D. J. (2021). Anxiety and depression in Canada during the COVID-19 pandemic: A national survey. *Canadian Psychological Association, 62*(1), 136–142. https://doi.apa.org/fulltext/2020-63541-001.html

Background: Anxiety and depression are the most prevalent mental health disorders among Canadians. It is speculated that there will be an increase in both incidence and prevalence of these disorders due to the COVID-19 pandemic.

Objective: The objective of this study was to determine the impact of COVID-19 on levels of anxiety and depression and on alcohol and cannabis consumption.

Method: A nationally representative sample of 1,803 Canadian adults (ages 18 years and older) responded to an online survey. Questions were asked pertaining to their level of anxiety and depression, previous diagnosis with either an anxiety or depressive disorder, and their alcohol and cannabis use.

Findings: The percentage of respondents who indicated their anxiety was high to extremely high increased from 5% to 20% and the number of respondents who reported depression increased from 4% to 10% since the beginning of COVID-19. Among those who reported using substances, 28% reported an increase in their consumption of alcohol, and there was a similar increase (29%) in the consumption of cannabis. Notably, one third of all respondents who reported having received a diagnosis of an anxiety or depressive disorder reported that their alcohol use increased (34% and 33%, respectively) during the pandemic. Further, two fifths of these individuals reported increased use of cannabis (47% and 41%).

Conclusion: The study findings demonstrated a substantive increase in the number of Canadians reporting high levels of anxiety and depressive symptoms and in their consumption of alcohol and cannabis during the pandemic. It is recommended that health providers conduct a detailed review of how individuals managed with their mood and substance use during the pandemic and beyond.

IN-A-LIFE 🏠

Clara Hughes (1972–)

PUBLIC PERSONA

Clara Hughes is a six-time Olympic medallist in cycling and speed skating. In 2006, when she stepped onto the Olympic podium in Torino, Italy, she became the first athlete to win multiple medals in both the Summer and Winter Games. Four years later, she proudly carried the national flag at the head of the Canadian team during the opening ceremony of the Vancouver Olympic Winter Games. Among others, her awards include Officer of the Order of Canada; Member of the Order of Manitoba; Inductee Canada Sports Hall of Fame; Star on Canada's Walk of Fame; Honorary Doctorate of Law, University of Manitoba;

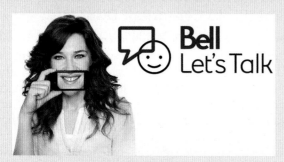

Credit: Photograph by Kent Kahlberg

Honorary Doctorate of Law, University of British Columbia; and Honorary Doctorate of Letters, University of New Brunswick (http://clara-hughes.com/about-clara/awards).

PERSONAL REALITIES

In her book, *Open Heart, Open Mind*, Hughes chronicles spending her teenage years misusing alcohol, tobacco, and other drugs. After years of intense competition, she shares her realization that her physical extremes, emotional setbacks, and partying habits were masking a severe depression. She has also shared that she struggled with an eating disorder (Arsenault, 2015). After winning the bronze medal in the last speed-skating race of her career, Hughes decided to retire, determined to transform her depression into something positive. She has since advocated for a variety of social causes, and in 2010, Hughes became a national spokesperson for Bell Canada's Let's Talk campaign, which is dedicated to breaking down the stigma of mental illness.

Sources: Arsenault, A. (2015, September 6). Olympian Clara Hughes reveals doping infraction. *CBC News*. http://www.cbc.ca/news/canada/olympian-clara-hughes-reveals-doping-infraction-1.3215617; Hughes, C. (2015). *Open heart, open mind*. Simon & Schuster.

---

concurrent disorders (Karapareddy, 2019; McKee, 2017). In a review of 24 international guidelines for concurrent disorder management, the conclusion was that guidelines generally supported combinations of treatments for individual disorders, but there was a small evidence base for concurrent disorders (Hakobyan et al., 2020).

Different models of care and treatment exist for persons with concurrent disorders: sequential (serial) treatment (whereby care is received in sequential treatment episodes in separate systems of care), **parallel care** (accessed for all disorders simultaneously, but in different systems, with varying degrees of coordination), and **integrated care** (where care is provided for both disorders by the same cross-trained team members in the same program, resulting in an integration of services). At the turn of the 21st century, Mueser and colleagues (1998) identified seven best practice components of integrated care these components still provide us with some guidance today:

- Integration of services (integrated care)
- Comprehensive approach to assessment and treatment
- Assertiveness (actively reaching out to persons with concurrent disorders)
- Reduction of negative consequences (e.g., harm reduction)

- Time-unlimited services (reflecting the chronic and severe nature of concurrent disorders)
- Adapting interventions to the person's stage of treatment
- Using multiple psychotherapeutic modalities

The advantages of integrated care have been increasingly validated through research. Some studies indicate that utilizing integrated care demonstrates better individual outcomes (Hakobyan et al., 2020) and improved clinical and social outcomes with comparable costs to standard care (Karapareddy, 2019). The optimal degree of integration should ensure that evidence-based safe and effective care is available, accessible, and affordable to each person suffering from a concurrent disorder. Early detection of the disorders, as well as primary, secondary, and tertiary prevention, warrants special attention.

Integrated treatment has been identified as a fundamental component to best practice guidelines for the treatment of concurrent disorders in Canada. In terms of which treatments ought to be offered, these include pharmacotherapy, psychoeducation, motivational interventions, social skills training, increasing healthy pleasures, cognitive–behavioural therapy, and contingency management (McKee, 2017).

Integrated care pathways are a structured multidisciplinary care plan that details essential steps in the care of individuals with concurrent disorders. These provide a more structured approach for combining psychotherapy and pharmacotherapy and deliver treatment in a coordinated way. A research study was conducted comparing integrated care pathways and treatment as usual for individuals with major depressive disorders and alcohol use disorders at the Centre for Addiction and Mental Health in Toronto. The study concluded that the structured care plan yielded significantly better outcomes in drinking patterns and severity of depressive symptoms and recommended expansion of this approach (Samokhvalov et al., 2017). Nurses are a vital member of multidisciplinary teams responsible for planning and implementing integrated care pathways.

Treatment Matching

The overarching principle in matching persons to the right level of care is to provide treatment at the least restrictive level of care that will be effective and safe. The concept of treatment matching has been formalized and is guided by a set of placement criteria. These provide separate placement criteria for individualized treatment plans through a multidimensional assessment that evaluates acute intoxication/withdrawal; biomedical conditions/complications; emotional, behavioural, or cognitive conditions/complications; readiness to change; relapse, continued use, or continued problem potential; and recovery environment. Based on this multidimensional assessment, treatment placement on one of five levels is recommended: Level 0.5 (early intervention), Level I (outpatient services), Level II (intensive outpatient/partial hospitalization services), Level III (residential/inpatient services), or Level IV (medically managed intensive inpatient services).

Indications for Hospitalization

Substance-related/addictive disorders and mental disorders are both risk factors for self-harm or suicide. Such risk has to be carefully and iteratively assessed, and attention should be given to detecting other risk factors, which include previous attempts at self-harm, any history of violence and/or trauma, lack of social support systems, and physical illness. (See Chapter 20 for detailed discussion on self-harm and suicidal behaviour.) Those at imminent and substantial risk of harm to self should be hospitalized to ensure safety. Other indications for hospitalization may include complicated withdrawal syndromes, or where interventions on a less restrictive level of care have failed to yield the necessary outcomes. Individual approaches should incorporate engagement, persuasion, active treatment, and relapse prevention (RP). Psychoeducation and support for treatment adherence will be important. Multimodal and integrated pharmacotherapy and behavioural approaches are key treatment options.

Implementing Interventions for Specific Concurrent Disorders

There is no single intervention that will work for every individual with a concurrent disorder, because each person may differ greatly with respect to severity, substance of abuse, mental disorder, and the individual's unique biologic, psychological, social, and spiritual considerations. Often several approaches can work together while others are deemed inappropriate. Treatment programs usually combine psychosocial interventions with other different approaches to provide a comprehensive plan based on the individual's needs. Nursing interventions vary depending on the nature of the current problems, the status and severity of the illnesses, and the individual's situation. Continuity of treatment is clearly important, but even more critical is the need to develop specific evidence-based treatments—pharmacologic and psychosocial interventions—for specific situations and specific individuals. The following section discusses the most salient examples of concurrent disorders that nurses will encounter during their practice.

Concurrent Substance Use and Mood Disorders

Mood disorders (e.g., major depressive disorder, persistent depressive disorder) represent some of the most common psychiatric disorders in the general population, and it is estimated that approximately 15% to 50% of those entering treatment for a substance use disorder have a lifetime diagnosis of at least one depressive disorder (Nunes & Wiss, 2014). Although bipolar disorder is less common than other mood disorders, the likelihood of having a substance use disorder is significantly elevated, with a prevalence of 40% (Nunes & Wiss, 2014; Yuodelis-Flores et al., 2019). Mood disorders and comorbid substance use represent an example of a common vulnerability as a result of genetic and/or environmental factors.

It is often challenging to distinguish between substance-induced mood symptoms and those associated with a bona fide mood disorder. To distinguish, it is useful to examine the onset of the conditions and to determine which condition preceded which or to investigate the persistence of mood symptoms during periods of sobriety and abstinence. It is often necessary to wait for a period of 4 weeks of sobriety/abstinence before diagnosing an independent mood disorder versus a substance-induced mood disorder. This poses obvious clinical concerns in terms of having to wait for several weeks prior to intervening. Suffering from a mood disorder and substance use disorder may increase the risk of suicide and shorten life expectancy, and it may also adversely impact the clinical course of either or both disorders.

Treatment of co-occurring depression with suitably matched antidepressant medication is helpful in reducing both substance abuse and depressive symptomatology. It should, however, not be considered stand-alone treatment and will unlikely resolve the addictive disorder, hence necessitating integrated care and treatment of both conditions. Similar to other studies of mood disorders, the placebo response rate is high. The selective serotonin reuptake inhibitors (SSRIs) are among the most favourable first-line options due to their tolerability and safety profile. However, in individuals with major depressive disorder and alcohol dependence, the use of SSRIs may be less effective (Hakobyan et al., 2020). The tricyclic antidepressants may be problematic in this population due to the sedating effects, the risk of overdose, and the risk of seizures. If SSRIs fail, alternative options include compounds like duloxetine (although not in alcohol-abusing persons), mirtazapine, venlafaxine, desvenlafaxine (serotonin and norepinephrine reuptake inhibitor, or SNRI), or bupropion.

Concurrent Substance Use and Anxiety Disorders

Anxiety disorders, symptoms of anxiety, and substance use disorders co-occur more commonly that what would be expected by chance alone (Hartwell et al., 2019). In the short term, it is reported that some substances may relieve symptoms of anxiety; but in the medium and long term, these very substances may worsen symptoms of anxiety. Similarly, the symptoms of anxiety may present during the course of chronic intoxication and withdrawal. Of the range of anxiety disorders, panic disorder is the single anxiety disorder most closely associated with addiction to alcohol, while generalized anxiety disorder (GAD) is the one most closely associated with dependence on substances other than alcohol (e.g., cannabis). The presence of GAD is also associated with a more rapid progression from first alcoholic beverage to addiction, as compared with individuals without anxiety disorder. For most persons with anxiety and an addictive disorder, it has been determined that the anxiety disorder generally preceded the development of the addictive disorder. The association between substance-related conditions and obsessive–compulsive disorder is considered the least robust of all the anxiety disorders.

CBT is considered the most effective treatment for anxiety co-occurring with an addictive disorder, and some benefits may be yielded from pharmacotherapy. In general, the use of benzodiazepines (or other substances with an abuse potential) should be avoided. There is limited evidence to guide treatment, but in general, the SSRIs or SNRIs may be considered helpful, along with psychotherapy (see Chapter 23).

Concurrent Substance Use and Posttraumatic Stress Disorders

Although PTSD affects less than 10% of the population, around 60% of persons who suffer from PTSD also suffer from an addictive disorder and are associated with less optimistic treatment outcomes (Saladin et al., 2019). The relationship between trauma, subsequent PTSD, and the development of a substance use disorder is complex and frequently complicates treatment. Persons suffering from PTSD may resort to self-medicating with substances to relieve or distract from the distressing emotions related to the symptoms of the illness. The use of cannabis for medical purposes ("medical marijuana") is not yet considered an evidence-based approach to the care and treatment of PTSD (Abizaid et al., 2019; National Academies of Science, Engineering, Medicine, January 2017). Treatment is offered by combining a first-line medication for PTSD (e.g., SSRI) with one of three modalities: prolonged exposure therapy (PE), cognitive processing therapy (CPT), or EMDR (eye movement desensitization and reprocessing therapy).

Concurrent Substance Use and Attention Deficit Hyperactivity Disorders

Attention deficit hyperactivity disorder is the most common behavioural disorder of childhood, and the most children who have ADHD continue to have symptoms in adulthood even though they may not meet the criteria for the disorder as an adult (see Chapter 30). Those with ADHD are more prone to develop addictive disorders, especially if ADHD remains untreated in the early stages. This is particularly the case for those with concurrent conduct disorder whereby the severity of impairment of each disorder is likely to increase (Levin & Mariani, 2019). The diagnosis of ADHD is complicated in persons who are already using substances because their use may mimic symptoms of ADHD and the latter is often underdiagnosed in clinical populations. Major depressive disorder, bipolar disorder, or psychotic disorders may also co-occur in those with ADHD and substance-related/addictive disorders, further complicating diagnostic uncertainty.

Attention placed on prevention, early identification, and care/treatment strategies can diminish the adverse consequences of ADHD. These include the trait of impulsivity and one of its most damaging consequences, namely, that of substance use and addiction. Stimulant medications (dextroamphetamine or methylphenidate) are the mainstay of treatment, and despite the abuse potential of these drugs, clinical evidence suggests that such treatment can be conducted safely and effectively. Nonstimulant medications such as atomoxetine, clonidine, and modafinil are also considered reasonable options. Precautions should be taken to avoid abuse when using medications that are associated with risk of abuse. Psychosocial interventions that are proven to yield benefits include contingency management and CBT.

Concurrent Substance Use and Psychotic Disorders

The rate of addiction is substantially elevated in those with psychotic disorder when compared with persons in the general population. Substance use may accelerate the onset of a psychotic disorder in a vulnerable individual, and cannabis has been determined to be an independent risk factor in the development of schizophrenia. Transient substance-induced psychotic features are not uncommon in persons intoxicated with substances (Ziedonis et al., 2019). The most obvious psychotic symptoms related to alcohol use occur during alcohol withdrawal. Symptoms typically emerge within 2 days from stopping consumption and often present with command hallucinations and/or agitation. Cannabis use may be associated with suspiciousness, confusion, and memory impairment, while the psychosis associated with cocaine use is typically associated with transient paranoia. Substance use may also worsen the symptoms and complicate the diagnostic certainty, course, and treatment of the illness.

A wide range of substances may mimic psychotic symptoms, during both intoxication and withdrawal. The first step in management is to ensure adequate safety and security. Following this, the concurrent treatment of psychotic symptoms and substance use is indicated. Special attention should be given to medication adherence, and the use of depot antipsychotics may have a special utility in ensuring such. The use of atypical antipsychotics appears to be superior to the use of typical/conventional antipsychotics in this regard, as the former appear to better target negative symptoms and are less prone to be associated with dysphoria. Atypical antipsychotics, such as clozapine, may work better in individuals with schizophrenia and substance use disorder (Hakobyan et al., 2020). Atypical antipsychotics are also associated with greater success in smoking cessation in persons with schizophrenia. Psychosocial approaches that have demonstrated effectiveness are motivational enhancement therapy, relapse prevention, and 12-step facilitation.

Concurrent Substance Use and Personality Disorders

Epidemiologic data have determined that most people who have a personality disorder also have a substance use disorder (Ross & Demner, 2019). Although antisocial personality disorder is the most commonly associated personality disorder with substance use disorders, the most challenging is likely borderline personality disorder. Both the addiction and the personality disorder are likely to result in complex and serious behav-

ioural problems, often with an associated risk of harm to self. It is also often associated with the co-occurrence of other mental disorders, for example, MDD, an eating disorder, or OCD. The category of concurrent personality disorders and substance use disorders pose some of the most vexing problems in care of this population.

Attention should first be paid to ensuring safety to self and to others. General principles of treatment include offering pharmacotherapy for comorbid conditions like MDD, OCD, or an eating disorder. No medication is indicated for any specific personality disorder. Behavioural interventions form the mainstay of treatment, specifically dialectical behavioural therapy (DBT). Applying the principles of DBT for the population of concurrent disordered individuals has demonstrated significant benefit by teaching cognitive self-control techniques that allow for turning themselves to abstinence (see Chapter 27).

▌ Nursing Management: Summary

Nurses working in nonpsychiatric inpatient and community settings may be the first healthcare contact for person individuals with concurrent disorders. Nurses must recognize that the stigma associated with both substance use and mental disorders can affect the person's readiness to address these illnesses. A helpful, knowledgeable, and nonjudgmental approach to the person may open a "window of opportunity" for seeking care and treatment. Because persons with concurrent disorders may have difficulty relating openly with others and trusting those in positions of authority, engaging the person in a way that concretely addresses presenting issues (e.g., acquiring social services, getting relief from psychiatric symptoms) can be particularly helpful. Note that assessment procedures that are protracted, complicated, and involve intimate personal questions may be discouraging to the individual. It may take some time and further engagement for the individual to be willing and able to provide an accurate history of substance use, severity of symptoms, and problems in living. Denial to oneself regarding these issues is a common defensive mechanism for persons with addiction (and in concurrent disorders); it may therefore be particularly difficult for them to always offer a reliable history. Medical records, other healthcare professionals, family members, and significant others may be of assistance to the person and the nurse in developing an accurate health history. See Box 33.2 Research for Best Practice on nursing care with inpatients.

Families of the individual with a concurrent disorder need education about concurrent disorders and guidance as to the best way to support their family member in recovery. Developing and sustaining a healthy lifestyle is an important aspect of recovery, and families can be particularly helpful in this area. Nurses can provide information at a level appropriate to the family, as well as the individual, on diet, exercise, sleep routine, stress

BOX 33.2 Research for Best Practice

UNDERSTANDING HELPFUL NURSING CARE FROM THE PERSPECTIVE OF MENTAL HEALTH INPATIENTS WITH A DUAL DIAGNOSIS: A QUALITATIVE DESCRIPTIVE STUDY

Brahim, L. O., Hanganu, C., & Gros, C. P. (2020). Understanding helpful nursing care from the perspective of mental health inpatients with a dual diagnosis: A qualitative descriptive study. *Journal of the American Psychiatric Nurses Association, 26*(3), 250–261. https://doi.10.1177/1078390319878773

Background: Nursing care for hospitalized individuals with dual diagnosis is understudied.

Objective: To determine which nursing interventions, attitudes, actions, and/or behaviours are considered helpful from the perspective of inpatients with dual diagnosis in a Canadian hospital.

Method: A qualitative–descriptive study employing semi-structured interviews with 12 adult patients.

Findings: Three themes of helpful nursing care were derived. These are promoting health in everyday life, including physical and psychosocial wellbeing; managing substance use in tandem with mental illness; and building therapeutic relationships through demonstrating caring, paying attention, and providing individualized care.

Conclusion: The study illuminates the importance of involving individuals receiving nursing care and draws attention to nursing's scope, complexity, and value.

management, and leisure activities. These are essential to a lifestyle that supports sobriety and prevents relapse. At times, families of persons with a concurrent disorder are no longer involved in their lives or are also living with substance use and/or mental health problems. Nurses need to assess the existing support system of the individual, as finding alternative supports and/or social services may need to be an immediate goal.

Psychoeducation regarding goal setting can give the individual a core strategy for making positive change. Access to crisis counselling is important, as is housing that allows for a situation supportive of recovery. Opportunities for a social network that reinforces sobriety and the maintenance of treatment plans for psychiatric symptoms will be important. Nurses can assist by referrals to local groups (e.g., 12-step programs, mental health drop-in clubs, partnership with volunteers) that aim to facilitate the development of such social networks. At an appropriate point in recovery, referral to vocational and employment guidance will be a priority. Relapse prevention is crucial to the care of the person in recovery from a concurrent disorder; patient education, whether offered on a one-to-one basis or in a group setting, is a key strategy. See Box 33.3 for recommended psychoeducational topics for relapse prevention.

Where Do We Go From Here?

In some settings, mental health and addiction systems continue to operate independently from each other and remain compartmentalized. As a result, the focus of treatment for people with concurrent disorders tends to be on one component of their concurrent disorder but not the other. Apart from research into the effectiveness of different treatment approaches, research into systems'

approaches is also direly needed. Universal education and training are needed for the workforce responsible for the care and treatment of those with concurrent disorders. The only reasonable solution to prevent those with concurrent disorders from "falling through the cracks" is to ensure integration of the national agendas for mental health and addiction. Unless we have a unified approach to all components of concurrent disorders, enjoying parity with regard to healthcare spending, our patients will not be able to reach their potential and thrive.

BOX 33.3 Psychoeducational Topics for Relapse Prevention

- Understanding addiction
- Effects and interaction of tobacco, alcohol, and other drugs in the body
- What is my relationship with tobacco, alcohol, and other drugs?
- How to live in a healthy way
- Leisure and relaxation
- Coping with stress
- Coping with anger
- Communicating with others
- Problem-solving strategies
- The relapse cycle
- Strategies for preventing relapse
- My plan for avoiding relapse
- My personal cues that relapse is imminent
- Dealing with crisis

Summary of Key Points

- *Concurrent disorders* are the term used when individuals suffer from at least *one* substance-related/addictive disorder as well as one (or more) *other* mental disorder. When these conditions co-occur, treatment should address both (or all) at the same time (integrated care or parallel treatment).
- Many individuals with co-occurring disorders, despite the associated challenges, do recover and live productive lives.
- An important reason why persons with addiction relapse to drug use is the presence of untreated mental illness. An important reason why persons with mental illness relapse is untreated addiction issues.
- When mental and substance-related/addictive disorders coexist, both disorders require specific and appropriate primary treatment.
- Both disorders should be considered "primary," and both should be treated at the same time.

- The specific content of primary treatment for each person with concurrent disorders must be individualized according to diagnosis, phase of treatment, level of functioning and/or disability, and assessment of level of care based on acuity, severity, medical safety, motivation, and availability of recovery support.
- The most effective approach for individuals is integrated care whereby healthcare professionals, programs, and resources are co-located and such services offered on a long-term basis with continuity of care across programs and time. Individuals with concurrent disorders benefit from a longitudinal care approach rather than episodic care.
- Psychoeducation regarding the effects of tobacco, alcohol, and other drug use; a healthy lifestyle; and relapse prevention is another key element of nursing care for persons with concurrent disorders, in addition to health education regarding their co-occurring mental disorder.

Thinking Challenges

1. You are performing an initial interview with a client who is seeking help for anxiety. Alex tells you that working from home and being isolated during the pandemic was particularly stressful and that life has still not returned to normal. You want to perform a fulsome assessment of the presenting problem.

   a. Why would you consider the possibility of a concurrent disorder with Alex?

   b. What questions would you ask to assess the presence of a substance use disorder?

   c. If you spot indications of a concurrent disorder, what are some steps to consider in the management of Alex's nursing care?

Visit thePoint to view suggested responses.
Go to **thePoint.lww.com/activate** and use the activation code found in the front of this text to unlock answers to the "Thinking Challenges" and other online resources.

Web Links

https://www.ccsa.ca Canadian Centre for Substance Abuse and Addiction is a nongovernmental organization that provides national leadership on substance use and solutions that address alcohol- and other drug-related harms. This is an excellent evidence-based resource for nurses and includes a number of publications on substances and addictions, including concurrent disorders in Canada.

https://www.porticonetwork.ca/web/knowledgex-archive/primary-care/resources-patients-families/resources-concurrent-disorders Portico: Canada's Mental Health & Addiction

Network lists several resources of relevance to PMH nurses in Canada, including *Concurrent Substance Use and Mental Health Disorder: An Information Guide* (available in both English and French) and *A Family Guide to Concurrent Disorders*.

http://www.camh.ca/en/education/about/AZCourses/Pages/default.aspx The Centre for Addiction and Mental Health (CAMH) is an excellent resource for individuals interested in learning more about concurrent disorders. In particular, CAMH offers a *Concurrent Disorders Core Online Course*, open to anyone, and a *Concurrent Disorder Certificate Program* designed for mental health and addictions' professionals.

Acknowledgment

The author thanks Sadie Deschenes, RN, MN, and doctoral candidate for her valuable review, literature search, and other contributions to the chapter.

References

Abizaid, A., Merali, Z., & Anisman, H. (2019). Cannabis: A potential efficacious intervention for PTSD or simply snake oil? *Journal of Psychiatry & Neuroscience, 44*(2), 75–78. https://doi.org/10.1503/jpn.190021

American Psychiatric Association. (2013). *Diagnostic and statistical manual of mental disorders* (5th ed.).

Arsenault, A. (2015). Olympian Clara Hughes reveals doping infraction. *CBC News.* http://www.cbc.ca/news/canada/olympian-clara-hughes-reveals-doping-infraction-1.3215617

Balhara, Y. P. S., Kuppili, P. P., & Gupta, R. (2017). Neurobiology of comorbid substance use disorders and psychiatric disorders: Current state of the evidence. *Journal of Addictions Nursing, 28*(1), 11–26. https://doi.org/10.1097/JAN.0000000000000155

Beaudette, J. N., & Stewart, L. A. (2016). National prevalence of mental disorders among incoming Canadian male offenders. *Canadian Journal of Psychiatry, 61*(10), 624–632.

Brahim, L. O., Hanganu, C., & Gros, C. P. (2020). Understanding helpful nursing care from the perspective of mental health inpatients with a dual diagnosis: A qualitative descriptive study. *Journal of the American Psychiatric Nurses Association, 26*(3), 250–261. https://doi.10.1177/1078390319878773

Brunette, M. F., Mueser, K. T., Babbin, S., Meyer-Kalos, P., Rosenheck, R., Correll, C. U., Cather, C., Robinson, D. G., Schooler, N. R., Penn, D. L., Addington, J., Estroff, S. E., Gottlieb, J., Glynn, S. M., Marcy, P., Robinson, J., & Kane, J. M. (2018). Demographic and clinical correlates of substance use disorders in first episode psychosis. *Schizophrenia Research, 194*, 4–12. https://doi.org/10.1016/j.schres.2017.06.039

Danda, M. (2020). Rethinking concurrent disorders: Implications and future directions for nursing practice. *Mental Health Practice, 23*(1), 28–33. https://doi.org/10.7748/mhp.2019.e1413

Dozois, D. J. (2021). Anxiety and depression in Canada during the COVID-19 pandemic: A national survey. *Canadian Psychological Association, 62*(1), 136–142. https://www.apa.org/fulltext/2020-63541-001.html

Drake, R. E., & Green, A. I. (2013). The challenge of heterogeneity and complexity in dual diagnosis awareness in everyday clinical practice. *Journal of Dual Diagnosis, 9*(2), 43–49. https://doi.org/10.1080/15504263.2013.779104

Hakobyan, S., Vazirian, S., Lee-Cheong, S., Krausz, M., Honer, W. G., & Schutz, C. G. (2020). Concurrent disorder management guidelines. Systematic review. *Journal of Clinical Medicine, 9*(8), 2406. https://doi.org/10.3390/jcm9082406

Hartwell, K. J., Orwat, D. E., & Brady, K. T. (2019). Co-occurring substance use and anxiety disorders. In S. C. Miller (Eds.), *The ASAM principles of addiction medicine* (6th ed., pp. 1389–1417). Wolters Kluwer.

Hughes, C. (2015). *Open heart, open mind.* Simon & Schuster Canada.

Kahn, S. (2017). *Concurrent mental and substance use disorders in Canada.* Statistics Canada. https://doi.org/10.1080/15504263.2018.1518553

Karapareddy, V. (2019). A review of integrated care for concurrent disorders: Cost effectiveness and clinical outcomes. *Journal of Dual Diagnosis, 15*(1), 56–66. https://doi.org/10.1080/15504263.2018.1518553

Levin, F. R., & Mariani, J. J. (2019). Co-occurring substance use disorder and attention deficit hyperactivity disorder. In S. C. Miller & R. Saitz (Eds.), *The ASAM principles of addiction medicine* (6th ed., pp. 1418–1435). Wolters Kluwer.

Margolese, H. C., Malchy, L., Carlos Negrete, J., Tempier, R., & Gill, K. (2004). Drug and alcohol use among patients with schizophrenia and related psychoses: Levels and consequences. *Schizophrenia Research, 67*, 157–166.

McKee, S. A. (2017). Concurrent substance use disorders and mental illness: Bridging the gap between research and treatment. *Canadian Psychology, 58*(1), 50–57. https://doi.org/10.1037/cap0000093

Menne, V., & Chesworth, R. (2020). Schizophrenia and drug addiction comorbidity: Recent advances in our understanding of behavioural susceptibility and neural mechanisms. *Neuroanatomy and Behaviour, 2*(1), e10. https://doi.org/10.35430/nab.2020.e10

Mental Health Commission of Canada. (2016). *Advancing the mental health strategy for Canada: A framework for action (2017–2022).*

Mueser, K. T., Drake, R. E., & Wallach, M. A. (1998). Dual diagnosis: A review of etiological theories. *Addictive Behaviours, 23*(6), 717–734.

National Academies of Sciences, Engineering, and Medicine. (2017). *The health effects of cannabis and cannabinoids: The current state of evidence and recommendations for research.* The National Academies Press. https://doi.org/10.17226/24625

National Institute on Drug Abuse. (2020). *Common comorbidities with substance use disorders research report.* https://www.drugabuse.gov/publications/research-reports/common-comorbidities-substance-use-disorders/why-there-comorbidity-between-substance-use-disorders-mental-illnesses

Nunes, E. V., & Wiss, R. D. (2014). Co-occurring addictive and mood disorders. In R. K. Ries & S. C. Miller (Eds.), *The ASAM principles of addiction medicine* (6th ed.). Wolters Kluwer.

Otasowie, J. (2020). Co-occurring mental disorder and substance use disorder in young people: Aetiology, assessment and treatment. *BJPsych Advances, 27*(4), 272–281. https://doi.org/10.1192/bja.2020.64

Ross, S., & Demner, A. R. (2019). Co-occurring personality disorders and addiction. In S. C. Miller & R. Saitz (Eds.), *The ASAM principles of addiction medicine* (6th ed., pp. 1436–1452). Wolters Kluwer.

Saladin, M. E., Teeters, J., Gros, D. F., Gilmore, A. K., Gray, K. M., Barrett, E. L., Lancaster, C. L., Killeen, T. K., & Back, S. E. (2019). Posttraumatic stress disorder and substance use disorder comorbidity. In S. C. Miller (Ed.), *The ASAM principles of addiction medicine* (6th ed., pp. 1452–1467). Wolters Kluwer.

Samokhvalov, A. V., Awan, A., George, T. P., Irving, J., Le Foll, B., Perrotta, S., Probst, C., Voore, P., & Rehm, J. (2017). Integrated care pathway for co-occurring major depressive and alcohol use disorders: Outcomes of the first two years. *American Journal on Addictions, 26*(6), 602–609. https://doi.org/10.1111/ajad.12572

Substance Abuse and Mental Health Services Administration. (2020). *Co-occurring disorders and other health conditions.* https://www.samhsa.gov/medication-assisted-treatment/medications-counseling-related-conditions/co-occurring-disorders

United States Department of Health and Human Services, Substance Abuse and Mental Health Services Administration. (2015). *Receipt of services for behavioral health problems: Results from the 2014 National Survey on Drug Use and Health.*

Xue, S., Husain, M. I., Zhao, H., & Ravindran, A. V. (2021). Cannabis use and prospective long-term association with anxiety: A systematic review and meta-analysis of longitudinal studies: Usage du cannabis et association prospective à long terme avec l'anxiété: une revue systématique et une méta-analyse d'études longitudinales. *The Canadian Journal of Psychiatry, 66*(2), 126–138. https://doi.org/10.1177/0706743720952251

Yuodelis-Flores, C., Goldsmith, R. J., & Ries, R. K. (2019). Substance-induced mental disorders. In S. C. Miller (Ed.), *The ASAM principles of addiction medicine* (6th ed., pp. 1287–1299). Wolters Kluwer.

Ziedonis, D. M., Fan, X., Bizamcer, A. N., Wyatt, S. A., Tonelli, M. E., & Smelson, D. (2019). Co-occurring addiction and psychotic disorders. In S. C. Miller & R. Saitz (Eds.), *The ASAM principles of addiction medicine* (6th ed., pp. 1402–1417). Wolters Kluwer.

CHAPTER 34

Care of Persons With Experiences of Abuse

Saima Hirani and Colleen Varcoe

LEARNING OBJECTIVES

After studying this chapter, you will be able to:

- Discuss the power dynamics underlying interpersonal forms of violence.
- Identify the prevalence and health effects of intimate partner violence, child abuse (or child maltreatment), and elder abuse in Canada.
- Explain the key elements of taking trauma- and violence-informed approach in practice.
- Take steps as a nurse to implement a trauma- and violence-informed approach to practice.

KEY TERMS

- child maltreatment/abuse • effects of abuse • elder abuse • intimate partner violence • intimate partner terrorism • neglect • patriarchy • situational couple violence • structural violence

KEY CONCEPTS

- strengths-based approach • trauma- and violence-informed care

In this chapter, nursing practice in relation to multiple forms of interpersonal abuse is considered, including intimate partner violence (IPV), child abuse (or child maltreatment), and elder abuse, with an emphasis on the implications for nursing. These forms of violence are prevalent in Canadian society, with profound impacts on mental health. Yet, the social responses to these patterns have been largely ineffective, in part because abuse is not understood as a widespread feature of society. The overall goal of this chapter is to strengthen the contribution of nursing to the wellbeing of people who have experienced abuse and to the wider social response to abuse.

The Social Context of Abuse

The term "abuse" is used because interpersonal violence is always an abuse of power. Abuses of power against individuals are shaped and sustained by wider social patterns of power inequity. In this chapter, power is understood, not as something people "have," but as being enacted in every relationship (among individuals, between individuals and within and by larger social structures). This is important because individuals are not simply victims or perpetrators; every person has agency situated within a larger society that shapes their circumstances, experiences and behavior.

The four-level social-ecological model, originally developed by Bronfenbrenner (1979), has been adapted by many researchers to understand the nuances of abuse and violence in various populations (Cardeli et al., 2019; Dekel et al., 2019; Kohli et al., 2015; Labrum & Solomon, 2015; Oriol et al., 2017). The understanding underlying this framework is that individuals are embedded within the multilayered domains of relationships, community, and society (see Fig. 34.1). Using this model helps to understand the factors influencing the prevalence and **effects of abuse** and the interrelations among individuals, families, communities, and society. It also helps to explain how factors and effects of abuse at one level impact other levels: individuals and their relationships are shaped by their community contexts and larger structural arrangements in society. The ecological framework is also useful to support the design of multifaceted interventions for prevention and reduction of violence at various levels (Centers for Disease Control and Prevention, 2022; World Health Organization [WHO], 2020a).

Key social patterns of power inequity that shape experiences of abuse include patterns of inequity based on gender, income, racism, age, and ability, among other forms of inequity. For example, consider Sam, a 47-year-old man seen in a forensic psychiatric setting as a consequence of probation conditions related to having knifed the family dog. Sam had previous interactions with police when neighbors complained about verbal abuse by Sam against his wife and two young children, but this is the first time he has faced charges. Sam is a veteran of the armed forces having served two tours of duty overseas on "peacekeeping" missions. On intake,

915

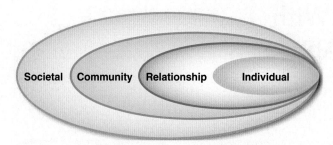

Figure 34.1 The social-ecological model: a framework for prevention. Source: Centers for Disease Control and Prevention. (2021). The social-ecological model: A framework for prevention. https://www.cdc.gov/violenceprevention/about/social-ecologicalmodel.html

the nurse learns that Sam has not been sleeping since his discharge from the forces 3 years ago; he is having nightmares and expresses anger that he cannot find work and that he is "no better off" than when he joined the forces 20 years ago and unable to find work. The nurse recognizes that Sam is exhibiting trauma symptoms and based on assessment of risk factors is deeply concerned about his potential for further violence. When asked about his wife and children, Sam makes racial slurs about them, deepening the nurse's concern.

Sam's situation demonstrates the complexity of patterns of social inequity. First, violence is gendered. As Hunnicutt (2020) argues, **patriarchy** (social systems in which cisgender men are in positions of power and cisgender women are largely excluded) is at the root of violence against women, but patriarchy and capitalism are entwined with impacts on people of all genders; together, they create social norms that dictate that "males must be both aggressive and economically successful" (p. 5). Men experience the highest levels of violence in most societies, whereas women bear the greatest burden of intimate and other forms of interpersonal violence. People who do not identify with the binary of male/female experience the highest levels of violence overall (Gehring & Knudson, 2005; James et al., 2016; Statistics Canada, 2020b). Gender interacts with other forms of inequity at all levels. For example, an online survey with Lesbian, Bisexual and Queer (LBQ) women living in Toronto, Canada, used the social ecological model and found a strong correlation between individual factors (sexual orientation, sexually transmitted infections [STIs], substance use, resilience, self-esteem); societal factors (stigma, social support, safer sex practices) and structural influences (access to STI testing and barriers to care) contributing to experiences of lifetime sexual assault (Logie et al., 2014). Furthermore, as part of a 2018 Survey of Safety in Public and Private Spaces, which asked Canadians about their experiences of "violent victimization and other unwanted sexual experiences while in public, online, or at work," Statistics Canada (2020b) reported that "gay, lesbian, bisexual, and other sexual minority people in Canada were almost three times more likely than heterosexual Canadians to report that

they had been physically or sexually assaulted" (p. 1). Refer to Figure 34.2.

Second, income inequities shape experiences of violence, with poverty often increasing exposure to violence, and decreasing resources to deal with the health effects of violence. As Hunnicutt (2020) explains, this is not simple resource deprivation; rather, socioeconomics shape life circumstances and cultural norms. So, for example, through values, norms, and opportunities, socioeconomic status shapes the likelihood of military service, and thus exposure to violence, and increases the mental distress of those who serve (Bareis & Mezuk, 2016; DiBiasio et al., 2014; Mariscal, 2007; McGlynn & Monforti, 2010).

Third, racism shapes experiences of violence in multiple ways. Systemic racism influences exposure to violence, and racial violence often intertwines with other forms of violence. For example, globally and in Canada, Indigenous women experience disproportionately high levels of **intimate partner violence**. In Canada, this disproportion has been repeatedly attributed to colonialism, racism, and the socioeconomic position of Indigenous women (Brownridge, 2008; Daoud et al., 2013; Pedersen et al., 2013). A systematic review showed that globally, experiences of IPV and mental disorders among Indigenous women are linked and exacerbated by poverty, discrimination, and problematic substance use (Chmielowska & Fuhr, 2017).

Age is also a key determinant of exposure to abuse. Again, it is not a simple matter of those who are very young or very old being more "vulnerable." Rather, how children and elders are valued, viewed, and treated in society shapes their disproportionate exposure to abuse. For example, Einboden et al. (2013) show how within capitalism, children are valued for their potential as human capital, investments in the future, or alternatively, as waste. Within late capitalist societies, children have increasingly been valued for their potential as productive citizens in a market economy and older persons viewed through the lens of the potential financial burden on society.

Finally, ability similarly shapes experiences of abuse. Women with disabilities have a much higher risk for IPV than women in the general population (Brownridge et al., 2008; Plummer & Findley, 2012), including both the types of violence perpetrated against women generally and abuse that targets the specific disability, and have been shown to have significantly more mental health symptoms related to IPV (Tutty et al., 2017). Again, these dynamics are likely due to more than vulnerability created by the specific disability, including the ways in which ability is valued in Western societies, especially as related to socioeconomic productivity.

In summary, interpersonal forms of violence and abuse are linked to structural forms of violence, that is, the ways societies are arranged to harm some people, such as through socioeconomic deprivation so that some people cannot access basic necessities of life—shelter, food, clean water, or through systemic racism,

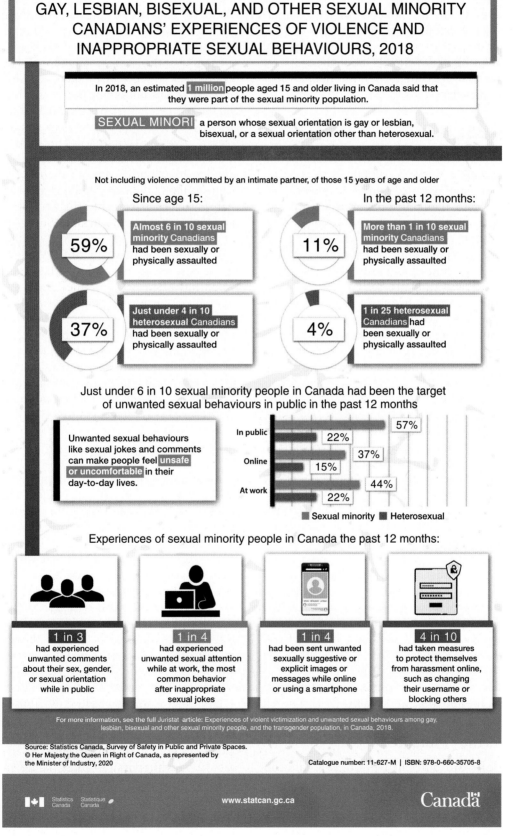

Figure 34.2 Gay, lesbian, bisexual, and other sexual minority Canadians' experiences of violence and inappropriate sexual behaviours, 2018. Source: Statistics Canada. (2020). Gay, lesbian, bisexual and other sexual minority Canadians' experience of violence and inappropriate sexual behaviours, 2018. Catalogue no: 11-627-M. Reproduced and distributed on an "as is" basis with the permission of Statistics Canada.

which impacts access to employment, education, housing, and other necessities. Interpersonal forms of abuse are abuses of power in relationships that are nested within the larger structures of communities and societies. Thus, approaches to understanding and supporting the mental health of individuals should be based on understanding the wider patterns of both interpersonal and **structural violence**.

Forms of Abuse

Family violence in Canada represents a serious public health issue. Family violence is committed by spouses, parents, children, and extended family members. Conroy (2021) reported that one in four victims (26%, or 102,316 victims) of police-reported violence were abused by a family member, and of this group, two thirds (67%) were female. Family violence is more than five times higher for women and girls when compared to men and boys; and similarly, sexual violence committed by family members is five and a half times higher for women and girls, when compared to men and boys. While police-reported family violence in Canada declined between 2009 and 2016, the year 2019 marked the third year in a row that saw an annual increase; up to 13% from 2016. In 2019, Saskatchewan, and Manitoba, had the highest rates of family violence among the Canadian provinces (i.e., 519/100,000 and 417/100,000, respectively), and nationally, reports of family violence are two times higher in rural areas (Conroy, 2021).

Interpersonal forms of abuse overlap and have cumulative health effects across the lifespan (Davies et al., 2015; Pereda & Gallardo-Pujol, 2014; Scott-Storey, 2011). That is, child maltreatment often cooccurs with interpersonal violence; elder abuse can be a continuation of IPV into older age; and sexual assault can be a feature of interpersonal violence (or can be perpetrated outside intimate partnerships). Each has profound effects on health that are cumulative. Further, the health effects of interpersonal forms of abuse are compounded by structural forms of violence, such as poverty and racism, which themselves have significant health effects (Paradies et al., 2015; Raphael, 2020). Overall, estimates of prevalence of all forms of abuse are likely underestimates given that reporting through police or research is limited by fear, intimidation, and shame.

Intimate Partner Violence

There are at least two different types of IPV. Johnson (2006) differentiated between two most common types **"intimate partner terrorism"** and **"situational couple violence,"** which are now thought to overlap and exist on a continuum from less to more severe (Eckstein, 2017; Love et al., 2020; Nevala, 2017). Intimate partner terrorism involves repeated acts of violence within

tactics of coercive control and intimidation used to elicit fear and terror. Intimate Partner Terrorism is reinforced by patterns of threats and/or acts of violence that often escalate in frequency and severity over time and result in the most severe health and social consequences for the victim. Situational couple violence results from arguments or situations that can escalate to physical acts but is not part of an intention to control the partner. Rather, occasional, mutual, lower intensity acts are attempts to deal with conflict, rather than to exert power and control over the partner through fear and intimidation. People of all genders can experience and perpetrate both forms of violence. Evidence, mostly from studies of women experiencing male IPV, suggests that greater coercive control is associated with greater harm including mental health effects (Hardesty et al., 2015).

Measuring the prevalence of IPV has been challenging because the way it is measured, including in Canada, which has often oversimplified the complexity of the experiences, measured experiences at single time points (rather than capturing patterns over time), and privileged physical abuse (Ford-Gilboe et al., 2016). Despite these limitations, evidence shows that IPV is very common globally, in Canada representing almost a third of all violent crime reported to police, with women overrepresented as victims of IPV, accounting for almost 8 in 10 victims (79%) (Statistics Canada, 2018).

Child Abuse/Maltreatment

Child maltreatment/abuse is typically categorized as physical, mental or emotional, and sexual abuse, and **neglect**, with children's exposure to interpersonal violence sometimes considered a form of abuse of children. Like other forms of abuse, the different types of child abuse often overlap and deprive children of their rights to health, development, survival, education, dignity, and protection from actual or potential harm (WHO, 2020b). Like adult forms of abuse, child maltreatment may be associated with coercive control. Importantly, neglect can encompass material or physical neglect arising from a lack of access to material resources that is not within caregiver control and neglect that is intentionally harmful within a context of coercive control.

Like other forms of abuse, child abuse has profound health effects, particularly on mental health (Afifi et al., 2014). Using Canadian population level data, Afifi and colleagues found that prevalence of any child abuse was 32%, with physical abuse being most common (26.1%), followed by sexual abuse (10.1%) and exposure to interpersonal violence (7.9%). All types of child abuse were associated with all mental health conditions, including suicidal ideation and suicide attempts and with more types of abuse experienced being associated with greater odds of mental health issues. The

General Social Survey-2014, conducted with Canadian adults who experienced childhood abuse, showed that the majority of childhood abuse victims reported having been physically and/or sexually abused between 1 and 6 times during their childhood (Burczycka & Conroy, 2017). Refer further to Chapter 29.

Elder Abuse

Approximately 17% of the total Canadian population represents seniors aged 65 years and older (Statistics Canada, 2020a), and in the next 20 years, Canada's seniors population is predicted to grow by 68% (Canadian Institute for Health Information, 2017). With this growing aging population, **elder abuse** is increasingly recognized as a significant problem in Canada. Abuse of older persons encompasses forms of interpersonal violence, such as IPV, that continue as people age, and forms of abuse and neglect that arise as people become increasingly vulnerable as they age. Such abuse may be physical, mental, emotional, sexual, or financial. In Canada in 2018, there were 12,202 senior victims (aged 65 and older) of violence reported to police; the abuse reported was more likely to be financial abuse than physical abuse (Statistics Canada, 2018). Canadian police reported data collected in 2015 indicated that six in ten senior victims were female and, overall, most senior victims were likely to have been abused by a family member, an older child, or a spouse (Burczycka & Conroy, 2017). Refer further to Chapter 31.

The Health Impacts of Abuse

Trauma is a response to any negative event that individuals find physically or emotionally harmful (American Psychiatric Association, 2013). Although the majority of violence is nonfatal, trauma related to abuse can be complex and often has significant consequences for individual, family, and community health. Research on the health effects of abuse indicates a range of short- and long-term effects on physical health, and mental health (Campbell et al., 2018; Lutwak, 2018).

Health Effects of Intimate Partner Violence

The overemphasis on physical violence has led nurses and other healthcare providers (HCPs) to focus on physical evidence of injuries in their recognition and assessment of the health effects of abuse. It has also led to those experiencing abuse having difficulty recognizing it as such in the absence of physical abuse. However, mental and emotional abuse, particularly in the context of coercive control, has profound effects on physical and mental health through the chronic stress of living with abuse and threats.

Physical Health

Research that focuses on women indicates the devastating effects of IPV on women's physical health (Davies et al., 2015; Dillon et al., 2013; WHO, 2013a). In terms of direct physical injuries, over 40% of women and about 15% of men experiencing IPV report injuries to head, neck, and face (Black et al., 2011; Smith et al., 2018). IPV has been considered one of the leading causes of injury among reproductive-aged women (Mendez-Figueroa et al., 2013). Data from a Canadian study revealed that physical injury was found to be significantly higher among women who experienced pregnancy violence than women who did not experience abuse during pregnancy (Taillieu et al., 2016). The direct consequences of IPV on female physical health include fractures, lacerations, head injuries, and STIs (Chisholm et al., 2017). Other reported physical health effects correlated with IPV are chronic pain, disability, fibromyalgia, gastrointestinal disorders, irritable bowel syndrome, sleep disorders, and general reductions in physical functioning/health-related life quality (Wathen, 2012). Importantly, these effects are not only the consequences of physical abuse. For example, Coker et al. (2000) found that women experiencing psychological IPV were significantly more likely to report poor physical and mental health. Psychological IPV was associated with a number of adverse health outcomes, including a disability preventing work, arthritis, chronic pain, migraine and other frequent headaches, STIs, chronic pelvic pain, and frequent gastrointestinal problems. Findings from the past 22 years of data showed an increased risk of cardiac diseases and type 2 diabetes mellitus among women who experience IPV (Chandan et al., 2020). A study with Canadian men who experienced lifetime violence showed a high prevalence of chronic pain (35.8%) strongly associated with the lifetime cumulative violence severity scores (Wuest et al., 2020), signaling the profound and complex health impacts of violence.

Mental Health

The experience of IPV is very stressful and exerts tremendous negative effects on mental health. A systematic review of 53 studies provided strong evidence suggesting that IPV is one of the chronic stressors contributing to poor mental health (Yim & Kofman, 2019). Severe trauma related to abuse can abruptly overwhelm the capacity to feel safe (Cooper, 1986) and cause long-term effects on individual's psychological health. Single or multiple traumatic experiences can overwhelm the human stress system, causing anxiety, sadness, and hopelessness (Zaleski et al., 2016). IPV affects individuals of all sexes and genders; however, women are more likely to experience depression and other mental health issues as a result of abuse (Gobinath et al., 2015; Lysova et al., 2019). Women who experienced IPV reported symptoms of poor mental health three times more often than women who did not have history of abuse (Gobinath et al., 2015; Smith et al., 2018).

The most commonly reported mental health issues among people who experience IPV are depression, anxiety, substance abuse, somatic symptoms, and posttraumatic stress disorder (PTSD) (Bacchus et al., 2018; Devries et al., 2013; Jordan et al., 2010). Not everyone who has experienced abusive trauma will develop symptoms consistent with a diagnosis of PTSD; however, most experience a cluster of symptoms such as anxiety, sadness, sleep problems, and nightmares, which are the common features of PTSD. Studies also report shame, guilt, humiliation, and poor self-esteem as mental health consequences of IPV for women. Exposure to IPV is also associated with high mortality due to femicide, homicide, and suicide (McLaughlin et al., 2012; Stöckl et al., 2013). (See Chapters 18, 22, 23, and 24 for further information.)

Some studies report the persistence of long-term mental health consequences on women even after women terminate their abusive relationships (Temple et al., 2010; Wathen, 2012). Indeed, in a study of 309 Canadian women, women of all ages and income levels remained in significantly worse mental and physical health than would be expected in the general population, even 7 years postseparation from an abusive partner (Ford-Gilboe et al., in press).

The effects of IPV also involve adverse social and economic outcomes that often pose negative impacts on individuals' and their families' mental health. Most people who experience violence consider the social impact of IPV a serious concern for their families. The commonly reported social effects of IPV are social isolation, exclusion from community activities due to stigma, child neglect, negative interactions among children, family and community members (Eriksson & Mazerolle, 2015; Roman & Frantz, 2013), lack of community support in the time of need, fragile family relationships, poor parental role modeling, lack of economic stability, and potential loss of economic resources (Kohli et al., 2015).

Health Effects of Child Abuse

Child abuse is linked to various poor health outcomes including in the physical, psychological, and social domains (Banyard et al., 2017). The health consequences for each child vary and depend on factors such as the child's age, types of experiences, and family environment (Child Welfare Information Gateway, 2019).

In addition to the immediate physical consequences of physical abuse such as bruises, cuts, broken bones, head injury, and infections (Jud & Trocmé, 2012), there is strong evidence suggesting long-term physical harm as a result of child maltreatment. A Canadian community health survey of 23,395 adults found a strong association between abuse in childhood and the severe physical health effects in adulthood such as arthritis, back problems, high blood pressure, headaches, chronic respiratory infections, cancer, stroke, bowel issues, and chronic fatigue (Afifi et al., 2016). Ongoing and cumulative childhood trauma can also result in severe and permanent disabilities due to traumatic brain injury (Bennett et al., 2016; Paek & Kwon, 2020). Findings from the Canadian Incidence Study (CIS) of Reported Child Abuse and Neglect—2008 also indicated an increased odds of child functional impairment as a result of child maltreatment (Cheung et al., 2020). Analysis of the CIS also showed that 6% ($n = 979$) of children required medical treatment and the severity of harm included death (Jud & Trocmé, 2012).

Sequential traumatic experiences in childhood can become significant risk factors for developing various forms of psychiatric conditions in later life (Afifi et al., 2014; Canadian Mental Health Association-BC Division, 2013). According to the Ontario Incidence Study of Reported Child Abuse and Neglect (OIS) conducted in 2018, 36% (13,559) of child abuse investigations indicated evidence of psychological harm (Fallon et al., 2020). Research shows that people who experience childhood abuse may have a higher risk of developing chronic stress (Lanius et al., 2017), depression (Negele et al., 2015), anxiety, PTSD (Boughner & Frewen, 2016), eating disorders (Caslini et al., 2016), and personality disorders (Kaplan et al., 2016; Mainali et al., 2020). Findings from a Canadian population survey reported 80% of attempted suicides were linked to a history of child abuse (Martin et al., 2016). Studies also show a serious risk and fear of revictimization among people who have experienced the trauma of sexual abuse (Das & Otis, 2016; Lanius et al., 2017; Lau & Kristensen, 2010).

Childhood trauma can have lifelong and intergenerational impacts (Buss et al., 2017; Van Wert et al., 2019). A prospective study conducted with 1,507 mothers concluded that children whose mothers had experienced childhood trauma showed more significant emotional challenges than children whose mothers had not (Giallo et al., 2020). Another study of 6,935 low-income children showed a positive association between child abuse and the risk of later perpetration (Ben-David et al., 2015). A number of epidemiological studies have shown that childhood abuse may also increase the risk of experiencing behavioral issues and substance abuse in adulthood (Cross et al., 2015; Farnia et al., 2020). Findings from a nationally representative Canadian survey of mental health conducted on 21,554 participants revealed higher odds of drug use among people with childhood abuse history (Fuller-Thomson et al., 2016). Research also demonstrates a strong association among PTSD, depression, and substance abuse (Machisa et al., 2017).

The association between childhood sexual abuse and engaging in delinquent behavior in later life has been documented. The risk of developing antisocial traits and criminal behavior is observed higher in children with experiences of abuse and neglect (Connolly, 2020; National Institute of Justice, 2017). Data from longitudinal studies of child abuse reported that the risk of violent and antisocial behavior is 1.7 times higher in people who were subjected to child sexual abuse than those who were not (Kozak et al., 2018). These relationships to violent and antisocial behavior suggest that child abuse also has community-level consequences (Rivara et al., 2019).

Health Effects of Elder Abuse

Similar to the health effects of abuse on other populations, various detrimental health effects of elder abuse have been reported in physical, psychological, and social spheres. A systematic review by Yunus and colleagues (2019) documented a wide range of morbidity outcomes related to elder abuse including physical problems such as chronic pain, headache, incontinence, allergy, gastrointestinal and digestive problems, sleeping problems, metabolic syndrome and disability, and psychological issues such as symptoms of depression and anxiety, psychological distress, stress, suicidal ideations and attempts, somatic symptoms, and social isolation. This review also highlighted higher risks of death as an emerging outcome of elder abuse. Another review of 63 papers identified additional physical impacts including bruises, cuts, malnutrition, and poor hygiene (Bhagat & Htwe, 2018).

Research indicates that elder abuse is more often financial than physical (National Initiative for The Care of The Elderly, 2016; Wong & Waite, 2017) and contributes to psychological and social deterioration for older people. In one study, older adults who reported abuse/neglect showed a higher proportion of depression (ranging from 28% to 37%) compared to those without any reported abuse history (18% to 20%) (Roepke-Buehler et al., 2015). The effects of elder abuse and neglect have been associated with other age-related vulnerabilities and dependence, such as problems with physical and mental health, serious financial and social dependence, substance use problems, and challenging relationships with caregivers (Storey, 2020). Strong empirical evidence indicates that preexisting depression (Santos et al., 2017; Sirey et al., 2015) and reduced cognitive functioning (e.g., dementia, confusion, reduced memory, etc.) in older adults are strong predictors of developing further psychological and emotional distress as a result of abuse (Friedman et al., 2017; Yan et al., 2015).

The Nursing Role: Recognizing and Responding to Abuse

Nurses can play a vital role in providing care to people who are impacted by trauma and violence. Nurses are likely to be the first contact for patients with history of abuse in various healthcare settings, for example,

emergency departments, medical–surgical units, psychiatric units, paediatric units, maternity care, long-term care, nursing homes, and primary healthcare settings. Research shows that women who experience IPV access health care more frequently than women with no history of abuse (Alvarez et al., 2016; Ansara & Hindin, 2010). A study of 6 clinics in Canada and 1 in United States observed that 1 in 3 women presented to the emergency department with trauma associated with IPV, and 1 in 6 women who presented to fracture clinics had experiences of IPV in the previous 12 months (EDUCATE Investigators, 2018). Nurses can create a safe environment by actively demonstrating a nonjudgmental stance, understanding that people who have a history of abuse want to be heard but face multiple challenges when accessing health care, including fear of being negatively judged. For example, a study conducted with women from rural and northern Canada described numerous barriers to accessing resources including poverty, distance or transportation issues, language barriers, cultural variances, feelings of shame and embarrassment, and lack of measures to insure confidentiality (Zorn et al., 2017). In these circumstances, women expect their HCPs to have knowledge, open mindedness, and patience while talking with them (Usta et al., 2012). Research has identified barriers that men with the history of IPV face while seeking professional help, such as gender stereotypes, risks to their masculinity, inadequate and biased responses by professionals, and subsequent feelings of dejection, lack of trust, and confidentiality concerns (Huntley et al., 2019; Machado et al., 2017).

Given the burden of traumatic experiences and their profound consequences on individuals, families, communities, and society, it is crucial for nurses and all HCPs to be well equipped with skills required to provide safe and effective care. Research suggests that despite being an important area of care, many HCPs lack understanding and skills in dealing with people who are experiencing on-going abuse or have previous experiences of abuse (Gutmanis et al., 2007; Kassam-Adams et al., 2015). A Canadian study, conducted with primary HCPs working with rural First Nations women, reported factors such as a lack of formal training, inadequate services for IPV, limited understanding of the context of Indigenous People's lives, and the challenges of maintaining confidentiality in small communities as key underlying reasons for their lack of preparedness to deal with IPV (Rizkalla et al., 2020). Further, organizational factors such as a lack of private space in healthcare settings, the high workload of HCPs, and lack of information about services contribute to inadequate responses toward abuse (Violence Evidence Guidance Action, n.d.). Evidence suggests that training HCPs to support patients with traumatic experiences can improve provider's confidence (Levine et al., 2020) and improve patient outcomes (Brown et al., 2013; Burton & Carlyle, 2015).

In order to provide a fair and appropriate care to all gender identities, guidelines by the Canadian Task Force on Preventive Health Care (2013) and the WHO (2013b) recommend taking measures based on the principles of trauma- and violence-informed care. When patients experience trauma- and violence-informed care, they feel more confident in the care they receive and better able to manage their own health, which predicts better health outcomes, including lower trauma symptoms, lower depressive symptoms, less disabling pain, and better quality of life (Ford-Gilboe et al., 2018). See also Chapter 18.

From Screening to Trauma and Violence Informed Care

Whereas the early literature on responding to violence advocated universal screening for violence (in which every person was asked about violence in every healthcare encounter), evidence has shown that such screening leads to improved recognition of such histories but does not lead to increased referrals or better outcomes (MacMillan et al., 2009; O'Doherty et al., 2015; Wathen et al., 2013, 2016). Currently, the WHO does not recommend universal screening, but rather recommends "case finding" in settings where a high prevalence of histories of violence are to be expected, such as substance use settings, mental health settings, and maternity care (García-Moreno et al., 2015; WHO, 2014), wherein HCPs are alert for and inquire about histories of abuse. However, given the high prevalence of violence, trauma- and violence-informed care is recommended *throughout* health care across the lifespan.

Trauma- and violence-informed care (TVIC) is an approach that extends the principles of trauma-informed care to ensure it encompasses experiences of violence and acknowledges the traumatic effects of abuse on individuals with a focus on their safety and recovery (Cleary & Hungerford, 2015; Covington, 2008; Elliot et al., 2005; Kassam-Adams et al., 2015). TVIC recognizes both interpersonal and structural forms of violence as causes of trauma; it helps care providers consider both the health effects of current experiences of abuse and the enduring effects of past experiences of abuse (Government of Canada, 2018; Ponic et al., 2016). Importantly, TVIC does not require that care providers know a person's history; rather, providers strive to make care safe for *all* persons by assuming that anyone might have such a history, or be currently experiencing abuse. The goal is a safe environment, not disclosure.

To take a TVIC approach, practice should be rooted in the following principles (Ponic et al., 2016).

1. Understand trauma, violence, and its impact on people's lives and behavior.
- Assume anyone may have a history of or be experiencing abuse.
- Believe patients' reported experiences.
- Actively listen and reflect.
- Express genuineness and concern.

- Recognize patients' strengths.

2. Create emotionally and physically safe environments for all clients and providers.
- Be nonjudgmental, express respect and acceptance
- Allow patients to express their feelings freely.
- Make observations and acknowledge nonverbal expressions.
- Provide clear and realistic information about services.
- Respond by offering comfort and support.

3. Foster opportunities for choice, collaboration, and connection.
- Support patients to make choices for their treatment/services.
- Take a collaborative approach.
- Encourage open communication without being judgmental.
- Reflect and summarize to ensure that you have heard correctly.

4. Use a strength-based and capacity building approach to support clients.
- Help people identify their strengths.
- Recognize the impact of their life circumstances and conditions.
- Help people realize that their reactions and emotions are normal.

KEY CONCEPT

Trauma- and violence-informed care is an approach to care that is grounded in an understanding of the impact of trauma and violence on individuals' lives and behaviours, situated in physically and emotionally safe environments, and offers strengths-based, capacity-building support that fosters coping and resilience.

Using a TVIC approach will often create a sufficiently safe environment for people to disclose their experiences; thus, nurses must develop confidence in responding to disclosures and providing care to people with known histories of abuse.

Nursing Assessment: Physical Examination and History Taking

Although universal screening for IPV is not justified by available evidence (O'Doherty et al., 2015; Wathen et al., 2016), an awareness of the prevalence of abuse and attentiveness in observing and listening with respectful direct questioning are warranted in all settings. All care, including assessment, should be based on the TVIC principles. When assessing patients with a history of IPV, child abuse, or elder abuse, and if the patient consents, a thorough head to toe assessment is indicated if the abuse is current or ongoing. Remembering that most abuse is not physical abuse, nurses should be aware of the following physical and clinical signs (Beach et al., 2016; Christian & Committee on Child Abuse and Neglect, 2015).

- Bruising
- Lacerations and injuries—look for injuries in perineal and genital areas in children and older people. There is a mnemonic called "TEN4" meaning look for signs of abuse on Torso, Ear, Neck and in children less than 4 years or 4 months of age (Gonzalez et al., 2020)
- Signs of child neglect (e.g., poor hygiene and health, malnourishment, developmental differences)
- Fractures
- Repeated injuries
- Pain (joint, muscle, and pelvic pain)

Many people who experience abuse present with signs of emotional and psychological disturbances (Mason et al., 2017). Nurses should be aware of the following signs:

- Fear
- Stress and anxiety
- Feelings of worthlessness or guilt
- Thoughts and/or attempts of suicide
- Nervous and ashamed
- Anger
- Hyperarousal
- Avoidance

Along with the physical examination, brief history taking is an important tool for assessment. Nurses should obtain a history from patients with care to limit harm. To mitigate the risk of retraumatization, avoid repeated history taking and follow the lead of the person in determining how much they wish to say. Effective therapeutic communication is the basis for comprehensive assessment and case finding for IPV. For example, in a Canadian study of nurse home visiting, researchers found that a combination of questions on parenting, safety, or relationships was an effective approach to engaging women who may be experiencing IPV (Jack et al., 2016).

In the case of sexual assault, whether within an intimate partner relationship or not, collection of forensic evidence is required if legal action will be taken. An expert trained nurse or physician is required to perform such assessment, and many healthcare settings have access to sexual assault teams, usually composed of a Sexual Assault Nurse Examiner (SANE) and a support/advocate person. Nurses in all settings should know the availability of and referral pathway to such services.

In case of child abuse, it is important to pay attention to the length of questions and level of language used. The WHO's guidelines (2019) for HCPs recommend asking open-ended questions with age-appropriate language. It is often effective to invite children to express their answers through different strategies such as drawing, writing, or using models. Children should

be interviewed separately in order to maintain their confidentiality and promote safety; however, offering the option of the support of an adult caregiver can be considered if it is clear that the caregiver is not a perpetrator of abuse toward that child.

If elder maltreatment or abuse is suspected, nurses should draw on their knowledge of normal aging and common health issues in older adults so they can differentiate between abuse and other issues (Fulmer et al., 2011). Nurses need to pay attention to indications that elders are being asked to do things against their will, such as signing documents, and conflicting statements between patients and their caregivers (Wang et al., 2015), taking care not to assume such discrepancies are due to compromised mental acuity in the elder.

Caring for People Who Experience Abuse: Taking a Strengths-Based Approach

Building on a TVIC approach, therapeutic responses to people experiencing abuse require a strengths-based approach (SBA). A strengths-based approach is required when a history of abuse is known or disclosed. This approach is based on a philosophy of working with individuals', families', and communities' strengths and positive attributes (Scerra, 2011), while concentrating on individuals' resilience, abilities, potentials, and resources (Grant & Cadell, 2009). The goal of strengths-based interventions is to support empowerment, including confidence and trust in one's own choices and abilities (Hammond, 2010). Evidence supports the use of SBA for cultivating hope and advancing self-determination in people who experience abuse (Chandhok & Anand, 2020). A study conducted in Ontario discovered hope, sense of self-esteem, and wish for a better life as key strengths drawn from women's experiences (Janes & Rodger, 2012).

Social support has been found to be a significant contributor to the strength of women who have experienced abuse (Machisa et al., 2018; Ogbe et al., 2020). A SBA acknowledges the pain of abusive experiences and helps people to focus on identifying their strengths and abilities (Anand, 2020). This requires establishing genuine rapport, using nonjudgmental communication, listening actively, offering support, and helping people to take control over their lives (Anand, 2017; Saleebey, 2013). A number of concepts such as empowerment, community connectedness, resilience, and acknowledgement and mobilization of internal and external resources are drawn upon to support achieving the desired outcomes by people who experience abuse-related trauma (Saleebey, 2013). The SBA has been found effective in providing care to those experiencing child abuse (Merdian et al., 2017) and elder abuse (Registered Nurses' Association of Ontario, 2014).

A **strengths-based approach** to nursing care, unlike a deficit approach that focuses on an individual's problems and health barriers, concentrates on an individual's assets, such as personal qualities (e.g., flexibility, experience, humour), interpersonal assets (e.g., family, support group membership), and external resources (e.g., local healthcare institute, visiting nurse services, accommodating employer).

According to the WHO's guidelines (2014), "first-line support" is the most important aspect of care for people who experience violence. This support focuses on four main areas (psychological needs, immediate physical needs, safety, and ongoing support) that require critical attention of nurses and other HCPs. WHO (2014) advises using the "LIVES" approach (Listen, Inquire, Validate, Enhance safety, and Support) to provide first-line care to people with a known history of abuse or who disclose (Fig. 34.3).

Listen

Active listening is a key to first-line support and a foundation to emotional recovery. Nurses should use nonjudgmental and compassionate listening without forcing individuals to talk. Active listening begins with recognition by nurses of their own understanding, experiences, values, and prejudices about abuse (Askew, 2016; Rob-

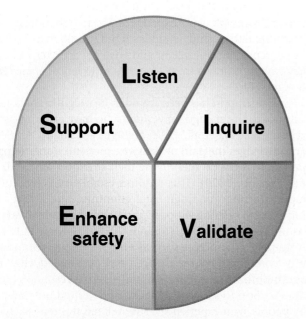

Figure 34.3 "LIVES" approach to provide first-line support to people experiencing abuse. World Health Organization (2014). Health care for women subjected to intimate partner violence or sexual violence. A clinical handbook, p.14. https://www.who.int/reproductivehealth/publications/violence/vaw-clinical-handbook/en/ Adapted with permission.

erts et al., 2019). Effective listening requires empathy as key to building trust, which involves paying attention to what patients have not said—that is, recognizing the nonverbal expressions and feelings behind their words (Abrahams, 2017). Nurses need to ask themselves: Am I actively listening to my patients? According to WHO (2014), active listening includes the following:

- Being calm and gentle—do not rush patients or force them to talk.
- Having eye-level communication that shows that you are listening and paying attention.
- Paying attention to verbal and nonverbal expression.
- Genuinely demonstrating that you understand the person's feelings (e.g., saying things such as "that must have been difficult…").
- Periodically offering assistance without taking control (e.g., saying: "How can I help you?").
- Providing them time to think and reflect—use silence generously while maintaining a stance of active listening. Abuse experiences are difficult to talk about, and people often assume they are too painful for providers to listen to.

Since many individuals accessing healthcare services will have a history of abuse, a sound knowledge regarding abuse, its related factors, and health effects is essential for all nurses practicing in any clinical setting or specialty.

Inquire

Inquiring about individuals' concerns using TVIC approach is therapeutic and can allow nurses to identify physical, psychological, and safety needs of people experiencing abuse (Bradbury-Jones et al., 2017). Inquiring can help patients to identify and recognize their own needs and ability to control their lives (Ford-Gilboe et al., 2011). According to the WHO (2014) guidelines, the following techniques and principles should be applied for safe inquiring:

- Invite patients to speak by asking: "What would you like to talk about?", "Can you tell me more about it?" Allow patients to choose whether they want to disclose and follow the lead of their communication.
- Use open-ended questions.
- Use reflective statements—"you seem concerned that…"
- Ask for clarification if needed—"Can you explain that…?"
- Help patients to share their needs and concerns— "Is there anything that you are worried about?," "It sounds like you are worried about…"
- Summarize what patients have shared—"you seem to be saying that…"
- Allow patients to make corrections if needed by asking—"does that sound correct?"
- Avoid asking "why" questions. Doing so may sound blaming and accusatory.

Validate

Validation is essential to offering support. Validation depends upon identification and acknowledgement of abuse as a problem underlying many health concerns (García-Moreno et al., 2015). HCPs should recognize that people experiencing abuse may experience multiple emotions including despair, hopelessness, guilt, shame, fear, loss of control, anxiety, and anger (Coyle et al., 2014; WHO, 2014). Validation means recognizing, understanding, and believing patients' feelings and concerns and affirming the person's worth (Hall, 2012). One study showed that women's trust with their HCPS was improved when they felt their HCPs cared about their feelings and understood their issues (Bacchus et al., 2016). According to WHO's guidelines (2014), the following are important principles to use in responding to people disclosing a history of abuse:

- Tell patients—"it is not your fault…," "it is okay to talk about it…"
- Recognize and accept your own feelings—it is okay to show patients that you are feeling distressed about what had happened.
- Acknowledge patients' feelings—"that must have been so painful"
- Offer help when resources are available.
- Affirm that the person's life is important and of value and that no one deserves to be abused.

Enhance Safety

Enhancing safety is an essential component of care for people who experience any form of abuse. It is important for nurses to help patients acknowledge that they do not have control over violence and their safety is foremost. A study conducted with women who experienced IPV reported that most women consider their children's basic needs and keeping their families united ahead of their own safety (Ivany et al., 2018). Another Canadian study reported that only one in five women who experience IPV access services for safety planning (Barrett & Pierre, 2011). Nurses should understand that planning for safety is a continual, long-term process and not a one-time event.

Nurses must ascertain whether patients are at immediate risk of harm, including for homicide, suicide, or other trauma (Campbell et al., 2009). Tools, including suicide assessment and danger assessment tools (Campbell et al., 2009; Danger Assessment, 2020), are available to assess risk for those experiencing abuse. Such assessments must be conducted in a private space. Explaining the reason for such assessments will help reduce fear and anxiety. People can be supported to assess their own situation and risks. For example, a Canadian study conducted by Ford-Gilboe et al. (2020) found that women experiencing abuse benefitted from an online health and safety resource that included such assessments (see Box 34.1).

BOX 34.1 Research for Best Practice

STUDY TITLE: LONGITUDINAL IMPACTS OF AN ONLINE SAFETY AND HEALTH INTERVENTION FOR WOMEN EXPERIENCING INTIMATE PARTNER VIOLENCE: RANDOMIZED CONTROLLED TRIAL

Ford-Gilboe, M., Varcoe, C., Scott-Storey, K., Perrin, N., Wuest, J., Wathen, C. N., Case, J., & Glass, N. (2020). Longitudinal impacts of an online safety and health intervention for women experiencing intimate partner violence: Randomized controlled trial. *BMC Public Health, 20,* 260. https://doi.org/10.1186/s12889-020-8152-8

Purpose: The objective of this study was to test the effectiveness of iCAN, an interactive, tailored, online safety, and health intervention on mental health and safety outcomes of Canadian women experiencing IPV.

Method: In a double blind randomized controlled trial, 462 Canadian adult women who experienced recent IPV were randomly assigned to receive either a tailored, interactive online safety and health intervention (iCAN Plan 4 Safety) or a static, nontailored version of this tool.

Findings: Women in both tailored and nontailored groups improved over time on primary outcomes of depression and PTSD and on all secondary outcomes

(helpfulness of safety actions, confidence in safety planning, mastery, social support, experiences of coercive control, and decisional conflict). Women in both groups reported high levels of benefit, safety, and accessibility of the online interventions, with low risk of harm, although those completing the tailored intervention were more positive about fit and helpfulness. The tailored intervention had greater positive effects for 4 groups of women, those with children under 18 living at home; reporting more severe violence; living in medium-sized and large urban centres; and not living with a partner, showing the importance of attending to diverse contexts and needs.

Implications for Nursing: The study findings support the importance of contextually relevant online health interventions for better mental health outcomes of Canadian women who experience IPV. iCAN intervention has shown potential to complement the existing resources and can be integrated in healthcare settings for positive health and safety outcomes of Canadian women experiencing IPV.

Nurses should help patients to make careful safety plans, especially when they think about leaving abusive partners, given that risk of further violence increases when doing so. For women with children, planning must include insuring children's safety. According to the WHO (2014) guidelines, a safety plan includes the following elements:

- Safe place: "where could you go, if you need to leave your home?"
- Transport: "how will you get there?"
- Children: "how will you insure your children's safety...?"
- Financial support: "how can you access money to support you and your children?"
- Other support: "can you tell someone you trust about the violence so they can help you in emergency?"

In the case of child abuse, safety planning will be most helpful to children if HCPs consider the individual needs of children, their age and developmental stage, physical and mental health status, and relationship with parents and guardians (Ministry of Justice, 2013).

Support

The degree of support provided to people with history of abuse varies with nurses' roles and clinical settings. People who experience abuse have needs beyond immediate health and safety needs, including shelter, financial assistance, legal aid, mental health care, and child care support. While nurses in settings such as Emergency Departments or primary care clinics will not be able to provide ongoing support, they can help people identify their needs and refer them to appropriate resources and support services. WHO (2014) endorses the following approaches to support:

- Explore what matters most to the person right now. What help they would like to have the most?
- Provide time to identify their needs.
- Support the person to consider their options.
- Explore their support systems.

- Help them identify any trusted person in their families or neighborhood.
- Connect them with other resources or support services available in the community.

Support may include referral for treatment of multiple psychological symptoms caused by trauma related to abuse. Several therapeutic approaches including cognitive behavioral therapy (CBT), interpersonal psychotherapy (IPT), and psychopharmacologic treatment have been found effective in treating depression and PTSD in patients with the history of abuse (Duberstein et al., 2018; Markowitz et al., 2017; Strangio et al., 2017). See Chapters 9 and 14 for further information. A meta-analysis examining the effects of psychotherapies on women with the history of childhood sexual abuse noted reductions in symptoms of depression and PTSD (Lu et al., 2020). These therapies have also showed positive outcomes for men with a history of childhood sexual abuse (O'Cleirigh et al., 2019). Nurses should be aware of these modalities, their availability, and how to refer people to them in their settings.

Documentation

Careful and accurate documentation of findings related to IPV, child, and elder abuse is a key responsibility of nurses. All observations made during physical examination and history taking should be documented including day and time of examination, location, number, and types of injuries using a body chart or map. Documentation can include taking photographs of injuries with patients' permission. Patients' comments should be quoted clearly and exactly. Documenting discrepancies between patients' statements and their caregivers or family members is also important (WHO, 2019). Nurses should avoid drawing conclusions based on situations, where there is no and/or lack of clear data to support the occurrence or past history of abuse (Lentz, 2011). When documenting the history and findings of abuse, it is important for nurses to understand the sensitivity of confidentiality and be vigilant about what and where to write the notes (WHO, 2014).

🍁 Summary of Key Points

- Abuse in any form against any person of any gender identity and at any developmental stage is a serious concern that requires awareness and a safe response by nurses and other healthcare providers.
- Interpersonal forms of violence and abuse are often embedded within structural inequities (e.g., poverty) that shape people's circumstances, experiences, and behavior (e.g., poverty stigma creating barriers to care access).
- Approaches to supporting the mental health of people who experience abuse should be based on

understanding the wider patterns of both interpersonal and structural violence.
- Interpersonal violence, including IPV, child abuse, and elder abuse, can have serious consequences on individuals' health and wellbeing.
- Nurses can play a key role in contributing to the wellbeing of people who have experienced abuse.

Nurses' therapeutic responses should be based on the principles of trauma and violence informed care so they can understand the prevalence of abuse, acknowledge the traumatic effects of abuse on individuals, and focus on their safety and recovery without retraumatizing them.

Thinking Challenges

1. Revisit the case from early in the chapter of Sam, the 47-year-old armed forces veteran in a forensic psychiatric setting as a consequence of breaching probation when he knifed the family dog. Describe what you and the team might explore in order to develop a strengths-based approach to helping Sam.
2. Contact with healthcare services can be an important opportunity for a person who is at risk for or is experiencing abuse. The communication between the person and a healthcare practitioner (HCP) at this time can be a significant factor in help seeking. Identify and describe five key points that can guide you as a HCP in these situations.
3. Outline what must be documented when assessing an individual in relation to interpersonal violence and/or abuse.

> Visit thePoint to view suggested responses.
> Go to thePoint.lww.com/activate and use the activation code found in the front of this text to unlock answers to the "Thinking Challenges" and other online resources.

 Web Links

https://cnpea.ca/en/ The Canadian Network for the Prevention of Elder Abuse provides information about issues related to abuse and neglect in later life, and advances policy development on issues related to the prevention of abuse in older adults across local, regional, provincial/territorial and, national levels.

https://www.redcross.ca/how-we-help/violence-bullying-and-abuse-prevention/educators/child-abuse-and-neglect-prevention The website of the Canadian Red Cross includes a section on violence, bullying, and abuse prevention resources, online courses, links to protective legislation, and information targeted to the work place, Indigenous Peoples, parents, youth, and organizations.

futureswithoutviolence.org For more than 30 years, FUTURE has provided a number of programs, policies, and campaigns to empower individuals and organizations working to end violence against women and children globally. Their vision is "a future without violence that provides education, safety, justice, and hope." Here, readers will find a number of excellent evidence-based resources, regarding children, youth, and teens; working with older adults; global violence prevention; and more. Readers can sign up for to be on their email list.

myplanapp.ca/en/ The free *myPlan Canada* app for those at risk or experiencing abuse can be found here. As noted on their website, "safety planning is the cornerstone of intimate partner violence interventions." Provincial services and supports are listed on their resources page. Nurses working with such individuals will find it helpful, as well.

https://rnao.ca/sites/rnao-ca/files/Booklet-RNAO-web.pdf The Registered Nurses Association of Ontario's pocket guide for *Preventing and Addressing Abuse and Neglect of Older Adults* is available at this site. Readers can find the full clinical best practice guideline *Preventing and Addressing Abuse and Neglect of Older Adults: Person-Centred, Collaborative, System-Wide Approaches* at https://rnao.ca/sites/rnao-ca/files/Preventing_Abuse_and_Neglect_of_Older_Adults_English_WEB.pdf Also of interest, as part of *Addressing abuse of older adults—RNAO Initiative*, readers will find a Best Practice Success Kit, compete with learning video, discussion guides, strategies to help nurses and other healthcare providers address abuse and neglect in older adults. For more information, see https://rnao.ca/bpg/initiatives/abuse-and-neglect-older-adults-pan-canadian-best-practice-guideline-initiative .

who.int/reproductivehealth/publications/violence/global-plan-of-action/en/ At this site is the WHO's *Global plan of action to strengthen the role of the health system within a national multisectoral response to address interpersonal violence, in particular against women and girls, and against children* (2016).

https://www.canada.ca/en/public-health/services/health-promotion/stop-family-violence.html Stop Family Violence is a one-stop source of information on family violence, with links to supports, resources, and services throughout Canada.

References

Abrahams, H. (2017). Listen to me: A reflection on practice in qualitative interviewing. *Journal of Gender-Based Violence, 1*(2), 253–259. https://doi.org/10.1332/239868017X15090095938377

Afifi, T. O., MacMillan, H. L., Boyle, M., Cheung, K., Taillieu, T., Turner, S., & Sareen, J. (2016). Child abuse and physical health in adulthood. *Health Reports, 27*(3), 10. https://www150.statcan.gc.ca/n1/en/pub/82-003-x/2016003/article/14339-eng.pdf?st=xHjriJLL

Afifi, T. O., MacMillan, H. L., Boyle, M., Taillieu, T., Cheung, K., & Sareen, J. (2014). Child abuse and mental disorders in Canada. *Canadian Medical Association Journal, 186*(9), E324–E332. https://doi.org/10.1503/cmaj.131792

Alvarez, C., Fedock, G., Grace, K. T., & Campbell, J. (2016). Provider screening and counseling for intimate partner violence a systematic review of practices and influencing factors. *Trauma, Violence and Abuse, 18*(5), 479–495. https://doi.org/10.1177/1524838016637080

American Psychiatric Association. (2013). *Diagnostic and statistical manual of mental disorders* (5th ed.).

Anand, M. (2017). Battered conjugality: Dynamics of intimate partner violence and social work practice. *Journal of Social Work Education, Research and Action, 3*(3), 35–56.

Anand, M. (2020). *Gender and mental health: Combining theory and practice.* Springer Nature.

Ansara, D. L., & Hindin, M. J. (2010). Formal and informal help-seeking associated with women's and men's experiences of intimate partner violence in Canada. *Social Science & Medicine, 70*, 1011–1018. https://doi.org/10.1016/j.socscimed.2009.12.009

Askew, I. (2016). *Health workers: Listening when women need it most.* World Health Organization-Media Center. https://www.who.int/mediacentre/commentaries/2016/health-workers-women/en/

Bacchus, L. J., Bullock, L., Sharps, P., Burnett, C., Schminkey, D., Buller, A. M., & Campbell, J. (2016). 'Opening the door': A qualitative interpretive study of women's experiences of being asked about intimate partner violence and receiving an intervention during perinatal home visits in rural and urban settings in the USA. *Journal of Research in Nursing, 21*(5–6), 345–364. https://doi.org/10.1177/1744987116649634

Bacchus, L. J., Ranganathan, M., Watts, C., & Devries, K. (2018). Recent intimate partner violence against women and health: A systematic review and meta-analysis of cohort studies. *BMJ Open, 8*(7), e019995. https://doi.org/10.1136/bmjopen-2017-019995

Banyard, V., Hamby, S., & Grych, J. (2017). Health effects of adverse childhood events: Identifying promising protective factors at the intersection of mental and physical well-being. *Child Abuse & Neglect, 65*, 88–98. https://doi.org/10.1016/j.chiabu.2017.01.011

Bareis, N., & Mezuk, B. (2016). The relationship between childhood poverty, military service, and later life depression among men: Evidence from the Health and Retirement Study. *Journal of Affective Disorders, 206*, 1–7. https://doi.org/10.1016/j.jad.2016.07.018

Barrett, B. J., & Pierre, M. S. (2011). Variations in women's help seeking in response to intimate partner violence: Findings from a Canadian population-based study. *Violence Against Women, 17*(1), 47–70. https://doi.org/10.1177/1077801210394273

Beach, S., Carpenter, C., Rosen, T., Sharps, P., & Gelles, R. (2016). Screening and detection of elder abuse: Research opportunities and lessons learned from emergency geriatric care, intimate partner violence, and child abuse. *Journal of Elder Abuse & Neglect, 28*(4–5), 185–216. https://doi.org/10.1080/08946566.2016.1229241

Ben-David, V., Jonson-Reid, M., Drake, B., & Kohl, P. L. (2015). The association between childhood maltreatment experiences and the onset of maltreatment perpetration in young adulthood controlling for proximal and distal risk factors. *Child Abuse & Neglect, 46*, 132–141. https://doi.org/10.1016/j.chiabu.2015.01.013

Bennett, T. D., Dixon, R. R., Kartchner, C., DeWitt, P. E., Sierra, Y., Ladell, D., Kempe, A., Runyan, D. K., Dean, J. M., & Keenan, H. T. (2016). Functional status scale in children with traumatic brain injury: A prospective cohort study. *Pediatric Critical Care Medicine: A Journal of the Society of Critical Care Medicine and the World Federation of Pediatric Intensive and Critical Care Societies, 17*(12), 1147. https://doi.org/10.1097/PCC.0000000000000934

Bhagat, V., & Htwe, K. (2018). A literature review of findings in physical and emotional abuse in elderly. *Research Journal of Pharmacy and Technology, 11*(10), 4731–4738. https://doi.org/10.5958/0974-360X.2018.00862.4

Black, M. C., Basile, K. C., Breiding, M. J., Smith, S. G., Walters, M. L., Merrick, M. T., Chen, J., & Stevens, M. R. (2011). *National intimate partner and sexual violence survey: 2010 summary report*. Centers for Disease Control and Prevention. https://www.cdc.gov/violenceprevention/pdf/nisvs_report2010-a.pdf

Boughner, E., & Frewen, P. (2016). Gender differences in perceived causal relations between trauma-related symptoms and substance use disorders in online and outpatient samples. *Traumatology, 22*(4), 288–298. https://doi.org/10.1037/trm0000071

Bradbury-Jones, C., Clark, M., & Taylor, J. (2017). Abused women's experiences of a primary care identification and referral intervention: A case study analysis. *Journal of Advanced Nursing, 73*(12), 3189–3199. https://doi.org/10.1111/jan.13250

Bronfenbrenner, U. (1979). *The ecology of human development*. Harvard University Press.

Brown, V. B., Harris, M., & Fallot, R. (2013). Moving toward trauma-informed practice in addiction treatment: A collaborative model of agency assessment. *Journal of Psychoactive Drugs, 45*(5), 386–393. https://doi.org/10.1080/02791072.2013.844381

Brownridge, D. A. (2008). Understanding the elevated risk of partner violence against Aboriginal women: A comparison of two nationally representative surveys of Canada. *Journal of Family Violence, 23*(5), 353–367. https://doi.org/10.1007/s10896-008-9160-0

Brownridge, D. A., Ristock, J., & Hiebert-Murphy, D. (2008). The high risk of IPV against Canadian women with disabilities. *Medical Science Monitor, 14*(5), PH27-32. http://search.ebscohost.com/login.aspx?direct=true&db=flh&AN=18443559&site=ehost-live

Burczycka, M., & Conroy, S. (2017). *Family violence in Canada: A statistical profile, 2015*. Statistics Canada. https://www150.statcan.gc.ca/n1/en/pub/85-002-x/2017001/article/14698-eng.pdf?st=Q4Ws1nqD

Burton, C. W., & Carlyle, K. E. (2015). Screening and intervening: Evaluating a training program on intimate partner violence and reproductive coercion for family planning and home visiting providers. *Family & Community Health, 38*(3), 227–239. https://doi.org/10.1097/fch.0000000000000076

Buss, C., Entringer, S., Moog, N. K., Toepfer, P., Fair, D. A., Simhan, H. N., Heim, C. M., & Wadhwa, P. D. (2017). Intergenerational transmission of maternal childhood maltreatment exposure: Implications for fetal brain development. *Journal of the American Academy of Child & Adolescent Psychiatry, 56*(5), 373–382. https://doi.org/10.1016/j.jaac.2017.03.001

Campbell, J. C., Anderson, J. C., McFadgion, A., Gill, J., Zink, E., Patch, M., Callwood, G., & Campbell, D. (2018). The effects of intimate partner violence and probable traumatic brain injury on central nervous system symptoms. *Journal of Women's Health, 27*(6), 761–767. https://doi.org/10.1089/jwh.2016.6311

Campbell, J., Webster, D., & Glass, N. (2009). The danger assessment: Validation of a lethality risk assessment instrument for intimate partner femicide. *Journal of Interpersonal Violence, 24*(4), 653–674. https://doi.org/10.1177/0886260508317180

Canadian Institute for Health Information. (2017). *Infographic: Canada's seniors population outlook: Uncharted territory*. https://www.cihi.ca/en/infographic-canadas-seniors-population-outlook-uncharted-territory#:~:text=Over%20the%20next%2020%20years,sits%20at%20about%206.2%20million

Canadian Mental Health Association-BC Division. (2013). *Childhood sexual abuse: A mental health issue*. https://www.heretohelp.bc.ca/infosheet/childhood-sexual-abuse-a-mental-health-issue

Canadian Task Force on Preventive Health Care. (2013). *Guideline: Screening for intimate partner violence and abuse of elderly and vulnerable adults: U.S. preventive services task force recommendation statement*. https://canadiantaskforce.ca/wp-content/uploads/2016/05/2013-domestic-abuse-en.pdf

Cardeli, E., Bloom, M., Gillespie, S., Zayed, T., & Ellis, B. H. (2019). Exploring the social-ecological factors that mobilize children into violence. *Terrorism and Political Violence*, 1–23. https://doi.org/10.1080/09546553.2019.1701444

Caslini, M., Bartoli, F., Crocamo, C., Dakanalis, A., Clerici, M., & Carrà, G. (2016). Disentangling the association between child abuse and eating disorders: A systematic review and meta-analysis. *Psychosomatic Medicine, 78*(1), 79–90. https://doi.org/10.1097/PSY.0000000000000233

Centers for Disease Control and Prevention. (2022). *The social-ecological model: A framework for prevention*. https://www.cdc.gov/violenceprevention/about/social-ecologicalmodel.html

Chandan, J. S., Thomas, T., Bradbury-Jones, C., Taylor, J., Bandyopadhyay, S., & Nirantharakumar, K. (2020). Risk of cardiometabolic disease and all-cause mortality in female survivors of domestic abuse. *Journal of the American Heart Association, 9*(4), e014580. https://doi.org/10.1161/JAHA.119.014580

Chandhok, G., & Anand, M. (2020). Practising strength-based approach with women survivors of domestic violence. In M. Anand (Ed.), *Gender and mental health* (pp. 237–249). Springer, Singapore. https://doi.org/10.1007/978-981-15-5393-6_16

Cheung, K., Taillieu, T., Tonmyr, L., Sareen, J., & Afifi, T. O. (2020). Previous reports of child maltreatment from the Canadian Incidence Study (CIS) 2008 of reported child abuse and neglect: An examination of recurrent substantiation and functional impairment. *Children and Youth Services Review, 108*, 104507. https://doi.org/10.1016/j.childyouth.2019.104507

Child Welfare Information Gateway. (2019). *Long-term consequences of child abuse and neglect*. https://www.childwelfare.gov/pubPDFs/long_term_consequences.pdf

Chisholm, C. A., Bullock, L., & Ferguson II, J. E. J. (2017). Intimate partner violence and pregnancy: Epidemiology and impact. *American Journal of Obstetrics and Gynecology, 217*(2), 141–144. https://doi.org/10.1016/j.ajog.2017.05.042

Chmielowska, M., & Fuhr, D. C. (2017). Intimate partner violence and mental ill health among global populations of Indigenous women: A systematic review. *Social Psychiatry Psychiatric Epidemiology, 52*(6), 689–704. https://doi.org/10.1007/s00127-017-1375-z

Christian, C. W., & Committee on Child Abuse and Neglect. (2015). The evaluation of suspected child physical abuse. *Pediatrics, 135*(5), e1337–e1354. https://doi.org/10.1542/peds.2015-0356

Cleary, M., & Hungerford, C. (2015). Trauma-informed care and the research literature: How can the mental health nurse take the lead to support women who have survived sexual assault. *Issues in Mental Health Nursing, 36*(5), 370–378. https://doi.org/10.3109/01612840.2015.1009661

Coker, A. L., Smith, P. H., McKeown, R. E., & King, M. J. (2000). Frequency and correlates of intimate partner violence by type: Physical, sexual, and psychological battering. *American Journal of Public Health, 90*, 553–559. https://doi.org/10.2105/ajph.90.4.553

Connolly, E. J. (2020). Further evaluating the relationship between adverse childhood experiences, antisocial behavior, and violent victimization: A sibling-comparison analysis. *Youth Violence and Juvenile Justice, 18*(1), 3–23. https://doi.org/10.1177/1541204019833145

Conroy, S. (2021). *Family violence in Canada: A statistical profile, 2019*. Statistics Canada no. 85-002-X. https://www150.statcan.gc.ca/n1/en/pub/85-002-x/2021001/article/00001-eng.pdf?st=-tRqUuMK

Cooper, A. M. (1986). Toward a limited definition of psychic trauma. In A. Rothstein (Ed.), *In the reconstruction of trauma: Its significance in clinical work* (pp. 41–56). International Universities Press.

Covington, S. S. (2008). Women and addiction: A trauma-informed approach. *Journal of Psychoactive Drugs, 5*, 377–385. https://doi.org/10.1080/02791072.2008.10400665

Coyle, E., Karatzias, T., Summers, A., & Power, M. (2014). Emotions and emotion regulation in survivors of childhood sexual abuse: The importance of "disgust" in traumatic stress and psychopathology. *European Journal of Psychotraumatology, 5*. https://doi.org/10.3402/ejpt.v5.23306

Cross, D., Crow, T., Powers, A., & Bradley, B. (2015). Childhood trauma, PTSD, and problematic alcohol and substance use in low-income, African-American men and women. *Child Abuse and Neglect, 44*, 26–35. https://doi.org/10.1016/j.chiabu.2015.01.007

Danger Assessment. (2020). https://www.dangerassessment.org

Daoud, N., Smylie, J., Urquia, M., Allan, B., & O'Campo, P. (2013). The contribution of socio-economic position to the excesses of violence and intimate partner violence among aboriginal versus non-Aboriginal Women in Canada. *Canadian Journal of Public Health, 104*(4), e278–e283. https://doi.org/10.17269/cjph.104.3724

Das, A., & Otis, N. (2016). Sexual contact in childhood, revictimization, and lifetime sexual and psychological outcomes. *Archives of Sexual Behavior, 45*(5), 1117–1131. https://doi.org/10.1007/s10508-015-0620-3

Davies, L., Ford-Gilboe, M., Willson, A., Varcoe, C., Wuest, J., Campbell, J., & Scott-Storey, K. (2015). Patterns of cumulative abuse among female survivors of intimate partner violence: Links to women's health and socioeconomic status. *Violence Against Women, 21*(1), 30–48. https://doi.org/10.1177/1077801214564076

Dekel, R., Shaked, O. Z., Ben-Porat, A., & Itzhaky, H. (2019). Posttraumatic stress disorder upon admission to shelters among female victims of domestic violence: An ecological model of trauma. *Violence and Victims, 34*(2), 329–345. https://doi.org/10.1891/0886-6708.VV-D-16-00200

Devries, K. M., Mak, J. Y., Bacchus, L. J., Child, J. C., Falder, G., Petzold, M., Astbury, J., & Watts, C. H. (2013). Intimate partner violence and incident depressive symptoms and suicide attempts: A systematic review of longitudinal studies. *PLoS Medicine, 10*(5), e1001439. https://doi.org/10.1371/journal.pmed.1001439

DiBiasio, E., Clark, M. A., & Rosenthal, S. R. (2014). Correlates of frequent mental distress among active and former military personnel. *Journal of Military & Veterans' Health, 22*(2), 4–13. http://ezproxy.library.ubc.ca/login?url=https://search.ebscohost.com/login.aspx?direct=true&db=aph&AN=101653702&site=ehost-live&scope=site

Dillon, G., Hussain, R., Loxton, D., & Rahman, S. (2013). Mental and physical health and intimate partner violence against women: A review of the literature. *International Journal of Family Medicine, 2013*, 313909. http://dx.doi.org/10.1155/2013/313909

Duberstein, P. R., Ward, E. A., Chaudron, L. H., He, H., Toth, S. L., Wang, W., Van Orden, K. A., Gamble, S. A., & Talbot, N. L. (2018). Effectiveness of interpersonal psychotherapy-trauma for depressed women with childhood abuse histories. *Journal of Consulting and Clinical Psychology, 86*(10), 868–878. https://doi.org/10.1037/ccp0000335

Eckstein, J. J. (2017). Intimate terrorism and situational couple violence: Classification variability across five methods to distinguish Johnson's violent relationship types. *Violence and Victims, 32*(6), 955–976. https://doi.org/10.1891/0886-6708.VV-D-16-00022

EDUCATE Investigators. (2018). Novel educational program improves readiness to manage intimate partner violence within the fracture clinic: A pretest–posttest study. *Canadian Medical Association Journal Open, 6*(4), E628–E636. https://doi.org/10.9778/cmajo.20180150

Einboden, R., Rudge, T., & Varcoe, C. (2013). Producing children in the 21st century: A critical discourse analysis of the science and techniques of monitoring early child development. *Health: An Interdisciplinary Journal for the Social Study of Health, Illness & Medicine, 17*(6), 549–566. https://doi.org/10.1177/1363459312472081

Elliot, D. E., Bjelajac, P., Fallot, R. D., Markoff, L. S., & Reed, B. G. (2005). Trauma-informed or trauma-denied: Principles and implementation of trauma-informed services for women. *Journal of Community Psychology, 33*(4), 461–477. https://doi.org/10.1002/jcop.20063

Eriksson, L., & Mazerolle, P. (2015). A cycle of violence? Examining family-of-origin violence, attitudes, and intimate partner violence perpetration. *Journal of Interpersonal Violence, 30*(6), 945–964. https://doi.org/10.1177/0886260514539759

Fallon, B., Filippelli, J., Lefebvre, R., Joh-Carnella, N., Trocmé, N., Black, T., MacLaurin, B., Helie, S., Morin, Y., Fluke, J., King, B., Esposito, T., Collin-Vézina, D., Allan, K., Houston, E., Harlick, M., Bonnie, N., Budau, K., Goodman, D., ... Stoddart, J. (2020). *Ontario incidence study of reported child abuse and neglect-2018 (OIS-2018)*. Child Welfare Research Portal. https://cwrp.ca/sites/default/files/publications/Ontario%20Incidence%20Study%20of%20Reported%20Child%20Abuse%20and%20Neglect%202018.pdf

Farnia, V., Salemi, S., Mordinazar, M., Khanegi, M., Tatari, F., Golshani, S., Jamshidi, P., & Alikhani, M. (2020). The effect of child-abuse on the behavioral problems in the children of the parents with substance use disorder: Presenting a model of structural equations. *Journal of Ethnicity in Substance Abuse*, 1–17. https://doi.org/10.1080/15332640.2020.1801547

Ford-Gilboe, M., Merritt-Gray, M., Varcoe, C., & Wuest, J. (2011). A theory-based primary health care intervention for women who have left abusive partners. *Advances in Nursing Science, 34*(3), 198–214. https://doi.org/10.1097/ANS.0b013e3182228cdc

Ford-Gilboe, M., Varcoe, C., Scott-Storey, K., Perrin, N., Wuest, J., Wathen, C. N., Case, J., & Glass, N. (2020). Longitudinal impacts of an online safety and health intervention for women experiencing intimate partner violence: Randomized controlled trial. *BMC Public Health, 20*, 260. https://doi.org/10.1186/s12889-020-8152-8

Ford-Gilboe, M., Varcoe, C., Wuest, J., Campbell, J., Pajot, M., Heslop, L., & Perrin, N. (in press). Trajectories of depression, post-traumatic stress and chronic pain among women who have separated from an abusive partner: A longitudinal analysis. *Journal of Interpersonal Violence*.

Ford-Gilboe, M., Wathen, C. N., Varcoe, C., Herbert, C., Jackson, B., Lavoie, J., Pauly, B. B., Perrin, N. A., Smye, V., Wallace, B., Wong, S. T., & Browne, A. J. (2018). How equity-oriented health care affects health: Key mechanisms and implications for primary health care practice and policy. *Millbank Quarterly, 96*(4), 635–671. https://doi.org/10.1111/1468-0009.12349

Ford-Gilboe, M., Wathen, C. N., Varcoe, C., MacMillan, H. L., Scott-Storey, K., Mantler, T., Hegarty, K., & Perrin, N. (2016). Development of a brief measure of intimate partner violence experiences: The composite abuse scale (Revised)—Short form (CASR-SF). *BMJ Open, 6*(12), 1–13. https://doi.org/10.1136/bmjopen-2016-012824

Friedman, L. S., Avila, S., Rizvi, T., Partida, R., & Friedman, D. (2017). Physical abuse of elderly adults: Victim characteristics and determinants of revictimization. *Journal of the American Geriatrics Society, 65*, 1420–1426. https://doi.org/10.1111/jgs.14794

Fuller-Thomson, E., Roane, J. L., & Brennenstuhl, S. (2016). Three types of adverse childhood experiences, and alcohol and drug dependence among adults: An investigation using population-based data. *Substance Use & Misuse, 51*(11), 1451–1461. https://doi.org/10.1080/10826084.2016.1181089

Fulmer, T., Sengstock, M. C., Blankenship, J., Caceres, B., Chandracomar, A., Ng, N., & Wopat, H. (2011). Elder mistreatment. In J. Humphreys & J. C. Campbell (Eds.), *Family violence and nursing practice* (pp. 347–366). New York, NY: Springer.

García-Moreno, C., Hegarty, K., Lucas d'Oliveira, A. F., Koziol-McLain, J., Colombini, M., & Feder, G. (2015). The health-systems response to violence against women. *Lancet, 385*(9977), 1567–1579. https://doi.org/10.1016/S0140-6736(14)61837-7

Gehring, D., & Knudson, G. (2005). Prevalence of childhood trauma in a clinical population of transsexual people. *International Journal of Transgenderism, 8*(1), 23–30. https://doi.org/10.1300/J485v08n01_03

Giallo, R., Gartland, D., Seymour, M., Conway, L., Mensah, F., Skinner, L., Fogarty, A., & Brown, S. (2020). Maternal childhood abuse and children's emotional-behavioral difficulties: Intergenerational transmission via birth outcomes and psychosocial health. *Journal of Family Psychology, 34*(1), 112. https://doi.org/10.1037/fam0000623

Gobinath, A. R., Mahmoud, R., & Galea, L. A. M. (2015). Influence of sex and stress exposure across the lifespan on endophenotypes of depression: Focus on behavior, glucocorticoids, and hippocampus. *Frontiers in Neuroscience, 8*, 420. https://doi.org/10.3389/fnins.2014.00420

Gonzalez, D., Mirabal, A. B., & McCall, J. D. (2020). *Child and abuse neglect*. StatPearls Publishing LLC. https://www.ncbi.nlm.nih.gov/books/NBK459146/

Government of Canada. (2018). *Trauma and violence-informed approaches to policy and practice*. https://www.canada.ca/en/public-health/services/publications/health-risks-safety/trauma-violence-informed-approaches-policy-practice.html

Grant, J. G., & Cadell, S. (2009). Power, pathological worldviews, and the strengths perspective in social work. *Families in Society, 90*(4), 425–430. https://doi.org/10.1606/1044-3894.3921

Gutmanis, I., Beynon, C., Tutty, L., Wathen, C. N., & MacMillan, H. L. (2007). Factors influencing identification of and response to intimate partner violence: A survey of physicians and nurses. *BioMed Central Public Health, 7*(1), 12. https://doi.org/10.1186/1471-2458-7-12

Hall, K. (2012). Understanding validation: A way to communicate acceptance. *Psychology Today*. https://www.psychologytoday.com/ca/blog/pieces-mind/201204/understanding-validation-way-communicate-acceptance#:~:text=Validation%20is%20a%20way%20of%20communicating%20that%20the%20relationship%20is,sensations%2C%20and%20behaviors%20as%20understandable

Hammond, W. (2010). Principles of strength-based practice. *Resiliency Initiatives, 12*(2), 1–7. https://greaterfallsconnections.org/wp-content/uploads/2014/07/Principles-of-Strength-2.pdf

Hardesty, J. L., Crossman, K. A., Haselschwerdt, M. L., Raffaelli, M., Ogolsky, B. G., & Johnson, M. P. (2015). Toward a standard approach to operationalizing coercive control and classifying violence types. *Journal of Marriage and the Family, 77*(4), 833–843. https://doi.org/10.1111/jomf.12201

Hunnicutt, G. (2020). Commentary on the special issue: New ways of thinking theoretically about violence against women and other forms of gender-based violence. *Violence Against Women, 27*(5), 708–716. https://doi.org/10.1177/1077801220958484

Huntley, A. L., Potter, L., Williamson, E., Malpass, A., Szilassy, E., & Feder, G. (2019). Help-seeking by male victims of domestic violence and abuse (DVA): A systematic review and qualitative evidence synthesis. *BMJ Open, 9*(6), e021960 https://doi.org/10.1136/bmjopen-2018-021960

Ivany, A. S., Bullock, L., Schminkey, D., Wells, K., Sharps, P., & Kools, S. (2018). Living in fear and prioritizing safety: Exploring women's lives after traumatic brain injury from intimate partner violence. *Qualitative Health Research*, 28(11), 1708–1718. https://doi.org/10.1177/1049732318786705

Jack, S. M., Ford-Gilboe, M., Davidov, D., MacMillan, H. L., & NFP IPV Research Team. (2016). Identification and assessment of intimate partner violence in nurse home visitation. *Journal of Clinical Nursing*, 26(15–16), 2215–2228. https://doi.org/10.1111/jocn.13392

James, S., Herman, J., Rankin, S., Keisling, M., Mottet, L., & Anafi, M. (2016). *The report of the 2015 US transgender survey*. www.transequality.org/sites/default/files/docs/USTS-Full-Report-FINAL.PDF

Janes, K. M., & Rodger, S. (2012). *Hearing women's voices: Understanding women's stories of violence from the perspective of strength*. https://ir.lib.uwo.ca/cgi/viewcontent.cgi?article=1628&context=etd

Johnson, M. (2006). Conflict and control: Gender symmetry and asymmetry in domestic violence. *Violence Against Women*, 12(11), 1003–1018. https://doi.org/10.1177/1077801206293328

Jordan, C. E., Campbell, R., & Follingstad, D. (2010). Violence and women's mental health: The impact of physical, sexual, and psychological aggression. *Annual Review of Clinical Psychology*, 6, 607–628. https://doi.org/10.1146/annurev-clinpsy-090209-151437

Jud, A., & Trocmé, N. (2012). *Physical abuse and physical punishment in Canada*. Child Canadian Welfare Research Portal Information Sheet # 122E. https://cwrp.ca/information-sheet/physical-abuse-and-physical-punishment-canada

Kaplan, C., Tarlow, N., Stewart, J. G., Aguirre, B., Galen, G., & Auerbach, R. P. (2016). Borderline personality disorder in youth: The prospective impact of child abuse on non-suicidal self-injury and suicidality. *Comprehensive Psychiatry*, 71, 86–94. https://doi.org/10.1016/j.comppsych.2016.08.016

Kassam-Adams, N., Rzucidlo, S., Campbell, M., Good, G., Bonifacio, E., Slouf, K., Schneider, S., McKenna, C., Hanson, C. A., & Grather, D. (2015). Nurses' views and current practice of trauma-informed pediatric nursing care. *Journal of Pediatric Nursing-Nursing Care of Children & Families*, 30(3), 478–484. https://doi.org/10.1016/j.pedn.2014.11.008

Kohli, A., Perrin, N., Mpanano, R. M., Banywesize, L., Mirindi, A. B., Banywesize, J. H., Mitima, C. M., Binkurhorhwa, A. K., Bufole, N. M., & Glass, N. (2015). Family and community driven response to intimate partner violence in post-conflict settings. *Social Science & Medicine*, 146, 276–284. https://doi.org/10.1016/j.socscimed.2015.10.011

Kozak, R. S., Gushwa, M., & Cadet, T. J. (2018). Victimization and violence: An exploration of the relationship between child sexual abuse, violence, and delinquency. *Journal of Child Sexual Abuse*, 27(6), 699–717. https://doi.org/10.1080/10538712.2018.1474412

Labrum, T., & Solomon, P. L. (2015). Physical elder abuse perpetrated by relatives with serious mental illness: A preliminary conceptual social–ecological model. *Aggression and Violent Behavior*, 25, 293–303. https://doi.org/10.1016/j.avb.2015.09.006

Lanius, R. A., Rabellino, D., Boyd, J. E., Harricharan, S., Frewen, P. A., & McKinnon, M. C. (2017). The innate alarm system in PTSD: Conscious and subconscious processing of threat. *Current Opinion in Psychology*, 14, 109–115. https://doi.org/10.1016/j.copsyc.2016.11.006

Lau, M., & Kristensen, E. (2010). Sexual revictimization in a clinical sample of women reporting childhood sexual abuse. *Nordic Journal of Psychiatry*, 64(1), 4–10. https://doi.org/10.3109/08039480903191205

Lentz, L. (2011). 10 tips for documenting domestic violence. *Nursing Critical Care*, 6(4), 48. https://doi.org/10.1097/01.CCN.0000398775.42472.da

Levine, S., Varcoe, C., & Browne, A. J. (2020). "We went as a team closer to the truth": Impacts of interprofessional education on trauma- and violence-informed care for staff in primary care settings. *Journal of Interprofessional Care*, 35(1), 46–54. https://doi.org/10.1080/13561820.2019.1708871

Logie, C. H., Alaggia, R., & Rwigema, M. J. (2014). A social ecological approach to understanding correlates of lifetime sexual assault among sexual minority women in Toronto, Canada: Results from a cross-sectional internet-based survey. *Health Education Research*, 29(4), 671–682. https://doi.org/10.1093/her/cyt119

Love, H. A., Spencer, C. M., May, S. A., Mendez, M., & Stith, S. M. (2020). Perpetrator risk markers for intimate terrorism and situational couple violence: A meta-analysis. *Trauma, Violence & Abuse*, 21(5), 922–931. https://doi.org/10.1177/1524838018801331

Lu, J. Y., Tung, T. H., Shen, S. A., Huang, C., & Chen, P. S. (2020). The effects of psychotherapy for depressed or posttraumatic stress disorder women with childhood sexual abuse history: Meta-analysis of randomized controlled trials. *Medicine*, 99(17), e19776. https://doi.org/10.1097/MD.0000000000019776

Lutwak, N. (2018). The psychology of health and illness: The mental health and physiological effects of intimate partner violence on women. *The Journal of Psychology*, 152(6), 373–387. https://doi.org/10.1080/00223980.2018.1447435

Lysova, A., Dim, E. E., & Dutton, D. (2019). Prevalence and consequences of intimate partner violence in Canada as measured by the National Victimization Survey. *Partner Abuse*, 10(2), 199–221. https://doi.org/10.1891/1946-6560.10.2.199

Machado, A., Santos, A., Graham-Kevan, N., & Matos, M. (2017). Exploring help seeking experiences of male victims of female perpetrators of IPV. *Journal of Family Violence*, 32(5), 513–523. https://doi.org/10.1007/s10896-016-9853-8

Machisa, M. T., Christofides, N., & Jewkes, R. (2017). Mental ill health in structural pathways to women's experiences of intimate partner violence. *PLoS One*, 12(4), e0175240. https://doi.org/10.1371/journal.pone.0175240

Machisa, M. T., Christofides, N., & Jewkes, R. (2018). Social support factors associated with psychological resilience among women survivors of intimate partner violence in Gauteng, South Africa. *Global Health Action*, 11(Suppl. 3), 1491114. https://doi.org/10.1080/16549716.2018.1491114

MacMillan, H. L., Wathen, C. N., Jamieson, E., Boyle, M. H., Shannon, H. S., Ford-Gilboe, M., Worster, A., Lent, B., Coben, J. H., Campbell, J. C., McNutt, L., & McMaster Violence Against Women Research Group. (2009). Screening for intimate partner violence in health care settings: A randomized trial. *Journal of the American Medical Association*, 302(5), 493–501. https://doi.org/10.1001/jama.2009.1089

Mainali, P., Rai, T., & Rutkofsky, I. H. (2020). From child abuse to developing borderline personality disorder into adulthood: Exploring the neuromorphological and epigenetic pathway. *Cureus*, 12(7), e9474. https://doi.org/10.7759/cureus.9474

Mariscal, J. (2007). The poverty draft. *Sojourners Magazine*, 36(6), 32–35. https://sojo.net/magazine/june-2007/poverty-draft

Markowitz, J. C., Neria, Y., Lovell, K., Van Meter, P. E., & Petkova, E. (2017). History of sexual trauma moderates psychotherapy outcome for post-traumatic stress disorder. *Depression and Anxiety*, 34(8), 692–700. https://doi.org/10.1002/da.22619

Martin, M. S., Dykxhoorn, J., Afifi, T. O., & Colman, I. (2016). Child abuse and the prevalence of suicide attempts among those reporting suicide ideation. *Social Psychiatry and Psychiatric Epidemiology*, 51(11), 1477–1484. https://doi.org/10.1007/s00127-016-1250-3

Mason, R., Wolf, M., O'Rinn, S., & Ene, G. (2017). Making connections across silos: Intimate partner violence, mental health, and substance use. *BMC Women's Health*, 17, 29. https://doi.org/10.1186/s12905-017-0372-4

McGlynn, A., & Monforti, J. L. (2010). *The poverty draft? Exploring the role of socioeconomic tatus in U.S. military recruitment of Hispanic students*. American Political Science Association, 1–14. https://ssrn.com/abstract=1643790

McLaughlin, J., O'Carroll, R. E., & O'connor, R. C. (2012). Intimate partner abuse and suicidality: A systematic review. *Clinical Psychology Review*, 32(8), 677–689. https://doi.org/10.1016/j.cpr.2012.08.002

Mendez-Figueroa, H., Dahlke, J. D., Vrees, R. A., & Rouse, D. J. (2013). Trauma in pregnancy: An updated systematic review. *American Journal of Obstetrics and Gynecology*, 209(1), 1–10. https://doi.org/doi:10.1016/j.ajog.2013.01.021

Merdian, H., Kettleborough, D., McCartan, K., & Perkins, D. E. (2017). Strength-based approaches to online child sexual abuse: Using self-management strategies to enhance desistance behaviour in users of child sexual exploitation material. *Journal of Criminal Psychology*, 7(3), 183–192. https://doi.org/10.1108/JCP-10-2016-0035

Ministry of Justice. (2013). *Safety planning with children and youth: A toolkit for working with children and youth exposed to domestic violence*. https://www2.gov.bc.ca/assets/gov/law-crime-and-justice/criminal-justice/victims-of-crime/vs-info-for-professionals/training/child-youth-safety-toolkit.pdf

National Initiative for the Care of The Elderly. (2016). *Into the light: National survey on the mistreatment of older Canadians 2015*. https://cnpea.ca/images/canada-report-june-7-2016-pre-study-lynnmcdonald.pdf

National Institute of Justice. (2017, October 12). *Pathways between child maltreatment and adult criminal involvement*. https://nij.gov/topics/crime/children-exposed-to-violence/Pages/pathwaysbetween-child-maltreatment-and-adult-criminalinvolvement.aspx

Negele, A., Kaufhold, J., Kallenbach, L., & Leuzinger-Bohleber, M. (2015). Childhood trauma and its relation to chronic depression in adulthood. *Depression Research and Treatment*, 2015, 650804. https://doi.org/10.1155/2015/650804

Nevala, S. (2017). Coercive control and its impact on intimate partner violence through the lens of an EU-wide survey on violence against women. *Journal of Interpersonal Violence*, 32(12), 1792–1820. https://doi.org/10.1177/0886260517698950

O'Cleirigh, C., Safren, S. A., Taylor, S. W., Goshe, B. M., Bedoya, C. A., Marquez, S. M., Boroughs, M. S., & Shipherd, J. C. (2019). Cognitive behavioral therapy for trauma and self-care (CBT-TSC) in men who have sex with men with a history of childhood sexual abuse: A randomized controlled trial. *AIDS and Behavior, 23*(9), 2421–2431. https://doi.org/10.1007/s10461-019-02482-z

O'Doherty, L., Hegarty, K., Ramsay, J., Davidson, L. L., Feder, G., & Taft, A. (2015). Screening women for intimate partner violence in healthcare settings. *Cochrane Database of Systematic Reviews, 2015*(7), CD007007. https://doi.org/10.1002/14651858.CD007007.pub2.77

Ogbe, E., Harmon, S., Van den Bergh, R., & Degomme, O. (2020). A systematic review of intimate partner violence interventions focused on improving social support and/mental health outcomes of survivors. *PLoS One, 15*(6), e0235177. https://doi.org/10.1371/journal.pone.0235177

Oriol, X., Miranda, R., Amutio, A., Acosta, H. C., Mendoza, M. C., & Torres-Vallejos, J. (2017). Violent relationships at the social-ecological level: A multi-mediation model to predict adolescent victimization by peers, bullying and depression in early and late adolescence. *PLoS One, 12*(3), e0174139. https://doi.org/10.1371/journal.pone.0174139

Paek, D., & Kwon, D. I. (2020). A review on four different paths to respiratory arrest from brain injury in children; implications for child abuse. *Journal of Forensic and Legal Medicine, 71*, 101938. https://doi.org/10.1016/j.jflm.2020.101938

Paradies, Y., Ben, J., Denson, N., Elias, A., Priest, N., Pieterse, A., Gupta, A., Kelaher, M., & Gee, G. (2015). Racism as a determinant of health: A systematic review and meta-analysis. *PLoS One, 10*(9), e0138511. https://doi.org/10.1371/journal.pone.0138511

Pedersen, J. S., Malcoe, L. H., & Pulkingham, J. (2013). Explaining aboriginal/non-aboriginal inequalities in postseparation violence against Canadian women: Application of a structural violence approach. *Violence Against Women, 19*(8), 1034–1058. https://doi.org/10.1177/1077801213499245

Pereda, N., & Gallardo-Pujol, D. (2014). One hit makes the difference: The role of polyvictimization in childhood in lifetime revictimization on a southern European sample. *Violence and Victims, 29*(2), 217–231. https://doi.org/10.1891/0886-6708.vv-d-12-00061r1

Plummer, S.-B., & Findley, P. A. (2012). Women with disabilities' experience with physical and sexual abuse: Review of the literature and implications for the field. *Trauma, Violence & Abuse, 13*(1), 15–29. https://doi.org/10.1177/1524838011426014

Ponic, P., Varcoe, C., & Smutylo, T. (2016). Trauma- (and violence-) informed approaches to supporting victims of violence: Policy and practice considerations. *Victims of Crime Research Digest, 9*, 3–15. https://www.justice.gc.ca/eng/rp-pr/cj-jp/victim/rd9-rr9/p2.html

Raphael, D. (2020). *Poverty in Canada: Implications for health and quality of life* (3rd ed.). Canadian Scholars Press.

Registered Nurses' Association of Ontario. (2014). *Preventing and addressing abuse and neglect of older adults: Person-centred, collaborative, system-wide Approaches.* https://rnao.ca/sites/rnao-ca/files/Preventing_Abuse_and_Neglect_of_Older_Adults_final_July31.pdf

Rivara, F., Adhia, A., Lyons, V., Massey, A., Mills, B., Morgan, E., Simckes, M., & Rowhani-Rahbar, A. (2019). The effects of violence on health. *Health Affairs, 38*(10), 1622–1629. https://doi.org/10.1377/hlthaff.2019.00480

Rizkalla, K., Maar, M., Pilon, R., McGregor, L., & Reade, M. (2020). Improving the response of primary care providers to rural First Nation women who experience intimate partner violence: A qualitative study. *BMC Women's Health, 20*(1), 1–13. https://doi.org/10.1186/s12905-020-01053-y

Roberts, S. J., Chandler, G. E., & Kalmakis, K. (2019). A model for trauma-informed primary care. *Journal of the American Association of Nurse Practitioners, 31*(2), 139–144. https://doi.org/10.1097/JXX.0000000000000116

Roepke-Buehler, S. K., Simon, M., & Dong, X. (2015). Association between depressive symptoms, multiple dimensions of depression, and elder abuse. *Journal of Aging and Health, 27*, 1003–1025. https://doi.org/10.1177/0898264315571106

Roman, N. V., & Frantz, J. M. (2013). The prevalence of intimate partner violence in the family: A systematic review of the implications for adolescents in Africa. *Family Practice, 30*(3), 256–265. https://doi.org/10.1093/fampra/cms084

Saleebey, D. (2013). *Strengths perspective in social work practice* (6th ed.). Pearson.

Santos, A. J., Nunes, B., Kislaya, I., Gil, A. P., & Ribeiro, O. (2017). Exploring the correlates to depression in elder abuse victims: Abusive experience or individual characteristics? *Journal of Interpersonal Violence, 36*(1–2), NP115–NP134. https://doi.org/10.1177/0886260517732346

Scerra, N. (2011, July). *Strengths-based practice: The evidence.* Uniting Care Children, Young People and Families. https://bluepeteraustralia.files.wordpress.com/2012/12/strengths-based-perspective.pdf

Scott-Storey, K. (2011). Cumulative abuse: Do things add up? An evaluation of the conceptualization, operationalization, and methodological approaches in the study of the phenomenon of cumulative

abuse. *Trauma, Violence & Abuse, 12*(3), 135150. https://doi.org/10.1177/1524838011404253

Sirey, J. A., Berman, J., Salamone, A., DePasquale, A., Halkett, A., Raeifar, E., Banerjee, S., Bruce, M. L., & Raue, P. J. (2015). Feasibility of integrating mental health screening and services into routine elder abuse practice to improve client outcomes. *Journal of Elder Abuse & Neglect, 27*(3), 254–269. https://doi.org/10.1080/08946566.2015.1008086

Smith, S. G., Zhang, X., Basile, K. C., Merrick, M. T., Wang, J., Kresnow, M., & Chen, J. (2018). *National intimate partner and sexual violence survey: 2015 data brief—Updated release.* Centers for Disease Control and Prevention. https://www.cdc.gov/violenceprevention/pdf/2015data-brief508.pdf

Statistics Canada. (2018). *Family violence in Canada: A statistical profile 2018.* https://www150.statcan.gc.ca/n1/pub/85-002-x/2019001/article/00018-eng.htm

Statistics Canada. (2020a). *Table 17-10-0005-01 Population estimates on July 1st, by age and sex.* https://doi.org/10.25318/1710000501-eng

Statistics Canada. (2020b). *Sexual minority people almost three times more likely to experience violent victimization than heterosexual people.* Catalogue No. 11-001-X, pp. 1–4. https://www150.statcan.gc.ca/n1/en/daily-quotidien/200909/dq200909a-eng.pdf?st=WJ8Yphi-

Stöckl, H., Devries, K., Rotstein, A., Abrahams, N., Campbell, J., Watts, C., & Moreno, C. G. (2013). The global prevalence of intimate partner homicide: A systematic review. *The Lancet, 382*(9895), 859–865. https://doi.org/10.1016/S0140-6736(13)61030-2

Storey, J. E. (2020). Risk factors for elder abuse and neglect: A review of the literature. *Aggression and Violent Behavior, 50*, 101339. https://doi.org/10.1016/j.avb.2019.101339

Strangio, A. M., Rinaldi, L., Monniello, G., Sisti, L. G., de Waure, C., & Janiri, L. (2017). The effect of abuse history on adolescent patients with feeding and eating disorders treated through psychodynamic therapy: Comorbidities and outcome. *Frontiers in Psychiatry, 8*, 31. https://doi.org/10.3389/fpsyt.2017.00031

Taillieu, T. L., Brownridge, D. A., Tyler, K. A., Chan, K. L., Tiwari, A., & Santos, S. C. (2016). Pregnancy and intimate partner violence in Canada: A comparison of victims who were and were not abused during pregnancy. *Journal of Family Violence, 31*(5), 567–579. https://doi.org/10.1007/s10896-015-9789-4

Temple, J. R., Weston, R., & Marshall, L. L. (2010). Long-term mental health effects of partner violence patterns and relationship termination on low-income and ethnically diverse community women. *Partner Abuse, 1*(4), 379–398. https://doi.org/10.1891/1946-6560.1.4.379

Tutty, L. M., Radtke, H. L., Ateah, C. A., Ursel, E. J., Thurston, W. E. B., Hampton, M., & Nixon, K. (2017). The complexities of intimate partner violence: Mental health, disabilities, and child abuse history for white, indigenous, and other visible minority Canadian women. *Journal of Interpersonal Violence, 36*(3–4), 1208–1232. https://doi.org/10.1177/0886260517741210

Usta, J., Antoun, J., Ambuel, B., & Khawaja, M. (2012). Involving the health care system in domestic violence: What women want. *The Annals of Family Medicine, 10*(3), 213–220. https://doi.org/10.1370/afm.1336

Van Wert, M., Anreiter, I., Fallon, B. A., & Sokolowski, M. B. (2019). Intergenerational transmission of child abuse and neglect: A transdisciplinary analysis. *Gender and The Genome, 3*, 1–21. https://doi.org/10.1177/2470289719826101

Violence Evidence Guidance Action. (n.d.). *Responding safely to intimate partner violence (IPV): We must do better than screening.* https://vega-project.mcmaster.ca/docs/default-source/pdf/responding-safely-to-intimate-partner-violence-ipv_-we-must-do-better-than-screening.pdf?sfvrsn=57f4b4c1_0

Wang, X. M., Brisbin, S., Loo, T., & Straus, S. (2015). Elder abuse: An approach to identification, assessment and intervention. *Canadian Medical Association Journal, 187*(8), 575–581. https://doi.org/581.10.1503/cmaj.141329

Wathen, N. (2012). *Health impacts of violent victimization on women and their children.* Research and Statistics Division Department of Justice Canada. https://www.justice.gc.ca/eng/rp-pr/cj-jp/fv-vf/rr12_12/rr12_12.pdf

Wathen, C. N., MacGregor, J. C. D., & MacMillan, H. L. (2016). *Research brief: Identifying and responding to intimate partner violence against women.* PreVAiL research network. http://projectvega.ca/documents/2016/11/prevail-ipv-brief-fall-2016.pdf

Wathen, C. N., MacGregor, J. C. D., Sibbald, S. L., & MacMillan, H. L. (2013). Exploring the uptake and framing of research evidence on universal screening for intimate partner violence against women: A knowledge translation case study. *Health Research Policy and Systems, 11*(13). https://doi.org/10.1186/1478-4505-11-13

Wong, J. S., & Waite, L. J. (2017). Elder mistreatment predicts later physical and psychological health: Results from a national longitudinal study. *Journal of Elder Abuse & Neglect, 29*(1), 15–42. https://doi.org/10.1080/08946566.2016.1235521

World Health Organization. (2013a). *Global and regional estimates of violence against women: Prevalence and health effects of intimate partner violence and non-partner sexual violence.* https://www.who.int/publications/i/item/9789241564625

World Health Organization. (2013b). *Responding to intimate partner violence and sexual violence against women WHO clinical and policy guidelines.* https://apps.who.int/iris/bitstream/handle/10665/85240/9789241548595_eng.pdf;jsessionid=A177B5522756D509DABB76C7EB2081BA?sequence=1

World Health Organization. (2014). *Health care for women subjected to intimate partner violence or sexual violence: A clinical handbook.* http://apps.who.int/iris/bitstream/10665/136101/1/WHO_RHR_14.26_eng.pdf?ua=1

World Health Organization. (2019). *Caring for women subjected to violence: A WHO curriculum for training health-care providers.* https://apps.who.int/iris/handle/10665/330084

World Health Organization. (2020a). *The ecological framework.* Violence prevention alliance. https://www.who.int/violenceprevention/approach/ecology/en/

World Health Organization. (2020b, 8 June). *Child maltreatment.* https://www.who.int/news-room/fact-sheets/detail/child-maltreatment

Wuest, J., O'Donnell, S., Scott-Storey, K., Malcolm, J., Vincent, C. D., & Taylor, P. (2020). Cumulative lifetime violence severity and chronic pain in a community sample of Canadian men. *Pain Medicine, 22*(6), 1387–1398. https://doi.org/10.1093/pm/pnaa419

Yan, E., Chan, K., & Tiwari, A. (2015). A systematic review of prevalence and risk factors for elder abuse in Asia. *Trauma, Violence, & Abuse, 16*(2), 199–219. https://doi.org/10.1177/1524838014555033

Yim, I. S., & Kofman, Y. B. (2019). The psychobiology of stress and intimate partner violence. *Psychoneuroendocrinology, 105,* 9–24. https://doi.org/10.1016/j.psyneuen.2018.08.017

Yunus, R. M., Hairi, N. N., Choo, W. Y. (2019). Consequences of elder abuse and neglect: A systematic review of observational studies. *Trauma Violence Abuse, 20*(2), 197–213. https://doi.org/10.1177/1524838017692798

Zaleski, K. L., Johnson, D. K., & Klein, J. T. (2016). Grounding Judith Herman's trauma theory within interpersonal neuroscience and evidence-based practice modalities for trauma treatment. *Smith College Studies in Social Work, 86*(4), 377–393. https://doi.org/10.1080/00377317.2016.1222110

Zorn, K. G., Wuerch, M. A., Faller, N., & Hampton, M. R. (2017). Perspectives on regional differences and intimate partner violence in Canada: A qualitative examination. *Journal of Family Violence, 32*(6), 633–644. https://doi.org/10.1007/s10896-017-9911-x

CHAPTER 35

Care of Persons Under Forensic Purview

Cindy Peternelj-Taylor

LEARNING OBJECTIVES

After studying this chapter, you will be able to:

- Describe the complexity of mental health challenges experienced by persons under forensic purview.
- Examine the issues that are critical to the development of therapeutic relationships in forensic settings.
- Consider the challenges and opportunities that exist for nursing given the diversity of settings in which forensic nurses practise.
- Analyze the issues inherent in professional role development for nurses practising in the forensic milieu.
- Evaluate the societal norms that affect contemporary care and treatment of persons under forensic purview.
- Discuss the strategies for ongoing education, research, and practice development in forensic nursing.

KEY TERMS

- boundary violations • compassionate release
- dynamic security awareness • forensic nursing
- relational security • static security

KEY CONCEPTS

- criminalization of persons with mental illness •
custody and caring • manipulation • othering • recovery
• vulnerable

In Canada, as in many Western countries, large numbers of vulnerable and at-risk individuals find themselves seeking mental health care under the auspices of the criminal justice system. This chapter focuses on persons under forensic purview: those who have violated the law in some way, including those remanded in custody while awaiting trial (charged but not yet sentenced); those who have been remanded in a secure forensic mental health facility for psychiatric evaluation and/or treatment; those who are found unfit to stand trial (UST) or not criminally responsible on account of a mental disorder (NCRMD); as well as those individuals who have been charged, sentenced by the courts to community supervision, or incarcerated in provincial, territorial, or federal correctional facilities. Nurses practising where the domains of criminal justice and health care intersect are typically referred to as *forensic* nurses, and their ability to provide competent and ethical care is often compromised by social and political animosity toward crime, criminality, and mental disorders.

Forensic nurses are responsible for providing mental health care and treatment to persons under forensic purview in a variety of secure institutional facilities, including forensic psychiatric units within general hospitals, forensic mental health (FMH) hospitals, jails, prisons, correctional facilities, and institutions for youth in custody. They are also involved in community-based court diversion schemes and community treatment orders (CTOs), and

they assist forensic clients with recovery and reintegration into the community. Practising "at the interface of justice and mental health where the patient population does not fit neatly into either department" (Martin et al., 2013, p. 172) can be particularly challenging for nurses. A variety of terms are used to refer to this evolving specialty area, including forensic psychiatric nursing, FMH nursing, community FMH nursing, and correctional or prison nursing. For simplicity, **forensic nursing** is used throughout this chapter and refers to nurses who integrate psychiatric and mental health nursing "philosophy and practice within a sociocultural context that includes the criminal justice system to provide comprehensive care to clients, families, and communities" (Peternelj-Taylor & Hufft, 2006, p. 379).

Criminalization of the Mentally Ill

Throughout Canada, jails, prisons, and custodial facilities for persons in conflict with the law have become "de facto psychiatric institutions" with "access to psychiatric care only [occurring] after they have been criminalized" (Chaimowitz, 2012, p. 5). In a 2020 scoping review addressing the mental health needs of justice-involved persons, the Mental Health Commission of Canada (MHCC) (2020) concluded that "the criminal justice system has become an inappropriate mental health 'system' of last resort" (p. xii). When compared to the

933

general Canadian population, mental health problems are up to three times more common among federal correctional populations (Centre for Addiction and Mental Health [CAMH], 2020). Mental health services within correctional facilities have not kept up with this dramatic increase, and in many facilities, treatment is often nonexistent or unsatisfactory when compared with the community standard (CAMH, 2020, Dupuis et al., 2013; Office of the Correctional Investigator [OCI], 2015).

The criminalization of persons with mental illness in Canada and globally has frequently been attributed to the deinstitutionalization movement that occurred in the 1960s and the 1970s, and although this movement at the time was seen as the *right* thing to do, inadequate community-based services and housing resulted in the overrepresentation of people with mental illness in the criminal justice system (Dvoskin et al., 2020; MHCC, 2020). Unfortunately, the ongoing failure of provincial, territorial, and federal governments to provide sufficient mental health funding to fully realize the goals of deinstitutionalization (e.g., independent living within the community) resulted in a fragmented mental health system with woefully inadequate community-based services (Chaimowitz, 2012). Individuals who experience chronic mental illness are often well known by the police, the courts, mental health services, emergency departments, jails, and correctional facilities. Critics conclude that for many individuals caught up in this web, their only crime is that they are "guilty of mental illness" (Kanapaux, 2004).

As outlined in the *Mental Health Strategy for Canada*, the overrepresentation of people with mental health problems and illnesses in the criminal justice system (whether on remand, in correctional custody, or in a forensic facility) needs to be reduced (Mental Health Commission of Canada [MHCC], 2012). Furthermore, those who are in the system need to be able to access appropriate services, treatments, and supports that are "consistent with professionally accepted standards" (MHCC, 2012, p. 47). In collaboration with the MHCC, a Correctional Service Canada Federal–Provincial/Territorial partnership developed the *Mental Health Strategy for Corrections in Canada* (Correctional Service Canada [CSC] Federal–Provincial/Territorial Partnership, 2012) to meet the needs of youth and adults with mental health problems and illnesses enmeshed with the criminal justice system. Seven key components of this strategy are highlighted in Box 35.1. Forensic nurses are critical to the adoption, implementation, and evaluation of this strategy.

BOX 35.1 Mental Health Strategy for Corrections in Canada: Key Elements

1. Mental Health Promotion
2. Screening and Assessment
3. Treatment, Services, and Support
4. Suicide and Self-Injury Prevention and Management
5. Transitional Services and Support
6. Staff Education, Training, and Support
7. Community Supports and Partnerships

From Correctional Service Canada, Federal–Provincial/Territorial Partnership. (2012). *Mental health strategy for corrections in Canada.* http://www.csc-scc.gc.ca/health/092/MH-strategy-eng.pdf

---

The Paradox of Custody and Caring

Forensic settings are controversial. They arouse strong convictions from various sectors who debate their proper place in society. Nursing practice within this domain is particularly complex because it brings together the "coupling of two contradictory socioprofessional mandates: to punish and to provide care" (Holmes, 2005, p. 3). This paradox is disconcerting because a clear distinction between these two mandates is not always easily demarcated. Forensic settings provide society with two fundamental services: social necessities and social goods. Social necessities are considered essential to a community's existence; conversely, social goods are perceived as kindnesses, and although not necessarily essential, they are of benefit to the community nonetheless. Forensic settings meet their social necessity mandate through social control of those in their care. The protection of the community at large is perceived as a direct consequence of the processes of confinement and control. Forensic settings also provide social goods in the form of health care to those who are confined. In essence, forensic nurses are charged with the predicament of providing social good (e.g., health care) within institutions dedicated to providing social necessities (e.g., confinement) (Peternelj-Taylor & Johnson, 1995).

This coexistence of social control and nursing care creates a paradox for nurses and other healthcare professionals (Holmes, 2005, 2007), one that is laden with clinical issues and moral dilemmas not commonly encountered in more traditional healthcare settings. This paradox requires special attention and discernment because it permeates every aspect of forensic nursing. It is likely the single factor that differentiates forensic nursing from mental health nursing in a more general sense (Peternelj-Taylor, 2000). It is within this paradox, where the competing demands for custody and caring are embraced, that the moral climate of forensic institutions is shaped (Austin, 2001) (Fig. 35.1).

KEY CONCEPT

Mental healthcare resource shortages and a fragmented mental health system have led to correctional facilities becoming psychiatric institutions by default. Criminalization of persons with mental illness occurs when persons with an untreated mental illness contravene the law and enter the justice system rather than the healthcare system.

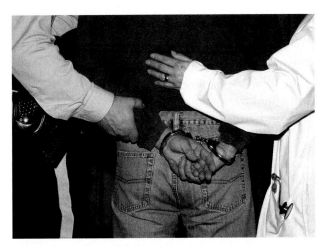

Figure 35.1 Custody and caring. (Courtesy of the Division of Media and Technology, University of Saskatchewan.)

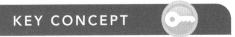

KEY CONCEPT

Nurses in forensic settings must meet the competing demands of custody (confinement and security) and caring (nursing care).

Forensic Nursing: A Model for Care

Nurses working with clients under forensic purview will find a familiar psychiatric and mental health nursing role, one that is "like 'stepping through the looking glass'—everything is the same, yet different" (Smith, 2005, p. 54). To illustrate the uniqueness of caring for this population, is presented a model of care. This model highlights the contextual and clinical practice issues affecting the articulation of a professional nursing role with persons under forensic purview, regardless of the setting. The five components of this model are the forensic client, nurse–client relationship, professional role development, treatment setting, and societal norms. Although each component of the model is discussed separately, in reality, the components are dynamic and interactive. Peternelj-Taylor and Hufft (2006) concluded that healthcare goals must be consistent with the reality of the client's life circumstances, as well as with the realities and the limitations of the setting in which nursing practice takes place. It may well be that not all forensic nurses will engage fully with each component of the model of care presented. However, the model as presented herein reflects the nature and scope of contemporary forensic nursing in Canada (Fig. 35.2).

Determinants of Health and the Forensic Client

As a group, persons under forensic purview present with a multitude of long-neglected physical and mental

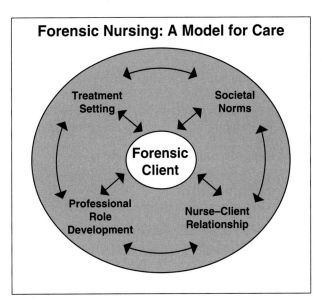

Figure 35.2 Forensic nursing: a model for care. (From Peternelj-Taylor, C. (2004). NURS 486—Forensic nursing in secure environments [Course material]. College of Nursing, University of Saskatchewan.)

healthcare challenges, often complicated by significant substance use problems. The health and psychosocial issues that they experience are often complex and multifaceted, contributing to the challenges encountered in their attempts to engage in treatment, relapse prevention, recovery, and reintegration. Frequently, their lives have been marked by illiteracy, poverty, and homelessness. Cultural and ethnic minorities, in particular, are overrepresented in correctional institutions (Kouyoumdjian et al., 2016a; Owusu-Bempah et al., 2021). Morbidity and mortality data suggest that those who are incarcerated experience higher rates of disease and disability when compared with nonincarcerated populations, which highlights the need for nursing leadership in primary, secondary, and tertiary levels of intervention. Persons under forensic purview frequently experience discrimination, stigmatization, and marginalization and often lack supportive relationships commonly associated with emotional and mental wellbeing (MHCC, 2020). Moreover, they are totally dependent on the system (whether it is the correctional system or the healthcare system) to meet their healthcare needs. Given the magnitude of these commingling issues, many forensic clients are at risk for dual, multiple, and overlapping sources of vulnerability. Yet, referring to those who have committed crimes against society as "vulnerable" seems somewhat contrary to conventional wisdom (Peternelj-Taylor, 2005).

Vulnerability and Vulnerable Populations

Broadly defined, vulnerability refers to a multifaceted concept that represents the commingling of resources, risk factors, and health status among a particular population or aggregate of people that places them at risk for altered health status (de Chesnay, 2020). As a concept, vulnerability is generally understood in one of two ways:

- From an individual viewpoint (vulnerability), which is concerned with such notions as "susceptibility" or "at risk for health problems"
- From an aggregate or group viewpoint (vulnerable populations), a public health perspective that focuses on those with a greater than average risk of developing physical, psychological, or social health challenges by virtue of their marginalized status, limited access to resources, and personal characteristics (de Chesnay, 2020)

Clearly, persons under forensic purview represent a significant portion of society's at-risk population. Therefore, understanding the concepts of vulnerability and vulnerable populations is essential to contemporary forensic nursing practice. Caution, however, should be exercised, because labelling someone as being a member of a vulnerable population can be perceived as patronizing by those receiving care, thereby further marginalizing those at risk (de Chesnay, 2020). Nurses are positioned at the interface of vulnerability and thus are challenged to engage in partnerships that encourage growth in their clients. Students and nurses alike can best work with vulnerable populations within FMH settings by learning how to actualize respect, significant to the development and maintenance of therapeutic relationships, even with unlikable clients (Rose et al., 2011).

KEY CONCEPT

Persons or populations are considered vulnerable when attributes, factors, or assigned status places them at greater risk for injury or poor health when compared with others.

Clients Experiencing Mental Illness

There is a great variation in the nature and severity of mental illnesses experienced by individuals who come into conflict with the law. In 1992, the Corrections and Conditional Release Act (Bill C-30) was proclaimed and led to the creation of review boards that are mandated to oversee the care and disposition of persons found UST or not criminally responsible on account of mental disorder (NCRMD) (Department of Justice, 2015). Under current Canadian law, an individual who comes into conflict with the law and is mentally ill can be found as follows:

- UST, when it is recognized that the accused is not fully capable of instructing legal counsel or not capable of understanding the nature and the consequences of a trial. In such situations, the judge has one of two choices: disposition for detention in hospital or a conditional discharge (the person, however, can later be found "fit" and tried in court and convicted, or deemed NCRMD).
- NCRMD is based on the accused person's mental state at the time the offence was committed. Although it is not a finding of guilt, the court or review board may give the following dispositions: detention in hospital, conditional discharge, or an absolute discharge. Individuals detained in a hospital are not required to submit to treatment; the disposition is meant to detain the person and make care available. If treatment is required, owing to the individual's deteriorating mental status, and the individual does not voluntarily agree to treatment, it is then provided as per provincial or territorial mental health acts.
- In some jurisdictions, instead of going to trial, court diversion schemes are options that may be exercised through mental health courts, drug treatment courts, or forensic assertive community treatment teams as correctional diversion (CAMH, 2020; Landess & Holoyda, 2017).

In all cases, the mentally disordered offender challenges the collective wisdom of both the healthcare system and the criminal justice system, creating a "crossover" of sorts, particularly when the individual has been found responsible for their crimes despite the mental illness. The incarceration experience represents a significant stressful life event, even for those who do not have a mental disorder; separation from family and friends, limitations on privacy, overcrowding, and fear of assault severely affect the individual's quality of life. For those with mental illness, prisons are dangerous places: they are often victimized by other offenders, they are at greater risk for engaging in self-harming behaviour and attempting suicide, and they are often confined in seclusion for their own protection. Unfortunately, such experiences can completely overwhelm the resources of individuals with mental illness. When compared with individuals in the community, incarcerated persons experience greater rates of schizophrenia, depression, bipolar disorder, anxiety disorders, and substance abuse disorders (Kouyoumdjian et al., 2016a). In a study on prevalence of mental disorders among incoming male federal offenders, Beaudette and colleagues (2015) found that 70% of male offenders met the diagnostic criteria for at least one mental disorder. Refer further to Box 35.2.

Suicide is the leading cause of death for persons under forensic purview, particularly those remanded or sentenced to a prison or correctional facility. A narrative review of related research studies has found that more than one in five persons in Canadian correctional facilities have attempted suicide (Kouyoumdjian et al., 2016a). Withdrawal from drugs or alcohol and the reality of incarceration or commitment to an FMH facility, coupled with comorbid mental disorders, may

BOX 35.2 Prevalence of Mental Health Disorders Among Male Federal Offenders at Intake

Mental Health Disorder	Prevalence Rate %
Alcohol or substance use disorders	49.6%
Antisocial personality disorder	44.1%
Anxiety disorders	29.5%
Mood disorders	16.9%
Borderline personality disorder	15.9%
Pathologic gambling	5.9%
Primary psychotic	3.3%

Source: Beaudette, J. N., Power, J., & Stewart, L. A. (2015). *National prevalence of mental disorders among federally-sentenced men offenders* (Research Report, R-357). Correctional Service Canada.

exacerbate a client's risk for suicide and thus warrants ongoing assessment, intervention, and evaluation by forensic nurses. Recognizing factors that may contribute to a client's vulnerability is critical. High-risk periods are considered those immediately following hospitalization, incarceration, release, or upon the receipt of bad news (Enggist et al., 2014; Olson, 2012).

Recovery

Recovery is a major tenet of the MHCC's (2012) *Mental Health Strategy for Canada*, one that can be particularly challenging for persons under forensic purview, especially following a serious offence. Moreover, although detention, hospitalization, and/or incarceration are opportunities for recovery, the person has to be an active participant in the recovery journey, which can be especially trying when the person is not voluntarily seeking treatment (McLoughlin et al., 2011). For persons under forensic purview, recovery is multifaceted and includes clinical recovery (symptom relief), functional recovery (life skills), social recovery (social inclusion), personal recovery (satisfying life living with illness), and offender recovery (redefinition of self). Of these, coming to terms with the offence clearly requires the active participation of the person (Drennan & Alred, 2012). Hope, empowerment, self-determination, and responsibility are considered the key principles of recovery (MHCC, 2012).

In 2015, the MHCC released comprehensive guidelines for recovery-oriented practice; unfortunately, specific strategies regarding how to adapt these guidelines to forensic or compulsory treatment settings are not addressed. Forensic nurses can, however, foster recovery in a number of ways: through supporting hope, engaging in respectful dialogue, strengthening the working alliance, attending to personal strengths, bridging security and therapy, and supporting personal responsibility (Clarke et al., 2016; Drennan & Alred, 2012). Recovery is possible and needs to underpin the nursing care of persons under forensic purview. The concept of success in the FMH system, from the perspective of service users and service providers, was examined by Livingston (2016), who concluded that success was seen as a dynamic multidimensional holistic process that a person works toward, and not simply an end state. Understanding success as a holistic multidimensional concept may assist nurses in their practice with FMH service users, as they work *with* them in their recovery journeys. More recently, Collingwood and colleagues (2021) explored the impact of equine interventions on forensic clients and staff engaged in a Horse Stables Program in Canada. Through qualitative interviews, four recovery-related themes emerged: (a) radical shift in environment; (b) opportunity for new roles; (c) building meaningful connections; and (d) expanding horizons. While not all persons under forensic purview will have opportunities to engage in equine therapies, programs such as these have the potential to promote recovery through the development of new skills and social relationships. Forensic nurses are often in key positions to work collaboratively with other disciplines in such ventures.

KEY CONCEPT

Recovery for persons under forensic purview includes clinical recovery through symptom relief, functional recovery through improving life skills, social recovery through community reintegration, personal recovery through achieving life satisfaction despite illness, and offender recovery through a redefinition of self.

Special Populations in the Forensic Setting

Although it could be argued that all persons under forensic purview have special mental health needs requiring the attention of special services and interventions by forensic nurses, groups more likely to require unique approaches include women, older adults, youth, cultural minorities, transgender offenders, and families.

The Female Forensic Client

In Canada, as in other Western countries, a marked increase in the number of women confined to forensic settings has been noted, even though they represent a small percentage of the overall forensic population (Blanchette & Brown, 2006). The OCI (2019) reported that since 2009, the number of women in custody under federal jurisdiction increased by 32.5%. Alarmingly, the number of federally sentenced Indigenous women increased by

73.8% in this same 10-year period. Nationally, Indigenous women represent the fastest growing group under federal jurisdiction, representing almost 41.4% of all federally incarcerated women, even though they represent only 4% of the female Canadian population.

In general, women most likely to find themselves within forensic settings are those who have grown up in poverty, have limited education and job skills, and have been exposed to violence, victimization, and discrimination. Women are often the primary caregivers for dependent children; as such, the fear of losing custody of their children is ever present (Blanchette & Brown, 2006; OCI, 2019). Female forensic clients are frequently victims as well as perpetrators of crime, having experienced physical, emotional, and sexual abuse as children and as adults, at the hands of fathers, husbands, boyfriends, acquaintances, and strangers (Green et al., 2005). Stanton and Rose (2020) recommend that nurses provide trauma-informed care and advocate for mental health treatment for women prerelease and postrelease. See Research for Best Practice, Box 35.3.

Common health concerns include significant substance use problems; higher rates of blood-borne infections such as HIV/AIDS and hepatitis B and C viruses; significant mental health concerns including anxiety-related disorders (e.g., posttraumatic stress disorder), concerns related to personality disorders (e.g., poor interpersonal functioning and complex and self-injurious behaviours), and serious mental illness (including depression and schizophrenia); pregnancy and gynaecologic problems; obesity; and chronic disorders such as diabetes, hypertension, epilepsy, and respiratory diseases (Green et al., 2005; Kouyoumdjian et al., 2016a; OCI, 2016).

The management of self-injurious behaviour among women under forensic purview is particularly challenging for forensic nurses. Mangnall and Yurkovich (2010), in a foundational study of deliberate self-harm in incarcerated women, reported that the most common method for self-harm was cutting, followed by carving arms, burning with an iron or with cigarettes, as well as swallowing glass shards, snipping veins with fingernail clippers, punching walls, or engaging in head-banging. In addition, although such behaviours typically result in immediate relief for the women, in practice, it is not uncommon for forensic nurses and correctional staff alike to be at odds with each other as they grapple with how to provide appropriate care for this group. In such cases, nursing typically assumes a therapeutic response, whereas corrections adopts a more punitive or custodial stance (Mangnall & Yurkovich, 2010; OCI, 2015, 2016).

In a comprehensive Canadian study addressing nonsuicidal self-injury (NSSI) in federally incarcerated women, Power and colleagues (2013) engaged

BOX 35.3 Research for Best Practice

EXPERIENCES OF WOMEN WHO ARE REINCARCERATED

Blair-Lawton, D., Mordoch, E., & Chernomas, W. (2020). Putting on the same shoes: Lived experiences of women who are reincarcerated. *Journal of Forensic Nursing, 16*(2), 99–107. https://doi.org/10.1097/JFN.0000000000000276

Purpose: Women throughout the world are discharged daily from correctional institutions. For many, their release is characterized by reimprisonment and subsequent rerelease into the community. This study examined the lived experiences of women who were imprisoned, released to the community, and returned to custody.

Methods: Utilizing a hermeneutic phenomenologic design, the researchers engaged 12 women (9 of whom were Indigenous) in face-to-face conversational interviews at a correctional centre located in the province of Manitoba. A qualitative thematic analysis, informed by van Manen's existentials (temporality/lived time, spatiality/lived space, relationality/lived human relations, and corporeality/lived body), provided a structure for the analysis.

Findings: Nine themes and 14 subthemes organized around the existentials illustrate the factors impacting on the participants' ability to avoid reimprisonment.

Interwoven throughout their accounts are lived experiences of personal and intergenerational trauma, painful childhoods, difficult relationships, substance misuse, gender discrimination, violence, and ineffective or absent personal and systemic supports. The phenomenon of "putting on the same shoes" represents a metaphor for their lives at the time of release—if they are not equipped to deal with release, if nothing has changed in their lives, they simply have "no other shoes to wear" and quickly default to what is familiar, which results in arrests and a return to custody.

Implications for Practice: The findings provide nurses with meaningful accounts of imprisoned women's lives—their stories, struggles, and strengths. Understanding their lived experiences is essential to the development, integration, and promotion of patient-centred trauma-informed supportive care. The researchers concluded that "It is vital that we listen to the voices of imprisoned women and work toward developing relevant resources and supports to combat the marginalized spaces that women often occupy" (p. 107).

participants in semistructured interviews focused on (a) reasons for self-injuring, (b) precipitating events, and (c) emotions experienced prior to, and after, the self-injury. While some common themes emerged in the data in relation to reasons (affect regulation), precipitating events (interpersonal conflict), emotions experienced prior to NSSI (anger and frustration), and emotions experienced after NSSI (relief), the researchers concluded that NSSI needs to be understood from a heterogeneous perspective and that effective treatment approaches need to consider the unique experiences of each individual woman.

Finally, approaches to self-injurious behaviour ultimately need to address underlying motivations versus simply trying to stop the behaviour (as in the custodial response). Dialectical behavioural therapy has been found to be a useful approach when working with women who engage in NSSI, in both outpatient and inpatient settings (Power et al., 2013).

The Older Forensic Client

For an increasing number of older Canadians, growing old in a prison or in a forensic psychiatric facility is a harsh reality. Forensic clients are considered to be "older" if aged 50 or more years. The transformation to being "older" is believed to be accelerated by 10 to 15 years within this group of clients (Hayes et al., 2012; Human Rights Watch [HRW], 2012). As of January 2019, 25% of federally incarcerated offenders were older than 50 years, and 5% were older than 65 years (McKendy et al., 2019).

Depending on the nature of imprisonment or hospitalization, persons under forensic purview may experience stressors related to general survival (particularly those who are incarcerated), coping with financial pressures, and withdrawal from drugs or alcohol, as well as the cumulative impact of high-risk behaviours, negative lifestyle practices, and inadequate health care, coupled

---

IN·A·LIFE

Rachel Fayter (1981—)

CONVICT, CRIMINOLOGY, AND ACADEMIC ACTIVIST

In 2008, I was 27 years old and halfway through a PhD program in Community Psychology when my life began spinning out of control. I had been involved in a series of long-term abusive relationships with violent men who had extensive criminal records and struggled with serious mental health issues and addiction to drugs and alcohol. By 2009, I was coping with fairly serious health problems of my own, and I survived a severe car accident that left me with chronic neck and back pain. My doctor at the time prescribed me OxyContin and Percocet, which I became addicted to, and quickly developed a tolerance requiring me to increase the amount of my doses.

Within 2 years my doctor retired, and his replacement suddenly cut off my prescription without warning or any support allowing me to taper off the medication. Within a few days, I experienced withdrawal so intense that I could not eat, sleep, or work whatsoever. I turned to the streets to find these same drugs. Opiates are an expensive habit, so I had to find ways to make extra money, such as selling marijuana. To make a long story short, I was arrested for "possession for the purpose of trafficking," was placed on house arrest for two and a half years, breeched my conditions, was arrested again, and subsequently spent three and a half years at Grand Valley Institution (GVI), a federal penitentiary

for women located in Kitchener, Ontario, until my statutory release date in June of 2017.

After losing everything, I was at an extremely low point in my life and did not think I would ever return to academia. After a few months at GVI, I enrolled in the *Walls to Bridges Collective,* a prison education program which brought students from Wilfrid Laurier University to study with incarcerated students inside the prison for a semester-long, for-credit university course. Joining this program completely changed my life! My involvement with the collective made prison more bearable and helped me to find a source of meaning in my life. It was through this program that I learned that the Department of Criminology was open to admitting someone with a criminal record and later discovered that my time in prison was considered an asset in this field.

While in prison, I witnessed a stream of human rights abuses, and as someone who values social justice and equity for marginalized groups, I decided to use my lived experience of prison as the basis for my doctoral thesis research. I began my PhD in criminology at Ottawa in September 2018. I currently hold a Social Sciences and Humanities Research Council doctoral fellowship that is funding my dissertation research on the strengths and resiliency of criminalized women. I share my experiences of the legal system to advocate for the rights and dignity of prisoners and criminalized people.

Source: Rachel Fayter, personal communication, May 11, 2021.

with psychosocial issues related to confinement and isolation (Beckett et al., 2003; HRW, 2012). Older forensic clients experience both physical and mental healthcare needs that set them apart from their younger counterparts, as well as those typical age-related problems experienced by their nonincarcerated peers. Common concerns evident in this population include cardiovascular diseases, pulmonary disorders, diabetes, arthritis, and cancer. Common mental health risks include stress, social isolation, major depressive disorder, alcohol use disorder, suicide, and, increasingly, neurocognitive disorders such as Alzheimer disease and other dementias (HRW, 2012; OCI, 2016). In short, those 50 years and older generally present with a high burden of disease.

In 2010, the Alzheimer Society of Canada predicted a "rising tide" of dementia within the general Canadian population in the coming years. Such increases in the general population will be felt by forensic and correctional authorities alike, given that many older incarcerated persons may be at risk for developing dementia while incarcerated (Gaston, 2018). Peacock and colleagues (2019) conducted an integrative review to synthesize the literature regarding the health and social care needs of older persons living in correctional facilities. Based on the articles reviewed, key findings included: (a) dementia was a concern for correctional populations, the need for dementia screening and programming for older persons, and recommendations for improved screening and care practices. Nurses who work in correctional settings in particular have opportunities to demonstrate leadership, collaborate with community-based interdisciplinary agencies, and advocate for improved services for older adults who are imprisoned (Peacock et al., 2018).

The healthcare needs of those under forensic purview clearly challenge traditional forensic and correctional resources and budgets, and questions related to the ability of these facilities to adequately care for older forensic clients are real (Beckett et al., 2003; HRW, 2012). Increasing numbers of older and infirm forensic clients face the grim possibility of dying while confined. Although **compassionate release** to community-based long-term care facilities, known in Canada as *Royal Prerogative of Mercy*, or parole by exception, is allowed under the Corrections and Conditional Release Act, ongoing fears about community safety, bed shortages in long-term care facilities, and the stigma surrounding the circumstances of the forensic client's hospitalization or incarceration are considered on an individual basis (Beckett et al., 2003; HRW, 2012). This option, however, is available to only a very few long-term and infirm forensic clients. In 2014–2015, the Parole Board of Canada denied all 28 formal requests (OCI, 2016). While accessing the numbers released from corrections for compassionate reasons are not readily accessible, it is known that during the pandemic, 12 parole by exception cases were granted in early 2020, and an additional 11 cases were

under review and pending decisions (Mahboob, 2020). While the Office of the Correctional Investigator continues to advocate for parole by exception for clients with terminal illnesses, the Office continues to express concern over how Medical Assistance in Dying (MAiD) is currently implemented in Canadian Prisons. Specifically, "the decision to seek MAiD is best made in the community, by parolees not inmates. Canada's correctional authority should not be seen to be involved in enabling or facilitating any king of death behind bars" (OCI, 2020, p. 4).

As a result, palliative care within forensic settings is a poignant reality. Meeting the needs of terminally ill forensic clients within secure environments is a time-consuming, resource-intensive, exhaustive effort fraught with perplexing moral dilemmas not commonly encountered in traditional healthcare settings (Stone et al., 2012). In many secure environments, in the United States in particular, the implementation of palliative care programming is accomplished through the use of prisoner/inmate caregivers under the supervision of forensic nurses (Loeb et al., 2013). To date, this approach to palliative care within correctional environments has not been adopted in Canada. Instead, nurses and other healthcare professionals grapple with the complex issues facing dying prisoners, in an effort to provide them with a "good death" (Burles et al., 2016).

The Youth Forensic Client

The Youth Criminal Justice Act, introduced in 2003, governs youth aged 12 to 17 who come into conflict with the law (Statistics Canada, 2009). As a group, youth under forensic purview are a vastly underserved population with greater than average mental health and substance use care needs, and because of this, they are particularly vulnerable to adverse outcomes (Vingilis et al., 2020). Studies consistently show that rates of anxiety disorders, attention deficit hyperactivity disorder (ADHD), depression, and substance use disorders are higher among youth in custody when compared with youth in the general population. Frequently, their behavioural problems associated with their criminal charges mask their overall healthcare needs and thwart treatment efforts. It is not uncommon for youth who find themselves in custody to experience symptoms consistent with a wide array of mental health disorders, even though they may not have a formal diagnosis as such. Additionally, youth frequently demonstrate health patterns related to their familial environments, because their families commonly struggle with mental and physical health problems and substance use issues, and present with criminal histories and records (Shelton & Pearson, 2005).

In Canada, in 2018–2019, the majority of youth (72%) entered correctional services under community supervision, whereas the number of youth admissions to correctional facilities totalled 14,578, a 15% decrease compared with 2017–2018. However, Indigenous youth continue to be disproportionately represented in the Canadian criminal justice system. In 2018, Indigenous youth only represented 8.8% of the youth population in Canada, yet represented 43% of youth admissions to correctional services in 2018–2019 (Malakieh, 2020). The statistics for overrepresentation of Indigenous youth are even more startling for female youths, who accounted for 60% of all female admissions to provincial and territorial correctional systems (Clark, 2019). High rates of foetal alcohol spectrum disorder (FASD), significant substance use issues, suicidal ideation, self-harm, histories of attempted suicide, and high rates of physical, sexual, and emotional abuse affect a large portion of the youth involved with a child protection agency at the time of their admission (Latimer & Foss, 2004). In a systematic literature review of FASD within correctional systems, Popova and colleagues (2011) concluded that individuals with FASD have a 19-fold greater risk of being incarcerated.

Appropriate assessment and rehabilitative accommodations for this group are necessary, given the cognitive disabilities associated with FASD. Tragically, most forensic nurses will come into contact with youth through the criminal justice system because very few hospitals are set up to deal with the complexity of needs experienced by youth who come into conflict with the law. However, confinement in and of itself will not facilitate improvement in the mental health of this vulnerable group. Efforts targeting prevention of mental health problems through the provision of services, treatments, and supports in the community are emphasized by the MHCC (2016), particularly when working with youth. Such initiatives are seen as an investment for the future and may prevent at-risk youth from involvement with the criminal justice system. Finally, intersectoral approaches that bring together justice, law, social services, education, and health care are necessary to address the complexity of issues facing at-risk youth. Forensic nurses are ideally situated to meet the needs of this group through engagement in interprofessional and intersectoral collaborations.

The Transgender Forensic Client

Correctional authorities throughout Canada have been challenged regarding the treatment, management, and housing of transgender persons. In 2015, provincial corrections in Ontario became the first jurisdiction in Canada to accommodate transgender persons based upon their self-identified gender, name, and pronouns, as well as their housing preference (Ontario Ministry of the Solicitor General, 2021). It is well understood that transgender persons are particularly vulnerable in prison because they are subjected to violence, bullying, sexual assault, and other forms of harassment, particularly if their housing placement is not compatible

with their gender identity or their gender expression. However, placing transgender females in women's correctional institutions is not without operational challenges, given that many females who are incarcerated have experienced trauma and sexual and physical violence (OCI, 2019). Additionally, males who are incarcerated may attempt to manipulate the system for their own personal gain. Such manoeuvring, although not a sizable problem, cannot be ruled out completely, whether in correctional systems or in secure FMH systems (Richards & Barrett, 2021). Within correctional systems, there are operational challenges that need to be addressed. For example, access to clothing, personal items, and private showers and toilets (Ontario Ministry of the Solicitor General, 2021); the need for enhanced security practices; concerns about searches (frisks and strip searches when necessary); and plans to safely integrate a transgender person into the environment are all necessary because social isolation and exclusion can affect the person's mental health and wellbeing (OCI, 2019). Forensic nurses working with transgender clients need to approach their work with respect, substantive knowledge, and sensitivity; in doing so they can be role models for others who may be "stuck in conventional attitudes and assumptions" (OCI, 2017, p. 17).

Culturally Diverse Clients

The ethnic diversity of Canada as a whole is reflected in the demographic profile of Canadian forensic facilities. However, as might be predicted, clients representing ethnic and racial minorities are disproportionately represented, particularly in correctional facilities. Ricciardelli and colleagues (2021) have observed that within criminalized populations, racial disparities have continually increased over the past 15 years. Federally sentenced visible minorities continue to be represented by Indigenous, Black, Asian, and other racialized groups, including foreign-born persons; comparable figures for hospitalization in forensic settings operated by the healthcare system are not readily available.

Indigenous People make up approximately 5% of Canada's adult population, but in 2020, the number of Indigenous incarcerated persons reached a new "historic high" surpassing the 30% mark, during a time when the overall federal incarcerated population declined (OCI, 2020). Overrepresentation of Indigenous persons within the criminal justice system is attributed to a number of complex factors related to the effects of colonization, assimilation, intergenerational trauma, cultural oppression, systemic discrimination, and cultural and socioeconomic marginalization, resulting in high rates of poverty, substance use, and victimization within families and communities of origin (Clark, 2019; Department of Justice, 2021). There has been a growing awareness among the health care and criminal justice systems of the need to provide culturally sensitive and appropriate programming. In the past, programs were developed on the assumption of sameness; this approach not only negated the forensic client's ethnic identity and culture of origin but also created barriers in the formation of therapeutic relationships and treatment programs, which ultimately interfered with successful community rehabilitation.

Families

In recent years, the needs of family members, the "forgotten clients" (Goldkuhle, 1999), have necessitated expanded roles for forensic nurses and community-based partnerships. Incarceration is a "family affair," and family members, children, and friends represent a hidden forensic population; they are not accounted for, and they are rarely discussed by policy makers or health service providers. Incarceration gives rise to family instability, as seen in unintended higher rates of female-headed households, family disruption, family breakup, forced kinship care, and foster care (Cooke, 2014). Young children can experience cognitive, mental, and behavioural problems that negatively affect their ability to learn; youth may forego personal health care, engage in risky behaviours, experiment with illicit substances, drop out of school, or experience early parenthood (Gifford, 2019).

Women whose partners are incarcerated are often raising children who are also at risk for early and repeated incarceration. The legacy of family violence is profound. Family members have often experienced various types of violence (e.g., child abuse, intimate partner violence, elder abuse), and children in particular are more likely to experience physical, emotional, and cognitive problems and engage in self-destructive patterns that increase their likelihood of spending time within the forensic system (i.e., prisons) when compared with children of nonincarcerated parents (Cooke, 2014).

All too often, forensic nurses assess their clients in isolation from their support systems, home environments, and daily routines, which is particularly problematic. Creating a forensic family genogram is helpful when working with forensic clients (Kent-Wilkinson, 1999). A genogram is both an assessment and an intervention tool, one that can assist nurses in identifying individual and family patterns (e.g., mental health history, criminal behaviour, substance abuse) and contribute to more comprehensive assessments, interventions, and appropriate community referrals for family members (see Chapter 16 for information regarding genograms).

Collaborating with family members is critical to the safe reintegration of the forensic client into the community. Gaining a more holistic understanding of the family may provide opportunities to enhance psychosocial interventions and contribute to family stability (Cooke, 2014). Working more closely with families is a role that is increasingly being embraced by forensic nurses,

particularly those affiliated with community-based FMH programs. Many factors affect the forensic client's care in, and readjustment to, the community, including family dynamics, stress, and the family's degree of involvement. Family members can be profoundly impacted by the offence. They receive little support and frequently experience shame and stigma (Pierce, 2011), in addition to guilt and remorse regarding the forensic client's criminal acts. In some cases, the behaviours of family members can sabotage treatment and reintegration plans, and nursing staff members often bear the brunt of sarcasm and hostility (Encinares & Golea, 2005).

Nurse–Client Relationship

Nursing by its very nature is relational; it is through the nurse–client relationship that nurses gain a deeper understanding and appreciation of the human condition. In fact, the ability to establish and maintain a therapeutic relationship with a forensic client is among the most important competencies required by forensic nurses (Peternelj-Taylor, 2002, 2004, 2012). In the forensic milieu, the emphasis of the therapeutic relationship as a primary intervention strategy is dependent on how the nurse's role is defined and on the context of the setting in which nursing practice takes place. For example, for forensic nurses practising in an inpatient forensic psychiatric unit, working in a sex offender treatment program, or counselling HIV-positive clients in a prison setting, the therapeutic relationship is fundamental to the identification and resolution of problems. In other areas of forensic nursing practice (e.g., an ambulatory care clinic in a correctional facility), the therapeutic relationship may be more in the background. Regardless of the setting or the nature of the relationship, it cannot be assumed that a therapeutic relationship will be present simply by virtue of one's nursing role (Peternelj-Taylor, 2004; Schafer & Peternelj-Taylor, 2003).

Engagement in a therapeutic relationship can be especially difficult for nurses when the client is accused (or convicted) of committing a morally reprehensible act; such a client may "evoke feelings of disgust, repulsion, and fear" (Jacob et al., 2009, p. 153). Clients may engage in threatening behaviours, break rules, and test boundaries, and they are often unappreciative of nurses' efforts in providing health care. Nurses, as members of society, are not immune to prevailing attitudes, beliefs, and stereotypes, and these may negatively colour their perceptions, therapeutic responses, and professional roles with forensic clients. The belief that every client has the potential to change and the right to treatment is one not shared by all forensic nurses (Peternelj-Taylor & Johnson, 1995). Martin (2001) warns that nurses "need to be cautious that their approach to patients does not reinforce the stigma and discrimination of the wider community" (p. 29).

To be successful, forensic nurses need to explore honestly and candidly their own preconceived ideas, attitudes, feelings, beliefs, and stereotypes regarding forensic clients. All too often, nurses can get caught up in the sensationalism that surrounds a particular forensic client (often fuelled by media hype), or the setting in which practice takes place, and ultimately, they can lose sight of the person in need of care. Furthermore, it is not uncommon for nurses who are employed in forensic settings to experience additional stressors unique to their work, which ultimately affects their ability to establish and maintain therapeutic relationships with the clients in their care. Some examples are issues related to personal safety (i.e., threat of violence by forensic clients) (Jacob et al., 2009), moral distress (Smith et al., 2021), understaffing (Cyr & Paradis, 2012), vicarious trauma (Newman et al., 2019), threats to professional identity (Goddard et al., 2019), and competing and conflicting expectations held between health care and correctional authorities (Lazzaretto-Green et al., 2011). Hammarström and colleagues (2019), in a study that addressed nurses' lived experiences in caring for clients in forensic psychiatry, concluded that strategies such as self-reflection, emotional regulation, and distancing when necessary may enable nurses to empathize with clients experiences and respond appropriately.

Common Relationship Issues Experienced by Forensic Nurses

Although barriers to therapeutic relationships can be found in all areas of nursing, it is the "special circumstance" (Austin, 2001) of forensic settings, where the moral climate is shaped by the divergent and competing demands for custody and caring, that contributes to forensic settings being described as "hotbeds" for potential problems. This is in part due to the complexity of healthcare needs experienced by forensic clients, the seductive pull of helping and the intensity of relationships that can develop, the professional isolation experienced by forensic nurses, and the cultural and philosophical differences that exist between forensic clients, forensic nurses, and other members of the treatment team (Cooke et al., 2019; Lazzaretto-Green et al., 2011; Schafer & Peternelj-Taylor, 2003). Forensic nurses, like all nurses, are moral agents, and as such, they are responsible for practising ethically with the clients in their care, regardless of the setting in which care is provided.

Othering

It is within these habitats of special circumstance that nurses meet forensic clients, and how the client is perceived is often illustrated by the language in which nurses frame their care. For example, are the clients seen as inmates, cons, psychopaths, murderers, psychos, or borderlines? Such labels not only evoke stereotypical images but, more importantly, cast the individual into the role of the "other," as illustrated in their verbal discourse and articulated in their written discourse

through their charting and documentation (Peternelj-Taylor, 2004). Such negative forms of engagement, known as *exclusionary othering*, can affect all aspects of nursing care and promote marginalization, stigmatization, and underinvolvement in a client's care (Canales, 2000, 2010). In a recent study utilizing a retrospective chart review, Martin and colleagues (2020) examined the style of documentation utilized by FMH nurses and found many negative themes in the documentation that discounted, pathologized, or paternalized the clients that the nurses were caring for. Such documentation can negatively influence and bias the perspectives of other staff members and affect the quality of care that is provided. *Inclusionary othering* on the other hand is promoted as a way of learning about the other as an individual and not simply as a crime or a label. Although this may be a tall order when working with forensic clients, nurses can learn about othering by gaining an appreciation for what it means to be othered (Canales, 2000, 2010). One way of coming to know the forensic client is through role-taking and trying to understand the world from the client's perspective, and to see the person and their crimes within their life as a whole, and within the context of forensic psychiatric care (Hörberg, 2018).

Forensic environments, by their very nature, contribute to what Jacob and colleagues (2021) refer to as structural othering, given the organizational culture, restrictive environments, and institutional policies and practices that historically have influenced how nurses engage in the nurse–client relationship. In forensic settings, exclusionary othering prevails, thereby limiting nurses' ability to engage in approaches that would facilitate inclusionary othering.

KEY CONCEPT

Othering is about the way one perceives and engages with another person. It can be exclusionary and negative (i.e., the other is different from and thus "less than" me) or inclusionary, tolerant, and accepting (i.e., the other is different from me, so I need to learn about his or her world view).

Boundary Violations

The complexities and uncertainties surrounding boundaries and **boundary violations** in practice can be difficult for forensic nurses to manage and lead to ongoing confusion in practice. The inability to differentiate the professional relationship from a social relationship by attempting to have one's personal needs met through the nurse–client relationship is consistently discussed as a precursor to boundary violations in the nursing literature (Peternelj-Taylor, 2012; Peternelj-Taylor & Schafer, 2008; Pilette et al., 1995. See Chapter 7. In forensic settings, nurses are often warned about getting "too close" to their patients while at the same time painted as "victims of circumstances" when boundaries are transgressed with a forensic client. However, it is important to remember that, from an ethical perspective, the nurse is the one responsible for managing boundaries within the nurse–client relationship, not the client. Mixed messages regarding treatment boundaries can be especially disconcerting for forensic clients, who frequently have problems with boundaries in general. Forensic healthcare professionals, including nurses, are most vulnerable to transgressing boundaries when they are experiencing major life stressors in their personal lives, such as changing life circumstances, relationship problems, bereavement, or personal caregiving responsibilities. During such times, they are also at risk of being "targeted" by forensic clients who are looking to exploit the therapeutic relationship for personal gain (Cooke et al., 2019; Faulkner & Regehr, 2011; Peternelj-Taylor, 2012).

Manipulation

The potential for manipulation is a very real factor in secure environments, one that requires thoughtful consideration by nurses in the provision of nursing care. As Austin (2001) notes, "cautioning, skepticism, and the questioning of patients' motives and actions are part of the daily experience of forensic nurses" (p. 13). Forensic clients can be powerful, dominant, intimidating, needy, charming, good-looking, and attentive, leading Gutheil and Brodsky (2008) to conclude that even the most ethical clinician can be tested by the manipulative behaviours of forensic clients. In some cases, individuals in forensic settings will attempt to manipulate or intimidate healthcare staff for some secondary gain, for example, additional medication or extra comfort items (blankets, pillows). Such items are often used to trade and barter with other incarcerated persons. Forensic clients may also engage in manipulative behaviours as a form of social diversion, which may lead to escape from the prison environment, and issues pertaining to safety cannot be ignored (Peternelj-Taylor, 2004; Smith et al., 2021).

Jacob (2014) notes that "the fact that patients are conceptualized as being con artists and manipulators inevitably affects the way care is delivered" (p. 50). When a forensic client is labelled a manipulator, nurses and others generally respond more punitively and fail to engage the client in a therapeutic dialogue surrounding the meaning of their behaviours; in such cases, the opportunity for mutual problem-solving around the manipulative behaviours is lost in the relationship (Peternelj-Taylor, 2004). To be successful, forensic nurses need to be astutely aware that there exists the potential for manipulation in all interactions with forensic clients, while simultaneously adhering to their professional responsibilities embedded within the therapeutic nurse–client relationship. In short, they have to negotiate the path between assuming the worst and recognizing that it can always happen (Schoenly, 2013; Smith et al., 2021).

KEY CONCEPT

Manipulation is a concern in secure environments because it can involve the use of deceit to reach a goal that could not be pursued openly (e.g., escape).

Professional Role Development

Historically, role development for forensic nurses has been difficult, owing to the myth that nurses who work with forensic clients are "second-class nurses" unable to secure employment elsewhere (Peternelj-Taylor & Johnson, 1995). Harris (2013) reported that the stigma experienced by FMH nurses impacted negatively on their adaptation to their professional roles. During this time of a global nursing shortage, recruitment and retention of forensic nurses can be particularly challenging for FMH and correctional administrators (Oates et al., 2020). Given the broad scope of forensic nursing as illustrated within this chapter, it should be evident that forensic nurses are highly skilled and knowledgeable professionals, committed to the health and wellbeing of the clients in their charge, as well as the community at large.

Professional Nursing Identity

The role of nurses as moral agents in their work with persons under forensic purview is one of the greatest challenges that nurses experience when working in forensic environments. Remaining true to their professional nursing roles and avoiding being seduced or co-opted into assuming custodial roles, where expectations and responsibilities seem more clearly defined, can be especially challenging, particularly when working in correctional facilities (Holmes, 2007; Peternelj-Taylor & Johnson, 1995; Smith, 2005). Tensions that exist between custody and caring in forensic environments make it "difficult to maintain the therapeutic culture known to nurses" (Jacob, 2014, p. 48). In forensic settings operated by the criminal justice system, forensic nurses must have a strong nursing identity in order to maintain their professional authority and responsibility, without succumbing to the temptation to align themselves with the correctional staff. However, forensic nurses who work within the healthcare system should also heed this lesson, for they too can assume a more custodial stance, especially when they believe that CTOs or dispositions in hospital are lenient forms of punishment. Thus, even when the care of forensic clients is the responsibility of the healthcare system, incongruent attitudes among healthcare staff may prevail. Lawson (2005) states that when we "set ourselves up as judge and jury" (p. 149), we minimize our ability to be therapeutic.

Professional Development for Forensic Nurses

In 1981, Petryshen published a classic paper entitled "Nursing the Mentally Disordered Offender." Since then, forensic nursing in Canada has undergone significant transformations in education, research, and practice developments related to the provision of nursing care to forensic clients.

Education

Forensic nursing content is slowly finding its way into undergraduate and graduate nursing curricula across the country, primarily through existing courses in psychiatric mental health or community health nursing. For example, the College of Nursing, University of Saskatchewan, offers an online senior elective nursing course entitled *Forensic Nursing in Secure Environments* in its undergraduate baccalaureate program, and students completing mental health clinicals have opportunities for clinical placements in both FMH settings and correctional environments. Terblance and Reimer-Kirkham (2020) discuss the unique opportunities that clinical placements in correctional environments offer undergraduate nursing students in both mental health and community health, emphasizing social justice, restorative justice, and the impact of poverty and marginalization on health. Given the complexity of healthcare challenges experienced by criminal justice–involved persons, secure forensic and correctional environments provide a fertile climate for educational experiences for undergraduate and graduate students (Peternelj-Taylor, 2020). Furthermore, continuing professional development for nurses who practise in forensic settings is also critical because it reinforces the therapeutic identity of nurses, assists with nursing policy development, and contributes to recruitment and retention in this specialized area of practice (Woods & Peternelj-Taylor, 2022).

Research

Embracing a research agenda in forensic nursing will guide nursing practice in this highly specialized area; provide new insights into primary, secondary, and tertiary health care (including recovery and reintegration into the community); and contribute to nursing science through the advancement of nursing knowledge regarding vulnerable populations in general (Peternelj-Taylor, 2005). Two research developments in this specialized area of practice include (a) the University of Ottawa's Research Chair in Forensic Nursing, established in 2009 to foster the development and dissemination of forensic nursing research and promote graduate student training, and (b) the Centre for Behavioural Science and Justice Studies, established in 2011, as an interdisciplinary collaboration between the University of Saskatchewan, the Correctional Service Canada, and the Saskatchewan Ministry of Justice–Corrections and Policing.

Recognizing the limited research conducted in Canada, regarding criminal justice–involved persons, Kouyoumdjian and colleagues (2016b, p. 1), utilizing a Delphi process, delineated a 10-year agenda for prison health research in Canada. Seven research priorities were identified:

- Diversion from and alternatives to incarceration
- Social and community reintegration
- Creating healthy environments in prisons
- Health care in custody
- Continuity of health care
- Substance use disorders
- Indigenous health

Nurses represent the largest group of healthcare professionals working with criminal justice–involved persons and are ideally situated to engage in research endeavours with colleagues interested in this distinctive environment. Studies addressing the health of clients under forensic purview, research regarding FMH and correctional healthcare systems, and advocacy projects are fundamental to the advancement of forensic nursing as a specialty and will contribute to evidence-based care for those under forensic purview.

Practice Developments

Forensic nurses may find guidance in the Canadian Federation of Mental Health Nurses' (2014) *Canadian Standards for Psychiatric–Mental Health Nursing*; however, standards to guide the unique needs of Canadian FMH nurses are nonexistent. Recognizing the need to build upon traditional mental health standards when working with persons under forensic purview, Martin and colleagues (2013) developed 16 standards to guide education, practice, and research in FMH nursing. Although written from an Australian perspective, these standards could easily cross international jurisdictions, as they capture the essence of FMH nursing in caring for clients under forensic purview. Furthermore, Canadian Correctional Nursing Standards are nonexistent, and nurses are expected to follow their provincial or territorial standards for nursing practice, which are generic in nature, and do not take into consideration the contextual nature of nursing practice with clients under forensic purview within correctional environments. Given these circumstances, Canadian correctional nurses have often turned to *Correctional Nursing: Scope and Standards for Practice*, published by the American Nurses Association (2021), to guide their correctional nursing practice.

In September 2006, the Canadian Forensic Nurses Association was formally organized by forensic nurses from across Canada to address the forensic nursing issues unique to Canada. The mission of the Association is "to promote trauma-informed, patient-centered, and evidence-based forensic nursing practice in Canada." Although this organization seeks to represent all forensic disciplines, most of the members work with victims of violence (e.g., those experiencing sexual assault, intimate partner violence).

Treatment Setting

Unlike more traditional practice settings, the interpersonal climate, organizational culture, and social context of FMH and correctional settings result in such environments being identified as among the most severe and extreme environments known to society. Power, control, and implicit authority are manifested in the physical and interpersonal environments of both correctional systems and mental healthcare systems and can be incompatible with the achievement of treatment goals (Austin, 2001; Holmes, 2005). Researchers have identified threats to professional identity, tensions between clinicians and correctional staff, and ethical and moral dilemmas common to the forensic and correctional milieu as particularly challenging (Simon et al., 2020; Smith et al., 2021).

Security Awareness

When working with forensic clients, issues surrounding safety and security are considered critical competencies, and nurses often struggle to find the right balance between their caring and custodial roles. The therapeutic treatment needs of their clients must always be considered within the context of maintaining security. Forensic settings (apart from community-based programs) are typically highly controlled environments, with the whereabouts of clients constantly monitored through a variety of institutional routines, mechanisms, rules, and regulations (Austin, 2001; Peternelj-Taylor & Johnson, 1995). Surveillance of staff and clients is deemed critical to the safe operation of all forensic facilities. Because of this, however, nursing staff members often experience additional stressors because they too are subject to the judgment of others: those who watch over are watched over in turn (Holmes, 2005).

Forensic nurses quickly become aware of three forms of security awareness: **static security** or physical security, dynamic or procedural security, and therapeutic and relational security (Quality Network for Forensic Mental Health Services [QNFMHS], 2015) (see Web Links). Static security awareness includes such things as the structural or environmental artifacts common to secure environments, for example, the use of two-way radios, personal protection alarms, video monitoring, electronic door locks, internal barriers, and perimeter fences or walls. **Dynamic security awareness**, on the other hand, is concerned with institutional policies, staffing patterns, and methods of operation. **Relational security** is concerned with knowing the client within the context of the environment, and having professional, therapeutic, purposeful relationships, with understood limits (QNFMHS, 2015). Finding the right balance between the security needs of the forensic setting (and the community at large) and the client's treatment needs is a balancing act at best. Practical points for competent and safe practice are found in Box 35.4.

In forensic settings operated under the jurisdiction of the healthcare system (e.g., forensic psychiatric hospitals

---

BOX 35.4 Tips for Security Awareness in Forensic Settings

- When working in institutional settings, never bring anything in or take anything out for a client, regardless of how insignificant the request may seem.
- Let coworkers know your whereabouts at all times; interview clients in designated interview rooms or in places visible to other staff members.
- When you are out working in the community, a "buddy system" is recommended. If you can't have a colleague accompany you, always share your itinerary, the anticipated length of your visits, and how you can be reached with a trusted colleague or manager.
- Observe policies and procedures related to security awareness specific to the forensic setting in which you are working. Ask questions in order to understand the rationale behind the policies.

- Do not share personal information about yourself, or other staff members, with clients.
- Clients may engage in sexually inappropriate banter or gestures. Report this immediately, no matter how embarrassed you may be.
- Be aware of the location of staff members in relation to clients. Use a buddy system (e.g., another staff member) when uncomfortable approaching a client, especially when entering the client's living space.
- Be alert for colleagues who may be struggling with managing professional boundaries, and make a point of discussing boundary maintenance on a regular basis during team meetings.
- In all cases, open communication is critical to safe and competent nursing practice. Report all suspicious behaviours as soon as possible.

and FMH units), forensic nurses assume broader roles in the maintenance of security. This can be particularly disconcerting because they may be expected to handcuff clients before a court visit or search them for contraband before and after personal visits (or absences from the unit) while at the same time engage them in a therapeutic nurse–client relationship. This overt attention to custodial roles can jeopardize the fragility of the developing therapeutic relationship, and systems often need to be in place that enable nurses from other units, or those not responsible for direct nursing care, to assist with these necessary custodial measures.

Risk Assessment and Management

Nurses practising in forensic settings work with clients with a proven capacity for violence. In recent years, risk assessment and management have become increasingly important competencies required of forensic nurses. Risk assessment is critical because it guides intervention and treatment. Simply stated, the greater the assessed risk, the higher the levels of intervention and supervision that are required; conversely, the lower the assessed risk, the lower the levels of intervention and supervision that are required, regardless of whether the forensic client is seeking treatment within a secure environment or a community treatment program (Woods, 2013). Although a detailed discussion of risk assessment and management is beyond the scope of this chapter, it is mentioned here because increasingly, forensic nurses, with additional training and experience, are using actuarial (or statistical) tools and structured clinical judgment to formulate treatment plans that increasingly include risk assessment and management (see Chapter 19). In an earlier review of the literature, Woods and Lasiuk (2008) concluded that forensic nurses should integrate the use of empirically guided approaches to risk, including actuarial measures and structured clinical approaches, along with their own subjective qualitative clinical assessments. However, reliance on clinical judgment alone, as noted in some settings, warrants further education and training in practice (Woods, 2013). More recently Maguire and colleagues (2018) found that when structured risk assessments were used, there was a greater likelihood of intervention, thereby emphasizing the importance of early intervention using the least restrictive measures.

Societal Norms

Humane care is defined by society, including the public, politicians, and the media. The continual expansion of correctional facilities, however, reveals society's failure to address complex health and social issues. For many, an attitude of "lock the door and throw away the key" prevails. There is a societal expectation that imprisonment will deter others from committing crimes, as well

as contribute to community safety. This can mean that prisons are more readily funded than other strategies to deal with poverty, homelessness, and mental illness. The impact of interpersonal violence and illicit drug-related activities on individuals and communities is not sufficiently addressed, nor is the limited healthcare services available to vulnerable and marginalized groups. Finally, attention must be paid to the Truth and Reconciliation Commission of Canada's (2015) recommendations regarding justice, in particular Recommendations 30 and 31 (see Box 35.5).

Understanding the comprehensive needs of individuals whose lives have become enmeshed within the criminal justice system requires an understanding of both the individual and the social determinants of health that are associated with mental health, mental illness, and criminal activity. Such an understanding provides for greater opportunities for the development of interventions and policies that may be effective at promoting mental health, preventing crime, and reducing the risk of repeat offending among those with a mental illness. Forensic nursing is uniquely positioned to intervene with the socially significant health issues associated with crime, incarceration, and release. Hospitalization and incarceration alike provide opportunities for effective mental health interventions that have the potential for secondary gains, such as improving public safety, decreasing healthcare costs, and decreasing recidivism (Kouyoumdjian et al., 2016a). Such interventions must be grounded in the conviction that caring for persons under forensic purview as vulnerable members of society is the appropriate and decent thing to do.

BOX 35.5 Truth and Reconciliation Commission of Canada: Calls to Action 30 and 31:

30. We call upon federal, provincial, and territorial governments to commit to eliminating the overrepresentation of Aboriginal people in custody over the next decade, and to issue detailed annual reports that monitor and evaluate progress in doing so.

31. We call upon the federal, provincial, and territorial governments to provide sufficient and stable funding to implement and evaluate community sanctions that will provide realistic alternatives to imprisonment for Aboriginal offenders and respond to the underlying causes of offending.

Source: Truth and Reconciliation Commission of Canada. (2015). Calls to Action. https://www2.gov.bc.ca/assets/gov/british-columbians-our-governments/indigenous-people/aboriginal-peoples-documents/calls_to_action_english2.pdf

Summary of Key Points

- The provision of nursing care to persons under forensic purview is a challenging and rewarding psychiatric and mental health nursing experience, one that balances the conflicting convictions of custody and caring.
- Components of care in forensic nursing include the forensic client, nurse–client relationship, professional role development, treatment setting, and societal norms.
- The ability to engage the forensic client in a therapeutic relationship is critical to competent forensic nursing care. Relationship issues experienced by forensic nurses include othering, boundary violations, and manipulation.
- Forensic nurses are uniquely situated to provide nursing care to forensic clients in a variety of community- and institution-based treatment settings.
- Intersectoral and interprofessional approaches that bring together justice, law, social services, education, and health care are deemed necessary to address the multitude of issues facing forensic clients, their families, and their communities.

Thinking Challenges

The Canadian Nurses Association (2017) outlines ethical responsibilities for registered nurses in relation to professional boundaries. Specifically:

> Nurses maintain appropriate professional boundaries and ensure their relationships are always for the benefit of the person. They recognize the potential vulnerability of persons receiving care and do not exploit their trust and dependency in a way that might compromise the therapeutic relationship. They do not abuse their relationship for personal or financial gain and do not enter into personal relationships (romantic, sexual, or other) with persons receiving care (p. 13).

1. What factors impact the development of a therapeutic relationship with clients under forensic purview?

2. How would you approach a colleague you believed was struggling to maintain professional boundaries?
3. What advice would you give someone about how to maintain boundaries in a therapeutic relationship?
4. Nurses can be overinvolved or underinvolved with forensic clients. What is the impact of underinvolvement in the nurse–client relationship?

> Visit thePoint to view suggested responses.
> Go to thePoint.lww.com/activate and use the activation code found in the front of this text to unlock answers to the "Thinking Challenges" and other online resources.

 ## Web Links

http://www.bcmhsus.ca/about/news-stories/stories/what-does-it-mean-to-be-%E2%80%98not-criminally-responsible%E2%80%99-for-a-crime The BC Mental Health and Substance Use Services has a very informative report addressing "not criminally responsible" for a crime, complete with Q & A, myths, and a brief video.

www.caefs.ca The Canadian Association of Elizabeth Fry Societies is made up of 24 self-governing community-based societies from across Canada that work with, and for, criminalized women and gender-diverse persons, including defending prisoners' rights, building capacity, and raising awareness.

www.csc-scc.gc.ca The Correctional Service Canada (CSC) contributes to the protection of society by actively assisting offenders (with sentences of over 2 years) in institutions of various security levels, and supervising those under conditional release in the community to become law-abiding citizens while exercising safe, secure, and humane control. CSC's website is a resource for Canadian policy, legislation, and research.

https://www.canadianforensicnurse.org/ The Canadian Forensic Nurses Association, was formally organized in 2006, to provide a forum for Canadian forensic nurses to discuss evidence-based practice unique to the diverse areas of forensic nursing in Canada.

https://www.forensicnurses.org/ The International Association of Forensic Nurses (IAFN) brings together nurses whose practice interfaces in some way with the law. The mission of the IAFN is to provide leadership in forensic nursing practice by developing, promoting, and disseminating information internationally about forensic nursing science.

www.iafmhs.org The mandate of the International Association of Forensic Mental Health Services is to enhance the standards of FMH services within an international context, to promote an international dialogue about all aspects of FMH, including violence and family violence, and to promote education, training, and research in FMH.

www.health.uottawa.ca/forensic-research The University of Ottawa's Research Chair in Forensic Nursing was established to foster the development and dissemination of forensic nursing research at the interface of the health and criminal justice systems. Research undertaken serves to inform healthcare decisions relevant to incarcerated persons and victims of criminal acts.

www.johnhoward.ca The John Howard Society of Canada is an organization of provincial and territorial societies with branches and offices aimed at understanding and responding to problems of crime and the criminal justice system, through advocacy, public education, and crime prevention.

www.oci-bec.gc.ca The Office of the Correctional Investigator has the authority to act as an ombudsman for federal offenders. The primary function of the office is to investigate and bring resolution to individual offender complaints.

www.prisonersofage.com This website features photographs, interviews, and documentaries with older inmates and correctional personnel and provides a glimpse into their lives, crimes, and the challenges they experience.

https://cfbsjs.usask.ca/ The Centre for Behavioural Science and Justice Studies at the University of Saskatchewan strives to build effective and sustainable working relationships between academic researchers and criminal justice professionals in the nonprofit, government, and Indigenous sectors. Centre researchers, including interdisciplinary affiliated university faculty members, and graduate students make evaluative and research-based contributions to science that directly benefit the programs and services of policing, corrections, justice, and nongovernmental criminal justice agencies.

https://nursing.usask.ca/ Since 1989, the College of Nursing, University of Saskatchewan, in collaboration with the Regional Psychiatric Centre, CSC, has hosted a biennial international nursing conference showcasing innovations in practice, education, research, administration, and policy development in the fields of correctional health and forensic mental health care in Canada and abroad.

https://www.icn.ch/sites/default/files/inline-files/A13_Nurses_Role_Detainees_Prisoners.pdf Here you will find the International Council of Nurses Position Statement on Nurses' roles in the care of detainees and prisoners.

https://www.rcpsych.ac.uk/docs/default-source/improving-care/ccqi/quality-networks/secure-forensic/forensic-see-think-act-qnfmhs/sta_hndbk_2nded_web.pdf?sfvrsn=90e1fc26_4 Here you will find the second edition of *Your Guide to Relational Security—See, Think, Act,* designed specifically for people who work in secure mental health services. Understanding relational security is fundamental to safe practice in forensic environments. The booklet contains assessment and reflection tools and is illustrated with vignettes from practice.

http://wallstobridges.ca/what-we-do/ As per their website, Walls to Bridges is an educational program that brings together incarcerated and nonincarcerated students to study postsecondary courses in jails and prisons across Canada. The program started in 2011 as a partnership between Grand Valley Institution for Women located in Kitchener, Ontario and the Faculty of Social Work at Wilfred Laurier University.

References

Alzheimer Society of Canada. (2010). *Rising tide: The impact of dementia on Canadian society.* http://www.alzheimer.ca/en/Get-involved/Raise-your-voice/Rising-Tide

American Nurses Association. (2021). *Correctional nursing: Scope and standards of practice* (3rd ed.).

Austin, W. (2001). Relational ethics in forensic psychiatric settings. *Journal of Psychosocial Nursing and Mental Health Services, 39*(9), 12–17.

Beaudette, J. N., Power, J., & Stewart, L. A. (2015). *National prevalence of mental disorders among federally-sentenced men offenders* (Research Report, R-357). Correctional Service Canada.

Beckett, J., Peternelj-Taylor, C., & Johnson, R. (2003). Growing old in the correctional system. *Journal of Psychosocial Nursing and Mental Health Services, 41*(9), 12–18.

Blair-Lawton, D., Mordoch, E., & Chernomas, W. (2020). Putting on the same shoes: Lived experiences of women who are reincarcerated. *Journal of Forensic Nursing, 16*(2), 99–107. https://doi.org/10.1097/JFN.0000000000000276

Blanchette, K., & Brown, S. L. (2006). *The assessment and treatment of women offenders: An integrative perspective.* John Wiley & Sons.

Burles, M. C., Peternelj-Taylor, C., & Holtslander, L. (2016). A 'good death' for all? Examining issues for palliative care in correctional settings. *Mortality, 21*(2), 93–111. https://doi.org/10.1080/13576275.2015.1098602

Canadian Federation of Mental Health Nurses. (2014). *Canadian standards for psychiatric-mental health nursing* (4th ed.). https://www.cna-aiic.ca/~/media/cna/page-content/pdf-en/code-of-ethics-2017-edition-secure-interactive

Canadian Nurses Association. (2017). *Code of ethics for registered nurses.*

Canales, M. K. (2000). Othering: Toward an understanding of difference. *Advances in Nursing Science, 22*(4), 16–31. https://doi.org/10.1097/00012272-200006000-00003

Canales, M. K. (2010). Othering: Difference understood? A 10-year analysis and critique of the nursing literature. *Advances in Nursing Science, 33*, 15–34. https://doi.org/10.1097/ANS.0b013e3181c9e119

Centre for Addiction and Mental Health. (2020). *Mental health and criminal justice policy framework.* https://www.camh.ca/-/media/files/pdfs---public-policy-submissions/camh-cj-framework-2020-pdf.pdf

Chaimowitz, G. (2012). Position paper: The criminalization of people with mental illness. *Canadian Journal of Psychiatry, 57*(2), 1–6.

Clark, S. (2019). *Overrepresentation of Indigenous people in the Canadian Criminal Justice System: Causes and responses.* Research and Statistics Division, Department of Justice Canada. https://www.justice.gc.ca/eng/rp-pr/jr/oip-cjs/oip-cjs-en.pdf

Clarke, C., Lumbard, D., Sambrook, S., & Kerr, K. (2016). What does recovery mean to a forensic mental health patient? A systematic review and narrative synthesis of the qualitative literature. *Journal of Forensic Psychiatry and Psychology, 27*(1), 38–54. https://doi.org/10.1080/14789949.2015.1102311

Collingwood, E., Messina, A., Dam, A., Bernard, T., Cockburn, L., & Penney, S. (2021). Experiences of recovery for Canadian forensic mental health patients and staff participating in a horse stables program. *The Journal of Forensic Psychiatry & Psychology, 32*, 641–657. https://doi.org/10.1080/14789949.2021.1881582

Cooke, B. K., Hall, R. C. W., Hatters Friedman, S., Jain, A., & Wagoner, R. (2019). Professional boundaries in corrections. *Journal of the American Academy of Psychiatry and the Law, 47*(1) 91–98. https://doi.org/10.29158/JAAPL.003825-19

Cooke, C. L. (2014). Nearly invisible: The psychosocial and health needs of women with male partners in prison. *Issues in Mental Health Nursing, 35*, 979–982. https://doi.org/10.3109/01612840.2013.873103

Correctional Service Canada, Federal–Provincial/Territorial Partnership. (2012). *Mental health strategy for corrections in Canada.* http://www.csc-scc.gc.ca/health/092/MH-strategy-eng.pdf

Cyr, J. J., & Paradis, J. (2012). The forensic float nurse: A new concept in the effective management of service delivery in a forensic program. *Journal of Forensic Nursing, 8*(4), 188–194. https://doi.org/10.1111/j.1939-3938.2012.01145.x

de Chesnay, M. (2020). Vulnerable populations: Vulnerable people. In M. de Chesnay & B. A. Anderson (Eds.), *Caring for the vulnerable: Perspectives in nursing theory, practice and research* (5th ed., pp. 3–15). Jones & Bartlett.

Department of Justice. (2015). *The review board systems in Canada: An overview of results from the mentally disordered accused data collection study.* Government of Canada. https://www.justice.gc.ca/eng/rp-pr/csj-sjc/jsp-sjp/rr06_1/p1.html

Department of Justice. (2021). *Understanding the overrepresentation of indigenous people in the criminal justice system.* Government of Canada. https://www.justice.gc.ca/socjs-esjp/en/ind-aut/uo-cs

Drennan, G., & Alred, D. (2012). Recovery in forensic mental health settings. In G. Drennan & D. Alred (Eds.), *Secure recovery: Approaches to recovery in forensic mental health settings* (pp. 1–22). Routledge.

Dupuis, T., MacKay, R., & Nicol, J. (2013). *Current issues in mental health in Canada: Mental health and the criminal justice system.* Background Paper (Publication No. 2013-88-E). Library of Parliament.

Dvoskin, J. A., Knoll, J. L., & Silva, M. (2020). A brief history of the criminalization of mental illness. *CNS Spectrums, 25*(5), 638–650. https://doi.org/10.1017/S1092852920000103

Encinares, M., & Golea, G. (2005). Client centered-care for individuals with dual diagnoses in the justice system. *Journal of Psychosocial Nursing and Mental Health Services, 43*(9), 29–36.

Enggist, S., Møller, L., Galea, G., & Udesen, C. (2014). *Prisons and health.* World Health Organization. http://www.euro.who.int/__data/assets/pdf_file/0005/249188/Prisons-and-Health.pdf

Faulkner, C., & Regehr, C. (2011). Sexual boundary violations committed by female forensic workers. *Journal of the American Academy of Psychiatry and the Law, 39*, 154–163.

Gaston, S. (2018). Vulnerable prisoners: Dementia and the impact on prisoners, staff, and the correctional setting. *Collegian, 25*, 241–242.

Gifford, E. J. (2019). How incarceration affects the health of communities and families. *North Carolina Medical Journal, 80*(6), 372–375. https://doi.org/10.18043/ncm.80.6.372

Goddard, D., de Vries, K., McIntosh, T., & Theodosius, C. (2019). Prison nurses' professional identity. *Journal of Forensic Nursing, 15*, 163–171. https://doi.org/10.1097/JFN.0000000000000239

Goldkuhle, U. (1999). Professional education for correctional nurses: A community-based partnership model. *Journal of Psychosocial Nursing and Mental Health Services, 37*(9), 38–44.

Green, B. L., Miranda, J., Daroowalla, A., & Siddique, J. (2005). Trauma exposure, mental health functioning, and program needs of women in jail. *Crime and Delinquency, 51*, 133–151.

Gutheil, T. G., & Brodsky, A. (2008). *Preventing boundary violations in clinical practice.* Guilford Press.

Hammarström, L., Häggström, M., Devik, S. A., & Hellzen, O. (2019). Controlling emotions-nurses' lived experiences caring for patients in forensic psychiatry. *International Journal of Qualitative Studies on Health and Well-Being, 14*(1), 1–11. https://doi.org/10.1080/17482631.2019.1682911

Harris, D. M. (2013). Working in forensic mental health. In P. Callaghan, N. Oud, J. H. Bjørngaard, H. Nijman, T. Palmstierna, R. Almvik, & B. Thomas (Eds.), *Proceedings of the 8th European Congress on violence in clinical psychiatry* (pp. 395–398). Kavanah, Dwingeloo & Oud Consultancy.

Hayes, A. J., Burns, A., Turnbull, P., & Shaw, J. J. (2012). The health and social needs of older male prisoners. *International Journal of Geriatric Psychiatry, 27*, 1155–1162. https://doi.org/10.1002/gps.3761

Holmes, D. (2005). Governing the captives: Forensic psychiatric nursing in corrections. *Perspectives in Psychiatric Care, 41*(1), 3–13. https://doi.org/10.1111/j.0031-5990.2005.00007.x

Holmes, D. (2007). Nursing in corrections: Lessons from France. *Journal of Forensic Nursing, 3*(3–4), 126–131. https://doi.org/10.1111/j.1939-3938.2007.tb00098.x

Hörberg, U. (2018). 'The art of understanding in forensic psychiatric care'—From a caring science perspective based on a lifeworld approach. *Issues in Mental Health Nursing, 39*(9), 802–809. https://doi/org/10.1080/01612840.2018.1496499

Human Rights Watch. (2012). *Old behind bars: The aging prison population in the United States.* http://www.hrw.org/reports/2012/01/27/old-behind-bars-0

Jacob, J. D. (2014). Understanding the domestic rupture in forensic psychiatric nursing practice. *Journal of Correctional Health Care, 20*(1), 45–58. https://doi.org/10.1177/1078345813505444

Jacob, J. D., Gagnon, M., & Holmes, D. (2009). Nursing so-called monsters: On the importance of abjection and fear in forensic psychiatric nursing. *Journal of Forensic Nursing, 5*(3), 153–161. https://doi.org/10.1111/j.1939-3938.2009.01048.x

Jacob, J. D., Gagnon, M., Perron, A., & Canales, M. K. (2021). Revisiting the concept of othering: A structural analysis. *Advances in Nursing Science, 44*, 280–290. https://doi.org/10.1097/ANS.0000000000000353

Kanapaux, W. (2004). Guilty of mental illness. *Psychiatric Times, XXI*(1). http://www.psychiatrictimes.com/p040101a.html

Kent-Wilkinson, A. (1999). Forensic family genogram: An assessment and intervention tool. *Journal of Psychosocial Nursing and Mental Health Services, 37*(9), 52–56.

Kouyoumdjian, F., Schuler, A., Matheson, F., & Hwang, S. (2016a). Health status of prisoners in Canada. *Canadian Family Physician, 62*, 215–222.

Kouyoumdjian, F. G., Schuler, A., McIsaac, K. E., Pivnick, L., Matheson, F. I., Brown, G., Kiefer, L., Silva, D., & Hwang, S. W. (2016b). Using a Delphi process to define priorities for prison health research in Canada. *BMJ Open, 6*, e010125. http://doi.org/10.1136/bmjopen-2015-010125

Landess, J., & Holoyda, B. (2017). Mental health courts and forensic assertive community treatment teams as correctional diversion programs. *Behavioral Sciences & the Law, 35*(5–6), 501–511. https://doi.org/10.1002/bsl.2307

Latimer, J., & Foss, L. C. (2004). *A one-day snapshot of Aboriginal youth in custody across Canada: Phase II.* Department of Justice Canada. http://www.justice.gc.ca/eng/rp-pr/cj-jp/yj-jj/yj2-jj2/index.html

Lawson, L. (2005). Furthering the search for truth and justice. *Journal of Forensic Nursing, 1*(4), 149–150. https://doi.org/10.1111/j.1939-3938.2005.tb00036.x

Lazzaretto-Green, D., Austin, W., Goble, E., Buys, L., Gorman, T., & Rankel, M. (2011). Walking a fine line: Forensic mental health practitioners' experience of working with correctional officers. *Journal of Forensic Nursing, 7*(3), 109–119.

Livingston, J. D. (2016). What does success look like in the forensic mental health system? Perspectives of service users and service providers. *International Journal of Offender Therapy and Comparative Criminology, 62*, 1–21. http://doi.org/10.1177/0306624X16639973

Loeb, S. J., Hollenbeak, C. S., Penrod, J., Smith, C. A., Kitt-Lewis, E., & Crouse, S. B. (2013). Care and companionship in an isolating environment: Inmates attending to dying peers. *Journal of Forensic Nursing, 6*, 35–44.

Maguire, T., Daffern, M., Bowe, S. J., & McKenna, B. (2018). Risk assessment and subsequent nursing interventions in a forensic mental health inpatient setting: Associations and impact on aggressive behaviour.

Journal of Clinical Nursing, 27(5-6), e971–e983. https://doi.org/10.1111/jocn.14107

Mahboob, T. (2020). Compassionate release should be prioritized over MAID in Canadian prisons, says expert. *The Sunday Magazine.* https://www.cbc.ca/radio/sunday/the-sunday-magazine-for-november-15-2020-1.5801033/compassionate-release-should-be-prioritized-over-maid-in-canadian-prisons-says-expert-1.5801035

Malakieh, J. (2020). *Adult and youth correctional statistics in Canada, 2018/2019.* Statistics Canada (no. 85-002-X). https://www150.statcan.gc.ca/n1/pub/85-002-x/2020001/article/00016-eng.htm

Mangnall, J., & Yurkovich, E. (2010). A grounded theory exploration of deliberate self-harm in incarcerated women. *Journal of Forensic Nursing, 6*, 88–95. https://doi.org/10.1111/j.1939-3938.2010.01072.x

Martin, T. (2001). Something special: Forensic psychiatric nursing. *Journal of Psychiatric and Mental Health Nursing, 8*, 25–32. https://doi.org/10.1046/j.1365-2850.2001.00349.x

Martin, T., Maguire, T., Quinn, C., Ryan, J., Bawden, L., & Summers, M. (2013). Standards of practice for forensic mental health nurses: Identifying contemporary practice. *Journal of Forensic Nursing, 9*(3), 171–178. https://doi.org/10.1097/JFN.0b013e31827a593a

Martin, K., Ricciardelli, R., & Dror, I. (2020). How forensic mental health nurses' perspectives of their patients can bias healthcare: A qualitative review of nursing documentation. *Journal of Clinical Nursing, 29*(13-14), 2482–2494. https://doi.org/10.1111/jocn.15264

McKendy, L., Biro, S. M., Stanley, D., & Keown, L. A. (2019). Older offenders in custody: Overall trends. *Research in Brief, /RIB-19-03.* https://www.csc-scc.gc.ca/research/rib-19-03-en.shtml

McLoughlin, K. A., Geller, J. L., & Tolan, A. (2011). Is recovery possible in a forensic hospital setting? *Archives of Psychiatric Nursing, 25*(5), 390–391. https://doi.org/ 10.1016/j.apnu.2011.04.007

Mental Health Commission of Canada. (2012). *Changing directions, changing lives: The mental health strategy for Canada.* http://strategy.mentalhealthcommission.ca/pdf/strategy-text-en.pdf

Mental Health Commission of Canada. (2015). *Guidelines for recovery-oriented practice.*

Mental Health Commission of Canada. (2016). *The mental health strategy for Canada: A youth perspective.* https://www.mentalhealthcommission.ca/sites/default/files/2016-07/Youth_Strategy_Eng_2016.pdf

Mental Health Commission of Canada. (2020). *The mental health needs of justice involved persons: A rapid scoping review of the literature.* https://www.mentalhealthcommission.ca/sites/default/files/2021-01/Justice_Scoping_Review_eng.pdf

Newman, C., Eason, M., & Kinghorn, G. (2019). Incidence of vicarious trauma in correctional health and forensic mental health staff in New South Wales, Australia. *Journal of Forensic Nursing, 15*(3), 183–192. https://doi.org/10.1097/JFN.0000000000000245

Oates, J., Topping, A., Ezhova, I., Wadey, E., & Rafferty, A. M. (2020). An integrative review of nursing staff experiences in high secure forensic mental health settings: Implications for recruitment and retention strategies. *Journal of Advanced Nursing, 76*(11), 2897–2908. https://doi.org/10.1111/jan.14521

Office of the Correctional Investigator (OCI). (2015). *Annual report of the Office of the Correctional Investigator 2014–2015.* http://www.oci-bec.gc.ca/cnt/rpt/pdf/annrpt/annrpt20142015-eng.pdf

Office of the Correctional Investigator. (2016). *Annual report of the Office of the Correctional Investigator 2015–2016.* http://www.oci-bec.gc.ca/cnt/rpt/pdf/annrpt/annrpt20152016-eng.pdf

Office of the Correctional Investigator. (2017). *Annual report: Office of the Correctional Investigator 2016-2017.* https://www.oci-bec.gc.ca/cnt/rpt/pdf/annrpt/annrpt20162017-eng.pdf

Office of the Correctional Investigator. (2019). *Annual report of the Office of the Correctional Investigator 2018-2019.* https://www.oci-bec.gc.ca/cnt/rpt/pdf/annrpt/annrpt20182019-eng.pdf

Office of the Correctional Investigator. (2020). *Annual report: Office of the Correctional Investigator 2019-2020.* https://www.oci-bec.gc.ca/cnt/rpt/pdf/annrpt/annrpt20192020-eng.pdf

Olson, R. (2012). *Prison inmate suicide—Why it matters.* Centre for Suicide Prevention. http://suicideinfo.ca/Library/Resources/iEinfoExchange/iE8PrisonInmateSuicide.aspx

Ontario Ministry of the Solicitor General. (2021). *Transgender inmate management policy.* https://www.ontario.ca/page/transgender-inmate-management-policy

Owusu-Bempah, A., Jung, M., Sbaï, F., Wilton, A. S., & Kouyoumdjian, F. (2021). Race and incarceration: The representation and characteristics of Black people in provincial correctional facilities in Ontario, Canada. *Race and Justice.* Published online April 8, 2021, https://doi.org/10.1177/21533687211006461

Peacock, S., Burles, M., Hodson, A., Kumaran, M., MacRae, R., Peternelj-Taylor, C., & Holtslander, L. (2019). Older persons with dementia in prison: an integrative review. *International Journal of Prisoner Health,* *16*(1), 1–16. https://doi.org/10.1108/IJPH-01-2019-0007

Peacock, S., Hodson, A., MacRae, R., & Peternelj-Taylor, C. (2018). Living with dementia in correctional settings: A case report. *Journal of Forensic Nursing, 14(*3), 180–184. https://doi.org/10.1097/JFN.0000000000000194

Peternelj-Taylor, C. (2000). The role of the forensic nurse in Canada: An evolving specialty. In D. Robinson & A. Kettles (Eds.), *Forensic nursing and multidisciplinary care of the mentally disordered offender* (pp. 192–212). Jessica Kingsley Publishers.

Peternelj-Taylor, C. (2002). Professional boundaries: A matter of therapeutic integrity. *Journal of Psychosocial Nursing and Mental Health Services, 40*(4), 22–29.

Peternelj-Taylor, C. (2004). An exploration of othering in forensic psychiatric and correctional nursing. *Canadian Journal of Nursing Research, 36*(4), 130–146.

Peternelj-Taylor, C. (2005). Conceptualizing nursing research with offenders: Another look at vulnerability. *International Journal of Law and Psychiatry, 28,* 348–359. https://doi.org/10.1016/j.ijlp.2004.05.002

Peternelj-Taylor, C. (2012). Boundaries and desire in forensic mental health nursing. In A. Aiyegbusi & G. Kelly (Eds.), *Professional and therapeutic boundaries in forensic mental health practice* (pp. 124–136). Jessica Kingsley Publishers.

Peternelj-Taylor, C. (2020). Special focus: Nursing in the correctional milieu. *Nursing Leadership, 33*(1), 1–7. https://doi.org/10.12927/cjnl.2020.26196

Peternelj-Taylor, C. A., & Hufft, A. G. (2006). Forensic nursing. In W. K. Mohr (Ed.), *Psychiatric-mental health nursing* (6th ed., pp. 377–393). Lippincott Williams & Wilkins.

Peternelj-Taylor, C., & Johnson, R. (1995). Serving time: Psychiatric mental health nursing in corrections. *Journal of Psychosocial Nursing and Mental Health Services, 33*(8), 12–19.

Peternelj-Taylor, C., & Schafer, P. (2008). Management of therapeutic boundaries. In A. Kettles, P. Woods, & R. Byrt (Eds.), *Forensic mental health nursing: Capabilities, roles and responsibilities* (pp. 309–331). Quay Books.

Petryshen, P. (1981). Nursing the mentally disordered offender. *Canadian Nurse, 77*(6), 26–28.

Pierce, S. (2011). The lived experience of parents of adolescents who have sexually offended: I am a survivor. *Journal of Forensic Nursing, 7,* 173–181. https://doi.org/10.1111/j.1939-3938.2011.01116.x

Pilette, P. C., Berck, C. B., & Achber, L. C. (1995). Therapeutic management of helping boundaries. *Journal of Psychosocial Nursing and Mental Health Services, 33*(1), 40–47.

Popova, S., Lange, S., Bekmuradov, D., Mihic, A., & Rehm, J. (2011). Fetal alcohol spectrum disorder prevalence estimates in the correctional system: A systematic literature review. *Canadian Journal of Public Health, 102*(5), 336–340. https://doi.org/10.1007/BF03404172

Power, J., Brown, S. L., & Usher, A. M. (2013). Non-suicidal self-injury in women offenders: Motivations, emotions, and precipitating events. *International Journal of Forensic Mental Health, 12,* 192–204. https://doi.org/10.1080/14999013.2013.832442

Quality Network for Forensic Mental Health Services. (2015). *Your guide to relational security: See, Think, Act* (2nd ed.). Royal College of Psychiatrists.

Ricciardelli, R., Bucerius, S., Tetrault, J., Crewe, B., & Pyrooz, D. (2021). *Correctional services during and beyond COVID-19* (pp. 490–516). FACETS. https://doi.org/10.1139/facets2021-0023

Richards, C., & Barrett, J. (2021). Supporting trans and non-binary people in forensic settings. In *Trans and non-binary gender healthcare* (pp. 61–69). Cambridge University Press.

Rose, D. N., Peter, E., Gallop, R., Angus, J. E., & Liaschenko, J. (2011). Respect in forensic psychiatric nurse-patient relationships: A practical compromise. *Journal of Forensic Nursing, 7,* 3–16. https://doi.org/10.1111/j.1939-3938.2010.01090.x

Schafer, P. E., & Peternelj-Taylor, C. (2003). Therapeutic relationships and boundary maintenance: The perspective of forensic patients enrolled in a treatment program for violent offenders. *Issues in Mental Health Nursing, 24,* 605–625. https://doi.org/10.1080/01612840305320

Schoenly, L. (2013). Safety for the nurse and the patient. In L. Schoenly & C. M. Knox (Eds.), *Essentials of correctional nursing* (pp. 55–79). Springer.

Shelton, D., & Pearson, G. (2005). ADHD in juvenile offenders: Treatment issues nurses need to know. *Journal of Psychosocial Nursing and Mental Health Services, 43*(9), 38–46.

Simon, L., Beckmann, D., Stone, M., Williams, R., Cohen, M., & Tobey, M. (2020). Clinician experiences of care provision in the correctional setting: A scoping review. *Journal of Correctional Health Care, 26*(4), 301–314. https://doi.org/10.1177/1078345820953154

Smith, S. (2005). Stepping through the looking glass: Professional autonomy in correctional nursing. *Corrections Today, 54–56,* 70.

Smith, S., Muse, M. V., & Phillips, J. M. (2021). Addressing moral distress in correctional nursing: A call to action. *Journal of Correctional Health Care, 27*(2), 75–80. https://doi.org/10.1177/1078345820953154

Statistics Canada. (2009). *Section A—Overview of issues: Mental health and the criminal justice system.* http://www.statcan.gc.ca/pub/85-561-m/2009016/section-a-eng.htm

Stanton, A. E., & Rose, S. J. (2020). The mental health of mothers currently and formerly incarcerated in jails and prisons: An integrative review on mental health, mental health treatment, and traumatic experiences. *Journal of Forensic Nursing, 16*(4), 224–231. https://doi.org/10.1097/JFN.0000000000000302

Stone, K., Papadopoulos, I., & Kelly, D. (2012). Establishing hospice care for prison populations: An integrative review assessing the UK and the USA perspective. *Palliative Medicine, 26,* 969–978. https://doi.org/10.1177/0269216311424219

Terblanche, L., & Reimer-Kirkham, S. (2020). Nursing leadership implications for clinical placements in corrections. *Nursing Leadership (Toronto, Ont.), 33*(1), 35–51. https://doi.org/10.12927/cjnl.2020.26193

Vingilis, E., Stewart, S., Hamilton, H. A., Seeley, J., Einarson, K. M., Kolla, N. J., Bondy, S. J., & Erickson, P. G. (2020). Pilot study of mental health and substance use of detained youths in Ontario, Canada. *Children and Youth Services Review, 116,* 105156. https://doi.org/10.1016/J.CHILDYOUTH.2020.105156

Woods, P. (2013). Risk assessment and management approaches on mental health units. *Journal of Psychiatric and Mental Health Nursing, 20,* 807–813. https://doi.org/10.1111/jpm.12022

Woods, P., & Lasiuk, G. (2008). Risk prediction: A review of the literature. *Journal of Forensic Nursing, 4*(1), 1–11. https://doi.org/10.1111/j.1939-3938.2008.00001.x

Woods, P., & Peternelj-Taylor, C. (2022). Correctional nursing in Canada's Prairie provinces: Roles, responsibilities, and learning needs. *The Canadian Journal of Nursing Research, 54,* 59–71. https://doi.org/10.1177/08445621211999282

Appendix A

Brief Psychiatric Rating Scale

Patient's name _____ Date _____ Interviewer's name _____

Hospital _____ Ward _____ Date of admission _____

Instructions: This form consists of 24 symptom constructs, each to be rated on a 7-point scale of severity ranging from "not present" to "extremely severe." If a specific symptom is not rated, mark "NA" (not assessed). Circle the number headed by the term that best describes the patient's present condition

NA Not Assessed	1 Not Present	2 Very Mild	3 Mild	4 Moderate	5 Moderately Severe	6 Severe	7 Extremely Severe

1.	Somatic concern	NA	1	2	3	4	5	6	7
2.	Anxiety	NA	1	2	3	4	5	6	7
3.	Depression	NA	1	2	3	4	5	6	7
4.	Guilt	NA	1	2	3	4	5	6	7
5.	Hostility	NA	1	2	3	4	5	6	7
6.	Suspiciousness	NA	1	2	3	4	5	6	7
7.	Unusual thought content	NA	1	2	3	4	5	6	7
8.	Grandiosity	NA	1	2	3	4	5	6	7
9.	Hallucinations	NA	1	2	3	4	5	6	7
10.	Disorientation	NA	1	2	3	4	5	6	7
11.	Conceptual disorganization	NA	1	2	3	4	5	6	7
12.	Excitement	NA	1	2	3	4	5	6	7
13.	Motor retardation	NA	1	2	3	4	5	6	7
14.	Blunted affect	NA	1	2	3	4	5	6	7
15.	Tension	NA	1	2	3	4	5	6	7
16.	Mannerisms and posturing	NA	1	2	3	4	5	6	7
17.	Uncooperativeness	NA	1	2	3	4	5	6	7
18.	Emotional withdrawal	NA	1	2	3	4	5	6	7
19.	Suicidality	NA	1	2	3	4	5	6	7
20.	Self-neglect	NA	1	2	3	4	5	6	7
21.	Bizarre behaviour	NA	1	2	3	4	5	6	7
22.	Elated mood	NA	1	2	3	4	5	6	7
23.	Motor hyperactivity	NA	1	2	3	4	5	6	7
24.	Distractibility	NA	1	2	3	4	5	6	7

Reprinted with permission from Lukoff, D., Liberman, R. P., & Nuechterlein, K. H. (1986). Symptom monitoring in the rehabilitation of schizophrenic patients. *Schizophrenia Bulletin, 12*(4), 578–602.

Appendix B

Simpson-Angus Rating Scale

1. GAIT: The patient is examined as they walk into the examining room; the gait, the swing of the arms, and the general posture all form the basis for an overall score for this item. This is rated as follows:

   0 Normal
   1 Diminution in swing while the patient is walking
   2 Marked diminution in swing with obvious rigidity in the arm
   3 Stiff gait with arms held rigidly before the abdomen
   4 Stooped shuffling gait with propulsion and retropulsion

2. ARM DROPPING: The patient and the examiner both raise their arms to shoulder height and let them fall to their sides. In a normal subject, a stout slap is heard as the arms hit the sides. In the patient with extreme Parkinson syndrome, the arms fall very slowly.

   0 Normal, free fall with loud slap and rebound
   1 Fall slowed slightly with less audible contact and little rebound
   2 Fall slowed, no rebound
   3 Marked slowing, no slap at all
   4 Arms fall as though against resistance, as though through glue

3. SHOULDER SHAKING: The subject's arms are bent at a right angle at the elbow and are taken one at a time by the examiner who grasps one hand and also clasps the other around the subject's elbow. The subject's upper arm is pushed to and fro, and the humerus is externally rotated. The degree of resistance from normal to extreme rigidity is scored as follows:

   0 Normal
   1 Slight stiffness and resistance
   2 Moderate stiffness and resistance
   3 Marked rigidity with difficulty in passive movement
   4 Extreme stiffness and rigidity with almost a frozen shoulder

4. ELBOW RIGIDITY: The elbow joints are separately bent at right angles and passively extended and flexed, with the subject's biceps observed and simultaneously palpated. The resistance to this procedure is rated. (The presence of cogwheel rigidity is noted separately.) Scoring is from 0 to 4, as in the Shoulder Shaking test.

   0 Normal
   1 Slight stiffness and resistance
   2 Moderate stiffness and resistance
   3 Marked rigidity with difficulty in passive movement
   4 Extreme stiffness and rigidity with almost a frozen shoulder

5. FIXATION OF POSITION OR WRIST RIGIDITY: The examiner holds the wrist in one hand and the fingers in the other hand, with the wrist moved to extension, flexion, and both ulnar and radial deviation. The resistance to this procedure is rated as in items 3 and 4.

   0 Normal
   1 Slight stiffness and resistance
   2 Moderate stiffness and resistance
   3 Marked rigidity with difficulty in passive movement
   4 Extreme stiffness and rigidity with almost a frozen shoulder

6. LEG PENDULOUSNESS: The patient sits on a table with the legs hanging down and swinging free. The ankle is grasped by the examiner and raised until the knee is partially extended. It is then allowed to fall. The resistance to falling and the lack of swinging form the basis for the score on this item.

   0 The legs swing freely
   1 Slight diminution in the swing of the legs
   2 Moderate resistance to swing
   3 Marked resistance and damping of swing
   4 Complete absence of swing

7. HEAD DROPPING: The patient lies on a well-padded examining table, and the head is raised by

the examiner's hand. The hand is then withdrawn, and the head is allowed to drop. In the normal subject, the head will fall upon the table. The movement is delayed in extrapyramidal system disorder, and in extreme parkinsonism, it is absent. The neck muscles are rigid, and the head does not reach the examining table. Scoring is as follows:

0   The head falls completely, with a good thump as it hits the table
1   Slight slowing in fall, mainly noted by lack of slap as the head meets the table
2   Moderate slowing in the fall, quite noticeable to the eye
3   The head falls stiffly and slowly
4   The head does not reach the examining table

8. GLABELLA TAP: The subject is told to open the eyes wide and not to blink. The glabella region is tapped at a steady, rapid speed. The number of times the patient blinks in succession is noted:

0   0 to 5 blinks
1   6 to 10 blinks
2   11 to 15 blinks
3   16 to 20 blinks
4   21 or more blinks

9. TREMOR: The patient is observed walking into the examining room and then is reexamined for this item:

0   Normal
1   Mild finger tremor, obvious to sight and touch
2   Tremor of hand or arm occurring spasmodically
3   Persistent tremor of one or more limbs
4   Whole body tremor

10. SALIVATION: The patient is observed while talking and then asked to open the mouth and elevate the tongue. The following ratings are given:

0   Normal
1   Excess salivation to the extent that pooling takes place if the mouth is open and the tongue raised
2   When excess salivation is present and might occasionally result in difficulty in speaking
3   Speaking with difficulty because of excess salivation
4   Frank drooling

Scoring: Each item is rated on a 5-point scale, with 0 meaning the complete absence of the condition and 4 meaning the presence of the condition in extreme form. The score is obtained by adding the items and dividing by 10.

Reprinted with permission from Simpson, G. M., & Angus, J. W. S. (1970). A rating scale for extrapyramidal side effects. *Acta Psychiatrica Scandinavica, 212*(Suppl), 11–19.

Appendix C

Abnormal Involuntary Movement Scale (AIMS)

	None	Minimal	Mild	Moderate	Severe
Facial and Oral Movements					
1: Muscles of facial expression (e.g., movements of forehead, eyebrows, periorbital area, cheeks; include frowning, blinking, smiling, grimacing)	0	1	2	3	4
2: Lips and perioral area (e.g., puckering, pouting, smacking)	0	1	2	3	4
3: Jaw (e.g., biting, clenching, chewing, mouth opening, lateral movement)	0	1	2	3	4
4: Tongue	0	1	2	3	4
Rate only increase in movement both in and out of the mouth, NOT inability to sustain movement					
Extremity Movements					
5: Upper (arms, wrists, hands, fingers)	0	1	2	3	4
Include choreic movements (i.e., rapid, objectively purposeless, irregular, spontaneous), athetoid movements (i.e., slow, irregular, complex, serpentine)					
Do NOT include tremor (i.e., repetitive, regular, rhythmic)					
6: Lower (legs, knees, ankles, toes) (e.g., lateral knee movement, foot tapping, heel dropping, foot squirming, inversion and eversion of the foot)	0	1	2	3	4
Trunk Movements					
7: Neck, shoulders, hips (e.g., rocking, twisting, squirming, pelvic gyrations)	0	1	2	3	4
8: Severity of abnormal movements	0	1	2	3	4
Global Judgment					
9: Incapacitation due to abnormal movements	0	1	2	3	4

10: Patient's awareness of abnormal movements		
Rate only the patient's report	No awareness	0
	Aware, no distress	1
	Aware, mild distress	2
	Aware, moderate distress	3
	Aware, severe distress	4

Global Judgment

11: Current problems with teeth and/or dentures	No	0
	Yes	1
12: Does the patient usually wear dentures?	No	0
	Yes	1

Examination Procedures for AIMS

Either before or after completing the examination procedure, observe the patient unobtrusively, at rest (e.g., in the waiting room). The chair to be used in this examination should be a hard, firm one without arms.

1. Ask the patient whether there is anything in the mouth (i.e., gum, candy, etc.) and if there is, to remove it.
2. Ask the patient about the *current* condition of the teeth. Ask the patient if they wear dentures. Do teeth or dentures bother the patient *now*?
3. Ask the patient whether they notice any movements in the mouth, face, hands, or feet. If yes, ask the patient to describe and to what extent they *currently* bother them or interfere with their activities.
4. Have the patient sit in the chair with hands on knees, legs slightly apart, and feet flat on the floor. (Look at the entire body for movements while in this position.)
5. Ask the patient to sit with the hands hanging unsupported. If male, between legs; if female and wearing a dress, hanging over knees. (Observe hands and other body areas.)
6. Ask the patient to open the mouth. (Observe the tongue at rest within the mouth.) Do this twice.
7. Ask the patient to protrude the tongue. (Observe the tongue at rest within the mouth.) Do this twice.
8. [a]Ask the patient to tap the thumb, with each finger, as rapidly as possible for 10–15 seconds; separately with right hand, then with left hand. (Observe facial and leg movements.)
9. Flex and extend the patient's left and right arms (one at a time). (Note any rigidity and rate on NOTES.)
10. Ask the patient to stand up. (Observe in profile. Observe all body areas again, hips included.)
11. [a]Ask the patient to extend both arms outstretched in front with palms down. (Observe trunk, legs, and mouth.)
12. [a]Have the patient walk a few paces, turn, and walk back to the chair. (Observe hand and gait.) Do this twice.

-----

[a]Activated movements.

Source: Guy, W. (1976). *ECDEU: Assessment manual for psychopharmacology (DHEW Publication No. 76–338)*. Department of Health, Education, and Welfare, Psychopharmacology Research Branch.

Appendix D

Simplified Diagnoses for Tardive Dyskinesia (SD-TD)

PREREQUISITES—The three prerequisites are as follows. Exceptions may occur.

1. A history of at least 3 months' total cumulative neuroleptic exposure. Include amoxapine and metoclopramide in all categories below as well.
2. **SCORING/INTENSITY LEVEL.** The presence of a **TOTAL SCORE OF FIVE OR ABOVE.** Also, be alert for any change from baseline or scores below 5 that have at least a "moderate" (3) or "severe" (4) movement on any item or at least two "mild" (2) movements on two items located in different body areas.
3. Other conditions are not responsible for the abnormal involuntary movements.

DIAGNOSES—The diagnosis is based upon the current exam and its relation to the last exam. The diagnosis can shift depending upon (a) whether movements are present or not, (b) whether movements are present for 3 months or more (6 months if on a semiannual assessment schedule), and (c) whether neuroleptic dosage changes occur and affect movements.

- **NO TD**—Movements **are not** present on this exam **or** movements are present, but some other condition is responsible for them. The last diagnosis must be NO TD, PROBABLE TD, or WITHDRAWAL TD.
- **PROBABLE TD**—Movements **are** present on this exam. This is the first time they are present, **or** they have never been present for 3 months or more. The last diagnosis must be NO TD or PROBABLE TD.
- **PERSISTENT TD**—Movements **are** present on this exam, **and** they have been present for 3 months or more with this exam or at some point in the past. The last diagnosis can be any except NO TD.
- **MASKED TD**—Movements **are not** present on this exam, **but** this is due to a neuroleptic dosage increase or reinstitution after a prior exam when movements were present. Also, use this conclusion if movements are not present due to the addition of a nonneuroleptic medication to treat TD. The last diagnosis must be PROBABLE TD, PERSISTENT TD, WITHDRAWAL TD, or MASKED TD.
- **REMITTED TD**—Movements **are not** present on this exam, **but** PERSISTENT TD has been diagnosed **and** neuroleptic dosage increase or reinstitution has occurred. The last diagnosis must be PERSISTENT TD or REMITTED TD. If movements reemerge, the diagnosis shifts back to PERSISTENT TD.
- **WITHDRAWAL TD**—Movements **are not seen while** receiving neuroleptics or at the last dosage level **but are seen within** 8 weeks following a neuroleptic reduction or discontinuation. The last diagnosis must be NO TD or WITHDRAWAL TD. If movements continue for 3 months or more after the neuroleptic dosage reduction or discontinuation, the diagnosis shifts to PERSISTENT TD. If movements do not continue for 3 months or more after the reduction or discontinuation, the diagnosis shifts to NO TD.

Instructions	Other Conditions (Partial List)
1. The rater completes the assessment according to the standardized exam procedure. If the rater also completes evaluation items 1–4, they must also sign the preparer box. The form is given to the physician. Alternatively, the physician may perform the assessment.	1. Age
	2. Blind
	3. Cerebral palsy
	4. Contact lenses
	5. Dentures/no teeth
	6. Down syndrome
2. The physician completes the evaluation section. The physician is responsible for the entire evaluation section and its accuracy.	7. Drug intoxication (specify)
	8. Encephalitis
	9. Extrapyramidal side effects (specify)
3. It is recommended that the physician examines any individual who meets the three prerequisites or who has movements not explained by other factors. Neurologic assessments or differential diagnostic tests that may be necessary should be performed.	10. Fahr syndrome
	11. Heavy metal intoxication (specify)
	12. Huntington chorea
	13. Hyperthyroidism
	14. Hypoglycaemia
	15. Hypoparathyroidism
4. File form according to policy or procedure.	16. Idiopathic torsion dystonia
	17. Meige syndrome
	18. Parkinson disease
	19. Stereotypies
	20. Sydenham chorea
	21. Tourette syndrome
	22. Wilson disease
	23. Other (specify)

Source: Sprague, R. L., & Kalachnik, J. E. (1991). Reliability, validity, and a total score cutoff for the Dyskinesia Identification System Condensed User Scale (DISCUS) with mentally ill and mentally retarded populations. *Psychopharmacology Bulletin, 27*(1), 51–58.

Appendix E

Hamilton Rating Scale for Depression

Clinic No. _____ Date _____ Rating No. _____ Code Number _____
Sex _____ Age _____ Patient's Name _____
Patient's Address _____ Tel _____

Item	Range	Score
1. Depressed mood	0–4	
2. Guilt	0–4	
3. Suicide	0–4	
4. Insomnia initial	0–2	
5. Insomnia middle	0–2	
6. Insomnia delayed	0–2	
7. Work and interest	0–4	
8. Retardation	0–4	
9. Agitation	0–4	
10. Anxiety (psychic)	0–4	
11. Anxiety (somatic)	0–4	
12. Somatic gastrointestinal	0–2	
13. Somatic general	0–2	
14. Genital	0–2	
15. Hypochondriasis	0–2	
16. Insight	0–4	
17. Loss of weight	0–2	
	Total score	
Diurnal variation (M.A.E.)	0–2	
Depersonalization	0–4	
Paranoid symptoms	0–4	
Obsessional symptoms	0–4	

The scale is designed to measure the severity of illness of patients already diagnosed as suffering from depressive illness. It is obviously not a diagnostic instrument because that requires much more information (e.g., previous history, family history, precipitating factors).

As far as possible, the scale should be used in the manner of a clinical interview. The first time, the interview should be conducted in a relaxed, free, and easy manner, giving the patients time to unburden themselves and giving them the opportunity to speak of their problems and ask whatever questions they wish. It may then be necessary to obtain further information by asking them questions. At subsequent assessments, the interview can be briefer and more to the point.

An observer rating scale is not a checklist in which each item is strictly defined. The raters must have sufficient clinical experience and judgment to be able to interpret the patients' statements and reticence about some symptoms and to compare them with other patients. They should use all sources of information (e.g., from relatives and nurses).

The scale consists of 17 items, the scores of which are summed to give a total score. These are four other items, one of which (diurnal variation) is excluded on the grounds that it is not an additional burden on the patient. The last three are excluded from the total score because they occur infrequently, although information on them may be useful for other purposes.

The method of assessment is simple. For some symptoms, it is difficult to elicit such information as will permit full quantification. If present, score 2; if absent, score 0; and if doubtful or trivial, score 1. For those symptoms where more detailed information can be obtained, the score of 2 is expanded into 2 for mild, 3 for moderate, and 4 for severe. In case of difficulty, the raters should use their judgment as clinicians.

Source: Hamilton, M. (1960). A rating scale for depression. *Journal of Neurology, Neurosurgery, and Psychiatry, 23,* 56.

Index

Note: Page numbers followed by "*b*" indicate boxed materials; page numbers followed by "*f*" indicate figures; page numbers followed by "*t*" indicate tables.

A

A Mind That Found Itself (Beers), 6
Ableism, 34
Aboriginal Community Wellness
    Strategies, 427
Aboriginal Health Care, 49–51
Aboriginal peoples, 46–51, 47*b*
    assimilation, 46–49
    colonialism, 46–49
    cultural diversity, 46
    historical trauma, 46–49
    indigenization of curricula, 50–51
    inhalant abuse, 675
    IRS system, 50
    mental health, 50
        and addiction, 48
        strategy, 51
    protective factors, 436–437
    residential schools, 48
    spirituality, 44
    strength-based approach, 51
    suicide, 48, 427*b*, 428
    trauma-informed care, 51
Abuse
    of children (*See* Child abuse)
    forms of, 918–919
        child maltreatment/abuse,
            918–919
        elder abuse, 919
        interpersonal, 918
        intimate partner violence, 918
    health impacts of, 919–921
        child abuse, 920–921
        elder abuse, 921
        intimate partner violence, 919–920
    nursing role, recognizing and
        responding to, 921–926
        documentation, 926
        physical examination and history
            taking, 922–923
        strengths-based approach, 923–926
        trauma- and violence-informed care,
            922
    social context of
        ability, 916
        age factor, 916
        four-level social-ecological model,
            915, 916*f*
        gender, 916, 917*f*

poverty, 916
racism, 916
types of, in Canada, 769, 769*t*
Acamprosate, 669
Accommodation, workplace, mental
    health, 349–350
Accountability, 234
Acetylcholine (ACh), 196
    sleep–wake disorders, 734, 735*t*
Acquired immunodeficiency syndrome
    (AIDS)
    dementia complex, 897
    substance-related disorders, 667–681
Actigraphy, 740
Active aging, 36
Active listening, 108
Activities of daily living training, 77
Activity enhancement, 580
Activity interventions, 235
Acute extrapyramidal syndromes, 266–268
Acute inpatient care, 78
AD. *See* Alzheimer disease (AD)
Adaptation, Roy's model, 159
Addiction treatment
    goals of, 662, 662*b*
    principles of, 660*b*, 662–663
Addictive disorders. *See* Substance-related
    disorders
ADHD (attention deficit hyperactivity
    disorder), 630, 641–642
    Rating Scale, 819*b*
Adler, Alfred, 160*t*, 162
Adler's Foundation for Individual
    Psychology, 160*t*, 162
Admission certificate, 127–128
Adolescents. *See also* Youth
    anxiety disorders in
        generalized anxiety disorder, 808–809
        separation anxiety disorder, 809–810
    assessment within age groups, 784–785
    bio/psycho/social/spiritual psychiatric
        nursing assessment, 785–796, 786*b*
    bipolar disorders in, 504
    clinical interview
        building rapport, 778–781, 778*b*
        interview techniques, 782–784, 783*b*
        observation, 781–782
    disruptive behaviour disorders,
        825–827

attention deficit hyperactivity
    disorder, 818–820
conduct disorder, 826–827
externalizing disorders, 825
internalizing disorders, 825
motor disorders, 827–829
oppositional defiant disorder, 825
girls positive self-identity, 602*b*
grieving in, 758*t*
history and hallmarks of, 804*b*
loss and, 759–760
physical and developmental challenges
    in, 763–765
sexual identity, 763–764
substance use, 764–765
Youth Health Promotion, 765
preventive interventions with, 770
rating scales, 784
sleep–wake disorders, 736
substance-related disorders, 667–681
trauma-and violence-informed care for,
    773–774, 773*b*
Adults
    grieving in, 758–760
    older (*see* Older adults)
Advice, leading groups, 308, 308*t*
Affect
    blunted, 220
    definition, 220
    expression of mood, 502
    flat, 220
Affective flattening/blunting, 451
Affective instability, 696–697
Affective interventions, 408
Affective lability, 478
Affliation programs, 10–11
Age friendly, 838*b*
Age-related memory alterations, 849
Aggression and violence, 453, 885–886.
    See also Abuse; Anger
    analysis and outcome identification
        for, 403
    assessment of
        in biologic domain, 406–407
        in psychological domain, 407–410
        in social domain, 410–412
        in spiritual domain, 412
    behaviours on, 396*t*
    characteristics and risk factors for, 401*t*

Aggression and violence (*Continued*)
clients etiologies for, 401*t*
continuum of care for, 415
definition of, 396–397
evaluation and treatment outcomes in, 415
interactional processes and, 412–413
models of
biologic, 397–398
interactional, 400
low serotonin syndrome, 398–399
neurochemical model, 398–399
psychological, 399–400
sociocultural, 400
nursing interventions for
for biologic domain, 406–407
planning and implementing, 404–406
for psychological domain, 408–410
for social domain, 410–412
for spiritual domain, 412
predictors of, 403
responding to assault and, 413–415, 414*t*
Aggression management, 77
Aggressor, 304
Agitated behaviour, 885–886, 890
Agitation, 453
Agoraphobia, 549–550, 549*b*, 560*b*
Agranulocytosis, 454–455
AIDS. *See* Acquired immunodeficiency syndrome (AIDS)
Akathisia, 267–268, 470
Alberta
Alberta Hospital, 8, 11
nurse education in, 11, 12*f*
training in, 7
Alcohol, 653, 655. *See also* Substance use disorders
addiction
aetiologic theories, 658–659
caffeine, 656–657
cannabis, 657
opioids, 657
societal costs, 657
tobacco, 657
withdrawal, 668–669, 669*b*, 670*b*
withdrawal symptoms, 665
Alcohol consumption, by older adults, 846
Alcohol use disorder, 669, 671*b*
Alcoholics Anonymous (AA), 659*b*, 666
Alcoholism, family history of mental disorders, 772–773
Allostasis, 545
Alogia, 451
Altruistic suicide, 432
Alzheimer, Alois, 872
Alzheimer disease (AD)
aetiology, 875–877, 875*f*
assessment of
biologic domain, 878–879
psychological domain, 882
social domain, 891
spiritual domain, 893
clinical course, 873, 873*t*
continuum of care, 894–896
diagnostic criteria, 873–874, 874*t*, 874*b*

epidemiology and risk factors for, 874–875
evaluation, 893–894
family response, 877–878
home visits and, 892
interprofessional treatment, 877
long-term care, 896
nursing care
biologic domain, 879
psychological domain, 886
social domain, 891
nursing care plan for, 895*b*
nursing interventions
biologic domain, 879–882
psychological domain, 886–891
social domain, 891–892
priority care issues, 877
treatment outcomes, 893–894, 894*f*
warning signs of, 873–874, 874*b*
Ambivalence, 478
motivational interviewing, 666
schizophrenia, 448–449
American Psychiatric Association (APA), 803
Amitriptyline, 580
Amphetamines
adverse reactions, 282–283
indications and mechanisms of action, 281
off-label use, 280
pharmacokinetics, 281–282
side effects, 282–283
toxicity, 282–283
Amygdala, 188
AN. *See* Anorexia nervosa (AN)
Anger. *See also* Aggression and violence
clinical vignette, 401
continuum of care, 415
definition, 395–396
evaluation and treatment outcomes, 415
experience of, 395, 395*b*
expression, facial, 395–396, 396*f*
management groups, 314
models of
biologic theories, 397–398
interactional theory, 400
physiologic and behavioural cues, 404*t*
psychological theories, 399–400
responding to assault, 413–415
sociocultural theories, 400
spiritual domain, 412
nursing management, 400–412
Anhedonia, 451, 678
Anima, 162
Animal models, 175
Animus, 162
Anomic suicide, 432
Anorexia nervosa (AN), 595–628
aetiology, 603–607, 603*f*
biochemical theories, 604
biologic theories, 603–604, 603*f*
family responses, 607
genetic theories, 604
neuropathologic theories, 604
psychological theories, 604–605
social theories, 606–607

spiritual theories, 607
assessment
biologic domain, 614
psychological domain, 622
clinical course, 596–597
continuum of care, 628
diagnostic criteria, 597–598, 598*b*
epidemiology, 599–603
age of onset, 599–600
comorbidity, 602–603
differences among people diagnosed with, 600, 601*b*
ethnic and cultural difference, 600–602
familial predisposition, 602
evaluation and treatment outcomes, 628
interdisciplinary treatment, 610–611, 611*t*
interventions
biologic domain, 621–622
psychological domain, 624–626
social domain, 626–627
neurobiology and neurochemistry of, 598–599
nursing care focus for
biologic domain, 621
psychological domain, 624
social domain, 626
spiritual domain, 627
nursing care plan, 615*b*
altered nutrition, 615*b*
clinical setting, 615*b*
distorted perception in body size and shape, 615*b*
impaired ability, 615*b*
nursing management, 614*b*
biologic domain, 614–622, 621*f*
psychological domain, 622–626, 622*b*, 625*b*, 626*t*, 626*b*
social domain, 626–627, 627*b*
spiritual domain, 627–628
pharmacologic interventions, 612
physiologic consequences of, 598–599, 599*b*
priority care issues, 612–614
risk factors, 607–610, 608*f*
biologic, 607–608
psychological, 608–609
social, 609–610
spiritual, 610
spiritual domain, 627–628
Anosognosia, 481
Anterograde amnesia, 512
Antianxiety medications, 882
Anticholinergic(s)
crisis, 486
side effects, nursing interventions, 493
signs and symptoms, 495
Antidepressants
agents, 882
bipolar disorders, 519*f*
mood stabilizing phases
discontinuation, 278
factors influencing, 274*b*
initiation, 278
maintenance, 278
stabilization, 278

novel drug development, 277b
Antioppressive and structural analysis strategies, 38, 38b
Antipsychotics
  agents, 881
  anticholinergic side effects, 265
  bipolar disorders, 525
  blood disorders, 266
  cardiovascular side effects, 264–265
  endocrine and sexual side effects, 265–266
  medication-related movement disorders
    acute extrapyramidal syndromes, 266–268
    akathisia, 267–268
    chronic syndromes, 268–269
    dystonia, 266
    pseudoparkinsonism, 267
    tardive dyskinesia, 268, 268b
  neuroleptic malignant syndrome, 266
  nursing interventions, 471t
  photosensitivity reactions, 266
  schizophrenia, 449b
  seizure disorder, 266
  side effects, 471t
  typical and atypical antipsychotics
    adverse reactions, 264–269
    chemical interactions, 263t
    drug formulations, 263–264
    indications and mechanisms of action, 262
    pharmacokinetics, 262–263, 263t–264t
    side effects, 261t, 264–269
    toxicity, 264–269
  weight gain, 270
Antisocial personality disorder (ASPD)
  aetiology, 718
  clinical course, 717–718
  comorbidity, 718
  nursing care, 718–720
  prevalence, 718
  psychoeducation, 719b
Anxiety, 161, 545, 588–589, 885. *See also* Generalized anxiety disorder (GAD); Obsessive-compulsive disorder (OCD); Panic disorder; Phobias; Posttraumatic stress disorder (PTSD)
  aetiologic theories
    genetic, 552
    neurobiology, 552–553
    neuroimaging data, 554
    neurotransmitters and neuropeptides, 553–554
    nursing management, 554–563
    psychodynamic theories, 554
  assessment
    occupational domains, 561–562
    psychological domain, 557–561
    social domains, 561–562
    spiritual domain, 562–563
  and concurrent addictive, 910
  continuum of care, 563
  due to COVID-19 pandemic, 907b
  evaluation and treatment outcomes, 563
  generalized anxiety disorder, 808–809

in interpersonal relations theory, 154
  interventions
    biologic domain, 554–557
    occupational domains, 562
    social domains, 562
  management, 889
  normal *vs.* abnormal response, 545
  nursing interventions, 559t
  in psychoanalytic theory, 161
  psychoeducation, 560
  rating scales, 567b
  separation anxiety disorder
    epidemiology and aetiology, 809
    nursing care, 809–810
    treatment interventions, 809
  symptoms, 546t
Anxiolytics, 562b, 683
Apathy, 478
Appearance, in mental status examination, 219
Appetite, in depressive disorders, 510
Apraxia, 850
Archetypes, 162
Aripiprazole (Abilify)
  dosage, half-life, and therapeutic blood level of, 264t
  side effects, 261t
Ascribed identity, 29–30, 50
ASPD. *See* Antisocial personality disorder (ASPD)
Assaultive ideation, 226
Assertive community treatment (ACT), 78, 409, 491, 936
Assertiveness, 402–403
Assessment, 208–228
  comprehensive, 209
  definition of, 209
  of family systems, 333
  focused, 213
  as process, 208–209
  techniques for, 213–216
    examination, 214
    interprofessional collaboration, 215–216
    interviewing, 214–215, 214b, 215b
    observation, 213
  types, 209–216, 209t–211t, 212b
Assimilation, cultural, 47
Association, cortex, 185
Athletes, eating disorders among, 610
Attachment, disorganized, 453–454, 791
Attachment theory
  bio/psycho/social/spiritual psychiatric nursing assessment of children and adolescents, 791
  bulimia nervosa, 632
  in children and adolescents, 757b
Attention
  definition, 818b
  in mental status examination, 221–223
Attention deficit hyperactivity disorder (ADHD), 630, 641–642, 818–820
  aetiologic factors, 818–819
  clinical observations, 818
  and concurrent addictive, 910–911
  diagnosis of, 818, 819b
  epidemiology, 818–819
  laboratory studies, 818
  longitudinal studies, 818

nursing care, 819–820, 820f
  psychosocial factors, 820
  treatment interventions, 819
Attitude toward interviewer, in mental status examination, 219–220
Atypical antipsychotics, 742t
Auditory hallucinations, schizophrenia, 478
Autism spectrum disorder (ASD), 814–817
  biopsychosocial domain, 816
  continuum of care, 816–817
  definition, 815b
  epidemiology and aetiology, 815, 815f
  nursing care, 815–817
Automatic thoughts, of cognition, 293, 295
Autonomic nervous system, 187–188, 190, 191f, 192t
Avoidant personality disorder, 721–722
Avolition, 481

B
Bandura, Albert, 165
Barager, Charles A., 7–8
Barker, Philip, 156–157
Basal ganglia, 185
Beck, Aaron T., 164t, 166
BED. *See* Binge-eating disorder (BED)
Bedlam, 2
Beers, Clifford, 6
Beginning stage of group development, 303–304
Behaviour changes, for older adults, 850
Behaviour control, ethics, 142–143
Behaviour therapy, 515
Behavioural experiments, 297–299
  modify symptoms, 298–299
Behavioural factors, in depressive disorders, 508
Behavioural interventions, 410
  for borderline personality disorder, 710
  enuresis, 829–830
Behavioural responses, 481
Behavioural theories, 163–165, 164t, 399
  applicability to psychiatric and mental health nursing, 166
  cognitive, 164t, 165–166
  reinforcement, 164t, 165
  stimulus–response, 163–165, 164t
Behaviourism, 165
Beliefs
  personal, understanding, 106
  religious, approaches to mental illness and, 46
Beneficence, 139
Benner, Patricia, 12–13, 156
Benzodiazepines, 581, 742t, 747
  adverse reactions, 279–280
  indications and mechanisms of action, 278
  panic disorder, 556
  pharmacokinetics, 278–279
  side effects, 252
  toxicity, 252–253
Benztropine mesylate (Cogentin), 472
Best interests, 126, 139, 146
  modified, 128

Best practice guidelines (BPGs), 231, 231b
Beta-amyloid plaques, 875
Bibliotherapy, 774–775
Bicetre, 3–4
Bidirectional feedback model, concurrent disorders, 906–907
Binge-eating disorder (BED), 636–643
  aetiology
    biologic theories, 639
    genetic, 639
    psychological and social theories, 639–640
    spiritual theories, 640
  clinical course, 636–637
  continuum of care, 643
  diagnostic criteria, 637
  epidemiology
    age of onset, 637
    comorbidity, 638
    complications, 638
    differences among people diagnosed with, 638
    ethnic and cultural difference, 638
    familial differences, 638
  evaluation and treatment outcomes, 643
  interdisciplinary treatment, 640–641
  nursing management
    biologic domain, 641–642
    psychosocial domain, 642, 642b
    spiritual domain, 643
    therapeutic relationship, 641
  priority care issues, 641
  psychoeducation, 642, 642b
  risk factors, 607–610, 608f, 640
  special populations, 637
Binge–purge cycle, 629–630, 629f
Bioavailability, 255
Biochemical theories
  anorexia nervosa, 604
  bulimia nervosa, 526b
Biogenic amines, 196–199
Biologic domain, 217
  assessment, 217 (See also specific disorders and conditions)
  bipolar disorder, 806
  brief psychotic disorder, 805
  conduct disorder, 826–827
  depressive disorders, 509, 807
  family assessment, 325–329
  genetic vulnerability, 788
  health history in, 217
  insomnia, 745–747
  motor disorder, 828
  neurologic examination, 788
  nursing interventions, 235–237, 438–439
    bipolar disorders, 519–537
    stress, 372–373
  obstructive sleep apnea, 749–750, 750f
  oppositional defiant disorder, 825
  physical examination in, 217, 218t–219t
  posttraumatic stress disorder, 813
  psychotic disorders, 805
  reactive attachment disorder, 812
  schizophrenia, 449–455, 449b, 451t
  stress, 372–373

Biologic model, 82–83, 83f
Biologic theories, 9, 159–160
  anorexia nervosa, 603–604, 603f
  somatic symptom disorder, 574–588
Biological foundations
  behavior
    epigenetics, 177
    genetics, 175–177
    population genetics, 176–177
    risk factors, 177
  central nervous system
    neuroanatomy, 183–190
    neurophysiology, 190–200
  neuroimaging methods, 180t
    structural neuroimaging, 180–182
    structure–function gap, 182–183
Biological treatment. See also specific disorders and conditions
  electroconvulsive therapy, 284
  light therapy (phototherapy), 284–285
  psychosocial issues, 285–286, 285b
  transcranial magnetic stimulation, 285
Biopsychosocial domain, autistic spectrum disorder, 816
Bio/psycho/social/spiritual boundaries, 112–114
Bio/psycho/social/spiritual interventions, 230–231, 232f, 366f
Bio/psycho/social/spiritual mental health nursing assessment
  assessment process, 841–844, 842b
  biologic domain, 844–846
    age-related increase in other health risks, 845–846
    assessment of, 846–848, 847b, 848b
    coronary artery changes, 844
    functional status, 847–848
    hearing and vision changes, 844–845
    musculoskeletal system, 845
    sexual health, 846, 847b
    sleep, change in, 846
  data collection techniques, 844, 845b
  definition, 841b
  psychological domain, 848–849
    behaviour changes, 850
    cognitive function, 848–850
    depression, 849–851
    memory, 849
    resiliency, 849
    stress and coping patterns, 851
    sucide risk assessment, 851
  social domain, 851–855
    assessment of, 854
    diversity, 853
    legal status, 855
    poverty, 853–854
    relationships, 852–853
    social connection, 852
    social support, 854
    social systems, 854–855
    spiritual domain, 855
Bio/psycho/social/spiritual model, 204, 204f, 777
Bio/psycho/social/spiritual psychiatric and mental health assessment, 216–227, 216f
  biologic domain and, 217

  health history in, 217
  physical examination in, 217, 218t–219t
  documentation for, 217
  psychological domain and, 217–226
    mental status examination and, 219–223, 219b, 220b
    responses to mental health problems and, 217
    risk assessment and, 223–226, 224f
    stress and coping patterns and, 223
  social domain and
    functional status and, 226–227
    gender identity, 212b
    spiritual assessment, 227
  types and sources of information for, 216–217
Bio/psycho/social/spiritual psychiatric nursing assessment
  adolescents, 785–796, 786b
  biologic domain, 787–788
  child abuse, 795–796
  children, 785–796, 786b
  psychological domain, 788–793
  social domain, 793–795
  spiritual domain, 795
Bio/psycho/social/spiritual self, 106
Biosocial learning theory, 701–702
Biperiden (Akineton), 267t
Bipolar disorders, 519–537
  aetiology, 523–524
  biologic domain, 806
  clinical course, 522
  continuum of care, 518–519, 537
  diagnostic criteria, 519–522, 520b
  epidemiology, 522
  evaluation and treatment outcomes, 531
  family response to, 524
  inpatient management, 537
  intensive outpatient programmes, 537
  interdisciplinary treatment, 524
  medical comorbidity, 523
  mixed features, 521–522, 525
  nursing interventions for
    biologic domain, 524–526
    psychological domain, 526–529
    social domain, 529–531
    spiritual domain, 531
  priority care issues, 524
  psychosocial domain, 806
  and related disorders, 805–806
  secondary mania, 522
  spectrum of care, 537
  treatment intervention, 805–806
Black, Indigenous, People of Colour (BIPoC), 853
Blocker, 304
Blunted affect, 220
BMI (body mass index), 597
BN. See Bulimia nervosa (BN)
Body dissatisfaction, 606b
Body image, 595–596
Body image distortion, 597–598, 598b
Body mass index (BMI), 597
Books (bCBT), 290
Borderline personality disorder (BPD), 630

aetiology
  biosocial theories, 701–702
  genetic factors, 699
  maladaptive schemas, 700, 700t
  psychological theories, 699–700
  psychosocial risk factors, 699
behavioural patterns in, 701b
clinical course of disorder
  affective instability, 696–697
  cognitive dysfunctions, 697–698
  dysfunctional behaviours, 698–699
  identity diffusion, 697
  unstable interpersonal relationships, 697
continuum of care, 714
evaluation and outcomes, 714
family response, 702–703
interdisciplinary treatment
  dialectical behaviour therapy, 692–693
  psychopharmacotherapy, 702
nursing care plan, 703–712, 715b
nursing management
  biologic domain, 703–705
  nursing care plan, 715b
  psychological domain, 706–712
  social domain, 712–714
  spiritual domain, 714
psychopharmacotherapy, 702
response patterns, 703b
Boundaries, in therapeutic
    communication, 112–114, 113b
Boundary violations, 113, 143, 713,
    943–944
Bradykinesia, 896–897
Brain
  in attention deficit hyperactivity
      disorder, 818
  plasticity, 179, 179t
Breathing control, panic disorder, 555
Brief intervention, 120, 121b, 663–664,
    681, 696
Brief psychotic disorder, 494, 804
British Columbia, Canadian suicide
    statistics, 424t
Brøset Violence Checklist (BVC), 403
Bulimia nervosa (BN), 628–636
  aetiology
    biochemical, 631
    biologic theories, 631
    genetic, 631
    neuropathologic, 631
    psychological and social theories,
        631–632
  behavioural techniques, 634–635, 635f
  clinical course, 629
  continuum of care, 636
  diagnostic criteria, 628
  epidemiology
    age of onset, 630
    comorbidity, 630
    differences among people
        diagnosed, 630
    ethnic and cultural differences, 630
    familial differences, 630
  evaluation and treatment outcomes,
      636
  interdisciplinary treatment, 632–633

nursing management
  biologic domain, 633
  psychosocial domain, 634–636
  spiritual domain, 636
  therapeutic relationship, 633
priority care issues, 633
psychoeducation, 635, 635b
risk factors, 607–610, 608f, 632
symptomatology, 629–630, 629f
Bullying, 433
Bullying, workplace, mental health,
    348–349, 348t
Bupropion, 680
Burnout, workplace, mental health, 351
Buspirone, 581
  adverse reactions, 280–281
  indications, 280
  mechanisms of actions, 280
  pharmacokinetics, 280
  side effects, 280–281
  toxicity, 280–281

C

Caffeine, 747
  substance-related disorders, 673–674
CAGE questionnaire, 663b
Calgary Family Assessment Model
    (CFAM), 333
Calgary Family Intervention Model
    (CFIM), 333
CAMIMH (Canadian Alliance on Mental
    Illness and Mental Health), 14
Campbell, Maria, 373
Camphor-induced seizures, 511
Canada Disaster Database (CDC), 380
Canada Health Act (CHA), 15
Canadian Alliance on Mental Illness and
    Mental Health (CAMIMH), 14, 99
Canadian Association of Schools of
    Nursing (CASN), 85
Canadian Collaborative Mental Health
    Initiative (CCMHI), 229–230
Canadian Data on Suicidality, 424
Canadian Federation of Mental Health
    Nurses (CFMHN), 85, 230
Canadian Index of Wellbeing (CIW), 21
Canadian Institute for Health
    Information [CIHI], 33
Canadian Journal for Nursing Research,
    12–13
Canadian Mental Health Association
    (CMHA), 10, 14, 776–777
Canadian mental health care. See
    Continuum of care
Canadian Multicultural Act of 1988, 29–30
Canadian Multiculturalism Policy, 43
Canadian National Committee for
    Mental Hygiene (CNCMH), 6
Canadian Nurses Association (CNA), 751
Canadian Nurses Association's Code of
    Ethics for Registered Nurses, 134
Canadian Psychiatric Association, 14
Canadian Standards of Psychiatric-Mental
    Health Nursing, 12–13, 77, 234
Cannabinoids, 200, 457, 674, 747,
    905–906
Cannabis, 457, 764–765
  substance-related disorders, 674

Capable wishes, 128
Cardiac arrhythmias, 473
Care, duty to provide, 383
Caregiver burden, 322–323
Caregiving context, bio/psycho/social/
    spiritual psychiatric nursing
    assessment of children and
    adolescents, 790–791
Caring
  custody and, paradox of, 934, 935f
  Watson's theory of, 156
Case management, 70, 71b
Case-based ethics, 137t, 139
Casuistry, 137t, 139
Catastrophic reactions, 885, 889
Catatonic excitement, schizophrenia, 453
Catharsis, 399
CBT. See Cognitive–behavioural therapy
    (CBT)
CCK (cholecystokinin), 631
  anxiety disorder, 555
Central nervous system (CNS)
  brain plasticity, 179, 179t
  chronobiology, 202
  diagnostic approaches
    biologic markers, 203
    electroencephalography, 203
    event-related potentials, 204
    evoked potentials, 204
    polysomnography, 203
  generalized anxiety disorder, etiologies,
      204, 204f
  neuroimaging methods, 180t
    functional neuroimaging, 182
    structural neuroimaging, 180–182
    structure-function gap, 182–183
  psychoendocrinology, 200–201
  psychoneuroimmunology, 201–202
Cerebrum
  left and right hemispheres, 183–188
  lobes of the brain, 184–185, 184f
  subcortical structures, 185–188, 186f
CFMHN Standard III, 230, 231b
CHA (Canada Health Act), 15
Charting by exception, 217
Chemical messengers, in depressive
    disorders, 508
Chemical restraint, 244
Child abuse, 769, 769t
  during COVID-19 pandemic, 769b
  evaluation of, 795–796
  forms of, 918–919
  health effects of, 920–921
  and neglect, 769–771, 769t
    emotional abuse, 769t
    neglect, 769t
    physical abuse, 769t
    sexual abuse, 769t
Child Behaviour Checklist (CBCL), 819b
Childhood, adverse experiences (ACES),
    369, 658
Childhood psychopathology, risk factors
  child abuse and neglect, 769–771, 769t
  homelessness, 768
  parent with substance abuse problem,
      772–773
  parents with mental illness, 771–772
  poverty, 767–768

Childhood sexual abuse, 609
Children. *See also* Youth
  anxiety disorders
    generalized anxiety disorder, 808–809
    nursing interventions, 559*t*
    separation anxiety disorder, 809–810
  bio/psycho/social/spiritual psychiatric
      nursing assessment, 785–796,
      786*b*
  bipolar disorders in, 504
  in care, 770–771
  clinical interview
    building rapport, 778–781, 778*b*
    discussion with, 782–783
    interviewing, 782–784, 783*b*
    observation, 781–782
  depressive disorders in, 504–505
  disruptive behaviour disorders,
      825–827
    conduct disorder, 826–827
    motor disorders, 827–829
    oppositional defiant disorder, 825
  grieving in, 758*t*
  history and hallmarks of, 804*b*
  obsessive–compulsive disorder,
      810–811
  preschool-aged, 759, 784–785
  rating scales, 784
  school-aged, 759, 778*b*
  sleep–wake disorders, 736
  somatic symptom disorder, 575
  trauma-and violence-informed care for,
      773–774, 773*b*
Chloral hydrate, 746–747
Chlorpromazine (Thorazine), 9
Cholecystokinin (CCK), 631
  anxiety disorder, 553
Cholinesterase inhibitors, 881
Chronobiologic theories, of bipolar
      disorders, 523
Chronobiology, 202
Cigarette smoking, 473
Circadian rhythm disorders, treatment of,
      752
Circadian rhythms, 732, 734*f*
Cisgender, 212
CIW (Canadian Index of Wellbeing), 21
Clarification, leading groups, 308*t*
Classic antihistamines, 742*t*
Classical conditioning, 165
Client education, 712–714
Client/family education, 241, 241*f*, 713.
      See also Psychoeducation
Clinical decision-making, 96
Clinical interview, 777–784
  as assessment technique, 214–215,
      214*b*, 215*b*
  with children and adolescents
    adolescents, 785
    building rapport, 778–781, 778*b*
    child and parent observation,
      781–782
    children's rating scales, 784
    discussion with child, 782–783,
      783*b*
    discussion with parents, 783–784
    interview technique, 782–784

preschool-aged children, 784–785,
      785*f*
  school-aged children, 785
Clomipramine (Anafranil), 273*t*
Closed group, 302
Clozapine (Clozaril), 454–455, 470*b*
Cluster B disorders, 630
CMHA (Canadian Mental Health
      Association), 10, 14
CNCMH (Canadian National Committee
      for Mental Hygiene), 6
CNS. *See* Central nervous system (CNS)
Cognition, 528, 861, 862*b*
  in bipolar disorders, assessment of,
      528
  in depressive disorders, assessment of,
      514
Cognitive appraisal, 240, 360–361, 364,
      398
Cognitive distortions, 296*b*, 626*t*
Cognitive dysfunction, in borderline
      personality disorder, 697–698
Cognitive functioning, 482–483
  in older adults, 848–850
Cognitive impairments, 457
  in schizophrenia, 479
Cognitive interventions, 240, 408–409
Cognitive neuroassociation model, 398
Cognitive processes, maladaptive, in
      borderline personality disorder,
      700
Cognitive reserve, 840, 849
Cognitive restructuring, 295, 295*b*
  automatic thoughts
    core beliefs, 297
    evaluating, 295–296
    identifying, 295
    intermediate beliefs, 294*f*, 297
    modification of, 297
    thinking errors, 296
Cognitive schemas, 293
Cognitive theories, 164*t*, 165–166, 292,
      399–400
  binge-eating disorder, 639–640
  bulimia nervosa, 632
  for depressive disorders, 515
  substance-related disorders, 674
Cognitive–behavioural formulation, 294*b*
Cognitive–behavioural groups, 312
Cognitive–behavioural therapy (CBT),
      291*b*, 559–561, 624–625, 693,
      908
  cognition levels
    automatic thoughts, 293
    core beliefs, 293
    intermediate beliefs, 293
    relationship, 293–294, 294*f*
  cognitive model, 291–293
  definition, 290
  on emotion and behaviour, 292*b*
  mindfulness, 299
  NCLEX, 291*b*
  panic disorder, 560
  principles of, 294*b*
    cognitive-behavioural formulation,
      294*b*
    educative, 294*b*

  goal oriented, problem focused, and
      change oriented, 294*b*
  inductive qualitative content
      analysis, 291
  time limitation, 294*b*
  psychotherapy, 290–291
  research for, 291*b*
  substance-related disorders, 666
  technology-supported delivery,
      290–291
  thinking errors, 296
  treatment strategies
    behavioural techniques, 297–299
    cognitive techniques, 295–297
Collaboration, 230*b*
  in assessment, 215–216
Collaborative care, 98–99
Collaborative mental health care models,
      75
Collective trauma, 369–371
Collective unconscious, 162
Colonialism, 47–48
Command hallucinations, 221
Common aetiology model, concurrent
      disorders, 906
Communication, 105–124
  action, 245
  blocks, 115
  disorders, 823–824
  group, 314
  nonverbal, 108–109, 111*f*
    group, 306–307
  with older adults, 840*b*
  open, 242
  patterns, family assessment, 325–329
  relational, 305–306
  self-awareness, 105
  triad, 711
  verbal, 106–108, 107*f*, 107*b*, 108*t*–110*t*,
      110*b*
Community
  action, 245
  assessment, with children and
      adolescents, 795
  bio/psycho/social/spiritual psychiatric
      nursing assessment of children
      and adolescents, 795
  care, 76–78, 490–491
  referrals, 73
  support, 76–78
  treatment
    anxiety, 563
    obsessive-compulsive disorder,
      566–568
    panic disorder, 547–549
    somatic symptom disorder, 585
Community mental health nursing, 10
Community resource base, 776–777
Community treatment orders (CTOs), 78,
      129–131, 132*f*
Community-based mental health
      promotion, new directions
      in, 776
Community-based residential
      services, 77
Community-based violence prevention,
      71

Comorbidity. *See specific disorders*

Compassion fatigue, 352

Compassionate release, 940

Competence
    apparent, in borderline personality
        disorder, 701*b*
    cultural, 53–54

Completed suicide, 422

Complicated grief, 759

Comprehensive approaches, mental4
        health promotion with children
        and adolescents, 776

Comprehensive assessment, 209

Comprehensive Behavioural Intervention
        for Tics (CBIT), for motor
        disorder, 829

Compulsions, 551

Compulsive personality disorder,
        722–723

Computed axial tomography, 181

Computer resources (cCBT), 290

Concentration, in mental status
        examination, 221–223

Concurrent disorders
    anxiety disorders and, 910
    assessment, 907
    attention deficit hyperactivity disorder
        and, 910–911
    care and treatment, 907–909
    development of, 906–907
    education and training, 912
    epidemiology of, 905–906
    indications for hospitalization, 909
    interventions, 909–911
        substance-related disorders (*see*
            Substance-related disorders)
    mood disorders and, 909–910
    nursing management, 911–912
    personality disorders and, 911
    posttraumatic stress disorder and, 910
    psychotic disorders and, 911
    research for, 912*b*
    treatment matching, 909

Conditional leave, 129

Conditioning, classical (Pavlovian), 164*t*,
        165

Conduct disorder, 723, 826–827

Confidentiality, 116–117, 144–145, 433

Conflict resolution, 238–239

Confrontation, leading groups, 308*t*

Confusion Assessment Method , 870*b*

Conners Parent Questionnaire, 819*b*

Conscientious objection, 135–136

Conscious mental processes, in
        psychoanalytic theory, 160–161

Consultation, 75

Consumer organizations, 13

Consumer self-help/survivor initiatives,
        73

Consumer-oriented interventions, 517

Content themes, 115, 115*b*

Continuous positive airway pressure
        therapy (CPAP), 749–750

Continuum of care, 66–80. *See also*
        specific disorders
    acute inpatient care, 78
    assertive community treatment, 78

case management and, 70, 71*b*

community treatment orders, 78

consumer self-help/survivor initiatives,
        73

coordination of care and, 70–71

crisis response systems and psychiatric
        emergency services, 73–74, 74*b*

definition of, 67–70

e-mental health, 78–79

housing and community support,
        76–78

integrated approach, 74

outpatient care, 75, 77*b*

patient services, 70–71

primary care, 74–75

psychosocial emergency preparedness
        and response, 74

recovery-oriented practice, 70, 72*b*

supported housing, 77

supportive employment, 77–78

Continuum of eating experiences,
        595–596, 595*f*

Conversion disorder, 589

Co-operative Commonwealth Federation,
        11–12

Coordinated/parallel care, 907–908

Coordination of care, 70–71

Coordinator, 304

Coping
    abilities, family assessment, 332
    assessment of, 223
        in bipolar disorders, 510
    mechanisms, 113–114
    patterns, 481, 483
    principles, 365–367
    problem-focused *vs.* emotion focused,
        365, 367*t*
    reappraisal, 365
    skills, borderline personality disorder,
        692*b*
    social functioning, 365, 366*f*
    stress and health illness, 358–359
    styles of (*See* Defence mechanisms)

CopingTutor, 481

Core beliefs, of cognition, 293–294,
        297

Cornell Scale for Depression in Dementia
        (CSDD), 850

Corrections and Conditional Release Act
        (Bill C-30), 936

Cortical dementia, 862

Corticotrophin-releasing hormone
        (CRH), 362–363, 553

Cortisol, 733–734

Counselling, 238

Countertransference, 161

COVID-19 pandemic, 344, 381–382
    anxiety and depression during, 907*b*
    child abuse during, 769*b*
    eating disorders, 613–614
    in older adults
        age-related decline, 839
        social support, 854
    psychiatric and mental health (PMH)
        nursing, 100–101
    substance use challenges during, 765

Craving, substance-related disorders, 655

Creativity and change, 155

CRH (corticotropin-releasing hormone),
        553

Criminal Code and Mental Disorders,
        133

Criminalization, of the mentally ill,
        933–934

Crisis
    balancing factors, 377, 378*f*
    community-based emergency housing,
        378–380
    deescalation, 73
    definition, 375–380
    developmental crisis, 376
    events, 368*b*
    intervention
        early, 377
        facilitating, 377
        preventive, for adolescents, 770
        problem focusing, 377
        Roberts' seven-stage, 378, 379*b*,
            380*f*
        self-reliance, 377
        stabilization, 377
    interventions, 73
    nursing care, 377–380
    prevention of relapse, 73
    response phases, 380–381
    response systems, 73–74, 74*b*
    short-stay hospitalization, 378–380
    situational crisis, 376
    stabilization, 73–74
    symptom reduction, 73
    telephone help lines, 378

Critical pathways, 96–97

CTO. *See* Community treatment orders
        (CTOs)

Cue elimination, 634–635

Cultural assessment, 226–227

Cultural beliefs, health, 43–44

Cultural brokering, 239

Cultural competence, 53–54

Cultural diversity, 43
    within Aboriginal peoples, 46–51
    diagnostic formulations and, 44–45
    family assessment, 330–332

Cultural humility, 55

Cultural identity, 43

Cultural safety, 55

Culture, 168
    and ethnicity
        bipolar disorders and, 522
        in depressive disorders, 522
        eating disorder, 600–602, 638

Cyclothymic disorder, 519

Cytokines in depressive disorders,
        508

D

DAR (data, action, and plan) method,
        217

Day treatment, bipolar disorders, 518

Death, loss and in childhood, 758–760

De-escalation, 243

Defence mechanisms, 113–114, 161

Deinstitutionalization, 10, 13

Delirium, 862, 862*b*
   aetiology, 864
   assessment of
      biologic domain, 866–867
      psychological domain,
         869–870
      social domain, 870–871
      spiritual domain, 871
   in children, 863
   clinical course, 862
   continuum of care, 871–872, 872*b*
   diagnostic criteria, 862–863
   emergency care for, 862
   epidemiology, 864
   evaluation and treatment outcomes,
      871
   hyperactive, 863
   hypoactive, 863
   interprofessional recognition and
      treatment, 866
   mixed variant, 870
   nursing diagnoses
      biologic domain, 866–869
      psychological domain, 869–870
      social domain, 870–871
   nursing interventions
      biologic domain, 867–869
      psychological domain, 870
      social domain, 871
   in older adults, 863
   postoperative, 863
   prevention, 864–866
   priority care, 866
   rating scales for, 870*b*
   risk factors, 864, 865*t*
Delirium rating scale (DRS), 870*b*
Delirium superimposed on dementia
   (DSD), 862–863
Delusion(s), 402, 408, 478, 482
   bizarre, 481
   nonbizarre, 494
Delusional disorder (DD), 494
Delusions, 478, 884–885, 888
Demara, Ferdinand Waldo, 720*b*
Dementia, 862*b*, 872–896
   Alzheimer type (*See* Alzheimer disease
      (AD))
   bio/psycho/social/spiritual
      interventions for persons with,
      893, 894*f*
   caused by, 897–899
      HIV infection, 897
      Huntington disease, 898
      prion disease, 898
      substance-/medication-induced
         dementia, 898–899
      traumatic brain injury, 897–898
   definition of, 404
   frontotemporal, 897
   with Lewy bodies, 896–897
   long-term care, 896
Dementia praecox, 458
Deontology, 137*t*, 138
Dependent personality disorder, 722
Depersonalization, 546*t*, 548*b*
Deprescribing, 846
Depression

due to COVID-19 pandemic, 907*b*
   management, 888–889
   in older adults, 849–851
   schizophrenia, 456
Depressive disorders, 806–808
   aetiology
      genetic factors, 506–507
      neurobiologic hypotheses, 507–508
      psychological theories, 508
      social theories, 508–509
   assessment
      biologic domain, 510–511
      psychological domain, 526–529
      social domain, 516–517
      spiritual domain, 517–518
   biologic domain, 807
   biologic treatments, 514–518
   Canada's indigenous populations,
      504–505
   clinical course, 503–504
   continuum of care, 518–519
   disruptive mood dysregulation
      disorder, 806
   epidemiology
      ethnic and cultural differences, 506
      risk factors, 506
   evaluation and treatment outcomes,
      518
   family response to, 509
   interdisciplinary treatment, 509
   light therapy, 512–513
   major depressive disorder, 806
   neuromodulatory therapies, 512
   nursing care, 807–808
   nursing diagnoses for
      biologic domain, 525
      psychological domain, 526–529
      social domain, 529
      spiritual domain, 518
   nursing management
      biologic domain, 510–511
      psychological interventions, 511
      social domain, 516–517
      spiritual domain, 517–518
   nutritional therapies, 513–514
   priority care issues, 509
   psychosocial domain, 807–808
   in special populations
      children and adolescents, 504
      COVID-19, 505
      indigenous and first nations
         populations, 504–505
      older adults, 504
   treatment interventions, 806
Depressive episode, 524–525
Derealization, 548*b*
Desmopressin, for enuresis, 829
Development, depressive disorders and,
   502
Developmental assessment, bio/psycho/
   social/spiritual psychiatric nursing
   assessment of children and
   adolescents, 788–790
Developmental delays, 757, 763, 768,
   814*b*
Developmental theories, 164*t*, 166–167
Deviant roles, 304

Diabetes mellitus, 457
Diagnostic and Statistical Manual of
   Mental Disorders, 5th ed., Text
   revision (DSM-5), 23–24, 24*b*,
   113–114, 216, 226, 448–449,
   452*b*, 502, 503*b*, 520*b*, 545, 573,
   597, 636, 644, 655, 688, 738,
   803, 904
Dialectical behaviour therapy (DBT),
   692–693
Dichotomous, in borderline personality
   disorder, 697
Dietary restraint, 630*b*
Diffusion tensor magnetic resonance
   Imaging (DTI), 181–182, 181*f*
Diphenhydramine (Benadryl), 746*t*
Disaster risk reduction, 382
Disasters
   assistance with stress management,
      387*b*
   definition, 380–388
   mental health and illness in, 384–386
   phases of, 375*f*, 384
   preparedness and response
      government, role of, 382
      individuals and families, role of, 384
      nurses, role of, 383–384
      United Nations, role of, 382
   psychological first aid, 385–386
   public health principles for, 385
   research for, 383*b*
   response to, 384–386
   types of, 385*t*–386*t*
   vulnerable populations
      children and adolescents, 387
      disabled persons, 388
      ethnic minorities, underrepresented,
         388
      indigenous peoples and disaster,
         386–387
      persons with existing mental
         disorder, 387–388
      relief workers, 388
   workplace mental health, 341–342
Discharge goals, 234
Discharge planning, 440
Discrimination, 51–52, 100
Disinhibited social engagement disorder,
   813
Disinhibition, 165
   in dementia, 886
Disliked member, groups, 310–311
Disorganized behaviour, 453–454
Disorganized communication, 478–479
Disorganized symptoms, schizophrenia,
   453
Disrupted attachments, bio/psycho/
   social/spiritual psychiatric nursing
   assessment of children and
   adolescents, 791
Disruptive behaviour disorders, 825–827
Disruptive mood dysregulation disorder,
   806
Disruptive personality disorder, 723–724
Dissociation
   in borderline personality disorder, 706
   management of, 710

Dissupport, stress, 364
Distraction, 236, 558
Divalproex sodium, 271–272, 407
Diversity
    among older adults, 853
    family assessment, 324–325
Divorce, 760–762, 761t
Documentation, 217
Domains of practice, 95–96
Dominator, 304
Dopamine, 196–197, 197f
Dopamine hyperactivity, 460–461
Dopamine hypothesis, schizophrenia, 460–461
Dorothea Lynde Dix, 4–5, 4f
Doxepin (Silenor), 746t
Drive for thinness, 599b
Drug abuse. See Substance-related disorders
Drug–drug interactions, 473–476
Duration of untreated psychosis (DUP), 450
Dynamic Appraisal of Situational Aggression (DASA), 403
Dynamic Nurse–Patient Relationship, The (Orlando), 154–155
Dysconnectivity hypothesis, 461–462
Dysfunctional thinking, in borderline personality disorder, addressing, 698–699, 709b
Dyskinesia identification system, 466, 467f
Dysphoric mood, 220
Dysthymic disorder, 504
Dystonia, 266
Dystonic reactions, 470–471

E

Early childhood intervention programs, 71
Early intervention programs, mental health promotion with children and adolescents, 775
Eating. See Nutrition
Eating Attitude Test, 622b
Eating disorders. See also Anorexia nervosa (AN); Binge-eating disorder (BED); Bulimia nervosa (BN)
    assessment tools, 622b
    boys and men, 601b
    classification, 644
    complications of, 600t
    COVID-19 pandemic, 613–614
    eating attitude test, 622b
    family and friends, 627b
    feminist ideology and, 605, 605b
    future directions, 644
    health, ideal body image, healthy eating and, 625b
    hospitalization criteria, 611t
    prevention, 643–644, 644t
    psychological characteristics, 598, 599b
    risk factors, 607–610, 608f
Echolalia, 478–479
Echopraxia, 481
    schizophrenia, 476

ECT (electroconvulsive therapy), 284
    for bipolar disorders, 495
    for depressive disorders, 511–512
Education. See also Psychoeducation nursing
    early, 6–7
    models of, 10–11
Ego, 161
Egocentrism, 785
Egoistic suicide, 432
Elder abuse
    forms of, 919
    health effects of, 921
Electroconvulsive therapy (ECT), 284
    for bipolar disorders, 468
    for depressive disorders, 511–512
Electroencephalography (EEG), 203, 729–730
Electronic media services, mental health promotion with children and adolescents, 775–776
Electrooculogram (EOG) testing, 738
Elicitation, 165
Elimination disorders
    encopresis, 830–831
    enuresis, 829–830
e-Mental health, 78–79, 100, 100f
Emergency care. See also specific disorders and conditions
    anorexia nervosa, 628
    panic disorder, 544–545
    schizophrenia, 490
    somatic symptom disorder, 585
Emergency preparedness and response, 382–384
Emotion(s). See also Feelings; specific emotions
    abuse, of children, 769t
    circuit, 397f
    definition of, 220, 696
Emotional dysregulation, in borderline personality disorder, 697
Emotional regulation, for borderline personality disorder, 710–711
Emotional vulnerability, in borderline personality disorder, 693
Emotions, 690
Empathic linkages, 106, 109–111, 154
Empathic listening, 214
Empathy, 112, 162–163
Employment, supportive, 77–78
Empowerment, 70, 78
    recovery orientation and, 239
Encopresis, 830–831
    epidemiology and aetiology, 830–831
    form of, 830
    nursing care, 831
Ending, or termination, stage of group development, 304
Endorphins, 675, 705
Engagement, 320, 327
Enmeshment, 607b
Enuresis, 829–830
    epidemiology and aetiology, 829
    nursing care, 830
    treatment interventions, 829–830
Epigenetics, 177

Epinephrine, 198
Equity, diversity, and inclusion (EDI), 344
Erikson, Erik, 166–167
Ethics
    approaches, 136–140, 137t
    of care, 137t, 139
    case-based, 137t, 139
    CNA code of, 134
    definition of, 133
    deontology and, 137t, 138
    everyday, 141
    feminist, 137t, 139–140
    health, 134
    human rights and, 137, 137t
    issues in psychiatric and mental health settings
        behaviour control, 142–143
        confidentiality and privacy as, 144–145
        dignity of patients, 142
        genetics, 145–146
        neurotechnology, 145
        psychiatric advance directives, 143
        relational engagement as, 143–144
        research and, 146–147
        seclusion and restraint as, 142–143
        social justice and, 146
    Kantian, 138
    moral dilemmas and, 141–142
    moral distress and, 141–142
    for nurses, 134
    practice environments, 141
    principlism and, 137t, 139
    relational, 137t, 140
    utilitarianism and, 137t, 138–139
    virtue, 137–138 , 137t
Ethics of care, 139
Ethnic assessment, 226–227
Euphoria, 519–521
Euphoric mood, 220
Euthymic mood, 220
Event-related potentials, 204
Evoked potentials (EPs), 204
Examination, as assessment technique, 214
Exercise interventions, 235
Existential anxiety scale (EAS), 563
Existential psychotherapy, 169
Existentialist therapy, 169
Exposure therapy, 561
Expressed emotion, 478–479
Extended family, 320–321
Externalizing disorders, 825
Extrapyramidal motor system, 188, 197
Extrapyramidal side effects, 470–471
Extrovert, 162

F

Factitious disorder. See also Somatic symptom disorder
    epidemiology, 590
    imposed on another, 590
    imposed on self, 589–590
    nursing interventions, 590
    nursing management, 590
    by proxy, 590

Families
  access to services, 324
  anorexia nervosa, 607
  assessment
    biologic domain, 329
    ecomap, 328–329, 328f
    engagement and, 327
    genograms and, 327–329
    mental health assessment, 326b
    psychological domain, 329–333
    social domain, 333–334
    spiritual domain, 334–335
  bipolar disorders and, 524
  bulimia nervosa, 632
  Canadian families, 320–322
  caregivers, 322–323
  communication patterns, 332
  concurrent disorders, 911–912
  cultural diversity, 330–332
  depressive disorders and, 515–516
  development, 330
  diversity of, 324–325
  financial status, 334
  formal and informal networks, 334
  intervention
    commendation, 337
    implementation, 337
    individual strengths, 337
    15-minute family interview, 336–337
    therapeutic questions in, 337
  life cycles, 330–332
  with low incomes, 332
  meetings, 323
  problem-solving skills, 332–333
  pyramid of family care framework, 335, 336f
  separation and divorce, 760–762, 761t
  social status, 334
  stigma, 324
  stress and coping abilities, 332
  systems, 333
Family Care Framework, pyramid of, 335, 336f
Family dynamics, 167–168
Family education, 483–484. See also
    Client/family education;
    Psychoeducation
Family interventions. See also specific
    disorders and conditions
  bipolar disorders, 529–531
  commendation, 337
  implementation, 337
  individual strengths, 337
  15-minute family interview, 336–337
  panic disorder, 563
  therapeutic questions in, 337
Family psychoeducation, 538
Family relationship, bio/psycho/social/
    spiritual psychiatric nursing
    assessment of children and
    adolescents, 793
Family therapy, 335
  applicability to psychiatric and mental
    health nursing, 168
  substance-related disorders, 667
Family-based interventions, 319
Family-based therapy (FBT), 624–625
Family-to-family interventions, 319

Fatalistic suicide, 432
Fear, 552–553
  conditioning, 552–553
Feelings
  anorexia nervosa, 624
  personal, understanding, 106
Female forensic clients, 937–939
Feminine psychology, 162
Feminism, eating disorders, 605b
Feminist ethics, 137t, 139–140
Financial status, of families, 334. See also
    Poverty
First episode psychosis, 450, 495
  nursing care plan, 487b
First-pass metabolism, 255
Fissures, 183
Flat affect, 220
Flight of ideas, in bipolar disorders, 520
Fluid imbalance assessment, 466
Fluoxetine (Prozac), 615, 633, 641–642
Flurazepam (Dalmane), 746t
Focused assessment, 213
Foetal alcohol spectrum disorder (FASD),
    824–825
Folie À deux, 494
Forensic psychiatric and mental health
    nursing
  client characteristics and
    cultural diversity and, 941–942
    experience of mental illness and,
      936–937, 937b
    families and, 942
    female, 937–939
    older forensic client, 939–940
    recovery, 937, 938b
    transgender, 941
    vulnerability, 935–936
    youth, 940–941
  criminalization of the mentally ill and,
    933–934
  model for care and, 935–947, 935f
  nurse–client relationship and, 942–944
    boundary violations, 943–944
    issues experiences by nurses and,
      943–944
    manipulation, 944
    othering, 943
    professional development and,
      944–946
    professional nursing identity and, 944
  paradox of custody and caring and,
    934, 935f
  security awareness and, 946–947, 946b
  societal norms and, 947, 947b
Formal group roles, 304
Formal operations, 759–760
Formal patient, 127, 128, 129f, 130f, 131
Formal support networks, 334
Fort McMurray Wildfire, 380–381, 381f
Frailty, 841, 863
Frankl, Victor, 855
Frankl, Viktor, 169
Freedom, 155–156
Freeze-hide response, 362
Freud, Sigmund, 160, 160t
Frontal lobe(s), 183f, 184, 185b
Frontal lobe syndrome, 185b
Frontotemporal dementia, 897

Fry, Elizabeth, 4–5
Functional neuroimaging, 180t, 182
Functional status, assessment of, 226–227
  of older adults, 839

G
GABA (gamma-aminobutyric acid), 553
Gabapentin (Neurontin), 271, 669
GAD (generalized anxiety disorder), 545,
    547, 910
Galactorrhoea, 473
Gambling disorders, 680–681, 724
Gamma-aminobutyric acid (GABA),
    192–193, 199, 553, 735t
Gay, lesbian, bisexual, or transgender
    (GLBT) sexual orientation, 428
Geel Lunatic Colony, 4
Gender, 168
  bipolar disorders and, 522
  bulimia nervosa, 630
  and sexual-based phobias, 33
  somatization, 574
  substance-related disorders, 653
  suicide, 427–428
  workplace, mental health, 343
Gender identity, 32–33
Gender-based exclusion, 33
Gendered depression, 507b
General medical conditions. See Mental
    illness
Generalized anxiety disorder (GAD), 545,
    547, 910
Generativity, 166–167
Genetic factors
  bipolar disorders and, 523–524
  bulimia nervosa, 631
  eating disorder, 604, 631, 639
Genetic theories
  anorexia nervosa, 604
  bulimia nervosa, 631
Genetic vulnerability, bio/psycho/social/
    spiritual psychiatric nursing
    assessment of children and
    adolescents, 788
Genetics, 145–146, 175–177
Genograms, family assessment,
    327–328
Genome, 175
Geriatric Depression Scale (GDS), 850,
    851b
Geriatric syndromes, 841, 844
Gerotranscendence, 166, 848
Gestalt therapy, 163
Ghrelin, sleep–wake disorders, 735t
Gilligan, Carol, 164t, 167
Glial cells, 190
Global mental health, 26, 26f
Glutamate, 199
Glutamate hypoactivity hypothesis, 461
Goals, initial, revised, discharge, 234
Grandiose delusions, schizophrenia, 452,
    494
Grey matter, 183
Grieving
  in childhood, adolescence, and
    adulthood, 758–760, 758t
  inhibited, in borderline personality
    disorder, 701b

Group(s)
  anger management, 314
  closed, 302
  cognitive–behavioural, 312
  cohesion, 307
  communication, 304–307, 314
  definitions and concepts, 301–308
  development, 303–304, 303t
  groupthink and decision making,
    307–308
  interactive, 306, 312–313
  leadership
    challenging behaviours, 310–311
    member selection, 309–310
    responsibilities and functions, 305t
    seating arrangement, 310
    skills, 308
    styles, typology, 309
    techniques, 308t
  medication, 313–314, 314b
  member roles, 304
  mental health promotion, 315
  norms and standards, 307
  nursing intervention, 313–314
  open, 302
  practices, 303
  psychoeducational, 311–312
  psychotherapy, 313
  reminiscence, 315
  self-care, 315
  self-help, 313
  size, 302–303
  skills, 301
  structured, 311–312
  support, 306, 307, 311, 313, 315, 316
  supportive therapy, 313
  symptom management, 314
  types of, 311–313
Group cohesion, 307
Group conflict, 311
Group dynamics, 301–302
Group leadership, 308–311
Group living, 77
Group themes, 306
Group therapy
  bulimia nervosa, 636
  for depressive disorders, 516
  substance-related disorders, 666
Groupthink, 307–308
Guided imagery, 236
Gynaecomastia, 473
Gyri, 183, 184f

H
Habit reversal therapy, 827, 829
Hallucinations, 221, 452b, 478, 480b,
  495, 885, 888
Hallucinogen, substance-related
  disorders, 674–675
HAM-D (Hamilton Rating Scale for
  Depression), 514
Hamilton rating scale, 558t
Hamilton Rating Scale for Depression
  (HAM-D), 514, 850
Harm reduction, education, 98, 439, 662,
  665–666
Harm reduction, substance-related
  disorders, 665–666

Harmonizer, 304
Hazards, workplace, mental health, 342
Health care delivery system, 99–100
Health care organization, 55
Health disparity, 54, 58, 311
Health ethics, 134
Health history, 217
Health promotion, 71–72
  McGill model of nursing, 157
Health services, Aboriginal populations,
  50
Health teaching. See Client/family
  education
Healthcare reform, 14–15
Healthy aging, 838b
Healthy workplaces, 344–347
  psychosocial factors in, 345t
  unsafe workplaces, 344, 346b
  work-life balance, 346–347, 346b
Hearing, age-related deficits in, 844–845
Helplessness, 429–430
Hierarchy of needs, 163, 163f
Highlighting, leading groups, 308t
Hippocampus, 187
Histamine, 199
Historical trauma, 369–371
Historical/Clinical/Risk-20 Version 3
  (HCR-20 V3), 403
History taking, for biologic domain
  ssessment, 217
Histrionic personality disorder, 720–721
Hoarding disorder, 551–552, 568
Holistic nursing care, expansion of, 12–13
Home visits, 244–245
Homelessness, in childhood
  andadolescence, 768
Homicidal ideation, 226
Hope, recovery orientation and, 239
Hopelessness, 429–430
Horney, Karen, 160t, 162
Horney's Feminine Psychology, 160t, 162
Hospital-based care, 585
Hospitalization. See also Inpatient care
  (hospitalization); Inpatient-
  focused care
  anorexia nervosa, 628
  anxiety, 554
  eating disorder, criteria, 611t
Housing services, 76–78
Hughes, Clara, 908b
Human genome, 175
Human rights, 126–133, 127t, 127b, 137t
Humanbecoming, 155–156
Humane treatment, 3–5
Humanistic theories, 162–163, 163f
Huntington disease, 898
Hydration interventions, 236–237
Hydrotherapy, 9
Hydroxyzine (Atarax), 746t
Hyperactive delirium, 863, 870
Hyperactivity
  attention deficit hyperactivity disorder,
    819
  definition, 818b
Hyperprolactinaemia, 473
Hypersexuality, 886
Hyperventilation, 555
Hypervigilance, schizophrenia, 454, 479
Hypnagogic hallucinations, 221

Hypnotic, substance-related disorders, 677
Hypoactive delirium, 863, 870
Hypochondriasis, 588
Hypocretin, sleep–wake disorders, 735t
Hypomanic episodes, 519
Hypothalamic-pituitary-adrenal (HPA)
  axis, 508
Hypothalamus, 187–188
Hysterical anorexia, 594–595

I
Ideation
  assaultive/homicidal, 226
  suicidal, 223
Identification, in psychoanalytic theory,
  161
Identity
  definition, 29–30
  diffusion, in borderline personality
    disorder, 697
  in Erikson's theory, 166
Identity-based exclusion, 31–36
  chronological age, 34–36
    children and youth, 34–35
    older adults, 35–36
  disability, 34
  gender and LGBTQI2SA+ identity,
    32–33
  mental illness diagnosis, 31
  racialized communities, 31–32
  socioeconomic status, 34
Illimitability, 155–156
Illness anxiety disorder, 588–589
Illusions, 221, 453, 884–885, 888
Immediate families, 320–321
Impaired driving, 665b
Impaired metacognition, 689–690
Impulse-control disorders
  intermittent explosive disorder, 723
  kleptomania, 723–724
  pyromania, 724
Impulsiveness, definition, 818b
Impulsivity
  in borderline personality disorder, 706
  personality disorder, 698
Impulsivity and destructive behaviour,
  690
Incivility, 348–349
Indian Act of 1876, 50
Indian Residential School (IRS), 48
Indicators, 234
Indigenous, 100, 246, 319, 331, 370–
  372, 386–387, 426–427, 433,
  455, 504, 505, 624
Individual role, group, 304
Inflammation, 876
Infodemic, 381
Informal group roles, 304
Informal support networks, 334
Information leading groups, 304
Information seeker, 304
Informed consent, 433–434
Inhalant-related disorders, 675
Inhibited grieving, in borderline
  personality disorder, 701b
Initial goals, 234
Inpatient care (hospitalization), 68, 77
  panic disorder, 563

Inpatient units, promotion of client safety on, 242–244
Inpatient-focused care
    schizophrenia, 490
    somatic symptom disorder, 588
Insight and judgment, 481
Insight, in mental status examination, 223
Insomnia, 846
    biologic domain, 745–747
    bio/psycho/social/spiritual outcomes, 743, 744f
    characteristics, 741–742
    definition, 743b
    factors and conditions related to, 742–743
    nursing management, 743–749
        BEARS Sleep Screening Questionnaire, 743, 744t
        care providers schedules, 744
        strategies for hospitalized and institutionalized patients, 744, 745b
    pharmacologic approaches to
        cannabis effect on sleep, 747, 747t
        historical perspective, 745
        present-day pharmacotherapy, 745–747, 746t
    psychological domain, 747–748
    sleep hygiene, 743, 743b
    social domain, 748
    spiritual domain, 748–749
    symptom, 741–742
    treatment, 742–743
Institutionalization. See Hospitalization; Inpatient-focused care
Institution(s) early, 2–3, 4f, 5t, 6–7
    life within, 6–7
Integrated care, 908
    pathways, 909
Integration into psychosocial treatment, 9
Intensive outpatient programs, 76
    for bipolar disorders, 537
Intensive residential services, 77
Interaction patterns, 306
Interactional theory, 400
Interactive groups, 312–313
Interdisciplinary approach, 610–611, 773
Intergenerational trauma, 50–51
Intermediate beliefs, of cognition, 294f, 297
Intermittent explosive disorder (IED), 723
Internalizing disorders, 825
Internet (iCBT), 290
Interoceptive awareness, 598–599, 599b
Interpersonal effectiveness skills, 693
Interpersonal psychotherapy (IPT), 624–625
Interpersonal Relations in Nursing (Peplau), 115, 154
Interpersonal relations models, 154–155
Interpersonal relationships, unstable, borderline personality disorder, 697
Interpersonal skills, for borderline personality disorder, 713
Interpersonal therapy (IPT), 666
    for depressive disorders, 515

metacognitive, 693–694
Interprofessional collaboration, 215–216
Intersectionality, 30, 30b, 30f
Intervention stage, of family systems, 333
Interventions. See specific disorders and conditions
Interviewing, 214–215, 214b, 215b. See also Clinical interview
Intimacy, fear of, in borderline personality disorder, 709
Intimate partner terrorism, 918
Intimate partner violence (IPV), 682, 915, 925b, 942
    forms of, 918
    health effects of, 919–920
        mental health, 919–920
        physical health, 919
Intoxication, 237, 266, 407, 408, 655, 664–665, 678, 682
Introvert, 162
Invalidating environment, borderline personality disorder, 702
Involuntary admission, 78, 127, 129, 131b
Involuntary hospitalization, 433–434
IPT (interpersonal therapy)
    for depressive disorders, 515
    metacognitive, 693–694
IRS (Indian Residential School), 48

J
Jet lag, 751–752
Job attitudes, workplace, mental health, 342
Job strain, workplace, mental health, 342
Journal(s), 12–13
Journal of Psychiatric Nursing, 12–13
Judgment, in mental status examination, 223
Jung, Carl Gustav, 160t, 162
Jung's Analytical Psychology, 160t, 162
Justice, 139

K
Kanner, Leo, 814
Kantian ethics, 138
Kindling theory, bipolar disorders and, 523
King, Imogene M., 157–158
Kleptomania, 723–724
Knowledge development, dissemination and application, 99
Knowledge resource base, 776–777

L
La Caridad y San Hipólito, order of, 2–3
Lactation, substance-related disorders, 682
Lamotrigine (Lamictal), 273
Languages. See also Speech; Verbal communication
    bio/psycho/social/spiritual psychiatric nursing assessment of children and adolescents, 789–790, 790t
Late adulthood, 839b. See also Older adults
Law and Psychiatric and Mental Health Care, 126–133

Leadership
    challenging behaviours, 310–311
    member selection, 309–310
    responsibilities and functions, 305t
    seating arrangement, 310
    styles, typology, 309
    techniques, 308t
Learning disorders, 823
Least restrictive environment, 433–434
Legal aspects. See Ethics
Legal issues
    basis for mental health treatment and, 5t, 6
    law and psychiatric and mental health care, 126–133
Legal status, of older adults, 855
Leininger, Madeleine, 169
Lesbian, gay, bisexual, transgender, queer, questioning, intersexual, or two-spirit (LGBTQI2SA+) youth, 428
Lethality, 429b, 435–436
Lewin, Kurt, 164t
Life expectancy, 837
Light therapy (phototherapy), 284–285, 512–513
Limbic midbrain nuclei, 188
Limbic system
    amygdala, 188
    hippocampus, 187
    hypothalamus, 187–188
    limbic midbrain nuclei, 188
    structures, 187f
    thalamus, 187
Lisdexamfetamine dimesylate (Vyvanse), 641–642
Listening
    active, 108
    passive, 108
Lithium
    interactions with medications and substances, 527t
    side effects, 526t–527t
Lithium (Eskalith), 531b
Lithium carbonate, 525–526
Locus coeruleus, 198, 198f
Logotherapy, 169
Loneliness
    definition, 852–853
    health problem of, 853
    risk factors for, 852–853
Low-income families, 332

M
"Mad houses,", 2
Magnetic resonance imaging (MRI), 181
Maintenance functions, group, 315–316
Maintenance of wakefulness test (MWT), 740
Major depressive disorder (MDD). See also Mood disorders
    children and adolescents, 806
Major depressive episode (MDE), 503
Maladaptive cognitive processes, 700, 700t
Maladaptive emotional response, 690
Males, eating disorder, 601b
Malingering, 589–590

Mandatory outpatient treatment (MOT), 129–131
Mania, 537
Manic episodes, 526b, 538
Manic-depressive disorders. *See* Bipolar disorders
MAOIs. *See* Monoamine oxidase inhibitors (MAOIs)
MAPS theories, 153
Marital therapy, for depressive disorders, 515–516
Marriage. *See also* Remarriage, children separation and divorce and, 760–762, 761t
Maslow, Abraham, 160t, 163, 163f
Maslow's Hierarchy of Needs, 163, 163f
Mass cluster, 432–433
Maturation, bio/psycho/social/spiritual psychiatric nursing assessment of children and adolescents, 789
Maturity fears, 604, 606b
Maximal mental disorder, 20
MDE (major depressive episode), 503
Medical Assistance in Dying, 133
Medicalization, 36–37
Medication groups, 313–314, 314b
Medication management, 237
Megavitamin therapy, 513
Melatonin, 733, 747
Memory, 494, 861, 862b, 882
 in depressive disorders, assessment, 514
 enhancement, 886–887
 in mental status examination, 221
 in older adults, 849
Memory and orientation, 479–481
Mental disorders. *See also* Mental illness; *specific disorders*
 diagnosis of
  DSM-5, 23–24, 24b
  labelling, 24–25
 early explanations of, 3
 mental health literacy, 25
 responses to, 217
Mental health
 and addiction, 48
 of Canadians, 25
 cultural roots of, 43
 family, 319, 325b
 global mental health, 26, 26f
 mental illness
  diagnosis of, 23–25
  mental health literacy, 25
 of older adults, 837–860
 recovery, 25
 research-based care, 25–26
 socioeconomic influences, 55–59
 well-being
  Canadian index of wellbeing, 21
  social progress index, 21–23
Mental Health Act, 6, 127–128, 128t
 admission certificate, 127–128
 competence of the person, 128
 formal patient, 127–128
 Formal Patient Certification process, 128, 129f
 Formal Patient Competency & Consent for Treatment Decisions, 128, 130f

involuntary admission, 127–129, 131b
 renewal certificates, 128
 review panel, 131
 substitute decision-making, 128
Mental health assessment
 in children and adolescents
  bio/psycho/social/spiritual model, 777
  bio/psycho/social/spiritual psychiatric nursing assessment, 785–796, 786b
  child and youth mental health framework, 777
  CMHA's Framework for Support, 776–777
  collection of, 777–785
 in older adults
  biologic domain, 844–846
  physiologic causes of changes, in mental status, 841, 842b
  psychological domain, 848–849
  social domain, 851–855
  spiritual domain, 855
Mental health care
 Aboriginal people, 46–51
 acceptability, 60
 accessibility, 60
 availability, 59–60
 continuum of, 66–80
 coordination of, 71–72
 cultural competence, 53–54
 cultural context of, 42–45
 cultural safety, 55
 diagnostic cultural formulations, 44–45
 discrimination, 51–52
 geographic context of, 59–61
 legal basis, 5t, 6
 mandatory outpatient treatment, 126, 129–131
 prejudice, 51
 primary care, 74–75, 76b
 recovery, 97, 169–170
 reform, 3–8, 14–15, 17, 126, 169, 683
 socioeconomic context of, 55–59
 stereotyping, 51
 stigma of, 52
Mental Health Commission of Canada (MHCC), 320, 342, 803–804
Mental health first aid, 385–386
Mental health legislation
 in Canada (*See* Mental Health Act)
 Canadian Nurses' Responsibility, 133
 and human rights, 126
Mental health literacy, 25
Mental health nursing practice, implications for, 38, 38b
Mental health problems, 477–478
Mental health promotion, 71–72, 72b, 756–802
 for bipolar disorders, 537
 in children and adolescents
  addressing risks and challenges, 770, 773–776
  factors for psychopathology and, 765–773
  mental health in children and adolescents and, 756–757

 promotion and prevention programs, 774–776
 stressors and, 757–765
 in older adults
  age category, 839
  ageism, 839
  functional status declines, 839
  maximum functioning and quality of life, 839
  psychological domain and, 848–849
  social domain and, 851–855
  spiritual domain, 855
  strategies, 839–841
 schizophrenia, 491
 somatic symptom disorder, 585–588
Mental health promotion activities, 537
Mental health promotion groups, 315
Mental health services, Aboriginal populations, 50
Mental health strategy, 51
 for Canada, 934, 934b
Mental health treatment, legal basis for, 5t, 6
"Mental Hygiene,", 6
Mental illness. *See also specific disorders*
 biologic view, 8
 Canadian families, 320–322
 caregivers, 320
 causes of, 3, 8
 connection and assessment, 328
 consultation, 335
 cultural roots of, 43
 diagnosis of, 23–25
 general education, 335
 life and economic impact of, 57
 mental health literacy, 25
 parents, 771–772
 prevention strategies, 71–72
 religious beliefs and approaches to, 46
 stigma of, 52, 324, 337
Mental status examination (MSE), 219–223, 219b, 220b
 bio/psycho/social/spiritual psychiatric nursing assessment of children and adolescents, 788
Mentalization-based treatment (MBT), 693
Mesolimbic pathway hyperactivity, schizophrenia, 461
Metabolic syndrome (MetS), 99, 265, 284, 456–457, 493, 523, 638
Metacognition, 689–690
Metacognitive interpersonal therapy (MIT), 693–694
Meteorologic-Hydrologic Disaster, 380–381
Methylphenidate (Ritalin)
 adverse reactions, 282–283
 indications and mechanisms of action, 281
 off-label use, 280
 pharmacokinetics, 281–282
 side effects, 282–283
 toxicity, 282–283
Meyer, Adolf, 8
MI (motivational interviewing), 119–120, 120b, 121b
Middle stage of group development, 304

Middle-old, 839
Mild cognitive impairment (MCI), 850, 872
Milieu therapy, 241–242, 516
Mindfulness, 299, 299b, 412
Mindfulness-based cognitive therapy, 515
Mindfulness-integrated CBT (MICBT), 299
Minority stress, 212b
Mixed episode, in bipolar disorders, 521–522
Mobile crisis response, 13, 73
Modafinil (Alertec; Provigil)
  adverse reactions, 282–283
  indications and mechanisms of action, 281
  off-label use, 280
  pharmacokinetics, 281–282
  side effects, 282–283
  toxicity, 282–283
Model for care, forensic nursing, 935–947, 935f
Modelling, 546, 641, 693, 696, 714, 762, 772, 824
Modern thinking, scientific thought
  Meyer and psychiatric pluralism, 8
  psychoanalytic theory, 8–9
  psychosocial treatment, integration biologic theories, 9
Monoamine oxidase inhibitors (MAOIs)
  adverse reactions, 275–277
  indications and mechanisms of action, 274–275
  pharmacokinetics, 275
  side effects, 275–277
  toxicity, 275–277
Monopolizing group time, 310
Mood, 514, 528
Mood and affect, 478
Mood disorders
  assessment of, 220
  and concurrent addictive, 909–910
  definition of, 220
Mood stabilizers, 742t, 882
  anticonvulsants
    adverse reactions, 272–273
    for bipolar disorder, 271
    clinical advantage, 271
    indications and mechanisms of action, 271–272
    pharmacokinetics, 272
    risk factor, 271
    side effects, 272–273
  lithium, 269–271
    adverse reactions, 270–271
    indications, 269–270
    mechanisms of action, 269–270
    side effects, 270–271
    toxicity, 270–271
Moral dilemmas, 141–142
Moral distress, 141–142
More for the Mind, 10
Motivational interviewing (MI), 119–120, 120b, 121b, 666
Motor disorders, 827–829
  aetiology, 827
  epidemiology, 827

nursing care, 827–829
treatment interventions, 827
MSE (mental status examination), 219–223, 219b, 220b
Multiple sleep latency test (MSLT), 740
Muscle relaxation, 556b
Myers-Briggs Type Indicator test, 162
Mystery, 155–156

N
Naltrexone, 669
Narcissistic personality disorder, 721
Narcolepsy, 752
Nardil (phenelzine), 274–275, 277
National Committee for Mental Hygiene, 6
National mental health strategy, 15–16, 15b
NCDs. *See* Neurocognitive disorders (NCDs)
NDRIs (norepinephrine-dopamine reuptake inhibitors), 742t
Neecham Confusion Scale, 870b
Needs
  hierarchy of, 163, 163f
  in interpersonal relations theory, 154
Negative symptoms, 453
  scale for assessment, 477
Neglect, of children, 769–771, 769t
Neo-Freudian models
  of Adler, 160t, 162
  of Horney, 160t, 162
  of Jung, 160t, 162
Nervous consumption, 594–595
Neuman, Betty, 158–159
Neuman systems model, 159
Neural connectivity, schizophrenia, 459–460
Neural diathesis–stress model, 459–460
Neuroactive steroids, 553–554
Neuroanatomy, 179t, 191f, 192t
  autonomic nervous system, 187–188
  cerebrum, 183–188, 183f
  extrapyramidal motor system, 188
  locus coeruleus, 188–189
  peripheral organ response, 192t
  pineal body, 188
Neurobehavioural disorder associated with prenatal alcohol exposure (ND-PAE), 824–825
Neurochemical model, 398–399
Neurocognition, 453
Neurocognitive disorders (NCDs)
  Alzheimer disease
    aetiology, 875–877, 875f
    biologic domain, 878–882
    clinical course, 873, 873t
    continuum of care, 894–896
    diagnostic criteria, 873–874, 874t, 874b
    epidemiology, 874–875
    evaluation, 893–894
    family response, 877–878
    interprofessional treatment, 877
    priority care issues, 877
    psychological domain, 882–891
    risk factors, 874–875
    social domain, 891–892

    spiritual domain, 893
    treatment outcomes, 893–894, 894f
  delirium
    aetiology, 864
    biologic domain, 866–869
    in children, 863
    clinical course, 862
    continuum of care, 871–872, 872b
    diagnostic criteria, 862–863
    epidemiology, 864
    evaluation, 871
    interprofessional recognition and treatment, 866
    older adults, 863
    prevention, 864–866
    priority care, 866
    psychological domain, 869–870
    risk factors, 864, 865t
    social domain, 870–871
    spiritual domain, 871
    treatment outcomes, 871
  dementia, 872
    HIV infection, 897
    Huntington disease, 898
    with Lewy bodies, 896–897
    prion disease, 898
    substance-/medication-induced dementia, 898–899
    traumatic brain injury, 897–898
  mild cognitive impairment, 872
  Parkinson disease dementia, 897
  vascular neurocognitive disorder, 896
Neurodevelopmental disorders, 814–825
  autism spectrum disorder
    biopsychosocial domain, 816
    continuum of care, 816–817
    epidemiology and aetiology, 815, 815f
    nursing care, 815–817
  communication disorders, 823–824
  foetal alcohol spectrum disorder, 824–825
  neurobehavioural disorder associated with prenatal alcohol exposure, 824–825
  specific learning disorders, 823
Neuroendocrine hypotheses, depressive disorder, 508
Neurofibrillary tangles, 875–876
Neurohormones, 188
Neuroimaging
  functional, 182
  methods of, 180t
  structural, 180–182
  structure-function gap, 182–183
Neuroleptic malignant syndrome (NMS), 266, 470
  diagnostic criteria, 475b
  signs and symptoms, 476
Neurologic examination, bio/psycho/social/spiritual psychiatric nursing assessment of children and adolescents, 788
Neuromodulatory therapies, 512
Neuropathologic theories
  anorexia nervosa, 604
  somatic symptom disorder, 576
Neuropeptide(s), 199–200
Neuropeptide hypotheses, 508

Neuropeptide Y (NPY), 735*t*
Neurophysiology
  categories, 190
  glial cells, 190
  neurons and nerve impulses, 190–192
  neurotransmitters, 195–200
    amino acids, 199
    biogenic amines, 196–199
    cholinergic, 196, 196*f*
    neuropeptides, 199–200
  receptors, 194–195
  synaptic transmission, 192–195
Neuroplasticity, 179, 194, 840
Neurosis, 9
Neuropsychiatric symptoms, 845, 881,
  883–885
Neurotechnology, 145
Neurotransmitters
  amino acids, 199
  biogenic amines, 196–199
    dopamine, 196–197, 197*f*
    epinephrine, 198
    histamine, 199
    norepinephrine, 197–198, 198*f*
    serotonin, 198–199
  categories, 192
  cholinergic, 196, 196*f*
  neuropeptides, 199–200
  synaptic transmission
    excitatory neurotransmitter, 192
    inhibitory neurotransmitter, 192
    lock-and-key analogy, 193
Nicotine, 678–680
Nicotine replacement therapy
  (NRT), 680
Nightingale, Florence, 154
Nihilistic delusions, schizophrenia, 452
N-Methyl-D-aspartate antagonists, 881
NMS. *See* Neuroleptic malignant
  syndrome (NMS)
Nonbenzodiazepine sedative–hypnotics,
  742*t*
Nonmaleficence ethics, 139
Nontherapeutic relationships, 118–119
Nonverbal communication, 108–109,
  111*f*, 306–307
Norepinephrine (NE), 197–198, 198*f*,
  553, 735*t*
Norepinephrine-and serotonin-selective
  reuptake inhibitors (NSSRIs), 556
Norepinephrine-dopamine reuptake
  inhibitors (NDRIs), 742*t*
Normalization, mental health promotion
  with children and adolescents, 774
Norms, 307
NPs (nurse practitioners), 59–60
Nuclear families, 320–321
Nurse practitioners (NPs), 59–60
Nurse–client relationship, 115–118,
  116*b*, 117*b*, 119*b*
  definition of, 115
  orientation phase, 115
  resolution phase of, 118, 119*b*
  testing of, 117
  working phase of, 117–118, 117*b*
Nurses, as health advocates, 682
Nurses fatigue, 351–352

Nursing care planning and
  implementation, 229–247, 230*b*
  documentation of goal achievement,
    234
  goals of nursing care, 233–234, 233*b*
  individual care goals, purposes of, 234
  nursing focus of care, 232–233, 233*b*
Nursing care plans, 715*b*. *See also* specific
  disorders conditions
  alcoholism, 659
  anorexia nervosa, 615*b*
  attention deficit hyperactivity disorder,
    821*b*
  bipolar disorder, 531*b*
  BPD, 715
  ineffective individual coping,
    535–536
  neurocognitive disorders, 895*b*
  schizophrenia, 452
  self-harm, 504, 520
  somatic symptom disorder, 586*b*
Nursing diagnosis. *See also specific*
  disorders and conditions
Nursing education, 53
  early, 6–7
  models of, 10–11
Nursing interventions, 234*b*. *See also*
  specific disorders and conditions
  for biologic domain, 235–237
    activity and exercise interventions,
      235
    hydration interventions, 236–237
    medication management, 237
    nutrition interventions, 236
    pain management, 237
    promotion of self-care activities,
      235
    relaxation interventions, 236
    sleep interventions, 235–236
    thermoregulation interventions, 237
  definition of, 234*b*
  Nursing Interventions Classification,
    234
  for psychological domain
    behaviour therapy, 240
    cognitive, 240
    conflict resolution, 238–239
    counselling, 238
    health teaching, 240–241
    psychoeducation, 240
    recovery orientation, 239
    reminiscence, 239–240
    video games, 238
  for social domain
    community action, 245
    home visits, 244–245
    milieu therapy, 241–242
    psychiatric units, 242–244
  for spiritual domain, 245–246
Nursing Interventions Classification
  (NIC), 234
Nursing journals, 12–13
  Nursing Mental Disease (Bailey), 8
Nursing roles, 53, 58–59
  recognizing and responding to abuse,
    921–926
    documentation, 926

physical examination and history
  taking, 922–923
  strengths-based approach, 923–926
  trauma- and violence-informed care,
    922
Nursing theories, 153–159
  existential and humanistic theoretic
    perspectives, 155–157
  interpersonal relations models,
    154–155
  of Nightingale, 154
  systems models, 157–159
Nutrition, 407
  counselling, 641
  regulation, somatic symptom disorder,
    580
Nutrition planning, 555
Nutrition regulation, 580
Nutritional balance, 705
Nutritional balance, for borderline
  personality disorder, 705
Nutritional interventions, 236
Nutritional planning, 564*f*
Nutritional therapies, 513–514

O

Object relations, in psychoanalytic
  theory, 161
Objective data, 216
Observation
  as assessment technique, 213
  promotion of client safety on, 243
Obsessions, 566
Obsessive–compulsive disorder (OCD),
  551, 722
  aetiology, 810–811
  assessment, 566–567
  clinical vignette, 566
  cognitive restructuring interventions,
    560
  community treatment, 567–568
  diagnostic criteria, 546
  epidemiology, 810–811
  exposure with response prevention,
    567
  family response, 567
  lifetime prevalence, 549
  nursing care, 811
  psychotherapeutic treatments, 567–568
  rating scales, 567*b*
  symptoms, 545
  Tourette syndrome, 811
  treatment, 567
  treatment interventions, 811
Obstructive sleep apnea (OSA), 729,
  749–751
  BANG and STOP mnemonics, 749,
    749*t*
  biologic domain, 749–750, 750*f*
  incidence, 749
  psychological domain, 750
  signs and symptoms of, 749
  social domain, 750–751
  spiritual domain, 751
Occipital lobes, 183*f*, 185
OCD. *See* Obsessive–compulsive disorder
  (OCD)

Older adults
  alcohol consumption, 846
  behaviour changes, 850
  bipolar disorders in, 524
  cognitive function, 848–850
  communication, 840b
  COVID-19 pandemic
    age-related decline, 839
    social support, 854
  delirium, 863
  depression, 849–851
  depressive disorders in, 504
  diversity, 853
  functional status, 839
  identity-based exclusion, chronological age, 35–36
  legal status, 855
  memory, 849
  mental health assessment
    biologic domain, 844–846
    physiologic causes of changes, in mental status, 841, 842b
    psychological domain, 848–849
    social domain, 851–855
    spiritual domain, 855
  mental health promotion
    age category, 839
    ageism, 839
    functional status declines, 839
    maximum functioning and quality of life, 839
    psychological domain and, 848–849
    social domain and, 851–855
    spiritual domain, 855
    strategies, 839–841
  pharmacotherapy, 847, 848b
  poverty, 853–854
  quality of life, 854
  relationship with, 852–853
  resiliency, 849
  schizophrenia, 454–455
  sleep, 846
  social connection, 852
  social support, 854
  social systems, 854–855
  somatic symptom disorder, 575
  in special populations, depressive disorders, 504
  spirituality, 855
  stresses and coping patterns, 851
Old-old, 839
Open communication, 242
Open group, 302
Operant behaviour, 165
Opioid, substance-related disorders, 675–677
Opportunity for All—Canada's First Poverty Reduction Strategy 2018, 853–854
Oppositional defiant disorder (ODD), 825
Optimal mental health, 20
Orem, Dorothea, 159
Orexin, sleep-wake disorders, 735t, 740
Orientation
  in mental status examination, 221
  modes

  feeling, 162
  intuition, 162
  sensation, 162
  thinking, 162
Orientation phase of nurse-client relationship, 116–117
  confidentiality in treatment, 116–117
  first meeting, 116
  testing the relationship, 117
Orlando, Ida Jean, 154–155
Orlistat, 641–642
Orthomolecular therapy, 513
Orthorexia, 595–596
Orthostatic hypotension, 472–473
Othering, 29, 943
Outpatient care, 441
Overcoming stigma, 100
Oxidative stress, 876

P

Pain management, 237, 580
Panic attacks, 548b
Panic disorder (PD), 545
  agoraphobia, 549–550, 549b
  assessment
    occupational domains, 561–562
    psychological domain, 557–561
    social domains, 561–562
    spiritual domain, 562–563
  continuum of care, 563
  DSM-5 diagnostic criteria, 548b
  evaluation and treatment outcomes, 563
  interventions
    biologic domain, 555
    occupational domains, 561–562
    social domains, 561–562
  panic attacks, 545
Panicogenic substance use, 555
Paradox, 155–156
Parallel care, 908
Paranoid personality disorder, 694
Paranoid schizophrenia, 492
Paraphrasing, leading groups, 308t
Parasuicidal behaviour, in borderline personality disorder, 702
Parasuicide, 421
Parent(s). *See also* Families
  discussion with, 783–784
  interviewing, in mental health assessment of children and adolescents, 782–784
  mental illness, 771–772
  separation and divorce and, 760–762, 761t
  substance abuse, 772–773
Parent-child interaction model, 781–782
Paresthesias, 548b
Parietal lobes, 182, 183f, 184
Parkinson disease dementia (PDD), 897
Parse, Rosemarie Rizzo, 155–156
Partial hospitalization programs (PHPs), 537
Passive listening, 108
Passivity, active, in borderline personality, 701b
Pathologic gambling, 937b

Patient- and family-centred care in Canada, 320, 321b
Patient education, 483
Patient-centred care, partnership, 71
Patient movement, 10
Patriarchy, 916
Pavlov, Ivan P., 163, 164t
Pavlovian conditioning, 163–165
PD. *See* Panic disorder (PD)
Peer support, 13, 14, 73, 78, 121, 334, 350, 462, 547, 644, 691
Pemoline (Cylert)
  indications and mechanisms of action, 281
  off-label use, 280
  pharmacokinetics, 281–282
Peplau, Hildegard, 12, 154
Perception, 221, 408
Perls, Frederick S., 160t, 163
Persecutory delusions, schizophrenia, 454
Person- and family-centred approach, 230b
Person resource base, 776–777
Persona, 162
Personal boundaries, 112
  establishing, in borderline personality disorder, 709–710
Personal fable, 758b
Personal Information Protection and Electronic Documents Act (PIPEDA), 144
Personality
  definition, 713
  psychoanalytic theory of, 161
Personality disorders (PD)
  aetiology, 689
  cluster A
    continuum of care, 696
    paranoid, 694
    schizoid, 695
    schizotypal, 695–696
  cluster B
    antisocial, 717–720
    borderline, 696–703
    histrionic, 720–721
    narcissistic, 721
  cluster C
    avoidant, 721–722
    dependent, 722
    obsessive-compulsive, 722–723
  common features and diagnostic criteria
    affectivity and emotional instability, 688–689
    cognitive schemas, 700
    emotional response, 690
    impulsivity and destructive behaviour, 690
    metacognition, 689–690
    self-identity and interpersonal functioning, 690
  comorbidities, 691–692
  contextual considerations, 690
  developmental stage, 690
  diagnosis, 688–689
  epidemiology, 689

features of, 689–690
gender, 690–691
recovery and treatment, 692–694
severity, 690–691
stigma and, 691
traits, 690
treatment of, 705
Personality theory, 161
Personality traits, 688
Perspectives in Psychiatric Care, 12–13
Pharmacologic assessment
for bipolar disorders, 525
in borderline personality disorder, 704
Pharmacotherapy. *See also specific disorders and conditions*
anorexia nervosa, 612
antidepressants for, 538
antipsychotics for, 515
bulimia nervosa, 633
for depressive disorders, medication administration for, 515
for enuresis, 829
medication groups, 313–314
medication management, 237
mood stabilizers for, 538
polypharmacy among older adults and, 847, 848b
for separation anxiety disorder, 809
substance-related disorders, 667
for Tourette disorder, 827
Phenelzine (Nardil), 273t, 274–275, 277
Phobias, 549–550, 549b
Phototherapy (light therapy), 284–285, 512–513
Physical care, teaching in bipolar disorders, 525
Physical functioning
somatic symptom disorder, 578–579
Physical restraint, 244
Piaget, Jean, 164t, 167
PIE (problem, implementation, and evaluation) method, 217
Pineal body, 188
Pituitary gland, 185–187
Plasticity, 179, 179t
PMH nursing. *See* Psychiatric and mental health (PMH) nursing
Polyglucosamine, 641–642
Polymorphism, 176
Polypharmacy, 845–846
Polysomnography, 203, 738, 739f
Population genetics, 176–177
Positive Mental Health Surveillance Framework, 21, 22f
Positive self-talk, 558–559
Positive symptoms, 454
assessment, scale for, 477
Positron emission tomography (PET), 182
Postoperative delirium, 863
Postpartum onset specifier, of mood disorders, 502
Posttraumatic stress disorder (PTSD), 368–369, 813–814, 814b, 910
Potency, 198, 251–253, 263, 264, 266, 674
Poverty, 34, 35b, 56–57
and Aboriginal mental health, 58
among older adults, 853–854

in childhood and adolescence, 767–768
and demographics:, 34, 35b
health disparity, 58
investment in mental health, 57
life and economic impact, 57
mental health and, 57
Powerlessness, 434
Preconscious, in psychoanalytic theory, 160–161
Predictability, ensuring, with autistic spectrum disorder, 816
Pregnancy, substance-related disorders, 682
Prejudice, 51
Preschool-aged children
clinical interview, 784–785
loss and, 759
Pressured speech, 220–221, 222b
Primacy of Caring (Benner), 156
Primary care, 74–75, 76b
Primary healthcare approach, 67, 74–75
Primary sources, 217
Principlism, 137t, 139
Prion disease, 898
Privacy Act, 144
Probing, leading groups, 308t
Problem solving, impaired, in borderline personality disorder, 698
Problem-oriented documentation, 217
Process recording, 114, 114b
Professional boundaries, 112–113, 113b
Progressive muscle relaxation, 555, 556b
Projection, 113–114
Projective
in borderline personality disorder, 699–700
identification, 699–700
Promotive factors, 223
Protective factors, 223–226
against childhood pathology, 762
for children of divorce and remarriage, divorce and, 761–762, 761t
Provincial Lunatic Asylum (New Brunswick), 5, 5t
Prozac (Fluoxetine hydrochloride), 634b
Pseudoneurologic symptoms, 589
Pseudoparkinsonism, 267
Psychiatric advance directives (PADS), 143
Psychiatric and mental health (PMH) nursing practice
addiction competencies, 85
biologic domain, 82–83, 83f
biologic theories, 159–160
biologic theories of, 159–160
care, 66
CASN/CFMHN entry-to-practice mental health and addiction competencies, 85, 85b, 86b, 87b
CCPNR Standards of Practice, 96
CFMHN Standards of Practice, 95–96
challenges, 99–101
clinical decision-making, 96
collaborative care, 98–99
continued evolution, 10–12, 12f
COVID-19 pandemic, 100–101
development of, 7–8, 7b

thought and, 8–9
domains of practice, 95–96
early views and, 7, 7b
e-Mental Health, 100
global community, 101
health care delivery system challenges, 99–100
humane treatment, 3–5
institutional care, 2–3
knowledge development, dissemination and application, 99
late 20th century, 12–16, 12f
modern thinking, 8–12
nursing theories of, 153–159
existential and humanistic theoretic perspectives, 155–157
interpersonal relations models, 154–155
systems models, 157–159
overcoming stigma and discrimination, 100
psychological domain, 83, 83f
psychological theories of, 160–167
behavioural theories, 163–165, 164t
cognitive theories, 164t, 165–166
developmental theories, 164t, 166–167
humanistic theories, 162–163
psychodynamic theories, 160–162, 160t
recovery, mental health care, 97
regional influences, 7–8
RPNRC entry-to-practice competencies, 88, 88b, 89b, 91b, 92b, 93b, 94b
scientific thought, 8–9
social domain, 83–84, 83f
social theories of, 167–169
family dynamics, 167–168
role theories, 168
sociocultural perspectives, 168–169
spiritual domain, 83f, 84
spiritual theories
applicability to psychiatric and mental health nursing, 169
of Frankl logotherapy, 169
of Yalom existential psychotherapy, 169
standards, 95–96
Standards of Professional Practice, 95–96
19th and early 20th centuries, 5–8
trauma-informed care, 97–98
Psychiatric disorders, 9. *See also* Mental disorders; Mental illness
anxiety disorders, 808–810
disruptive behaviour disorders, 825–827
elimination disorders, 829–831
gender dysphoria, 792
neurodevelopmental disorders, 814–825
schizophrenia, 804–805
Tourette disorder, 827–829
Psychiatric hospitals, 7
Psychiatric nurse, 11
Psychiatric Nurses Association of Canada, 11–12
Psychiatric nursing textbooks, first, 8

Psychiatric pluralism, 8
Psychiatric units, 242–244
Psychiatrization, 36, 39
Psychoanalysis, 160–161, 160t
Psychoanalytic movement, 8–9
Psychoanalytic theories, 399. *See also*
    Neo-Freudian models;
    Psychoanalytic theories
  anxiety and defence mechanisms, 161
  of borderline personality disorder,
    699–700
  object relations and identification in,
    161
  personality in, 161
  psychoanalysis and, 161
  sexuality in, 161
  transference and countertransference
    in, 161
  unconscious in, 160–161
Psychodynamic theories, 160–162, 160t.
    See also Neo-Freudian models;
    Psychoanalytic theories
  anxiety, 544–545
  applicability to psychiatric and mental
    health nursing, 163
  humanistic theories, 162–163, 163f
  interpersonal relations models, 160–
    162
Psychoeducation, 240, 324, 335
  anorexia nervosa, 626b
  anxiety and panic, 553
  for bipolar disorders, 529, 531b
  eating disorders, 626b
  mental health promotion with
    children and adolescents, 774–
    775
  schizophrenia, 483–484
Psychoeducational groups, 311–312
Psychoeducational topics, for relapse
    prevention, 912, 912b
Psychoendocrinology, 200–201
Psychological domain
  assessment of, 217–226
    in children and adolescents, 788–
      793
    mental status examination and,
      219–223, 219b, 220b
    responses to mental health problems
      and, 217
    risk assessment and, 223–226, 224f
    stress and coping patterns and, 223
  attachment theory, 791
  caregiving context, 790–791
  developmental assessment, 788–790
  disrupted attachments, 791
  family assessment, 325–329
    communication patterns, 332
    cultural diversity, 330–332
    family development, 330
    family life cycles, 330–332
    problem-solving skills, 332–333
    stress and coping abilities, 332
  insomnia, 747–748
  languages, 789–790, 790t
  maturation, 789
  mental status examination, 788
  obstructive sleep apnea, 750
  psychosocial development, 789

risk assessment, 792–793, 794b
secure attachments, 790–791
self-concept, 791–792, 792f
Psychological first aid (PFA), 385–386
Psychological model, 83, 83f
Psychological theories, 160–167
  anorexia nervosa, 604–605
  applicability to psychiatric and mental
    health nursing, 168
  behavioural theories, 163–165, 164t
  binge eating disorder, 639–640
  of bipolar disorders, 524
  of borderline personality disorder,
    699–700
  bulimia nervosa, 631–632
  cognitive theories, 164t, 165–166
  of depressive disorders, 508
  developmental theories, 164t, 166–167
  humanistic theories, 162–163
  psychodynamic theories, 160–162,
    160t
  schizophrenia, 478–479
  somatic symptom disorder, 576–577
  substance-related disorders, 658–659
Psychomotor activity, in mental status
    examination, 219
Psychoneuroimmunology, 201–202, 508
Psychopharmacologic drugs
  pharmacodynamics
    carrier proteins, 251, 251f
    efficacy and potency, 251–253,
      253t–254t
    enzymes, 251
    ion channels, 250
    receptors, 249–250, 250f
    toxicity, 252–253
  pharmacokinetics
    absorption and routes of
      administration, 254–256, 255t
    distribution, 256, 256t
    excretion, 258
    individual variations in drug effects,
      258–259
    metabolism, 257
  treatment phases
    discontinuation, 260–261
    initiation, 259
    maintenance, 260
    stabilization, 260
Psychopharmacologic interventions,
    580–581
Psychopharmacological therapies, 439
Psychopharmacology, 249b
Psychosis. *See* Delusional disorder;
    Psychotic disorders;
    Schizoaffective disorder;
    Schizophrenia; Schizophreniform
    disorder
Psychosis Symptom Severity scale, 226
Psychosocial development
  bio/psycho/social/spiritual psychiatric
    nursing assessment of children
    and adolescents, 789
  Erikson's theory of, 166–167
Psychosocial domain
  attention deficit hyperactivity disorder,
    820
  bipolar disorder, 806

brief psychotic disorder, 805
conduct disorder, 827
depressive disorders, 807–808
motor disorder, 828–829
oppositional defiant disorder, 825
posttraumatic stress disorder,
  813–814
psychotic disorders, 805
reactive attachment disorder, 813
Psychosocial emergency preparedness
    and response, 75
Psychosocial rehabilitation models, 8
Psychosocial treatment, integration of
    biologic theories into, 9
Psychosocially oriented ideas, 8
Psychosurgery, 9
Psychotherapy. *See also specific types of
    psychotherapy*
  for bipolar disorders, 529
  groups, 313
  transference and countertransference
    in, 161
Psychotic disorders. *See also* Delusional
    disorder; Schizoaffective disorder;
    Schizophrenia; Schizophreniform
    disorder
  concurrent disorders, 911
Psychotic episodes, in borderline
    personality disorder, 706
Pyridoxine, 513–514
Pyromania, 724

Q
Quaker(s), 3–4
Quaker Friends Asylum, 3–4
Quality of life of older adults, 854
Questioning, leading groups, 308t

R
Racial microaggressions, 32
Racism, 31, 32, 37, 44, 48, 51, 52b, 53,
    54b, 55, 66, 100, 371, 432, 609,
    915, 916, 918
Ramelteon (Rozerem), 746t
Rapid cycling, 525
Rapid eye movement (REM), 729–730
Rapport, 111–112
  building with children and
    adolescents, 778–781, 778b
Rating scales, for children, 784
REACH (Real Education About Cannabis
    and Health), 765, 766f
Reactive attachment disorder (RAD),
    812–813
Real Education About Cannabis and
    Health (REACH), 765, 766f
Recent Life Changes Questionnaire
    (RLCQ), 359, 360t
Reclamation, 156
Recognition seeker, 304
Recorder, 304
Recovery
  mental health care, 97
  orientation, 239
Recovery-oriented, trauma-informed
    mental health care, 142–143
Refeeding syndrome, 621

Reflecting behaviour, leading groups, 308t
Reflecting feelings, leading groups, 308t
Regional variations in canada, 424
Registered nurse, title of, 11
Registered Nurses Association, 8
Registered Nurses Association of Ontario (RNAO), 231, 232b
Registered Psychiatric Nurse Regulators of Canada (RPNRC), 88, 88b, 89b, 91b, 92b, 93b, 94b
Regressed behaviour, schizophrenia, 454
Rehabilitative services, 10
Reinforcement theories, 164t, 165
Reinier van Arkel asylum, 2
Reintegration, 76, 935, 942, 945
Relapse, 73, 77
Relapse prevention, 912, 912b
Relational communication, 305–306
Relational engagement, 143–144
Relational ethics, 137t, 140, 140b
Relational security, 946
Relationship
    nontherapeutic, 105, 118–119
    in older adults, 852–853
    therapeutic, 83, 88b–89b, 105–123, 161, 285, 299, 412, 515, 582, 633, 641, 719
Relaxation, 580
Relaxation strategies, 298–299, 298b
Relaxation techniques, 236, 555, 556b, 748, 748b
    panic disorder, 555
    somatic symptom disorder, 580
Religion. *See also* Spiritual *entries*
    in Canada, 45
    as cultural system, 45–46
Religious orders, 2–3
Remarriage, children, 761–762
Reminiscence therapy, 315
Remote areas, role of nurses in, 59–60
Remote CBT, 290
Renewal certificate, 128, 131
Repeating, leading groups, 308t
Repetitive behaviour, 890
Repetitive transcranial magnetic stimulation (rTMS), 285, 512
Residential school syndrome, 43, 47
Residential services
    intensive, 77
    respite, 72
Resiliency, 767
    in older adults, 849
Resolution phase of nurse-client relationship, 118, 119b
Respect for autonomy, 139
Respite programs, 72
Respondent behaviour, 165
Responsive behaviours, 885–886
Restlessness, 885–886, 889–890
Restraints, 243–244, 411–412
Retirement community, 854
Retrograde memory loss, 512
Review panel, 131
Revised goals, 234
Rights, of persons with mental illness, 52
Rigidity of families, anorexia nervosa, 607

Risk assessment
    bio/psycho/social/spiritual psychiatric nursing assessment of children and adolescents, 792–793, 794b
    in bipolar disorders, 528
Risk/rescue ratio, 429, 429b
Risperidone (Consta; Risperdal; Risperdal M-Tab), 468, 473
Riverview Hospital, 11, 12f
RLCQ (Recent Life Changes Questionnaire), 359, 360t
Roberts' seven-stage crisis intervention model, 378, 379b
Rogers, Carl, 160t, 162–163
Rogers' client-centred therapy, 162–163
Rogers, Martha, 159
Role overload, 347
Role theories, applicability to psychiatric and mental health nursing, 167
Roy, Callista, 159
rTMS (repetitive transcranial magnetic stimulation), 512

S
Safety interventions
    acute stress disorder, 816
    for safety promotion on inpatient units, 242
Saint Dymphna Guesthouse, 4
Salpetrière, 3–4
San Hipólito, 2–3
Saskatchewan
    nurse education in, 11–12
    standard of practice in, 96
SCA. *See* Schizoaffective disorder
Scale for the assessment of negative symptoms (SANS), 477
Scale for the assessment of positive symptoms (SAPS), 477, 477b
Schizoaffective disorder, 491–494
Schizoid personality disorder (SZPD), 695
Schizophrenia
    acute illness period, 449–451
    aetiology
        biologic theories, 463–490
        bio/psycho/social/spiritual, 491f
        familial patterns, 459
        genetic factors, 459
        neuroanatomic factors, 460
        neurochemical factors, 460–461
        neurodevelopment, 462
        neurotransmitters, pathways, and receptors, 460, 460f
        polygenic nature, 459
        psychological theories, 463
        social theories, 484–486
    assessment
        biologic domain, 463
        psychological domain, 477–484
        social domain, 484–486
        spiritual domain, 486–490
    in children, 454
    continuum of care, 486
    diagnostic criteria, 451–454
    disorganized behaviour, 453–454
    disorganized thinking, 453

disturbed thoughts and sensory perceptions, 482
    epidemiology
        age of onset, 455–456
        comorbidity, 456–457
        ethnic and cultural difference, 495
        familial difference, 459
        gender differences, 456
        risk factors, 455
    evaluation and treatment outcomes, 490–491
    eye and, 462
    family response to disorder, 462–463
    fostering recovery, 451t
    interaction of genes and environment, 459–460
    interdisciplinary treatment, 462
    maintenance and recovery period, 451
    negative symptoms, 453
    neurocognitive impairment, 453–454
    nurse–patient relationship, 482
    nursing care plan, 464b
    nursing diagnoses
        activity, exercise, and nutritional interventions, 468
        extrapyramidal side effects, 470–473
        monitoring and administering medications, 468–470
        pharmacologic interventions, 468
        self-care activities, 466–468
        thermoregulation interventions, 468
    nursing interventions
        biologic domain, 463–490
        psychological domain, 481
        social domain, 484–486
        spiritual domain, 486–490
    nursing management, 463–491
    in older adults, 454–455
    paranoid, 487
    pharmacologic assessment, 466
    positive symptoms, 452
    priority care issues, 462
    and psychiatric disorders, 804–805
    rating scales, 477b
    recovery, 449b
    relapses, 451
    self-monitoring and relapse prevention, 482
    spiritual domain, 486–490
    stabilization period, 451
    subtypes, 492
Schizophrenia Society of Canada, 13
Schizophreniform disorder, 494
Schizotypal personality disorder (STPD), 695–696
School functioning, bio/psycho/social/spiritual psychiatric nursing assessment of children and adolescents, 793–795
School phobia, 810
School-aged children
    loss and, 759
    semistructured interview with, 778b
Science of caring, 156
Scientific thought, evolution, 8–9
Screening, 663–664

Seasonal depression, of mood disorders, 513
Seating arrangement, groups, 310
Seclusion, 243, 411–412
Secondary mental disorder model, concurrent disorders, 906
Secondary sources, 217
Secondary substance use disorder model, concurrent disorders, 906
Secure attachments, bio/psycho/social/spiritual psychiatric nursing assessment of children and adolescents, 790–791
Security
    relational, 946
    static, 946
Security awareness, dynamic, 946–947
Security awareness, forensic nursing, 946–947, 946b
Sedation, 473
Sedative-related disorders, 677
Selective serotonin reuptake inhibitors (SSRIs), 273t, 612, 742t, 809
    adverse reactions, 275–277
    anorexia nervosa, 614b
    concurrent disorders, 910
    panic disorder, 556
    pharmacokinetics, 275
    side effects, 276
    toxicity, 276
Self-actualization, 163, 768
Self-awareness
    bio/psycho/social/spiritual self and, 106
    understanding personal feelings and beliefs and changing behaviour and, 106
Self-care
    groups, 315
    Orem's theory of, 235
    promotion of, 235
Self-compassion, 609
Self-concept, 481
    bio/psycho/social/spiritual psychiatric nursing assessment of children and adolescents, 791–792, 792f
Self-disclosure, 107–108, 108t
Self-efficacy, 165–166
Self-esteem, in borderline personality disorder, 713
Self-harm and suicidal behaviour
    aetiology, 430
        biologic theories, 430–431
        bio/psycho/social/spiritual, 429f, 434–440
        psychological theories, 431–432
        social theories, 432
        spiritual theories, 432–433
        suicidality, 434
    Canadian data, 424
    and Canadian military, 424–425, 425b
    Canadian Suicide Statistics, 424t
    definition, 421
    economic costs, 423
    effects of, 422–424
    epidemiology
        Aboriginal peoples, 427
        age, 430

gender, 427–428
        indigenous people, 426–427, 427b
        regional variations, 424
    evaluation and treatment outcomes, 440–442
    global rates, 424
    impact on nurses, 442
    legal considerations, 433
        confidentiality, 433
        informed consent, 433–434
        involuntary admission, 421
    lived experiences, 423–424
    long-term outcomes, 442
    nursing assessment
        acute care treatment, 438
        assessment and reassessment, 437
        comprehensive assessment, 434–435, 435b
        contracting for safety, 438
        documentation, 437
        inpatient care and acute treatment, 438–439
        method and access, 437
        planning and implementing nursing interventions, 437–438
        protective factors, resources, and support, 436–437
        tools, risk assessment, 434–435, 436b
    nursing interventions, 425
        biologic domain, 438–439
        moral distress and moral injury, 442
        planning and implementing, 437–438
        psychological domain, 439
        social domain, 440
        spiritual domain, 440
    outpatient care plan, 441
    prevention, 423
    referrals, resources, and additional support, 440–441
    risk and protective factors for, 423
    short-term outcomes, 441–442
    stigma and, 422
    suicidality and specific populations, 422–425
    survivors effect, 422
    survivors of suicide loss, 422
Self-help groups, 13, 313
Self-identity, 29–30, 690
    impaired, in personality disorders, 690
Self-injurious behaviours, in borderline personality disorder, 698
    physical indicators, 704
Self-invalidation, in borderline personality disorder, 701
Self-management skills, 693
Self-monitoring, 634–635
Self-report scales, panic disorder, 557
Self-system, 154
Sensitization, bipolar disorders and, 523
Sensorium, in mental status examination, 221–223
Sensory impairment, 407
Separation anxiety disorder
    epidemiology and aetiology, 809
    nursing care, 809–810
    treatment interventions, 809

Separation-individuation, in borderline personality disorder, 699–700
Serotonin (5-HT), 198–199, 556, 735t
Serotonin hyperfunction hypothesis, 461
Serotonin syndrome, low, 398–399
Serotonin–norepinephrine reuptake inhibitors (SNRIs), 742t
    panic disorder, 556
Sexual abuse
    anorexia nervosa, 609
    of children, 769t
Sexual Assault Nurse Examiner (SANE), 923
Sexual identity, associated with adolescence, 763–764
Sexuality, in psychoanalytic theory, 161
Shadow, Jungian concept of, 162
Short-term assessment of risk and treatability (START), 403
Short-term retrograde amnesia, 512
Sibling relationships, 762
Side effects, 252, 254t
Simple relaxation techniques, 236
Single photon emission computed tomography (SPECT), 182
Sisters of Mercy, 2–3
Situational couple violence, 918
Skills groups, for dialectical behaviour therapy, 693
Skinner, B.F., 164t, 165
Sleep
    architecture, 730
    brain activity, 731, 733f
    definition, 729–731
    dementia and, 880
    efficiency, 730
    hygiene, 743, 743b
    hypnogram, 730, 731f
    interventions, 235–236
    latency, 730
    neurobiology of, 734, 735t
    for older adults, 846
    REM and NREM, 730–732
    restriction therapy, 748
    stages, 731, 732t
    terrors, 752
Sleep disturbance, in depressive disorders, 537
Sleep enhancement, 705
Sleep pattern, panic disorder, 555
Sleep patterns, 555
Sleep restriction therapy, 748
Sleep-state misperception, 747
Sleep–wake assessments, 738–740, 739f, 740f
Sleep–wake cycles, 705, 732–733
Sleep–wake disorders
    actigraphy, 740
    assessments
        EEG, 738–739, 740f
        orexin, 740
        polysomnography, 738, 739f
        respiratory and cardiac, 740
    common circadian rhythm
        jet lag, 751–752
        narcolepsy, 752
        shift workers, 751, 751b
        sleep terrors, 752

treatments of, 752
comorbid mental illnesses and mental health problems, 741
consequences of inadequate sleep, 737, 737*f*
dreaming, 731–732, 733*f*
epidemiology, 738
historical perspectives, 729–730
impaired sleep substance use, 737*f*, 738
insomnia (*See* Insomnia)
maintenance of wakefulness test, 740
morbidity and impaired function, 737*f*, 738
multiple sleep latency test, 740
obstructive sleep apnea, 749–751
overview of, 738–741
process C and S
  circadian rhythms, 732, 734*f*
  hormones flucation, 733–734
  neurologic perspective, 734–736, 735*t*
  sleep–wake cycle, 732–733
sleep diary, 740–741 (*See* Sleep)
sleep pattern changes
  adolescents, 736
  children, 736
  cultural and racial factors, 737
  older adults, 736–737
  women, 736
sleep questionnaires, 741
Sleep–wake disturbances, 878
Slow-wave sleep (SWS), 280, 730, 747*t*
SNAP-IV, 819*b*
SOAP method, 217
Social anxiety disorder (SAD), 547
Social change
  Dix, Dorothea Lynde, 3–4, 3*b*, 4*f*
  during late 20th century, 12–16, 12*f*
  moral treatment, 3–4
  during 19th and early 20th centuries, 5–8, 5*f*
Social comparison theory, 606, 606*b*
Social connection, of older adults, 852
Social determinants of health (SDoH), 32, 33*b*, 51, 56
Social domain
  assessment of (*See also specific disorders and conditions*)
  in children and adolescents, 793–795
  community, 795
  family assessment, 333–334
    family systems, 333
    formal and informal support networks, 334
    perspectives on understanding families, 333–334
    social and financial status, 334
  family relationship, 793
  insomnia, 748
  nursing interventions for (*See specific disorders and conditions*)
  obstructive sleep apnea, 750–751
  school functioning, 793–795
  spiritual assessment, 227
  stresses and coping behaviours, 795
Social exclusion, 30, 30*b*
  global responses to, 37

Social isolation, 36, 424, 426, 438, 509, 816
Social justice, 146
Social model, 83–84, 83*f*
Social phobia, 547
Social Progress Index (SPI), 21–23
Social skills training, 77
  for mental health promotion, in children and adolescents, 774
Social support
  in borderline personality disorder, 712–713
  of older adults, assessment of, 854
Social systems
  of older adults, 854–855
  schizophrenia, 484
Social theories, 167–169
  anorexia nervosa, 606–607
  binge eating disorder, 639–640
  of bipolar disorders, 524
  bulimia nervosa, 631–632
  of depressive disorders, 524
  family dynamics, 167–168
  role theories, 168
  sociocultural perspectives, 168–169
  somatic symptom disorder, 577
  substance-related disorders, 659
Societal norms, forensic nursing, 947, 947*b*
Sociocultural perspectives, 168–169
Sociocultural risk factors, anorexia nervosa, 609–610
Sociocultural theories, 168–169, 400
Solubility, 263
Somatic delusions, 459
Somatic symptom disorder
  aetiology
    biologic theories, 576
    psychological theories, 576–577
    social theories, 577
  children, 575
  clinical course, 574
  comorbidity, 576
  continuum of care, 585
  conversion disorder, 589
  diagnostic criteria, 574–575
  epidemiology, 575–576
  evaluation and treatment outcomes, 585
  gender, ethnic and cultural differences, 575–576
  hypochondriasis, 588
  illness and anxiety disorder, 575
  interdisciplinary treatment, 577
  mental health promotion, 585–588
  nursing care plan
    biologic domain, 580–581
    chronic low self-esteem, 586
    clinical settings, 586*b*
    ineffective therapeutic regimen management, 587
  nursing management
    biologic domain, 577–581
    characteristics, 578*f*
    interventions, 590
    psychological domain, 581–583
    social domain, 583
    spiritual domain, 584

  therapeutic approach, 590
  older adults, 575
  psychoeducation, 583*b*
  psychological domain, 581–583
  risk factors, 577
  somatization, 574
  in special populations, 575
  and stress, 579
Somatic Symptom Disorder—B Criteria Scale (SSD-12), 575
Somatization, 574
Source-oriented documentation, 217
Specialist supportive clinical management (SSCM), 624–625
Specific learning disorders, 823
Spectrum of care, for bipolar disorders, 537
Speech, 220–221
  patterns, 478
Specificity, 250, 361, 544, 843–844
Spiritual assessment, 227. *See also specific disorders and conditions*
Spiritual domain, 795
  bio/psycho/social/spiritual psychiatric nursing assessment of children and adolescents, 795
  family assessment, 334–335
  insomnia, 748–749
  obstructive sleep apnea, 751
Spiritual interventions, 245–246
Spiritual model, 83*f*, 84
Spiritual theories
  anorexia nervosa, 607
  applicability to psychiatric and mental health nursing, 169
  eating disorders, 607
  of Frankl logotherapy, 169
  of Yalom existential psychotherapy, 169
Spirituality. *See specific disorders and conditions*
  bulimia nervosa, 632
  in children and adolescents, 831
  definition, 84
  eating disorder, 607
  mood disorder, 517
  older adults, 855
  substance-related disorders, 659
SSRIs. *See* Selective serotonin reuptake inhibitors (SSRIs)
Stabilization, 73–74, 260, 278, 377, 451, 463, 470
Standards, 307
Stereotypic behaviour, 814
Stereotyping, 51
Stereotypy, 481
  schizophrenia, 454
Stigma, 52
  bipolar disorder, 530*b*
  of mental illness, 324
  and suicide, 421–422
Stimulant-related disorders, 677–678
Stimulants, 281–283. *See also specific drugs*
Stimulation, 410
Stimulus control therapy, 748

Strengths-based approach, 51, 923–926, 924*b*
  active listening, 924, 924*f*
  enhance safety, 925–926, 925*b*
  inquiring about individuals' concerns, 924
  support, 926
  validation, 925
Stress, 358–375, 459–460, 481, 483, 907
  assessment of individuals affected of children and adolescents, 795
  assessment of individuals affected by, 223
    biologic, 362
    social, 364
    spiritual, 374
  in bipolar disorders, assessment of, 537
  cognitive appraisal, 360–361
  collective trauma and historical trauma, 369–371
  concept, evolution, 358–361
  coping, and adaptation model, 366*f*
  emotional responses to, 364–367, 365*t*
  evaluation and treatment outcomes, 374–375
  family assessment, 332
  intergenerational transmission of trauma, resilience and, 369
  Neuman systems model, 158–159
  nursing care of individual, 372
  nursing interventions for
    psychological domain, 373–374
    social domain, 374
    spiritual domain, 374
  nursing interventions for biologic domain, 372–373
  person-environment transaction, 359–361
  as physiologic response, 359
  responses
    allostasis, 361–362
    to collective and historical trauma, 370–371
    flow, 362
    freeze-hide, 362
    physiological, 362–364, 363*f*
    tend and befriend, 362
  social network and, 364
  social support and, 364
  somatic symptom disorder and, 579
  spiritual domain, 374
  as stimulus, 359
  stressors, in childhood
    divorce, 760–762, 761*t*
    family, 757
    grief and loss, 758–760, 758*t*
    physical and developmental challenges, 763–765
    physical illness, 762–763
    residential community, 757
    separation and divorce, 760–762, 761*t*
    sibling relationships, 762
  trauma, and illness, 367
  trauma-informed care, 371–372

  traumatic stressor, 368
    acute stress disorder, 368
    posttraumatic stress disorder, 368–369
  workplace, mental health, 347
Stress and coping, 528
Stress and coping skills, in dementia, 886
Stresses and coping behaviours, bio/psycho/social/spiritual psychiatric nursing assessment of children and adolescents, 795
Stresses and coping patterns, with older adults, 851
Structural neuroimaging, 180–182, 180*t*
Structural othering, 29
Structural stigma, 31
Structural violence, 918
Structured groups, 311–312
Structured interaction, 242
Structure-function gap, 182–183
Structures, 187*f*
Subcortical dementia, 862
Subjective data, 216
Substance use
  physical and developmental challenges in adolescents, 764–765
  problem with parents, 772–773
Substance use disorders (SUD), 682
Substance use, schizophrenia, 457
Substance-associated suicidal behaviour, 905
Substance-/medication-induced psychotic disorder, 494
Substance-related and addictive disorders, 439
Substance-related disorders
  addiction treatment
    goals of, 660*b*, 662
    principles of, 660*b*, 662–663
  aetiologic theories
    biologic, 658
    psychological, 658–659
    social, 659
    spiritual, 659, 659*b*
  alcohol
    caffeine, 656–657
    cannabis, 657
    opioids, 657
    societal costs, 657
    tobacco, 657
    withdrawal, 668–669, 669*b*
  alcoholics anonymous, 659*b*
  care, levels of, 662*b*
  definition, 654
  diagnostic criteria
    clinical course, 656
    non-substance related disorders, 656
    substance classes, 656
  epidemiology, 656
  interdisciplinary treatment recommendations
    addiction treatment, 660*b*, 662
    brief intervention and referral, 663–664
    cognitive-behavioural therapy, 666
    family therapy, 667

    group therapy, 666–667
    harm reduction, 665–666
    intoxication and withdrawal, 664–665
    matching treatment principle, 662–663
    motivational interviewing, 666
    multidimensional assessment, 664
    pharmacotherapy, 667
    psychosocial interventions, 666–667
    relapse prevention, 667
    screening, 667
    therapeutic alliance, 662
    toxicology testing/drug screening, 667
    twelve-step recovery programs, 666
  neurobiology, 654–655
  nurse, health advocate, 683
  nursing care plan
    discomfort related to, tobacco withdrawal, 673
    risk related to, alcohol withdrawal, 668–669
    setting, 671–672
  nursing interventions
    alcohol-related disorders, 668–669
    amphetamine, 674–675
    caffeine-related disorders, 673–674
    cannabis-related disorders, 674
    gambling disorder, 680–681
    hallucinogen-related disorders, 674–675
    hypnotic and anxiolytic-related disorders, 677
    inhalant-related disorders, 675
    opioid-related disorders, 675–677
    sedative-related disorders, 677
    stimulant-related disorders, 677–678
    tobacco-related disorders, 678–680
  in parents, 772–773
  prevention, 659–660
  special populations
    concurrent disorders, 682
    HIV/AIDS, 674
    nurses, 682
    postsecondary education students, 681
    pregnancy and lactation, 682
    youth, 681
Substance-related/addictive disorders. *See also* Concurrent disorders
  examples of, 904
SUD (substance use disorders), 662
Suggestions, leading groups, 308*t*
Suicidal behaviour
  aetiology, 430
    biologic theories, 430–431
    bio/psycho/social/spiritual, 429*f*, 434–440
    psychological theories, 431–432
    Schneidman's common characteristics, 430*b*
    social theories, 432
    spiritual theories, 432–433
  suicidality, 430

attempts, 223
Canadian data, 424
and Canadian military, 425b
Canadian Suicide Statistics, 424t
definition, 421–422
in depressive disorders, assessment of, 514
economic effect, 423
effects of, 422–424
epidemiology
  Aboriginal peoples, 427
  age, 425–426
  first responders, 428
  gay, lesbian, bisexual or transgender sexual orientation, 428
  gender, 427–428
  indigenous people, 426–427, 427b
  inmates, 428
  LGBTQI2SA+, 428
  regional variations, 424
evaluation and treatment outcomes, 440–442
impact on nurses, 442
legal considerations, 429–430
  confidentiality, 433
  informed consent, 433–434
  involuntary admission, 421
nursing assessment
  assessment and reassessment, 437
  comprehensive assessment, 434–435, 435b
  contracting for safety, 438
  documentation, 437
  inpatient care and acute treatment, 438–439
  method, 437
  planning and implementing nursing interventions, 437–438
  protective factors, resources, and support, 436–437
  tools, risk assessment, 436b, 440
nursing interventions, 434
  biologic domain, 438–439
  planning and implementing, 437–438
  psychological domain, 439
  social domain, 440
  spiritual domain, 440
prevention, 423
rates of, 424
regional variations in canada, 424
and religion, 432
risk and protective factors for, 423
risk assessment, 223–226, 851
  in borderline personality disorder, 698–699
stigma and, 428
suicidal ideation, 223
suicidality and specific populations, 424–425
survivors effect, 422
Suicidal ideation
  definition, 421
  rates of, 424
Suicidal plan, definition, 421
Suicide
  and the Canadian Military, 425b

under forensic purview, 936–937
Suicide attempt, 422
  definition, 438
Suicide cluster, 432–433
Suicide contagion, 432–433
Suicide pact, 432
Sulci, 183, 183f
Summarizing, leading groups, 308t
Superego, 161, 162
Support groups, 775
Support, leading groups, 308t
Support networks, 440
Supported employment (SE), 350, 450
Supported housing, 77
Supportive employment services, 77–78
Supportive therapy groups, 313
Suprachiasmatic nuclei (SCN), 732
Suspiciousness, 884–885, 888
Suvorexant (Belsomra), 746t
Symbolism, 114–115
Symptom expression, 174
Symptom management groups, 314
Synaptic transmission, 192–195
Systematic desensitization, 561
Systems models, 157–159

T
Tangentiality, 478–479
Tardive akathisia, 471–472
Tardive dyskinesia, 268, 268b, 471–472, 471t, 472b
Tardive dystonia, 471–472
Target symptoms, 252
Task functions, group, 304, 315–316
TCAs. *See* Tricyclic antidepressants (TCAs)
Teaching. *See* Client/family education
Telehealth, 60, 121–122, 143
Telephone (tCBT), 290
Temazepam (Restoril), 746t
Temperament
  antisocial personality disorder and, 717–720
  definition, 687
Temporal lobes, 183f, 184
Termination stage
  of family systems, 333
  of group development, 304
Thalamus, 187
The FICA History Tool—, 855
The Leyton Obsessional Inventory, 567b
Therapeutic alliance. *See also specific disorders and conditions*
  anorexia nervosa, 614
Therapeutic communication, 106–107, 107b
  analyzing interactions and, 114–115, 114b
  defence mechanisms iln, 113–114
  empathic linkages and, 106, 109–111
  empathy in, 112
  listening and, 108
  nonverbal, 108–109, 111f
  nurse–client relationship, 115–118, 116b, 117b, 119b
  personal boundaries in, 112
  principles of, 107b

professional boundaries in, 112–113, 113b
rapport in, 111–112
selecting techniques for, 111
self-disclosure in, 107–108, 108t
silence and, 108
strategies, 119–122
and technology, 121–122
validation in, 112
verbal, 106–108, 107f, 107b, 108t–110t, 110b
Therapeutic index, 252
Therapeutic relationship. *See also specific disorders and conditions*
  in depressive disorders, assessment of, 515
Therapeutic factors, 307, 314, 315
Thermoregulation interventions, 237
Thinking errors, in cognitive restructuring, 296
Thorndike, Edward L., 164t, 165
Thought(s)
  assessment of, 221, 222b
  content of, 221, 222b, 514
  dichotomous, in borderline personality disorder, 697
  disturbances of, in bipolar disorders, 522
  dysfunctional, challenging, 698–699, 701b
  processes, 221, 222b
  stopping, borderline personality disorder, 711
Thought disturbances, 528
Thought patterns, 557–558
Thought processes, 478, 850–851
Threats of suicide, 223
TIC (trauma-informed care), 51, 97–98, 371–372, 827–829
Tidal model, 156–157, 157b
Tiredness, in depressive disorders, 510
Tobacco. *See* Nicotine
Tobacco-related disorders, 678–680
Tolerance, 251–252
Tolman, Edward Chace, 164t
Topiramate, 669
Topiramate (Topamax), 273
Toronto Psychiatric Hospital, 6
Tourette syndrome (Tourette disorder). *See also* Motor disorders
  in children and adolescents
    aetiology, 827
    epidemiology, 827
    nursing care, 827–829
    treatment interventions, 827
Toxicology testing, for substance-related disorders, 667
Training School for Nurses, 7–8
Traits, 138, 176, 271, 395, 426, 603, 609, 629, 631, 687, 689, 691, 718
Transaction, 157–158
Transcultural health care, 169
Transference, 161
Transgender forensic client, 941
Transient postictal disorientation, 512
Transition times, family assessment, 330

Transitional relationship model (TRM), 120–121
Trauma, 433, 907, 919
    acute stress disorder, 813–814
    disinhibited social engagement disorder, 813
    historical, 46–49
    posttraumatic stress disorder, 813–814
    reactive attachment disorder, 812–813
    and stressor-related disorders, 811–814
Trauma- and stressor-related disorders, 368–369
Trauma- and violence-informed care (TVIC), 922
Trauma-informed care (TIC), 51, 97–98, 371–372
Travelbee, Joyce, 155
Trazodone (Desyrel), 746t
Triazolam (Halcion), 746t
Tricyclic antidepressants (TCAs), 580, 742t
    cardiotoxicity, 276
    for enuresis, 829
    indications, 274–275
    mechanisms of action, 274–275
    panic disorder, 556
    pharmacokinetics, 275
    side effects, 275–277
Triple stigmatization, 53
TRM (transitional relationship model), 120–121
Truth and Reconciliation Commission of Canada, 947, 947b
Tryptophan (5-HTP), 513
Typical antipsychotics, 742t
Tyramine-restricted diet, 277t
"Tyranny of the should,", 162

U

Unconditional positive regard, 162–163
Unconscious
    collective, 162
    in psychoanalytic theories, 160–161
Unconscious mental processes, in psychoanalytic theory, 160–161
Underemployed, 343
Unemployment, 343
Unipolar disorders. See Depressive disorders
United Nations Office for Disaster Risk reduction's (UNDRR) role, 382
United Nations, role of, 382
Unrestricted eating, 595–596, 595f
Unsafe workplace, 344, 346b
Utilitarianism, 137t, 138–139

V

Vagus nerve stimulation (VNS), 511
Validation, 242
    communication concepts, 112
    milieu therapy, 242
Validation therapy, 886

Varenicline, 680
Vascular neurocognitive disorder, 896
Verbal communication, 106–108, 107f, 107b, 108t–110t, 110b. See also Languages; Speech
    group, 309
    self-disclosure in, 107–108, 108t
    techniques, 108, 109t, 110b
Victimization, 433
Video link (vCBT), 290
Vincent de Paul, 2–3
Violence, 433. See also Aggression and violence
    predictors of, 403
    prevention of, 403
    workplace, mental health, 347–349, 352
Virtue ethics, 137–138, 137t
Vision changes, age-related, 844–845
Visual hallucinations, schizophrenia, 452
Visuospatial impairments, 882, 887–888
VNS (vagus nerve stimulation), 511
Vulnerability
    emotional, in borderline personality disorder, 701b
    forensic nursing, 935–936
    genetic, of children adolescents, 788
    schizophrenia, 459–460

W

Wakefulness, 734
Walden II (Skinner), 165
Wandering behaviour, 890
Watchful eating, 595–596, 595f
Watson, Jean, 156
Watson, John B., 164t, 165
Waxy flexibility, 481
    schizophrenia, 454, 481
Weight cycling, 607
Weight gain
    antipsychotics, 270
    schizophrenia, 457, 468
    side effects, psychiatric medications, 254t
    substance-related disorders, 674
Werther effect, 432–433
Western society, 400
Wisdom, practical, 138
Women
    incarcerated, 938–939
    sleep–wake disorders, 736
Word salad, 478–479
Work culture, 344
Working from home, 344
Working phase of nurse-client relationship, 117–118
Working stage of group development, 304
Work–life balance, 346–347, 346b
Work–life conflict, 346–347, 346b
Workplace, mental health
    health problems and disorders, 349–350
        accommodation, 349–350

    symptoms, 349, 350t
    work and persons living, 350
healthy workplaces, 344–347
    psychosocial factors in, 345t
    unsafe workplaces, 344, 346b
    work-life balance, 346–347, 346b
nurse
    burnout, 351
    compassion fatigue, 352
    COVID-19 pandemic, 352–353, 353b
    fatigue, 351–352
    job strain, 346–347
    recommendations for, 351–352, 351t
    violence, 352
threats
    bullying, 348–349, 348t
    burnout, 347
    emergencies/disasters, 349
    stress, 347
    violence, 347–349
work
    changing nature of, 343–344
    equity, diversity, and inclusion, 344
    and gender, 343
    unemployment, 343
Workplace violence, 347–349, 352
World Federation for Mental Health (WFMH), 101
World Suicide Prevention Day, 423b
World Suicide Report (WSR), 423b
Worry, 562

X

Xenophobia, 549b

Y

Yale-Brown Obsessive Compulsive Scale (Y-BOCS), 567b
Yale-Brown-Cornell Eating Disorder Scale (YBC-EDS), 622b
Yalom, Irving, 169
Y-BOCS (Yale-Brown Obsessive Compulsive Scale), 567b
Young-old, 839
Youth. See also Children; Clinical interview
    forensic nursing, 940–941
    mental health assessment of, 756–802
Youth Health Promotion, 765

Z

Zeitgebers, 202, 732
Ziprasidone (Zeldox), 468, 474
Zolpidem (Ambien), 746t
    adverse reactions, 280–281
    indications and mechanisms of action, 280
    pharmacokinetics, 280
    side effects, 280–281
    toxicity, 280–281
Zoophobia, 549b
Zopiclone (Imovane), 746t
Zyban, 276